Students' Paste:

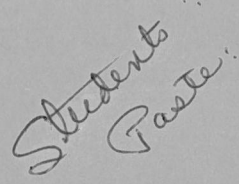

Errata Sheet for DOLAN: CRITICAL CARE NURSING: CLINICAL MANAGEMENT THROUGH THE NURSING PROCESS

**pp. 26–27 and 29–30:** The placement of the two sample care plans should be switched.

**p. 203:** Under Nursing Diagnosis #6, the statement "Assure patient that speech will improve over time and with rehabilitation" should appear within the Nursing Interventions column.

**p. 215:** There should be no rule between Nursing Diagnoses #1 and #2.

**p. 357:** The first lines of the Chapter Outline should be as follows:

> BODY METABOLISM AND ENERGY UTILIZATION
> PANCREAS: STRUCTURE AND FUNCTION
> METABOLIC STATES: ABSORPTIVE AND POSTABSORPTIVE STATES

**p. 379:** There should be no rule between Nursing Diagnoses #6 and #7. The Nursing Interventions and Rationales listed for #7 apply equally to #6 as well.

**p. 463:** The last two lines in the Nursing Diagnoses column for Nursing Diagnosis #2 should read "*hypo*kalemia (<3.5 mEq/liter)."

**p. 569:** The alveolar gas equation (in the left-hand column) should read as follows:

$$PAO_2 = FIO_2\,(P_B - PH_2O) - \frac{PaCO_2}{RQ}$$

**pp. 670–671:** The last line on p. 670 and the first two lines on p. 671 should read as follows:

> These conditions cause a shift of the oxygen dissociation curves (see Fig. 28–15) to the left, decreasing the concentration of oxygen released to the tissues.

**p. 809:** Under the "Rate" column in Fig. 40–27 (Atrial Fibrillation), the Ventricular rates should read as follows:

> Ventricular 100 controlled
> $>$100 uncontrolled

**p. 876:** The figure on this page should be Figure 42–4. Its legend should read: "Technique of PTCA. See text for description."

**p. 1283:** The figure referenced under "Feedback Mechanisms" should be Figure 61–3.

# CRITICAL CARE NURSING
## CLINICAL MANAGEMENT THROUGH THE NURSING PROCESS

# CRITICAL CARE NURSING

## CLINICAL MANAGEMENT THROUGH THE NURSING PROCESS

**JOAN T. DOLAN, M.S., R.N., C.S., CCRN**
Clinical Nurse Specialist
Massapequa General Hospital
Seaford, New York

President, Joan T. Dolan and Associates, Ltd.
Great River, New York

Formerly, Clinical Assistant Professor
Department of Adult Health Nursing
School of Nursing
State University of New York at Stony Brook
Stony Brook, New York

ILLUSTRATIONS BY KATHLEEN GEBHART
Media Services–Medical Illustration
State University of New York at Stony Brook
Stony Brook, New York

F. A. DAVIS COMPANY • PHILADELPHIA

Printed in the United States of America

Last digit indicates print number: 10 9 8 7 6 5 4 3 2 1

NOTE: As new scientific information becomes available through basic and clinical research, recommended treatments and drug therapies undergo changes. The author(s) and publisher have done everything possible to make this book accurate, up-to-date, and in accord with accepted standards at the time of publication. However, the reader is advised always to check product information (package inserts) for changes and new information regarding dose and contraindications before administering any drug. Caution is especially urged when using new or infrequently ordered drugs.

Library of Congress Cataloging-in-Publication Data
Dolan, Joan T.
Critical Care Nursing: Clinical Management through the Nursing Process / by Joan T. Dolan.
p. cm.
Includes bibliographical references.
ISBN 0-8036-2691-6
1. Intensive care nursing. I. Title.
[DNLM: 1. Critical Care—nursing. 2. Nursing Process. WY 154 D659c]
RT120.I5D65 1990
610.73'61—dc20
DNLM/DLC
for Library of Congress
89-25878
CIP

# Dedication

To my family, Joe, Joseph, and Mary Krista—
my source of strength, my love, my life.

*I do not wish the public to read entirely without effort*
*what I have written not entirely without effort*

Petrarch (1304–74)

# Foreword

It is an honor to be asked to write the foreword to this text on critical care nursing, which will undoubtedly be a strong positive influence on the education and clinical practice of both current and future critical care nurses.

Although the arena of critical care with its expanded nursing care demands continues to grow, the educational preparation of qualified nurses has lagged behind. The inclusion of critical care nursing subject matter in undergraduate nursing programs today remains inconsistent.[1] The preparation of critical care nurses is all too often only a catch-as-catch-can compendium obtained through the diligent efforts of the self-motivated nurse.

Those of us who were around in the early stages of critical care received on-the-job training from each other as well as our medical cohorts who were learning in the same manner—in the heat of the battle. It is no wonder that it took so many years for us to retrace our steps to determine the rationale—scientific or otherwise—of many of our actions and interventions.

As one who learned the hard way, I cannot help but be a bit envious of those who can now use this excellent text that unifies theoretical knowledge with clinical practice, integrating the science and the art of nursing. The logical progression from physiology to pathophysiology to environmental responses and interactions provides the warp and woof of the complex tapestry known as the nursing process. The final product is intricately woven, compiling all the elements of critical care for the student as well as the experienced practitioner. Its comprehensive knowledge base and clear design make this book useful in formal curriculum; its numerous tables make it useful as a quick and handy reference for the practicing nurse.

Joan Dolan had a vision. She saw the richness and order of this weaving, this unification of art and science. We in critical care can all be grateful for her resolve in the pursuit of her vision. The years of work that went into the preparation of this text, and the years of experience that form the background for it, have come to fruition in a work of greater magnitude than even she envisioned.

This is a book about human beings—about those who are in life-and-death crises, about patients, about families, about nurses—a book about human beings caring for other human beings. We can be proud.

Elaine Kiess Daily, R.N., B.S.
Clinical Cardiovascular Research Nurse
University of California at San Diego
San Diego, California

1. Tanner, CA, Hartshorn, J, and Rosenfeld, P: Critical care nursing in baccalaureate programs. Nursing and Health Care 10:483, 1989.

# Preface

In today's health care scene, individuals increasingly are requiring sophisticated, intensive, and humanistic nursing care, whether faced with a life-threatening crisis or the exacerbation of a chronic illness. Yet there is growing concern about this nation's ability to meet the needs of patients afflicted with life-threatening illness or injury. The shortage of nurses in general, and critical care nurses in particular, is profoundly affecting the delivery of care in critical care units throughout this country. Furthermore, although a critical care component is being incorporated into the curricula of nursing programs across the country, there is nevertheless a significant need for critical care educational programs, both in academic and in clinical settings. It is this need that *Critical Care Nursing: Clinical Management Through the Nursing Process* attempts to address.

The idea for this text was conceived when I was teaching a critical care course in a tertiary hospital setting and I determined that there was a need for a text designed for the classroom setting that could also serve as a comprehensive reference for clinical practice. A text was needed that blended theoretical concepts with clinical practice, structure with function, physiology with pathophysiology, internal and external environmental interactions, humanness and professionalism, all within the framework of the nursing process.

This text is designed to meet the educational needs of nursing students in critical care nursing or advanced medical-surgical nursing courses at either the undergraduate or graduate level. Its thorough review of anatomy and physiology and its integration of these topics with selected, commonly encountered pathophysiology, make this text especially well-suited for curricula in schools of nursing.

The book is also intended for use by practicing critical care, emergency, and medical-surgical nurses. Its extensive illustrations, tables, glossary, and indexing provide a concise synopsis of significant information available at one's fingertips. It is also well-suited for courses related to in-service training and continuing education. Furthermore, this text is a valuable resource for preparation for the CCRN certification examination, because its scope of coverage reflects to a great extent that of the AACN Core Curriculum.

The content of the text covers the major organ systems including the nervous, endocrine, renal, respiratory, cardiovascular, gastrointestinal, immune, and hematologic systems. These systems are addressed in this order based on their *regulatory* functions. Since the nervous system is the major system regulating and controlling body physiology, it is addressed first. The endocrine system, likewise exhibiting considerable control of body function, follows. The renal and respiratory systems, both contributing to the regulation of body functions (e.g., fluid, electrolyte, and acid-base balance) are presented next, followed by the support systems: cardiovascular, gastrointestinal, immune and hematologic.

In addition, topics of significance to critical care are addressed including:

- Oncologic critical care nursing
- Trauma (including cardiothoracic, abdominal and orthopedic)
- Burns
- Shock states (including septic and anaphylactic)
- Acute poisoning
- Psychosocial considerations in the care of the critically ill patient and family
- Patient/family education: principles of teaching/learning applied to critical care nursing
- Ethical and legal principles affecting decision making in critical care nursing.

This text uses as its framework Gordon's functional health patterns in the discussions of patient assessments, formulation of nursing diagnoses, and development of nursing care plans. Nursing diagnoses as defined by NANDA are used almost exclusively throughout the text. Nursing care plans are based on these identified nursing diagnoses.

This text is divided into units—the units are each devoted to a major organ system. Each unit's format (with the exception of that for the endocrine system) includes the following:

- **Anatomy and physiology**—The first chapter of each of these units begins with a thorough review of anatomy and physiology, emphasizing the relationship between structure and function. Special attention is given to microscopic structure, as it is at this level that function is realized.
- **Assessment**—The second chapter reviews pertinent information on the assessment of the organ system. The discussion of assessment uses as its framework Gordon's functional health patterns and includes the clinical history and the physical examination. A description of pertinent diagnostic tests/studies and implications for nursing care are also included.
- **Monitoring**—This chapter includes information on monitoring techniques including implications for nursing care (e.g., intracranial pressure monitoring, cardiac monitoring, and hemodynamic monitoring).
- **Therapeutic modalities**—The discussion of assessment and monitoring is followed by attention to those therapeutic modalities pertinent to treatment of a disruption/impairment of organ function (e.g., oxygen therapy, suctioning techniques, cardiac pacing and intra-aortic balloon pumping). Sample procedures are provided to assist the nurse to gain further insight into the skills pertinent to critical care nursing.
- **Pathophysiology**—Several chapters in each organ system are included to present pertinent, commonly seen pathophysiologic disorders/disease/syndromes (herniation syndromes, acute head injury, and so forth). The discussion of anatomy and physiology provides a basis for understanding the pathophysiology underlying insults to a specific organ system. To assist the reader to appreciate the significance of dysfunction, cross-referencing is provided to illustrations and discussions of normal physiology. Discussions of specific diseases largely include etiology, pathophysiology, clinical presentation, diagnosis, treatment, and nursing management.
- **Nursing management**—The nursing management of specific disease entities is presented through the use of Care Plans that can be applied clinically by the nurse. They include nursing diagnoses, desired patient outcomes, nursing interventions and rationales. Use of rationales for nursing interventions enables basic physiologic principles to be integrated with, and provide the basis for, specific nursing actions. Cross-referencing to illustrations and discussions of normal physiology within the same unit, as well as to other units, assists the reader to view the individual as a whole (that is, in terms of total body processes: physiologic, psychologic, emotional, and social). This educational process is facilitated

by extensive cross-referencing between and among Care Plans throughout the text as well as to the numerous other tables.

Using the care plan format assists the reader to appreciate the process involved in determining specific nursing diagnoses and shows how these diagnoses relate to desired patient outcomes, nursing interventions, and the language used to define these parameters. Specifically:

— Each nursing diagnosis is related to specific etiology or etiologies amenable to nursing interventions.
— Each desired patient outcome is stated in measurable terms and describes the outcome to be achieved by the patient.
— Nursing interventions are written in terms that reflect specific actions taken by the nurse.
— Rationales assist to integrate underlying physiologic principles.

- **Case studies**—Case studies of selected pathophysiologic disorders are presented sporadically throughout the text. Each one focuses the reader on an actual clinical scenario thereby integrating the underlying physiologic principles and concepts with the clinical circumstance.

The Sample Care Plans accompanying each case study allow the reader to identify the specific assessment data that provide the basis for the nursing diagnoses. The initial nursing diagnoses and their etiologies are listed and developed as part of the Sample Care Plan. They include desired patient outcomes, nursing interventions and rationales. In this way, the language of nursing process is reflected in the nursing care plan. Additional nursing diagnoses and their etiologies based on the assessment data presented in the case study are also listed to enable readers to develop their own care plans.

The inclusion of Sample Care Plans in conjunction with case studies enables the reader to apply information gleaned from the extensive Care Plans presented in the text that deal with the same disease/syndrome. These Care Plans provide a handy reference for the practicing nurse.

The nature of the information presented in Unit Three, the Endocrine System, has necessitated some variation in its format as compared with that of the units on other major organ systems. This unit's initial chapter discusses the characteristics and features common to all endocrine glands, and its second chapter covers the assessment of endocrine function. Each subsequent chapter in the endocrine unit then addresses a particular endocrine gland, its underlying structure and function, and select pathophysiology.

In the book's introductory unit, Chapter 1 introduces the reader to critical care nursing and its scope of practice. Chapter 2 defines the components of nursing process and how this process is integrated into the discussions of nursing care, including use of the Care Plans and Sample Care Plan format. The language of process and nursing diagnosis is emphasized especially because it provides the tools for care plan development and documentation and the critical thinking component that is needed in the nursing process. Chapter 3 deals with the psychosocial implications in the care of the critically ill patient and family. An examination of the functional health patterns is especially important here. Included in this chapter is an especially helpful tool (Table 3-1) concerned with a summary of nursing interventions to meet the needs of families of ICU patients. Chapter 4 is concerned with patient and family education, a major nursing function. Discussion includes goals of education, principles of adult learning, key factors in assessing learning needs, program development, and usefulness of contracting as a strategy for patient education. Finally, Chapter 5 looks at a critical illness from the perspective of the patient and family. Two scenarios are presented as seen through the eyes of the patient. Laughing, crying, feeling, touching, and sharing—the humanness of being and the dignity and worth of each patient and family are the focus of this chapter.

Following the units presenting organ systems, Unit Twelve consists of two chapters. Chapter 69 looks at critical care nursing from the perspective of the nurse. It focuses on the nurse's own feelings, concerns, satisfactions, and frustrations—the humanness of the nurse as he/she tries to meet the needs of the critically ill patient and family. This chapter is all about critical care nurses caring about their patients and each other, and sharing feelings. Chapter 70 concentrates on the ethical and legal principles affecting decision-making in critical care. Selected ethical theories and their application are discussed. The distinction is made between ethics and the law, and laws affecting the practice of nursing are examined. Specific legal concerns are discussed (consents, do-not-resuscitate, and so forth).

At the end of the text are a number of valuable reference aids: a glossary and Appendix A through F. Of these, two warrant special mention. The first, Appendix A, presents drugs that are commonly used in the critical care setting. It contains an introduction to important concepts in pharmacokinetics as well as a large number of up-to-date monographs on individual drugs. The second special appendix (Appendix E) is a monograph on cardiovascular assessment using the NANDA taxonomy, which is based on a framework of nine human response patterns. The inclusion of this monograph provides the reader with an interesting counterpoint to the functional health pattern assessment framework used throughout the text.

In today's health care system, where hospital settings are increasingly focusing on the care of the very sick patient and the patient's family, the need for critical care nurses capable of providing sophisticated, timely, and humanistic care is greater than ever. Whether in the classroom or at the patient's bedside, it is hoped that this text can help to improve the quality of patient care.

Joan T. Dolan, M.S., R.N., C.S., CCRN

# Acknowledgments

The publication of this book reflects the contributions of many. I am especially indebted to the late Elizabeth Meise, my former director of nursing at Southampton Hospital, Southampton, New York, whose confidence in my capabilities never faltered; to Dolores Zebrowski of Sag Harbor, New York, my teacher and mentor, whose love for the sciences was instilled in me; and to Ellen T. Fahy, Dean of the School of Nursing, University of Minnesota, Minneapolis, for her encouragement and guidance in helping to shape the scope of my practice. The late Maynard Dewey, who was Chairman of the Department of Anatomical Sciences at Stony Brook, always had time to share ideas and to answer yet another question. I am indebted to Pura Pantojas, Deputy Director, Division of Nursing at University Hospital at Stony Brook, where the book was conceived; to Lenora McLean, Dean of the School of Nursing at Stony Brook; to my colleagues in the Department of Adult Health Nursing, School of Nursing, State University of New York at Stony Brook; and to Eugenia Gearon, Director of Nursing Administration, Massapequa General Hospital, Seaford, New York, where the book reached fruition, for their assistance and encouragement.

I am grateful to my colleagues in the intensive care units at the University of California at San Diego Medical Center and at Massapequa General Hospital, for their steadfast assistance and enthusiasm in contributing to the many technical aspects of the text. A special thank you is extended to Kevin Kelly for his insightful suggestion.

Zena Gordon played a pivotal role in pulling the book together and charting a course that has led to its completion, and I am forever grateful for her talents, resolve and foresight. A special thank you to Alan Sorkowitz, who followed that course meticulously and tenaciously, and under whose guidance and fastidiousness the project has become reality.

Words cannot express my indebtedness to Barbara Baker, whose untiring fingers labored faithfully and unhesitantly to get the typing done. It is mainly through her dedication, commitment, and perseverance that the clerical aspects of this project were accomplished. The contribution of Kathleen Gebhart extends beyond the limits of the illustrations she has done for this book—both she and Barbara Baker have contributed a part of themselves to its nuts and bolts and its intrinsic value.

To my colleagues everywhere, a special thank you because you have helped to shape the very heart and soul of what it is that we do as nurses.

**J.T.D.**

# Contributors

**Mary Amendolari, R.N.**
Nursing Care Coordinator
Intensive Care Unit
Massapequa General Hospital
Seaford, New York

**Lorraine Brown, M.S.N., R.N.C.**
Assistant Director Nursing/Clinical Nurse Specialist
Massapequa General Hospital
Seaford, New York

**Christine M. Chmielewski, M.S., CNN**
Clinical Specialist
Transplant Department
Hospital of the University of Pennsylvania
Philadelphia, Pennsylvania

**Margaret Connelly-Duffy, M.S., R.N., CCRN**
Unit Educator, Coronary Care Unit
University Hospital
Health Sciences Center
State University of New York at Stony Brook
Stony Brook, New York

**Adrienne Coppola, R.N.**
Nursing Care Coordinator
Intensive Care Unit
Massapequa General Hospital
Seaford, New York

**Elaine Kiess Daily, B.S., R.N.**
Clinial Cardiovascular Research Nurse
University of California at San Diego
San Diego, California

**Raymond J. Dattwyler, M.D.**

Assistant Professor
Immunology Division, Department of Medicine
Health Sciences Center
State University of New York at Stony Brook
Stony Brook, New York

**Maria Elayne DeSimone, M.S., R.N.C., ANP**

Clinical Assistant Professor
School of Nursing
Health Sciences Center
State University of New York at Stony Brook
Stony Brook, New York

**Robert DiBartolo, M.A., P.T.**

Private Practice
Miller Place, New York

**Janet Donnard, B.S.N., R.N., ONC**

Intensive Care Unit, Assistant Head Nurse
Fox Chase Cancer Center
Philadelphia, Pennsylvania

**Frances Dooley, M.S., R.N., C.N.A., CCRN**

Private Practice
Massapequa, New York

**Carol Evans, M.S.N., R.N.**

Staff Development Coordinator
The Lower Bucks Hospital
Bristol, Pennsylvania

**Lorraine Fallon, M.S.N., R.N., CEN, CCRN**

Instructor, Our Lady of Lourdes School of Nursing
Camden, New Jersey
Staff Nurse, Emergency Department
Memorial Hospital of Burlington County
Mount Holly, New Jersey

**Joanne M. Farley, M.S.N., R.N., CCRN**

Clinical Nurse Specialist/Critical Care
Hahnemann University Hospital
Philadelphia, Pennsylvania

**Marc George Golightly, Ph.D.**

Section Head, Immunology
Health Sciences Center
State University of New York at Stony Brook
Stony Brook, New York

## Ginny Wacker Guido, J.D., M.S.N., R.N.

Associate Professor
School of Nursing
The University of Texas
Health Sciences Center at Houston
Houston, Texas

## Gail Habicht, Ph.D.

Professor
Department of Pathology
Health Sciences Center
State University of New York at Stony Brook
Stony Brook, New York

## K. Sue Hoyt, M.N., R.N., CEN

Associate Director, Trauma Research and Education Foundation
San Diego, California

## Thomas E. Kearney, Pharm.D.

Executive Director,
San Francisco Bay Area Regional Poison Control Center
San Francisco General Hospital
San Francisco, California

## Sheila M. Keller, M.S.N., R.N.

Instructor
St. Agnes Medical Center School of Nursing
Philadelphia, Pennsylvania

## Donna Kemp, M.N., R.N., CCRN

Neonatal Consultant
San Diego, California

## Janet M. Kennedy, M.S.N., R.N.

Vice President/Nursing
Staff Builders Health Care Services
Lake Success, New York

## Ellen McErlean, M.S.N., R.N., CCRN

Clinical Instructor
Cardiothoracic Nursing
Cleveland Clinic Foundation
Cleveland, Ohio

## Mary Meisel, M.S., R.N.

Surgical Clinical Nurse Specialist
Fairview Southdale Hospital
Edina, Minnesota

## Steven B. Meisel, Pharm.D.

Assistant Director for Clinical Services
Pharmacy Department
Fairview Southdale Hospital
Edina, Minnesota

## Frederick Miller, M.D.

Pathologist-in-Chief
Department of Pathology
Health Sciences Center
State University of New York at Stony Brook
Stony Brook, New York

## Gene D. Morse, Pharm.D.

Associate Professor of Pharmacy
Erie County Medical Center
State University of New York at Buffalo
Buffalo, New York

## JoAnn Murray-Schluckebier, B.S.N., R.N.

Transplant Coordinator
Albert Einstein Medical Center
Philadelphia, Pennsylvania

## Patricia Markman Naji, M.S.N., R.N., CCRN

Instructor, School of Nursing
University of Pennsylvania
Staff Nurse, Cardiothoracic-Surgical Intensive Care Unit
Hospital of the University of Pennsylvania
Philadelphia, Pennsylvania

## Patricia M. Orr, M.B.A., R.N., C.N.A., CCRN

Director of Nursing, Critical Care
St. Agnes Medical Center
Philadelphia, Pennsylvania

## Barbara J. Riegel, M.N., R.N., C.S.

Clinical Nurse Researcher
Critical Care Division
Sharp Memorial Hospital
San Diego, California

## Deborah Rodzwic, R.N., M.S.N., O.C.N.

Oncology Clinical Nurse Specialist
Mt. Sinai Hospital
Hartford, Connecticut

## Gary Sparger, M.S.N., R.N., CEN, MICN

Coordinator, Trauma/Emergency Clinical Nurse Specialist
California State University
Long Beach, California

**Carol A. Stephenson, Ed.D., R.N.**
Associate Professor
Harris College of Nursing
Texas Christian University
Fort Worth, Texas

**Laura Worthington Toledo, M.S., R.N.**
Consultant, Post-Anesthesia and Critical Care
San Diego, California

**Merri D. Walkenstein, M.S.N., R.N.**
Staff Development Instructor
Fox Chase Cancer Center
Philadelphia, Pennsylvania

**Patricia Wallace, M.S.N., R.N., CCRN**
Clinical Nurse Specialist
Medical Intensive Care Unit
Hospital of the University of Pennsylvania
Philadelphia, Pennsylvania

**Wayne Waltzer, M.D.**
Associate Professor
Department of Urologic Surgery
Health Sciences Center
State University of New York at Stony Brook

**Cathy Rodgers Ward, M.S., R.N., CCRN**
Nurse Manager, Cardiothoracic ICU
UCLA Medical Center
Los Angeles, California

**Jeannette Waterman, M.S.N., R.N.**
Nursing Instructor, Our Lady of Lourdes School of Nursing
Clinical Assistant Professor II
Camden County College
Camden, New Jersey

**Kathleen D. White, M.S., R.N., CCRN**
Director, Critical Care Institute
University Hospital
Health Sciences Center
State University of New York at Stony Brook
Stony Brook, New York

**Gayle R. Whitman, M.S.N., R.N., CCRN**
Director, Cardiothoracic Nursing
Cleveland Clinic Foundation
Cleveland, Ohio

# Consultants


**Carole Biggins, B.S.N., R.N.**
Nurse Clinician
Intensive Care Unit
Massapequa General Hospital
Seaford, New York

**Catherine Spearing Bolgiano, M.S.N., R.N., C.S.**
Pulmonary Clinical Nurse Specialist
University of Maryland Medical System
Baltimore, Maryland

**Eleanor F. Bond, Ph.D., R.N.**
Assistant Professor
University of Washington
School of Nursing
Seattle, Washington

**Ora James Bouey, M.A., R.N.**
Associate Professor and Director of Professional Resource Development
School of Nursing
State University of New York at Stony Brook
Stony Brook, New York

**Dorothy J. Brundage, Ph.D., R.N., FAAN**
Associate Professor of Nursing
Duke University School of Nursing
Durham, North Carolina

**Vicki L. Byers, Ph.D., R.N., CNRN**
Assistant Professor
University of Texas
Health Science Center
San Antonio, Texas

**Judy Donlen, M.S.N., R.N.**
Assistant Director of Nursing Education
Children's Hospital of Philadelphia
Philadelphia, Pennsylvania

**Deanna Epley, M.S.N., M.Ed.**
Assistant Professor
Barry University
Miami, Florida

**Dorrie Fontaine, D.N.Sc., R.N., CCRN**
Assistant Professor
Trauma/Critical Care Nursing
University of Maryland
School of Nursing
Baltimore, Maryland

**Eugenia Gearon, M.P.S., R.N., C.N.A.**
Director, Nursing Administration
Massapequa General Hospital
Seaford, New York

**Barbara Gleeson, M.S.N., R.N., CCRN**
Cardiac Rehabilitation
Clinical Nurse Specialist
Presbyterian Medical Center of Philadelphia
Philadelphia, Pennsylvania

**Susan Stabler Haas, M.S.N., R.N.**
Coadjutant Nursing Instructor
Delaware County Community College
Media, Pennsylvania

**Barbara Herlihy, Ph.D.**
Professor, Nursing and Natural Sciences
Incarnate Word College
San Antonio, Texas

**Jeremiah T. Herlihy, Ph.D.**
Associate Professor of Physiology
University of Texas Health Science Center at San Antonio
San Antonio, Texas

**Sheryl A. Innerarity, Ph.D., R.N.**
Clinical Assistant Professor
University of Texas at Austin
Austin, Texas

**Brenda S. Jackson, Ph.D., R.N.**
Associate Professor and Dunlap Chair
Division of Nursing
Incarnate Word College
San Antonio, Texas

**Merrilyn Finn Katz, M.S., R.N.**
Assistant Professor
School of Nursing
University of Maine at Fort Kent
Fort Kent, Maine

**Patricia Kennedy, B.S., R.N.**
Assistant Director of Nursing
Massapequa General Hospital
Seaford, New York

**Karen M. Kleeman, Ph.D., R.N., C.S.**
Associate Professor
University of Maryland
School of Nursing
Baltimore, Maryland

**Sister Kathleen Krekeler, Ph.D., R.N.**
Professor of Nursing
St. Louis University School of Nursing
St. Louis, Missouri

**Judith (Ski) Lower, M.S., CNRN, CCRN**
Head Nurse
Neuro Critical Care Unit
Johns Hopkins Hospital
Baltimore, Maryland

**Celeste Smith Makrevis, M.S.N., R.N.**
Kaiser-Permanente Medical Center
Department of Education and Training
Santa Clara, California

**Paula Manchester, Ph.D., R.N.**
Consultant in Health Services
Research and Educational Planning
President, Community Care Companions, Inc.
Setauket, New York

**Margaret Masselli, M.S.N., R.N., CCRN**
Staff Nurse Intensive Care Unit
Veterans Administration Medical Center
Northport, New York
Adjunct Clinical Assistant Professor
School of Nursing
Health Sciences Center
State University of New York at Stony Brook
Stony Brook, New York

**Linda S. Mayer, M.N., R.N.**
Clinical Nurse Specialist, Pulmonary
University of Kansas Medical Center
Kansas City, Kansas

**Ellen McAvoy, M.A., R.N.**
Clinical Instructor
Massapequa General Hospital
Seaford, New York

**Terry B. McGoldrick, M.S.N., R.N., C.N.A.**
Information Systems Coordinator
Albert Einstein Medical Center
Philadelphia, Pennsylvania

**Lenora J. McLean, Ed.D., R.N.**
Dean, School of Nursing
Health Sciences Center
State University of New York at Stony Brook
Stony Brook, New York

**Mary Frances Moorhouse, R.N., C.C.P., CCRN, CRRN**
Nurse Consultant, Critical Care
TNT-RN Enterprises and Fortis Corporation
Colorado Springs, Colorado

**Gene D. Morse, Pharm.D.**
Associate Professor of Pharmacy
Erie County Medical Center
State University of New York at Buffalo
Buffalo, New York

**Gene E. Mundie, Ed.M., R.N.**
Associate Director of Nursing
University Hospital
Health Sciences Center
State University of New York at Stony Brook
Stony Brook, New York

**Nina Spatafora Newton, M.A., R.D.**
University Hosptial
Health Sciences Center
State University of New York at Stony Brook
Stony Brook, New York

**Harold I. Palevsky, M.D.**
Assistant Professor of Medicine
Pulmonary Section/Department of Medicine
University of Pennsylvania School of Medicine
Philadelphia, Pennsylvania

**Pura Pantojas, Ed.M., R.N., C.N.A.A.**
Deputy Director
Division of Nursing
University Hospital
Health Sciences Center
State University of New York at Stony Brook
Stony Brook, New York

**Marcia Pencak, M.S., R.N.**
Assistant Unit Leader
Rush-Presbyterian St. Luke's Medical Center
Chicago, Illinois

**Karen J. Pickett, M.S., R.N.**
Instructor, Critical Care Nursing
Northern Illinois University
DeKalb, Illinois

**Rosemary C. Polomano, M.S.N., R.N.C.S.**
Oncology/Pain Clinical Nurse Specialist
Hospital of the University of Pennsylvania
Philadelphia, Pennsylvania

**Edith McCarter Randall, M.S.N., R.N., CCRN**
Trauma Nurse Coordinator
Thomas Jefferson University Hospital
Philadelphia, Pennsylvania

**Theresa S. Richmond, M.S.N., R.N., CCRN**
Trauma Specialist, Trauma Service
Thomas Jefferson University Hospital
Clinical Instructor, College of Allied Health Sciences
School of Nursing
Thomas Jefferson University
Philadelphia, Pennsylvania

**Renee A. Ryan, M.S., B.S.N., R.N.**
Assistant Director, Nursing Education
Ona M. Wilcox School of Nursing
Middletown, Connecticut

**June L. Stark, B.S.N., R.N., CCRN**
Associate Director of Education: Critical Care
New England Medical Center Hospitals
Boston, Massachusetts

**Frances L. Stier, M.S.N., R.N.C.**
Clinical Nurse Educator
University Medical Center
Tucson, Arizona

**Mary Troyer, M.S.N., R.N.**
Supervisor, In-service Education
Brackenridge Hospital
Austin, Texas

**Maria Vasselman, M.S.N., R.N.**
Quality Assurance Coordinator
Massapequa General Hospital
Seaford, New York

**Linda J. Waite, M.N., R.N., CCRN**
Clinical Supervisor
Marquette University
College of Nursing
Milwaukee, Wisconsin

**Norma Neahr Wilkerson, Ph.D., R.N.**
Associate Professor of Nursing
University of Wyoming
School of Nursing
Laramie, Wyoming

**Janice M. Zeller, Ph.D., R.N.**
Professor, Department of Medical Nursing
Associate Professor
Department of Immunology/Microbiology
Rush-Presbyterian St. Luke's Medical Center
Chicago, Illinois

**William Zirker, M.D., M.P.H.**
Assistant Professor, Clinical Medicine
School of Medicine
State University of New York at Stony Brook
Stony Brook, New York

# Table of Contents

# Abbreviations Used in This Book

| | |
|---|---|
| $AaDO_2$ | Alveolar-arterial oxygen gradient |
| AAPCC | American Association of Poison Control Centers |
| a/A ratio | Arterial/alveolar ratio |
| Ab | Antibody |
| ABGs | Arterial blood gases |
| ABO | Blood groups |
| ACh | Acetylcholine |
| AChR | Acetylcholine receptor |
| ACTH | Adrenocorticotropic hormone |
| ADH | Antidiuretic hormone |
| ADL | Activities of daily living |
| ADP | Adenosine diphosphate |
| AHA | American Heart Association |
| AIDS | Acquired immunodeficiency disease (Acquired immune deficiency syndrome) |
| ALG | Anti-lymphocyte globulin |
| ALS | Amyotrophic lateral sclerosis |
| ALT | Alanine aminotransferase (SGPT) |
| AMI | Acute myocardial infarction |
| An | Antigen |
| AP | Action potential |
| ARDS | Adult respiratory distress syndrome |
| ARF | Acute renal failure |
| ARF | Acute respiratory failure |
| AST | Aspartate aminotransferase (SGOT) |
| ATN | Acute tubular necrosis |
| ATP | Adenosine triphosphate |

| | |
|---|---|
| BMR | Basal metabolic rate |
| BSA | Body surface area |
| BUN | Blood urea nitrogen |
| CABG | Coronary artery bypass graft |
| CAD | Coronary artery disease |
| cAMP | Cyclic AMP (adenosine monophosphate) |
| CAPD | Continuous ambulatory peritoneal dialysis |
| CAVH | Continuous arteriovenous hemofiltration |
| CBC | Complete blood count |
| CCK | Cholecystokinin |
| cGMP | Cyclic GMP (guanosine monophosphate) |
| CHF | Congestive heart failure |
| CI | Cardiac index |
| CK (CPK) | Creatinine phosphokinase |
| CMV | Cytomegalovirus |
| CNS | Central nervous system |
| CO | Cardiac output |
| COPD | Chronic obstructive pulmonary disease |
| CPAP | Continuous positive airway pressure |
| CPE | Cardiogenic pulmonary edema |
| CPP | Cerebral perfusion pressure |
| CRF | Chronic renal failure |
| CRH | Corticotrophic releasing hormone |
| CSF | Cerebrospinal fluid |
| CT | Calcitonin |
| CT Scan | Computerized axial tomography |
| CV | Cardiovascular |
| CVA | Cerebrosvascular accident |
| $CvO_2$ | Oxygen content of mixed venous blood |
| CVP | Central venous pressure |
| CXR | Chest x-ray |
| DCT | Distal convoluted tubule |
| DI | Diabetes insipidus |
| DIC | Disseminated intravascular coagulation |
| DKA | Diabetic ketoacidosis |
| DNA | Deoxyribonucleic acid |

| | |
|---|---|
| DPG | 2,3-diphosphoglycerate |
| DTR | Deep tendon reflexes |
| DVT | Deep venous thrombosis |
| ECF | Extracellular fluid |
| ECG | Electrocardiogram |
| ECV | Extracellular fluid volume |
| EEG | Electroencephalogram |
| EMG | Electromyography |
| EOM | Extra ocular movements |
| ERV | Expiratory reserve volume |
| ESR | Erythrocyte sedimentation rate |
| ESRD | Endstage renal disease |
| f | Respiratory rate (breathing frequency) |
| FBS | Fasting blood sugar |
| FDP (FSP) | Fibrin degradation products (fibrin split products) |
| FEV | Forced expiratory volume |
| $FEV_1$/FVC | Forced expiratory volume/forced vital capacity |
| $FIO_2$ | Fraction of inspired oxygen |
| FRC | Functional residual capacity |
| FSH | Follicle stimulating hormone |
| FHF | Fulminating hepatic failure |
| GCS | Glasgow coma scale |
| GFR | Glomerular filtration rate |
| GH | Growth hormone |
| GHIH | Growth hormone inhibiting hormone |
| GHRH | Growth hormone releasing hormone |
| GI | Gastrointestinal |
| GnRH | Gonadotrophic releasing hormone |
| GVHD | Graft-versus-host disease |
| HBD | Hydroxybutyrate dehydrogenase |
| HC1 | Hydrochloric acid |
| $HCO3^-$ | Bicarbonate |
| Hct | Hematocrit |
| HDL | High-density lipoprotein |
| HDPM | Hemodynamic pressure monitoring |
| Hgb | Hemoglobin |

| | |
|---|---|
| HHNK | Hyperglycemic hyperosmolar nonketotic (coma) |
| HIV | Human immunodeficiency virus |
| HLA | Human leukocyte antigens |
| HPI | History of present illness |
| $HPO_4$ | Phosphate |
| HR | Heart rate |
| IABP | Intraaortic balloon pump |
| IC | Inspiratory capacity |
| ICF | Intracellular fluid |
| ICP | Intracranial pressure |
| ICPM | Intracranial pressure monitoring |
| ICS | Intercostal space |
| ICV | Intracellular fluid volume |
| IDDM | Insulin dependent diabetes mellitus |
| IDL | Intermediate density lipoprotein |
| Ig | Immunoglobulin (IgG, IgM, IgA, IgE, IgD) |
| IL-1, IL-2 | Interleukin-1, interleukin-2 |
| IMV | Intermittent mandatory ventilation |
| IPPB | Intermittent positive pressure breathing |
| IRV | Inspiratory reserve volume |
| IVP | Intravenous pyelography (Excretory urography) |
| JGA | Juxtaglomerular apparatus |
| KC1 | Potassium chloride |
| LAD | Left anterior descending coronary artery |
| LAP | Left atrial pressure |
| LBBB | Left bundle branch block |
| LCX | Left circumflex coronary artery |
| LDH | Lactic dehydrogenase |
| LDL | Low density lipoprotein |
| LH | Leuteinizing hormone |
| LLQ | Left lower quadrant |
| LMCA | Left main coronary artery |
| LMN | Lower motor neuron |
| LOC | Level of consciousness |
| LUQ | Left upper quadrant |
| LVAD | Left ventricular assist device |
| LVEDP | Left ventricular end-diastolic pressure |

| | |
|---|---|
| LVEDV | Left ventricular end-diastolic volume |
| LVH | Left ventricular hypertrophy |
| LVSWI | Left ventricular stroke work index |
| MAC | Midarm circumference |
| MAMC | Midarm muscle circumference |
| MAP | Mean arterial pressure |
| MAST | Military antishock trousers |
| MCL | Mid clavicular line |
| $MCL_1$ | Modified chest lead ($V_1$) |
| MDF | Myocardial depressant factor |
| mEq | Milliequivalent |
| MHC | Major histocompatibility complex |
| MI | Myocardial infarction |
| mOsm/kg | Osmolality |
| MOV | Minimal occlusive volume |
| MR | Mitral regurgitation |
| MRI | Magnetic resonance imaging |
| MSH | Melanocyte-stimulating hormone |
| MVA | Motor vehicle accident |
| $MVO_2$ | Myocardial oxygen consumption |
| MVV | Maximal voluntary ventilation |
| $NaHCO_3$ | Sodium bicarbonate |
| NANDA | North American Nursing Diagnosis Association |
| NCPE | Noncardiogenic pulmonary edema |
| NFP | Net filtration pressure |
| $NH4^+$ | Ammonium ion |
| NIDDM | Noninsulin dependent diabetes mellitus |
| NIF | Negative inspiratory force |
| NMJ | Neuromuscular junction |
| NPO | Nothing by mouth |
| NSR | Normal sinus rhythm |
| NTG | Nitroglycerin |
| $1,25\text{-}(OH)_2D$ | 1,25-dihydroxycholecalciferol |
| OKT-3 | Monoclonal antibody |
| PA | Pulmonary artery |
| $PACO_2$ | Alveolar carbon dioxide concentration |
| $PaCO_2$ | Arterial carbon dioxide concentration |

| | |
|---|---|
| PAedp | Pulmonary artery end-diastolic pressure |
| $PAO_2$ | Alveolar oxygen concentration |
| $PaO_2$ | Arterial oxygen concentration |
| PAP | Pulmonary artery pressure |
| PASG | Pneumatic antishock garment |
| PAW | Pulmonary artery wedge (PCWP) |
| $P_B$ | Barometric pressure |
| PCD | Post-cardiotomy delirium |
| $PCO_2$ | Partial pressure of carbon dioxide |
| PCT | Proximal convoluted tubule |
| PCWP | Pulmonary capillary wedge pressure |
| PEEP | Positive end-expiratory pressure |
| $P_E$ Max | Maximal expiratory pressure |
| PERRLA | Pupils equal, round, reactive to light and accommodation |
| $PGE_2$ | Prostaglandin $E_2$ |
| pH | Hydrogen ion concentration |
| PH (PTH) | Parathormone (Parathyroid hormone) |
| PIH | Prolactin inhibiting hormone |
| $P_I$ Max | Maximal inspiratory pressure |
| PIP | Peak inspiratory pressure |
| PMH | Past medical history |
| PMNs | Polymorphonuclear leukocytes |
| PND | Paroxysmal nocturnal dyspnea |
| PNS | Peripheral nervous system |
| $PO_2$ | Partial pressure of oxygen |
| PRH | Prolactin releasing hormone |
| PT | Prothrombin time |
| PTCA | Percutaneous transluminal coronary angioplasty |
| PTT | Partial thromboplastin time |
| $PvCO_2$ | Carbon dioxide concentration in mixed venous blood |
| $PvO_2$ | Oxygen concentration in mixed venous blood |
| PVR | Pulmonary vascular resistance |
| Q | Flow |
| RAP | Right atrial pressure |
| RAS | Reticular activating system |
| RBBB | Right bundle branch block |
| RCA | Right coronary artery |

| | |
|---|---|
| REF | Renal erythropoietic factor |
| RES | Reticuloendothelial system |
| RIND | Reversible ischemic neurologic deficit |
| RLQ | Right lower quadrant |
| RME | Resting metabolic expenditure |
| RML | Right middle lobe |
| RMP | Resting membrane potential |
| RNA | Ribonucleic acid |
| ROM | Range of motion |
| R/T | Related to |
| RUQ | Right upper quadrant |
| RV | Residual volume |
| RVEDP | Right ventricular end-diastolic pressure |
| RVF | Right ventricular failure |
| RVH | Right ventricular hypertrophy |
| RVP | Right ventricular pressure |
| $SaO_2$ | Percent saturation of hemoglobin |
| SIADH | Syndrome of inappropriate secretion of antidiuretic hormone |
| SIMV | Synchronized intermittent mandatory ventilation |
| SGOT | Serum glutamic oxaloacetic transaminase |
| SGPT | Serum glutamic pyruvic transaminase |
| SLE | Systemic lupus erythematosus |
| SLIDT | Assessment tool (see Table 7–1) |
| SOB | Shortness of breath |
| sp.gr. | Specific gravity |
| SV | Stroke volume |
| SVCS | Superior vena cava syndrome |
| SVI | Stroke volume index |
| $SvO_2$ | Mixed venous blood oxygen tension (saturation) |
| SVR | Systemic vascular resistance |
| SVT | Supraventricular tachycardia |
| $T_3$ | Triiodothyronine |
| $T_4$ | Thyroxine |
| TBG | Thyroid binding globulin |
| TBPA | Thyroid binding prealbumin |
| TBW | Total body water |
| TIA | Transient ischemic attacks |

| | |
|---|---|
| TLC | Total lung capacity |
| Tm | Maximal rate of mediated transport of a substance across a plasma membrane |
| TPN | Total parenteral nutrition |
| TRH | Thyrotrophic releasing hormone |
| TSH | Thyrotropic stimulating hormone |
| UMN | Upper motor neuron |
| $\dot{V}_A$ | Alveolar minute ventilation |
| VC | Vital capacity |
| $V_D(V_D/V_T)$ | Anatomic deadspace volume |
| $\dot{V}_E$ | Minute ventilation |
| VLDL | Very low density lipoprotein |
| VMA | Vanillylmandelic acid |
| VSD | Ventricular septal defect |
| $\dot{V}/\dot{Q}$ | Ventilation/perfusion ratio |
| $V_T$ | Tidal volume |
| WBC | White blood count |
| WPW | Wolff-Parkinson-White syndrome |

# UNIT ONE

# Overview of Critical Care Nursing

The human being is in a continuous, ongoing interaction of the self and the environment wherein energies are focused on maintaining individual life processes—physiologic, psychologic, and social—in a state of dynamic equilibrium. Each individual brings to this interaction unique human intellect, feeling, and creativity, and there emerges a new level of humanness.

As part of the human experience, the integrity of the individual and family may be disrupted by a critical illness or catastrophic event. At such times, the personalized, humanistic, and caring behaviors of critical care nurses and other health-care providers assist the individual to restore life processes to a state of dynamic equilibrium. It is through such involvement that each individual may evolve to a new level of consciousness regarding health and wellness, and a concern for one another.

In the chapters that follow, the role of the critical care nurse in this nurse–patient–environment interaction is examined closely. As discussed in Chapter 1, critical care nurses assist critically ill patients and their families to mobilize their resources in support of the integrity of the individual and interpersonal relationships. In Chapter 2, the nursing process that underlies nursing practice is discussed. It is through the process that is nursing that individual life processes are promoted and desired patient outcomes are achieved. The components of the nursing process are examined, and the foundation for the use of nursing care plans, both clinically and as presented in this text, is established.

In Chapter 3, stressors experienced by patients and their families in the intensive care environment are identified. The reactions of these individuals to stress are examined, and nursing interventions to counteract stress are discussed. A psychosocial assessment of patients and families is presented with case studies.

Patient and family education, the focus of Chapter 4, is a critical aspect of nursing care of the critically ill patient and family because it affords the opportunity for all individuals to gain new insight into self and environment, health and wellness. Principles of adult learning, program development, teaching plan preparation, and contracting are presented in this chapter.

In Chapter 5, the examination of depersonalization, dehumanization, and caring behaviors serves as a stepping stone to the chapters that follow, in which nursing care of critically ill patients with a variety of health problems is examined. **Perhaps most** important of all, as presented in this chapter, the focus of this unit and subsequent units, be it nurse, patient, or family, is on "being human."

## UNIT OUTLINE

CHAPTER 1

# Critical Care Nursing: An Introduction

In the ordinary course of life, the integrity of individual developmental processes and personal interaction with the environment may be disrupted and function may be compromised. Whether the dysfunction springs from a life-threatening crisis or from an exacerbation of a chronic disease, the critically ill person requires sophisticated intervention to restore life processes to their dynamic equilibrium. The goal of critical care nursing is to provide essential individualized care directed toward the survival of the person and the achievement of optimal physiologic, psychologic, emotional, and social potential. Restoration of individual life processes to dynamic equilibrium requires that the *process that is nursing* promote these life processes in the manner best calculated to achieve desired goals and outcomes.

A major pathophysiologic/psychologic insult to individual life processes and functions commonly places an extraordinary strain on the body's normal regulatory mechanisms, undermining the emotional and psychologic stability of the affected person and the person's family. It is in this situation that the critical care nurse not only helps to restore those processes vital to life, but also maintains life-sustaining functions until the individual is once more able to assume responsibility for personal interactions with the environment. Pathophysiology is seen within the context of cellular change and the effects of such change on the developmental processes of the individual as a whole and on his or her ongoing environmental interactions.

In approaching the individual as a whole, the critical care nurse bridges the gap between modern technology and the needs of the critically ill. The nurse strives to maintain the integrity of the individual in the face of an increasingly mechanistic environment, recognizing that individual responses to the environment largely reflect such integrity. Skilled nursing interventions aim to assist critically ill individuals and their families to mobilize their resources to support the integrity of individual and interpersonal relationships and to strengthen individual–environment interaction.

The critical care nurse serves as a catalyst in the healing process, making complex and timely judgments and decisions and taking actions for which the nurse remains accountable. The rationale for such decisions is based on a thorough knowledge of the health and behavioral sciences, fully developed skills, and the ability to evaluate one's own responses and limitations. This knowledge base is upgraded continuously by new clinical and educational experiences that reinforce the critical care nurse's professional practice and autonomy.

The nursing process is a scientific approach to decision-making through assessing, diagnosing, planning, implementing, and evaluating. Accurate documentation of the care process facilitates communication among health-care providers and may also serve as a measure of the quality of the health care given.

With the implementation of prospective payment plans designed to contain health-care costs and the consequent changes in health-care delivery, it is essential that the nurse document care in a manner that reflects the appropriateness and effectiveness of skilled nursing interventions. This requires an awareness of the intellectual process involved in providing care, together with an appreciation of the need to document this process in clear, concise language. Thus the critical care nurse defines what is done when care is provided, while also noting whether or not such care brings about a positive change in the patient's responses and clinical outcomes.

Today's critical care nurse is challenged by our ever-expanding knowledge of physiologic, psychologic, and sociologic interactions. These advancements, accompanied by complex technological innovations, require that the critical care nurse function at a highly sophisticated level when caring for the critically ill patient, family, and/or significant others. Standards of critical care nursing assist nurses to define their practice because such standards make the profession's expectation regarding quality patient care very explicit.

The American Association of Critical-Care Nurses (A.A.C.N.), which recognizes the complexity of nursing management of the critically ill, has been innovative in the promotion of competent critical care nursing practice. Through its ongoing activities, the A.A.C.N. strives to meet the educational needs of critical care nurses to ensure a high standard of care for all patients, their families, and/or significant others.

Comprehensive care of superior quality is possible only when there are participation and communication among all concerned health professionals. Often, it is the critical care nurse who serves as coordinator and collaborator, encouraging each caregiver to appreciate and to respect the contribution of other team members. This creates a climate in which the team can function with maximum efficiency as reflected by the achievement of desired patient outcomes.

The chapters that follow are designed to assist the critical care nurse to grasp the body of knowledge essential to practice. The study of human systems emphasizes the relationships between structure and function, physiology and pathophysiology, and internal and external environmental interactions. Case studies suggest the application of this knowledge to clinical situations. Nursing care plans based on nursing diagnoses and decision-making rationales demonstrate how clear and concise documentation reflects the actual care process. In this manner, the professional role of the critical care nurse is shown to be vital to the well-being of the critically ill patient.

CHAPTER 2

# Application of Nursing Process to Critical Care Nursing Practice

## CHAPTER OUTLINE



## LEARNING OBJECTIVES

**At the end of this chapter, you should be able to:**

1. Define nursing.
2. Define nursing process and its essential components.
3. Define nursing diagnosis and its language.
4. Describe the classification of nursing diagnoses developed by the North American Nursing Diagnosis Association (NANDA).
5. Analyze the format and language of nursing process.
6. Differentiate criteria for patient outcomes and their documentation.
7. Discuss the characteristics of nursing interventions, and implications for documentation.
8. Distinguish between independent and collaborative nursing activities.
9. Review Nursing Care Plan: Nursing Diagnoses, Desired Patient Outomes and Nursing Interventions.

## NURSING PRACTICE: NURSING PROCESS DEFINED

"Nursing is the diagnosis and treatment of human responses to actual or potential health problems."[1] The fundamental basis of nursing practice is PROCESS. Every aspect of practice is affected by an understanding and utilization of nursing process.

Nursing process is an organized approach to problem-solving and decision-making that describes the intellectual activity of the nurse. It is the accepted methodology for nursing practice.

## NURSING PROCESS: A 5-STEP PROCESS

Nursing process involves 5 steps: assessing, diagnosing, planning, implementing, and evaluating.

### Assessing

Assessing involves a thorough, ongoing, comprehensive collection of subjective and objective data of the patient–family–environment interaction. Such data are obtained via history-taking, observation, physical examination, laboratory data, x-rays, and other diagnostic studies. Use of *functional health patterns*[2] (see Appendix C) assists in eliciting information of concern to nursing. The patient's database should reflect those data that form the basis for nursing diagnoses.

### Diagnosing

Diagnosing involves the identification of the patient's actual or potential health problem, and the etiology, or cause, of the problem that nurses can independently treat. Nursing diagnosis is a *pivotal* component of nursing process. On the one hand it is the judgment, conclusion, or decision determined by the nurse as a result of the assessing and problem-solving process. It reflects the process involved in gathering, analyzing, and interpreting the assessment data.

On the other hand, nursing diagnosis provides the basis from which patient outcomes are derived and a plan of appropriate nursing interventions is developed and implemented. Put another way, nursing diagnosis emerges from the collection, analysis, and interpretation of assessment data, and provides the framework from which the patient's plan of nursing care evolves.

### Planning

Planning involves the determination of desired patient outcomes and nursing interventions based on the nursing diagnosis. The nurse supports the individual in self-advocacy for the optimal level of health desired. The nurse motivates the patient, family, and/or significant others to become actively involved in the "care process." The nurse–patient–family interaction assists in determining priority of nursing diagnoses and setting patient goals and outcomes that clearly communicate the nature of the actual or potential health problem. Ideally, patient outcomes should reflect the patient's input in determining realistic and measurable outcomes.

### Implementing

Implementing involves the specific nursing interventions and activities delineated in the patient's care plan and designed to treat the etiology (cause) of the patient's problem defined in the nursing diagnosis.

### Evaluating

Evaluating involves an appraisal of the effectiveness of the nursing interventions in resolving the patient's problem as defined in the nursing diagnosis. A comparison is made of the actual patient outcomes in response to nursing interventions and those outcomes predicted in the patient's care plan.

Reassessment of the patient's status and nursing diagnoses is necessary to determine the effectiveness of nursing interventions. Revisions of the patient's care plan and its implementation are based on the reassessment of the patient and the nursing diagnoses.

## KNOWLEDGE: THE RATIONAL BASIS FOR DECISION-MAKING

Nursing diagnoses are formulated based on the analysis of the assessment data obtained. The analysis and interpretation of the assessment data require that the nurse integrate theoretical and experimental knowledge in clinical applications. The integration of such knowledge within the clinical setting provides the *rational basis for decision-making*.

The activities inherent in the "care process" require that each nurse expand his or her knowledge base and develop more sophisticated skills in assessment, problem-solving, decision-making, and management. The nurse must become disciplined to think through the process, to identify the components of the process as they occur in practice, and to document that process in a language that reflects the functions that are nursing.

## NURSING PROCESS: THE LANGUAGE

The language of process is unique because it reflects the nurse's practice; it is used to verbalize what one is doing and why something is being done. Nurses need to communicate the "care process" to colleagues and fellow health-care providers as it evolves, and in a precise and concise manner. Language must be clear and consistent so other health-care providers will know what to expect of nursing and so that nurses will know what to expect of each other.

### Nursing: A Diagnosis-Based Practice

Nursing, as a *diagnosis-based practice*, demands that nurses become expert at assessing patient's needs and problems, formulating nursing diagnoses based on that assessment, evolving and implementing a plan of care, and documenting this "care process" in a manner reflective of the professional, skilled nursing care rendered. It is only by documenting nursing activities that professional practice can be validated and financially rewarded.

### Nursing Diagnosis: Defined

Simply defined, a nursing diagnosis reflects a patient's problem or unhealthful response, and the problem's etiology that nurses can treat independently. It is a definitive statement of an actual or potential problem, alteration, or deficit in the life processes (physiologic, psychologic, and sociologic) of an individual.

### Nursing Diagnosis: A Two-Part Statement

The nursing diagnosis consists of two parts, the problem and its etiology. The *problem* reflects the patient's actual or potential unhealthful response; the *etiology*, if known, reflects the cause of the unhealthful response or problem that is amenable to independent nursing intervention. Use of the phrase "related to" (R/T) suggests a relationship between the patient's unhealthful response and its etiology, or cause. This phrase has been legally recommended because it avoids implying an actual cause-and-effect relationship.

The nursing diagnosis should be specific because it provides the framework for developing the plan of care. The *problem* portion of the nursing diagnosis predicts what the *patient outcomes* should be; there is a direct relationship between the patient's problem and the desired outcomes. The *etiology* portion of the nursing diagnosis dictates what *nursing interventions* must be implemented if the patient's outcomes are to be achieved and the problem is to be resolved.

Determining the etiology of the patient's problem helps individualize patient care, that is, no two patients with a similar problem can be expected to have the same underlying etiology or require the same nursing interventions to treat it. It necessitates that interventions required to treat the cause of the patient's problem be within the scope of nursing's independent functions. The nurse must determine if such interventions can be performed independently.

### Nursing Diagnosis: Descriptive Categories

Nursing diagnosis may be described as actual, potential, or possible. An *actual* nursing diagnosis reflects a patient's problem or unhealthful response that *is present* as indicated by specific signs and symptoms, or defining characteristics. A *potential* nursing diagnosis suggests that a patient's problem or unhealthful response *may occur* unless preventive nursing measures are initiated. While specific symptomatology or defining characteristics may not be evident, risk factors can usually be identified that suggest the necessity of implementing preventive nursing interventions. A *possible* nursing diagnosis suggests that a patient's problem or unhealthful response *may be present*, but the symptomatology or defining characteristics may not be apparent or discernible. The nurse must obtain additional information to either confirm or rule out the diagnosis.

### Classification of Nursing Diagnoses

For nearly 20 years, the efforts of the North American Nursing Diagnosis Association (NANDA) in developing a classification of nursing diagnoses have been highly instrumental in moving the profession of nursing toward the development of a language that communicates its unique functions. As of 1989, NANDA's list contained more than 80 approved nursing diagnostic categories (see Appendix B), which reflected the patient's actual, potential, or possible problem (i.e., the *first* part of the 2-part nursing diagnosis statement). The addition of the etiology of the problem (i.e., the *second* part of the nursing diagnosis statement) completes the formulation of the nursing diagnosis and individualizes the diagnosis for the particular patient.

Nurses are encouraged to use these nursing diagnostic categories in their daily practice when formulating nursing diagnoses. Clinical applications and study of these diagnoses must be promoted so that the language of nursing diagnosis and the functions it reflects can be refined and validated.

Nurses need not feel restricted to the use of NANDA's list but rather should be motivated to develop in practice other nursing diagnoses, which can be submitted for possible inclusion in NANDA's list. In this way, nurses are able to share their ideas, experiences, logic, and creativity. The procreation of nursing's language, along with an ever-increasing awareness of the intellectual activity involved in its process and implementation, is every nurse's professional responsibility.

## Integration of Knowledge and the Language of Nursing Process

There is another dimension to be considered with respect to the language of nursing process. Often, such terms as "turning and positioning" are used to describe nursing actions. In this regard, the underlying physiologic principle dictating the turning and positioning of the patient is to "maximize mobility to maintain tissue perfusion, decrease the possibility of atelectasis, or prevent a deep venous thrombosis with its concomitant risk of pulmonary embolism." With this latter statement more is communicated than just "turning and positioning." You are *thinking* about what you are doing and you are documenting it. You are integrating your theoretical and experimental knowledge base within the conceptual framework of the interacting whole individual, with respect to both the internal environment (cellular interaction) and the external environment (person–environment interaction). Documentation of such intellectual activities reflects the professional practice of the nurse and becomes the basis for reimbursement of professional service rendered.

## Criteria for Patient Outcomes and Their Documentation

Patient outcomes evolve from, and are *predicted* by, the problem portion (first part) of the nursing diagnosis. Use of precise terminology (language) in formulating and documenting patient outcomes facilitates consistency and continuity in the patient's overall care. It communicates the patient's status to all health-care providers involved in the patient's care. Criteria for patient outcomes and their documentation are listed in Table 2–1. (Note that because time frames need to be individualized for each patient, such time frames are not incorporated into the Nursing Care Plans presented in this text.)

## Characteristics of Nursing Interventions

Nursing interventions evolve from the etiology portion (second part) of the nursing diagnosis. Several characteristics of nursing interventions and their documentation should be noted, and these are listed in Table 2–2. (Note that specific dates and times are not included in the Nursing Care Plans presented in this text because they need to be individualized for the specific patient.)

TABLE 2–1
**Criteria for Patient Outcomes**

Patient outcomes should:
1. Be written as the patient's behaviors or goals. Patient outcomes reflect those human responses (physiologic, psychologic, and emotional) that must occur if the patient's problem is to be resolved. Patient outcomes do not reflect goals that the nurse will achieve. The nurse's role is to support and assist the patient to identify and use his/her capabilities and coping mechanism more effectively in dealing with the problem.
2. Be written in precise and concise terms using *action verbs.*
3. Provide *direction* for care.
4. Specify an appropriate time frame within which the patient is reassessed and the care plan is reevaluated. This serves to determine the effectiveness of the nursing interventions in assisting the patient to achieve the desired outcome(s). (Because time frames need to be individualized for each patient, Nursing Care Plans presented in this text do not incorporate specific time frames.)
5. Be realistic.
6. Be measurable. It is crucial that patient outcomes be stated in measurable terms so that nurses caring for the patient can use the same criteria to evaluate the patient's response to therapy.

TABLE 2–2
**Characteristics of Nursing Interventions**

1. Determining nursing interventions requires that the nurse have a strong theoretical and experiential knowledge base.
   The nurse must be able to establish appropriate rationales for each nursing intervention implemented.
2. Nursing interventions need to be specific; their implementation is directed toward treating the cause and resolving the patient's problem.
3. Nursing interventions prescribe nursing treatments, that is, what it is the nurse must do to treat the etiology (cause) of the patient's problem. Behaviors described by nursing interventions reflect those of the nurse and not necessarily those of the patient.
   Clear and concise documentation of nursing interventions on the patient's care plan is essential to communicate the activities and behaviors of the nurse to colleagues and other health-care providers.
4. In writing nursing interventions, the care plan needs to be revised systematically in terms of patient responses and outcomes. Decisions can then be made as to when specific interventions should be revised, updated, renewed, or discontinued. Specific dates and time frames should be documented accordingly. (Note that specific dates and times are not included in the Nursing Care Plans presented in this text because they need to be individualized for the specific patient.)
5. Each documented nursing intervention should be dated and signed by the nurse. The nurse's signature is particularly important in terms of accountability and in the sharing of information (feedback), including clarification of goals and rationales underlying care.

### *Nursing Practice: Independent and Collaborative Nursing Functions*

Nursing practice involves nursing functions that can be classified as independent or collaborative. *Independent* nursing functions include those activities that nurses are licensed to perform. In performing these functions, the nurse has complete autonomy with respect to diagnosing and treating a particular patient problem and does not require the direction of another health-care provider. The nurse is directly responsible and accountable for decisions made and actions taken.

*Collaborative* nursing functions are those in which the nurse works together with other health-care providers (usually physicians) to treat certain pathophysiologic, psychologic, and emotional problems. Activities may be performed by the nurse under the direction of another health-care provider. While the nurse may be indirectly responsible as a decision-maker, he or she remains accountable for actions taken.

In caring for critically ill patients in the intensive care setting, the critical care nurse often engages in many *inter*dependent patient care activities while collaborating with a variety of health-care providers, including physicians, respiratory therapists, nutritionists, social workers, spiritual advisors, and others.

## NURSING CARE PLANS: NURSING DIAGNOSES, DESIRED PATIENT OUTCOMES, AND NURSING INTERVENTIONS

Documentation of the patient's nursing care plan reflects the culmination of the problem-solving/decision-making activities of the professional nurse. Such documentation demonstrates the ability of the nurse to apply nursing knowledge to clinical situations and to integrate this knowledge in the implementation of the components of nursing process.

The nursing care plan format is used throughout this text to afford the reader the opportunity to examine the interrelatedness of the components of process and to appreciate how documentation of the language of process (i.e., nursing diagnoses, desired patient outcomes, and nursing interventions) ultimately reflects those functions and activities within the realm of professional nursing practice.

Nursing diagnoses used in each Nursing Care Plan reflect the 2-part nursing diagnosis statement described earlier in this chapter; patient outcomes and nursing interventions are written in the manner described in Tables 2–1 and 2–2, respectively. Rationales underlying nursing interventions are included as part of the Nursing Care Plans to assist the nurse to integrate theoretical and experimental knowledge in specific clinical circumstances.

Each Nursing Care Plan included in the text is presented in table form consisting of four columns (see Sample Care Plan: Patient with Acute Spinal Cord Injury at the end of the chapter). The first column lists the most pertinent nursing diagnoses associated with a specific pathophysiologic condition. Nursing diagnoses used throughout the text largely incorporate the diagnostic categories included in NANDA's list (see Appendix B).

The second column of the care plan includes desired patient outcomes predicted by the problem portion (first part) of each nursing diagnosis listed. Nursing interventions to treat the stated etiology (second part) are included in the third column of the care plan format. Appropriate rationales underlying specific nursing interventions are presented in the final column. (Note that specific dates and time frames for desired patient outcomes and nursing interventions are not included in the Nursing Care Plans presented in this text because they need to be individualized for each patient.)

## CASE STUDIES

Case studies are also incorporated into the text to provide the reader with the opportunity to apply nursing knowledge to specific clinical situations and to work through the components of nursing process. Nursing diagnoses are formulated based on the assessment data provided, and priority nursing diagnoses are incorporated into the nursing care plan developed for each case study. Sample nursing care plans developed for each case study reflect the language of nursing process, including nursing diagnoses, desired patient outcomes, nursing interventions, and their rationales.

## CASE STUDY WITH SAMPLE CARE PLAN: PATIENT WITH ACUTE SPINAL CORD INJURY

R.T., a well-nourished, muscular, 21-year-old white male, sustained cervical spinal injury when thrown from his motorcycle while on his way to morning classes at the university, at approximately 8:45 a.m. He was admitted to the Emergency Room of University Hospital at 9:45 a.m., where a diagnosis of transection of the spinal cord at cervical C-6 vertebral level was made. Following stabilization of his condition, Mr. T. was taken to the operating room for insertion of Crutchfield tongs.

7/16: 3:00 p.m. Upon arrival in the intensive care unit, initial assessment reveals the patient on a Stryker frame with Crutchfield tongs maintained with 15 lb of cervical traction; the patient is aligned appropriately. Mr. T. is lethargic, but arousable; oriented to person and place, but not time; pupils equal in size, round, and reactive to light and accommodation (PERRLA). The extremities are flaccid with no sensation or movement.

Vital signs on admission to the unit: blood pressure 90/60, heart rate 56, regular sinus rhythm, temperature 97.6 (R). Skin pale, cool, and dry; patient complains of chilling. Intravenous fluid administration of 0.9% normal saline infusing at 100 ml/hour. Respiration: patient on room air, breathing shallow at rate of 24/minute. Arterial blood gases drawn: $PaO_2$ 80 mmHg, $PaCO_2$ 44 mmHg, pH 7.35. Breath sounds diminished. Gastrointestinal: abdomen soft, nondistended, without bowel sounds. The patient is currently receiving nothing by mouth (NPO). Nasogastric tube to suction. Renal/urinary: straight catheterization in recovery room at 2:30 p.m. with 400 ml urine obtained. Urine specimen sent for culture/sensitivity. There is no evidence of bladder distention.

Mother at her son's bedside; Mr. T's surgeon spoke briefly with the patient and family, briefing them on the patient's current status and expectations.

### Initial Nursing Diagnoses

1. Ineffective breathing pattern: alveolar hypoventilation, related to neuromuscular impairment.
2. Ineffective airway clearance, related to compromised cough/gag reflexes.
3. Cardiac output, alteration in: decreased, re-

## SAMPLE CARE PLAN FOR THE PATIENT WITH SPINAL CORD INJURY

| Nursing Diagnoses | Desired Patient Outcomes | Nursing Interventions | Rationales |
|---|---|---|---|
| ***Nursing Diagnosis #1***<br>Ineffective breathing pattern: alveolar hypoventilation, related to:<br>1. Altered ventilatory mechanics: hypoventilation associated with paralysis of intercostal and abdominal muscles. | Patient will:<br>1. Demonstrate effective minute ventilation with trend of improving:<br>• Tidal volume $>7-10$ ml/kg<br>• Respiratory rate $<25$/min.<br>2. Achieve a vital capacity of $>15-25$ ml/kg.<br>3. Verbalize ease of breathing. | • Perform a comprehensive respiratory assessment:<br>○ Airway patency; rate, rhythm, depth of breathing; chest and diaphragmatic excursion; use of accessory muscles; breath sounds and presence of adventitious sounds. | • Major goal of airway management is to establish/maintain adequate alveolar ventilation.<br>○ Increased rapid, shallow respirations may signal deterioration of respiratory function. |
| | | • Assess neurologic status: mental status, level of consciousness, status of protective reflexes (cough, gag, swallowing). | • Hypoxia may be reflected by changes in mental status or behavior (restlessness, irritability). |
| | | • Monitor serial pulmonary function tests: tidal volume, vital capacity. | • Serial monitoring enables trends to be identified in pulmonary function. |
| | | • Assess ability to cough and handle secretions. | • Loss of intercostal and abdominal muscles compromises the patient's ability to cough effectively. |
| ***Nursing Diagnosis #2***<br>Ineffective airway clearance, related to:<br>1. Ineffective cough associated with paralysis of intercostal and abdominal muscles.<br>2. Immobility. | Patient will:<br>1. Demonstrate a secretion-clearing cough.<br>2. Maintain arterial blood gas values:<br>• $PaO_2 > 80$ mmHg<br>• $PaCO_2 \sim 35-45$ mmHg<br>• pH $7.35-7.45$ | ○ Monitor quality, quantity, color, and consistency of sputum; obtain specimen for culture/sensitivity. | ○ Loss of protective reflexes places patient at increased risk of developing aspiration pneumonia. |
| | | • Implement measures to ensure adequate respiratory function: | • Airway obstruction frequently occurs with spinal cord injury or injuries involving head and neck. |
| | | ○ Establish and maintain patent airway.<br>○ Monitor serial arterial blood gases; establish baseline function.<br>○ Initiate oxygen therapy to maintain arterial blood gases within acceptable range. | ○ Hypoxemia in the spinal cord-injured patient is most commonly associated with retained secretions. |
| | | ○ Initiate measures to handle secretions; provide humidified oxygen; maintain hydration; nasotracheal suctioning only when necessary. | ○ Suctioning increases risk of infection; suctioning-associated vagal stimulation may precipitate bradycardia in the spinal cord-injured patient who may already be bradycardic. |
| | | ○ Initiate chest physiotherapy when overall condition is stabilized: postural drainage; percussion and vibration; deep breathing and coughing exercises. | ○ Loosens and dislodges secretions and enhances movement of secretions toward trachea where they may be accessible to removal by coughing/suctioning. |
| | | ○ Instruct in use of incentive spirometry. | ○ Use of incentive spirometry encourages deep breathing, reducing risk of atelectasis. |
| | | ○ Use a calm, reassuring approach: anticipate needs, offer explanations, be accessible to patient/family. | ○ Anxiety is a major problem in the spinal cord-injured patient. |

| | | | |
|---|---|---|---|
| ***Nursing Diagnosis #3***<br>Cardiac output, alteration in: decreased, related to:<br>1. Loss of systemic vasomotor tone (neurogenic shock). | Patient's vital signs will stabilize:<br>• BP > 90 mmHg systolic (or within 10 mmHg of baseline)<br>• Heart rate ~60/min.<br>• Body temperature 98.6°F. | • Assess cardiovascular function and presence of neurogenic (spinal) shock:<br>○ Blood pressure, pulse, body temperature; skin temperature.<br>○ Cardiac monitoring for dysrhythmias.<br>○ Hydration status.<br><br>• Implement measures to stabilize cardiopulmonary function:<br>○ Initiate prescribed intravenous therapy ~75–100 ml/hr.<br>○ Monitor intake and output.<br>○ Initiate measures to minimize orthostatic hypotension: apply antiembolic stockings; abdominal binder.<br>○ Elevate lower extremities at regular intervals. | • Spinal cord injury ($T_{4-6}$ and above) precipitates spinal shock with loss of sympathetic autonomic reflexes: loss of systemic tone leads to hypotension; unopposed parasympathetic tone predisposes to bradycardia; interruption of sympathetic innervation underlies hypothermia with impaired temperature regulation.<br><br>○ Orthostatic hypotension results from venous stasis associated with impaired vasomotor tone and skeletal muscle paralysis. |
| ***Nursing Diagnosis #4***<br>Urinary elimination, alteration in, related to:<br>1. Loss of voluntary control of micturition.<br>2. Compromised micturition reflex. | Patient will maintain:<br>• Urine output > 30 ml/hr.<br>• Weight within 5% of baseline.<br>• Balanced intake and output.<br>• Stable serum electrolytes, BUN, and creatinine.<br>• Infection-free urinary tract. | • Monitor renal and hydration status:<br>○ Specific parameters to assess include body weight (daily), intake/output, serum electrolytes, BUN and creatinine, hematology profile (Hct, Hgb).<br><br>○ Implement straight catheterization protocol using aseptic technique noting amount, color, clarity, and specific gravity of urine.<br>○ Assess for bladder distention at regular intervals and straight catheterize PRN. | • Urinary retention predisposes to complications, such as urinary tract infection, and autonomic dysreflexia.<br>• Accurate intake/output and daily weight assist in determining adequacy of renal/urinary function, and fluid balance.<br>• Adequate hydration functions to prevent urinary infection and urinary calculi.<br>○ Adequate renal perfusion maintains filtration and renal function; hemoconcentration may predispose to electrolyte imbalance; increased blood viscosity may cause thromboembolic complications. |

*(continued)*

## SAMPLE CARE PLAN FOR THE PATIENT WITH SPINAL CORD INJURY *(Continued)*

| Nursing Diagnoses | Desired Patient Outcomes | Nursing Interventions | Rationales |
|---|---|---|---|
| ***Nursing Diagnosis #5***<br>Skin integrity, impairment of, related to:<br>1. Immobility.<br>2. Sensory loss. | Patient will maintain:<br>• Intact skin with good turgor.<br>• Body weight within 5% of baseline. | • Maintain skin integrity.<br>○ Assess skin carefully q2h for signs of compromised circulation especially at pressure points.<br>• Initiate therapeutic regimen:<br>○ Turn/position q2h; document rotation of positions.<br>○ Maintain proper body alignment. | • Pressure ulcer develops when there is lack of movement and distribution of weight; pressure is most concentrated between bone and skin surfaces that support body weight.<br>• Implementation of therapeutic regimen maximizes tissue perfusion, prevents venostasis and tissue ischemia.<br>○ Maintenance of proper body alignment prevents further neurologic damage. |
| | | ○ Passive ROM exercises. | ○ Passive ROM exercises help to maintain muscle tone and to improve circulation. |
| | | ○ Use of footboard, splints, sheepskin or air mattress, elbow/heel pads.<br>○ Administer lotion to pressure points.<br>○ Monitor and evaluate response to therapy. | |
| | | • Consult with nutritionist to initiate necessary nutritional regimen. | • Breakdown of body proteins (gluconeogenesis) impairs tissue healing and places the patient at increased risk of pressure ulcer development and infection. |

lated to loss of systemic vasomotor tone (neurogenic or spinal shock).

4. Urinary elimination, alteration in, related to loss of voluntary control and compromised micturition reflex.
5. Skin integrity, impairment of: potential, related to immobility and sensory loss.

The above nursing diagnoses are documented on the preceding Sample Nursing Care Plan. Additional nursing diagnoses may include:

6. Anxiety, related to unfamiliar environment and disorientation associated with loss of sensory function/perception.
7. Comfort, alteration in: increased sound conduction via Crutchfield tongs; feeling of chilliness/diaphoresis.
8. Bowel elimination, alteration in: constipation, related to loss of voluntary control and compromised defecation reflex.
9. Nutrition, alteration in: less than body requirements.
10. Sleep pattern disturbance, related to disrupted motor/sensory function; intensive care environment; anxiety.
11. Self-concept, disturbance in, related to feelings of powerlessness; dependence on others to satisfy needs.
12. Self-care deficit, related to impaired motor/sensory capabilities.
13. Coping, ineffective individual/family.
14. Knowledge deficit regarding ramifications of catastrophic spinal cord injury and rehabilitation.
15. Grieving, related to loss of motor/sensory capabilities.
16. Social isolation, related to immobility and prolonged hospitalization.

## REFERENCES


1. American Nurses' Association: Nursing: A Social Policy Statement. American Nurses' Association, Kansas City, Mo, 1980, p 9.
2. Gordon, M: Nursing Diagnosis Process and Application, ed 2. McGraw-Hill, New York, 1987.

CHAPTER 3

# Psychosocial Implications in Care of the Critically Ill Patient and Family

*Mary Meisel*

## CHAPTER OUTLINE



## LEARNING OBJECTIVES

**At the end of this chapter, you should be able to:**

1. Define stress and theories of stress.
2. List the needs of critically ill patients.
3. Identify patient stressors in the ICU.
4. Describe patient reactions in the ICU.
5. State the needs of the family of the critically ill patient.
6. Identify stressors of families.
7. Describe the needs of families.
8. Describe reactions of families to stress.
9. Define essential components of the psychosocial assessment of critically ill patients and their families.
10. List pertinent nursing diagnoses associated with psychosocial function/dysfunction.

## THE CRITICALLY ILL PATIENT

An intensive care unit (ICU) can be a very intimidating place for a patient. Shrill alarms sound seemingly without reason, lights flash from machines intermittently, and unpleasant odors permeate the air. While ICU nurses feel comfortable amidst the advanced technology and flashing screens, patients and their families can make little sense of this strange and overwhelming environment. It is difficult for patients and families to know who they are talking to when all the ICU staff members are dressed alike in surgical scrub uniforms. Overall, the experience of being admitted to an ICU or having a family member admitted is unsettling and frightening for both the patient and the family.

The ICU nurse can demystify the ICU for the patient and family by assessing their needs and concerns regarding the ICU environment, and by assessing how well the patient and the family are coping with the situation. From the assessment, the nurse diagnoses, plans, and intervenes with patients and families to meet their needs, and evaluates the effectiveness of these nursing interventions in terms of patient/family outcomes. A nurse who ascribes to the concept of total patient care must include both the patient and the patient's family in that plan of care.

The beginning of this chapter discusses the ICU patient's stressors and reactions to stress, and nursing interventions to counteract that stress. Stressors of ICU patients' families and their reactions to those stressors are then discussed. A psychosocial assessment of patient and family is presented with case studies.

## Critically Ill Patient and Stress

Patients in the ICU come from a variety of sociocultural and intellectual backgrounds and have various disease and surgical diagnoses that differ in severity. Despite these differences, all ICU patients experience stress as a result of their admission to the ICU. The amount of stress patients experience depends on their past experiences with illness, their perception of the threat of their present illness to their lives, self-images, and integrity, and the coping methods and support systems available to them.

### *Physiologic Theory of Stress*

Various theories of how stress affects people have been proposed. Selye's theory concentrates on the body's physiologic response to stimuli or stressors, rather than on an individual's psychologic response to stress. Selye defines stress as "a state manifested by a specific syndrome which consists of all the non-specifically induced changes within a biological system," or more simply, ". . . the rate of wear and tear in the body caused by life at any one time."[1] According to Selye, a stressor is that which produces stress.[1] A stressor can be physiologic, psychologic, cultural, sociologic, or environmental.

Selye's general adaptation syndrome (GAS) describes the individual's adaptation to stressors. The syndrome consists of three stages. The first is the alarm stage in which the individual experiences a sudden exposure to a noxious stimulus (stressor) to which the individual is not adapted. The second is the resistance stage, which involves the individual's full adaptation to the stressor along with a concurrent decrease in resistance to other stimuli. The final stage, the stage of exhaustion, occurs if the stressor is prolonged and severe. This stage can result in death because an individual is not infinitely capable of adapting to a stressor.

Selye describes the stress response as a "fight or flight" reaction associated with release of epinephrine and characterized by an increase in blood pressure, increased cardiac output, increased heart rate and respirations, increased blood glucose, pupillary dilation, decreased renal perfusion, and increased muscle tension in the affected individual (see Tables 6–10 and 6–11). Many of these signs can be observed in newly admitted ICU patients and their families. Prolonged stress can alter an individual's biologic function and has been associated with the development of hypertension, peptic ulcers, asthma, allergies, and cancer.

### *Psychologic Theory of Stress*

Lazarus[2] views stress as a transaction between the environment and the person. The person appraises the transaction and interprets the significance of the stress and the effect it may have on the person's well-being. According to Lazarus, individuals cope with the stress by changing themselves or adapting to the environment.

The same stressor will not affect everyone equally. Stress is determined by the person's perception of the stress, rather than the stressful situation itself. If patients admitted to rule out a myocardial infarction perceive themselves to be "well" and do not view hospitalization as a threat, they will not appear to be as stressed as patients who view an ICU admission as a threat to their lives and integrity.

### *Stress and Illness*

Stress may increase a person's susceptibility to illness, especially if the person experiences several stressors at the same time. Any life event may be stressful if it causes change in, and demands readjustment of, a person's normal routine. The more stressful the life event present in a person's life at a given time, or the presence of more than one stressor, increases the individual's chance of becoming ill.

People who are admitted to an ICU experience many stressors. A major stressor is the medical and/or surgical reason for their admission. Patients also experience a feeling of loss of control of their situation, separation from family and significant others, and fear and anxiety related to the overwhelming technical environment of the ICU.

Just as people react differently to the same stressors, so people will differ in their reaction to their ICU admission. A person's reaction to illness depends on the type of illness, whether there is a stigma attached to the illness, or if it is an acute or a chronic illness. The severity of the illness and the prognosis and course of treatment involved also influence the person's reaction. Patients' prior physical and psychologic health, availability of a support system, past experiences with illness, sociocultural beliefs, and personality characteristics will affect their reaction to their present illness.

## Needs of Critically Ill Patients

Maslow's[3] conceptual hierarchy of basic human needs forms a staircase, with physiologic needs acting as the base (Fig. 3-1). The level of needs changes from basic physiologic requirements to emotional needs, and ends with aesthetic needs at the top of the staircase.

All humans have basic *physiologic* needs, which include the need for oxygen, fluids, sleep, food, and sexual activity. *Safety* needs include both environmental and psychologic requirements. Environmental needs refer to adequate shelter from the elements and protection from harm and attack. Laws are an example of psychologic needs that help a person feel safe and secure.

*Love and belonging* needs are the next level in Maslow's hierarchy. Meaningful relationships with other people, not just sexual relationships, love of a cause, and membership in a group are examples of love and belonging needs.

*Self-love or liking* is important in developing self-esteem. Having self-esteem allows a person to feel good about himself/herself and helps to provide meaning in a person's life.

Maslow calls *self-actualization* "being true to oneself." People attempt to achieve self-actualization by fulfilling their potential through their actions and feelings.

The need to *know and understand* involves an individual's quest for knowledge for its own sake. *Aesthetic* needs are the highest need level in Maslow's hierarchy. These needs refer to awareness of the beauty of nature and the appreciation of fine arts.

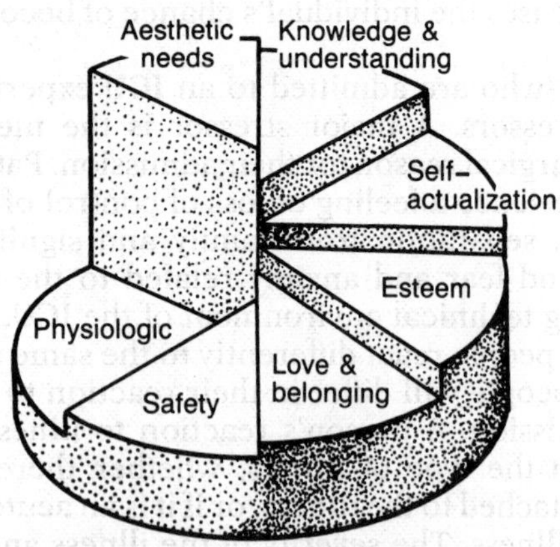


**Figure 3-1.** Maslow's Hierarchy of Needs. (Adapted from Ellis, JR and Nowlis, EA: Nursing: A Human Needs Approach. Houghton Mifflin, Boston, 1977, p 34.)

According to Maslow, the needs at the bottom of the staircase must be met and fulfilled before an individual can seek to satisfy an upper level need. There is flow and overlap between/among need levels.

Patients admitted to an ICU are experiencing biologic crises. Survival is their immediate need. ICU staff members strive to meet patients' physiologic needs by using modern technology and drugs to counteract the biologic crises. Safety needs are also attended to by the use of side rails, restraints, and sedatives to protect patients from injury.

Patients' love and belonging needs are normally provided through their relationship with their family or significant others. Patients in an ICU are physically isolated from family and significant others through limited visiting hours and age restrictions. Just when patients need their support system the most, it is limited through rules and regulations. ICU nurses can establish relationships with patients based on mutual trust, but patients still need the support of family and friends. A critically ill patient "is able to derive strength from his family to sustain him through his biological crisis."[4] The ICU staff members strive to meet a patient's physiologic and safety needs, but it is the patient's family and significant others who try to meet the love and belonging needs.

A patient's self-esteem needs can be partially met by nurses who encourage patients to participate in their own care. The need to know may be met by providing patients with information regarding their prognosis and treatment. Self-actualization needs and aesthetic needs are difficult for the nurse to provide in the ICU, and usually a patient's physiologic safety and love and belonging needs take priority.

## Patient Stressors in the ICU

The ICU environment provides unique stressors not found in other hospital units. Stressors that affect ICU patients can be physiologic, psychologic, emotional, social, and even cultural. Several of the common ICU stressors are described below.

### *Communication*

Communication between staff members as to the staff members' personal lives is ranked very high as a stressor by ICU patients.[5] It is also distressing for patients to overhear conversations between staff members regarding the patients' prognosis and treatment. Whether such conversations are understood or misinterpreted by patients, they may experience emotional distress as a result. The ICU staff should refrain from personal conversation when performing patient care. Equally as distressing as listening to inappropriate conversation is when patients fail to receive adequate communication from a nurse regarding procedures the patients are undergoing. Concise explanations can ease a patient's fears and help develop a trusting relationship between the patient and staff.

#### Pain and Analgesic Medications

Experiencing pain can be both physiologically and psychologically stressful for a patient. Analgesic medications can cloud a patient's judgment and produce hallucinations, as well as relieve pain and cause euphoria. This can result in anxiety and confusion for the patient, which further increase his/her stress. Nurses can provide explanations to patients and families regarding these possible side effects of medications, and in so doing can help them to understand what is happening.

#### Immobilization

Immobilization and claustrophobia are among the most stressful elements for a surgical ICU patient.[5] Even patients without actual physical restraints feel tied down by nasogastric tubes, intravenous lines, indwelling catheters, and endotracheal tubes. Patient restraints should be used only when necessary to ensure patient safety. Repeated explanations to patient and family of the function of restraints are necessary to decrease the patient's and family's anxiety.

#### Depersonalization

Patients also experience stress if the ICU staff depersonalizes the care to the patient by referring to a patient by diagnosis rather than by name. The patient becomes an object and is not recognized as a thinking, feeling human being. Nurses can enhance a trusting nurse–patient relationship and minimize depersonalization of patients by introducing themselves by name to the patient and family at the beginning of the shift and addressing patients by their preferred names.

#### Noise

The noise level of an ICU is very high, with the monotonous cycling of ventilators, unexpected cardiac monitor alarms, and staff conversations. Noise is a source of sensory overload for ICU patients. Patients can adapt to some types of rhythmic noise, such as a ventilator cycling. Unexpected noise, however, may initiate a startle reflex in the patient. The startle reflex will stimulate the sympathetic nervous system and initiate the stress response. Soon after the stressor is discontinued, the body will regain homeostasis.

The two main noise sources identified by ICU patients are conversations among staff nurses and noise from equipment. Patients are unable to adapt to sudden or unrhythmic noise such as staff conversations, because of the unexpected nature of such noise. To reduce the noise level in the ICU, nurses should limit noisy activities, such as personal conversation, when they are near a patient who is resting. If possible, soften ventilator alarms and telephone rings.

#### Sleep Deprivation

Sleep deprivation is partly a result of the high noise level in the ICU. Invasive procedures can also disrupt sleep. Sleep deprivation results not only from diminished hours of sleep but also from inconsistent and poor quality sleep. Twenty-four-hour lighting and rooms without windows contribute to sleep deprivation by altering the human biologic clock that regulates sleep patterns by light/dark cycles and periods of rest. ICU patients lose track of whether it is day or night. Frequent monitoring of a patient's vital signs interrupts a patient's sleep and causes sleep deprivation by as early as the second sleepless night.

Signs of sleep deprivation include impaired intellectual functioning, labile affect, anxiety, agitation, depression, confusion, disorientation to time and place, and impaired cognitive functioning. Fortunately, most symptoms of sleep deprivation resolve within 48 hours after an ICU patient is transferred to a general care floor.[6]

Nursing interventions to combat sleep deprivation include dimming the lights around the patient's bed at night and limiting vital sign checks of a stable patient to every 4 to 8 hours during the night as per physician's orders. The nurse can coordinate the patient's care to allow for uninterrupted rest periods and administer medications to induce sleep to help the patient rest.

#### Sensory Deprivation and Sensory Overload

Two other environmental stressors in the ICU are sensory deprivation and sensory overload.

Sensory deprivation for a patient can result from the monotony of the background noise of an ICU, isolation from family and significant others, being in an unfamiliar environment, and physical restraints or feeling tied down with tubes. Despite the multiple stimuli in an ICU, sensory deprivation can occur if the stimuli are not familiar or meaningful to a patient. Signs of sensory deprivation include restlessness, anxiety, and worry. Imagine a newly diagnosed quadraplegic, who must lay flat with cervical traction, unable even to scratch an ear. It is easy to see how sensory deprivation can occur.

Sensory overload can result from the same stimuli that cause sleep deprivation: high noise levels, constant lighting, and interruptions of normal sleep–awake cycles. The patient's senses are assaulted by numerous visual, auditory, olfactory, and painful tactile stimuli. The combination of stimuli and stressors can cause a patient to feel anxious, restless, and fearful. "The nurse has been pinpointed as the primary source of sensory overload in the ICU."[7]

By providing meaningful stimuli for the patient the nurse can combat sensory overload/deprivation. Clocks, calendars, television, cassettes, radios tuned to the patient's favorite station, and family visits can provide meaningful stimuli for the patient. The radio or television should not be played for prolonged periods or sensory overload can occur.

### *Witnessing a Cardiac Arrest*

While it is commonly assumed that a patient who witnesses a cardiac arrest will experience stress as a result, some patients have denied feeling any fear as a result of the incident, and they did not identify themselves with the patient who arrested.[8]

## Patient Reactions in the ICU

As previously mentioned, a patient's reaction to illness/surgery and subsequent admission to an ICU depends on past experience with illness and hospitalization, personality characteristics, severity of the illness/injury, whether the illness is an acute episode or chronic event, the patient's support system, cultural background, and level of knowledge regarding the illness/surgery.

Commonalities in patients' reactions can be observed despite the variety of factors that influence the reactions. Each reaction is described briefly below. Every patient will not demonstrate all these reactions.

### *Denial*

The first reaction many ICU and coronary care unit (CCU) patients experience is denial. Denial occurs when a person "refuses to acknowledge or attempts to deny some anxiety-provoking aspect of self, or external reality."[9] A sign of denial is an "inability to appreciate the significance of stimuli" and may include an "insensitivity to changes in body."[10] The person may also distort or minimize meanings to "the point where real meanings are clouded over."[10]

A person can control the meaning of an experience by denying that it exists and thus decrease or neutralize the anxiety aroused by the experience. An example of denial is a patient experiencing chest pain with radiation down the left arm, who delays seeking medical assistance because "I thought the pain would go away" or "I thought it was gas." *Avoidance* is closely related to denial, but differs in that patients make a deliberate effort not to think about the threat to their health, although they accept the reality of the threat. Patients who change the subject of conversation whenever it touches on their illness may be using avoidance to cope.

Contradicting the patient's view of his/her illness is not an appropriate nursing intervention. The use of denial helps protect the patient from the pain of reality. Studies have shown decreased mortality in myocardial infarction patients who use denial as a coping mechanism as opposed to patients who do not use denial.[8,11] The nurse must be patient and must continually reassess the patient's need for accurate information regarding the diagnosis. Patients may use denial throughout their entire ICU stay.

### *Anxiety*

Anxiety is a common reaction to any stressful situation. It can be defined as an uneasiness due to an impending or anticipated threat. An ICU patient who views hospitalization as a threat will become anxious. Anxiety can range from mild anxiety to panic. An anxious patient may react by fidgeting, being restless, asking the same question repeatedly, talking incessantly, or using inappropriate humor. Some anxious patients may react by withdrawing and limiting conversation. If withdrawal continues, apathy and depression can result. The patient may require counseling to overcome the depression.

The majority of ICU patients experience anxiety at some level. Nursing interventions for easing a patient's anxiety include providing the patient with explanations regarding treatments and procedures, allowing the patient to verbalize concerns and fears, and listening in a nonjudgmental manner. If necessary, discuss the possibility of the use of antianxiety medications with the patient's physician, or obtain a psychiatric consultation if the patient's anxiety is severe.

### *Demonstrating a Need for Control*

Control is a coping mechanism where optimal controls "slow down recognition processes and so provide tolerable doses of new information and emotional responses."[10] Control can be viewed as "the tendency to believe and act as if one can influence the course of events."[12] An example of a controlling person is one with a type A behavior pattern who wants to conduct business from an ICU bed via telephone, even while experiencing chest pain.

Other patients may try to maintain control over their situation and the ICU environment by asking questions or refusing treatments they do not want or understand. Even the alert patient who deliberately removes an endotracheal tube, intravenous line, or Foley catheter may be trying to demonstrate control over the ICU environment.

The nurse can provide the patient with opportunities to make decisions regarding patient care. If a patient refuses a treatment or medication, do not attempt to force the issue. Contact the patient's physician and convey the patient's reasons for the refusal. The patient needs a strong advocate, and that advocate is the patient's nurse.

### Feelings of Powerlessness

Closely related to control are feelings of powerlessness. Powerlessness is "the perception on the part of the individual of a lack of personal or internal control over events in a given situation."[13] This definition limits feelings of powerlessness to a specific situation and emphasizes that it is the individual's perception of a lack of control, not the situation itself, that leads to feelings of powerlessness.

*Passivity* is closely related to powerlessness and is the opposite of demonstrating control. Passive patients seem to allow events to control them, rather than exerting control over the events. An ICU patient who never questions any treatments and follows all directions may be the model of an ideal patient or may be feeling powerless to change the situation, and thus reacts passively. As with patients who feel a lack of control, allow patients who feel powerless to make decisions about, and participate in, their care and treatment.

### Anger

Patients whose reaction to hospitalization is anger may have feelings that malpractice or mistreatment has occurred. A patient who undergoes repeated blood drawing or CVP line insertion attempts may have reason to be angry if a repeated attempt is required as a result of a practitioner's lack of skill in performing a procedure. The patient is angry at having no control over the situation.

Anger may mask anxiety and act as a relief valve for a patient who is "fed up" with treatments and procedures. Anger may also be a result of a patient's distrust of the ICU staff. Salyer and Stuart[14] found that patients will react negatively by demonstrating anger or hostility when a nurse's action is perceived as negative to the patient, such as a nurse who criticizes a patient or is silent during administration of patient care.

Anger can also be a cover-up for fear. Patients fear pain, disfigurement, and death in the ICU. Allow patients to express their anger and try to correct any legitimate complaints voiced. Try not to take the patient's anger personally.

### Regression

ICU patients relinquish much of the control over their bodies when in an ICU. A patient may react by regressing to a former level of development. Patients capable of assisting with morning care may want a relative to help brush their hair or feed them. The family needs to understand that the regression is common and temporary.

Many patient reactions, such as regression, anger, and denial, have a negative connotation. Some patients' reactions are surprising. Humor can be used effectively as a coping mechanism. Patients may be able to face fear more easily if they can laugh at it. Inappropriate humor, such as sexual comments or innuendo, may be the patient's way of masking fear or perhaps anger at the staff. If the nurse is the recipient of inappropriate humor, a statement such as, "Mr. Jones, your remark is inappropriate and offensive to me. Please refrain from that language," is appropriate.

Patients may react to illness by using prayer and clergy for comfort and by verbalizing their fears and concerns to sympathetic relatives or ICU staff. Patients sometimes have a need to relive the precipitating event of the hospitalization and a need just to talk. A nurse can help a patient by listening and allowing the patient to talk.

### ICU Syndrome

A severe patient reaction to ICU is the development of ICU syndrome. This syndrome can be defined as "an altered emotional state occurring in a highly stressful environment, which may manifest itself in various forms such as delirium, . . . psychosis or neurosis."[15] Patients who have had severe trauma, lengthy anesthesia, or long surgical procedures have a greater chance of developing ICU psychosis or syndrome.

The common characteristics of ICU syndrome are similar to those observed in sleep deprivation, and sleep deprivation contributes to the development of ICU psychosis. These characteristics are decreased abilities to maintain attention, clouding of consciousness, memory problems, orientation difficulties, and labile affect.[15] Patients in CCUs tend to suffer less from ICU syndrome than patients in medical and surgical ICUs.[11]

The environmental stressors mentioned earlier all can contribute to the development of ICU syndrome, such as loss of day–night orientation, high noise level, isolation, medications, immobilization, sleep deprivation, depersonalization, and staff communications. The nursing interventions discussed under the sections entitled "Noise," "Sleep Deprivation," and "Sensory Deprivation and Sensory Overload" (above) are appropriate to use with ICU syndrome. Families need to be informed regarding the patient's unusual behavior during ICU syndrome. Use patient restraints and administer sedatives as necessary to ensure the patient's safety.

Some neurologic illnesses and trauma will alter a

patient's personality and reaction to the ICU environment. A patient with a closed head injury reacts in a varied and unpredictable manner. Medications, including morphine, phenothiazines, cimetidine, and lidocaine, can also alter a patient's reaction to the ICU. The nurse has to assess the impact of drugs and the type of injury to judge their effects on a patient's reaction.

## THE FAMILY OF THE CRITICALLY ILL PATIENT

A family is "a basic societal unit in which members have a commitment to nurture each other emotionally and physically."[16] The family has been described as "a system, a complex network of interdependent interactions among family members which fulfills needs and achieves equilibrium."[17]

A family can be viewed as an open system. Any change or disturbance in a part of the system will create a change or disturbance in the whole system.[18] Therefore, any stress on one family member will affect the whole family. Illness of a family member is a common situational stress that a family could experience. The family may view a member's illness as a threat to the family's equilibrium and integrity, especially if hospitalization is required. Nonhospitalized family members may have to assume the family roles of the sick member. The needs met through the relationship with the sick member may not be satisfied while the patient is hospitalized.

The illness (stressor) may precipitate a crisis in the family, especially if the stressor is a new stimulus that the family has not dealt with previously. Not all families will react similarly to the same stressor. Therefore, every illness and hospitalization may not cause a family to experience a crisis. But if the family views the illness as a threat to the family's integrity, a crisis can develop.

A crisis occurs when a person is confronted with a problematic situation for which his/her typical way of operating in the world and the usual supports are not sufficient.[18] "A crisis effects a temporary disruption of an individual's normal patterns of living, and is characterized by high levels of tension."[19] The interactional patterns reach a temporary state of disequilibrium in a family crisis. A period of disorganization ensures a period of upset, during which many abortive attempts at solution are made.[20]

The disorganization a family experiences will be in its function and structure. Initially, family members may be immobilized by feelings of disbelief, shock, fear, helplessness, and anxiety.[21] The family will begin to feel the loss of the predictable functions of the hospitalized relative.[22] Basic emotional and physical needs of the family members may be unmet, as they attempt to resolve the disorganization that one member's hospitalization has precipitated. Unmet needs produce stress in the family.[23]

If a family's needs are not met, they may be unable to "provide an ongoing social system for the patient during the crisis."[24] The well family members may experience anxiety as their attempts at resolving the disorganization fail because they lack the problem-solving skills to deal with the crisis.

"Interactions between members in a family system are circular. The behavior of one member affects the behavior of another."[25] Family members can transfer their anxiety to the patient, thereby increasing the patient's stress.[24] The patient, especially in ICU, is struggling to overcome a biologic crisis and does not need the added stress of a family's anxiety. When the stress a family experiences decreases, the amount of support the family can offer the patient increases.[26] Cobb[27] states that "support from the patient's family is crucial to the patient's survival."

Critical care nurses need to be aware of the relationship between their patient's recovery and the family members' support. The needs of the family have to be met in order to reduce the family's stress.[26] The nurse needs to assess the family's potential for crisis and develop interventions that will enable the family to support the patient and regain its equilibrium and continue to grow. During a crisis, a person is more open to suggestions and to help; therefore, nursing interventions have fertile ground in which to work.[28] Successful intervention may help the family to regain their previous level of function and, perhaps, improve their coping ability. The needs of the family may change as time passes, so the nurse has to reassess the family to plan interventions accordingly.

### Stressors of Families

The stressors of families of ICU patients are slightly different from patient stressors. Families experience physical isolation from their relative in ICU and perhaps emotional isolation from other well family members, if the family support system is not strong enough to allow members to comfort each other. Families fear death or permanent disability of the ill member, fear that the injury will cause the relative chronic pain, and fear the loss of a "healthy" family member. Well members also have to absorb the role responsibilities of the ill member, if the ill member is financially responsible for the family, the illness will take a toll on family finances.

The ICU environment also stresses the family. Members are confronted with machines that sound alarms seemingly without cause, numerous intravenous lines, and other "tubes." If a patient is intubated or in an altered neurologic state, the difficult or impossible communication between patient and family can cause stress for the family. Families have to put trust in strangers and hope that the ICU staff is competent. Restricted visiting hours, crowded ICU rooms, and the hurried ICU atmosphere can make families feel unwelcome in the ICU. Relatives may be reluctant to touch the patient for fear of dislodging a tube or disturbing the patient's sleep.

The ICU waiting room can provide additional stressors if it is crowded, smoky, and far from vending machines and restrooms. The family may not want to leave the waiting room to eat for fear of missing a doctor's visit or change in their relative's condition. Because a family's support is vital to an ICU patient's recovery, the ICU staff needs to be aware of these stressors and the needs of family members.

## Family Needs

When a family member is critically ill, well members concentrate all their energy on the patient, at the expense of their own physiologic needs. With the patient's admission to the ICU, families will forgo sleep, forget to eat, and push themselves to the point of exhaustion. The well members' primary concern is for the patient to survive the current biologic crisis; all the family's other needs are pushed aside.

In the past 10 years, research regarding the needs of family members of ICU patients has blossomed. Hampe's[29] pioneer study of the needs of spouses of terminally ill patients in 1975 identified eight personal needs of the spouses (the death of their spouse did not change these needs):

1. Need to be with the dying person.
2. Need to be helpful to the dying person.
3. Need for assurance of the comfort of the dying person.
4. Need to be informed of the mate's condition.
5. Need to be informed of the impending death.
6. Need to ventilate emotions.
7. Need for comfort and support of family members.
8. Need for acceptance, support, and comfort from health professionals.

Dracup and Breu[30] used the results of Hampe's study to develop a special care plan for the spouses of critically ill CCU patients based on the eight needs identified by Hampe's subjects. The interventions included flexible visiting hours for the spouses, the patient's primary nurse calling the spouse at home twice daily with condition reports, and arranging to meet with the spouse for 15 minutes every day for the nurse to answer any questions the spouse may have and to provide emotional support. The results of their study indicated that spouses who received the special interventions felt that more of their needs were met by the nursing staff than spouses who received the CCU's usual nursing interventions.

Molter's[31] study in 1970 was another milestone in the research of the identification of family members needs. In her study, Molter found that the families of ICU patients may have specialized needs. The subjects included not only the spouse of the patient, but also parents, children, siblings, and even a niece. She also interviewed more than one family member per patient.

The top ten ranked needs in Molter's study were:

1. To feel there is hope.
2. To feel that hospital personnel care about the patient.
3. To have the waiting room near the patient.
4. To be called at home about changes in the condition of the patient.
5. To know the prognosis.
6. To have questions answered honestly.
7. To know specific facts concerning the patient's progress.
8. To receive information about the patient once a day.
9. To have explanations given in terms that are understandable.
10. To see the patient frequently.

The subjects were also asked to list who they felt were meeting their needs. The results showed that the subjects felt nurses met the majority of the families' needs overall and that physicians met most of their top ten needs, which included the need for information regarding the patient's prognosis and treatments. The needs that nurses met were related to the physical comfort and emotional support of the patient. In both Hampe's and Molter's studies, family members stated that they felt the nurse should be responsible only for the patient's needs and not the family's needs.

The literature indicates that family members of ICU patients have specific needs. Among the most important needs are to have knowledge and information regarding the patient's prognosis and treatment, to feel that the patient is receiving the best care, and to visit the patient frequently. The establishment of good communication and a trusting relationships among the patient, family, and ICU staff would be the first step in meeting these family needs by the ICU nurse.

## Family Reactions

Most families experience shock and fear when a relative is admitted to an ICU. The patient's admission is usually sudden and unexpected and can precipitate a crisis in the family, especially if the family members have little experience in dealing with hospitalization. Family members may feel guilty and angry if they feel that they are partially responsible for the patient's injury or illness. Like the patient, the family feels physically isolated and powerless to help their relative. The family has little control over the patient's environment or treatment.

Families react to their feelings of helplessness and powerlessness differently. Geary[32] has identified five common coping mechanisms families use to deal with a relative's hospitalization. According to Geary, a coping mechanism is "any behavior or mental processes used to attempt to come to terms with illness in the family."[32]

### Minimization

Minimization is the first and most prevalent coping mechanism described by Geary. It is characterized by reducing or attempting to ignore the significance of an event. One example of minimization is the family who takes on a cheerful demeanor while visiting the patient or talking with the nurse in hopes of reducing the significance of the hospitalization.

A family member who does not remember information regarding a patient's condition, or cannot understand repeated explanations, may be minimizing the patient's situation by ignoring explanations and information.

### Intellectualization

Intellectualization is another coping mechanism. Family members who use this mechanism appear overly rational and minimize any feelings they are experiencing. A family member who wants to know every function of a ventilator, but who fails to be concerned about the patient's ventilator dependence, may be using intellectualization.

### Repetition

Every ICU nurse has had the experience of a family member repeatedly asking the same questions or repeating the same story over and over. It is not clear if family members who use repetition as a coping mechanism are trying to convince themselves of something or just need to ventilate their anxiety.

### Acting Strong

The family member who presents a strong, competent attitude seems to indicate an ability to deal well with the relative's illness. The family member may be trying to demonstrate that he has strong inner resources and can take over the ill member's role if he dies or has a long rehabilitation.

### Remaining Near the Patient

Family members may react to the patient's illness by keeping a vigil at the patient's bedside or remaining in the waiting room for 24 hours a day. Some families feel that leaving the hospital for a while indicates a lack of hope for the patient's recovery. Ethnic customs and mores can influence a family's reaction to separation from the patient. Some cultures feel that the family's presence either at the patient's bedside or in the waiting room is essential for the patient's recovery.

Somatic complaints may be experienced by some family members, including restlessness, interrupted sleep pattern, weight loss, feelings of depression, and diminished appetite.

Another reaction family members may demonstrate is turning to others for support, such as friends, relatives, and ICU staff. Families need to feel there is hope for the patient's recovery or, in cases of patients with terminal illnesses, that their relative won't suffer and will die peacefully.

Regardless of the coping methods a family uses, the family's goal is to manage the stressful hospitalization the best that they can. Nurses need to recognize that the family is under stress and trying to cope. The nurse needs to assess how effective a family's coping efforts are and to intervene to support or reinforce their coping efforts.

Bowman[24] divided Molter's[31] need statements into three categories — cognitive needs, emotional needs, and physical needs — and then developed nursing interventions for some of the needs in each category. Table 3–1 is a summary of nursing interventions to meet the needs of families of ICU patients.

## PSYCHOSOCIAL ASSESSMENT OF CRITICALLY ILL PATIENTS AND THEIR FAMILIES

One of the most difficult, and often the most neglected, patient/family assessment is the nurse's assessment of the patient's and family's *psychosocial functioning*. The ICU patient is in a biologic crisis and many times the ICU staff members concentrate their energy on supporting the patient's physiologic needs and on resolving the patient's biologic crisis. It is easy to forget that in the center of all the machines, intravenous lines, and various tubes lies a person who is experiencing fear and anxiety. The ICU nurse is responsible not only for supporting the patient's physiologic functioning, but also for assessing and supporting the patient's emotional and social needs.

A psychosocial assessment of a patient involves observation of a patient's behavior. A patient's facial expressions and body language can indicate unvoiced anxiety and fear, depression, and even

TABLE 3-1

**Summary of Nursing Interventions to Meet the Needs of Families of ICU Patients***

**Cognitive Needs**

1. To Know Specific Facts About the Patient's Progress.
   - Avoid using generalizations such as "he's much better" or "things are about the same today."
   - Use the same simple terms each day to discuss progress and concerns (e.g., heart rhythm, blood pressure, level of pain, level of oxygen in the blood, not responding/very groggy/sleepy/awake, and so forth). This permits families to focus their attention on the same frame of reference and, when applicable, to put closure on the topic.
   - Relate progress to the illness as you have described it initially.
   - Use nursing care plan to communicate phrases and areas of concern being discussed so that all staff members use the same terminology.
2. To Know the Probable Outcome.
   - Be as realistic as possible, but be aware of family's coping mechanisms (such as denial) as well as their need for hope.
   - Establish short-term goals so that positive change can be identified.
   - If patient's prognosis is poor, allow adequate time to spend with the family so that feelings or questions can emerge. Establish times to meet with the family again.
   - Verbally recognize and accept family's desire for certainty in an ambiguous situation.
3. To Know Exactly What Is Being Done for the Patient (How the Patient Is Being Treated Medically, Why Things Are Being Done for the Patient).
   - Briefly describe each line and/or monitoring device, including IVs, urinary catheters, arterial lines, nasogastric tubes, $O_2$ devices, and so forth.
   - Encourage questions.
   - Remember that one explanation may not be enough; high anxiety is a barrier to learning.
   - Use simple terminology such as "breathing tube," "cardiogram," or "special intravenous" rather than endotracheal tube, electrocardiogram, or Swan-Ganz catheter.
   - Base explanations of treatment on patient's illness as you have described it initially. Reinforce explanations of pathophysiology as needed.
   - Promote continuity through nursing care plan.
4. To Have Questions Answered Honestly.
   - Be specific; discuss all issues as they relate to the patient as a unique individual.
   - Maintain good communications with physicians so that you are aware of what they have told the family. Discuss with them any information they feel should be withheld to determine rationale.
   - Use nursing care plan for consistency. Families quickly become aware of evasive answers. Consistency decreases anxiety and feelings of dehumanization and promotes cooperation.
5. To Have Explanations Given in Understandable Terms.
   - Assess family's knowledge base and previous experience with patient's condition.
   - Determine family's priority for learning; what do they want to know immediately.
   - Provide basic pathophysiology slowly, allowing time for questions. Repeat pathophysiologic concepts when discussing treatments or progress.
   - Divide informational sessions so that family is not overwhelmed. Establish times at which you will meet with them again to answer questions or provide additional explanations.
   - Remember that high anxiety is a barrier to learning; explanations usually have to be repeated.
   - Respond positively to questions, recognizing their right to understand what is happening.
6. To Have Explanations About the Environment Before Going into ICU for the First Time.
   - Use time before patient arrives on unit to meet with family.
   - Remember that the environment *is* frightening, not only equipment surrounding patient, but also the equipment used for other patients in the area.
   - While describing equipment, reinforce that much of it is present for prevention and early detection of problems.
   - Verbally recognize family's feelings and reassure them that these are normal and acceptable.
   - Be with family during their first visit to provide additional explanations and support.
   - For planned admissions (e.g., post surgery):
     Establish guidelines in teaching for discussion of environment.
     Provide patient and family tours of ICU if desired.
     Have ICU nurse who will be assigned to patient immediately postoperatively meet with family before surgery.

**Emotional Needs**

1. To Be Assured That the Best Possible Care Is Being Given to the Patient.
   - Emphasize that nurses and physicians are experienced and have special training to provide expert care.
   - Verbally recognize family's anxiety. Reassure them that such feelings are normal and that they do not have to hide these feelings.
2. To Be Called at Home About Changes in the Patient's Condition.
   - Establish guidelines with family about who is to be called and in what time frame.
   - Always ensure that the family knows about any significant change in patient's status before first visit of the day. If they are not informed about a change for the better, families frequently assume they will not be notified of other changes.
3. To Receive Information About the Patient Once Each Day.
   - Set aside one period during the day, as early as possible, during which progress reports are given.
   - Assess whether this time is adequate and follow up as needed, particularly if patient's condition changes.
   - Be aware if family needs to have physicians' explanations clarified or amplified.
4. To See the Patient Frequently.
   - Review policy for visiting hours to determine if they meet family needs; adjust as permitted by current situation in ICU.
   - If a visit must be delayed, explain reason clearly; make sure that the family does not believe the delay is due to a crisis unnecessarily.
   - Provide time for patient and family to be alone together.

*(continued)*

TABLE 3-1
**Summary of Nursing Interventions to Meet the Needs of ICU Patients *(Continued)***

**Emotional Needs**

5. To Feel That Hospital Personnel Care About the Patient.
   - Use information gained during family assessment to anticipate concerns.
   - Listen to family's concerns, demonstrating that staff sees patient as an individual. Seek advice from the family about meeting patient needs.
   - Tell the family what patient communicates.
   - Focus on sensations patient will feel and possibly communicate to the family so that these do not come as a surprise (e.g., sore throat following endotracheal tube, fragility of chest wall post CABG, noisy environment, and so forth).
   - Remember that family members may focus on small details such as patient's position, cleanliness, or bedding because these are within their normal range of control.
   - Remember that family members may take out their feelings of grief, guilt, or anger on nursing staff; be patient.
6. To Talk About the Possibility of the Patient's Death. To Feel There Is Hope.
   - Determine family's perception of situation.
   - Anticipate and recognize signs of anticipatory grieving. Provide open-ended questions to encourage them to express their feelings.
   - Provide concrete information about patient's status slowly, assessing family's response. False reassurance and the opposite extreme, abrupt confrontation with reality, may hinder appropriate coping.
   - Meet jointly with physician and family to discuss use/non-use of extraordinary measures or advanced life support systems.
   - Be aware of how comfortable you are when discussing a patient's death. If unable to meet family needs by yourself, arrange for another member of the health team to meet with family.
   - If there is no *real* contraindication, allow family to spend additional time with dying patient.

**Physical Needs**

1. To Help with the Patient's Physical Care.
   - Anticipate that family may be reluctant to touch patient because of equipment and yet want/need to touch him/her for reassurance. Small directed activities meet both these concerns.
   - Allow family to do small things for patient (e.g., providing ice chips, wiping face, washing old blood off hands, and so forth).
   - If there is no *real* contraindication, allow family member to provide parts of morning care.
2. To Visit Anytime.
   - Discuss visiting regulations with family.
   - Be flexible if special arrangements need to be made because of other responsibilities.
   - Recognize that this need will probably diminish over a few days as families become aware that visiting hours are adequate and that they *will* be permitted to see patient frequently.
3. To Have the Waiting Room Near ICU. To Have a Telephone Near the Waiting Room.
   - If these are not available in your hospital, be aware of potential stress for families. Discuss possible alternative arrangements.
   - Discuss the need for family members to get adequate rest so that they will be able to support patient later in hospitalization and to minimize extended stays by family in waiting room.
4. To Have a Place to Be Alone in the Hospital.
   - Direct family to hospital chapel if available.
   - Determine if there is space available nearby, currently being used for another purpose, that could be used by family for periods of privacy.
   - If weather is pleasant, encourage family to exercise outdoors during the day.

* From Bowman,[24] with permission.

anger. Observe patients for signs of anxiety such as facial grimacing, restlessness, picking at bedsheets, clenching hands, and crying. Fearful and anxious patients may repeat questions, use inappropriate humor, or be silent. Intubated patients may communicate fear through wide-eyed looks and pulling at their tubes.

Because the family's support of a patient can help the patient overcome a biologic crisis, it is important for the nurse to assess how supportive a patient's family is and to plan interventions that encourage family support. Observe the quality of the patient–family interactions. Questions regarding the patient's marital status and living arrangements can provide clues to the strength of his/her support system.

Other important information is the patient's past hospital experiences (especially past ICU experiences) and the coping methods the patient used to handle previous hospitalizations. This information can give the nurse clues as to how the patient may react with this hospitalization. Any past history of emotional instability or use of street drugs and alcohol by the patient can help a nurse plan interventions to protect the patient's safety. Discovering if the patient has recently undergone any major life changes will help the nurse understand the patient's current stress level.

Patients' vital signs can also provide clues to their emotional status. Patients experiencing emotional distress may exhibit an increased blood pressure and cardiac output, increased pulse and respiratory rate, and dilated pupils as a result of increased epinephrine secretion. Their blood glucose and cholesterol levels can also rise.

Specific questions ICU nurses can ask patients and/or the patients' families include:

1. What are the family's living arrangements?
2. Has the patient been hospitalized previously? If yes, what was the experience like? What helped the patient/family deal with the hospitalizations?
3. What family does the patient have? Where do they live?
4. What questions or concerns does the patient/family have?

ICU nurses, using these questions as guidelines, can expand their inquiries into potential problem areas. For example, if a young mother states she has an infant at home, the nurse can ask who is taking care of the child and then determine the need for social services assistance.

To perform a psychosocial assessment, an ICU nurse needs to use the same skills used for any patient or family assessment. Good communication skills are essential for gathering data. Empathic, objective listening and the ability to ask open-ended questions are skills that a nurse must possess. Nurses can use their senses of touch, hearing, sight, and smell to gather objective and subjective data. Observing a patient's behavior can provide clues as to how that patient is feeling and coping with illness. The ICU nurse must also understand the importance of the patient's emotional and social status and how the patient's family and support system can positively influence a patient's recovery.

After collecting subjective and objective psychosocial patient data, the nurse proceeds to make a nursing diagnosis based on that data. Examples of nursing diagnoses associated with psychosocial functioning include:[33]

- Anxiety
- Communication, impaired, verbal
- Coping, ineffective family (specify compromised or disability)
- Coping, ineffective individual
- Fear (specify)
- Grieving (specify anticipatory or dysfunctional)
- Powerlessness
- Rest/activity pattern: ineffective
- Role disturbance
- Self-concept, disturbances in: body image, self-esteem, role performance, personal identity
- Sleep pattern disturbance
- Social isolation
- Spiritual distress

Based on the nursing diagnosis, the nurse plans the nursing interventions to be used to achieve the patient outcomes. All interventions need to be evaluated for their effectiveness and revised if the patient outcome is not achieved.

Family members' needs and concerns should be assessed by the nurse. The family can provide the nurse with information regarding the patient if the patient is unable. The family can be observed for their methods of coping with their family member's illness and for the amount of support they offer the patient. The nurse can ascertain who in the family fills what roles and which family member has assumed the responsibilities of the sick patient's role(s). The nurse can gather data about the patient's family through observing questioning, and listening.

The two short case studies with sample care plans that follow illustrate the use of nursing diagnoses concerned with psychosocial function.

## CASE STUDY WITH SAMPLE CARE PLAN: RULE-OUT MYOCARDIAL INFARCTION (MI)

C.M., a 54-year-old white male, experienced acute onset of midsternal chest pain with left arm radiation while shoveling snow. He was brought to the Emergency Room (ER) of University Medical Center via ambulance at 10:00 a.m.

Mr. M. was directly admitted to the Coronary Care Unit (CCU), where he was attached to a cardiac monitor, and continued to receive intravenous fluid (IV) at 25 ml/hour and oxygen at 3 liters/minute via nasal cannula. Mr. M. received 3 sublingual nitroglycerin tablets in the ER and 5 mg of IV morphine. His chest pain has subsided.

The CCU nurse completing Mr. M.'s admission form observes that he answers questions rapidly and repeats phrases several times, such as "I could not believe I was having chest pain. I thought it was indigestion." Mr. M.'s eyes dart all around the floor, and he makes limited direct eye contact with the nurse. He fidgets with the sheets and keeps folding and unfolding his arms. The nurse records several of Mr. M.'s statements in the admission note. "I've never been sick a day in my life. This is the first time I've been in a hospital. I feel so nervous. What is that beeping sound? Is my heart OK? Both my father and my brother died of heart attacks in their 50s. Did I have a heart attack?" Mr. M.'s blood pressure is 154/92, pulse 100; he is in sinus rhythm with a rare PVC, and his respirations are 20. His skin is cool and clammy. His wife is present in the room and sits quietly in a chair by her husband's bed.

### Nursing Diagnoses

1. Psychosocial anxiety, related to unfamiliar environment.
2. Fear of dying, related to familial history of myocardial infarction.

## SAMPLE CARE PLAN FOR THE PATIENT/FAMILY WITH PSYCHOSOCIAL DYSFUNCTION WITH CLOSED HEAD INJURY

| Nursing Diagnoses | Desired Patient Outcomes | Nursing Interventions | Rationales |
|---|---|---|---|
| ***Nursing Diagnosis #1***<br>Anxiety, related to unfamiliar environment | Patient will:<br>1. Verbalize a decrease in anxiety.<br>2. Appear less anxious.<br>3. Maintain stable vital signs:<br>• BP within 10 mmHg of baseline<br>• Heart rate < 100/min<br>• Respiratory rate/rhythm < 25/min eupneic | • Encourage patient to verbalize concerns, and actively listen. | • By verbalizing anxiety, it helps the patient to recognize existence of anxiety, and makes the anxiety less threatening and easier to deal with. |
| | | • Demonstrate an empathic and caring attitude. | • An empathic attitude and active listening help demonstrate that the nurse respects the patient, and begins to develop a trusting nurse/patient relationship. |
| | | • Observe for behavioral clues that anxiety is decreasing (i.e., more direct eye contact, less rapid speech, slower body movements). | • Behavior gives clues to underlying anxiety. Body language can be observed for presence of anxiety.<br>• Rapid speech and repeated questions can be a sign of anxiety. |
| | | • Monitor vital signs: blood pressure, pulse, and respiratory rate/rhythm. | • Somatic signs of the stress response are seen in increased blood pressure, pulse, and cool, clammy skin, as epinephrine is released and blood is rerouted to major organs. |
| | | • Monitor response to prescribed analgesia therapy (e.g., morphine, nitroglycerin, and/or sedatives to reduce and minimize chest pain).<br>○ Antianxiety agents (e.g., Valium) may also be indicated. | • The effectiveness of analgesic and antianxiety medication in relieving pain and anxiety should be carefully monitored. |
| | | • Decrease noise level (e.g., by shutting doors between patient rooms, encouraging a quiet rest period during each shift, and organizing patient care to provide frequent rest periods). | • The stress response is harmful to the hypoxic (ischemic) heart and could lead to an extension of the infarct. |
| | | • Orient patient/family to surrounding and protocols. | |

| | | | |
|---|---|---|---|
| ***Nursing Diagnosis #2***<br>Ineffective coping: family, related to:<br>1. Catastrophic illness<br>2. Necessary changes in lifestyle | Patient/family will demonstrate acceptance of illness by:<br>1. Discussing impact of illness on lifestyle.<br>2. Initiating appropriate changes in lifestyle to maintain level of health desired.<br>Cessation of cigarette smoking by patient and spouse<br>Reducing level of stress in daily activities | • Encourage spouse to visit frequently if desired.<br>• Encourage patient's spouse to use self as a support for the patient. Provide support to the spouse and assist in identifying effective coping mechanisms.<br>• Strengthen spouse's ability to support patient by:<br>○ Listen empathically.<br>○ Include spouse in patient's care.<br>○ Praise the efforts of the spouse in supporting patient. | • Family support positively affects the patient's status and outcome; interaction with loved ones helps to reduce anxiety in all family members and helps in coping.<br>• Family support of patients can influence their recovery process. |
| ***Nursing Diagnosis #3***<br>Fear of death, related to familial history of myocardial infarction | Patient will verbalize concerns and fears. | • Strengthen patient/family/nurse relationship.<br>○ Exhibit empathic attitude.<br>○ Listen actively.<br>○ Encourage patient to verbalize concerns and fears.<br>• Consult with patient's physician sharing familial history ascertained.<br>○ Share approach to therapy.<br>○ Jointly inform patient and spouse about diagnosis, course of treatment, and prognosis for recovery.<br>• Offer patient/family positive information regarding the patient's recuperative progress as patient's condition improves. Avoid offering false reassurance.<br>• Encourage patient to discuss fears with spouse. Support patient and spouse in reassessing goals and planning beyond discharge. | ○ An empathic attitude and active listening help to demonstrate that the nurse respects the patient, and begins to develop a trusting nurse/patient/family relationship.<br>○ Verbalization of fear and concerns allows patient to acknowledge fear and, thus, to begin to deal with it.<br>• Collegial interaction ensures continuity of care; reassures patient/family.<br>• Information from members of health team gives facts that patient/family can deal with. This may assist them in handling fears and reassessing lifestyle.<br>• Reassurance regarding improvement in patient's condition helps to reduce fear. |

## CASE STUDY WITH SAMPLE CARE PLAN: CLOSED HEAD INJURY

The Smiths' only child, 19-year-old Cory, a white male, sustained a severe closed head injury 2 days ago in a motorcycle accident. Cory is in a deep coma and unresponsive to painful stimuli. His prognosis is grim, and the Smiths have been told that Cory has a minimal chance of regaining consciousness.

Mr. Smith appears calm, but the nurse observed that he asked more questions about the ventilator and hemodynamic monitoring than about Cory's condition. He states that his wife does not work and that he handles all the financial concerns in the family. "My insurance should easily cover all of Cory's expenses." He never touches Cory or sits by the bedside. Mr. Smith's visits are brief and infrequent.

Mrs. Smith insists on sitting by Cory's bed at all times. She leaves the patient's room only when asked to and has slept in the family lounge since Cory's admission. When a nurse suggested she go home and sleep, she stated, "Cory's all I got and I'm going to stay with him until he wakes up." She will ask every person who takes care of Cory the same questions, which makes the nursing staff feel as if she is checking up on them. She and her husband, when in the patient's room together, rarely converse or touch each other. Mr. Smith leaves the hospital at night. No other relatives have visited Cory or have called.

### Nursing Diagnoses

1. Coping, ineffective, compromised.
2. Social isolation.

## REFERENCES


1. Selye, H: The Stress of Life. McGraw-Hill, New York, 1956, pp 54, 64.
2. Lazarus, RS: Stress, Appraisal and Coping. Springer, New York, 1984.
3. Maslow, AH: Motivation and Personality, ed 2. Harper & Row, New York, 1970, pp 35–58.
4. Roberts, S: The role of the family in critical care. In Behavioral Concepts and the Critically Ill Patient, Prentice-Hall, Englewood Cliffs, NJ, 1976, p 352.
5. Ballard, KS: Identification of environmental stressors for patients in a surgical intensive care unit. Issues in Mental Health Nursing 3(1–2):89, 1981.
6. Luce, C: Current Research on Sleep and Dreams. US Department of Health, Education and Welfare, Public Health Services Publication No. 1389. National Institutes of Health, Bethesda, 1965, pp 10–15, 22–24.
7. Mackinnon-Kessler, S: Maximizing your ICU patient's sensory perception environment. Canadian Nurse 79(5):41, 1983.
8. Hackett, TP, Cassem, NH, and Wishnie, HA: The coronary care unit: An appraisal of its psychologic hazards. N Engl J Med 279(25):1365, 1968.
9. Haber, J, Leach, AM et al: Comprehensive Psychiatric Nursing, ed 2. McGraw-Hill, New York, 1982.
10. Horowitz, M: Psychological response to serious life events. In Hamilton, V and Warburton, D (eds): Human Stress and Cognition. Wiley, New York, 1980.
11. Hackett, TP and Cassem, NH: Psychological management of the myocardial infarction patient. Human Studies 1(3):25, 1975.
12. Kobasa, S: The hardy personality: Toward a social psychology of stress and health. In Sanders, GS and Suls, J (eds): Social Psychology of Health and Illness. Lawrence Erlbaum, New Jersey, 1982, pp 3–32.
13. Roy, Sr C: Introduction to Nursing: An Adaptation Model. Prentice-Hall, Englewood Cliffs, NJ, 1976, p 224.
14. Salyer, J and Stuart, BJ: Nurse–patient interaction in the intensive care unit. Heart Lung 14(1):20, 1985.
15. Kleck, HG: ICU syndrome: Onset, manifestations, treatment, stressors and prevention. Crit Care Q 6(4), 1984, pp 21–28.
16. Smilkstein, G: The cycle of family function: A conceptual model for family medicine. J Fam Pract 11:223, 1980.
17. Ruben, HL: Family crisis. Am Fam Physician 11:132, 1975.
18. Parad, HJ and Caplan, G: A framework for studying families in crisis. In Parad, HJ (ed): Crisis Intervention: Selected Readings. Family Services Association of America, New York, 1965, pp 53–72.
19. Umana, RF, Gross, ST, and McConville, MT: Crisis in the Family: Three Approaches. Gardner Press, New York, 1980.
20. Caplan, G: An Approach to Community Mental Health. Grune & Stratton, New York, 1961.
21. Gardner, D and Stewart, N: Staff involvement with families of patients in critical care units. Heart Lung 7(1):105, 1978.
22. Braulin, J, Rook, J, and Sills, GM: Family in crisis: The impact of trauma. Crit Care Q 5(3), 1982, pp 38–46.
23. Orlando, IJ: Dynamic Nurse–Patient Relationship. GP Putnam's Sons, New York, 1961.
24. Bowman, CC: Identifying priority concerns of families of ICU patients. Dimensions of Critical Care Nursing 3(5):313, 1984.
25. Levitt, MB: Nursing and family-focused care. Nurs Clin North Am 19(1):83, 1984.
26. Bozett, FW and Gibbons, R: The nursing management of families in the critical care setting. Critical Care Update 10(2):22, 1983.
27. Cobb, S: Social support as a moderator of life stress. Psychosom Med 38:300, 1976.
28. Brose, C: Theories of family crisis. In Hymovich, DP and Barnard, MU (eds): Family Health Care. New York, McGraw-Hill, 1979.
29. Hampe, SO: Needs of the grieving spouse in a hospital setting. Nurs Res 24(2):116, 1975.
30. Breu, C and Dracup, K: Helping spouses of critically ill patients. Am J Nurs 78(1), 1978, pp 51–53.
31. Molter, NC: Needs of relatives of critically ill patients: A descriptive study. Heart Lung 8(2):332, 1970.
32. Geary, MC: Supporting family coping. Supervisor Nurse 10(3), 1979, pp 52–53, 57–59.
33. Kim, MJ, McFarland, GK, and McLane, AM: Pocket Guide to Nursing Diagnoses. CV Mosby, St Louis, 1989.

## SAMPLE CARE PLAN FOR THE PATIENT/FAMILY WITH PSYCHOSOCIAL DYSFUNCTION WITH MYOCARDIAL INFARCTION

| Nursing Diagnoses | Desired Patient Outcomes | Nursing Interventions | Rationales |
|---|---|---|---|
| ***Nursing Diagnosis #1***<br>Coping: Ineffective-compromised | Patient's parents will:<br>1. Verbalize questions and concerns regarding son's condition.<br>2. Approach patient at bedside and hold hands.<br>3. Reduce the number of repetitive questions.<br>4. Leave the hospital for 1 hour/day, and sleep at home. | • Exhibit an empathic attitude; offer to listen, and encourage patient to verbalize concerns when ready to do so. | • The nurse is accessible to the patient's parents and offers a listening ear. This helps to nurture the patient/parent/nurse relationship.<br>◦ Family members who intellectualize may do so because, at least initially, they may be unable to discuss feelings with others.<br>◦ Nurturing this relationship may eventually assist family members in coping. |
| | | • Explain to parents that touching the patient is perfectly okay.<br>◦ Encourage them to sit at bedside and reassure that they will not disturb the patient's equipment/machinery. | |
| | | ◦ Encourage questions and make necessary explanations. | ◦ Explanations may correct misconceptions on the part of the patient's parents. |
| | | • Approach patient's mother with concern and state, "It sounds like you are having a difficult time" after she asks repetitious questions. | • Patient's mother may be using repetition to mask anxiety; offering to listen may help her verbalize and deal with her anxiety. |
| | | • Alert other health-care providers that asking repetitious questions may reflect the patient's mother's underlying anxiety. | • Incorporating this information into the patient's care plan will help to ensure continuity of care. |
| | | • Explain to patient's parents that when they go home at night, they will be called immediately if there is a change in the patient's condition. | • The patient's mother may need "permission" to leave the hospital, fearing that by leaving she shows a lack of hope for her son. |

| | | | |
|---|---|---|---|
| | | ○ Provide the family with the ICU telephone number, and encourage them to call when they feel apprehensive.<br>○ Explain the need for the parents to take care of themselves so as to avoid illness during this time of stress.<br>○ Treat patient and family with respect and demonstrate competence. | ○ Treating patient and family with respect and demonstrating competence may help to ease the anxiety experienced by the patient's parents. |
| | | • Encourage the patient's mother to visit frequently; provide necessary explanations at those times when she may be asked to leave the patient's room. | • Allowing mother to visit and providing necessary telephone numbers may help to decrease anxiety.<br>• Providing explanations as to the patient's care may allay anxiety when the patient's mother is asked to leave the patient's room. |
| ***Nursing Diagnosis #2***<br>Social isolation | Patient's parents will:<br>1. Converse daily with each other.<br>2. Use family and friends to help with home maintenance and as support for themselves. | • Ascertain if other relatives or friends are aware of the patient's injury.<br>○ Inquire as to how they are managing in health and home maintenance.<br>• Encourage patient's parents to use and to share with other family members and friends. | • In time of crisis, family members may become disorganized and need support of friends and family in order to cope with the crisis. |
| | | • Advise family of the availability of the hospital chaplain.<br>○ Inquire if they would appreciate a visit from their own minister. | • Many people find comfort in religion and prayer; such activities can provide positive support. |
| | | • Reinforce staff support to patient/family<br>○ Be accessible; listen attentively.<br>○ Take time to care. | • In a family lacking external support system, the ICU staff and other patients' families can be a source of comfort and support.<br>• Family members who cannot support each other will have limited resources with which to support the patient in this biologic crisis. |

CHAPTER 4

# Patient/Family Education: Principles of Teaching/ Learning Applied to Critical Care Nursing

*Carol A. Stephenson*

## CHAPTER OUTLINE



## LEARNING OBJECTIVES

**At the end of this chapter, you should be able to:**

1. Specify the goal of education of patient and family during the critical phase of illness.
2. State the principles of adult education that facilitate the teaching/learning process.
3. Give examples of how learning can be assessed and evaluated.
4. Identify factors that reduce learning.
5. Describe how the use of the nursing diagnosis "knowledge deficit" can be applied clinically.
6. Identify key factors in assessing learning needs.
7. Review the underlying purpose(s) for developing an educational program.
8. Describe the significance of stating specific objectives (goals or patient outcomes) in developing a teaching program.
9. State an objective using measurable terminology.
10. Define the usefulness of contracting as a strategy for patient education.

## PHILOSOPHY OF PATIENT AND FAMILY EDUCATION APPLIED TO CRITICAL CARE NURSING

The citizens of our society have come to expect the best and most advanced health care to be available to them when they are ill. As a result, many persons are treated in critical care units. The events that occur in these units, while usually life-saving, can add to the stress of the catastrophic illness for the patient and for his/her significant others. The persons involved are often glad that everything possible is being done for the ill family member, but they have little understanding of exactly what is being done or why. This can lead to unanswered questions, anger, and hostility because of lack of understanding or inappropriate expectations, and poor cooperation because they don't know either how or why to cooperate. Education of the patient and his/her family, therefore, becomes a necessity during the critical care experience.

### Goal of Education During the Critical Phase of Illness

Education in the critical care area should follow the same principles as education in other areas of health and illness. People still have the same learning strategies and the same barriers to learning when they are critically ill that they have during other times in their lives. However, because of the nature of the crisis, the barriers to learning are often much higher than they are in other situations. Therefore, it is inappropriate to dwell on long-term goals and teaching during catastrophic illness. Teaching in the critical care area should be aimed at what the patient and his/her significant others need to know at the present moment to cooperate or function, and to answer questions and impart basic understandings of the processes and technology involved.

In the critical care area, just as in other areas of patient teaching, the nurse should remember that teaching and learning are not synonymous. Just because the nurse has taught does not mean the patient has learned. Learning can be said to have occurred when a behavior change has occurred as a result of the material that has been taught. It is also important to realize that every instance of information giving is not a teaching/learning experience. If there are no goals for the experience or if teaching is not approached in a way that is optimal for learning, it is not a teaching/learning experience.

### Principles of Adult Education

A large porportion of critically ill patients are adults. The parents of children and the significant others of critically ill adults are also usually adults. Therefore, some principles of adult learning can be applied to teaching in the critical care unit.

#### Adult Learning: A Volitional Activity

The first consideration with regard to adult learning is that adults consider their learning experiences to be voluntary. Just as is true in any educational setting, patients have a right to choose to learn or not to learn. Even though the health-care provider knows how much difference the information and resulting behavior changes could make in the health of a patient, there is no way to mandate learning or behavior changes. The nurse may work on motivating strategies to try to get the patient to want to learn, but the bottom line is that the patient will choose to learn or not to learn and there is nothing the health-care provider can do about it. The patient may listen politely as the information is given and even actively participate in the learning experience. In the long run, however, the individual will decide whether to incorporate the information into his/her knowledge base and act on it. The health-care provider needs to respect the individual's choices in the matter and not downgrade care or respectful behaviors as a result.

#### A Trusting Relationship: Basis for Learning

When working with adults, the teacher has no actual authority over the student. There are no grades to be given and no deadlines for papers, projects, and the like. There is some perceived authority of the health-care provider over the patient while the patient is in the health-care setting, but this authority is lost when the patient leaves the health-care setting. The nurse, therefore, must make the development of a collegial, trusting relationship an extremely high priority with regard to patient/family education. It is hoped that having this type of relationship will facilitate the client's learning.

#### Past Experiences: Impact on Learning

Adult patients bring more maturity and experience to the learning situation than do children and teenagers. This may be a positive or a negative factor in terms of the present learning situation. Past experiences will alter the adult patient's expectations of any learning experience. Such experiences may reduce the patient's expectations that learning can occur. Often, however, past experiences have led the person to have higher expectations of any learning experience than would a child or a teenager. The nurse needs to be certain that the learning encounter is seen by patients as worthy of their time and effort, and that it is productive of useful information or skills.

With regard to maturity, many adults will be better able to solve problems and see important concepts and relationships than youngsters are able to do. For some, however, the years of maturing have simply intensified poor interpersonal skills and learning habits. Some will be completely closed to new learning experiences, believing they already know what they need to know about the topic. Others may believe they are unable to learn.

Children attending school usually do so because it is required. They have no specific goal for the educational experience except to do exactly what is expected of them. Adults, however, will learn better if they have specific goals for learning. They need to know why the learning experience is occurring and what is to be achieved by it. Adults will learn even more readily if they participate in stating the goals for the learning experience. In other words, adults define what they want to know or accomplish, and learning is aimed directly at meeting that goal. This will lead to much more productive learning than when the nurse is armed with a sheet of paper that specifies that "every person with this disease needs to know these things," and provides information without regard for the patient's priorities.

In the critical care area, the nurse should be sensitive to cues from the patient and the family that specify learning goals and should seek information as to the meaning of these cues. For example, a patient returns from emergency neurosurgery with his/her face appearing bruised and battered and having two black eyes. The family may express much concern over the appearance of the patient's face. This can be translated into a goal regarding gaining information about the cause of the altered facial appearance. The nurse can then explain about the frame that supported the patient's face during surgery and about the blood pooling that resulted, and relate these understandings to the altered facial appearance. The nurse can then follow up with information about how and when the bruising might resolve. This type of teaching will achieve the family's immediate goals related to that concern.

Few adults seek learning for the sake of learning. They wish their learning experiences to be practical and meaningful. Before teaching, the nurse should be certain that the information to be given has meaning and practicality for the patient. This can usually be determined by a careful assessment prior to teaching.

For some adults, any learning experience is traumatic. If they have had unpleasant educational experiences in the past, they are likely to react to any new learning experience as a traumatic one. The fact that this learning takes place in the presence of a crisis such as critical illness or injury only makes the experience that much more traumatic. The nurse should be alert to verbal and nonverbal cues being given by the patient and family, which may signal that the learning experience is stressful for them. The teaching approaches should then be modified accordingly.

#### *Computerized Learning: Some Pitfalls*

A common method of learning in our society today is through the use of computerized materials. Many adults do not feel comfortable with these and do not know how to use the equipment. Hence, they do not learn as well as by other methods. In addition, it is often difficult to individualize computerized materials to match a specific patient's needs. If computerized materials are to be used, it is necessary to be certain that the patient can use them without feeling incompetent or threatened and to provide appropriate support during the learning experience.

#### *Use of Senses: Enhances Learning*

The more senses that are involved, the better the patient will learn. A person who hears the concept, sees an illustration or a film of it, and practices and discusses it will retain it much better than one who only hears the concept.

#### *Familiarity Reinforces Learning*

Adult learning will be more effective when it relates to or builds on familiar concepts. The nurse should get to know patients well enough to be able to use concepts that will be familiar to them, and to build on familiar knowledge when teaching new concepts. The nurse who can develop analogies with whatever concepts patients are familiar with will be more successful than the nurse who uses the same explanations for all patients.

#### *Learning Process: Simple to Complex*

Learning is enhanced when it proceeds from the simple to the complex. The learning experience should be planned as much as possible so that the simplest concepts are taught first. These concepts can then be used as a base for teaching the more complicated aspects of the topic. Teaching the simpler information first builds success, motivation, and self-confidence.

The teaching/learning environment is important for adult learners. They seem to learn best in a comfortable and informal setting. The situation should be as pleasant as possible. Accommodations should be made as necessary for visual and hearing deficits.

## Factors That Reduce Learning

Some of the factors that reduce learning relate directly to the previously described principles of adult learning.

#### *Poor Motivation*

If patients see the learning as impractical or unnecessary, or if they view it as being in competition with their own belief structure, they will probably be poorly motivated to learn. It is essential that adults want to learn the material and that they believe it to be valuable.

A nurse once discovered the importance of this while attempting to teach an anemic patient about foods high in iron. The patient was openly hostile to a discussion of iron-rich foods. Finally, the nurse asked why the patient was not interested in the discussion. He explained that he regularly listened to a certain radio program (presented by a food faddist), and from that program, he learned that apples are rich in iron. The evidence presented was the fact that when left open to air, apples turn brown. The faddist explained that the brown is iron. This patient, therefore, ate apples or applesauce daily and was absolutely convinced that he was eating a diet rich in iron!

### Low Self-Esteem and Increasing Age

Low self-esteem and increasing age can affect learning. Increasing age tends to reduce openness to new ideas. Some persons believe they are "too old to learn" or that they are incapable of learning. The nurse may be put in the position of having to convince patients that they are capable of learning before they will tackle the learning experience.

### The Issue of Literacy

A related problem is literacy. The nurse should not assume that an adult patient can learn with written materials. The patient's reading skills may be so poor that this is not possible. All written material should be read and discussed together. The most important aspects should be pointed out and underlined or highlighted. This is not to say that written materials should not accompany teaching as an aid to recall. Actually, they are invaluable references for almost all patients. It is rather to caution the nurse that not everyone will be able to read and understand written materials.

### Individual's Belief System: Impact on Motivation and Learning

The patient's belief system about whether recommended actions can make a difference is critical to learning. Many persons do not adhere to their therapeutic program simply because they do not believe their actions make a difference or because they do not believe they are at risk. A common example: Few persons today would tell you that they truly do not believe that smoking cigarettes is hazardous to the health of most persons. However, those persons who smoke will often say that they do not perceive themselves to be at risk for the known hazards of smoking. They say they have smoked for a given number of years and nothing has happened yet. As a result, they keep on smoking.

Others perceive themselves somewhat as victims. They are ill and they say they don't know why; they also say that whatever is going to happen will happen whether or not they cooperate with their care, take their medicines, do their exercises, and the like. With this attitude, why bother to buy medicine, cooperate with therapy, or keep appointments?

### Anxiety, Fear, and Pain: Impact on Learning

Anxiety, fear, and discomfort all reduce the individual's ability to pay attention and perceive what is going on in the learning experience. If any of these are present, they can be so overwhelming that the patient may recall nothing else that happened during a given period of time. These factors need to be dealt with and relieved before trying to teach a patient. However, if relieving discomfort involves the use of drugs that reduce perception and cognitive abilities, patients, although they are happier and more comfortable, may be just as unable to learn as they were prior to pain relief.

### Self-Pride: Impact on Learning

Pride is another problem in teaching adults. It is not uncommon for adults to attempt to conceal their lack of knowledge because to admit it would cause "loss of face" or injury to their pride. Such persons would rather do without the knowledge than admit their need for it. The nurse can often deal with this by providing privacy for the learning experience or by presenting a topic in terms such as "a lot of people say this is a problem for them . . . Have you found it to be a problem for you?" Sometimes, group classes help to deal with this problem because one patient will ask a question or admit a problem that another patient may be too proud to admit.

Some persons have developed poor learning skills. They may not have learned how to learn or how to use the resources that are available to them. If the nurse finds this to be the case, it may be necessary to do some remedial teaching about how to learn before teaching the intended content.

### Unrealistic Goals or Expectations

Another poor learning skill that many have is unrealistic goals or expectations of themselves. As a result, they are quite frustrated when they cannot achieve their self-imposed goals. The nurse will have to assist these patients to revise their goals so as to be realistic. This is often difficult because such revisions may be viewed as a sign of incompetence.

The relationship between the patient and the

nurse greatly affects learning. Some patients are openly hostile to the idea of being taught anything. Others simply do not trust the nurse to be able to teach them. A great number of factors contribute to these situations. The nurse must assess and deal with them as well as possible. In some cases, it simply is not possible to teach the patient. In others, teaching is possible only after a rapport has been established. In yet others, another person such as a physician or a different nurse may be able to relate to the patient better. Because the ultimate goal is teaching patients what they want and need to know, all possible alternatives should be explored. Certainly, the nurse should approach each patient with an attitude of respect, regardless of his/her individual behaviors.

## Nursing Diagnosis: Knowledge Deficit

When doing nursing care plans related to patient education, the accepted nursing diagnosis is "knowledge deficit." The cause of the knowledge deficit varies with the patient. Some may never have had access to the knowledge before or may have forgotten or misinterpreted it. Others may have been taught poorly or at a time when they were not able to learn. Still others may be receiving competing or conflicting information from family and acquaintances. For some patients, the knowledge or related behaviors may be in direct conflict with their belief systems and usual practices.

Some sample information related to this nursing diagnosis is presented in Table 4-1. It is intended

TABLE 4-1
**Nursing Diagnosis: Knowledge Deficit**

| Nursing Diagnosis | Desired Patient Outcomes | Nursing Interventions | Evaluation Strategies |
|---|---|---|---|
| *Knowledge Deficit*<br>Defining characteristics:<br>• Verbalization or performance indicates inadequate knowledge or skill, misunderstandings.<br>• Poor utilization of previously taught information.<br>• Poor compliance or adherence.<br>• Evidence of cognitive impairment.<br>• Verbalizes questions or requests for information. Complains about lack of information.<br>• Poor knowledge of or utilization of resources.<br>• Hostility or unwillingness to participate in learning experience. | • Correctly completes verbal or written post-test on information that has been taught.<br>• Follow-up visits yield data that information is being used or followed appropriately.<br>• Consistently and correctly performs skills that have been taught.<br>• Verbalizes that his/her priorities have been met and questions have been answered.<br>• If cognitively impaired, family is taught and verbalizes or demonstrates understanding.<br>• Verbalizes plans to use the material that is taught. | • Assess patient and family's learning needs carefully. Check present knowledge, skills, beliefs.<br>• Adhere to teaching/learning principles.<br>• Include family or significant others in teaching.<br>• Include frequent return demonstrations, post-tests, validation of learning. Give support and reteach PRN.<br>• Use frequent repetition.<br>• Teach by example.<br>• Make appropriate referrals to resource agencies.<br>• Break learning into small parts, which are taught in a logical order and form.<br>• Build success and praise into the experience.<br>• Do not punish for failure.<br>• Save long-term teaching for a time when the situation is no longer critical.<br>• Incorporate learned materials or skills into daily hospital routine.<br>• Use varied but appropriate learning strategies.<br>• If patient is hostile or noncompliant, try to find out why and deal with the problem before teaching. Do not force teaching on patient.<br>• If cognitively impaired, limit teaching of patient to what he/she needs to know to function or what he/she seems to want to know. | • Verbal or written post-test.<br>• Informal follow-up and discussion to check understanding.<br>• On follow-up visits, review understanding, practices, and adherence.<br>• Allow patient and family to do return demonstrations and practice skills frequently.<br>• Ask patient if priorities have been met and questions have been answered.<br>• Teaching of cognitively impaired patient is limited to necessary material. Family is taught more.<br>• Ask patient to describe plans to use material.<br>• The same questions are not repeated often or the same unsafe practices are not repeated. |

only as a starting point for the nurse in preparing nursing care plans. Much individualization will be necessary.

## Assessment of Learning Needs

It is very important that patient education *not* be done on the basis of what the health-care provider *believes* the patient needs to know. If formal teaching is to be done, a complete learning assessment should be done first.

To accomplish this, the nurse should spend time with the patient and family discussing what they know about the topic and what questions they have. It is very helpful to ask what the patient and family want to know and learn. Teaching may reinforce and build on what they already know. It can also be a time to recognize and reinforce positive health behaviors. It is helpful to attempt to discover what support systems and resources the patient has available, as well as areas in which support or resources are clearly lacking. The nurse should also assess for the presence or absence of key factors as discussed in the section entitled "Principles of Adult Education" (above), and barriers to learning such as lack of motivation, unreadiness to learn, hostility, the presence of pain or anxiety, and the like. These are just as important to deal with as knowledge deficit.

### *Non-Critical Care Setting*

In the non-critical care situation, the focus of the assessment may be different than it is when the patient is critically ill. During the crisis, the patient and family need to focus their energies on coping with the present. This is not the time for long-range planning or discharge teaching. Rather, it is the time for discovering present fears and anxieties as well as what information the patient and significant others want and need during the crisis. After the patient is out of the critical phase of illness, a reassessment can be performed and a new, longer-range teaching plan can be developed. The importance of setting priorities in terms of teaching/learning is illustrated in the following mini-case study.

## MINI-CASE STUDY: PATIENT WITH SPINAL CORD INJURY

Mr. H., age 32, is in the ICU 24 hours post trauma. He has a spinal cord injury without a neurologic deficit. He is on a kinetic bed, which rotates him constantly side to side 60 degrees, and he has Crutchfield tongs to his head. The tongs are attached to traction weights. He is NPO with a nasogastric tube in place. Mr. H. is alert and oriented but says very little. He is wide-eyed and his face appears anxious. He holds his body stiffly and clutches the sides of the bed as it turns as though to keep himself from falling.

Mindy, a senior nursing student, is assigned to care for Mr. H. When she presents her nursing care plan to her instructor, it shows the following:

**Nursing Diagnosis:** Altered nutrition: excess, related to excess intake, resulting in moderate obesity.

**Goal:** Within 2 days,

1. Patient will state a specific goal for weight loss.
2. Patient and wife will identify and describe an appropriate diet.

**Nursing Interventions:**

1. Discuss obesity with patient and the need to lose weight.
2. Teach appropriate diet.
3. Help patient set goals for weight loss.

Although the format is acceptable, this nursing care plan has several problems. First, the student (who was quite thin) imposed her priorities on the patient and his wife. Second, even if she did the teaching this time, the patient and his wife wouldn't hear it. In fact, the student's lack of sensitivity might greatly reduce her rapport with them on a long-term basis.

How much better it would have been if Mindy, after introducing herself, had approached the situation something like this:

Mindy: Mr. H., you don't look very comfortable to me. Is there a problem I can help you with?
Mr. H.: No, I'm not comfortable. I hurt all over. I'm afraid I'll fall out of this contraption if I go to sleep.

At this point, Mindy has a choice. She could, as many nurses do, "reassure the patient"—"Oh, don't be silly. Nobody has fallen out of one of these beds yet. You just relax and let us take care of everything." However, this is not teaching and would do little toward meeting the needs of the patient.

A better choice is to discuss the two problems that have been brought up: the pain and the fear of falling. The conversation might go like this:

Mindy: Are you having a great deal of pain right now?
Mr. H.: I sure am.
Mindy (looking at chart): I see you haven't had a shot for pain for 8 hours. You can have it every 3 hours if you need it.
Mr. H. Nobody told me that.
Mindy: I'll get you a shot now. You tell the nurses when you are hurting so they can try to keep you more comfortable. They need your help to know how you are feeling.
Mr. H.: I didn't know I could ask for a shot. I

thought the nurses would know what to do and when.

Mindy: No, they need you to tell them what you are feeling and when you need something.

This portion of the interaction is brief, but Mindy has informally taught Mr. H. something quite valuable about communication in the hospital. With this understanding, Mr. H. can more readily participate in decision-making regarding his care. It will be relatively easy to evaluate his learning by observing his communication behaviors over the next few days.

After Mr. H. is comfortable from the medication, Mindy can then address the fear of falling:

Mindy: Mr. H., you said you are afraid of relaxing because you might fall out of the bed.

Mr. H.: I sure am. You must know what you're doing, but this is a scarey contraption you've got me in.

Mindy: Would it help if I explain the bed and your traction to you? I can show you why you're on it and how you are protected from falling.

Mr. H.: I really need that. Could my wife come in and learn about the bed, too?

Mindy could then call in Mrs. H. and explain Mr. H.'s traction and bed to them in clear, simple terms. She could explain why the bed is necessary, how it is better right now than a "regular" bed, and the bed's safety features. She could later evaluate this discussion in several ways: by asking Mr. and Mrs. H. if they have questions after she finished; by asking them to explain key points back to her; and, most importantly, by observing whether Mr. H. is able to relax and stop clinging to the bed as it rotates. Mindy would then document her teaching and its results in her nurse's notes as follows:

1630—Appears anxious and uncomfortable. Clinging to the bed constantly. Body rigid. In response to questioning, states he is in pain and afraid of falling. Medicated for pain. Discussed the need for him to keep nurses informed of pain and other subjective problems. Explained purpose of traction and bed to patient and wife. Pointed out safeguards to prevent falling. They expressed understanding.

1800—Apparently sleeping. Appears relaxed.

Just because Mindy did this teaching today does not mean it won't need repeating tomorrow. As stated earlier, pain, fear, and anxiety reduce perception and information retention. Simple explanations may need to be given on a daily basis or even several times a day. This does not mean the teaching should not be done or is unsuccessful.

Perception is reduced even more if the patient's cognitive abilities are reduced either by medication or disease, trauma, or surgery. The patient may have the ability to understand simple explanations at the time, but may forget the information within the hour. Major teaching in this case should be done for the family; the patient needs to be taught only what is absolutely necessary for immediate care activities. For example, the family of a patient who has had a cerebral vascular accident (CVA, or stroke) should be taught about what a stroke is, its general treatment, the expectations for rehabilitation, and the like. However, the stroke-injured patient does not have the cognitive abilities to deal with this type of teaching. Teaching should be confined to the patient's immediate needs, such as how to scan the environment to compensate for visual field losses or how to support the affected arm and leg when turning.

## PROGRAM DEVELOPMENT

### Program Purposes

There are two overall purposes for developing teaching programs. One is to develop a generic program, which includes all the information that a patient with a particular problem would be likely to need to know (such as a cardiac rehabilitation program). Once this program is developed, its component parts can be used one at a time with particular patients to supplement knowledge and skills until they have learned what is necessary and essential. This is an excellent way to plan programs to be used on units that have many patients with similar problems (such as cardiac units, diabetic units, orthopedic surgery units, pulmonary medicine units, and the like). Patients in these types of units often have similar learning needs. Once the program is well developed, it is easy for an individual nurse to adapt it to an individual patient.

This type of program is not always successful in the critical care unit, however. As has been pointed out, the patients and their families are stressed to the point where long-term learning and planning are not possible. It is often much more appropriate to plan individual learning programs directed at the particular needs of individual patients and their families.

If the unit is a specialized one that receives many similar patients, it may be helpful to plan *mini-programs* to address common problems of patients and families. If this is done, the nurse does not have to generate a completely new teaching program each time it is needed. For example, a news article on premature infant ICUs focused on one of the parents. It states, "By the time their son was able to come home . . . (the mother) had become an expert on the problems of premature babies. She speaks knowledgeably of transcutaneous oxygen monitors and eye problems that often affect the babies. 'They sent me through a whole medical course,' she says, 'but understanding what was going on was the only thing that saved me.'"[1]

It is conceivable that such a unit might have some prepared materials and simple diagrams or displays regarding such topics as transcutaneous monitors, ventilators, infant hyperalimentation, why a premature infant looks the way he/she does, and parenting needs of premature infants. There would be no point in generating this information from scratch for each parent whose child is admitted to the unit. Individual needs could be added to the teaching plan for each parent. Individualization would also attend to the fact that many other parents might not want or be able to comprehend as much information as this mother did.

## Negotiating and Writing Objectives

Once the assessment is done, the nurse and the patient can ask, "What does he/she need to know and how will we both know when it is known?" It is critical that the patient be able to specify what learning is important. If nurses teach only what meets their priorities, they may risk losing the patient's desire to learn. Also, by knowing what the patient already knows and does well, nurses can avoid undermining the patient's intelligence and wasting time by reteaching that material. Teaching the information that is priority knowledge for the patient first will increase the desire to learn and assure patient satisfaction that learning needs are being met. Together, the nurse and patient can set measurable objectives and target dates for their achievement. After that, learning experiences can be planned to meet the objectives.

Evaluation will be the last part of the plan and should be based directly on the objectives. Sometimes, the planning may be done formally and the nurse will return at another time to teach. In the critical care unit, however, it is often appropriate to do the teaching as soon as the objective has been stated formally or informally. It is important to know what the objective or goal is so that both the nurse and the patient know what is to be achieved by the interaction. With a clearly stated objective, they will both know when they have achieved it. Without such an objective, they may have differing opinions on what, if anything, was achieved. The objectives will also be a valuable aid to selecting teaching content, strategies, and instructional aids.

### *Domains of Learning*

Objectives can be written in any of the three recognized domains of learning. The *cognitive* or *thinking* domain is concerned with intellectual abilities such as remembering, analyzing, evaluating, and creative thinking. The *affective* domain, which is used less in patient teaching but in some cases may be vitally important, is related to feelings and emotions about the topic in question. Finally, the *psychomotor* domain relates to the performance of skills that require the coordination of body muscles. In other words, this is the doing part of learning.

### *Statement of the Objective: Specific Components*

The statement of the objective will have four parts. First, there will be a description of the learner. This may simply be "the patient with pulmonary disease" or a like statement. It must be specific enough to say that the learner in this case is different from "anyone, anywhere." The material to be taught is for a person with a specific learning need, not just for anyone. Second, there will be a statement about what will be performed or a statement of the behavior to be exhibited if learning has taken place. Third, there will be a description of the conditions under which that performance will occur. Finally, there will be a standard of accuracy (criterion statement) or how well the performance must be done to be acceptable.

### *Writing Objectives: Measurable Terminology*

The performance statement must be in *observable* behavioral terms. Often, as health-care providers, we may think we are giving good directions, but in actuality, the patient does not have enough information to accomplish the task or objective. For example, how often do health-care providers ask patients to "drink plenty of fluids"? This may mean 4 cups of coffee a day for some patients and continual fluid ingestion for others. How much more easily the patient would be able to comply with directions such as "drink eight 8-ounce glasses of fluid a day" or "drink one-half glass of fluid every hour." Terms that cannot be observed or measured are not helpful in aiding the nurse or the patient to know when learning has been achieved.

The statement must be in terms of learner behaviors, not teacher behaviors. For example, a statement such as "to teach the importance of high fluid intake" is a teacher behavior or patient outcome. A statement of learner behavior might be "to list three reasons for a fluid intake of 2500 ml per day" or "to ingest 2500 ml of fluids per day." Each objective should include only one statement of a behavior.

The performance statement should avoid ambiguous and unmeasurable terms such as:

| | | |
|---|---|---|
| to know | to understand | to appreciate |
| to grasp the significance of | to enjoy | to believe |
| | to have faith in | to want |

| | | |
|---|---|---|
| to perceive | to like | to master |
| to become | to learn | to feel |

The acceptable terms for performance could include many specific terms, only some of which are included here:

| | | |
|---|---|---|
| to write | to define | to list |
| to identify | to indicate | to state |
| to compare | to compute | to contrast |
| to describe | to differentiate | to discuss |
| to distinguish | to classify | to apply |
| to calculate | to demonstrate | to practice |
| to solve | to use | to analyze |
| to explain | to summarize | to integrate |
| to plan | to organize | to assess |
| to evaluate | to rank | to measure |

Stating the conditions under which the performance will take place will include terms such as the following:

| | | |
|---|---|---|
| Given | Using | Following |
| Provided with | Starting with | Beginning with |

Finally, the performance standard will describe an acceptable performance. It may include a statement such as "with 80% accuracy," "within 30 minutes," or the like.

Some sample objectives are listed below:

1. Given a diagram of the lungs, the patient will, with 90% accuracy, identify the structures.
2. Provided with a blank injection rotation diagram, the diabetic patient will plan an appropriate site rotation schedule within 30 minutes.

### *Preparing a Teaching Plan*

The nurse can ask several questions as he/she prepares a teaching plan. These include the following:

1. What are the characteristics of the patient?
2. What are the patient's learning priorities?
3. What does the patient need to know?
4. What is my educational purpose?
5. How can I determine if learning has occurred?

The above questions can be used to aid the nurse in developing a set of objectives for the learning experience. The objectives should be as precise as possible so they will be useful as a teaching guide for the nurse and a learning guide for the patient. The following sample objectives might be used in a master teaching plan in an intensive care unit where many patients who have emphysema are admitted. It could be individualized according to the learning priorities and prior knowledge of each patient and family.

Given a brief discussion, visual aids, and written materials, the patient or his/her family will be able to do the following with 100% accuracy:

1. Identify emphysema by name and general description.
2. Describe the pathology of emphysema.
3. State how the emphysematous lungs differ from normal lungs in terms of structure and function.
4. List the major causes of emphysema.
5. Describe the major symptoms of emphysema and relate these to the client's symptoms.
6. Very generally, describe the care of emphysema. (Care would be taught more specifically at another time when the crisis period is over.)

A simple teaching plan could then be built on these objectives. It would include four columns: the objectives, the content related to the objectives, the teaching strategies and resources, and, finally, the methods of evaluation. See Table 4–2 for an example of a teaching plan.

### *Evaluation Process*

The methods of evaluation would directly relate back to the objectives. In some way, the nurse would evaluate attainment of an objective by asking the patient to do whatever the objective states. For example, if the objective says, "list . . . ," the patient could be asked to list the material verbally or in writing. If the objective asks the patient to "describe . . . ," this could be done verbally during a discussion or in writing. If the objective asks the patient to "perform . . . ," the evaluation would be done by watching the patient perform the task and evaluating it according to accuracy of performance.

In an earlier example of a *performance* objective, the patient was asked "to ingest 2500 ml of fluids per day." A simple way to evaluate the accomplishment of this objective or goal is to look at the patient's intake sheet for the 24-hour period. If the intake was 2500 ml or more, the goal was accomplished. If the intake was less than 2500 ml, the nurse should seek the reasons why the goal was not accomplished. Perhaps the patient was NPO for several hours for diagnostic tests. In this case, the best route might be to reevaluate the intake the next day. Perhaps he/she did not understand the teaching or did not like the idea of taking in so many fluids. In this case, the nurse must go back to the original goal and teaching strategies and find another way to motivate the patient to drink; or to help the patient learn why fluids are so important; or how to stagger the intake so he/she is drinking small amounts frequently instead of trying to ingest larger amounts at longer intervals. The evaluation process, therefore, not only helps the nurse know that teaching has been effective, but is a guide to the need for reteaching or revision of teaching techniques and strategies.

In addition to all of the teaching principles listed so far, nurses should remember that they teach by example as well as by planned verbal interactions.

TABLE 4–2
**Sample Teaching Plan: "What Is Emphysema?"**

| Objective* | Content | Teaching Strategy/ Resources | Evaluation Strategy |
|---|---|---|---|
| Identify emphysema by name and general description. | Emphysema and chronic bronchitis are two diseases ordinarily grouped under the title of chronic obstructive lung disease (COPD). Although they often occur together, a person may have predominately one disease or the other. | Individualize discussion according to the patient's primary disease. | Ask patient to name his/her disease process. |
| Name the major pertinent respiratory structures and cite the changes in emphysema. | Structure and function of normal lungs:<br>• Purpose of breathing—to get oxygen into the body.<br>• Oxygen provides energy for body functions.<br>• The lungs eliminate the waste product of oxygen use, carbon dioxide.<br>Major pertinent respiratory structures:<br>• Airways, alveoli, diaphragm.<br>• Lungs are elastic spongy tissue.<br>• Airways are hollow, branching tubes like upside-down trees.<br>• Alveoli are air sacs.<br>• Alveoli help keep the airways open during exhalation.<br>• Oxygen and carbon dioxide pass through alveolar walls to and from blood.<br>• Diaphragm is major muscle of respiration.<br>Pathology of emphysema:<br>• Walls of alveoli tear or are destroyed.<br>• There is less area for oxygen exchange.<br>• Airways tend to collapse on expiration.<br>• Airway collapse leads to air trapping and reduced ability to use the diaphragm.<br>• This increases the work of breathing and reduces body oxygen levels. | *Medical Illustrations of Common Disorders of the Respiratory Tract.* Normal airway and lung diagram; emphysema diagram (Lilly publication). An illustration of the diaphragm and its location. | Ask patient to name the pictured lung structures and identify briefly the changes that occur in emphysema. |
| Describe the general care of emphysema. | The disease can be controlled, not cured.<br>• Medications:<br>○ To open airways (bronchodilators).<br>○ To reduce inflammation (steroids).<br>○ To treat infection (antibiotics).<br>○ To improve oxygenation (oxygen).<br>○ To reduce water retention if necessary (diuretics). | As each drug is administered, state briefly what its name is and the major purpose for which it is given. | After the drug has been given and discussed several times, name the drug when administering it and ask the patient to name its purpose. |

* Both content and depth would be varied according to the patient's condition and ability to learn.

For example, what is the patient really going to believe if the nurse who is teaching about the hazards of smoking and why it should be stopped has tobacco-stained fingernails and smells heavily of smoke himself/herself? The nurse who follows a healthy diet and exercise program will teach more by example when discussing these topics than the nurse who is obviously overweight and out of condition. In teaching adults, health-care providers cannot get by with imparting a message such as "do as I tell you—not as I do."

To summarize the planning of objectives and teaching strategies, an instructional objective should describe the intended learning outcome or behaviors rather than summarizing teaching content. The objectives will be stated in terms of learner behaviors rather than teacher behaviors. For most teaching programs, there will be a series of objectives rather than just one objective. The objective statements should include four parts as previously described. These objective statements then become the guide for selecting teaching content and strategies and for selecting evaluation strategies. Finally, the learner should have a copy of the objectives so that he/she knows what is to be learned. All teaching and the evaluation of its outcomes should be documented in the patient's record.

The teaching plan in Table 4-2 was selected as an example of information that many critically ill patients want and that could be taught relatively easily and quickly. Once the assessment has been done and the nurse has found that the patient and his/her significant others do not understand the nature of the illness but would like to do so, the teaching could be done at the earliest opportunity when the patient is awake and relatively comfortable, and interruptions are unlikely. The nurse could take the visual aids and resource materials to the bedside, sit down with the patient and significant others, and inform them of what it is they should understand regarding the nature of the illness and encourage them to ask questions.

Nurses should not use the content column of the teaching plan verbatim but should use it as a guide to discuss the disease in their own words. Nurses should allow the patient and significant others time to look at the visual aids and ask questions. When summarizing the care portion of the teaching, nurses can relate the care right back to what has already been said, for example, "there is aminophylline in this IV you are receiving. This drug will open up your airways and help you to breathe more easily. It should relieve some of your shortness of breath and your need to sit up to breathe. It will also help you to clear your airways because they will be more open when you cough."

The nurse can evaluate learning immediately after the teaching presentation or on an ongoing basis for the next few days. For example, when changing the IV aminophylline, the nurse might say, "I have your new bag of aminophylline here. Tell me what you remember about the reason you are receiving it." The client's answer will alert the nurse as to whether reteaching is necessary.

### *Contracting*

Contracting, a strategy for patient education, involves the writing of a contract between patient and nurse. The contract specifies behaviors to be done by the patient and a reward or reinforcer that will be received as a result. The idea of contracting is based on the theory that if a positive reinforcer is received soon after a behavior, the person will be more likely to perform the behavior again.[2] As with any other type of patient education, contracting should be based on a thorough assessment of behaviors, knowledge, and beliefs. It is not done until the nurse and the patient have mutually agreed on the patient's learning priorities.

Contracting can be helpful for a variety of reasons. First, it removes any doubt by the patient as to what behavior is expected. Objectives for the contract are stated very specifically so that both patient and nurse know exactly what the patient is expected to do, under what conditions, and when.

In some cases, patients are more willing and able to adhere to the treatment program if they are working for a reward or a reinforcer. The reinforcer should be meaningful to and, ideally, selected by, the patient.

The use of contracts can make the reinforcement of correct behaviors more consistent. Health-care providers may feel they frequently reinforce patient behaviors by praise, recognition of effort, and the like. Actually this is not usually done systematically, so the patient doesn't expect the praise or other reinforcer to occur every time the behavior is done. With contracting, the nurse and patient agree on the behavior and the reinforcer ahead of time. Then, the reinforcer is given without fail when the behavior is exhibited.[3]

Another advantage of using contracts is to give the patient optimal credit for maintaining his/her health. All too often, the health-care providers are quick to place blame on the patient when health is not maintained or improved, but if it is improved, the treatment or health-care providers get the credit.[4]

Contracting also reduces the likelihood that the patient will be scolded or punished as the result of poor health behaviors. If poor behaviors occur, nothing is said. The reinforcer simply is not given.

**Writing a Contract.** After assessing the patient's beliefs and behaviors, the patient and the nurse should decide on the patient's learning priorities. The learning can then be broken down into smaller bits, each of which can be accomplished rather quickly. The behaviors for the first step will be on

I,________________________________, will ______________

________________________________, in return for ____________

________________________________.

Signed ______________

Signed ______________

Date ______________

[*Note:* This part of the page is left blank so that the client and nurse can identify bonuses or future successive approximations. It is also used to record information the client might want, such as blood pressure, weight, diet suggestions, telephone numbers, and so on.]

**Figure 4–1.** A sample contract. (From Steckel,[2] p 44, with permission.)

the first contract. These will be stated so that they are well defined, observable, and measurable. A date by which the behavior will be displayed should be specified. The reinforcer or privilege should be clearly specified as should a description of what will occur when the contract is not fulfilled (if this is appropriate). In some cases, a bonus clause may be added as a reward for extra accomplishments. Any record keeping that is to be done should also be specified in the contract.[5] Steckel has developed a very simple contract form (Fig. 4–1).

**A Contracting Vocabulary.** Definitions of terms pertaining to contracting are presented below, based on Steckel[2]:

Contract—An agreement between a patient and a health-care provider, which specifies a behavior to be done, a date by which it is to be done, and a reinforcer to be received as a result.

Reinforcer—A tangible or intangible consequence that strengthens a behavior.

Negative reinforcer—A consequence whose removal strengthens a behavior. It is not a punishment.

Strengthening a behavior—Increasing the chance that behavior will be repeated.

Consequence—The result of a behavior.

Reward—A pleasant experience but one that does not necessarily strengthen a behavior.

## MINI-CASE STUDY: PATIENT WITH SEVERE BURNS

M.S. was a 15-year-old girl recovering from severe burns of her hands and arms. Despite the use of analgesics, physical therapy was very painful for her. As a result, she was so combative and uncooperative that little was being accomplished in the therapy sessions. During a discussion with M. and her mother, the nurse discovered that M. wanted some cassette tapes of a certain rock star very badly. With that in mind, M., her mother, and the nurse formulated a plan: Each day that M. cooperated with the physical therapist rather than fighting, a check would be put on a graph, which was taped to the wall of her room. Five consecutive checks would earn her a tape, to be purchased by her mother. If she missed a day of being cooperative, nothing would be said. Instead, she would start again at the next session to work toward her goal of 5 consecutive checks.

M.'s contract would look like this:

> I, M______ S______, will earn five consecutive checks for cooperating with my physical therapy exercises in return for a rock tape of my choice to be purchased by my mother.
>
> Signed—M______ S______
> Signed—C. S______, RN
> Date—November 13, 1989

As a result of the contract, M. was much more cooperative and began to make progress with her therapy. After using this contract several times, a new contract was written, which required more consecutive checks and which changed the reinforcer to something else M. wanted. Notice that the contract did not specify that the physical therapy sessions produced results, only that M. cooperated. Whether it is weight loss, respiratory function, or anything else, results are often not predictable enough to use in contracts. Behaviors that would lead to the desired results are more predictable and easier to count. Certainly the behavior should be reinforced regardless of the results.

Reinforcers do not have to be objects or things. They may be intangibles such as spending time with a special person, discussion of a topic of the client's choice, reading a story together, and the like. A thorough discussion of contracting may be found in the book, *Patient Contracting*, by Steckel.[2]

## PATIENT EDUCATION RESOURCES

Many resources are available for patient education. The more familiar nurses are with educational principles and materials, the more effective they can be as educators. If nurses are using prepared or purchased materials, they should evaluate them carefully as to appropriateness and usability. The materials should be modified as necessary to meet the needs of the individual patient teaching situation.

A reading list of resources is included at the end of this chapter. This is only a sampling of materials available. Some of the materials might seem old at first glance, but they are classics and can be extremely helpful. Visual aids and pamphlets can often be obtained at low cost or at no cost from drug companies and voluntary agencies such as the American Heart Association, American Lung Association, American Cancer Society, and American Diabetes Association.

## CHAPTER SUMMARY

Patient and family education is an integral part of nursing care in every setting. When the educational process is conducted in the critical care setting, the basic principles of teaching and learning apply. Some of the principles become extremely important in such settings. A person's ability to learn and retain information is impeded greatly by anxiety, fear, pain, drugs, and the like. As a result, teaching in the critical care setting should be confined to information that the patient and significant others need to know at the time.

Long-term teaching and plans for care should be delayed until the patient is out of the critical care area. Even when teaching is confined to the urgent learning needs of those in the critical care setting, retention and compliance may be poor. As a result, repetition becomes quite important. Nurses continually assess critical knowledge and behaviors and should be willing to repeat the teaching of critical material as often as necessary. To aid patient education, it is a good idea for a unit to prepare teaching materials, visual aids, and resources for teaching topics that are used frequently. These can then be easily individualized to any patient situation.

## REFERENCES

1. Sanz, C: The reality behind the miracle babies. Dallas Morning News, Nov 1987, p 10C.
2. Steckel, S: Patient Contracting. Appleton-Century-Crofts, Norwalk, Conn, 1982.
3. Ibid, p 152.
4. Ibid, p 48.
5. Stuart, RB: Behavior contracting with Families of delinquents. J Behav Ther Exper Psychiatry 2(1):1–11, 1971.

## SUGGESTED READINGS

Barber, C and Langfitt DE: Teaching the Medical–Surgical Patient: Diagnostics and Procedures. Appleton-Century Crofts, Norwalk, Conn, 1983.

Guinee, KK: Teaching and Learning in Nursing. Macmillan, New York, 1978.

Kemp, JE: Instructional Design Process. Harper & Row, New York, 1985.

Mager, RF: Measuring Instructional Results, ed 2. DF Lake, Belmont, Calif, 1984.

Mager, RF: Developing Attitude Toward Learning. DF Lake, Belmont, Calif, 1984.

Mager, RF: Preparing Instructional Objectives. DF Lake, Belmont, Calif, 1984.

Pohl, ML: The Teaching Function of the Nursing Practitioner. Wm C Brown, Dubuque, Iowa, 1981.

CHAPTER 5

# Being Human

*Lorraine Brown*
*Frances Dooley*

## CHAPTER OUTLINE



## A CASE STUDY IN DEPERSONALIZATION

Depersonalization—the feeling that one is not human, but, rather, an illness to be treated—occurs because health-care providers are so involved with saving the patient's life that the patient's humanness is ignored.

> The sirens roared and the lights flashed as the ambulance raced through the traffic-laden streets of the east side of Manhattan to the Hospital Center. Within minutes I was strapped onto a stretcher, which crashed through two steel doors into a land of mystique and staring eyes. Four white-uniformed personnel mumbled an introduction as they simultaneously attached wires to my 4 limbs, took my blood, and slapped 3 round disks to my roughly exposed chest. As my eyes darted around this noise-filled room, the already increasing tightness in my chest was now accompanied by a dry throat and the sweats.
>
> Overwhelmed with fear and anticipation, I lay motionless as my body became the center of various unfamiliar activities. The blurred faces and muffled voices of the doctors and nurses continued around me as I became suddenly aware I had been wheeled into the Heart Room. The lights, beeps, and bells seemed to be penetrating my already overwhelming thoughts of death and fears of the unknown. These white-clothed experts kept referring to me as the new massive MI with occasional PVCs in Room 3.
>
> Two doctors came into my room and immediately focused their eyes on what appeared to be a small TV set, which showed my heart beats. A nurse entered, rambled her name, put a needle in my arm, connected a tube feeding into two bottles, and said this is an IV.
>
> Somehow, I didn't feel like I was part of my body, and I still did not know what was happening to me. The foreign terms, strange noises, and unfamiliar faces made me very nervous and afraid. Several questions paraded through my mind: Was I going to die? Did I have a heart attack? Did anyone call my wife? Should I tell someone I still have that pain in my chest? Does anyone here know my name? What is an EKG? MI? PVC? IV? Why does everyone use initials? Why doesn't someone sit down and tell me what is going on? Why is everyone rushing around to get things done? I just wanted to shout out, "Hey, my name is Joe, I am 48 years old and a New York City fireman, and I am afraid!"

The above account is a patient's assessment of the initial phase of his myocardial infarction within the environment of an emergency room. The critically ill patient arrived in a state of crisis, and the emphasis was placed on the equipment, procedures, and physiologic condition.

As the patient underwent intensive treatment, he

appeared to develop an astuteness to what was happening around him. This sensitivity increased when he believed his survival was dependent on equipment and fast-paced personnel. Attachment to machinery provided comfort to the patient who was faced with the threat of death, but it also caused the patient to experience himself as an object who had lost his value as a human being. A setting that will keep the patient human, as well as functioning efficiently, is of great importance when the person is detached from his normal environment.

This environmentally shocked patient was further stressed by the impersonal hustle and bustle of the health professionals. An individual patient such as Joe does not equate himself with his myocardial infarction. If he did, then treating his illness would satisfy his humanistic needs. The caregivers perceived Joe's illness as something he was, not something he had.

The patient was being perceived as a myocardial infarction with presenting ectopic beats instead of as a human being who was ill. Although grateful for the attention given to his physical condition, he was resentful toward those caregivers who had failed to recognize him as a person.

In the initial emergency phase of the illness, Joe is faced with an abrupt alteration in his life. Being unprepared to face this situation renders him helpless and adds to his already overwhelmed emotional state. His feeling of loss of control imposes severe psychologic stress, and he submits to treatment in a nonquestioning complacent manner.

This critical situation rendered Joe into a state of profound numbness. He experienced a sense of unreality, a strangeness of being outside of his body. He felt his immediate and familiar presence in jeopardy, and what lay ahead seemed ambiguous to him.

Joe's socioemotional needs were dramatically pushed aside for physiologic needs. The health professionals were so involved with life-saving technical procedures that the humanness of Joe was ignored. The behavioral "me" aspect of Joe as an individual was removed, and he was perceived as an illness rather than a person. Sensation and emotion were nondiscernible for Joe. The numbness and strangeness Joe experienced is a common state shared by many critically ill patients—depersonalization.

## A CASE STUDY IN DEHUMANIZATION

Frequently accompanying the state of depersonalization is the process of *dehumanization*. This process of human reduction begins subtly when the critically ill patient enters the intensive care unit. It continues to increase with the number of health-care providers perceiving the individual as a patient rather than as a human being. Dehumanization, conscious or unintentional, demotes the person to an object or thing as seen in the following case study.

> When I first came to, the tubes were everywhere. They were in my mouth, they were in my chest, my neck, my arm, and even in my penis. I hurt all over. There were noises and unfamiliar pieces of equipment all around me. I still didn't know what had happened, and no one cared to tell me. I tried to communicate, but they just kept saying, "Don't worry, you are all right. You are out of the OR. You are in the ICU."
>
> There were two female nurses by my bed; they were looking at papers and talking about tubes. Suddenly they yanked the sheets down to my knees. They told me that they wanted to check my abdominal dressing and my Foley. They did not introduce themselves or explain things. They didn't even cover my private area. I felt so embarrassed, but I was too afraid to move because my arm was strapped down to a board.
>
> After examining my exposed body, they said I had to turn on my side. I tried to resist because they were hurting me, but the two of them just pulled and pushed until they were satisfied with my position and assured me that I would be more comfortable.
>
> The next day the tube in my mouth came out. I thought things were getting better. I started eating spoonfuls of Jello. Suddenly the thought occurred to me, how was I going to go to the bathroom? When I asked the nurse she said, "Don't worry about it."
>
> Here I was with tubes all over. I knew I couldn't get out of bed, and I needed to answer this worry. Why didn't anyone care? My anger started to rage. Why didn't anyone listen to me? When the time finally came, the nurse said, "Don't worry about it. Just go in the bed if you have to." How could they make me do this? I could not face anyone. I just wanted to sleep. I kept my eyes closed just wanting desperately to be somewhere else.
>
> That evening when dinner came, I threw the tray on the floor and ordered everyone to leave me alone. I had had enough! I just wanted to shout, "My name is Charlie, I'm only 20 years old and I don't know what happened to me."

This patient is experiencing the process of dehumanization. The high-tech machinery, sophisticated environment, and lack of primary caring and concern on the part of the health-care providers all help to promote this process. Failure to recognize the patient's beliefs, values, perceptions, and expectations further damaged this already helpless individual. A seriously ill patient hence becomes childlike, with a tendency to look for omnipotence and infallibility in the caregivers. Charlie is seriously ill. He feels damaged and hurt, and no one takes the time to explain what has happened to him. He is not given the opportunity to verbalize his feelings, and he becomes enmeshed in feelings of hopelessness. He begins to experience himself as an object who has lost his value as a human being.

Dehumanization strips the person of human capacity, and it can occur whenever another person or group becomes responsible for making ongoing daily decisions regarding the comfort and welfare of another. The integrity and uniqueness of the individual are lost.

Charlie perceives himself as a helpless child unable to make any decisions regarding even basic activities of daily living. When subjected to this process, Charlie experienced one of the most common emotional responses, anger. Initially, Charlie suppresses his anger for fear of rejection and retaliation by his caregivers. He withdraws into sleep. Charlie is already in a physiologic crisis, and his adjustment is further hampered by a loss of self-identity and a threat of abandonment.

Charlie's caregivers are expected to make things better for him, but because of their lack of humanistic caring, he becomes more angered and unable to cope with his physiologic crisis. The primary physical care delivered fails to offer satisfaction to Charlie in his time of crisis.

In the scenarios just presented, one can see how the onset of critical illness disrupts the dynamic equilibrium of the individual's life processes. As vividly portrayed in the experiences of Joe and Charlie, the inability of the individual to cope effectively with and to manage a physiologic and emotional crisis is often undermined by the state of depersonalization and the process of dehumanization.

As a result of the incapacitating nature of critical illness, critically ill patients experience a loss of self-worth and self-esteem; they are stripped of their sense of independence and privacy; and they feel isolated from their family and significant others. These patients are dependent on the knowledge, skills, and dedication of the ICU team to meet their complex and intimate needs. Their very lives are entrusted to virtual strangers, which adds to their high level of stress and fear. Patients usually want to experience self-worth and protect their own personal identity and integrity. The nurse must allow patients to resolve these aspects of this human struggle as they face the life-threatening event.

Critical care nurses must be able to recognize clues to these problems, to identify patients at risk, and to be prepared to intervene to alleviate and/or prevent their occurrence. In the discussion that follows, emphasis will be placed on some behaviors the nurse can use in fostering a more personalized and humanistic approach in caring for critically ill patients.

## CARING BEHAVIORS

Caring is vital in the achievement of wellness. It is as important as curing and is proclaimed on a national level (i.e., American Nurses' Association's *Social Policy Statement*) as the essential concept underlying nursing practice. The art of caring fosters nursing the "me" quality of patients. Nurses focus on patients as people rather than as illnesses. The thinking, feeling, and sensing human being becomes the central focal point of nursing care.

Personalized humanistic care is provided by the caring behaviors of the caregivers. Along with technological skills, caring behaviors must be recognized, developed, and integrated into our daily practice as professional nurses. These caring behaviors should be incorporated into the care of the critically ill patient upon admission to the intensive care setting.

### Communicating

A simple yet easily overlooked behavior on the part of the nurse is an introduction, including the nurse's name and a recognition by the nurse of each patient's choice of names. In the process of this social exchange, an extension of hands to affirm the introduction is well received by each individual as a respect for his/her personal worth, and is necessary to establish a nurse–patient bond.

In most critical care areas, first names are used by the nurses to foster a close relationship with patients. The admitting nurse initiates the care for the patient and is the professional in whom patients must first place their trust to safeguard their well-being. Time is of the essence in developing a therapeutic relationship to stabilize the patient's disequilibrium brought on by a life-threatening event.

Effective, ongoing communication between nurses and their patients is essential as patients progress through the course of their illness. Communication is the most significant mode of activity through which patients can affect their environment from the supine position. It is vital that the communication be meaningful to the patient. In the first case study, the health-care professionals used medical jargon, abbreviations, and unfamiliar terms, and failed to offer explanations. Joe's inability to understand and to question his caregivers further overwhelmed him as he faced his physiologic crisis. Likewise in the second case study, Charlie awakens and desperately seeks an explanation as to his present circumstance. The responses of the nurses failed to offer any meaning to his confused, fearful state.

The nurses should have attempted to make their communication meaningful. Use of understandable terminology, simple explanations of procedures, and an introduction and orientation to an unfamiliar environment could have assisted both Joe and Charlie in dispelling their fears and confusion.

## Touching

As seen in both case studies described earlier, nurses failed to establish a therapeutic relationship with their patients. No time was devoted to establishing a personal approach by introducing themselves by name and inquiring from the patients what they wished to be called. A single act of human touch, for example, a warm hand shake or gentle squeeze, would have been helpful in establishing a trusting relationship and fostering the personalization of the patient. Personalization reflects a greater sense of one's own identity, and feeling comfortable with oneself and being in touch with one's feelings.

In addition, a warm caring touch of Joe's shoulder or head would have improved the potential for sincere nurse–patient communication. He was feeling very nervous and afraid as people hurried around him performing various procedures. A simple touch, which serves to reassure an individual of his self-worth, could have allayed Joe's fears and imparted a sign that someone cared. The distance of the health-care workers in Joe's case made him sense only blurred faces and muffled voices, and he couldn't become a part of the experience.

In Charlie's case, the nurses made physical contact with him, but the contact lacked human touch qualities. Touch should be a deliberate action to convey understanding and acceptance. When possible, touch should be accompanied with eye contact. Touch is a necessary building block in forming a trusting relationship.

## Valuing

The development of an interpersonal relationship through communication serves as a basis for nurses in forming judgments and making decisions. A recognition of who their patients really are and the patients' right to participate in their own care will enable nurses to be more alert to patients' behavioral cues. Patients need to know that they are valued by the caregivers, and that their behavior and verbalization will be acknowledged as significant to them.

Failure to recognize the person of Joe can clearly be seen in the first example. Who was he? What role did he play in his family, community, and society in general? Joe's identity as an individual, and his feelings, needs, and concerns were pushed aside as the attentions of the caregivers focused on his physiologic instability. Joe, being afraid and isolated from his wife, needed someone to value his feelings, needs, and concerns. If only someone would have called his wife. As for Joe himself, he was so overwhelmed by the activities of his caregivers, he dared not make this request. Upon the initial encounter with Joe, the critical care nurse should have inquired if there was anyone who could be called or contacted on Joe's behalf. In addition, Joe's nonverbal behavior should have alerted the professional nurse to his fear and the need to have a loved one nearby.

## Listening

Greater emphasis must be placed on listening to patients and responding to their cues and clues. Listening is a sensory skill essential for effective, therapeutic communication. When nurses listen to their patients, they should do so at a conscious level. They should reach out to their patients and become sensitized to their inner world. In caring for patients, nurses voluntarily enter a world of thoughts and feelings many times foreign to their own world. Without losing their objectivity, nurses should listen carefully to patients and try to place themselves into their patients' frame of reference.

In reviewing Charlie's experience, it becomes obvious that the nurses failed to place themselves into his world. They failed to realize that here is a 20-year-old youth who has no idea what has happened to him and is frightened by the overwhelming technological and impersonal invasion of his body and person. At first, Charlie cannot verbalize his feelings and misgivings, and the nurses caring for Charlie fail to recognize his tense, motionless state. From Charlie's perspective, they seem to blatantly disregard his need for modesty and his need to protect his identity and integrity as a man.

## Perceiving

Had the nurses truly and consciously listened to Charlie's questions and perceived his feelings, they may have tried to communicate more effectively and diligently with him. They may have encouraged him to express his thoughts and feelings and to formulate realistic expectations about his care and progress. Charlie needed to know what was happening to him. Unable to ask and not given the opportunity to do so, his anticipatory fear led him further into emotional turmoil.

The eruption of anger easily may have been prevented if the nurses had accurately perceived Charlie's reaction to a threatening and perplexing environment. The nurses should have included Charlie in the planning of his care, allowing him to make certain decisions. For example, allowing Charlie to decide which side to be positioned on or seeking his permission to uncover his body to check his dressing and Foley catheter would have helped to maintain Charlie's feelings of control and self-worth.

## Involving

For nurses to know a patient well enough to provide individualized care, they must allow themselves to become involved with the patient and his/her world. Involvement is reaching out, touching, and hearing the inner being of another. Nurses obtain knowledge about the patient by recognizing and perceiving that the patient's verbal and nonverbal expressions are reflective of underlying thoughts and feelings, which are in essence the patient's reality. Acceptance of the patient and his/her reality with unconditional positive regard conveys to the patient that he/she is recognized and respected as a separate and distinct person, having the right to his/her own feelings whether or not the nurse agrees with them.

## Empathizing

The ability to perceive the feelings of another person accurately is known as empathy. Empathic communication needs to be expressed in the language and feeling tone of patients. When nurses actively respond, patients have a greater sense of being understood. This provides an opportunity for correction of any perceptual errors. This empathic communication is vital in the personalization process.

## SUMMARY

As we have seen through the case studies of Joe and Charlie, and the analysis of their experiences, caring behaviors on the part of the nurses might have made a difference. Such behaviors identified in the above discussion included communicating, touching, valuing, listening, perceiving, involving, and empathizing. Through these behaviors, nurses are able to deliver personalized humanistic care and to prevent the state of depersonalization and the process of dehumanization in their patients.

Caring affects both those who care and those being cared for. Thus it is important to demonstrate our caring behaviors to our patients and their significant others. At times, caring can be painful as well as satisfying to the nurse who enters the tormented or tragic world of a patient. Cradling a dying infant and sharing the grief of the parents; stroking the forehead of a severely burned victim, hoping it offers some comfort as he writhes in pain from the extensive body dressing changes; having to care for the teenager who has been suddenly paralyzed as a result of a motor vehicle accident and is enmeshed in feelings of hopelessness and despair, certainly challenge the caring nurse who attempts to instill a ray of hope for the future. To fight the battle of AIDS with a patient only to face it over and over again until the struggle becomes futile and death prevails is certainly a heart-breaking experience for the critical care nurse. To be hugged with gratification by the loved ones of a cancer patient who has finally achieved peace in a dignified death is surely a moving experience for the nurse.

We feel with our patients and their loved ones—the pain, the anger, the sorrow, the joy, and hopefully the peace. We cry, we laugh, we touch, and we share a part of ourselves with each other as we face the challenge of critical care nursing. Loretta Zderad[1] summarizes this sensitive caring focus in nursing by her statement:

> To truly treat another as a unique individual, to see him as a subject rather than to look on him as an object, to be able to do with him rather than to him, it is necessary to grasp his perspective, to see his world as he does.

## REFERENCE

1. Zderad, L: Empathetic nursing: Realization of a human capacity. Nurs Clin North Am 4(4):655, 1969.

## SUGGESTED READINGS

American Nurses' Association: Nursing: A Social Policy Statement. American Nurses' Association, Kansas City, Mo, 1980.
Cawley, M: No cure, just care. Am J Nurs 74:2011, 1974.
Hein, E: Listening. Nursing '75, 5(3):93, March 1975.
Kalish, B: What is Empathy? Am J Nurs 73(3):1548, Sept 1973.
Qamar, S: The stress–carative model of nursing practice. Focus on Critical Care 13(6):15, 1986.
Roberts, S: Behavioral Concepts and the Critically Ill Patient, ed 2. Appleton-Century Crafts, Norwalk, Conn, 1986.
Roberts, S: Psychological equilibrium. In Kinney, M (ed): AACN's Clinical Reference for Critical Care Nursing. McGraw-Hill, New York, 1981, p 331.
Wright, J: Self-perception alterations with coronary artery bypass surgery. Heart Lung 16(5):483, Sept 1987.
Zderad, L: Empathetic nursing: Realization of a human capacity. Nurs Clin North Am 4(4):655, 1969.

# UNIT ONE

# Bibliography

American Nurses' Association: Nursing: A Social Policy Statement. Kansas City, Mo, American Nurses Association, 1980.

Ballard, KS: Identification of environmental stressors for patients in a surgical intensive care unit. Issues in Mental Health Nursing 3(1–2):89–108, 1981.

Bowman, CC: Identifying priority concerns of families of ICU patients. Dimensions of Critical Care Nursing 3(5):313–319, 1984.

Bozett, FW, and Gibbons, R: The nursing management of families in the critical care setting. Critical Care Update 10(2):22, 1983.

Braulin, J, Rook, J, and Sills, GM: Family in crisis: The impact of trauma. Crit Care Q 5(3):38–46, 1982.

Brose, C: Theories of family crisis. In Hymovich, DP and Barnard, MU (eds): Family Health Care. McGraw-Hill, New York, 1979.

Breu, C and Dracup, K: Helping spouses of critically ill patients. J Nurs 78(1):51, 1978.

Caplan, G: An Approach to Community Mental Health. Grune & Stratton, New York, 1961.

Cobb, S: Social support as a moderator of life stress. Psychosom Med 38:300, 1976.

Gardner, D and Stewart, N: Staff involvement with families of patients in critical care units. Heart Lung 7(1):105, 1978.

Geary, MC: Supporting family coping. Supervisor Nurse 10(3):52–59, 1979.

Gordon, M: Nursing Diagnosis Process and Application, ed 2. McGraw-Hill, New York, 1987.

Haber, J, Leach, AM, et al: Comprehensive Psychiatric Nursing, ed 2. McGraw-Hill, New York, 1982.

Hackett, TP and Cassem, NH: Psychological management of the myocardial infarction patient. Journal of Human Studies 1(3):25, 1975.

Hackett, TP, Cassem, NH, and Wishnie, HA: The coronary care unit: An appraisal of its psychologic hazards. N Engl J Med 279(25):1365–1370, 1968.

Hampe, SO: Needs of the grieving spouse in a hospital setting. Nurs Res 24(2):116, 1975.

Horowitz, M: Psychological response to serious life events. In Hamilton, V and Warburton, D (eds): Human Stress and Cognition. Wiley, New York, 1980.

Kim MJ, McFarland, GK, and McLane, AM: Pocket Guide to Nursing Diagnoses. CV Mosby, St Louis, 1989.

Kleck, HG: ICU syndrome: Onset, manifestations, treatment, stressors and prevention. Crit Care Q 6(4):21–28, March 1984.

Kobasa, A: The hardy personality: Toward a social psychology of stress and health. In Sanders, GS and Suls, J (eds): Social Psychology of Health and Illness. Lawrence Erlbaum, New Jersey, 1982.

Lazarus, RS: Stress Appraisal and Coping. Springer, New York, 1984.

Levitt, MB: Nursing and family-focused care. Nurs Clin North Am 19(1):83, 1984.

Luce, C: Current Research on Sleep and Dreams. US Department of Health, Education and Welfare, Public Health Services Publication No. 1389. National Institutes of Health, Bethesda, Md, 1965.

Mackinnon-Kessler, S: Maximizing your ICU patient's sensory perception environment. Canadian Nurse 79(5):41, 1983.

Maslow, AH: Motivation and Personality, ed 2. Harper & Row, New York, 1970.

Molter, NC: Needs of relatives of critically ill patients: A descriptive study. Heart Lung 8(2):332, 1970.

Orlando, IH: Dynamic Nurse–Patient Relationship. GP Putnam's Sons, New York, 1961.

Parad, HJ and Caplan, G: A framework for studying families in crisis. In Parad, HJ (ed): Crisis Intervention: Selected Readings. Family Services Association of America, New York, 1965.

Roberts, S: The Role of the Family in Critical Care, Behavioral Concepts and the Critically Ill Patient. Prentice-Hall, Englewood Cliffs, NJ, 1976.

Roy, Sr C: Introduction to Nursing: An Adaptation Model. Prentice-Hall, Englewood Cliffs, NJ, 1976.

Ruben, HL: Family crisis. Am Fam Physician 11:132, 1975.

Salyer, J and Stuart, BJ: Nurse–patient interaction in the intensive care unit. Heart Lung 14(1):20, 1985.

Sanz, C: The reality behind the miracle babies. Dallas Morning News, Nov 1987, p 10c.

Selye, H: The Stress of Life. McGraw-Hill, New York, 1978.

Smilkstein, G: The cycle of family function: A conceptual model for family medicine. J Fam Prac 11:223, 1980.

Steckel, SB: Patient Contracting. Appleton-Century-Crofts, Norwalk, Conn, 1982.

Stuart, RB: Behavioral contracting within families of delinquents. J Behav Ther Exp Psychiatry 2(1):1–11, 1971.

Umana, RF, Gross, ST, and McConville, MT: Crisis in the Family: Three Approaches. Gardner Press, New York, 1980.

Zderad, L: Empathetic nursing: Realization of a human capacity. Nurs Clin North Am 4(4):655, 1969.

# UNIT TWO

# Nervous System

The human body is a complex organism composed of many different kinds of cells and the extracellular fluid that surrounds them. The activities of these cells must be coordinated so that optimal functioning is achieved and a state of dynamic equilibrium is maintained.

This coordination requires that the human body be capable of perceiving and acknowledging changes in its environment and of responding appropriately. It requires a unique communication system in which the activities of the cells are regulated and integrated in such a way that any change occurring in the environment automatically initiates actions to minimize that change. This ability of cells to respond is modulated by a variety of regulatory and compensatory mechanisms, which ensure maintenance of an equilibrated state. Thus, the body receives information from a variety of sensory organs, sorts it out, integrates and evaluates it to determine the appropriate response, and then directs the cells to carry out this response.

Most of the communicative and regulatory functions of the body are mediated by two major organ systems — the nervous system and the endocrine system (see Unit Three). The chapters in Unit Two examine the intricate relationship between structure and function within the human nervous system. Such information establishes a basis for understanding the pathophysiology underlying insults to the nervous system, and the implications for nursing care.

The discussion of pathophysiology includes acute head trauma, herniation syndromes, cerebrovascular disorders, spinal cord injury, meningitis, seizures, Guillain-Barré syndrome, myasthenia gravis, and amyotrophic lateral sclerosis.

Nursing care of the patient with compromised neurologic function is examined in terms of nursing process, including the use of pertinent nursing diagnoses. Nursing care plans are presented based on nursing diagnoses and include specific patient outcomes and nursing interventions and their rationales.

## UNIT OUTLINE

CHAPTER 6

# Anatomy and Physiology of the Nervous System

## CHAPTER OUTLINE



## LEARNING OBJECTIVES

**At the end of this chapter, you should be able to:**

1. Outline the major divisions of the nervous system.
2. Describe the functional unit of the nervous system, the neuron.
3. State the major factors involved in establishing and maintaining the resting membrane potential.
4. Identify the electrochemical phenomena underlying the action potential, threshold potential, and refractory periods.
5. Describe the functional anatomy of the synapse and the role of neurotransmitters.
6. Describe the structural support systems of the brain including the skull, cranial vault, and the meninges.
7. Review the functional support systems of the brain including the ventricular system, cerebrospinal fluid, and blood circulatory systems.
8. Delineate brain structures and their functions.
9. Associate metabolic needs of neural tissue with autoregulation and cerebral perfusion pressure.
10. Relate compensatory mechanisms to the maintenance of intracranial pressure within physiologic range.
11. Describe the structure of the spinal cord including spinal nerves and plexi.
12. Differentiate between ventral and dorsal spinal cord roots.
13. Identify the functional components of the reflex arc.
14. Trace the circuitry of primary sensory and motor pathways.
15. Describe the structure and function of the autonomic nervous system.

## MAJOR DIVISIONS OF THE NERVOUS SYSTEM

The nervous system consists of two major divisions, the *central nervous system* and the *peripheral nervous system* (Table 6–1). The central nervous system (CNS) is composed of the brain and spinal cord; the peripheral nervous system (PNS) consists of all the nerves outside of the brain and spinal cord, including 12 pairs of *cranial* nerves and 31 pairs of *spinal* nerves.

The peripheral nervous system is further divided

TABLE 6-1
**Divisions of the Nervous System**

I. Central nervous system (CNS)
 A. Brain
 B. Spinal cord
II. Peripheral nervous system (PNS)
 A. Afferent division
 B. Efferent division
  1. Somatic nervous system
  2. Autonomic nervous system
   a. Sympathetic division
   b. Parasympathetic division

into the *afferent* and *efferent* divisions. Afferent, or sensory, nerves transmit information received from specialized *receptors* in peripheral and deep structures of the body *toward* the central nervous system (i.e., the brain and spinal cord); efferent, or motor, nerves transmit information *away* from the brain and spinal cord to structures throughout the body, including skeletal muscle, cardiac muscle, and smooth muscles of visceral organs and glands. These structures are called *effectors* because it is through them that the response of the central nervous system is realized.

The efferent division of the peripheral nervous system is further divided into the *somatic* nervous system and the *autonomic* nervous system. Nerves of the somatic nervous system are concerned with the interaction of the body with the external environment. These nerves innervate skeletal muscle cells.

The autonomic nervous system is divided into the *sympathetic* and *parasympathetic* divisions. Activated by centers in the brain (hypothalamus and brainstem), these two divisions are anatomically and physiologically distinct, and largely exert opposing or antagonistic effects on specific organs of the body that they reciprocally innervate. Nerves of the autonomic nervous system are concerned primarily with visceral functions and interaction with the internal environment. These nerves innervate cardiac muscle, smooth muscle, and glands.

## FUNCTIONAL MICROANATOMY OF THE NERVOUS SYSTEM

### Cell Types

#### *Neuron — The Functional Unit*

The *neuron* is the functional unit of the nervous system. Neurons are among the most highly specialized cells within the human body, and although they occur in many different forms and sizes, they all have three basic fundamental properties. These include the capacity to react to stimuli, to initiate and conduct action potentials in response to stimuli, and to enable a response to occur by influencing other neurons, muscles, or glands.

**Structural Components.** Each neuron consists of three major structural components: the cell body, dendrites, and axon (Fig. 6-1). Dendrites and axons are collectively referred to as *nerve fibers*.

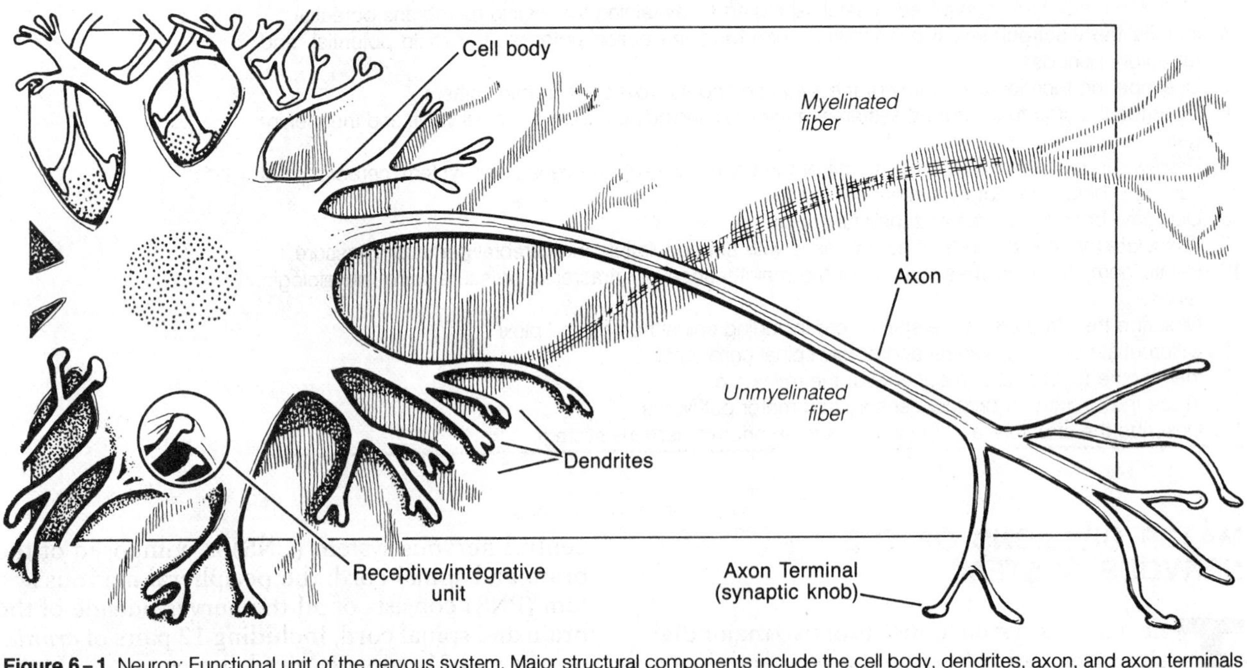


**Figure 6-1.** Neuron: Functional unit of the nervous system. Major structural components include the cell body, dendrites, axon, and axon terminals (synaptic knobs). The neuron consists of receptive/integrative units comprised of dendrite-cell body complexes. These units function to process incoming information. Two types of neurons include myelinated and unmyelinated neurons: myelinated fibers are covered with myelin (i.e., a lipid-protein substance); unmyelinated fibers are without myelin.

*Dendrites* are generally short, highly branched cytoplasmic extensions of the cell body, which receive incoming information (in the form of nerve impulses) and conduct it *toward* the cell body. The dendrite-cell body complex can be thought of as the *receptive/integrative unit* of the neuron (see Fig. 6–1). Dendrites provide most of the receptor surface for incoming information from other neurons. This information is processed within the dendrite-cell body complex in such a way that the net response of the neuron reflects the integration of numerous, often conflicting bits of information received from other neurons.

The *axon* is usually a single process arising from the cell body, and conducts information *away* from the cell body to the *axon terminals (synaptic knobs)* (see Fig. 6–1). Some axons are covered with a lipid-protein substance called *myelin*, which functions to insulate the axonal membrane and influences the speed of impulse conduction. Myelin is deposited along the axons in a circular manner so as to surround the axon with an outer enveloping layer called the *myelin sheath*. The myelin sheath is not a continuous layer but is segmented or interrupted at regular intervals called *nodes of Ranvier*. The presence of such nodes facilitates rapid impulse transmission via *saltatory conduction*.

Nerve fibers that have a myelin sheath are called *myelinated* fibers and make up the white matter of the CNS. The term white reflects the high lipid content in myelin. Nerve fibers without a myelin sheath are called *unmyelinated* and make up the gray matter within the CNS (see Fig. 6–1).

### *Neuroglial Cells*

Neuroglial cells are specialized, non-nervous connective tissue cells within the central nervous system, which function to sustain neurons metabolically, provide structural support, and help to regulate ionic concentrations in extra-cellular fluid.

Several types of neuroglial cells have been identified, and these include *astroglia, microglia, oligodendroglia*, and *ependymal* cells. The latter two cell types deserve special mention. *Oligodendroglia* are glial cells responsible for myelin production within the CNS and for establishing and maintaining the myelin sheaths of myelinated axons. (Their counterparts in the peripheral nervous system are called *Schwann's cells*.) *Ependymal* cells are glial cells that line the ventricles and choroid plexuses, and are thought to be involved in production of cerebrospinal fluid. These cells play a role in establishing and maintaining the blood–brain barrier (see Fig. 6–11).

Neuroglial cells are of clinical importance in that 40% to 50% of intracranial tumors are derived from glial cells *(gliomas)*. These cells, unlike neurons, can undergo mitosis. Glial scars after brain injury or surgery may result in focal seizures.

## Electrochemical Physiology: Membrane Potentials

### *Resting Membrane Potential*

Intracellular and extracellular fluids contain electrolytic solutions that have the same concentrations of positively and negatively charged ions. Intracellularly, there are a slightly greater number of negatively charged ions that accumulate along the inner surface of the plasma membrane; extracellularly, there are a slightly greater number of positively charged ions that accumulate along the outer surface of the plasma membrane. The electrochemical attraction of these ions, separated as they are across the membrane, accounts for the membrane *potential* and the cell is said to be *polarized* (Fig. 6–2*A*).

The membrane potential is determined primarily by 2 factors: the difference in the electrochemical gradients between intracellular and extracellular fluids, largely involving potassium and sodium ions, respectively; and the selective permeability of the plasma membrane to potassium in its resting state.

Normally, the intracellular concentration of potassium ions is approximately 140 mEq/liter, while the extracellular concentration ranges between 3.5–5.5 mEq/liter. Conversely, the intracellular concentration of sodium ions is approximately 14 mEq/liter, while the extracellular concentration is about 142 mEq/liter.

Under these conditions, potassium ions diffuse out of the cell along electrochemical gradients

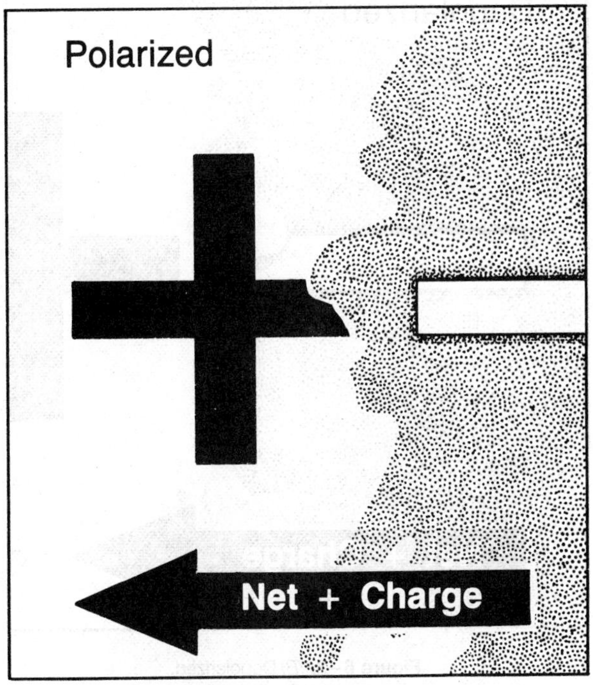


**Figure 6–2.** *(A)* Polarized.

leaving behind charged proteins, organic phosphates, sulfates, and other ions that are too large to diffuse through the membrane. Thus, the intracellular potential becomes increasingly negative while that of the extracellular fluid becomes increasingly positive, until an electrochemical equilibrium potential is reached.

To a lesser extent, the sodium/potassium pump located within the plasma membrane also contributes to the resting membrane potential by helping to maintain electrochemical gradients.

### Action Potential

**Depolarization.** An *action potential* occurs in response to a stimulus and results from a rapid, transient change in membrane ion permeability. There is a several hundredfold increase in the membrane permeability to sodium, which allows sodium ions to rush through open sodium channels along electrochemical gradients and into the cell. During this phase more positive charge enters the cell in the form of sodium ions than leaves in the form of potassium ions. This eventually *reverses* the *polarity* of the membrane potential, becoming positive on the inside and negative on the outside of the membrane. This phase of the action potential characterized by a reversal of polarity in conjunction with an increase in membrane permeability to sodium is called *depolarization* (Fig. 6–2*B*).

**Repolarization.** Action potentials in nerve cells last about 1 millisecond. The rapid return of the membrane potential to its resting level is facilitated as follows: (1) the membrane again becomes impermeable to sodium as sodium ion channels close; and (2) most importantly, there is a simultaneous increase in potassium permeability. Moving along electrochemical gradients, potassium passively diffuses out of the cell. It is this movement of potassium ions out of the cell that returns the membrane potential to its resting state, and the membrane is said to be *repolarizing*. Repolarization is completed when resting membrane permeability is restored and the resting membrane potential is re-established (Fig. 6–2*C*).

### Threshold Potential

Not all stimuli depolarize the plasma membrane sufficiently to trigger an action potential. Action potentials occur only when membrane permeability to sodium is sufficiently increased (i.e., enough sodium channels open) to enable positive sodium ions to rush into the cell along electrochemical gradients. This results in a net movement of positive charge inward, and the membrane potential becomes less negative (i.e., it moves toward zero). The membrane is said to be depolarized. The potential at which this net inward movement of positive charge occurs is called the *threshold potential.*

Once threshold potential is reached, the action potential that occurs reaches a *maximal* potential. Action potentials either occur maximally, as determined by the electrochemical conditions across

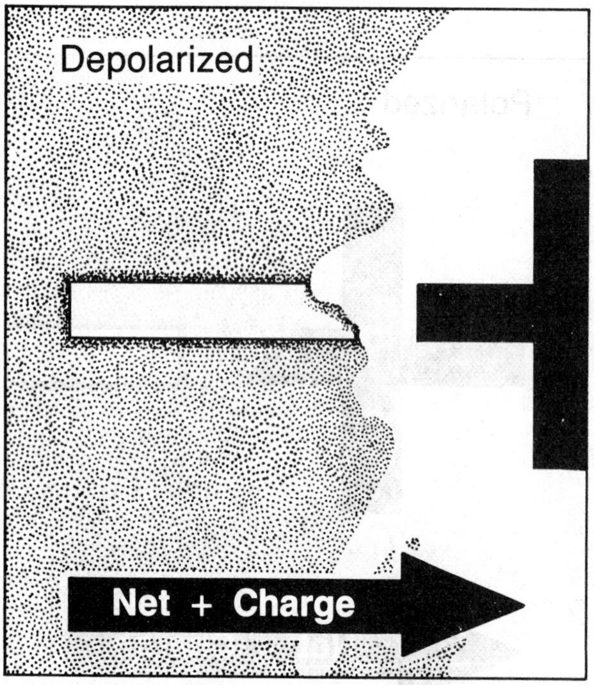


**Figure 6–2.** *(B)* Depolarized.

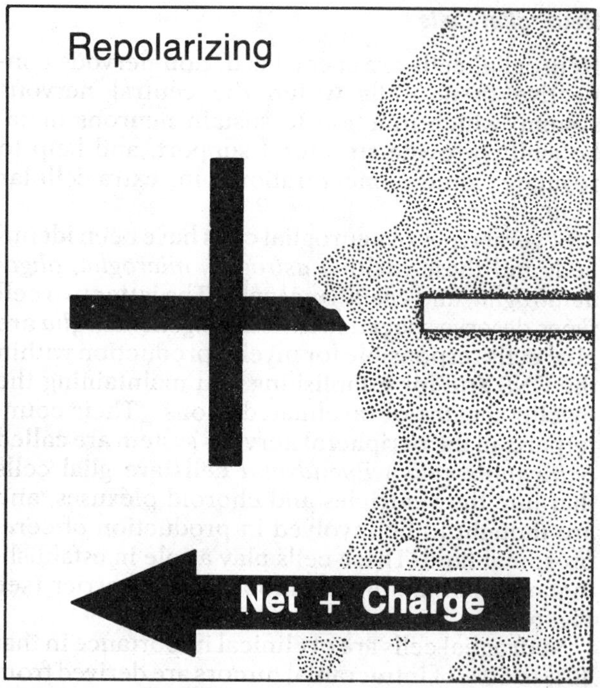


**Figure 6–2.** *(C)* Repolarizing.

the membrane, or they do not occur at all. This is referred to as the *all or none phenomenon.*

### Refractory Periods

Once an action potential occurs, a second action potential cannot be generated for a certain period of time, during which the plasma membrane remains unresponsive to stimuli. This is referred to as the *refractory* period.

The *absolute* (effective) refractory period is the time during an action potential when a second stimulus, no matter how strong, will not produce a second action potential.

Following the absolute refractory period there is an interval during which a second action potential can be fired, but only if the strength of the stimulus is greater than the usual threshold level. This is the *relative* refractory period.

### Action Potential Propagation

**Local Current Flow.** Once triggered, a particular action potential does not itself travel along the plasma membrane. Rather, because of *local current flow,* which occurs between regions of different electric potential, each action potential is able to depolarize adjacent membrane to threshold potential, thus generating a new action potential (Fig. 6–3). The new action potential, in turn, produces local currents of its own, which depolarize the region adjacent to it, generating yet another action potential. In this manner action potential propagation occurs along the plasma membrane.

Propagation of action potentials is always *away* from the site of the stimulus because areas of the membrane having just undergone an action potential are *refractory.* In most nerve cells, propagation of action potentials is unidirectional (i.e., action potentials are initiated at one end of the cell and propagate toward the other end).

**Saltatory Conduction.** In addition to local current flow, action potentials are also propagated via *saltatory conduction.* As mentioned earlier, this type of conduction occurs along myelinated axons where the myelin sheath is interrupted by the nodes of Ranvier. The action potential jumps from one node to the next as it propagates along the axon, thus increasing the speed of impulse conduction (see Fig. 6–3).

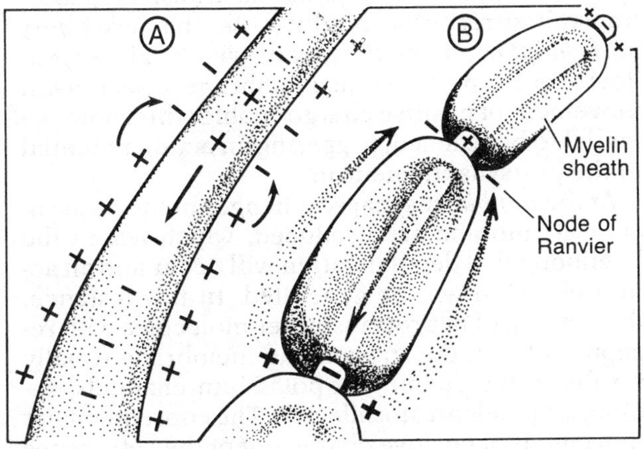


**Figure 6–3.** Action potential conduction. *(A)* A neuron with an unmyelinated axon depicting local current flow. *(B)* A neuron with a myelinated axon depicting saltatory conduction. The *minus (—) sign* within the neurons signifies the difference in potential across the membrane, with the inside of the cell negatively charged with respect to the outside. *Solid arrows* outside the neurons indicate the direction in which the nerve impulses are propagated.

### Synapse

Information is communicated throughout the nervous system by both electrical and chemical processes. As we have just seen, impulses are conducted along the nerve fiber electrically via local current flow or saltatory conduction. Transmission of impulses from one neuron to the next occurs via a synapse. There are 2 types of synapses: *electrical* and *chemical.* Chemical synapses predominate.

A *synapse* is a strategic, anatomically specialized junction between 2 neurons at which the electrical activity in one neuron influences the activity of the second neuron. At chemical synapses this activity is communicated by a chemical "messenger" called a *neurotransmitter.*

Structurally, the synapse consists of the *synaptic knob (axon terminal)* of the *presynaptic* neuron, and the *subsynaptic membrane* of the *postsynaptic* neuron, separated by a small space called the *synaptic cleft* (Fig. 6–4). The synaptic cleft is sufficiently wide to prevent the direct propagation of electrical current from the presynaptic neuron to the postsynaptic neuron. Rather, such activity is transmitted across the synaptic cleft *chemically* by a neurotransmitter released from the synaptic knob.

Structurally, the *synaptic knob* is well suited for its strategic role in interneuronal communication by chemical means. It contains mechanisms necessary for the following key functions: synthesis of neurotransmitter, storage of neurotransmitter in presynaptic vesicles, release of neurotransmitter from these vesicles into the synaptic cleft (see Fig. 6–4), and reuptake and/or metabolism of neurotransmitter.

In response to an action potential, which spreads over the synaptic knob depolarizing its membrane, small quantities of neurotransmitter are released into the synaptic cleft from *presynaptic vesicles,* which merge with the plasma membrane. Calcium is considered to be the link between depolarization of the presynaptic membrane by an arriving action potential and neurotransmitter release.

Once released, the neurotransmitter molecules

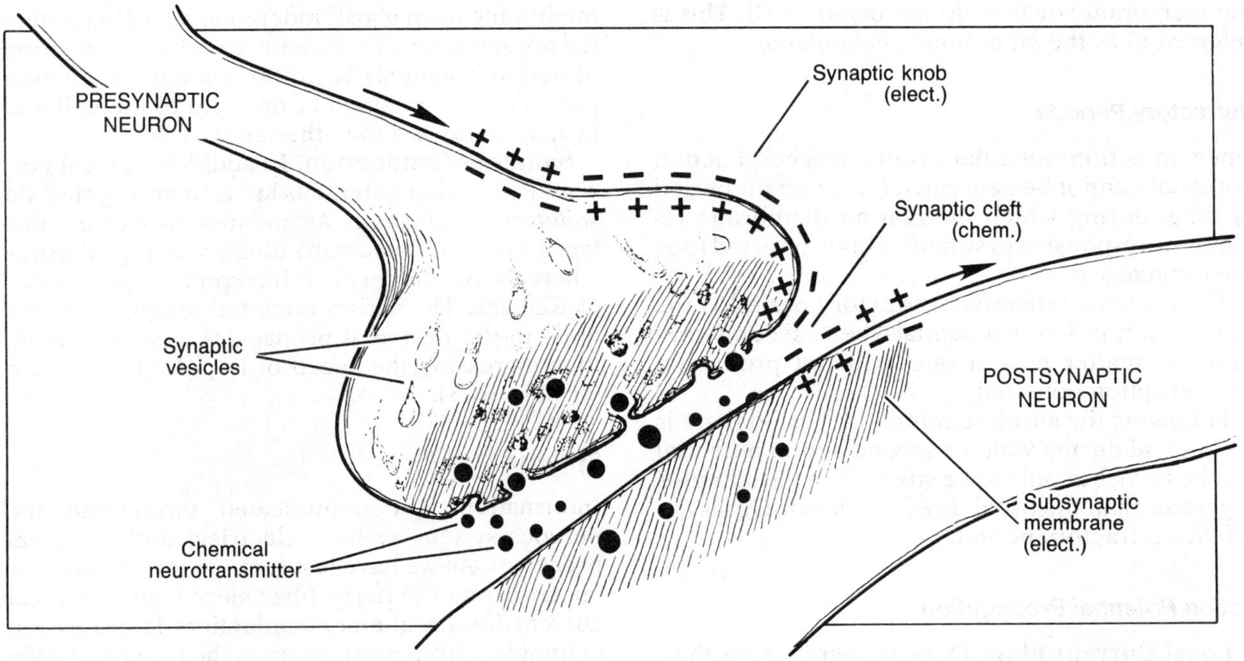


**Figure 6 – 4.** Diagram of synapse, a specialized junction between two neurons separated by a synaptic cleft. The presence of the synaptic cleft requires that the transfer of information between these two neurons occurs via the secretion of a chemical neurotransmitter.

diffuse across the cleft and bind in a transient manner and very specifically to receptor sites on the *subsynaptic plasma membrane* of the postsynaptic neuron. A neurotransmitter binding to its specific receptor causes an immediate change in the permeability characteristics of the subsynaptic membrane by opening specific ion channels. The type of receptor and the type of channel the receptor controls largely determine the effects, whether excitatory or inhibitory, that the neurotransmitter has on the postsynaptic neuron.

The synaptic activity is terminated very quickly when the neurotransmitter leaves the postsynaptic receptor. Ion channels close, terminating the postsynaptic membrane potential.

Neurotransmitter is removed from the synaptic cleft by one of the following mechanisms: diffusion of neurotransmitter away from the receptor site, active re-uptake of the neurotransmitter back into the synaptic knob, and metabolic inactivation of the neurotransmitter.

It is apparent that because neurotransmitter is stored on the *pre*synaptic side of the synaptic cleft and the receptor sites occur on the *post*synaptic side, chemical synapses operate in *one* direction only. This also explains why action potentials move along multineuronal pathways in one direction.

A *synaptic delay* occurs between the arrival of an action potential at the synaptic knob and the transmembrane potential changes in the subsynaptic membrane of the postsynaptic neuron. This largely reflects the time required for release of neurotransmitter from the presynaptic vesicles.

**Excitatory and Inhibitory Synapses.** Whether a synapse is excitatory or inhibitory is determined largely by the type of receptor on the postsynaptic membrane to which the neurotransmitter binds and the type of membrane ion channels the receptor controls.

At the *excitatory* synapse, the response of the postsynaptic membrane to the neurotransmitter is *depolarization*, bringing the membrane potential *closer* to threshold. This is usually accomplished by the opening of sodium ion channels in the subsynaptic membrane in response to transient neurotransmitter-receptor binding. As this *excitatory postsynaptic potential* spreads via local current flow over the postsynaptic membrane, a net *inward* movement of positive charge enables threshold potential to be reached, triggering an action potential in the postsynaptic neuron.

At the *inhibitory* synapse, changes in the postsynaptic membrane are produced, which lessen the likelihood that depolarization will occur and an action potential will be generated. In this instance, the binding of neurotransmitter molecules with receptor sites in the subsynaptic membrane usually results in the opening of potassium channels; sodium channels are not affected. The consequent net movement of positive charge *out* of the cell causes the membrane potential to move *away from threshold,* and *hyperpolarization* of the membrane is said to occur. An *inhibitory postsynaptic potential,* therefore, *prevents* the triggering of an action potential in the postsynaptic neuron.

**Neurotransmitters.** Neurotransmitters are the

TABLE 6–2
**Classes of Neurotransmitters**

I. Acetylcholine
II. Monoamines
  A. Catecholamines
    1. Dopamine
    2. Epinephrine
    3. Norepinephrine
  B. Histamine
  C. Serotonin (5-hydroxytryptamine)
III. Amino acids
  A. Aspartate
  B. Gamma-amino butyric acid (GABA)
  C. Glutamate
  D. Glycine
IV. Peptides
  A. Angiotensin II
  B. Bradykinin
  C. Endorphins
  D. Enkephalins
  E. Hormones

chemical messengers by which presynaptic neurons can influence postsynaptic neurons at chemical synapses. Neurotransmitters are also the vehicle by which efferent neurons influence *effector* cells (skeletal, cardiac and smooth muscles, and glands). Although there are many different neurotransmitter substances, they are highly specific, and in many instances neurons are identified by the type of neurotransmitter they release at their synapses, or at neuromuscular junctions.

In a few instances, more than one neurotransmitter may be released from the synaptic knob. Such neurotransmitters may have a *synergistic* effect on each other. More commonly, all synaptic knobs (axon terminals) on a given neuron probably release the same neurotransmitter. It is also possible for a given neurotransmitter to produce excitation at one synapse and inhibition at another. These considerations, coupled with the infinitesimal number of synapses within the nervous system, help to explain the degree of sophistication of integration and communication unique to the human body. Table 6–2 lists some of the more commonly known neurotransmitters.

# FUNCTIONAL ANATOMY OF THE BRAIN

## Structural and Functional Support Systems

### Skull and Cranial Vault

The brain is enclosed within the cranium, that portion of the bony framework of the skull that provides a protective vault for this vital organ. The bony structure of the cranium consists of an outer and inner table of *compact* bone with a layer of *cancellous* (interwoven) bone in between. Such structure increases strength without increasing weight. A number of very small openings, or *foramina,* in the base of the skull allow for entrance and exit of blood vessels and cranial nerves. There is one large opening, the *foramen magnum,* where the brainstem connects with the spinal cord.

The floor of the cranial vault is divided into the anterior, middle, and posterior *fossae,* or compartments, which conform to and house the frontal lobe, temporal lobe, and brainstem and cerebellum, respectively (Fig. 6–5). The *anterior* fossa is formed largely by the frontal bone, except for a tiny midline section formed by the ethmoid bone. This bone contains the *cribriform plate,* which contains many openings traversed by olfactory nerve fibers.

The anterior fossa is separated from the middle fossa by the sphenoid bone. The *middle* fossa is bounded largely by the sphenoid and temporal bones. The *sella turcica,* which houses the *pituitary gland (hypophysis),* occurs in the midline. The *optic foramina* occur under the lesser wings of the sphenoid bone.

The *petrous* portion of the temporal bone provides the boundary between the middle and posterior fossae. The *posterior* fossa is the largest and is formed primarily by occipital bone. The *foramen magnum* is the most conspicuous foramen.

It is important to appreciate the structural relationship between the brain and the bony cranium that encases it because significant clinical implications may occur when the integrity of this relationship is altered by injury or pathology. While the cranium protects the brain, it can also confine it. In the face of an insult to the brain (e.g., cerebral hemorrhage, cerebral edema), the cranium functions as a rigid container unyielding to brain expansion except via the foramen magnum (see Fig. 6–5). This unique relationship between the cranium and its contents provides the pathophysiologic basis underlying *herniation syndrome.* Herniation syndromes are discussed in Chapter 8.

Significant clinical implications are associated with the patient admitted with possible *basal* skull fracture. As depicted in Figure 6–5, bony, seemingly sharp ridges occur in the base of the skull formed by the lesser wings of the sphenoid bone and angular elevations of the petrous bones. These ridges have the potential of causing considerable damage to the brain when injurious forces applied to the head cause the brain to be thrown up against these ridges. This often results in a "shearing-type" injury to the base of the brain.

Fractures of basal skull bones and associated lacerations to brain coverings (meninges) and blood vessels may result in leakage of cerebrospinal fluid from the nose and/or ear, and bleeding into the cranial bones. Clinical implications related to assessment and management of such conditions are discussed in Chapters 7 and 10.

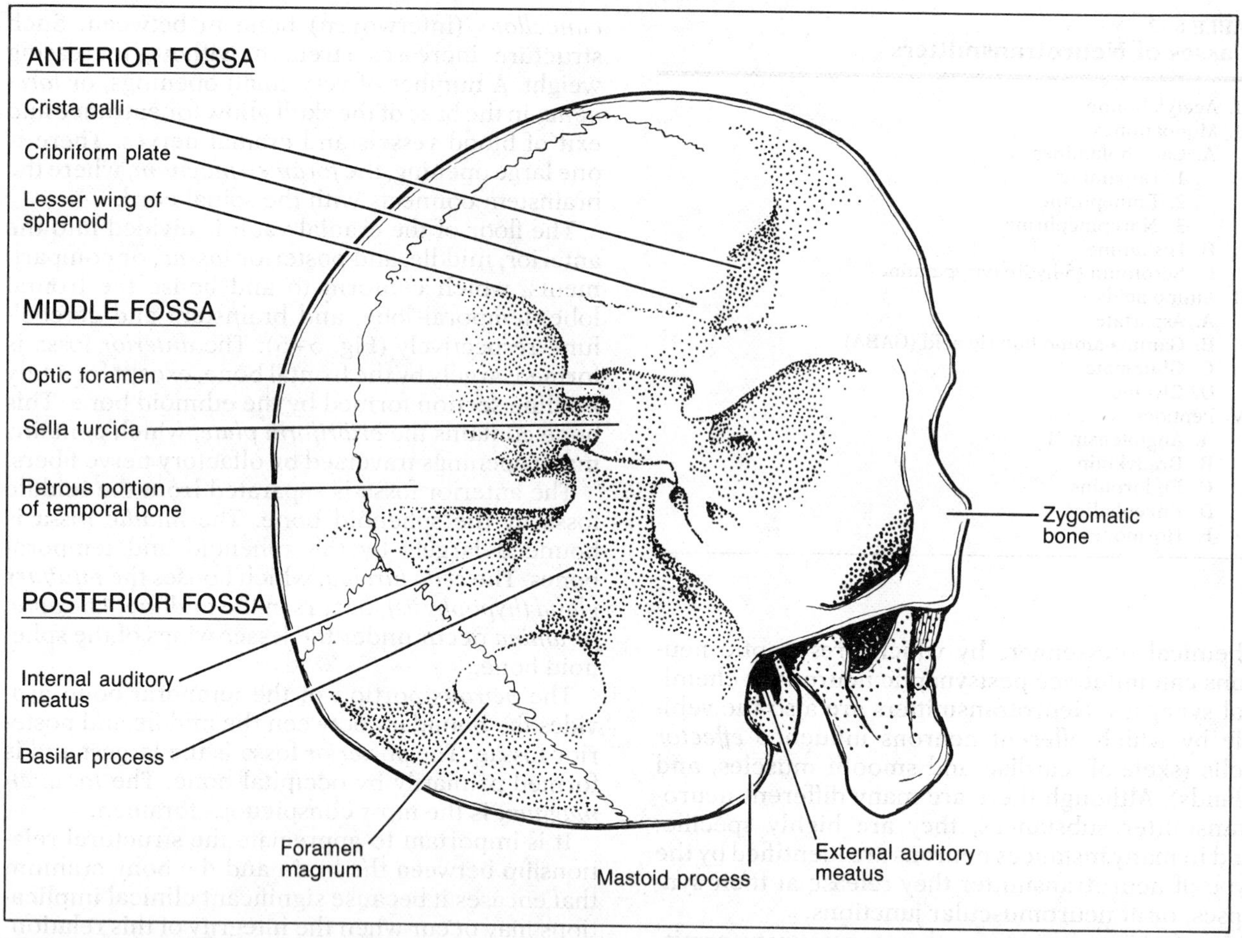


**Figure 6–5.** Intact skull and cranial vault. The floor of the cranial vault is divided into the anterior, middle, and posterior fossae (or compartments), which conform to and house the frontal lobe, temporal lobe, brainstem, and cerebellum, respectively. The intact skull has only one large opening, the foramen magnum. Expansion of the contents within the rigid skull (e.g., brain parenchyma, blood, and cerebrospinal fluid) is very limited except via the foramen magnum. Sharp ridges are formed by the lesser wings of the sphenoid bone and angular elevation of the petrous portion of the temporal bone. These have the potential of causing a "shearing-type" injury to the base of the brain should forces applied to the head thrust the brain up against these bony ridges.

### Meninges

The *meninges* are connective tissue membranes, which cover and surround the brain and spinal cord to support and protect these soft, delicate tissues. There are three separate and continuous layers of tissue: the dura mater, arachnoid mater, and pia mater.

The *dura* mater, the tough, fibrous outermost membrane, occurs in two layers. The outer, periosteal layer is continuous with the inner table of the bony cranium; the thick inner layer follows the contour of the skull except at sites of certain major fissures. In these locations the dura mater is a sturdy sheath that compartmentalizes major areas of the brain. The *falx cerebri* is the sturdy midline sheath located in the *longitudinal fissure* between the cerebral hemispheres (Fig. 6–6). The *falx cerebelli* is the dural sheath that separates the two cerebellar hemispheres. The *tentorium cerebelli* is a smaller fold of dura, which extends between the cerebral hemispheres and the cerebellum to form a "tent" over the cerebellum. A *notch,* or opening, within the tentorium accommodates the brainstem.

The *arachnoid* mater, a thin, delicate fibroelastic tissue, loosely encloses the brain but does not dip into its sulci and fissures. As this membrane skips from crest to crest over the surface of the brain, it gives rise to several large spaces called *cisterns.* The *cisterna magnum* is located between the hemispheres of the cerebellum and medulla, and the *lumbar cistern* is located in the lumbar region of the vertebral column. Both of these enlarged spaces are accessible for aspiration of cerebrospinal fluid.

The *pia* mater, a thin, delicate membrane, is attached intimately to the brain surface following every sulcus and fissure. This membrane functions to hold the brain and spinal cord substance together; it is a very vascular membrane through which pass the cerebral blood vessels that nourish

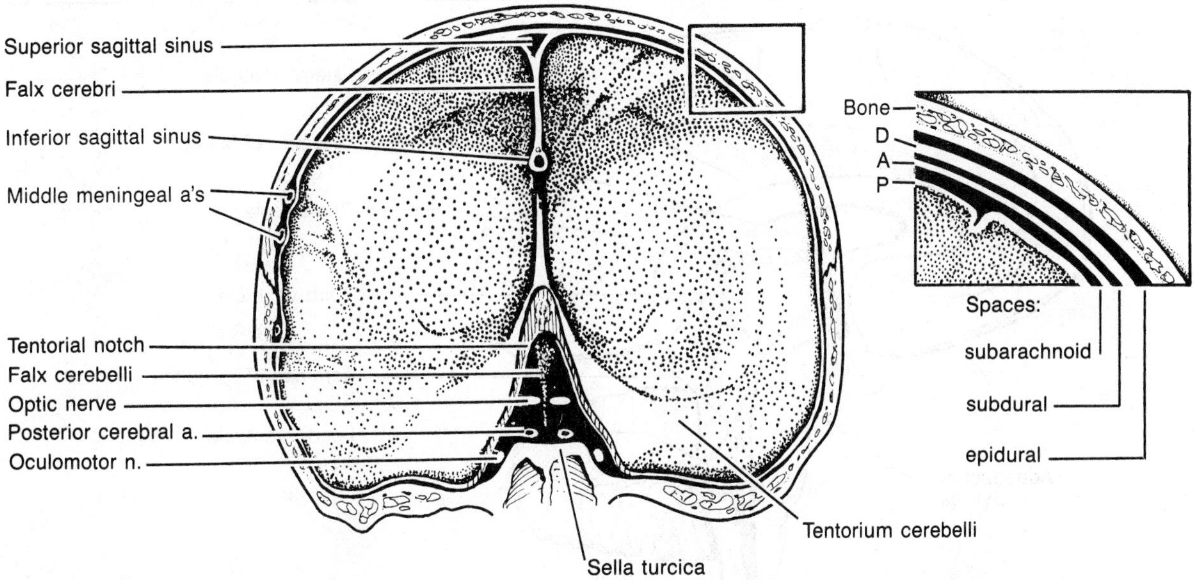


**Figure 6–6.** The meninges (connective tissue coverings) in a coronal section of the head with unobstructed view of the posterior wall of the cranial cavity. The meninges that surround the brain consist of three separate and continuous layers (D = dura mater, A = arachnoid mater, P = pia mater). Sturdy dural sheaths divide the brain vertically in the midline. The tentorium cerebelli is a dural fold, which extends horizontally between the cerebral hemispheres and the cerebellum so as to form a "tent" over the cerebellum. Potential spaces occur between the meningeal layers. These spaces are significant clinically, in that bleeding into these spaces leads to hematoma formation.

the brain tissues; and it functions as part of the *blood–brain barrier* (discussed below).

The unique interrelationship of the meninges is responsible for the "spaces" within the cranial cavity. The *epidural (extradural)* space is a potential space occurring between the periosteal dura and the bone itself (see Fig. 6–6). The *subdural* space occurs between the layers of dura and arachnoid mater. A venous vasculature traverses throughout this space. The *subarachnoid* space occurs between the arachnoid and pia mater. It contains numerous blood vessels and is the space throughout which cerebrospinal fluid circulates and is reabsorbed.

### Ventricular System

The *ventricular system* includes a series of interconnected cavities within the brain, which are lined with ependymal cells and filled with cerebrospinal fluid. Two *lateral* ventricles, one in each cerebral hemisphere, communicate with the *third* ventricle via the *foramen of Monro* (Fig. 6–7). The third ventricle communicates with the *fourth* ventricle via the *aqueduct of Sylvius*. The fourth ventricle gives rise to the *central canal* of the spinal cord and contains the *foramina of Luschka and Magendie*.

**Formation, Circulation, and Reabsorption of Cerebrospinal Fluid.** Cerebrospinal fluid is essentially a plasma filtrate formed from the blood in the *choroid plexuses* located in portions of the lateral, third, and fourth ventricles (see Fig. 6–7). Cerebrospinal fluid is a crystal clear, colorless fluid, which normally is almost completely devoid of protein but contains *glucose*. The presence of glucose helps to differentiate it from mucous drainage from the nose in the scenario of head injury or brain surgery. Mucus contains no glucose. Other characteristics of cerebrospinal fluid are listed in Table 6–3.

In the average adult, cerebrospinal fluid is formed at the rate of approximately 400–600 ml/day. At any given moment the volume within the cranium is approximately 100–150 ml. Because the cranium is a rigid, unyielding container, cerebrospinal fluid must be removed from the cranial cavity at about the same rate as it is formed in order to maintain intracranial pressure within normal limits. The normal pressure of cerebrospinal fluid in the lateral recumbent position is in the range of 60–180 $mmH_2O$.

Cerebrospinal fluid flows from its origin in the choroid plexuses through the interconnected ventricular system into the cisterns and subarachnoid spaces occurring within and surrounding the brain and spinal cord (Fig. 6–8).

Eventually, cerebrospinal fluid is reabsorbed into the blood via the *arachnoid granulations (villi)*. These are projections of arachnoid tissue that provide for unidirectional flow of cerebrospinal fluid from the subarachnoid space into the blood.

**Functions of Cerebrospinal Fluid.** Cerebrospinal fluid plays a critical role in the maintenance of normal neuronal function. It provides a protective fluid "cushion" for all components of the cen-

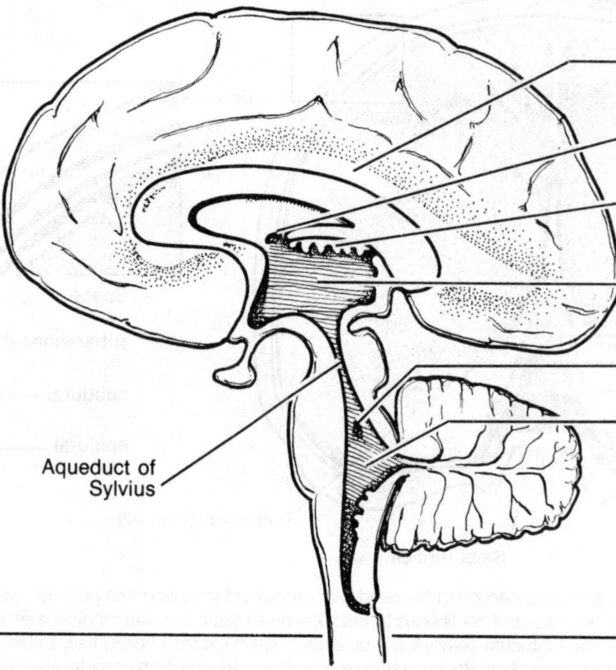


**Figure 6-7.** The ventricular system consists of a series of interconnected cavities within the brain, which contain cerebrospinal fluid.

TABLE 6-3
**Cerebrospinal Fluid: Normal Laboratory Values**

| Laboratory Tests | Normal Values (Adult) |
|---|---|
| Appearance | Crystal clear, colorless |
| Pressure (lateral recumbent) | 70-180 $mmH_2O$ (initial) |
| Protein: | |
| Lumbar | 15-45 mg/100 ml |
| Ventricular | 5-15 mg/100 ml |
| Glucose | 50-75 mg/100 ml |
| Electrolytes: | |
| Sodium | ~141.0 mEq/liter |
| Potassium | ~3.3 mEq/liter |
| Chloride | 120-130 mEq/liter |
| pH | 7.32-7.35 |
| Specific gravity | 1.007 |
| Cell count: | |
| RBCs | None |
| WBCs | 0-5 $mm^3$ |
| Gram stain | Negative |
| Culture and sensitivity | No growth of organisms |

tral nervous system; it acts as a medium for the exchange of some nutrients and end-products of neural metabolism; it is a vital link in the regulation of the chemical environment of the central nervous system; it may serve as a channel for the transport of substances within the brain parenchyma; and it plays a vital compensatory role in maintaining intracranial pressure within normal limits (see Chap. 8).

### *Cerebral Circulatory System*

A constant, copious blood supply to the brain is required for normal cerebral function because the brain has little metabolic and energy reserves. Interruption of blood supply to the brain for only a few minutes may result in irreparable damage to neural tissue.

**Arterial Vasculature.** The major arterial blood supply to the brain is derived from two sources: the *vertebral* arteries and the *internal carotid* arteries. There is a branching anastomosing network of collateral vessels with considerable overlapping of distribution to ensure adequate blood supply to neural tissue. At the base of the cranial cavity the *circle of Willis* connects the vertebral and internal carotid circulations. As depicted in Figure 6-9, there is considerable variation in the actual structure of the circle of Willis throughout the population.

***Vertebral Circulation.*** The vertebral arteries ascend from the subclavian arteries, through the transverse foramina of the cervical vertebrae to enter the cranial cavity via the foramen magnum. These arteries give off branches to the spinal cord, medulla, and cerebellum, before joining to form the *basilar* artery (see Fig. 6-9).

The basilar artery, in turn, sends branches to several regions of the brain (brainstem, cerebellum, diencephalon, internal ear) before bifurcating and terminating as the *posterior cerebral* arteries.

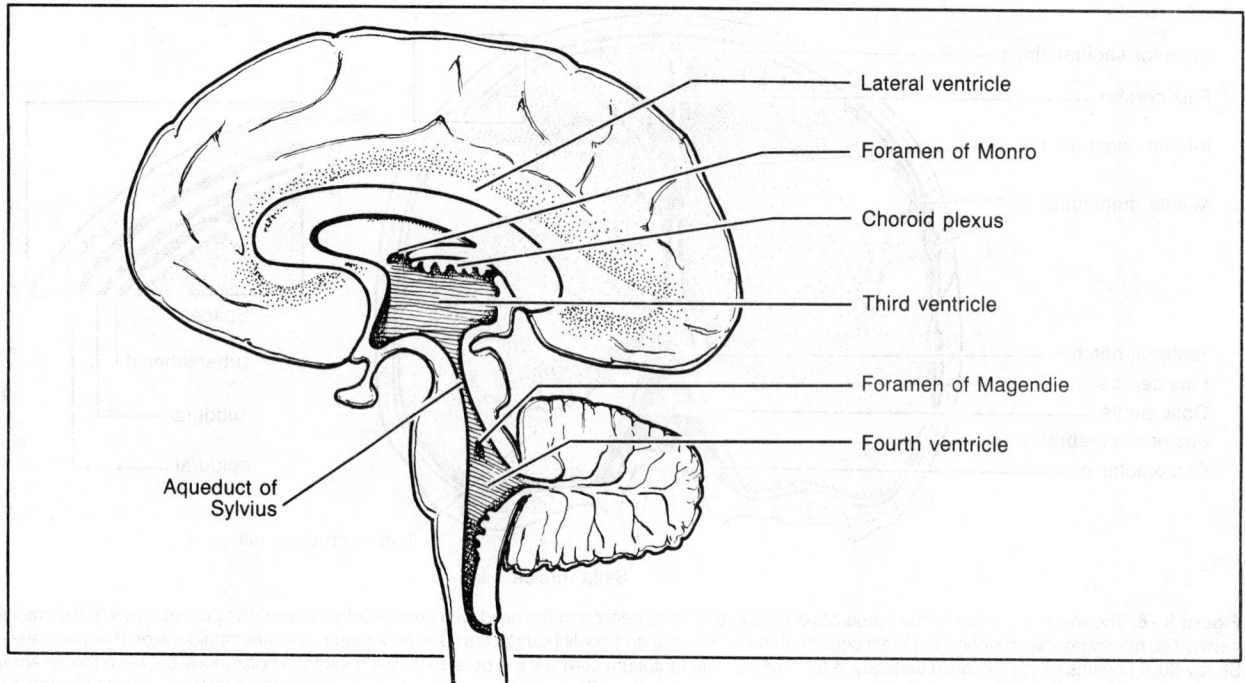

The posterior cerebral arteries supply inferior

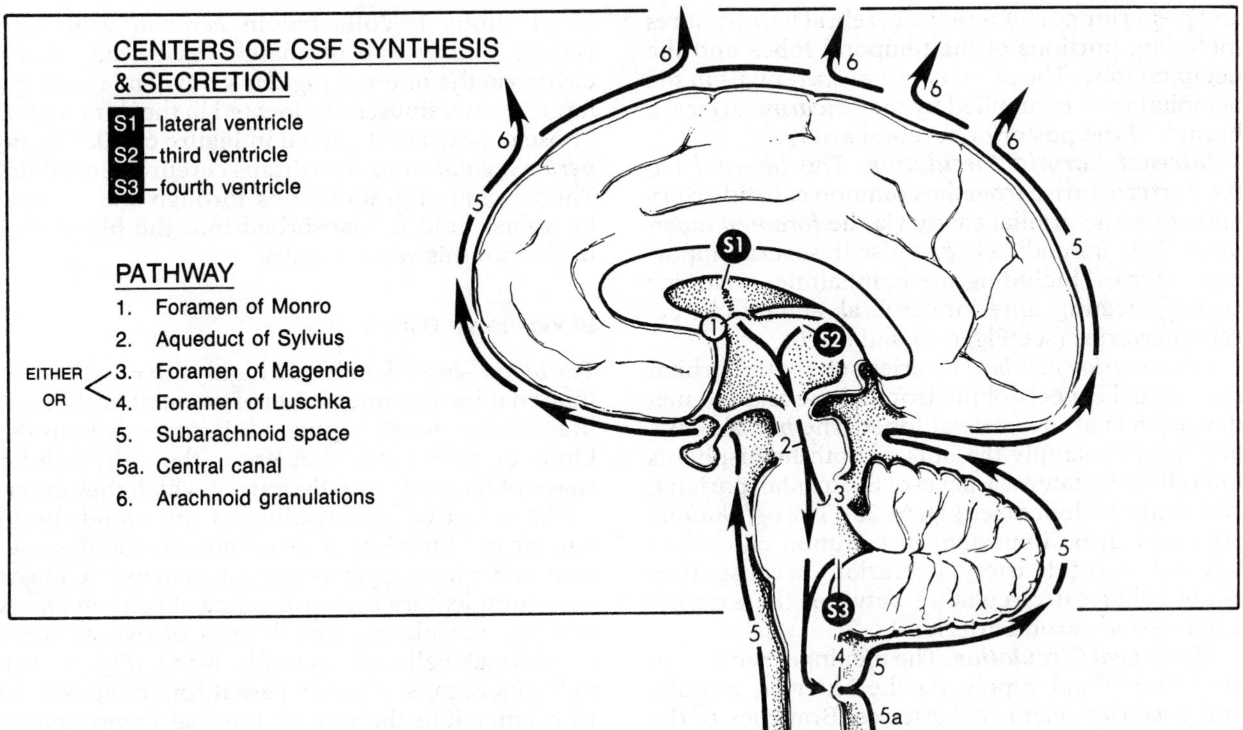


**Figure 6-8.** Formation, circulation, and reabsorption of cerebrospinal fluid. Cerebrospinal fluid is synthesized within the choroid plexus (see Fig. 6-7) and circulates via the interconnected ventricular system throughout the subarachnoid spaces occurring within and surrounding the brain and spinal cord. Eventually, cerebrospinal fluid is reabsorbed via the arachnoid granulations in the superior saggital sinus.

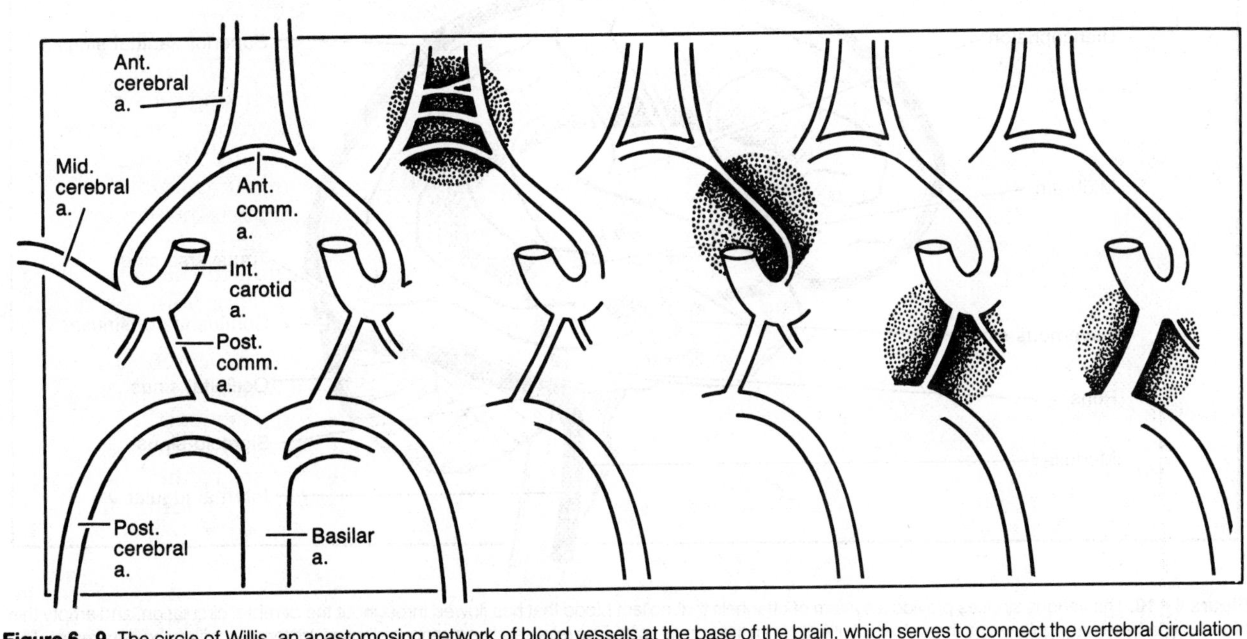


**Figure 6-9.** The circle of Willis, an anastomosing network of blood vessels at the base of the brain, which serves to connect the vertebral circulation with the internal carotid circulation. Considerable variation in the structure of the circle of Willis occurs throughout the population. Several types of variations are indicated here.

and posterior portions of the cerebral hemispheres including portions of the temporal lobes and the occipital lobe. The *primary visual cortex* within the occipital lobe is supplied by the *calcarine* artery, a branch of the posterior cerebral artery.

***Internal Carotid Circulation.*** The *internal carotid* arteries arise from the common carotid artery and enter the cranial cavity via the *foramen lacernum.* They immediately give rise to several important arteries, including the ophthalmic, posterior communicating, anterior cerebral, and middle cerebral arteries (see Fig. 6–9 and 6–20).

The *anterior cerebral* arteries supply the orbital and medial aspects of the frontal lobe and the medial aspects of the parietal lobes. The *middle cerebral* arteries supply the bulk of both hemispheres including the lateral aspects of the frontal, parietal, and temporal lobes (see Fig. 6–20). The *ophthalmic* arteries can be important in common carotid or internal carotid artery occlusion because they allow collateral circulation between the *external* and *internal* carotid arteries.

***Meningeal Circulation.*** The meninges receive an abundant blood supply via the anterior, middle, and posterior *meningeal* arteries. Branches of the *middle meningeal* artery, which arises from the external carotid artery, fan out over the lateral surfaces of dura covering the brain and are snugly nestled between the periosteal dura and inner table of compact bone (see Fig. 6–6).

**Venous Sinuses.** After flowing through the brain, blood is collected in *cerebral veins* and *venous sinuses* and ultimately leaves the cranial cavity via the *internal jugular* veins. The relatively large venous sinuses are located in the dura mater. Those of note are depicted in Figure 6–10. The *superior sagittal sinus* also drains cerebrospinal fluid. The arachnoid granulations through which cerebrospinal fluid is reabsorbed into the blood protrude into this venous sinus.

### Blood–Brain Barrier

The *blood–brain barrier* is a highly selective barrier that enables the internal environment within the brain to be closely regulated. It controls both the kinds of substances that enter the extracellular space of the brain and the rate at which they enter.

The selective permeability of the blood–brain barrier is a function of its unique anatomic structure and physiologic transport systems. A major structural feature is the presence of *tight junctions* wherein the plasma membranes of two adjacent ependymal cells are actually fused (Fig. 6–11). Substances must actually pass through the cells to gain entry into the brain's internal environment. *Gap junctions,* tiny channels between adjacent cells, provide for further selectivity. Tight junctions also occur between adjacent endothelial cells, which line capillaries within the cerebral vasculature.

The blood–brain barrier is highly permeable to

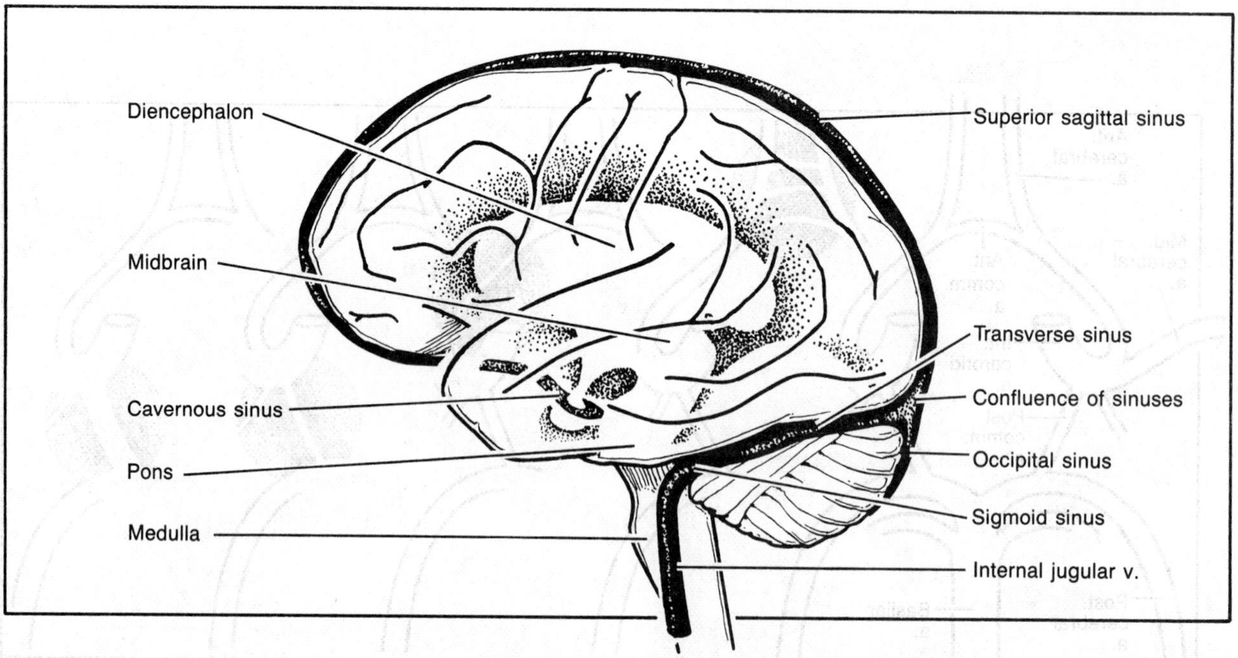


**Figure 6–10.** The venous sinuses provide a system of channels that collect blood that has flowed throughout the cerebral circulation, and empty this blood into the internal jugular veins through which it exits from the cranial vault. The relatively large venous sinuses are located within the dura mater. The superior sagittal sinus also drains cerebrospinal fluid. The arachnoid granulations responsible for the reabsorption of cerebrospinal fluid are located within the superior sagittal sinus. (See Fig. 6–8.)

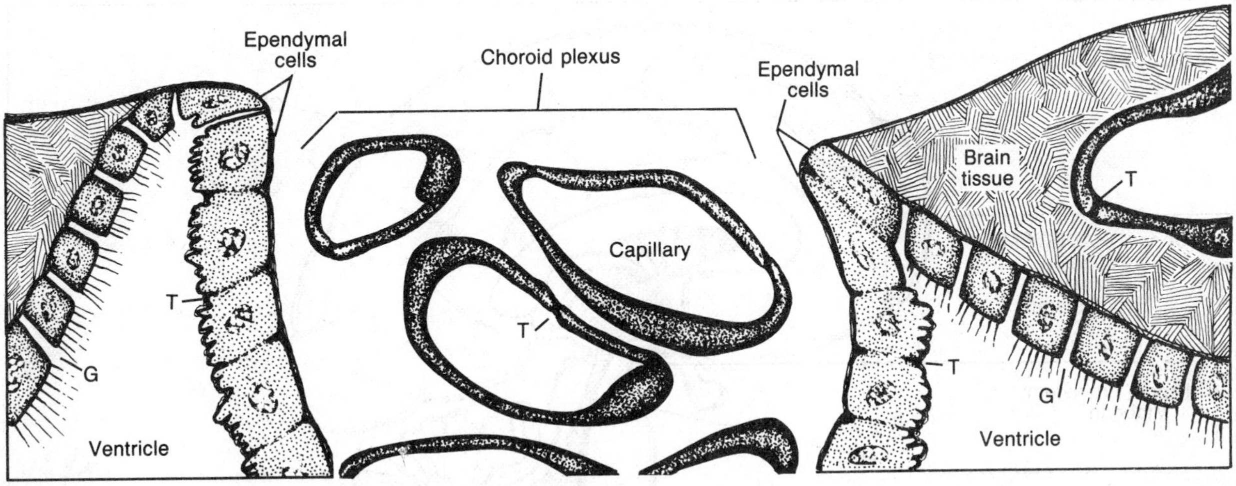


**Figure 6–11.** The blood–brain barrier is a highly selective cellular membrane, which enables the internal environment within the brain to be closely regulated. Structurally, it is characterized by the presence of specialized junctions between epithelial cells, including tight junctions (T) and gap junctions (G). Tight junctions occur when the plasma membranes of two adjacent cells are fused, as for example, between ependymal cells lining the ventricles, or between adjacent endothelial cells lining cerebral capillaries. The presence of tight junctions necessitates that substances must pass *through* these cells to gain entry into the brain's internal environment. Gap junctions, specialized channels between adjacent cells, provide a second mechanism contributing to further selectivity of substances allowed to enter the brain's internal environment via the blood–brain barrier.

water, carbon dioxide, oxygen, most lipid-soluble substances (e.g., alcohol and anesthetics), and small molecular substances. Its selectivity prevents movement of many drugs, toxic substances, plasma proteins, and large molecules. The barrier is slightly permeable to movement of electrolytes (sodium, potassium, and chloride), but active transport mechanisms ensure necessary rapidity of movement to provide a stable internal environment.

Clinically, knowledge regarding the blood–brain barrier is essential in terms of fluid and drug administration. The underlying basis for the use of osmotic diuretics (e.g., Mannitol) is that the blood–brain barrier is largely impermeable to movement of these large molecular substances. Because water readily passes through the barrier, these hypertonic solutions readily draw water from the brain's internal environment into the systemic blood circulation.

## Brain Structures and Function

The brain has 3 major divisions: the forebrain, brainstem, and cerebellum (Table 6–4). The forebrain is comprised of the cerebrum and upper brainstem, which includes the diencephalon. The diencephalon is, in turn, comprised of the thalamus and hypothalamus. The remaining brainstem consists of the midbrain, pons, and medulla (Fig. 6–12). A review of the functional anatomy of specific brain structures is presented in Table 6–5. Primary functional areas of the cerebral cortex are depicted in Figure 6–13.

TABLE 6–4
**Divisions of the Brain**

- I. Forebrain
  - A. Cerebrum
    - 1. Cerebral hemispheres
  - B. Diencephalon (upper brainstem)
    - 1. Thalamus
    - 2. Hypothalamus
- II. Brainstem
  - A. Midbrain
  - B. Pons
  - C. Medulla
- III. Cerebellum

### *Reticular Formation*

Operating throughout the entire brainstem is a core of tissue called the *reticular formation*. It consists of intricate networks of highly branched neurons, which extend from the medulla upward through the diencephalon into subcortical areas (Fig. 6–14). It is a highly strategic region in that neurons of the reticular formation receive and integrate information from many afferent pathways as well as from many other regions of the brain. As a result of such integration the reticular formation influences and, in turn, is influenced by many different systems, somatic and autonomic, sensory and motor.

Although functions of the reticular formation cannot be clearly identified as separate and apart from the overall integrated activities of the various regions of the brain, the influence of the reticular formation on certain bodily activities and responses has been recognized, and some of these are listed in Table 6–5.

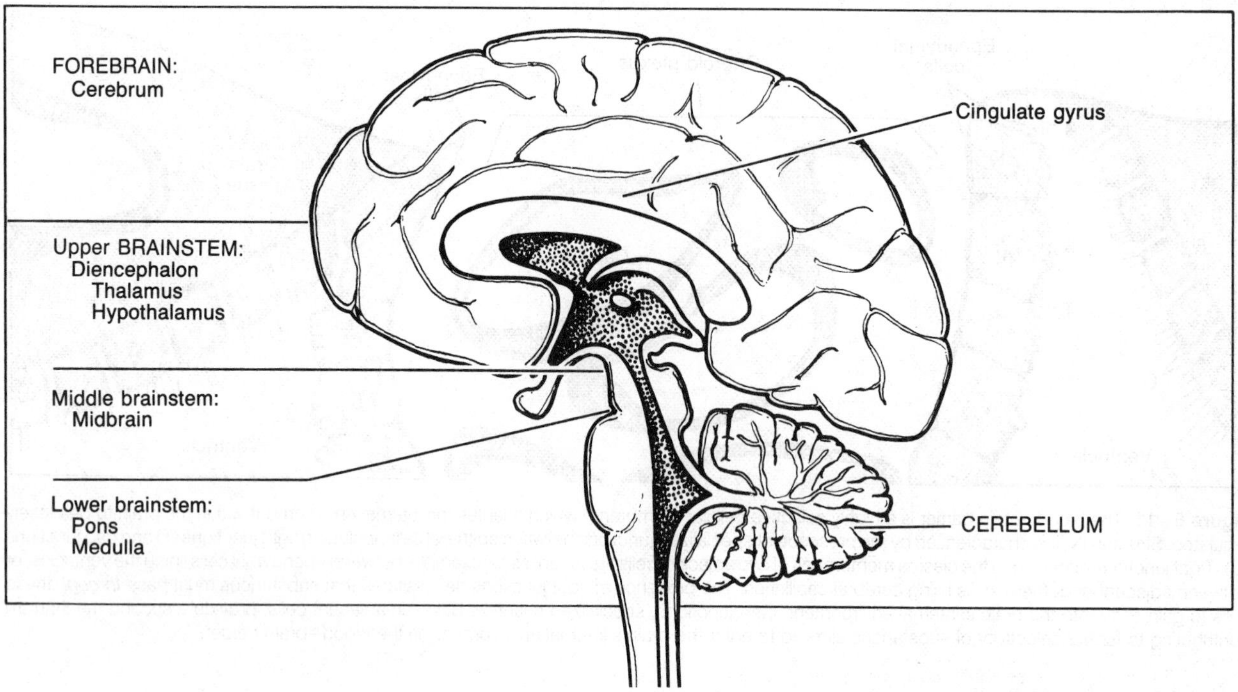


**Figure 6–12.** The gross structure of the brain is comprised of three major divisions: the forebrain, brainstem, and cerebellum. The forebrain consists of the cerebrum (center of intellectual activity and regulation of sensory and motor activity); the upper brainstem, which includes the diencephalon (the diencephalon, in turn, is comprised of the thalamus [central sensory relay center] and hypothalamus [center of autonomic regulation]). The remaining brainstem consists of the midbrain and lower brainstem (central nerve tracts between cerebral hemispheres and spinal cord); the lower brainstem, in turn, is comprised of the pons and medulla (center of control of vital functions [e.g., respiratory physiology, vasomotor control]).

The *reticular activating system* (RAS), an ascending neuronal pathway, conducts impulses upward through the reticular formation to the thalamus and subcortical areas. It *activates* or arouses higher cortical functions via its thalamocortical connections and, therefore, plays a role in controlling consciousness and the sleep–wakefulness cycle. A discussion regarding the physiology of consciousness is presented in Chapter 7.

Many areas of the brain operate together to produce appropriate, coordinated responses. For example, activity in Wernicke's area (temporal lobe), concerned with formulating words or phrases (language), must be coordinated with the activity in Broca's area (frontal lobe), which is responsible for articulating or speaking.

Various areas of the cerebral cortex, identified as having specific primary motor and sensory function, do not in and of themselves necessarily process all components of a given function or response. For example, different aspects of the sensation of vision (e.g., color, contour, movement) are carried in paralled pathways and processed simultaneously and more or less independently in different parts of the cerebral cortex. In this case the primary visual cortex (occipital lobe) functions to reintegrate all this incoming information from various regions of the brain to produce the conscious sensation of sight.

### *Cranial Nerves*

The 12 pairs of cranial nerves are the *peripheral* nerves of the brain and brainstem. With the exception of cranial nerves I and II, which strictly speaking are not peripheral nerves but rather *fiber tracts* within the brain, all the other cranial nerves (III through XII) have their origin in the brainstem.

The cranial nerves occur in a *rostral* to *caudal* (head to toe) sequence, which is reflected in their numbering. The *olfactory* nerve is anatomically uppermost or superior to all other cranial nerves and is designated as cranial nerve I. Slightly caudal, or inferior, to this nerve lies the *optic* nerve *(optic chiasm)*, designated as cranial nerve II. These two cranial nerves do not originate in the brainstem as do all the other cranial nerves. Cranial nerve III *(oculomotor)* originates at the midbrain, followed by the remaining cranial nerves, which arise sequentially from the pons and medulla and are numbered accordingly.

The relationship of the cranial nerves to surrounding structures is of critical importance. The close approximation of the optic chiasm to the pituitary gland in the sella turcica and the relationship of cranial nerve III at the midbrain to the tentorium cerebelli (tentorial notch) are two examples wherein intracranial pathology and dysfunction may be detected by ongoing assessment of cranial

TABLE 6–5
**Structures of the Brain: Functional Anatomy**

| Structure | Description | Function |
|---|---|---|
| • Cerebrum (see Fig. 6–12) | • Largest and most prominent component of the brain.<br>• Divided by the *longitudinal fissure* into right and left hemispheres. The hemispheres are joined by and communicate with one another via a band of *commissural* nerve fibers called the *corpus callosum.* Each hemisphere, for the most part, innervates the contralateral (opposite) side of the body. | • Regulates sensory and motor activities, and other activities having to do with memory, intelligence, reasoning, language, and personality.<br>○ Left hemisphere largely influences symbolic language.<br>○ Right hemisphere integrates spatial (dimensional and perceptual) information. |
| • Cerebral cortex | • Constitutes the outer gray surface of the brain and is marked by many convolutions. The convolutions consist of *gyri* (ridges) and *sulci* (indentations), which provide for a tremendous surface area in an otherwise tight, rigid, and restrictive cranial vault. The cerebral cortex is divided into lobes: | • The most complex integrating area of the nervous system.<br>○ Operates to produce coordinated function. |
| | ○ *Frontal* lobe (see Fig. 6–13). | ○ Operates in all cognitive and perceptive functions.<br>○ Plays a role in reasoning, abstract thinking, creativity, memory, personality, and behavior. |
| | ○ *Pre-central gyrus.* | ○ Contains primary motor area concerned with voluntary muscle movement. |
| | ○ *Broca's speech area* lies adjacent to motor areas controlling muscles of face, tongue, jaw, and throat; located within left cerebral hemisphere in most individuals.<br>Dysfunction in this area can cause an *expressive dysphasia (aphasia)* (i.e., difficulty or inability in formulating and articulating words). Patients with expressive dysphasia have great difficulty expressing their needs. | ○ Plays a significant role in language; involved in the articulation of speech. |
| | ○ *Temporal* lobe (see Fig. 6–13).<br>○ *Wernicke's* area. Connected to Broca's area by association nerve fibers. In Broca's area the precise motor responses are programmed so that the phrase that arises in Wernicke's area can be spoken or articulated.<br>Dysfunction in this area can result in *receptive* dysphasia (aphasia) (i.e., the inability to comprehend or understand language). | ○ Sensory receptive area for auditory stimuli.<br>○ Involved in formulation of language, i.e., what phrase is to be said, which, in turn, is then articulated via Broca's speech center.<br>○ Plays a major role in comprehension of spoken word and in reading and writing.<br>○ Memory storage and retrieval. |
| | ○ *Parietal lobe.*<br>○ *Post-central gyrus.* All sensory information is funneled to the post-central gyrus from the thalamus. Sensory information is received and interpreted from a variety of sensory receptors throughout the body (see Table 6–8). | ○ Contains the primary sensory area enabling conscious awareness and interpretation of sensory stimuli. |
| | ○ *Occipital* lobe: The primary visual area is comprised of a number of subdivisions, each responding to a functionally distinct aspect of the visual stimulus (e.g., color of stimulus, direction of movement, or contours of objects, among others). | ○ Contains primary visual area for integrating different aspects of visual information. This enables the conscious sensation of sight to be produced. |
| • Subcortical areas | ○ *Limbic* system: This is not a single area of the brain but reflects an interconnected group of structures located within portions of the frontal and temporal lobes, thalamus, and hypothalamus. Some of these structures include the *cingulate gyrus, amygdala,* and *hippocampus.* | ○ Associated with short-term memory, learning, and emotional behavior (fear, rage, sexual behavior).<br>○ Connects areas of higher brain functioning with more primitive areas, and areas of autonomic and endocrine activities. |
| | ○ *Basal ganglia:* Areas of gray matter embedded within the subcortical white matter having multiple connections throughout CNS including cerebral cortex, diencephalon, brainstem, reticular formation, and cerebellum. | ○ Function to coordinate motor activity to ensure fine, discrete, and coordinated movements. |

*(continued)*

TABLE 6–5
**Structures of the Brain: Functional Anatomy *(Continued)***

| Structure | Description | Function |
|---|---|---|
| • Diencephalon (upper brainstem) (see Fig. 6–12) | • Uppermost portion of brainstem, which actually forms the inner core of the cerebrum. It consists of thalamus and hypothalamus. | |
| | ○ *Thalamus.* *Third ventricle* located in this area. | ○ Functions as a major relay station and integrating center for all incoming sensory information from spinal cord and brainstem on its way to cerebral cortex. |
| | ○ An anatomic and functional relationship exists between the thalamus, cerebral cortex, basal ganglia, and cerebellum. | ○ Plays a key role in refining motor responses. |
| | ○ *Hypothalamus:* Lies below the thalamus; contains *hypothalamic-pituitary stalk,* which directly links the nervous system to the endocrine system. | ○ Major control area for regulating activities of the internal environment.<br>○ Monitors and controls autonomic activities.<br>○ Involved in regulation of body water and electrolytes, body temperature, thirst, hunger, sexual and emotional behavior. |
| • Brainstem | • Literally constitutes the stalk of the brain (see Fig. 6–12). | • Enables sensory input and motor output to be relayed between spinal cord and higher brain centers.<br>○ Gives rise to all cranial nerves, excluding olfactory and optic nerves. |
| | ○ *Midbrain:* Located between diencephalon and pons. *Aqueduct of Sylvius* passes through this area, connecting the third and fourth ventricles. | ○ Contains afferent and efferent pathways concerned with motor coordination, and visual and auditory reflexes. |
| | ○ *Edinger-Westphal nucleus:* Parasympathetic nerve fibers leave midbrain via oculomotor nerve (cranial nerve III) and travel to each orbit to stimulate muscles of the iris to contract. This results in pupillary constriction. Interruption in parasympathetic innervation to the iris results in pupillary dilation. | ○ Contains autonomic parasympathetic reflex centers for pupillary constriction.<br>○ Gives rise to cranial nerve III. |
| | ○ Pons: The "bridge" that connects the cerebellum with the brainstem. | ○ Conductive pathway for all ascending and descending nerve tracts. |
| | ○ *Pneumotaxic* and *apneustic* area. | ○ Play a fundamental role in respiration. |
| | ○ Contains nuclei of cranial nerves: trigeminal, abducens, facial, and acoustic. | ○ Gives rise to cranial nerves V, VI, VII, and VIII. |
| | ○ *Medulla:* Site of transition from the brainstem to spinal cord. | ○ Conductive pathway for all ascending and descending nerve tracts. |
| | ○ Site of decussation of corticospinal motor pathways, resulting in innervation of contralateral sides of the body by each cerebral hemisphere. | ○ Contains major reflex centers controlling vital activities related to cardiac, vasomotor, respiratory, sneezing, coughing, swallowing, salivating, and vomiting functions. |
| | ○ Contains nuclei of cranial nerves: glossopharyngeal, vagus, accessory, and hypoglossal. | ○ Gives rise and cranial nerves IX, X, XI, and XII. |
| • Reticular formation | • An extensive network of fine, highly branched neurons extending throughout the core of the brainstem and ascending through the diencephalon into subcortical areas. A strategic region enabling impulses from various regions of the brain (cerebral cortex, basal ganglia, ascending and descending nerve tracts, cerebellum, nuclei of cranial nerves, and spinal cord) to converge and interact (see Fig. 6–14). | • Acts to facilitate, modify, or inhibit impulse transmissions. |
| | ○ *Sensory:* Linked functionally to thalamus. | ○ Receives and integrates information from afferent pathways as they ascend through the brainstem; relays some of this information to thalamus. |
| | ○ Incredibly widespread networks of neuronal connections provide alternate pathways and mechanisms. | ○ Permit qualities such as modality and localization of sensation to be discerned more clearly.<br>○ Enhances ability to associate and discriminate sensory information.<br>○ Maintains degree of alertness or excitability required for sensory perception.<br>○ Actively involved in the maintenance of equilibrium, proprioception, and audition functions. |

TABLE 6-5
**Structures of the Brain: Functional Anatomy *(Continued)***

| Structure | Description | Function |
|---|---|---|
| | ○ *Motor:* A balance between excitatory and inhibitory influences contributes to normal tone of skeletal muscles. | ○ Exerts both an excitatory and inhibitory effect on motor function.<br>○ Provides continuous impulses to muscles in order to support the body against gravity; maintains posture. |
| | ○ *Reticular activating systems:* An ascending neuronal pathway within the reticular formation with extensive thalamocortical connections. It is considered to be instrumental in activating or arousing higher cortical function. | ○ Plays a role in controlling consciousness and the sleep-wakefulness cycle.<br>○ Influences attentiveness to specific tasks. |
| • Cerebellum (see Fig. 6-12) | • This structure is located within the posterior fossa where it is separated from the cerebral hemispheres by a dural fold called the *tentorium cerebelli.*<br>• Chiefly involved with skeletal muscle function. | • Functions to maintain balance.<br>• Coordinates skeletal muscle activity to provide for smooth, directed movements.<br>• Maintains upright posture.<br>• Plays a major role in coordinating movements of speech. |

nerve function. In the patient who has sustained an insult to intracranial structures, the response to therapeutic modalities can be evaluated through the assessment of cranial nerve function. Assessment of cranial nerves is discussed in Chapter 7 (see Table 7-3). Details regarding the cranial nerves and their function are included in Table 6-6.

## Brain Physiology

### *Intracranial Pressure (ICP)*

The volume of blood, cerebrospinal fluid, and brain tissue enclosed within the intracranial cavity determines intracranial pressure. The approximate per-

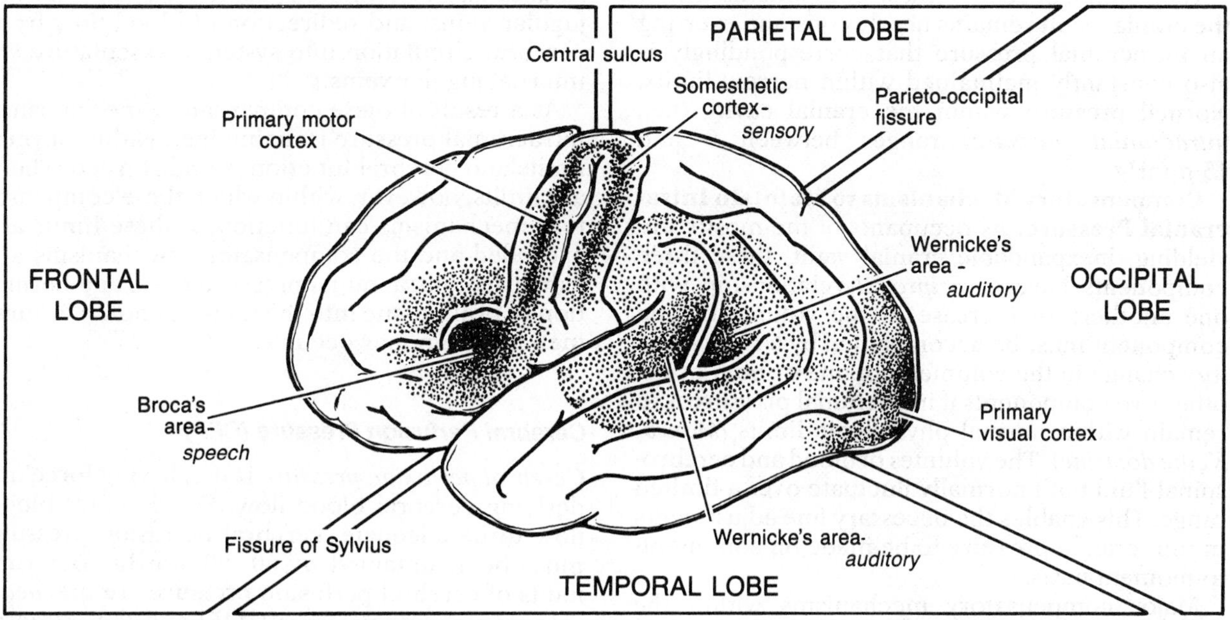


**Figure 6-13.** Primary functional areas of cerebral cortex. Frontal lobe contains Broca's speech center (articulation of language) and primary motor cortex; parietal lobe contains the primary sensory area (i.e., somesthetic cortex; see Fig. 6-20); the temporal lobe contains the sensory receptive area for auditory stimuli and Wernicke's area, a more diffuse area concerned with the formulation of language; and the occipital lobe, which contains the primary visual cortex.

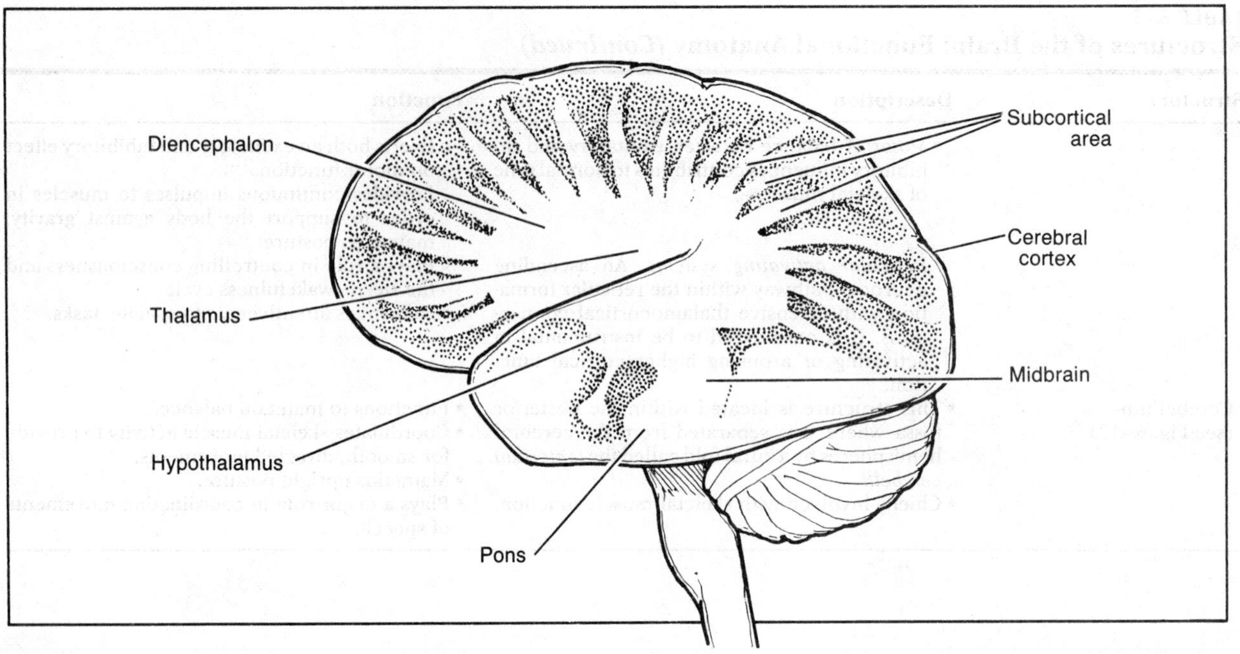


**Figure 6-14.** The reticular formation consists of intricate networks of highly branched neurons, which extend from the medulla upward through the diencephalon into the subcortical areas. While the reticular formation is not defined structurally, it is a highly strategic region in that neurons comprising the reticular formation receive and integrate information from many different pathways within the brain and spinal cord. These neurons, in turn, influence other networks of neurons including sensory, motor, somatic, and autonomic.

centage of total intracranial volume contributed by each of these substances is as follows:

| | |
|---|---|
| Blood | 2–10% |
| Cerebrospinal fluid | 9–11% |
| Brain tissue | ~ 88% |

The volume of each of these components within the cranial vault remains nearly constant, exerting an intracranial pressure that correspondingly is also constantly maintained within narrow limits. Normal pressure within the cranial cavity (i.e., *intracranial pressure*) ranges between 0 and 15 mmHg.

**Compensatory Mechanisms to Maintain Intracranial Pressure.** As occupants of the mostly unyielding, inexpandable cranial vault, these three components have a *reciprocal* relationship with one another; an increase in the volume of one component must be accompanied by a *compensatory* change in the volume(s) of one or both of the other two components if intracranial pressure is to remain within normal physiologic limits *(Monro-Kellie doctrine)*. The volumes of blood and cerebrospinal fluid both normally fluctuate over a limited range. This enables the necessary fine adjustments in intracranial pressure to be made on a moment-to-moment basis.

Major compensatory mechanisms within the brain that function to maintain intracranial pressure within its normal physiologic range include the following: the limited expansiveness of the dura mater, which can accommodate cerebrospinal fluid as it leaves the subarachnoid space; an increase in the flow of cerebrospinal fluid into the subarachnoid space and central canal of the spinal cord; a decrease in formation and/or increase in reabsorption of cerebrospinal fluid into the venous sinuses and systemic circulation via the internal jugular veins; and redirection of blood flow from cerebral circulation into systemic vasculature via internal jugular veins.

As a result of these compensatory mechanisms, intracranial pressure is maintained within normal limits and cerebral function is undisturbed. There are limits, however, within which these compensatory mechanisms can function. If these limits are exceeded and the compensatory mechanisms are exhausted, intracranial pressure rises, and herniation of brain tissue into the tentorial notch or foramen magnum may occur.

### *Cerebral Perfusion Pressure (CPP)*

*Cerebral perfusion pressure* is the driving force underlying cerebral blood flow. For cerebral blood flow to be adequate, cerebral perfusion pressure must be maintained at 60–90 mmHg. Determinants of cerebral perfusion pressure are the *mean arterial systemic pressure (MAP)* and the *intracranial pressure (ICP)* expressed as follows:

$$CPP = MAP - ICP$$

TABLE 6–6
**Cranial Nerves**

| Cranial Nerve | Type | Central Connection | Peripheral Connection | Function |
|---|---|---|---|---|
| I. Olfactory | Sensory (afferent) | Olfactory tract and bulb | Olfactory epithelium in upper nasal cavity | Smell Perception/interpretation in medial temporal lobes |
| II. Optic | Sensory | Optic chiasm and tract | Ganglion cells of retina | Sight Perception/interpretation in occipital lobe |
| III. Oculomotor | Motor (efferent) | Midbrain | Extrinsic eye muscles: superior, inferior, and medial recti, and inferior oblique, levator palpebrae muscle | Movement of eyes; elevation of upper eyelid |
| | Autonomic (parasympathetic) | Midbrain (Edinger-Westphal nucleus) | Intrinsic eye muscles; ciliary and pupillary muscles | Pupillary constriction; accommodation |
| IV. Trochlear | Motor | Midbrain | Extrinsic eye muscle: superior oblique | Movement of eyes |
| V. Trigeminal | Sensory | Pons | Skin and mucous membranes of face and mouth | General sensation to face via three branches: ophthalmic, maxillary, and mandibular branches; includes sensation to cornea and mucosa of nose and mouth |
| | Motor (mandibular division) | Pons | Muscles of mastication | Mastication; jaw clenching and lateral jaw movement |
| VI. Abducens | Motor | Pons | Extrinsic eye muscle: lateral rectus | Movement of eyes |
| VII. Facial | Sensory | Medulla | Tastebuds of anterior two thirds of tongue | Taste—sweet and salty "Taste-center" in temporal lobe |
| | Motor | Caudal pons | Muscles of facial expression | Facial expression |
| VII. | Autonomic (parasympathetic) | Medulla | Salivary glands (sublingual, submaxillary) and lacrimal glands | Secretion of saliva and tears |
| VIII. Acoustic | | | | |
| Cochlear | Sensory | Medulla | Organ of Corti in inner ear | Hearing Perception/interpretation in temporal lobe |
| Vestibular | Sensory | Medulla | Receptors in semicircular canals, utricle, and saccule | Equilibrium |
| IX. Glossopharyngeal | Sensory | Medulla | Taste buds in posterior one third of tongue; soft palate | Taste—sour and bitter "Taste center" in temporal lobe |
| | Sensory | Medulla | Cutaneous receptors; mucous membrane pharyngeal area; carotid sinus | General sensations from external ear and surrounding area; pain and temperature. Involved in reflex control of blood pressure and respirations |
| | Motor | Medulla | Muscles of pharynx | Swallowing and phonation, gag reflex |
| | Autonomic (parasympathetic) | Medulla | Salivary gland (parotid) | Salivary secretion |

(continued)

TABLE 6–6
**Cranial Nerves *(Continued)***

| Cranial Nerve | Type | Central Connection | Peripheral Connection | Function |
|---|---|---|---|---|
| X. Vagus | Sensory | Medulla | Cutaneous receptors | General sensations from skin in area surrounding ear; pain and temperature |
| | Sensory | Medulla | Receptors from thorax and abdomen | Sensory from visceral structures |
| | Motor | Medulla | Muscles of pharynx and larynx | Swallowing and control of larynx; protective reflexes: cough and gag |
| | Autonomic (parasympathetic) | Medulla | Smooth muscle and glands of thorax and abdomen | Regulation of smooth and cardiac muscle, and glands; carotid reflex |
| XI. Accessory | Motor | Medulla | Muscles of pharynx and larynx (distributed with vagus) | Swallowing and control of larynx |
| | Motor | Upper cervical cord segments (C-1—C-5) | Sternocleidomastoid and trapezius muscles | Movement of head and shoulders |
| XII. Hypoglossal | Motor | Medulla | Extrinsic and intrinsic muscles of tongue | Movement of tongue necessary for swallowing and phonation |

Any factor that *decreases* mean arterial pressure or *increases* intracranial pressure will cause a corresponding decrease in cerebral perfusion pressure. If cerebral perfusion pressure is reduced to the level of intracranial pressure, cerebral blood flow ceases.

### *Metabolic Needs of Neural Tissue*

To maintain a state of excitability so vital to impulse initiation and propagation, neural tissue is highly active metabolically. Because energy stores within neurons are limited, there is a high and constant demand for oxygen and glucose. Any state that increases the demand of neural tissue for oxygen and glucose or decreases the blood supply of these vital substrates may alter cellular metabolism and place neural tissue at risk of developing ischemia, injury, or necrosis. Fever, for example, increases metabolic demands of neural tissue by as much as 10% for every *1 F.* rise in temperature. An increase in metabolic rate not only increases the demand for oxygen and glucose, but is associated concomitantly with increased levels of end-products of metabolism, including carbon dioxide and hydrogen ion concentrations.

### *Autoregulation*

Autoregulation refers to the inherent ability of tissues to self-regulate their blood flows. Within the cerebral circulation, autoregulation functions to maintain cerebral perfusion pressure and, thus, cerebral blood flow, regardless of systemic arterial pressure. This ensures that the metabolic needs of neural tissue will be met.

## Major Factors Influencing Cerebral Blood Flow

### *Metabolic Factors*

*Carbon Dioxide, Oxygen, and Hydrogen Ion Concentrations.* Three metabolic factors have a potent effect on cerebral blood flow: carbon dioxide, oxygen, and hydrogen ions. Cerebral *vasodilation* occurs in response to an increase in the carbon dioxide concentration in arterial blood and results in a substantial increase in cerebral blood flow. Hypoxia also leads to cerebral arteriolar *dilation* and an increase in cerebral blood flow. An increase in hydrogen ion concentration associated, for example, with hypercapnia and/or lactic acidemia is another potent stimulus for cerebral vasodilation.

The resultant increase in cerebral blood flow in each of these circumstances is significant because it facilitates removal of carbon dioxide and acidic end-products of metabolism from cerebral tissues. In the normal brain, or the brain not under increased pressure, the fine moment-to-moment adjustments of cerebral vascular resistance made in response to these substances help to ensure that blood flow is adequate to meet the nutrient and oxygen needs of neural tissue.

*Glucose.* To meet cerebral metabolic needs adequately, serum glucose levels must be maintained at 70–110 mg/100 ml. A reduction in these levels below 70 mg/100 ml may predispose to an increase in cerebral blood flow.

*Serum Osmolality.* Serum osmolality (i.e., a measure of the number of osmotically active particles dissolved in a specific volume of fluid) must be maintained between 285–295 mOsm/kg. Alterations in serum osmolality are frequently associated with abnormal metabolic states (e.g., diabetic ketoacidosis; hyperosmolar hyperglycemic, nonketotic coma [HHNK]; hepatic encephalopathy) and can disrupt cerebral blood flow, leading to neurologic dysfunction.

*Body Temperature. Cellular metabolic activity* is perhaps the most important factor influencing cerebral blood flow at the tissue level. Any increase in metabolic activity (e.g., fever) ultimately leads to an increase in cerebral blood flow. This is necessary to increase availability of oxygen and glucose to these highly active cells and to enhance removal of carbon dioxide and other metabolic end-products.

#### Hemodynamic Factors

*Systemic Arterial Blood Pressure.* Autoregulatory mechanisms within the brain function to maintain cerebral blood flow within normal physiologic limits despite wide variations in arterial blood pressure. Systemic arterial blood pressure may fluctuate over a range of 60–150 mmHg without any significant change in cerebral blood flow.

A mean arterial pressure (MAP) of ~100 mmHg is desired to maintain adequate cerebral perfusion pressure. At *higher* mean pressure, cerebral *vasoconstriction* occurs to limit the amount of blood perfusing the brain; at *lower* mean pressures, cerebral *vasodilation* occurs to increase cerebral perfusion. In this way, cerebral perfusion pressure and cerebral blood flow are preserved.

*Cardiac Contractility.* A cardiac output sufficient to maintain mean systemic arterial blood pressure at approximately 100 mmHg is essential. Normal cardiac output ranges between 4–8 liters/min.

### Autonomic Nervous System Influence

Sympathetic stimulation causes slight vasoconstriction of cerebral blood vessels; the parasympathetic effect is to promote slight vasodilation of these vessels.

Specialized receptors also function to maintain a constant blood flow to the brain. *Baroreceptors,* especially sensitive to stretch and located in the carotid sinus and aortic arch, continuously monitor systemic arterial blood pressure. When systemic blood pressure falls, these receptors react quickly to reflexly stimulate respiratory and vasomotor centers in the medulla. *Chemoreceptors* located in the carotid body and great vessels react similarly when levels of carbon dioxide and hydrogen ion concentrations in arterial blood increase and/or arterial oxygen tension decreases.

A severe drop in systemic blood pressure evokes the *cerebral ischemic reflex* wherein neurons in the medulla respond via increased sympathetic innervation to the heart. The response is an increase in contractility and cardiac output.

A summary of the major factors influencing cerebral blood flow is presented in Table 6–7.

## FUNCTIONAL ANATOMY OF THE SPINAL CORD

The spinal cord provides the connections between impulses coming from *re*ceptors and those going to *ef*fectors. In this way the spinal cord functions as a communication system wherein cells sensitive to changes in the environment are linked with cells responsible for carrying out the appropriate responses to minimize those changes. The spinal cord distributes responses of cerebral activities appropriately throughout the peripheral nervous system, and thus facilitates the expression of cerebral function.

### Structural and Functional Support Systems

#### Vertebral Column and Ligaments

The vertebral column functions to support the skull and to provide protection for the spinal cord and spinal nerves. It bears the weight of the entire upper portion of the body including head, neck, trunk, and arms. *Intervertebral foramina* occurring between adjacent vertebrae accommodate the spinal nerves as they leave the spinal cord (Fig. 6–15).

There is an extensive attachment of ligaments and muscles to the vertebral processes of the uniquely structured vertebrae. This provides support to the vertebral column and, together with the *intervertebral disks,* allows for substantial stability and flexibility of the spinal column. Ligaments provide for safe, smooth movement of the head and neck and a considerable degree of movement of the entire vertebral column.

#### Meninges

The spinal cord is encased within the *spinal foramen (spinal canal)* of the vertebral column, which conforms to the variations in size and diameter of the spinal cord and protects and supports it. Protection is also afforded by the meningeal connective tissue sheaths, which are largely continuous with those surrounding the brain.

There occurs a distinct *epidural space* between

TABLE 6-7
## Summary of Major Factors Influencing Cerebral Blood Flow

| | |
|---|---|
| **Metabolic Factors** | |
| Serum carbon dioxide levels ($PaCO_2$) | • Carbon dioxide is a potent stimulus for cerebral vasodilation. Elevated levels of carbon dioxide ($PaCO_2$ >40–45 mmHg) cause vasodilation with an increase in cerebral blood flow.<br>• Ideally, in patients at risk of developing an increase in intracranial pressure, $PaCO_2$ is maintained at ≦30 mmHg. |
| Serum oxygen levels ($PaO_2$) | • Cerebral vasodilation with an increase in cerebral blood flow occurs with lower oxygen tension ($PaO_2$ <60 mmHg).<br>• To adequately meet cerebral metabolic needs $PaO_2$ should be maintained at >80 mmHg. |
| Hydrogen ion concentration | • An increase in hydrogen ion concentration (↓ pH) is a potent stimulus for cerebral vasodilation with an increase in cerebral blood flow. |
| Serum glucose levels | • To adequately meet cerebral metabolic needs serum glucose levels must be maintained at 70–110 mg/100 ml. While hypoglycemia per se does not increase cerebral blood flow, it does reduce the "fuel" available for cellular activities. |
| Serum osmolality | • Serum osmolality must be maintained between 285–295 mOsm/kg. Alterations in serum osmolality may reflect an alteration in cellular integrity with hyperosmolality (dehydration) or hypo-osmolality (edema).<br>• Hyperosmolar therapy may be prescribed to treat cerebral edema. |
| Body temperature | • For every degree rise in body temperature, metabolic demands of neural tissue increase by 10%.<br>• Body temperature should be maintained at 98.6°F (37°C) unless hypothermia therapy is prescribed. |
| Seizure activity | • Seizures increase the metabolic rate of nerve cells twofold and threefold, which in turn increases need for oxygen and glucose, and removal of carbon dioxide and other metabolic end-products. |
| **Hemodynamic Factors** | |
| Systemic arterial blood pressure | • To ensure a cerebral perfusion pressure of >60 mmHg, mean arterial pressure should be maintained at ~100 mmHg.<br>• Autoregulatory mechanisms maintain intracranial pressure over a wide range of mean arterial pressures (60–150 mmHg).<br>• At mean systemic pressures >150 mmHg or <60 mmHg, loss of local cerebral autoregulatory capability begins to occur and cerebral blood flow becomes passively dependent on systemic blood pressure.<br>• At high arterial blood pressures, cerebral vasoconstriction occurs; at lower pressures, cerebral vasodilation occurs. |
| Cardiac contractility | • Cardiac output must be maintained between 4–8 liters/min to ensure a mean arterial blood pressure ~100 mmHg. |
| Blood viscosity | • An increase in blood viscosity increases resistance to blood flow, which may predispose to an increase in blood pressure. |
| **Autonomic Nervous System Influence** | |
| Sympathetic innervation | • Sympathetic effect causes slight vasoconstriction of cerebral blood vessels. |
| Parasympathetic innervation | • Parasympathetic effect causes slight vasodilation of cerebral blood vessels. |
| Baroreceptors | • Sense organs, especially sensitive to stretch and located in carotid sinus and aortic arch, continuously monitor and respond to changes in systemic arterial blood pressure. |
| Chemoreceptors | • Sense organs in carotid body and great vessels continuously monitor and respond to changes in serum levels of oxygen, carbon dioxide, and pH. |
| **Reflexes** | |
| Cerebral ischemic reflex | • This reflex is evoked by a severe drop in systemic arterial blood pressure. A medullary response mediated via sympathetic pathways increases cardiac contractility and cardiac output. The end result is a rise in systemic blood pressure. |
| Cushing reflex | • This reflex is evoked in response to a decrease in cerebral perfusion pressure and cerebral ischemia. It functions to slow heart rate, which increases the stroke volume; it raises systolic blood pressure to levels adequate to perfuse the brain.<br>• A widening pulse pressure results from the increasing systolic blood pressure and decreasing diastolic pressure.<br>• Cushing's triad includes:<br>↑ systolic BP with widening pulse pressure<br>↓ heart rate<br>abnormal respiratory function. |

the spinal dura and bony surface of the vertebral column. This space is filled with fatty substance and blood vessels, which serve to protect and nourish the cord. The *subarachnoid space* is continuous with that surrounding the brain. It is filled with cerebrospinal fluid, which provides a protective cushion around the spinal cord. Cerebrospinal fluid also circulates throughout the *central canal* of the spinal cord. In the event of a rise in intracranial pressure, the subarachnoid space and central canal within the cord can accommodate an increased quantity of cerebrospinal fluid, which may help ini-

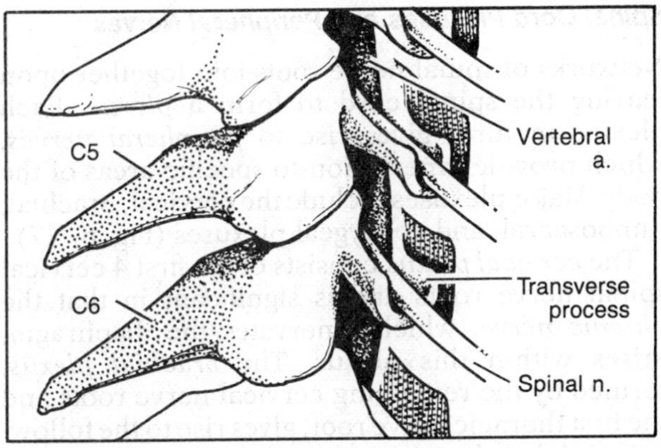


**Figure 6-15.** Intervertebral foramina occurring between adjacent cervical vertebrae. These vertebrae accommodate the spinal nerves as they leave the spinal cord via grooves within the vertebrae. The vertebral artery is depicted ascending via the transverse foramina in the transverse processes of the cervical vertebrae.

tially to *compensate* for the increase in intracranial pressure.

The pia mater is closely applied to the spinal cord. It continues caudally beyond the conus medullaris as a connective tissue filament, the *filum terminale,* which eventually attaches to the coccyx bone where it serves to anchor the cord. The *dentate ligaments,* extending from the pia to the dura, serve to anchor the cord laterally and keep it centered within its bony encasement.

### *Blood Supply to Spinal Cord and Vertebral Column*

There is not an extensive blood supply to the spinal cord and vertebral column. The intervertebral disks are especially limited in their blood supply. The two major arteries nourishing the spinal cord are the *anterior* and *posterior spinal* arteries, which arise from the vertebral arteries. The spinal arteries are reinforced by smaller *radicular* arteries, which arise from the thoracic and abdominal aorta and enter the spinal column via the intervertebral foramina. Interconnections between these vessels and those from the vertebral system exist, but, unlike the brain, collateral circulation to the spinal cord is not well developed. Venous drainage of the vertebral column and spinal cord follows the arterial distribution very closely.

## Spinal Cord Structure and Function

The spinal cord is continuous with the medulla and extends from the foramen magnum to the upper border of the second lumbar vertebra (in adults) where it terminates as the *conus medullaris.* Spinal nerve roots descend below the conus medullaris and are known collectively as the *cauda equina.*

Thirty-one pairs of spinal nerves exit from successive levels or segments of the spinal cord via the intervertebral foramina. These include 8 pairs of cervical nerves, 12 pairs of thoracic nerves, 5 lum-

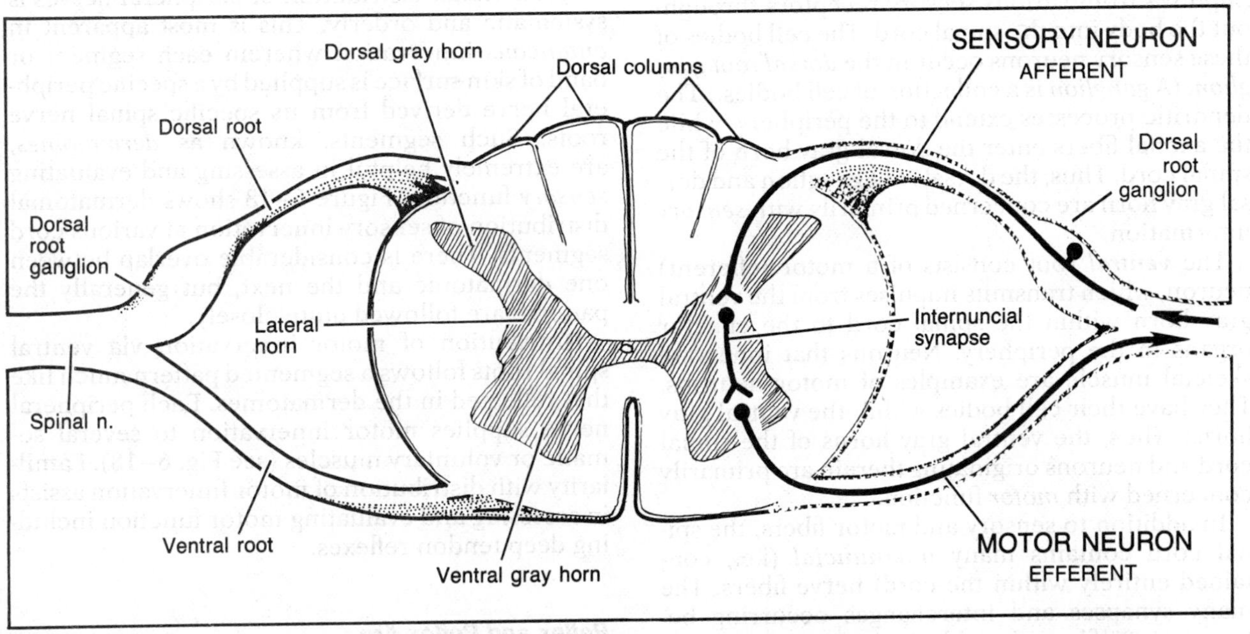


**Figure 6-16.** Spinal cord in cross-section. There is a characteristic centrally placed area of gray matter occurring in the shape of an H. The projections of gray matter are divided into the dorsal and ventral gray horns; lateral projections (i.e., lateral horn) can be observed in sections of the thoracolumbar cord. Surrounding the gray matter is the white matter of the cord comprised of columns of ascending and descending nerve fibers. A spinal nerve is depicted as being comprised of a dorsal root (sensory) and a ventral root (motor). Sensory information is carried into the dorsal spinal cord from peripheral areas of the body by the sensory, or afferent, neuron; it is characterized by a dorsal root ganglion, which contains cell bodies of all incoming sensory neurons.

bar nerves, 5 sacral nerves, and 1 pair of coccygeal nerves.

### Spinal Cord in Cross-Section

A significant feature in a cross-section of the spinal cord is the presence of a centrally placed area of *gray* matter occurring in the shape of an H (Fig. 6–16). These projections are known as the *dorsal* and *ventral gray horns.* They consist primarily of neuronal cell bodies, synapses, unmyelinated nerve fibers, and glial cells. For example, cell bodies of motor (efferent) neurons innervating skeletal muscle lie in the ventral horns. In the thoracolumbar cord, lateral projections of gray matter, the *lateral (intermediolateral)* horns, occur, which contain cell bodies of autonomic neurons innervating smooth and cardiac muscle and glands.

Surrounding the gray matter is the *white matter* of the cord, which contains bundles of longitudinal ascending or descending myelinated nerve fibers, as well as fibers entering or leaving the cord. The presence of myelin surrounding these fibers accounts for the "white" appearance.

### Spinal Nerves: Dorsal and Ventral Roots

Each spinal nerve is a *mixed* nerve, formed from the union of its dorsal (sensory) root with its ventral (motor) root (see Fig. 6–16). The *dorsal* root consists of a sensory (afferent) neuron, which transmits impulses from various sensory receptors throughout the body into the spinal cord. The cell bodies of these sensory neurons occur in the *dorsal root ganglion.* (A *ganglion* is a collection of cell bodies.) The dendritic processes extend to the periphery, while the axonal fibers enter the dorsal gray horn of the spinal cord. Thus, the dorsal root ganglion and dorsal gray horn are concerned primarily with *sensory* information.

The *ventral* root consists of a motor (efferent) neuron, which transmits impulses from the ventral gray horn within the spinal cord to the effector organs in the periphery. Neurons that innervate skeletal muscle are examples of motor neurons. They have their cell bodies within the ventral gray horns. Thus, the ventral gray horns of the spinal cord and neurons originating therein are primarily concerned with *motor* function.

In addition to sensory and motor fibers, the spinal cord contains many *internuncial* (i.e., contained entirely within the cord) nerve fibers. The many synapses and interchanges occurring between nerve fibers throughout the central nervous system allow for the high degree of processing and integrating of information characteristic of the human nervous system.

### Spinal Cord Plexuses and Peripheral Nerves

Networks of spinal nerve roots join together upon leaving the spinal cord to form a *plexus.* Each plexus, in turn, gives rise to *peripheral nerves,* which provide innervation to specific areas of the body. Major plexuses include the cervical, brachial, lumbosacral, and coccygeal plexuses (Fig. 6–17).

The *cervical plexus* consists of the first 4 cervical spinal nerve roots and is significant in that the *phrenic nerve,* which innervates the diaphragm, arises within this plexus. The *brachial plexus,* formed by the remaining cervical nerve roots and the first thoracic nerve root, gives rise to the following peripheral nerves: the *median, radial, ulnar,* and *musculocutaneous.* These nerves provide innervation to the upper extremities.

Spinal nerve roots from the lumbar and sacral portions of the cord overlap to form the *lumbosacral plexus.* Important peripheral nerves that arise from this plexus include the *femoral* and *saphenous nerves,* which supply in part the pelvis and hip areas and anterior portion of lower extremities. The *sciatic nerve,* which arises from the sacral portion of the lumbosacral plexus, innervates the posterior thigh muscles. The *peroneal* and *tibial nerves,* branches of the sciatic nerve, innervate most of the lower leg and foot. The *pudendal nerve,* which also arises from the lumbosacral plexus, provides innervation to the perineum.

### Peripheral Nerve Distribution

The functional distribution of peripheral nerves is systematic and orderly. This is most apparent in *cutaneous* innervation wherein each segment or band of skin surface is supplied by a specific peripheral nerve derived from its specific spinal nerve roots. Such segments, known as *dermatomes,* are extremely helpful in assessing and evaluating *sensory* function. Figure 6–18 shows dermatomal distribution of sensory innervation at various cord segments. There is considerable overlap between one dermatome and the next, but generally the patterns are followed quite closely.

Distribution of motor innervation via ventral spinal roots follows a segmented pattern much like that reflected in the dermatomes. Each peripheral nerve supplies motor innervation to several somatic or voluntary muscles (see Fig. 6–18). Familiarity with distribution of motor innervation assists in assessing and evaluating motor function including deep tendon reflexes.

### Reflex and Reflex Arc

The *reflex* is the basis of nervous system function. It is a predictable and stereotyped response to a stimulus; a specific stimulus will evoke the same

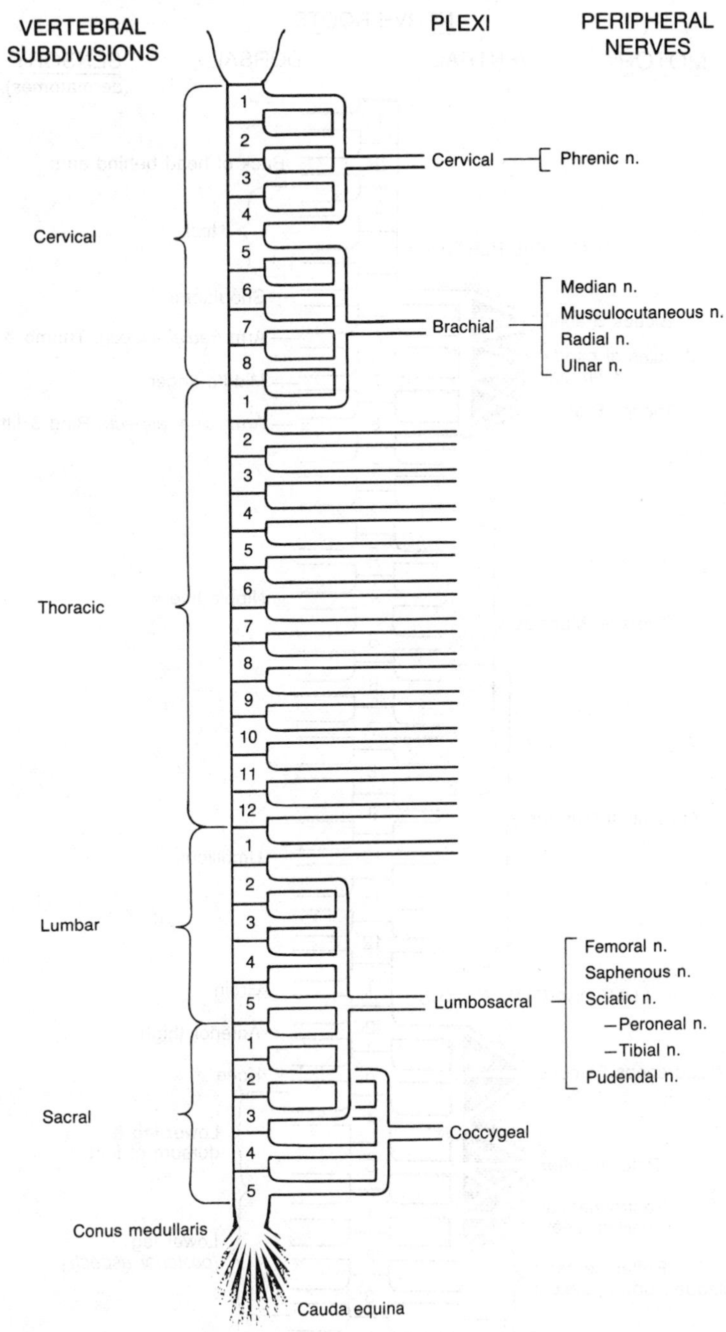


**Figure 6–17.** Spinal cord plexuses and peripheral nerves. Major vertebral subdivisions include cervical, thoracic, lumbar, and sacral vertebrae. Spinal nerves leave via intervertebral foramina between adjacent vertebrae (see Fig. 6–15). Networks of spinal nerve roots join together upon leaving the spinal cord to form a plexus. Each plexus, in turn, gives rise to peripheral nerves. Major plexuses include the cervical, brachial, lumbosacral, and coccygeal plexuses. There is some overlap between lumbosacral and coccygeal nerve roots. Major peripheral nerves associated with each plexus are identified.

response each time it is applied. Reflex actions underlie virtually everything we do including the volitional functions of skeletal muscles and the autonomic functions of cardiac and smooth muscle, and glands.

The *reflex arc* in its simplest form consists of two neurons: a *sensory neuron,* which carries impulses from receptors into the central nervous system, and a *motor neuron,* which transmits the neuronal response to the effector organ(s). This type of reflex arc involves 1 synapse *(monosynaptic)*. More commonly, 1 or more *internuncial neurons* are interposed between the sensory and motor neurons *(polysynaptic)* (see Fig. 6–16). This increases synaptic interactions not only at the entry segment of the spinal cord, but up and down the cord and into higher centers of the brain as well.

Such an arrangement is critical because it allows reflex actions to occur within the spinal cord independent of higher brain center activity. Many responses occur automatically at this level enabling the individual to focus attention on more sophisticated cognitive activities and functions. The multitude of internuncial connections and

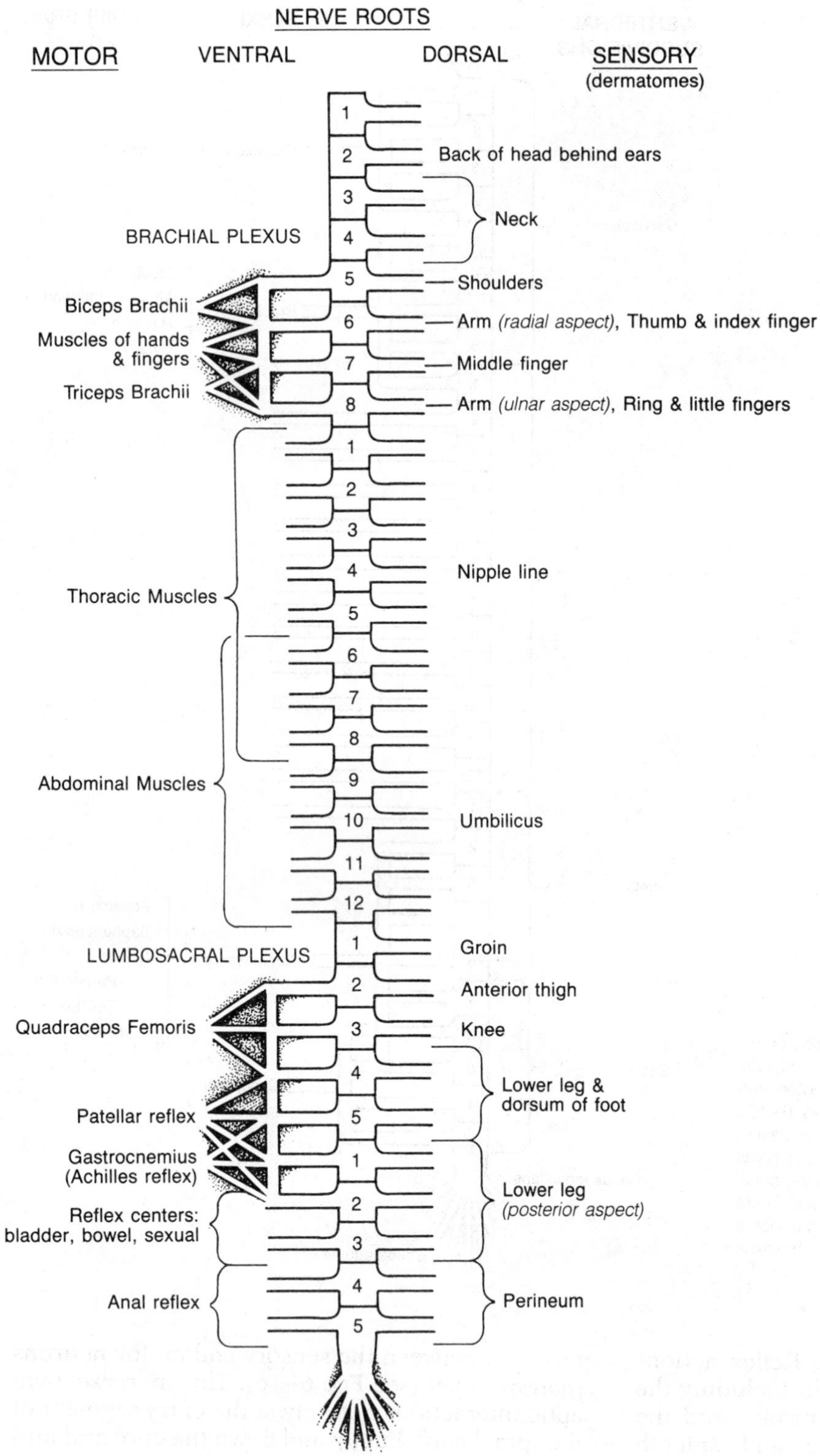


**Figure 6–18.** Peripheral nerve distribution. Distribution of sensory innervation occurs via a segmented pattern wherein each segment or band of skin surface is supplied by a specific peripheral nerve derived from its specific spinal nerve roots. Such segments are referred to as dermatomes. Specific dermatomes and their dorsal roots are identified. Distribution of motor innervation, which occurs via ventral nerve roots, follows a similar segmented distribution.

synaptic interactions provides for an infinite number and variety of human responses.

Major categories of reflexes include the *stretch or deep tendon reflexes, cutaneous or superficial reflexes,* and *brainstem reflexes.* A discussion of these reflexes is presented in Chapter 7. Spinal cord activities also involve *autonomic reflexes* concerned with visceral functions as, for example, control of vasomotor tone and smooth muscle tone of abdominal viscera. Reflex centers concerned with urinary bladder and rectum emptying are located in the sacral portion of the spinal cord. These reflexes are discussed in Chapter 12.

### Nerve Tracts — Nomenclature

A *nerve tract* (also termed *column* or *lemniscus*) is a bundle of nerve fibers that occurs within the *white* matter of the spinal cord. Specific bundles of such fibers generally have the same *origin, termination,* and *function.* There are *ascending,* or *sensory,* tracts, which carry information up the spinal cord to the brain; *descending,* or *motor,* tracts, which carry impulses from the brain to motor neurons within the spinal cord; and *associative (intersegmental)* tracts, which may be ascending or descending within the spinal cord segments.

Nerve tracts are named to denote origin and termination of their fibers. *Origin* refers to the location of the cell bodies of these nerve fibers; *termination* refers to the point where the axonal endings of these nerve fibers occur. Simple analysis of tract names determines location and function. Thus, a *spinothalamic tract* has its origin in the *spinal cord* and its termination in the *thalamus.* This tract is, therefore, an ascending neuronal pathway carrying *sensory* information from the spinal cord to the brain. The *corticospinal tract* has its origin in the cerebral *cortex* and its termination in the *spinal cord.* This tract is a descending neuronal pathway carrying *motor* responses from the brain to the spinal cord.

Specific nerve tracts and their functions are discussed in the sections on sensory and motor function, which follow.

### Sensory Function — Receptors and Circuitry

**Receptors.** All input into the central nervous system is provided by *sensory receptors* and/or *free nerve endings* of afferent (sensory) neurons, which detect and respond to a variety of sensory stimuli including touch, pain, heat, cold, and proprioception (position sense), among others. Each afferent fiber carries information about *1* such *stimulus* or *modality.* Sensory impulses thus generated may be incorporated into spinal reflexes and/or relayed over distinct ascending sensory pathways to the brainstem and higher cortical areas. Sensation occurs when the reticular activating system and the cerebral cortex are sufficiently aroused to process, integrate, interpret, and respond to incoming sensory information.

Sensory receptors are located throughout the body. These receptors can be classified as *mechanoreceptors, interoceptors,* and *special* receptors. A list of specific receptors and their functions is presented in Table 6–8.

**Circuitry.** The sensation one experiences is determined by the nature of the initial stimulus, the circuitry of the specific sensory pathway or nerve tract, and the perceptive areas within the brain to which the particular pathway is directed.

The circuitry of each sensory pathway consists of a series of *3 neurons* (Fig. 6–19). The *first-order* neuron arises at the peripheral receptor and conducts the impulse via its axon into the central nervous system. Its cell body lies in the dorsal root ganglion. A synapse occurs between the axon terminals of the first-order neuron and the *second-order* neuron, which arises within the spinal cord or medulla. After synapsing, the second-order neuron

TABLE 6–8
**Classification of Sensory Receptors**

| | |
|---|---|
| I. Mechanoreceptors | These receptors detect sensations of pressure, touch, vibration, and kinesthesia (inability to perceive direction or extent of movement). |
| A. Exteroceptors | Superficial or cutaneous sensations (epidermis and dermis). |
| Epidermis | Free nerve endings — pain, tactile, and temperature sense. |
| | Merkel's disk — tactile. |
| Epidermis | Ruffini's end organ — touch, pressure, position sense. |
| Dermis | Meissner's corpuscles — tactile. |
| Connective tissue | Pacinian's corpuscle — vibratory sense, touch, pressure. |
| B. Proprioceptors | Endings in muscle, tendon, joints, for deep sensations. |
| | Muscle spindle — stretch. |
| | Golgi tendon receptors — tension. |
| II. Interoceptors | Special receptors in visceral organs. |
| A. Chemoreceptors | Carotid and aortic bodies — arterial carbon dioxide and oxygen levels. |
| | Osmoreceptors in hypothalamus — osmolality of blood. |
| B. Baroreceptors | Sensitive to stretch. |
| | Vasomotor reflexes in carotid sinus. |
| | Respiratory reflex (Hering-Breuer reflex) stretch receptors, which help to prevent overexpansion of lungs. |
| C. Nociceptors | Free nerve endings in viscera — pain. |
| D. Thermoreceptors | Cold receptors. |
| III. Special receptors | Olfactory epithelium — small taste buds — gustatory. |
| | Organ of Corti of inner ear — audition. |
| | Rods and cones of retina — vision. |
| | Hair cells in semicircular canals — equilibrium. |

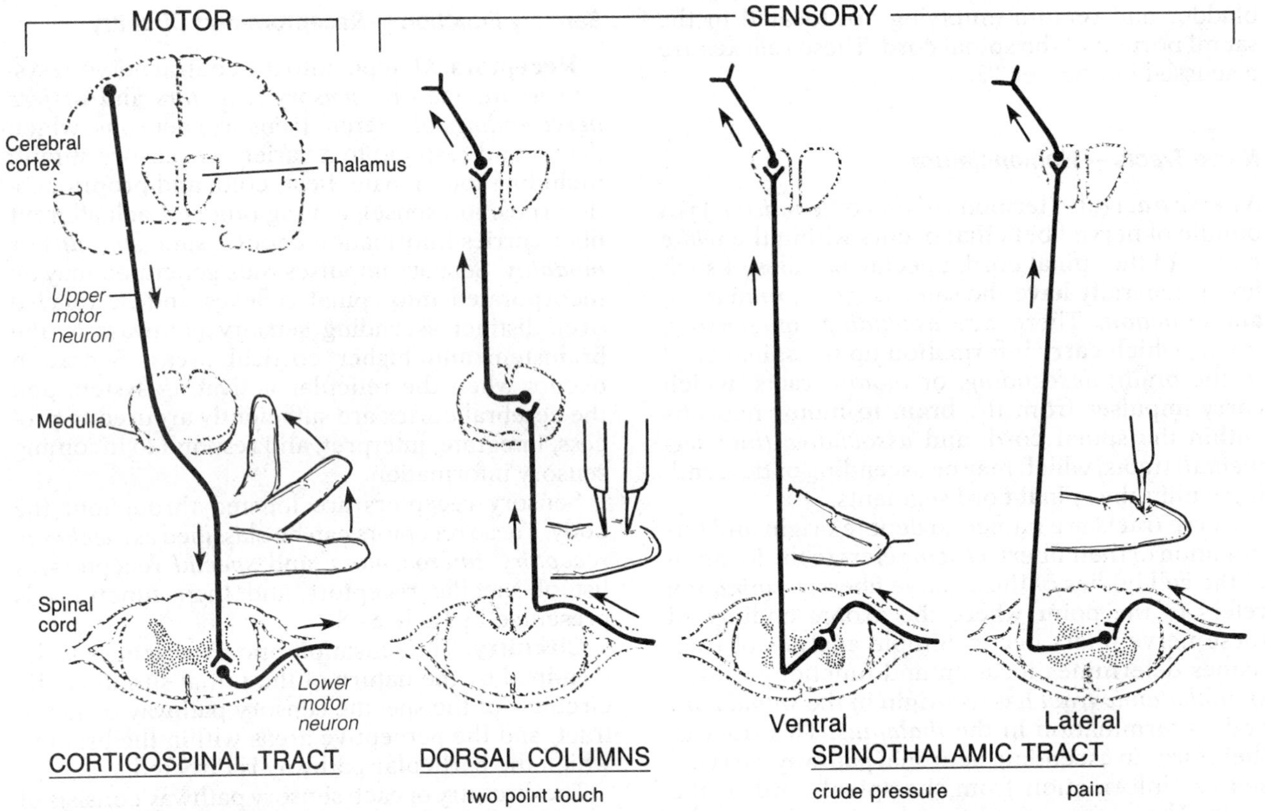


**Figure 6–19.** Circuitry of sensory and motor tracts.

*decussates* (crosses to the other side) and conveys the impulse via nerve tracts in the white matter of the cord to the thalamus. The thalamus is the major relay station for all incoming sensory information providing for an almost infinite number of connections and interactions with other nerve fibers. The *third-order* neuron, after synapsing with the second-order neuron in the thalamus, conducts the impulse to the primary sensory area within the cerebral cortex.

All primary sensory pathways ascend to reach the cerebral cortex, and they all cross to the opposite side (decussate) at some level of the spinal cord or medulla. Thus, the left side of the body is represented within the right cerebral hemisphere, and vice versa. Arrangement of the ascending nerve tracts within the white matter of the spinal cord serves to provide for a certain amount of modality separation. The *dorsal columns,* for example, carry impulses concerned primarily with proprioception, touch, and movement; the *lateral tracts* carry impulses concerned with pain and temperature.

Distribution of sensory innervation within the central nervous system can be divided into *special senses,* which include sight, hearing, taste, and smell, and *general somatic senses,* which convey information regarding pressure, touch, proprioception, temperature, and comfort. Primary receiving areas for each of these senses occur within the cerebral cortex. The primary areas for the special senses are listed in Table 6–5 (see Fig. 6–13). Pathways for the general somatic senses terminate in the somatosensory area of the cerebral cortex located in the *post-central gyrus* of the parietal lobe. This area is often called the *somesthetic cortex* because it provides a representation of senses from various segments of the body (Fig. 6–20).

**Somesthetic Cortex.** Regions of the body receiving a large amount of innervation receive a correspondingly larger topographic representation on the surface of the cortex. Thus, fingers (including the thumb), the lips, and tongue, having many peripheral cutaneous receptors with a high degree of sensory acuity and discrimination, receive greater cortical representation. Representation of the lower extremities, back, and lower trunk occurs over the *medial* surface of the cortex, while that of the hands and face is distributed over the *lateral* surface (see Fig. 6–20).

### Sensory Pathways

***Dorsal Columns (Dorsal Lemniscal System).*** The *dorsal columns* are the nerve tracts responsible for conveying information to the brain related to fine, 2-point touch discrimination, vibratory sense, proprioception, and movement. Impulses originating in peripheral mechanoreceptors (see Table 6–8) in response to external stimuli are conducted to the

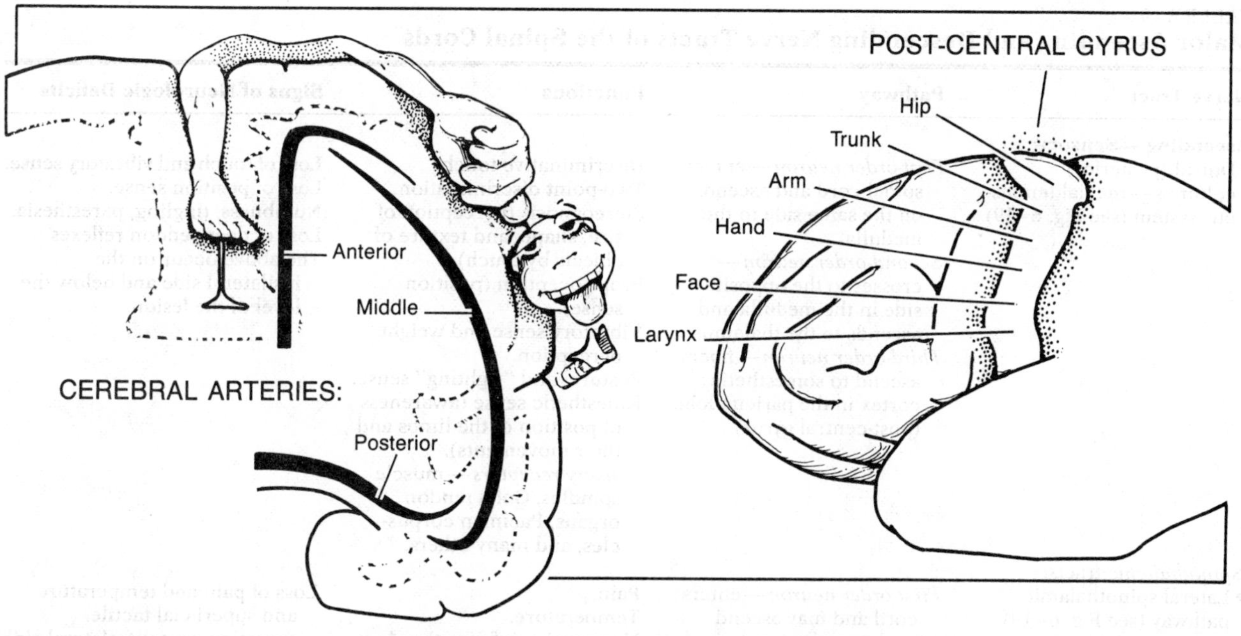


**Figure 6-20.** Somesthetic cortex refers to the topographic representation on the surface of the cortex (primary sensory cortex) of regions of the body receiving innervation. The regions of the body receiving a large amount of innervation (e.g., tongue, lips, thumb, fingers) receive a correspondingly larger topographic representation over the surface of the cortex; areas of the body receiving less innervation (e.g., lower extremities, back, and trunk) receive a correspondingly smaller representation. Note that representation of the hands and face is distributed over the lateral surface of the cortex, an area receiving its blood supply via the *middle* cerebral artery; the medial aspect of the cortex concerned with innervation to the back, trunk, and lower extremities receives its blood supply via the *anterior* cerebral artery; the visual cortex within the occipital lobe is nourished via the *posterior* cerebral artery. Knowledge of this topographic representation and blood supply is helpful in pinpointing the location of a brain lesion, based on history and physical findings.

cerebral cortex via the three-order neuronal system. Specific to this system is that the first-order neurons enter the cord and ascend directly to the medulla via the dorsal columns on the *ipsilateral* (same) side as the initial stimuli. It is at the level of the medulla that these nerve fibers synapse with the second-order neuron. Second-order neurons decussate in the medulla and ascend to the thalamus where they synapse with third-order neurons. These neurons conduct impulses to the somesthetic cortex (see Fig. 6-19 and Fig. 6-20).

***Lateral Spinothalamic Tract.*** The *lateral spinothalamic* tract is associated with the modalities of pain and temperature. Impulses originating in peripheral receptors or free nerve endings (pain) are conducted to the cerebral cortex via the three-order neuronal system. In contrast to the dorsal columns, the first-order neurons of this system enter the dorsal gray horn where they synapse with second-order neurons. Second-order neurons then cross the cord to the opposite side (decussate) at the *same* level of entry into the cord, or within the segments of cord immediately above or below the level of entry. The second-order nerve fibers ascend the cord via a *lateral* tract and travel directly to the thalamus where synapsis with the third-order neuron occurs (see Fig. 6-19).

***Ventral Spinothalamic Tract.*** The *ventral spinothalamic* tract is associated with pressure and crude touch sensations. Its circuitry is similar to that of the lateral spinothalamic tract in that the nerve fibers decussate at the *same* level of entry into the cord. Upon decussation, however, these fibers ascend the cord via a *ventral (anterior)* tract to synapse with the third-order neuron in the thalamus (see Fig. 6-19).

Although distinct individual fiber tracts have been identified, there occurs a tremendous amount of processing of incoming information between various ascending and descending pathways within the cord. This enables most responses of the body to occur at subconscious and/or reflex levels, leaving the highest centers of the brain free to deal with the more relevant, sophisticated, and important information and concerns. Specific details regarding major ascending and descending tracts are listed in Table 6-9.

### *Motor Function — Circuitry and Effectors*

**Primary Motor Cortex.** The *primary motor cortex* occurs within the frontal lobe, specifically the *pre-central gyrus,* which lies just anterior to the *central sulcus* (see Fig. 6-13). It contains the giant, pyramidal cell bodies of the upper motor neurons and is concerned largely with movement of voluntary (skeletal) muscles. Representation of innervation within the motor cortex closely follows that of the somesthetic cortex (see Fig. 6-20). Areas of the body involved in highly sophisticated and intricate

TABLE 6-9
**Major Ascending and Descending Nerve Tracts of the Spinal Cords**

| Nerve Tract | Pathway | Functions | Signs of Neurologic Deficits |
|---|---|---|---|
| **Ascending—Sensory:** | | | |
| • Dorsal (posterior) columns—medial lemniscus system (see Fig. 6-19) | *First-order neuron*—enters spinal cord and ascends on the same side to the medulla.<br>*Second-order neuron*—crosses to the opposite side in the medulla and ascends to the thalamus.<br>*Third-order neuron*—fibers ascend to somesthetic cortex in the parietal lobe (post-central gyrus). | Discriminative touch.<br>Two-point discrimination.<br>Stereognosis (perception of size, shape, and texture of objects by touch).<br>Proprioception (position sense).<br>Vibratory sense and weight perception.<br>Postural and "righting" sense.<br>Kinesthetic sense (awareness of position of the limbs and their movements).<br>*Sensory receptors*—muscle spindles, Golgi tendon organs, Pacinian corpuscles, and many others. | Loss of touch and vibratory sense.<br>Loss of position sense.<br>Numbness, tingling, paresthesia.<br>Loss of deep tendon reflexes.<br>The above occur on the ipsilateral side and below the level of the lesion. |
| *Spinothalamic* tracts: | | | |
| • Lateral spinothalamic pathway (see Fig. 6-19) | *First-order neuron*—enters cord and may ascend or descend several segments before synapsing with second-order neuron in dorsal gray horn.<br>*Second-order neuron*—crosses to contralateral side and ascends to thalamus.<br>*Third-order neuron*—relays impulse from thalamus to somesthetic cortex. | Pain.<br>Temperature.<br>Nociceptive information.*<br>*Sensory receptors*—free nerve endings. | Loss of pain and temperature and superficial tactile sensation on contralateral side below the level of the lesion. |
| • Ventral (anterior) spinothalamic pathways (see Fig. 6-19) | *First-order neuron*—enters cord and synapses with the second-order neuron in the posterior horn.<br>*Second-order neuron*—crosses cord and ascends to the thalamus.<br>*Third-order neuron*—relays impulse from thalamus to somesthetic cortex. | Tactile sensation.<br>Nociceptive information.* | Loss of pain and temperature and superficial touch on contralateral side below the level of the lesion. |
| *Spinocerebellar* tracts: | | | |
| • Dorsal (posterior) spinocerebellar pathway | *First-order neuron*—enters cord and synapses with second-order neuron in dorsal gray area of cord.<br>*Second-order neuron*—ascends on ipsilateral side via dorsal lateral spinocerebellar tract to cerebellum.<br>*NOTE:* This is a two-neuron pathway. | Unconscious proprioceptive information from lower part of body and lower extremities.<br>Fine coordination of individual muscles concerned with postural adjustments.<br>Sensations of touch and pressure.<br>*Sensory receptors*—stretch receptors including muscle spindle and Golgi tendon organs, exteroceptive receptors (touch and pressure) | There may be no abnormal signs unless there is involvement of the cerebellum.<br>With cerebellum involvement, the following may appear:<br>Nystagmus<br>Uncoordinated movement of lower extremities<br>Intention tremors<br>Hypotonia<br>Decreased deep tendon reflexes |
| • Ventral (anterior) spinocerebellar pathway | *First-order neuron*—enters cord and synapses with second-order neuron in dorsal gray area. | Conveys to the cerebellum information related to pain, tactile and pressure receptors. | |

*(continued)*

TABLE 6–9
**Major Ascending and Descending Nerve Tracts of the Spinal Cords *(Continued)***

| Nerve Tract | Pathway | Functions | Signs of Neurologic Deficits |
|---|---|---|---|
| | *Second-order neuron*—crosses cord immediately and ascends via the ventral spinocerebellar tract directly to cerebellum. *NOTE:* This is a two-neuron pathway. | Spinocerebellar tracts monitor ongoing activity of muscle groups and contribute to a smooth, well-coordinated performance. | |
| **Descending—Motor:** | | | |
| *Corticospinal* tracts: | | | |
| • Lateral corticospinal tract (see Fig. 6–19) | *Upper motor neuron* (UMN)—cell bodies of UMN occur in premotor, motor cortex of precentral gyrus, and sensorimotor cortex of post-central gyrus. Approximately 85–90% of these fibers cross to contralateral side at the level of the medulla. These fibers descend the cord as part of the lateral corticospinal tract. | Primarily concerned with skilled movement of muscles in the extremities. Integrated movements of limbs; facilitates activity of extensor muscles while inhibiting activity of flexor muscles. | Upper motor neuron paralysis<br>• Affects groups of muscles rather than individual fibers†<br>• Spasticity and hyperactivity of deep tendon reflexes<br>• Slight muscle atrophy due to disuse<br>• Babinski's sign<br>• No fasciculations |
| • Ventral (anterior) corticospinal tract | Upper motor neuron—cell bodies of UMN in pre-motor, motor cortex (precentral gyrus), and sensorimotor cortex (post-central gyrus). Approximately 10–15% of these fibers descend the cord on the ipsilateral side and cross to the opposite side within a spinal cord segment. | Primarily concerned with voluntary muscles of the trunk. | |
| *Extrapyramidal pathways:* | | | |
| • Rubrospinal tract | Motor fibers arise from the *red nucleus* within the brainstem and function via *alpha* and *gamma* motoneurons to excite flexor muscle groups while inhibiting the activity of the extensor groups. These fibers cross immediately to the opposite side and descend the cord. | Major functions include a facilitatory or inhibitory influence on the maintenance of muscle tone, reflexes, and muscular activity concerned with posture and equilibrium, unconscious integration and coordination of muscular movement. | Muscular rigidity.<br>Involuntary tremor at rest.<br>*Athetosis*—a succession of slow, involuntary, writhing movements of hands and fingers (sometimes toes and feet) including flexion, extension, pronation, and supination. |
| • Vestibulospinal tract | Motor fibers arise from vestibular nuclei within the brainstem. | These tracts function to maintain posture and equilibrium by influencing anti-gravity muscle groups. Medial pathway also influences cranial nerve nuclei (III, IV, VI) concerned with extraocular movement; coordinates head and eye movements. | |
| Medial | • Decussate and descend the cord on the opposite side | | |
| Lateral | • Fibers remain uncrossed | | |
| • Reticulospinal tract | Motor fibers arise from pontine and medullary areas of brainstem and remain largely uncrossed. | These tracts function to influence muscle activities related to posture and maintenance of muscle tone. | |

*(continued)*

TABLE 6-9
**Major Ascending and Descending Nerve Tracts of the Spinal Cords *(Continued)***

| Nerve Tract | Pathway | Functions | Signs of Neurologic Deficits |
|---|---|---|---|
| Medial<br>Lateral | • Facilitates extensor reflexes while inhibiting flexors<br>• Excites flexor reflex while inhibiting extensors | Transmit impulses to the autonomic nervous system via spinal cord fibers which synapse with the preganglionic fibers of sympathetic and parasympathetic branches of autonomic nervous system. | |
| • Tectospinal tract | Motor fibers arise in the midbrain, decussate and descend the cord to terminate in the cervical cord segments. | These tracts function to influence activity of head and neck muscles in movements of the head associated with visual and auditory stimuli. | |

* Note that *both* the lateral and ventral spinothalamic tracts are thought to mediate the same sensations.
† Compare with lower motor nerve paralysis.

function (fingers, thumbs, lips) receive a predominant portion of representation within the motor cortex.

### Circuitry—Somatic Division (Skeletal Muscle)

***Corticospinal Pathways (Pyramidal System).*** The brain exerts its influence on skeletal muscle throughout the body via *descending motor pathways.* The *corticospinal pathways* are descending motor pathways that function to provide for fine, smooth, and controlled movement of the extremities by exerting an *excitatory* influence on flexor muscle groups, while exerting an *inhibitory* effect on extensor muscles. These descending pathways consist of a series of 2 neurons: the upper motor neuron and the lower motor neuron.

*Upper Motor Neuron.* The *upper motor neuron* originates and terminates within the central nervous system. Its large pyramid-shaped cell body occurs within the motor cortex. Its axon terminals synapse directly with a lower motor neuron or with internuncial neurons, which in turn synapse with lower motor neurons within the spinal cord. The influence of the upper motor neuron on the lower motor neuron is modulated by input from the somesthetic cortex, basal ganglia, reticular activating system, and cerebellum, as well as by ascending sensory fiber tracts, which occur between the spinal cord and the thalamus.

Approximately 85% of corticospinal fibers decussate to the *contralateral* (opposite) side at the level of the medulla. These fibers descend the cord via the *lateral corticospinal* tracts (see Fig. 6-19). The remaining uncrossed corticospinal fibers descend the cord via the *ventral corticospinal* tracts, eventually crossing to the contralateral side at some level within the spinal cord.

*Lower Motor Neuron.* The other major neuron in this descending motor pathway is the *lower motor neuron,* also called the *final common pathway.* This latter term reflects the fact that the lower motor neurons are the *only* neurons in the body that innervate skeletal muscle. Unlike the upper motor neuron, which resides completely within the central nervous system, the lower motor neuron originates in the central nervous system with its large cell body in the ventral gray horn; it terminates at the *neuromuscular junction (motor end plate)* of individual skeletal muscle fibers.

In addition to their large cell bodies, the lower motor neurons to the extremities have long, heavily myelinated axons, which enable impulses to be transmitted at tremendously high velocities, rapidly initiating muscular activity.

The ultimate message delivered to the lower motor neuron and expressed via skeletal muscle activity represents the *sum* of all excitatory and inhibitory impulses arising from many sensory and motor areas throughout the central nervous system.

*Neuromuscular Junction.* Each skeletal muscle fiber has *1* specialized area within its membrane called the *motor end plate.* It is here that an axon terminal of the lower motor neuron articulates with specific receptors on the individual muscle fiber. This enables the electrical activity within the neuron to be transmitted to the muscle fiber in chemical form via a neurotransmitter, evoking a specific motor response. This junction of nerve with skeletal muscle fiber is called the *neuromuscular junction.* The neurotransmitter secreted here is *acetylcholine.*

***Extrapyramidal Pathways.*** Because the corticospinal pathways project directly from the cerebral cortex to the spinal cord, they are frequently referred to as *direct* pathways. A number of other descending motor pathways are classified as *indi-*

*rect* because of their multiple synapses and connections with other neuronal pathways throughout the central nervous system. They arise from cortical and subcortical areas of the brain, basal ganglia, cerebellum, and various areas within the brainstem including the thalamus, substantia nigra, red nucleus, and reticular formation. These pathways do not decussate at the medulla as do corticospinal (pyramidal) pathways, and they have been labeled *extrapyramidal* pathways.

Extrapyramidal pathways modulate the activities of the pyramidal system. Working in synchrony with the cerebellum, these pathways help to regulate and maintain activites related to muscle tone, posture, proprioception, equilibrium, and reflexes. Their excitatory and inhibitory influences are indispensable in performing fine, discrete, volitional movements.

The final pathways for the conduction of motor impulses via extrapyramidal tracts have their origin within the brainstem and termination in the spinal cord. Specific extrapyramidal tracts include the rubrospinal tract, vestibulospinal tract, reticulospinal tract, and tectospinal tract. (Refer to Table 6-9 for specific details regarding these tracts.)

**Circuitry—Autonomic Division (Cardiac and Smooth Muscle, and Glands).** The *autonomic* division of the nervous system is concerned with innervation of cardiac muscle, smooth muscle, and glands. Because these tissues participate as effectors in most bodily functions, it follows that the autonomic nervous system plays a significant role in the regulation and maintenance of the activities of the internal environment in a dynamic equilibrium.

***Sympathetic and Parasympathetic Systems.*** The autonomic division is comprised of the *sympathetic* and *parasympathetic* systems. These systems coordinate and control many vital activities, including maintenance of blood pressure, heart rate, digestive processes, respiratory and excretory functions, body temperature, and emotional behavior. Many of these functions occur below the level of consciousness; most involve reflex activity. The activities of one system tend to be balanced by activities of the other.

TABLE 6-10
**Responses of Effector Organs to *Adrenergic** Innervation**

| Organ | Alpha Receptors | Beta$_1$ Receptors | Beta$_2$ Receptors |
|---|---|---|---|
| *Heart* | | Stimulation of these receptors increases: | |
| SA node | | Myocardial contractility | |
| Atria | | Conduction velocity | |
| AV node | | Automaticity | |
| Ventricles | | Heart rate | |
| | | In the ventricles, an increase in the rate of idioventricular pacemakers may occur. | |
| *Arterioles*† | | | |
| Coronary | Vasoconstriction + | | Vasodilation ++ |
| Skeletal muscle | Vasoconstriction ++ | | Vasodilation ++ |
| Cerebral | Vasoconstriction (slight) | | |
| Pulmonary | Vasoconstriction + | | Vasodilation |
| Abdominal viscera | Vasoconstriction +++ | | Vasodilation |
| Renal | Vasoconstriction +++ | | Vasodilation |
| Skin-mucosa | Vasoconstriction | | |
| Salivary glands | Vasoconstriction | | |
| *Veins* | | | |
| Systemic | Vasoconstriction ++ | | |
| *Lungs* | | | |
| Bronchial muscle | | | Relaxation (bronchodilation) |
| *Intestinal* | | | |
| Smooth muscle | Relaxation | | Relaxation |
| *Uterus* | Contraction | | |
| *Ureter* | Contraction | | |
| *Metabolism* | | Beta stimulation | |
| | | Lipolysis | |
| | | Muscle glycogenolysis | |
| | | Insulin secretion | |

* *Dopaminergic* receptors may be found in renal, mesenteric, splanchnic, cerebral, and coronary arteries. Vasodilation and increased blood flow to these vascular beds occurs following dopaminergic stimulation. Only *dopamine* is presently known to activate this receptor.

† Almost all arterial beds have both alpha and beta receptors, and some additionally possess dopaminergic receptors. The *net* physiologic response depends almost entirely on the amount of stimulation being received by each receptor at any given time.

\+ Reflects degree of vasoconstriction or vasodilation, with + <++ <+++.

The sympathetic and parasympathetic systems differ in several respects: (1) anatomic distribution of nerve fibers, (2) neurotransmitters secreted at postganglionic synapses, and (3) antagonistic physiologic effect on most organs they dually innervate.

Anatomically, nerve fibers of both the sympathetic and parasympathetic motor pathways consist of a series of *2* neurons termed the *preganglionic neuron* and the *postganglionic neuron*. The preganglionic neuron has its cell body and dendrites within the central nervous system. Its efferent fibers terminate in the *autonomic ganglia,* cell clusters that occur outside the central nervous system. The postganglionic neuron has its cell body and dendrites within the autonomic ganglia, and its axon terminals directly innervate the effector organ, that is, smooth or cardiac muscle, or glands (e.g., adrenal medulla).

Cell bodies of preganglionic *sympathetic* neurons occur in the *lateral* gray horn of the thoracic and lumbar cord; thus, this system is also termed the *thoracolumbar* system. Cell bodies of preganglionic *parasympathetic* neurons occur in the brainstem and sacral cord, thus, this system is also labeled the *craniosacral* system.

Axons of preganglionic sympathetic neurons exit the spinal cord via the ventral roots of spinal nerves. These fibers then leave the spinal nerve to enter the chain of autonomic ganglia via a white *ramus* (connecting pathway). The *chains* of autonomic ganglia lie close to and on either side of the spinal cord. These chains extend from the cervical to sacral cord and constitute the *sympathetic trunk.* It is within the ganglia that the preganglionic neuron synapses with the postganglionic sympathetic neuron. The postganglionic neuron ultimately travels to the effector organ, which it innervates.

Axons of preganglionic parasympathetic neurons depart the brainstem via cranial nerves III, VII, IX, and X, and the sacral segments of the spinal cord via the spinal nerves. These neurons travel directly to ganglia at or near the effector organ. Here they synapse with the postganglionic parasympathetic neuron, which, in turn, innervates the effector organ.

In both sympathetic and parasympathetic systems, *acetylcholine* is the neurotransmitter released at *all* ganglionic synapses between pre- and postganglionic nerve fibers. In the parasympathetic system, the neurotransmitter between the postganglionic fibers and effector organ is also acetylcholine, and these fibers are called *cholinergic* fibers. In the sympathetic system, the neurotransmitter between postganglionic fibers and effector organ is predominantly *norepinephrine (noradrenaline),* and these fibers are called *adrenergic* fibers.

*Neurotransmitters—Receptor Specificity.* There are several different types of receptors for each neurotransmitter. For example, acetylcholine recep-

TABLE 6-11
**Autonomic Nervous System: Effect of Dual Innervation on Effector Organs**

| Effector Organ | Effect of Sympathetic Stimulation | Effect of Parasympathetic Stimulation |
|---|---|---|
| Eye | | |
| Pupil | Dilation (mydriasis) | Contraction (miosis) |
| Ciliary muscle | Relaxation | Contraction |
| Glands | | |
| Lacrimal | ↓ Secretion | Stimulates secretion |
| Salivary | Scanty, viscous secretion | Profuse, watery secretion |
| Lungs | | |
| Bronchioles | Bronchodilation | Bronchoconstriction |
| Heart | ↑ Rate | ↓ Rate |
| | ↑ Conduction velocity | ↓ Conduction velocity |
| | ↑ Contractility | ↓ Contractility |
| Gastrointestinal tract | | |
| Lumen | ↓ Peristalsis and tone | ↑ Peristalsis and tone |
| Sphincters | ↑ Tone (usually contraction) | ↓ Tone (usually relaxation) |
| Secretions | May inhibit secretions | Stimulates secretions |
| Adrenal medulla | Secretion of epinephrine and norepinephrine | No significant effect |
| Urinary bladder | | |
| Detrusor muscle | Relaxation (usually) | Contraction |
| Internal sphincter | Contraction | Relaxation |
| Blood vessels | | |
| Coronary | Vasodilation | Minimal effect |
| Skeletal muscle | Vasodilation | Minimal effect |
| Splanchnic | Vasoconstriction | Minimal effect |
| Skin | Vasoconstriction | Minimal effect |
| Blood | | |
| Glucose | Increased | |
| Free fatty acids | Increased | |

tors at all synapses between preganglionic and postganglionic autonomic fibers are called *nicotinic* receptors because they respond to the drug, nicotine. Likewise, receptors at neuromuscular junctions in the somatic division (skeletal muscle) are also of the nicotinic type. In contrast, acetylcholine receptors (parasympathetic system) on cardiac muscle, smooth muscle, and glands are of the *muscarinic* type (i.e., they respond to the drug, muscarine).

Similarly, there are two classes of adrenergic receptors in the sympathetic system, namely, *alpha-adrenergic* and *beta-adrenergic* receptors. Beta-adrenergic receptors are further classified as $Beta_1$ and $Beta_2$ receptors. *Dopamine* has been identified as another neurotransmitter within the sympathetic system, and *dopaminergic* receptors are specific for dopamine. Responses of effector organs to adrenergic innervation are listed in Table 6–10. Refer to Table 6–2 for a list of neurotransmitters that have been identified.

*Dual Innervation.* Most organs of the body, including the heart, many glands, and smooth muscles, are innervated by both the sympathetic and parasympathetic postganglionic fibers. Thus, they receive *dual innervation.* Most commonly, these two systems have opposing or antagonistic effects on most organs of the body. The effects of dual innervation on some effector organs are listed in Table 6–11.

Activities of the autonomic nervous system are largely modulated and regulated by centers in the hypothalamus, medulla, and reticular formation. Areas within the cerebral cortex may also influence autonomic responses.

*Innervation of Adrenal Medulla.* The adrenal medulla functions as part of an autonomic reflex arc. In this instance, the afferent or sensory limb is *neural* in nature. Innervation of this gland occurs via *pre*ganglionic sympathetic fibers, which originate in the thoracic segments of the cord and travel directly to the adrenal medulla where they synapse with specialized cells contained therein. The cells respond by secreting epinephrine (predominantly) and norepinephrine directly into the circulating blood, and these substances affect cells widely dispersed throughout the body. Thus, the efferent or motor limb of this reflex arc is *hormonal.* The unique structure of this autonomic reflex arc demonstrates the close interaction between the nervous and endocrine systems in regulating body functions.

## SELECTED READINGS


Barr, ML: The Human Nervous System: An Anatomical Viewpoint, ed 5. JB Lippincott, Philadelphia, 1988.

Carpenter, MB: Core Text of Neuro Anatomy, ed 3. Williams & Wilkins, Baltimore, 1985.

Cormack, DH: Ham's Histology, ed 9. JB Lippincott, Philadelphia, 1987.

Daube, JR, et al: Medical Neurosciences, ed 2. Little, Brown & Co, Boston, 1986.

Gilman, S and Newman, SW: Manter and Gatz's Essentials of Clinical Neuroanatomy and Neurophysiology, ed 7. FA Davis, Philadelphia, 1987.

Hickey, J: The Clinical Practice of Neurological and Neurosurgical Nursing, ed 2. JB Lippincott, Philadelphia, 1986.

Krause, WJ and Cutts, JH: Concise Text of Histology, ed 2. Williams & Wilkins, Baltimore, 1986.

Pansky, B, Allen, DJ, and Burd, GC: Review of Neuroscience, ed 2. Macmillan, New York, 1988.

Rudy, E: Advanced Neurological and Neurosurgical Nursing. CV Mosby, St. Louis, 1984.

CHAPTER 7

# Neurologic Assessment: Assessment of the Patient with an Altered Level of Consciousness

## CHAPTER OUTLINE



## LEARNING OBJECTIVES

**At the end of this chapter, you should be able to:**

1. Describe essential aspects of the clinical history as they pertain to neurologic function and dysfunction.
2. Elicit assessment data based on knowledge of functional health patterns.
3. Discuss the physiology of consciousness and the significance of the level of consciousness as an important indicator of neurologic function.
4. Delineate the components of mentation and their significance as indicators of the level of brain function.
5. Discuss how assessment of cranial nerves assists in evaluating the integrated human functions concerned with sensation and movement.
6. Establish the clinical significance of assessing somatic and cortical sensory modalities.
7. Review the significance of assessing cerebellar, motor, and reflex activity in evaluating integrated human functions concerned with movement.
8. Describe specific parameters to be assessed in the patient with an altered state of consciousness, which assist in localizing lesions and evaluating the level of brain function.
9. List commonly used neurodiagnostic tests and procedures and implications for nursing care.

The nervous system plays a major role in the communicative and regulatory functions of the body and is at the very core of our functioning as human beings. Consequently, assessment of neurologic function is an integral part of any evaluation of total body function and a person's ability to cope with the activities of daily living physiologically, psychologically, and socially.

In the critical care setting, neurologic dysfunction, whether the cause or consequence of multisystem problems, has significant implications for nursing care. The potential for rapid deterioration in body functions and irreversible damage to fragile nerve tissue makes survival of the individual and the quality of life post-recovery especially dependent on skilled nursing care.

The purpose of the neurologic assessment is to assist in determining: (1) the presence or absence of nervous system dysfunction; (2) the location, type, and extent of the lesion or insult; (3) the impact of the neurologic dysfunction on the individual's self-care capabilities; and (4) the degree to which the healthy portion of the patient's nervous system can be used for rehabilitation. Such data provide the foundation for diagnosing and planning patient care.

Performing a neurologic assessment can be a perplexing and formidable challenge. Many of the signs and symptoms of neurologic dysfunction are subjective (e.g., pain), while others are objective and behavior based (e.g., expressive aphasia, that is, the inability to express thoughts appropriately both in words and in writing). Changes in neurologic function are often subtle and elusive; commonly, the patient is unarousable or unresponsive.

Data gathering must be organized, systematic, and objective. It requires attentive listening and astute observation skills. The nurse must master techniques necessary to evaluate the various aspects of neurologic function (e.g., general cerebral, cranial nerve, and sensorimotor functions). Standard neurologic check sheets with clearly defined grading scales can be used to verify objective data.

To assist the nurse in diagnosing, planning, and evaluating patient care, baseline neurologic function must be established and all data must be correlated over time. Frequently, a *trend* is more significant than any one piece of data. The results of the initial and ongoing history taking, physical examination, and diagnostic studies must be integrated, analyzed, and interpreted. Such information provides the basis for diagnostic decision-making and therapeutic intervention; it assists in evaluating the patient's response to therapy, and it lays the foundation for patient/family rehabilitation.

The major components of the patient's assessment include relevant clinical history, physical examination, and ancillary diagnostic studies and techniques.

## CLINICAL HISTORY

The single most important source of information necessary to evaluate any specific neurologic problem, as well as overall function, is the clinical history. The history, carefully elicited from the patient and/or those familiar with the patient, is the key to nursing diagnosis. The history provides important clues, which guide subsequent observation and examination.

When initiating the neurologic assessment, the nurse must determine the patient's level of consciousness and mentation. This can be done by asking the patient the following questions: Who are you? Where are you? What is the date/time? Why are you here? If a patient is ventilated or has an altered level of consciousness, his or her behavior should be observed, (e.g., opening eyes when name is mentioned or when touched; or responding by blinking eyes or smiling). Orientation to person, place, date, and time reflects consciousness; use of language and memory reflects intact mentation; appropriate behavioral responses may reflect awareness and understanding.

The thoroughness of the initial history and examination will depend on the patient's immediate status. If the patient is experiencing any distress (e.g., dyspnea, pain), the history and physical examination should be modified accordingly. The patient's mental and emotional status should be observed throughout the history taking and examination for possible subtle clues about the underlying concern or problem and the patient's perception of what is happening.

### Components of Clinical History

#### *Chief Complaint*

The chief complaint is the major reason why the patient has sought health care at this point in time. The patient should be encouraged to describe the presenting symptom in his/her own words. If possible, a time frame should be established. For example, the patient may state: "I had a severe headache that lasted about an hour." For patients who have an altered level of consciousness or are unable to speak (e.g., the ventilated patient), it may be necessary to elicit information about the patient's status from family members or significant others.

#### *History of Present Illness*

The history of present illness assists in eliciting the details surrounding the chief complaint. It should include a clear description of the initial symptoms and the patient's best approximation of the date/time of onset, the course or progress since onset, the current or immediate status of the presenting problem, and the patient's overall status.

The "SLIDT" assessment tool (Table 7–1) can be used to elicit and clarify specific information regarding the nature and characteristics of the presenting symptom.

**Questions to Be Asked.** Describe the initial symptom. When did it start? What is it like? Did it develop suddenly or gradually? What was the patient doing at the time? Has the condition improved or deteriorated? Does it come and go, or is it constant? Were there any precipitating factors, such as infection (sinusitis, upper respiratory infection, ear or tooth infections) or trauma affecting the nervous and/or musculoskeletal systems? Has there been any recent unusual physical, mental, or emotional stress?

TABLE 7-1
**Assessment Tool: SLIDT***

S = Severity—How severe or intense is the symptom?
L = Location—Where is it located? Does it radiate to other parts of the body?
I = Influencing factors
*Precipitating*—What causes or predisposes to the symptom?
*Ameliorating*—What relieves symptoms?
*Aggravating*—What makes it feel worse?
*Associated*—What else happens at the same time (e.g., nausea, vomiting, blurred vision)? What is the setting in which it occurs (e.g., home, workplace, during exercise, or at rest)?
D = Duration—Timing of symptom in terms of events and patterns surrounding the patient. When does it occur? How long does it last? Does it come and go?
T = Type—The quality or characteristics of the symptom. What does it feel like (e.g., "throbbing," "constricting," "pounding like a sledgehammer," "knife-like")?

* This assessment tool can be applied to a variety of symptoms, including pain, bleeding, cough, and sputum production.

If trauma to the head occurred, was the patient unconscious, and if so, how long? Were there seizures? Was there bleeding from ear, nose, or mouth? Were there subsequent headaches, memory loss, or changes in behavior or personality? Has the patient experienced vertigo, dizziness, tinnitus, or loss of balance? Have there been problems with speaking, hearing, or seeing? Has the patient experienced alterations in sensations (e.g., numbness, tingling, pain)? Has the patient experienced muscle weakness or paresis? Is there difficulty in walking, or carrying out activities of daily living? Has there been any changes in digestive, urinary, or bowel functions?

It is important to speak with a patient's relatives and friends if possible. They may be able to verify or corroborate information elicited from the patient; or they may provide more accurate and more objective information regarding the patient's personality and behavior. Important facts may be unveiled that the patient is unaware of, or has deemphasized, overemphasized, or completely forgotten.

### Past Medical History

It is important to establish a relationship between past illnesses and current problems. Is there a history of traumatic injury? For example, if an elderly patient who sustained a Colles' fracture (fractured wrist) in a fall 6 months ago is presently admitted with a seizure disorder, are these 2 events related?

Has the patient been hospitalized previously? If so, when, how long, and for what reason? Is there a history of transient ischemic attacks (TIAs), or stroke? Hypertension? Other cardiovascular disorders? Is there evidence of pulmonary disease? Hypoxemia associated with chronic cardiopulmonary disease might underlie complaints of neurologic dysfunction (e.g., confusion, lethargy). Is the patient anemic? Has the patient recently experienced an infectious disease? Have there been other recent stressors (personal, social, economic, or occupational) in the patient's life? Has there been recent travel abroad?

Is there a history of birth trauma or congenital anomaly? What childhood diseases has the patient experienced? Immunizations, and reactions, if any? Has the patient had a previous neurologic assessment? If so, what was done, when, and for what reason? Who prescribed the testing procedures, where were they performed, and what were the results?

### Family History

Neurologic and neuromuscular dysfunction is often related to congenital or hereditary diseases. Is there a history of congenital or hereditary disease in the family? Down's syndrome? Epilepsy or other seizure disorder? Huntington's chorea? Is there a history of neuromuscular disease in the family? Muscular dystrophy? Myasthenia gravis? Multiple sclerosis?

Cerebrovascular diseases are often implicated as underlying causes of neurologic dysfunction. Is there a family history of strokes, coronary artery disease, or cardiac myopathies? Is there a history of hypertension? Endocrine disorders, diabetes mellitus, pituitary or thyroid disorders? Renal disease? Alcoholism? Drug abuse? Psychologic, mental, or emotional disorders? Suicidal tendency?

### Functional Health Patterns[1]

It is especially important to consider how the patient who is experiencing neurologic dysfunction functioned prior to illness, and how the underlying neurologic problem might affect the patient's lifestyle and potential for recovery and rehabilitation. (See Appendix C for a description of the functional health patterns.)

**Health Perception—Health Management.** It is important to ascertain the patient's overall health status: What has been the patient's previous health status? Has there been any recent physical, mental, or emotional stress? Any significant changes in lifestyle? Is there chronic illness? Have the patient's capabilities for self-care changed? Who does the patient live with? What are the patient/family attitudes regarding health? What do they consider to be an optimal level of health?

What are the patient/family attitudes and behaviors regarding drug use or abuse? This should include prescription as well as over-the-counter drugs, recreational drugs (e.g., cocaine, marijuana), alcohol, and cigarette smoking. What are patient/family attitudes regarding pain and pain relief?

Does the patient have seizure disorder? If so, how does the patient describe the seizure activity? When did it begin? What were the circumstances surrounding its occurrence? How does the patient/family feel about the condition? Does the patient take anticonvulsant therapy?

Is there a history of psychologic dysfunction? Depression, apathy, mental sluggishness? Anxiety? Does the patient take tranquilizers or antidepressants? Who prescribed the medication, and why?

Has the patient previously experienced a stroke or other cerebrovascular disorder? If so, are there any lasting sequelae? How do they impact on the patient's activities of daily living? Is the patient taking anticoagulant medication? Is there the potential for drug interactions? Does the patient know what medications are being taken, and why?

**Nutritional — Metabolic.** Is is important to establish baseline body weight. Has there been a recent loss or gain in weight? How much over how long a period of time? Has there been a recent loss in stamina? Does the patient tire easily? When was this first noticed? What was happening with the patient at that time? It is especially important to establish a database regarding the patient's eating habits, likes and dislikes, and a typical daily diet. Have there been any recent changes in chewing and swallowing capabilities? Difficulty handling saliva? Drooling? Attitudes regarding the importance of good nutrition should be explored.

Does the patient have an endocrine disorder? Hormonal disturbances may alter neurologic status. Is there a pituitary disorder? Diabetes mellitis? Thyroid dysfunction? Hypoglycemia or diabetic ketoacidosis can cause confusion, seizures, and unconsciousness. Hyperthyroidism may precipitate extreme anxiety, hyperactivity, and tremors; hypothyroidism causes mental sluggishness, lethargy, apathy, and weakness.

**Elimination.** Has the patient experienced any recent changes in urinary routine or habits? Is there frequency or urgency of urination, or incontinence? When did the incontinence begin? What were the circumstances surrounding its occurence? Is there a history of renal disease? Uremia, associated with chronic renal failure, may cause confusion, convulsions, and coma.

Has the patient experienced any recent changes in bowel routine or habits? Or has a recent cerebrospinal insult compromised bowel function? It is important to establish a database regarding the patient's usual bowel habits because such information may be useful to bowel retraining and rehabilitation. Important information to elicit includes frequency of bowel movement, time of day, diet, problems of constipation, diarrhea, incontinence, and use of laxatives.

**Activity — Exercise.** Has the patient experienced recent difficulties in performing activities of daily living? If so, what were the nature of the difficulties and possible underlying cause? Are there limitations involved in dressing, feeding, or bathing? When walking, is there a gait problem? It is important to explore how the current illness might affect the patient's ability to participate in activities of daily living and recreational and work-related activities. Potential problems for rehabilitation should be ascertained and documented, so that they may be addressed in planning care. Discharge planning considerations begin when the patient is admitted to the hospital.

**Cognitive — Perceptual.** Has the patient experienced recent difficulties in concentrating or problem-solving? Is there difficulty recalling recent or remote experiences? Have changes occurred in the patient's sensory perception — visual, auditory, tactile, taste, and smell? Have changes occurred in the patient's ability to read, speak, and understand language?

What is the patient/family understanding as to the underlying disease and ramifications it may have in terms or lifestyle? Is there a readiness to learn?

**Sleep — Rest.** The patient's sleeping pattern should be ascertained, including the hour of retiring and the number of hours of sleep daily. Does the patient experience insomnia? If so, under what circumstances? Does the patient use prescription or over-the-counter sleeping medications? Does the patient incorporate rest periods into daily routine? What does the patient do to relax?

**Role — Relationship.** What are the patient's perceptions as to major roles and responsibilities? Who is the bread-winner and decision-maker in the family? How does the patient view family dynamics? How might the patient's illness affect family dynamics and the patient's livelihood?

**Coping — Stress Tolerance.** How do the patient and family cope with stress? How does the patient usually deal with problems? How does the patient/family view this illness and its impact on their lifestyle? How are they coping at present? What are the family resources, strengths, and weaknesses? In the event of catastrophic illness (e.g., acute head injury), what health-care and financial resources are available to the patient and family?

**Self-Perception and Self-Concept.** Often neurologic dysfunction causes changes in the patient's body image (e.g., sexuality in quadriplegics). The patient's response to these changes will need to be examined over time as the patient indicates a readiness to deal with the problem or concern.

**Value — Belief.** A pivotal aspect of care for patients with neurologic dysfunction, especially those with permanent sequelae (e.g., hemiparesis in the stroke patient, or paralysis associated with spinal cord injury), is to explore and examine with the patient and family some of the following concerns: What are their short- and long-term goals? Are they realistic? Attainable? How does the illness compromise efforts to attain these goals? How might these goals be achieved despite any disabilities? What options are open to the patient/family? Are they aware of these options? Are they familiar with available resources?

## NEUROLOGIC EXAMINATION

## General Cerebral Functions

### *Consciousness*

Changes in the level of consciousness can be the most sensitive indicator of level of neurologic function. The functional components of consciousness are arousal (alertness) and awareness (content) of self and environment. *Arousal* is largely subserved by brainstem activity including that of the reticular activating system (RAS), which consists of the brainstem reticular core and its projections to the diencephalon and subcortical areas (see Fig. 6–14). The reticular activating system functions to alert the cerebral hemispheres to incoming sensory information. Arousal is demonstrated clinically by eye opening.

*Awareness*, or content, requires an intact cerebral cortex and association fibers. Either cerebral hemisphere alone is sufficient to maintain consciousness, providing the reticular activating system is intact. Coma ensues when function of both hemispheres is impaired or when there is brainstem injury involving the reticular activating system. Clinically, awareness is demonstrated by verbal and motor responses, which have their origin within the cortical areas.

The state of consciousness depends on the close interactions between components of the brainstem (arousal) and the intact cerebral hemisphere(s) (awareness). The diffuse anatomic and functional interrelationship of these structures accounts for the fact that, should brain dysfunction occur, the *earliest* evidence of such dysfunction will be reflected by changes in the level of consciousness.

Arousal is assessed by observing eye opening. Do the patient's eyes open spontaneously when the nurse approaches the bedside, prior to, or upon being spoken to? If there is no eye opening and the patient does not respond to verbal or auditory stimuli, a painful stimulus can be applied to determine if the arousal mechanism is intact.

Awareness is assessed by determining the patient's orientation to self and environment. This can be accomplished by asking the questions: What is your name? Where are you? What is the date/time? Evaluating the status of verbal and motor responses assists in assessing awareness. Awareness can be evaluated more closely by tests of mental status described in the section that follows.

In critically ill patients whose conditions are unstable, or who have the potential for rapid deterioration in neurologic function, the Glasgow Coma Scale can be used as an adjunct to assessing neurologic function.

**Glasgow Coma Scale.** The Glasgow Coma Scale (GCS)[2] is a simple, systematic adjunct assessment tool with defined grading scales used to verify objective data. This scale provides a useful means of detecting trends in neurologic status. When used in conjunction with an evaluation of brainstem function (e.g., respiratory pattern, pupillary responses, eye movements, and motor responses), this scale assists in monitoring the status of protective reflexes (cough, gag, and epiglottal closure) and the patient's airway. The Glasgow Coma Scale assesses eye opening, best verbal response, and best motor response (Table 7–2).

***Eye Opening.*** Eye opening is scored as 1 of 4 responses. Eyes open *spontaneously* when the nurse approaches the bedside; eyes open to *speech* if the patient's eyes open when the nurse verbalizes; eyes open to painful stimuli, such as pinching; and eyes do not open at all.

***Best Verbal Response.*** The *oriented* patient is able to respond appropriately to questions related to identification of self, place, and date/time. The *confused* patient is capable of producing language but is not oriented. *Inappropriate* words indicate the patient has occasional utterances including cursing, which are frequently provoked in response to physical rather than verbal stimuli. *Incomprehensible* sounds include groans and other indistinct mumbling without any identifiable words, which indicate decreased cerebral function. No verbal response, even with painful stimuli, suggests brainstem dysfunction.

***Best Motor Response.*** Best motor responses are scored as 1 of 6 responses involving the arms. The

TABLE 7–2
**Glasgow Coma Scale: Assessment of Arousal***

| Response | Grading Scale | Score |
|---|---|---|
| Eyes open | Spontaneously | 4 |
| | To speech | 3 |
| | To pain | 2 |
| | None | 1 |
| Best verbal response | Oriented | 5 |
| | Confused | 4 |
| | Inappropriate words | 3 |
| | Incomprehensible sounds | 2 |
| | None | 1 |
| Best motor response | Obeys commands | 6 |
| | Localizes | 5 |
| | Flexion withdrawal | 4 |
| | Abnormal flexion | 3 |
| | Abnormal extension | 2 |
| | None | 1 |

* Maximum score 15; minimum score 3.

patient who *obeys* a command can appreciate directions or instructions whether given verbally, in writing, or by gesture. *Localizes* pain requires that the patient make an appropriate or purposeful attempt to remove the stimulus. *Flexion withdrawal* suggests that the patient cannot localize the stimulus but will at least flex the arm when a painful stimulus is applied (e.g., pressure on a fingertip). *Abnormal flexion* in response to a painful stimulus involves flexion at elbow and internal rotation of wrists. *Abnormal extension* involves extension of arm at elbow with adduction and internal rotation at the shoulder. *None* involves the patient not responding at all. (See Fig. 7–4.)

A maximum score of 15 reflects a fully alert, oriented patient, who follows commands; a minimum score of 3 indicates a completely unresponsive, unarousable patient. An advantage in using the Glasgow Coma Scale is that it is easily standardized and consistently reproducible by different health-care providers. Such terms as alert, obtunded, stuporous, and comatose are commonly used to describe the level of consciousness, but these lack precise definitions and are subject to considerable variations and inconsistencies in their usage by health professionals. They are mentioned here only to emphasize their inadequacies in describing the patient's level of consciousness and to discourage their use in the clinical setting.

Although use of the Glasgow Coma Scale is helpful in recognizing trends in the patient's responses, its use should not supplant descriptive documentation of observed responses. The scale is most useful in assessing the head-injured patient. Once scores of 10–15 are achieved, the scale offers very little information regarding the patient's neurologic status.

Some practical problems are associated with the use of the Glasgow Coma Scale in evaluating patients with an altered level of consciousness.[3] For example, eyelids may remain open after they have been drawn back, or swelling may prevent eyelid opening. Verbal response may be impaired by dysphasia or deafness; the presence of an endotracheal tube may interfere with communication. Motor activity refers to responses of the upper extremities; a flexion withdrawal response by lower extremities may reflect neural activity at the level of the spinal cord.

### *Mentation*

Mentation involves an integration of those processes concerned with memory, thought, language, emotions, and spatial perception.[4] An assessment of mental status provides a measure of the integrity of the cerebral cortex and subcortical areas. Specific tests to assess these functions are discussed below.

**Memory.** Recent memory and remote memory depend on an intact integration of functions of the reticular activating system, limbic system, and cerebral cortex. Recent memory can be tested by the retention of digits (e.g., 42579), working from shorter to longer series. Ask the patient to repeat a series of numbers forward and then backwards. For critically ill patients, it may be more appropriate to use a simpler test, such as repeating objects (e.g., dog, cat, car). Remote memory (i.e., long-term memory) can be tested by asking the patient his/her date and place of birth.

**Thinking.** *Thinking* is the sum total of the patient's intellectual and cognitive capabilities, and its assessment provides an estimate of the intactness of the cerebral cortex. Aspects of thinking that can be assessed include the patient's *knowledge base* (e.g., current president, current events); capacity for *calculation* (e.g., have the patient add 2 digits, multiply 2 digits, and count backward from 100 by 7's); *abstract reasoning* (e.g., ask the patient to explain the meaning of a familiar slogan, such as "A stitch in time, saves nine"); and *problem-solving ability* (e.g., ask the patient what he would do if a ball rolled into the street in the path of his approaching car).

**Language.** *Language* is a highly complex mental function involving the use of symbols to convey meaning by speaking, reading, and writing. Many areas of the brain operate together to produce appropriate, spontaneous language. For example, Broca's area is critical to the actual production of speech; Wernicke's area functions in speech comprehension (e.g., following a command). Association fibers between these two areas facilitate the integration of their activities (see Table 6–5). The left cerebral hemisphere is language-dominant in most people.

The patient's speech is assessed for spontaneity and content during history taking. Comprehension of language is evaluated to some extent by the patient's ability to follow directions. Comprehension can also be assessed by having the patient read a paragraph from a newspaper or book out loud and then explain the meaning of the passage. The patient can be asked to write what the nurse dictates (e.g., "Many flowers bloom in spring"). A language deficiency is the inability to communicate through speech, writing, or signs (e.g., following a command). *Dysphasia* is difficulty in understanding and communicating using words; *aphasia* is the inability to understand and communicate through word usage.

**Spatial Perception.** Spatial perception is a function subserved predominantly by the right cerebral hemisphere in most individuals. It involves the recognition of space and shape. *Gnosia* is the ability to recognize objects via the senses (i.e., visual, auditory, tactile). For example, tactile spatial perception can be assessed by putting objects into the patient's hand (e.g., paper clip, coin) and having the patient identify them without looking at them. Visual perception is tested by showing the patient a picture (e.g., a square or triangle), putting the picture away, and then asking the patient to draw the picture. Auditory perception can be tested by asking the patient to repeat a sentence such as "The cat chased the squirrel up the tree" and to explain its meaning. *Agnosia* is the inability to recognize objects through any of the special senses in the presence of an intact sensory system and sensorium.

**Emotion (Feeling).** The patient's emotional status is subserved largely by the limbic system with modulation of primitive or undifferentiated emotional behavior by the frontal lobes. Critically ill patients are frequently highly sedated and may experience an altered level of consciousness; others may exhibit changes in mood and affect, and these patients should be observed closely. Is the affect natural and even, or is the patient irritable, angry, anxious, depressed, apathetic, or euphoric? Ask the patient to describe his/her mood, and observe the facial expression and body language. Consider the appropriateness of the patient's responses to the situation. These very same considerations can also be applied to the patient's family or significant others.

## Cranial Nerve Function

Assessment of cranial nerves provides a guide as to the integrity of the brainstem. (Table 6-6 lists the central and peripheral connections of cranial nerves; circuitry [i.e., reflex arcs] of brainstem reflexes is presented in Table 7-6). Cranial nerves can be assessed while evaluating the integrated human functions of seeing, hearing, feeling, smelling, tasting (sensation), speaking, eating, and expressing (movement).[5] Assessment of cranial nerves is presented in Table 7-3.

Only certain cranial nerves can be tested in critically ill patients who may be sedated or who may have an altered level of consciousness. This is accomplished by assessing brainstem reflexes. Brainstem reflexes of importance are listed in Table 7-6. Further discussion of these reflexes is presented below in the sections entitled "Brainstem Reflexes" and "Patient with Altered Level of Consciousness."

## Sensation

The sensory division of the nervous system consists of the special senses, somatic senses, and cortical and discriminatory sensations. Assessment of special senses (i.e., smell, sight, hearing, and taste) is discussed in the section entitled "Cranial Nerve Function" (above); evaluation of somatic senses and cortical sensations is addressed here.

The *somatic* sensations include light touch, crude pressure, pain, temperature, proprioception, and vibration. Circuitries of these sensory pathways are depicted in Figure 6-19; primary cortical representation of sensory innervation (somesthetic cortex) is shown in Figure 6-20.

Sensory phenomena are largely subjective. Thus, the results of sensory testing depend on the patient's perception and interpretation of the stimuli, and on his or her consequent verbal response. These tests to evaluate sensory function require a cooperative patient and may be inappropriate for some critically ill patients. Much depends on the patient's cooperation and on the technique of the examiner.

Throughout the assessment of sensory function, the examiner should:[6]

1. Note the patient's ability to perceive the sensation being tested.
2. Compare both sides of the body and corresponding extremities.
3. Compare sensitivity of the distal and proximal parts of each extremity for each form of sensation (e.g., sensitivity to a wisp of cotton, a pinprick, and to vibration).
4. Try to determine whether the senory changes involve one entire side of the body, are dermatomal in distribution, or are confined to the peripheral nerves.
5. Ask the patient to keep his/her eyes closed during the testing.
6. Avoid giving verbal or tactile cues.

### *Assessment of Somatic Senses*

**Light Touch—Superficial Tactile Sensation.** To assess: Lightly touch the patient with a wisp of cotton. Ask the patient to say "now" when he/she feels the stimulus, to name the area stimulated, and to state the nature of the stimulus. Compare the sensitivity of the proximal part of each extremity to the distal part.

**Pain.** To assess: Repeat procedure as in light touch, but use a pin. Apply only a sufficient stimulus to generate a response. Pain and temperature modalities are carried in the same pathways so only pain sensation needs to be assessed in a screening examination.

**Vibration.** To assess: Place vibrating tuning fork to bony prominences of each of the 4 extremities testing distal aspects (fingers and toes) first. Ask the patient if he/she feels the vibration, where it is felt, and when the vibration stops. To differentiate vibrating sense from pressure, place a nonvibrating fork on a bony prominence and repeat the questions.

**Proprioception.** (Awareness of posture and movement, and knowledge of position in space). To assess: Ask the patient to indicate the direction of movement and final position of a finger or toe. The

TABLE 7–3
## Assessment of Cranial Nerves and Integrated Human Functions

1. **Smelling:** Cranial nerve I, olfactory (Fig. A)
   To assess: (1) establish patency of nasal passages; (2) with his/her eyes closed, ask the patient to identify familiar odors such as coffee, tobacco, or spice. Each side of nose is tested separately.

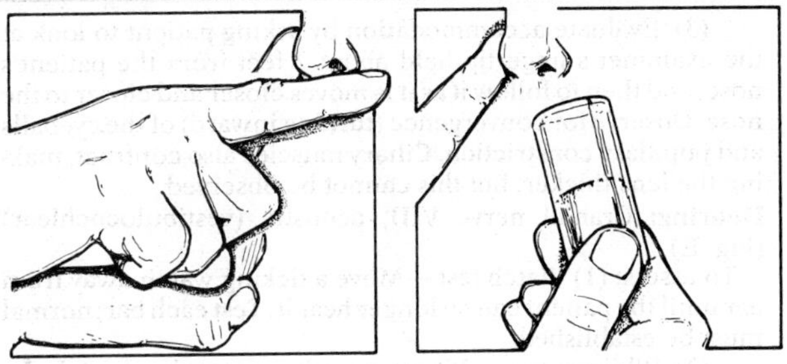

A

2. **Seeing:**
   A. Visual acuity and visual fields: Cranial nerve II, optic (Fig. B)
   To assess: (1) Ask the patient to read Snellen chart or newsprint, testing one eye at a time. If corrective lenses are worn, test both eyes with and without corrective lens. Ability to read newsprint comfortably at arm's length is optimal. If the patient is unable to read, ask the patient to identify the number of fingers you hold up. (2) Divide visual field for each eye into six quadrants. The stimulus, a moving finger or cotton-tipped applicator, is presented from the periphery of each quadrant while the patient is instructed to close one eye and to look at the examiner's nose with the other. The examiner closes one eye opposite to the patient's closed eye. The patient is instructed to say "now" as soon as he/she sees the stimulus come into view. The test is performed for each eye. This method of testing is called *visual fields by confrontation.* It is especially helpful in assessing the patient with a cerebral vascular accident (stroke) who commonly experiences a visual field deficit.

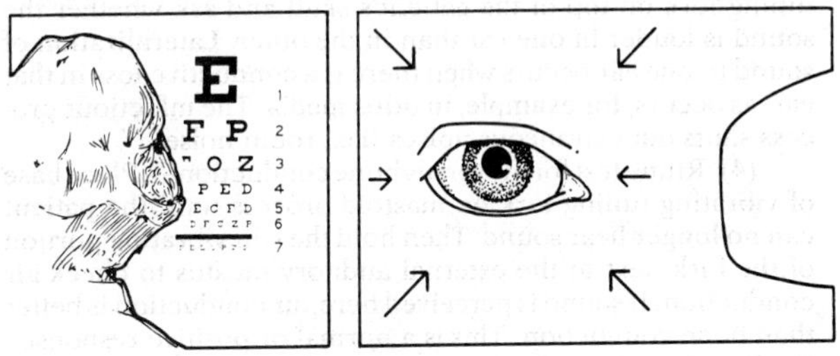


B

   B. Extraocular movements: Cranial nerves III, oculomotor; IV, trochlear; and VI, abducens (Fig. C)
   To assess: (1) With his/her head held still, ask the patient to follow the movement of a pencil or examiner's finger as it is moved in all directions of gaze. It is important to move the stimulus to the extremes of each direction of gaze. The examiner looks for eye movement up and down, and in toward nose (III and IV); and lateral movement toward the ear (VI). The patient is also observed for nystagmus (i.e., rapid jerking of the eyes when they are tracking an object) with direction of the nystagmus based on the fast component. Incoordination of eye movements suggests cerebellar dysfunction. Note any complaints of blurred vision or diplopia (double vision).
   C. Corneal reflex: Cranial nerves V, trigeminal; and VII, facial (Fig. C)
   To assess: Test the corneal reflex by observing whether the patient blinks in response to a light touch with a wisp of cotton on the cornea. Avoid striking only the sclera.

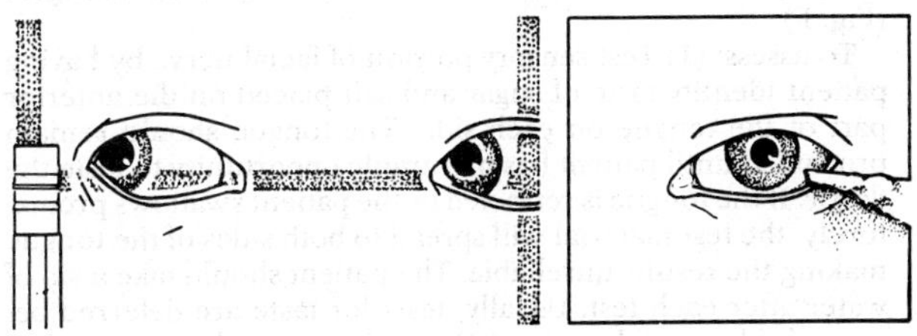

C

   D. Direct and consensual light reflex and accommodation: Cranial nerves II, Optic; and III, oculomotor (Fig. D)
   To assess: (1) Examine pupils, noting size, shape, and equality before testing for reactivity. Many individuals (about 17%) have unequal pupils. It is important to ascertain if the patient has had prior eye surgery, which may account for unequal, unusually shaped pupils. Drugs can affect pupillary responsiveness. A drug history is essential. Pupillary size may be recorded in millimeters, or as constricted, normal, or dilated.
   (2) Evaluate pupillary light reflexes by noting pupillary constriction in response to a light shown into each eye from the side. Shine the light into one eye and observe the pupillary response in that eye. Next, shine the light into the same eye and observe the pupillary response in the *other* eye. When one eye is stimulated, the pupil of the other eye should also constrict (i.e., consensual light reflex). Decussation (i.e., crossing) of optic nerve fibers at the optic chiasm provides the structural basis for the direct and consensual reflex. To discern pupillary reactivity in extremely pinpoint pupils, darkening the room may help.

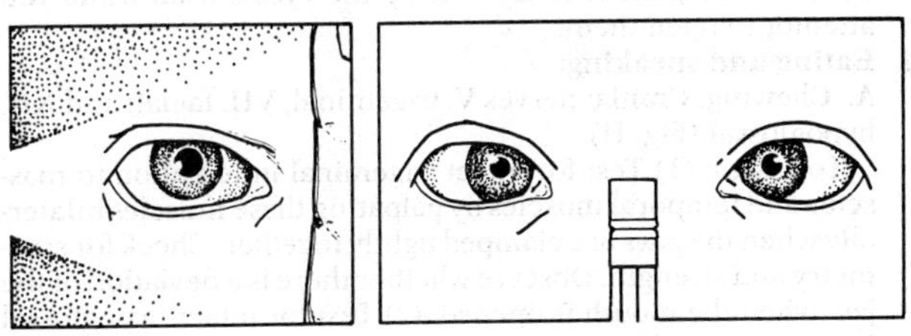

D

*(continued)*

TABLE 7–3
## Assessment of Cranial Nerves and Integrated Human Functions *(Continued)*

(3) Evaluate accommodation by asking patient to look at the examiner's fingertip held about 2 feet from the patient's nose, and then to follow it as it is moves closer and closer to the nose. Observe for convergence (turning inward) of the eyeballs and pupillary constriction. Ciliary muscles also contract, making the lens thicker, but this cannot be observed.

3. **Hearing:** Cranial nerve VIII, acoustic (vestibulocochlear) (Fig. E)
   To assess: (1) Watch test—Move a ticking watch away from ear until the patient can no longer hear it. Test each ear; normal must be established.
   (2) Whisper test—Whisper softly into each ear. Ask the patient to repeat what was said.
   (3) Weber test for lateralization—Place base of vibrating tuning fork on top of the patient's skull and ask whether the sound is louder in one ear than in the other. Lateralization of sound to one ear occurs when there is a conductive loss in that ear, as occurs, for example, in otitis media. The infectious process shuts out extraneous noises (i.e., room noise).
   (4) Rinne test for air versus bone conduction—Place base of vibrating tuning fork on mastoid process until the patient can no longer hear sound. Then hold the still vibrating portion of the fork next to the external auditory meatus to check air conduction. If sound is perceived here, air conduction is better than bone conduction. This is a normal or positive response.
4. **Feeling:** Tactile and pain sensation of face: Cranial nerve V, trigeminal (Fig. F).
   To assess: (1) Ask patient to close eyes and then alternately test for light touch (cotton wisp) and pain sensation (pin prick) on both sides of the face including forehead, cheeks, and jaw. Failure to feel tactile sensation is termed *anesthesia;* failure to feel pain is *analgesia.*
5. **Tasting:** Cranial nerves VII, facial; and IX; glossopharyngeal (Fig. F)
   To assess: (1) Test sensory portion of facial nerve by having patient identify taste of sugar and salt placed on the anterior part of the tongue on each side. The tongue should remain protruded until patient has had ample opportunity to taste the flavor. If the tongue is retracted or the patient swallows prematurely, the test material will spread to both sides of the tongue making the results unreliable. The patient should take a sip of water after each test. Usually, tests for taste are deferred because both cranial nerves VII and IX are evaluated in other ways.
6. **Expressing:** Cranial nerve VII, facial (Fig. G)
   To assess: (1) To test facial nerve ask patient to imitate you as you raise your eyebrows, wrinkle your forehead, frown, smile, and blow out your cheeks. Observe for any asymmetry of the face, such as flattening of the nasolabial fold or drooping of the lower lip on either side. (2) To test strength of the eyelid muscles, ask the patient to try to keep the eyes closed while you attempt to open them.
7. **Eating and speaking:**
   A. Chewing: Cranial nerves V, trigeminal; VII, facial; and XII, hypoglossal (Fig. H)
   To assess: (1) Test for intact trigeminal innervation to masseter and temporal muscles by palpating these muscles bilaterally when the jaws are clamped tightly together. Check for symmetry and strength. Observe whether there is a deviation of the jaw when the mouth is opened. (2) Test for intact hypoglossal innervation to the tongue by observing for any lateral deviation when the tongue is protruded, atrophy, or tremor. Strength of

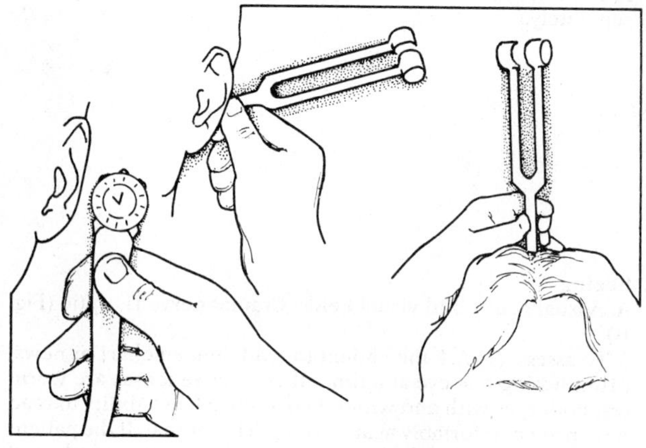

E

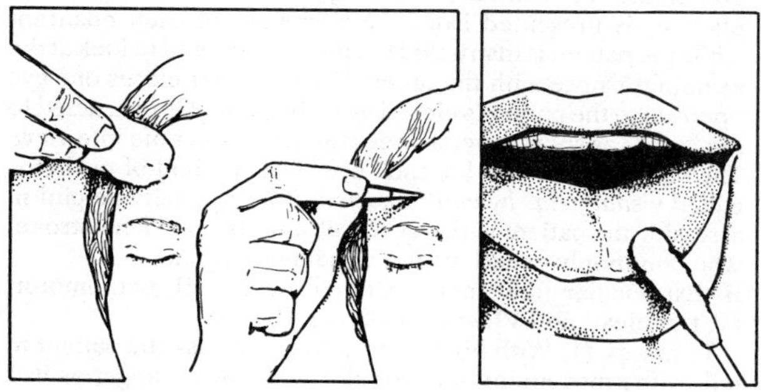

F

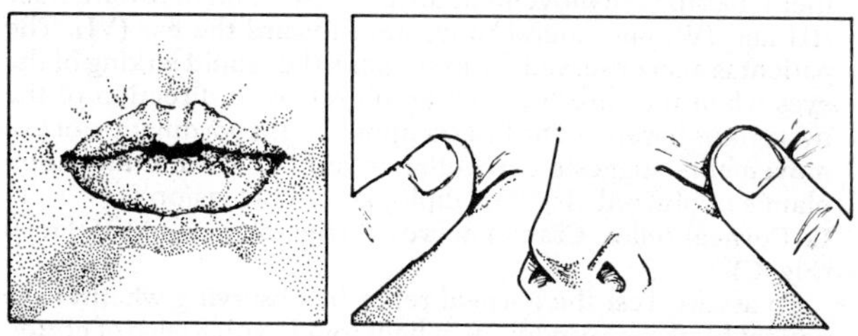

G

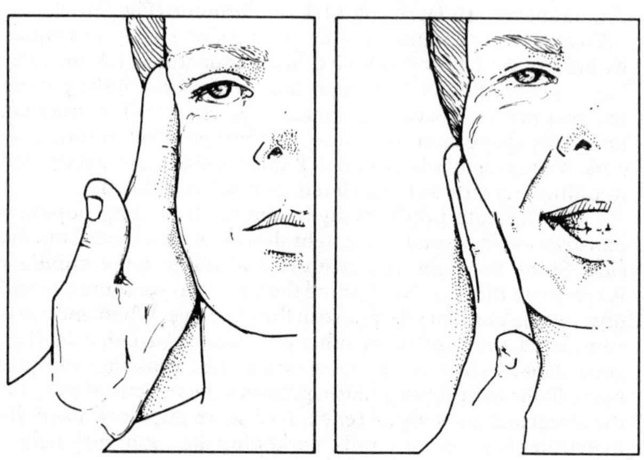

H

TABLE 7-3
**Assessment of Cranial Nerves and Integrated Human Functions *(Continued)***

the tongue is tested by asking the patient to protrude and move it from side to side against the resistance of a tongue depressor (Fig. I).

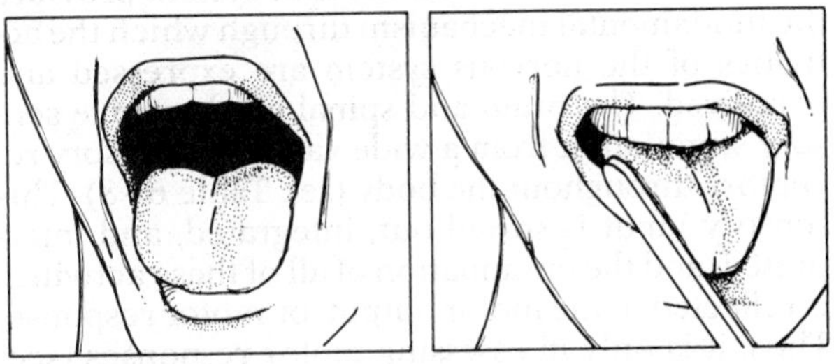
I

B. Swallowing: Cranial nerves VII, facial; IX, glossopharyngeal; X, vagus; and XII, hypoglossal (Fig. J)
To assess: (1) Observe the patient's ability to swallow food and liquid. If the patient swallows without difficulty, these nerves may be considered to be intact.

C. Speaking: Cranial nerves VII, facial; IX, glossopharyngeal; X, vagus; and XII, hypoglossal
To assess: (1) Evaluate the ability of the patient to articulate word sounds. Specifically, "me, me, me" (VII), "ga, ga, ga" (IX and X), "la, la, la" (XII). Normal articulation suggests that all four cranial nerves and the cerebellum are intact.
(2) Evaluate phonation by asking the patient to say "ah," and observe for elevation of uvula and soft palate. This procedure tests the integrity of cranial nerve X (Fig. J).
(3) Assess pharyngeal gag reflex by touching each side of the pharynx with a tongue depressor. The palatal reflex is tested by stroking each side of the uvula. The side touched should rise. These tests evaluate function of cranial nerves IX and X (Fig. J).

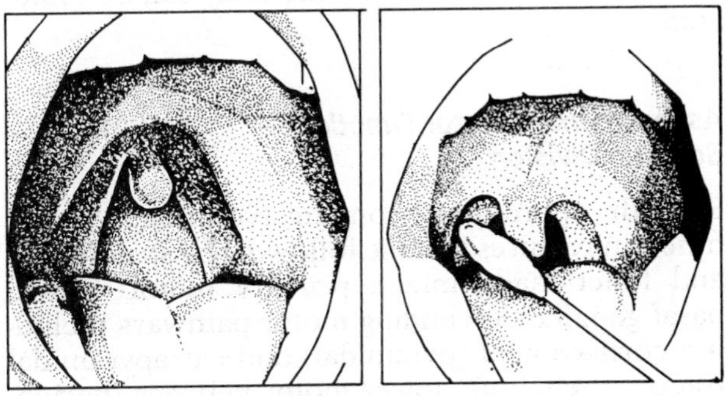
J

8. **Muscle strength:** Cranial nerve XI, accessory (Fig. K)
To assess: (1) Palpate and test sternocleidomastoid muscle for strength. Ask patient to turn head against resistance offered by the examiner's hand. Palpate the opposite sternocleidomastoid muscle. Repeat procedure bilaterally. (2) Palpate and note strength of trapezius muscle while shoulders are shrugged or arms are raised against resistance.

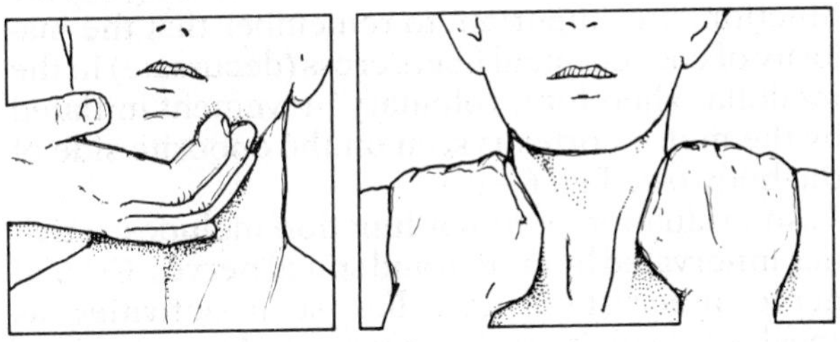
K

examiner should carefully grasp the *sides* of the fingers and toes to avoid pressure on the skin, which might provide the patient with a clue as to the direction of movement. Another test for proprioception is the Romberg test (see section entitled "Cerebellar Function").

**Deep Pressure.** To assess: Squeeze the muscle across the shoulders, or the Achilles tendon, and note sensitivity.

### *Assessment of Cortical Sensations*

Several types of cortical and discriminatory sensations involve complex somatic sensory impressions requiring cortical interpretation. Assessment tests are performed with the patient's eyes closed.

**Two-Point Discrimination.** To assess: Touch various parts of the body with two sharp objects (e.g., pins). Ask each time if the patient feels 1 or 2 points. The distance at which the patient can distinguish 1 from 2 distinct points varies in different parts of the body. Fingertips and the lips are especially sensitive. Any impairment of 2-point discrimination may reflect a problem along the sensory pathways beginning with the peripheral receptor and ending in the somesthetic cortex.

**Stereognosis.** (Ability to recognize form of solid objects by touch). To assess: Ask the patient to identify a familiar object by touch (see section entitled "Spatial Perception," above). Stereognosis requires intact touch and motor function (the latter allows for the manipulation of the object).

**Graphesthesia.** (Ability to recognize numbers, words, or symbols traced upon the skin). To assess: Ask the patient to recognize letters or numbers written on the palms of the hands.

**Sensory Extinction Phenomenon.** To assess: Touch 2 points simultaneously on opposite sides of the body in identical areas. The patient should be able to perceive that he/she has been touched on *both* sides.

## Movement

The motor division of the nervous system provides the fundamental mechanism through which the activities of the nervous system are expressed and perceived. The brain and spinal cord receive sensory stimulation from a wide variety of sensory receptors throughout the body (see Table 6–8). This sensory input is sorted out, integrated, and interpreted, and the culmination of all of these activities is reflected in the motor output, or motor response. Thus, it is only in assessing motor responses (seeing, speaking, eating, expressing, walking) that the effect of sensory stimuli on the body can be evaluated.

### Assessment of Motor Function—Somatic Division

Smooth, coordinated somatic (voluntary) motor function requires that the following be structurally and functionally intact: primary motor cortex, basal ganglia, descending motor pathways including corticospinal (pyramidal) and extrapyramidal tracts, cerebellum, lower motor neurons (peripheral nerves), neuromuscular junctions, and individual skeletal muscle fibers. When assessing motor function, it is important to remember that the majority of corticospinal fibers cross (decussate) in the medulla. Therefore, voluntary movement initiated by the motor cortex is seen on the opposite side of the body (see Fig. 6–19).

An evaluation of motor function includes activities innervated by cranial and spinal nerves. Cranial nerve innervation underlies such activities as speaking, eating, and expressing. Assessment of these activities is discussed in the section entitled "Cranial Nerve Function." The emphasis here is to examine motor activities innervated by spinal nerves. Specifically addressed is the status of skeletal muscle, cerebellar function, and reflexes, all of which underlie the functional activities of walking and moving.

#### Skeletal Muscle Testing

***Muscle Size.*** To assess: Inspect and palpate the patient's muscles while at rest for size, consistency, and possible atrophy. A tape measure may be used to compare corresponding parts of the upper arms, thighs, and calves for size. Compare fine muscles of each hand to assess for wasting, fasciculations (twitchings), and fine tremors of a single motor unit.

***Muscle Tone.*** To assess: Palpate the patient's muscles at rest and note the resistance to passive movement. Assess for spasticity (i.e., increased resistance to passive muscle stretch), rigidity, stiffness of extremities when passively moved, or flaccidity (i.e., decreased resistance to passive muscle stretch).

***Muscle Strength.*** To assess: Ask the patient to move each of the major muscles first without resistance, and then against the resistance offered by the examiner. Compare corresponding muscles on each side. (Examination of sternocleidomastoid and trapezius muscles is discussed in the section entitled "Cranial Nerve Function.") A *universal* system for recording muscle strength utilizes a scale rating from 0 to 5

0 = no contraction
1 = trace (flicker) of contraction
2 = active movements without gravity
3 = active movements against gravity
4 = active movements against gravity and resistance
5 = usual (normal) strength

***Involuntary Movements.*** To assess: Inspect for irregular, spasmodic choreiform movements (i.e., marked by involuntary muscular twitchings of the limbs and/or face), rapid myoclonic contractions, tics, or tremors. A *resting* tremor is diminished by voluntary movement; an *intention* tremor is accentuated by voluntary movement. Strictly defined, a resting tremor is one that is present when the involved part is at rest, but absent or diminished when active movements are attempted; an intention tremor occurs when active, voluntary motion is attempted.

### Cerebellar Function: Coordination of Movement and Balance

**Balance.** To Assess:

(1) *Romberg test*—Ask the patient to stand erect with feet together, first with eyes open, and then with eyes closed. If the patient sways or falls after closing eyes, the test is *positive*. This is a test for proprioception (i.e., position sense). When the patient's eyes are open, visual cues aid in maintaining balance; when the eyes are closed, maintenance of balance relies largely on proprioceptive input.

(2) *Gait*—Ask the patient to walk naturally with eyes open and then closed; ask patient to walk in tandem fashion (i.e., heel-to-toe). Observe gait for arm swing, rhythm, symmetry, and coordination. The examiner should remain near the patient during these tests in case the patient should begin to fall.

Tests for balance and gait depend on the ability of the patient to perform volitional movements. Such activity is beyond the capability of most critically ill patients. These tests are included here to assist the reader to appreciate the major components of the overall neurologic assessment.

**Coordination.** To assess: *Finger-to-nose tests* (1)

Ask the patient to touch his/her finger to the nose, first with one hand and then with the other. The test is repeated with the eyes closed. (2) With eyes open, ask the patient to place his/her finger on the nose and then on the examiner's finger as the examiner changes the position of his/her finger. This action can be repeated with increasing rapidity as the examiner moves his/her own finger.

To assess: *Alternating movements* (1) Ask the patient to touch his/her fingers to thumb in rapid succession. (2) Ask the patient to pat his/her knees with the palms and the backs of the hands, by pronating and supinating. All tests are performed for both hands.

To assess: *Heel-to-shin test* (1) Ask the patient to run his/her heel down the shin, alternately first with one leg and then the other; ask the patient to point to the examiner's hand with each big toe, and to make a "figure 8" in the air with each foot.

Observe whether the movements are executed accurately, smoothly, and without tremor or ataxia (wide-based staggering), which suggests cerebellar or dorsal column disorder. The rapidity of performance should be observed. Not all of the tests described need to be performed to assess cerebellar function. A test of upper extremity performance and one of lower extremity performance may be sufficient in screening examination.

### Reflexes

Reflex activity underlies virtually everything we do. Assessment of reflexes helps to localize lesions of the nervous system. In the patient with an altered state of consciousness, brainstem and autonomic reflexes provide critical clues to the status of protective reflexes (i.e., cough, gag, epiglottal closure) and the need to safeguard the airway. (See following section.) Spinal reflexes that remain intact can be used as the basis to attain autonomic control of bladder and bowel function in patients sustaining acute spinal cord injury (See Chap. 12.) (See Fig. 6-16 for a schematic depiction of a reflex arc.)

Major categories of reflexes include the stretch or deep tendon reflexes (DTR), cutaneous or superficial reflexes, and brainstem reflexes.

**Deep Tendon Reflexes (DTR).** To assess: Elicit a reflex response by briskly striking a muscle or tendon (use a reflex hammer), which stimulates the muscle spindle stretch receptors. The expected motor response to this stretch stimulus is an action to reduce the stretch (i.e., contraction of the appropriate muscles). The presence of muscle stretch indicates that all components of the reflex arc are intact. Table 7-4 lists the important deep tendon reflexes and their assessment. A scale of 0 to 4 is used to quantify the degree of the reflex (0 = absent; 1 = present but diminished; 2 = normal; 3 = increased, but not pathologic; 4 = markedly hyperactive).

**Cutaneous or Superficial Reflexes.** To assess: Stroke skin with a moderately sharp object (but not sharp enough to break the skin), and observe response of related muscles. These reflexes have reflex arcs wherein the sensory receptors are in the skin rather than in muscle fibers. Examples of important cutaneous or superficial reflexes and their assessment are listed in Table 7-5.

**Brainstem Reflexes.** Most brainstem reflexes are tested in the routine examination of the cranial nerves. (See section entitled "Cranial Nerve Function.") Familiarity with the level of the reflex arcs and the cranial nerves involved is helpful in evaluating brainstem function. Table 7-6 lists some of the important brainstem reflexes, their assessment, and the cranial nerves involved in the reflex arcs.

### Pathologic Reflexes

***Babinski's Sign.*** To assess: Elicit reflex by briskly stroking lateral aspect of the sole and across the ball of the foot using a semi-sharp object (e.g., car key). A normal response is plantar flexion of the toes. An abnormal response (i.e., Babinski's sign) is dorsiflexion of the big toe, with or without fanning of the other toes (Fig. 7-1). The presence of Babinski's sign reflects corticospinal tract dysfunction.

TABLE 7-4
**Deep Tendon Reflexes**

| Reflex | Elicited by | Normal Response | Spinal Cord Segment |
|---|---|---|---|
| Biceps | Tapping biceps tendon | Flexion at elbow | Cervical 5 and 6 |
| Triceps | Tapping triceps tendon | Extension at elbow | Cervical 6, 7, and 8 |
| Brachioradialis | Tapping styloid process of radius | Flexion of elbow and pronation of forearm | Cervical 5 and 6 |
| Patellar (knee jerk) | Tapping patellar tendon | Extension at knee | Lumbar 2, 3, and 4 |
| Achilles | Tapping Achilles tendon | Plantor flexion of foot | Sacral 1 and 2 |

TABLE 7-5
**Cutaneous or Superficial Reflexes**

| Reflex | Elicited by | Normal Response | Spinal Cord Segment |
|---|---|---|---|
| Epigastric | Stroking downard from nipples | Dimpling of epigastrium on the side stimulated | Thoracic 7 to 9 |
| Abdominal | | | |
| Upper | Stroking skin over lower costal margins toward midline | Umbilicus moves up and toward area being stroked | Thoracic 7 to 9 |
| Midabdominal | Stroking laterally from flanks to midline at umbilicus | Umbilicus moves toward side being stroked | Thoracic 9 to 11 |
| Lower | Stroking from iliac crests toward the midline | Umbilicus moves down and toward side being stroked | Thoracic 11 and 12 |
| Cremasteric | Stroking medial surface of upper thigh | Ipsilateral elevation of testicle | Thoracic 12 and Lumbar 1 |
| Gluteal | Stroking skin of buttocks | Skin tenses at gluteal area | Lumbar 4 and 5 |
| Plantar | Scratch sole of foot on lateral surface from heel to toes | Plantar flexion of toes | Lumbar 4 and 5 |
| Bulbocavernous | Pinching dorsum of glans | Tensing of bulbous urethra | Sacral 3 and 4 |
| Superficial anal | Pricking perineum | Tensing of external anal sphincter | Sacral 4 and 5, Coccygeal |

***Signs of Meningeal Irritation***

1. *Nuchal rigidity:* The patient is unable to flex chin on chest. Passive flexion of the neck is limited by involuntary muscle spasm.
2. *Spinal rigidity:* Spasms of spinal muscles (erector spinae) limit movement of the spine. *Opisthotonos* is a condition of extreme spasm (tetanic contraction) producing rigid hyperextension of the entire spine; the head is forced backwards and the trunk is thrust forward.
3. *Kernig's sign:* With the patient supine, passively flex the patient's hip to 90 degrees while also flexing the patient's knee to 90 degrees. While maintaining the hip in the flexed position, attempt to extend the patient's knee. Production of pain in the hamstrings and resistance to further extension are reliable signs of meningeal irritation. This response may also occur with herniated disk or tumors of the cauda equina (see Fig. 6-17).
4. *Brudzinski's sign:* With the patient supine and

TABLE 7-6
**Brainstem Reflexes**

| Reflexes | Elicited by | Normal Response | Cranial Nerves/ Reflex Arcs |
|---|---|---|---|
| ***Pupillary*** | | | |
| Direct reaction | Shine bright light into eye | Pupillary constriction of ipsilateral eye | Afferent: II<br>Efferent: III |
| Consensual reaction | Shine bright light into eye | Pupillary constriction of contralateral eye | Afferent: II<br>Efferent: III |
| Pupillary constriction—response via parasympathetic fibers of III | | | |
| Pupillary dilation—response via sympathetic fibers Cervical 8, Thoracic 1 and 2 | | | |
| ***Corneal*** | Touching cornea with a wisp of cotton | Blinking of eyelids | Afferent: II, V<br>Efferent: III |
| ***Reflex Eye Movements*** | | | |
| Oculocephalic (doll's eye) | Holding both eyelids open, briskly rotate head first to one side, and then to the other | Conjugate eye deviation: if head is turned to left, eyes linger with deviation to right | Afferent: VIII<br>Efferent: III, VI |
| Oculovestibular (caloric stimulation) | Introduction of ice water into ear canal | Nystagmus with slow component toward irrigated ear and fast component away from irrigated ear | Afferent: VIII<br>Efferent: III, VI |
| ***Pharyngeal*** | | | |
| Gag | Stroking the pharynx | | Afferent: V, IX, X<br>Efferent: IX, X |
| Swallowing (pharyngeal stage) | Voluntary movement of food to posterior pharynx | | Afferent: V, IX<br>Efferent: V, IX, X |

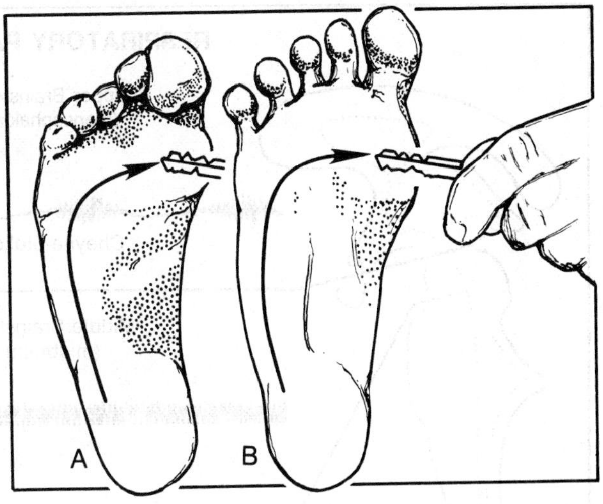


**Figure 7-1.** Plantar reflex elicited as indicated. *(A)* Normal response is the plantar flexion of the toes. *(B)* Abnormal response (i.e., the Babinski's sign) is dorsiflexion of the big toe, with or without fanning of the other toes.

the limbs extended, passively flex the patient's neck. Involuntary flexion of the hip and knees is a positive sign of meningeal irritation.

### *Assessment of Motor Function: Autonomic Division*

**Patient with Altered Level of Consciousness.** Evaluation as to the level of brain function in the patient with an altered state of consciousness is essential to localize (i.e., establish level of) the lesion, and to determine the direction in which the pathologic process is evolving. Such evaluation depends on the ongoing assessment of reflex responses and autonomic functions. Physiologic parameters assessed include the level of consciousness, vital signs (e.g., blood pressure, heart rate, body temperature), respiratory pattern, size and reactivity of pupils, ocular movements, and postural motor responses. Assessment of the level of consciousness, including the use of the Gasgow Coma Scale, was discussed previously in the section entitled "General Cerebral Functions." The other parameters are discussed here.

***Vital Signs.*** Cardiovascular functions, including systemic blood pressure and heart rate, are controlled by the vasomotor center in the lower pons and upper medulla. These parameters are regulated to ensure a cerebral perfusion pressure sufficient to satisfy the metabolic needs of fragile brain tissue. Ongoing assessment of mean arterial pressure is especially important in this regard. Dysrhythmias associated with structural changes (e.g., compression of brainstem), or metabolic disturbances (e.g., blood gas alterations) commonly occur, requiring close monitoring of heart rate and rhythm.

One must be cautioned about overreliance on vital signs, especially in patients at risk of developing an increase in intracranial pressure with potential brain herniation (e.g., severe head injury). An increase in systolic blood pressure, widening pulse pressure, slow bounding pulse, and alterations in respiratory pattern (Cushing reflex) signal a grave prognosis. It must be emphasized that these signs are *late* findings. They are associated with compression of vital centers in the lower brainstem and occur too late to prevent herniation and irreversible brain damage. In this clinical circumstance early initiation of intracranial pressure monitoring is essential (see Chap. 8).

Changes in body temperature significantly affect neurologic function. An increase in body temperature increases the metabolic requirements of neural tissue. *Hyperpyrexia* may reflect pathology involving the hypothalamus, or it may be indicative of infection in another part of the body. Measures should be implemented to maintain body temperature within the normal range. Hypothermia may be initiated as a therapeutic modality.

Major factors influencing cerebral blood flow (presented in Table 6-7) must be considered in the neurologic assessment.

***Respiratory Patterns.*** Plum and Posner define breathing as a "sensorimotor act integrated by nervous influences that arise from nearly every level of the brain and upper spinal cord."[7] Regulation of breathing is an interplay of metabolic and neurogenic factors occurring at these various levels. The significance of this dual control mechanism is that pathology predisposing to the altered state of consciousness may involve structural lesions and/or metabolic disturbances, and frequently an overlapping of both.

In the patient with an altered state of consciousness, specific patterns of breathing may signify a change in the patient's status and may have localizing features reflecting the level of brain function.

*Cheyne-Stokes Respiration.* This is one of the most common and often earliest abnormal patterns

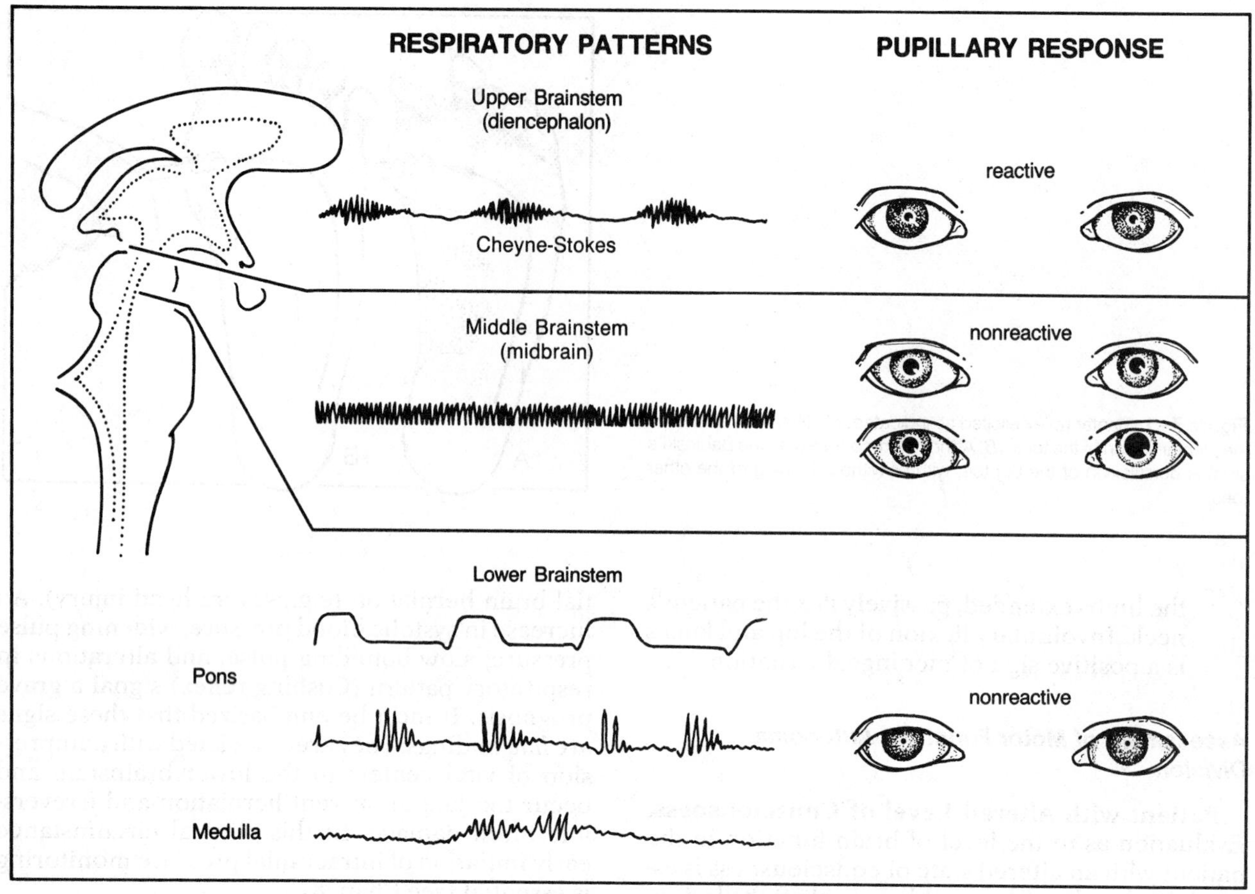


**Figure 7-2.** The presence of abnormal respiratory patterns and pupillary responses in the patient with an altered state of consciousness assists in localizing the level of brainstem function and/or signifying changes in the patient's underlying status.

of breathing. It reflects the presence of bilateral deep hemispheric or diencephalic lesions (upper brainstem). It is characterized by a periodic pattern of breathing in which respiratory excursion waxes and wanes, with phases of hyperpnea alternating with apnea. There is a characteristic pattern of crescendo-decrescendo breathing followed by a period of apnea (Fig. 7-2).

During the hyperpneic phase an abnormally increased ventilatory response to carbon dioxide stimulation occurs, reducing the carbon dioxide stimulus (metabolic). Apnea results and is maintained because of the abnormally decreased ventilatory stimulus (neurogenic). The stimulation to respiration does not return until there is sufficient accumulation of carbon dioxide to trigger chemoreceptors and initiate the next cycle.

*Central Neurogenic Hyperventilation.* This pattern reflects brainstem function at the level of the midbrain (see Fig. 6-12). It is characterized by a pattern of deep, rapid, and sustained hyperpnea, with consequent hypocapnia (i.e., an abnormally low tension of carbon dioxide in circulating blood) (see Fig. 7-2). The diagnosis of central neurogenic hyperventilation is made in the clinical scenario of a high respiratory rate (25-40/minute), accompanied by arterial blood gas values indicating an elevated $PaO_2$ (i.e., oxygen tension in circulating blood), and a lowered $PaCO_2$ (i.e., carbon dioxide tension in circulating blood), with commensurate elevated blood pH, in a patient breathing room air. The underlying pathophysiology suggests that there is an abnormally low threshold for stimulation by carbon dioxide.

*Apneustic Breathing.* The characteristic feature of this pattern is the long pause that occurs at full inspiration. The apneustic center occurs in the lower pons and is not very well defined.[8] Impulses generated here attempt to prevent turn-off of inspiration. Normally, these signals are overridden by those of the pneumotaxic center, which functions to limit inspiration. If impulses from the pneumotaxic center are interrupted, signals from the apneustic center are unopposed, resulting in a sustained inspiratory breathing pattern. Thus, apneustic breathing can be a very valuable localizing sign in terms of the level of brain function (see Fig. 7-2).

*Cluster Breathing.* This pattern is associated with lesions of the pons. It is described as clusters of breaths occurring in a disorderly sequence with irregular pauses between each cluster. Onset of this type of breathing signals the occurrence of brain herniation (see Chap. 8).

*Ataxic Breathing (Biot's Respirations).* This breathing pattern reflects a depth and rate of breathing that are completely irregular and random, often slow with periods of apnea. There is loss of the "to-and-fro" pattern of breathing suggestive of involvement of the reticular formation at the level of the medulla. It differs from Cheyne-Stokes respirations in terms of its irregularity. Lesions in the posterior fossa (cerebellum), particularly rapidly expanding lesions (e.g., cerebellar or pontine hemorrhage), may precipitate this type of breathing. Complete respiratory assistance is initiated as alveolar ventilation becomes compromised.

***Protective Reflexes.*** An important component of the respiratory assessment in the patient with an altered state of consciousness is an evaluation of the status of the *protective* reflexes (e.g., cough, gag, epiglottal closure). Innervation of these reflexes occurs via neurons located in the "respiratory centers" of the pons and medulla. Loss of these reflexes presents an imminent threat to life with loss of airway and respiratory arrest. Immediate intubation, with initiation of mechanical ventilation, is imperative. Efforts also need to be taken to prevent aspiration of secretions. Serial arterial blood gas studies assist in assessing the effectiveness of the ventilatory effort.

***Pupillary Size and Reactivity.*** Pupillary size and reactivity to light provide key information related to structural disturbances of the diencephalon, midbrain, and pons. Such information is significant because areas of the brainstem controlling arousal (reticular activating system) lie adjacent to those areas controlling pupillary activity. Consequently, evaluating pupillary changes provides a guide to localizing brainstem lesions causing coma and/or determining the level of brainstem function.

Of critical importance is the circuitry of autonomic fibers to each eye. Innervation of the eye by parasympathetic and sympathetic fibers occurs over separate and distinct pathways, which assist in localizing lesions and determining the level of brain function. Parasympathetic fibers arise within the Edinger-Westphal nucleus located at the midbrain. These fibers leave the midbrain along with the oculomotor nerve (III) at a point adjacent to the *tentorial notch* (i.e., the opening in the meningeal fold, the falx tentorium, which accommodates the brainstem). (See Fig. 6–6.) From here the third nerve and parasympathetic fibers proceed directly to the orbit.

Sympathetic fibers arise from nuclei in the hypothalamus and descend through the brainstem as *pre*ganglionic fibers to the lower cervical/upper thoracic spinal cord segments. Upon synapsing in the sympathetic ganglia, *post*ganglionic fibers ascend along with the internal carotid artery, eventually to reach the orbit.

Parasympathetic innervation to the eye stimulates contraction of the pupilloconstrictor muscle fibers of the iris, and the pupil becomes smaller *(miosis)*. Sympathetic innervation stimulates contraction of the pupillodilator muscle fibers of the iris, and the pupil becomes larger *(mydriasis)* (see Table 6–11). Both systems are continually active, and the resulting pupillary size reflects a balance between these two innervations.

If either the parasympathetic or sympathetic pathway is disrupted, the activity of the unopposed system becomes maximally expressed. Thus, altered sympathetic innervation results in *pinpoint* pupils (1.5–2.5 mm); altered parasympathetic innervation causes widely *dilated* pupils (8–9 mm). If innervation from both systems is disrupted, pupils become mid-sized (4–5 mm) and react sluggishly or become unreactive to light stimulus (i.e., fixed).

***Pathologic Pupillary Responses.*** A variety of abnormal pupillary responses can occur depending on the underlying pathophysiology. The localizing implications of pupillary abnormalities, in terms of levels of brain function in the patient with an altered level of consciousness, have been well documented by Plum and Posner.[9] Bilateral pressure applied to the diencephalon and upper brainstem during early rostral to caudal (i.e., head to toe) deterioration in brain function produces symmetrically constricted pupils, but the light reflex remains intact (see Fig. 7–2).

In this instance, it is also important to appreciate that metabolic disturbances can result in similar pupillary responses. Plum and Posner suggest that "because pupillary pathways are relatively resistant to metabolic insult, the presence or absence of the light reflex is the single most important physical sign potentially distinguishing structural from metabolic coma." In coma precipitated by metabolic disturbances, the pupils retain the light reflex.

Midbrain involvement is reflected in some definitive pupillary abnormalities. Midposition (4–5 mm) fixed (i.e., unreactive) pupils that are frequently unequal and slightly irregular in shape are caused by midbrain lesions, which interrupt both parasympathetic and sympathetic innervation of the eye (e.g., in transtentorial herniation, midbrain hemorrhages or infarctions, or tumors).

A dilated ("blown") (8–9 mm) pupil, which reacts sluggishly or is fixed, occurs with unilateral compression of the oculomotor nerve where it leaves the midbrain at the tentorial notch. The consequent compression of parasympathetic fibers interrupts stimulation to the eye on the same side. This results in unopposed sympathetic stimulation and, thus, the "blown" pupil (see Fig. 7–2). A unilateral fixed and dilated pupil in the patient at risk of developing an increase in intracranial pressure (e.g., acute head injury) indicates that brain herniation is occurring. This constitutes a *neurologic emergency* requiring immediate and aggressive treatment if compression of vital centers within the pons and medulla is to be averted.

Lesions of the pons may interrupt sympathetic pathways that descend through the brainstem to the spinal cord before ascending to the orbit. Pupils in this circumstance are *pinpoint* due to unopposed parasympathetic innervation, and they may be reactive (see Fig. 7-2).

Anoxia and ischemia (cardiac arrest) usually cause widely dilated fixed pupils. Anoxic pupillary dilation lasting longer than a few minutes yields a very grave prognosis, usually of irreversible brain damage.

***Ocular Movements.*** Ocular movements are controlled by brainstem structures; thus, evaluation of these motor responses may help determine the level of brainstem function in the patient with an altered state of consciousness.

Extraocular movements involve three cranial nerves: oculomotor (III), trochlear (IV), and abducens (VI). (See section entitled "Cranial Nerve Function.") While the patient with an altered state of consciousness is unable to cooperate in the examination of these nerves, if the brainstem is intact, spontaneous roving eye movements should be *conjugate* (i.e., both eyes move together so that only one image is perceived), and they cover the full range of gaze.

*Reflex Eye Movements.* Reflex eye movements include the oculocephalic and oculovestibular reflexes. The reflex arc for both of these reflexes involves the following cranial nerves: acoustic (vestibulocochlear; VIII) as the afferent limb and the oculomotor (III) and abducens (VI) as the efferent limb. Abnormal reflex eye movements indicate brainstem dysfunction below the midbrain (see Fig. 6-12).

1. *Oculocephalic reflex (doll's eye phenomenon).* To assess: Hold the comatose patient's eyelids open, and briskly rotate the patient's head horizontally, first to one side, and then to the other from the midline. Observe the position of the eyes in relation to the head. The normal response is for the eyes initially to move in the direction opposite to the head turning, and then, within a few seconds, to move back to midline. If the reflex is not functioning, the eyes will move with the head as though painted on or fixed in place. Likewise, if the head is moved up and down vertically, the eyes will normally linger in the position opposite to the direction in which the head is moved. Pupils that move in the same direction as the head, as though painted on, are abnormal (Fig. 7-3). All tests for reflex eye movements should be deferred until x-rays rule out cervical spinal injury.

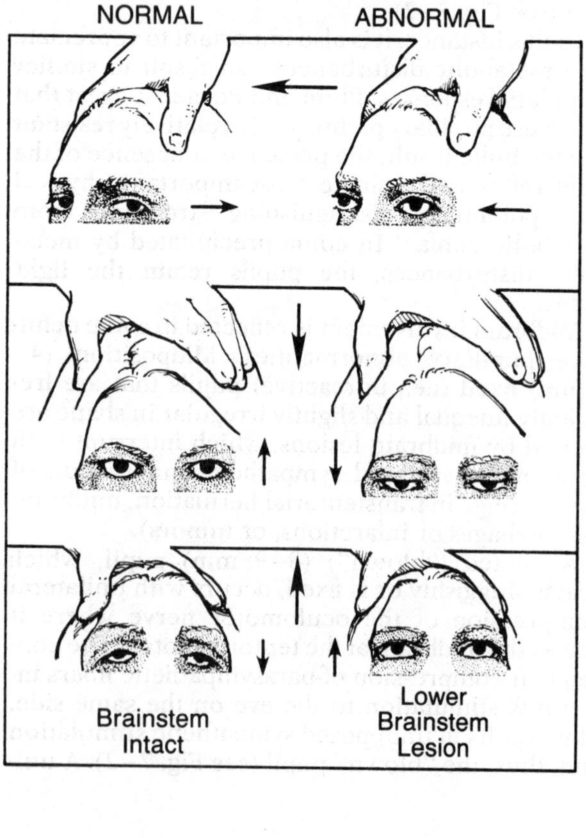


**Figure 7-3.** Oculocephalic reflex (doll's eye phenomenon).

Assessment of *horizontal* ocular movement: Normal response—With eyelids held open, the eyes should be observed initially to linger in the *opposite* direction to which the head is turned, eventually to return to the midline. Abnormal response—the eyes are observed to move in the *same* direction in which the head is turned. Both directions should be tested.

Assessment of *vertical* ocular movement. Head flexed (i.e., chin to chest): Normal response—The eyes will linger in the *opposite* direction in which the head is moved (i.e., looking up). Abnormal response—the eyes are observed to look downward in the *same* direction in which the head is moved.

Head hyperextended (i.e., facing the ceiling): Normal response—The eyes are observed to linger in a downward gaze in *opposite* direction to which the head is moved. Abnormal response—the eyes are observed to move in the *same* direction in which the head is moved (i.e., looking up at the ceiling).

2. *Oculovestibular reflex.* To assess: The *caloric stimulation* test is used to evaluate the oculovestibular reflex. The auditory canal is examined carefully before the test is performed to ensure that the tympanic membrane is intact. The head is raised to about 30 degrees, and up to 120 ml of ice water is slowly introduced into the auditory canal of the compromised patient. In the normal response (intact brainstem), the eyes will exhibit a horizontal nystagmus with the slow conjugate component moving toward the irrigated ear and the rapid component moving away from the irrigated ear.

The oculovestibular reflex is significant in that it may be preserved somewhat longer than the oculocephalic reflex in the presence of brainstem pathology. These tests should never be performed in a patient with possible cervical spine injury. These tests are included with other brainstem reflexes in Table 7–6.

***Postural Responses.*** Motor function in patients with an altered level of consciousness can be assessed by applying a noxious stimulus (e.g., pressure on fingertip, supraorbital pressure, or compression of sternum) and observing the response. One of 3 patterns of movement may be evoked in response to such stimuli: appropriate, inappropriate, or flaccidity.

*Appropriate* responses include purposeful movement to push the stimulus away, or the withdrawal of the limb. A facial grimace or groan may accompany the motor response. Such responses imply the presence of functioning sensory pathways and intact or partially intact descending motor pathways (corticospinal tracts).

*Inappropriate* motor responses include flexor spasms and extensor spasms. The pattern of these abnormal responses varies according to the site and severity of brain involvement. An abnormal *flexor* response in the arm with extension of the leg is often referred to as *decorticate* posturing or rigidity. When fully developed, this response is characterized by flexion of the arm, wrist, and fingers, with adduction in the upper extremity (Fig. 7–4). There are extension, internal rotation, and vigorous plantar flexion of the lower extremity. This reflects a lesion in the cerebral hemisphere, basal ganglia, and/or diencephalon, which interrupts corticospinal pathways.

Abnormal *extensor* responses in upper and lower extremities is termed *decerebrate* posturing or rigidity. When fully developed, this response is characterized by stiffly extended, adducted, and hyperpronated arms (see Fig. 7–4); and stiffly extended legs with the feet plantar flexed. Frequently, the patient is also opisthotonic with clenched teeth.

*Flaccidity* suggests an absence of motor activity and reflects dysfunction of central motor mechanisms in the pontine reticular formation or, possibly, peripheral denervation.

Clinically, the examination of motor function in the patient with an altered state of consciousness provides valuable information as to the level of the lesion and may serve as a guide to the progress of the illness. Abnormal flexor and extensor responses can shift back and forth from one combination to the other. Decerebrate posturing carries with it a more ominous prognosis. Its appearance during the course of rostral-caudal (head to toe) deterioration in brain function, as diencephalic dysfunction (decorticate) evolves into the stage of midbrain

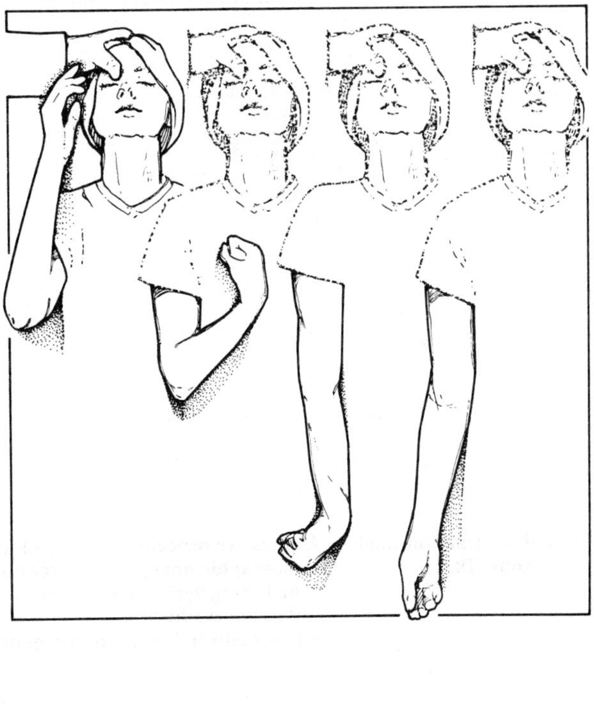

**Figure 7–4.** Motor responses to a painful stimulus (e.g., supraorbital pressure) in the patient with an altered state of consciousness. Appropriate response is to push the stimulus away; inappropriate responses include abnormal flexor response, abnormal extensor response, and flaccidity. These responses reflect varying degrees of responsiveness decreasing from left to right.

TABLE 7–7
**Diagnostic Studies and Procedures for Neurologic Dysfunction**

| Test | Description/Purpose | Clinical Significance/Nursing Implications |
|---|---|---|
| ***Lumbar Puncture*** | Performed to: (1) Measure CSF pressure (normally 50–200 $cmH_2O$). Opening CSF pressure relatively equivalent to intracranial pressure in most patients.<br>(2) Sample CSF (normal constituents listed in Table 6–3).<br>(3) Inject medication or contrast media.<br>*Procedure:* A hollow needle is inserted into subarachnoid space at lumbar 3-4 or lumbar 4-5 spinal segment. | *Patient preparation:* Explain the purpose of test and procedure involved; position to be assumed (side-lying position with head and knees maximally flexed); need to avoid sudden movement or coughing; expectations about what the patient may expect to feel during and after procedure.<br>*Post-procedure care:* Patient is advised to remain flat for 8–10 hours to prevent headache; fluids are encouraged.<br>• Clinically, presence of blood in CSF may indicate subarachnoid hemorrhage, brain laceration.<br>• CSF glucose level approximately two-thirds that of serum glucose; a blood sugar should be drawn in conjunction with lumbar puncture.<br>• *Contraindications:* Patients with incipient brain herniation and/or posterior fossa lesions; acute head injury. |
| Queckenstedt test | Performed to detect subarachnoid obstruction (e.g., spinal tumor; vertebral compression fracture).<br>• Performed in conjunction with lumbar puncture; involves manual compression of jugular veins for about 10 seconds. | Normally a rapid rise in CSF pressure occurs during compression, with a rapid fall to normal upon release. |
| ***Radiology Studies*** | | |
| Skull x-rays | May reveal: skull fractures or abnormalities of cranial vault; intracranial calcification; dense vascular markings; presence of tumor or congenital anomaly; possible detection of an increase in intracranial pressure. | *Patient preparation:* Explain purpose of test and procedure involved including the need for several different radiologic views; emphasize that the procedure is painless with minimal exposure to radiation; remove all hair pins, jewelry, or other metal objects. |
| Spine x-rays | Used to identify vertebral fracture or dislocation, which may be impinging on the spinal cord or its nerve roots. | Same as above. |
| ***Contrast Studies*** | | |
| Cerebral angiography | An invasive procedure requiring the injection of radiopaque dye into the cerebral circulation via the carotid or vertebral arteries (also via femoral or brachial), during which time serial radiographs are taken.<br>• Useful in the diagnosis of abnormalities of cerebral vasculature; or findings obtained by CAT scan or radionuclide studies. | *Patient preparation:* Requires thorough explanations to patient/family regarding indications and expectations of the procedure (i.e. insertion site, warm flush feeling when contrast is injected, post-procedure care).<br>• It is essential to establish if patient has had previous allergic reaction to contrast media or if the patient is allergic to iodine-containing foods or medications; or if patient is taking anticoagulant (if so, why?).<br>• Patient should be well hydrated to facilitate elimination of dye via kidneys.<br>*Post-procedure care:* Monitor every 15 to 30 minutes until stable; assess for bleeding, swelling, or redness at insertion site; assess extremity distal to insertion site for signs of altered circulation caused by vessel spasm or occlusion (skin color, temperature, and peripheral pulses).<br>• Encourage fluids to flush out contrast media.<br>• *Complications:* Dysrhythmia, allergic reaction to contrast medium, bleeding at insertion site, infection.<br>• Clinically: Confirm presence of cerebrovascular abnormalities including aneurysm, arteriovenous malformations, vessel thrombosis, stenosis, or occlusion; alteration in blood flow characteristic of arteriovenous malformation, or associated with tumor; and vascular changes associated with hematoma formation, cyst, edema, herniation, and arterial spasm. |
| Digital subtraction angiography (DSA) | An invasive procedure that produces enhanced radiographic images of extracranial vasculature including vessel size; patency and degree of stenosis or occlusion.<br>• Especially indicated in studies of carotid or renal | See patient preparation above. Make necessary explanations regarding procedure; patient should understand the need to remain motionless while radiographs are being taken.<br>• Ascertain history of previous contrast studies |

TABLE 7–7
## Diagnostic Studies and Procedures for Neurologic Dysfunction *(Continued)*

| Test | Description/Purpose | Clinical Significance/Nursing Implications |
|---|---|---|
| | artery disease, thrombotic or embolic disease of great vessels, and in detection of aneurysms and other vascular abnormalities.<br>• Uses a computer system in combination with a fluoroscopy apparatus capable of intensifying images.<br>• Computer converts images into digital form and "subtracts" data compiled on plain radiography from that compiled on contrast radiographs after injection of contrast dye. | and any reaction to contrast dye used; or allergies to foods or drugs; what other medications is the patient taking and why? Patient should be well hydrated.<br>*Post-procedure care and complications:* See cerebral angiography, above. |
| Myelography | An invasive procedure involving injection of contrast dye or air via puncture into spinal subarachnoid space followed by fluoroscopic or serial radiographic study. | *Procedure and preparation:* See lumbar puncture; above.<br>*Post-procedure care:* Depending on contrast medium used, the patient may be advised to lie flat or with head slightly elevated for several hours. If a water-soluble medium is used (e.g., metrizamide) the patient's head is elevated 30 degrees for about 8 hours. The head elevation prevents the contrast medium from irritating cerebral cortex. It is absorbed into the bloodstream and eventually excreted by the kidneys.<br>• Clinically, reveals distortions of spinal cord, spinal meninges, or intervertebral disks. Used to detect suspected spinal lesions such as tumors, cysts, herniated disks, or other lesions that may partially or totally block CSF circulation. |
| ***Computerized Axial Tomography*** | | |
| CAT scan (CT scan) | This study may be noninvasive or invasive (intravenous injection of contrast medium). It permits rapid, detailed screening for hematomas or other traumatic lesions, with minimum exposure to radiation.<br>• A computerized picture is derived from the scanning of successive layers by a narrow x-ray beam. It provides a cross-sectional view of the brain, distinguishing densities. Lesions appear as variations in tissue density, differing from normal tissue. | *Patient preparation:* Explain the purpose of the test, procedure involved, and expectations of the patient. It is important for the patient to remain motionless during the procedure. Sedation should be administered if necessary.<br>• If contrast dye is to be injected, screen for possible allergies (drug or food).<br>• Encourage fluids if contrast dye is used.<br>• Clinically, CAT scan plays a strategic role in the *initial* diagnosis of most intracranial or spinal abnormalities, including neoplastic or vascular lesions; intracerebral hemorrhage or hematoma formation; hydrocephalus; ventricular anomalies; brain infection; or abscess. Use of contrast dye helps to define abnormalities. |
| ***Nuclear Medicine Tests*** | | |
| Brain scan | This study employs a technique involving the intravenous administration of a radionuclide. The gamma rays emitted by the radionuclide are then detected by a scanner, which converts them into images and displays them on a screen.<br>• The final image reflects the uptake and distribution of the radionuclide. Any alteration in the blood–brain barrier enables the radionuclide to accumulate in the affected area.<br>• This study assists in locating areas of ischemia, infarction, hematoma, intracerebral hemorrhage, and tumors. In these areas there is an increase in radionuclide uptake.<br>• Evidence of brain abscess or infection is indicated by a decreased uptake of the radionuclide. | *Patient preparation:* Explain purpose of the test and procedure involved. Assure patient that the amount of radionuclide administered is small, and that it has a very short half-life, so there is a minimal hazard of radiation.<br>• Determine whether patient has any allergies.<br>• Clinically, this study is used to locate intracranial masses, vascular lesions, brain abscess, or communicating low pressure hydrocephalus. It may also confirm the presence of a CSF leak in basal skull fractures. |
| Positron-emission tomography (PET) | This technique maps the brain's metabolic activity produced by the interaction of an injected radioactively-tagged biochemical (e.g., glucose or oxygen) and charged electrons in the brain. The biochemical is administered intravenously or via inhalation. A scanner detects the tissue uptake of the radioactive substance, and a computer produces a color composite indicating distribution of the radioactive material corresponding to cellular metabolism and cerebral blood flow. | *Patient preparation:* Same as for brain scan, above.<br>• Clinically, this study provides a measure of metabolism and cerebral blood flow; it may also detect structural abnormalities (e.g., vascular disorders, tumors); or it can be used to investigate behavioral abnormalities that have a possible physiologic basis (e.g., schizophrenia).<br>• This study is unlike x-rays and CAT scans in that it shows how the organ is functioning. |

*(continued)*

TABLE 7-7

**Diagnostic Studies and Procedures for Neurologic Dysfunction *(Continued)***

| Test | Description/Purpose | Clinical Significance/Nursing Implications |
|---|---|---|
| ***Nuclear Medicine Tests*** | | |
| Magnetic resonance imaging (MRI) | A noninvasive procedure that provides greater tissue discrimination without the risk of ionizing radiation.<br>• This method uses two kinds of magnetism rather than x-rays. The patient is placed within a giant magnetic field, which aligns protons of hydrogen ions in body cells. Following burst of radiofrequency magnetism, the protons realign, and the resulting change in the magnetic field is processed by a computer. | *Procedure:* See Chapter 39.<br>*Patient preparation:* Explain purpose of test, procedure involved, and expectations of patient.<br>• All metal objects must be removed from the patient's body; the procedure is contraindicated in patients with previous surgery where metal hemostatic or aneurysm clips were inserted. This test is contraindicated in patients with pacemakers.<br>• MRI is useful in evaluating cerebral edema, hemorrhage, infarction, bone lesions, and blood vessels.<br>• Risk factors for this new technique are not well defined.<br>• Clinically, this test may also be helpful in detecting small lesions or differentiating between healthy and ischemic or infarcted tissues. |
| ***Electrophysiologic Tests*** | | |
| Electroencephalogram (EEG) | In this study, electrodes applied to the scalp produce a graphic recording of the electrical impulses generated within the cerebral cortex.<br>• This study is used to diagnose areas of abnormal electrical activity within the cerebral cortex. | *Patient preparation:* Explain purpose of tests, procedure involved, and expectations of patient. Emphasize that the patient will not experience an electrical shock.<br>• Patient's scalp should be clean and free of hairspray or creams.<br>• If the procedure is done at bedside, electrical devices surrounding the patient should be removed, if possible, to minimize electrical interference.<br>• Clinically, this procedure is helpful in the diagnosis and management of seizure disorders; localization of structural abnormalities (e.g., tumors, abscesses, vascular anomalies); and investigation of metabolic alterations and sleep disturbances.<br>• This procedure is also used in organic brain syndrome, coma, and brain death to detect characteristic patterns of electrical activity or the absence of electrical activity. |
| Cortical evoked potentials | These studies measure the electrical potential or activity that occurs along specific neuronal pathways in response to visual, auditory, or somatosensory (tactile) stimuli. By measuring such potentials, the integrity of visual, auditory, and somatosensory pathways can be evaluated.<br>• This technique uses a special device, which senses cerebral cortical electrical activity via surface electrodes attached to standard sites. These potentials, evoked in response to specific stimuli, are then intensified by a computer and graphically displayed for accurate measurement. | *Patient preparation:* Tests can be performed at patient's bedside on conscious or unconscious patients. If conscious, patients need to be instructed to remain motionless as much as possible to minimize interference of musculoskeletal-derived electrical potentials. Skin or hair should be clean and free of oils, creams, or hairspray.<br>• Depending on modality being tested, the patient can expect to receive a series of stimuli, such as flashing lights or a pattern of identifiable shapes (visual), clicking sounds delivered to the ear (auditory), or electrical stimulation of the skin (tactile-somatosensory).<br>• The patient should be assured that no electrical shock or pain will be experienced.<br>Clinically:<br>• Visual evoked potentials (responses): Assist in evaluating post-traumatic injury.<br>• Auditory evoked potentials (responses): Assist in localizing auditory lesions and evaluating the integrity of the brainstem and the sequential auditory pathways located therein; useful in diagnosing posterior fossa lesions and multiple sclerosis; helpful in determining the reversibility of coma. |

TABLE 7-7
**Diagnostic Studies and Procedures for Neurologic Dysfunction *(Continued)***

| Test | Description/Purpose | Clinical Significance/Nursing Implications |
|---|---|---|
| ***Electrophysiologic Tests*** | | |
| | | • Somatosensory evoked potentials (responses): Assist in diagnosing peripheral nerve disease and lesions in the brain and spinal cord (e.g., demyelinating disease). Recordings are made via surface electrodes placed in the scalp overlying somesthetic cortical area (i.e., post-central gyrus, parietal lobe).<br>• All methods are useful in monitoring for neurologic injury before, during, and after surgery involving nerve tissue. |
| Electromyography (EMG) | This study records the electrical activity of select groups of muscles at rest and during voluntary contraction. It is useful in localizing lesions and differentiating primary disease of muscle fibers or neuromuscular junction from lower motor neuron disease.<br>• The test is not definitive as to underlying disease but assists in determining approach to more specific diagnostic workup. | *Patient preparation:* Explain purpose, of test, procedure, and expectations of the patient. Emphasize that the test is similar to an electrocardiogram except a needle will be inserted into specific muscle groups.<br>• Clinically, EMG is a useful diagnostic technique in muscular dystrophies, amyotrophic lateral sclerosis, myasthenia gravis, and peripheral denervation conditions. To differentiate muscle disorder from denervation disorders, it is necessary for results of EMG studies to be correlated with patient's history, clinical status, and other neurologic tests. |

dysfunction, may herald impending brain herniation.

In terms of documentation, it is more desirable to describe abnormal motor responses as abnormal flexor, abnormal extensor, or absent (flaccid), designating the specific limbs involved, rather than to use the terms decorticate or decerebrate.

## ANCILLARY DIAGNOSTIC STUDIES AND TECHNIQUES

The diagnosis of neurologic dysfunction initiated with the patient's history and neurologic examination can be verified by sophisticated diagnostic studies and techniques. Digital subtraction angiography, positron emission tomography, nuclear magnetic resonance (magnetic resonance imaging), and electrophysiology studies are major advances in neurodiagnostic testing.

Health-care professionals must familiarize themselves with these investigative techniques: What are they? How are they performed? What patient preparation is required? What is their clinical significance? Table 7-7 briefly summarizes new as well as precedent neurodiagnostic tests and procedures most commonly performed on critically ill patients with neurologic dysfunction, including some implications for nursing care.

## REFERENCES

1. Gordon, M: Nursing Diagnosis Process and Application, ed 2. McGraw-Hill, New York, 1987.
2. Jones, C: Glasgow Coma Scale. Am J Nurs 79(9):1551, 1979.
3. Brown, JD: Acute disturbances of consciousness. In Sibbald, WJ (ed): Synopsis of Critical Care, ed 3. Williams & Wilkins, Baltimore, 1988, p 163.
4. Mitchell, PH, et al: Neurological Assessment for Nursing Practice. Reston Publishing, Reston, Virginia, 1984, p 35.
5. Mitchell, PH, et al: Neurological Assessment for Nursing Practice. Reston Publishing, Reston, Virginia, 1984, pp 41, 58.
6. DeJong, RN, et al: Essentials of the Neurological Examination. Smith Kline Corporation, Philadelphia, 1979, pp 36-42.
7. Plum, F and Posner, J: The Diagnosis of Stupor and Coma, ed 3. FA Davis, Philadelphia, 1980, p 32.
8. Guyton, A: Textbook of Medical Physiology, ed 7. WB Saunders, Philadelphia, 1986, p 506.
9. Plum, F and Posner, J: The Diagnosis of Stupor and Coma, ed 3. FA Davis, Philadelphia, 1980, p 46.

## SUGGESTED READINGS

Nikas, DL: Neurologic assessment of altered states of consciousness, Part I. Focus on Critical Care 10(5):10, 1983.
Nikas, DL: Neurologic assessment of altered states of consciousness, Part II. Focus on Critical Care 10(6):10, 1983.
Nikas, DL: Neurologic assessment of altered states of consciousness, Part III. Focus on Critical Care 11(1):54, 1984

CHAPTER 8

# Nursing Management of the Patient with Intracranial Pressure Monitoring: Brain Herniation Syndrome

## CHAPTER OUTLINE



## LEARNING OBJECTIVES

**At the end of this chapter, you should be able to:**

1. State the purpose of intracranial pressure monitoring and indications for its use.
2. List clinical signs and symptoms of increased intracranial pressure.
3. Examine intracranial volume-pressure relationships and their clinical significance.
4. Describe methods for measuring intracranial pressure.
5. Analyze and interpret intracranial pressure waveforms and digital readouts in terms of intracranial volume-pressure dynamics.
6. Describe pathophysiologic mechanisms underlying the phenomenon of brain herniation.
7. Distinguish supratentorial and infratentorial herniations.
8. Contrast central herniation syndrome with uncal herniation syndrome of brain dysfunction.
9. Incorporate underlying physiologic principles into the nursing management of the patient with increased intracranial pressure.

## LEARNING OBJECTIVES—*CONTINUED*

10. Delineate the nursing process in the management of the patient with an increase in intracranial pressure including:
    Assessment
    Nursing diagnosis
    Planning: Desired patient outcomes
    Nursing interventions

# INTRACRANIAL PRESSURE MONITORING

## Purpose and Clinical Significance

Intracranial pressure is defined as the pressure within the intracranial cavity, which is exerted by the volumes of blood, cerebrospinal fluid, and brain parenchyma contained within the cavity. Intracranial pressure monitoring (ICPM) measures intracranial pressure. In the scenario of intracranial hypertension (i.e., an increase in intracranial pressure), such monitoring is clinically significant because changes detected during continuous monitoring of intracranial pressure reflect the status of intracranial pressure dynamics *early*, before such changes become clinically evident.

Under ordinary circumstances, compensatory and autoregulatory mechanisms maintain intracranial pressure within the normal range (0–15 mmHg). These mechanisms involve the interplay of forces generated within the cranial vault by the volumes of cerebrospinal fluid, blood, and brain tissue. (See Chap. 6 for further discussion of compensatory and regulatory mechanisms.)

Briefly, initial compensatory changes involve a reduction in the formation and secretion of cerebrospinal fluid and an increase in its reabsorption. The distensibility of the dura and the pliability of brain tissue also accommodate an increase in intracranial volume early on. The reciprocal relationship between the volumes of cerebrospinal fluid and blood within the cranial vault is a major compensatory mechanism. When the volume of one increases, the volume of the other decreases and, in so doing, maintains intracranial pressure within normal limits.

Autoregulatory mechanisms involve the intrinsic capacity of cerebral blood vessels to respond to changes in the brain's environment. The cerebral vasculature can maintain cerebral perfusion pressure, despite wide fluctuations in mean arterial blood pressure (>60 or <150 mmHg).

### *Signs and Symptoms of Increased Intracranial Pressure*

An increase in intracranial pressure may have adverse effects on cerebral structures and function. These include the mechanical deformation or shift of cerebral contents within the confines of the rigid cranial vault, and an alteration in cerebral blood flow. These underlying pathophysiologic phenomena create a decrease in cerebral perfusion pressure leading to ischemia and an alteration in cellular metabolism. Clinically, these changes are demonstrated by the appearance of a wide range of neurologic deficits, as well as systemic changes within the body as a whole.

Generalized signs and symptoms of increased intracranial pressure may include changes in the level of consciousness, memory loss, or alterations in thought processes. Nonspecific changes may include headache, nausea, vomiting, and diplopia (i.e., double vision). The patient may experience sensory loss and paresthesias; alterations in motor function may be exhibited by the presence of paresis or plegia. Changes in pupillary size and reactivity, alterations in body temperature, and seizure activity may also become evident. In a smaller sample of the population (about 20–30%), papilledema (i.e., edema of the optic disk) may be the only neurologic sign of underlying pathophysiology until intracranial pressure rises high enough to impair cerebral blood flow. When signs and symptoms occur, they usually do so only after pathologic changes have occurred. Their appearance does not definitively reflect the magnitude of the pressure elevation.

In addition to its effect on brain metabolism and function, intracranial hypertension has been implicated in the dysfunction of other major organ systems.[1] Gastrointestinal bleeding in conjunction with intracranial pathology is widely known. Ulceration may result from an increase in hydrochloric acid secretion and/or a disruption in the integrity of the gastric mucosal barrier. Although the precise role played by intracranial hypertension in the pathogenesis of the ulcerative process remains undefined, its potential occurrence in patients sustaining insults to the central nervous system underlies the importance of initiating early antacid therapy and/or use of histamine$_2$-receptor antagonists (e.g., ranitidine).

Changes in cardiopulmonary function associated with intracranial hypertension may include a variety of electrocardiographic abnormalities (e.g., T wave changes, ST segment elevation or depression, or the appearance of Q waves in both standard and precordial leads), as well as the appearance of cardiac dysrhythmias (e.g., bradycardia, atrial fibrillation). These changes have been associated with metabolic disturbances (e.g., hypercapnia, hypoxemia, hypokalemia) and with altered autonomic function (i.e., sympathetic and parasympathetic function).

Specific vasomotor reactions occurring in response to severely elevated intracranial pressure have been identified. The classic Cushing triad consists of elevated systolic blood pressure with widening pulse pressure (i.e., the difference between systolic and diastolic pressures), bradycardia, and altered respiratory rate and rhythm. These are *late* signs, which usually reflect the presence of irreversible brain pathology, and their appearance signals a grave prognosis. Thus, under these circumstances, a thorough and meticulous ongoing neurologic assessment is more important than the monitoring of vital signs or the Cushing triad, and assessment of overall body function is of the utmost urgency.

### *Uses of Intracranial Pressure Monitoring*

Continuous ICPM is used to facilitate: (1) early diagnosis via the assessment of intracranial pressure dynamics, and (2) treatment, including timely initiation of pressure-reducing measures and evaluation of the patient's response to these therapeutic measures. Timely intervention afforded by ICPM may improve prognosis as reflected by retained and potential function and reduced residual sequelae. ICPM serves as a guide for nursing care so that sudden rises in intracranial pressure can be prevented. Various procedures (e.g., suctioning, bathing, and so forth) can be scheduled at different times so the patient is not harmed by their cumulative effects. ICPM provides the only reliable means to determine, early in the course, the presence and degree of elevation of intracranial pressure. When used in conjunction with the total patient assessment, ICPM is invaluable.

## Indications for Intracranial Pressure Monitoring

ICPM is indicated for the patient who has, or is at risk of developing, an increase in intracranial pressure. Whenever a change is anticipated in intracranial volume, be it brain mass (e.g., cerebral edema or space-occupying brain lesions), blood (e.g., bleeding with associated head trauma, cerebral hemorrhage, or an increase in cerebral blood flow), or cerebrospinal fluid (e.g., overproduction or decreased reabsorption), ICPM is indicated. Most importantly, ICPM can help to prevent or avert the occurrence of catastrophic secondary effects (e.g., ischemia, injury, infarction, or development of cerebral edema) in what at the onset appeared to be an innocuous primary insult. ICPM is avoided if it would not make a difference in patient outcome.

### *Cerebral Edema*

Cerebral edema is one of the major causes of increased intracranial pressure. It is simply defined as an increase in water content of the brain parenchyma. Cerebral edema results from direct traumatic or penetrating injury to brain tissue or from massive tissue damage, such as might occur in cerebral infarction. Secondarily, cerebral edema may be precipitated by underlying pathophysiologic processes including cerebral ischemia, anoxia, and hypercapnia.

Three types of cerebral edema have been described: vasogenic, cytotoxic, and interstitial edema.

**Vasogenic Edema.** Vasogenic edema is the most common source of fluid accumulation within the brain. It is essentially an *extra*cellular edema, which results from damage to cerebral capillaries causing disruption of the blood–brain barrier (see Fig. 6–11). The breakdown of capillary permeability allows transudation (i.e., passage of fluid or solute through a membrane by hydrostatic or osmotic pressure gradients) of protein into the extracellular space, which is followed by an influx of water from the intravascular space into the brain interstitium. Vasogenic edema may be caused by trauma, ischemia, tumor, infection, or brain abscess.

**Cytotoxic Edema.** Cytotoxic edema is *intra*cellular—fluid accumulates within cells, predominantly the glial astrocytes. An increased permeability of capillary endothelial cells to water is a factor, resulting in an overall increase in water content within the brain. The underlying pathophysiologic mechanism is thought to involve alterations in ionic transport mechanisms within cellular membranes. Inhibition of the ATPase Na–K (sodium–potassium) pump may be involved, allowing potassium to leave the cell while sodium, chloride, and water enter it, causing the cell to swell. Failure of the Na–K pump is a primary consideration in the presence of hypoxia and ischemia. Conditions that cause brain hypoxia and/or ischemia (e.g., trauma, cerebral hemorrhage), as well as hypo-osmolality, may predispose to cytotoxic edema. Reye's syndrome has been associated with this form of edema.

**Interstitial (Hydrocephalic) Edema.** Interstitial or hydrocephalic edema is associated with obstructive hydrocephalus. (Hydrocephalus is a condition marked by excessive accumulation of fluid within the brain.) A buildup of cerebrospinal fluid pressure in the ventricular system causes transudation of cerebrospinal fluid through the ependymal layer into the periventricular white matter. The location of the edema fluid is *extra*cellular. Infection and brain tumor, among others, may predispose to interstitial edema.

The pathophysiologic effects of cerebral edema result primarily from an increase in intracranial pressure. The clinical presentation of cerebral edema may be profound and depends on the rapidity of formation and the extent to which brain tissues are involved. When intracranial pressure rises, signs and symptoms may become severe. Changes in the level of consciousness occur early, followed by alterations in the other major variables, namely, the rate and pattern of respiration, size and reactivity of the pupils, ocular movements, and skeletal motor responses. (For a review of the assessment of these parameters, see Chap. 7.)

## Intracranial Volume–Pressure Relationships

To effectively monitor and manage the patient with, or at risk of developing, an increase in intracranial pressure, one must understand intracranial volume–pressure relationships. The rigid cranium, while protecting the brain against external injury, also imposes constraining volume–pressure relationships so that effective brain compliance (i.e., the degree of brain compressibility) drops dramatically as cranial volume increases. The volume of fluid that can be displaced from the cranial vault (i.e., compensatory mechanisms involving cerebrospinal fluid and blood) is also limited. If the volume within the cranium continues to expand, the intracranial pressure rises at a precipitous rate. Stated another way, the rigid cranium produces a rapid rise in intracranial pressure as the brain swells following illness or injury.

### Volume–Pressure Curve

The volume–pressure curve relates changes in volume and pressure (Fig. 8–1). As the intracranial volume increases (in the initial stage), intracranial pressure remains within the normal physiologic limits (i.e., 0–15 mmHg) because normal compensatory mechanisms (e.g., displacement of cerebrospinal fluid and blood) are operant (gradual slope of curve).

However, the brain has only a small margin for compensation. When a rapidly expanding volume within the cranial vault (e.g., cerebral hemorrhage) becomes greater than that volume displaced from the vault, the compensatory mechanisms normally operant are exceeded and intracranial pressure rises (steep slope of curve).

If intracranial pressure is already elevated and compensatory mechanisms are compromised, a relatively minor increase in intracranial volume can precipitate a major rise in intracranial pressure. This relationship can be demonstrated clinically (see Fig. 8–1, Evaluation of Compliance). A

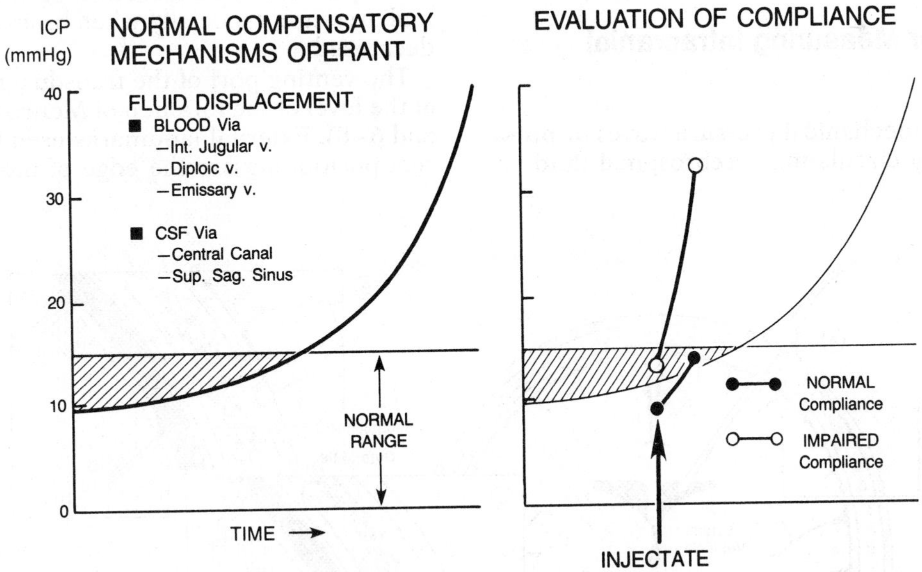


**Figure 8–1.** Intracranial volume–pressure curve. This curve relates changes in volume and pressure and reflects the degree of brain compressibility, or compliance. *(Left panel)* The normal intracranial volume–pressure curve reflects the presence of intact or operant compensatory mechanisms, thus maintaining intracranial pressure within the normal physiologic range (0 to 15 mmHg) in the face of changes in intracranial volume. *(Right panel)* Evaluation of brain compliance. When baseline intracranial pressure is within the normal range, a rise in intracranial pressure of 2 mmHg or less in response to the injectate (•–•), indicates compensatory mechanisms are operant (i.e., normal compliance); when the intracranial pressure baseline is initially high (○–○), a relatively small increase in volume (injectate) can cause potentially dangerous increases in intracranial pressure (i.e., impaired compliance). In this circumstance, compensatory mechanisms are impaired or no longer operant.

baseline intracranial pressure is measured following which the physician injects 1 ml of normal saline or Ringer's lactate (injectate) into the system via an intracranial pressure monitoring line over a 1-second period of time.

When the baseline intracranial pressure is within the normal range (0–15 mmHg), a rise in intracranial pressure of 2 mmHg or less in response to the injectate indicates compensatory mechanisms are intact (i.e., brain compliance is high). When the baseline intracranial pressure is initially high or elevated, a relatively small increase in volume (injectate) can cause potentially dangerous increases in intracranial pressure (i.e., brain compliance is low). (For a review of compensatory and autoregulatory mechanisms, see Chap. 6.)

Knowledge of intracranial volume–pressure relationships and compliance is critical to patient management. The ultimate concern is to maintain cerebral perfusion pressure within a range that ensures adequate cerebral blood flow. Plum and Posner suggest that in the normal brain, cerebral perfusion pressure must drop below 40 mmHg before cerebral blood flow is compromised, because of the normal compensatory and autoregulatory mechanisms.[2] In the damaged brain, the cerebral perfusion pressure at which cerebral circulation is impaired is not so easily determined. Furthermore, depending on the underlying pathology, variations in cerebral perfusion pressure may occur from one region of the brain to the next. (For a review of cerebral perfusion pressure, its determinants, and its clinical significance, see Chap. 6.)

## Methods for Measuring Intracranial Pressure

In ICPM, the mechanical pressure waves or pulsations of freely circulating cerebrospinal fluid are converted into electrical impulses via a sensor or transducer. These electrical impulses, in turn, are converted into visual waveforms and digital readouts by an oscilloscope or chart recorder.

Theoretically, because pressure exerted by fluids is distributed equally in all directions, measurement of cerebrospinal fluid is considered to be an acceptable indicator of overall intracranial pressure. It should be appreciated that pressure gradients may exist between intracranial compartments, and in these cases, the pressure of cerebrospinal fluid may not accurately reflect overall intracranial pressure. ICPM can only be employed effectively if cerebrospinal fluid is circulating freely and pressure exerted by cerebrospinal fluid is transmitted freely from one intracranial compartment to the next.

Three methods are employed in ICPM: intraventricular, subarachnoid, and epidural.

### *Intraventricular Method*

The intraventricular method of ICPM uses a catheter, which is introduced via a burr hole in the skull and placed within the anterior (most commonly) or occipital horn of the ventricle (Fig. 8–2*A*). The catheter is connected to the transducer via stopcocks and pressure tubing. Sterile normal saline without preservative is used as the fluid column between cerebrospinal fluid and the diaphragm of the transducer dome. A continuous fluid flush device is not used for ICPM because the addition of even a small amount of fluid into the system can cause potentially dangerous increases in intracranial pressure, especially when brain compliance is decreased.

The venting port of the transducer is positioned at the level of the foramen of Monro (see Figs. 6–7 and 6–8). External landmarks used to ensure correct positioning are the edge of the eyebrow and

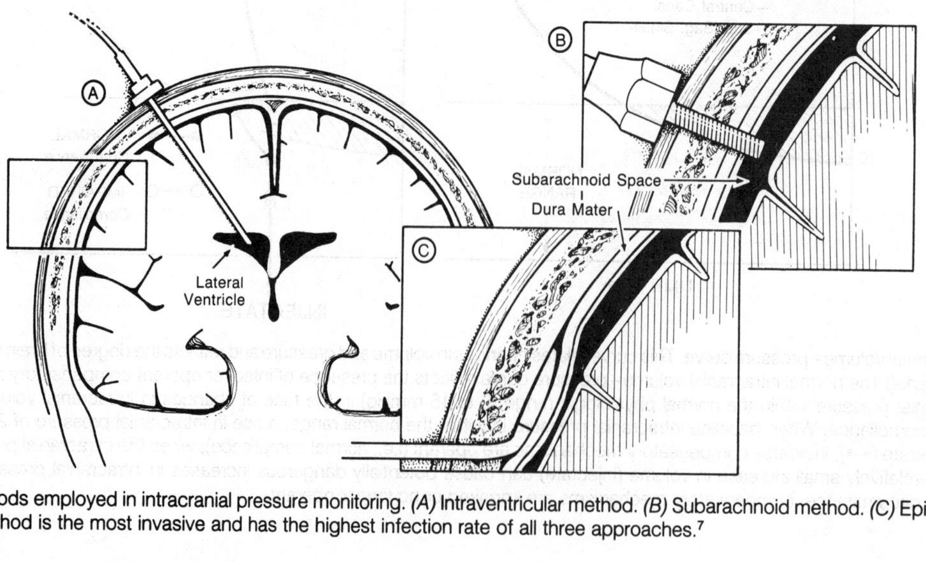


**Figure 8–2.** Methods employed in intracranial pressure monitoring. *(A)* Intraventricular method. *(B)* Subarachnoid method. *(C)* Epidural method. The intraventricular method is the most invasive and has the highest infection rate of all three approaches.[7]

tragus of the ear. A carpenter's level can be used to verify that the transducer is level with the foramen of Monro. Proper positioning of the transducer is critical when monitoring intracranial pressure. For every inch of discrepancy between the level of the transducer (venting port) and pressure source (foramen of Monro), there is an error of about 2 mmHg. Because the intracranial pressure system is a *low* pressure system (0–15 mmHg), a discrepancy of 2 mmHg may have considerable significance in terms of patient management. Some of the advantages, disadvantages, and nursing considerations of this approach are presented in Table 8–1.

#### Subarachnoid Method

The subarachnoid method uses a subarachnoid screw, which is inserted via a burr hole in the skull and placed so that the tip rests in the subarachnoid space (see Fig. 8–2*B*). The cerebrum is not penetrated, and pressures generated by cerebrospinal fluid are measured directly. The transducer may be attached directly to the screw, or may be connected via pressure tubing in the manner described for the intraventricular method. Table 8–1 lists some advantages, disadvantages, and nursing considerations of this method.

#### Epidural Method

Unlike the intraventricular method, or possibly the subarachnoid method, where a fluid column is used as a sensor, epidural methods use other types of sensors, which are placed within the epidural (extradural) space between the dura and skull via a small burr hole. One method uses a tiny balloon with radioisotopes; another uses a radiotransmitter; and still another uses a fiberoptic sensor (see Fig. 8–2*C*). A cable connects the sensor to the monitor and recorder.

### Intracranial Pressure Monitoring Waveforms: Analysis and Interpretation

ICPM reflects the status of intracranial pressure dynamics, which fluctuate continuously. Normal intracranial pressure ranges from 0–15 mmHg, with less than 10 mmHg being ideal and 15 mmHg reflecting the upper limit of normal. Activities involving coughing or straining (Valsalva's maneuver) may increase intracranial pressure momentarily to as high as 100 mmHg.

In the setting of a severe insult to the brain (e.g., head trauma), intracranial pressure may be labile with rapid changes and elevations, which are not well tolerated. Symptoms may appear at pressures of 20–25 mmHg. This is in sharp contrast to the clinical circumstance of certain brain tumors, in which increases in intracranial pressure, occurring gradually over time, are, thus, better tolerated.

#### "Normal" Intracranial Pressure Waveform

A "normal" intracranial pressure waveform is similar to the arterial waveform of hemodynamic pressure monitoring and reflects the cardiovascular dynamics that occur with each beat (see arterial waveform configuration, Fig. 41–8). The proximity of circulating cerebrospinal fluid to arterial pulsations as they occur within the vasculature of the choroid plexuses accounts for the configuration of the intracranial waveform.

The amplitude of the "normal" intracranial pressure waveform (i.e., the distance between its high [systolic] and low [diastolic] pressure points) reflects the pulse pressure. When intracranial pressure is within the normal range (0–15 mmHg), cardiac dynamics, as reflected by the arterial pulsations, produce only slight variations between the high and low pressures. Intact intracranial compliance, reflective of compensatory shifts in blood and cerebrospinal fluid, accounts for these minimal pressure variations.

As the intracranial pressure rises, compensatory mechanisms become compromised and intracranial compliance is reduced. With the reduction in compliance, the brain is less able to compensate for volume changes, and the consequent changes in pressure are reflected on the ICPM recording by a widening of the amplitude, and, thus, the pulse pressure (Fig. 8–3).

If the ICPM waveforms are carefully and serially scrutinized, a trend reflecting a *widening* of the pulse pressure in conjunction with a *rising* intracranial pressure may become obvious. Such a trend is ominous and usually is evoked in response to a decrease in cerebral perfusion pressure and cerebral ischemia. Timely and aggressive pressure-reducing interventions may be indicated.

In this way, the ICPM waveform reflects underlying physiologic responses related to a rise in intracranial pressure, and it should be analyzed and interpreted as part of the patient's total assessment.

#### Abnormal Intracranial Pressure Waveforms

**A Waves (Plateau Waves).** A Waves, also called plateau waves because of their distinctive pattern (see Fig. 8–3), are the most clinically significant waveforms. They are associated with cerebral ischemia and represent a serious risk to the maintenance of intracranial pressure within acceptable physiologic limits ($<$15 mmHg). The appearance of plateau waves may be sudden, paroxysmal, and transient, and they usually occur in patients whose baseline intracranial pressure is already elevated ($>$15–20 mmHg). The amplitude of these plateau waves, and thus the pulse pressure, may range between 50–100 mmHg, and they have a duration of 5–20 minutes.

Signs and symptoms related to the onset and peak of plateau waves include alterations in level of con-

TABLE 8–1
## Summary of Methods Used in Intracranial Pressure Monitoring

| Method | Purpose | Advantages | Disadvantages | Nursing Considerations |
|---|---|---|---|---|
| *Ventricular:* Catheter in anterior or occipital horns of lateral ventricle. (Anterior horn most commonly used.) | 1. Measure ICP.<br>2. Provide sample of CSF for analysis.<br>3. Drain off CSF to reduce ICP.<br>4. Instill contrast medium or drugs.<br>5. Evaluate volume–pressure relationship (compliance). | 1. Direct ICP measurement is most accurate.<br>2. Direct access to CSF to:<br>a. obtain sample of CSF for analysis.<br>b. drain off CSF to reduce ICP.<br>3. Access to determine volume–pressure response (compliance).<br>4. Access for instillation of drugs. | 1. Complexity of insertion if ventricles are:<br>a. small in size.<br>b. shifted or compressed.<br>2. Risk of infection.[7]<br>3. Leakage of CSF.<br>4. Hemorrhage as catheter is placed through brain tissue. | 1. Use baseline position for level of transducer to obtain consistent data.<br>a. Venting port of transducer positioned at level of foramen of Monro.<br>(1) External landmarks include edge of eyebrow or tragus of ear.<br>b. All stopcocks must be in accurate position to avoid excessive drainage of CSF and sudden drop in ICP.<br>(1) For each inch of discrepancy between level of transducer and pressure source, there is an error of 2 mmHg.<br>c. Recalibrate the transducer and monitoring equipment as indicated.<br>d. Assess catheter patency frequently. A dampened waveform may be produced if there is compression of the catheter tip by the ventricular walls or blood in the CSF. If catheter becomes obstructed, notify physician (as per hospital protocol).<br>e. Observe for any sudden changes in ICP.<br>2. Correlate ICP data with total assessment of patient. Remember ICPM is another assessment technique. It is only significant when evaluated in terms of the status of the whole patient.<br>3. Monitor closely for infection with this most invasive ICPM approach (see Chap. 7). |

| | | | | |
|---|---|---|---|---|
| | | | | 4. Expect catheter placement to be difficult if brain is shifted or the ventricles are small or compressed. ICPM must be done in conjunction with CAT scanning.<br>5. Avoid taking pressure measurements when the patient is moving, coughing, using abdominal muscle to breath, or has his/her head turned to one side. These activities may cause ICP to increase. |
| *Subarachnoid:* Screw is placed in subarachnoid space through burr hole in skull. Transducer may be attached directly to the screw or connected via pressure tubing in the manner described for the intraventricular method. | 1. Measure ICP.<br>2. Provide access for ICP drainage.<br>3. Evaluate volume–pressure relationship (compliance). | 1. Direct ICP measurement.<br>2. Assess to evaluate volume–pressure response (compliance).<br>3. Ease and speed of insertion.<br>4. Lower risk of infection than in ventricular monitoring. | 1. Risk of infection.<br>2. Measurements may be inaccurate if screw becomes occluded with brain tissue, meninges, or bone fragments from drilled burr hole.<br>3. Unable to instill contrast medium.<br>4. Skull must be completely intact (no fractures).<br>5. Leakage of CSF. | 1. If waveform wanders from baseline, assess patency of screw. If screw becomes occluded, notify physician.<br>2. Recalibrate transducer/monitor as indicated.<br>3. Monitor for signs of infection and signs of meningeal irritation (see Chap. 7). |
| *Epidural*<br>1. Epidural placement of a tiny balloon with radioisotopes or radiotransmitters in the epidural space via burr hole in the skull.<br>2. Epidural fiberoptic sensing device directly connected to bedside monitor.<br>3. Completely implantable epidural transducer—potential for telemetric monitoring. | 1. Measure ICP. | 1. Easy and quickly inserted into epidural space.<br>2. Less invasive; dura is not penetrated.<br>3. No uncontrolled loss of CSF.<br>4. No alterations of pressure monitoring due to plugging or obstruction of sensing device.<br>5. No insertion difficulties related to ventricular size, compression, and displacement.<br>6. Allows greater mobility: transporting patients is easier.<br>7. Allows for long-term use (10 to 14 days) or as long as the dura remains intact. | 1. Accuracy of epidural pressure monitoring questioned.<br>2. No access for sampling or drainage of CSF.<br>3. Cannot be recalibrated if environmental factors change.<br>4. Pressure readings may be inaccurate if the dura is compressed, is thickened, or has an increased surface tension. | 1. Check to ensure connecting tube is inserted properly into bedside montior.<br>2. Calibrate prior to insertion; discard sensor or transducer if readouts are inaccurate. |

ICP = intracranial pressure; CSF = cerebrospinal fluid; ICPM = intracranial pressure monitoring.

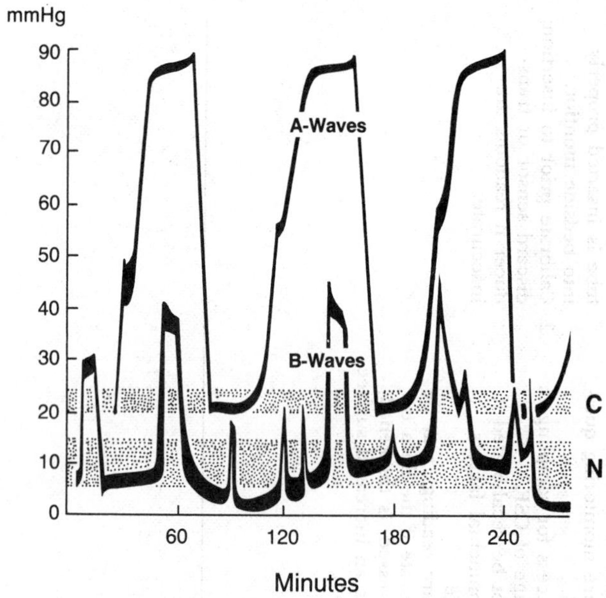


**Figure 8-3.** Intracranial pressure waveforms. Waveforms reflect pressure in mmHg and time in minutes. Two abnormal waveforms are depicted, including A waves and B waves. A waves reflect intracranial pressure in the range of 50 to 100 mmHg. They have a duration of 5 to 20 minutes or longer. Their waveforms have a distinctive plateau and they are referred to as "plateau" waves. B waves occur as sharp, peaked (saw-tooth pattern) rhythmic oscillations, which may reach a peak pressure of 50 mmHg. They have a duration of 1/2 to 2 minutes. N refers to "normal" intracranial pressure waveforms and reflects a pressure within the range of 0 to 15 mmHg. C refers to the pressure waveform for C waves. C waves are usually rapid, rhythmic waves with an amplitude of about 20 mmHg. They occur every 4 to 8 minutes.

sciousness and respiratory rate and pattern; headache, nausea, and vomiting (projectile); altered pupillary responses to light stimulus; altered motor responses (e.g., paresis, decorticate and decerebrate posturing); and changes in vital signs, although these latter signs are not always a consistent finding.

It is important to appreciate that plateau waves can occur without any accompanying changes in behavior reflective of cerebral dysfunction. In fact, the increase in intracranial pressure may be substantial without any clinical signs or symptoms as to its presence. In these instances, ICPM and a clinically astute nurse may provide the only clues to the presence of underlying pathophysiology.

Plateau waves have been well correlated physiologically with later stages of a prolonged increase in intracranial pressure *(cerebral hypertension)*, which predisposes to cerebral ischemia, cellular hypoxia, and possibly infarction with necrosis of selected tissues. Their appearance signals that compensatory and autoregulatory mechanisms are no longer successful in controlling intracranial pressure. This loss of compliance resulting in elevated, sustained plateau waves is an ominous sign, and aggressive therapy needs to be provided on an emergency basis.

**B Waves.** B waves occur as sharp, peaked (saw-tooth pattern) rhythmic oscillations, which reach an amplitude of as much as 50 mmHg and occur as frequently as every 1/2 to 2 minutes (see Fig. 8-3). The elevated pressures are not sustained, and the rhythmic fluctuations appear to reflect respiratory and cardiovascular dynamics. A decreased arousal or wakefulness state appears to be associated with the occurrence of B waves.

The clinical significance of B waves is not well established, but they are seen more commonly in patients with unstable intracranial pressure. Their appearance suggests a decrease in intracranial compliance and may signal that the patient's condition is deteriorating. B waves may precede A waves and require thorough, ongoing assessment, particularly if they appear with increasing frequency.

**C Waves.** C waves, also known as Traube-Hering-May waves, are rapid, rhythmic waves with an amplitude of approximately 20 mmHg. They occur every 4 to 8 minutes, and the waveform reflects respiratory and cardiovascular dynamics.

## Intracranial Hypertension: Nursing Care Considerations

In caring for the patient with central nervous system pathology who has, or is at risk of developing, an increase in intracranial pressure (i.e., intracranial hypertension), it is essential for the nurse to appreciate those activities that can elevate intracranial pressure. Such knowledge is necessary so that patient care activities can be spaced to minimize any elevation in intracranial pressure. In one descriptive study,[3] the effects of specific occurrences during patient care on intracranial pressure were examined and categorized under nursing (health) care activities, patient-initiated activities, and environmental stimuli.

Nursing care activities associated with an increase in intracranial pressure included turning the patient to the left and to the right, repositioning of extremities and placement into an appropriate alignment, and flexion of the head, for example, during turning. Turning done rapidly and at angles ranging from 45–90 degrees was associated with an increase in intracranial pressure. Slower turning and maintenance of the body in proper alignment during turning may help to minimize any increase in intracranial pressure. Elevation of the head of the bed was associated with a decrease in intracranial pressure. Maintenance of the patient in this position facilitates venous drainage from the cranial vault via gravity.

Other nursing care activities associated with an increase in intracranial pressure included bathing, instilling eyedrops, starting or manipulating an intravenous line, drawing blood from an arterial line, irrigating and dressing wounds, taking a rectal temperature, and providing oral care. Major elevations in intracranial pressure were associated with suctioning and resultant coughing. This obviously poses a major concern because the need for suctioning is unavoidable. Hyperinflation of the lungs with 100% oxygen prior to and after each suction pass and meticulous suctioning technique (see Table 32–4) may reduce the risk of hypoxemia and minimize any elevation in intracranial pressure. Use of a kinetic bed, if available, may assist in the prevention of pooling of pulmonary secretion within the pulmonary circuit, thus facilitating their removal; it also helps to maximize tissue perfusion, thus decreasing the risk of decubitus formation especially during long-term care.

Patient-initiated activities resulting in elevation of intracranial pressure included flexion of extremities, flexion/rotation of the neck, and coughing. Increased muscle tone associated with decerebrate posturing also increased intracranial pressure, probably as a result of increased intrathoracic pressures and flexion of the neck. Nursing measures, such as supporting the sides of the head to prevent rotation and timely suctioning to prevent unnecessary coughing, may help to prevent an increase in intracranial pressure.

The role played by environmental factors in elevating intracranial pressure was not so well defined. Nevertheless, emotional stress and conversation about the patient's condition at the bedside are considered to be factors contributing to an increase in intracranial pressure. Environmental noise should be kept to a minimum; rest periods during which the patient is undisturbed should be provided; and conversation in the patient's presence whether about the patient, or plain "chit-chat" between staff members, should be avoided.

## CONSEQUENCES OF INCREASED INTRACRANIAL PRESSURE—BRAIN HERNIATION

Brain herniation refers to the shifting of intracranial structures from a compartment of high pressure to one of lower pressure. It is most commonly associated with craniocerebral trauma and usually requires emergent treatment to avert an increase in intracranial pressure and consequent decrease in cerebral perfusion pressure and cerebral blood flow.

### Pathophysiology

Pathophysiologic mechanisms underlying the evolution of brain herniation are described as occurring at three stages: primary, secondary, and tertiary.[4] Primary stage involves the actual mechanical injury or insult to brain tissue and/or its connective support systems. The secondary stage reflects pathology to brain tissue occurring as an indirect result of the primary insult and commonly involves intracerebral hemorrhage, hematoma formation, and cerebral edema. The tertiary stage involves the loss of autoregulatory and compensatory mechanisms and brain compliance, resulting in an increase in intracranial pressure.

As intracranial pressure rises, the cerebral vasculature becomes compressed, impairing blood flow. This predisposes to cerebral ischemia, cellular hypoxia, and cerebral edema, and the vicious cycle leading to herniation with infarction and necrosis of brain tissue is perpetuated. If timely and aggressive pressure-reducing measures are not initiated the patient will die (Fig. 8–4).

### Treatment and Management

The primary goal of medical and nursing management is to intervene at the primary stage to treat and/or prevent secondary and tertiary events from occurring. The significance of the herniation process, when it occurs, is that a potentially *reversible* process is converted to an irreversible and catastrophic one.

Nursing care includes: (1) monitoring for signs and symptoms of increasing intracranial pressure; (2) maintaining the integrity of the intracranial pressure monitoring system; and (3) implementing measures to prevent and/or reduce intracranial pressure. Specific therapeutic interventions include efforts to increase drainage of blood and cerebrospinal fluid from the cranial vault via gravity. Maintenance of proper body positioning and alignment in this regard was mentioned earlier.

Cerebral blood flow may be decreased by controlled hyperventilation (to maintain $PaCO_2$ between 25–35 mmHg), and by prevention of a buildup of tracheobronchial secretions. Secretion buildup reduces alveolar ventilation and leads to hypercapnia. Hypercapnia, in turn, causes cerebral vasodilation, resulting in an increased cerebral blood flow.

Efforts to limit or decrease cerebral edema may be initiated. Therapies usually include the adminis-

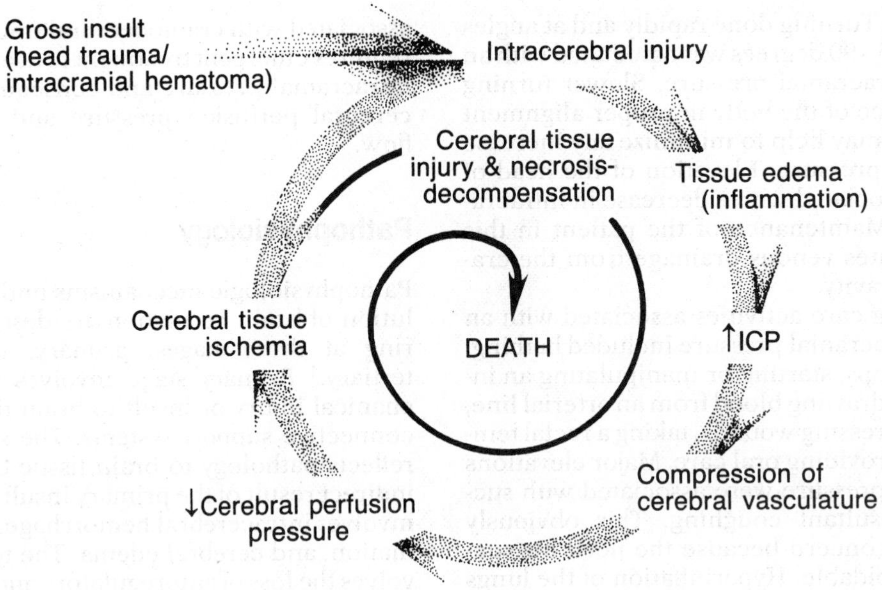


**Figure 8-4.**

tration of a diuretic (e.g., furosemide) and hyperosmolar agents (e.g., mannitol). These agents decrease total body water. Corticosteroid therapy (e.g., dexamethasone, methylprednisolone) is usually prescribed to stabilize cellular membranes, as well as for the anti-inflammatory effect exhibited by steroids. Although a definitive cause and effect relationship has not been established, ranitidine, a histamine$_2$-receptor antagonist, is usually administered in conjunction with corticosteroid therapy to reduce the risk of gastrointestinal bleeding. This is especially important because, as mentioned earlier, patients sustaining insults to the central nervous system resulting in intracranial hypertension are already at high risk of developing gastrointestinal ulceration. Gastric pH should be monitored hourly and should be maintained at greater than 4.5.

Fluid intake is usually restricted to 1200–1500 ml/day, with meticulous monitoring of intake and output, serum electrolytes, serum osmolality, total serum proteins, hematology profile, and urine specific gravity.

Measures to reduce cellular metabolism are usually implemented because any reduction in metabolism reduces the need for metabolic substrates and the removal of waste products of metabolism, thus decreasing cerebral blood flow. Comfort measures are employed to reduce pain and anxiety; anticonvulsant therapy may be initiated to reduce the risk of seizures and their concomitant effect of increasing tissue demand for oxygen and nutrients; and body temperature is maintained within normal limits to prevent shivering. For every 1°F increase in body temperature, the metabolic rate increases by 10%.

Nursing activities are planned to avoid a cumulative increase in intracranial pressure. Suctioning should only be performed when clinically indicated as determined, for example, by an increase in restlessness, an increase in adventitious sounds (e.g., crackles, wheezes, rhonchi), and triggering of ventilator alarms. The immediate environment should remain quiet, with a minimum of stimuli. (Table 8–2, Nursing Care Plan for the Patient with Increased Intracranial Pressure, provides a detailed list of nursing interventions and their rationales.)

## INTRACRANIAL COMPARTMENTS: SUPRATENTORIAL AND INFRATENTORIAL

Structurally, the cranial vault can be described as consisting of two compartments separated by the dural fold, the tentorium cerebelli (see Figs. 6–6 and 8–6). The supratentorial compartment occurs superior to, or above, the tentorium. It consists of the anterior and middle fossae, which house the cerebral hemispheres, basal ganglia, and diencephalon. The infratentorial compartment lies inferior to, or below, the tentorium. It consists of the posterior fossa, which contains the cerebellum and brainstem (see Fig. 6–5). These two compartments

## TABLE 8–2. CARE PLAN FOR THE PATIENT WITH INCREASED INTRACRANIAL PRESSURE

| Nursing Diagnoses | Desired Patient Outcomes | Nursing Interventions | Rationales |
|---|---|---|---|
| ***Nursing Diagnosis #1***<br>Alteration in cerebral tissue perfusion, related to:<br>1. Increased intracranial pressure associated with cranial and/or cerebral insult (head injury, hematoma formation, cerebral hemorrhage, cerebral edema). | Patient will:<br>1. Maintain cerebral perfusion pressure (CCP) >60 mmHg.<br>• Intracranial pressure (ICP) <15 mmHg.<br>• Mean arterial blood pressure (MAP) ~80–100 mmHg or baseline (for patient). | • Monitor continuously for signs and symptoms of increasing ICP. | • Continuous monitoring is necessary as patient responses related to intracranial pressure can change rapidly from moment to moment. |
| | | ◦ Establish baseline parameters. | ◦ Baseline measurements can be used to compare subsequent responses. |
| | | ◦ Determine arousability and assess for changes in level of consciousness and mentation: restlessness, agitation, irritability; disorientation, inattentiveness; disturbed thought processes, loss of memory; inability to answer questions or follow commands. | ◦ Arousability reflects functioning of reticular activating system within brainstem.<br>◦ Level of consciousness provides earliest clinical evidence of a change in intracranial volume/pressure dynamics. It reflects the status of cerebral hemispheres and diencephalon. |
| | | ◦ Assess for sensory function:<br>– *Special senses:* visual acuity and visual fields; hearing.<br>– *Somatic senses:* touch, pressure, pain, temperature, proprioception, vibration. | ◦ Assessment of sensory function affords an evaluation of sensory pathways and functioning of primary sensory center (postcentral gyrus, parietal lobe). |
| | | ◦ Assess for motor function (somatic): appropriate or inappropriate responses (decorticate or decerebrate posturing, flaccidity); muscle strength, tone, deep tendon reflexes. | ◦ Appropriate motor responses and deep tendon reflexes reflect intact sensory pathways and total or partial intact motor pathways and neuromuscular junctions. |
| | | ◦ Assess for motor function (autonomic): respiratory rate and pattern; pupillary size and reactivity; ocular movements: dysconjugate gaze, nystagmus; oculocephalic and oculovestibular reflexes (doll's eyes phenomenon and caloric tests). | ◦ Pupillary responses reflect status of midbrain and pons. In the patient with an altered state of consciousness who has fixed, moderately dilated pupils, ocular reflexes may provide the only clinical data reflective of the level of brainstem function. |
| | | ◦ Assess cranial nerves and status of protective reflexes. | ◦ Increasing ICP causes pressure on brainstem, disrupting cranial nerve function (IX and X) and compromising protective reflexes (gag, cough, epiglottal closure). This places airway in great danger. |
| | | ◦ Assess for headache, nausea, vomiting, papilledema, diplopia, blurred vision, seizures. | ◦ Many signs/symptoms of early rise in ICP tend to be nonspecific. |
| | | ◦ Assess vital signs: mean arterial blood pressure, pulse pressure, heart rate. | ◦ A rise in blood pressure, widening pulse pressure, and slow, bounding heart rate are classic, *late*-occurring signs of increasing ICP. |

*(continued)*

**TABLE 8-2. CARE PLAN FOR THE PATIENT WITH INCREASED INTRACRANIAL PRESSURE *(Continued)***

| Nursing Diagnoses | Desired Patient Outcomes | Nursing Interventions | Rationales |
|---|---|---|---|
| *Nursing Diagnosis #1 (cont.)* | | | |
| | | • Maintain intracranial pressure monitoring (ICPM) system. | • ICPM is a highly invasive technique with a high risk of infection. |
| | | ◦ Take measures to reduce risk of infection: wash hands meticulously, use aseptic technique at all times. | |
| | | ◦ Maintain integrity of ICPM system: | ◦ Maintaining a closed system and avoiding disconnections reduce the risk of infection. |
| | | – Check for leaks or air and ensure all stopcocks are in their appropriate positions. | |
| | | ◦ Flush system as per protocol if appropriate for method in use. | ◦ Introduction of any fluid into the system for whatever reason can be *very dangerous* in the compromised patient. If done, it should only be done with continuous ICPM. Such activities are usually the responsibility of the patient's physician; nurses do *not* routinely inject fluid into the ICPM system. |
| | | – Turn off stopcock to patient if it is absolutely necessary to disconnect the system. | |
| | | ◦ Avoid rapid or prolonged drainage of cerebrospinal fluid (CSF); follow unit protocol. | ◦ Aspiration of CSF is a critical procedure, which can markedly reduce ICP, especially when intracranial volume is increased and compliance is significantly reduced. Risk of infection is a major disadvantage of this pressure-reducing measure. It can also precipitate a collapse of the ventricle or cause brain tissue to be sucked into the monitoring catheter or other device (subarachnoid screw).<br>– Excessive loss of CSF in the presence of increased ICP can alter intracranial pressure dynamics and precipitate herniation. |
| | | – Protect ICPM system when moving or positioning patient, or if patient is restless or agitated. | |
| | | ◦ Perform insertion site care as per unit protocol. | ◦ Reduce risk of infection. |
| | | ◦ Obtain the record pressure measurements: | ◦ Avoid treatment of increased ICP without *accurate* pressure measurements. |
| | | ◦ Confirm accurate placement of transducer; use carpenter's level for accuracy. | ◦ The venting port of transducer should always be at pressure source, the foramen of Monro. Use edge of eyebrow and tragus of ear as guidelines. |

| | |
|---|---|
| – Balance and recalibrate system if appropriate for method in use. | – For every inch that the measurement is off, approximately 2 mmHg is added or subtracted from the digital readout. This is significant in a low pressure system and must be avoided. |
| ○ Observe for fluctuation of CSF column. | ○ Reflects cardiovascular dynamics and indicates proper placement of catheter or screw. |
| ○ Obtain baseline waveform configuration and digital readout. | ○ Establishes measure with which to compare subsequent data. |
| ○ Monitor pressure waveform and digital readouts continuously. | ○ Waveform configuration and amplitude can reflect patency of system, rise in ICP, and status of intracranial compliance. |
| – Be consistent in taking ICP readings.<br>– Calculate and record cerebral perfusion pressure hourly. | |
| ○ Analyze waveforms and pressure readings and identify trends. | ○ *Trends* are more significant in determining status of ICP and intracranial compliance. |
| ○ Troubleshoot the system if unable to obtain a waveform, or if the waveform is dampened. | ○ Refer to Table 8–5 for troubleshooting guidelines. |
| • Implement measures to prevent rise in and/or reduce ICP. | |
| ○ Maintain proper positioning: elevate head of bed 30 to 45 degrees; avoid using pillows. | ○ Allows for optimal venous drainage from cranium via gravity; prevents compromise of cerebral blood flow. |
| ○ Maintain body alignment in midline, and avoid neck flexion or head rotation. | ○ Prevents jugular vein compression or obstruction. |
| ○ Avoid hip flexion.<br>– Maintain head–neck alignment when turning. | ○ May increase intra-abdominal pressure and impede cerebral drainage via jugular veins and vena cavae. |
| ○ Prevent increase in cerebral blood flow. | ○ Increase in cerebral blood volume may compromise compensation and compliance in the patient with increased ICP. |
| ○ Initiate controlled hyperventilation:<br>– Maintain $PaCO_2$ 25–35 mmHg, $PaO_2$ >80 mmHg.<br>– Monitor arterial blood gas. | ○ Reduced $PaCO_2$ *(hypocapnia)* causes cerebral *vasoconstriction* and thus lowers cerebral blood volume. A reduction in cerebral blood volume augments compensatory mechanisms or compliance. |
| ○ Minimize cellular metabolism:<br>– Relieve pain and anxiety. | ○ Reduction in cellular metabolism decreases need for metabolic substrates (e.g., oxygen and glucose), while reducing the amount of metabolic waste products (e.g., carbon dioxide and hydrogen ions). The end result is a decrease in cerebral blood flow and intracranial pressure. |

*(continued)*

**TABLE 8–2. CARE PLAN FOR THE PATIENT WITH INCREASED INTRACRANIAL PRESSURE *(Continued)***

| Nursing Diagnoses | Desired Patient Outcomes | Nursing Interventions | Rationales |
|---|---|---|---|
| ***Nursing Diagnosis #1 (cont.)*** | | ○ Plan nursing care activities so as to avoid a *cumulative* increase in ICP. | ○ A potential increase in ICP can occur when nursing care activities are implemented in close succession. |
| | | ○ Identify activities that cause a change in ICP (e.g., coughing, suctioning, positioning).<br>– Incorporate planned rest periods into daily nursing care spaced between those procedures known to increase ICP. | ○ Provides a guide for planning nursing care. |
| | | ○ Administer prescribed sedatives or analgesics prior to procedures that may cause an increase in ICP. | ○ These measures may prevent an inordinate increase in ICP. |
| | | ○ Avoid discussing patient's condition at the bedside or within earshot of the patient. | ○ Such conversations, if overheard, could be upsetting to the patient and may predispose to an increase in ICP. |
| | | ○ Teach the responsive patient to avoid excessive coughing, Valsalva's maneuver (straining), isometric exercises, or pushing against bed rails; avoid use of footboard or restraints. | ○ These activities increase intrathoracic and intra-abdominal pressures, which can impede outflow of blood from cranium. |
| | | ○ Assess for bladder distention, paralytic ileus, constipation.<br>– Maintain quiet environment with a minimum of stimuli; gently stroke the patient and speak with a soothing tone of voice. | ○ These conditions may cause abdominal distention, thus increasing intra-abdominal pressures and limiting diaphragmatic excursion. |
| ***Nursing Diagnosis #2***<br>Airway clearance ineffective, related to:<br>1. Compromised cough.<br>2. Immobility with pooling of secretions. | Patient will:<br>1. Maintain intact airway and protective reflexes.<br>2. Demonstrate secretion-clearing cough.<br>3. Have breath sounds clear on auscultation. | • Prevent accumulation of tracheobronchial secretions. | • Accumulation of secretions reduces alveolar ventilation; a consequent *hypercapnia* causes an increase in cerebral blood flow, which increases ICP. |
| | | ○ Perform suctioning *only* when indicated by auscultation of breath sounds or excessive coughing.<br>• Suction only briefly (<10 seconds). | ○ Suctioning stimulates cough reflex and Valsalva's maneuver; a consequent increase in intrathoracic pressure reduces venous outflow from the brain via jugular veins and vena cava. |
| | | ○ Pre-oxygenate and hyperventilate with 100% oxygen before suctioning; repeat after suctioning. | ○ Proper suctioning technique minimizes the risk of hypoxemia. |
| ***Nursing Diagnosis #3***<br>Potential for fluid and electrolyte imbalance, related to: | Patient will:<br>1. Maintain baseline body weight. | • Limit or decrease cerebral edema:<br>○ Administer diuretic (furosemide) and hyperosmolar agents (Mannitol, urea) as prescribed. | • Fluid restriction coupled with pharmacologic therapy helps to decrease extracellular |

| | | | |
|---|---|---|---|
| 1. Osmotic diuretic therapy.<br>2. Diabetes insipidus. | 2. Balance fluid intake with output.<br>3. Maintain baseline laboratory values.<br>• Serum electrolytes, BUN, creatinine, serum protein, serum osmolality.<br>• Urine specific gravity—0.010 to 0.025. | – Monitor response to therapy.<br>○ Administer prescribed corticosteroid therapy (dexamethasone or methylprednisolone)<br>– Monitor response to therapy.<br>○ Restrict fluid intake (usually 1200–1500 ml/day).<br>○ Meticulously record intake and output (hourly).<br>– Weigh patient daily if not contraindicated.<br>○ Monitor urine specific gravity.<br>○ Monitor serum electrolytes and replace as prescribed.<br>○ Monitor serum osmolality and maintain at 305–315 mOsm/kg. | fluid volume that may contribute to edema formation. A mild dehydrated state is usually maintained.<br>○ Corticosteroids are thought to ameliorate cerebral edema, which occurs secondarily to the primary craniocerebral insult.<br>○ Intake/output includes intravenous medications (IV piggybacks) and CSF.<br>○ A Foley catheter is usually inserted to reduce patient activity and to monitor urine output. Physician should be notified if urine output is $<30$ or $>200$ ml/hr for 2 consecutive hours.<br>○ Craniocerebral insults frequently predispose to diabetes insipidus.<br>○ Increased serum osmolality helps to draw fluid from brain interstitium and reduce cerebral edema. |
| ***Nursing Diagnosis #4***<br>Potential for physiologic injury, related to seizures. | Patient will remain seizure free on anticonvulsant medications. | • Prevent seizure activity by administering prescribed anticonvulsant therapy.<br>– Monitor patient's response to anticonvulsant therapy.<br>○ Maintain normothermia and prevent shivering. | • Seizure activity greatly increases the demand for oxygen and glucose and, thus, cerebral blood flow.<br>○ Pyrexia causes cerebral vasodilation with increased blood flow. For every 1°F increase in body temperature, metabolic rate increases by 10%. |
| ***Nursing Diagnosis #5***<br>Potential for physiologic injury, related to gastrointestinal bleeding associated with stress, and possibly corticosteroid therapy. | Patient will:<br>1. Remain without gestrointestinal bleeding:<br>• Absence of blood in gastric contents and stool.<br>• Stable hematocrit, hemoglobin, and RBC values.<br>2. Maintain gastric pH $>4.5$. | • Initiate therapy to reduce the risk of gastrointestinal bleeding.<br>– Administer prescribed histamine$_2$-receptor antagonists: ranitidine (Zantac) is used most commonly.<br>– Initiate antacid prophylaxis therapy as prescribed.<br>○ Monitor acidity of gastric pH every 1 to 2 hr. | • Patients under extreme stress who receive corticosteroids seem to be at higher risk of developing gastrointestinal bleeding.<br>○ Ideal gastric pH is greater than 4.5. |
| ***Nursing Diagnosis #6***<br>Potential for infection, related to:<br>1. Invasive monitoring technique. | Patient will:<br>1. Maintain normal body temperature ~98.6°F (37°C). | • Implement measures to reduce risk of infection. | • An increase in body temperature of 1°F can increase cerebral cellular metabolism by 10%. |

*(continued)*

## TABLE 8-2. CARE PLAN FOR THE PATIENT WITH INCREASED INTRACRANIAL PRESSURE *(Continued)*

| Nursing Diagnoses | Desired Patient Outcomes | Nursing Interventions | Rationales |
|---|---|---|---|
| ***Nursing Diagnosis #6 (cont.)*** | | | |
| 2. Compromised protective reflexes (gag, cough, epiglottal closure).<br>3. Compromised immune response (stress, corticosteroid therapy).<br>4. Altered nutrition (see Table 49-7). | 2. Maintain white blood count at baseline level.<br>3. Remain without other evidence of infection (e.g., cough productive of thick, tenacious sputum; cloudy appearing urine; pain, redness, and swelling at invasive monitoring and intravenous sites). | ○ Maintain sterile technique for all procedures involved in ICPM. | ○ ICPM is a highly invasive diagnostic approach placing the patient at serious risk of infection (e.g., meningitis, encephalitis). |
| | | ○ Maintain aseptic technique for all invasive procedures:<br>○ Endotracheal/tracheostomy tube care and management.<br>– Foley catheter care.<br>– All invasive lines: pulmonary artery catheter; triple lumen catheters (CVP or central lines); all peripheral intravenous lines. | ○ Artificial airways compromise the normal physiologic functions of the respiratory tract including the warming, filtering, and humidifying of inhaled gases. |
| | | ○ Prevent urinary retention. | ○ The physiologically compromised patient is at risk of urinary infection. |
| | | – Monitor the following parameters: temperature; all intravenous sites for signs of redness, swelling, warmth, pain, and tenderness.<br>– Assess for wound drainage—quantity and quality.<br>– Monitor cough and sputum production.<br>– Monitor WBC profile. | |
| | | ○ Assess for signs of meningeal irritation: increased restlessness; presence of Kernig or Brudzinski signs; status of protective reflexes: cough, gag, epiglottal closure. | ○ Status of protective reflexes needs to be monitored because aspiration is a common risk in the compromised patient. |
| | | ○ Obtain culture and sensitivity on body discharges, secretions, wounds, and puncture sites.<br>– Initiate prescribed antibiotic therapy and monitor response to therapy. | ○ Cultures and sensitivity ensure that the appropriate antibiotic is prescribed. |
| | | ○ All staff caring for compromised patient should execute meticulous handwashing; visitors should be taught to do likewise. | |
| | | ○ Monitor nutrition status. | ○ Neurologically compromised patients are at risk of malnutrition; an appropriate dietary regimen should be initiated as early as possible. |
| | | ○ Hyperalimentation should be initiated early in treatment. | ○ Hyperalimentation provides necessary protein for tissue repair and rebuilding; necessary carbohydrates and lipids for energy; and necessary minerals and vitamins for cellular metabolism. |

are continuous with one another at the tentorial notch, or opening in the tentorium, which accommodates the brainstem.

## Supratentorial Herniations

There are three patterns of supratentorial herniation: cingulate, central or transtentorial, and uncal herniation. In each case, the significance of supratentorial shifts and displacements is that they compress blood vessels and brain parenchyma, causing cerebral ischemia and edema. This, in turn, further increases intracranial pressure.

### *Cingulate Herniation*

Cingulate herniation describes an expanding hemispheric lesion that shifts medially across the midline, forcing the cingulate gyrus under the falx cerebri (Fig. 8–5). Shifting of the falx can cause compression and displacement of the great vein and branches of the ipsilateral (i.e., same side) anterior cerebral artery. This results in disruption of cerebral blood flow to the medial aspects of the cerebral hemisphere (see Fig. 6–20).

### *Central, or Transtentorial, Herniation*

Central, or transtentorial, herniation is characterized by a rostral to caudal (i.e., head to toe) progression of events wherein a downward displacement of the cerebral hemispheres and basal ganglia compress the diencephalon and eventually displace the upper brainstem and midbrain through the tentorial notch (Fig. 8–6).

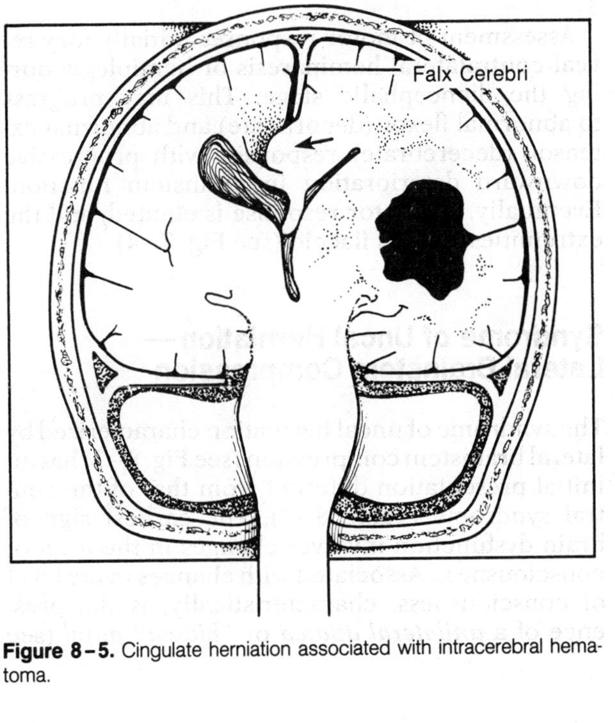


**Figure 8–5.** Cingulate herniation associated with intracerebral hematoma.

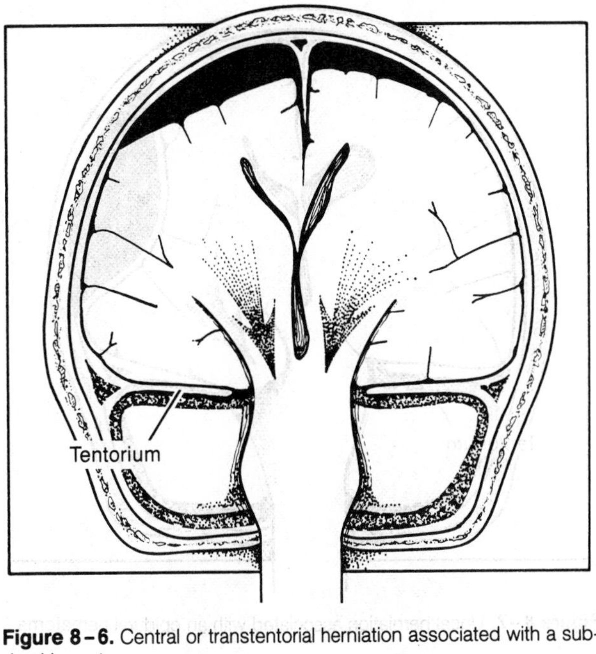


**Figure 8–6.** Central or transtentorial herniation associated with a subdural hematoma.

In the course of these events, other structures at the tentorial notch may be compromised. These include the oculomotor nerve (III), the posterior cerebral artery, the aqueduct of Sylvius, and subarachnoid space. Compression of these structures can, respectively, disrupt pupillary size and reactivity, cause ischemia and infarction of the occipital lobe, and interfere with the circulation and absorption of cerebrospinal fluid. Such pathophysiologic changes underlie clinical clues as to the level of brainstem function. A continuing increase in intracranial pressure reflects the brain's compromised compensatory mechanisms and reduced compliance.

### *Uncal Herniation*

Uncal herniation is most commonly associated with an expanding lesion of the lateral middle fossa, which causes the basal medial edge, or uncus, of the temporal lobe to be forced down into the tentorial notch (Fig. 8–7). As the swollen uncus protrudes into the notch, it impinges on the oculomotor nerve and posterior cerebral artery. Lateral displacement of the diencephalon and midbrain to the side opposite that of the uncal herniation may also occur.

## Infratentorial Herniations

Lesions occurring below the tentorium in the posterior fossa involve the cerebellum and lower brainstem. Underlying pathologic mechanisms in-

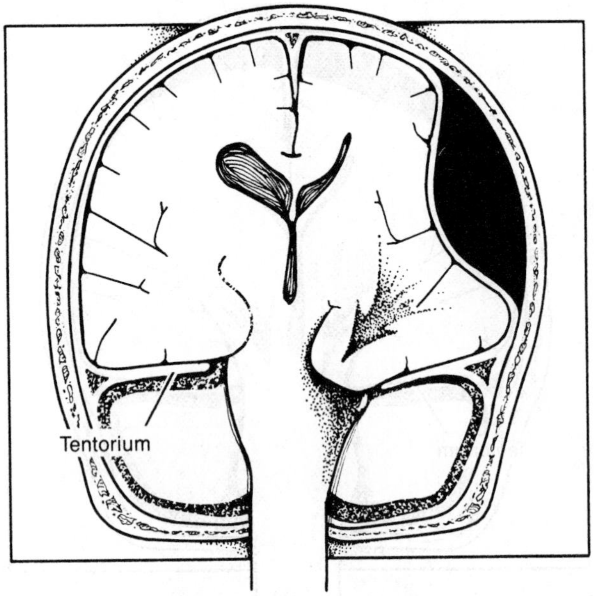


**Figure 8-7.** Uncal herniation associated with an epidural hematoma.

clude direct compression of lower brainstem (pons and medulla); upward transtentorial herniation with midbrain compression, and downward herniation into the foramen magnum.[5]

## HERNIATION SYNDROMES AND BRAIN DYSFUNCTION

To distinguish the course of one type of supratentorial mass lesion from another, Plum and Posner[6] describe two clinically distinct syndromes, namely, *central* and *uncal* herniation syndromes. Although these two syndromes may be clinically distinct early in their pathologic progression, once there is involvement of the midbrain-upper pons, their clinical pictures merge (i.e., the clinical signs of progressive uncal herniation become indistinguishable from those of central herniation syndrome).

The clinical manifestations of brain dysfunction are reflected by changes in the following parameters: level of consciousness and mentation, respiratory rate and pattern, pupillary size and reactivity, ocular movements, oculocephalic and oculovestibular reflexes, and sensorimotor responses. In the scenario of increased intracranial pressure and brain herniation, each of these parameters is described as occurring in four stages: early diencephalic, late diencephalic, midbrain-upper pons, and lower pons-upper medulla.

### Central Syndrome of Rostral to Caudal Deterioration in Brainstem Function

The *earliest* clinical sign of the central syndrome of rostral to caudal deterioration in brainstem function is an *alteration in the level of consciousness.* This occurs during the early diencephalic stage (Table 8-3). As the level of brainstem function deteriorates to the late diencephalic stage, the patient becomes stuporous and eventually slips into a coma at the midbrain stage.

Referring to Table 8-3, the respiratory pattern can be seen to be eupneic during the early diencephalic stage with perhaps an occasional deep sigh or yawn. Cheyne-Stokes pattern of respirations may be seen at the late diencephalic stage, progressing to central neurogenic hyperventilation characteristic of the midbrain-upper pons stage (see Fig. 7-2).

Pupils initially are pinpoint but reactive during the diencephalic stages. When the deterioration of brainstem function reaches the midbrain, pupils become moderately dilated, irregularly shaped, and unreactive (fixed) (see Fig. 7-2).

Roving ocular movements may vary from conjugate (movement of both eyes together) to dysconjugate (movement of eyes separately in different directions) during the late diencephalic stage. Oculocephalic and oculovestibular reflexes usually remain intact until the midbrain-upper pons stage. At this level the oculocephalic reflexes (doll's eye maneuver) may be abnormal or absent. Oculocephalic reflexes, which reflect brainstem function, are commonly used in determining brain death. Oculovestibular reflexes are preserved somewhat longer than the oculocephalic reflexes (see Fig. 7-3).

Assessment of motor responses initially may reveal contralateral hemiparesis or hemiplegia during the diencephalic stage. This may progress to abnormal flexor (decorticate) and abnormal extensor (decerebrate) responses with progressive downward deterioration in brainstem function. Eventually, no motor response is elicited, and the extremities remain flaccid (see Fig. 7-4).

### Syndrome of Uncal Herniation—Lateral Brainstem Compression

The syndrome of uncal herniation characterized by lateral brainstem compression (see Fig. 8-7) has an initial presentation different from that of the central syndrome (Table 8-4). The earliest sign of brain dysfunction involves changes in the level of consciousness. Associated with changes in the level of consciousness, characteristically, is the presence of a *unilateral dilated* or *"blown" pupil* (see

TABLE 8-3
**The Central Syndrome of Rostral to Caudal Deterioration**

| Clinical Signs | Early Diencephalon | Late Diencephalon | Midbrain-Upper Pons | Lower Pons-Upper Medulla | Medulla |
|---|---|---|---|---|---|
| Level of consciousness | Difficulty in concentration, loss of memory of recent events; agitation; drowsiness | Stupor → Coma → | Deep coma → | Same → | Same |
| Respiratory pattern | Eupneic, deep sighs, yawns → | Cheyne-Stokes → | Sustained, regnlular, hyperventilation → | Eupneic, shallow, and rapid (>20/minute) → | Ataxic (irregular in rate and amplitude) |
| Pupillary size and reactivity | Bilateral small and reactive (requires close scrutiny with bright light); pupil size 1 to 3 mm → | Same → | Moderately dilated (3 to 5 mm); irregular in shape and fixed | Mid-position, pinpoint (<3 mm) and fixed | Dilated and fixed |
| Oculocephalic/oculovestibular responses | Conjugate or slightly divergent roving eye movements → | Same, with impairment of upper conjugate gaze | Doll's eye maneuver impaired (eyes move in the direction the head is turned; may be dysconjugate) (Oculovestibular reflexes are preserved somewhat longer than oculocephalic reflexes.) | Oculocephalic reflexes, no response → | Absent |
| | Doll's eye maneuver → | Same, but easier to obtain | | | |
| | Full conjugate lateral gaze *opposite* to direction of turning | | | | |
| Motor responses | Bilateral signs of corticospinal and extrapyramidal dysfunction: | | | | |
| | Contralateral hemiparesis or hemiplegia → | Same, with addition of ipsilateral rigidity (paratonic resistance) | Usually motionless; extension of both arms and legs, particularly on side opposite to primary lesion | No purposeful movement; or possible flexor response in lower extremity to noxious stimuli | Flaccid |
| | Purposeful response to noxious stimuli → | Legs extended, arms rigidly flexed | | | Terminal stage |
| Babinski's sign | Absent | Bilateral | Bilateral extensor plantar responses | | |

Fig. 7-2). Function of the diencephalon may be spared, at least initially, and it is possible that some patients may present with a "blown" pupil and still remain arousable and aware. Other than an altered state of consciousness, the dilated, sluggishly reactive pupil may be the only sign that pathology exists at the level of the midbrain in the progression of uncal herniation. Respirations may be eupneic, ocular reflexes may remain intact, and motor responses are usually appropriate.

The major concern regarding uncal herniation is that once the pupil "blows," the course of brainstem compression proceeds rapidly, and function deteriorates precipitously. The patient may progress from a state of consciousness to one of deep coma in minutes to within several hours. The respi-

TABLE 8-4
**Syndrome of Uncal Herniation—Lateral Brainstem Compression**

| Clinical Signs | Early-Focal Neurologic Deficits | Diencephalon-Midbrain | Midbrain-Upper Pons | Lower Pons-Upper Medulla | Medulla |
|---|---|---|---|---|---|
| Level of consciousness | May be arousable → Perhaps some restlessness | Rapid deterioration (once signs of herniation appear) (stupor to coma) → | Deep coma → | Same → | Same |
| Respiratory pattern | Eupneic | Sustained, regular hyperventilation → | Same → | Eupneic, shallow, and rapid (>20/minute) → | Ataxic (irregular in rate and amplitude) |
| Pupillary size and reactivity | Unilateral dilated pupil; sluggishly reactive → | Unilateral dilated pupil, constricts sluggishly | Ipsilateral pupil widely dilated and fixed | Pupil opposite the one originally dilated may: (1) dilate widely and fix; (2) enlarge to fix in mid-position. | Dilated and fixed |
| Oculocephalic/oculovestibular responses | Intact | Once pupil dilates, external oculomotor ophthalmoplegia appears. | Impairment of oculomotor function persists, rapidly becomes sluggish, and disappears. | No response → | Absent |
| Motor responses | Appropriate response to noxious stimuli → | Purposeful movement to noxious stimuli; contralateral paratonic resistance or rigidity | Hemiplegia develops ipsilateral to the expanding supratentorial lesion. | Extensor posturing | Flaccid<br>Terminal stage |
| Babinski's sign | | Contralateral extensor plantar reflex | Bilateral extensor plantar responses | | |

ratory pattern may progress to sustained regular hyperventilation. Oculocephalic and oculovestibular reflexes become sluggish and impaired, and eventually disappear. Motor function progresses from purposeful movement to ipsilateral hemiplegia, eventually to assume abnormal flexor and abnormal extensor responses, described in central herniation syndrome. It is at this point that the clinical signs of central and uncal herniation syndromes become indistinguishable. Often, signs of both syndromes are reflected in the same patient.

Familiarity with the clinical manifestations reflective of underlying brainstem pathology is essential to: (1) evaluate the level of brainstem function and potential threat to vital respiratory and vasomotor centers, (2) determine the direction in which the pathologic process is progressing, and (3) assess the patient's response to therapeutic interventions.

## NURSING MANAGEMENT OF THE PATIENT WITH INCREASED INTRACRANIAL PRESSURE

Primary nursing responsibilities in the care of the patient with, or at risk of developing, an increase in intracranial pressure are: (1) to assess for and identify early signs of increasing intracranial pressure and (2) to implement measures to reduce intracranial pressure, maintain optimal cerebral perfusion pressure and cerebral blood flow, and minimize and/or prevent secondary injury associated with cerebral ischemia, cerebral hypoxia, and cerebral edema. A potentially reversible insult or process must *not* be allowed to become irreversible and catastrophic.

It is important to appreciate that while intracranial pressure monitoring is invaluable in the *early* diagnosing and monitoring of an increase in intracranial pressure, it is only one important parameter of the patient's total assessment. The nurse must be able to analyze and interpret data obtained via intracranial pressure monitoring, and to evaluate the significance of those data in terms of the patient's total body function.

The nurse must obtain accurate pressure measurements and be consistent in taking pressure readings. The head, for example, should always be at the same level in relationship to the transducer (i.e., at the level of the foramen of Monro). The nurse must be able to analyze pressure recordings and identify trends. Isolated readings are less meaningful than repeated or serial readings.

Patient activities (e.g., coughing, moving, posturing) may produce momentary elevations in intracranial pressure readings, and such readings may reflect normal compensatory volume/pressure responses and normal compliance. Changes in intracranial pressure fluctuate with cardiovascular dynamics and with changes in intrathoracic and intra-abdominal pressures reflected via the vena cavae and internal jugular veins. An appreciation of these interrelationships can help the nurse plan patient care.

TABLE 8-5
**Intracranial Pressure Monitoring: Troubleshooting the System**

| Problem | Cause | Intervention |
|---|---|---|
| Absent, dampened, or drifting waveform | • Transducer stopcock turned off to patient. | • Turn stopcock to appropriate positon. |
| | • Transducer connected incorrectly; loose connections. | • Check all connections; be sure appropriate connector for amplifier is in use. |
| | • Air between transducer diaphragm and pressure source. | • Eliminate air bubbles with sterile normal saline or Ringer's lactate; tighten all connections. |
| | • Occlusion of intracranial measurement device (sensor) with blood or brain tissue; or by catheter tip pushing against ventricular wall. | • Flush intracranial device as per prescribed protocol; 0.25 ml sterile normal saline is frequently used. Note: nurses do *not* routinely inject fluid into the ICPM system. |
| | • Compression of monitor cable, kinking or compression of catheter tubing, or patient movement (artifact). | • Avoid kinking of catheter tubing as patient is moved or positioned in bed. |
| | • Incorrect gain setting for pressure, or patient having plateau waves (A waves). | • Adjust gain setting for higher pressure setting. |
| | • Trace turned off. | • Turn power on to trace: monitor and transducer should have ample time to warm up prior to use. |
| False high pressure | • Transducer below level of pressure source. | • Place venting port of transducer at level of foramen of Monro. For every inch the transducer is below the pressure source, there is an error of approximately 2 mmHg. |
| | • Transducer incorrectly balanced. | • Correctly position transducer and rebalance. Transducer should be balanced every 8 hr, and repositioned as necessary to ensure reliable measurements.<br>• Avoid initiating treatment for increased ICP unless readouts are reliably accurate. |
| | • Monitoring system incorrectly calibrated. | • Repeat calibration procedure. |
| | • Air in system. Air may attenuate or amplify pressure signal. | • Remove air from monitoring line. |
| False low pressure readings | • Complete occlusion of catheter or screw device. | • Flush monitoring device. |
| | • Air bubbles between transducer and pressure source, loose connections. | • Eliminate air bubbles with sterile normal saline or Ringer's lactate. Tighten all connections. |
| | • Transducer above the level of the pressure source. | • Place venting port of transducer at level of foramen of Monro. For every inch the transducer is above the level of the pressure source there will be an error of approximately 2 mmHg. |
| | • Zero and/or calibration incorrect. | • Re-zero and calibrate monitoring system. |

*Note:* Troubleshooting and assessment of the entire monitoring system should be done frequently; the pressure waveform and digital readouts need to be evaluated in terms of other assessment data reflective of the patient's overall status.

Specifically, those patient care activities that cause changes in intracranial pressure must be identified. Such activities as coughing, suctioning, and positioning may cause momentary increases in intracranial pressure, and their implementation should be spaced apart. Planned rest periods should be incorporated into daily care, and the environment should remain as quiet as possible. The responsive patient should be taught to avoid excessive coughing, Valsalva's maneuver, isometric exercises, or pushing against side rails or footboard. The patient should be assessed for bladder distention, paralytic ileus, and constipation.

A sustained increase in intracranial pressure (>20–25 mmHg) for an extended period of time (15–20 minutes) suggests a loss of compensation and brain compliance. Under these circumstances, the nurse must recognize the clinical significance of the cerebral hypertension and act in a timely and aggressive manner to initiate prescribed treatments and nursing measures designed to reduce the intracranial pressure. (Specific therapeutic pressure-reducing measures and their nursing implications are discussed in Chapter 9.)

## Intracranial Pressure Monitoring: Maintaining the Integrity of the System

A major responsibility assumed by critical care nurses caring for the neurologically compromised patient is to prevent infection. Scrupulous aseptic technique is absolutely essential when working with an intracranial pressure monitoring system. A leak or breakdown in the integrity of the system requires immediate intervention to stop and/or control the leak, and to re-establish and maintain sterility of the system.

The intracranial pressure monitoring system requires frequent checks to ensure that all stopcocks are in their appropriate positions. Inadvertent introduction of even small amounts of fluid may have profound deleterious effects on the patient in whom intracranial pressure is already elevated. Leaks in the system resulting in inadvertent drainage of cerebrospinal fluid may result in a significant lowering of intracranial pressure, causing brain tissue to be sucked up against the catheter or screw. The ventricles may collapse, precipitating a shift in intracranial contents.

The nurse must be vigilant for potential problems that may occur with use of invasive pressure monitoring. Treatment of increases in intracranial pressure and an evaluation of the patient's response to that treatment must be based on clearly established and accurate pressure measurements.

## Nursing Diagnoses, Desired Patient Outcomes, and Nursing Interventions/ Rationales

Specific nursing diagnoses, desired patient outcomes, and nursing interventions concerned with the management of the patient with, or at risk of developing, an increase in intracranial pressure are presented in Table 8–2. Physiologic principles underlying nursing interventions are incorporated into the rationales for decision-making. Guidelines for troubleshooting the invasive intracranial pressure monitoring system are included in Table 8–5.

## REFERENCES

1. Muwaswes, M: Increased intracranial pressure and its systemic effects. Journal of Neurosurgical Nursing 17(4):238, 1985.
2. Plum, F and Posner, J: The Diagnosis of Stupor and Coma, ed. 3. FA Davis, Philadelphia, 1980, p 95.
3. Boortz-Marx, R: Factors affecting intracranial pressure: A descriptive study. Journal of Neurosurgical Nursing 17(2):89, 1985.
4. Epstein, FB and Hamilton, GC: Initial approach to the brain-injured patient. Crit Care Q 5(4):14, 1983.
5. Plum, F and Posner, J: The Diagnosis of Stupor and Coma, ed. 3. FA Davis, Philadelphia, 1980, pp 153–160.
6. Plum, F and Posner, J: The Diagnosis of Stupor and Coma, ed. 3. FA Davis, Philadelphia, 1980, pp 103–109.
7. Smith, KA: Head trauma: Comparison of infection rates for different methods of intracranial pressure monitoring. Journal of Neurosurgical Nursing 19(6):310–314, 1987.

CHAPTER 9

# Therapeutic Modalities in the Treatment of the Patient with Neurologic Dysfunction

## CHAPTER OUTLINE

MANAGEMENT OF THE PATIENT WITH INCREASED INTRACRANIAL PRESSURE
Treatment of Intracranial Hypertension

## LEARNING OBJECTIVES

**At the end of this chapter you should be able to:**

1. State the physiologic principles underlying the maintenance of ventilatory function in the patient with a craniocerebral insult.
2. Describe how the appropriate positioning of the patient with, or at risk of developing, increased intracranial pressure reduces and/or prevents intracranial hypertension.
3. Report on how Valsalva-type maneuvers can cause an increase in intracranial pressure.
4. Describe why administration of morphine sulfate is an adjunct to therapy in the responsive, "pavulonized" patient.
5. Analyze the hemodynamic mechanisms at work in patients with compromised autoregulatory mechanisms and reduced brain compliance.
6. Describe the physiologic basis for maintaining the patient with an acute craniocerebral insult in a slightly dehydrated state.
7. Discuss why an intact blood–brain barrier is necessary for the optimal benefit of hyperosmolar therapy.
8. List important nursing considerations associated with corticosteroid therapy in the patient with intracranial hypertension.
9. Report on the physiologic considerations underlying the nursing management of the patient in barbiturate coma.
10. Implement the nursing process in the management of the patient with craniocerebral surgery:
    Assessment
    Nursing diagnosis
    Planning: Desired patient outcomes
    Nursing interventions

## MANAGEMENT OF THE PATIENT WITH INCREASED INTRACRANIAL PRESSURE

The major goals in the nursing management of the patient with increased intracranial pressure (i.e., intracranial hypertension) are: (1) to reduce intracranial pressure to within normal physiologic limits (0–15 mmHg);(2) to maintain cerbral perfusion pressure (>60 mmHg) and cerebral blood flow; and (3) to protect the patient from any further episodes of increased intracranial pressure, which can precipitate secondary pathophysiologic changes such as cerebral ischemia, cellular hypoxia, and cerebral edema. Without timely, appropriate, and aggressive intervention, should the patient survive, these secondary changes can predispose to permanent neurologic sequelae or disabilities, seriously disrupting the quality of life for the patient, family, and significant others.

In the acute setting, prognosis appears to be related to the *control* of intracranial pressure. Patients experiencing an increase in intracranial pressure (> 30 mmHg) on a consistent basis or for extended periods of time (20–30 minutes) rarely do well. A reasonable approach in the care of these patients is to initiate treatment to maintain *baseline* intracranial pressure at less than 20–25 mmHg, and cerebral perfusion pressure at greater than 60 mmHg. Ideally, intracranial pressure should be maintained at less than 15 mmHg, and cerebral perfusion pressure at approximately 80–90 mmHg.

Currently, a number of therapeutic approaches are available to treat intracranial hypertension. Surgical decompression affords direct evacuation of a mass intracranial lesion. Drainage of cerebrospinal fluid via an intraventricular catheter helps to reduce intracranial volume. Proper patient positioning also helps to reduce intracranial volume by facilitating drainage of blood and cerebrospinal fluid from the cranial vault by gravity.

A reduction in cerebral blood flow can be achieved by controlled hyperventilation. Measures that reduce cellular metabolism also assist in reducing cerebral blood flow. These measures include use of analgesics, antipyretics, and anticonvulsants; hypothermia; and barbiturate coma. Cerebral edema may be limited by administering diuretics, hyperosmolar agents, and corticosteroids. Fluid restriction also assists by maintaining the patient in a slightly dehydrated state.

More recently, calcium antagonists have been used to manage cerebral ischemia associated with cerebral vasospasm. Use of histamine$_2$ antagonists and antacid therapy help to prevent gastrointestinal injury caused by stress ulcerations.

The critical care nurse is largely responsible for implementing the plan of care; monitoring and reassessing the patient continuously to evaluate the patient's response to therapeutic measures; and constantly watching for subtle signs of a deterioration in the patient's condition, which may warrant timely and aggressive intervention to minimize underlying pathology.

## Treatment of Intracranial Hypertension

### *Surgical Decompression*

In the patient who has sustained an acute craniocerebral insult, immediate surgical decompression via craniotomy or burr holes may be indicated to evacuate a rapidly expanding intracranial mass lesion (e.g., epidural hematoma) and to relieve the consequent intracranial hypertension (i.e., increased intracranial pressure). Surgical intervention alleviates and/or prevents a precipitous rise in intracranial pressure, which might otherwise predispose to *brain herniation* with irreversible brain damage and death. Intracranial volume and pressure may be reduced surgically by arresting hemorrhaging, removing clots (e.g., hematomas), and elevating depressed skull fractures.

**Nursing Diagnoses, Patient Outcomes, and Nursing Interventions/Rationales in the Care of the Patient with Craniocerebral Surgery.** The postoperative management of the patient who has had craniocerebral surgery is especially challenging because a wide spectrum of complications are possible.[1] Some selected postoperative complications include an altered state of consciousness, cerebral edema, intracranial bleeding, cerebral ischemia and infarction, hydrocephalus, tension pneumocephalus, and intracranial hypertension. Table 9–1 presents specific nursing diagnoses, patient outcomes, and nursing interventions concerned with the postoperative care of the craniocerebral surgery patient.

### *Cerebrospinal Fluid Drainage*

Cerebrospinal fluid (CSF) is sometimes drained to reduce intracranial volume and relieve intracranial pressure, especially in patients with reduced brain compliance. Usually a ventricular catheter is used, and intracranial pressure is carefully monitored. Cerebrospinal fluid shunting procedures (e.g., ventriculo-peritoneal) may also be surgically performed to establish long-term shunting of CSF from the intracranial cavity. Such procedures may be performed to relieve *obstructive hydrocephalus.*

A major complication of CSF drainage is infection. Strict aseptic technique must be used at all times, and the integrity of the system must be maintained.

### *Maintenance of Ventilatory Function*

A major nursing responsibility is the prevention of hypercapnia ($PaCO_2 > 45$ mmHg) and hypoxemia ($PaO_2 < 60$ mmHg). Both hypercapnia and hypoxemia have a potent *vasodilatory* effect on cerebral blood vessels. Vasodilation increases the volume of blood within the cerebral vasculature, which, in the absence of autoregulatory and compensatory control, precipitates a rise in intracranial pressure.

On the contrary, hypocapnia ($PaCO_2 < 30$–35 mmHg) is a potent stimulus for cerebral *vasoconstriction,* which functions to decrease the volume of blood within the cerebral vasculature. A reduction in cerebral blood volume helps to reduce

**TABLE 9–1. CARE PLAN FOR POSTOPERATIVE PATIENT WITH CRANIOCEREBRAL SURGERY**

| Nursing Diagnoses | Desired Patient Outcomes | Nursing Interventions | Rationales |
|---|---|---|---|
| ***Nursing Diagnosis #1*** Alteration in cerebral perfusion pressure, related to:<br>1. Cerebral edema.<br>2. Potential intracranial bleeding with hematoma formation.<br>3. Compromised cardiovascular function. | Patient will:<br>1. Maintain<br>• Cerebral perfusion pressure > 60 mmHg.<br>• Intracranial pressure < 15 mmHg.<br>• Mean arterial blood pressure ~ 80 mmHg.<br>2. Exhibit intact level of consciousness and mentation; open eyes when name is called; be oriented to person and place.<br>3. Follow commands; differentiate pin prick from crude pressure. | • Refer to Table 8–2 for a presentation of the following nursing interventions/rationales:<br>○ Monitor for signs and symptoms of increasing intracranial pressure.<br>○ Maintain intracranial pressure monitoring system.<br>○ Implement measures to prevent and/or reduce intracranial pressure.<br>○ Maintain optimal positioning.<br>○ Prevent increase in cerebral blood flow.<br>○ Limit or decrease cerebral edema.<br>○ Minimize cellular metabolism.<br>○ Plan nursing care activities to prevent cumulative increase in intracranial pressure. | |
| ***Nursing Diagnosis #2*** Breathing pattern ineffective, related to:<br>1. Brainstem compression associated with cerebral edema (especially following *infra*tentorial craniotomy).<br>2. Respiratory depression associated with anesthesia, analgesia, and muscle relaxants. | Patient will demonstrate effective breathing pattern:<br>1. Respiratory rate < 25/min.<br>2. Rhythm and depth eupneic.<br>• Tidal volume > 7–10 ml/kg.<br>• Vital capacity > 12–15 ml/kg.<br>3. Adequate alveolar ventilation and gas exchange:<br>• $PaCO_2$ < 30–35 mmHg.<br>• $PaO_2$ > 80 mmHg.<br>• pH 7.35–7.45. | • Assess respiratory function hourly.<br>○ Assess spontaneous respiratory effort: rate, depth, rhythm; use of accessory muscles; dyspnea, tachypnea; hyper- or hypoventilation.<br>○ Monitor arterial blood gases.<br>• Implement measures to improve breathing pattern.<br>○ Maintain patient in semi-Fowler's position.<br>○ Maintain nasogastric decompression as indicated.<br>○ Maintain mechanical ventilation and oxygenation.<br>– Assess tidal volume and vital capacity. | • Adequate ventilation and oxygenation are imperative because hypercapnia and hypoxia cause cerebral vasodilation. In the patient with reduced intracranial compliance, an increase in cerebral blood flow may precipitate a significant rise in intracranial pressure.<br>○ Reflect adequacy of ventilation and oxygenation.<br>○ Permits maximal chest excursion and facilitates drainage of blood and cerebrospinal fluid from cranial vault via gravity.<br>○ Prevents abdominal distention, which can compromise diaphragmatic excursion; minimizes danger of aspiration.<br>○ See Tables 32–5 through 32–9. |

*(continued)*

**TABLE 9–1. CARE PLAN FOR POSTOPERATIVE PATIENT WITH CRANIOCEREBRAL SURGERY *(Continued)***

| Nursing Diagnoses | Desired Patient Outcomes | Nursing Interventions | Rationales |
|---|---|---|---|
| ***Nursing Diagnosis #3***<br>Airway clearance ineffective, related to:<br>1. Compromised cough.<br>2. Thick, tenacious secretions. | Patient will:<br>1. Maintain patent airway.<br>• Normal breath sounds on auscultation.<br>• Absence of adventitious sounds (crackles, rhonchi, wheezes).<br>2. Demonstrate secretion-clearing cough (unless contraindicated by intracranial hypertension). | • Assess respiratory function hourly. | • Hypercapnia and hypoxia increase cerebral blood flow. |
| | | ∘ Assess airway patency: status of protective reflexes: cough, gag, epiglottal closure. | ∘ Compromised protective reflexes place patient at risk of aspirating tracheobronchial secretions. |
| | | ∘ Auscultate breath sounds bilaterally.<br>∘ Assess characteristics of sputum (e.g., color, tenaciousness, amount). | ∘ Presence of rales (crackles), wheezes, or rhonchi suggests increased pulmonary secretions (e.g., pulmonay edema, infection) or inability to mobilize or clear secretions. Patient is at increased risk of developing a pneumonia. |
| | | ∘ Assess hydration status. | ∘ Dehydration causes tracheobronchial secretions to become thick, tenacious, and difficult to clear. |
| | | • Implement measures to maintain airway patency:<br>∘ Humidify inspired air. | |
| | | ∘ Initiate suctioning of tracheobronchial secretions *only* when indicated; assess effect of suctioning on patient's intracranial pressure. | ∘ Suctioning stimulates cough reflex and Valsalva's maneuver; these responses are associated with an increase in intracranial pressure.<br>∘ See Table 32–4. |
| | | ∘ Follow appropriate suctioning technique, minimize suctioning time; hyperventilate with 100% oxygen via resuscitator prior to and between each pass, and after suctioning.<br>– Monitor hydration status. | ∘ Reduces risk of developing hypercapnia and hypoxemia; minimizes risk of increasing intracranial pressure. |
| | | ∘ Turning and positioning measures. (Refer to Table 8–2, Care Plan for nursing activities to avoid a cumulative increase in intracranial pressure.) | ∘ Movement of the patient is guided by the status of intracranial pressure; turning the patient should be avoided when intracranial pressure is unstable. |
| ***Nursing Diagnosis #4***<br>Alteration in comfort: Headache, related to:<br>1. Meningeal irritation.<br>2. Surgical scalp incision.<br>3. Anxiety. | Patient will:<br>1. Verbalize and/or indicate comfort.<br>2. Demonstrate relaxed facial expression and demeanor.<br>3. Maintain intracranial pressure $<15$ mmHg. | • Assess patient for signs of pain and discomfort.<br>∘ Symptoms may include: restlessness, agitation; clenched fist, tense facial expression; photophobia.<br>∘ Signs of discomfort may be reflected by increase in intracranial pressure, heart rate, blood pressure, and respiratory rate. | • The patient must be as comfortable as possible to prevent any increase in intracranial pressure. Pain, fear, anxiety, and muscle tenseness or rigidity can precipitate a rise in intracranial pressure and must be avoided. |

| | | | |
|---|---|---|---|
| | | • Implement measures to reduce discomfort.<br>◦ Administer analgesic or sedative as prescribed. Evaluate patient's response to medication.<br>◦ Position patient to relieve muscle tension and pressure on bony prominences.<br><br>◦ Make sure dressing is not too tight and constricting.<br>◦ Provide quiet environment. Minimize environmental stimuli: dim lights, reduce noise level, restrict visitors if necessary.<br>◦ Provide periods for uninterrupted sleep.<br>◦ Provide touch therapy; speak softly in a soothing voice.<br>– Reassure patient you are there to anticipate and fulfill his/her needs.<br>– Provide appropriate explanations.<br>◦ Employ diversional and comfort measures (e.g., soft music, mouth care, back rub, passive movement of extremities). | • Nursing activities that limit sensory overload, prevent sleep deprivation and provide reassurance help to minimize changes in the patient's intracranial pressure status; such care minimizes cellular metabolic activities, reducing demand for oxygen and glucose, and thus the need for increase in cerebral blood flow.<br>◦ Brain tissue itself is without free pain endings; pain experienced by patients is usually related to meningeal irritation and/or injury to scalp where free nerve endings are numerous. |
| ***Nursing Diagnosis #5***<br>Alteration in fluid and electrolyte balance.<br>1. Fluid volume excess related to:<br>• Cerebral edema.<br>• SIADH.<br>2. Fluid volume deficit related to:<br>• Diuretic therapy.<br>• Diabetes insipidus.<br>3. Altered electrolytes related to:<br>• Diuretic therapy.<br>• Corticosteroid therapy.<br>• Acid–base imbalance. | Patient will:<br>1. Maintain hemodynamic function.<br>• Mean systemic blood pressure ~80–100 mmHg.<br>• Heart rate at patient's baseline; rhythm regular, without dysrhythmias.<br>2. Maintain balanced intake and output.<br>• Stable baseline daily weight (unless contraindicated).<br>• Urine output >30 ml and <200 ml/hr.<br>• Urine specific gravity 1.010–1.025.<br>3. Demonstrate good skin turgor and moist mucous membranes. | • Refer to the appropriate tables in Chapters 23 and 30.<br>• Monitor for signs and symptoms of diabetes insipidus: polyuria, polydipsia, and urine specific gravity <1.005; monitor fluid intake and output, weight; serum electrolytes and osmolality.<br>◦ Monitor for signs and symptoms of dehydration.<br><br>• Implement measures to:<br>◦ Maintain adequate fluid intake to prevent dehydration.<br>◦ Administer prescribed medications: vasopressin replacement therapy; agents that enhance ADH secretion (e.g., chlorpropamide, carbamazepine). | • Diabetes insipidus may occur secondary to craniocerebral trauma, infection (e.g., meningitis), or pituitary tumors.<br>◦ Cerebral edema related to trauma or surgery may impair synthesis and release of antidiuretic hormone temporarily resulting in polyuria within 24–48 hr. As cerebral edema subsides, symptoms also regress and diminish.<br>• For information related to the diagnosis, treatment, and nursing management of diabetes insipidus, see Chapter 16. |

(continued)

**TABLE 9-1. CARE PLAN FOR POSTOPERATIVE PATIENT WITH CRANIOCEREBRAL SURGERY *(Continued)***

| Nursing Diagnoses | Desired Patient Outcomes | Nursing Interventions | Rationales |
|---|---|---|---|
| ***Nursing Diagnosis #5 (cont.)*** | | | |
| | 4. Maintain laboratory parameters within acceptable range.<br>• Serum electrolytes, BUN, and creatinine.<br>• Hematocrit, hemoglobin.<br>• Serum osmolality.<br>• Arterial blood gas studies; acid–base balance intact. | | |
| ***Nursing Diagnosis #6***<br>Potential for injury: Seizures, related to:<br>1. Cerebral ischemia and injury associated with surgical manipulation. | Patient will:<br>1. Not have any seizures. (See Chap. 13.) | • Assess characteristics of seizure activity.<br>○ Specific signs: onset (what triggers the seizure, type, locality, presence of aura, duration of seizure); type of movement: tonic, clonic, flaccid; associated changes in level of consciousness; pupillary size and reactivity; extraocular movements; associated vomiting or incontinence (urinary, fecal).<br>• During seizure activity:<br>○ Maintain safe environment.<br>○ Remain with patient but do not restrain; provide reassurance.<br>○ Do not force airway or other objects between clenched teeth.<br>○ Keep resuscitative equipment at bedside. | • Seizure activity can precipitate a significant increase in intracranial pressure; it increases cellular metabolism and the demand for metabolic substrates—oxygen and glucose; it raises body temperature.<br>○ Postoperative seizure activity may be precipitated by hypoxia, hyperventilation, hyperpyrexia, meningeal irritation, and bladder distention. |
| | | • Implement measures to prevent seizure activity.<br>○ Avoid problems that cause an increase in intracranial pressure (e.g., headache, anxiety, hypoxia, hyperventilation, urinary retention, fecal impaction, hyperpyrexia).<br>○ Monitor for signs of meningeal irritation (see Nursing Diagnosis #7). Initiate and maintain seizure precautions: oral airway; padded side rails and headboard; keep bed in low position with side rails in up position.<br>○ Administer prescribed anticonvulsant therapy. | • A rise in intracranial pressure may precipitate seizure activity associated with cerebral ischemia. |

| | | | |
|---|---|---|---|
| | | ○ Evaluate patient's response to anticonvulsant therapy.<br>– Obtain serum levels of phenytoin.<br>– Be familiar with effect of phenytoin on cardiovascular hemodynamics and adverse drug reactions. | ○ Diazepam, phenytoin, and barbiturates are commonly used to prevent and/or treat seizures. For specific information related to dose, route of administration, adverse reactions, and nursing implications for each of these drugs, see Appendix A. |
| ***Nursing Diagnosis #7***<br>Potential for infection: Meningitis (see Chap. 13), related to:<br>1. Craniocerebral trauma.<br>2. Surgical disruption of integrity of the meninges.<br>3. Iatrogenic causes via invasive procedures. | Patient will:<br>1. Maintain body temperature ~98.6°F (37°C).<br>2. Remain free of signs of meningeal irritation (nuchal rigidity, headache, photophobia, positive Kernig and Brudzinski's signs).<br>3. Demonstrate normal cerebrospinal fluid analysis (WBC and protein levels); serum WBC within normal range. | • Monitor for signs and symptoms of infection.<br>○ Assess for meningeal irritation: hyperpyrexia, chills, nuchal rigidity, photophobia, persistent headache, positive Kernig's sign (i.e., inability to extend lower leg when hip is flexed), positive Brudzinski's sign (i.e., flexion of hips and knees when head is flexed on chest).<br>○ Assess for otorrhea and rhinorrhea.<br>○ Use of Dextrostix to test for presence of glucose.<br>– Observe for clear halo around serosanguineous drainage from ear, nose, or dressing.<br>– Observe for excessive swallowing or complaints of postnasal drip.<br>○ Assist with lumbar puncture.<br>– Observe color of cerebrospinal fluid.<br>– Record cerebrospinal pressure. | • See Table 49–7.<br><br>○ Meningeal tears often accompany basal skull fractures.<br>○ Presence of glucose in nonbloody drainage from nose or ear suggests cerebrospinal leak. Nasopharyngeal secretions do not contain glucose.<br><br>○ Presence of elevated levels of WBCs and protein in cerebrospinal fluid strongly suggests meningitis. |
| | | • Implement measures to prevent infection.<br>○ Specific nursing actions include: strict handwashing, sterile technique in managing all invasive procedures (e.g., intracranial pressure monitoring, ventricular shunts), sterile technique employed for all dressing changes (as per unit protocols).<br>○ If rhinorrhea or otorrhea are present:<br>○ Caution patient not to cough, sneeze, blow the nose, or perform a Valsalva's maneuver (e.g., straining at stool).<br>– Instruct patient not to put fingers into ears or nose, and to lie quietly.<br>– Allow free flow of drainage directly onto sterile pad; change pad as soon as it becomes damp.<br>○ Have patient assume a position that facilitates free drainage (e.g., semi-Fowler's position) in the presence of rhinorrhea. | • Disciplined aseptic technique is essential to prevent meningitis.<br><br>○ These activities increase intracranial pressure and can place further stress on the dural tear.<br><br>○ Free flow of drainage prevents pooling, which might otherwise provide a medium for bacterial colonization. |

*(continued)*

## TABLE 9-1. CARE PLAN FOR POSTOPERATIVE PATIENT WITH CRANIOCEREBRAL SURGERY *(Continued)*

| Nursing Diagnoses | Desired Patient Outcomes | Nursing Interventions | Rationales |
|---|---|---|---|
| ***Nursing Diagnosis #7 (cont.)*** | | | |
| | | ◦ Provide quiet environment; minimize stimuli. | ◦ Reduces risk of aggravating underlying dural tear. |
| | | • Administer prescribed course of antibiotics.<br>◦ Evaluate response to therapy:<br>– Monitor temperature, WBC profile.<br>– Monitor neurologic function and signs of meningeal irritation.<br>– Monitor intracranial pressure. | ◦ Administration of corticosteroids to reduce cerebral edema may compromise the immune response, placing patient at greater risk of developing an infection. Ongoing assessment for signs of infection must be diligent; aseptic technique must be impeccable. |
| | | • Provide reassurance to patient and family. | |
| ***Nursing Diagnosis #8***<br>Potential for alteration in body temperature, related to:<br>1. Cerebral edema with altered hypothalamic function.<br>2. Infection. | Patient will:<br>1. Maintain optimal body temperature ~98.6°F (37°C). | • Monitor body temperature every 1–2 hr if unstable.<br>◦ Assess for signs and symptoms of hyperpyrexia (e.g., hot, dry skin; parched tongue; cool extremities; delirium). | • Hyperpyrexia increases cerebral metabolism and cerebral blood flow; an increase in intracranial pressure may result from the consequent increase in intracranial blood volume. |
| | | • Obtain specimens of body fluid (e.g., blood, urine, sputum, wound drainage) for culture and sensitivity.<br>• Inspect all invasive sites and wounds for signs of infection (e.g., redness, warmth, swelling, pain; amount and characteristics of wound drainage).<br>• Implement measures to reduce body temperature.<br>◦ Administer prescribed antibiotic and antipyretic therapy.<br>– Evaluate patient's response to therapy by monitoring body temperature and WBC profile.<br>◦ Provide comfort measures.<br>– Remove excess clothing and blankets.<br>– Maintain room temperature at ~20°C (68°F).<br>– Apply ice bags to groin and axilla; tepid bath.<br>◦ Provide diligent wound care.<br>– Wash hands thoroughly. | • In the scenario of a spiking body temperature (~39°C–41°C [102.2°F–105.8°F]), obtain culture of body fluids prior to initiating prescribed antibiotic therapy. |

| | | | |
|---|---|---|---|
| | | – Monitor all invasive sites and wounds for signs/symptoms of infection.<br>– Provide wound care and dressings using aseptic technique; damp dressings should be changed promptly, and dry dressings should be applied as per unit protocol.<br>• Implement hypothermia therapy as prescribed.<br>• Offer reassurance to patient and family. | • When inducing an increase or decrease in body temperature, the change in temperature should not exceed 1°F (0.56°C) per 15–20 minutes. |
| ***Nursing Diagnosis #9***<br>Potential for physiologic injury: Gastrointestinal bleeding associated with stress and corticosteroid therapy. | Patient will remain without gastrointestinal bleeding:<br>1. Hematocrit stable.<br>• Male 45%–52%.<br>• Female 37%–48%.<br>2. Hemoglobin stable.<br>• Male 13–18 g/100 ml.<br>• Female 12–16 g/100 ml.<br>3. Nasogastric drainage.<br>• Negative for occult blood.<br>• pH >4.5.<br>4. Stool negative for occult blood.<br>5. Vital signs stable.<br>• Blood pressure and heart rate at patient's baseline level. | • See Table 49–6. | |
| ***Nursing Diagnosis #10***<br>Alteration in nutrition: Less than body requirements, related to:<br>1. Stress (craniocerebral insult).<br>2. Compromised or absent protective reflexes (e.g., cough, gag, epiglottal closure).<br>3. Altered state of consciousness. | Patient will receive adequate nutritional intake.<br>• Stable baseline body weight.<br>• Balanced intake and output.<br>• Stable laboratory parameters: serum protein (albumin) 3.5–5.0 g/100 ml, BUN, creatinine.<br>• Positive nitrogen balance. | • Consult with nutritionist to assess metabolic needs.<br>○ See Tables 53– 1: Components of a Dietary History<br>53– 7: Protein Measurements<br>53– 9: Correction Factors for Predicting Energy Requirements in Hospitalized Patient<br>53–10: Caloric Requirements of the Critically Ill<br>53–14: Large Bore vs. Small Bore Feeding Tubes<br>53–15: Method of Enteral Administration<br>53–18: Mechanical Complications Associated with Enteral Feeding Tubes<br>53–25: Special Considerations for Specific Disease States | |

*(continued)*

**TABLE 9–1. CARE PLAN FOR POSTOPERATIVE PATIENT WITH CRANIOCEREBRAL SURGERY *(Continued)***

| Nursing Diagnoses | Desired Patient Outcomes | Nursing Interventions | Rationales |
|---|---|---|---|
| ***Nursing Diagnosis #11***<br>Alteration in self-concept, related to:<br>1. Changes in body image associated with physical appearance (e.g., shaved head) or neurologic deficits (e.g., loss of sensorimotor function).<br>2. Loss of self-esteem (i.e., dependence on others to achieve activities of daily living).<br>3. Alterations in role and personal identity.<br>4. Stigma of seizure disorder. | Patient will:<br>1. Verbalize positive feelings about self.<br>2. Maintain interpersonal relationships with family members and significant others.<br>3. Participate in decision-making process regarding care.<br>4. Initiate activities related to self-care. | • Encourage verbalization regarding patient's perceptions of changes in appearance and body function.<br>∘ Observe nonverbal behavior reflective of underlying feelings and concerns.<br>∘ Listen to patient's concerns.<br>∘ Provide information and explanations regarding patient's status and prognosis. Clarify misconceptions.<br>∘ Ascertain patient/family expectations and understanding regarding impact of illness on family lifestyle.<br>∘ Facilitate communication between patient, family, and significant others.<br>• Assist patient/family to identify coping patterns/strengths and weaknesses.<br>• Assess patient/family's readiness to participate in decision-making process regarding care. | • Assists patient to increase self-awareness and to recognize and vent feelings of fear, anger, or frustrations.<br>∘ Often what the patient doesn't say is reflected in the body language. |
| | | • Involve patient in making choices and decisions regarding self-care.<br>∘ Readily identify and praise patient's accomplishments. Identify improvements in bodily functions as they occur. | • Assists patient in maintaining a sense of control over his/her life.<br>∘ Positive reinforcement nurtures self-motivation. |
| | | • Assist patient/family in initial goal setting.<br>∘ Refer to social worker.<br>– Identify community resources.<br>– Encourage use of community support groups (e.g., head injury support groups). | • Depending on underlying problem, a craniocerebral insult or injury can be catastrophic in terms of health-care costs, productivity, and quality of life for all concerned.<br>∘ Early referral to social worker and community agencies should be initiated. |

and/or maintain intracranial pressure within the normal physiologic range (0–15 mmHg).

**Maintenance of Patent Airway.** A major nursing responsibility is to ensure that the patient has a patent airway so that hypercapnia and hypoxemia can be prevented. A thorough assessment of respiratory function is necessary to determine patency of the airway and the response of the patient to the ventilatory regimen.

In the responsive patient, the respiratory assessment might be guided by the following questions: Is the patient alert and oriented to person, place, and time? Is the patient restless? Is the patient cooperative? Does he/she follow verbal commands? Can the patient cough and deep breathe effectively? Can the patient swallow? Is the gag reflex intact? What are the tracheobronchial secretions like? Can the patient handle the secretions effectively? What is the work of breathing like? Are accessory muscles used in breathing? Is there ventilatory dyscoordination? Is the patient hemodynamically stable? What is the hydration status?

Rate, depth, and pattern of breathing should be assessed. Auscultation of anterior and posterior thorax may help to evaluate the degree of lung expansion; and detection of adventitious sounds (rales or crackles, rhonchi, wheezes) may provide clues to underlying pathology (e.g., pneumonia, pneumothorax, pulmonary edema). Arterial blood gases should be assessed at regular intervals to evaluate the effectiveness of the ventilatory effort. Serial assessment of tidal volume and vital capacity also assists in assessing ventilatory capacity.

***Endotracheal Suctioning.*** Suctioning of the intubated patient maintains a patent airway and reduces the risk of pulmonary complications. Pneumonia, for example, associated with pooling and buildup of pulmonary secretions is a major complication in head-injured patients. In the patient with unstable intracranial pressure, suctioning is especially critical to avert a reduction in alveolar ventilation associated with secretion buildup, with consequent hypercapnia and hypoxemia.

Suctioning may increase the sympathetic nervous system response manifested clinically by an increase in blood pressure and heart rate. The consequent increase in cerebral perfusion and cerebral blood flow may, in turn, increase intracranial pressure. Parasympathetic stimulation (e.g., vagal response) may also be triggered by suctioning, as is the Valsalva's maneuver. The increase in intrathoracic pressures associated with Valsalva's maneuver may contribute to an increase in intracranial pressure by impeding normal venous drainage from the cranial vault via the jugular veins into the superior vena cava. In the absence of autoregulatory and compensatory controls, all of these responses triggered by endotracheal suctioning can induce a considerable increase in intracranial pressure, which may persist after the procedure is completed.

Cognizant of the perils of suctioning on intracranial pressure, yet appreciative of the need for timely and effective suctioning to prevent pulmonary complications, the nurse must use appropriate suctioning technique. Each suctioning pass should be limited to 10 seconds, and suctioning should only be performed when clinically necessary (e.g., a buildup of pulmonary secretions as indicated by the presence of adventitious breath sounds on auscultation, an increase in $PaCO_2$ and decrease in $PaO_2$ on arterial blood gas analysis, and/or triggering of ventilator alarm system).

Prior to suctioning, the lungs should be hyperventilated with 100% oxygen using a hand-held resuscitator. High percentage oxygenation over several inflations helps to reduce the degree of hypoxemia and the risk of cardiac dysrhythmias that may occur as a result of the suctioning procedure. Hyperventilation using a hand-held resuscitator, performed on an hourly basis, also serves to inflate alveoli and prevent atelectasis.

Because suctioning highly influences intracranial pressure, it should be done when the patient is at rest and the intracranial pressure is at baseline. Monitoring of the intracranial pressure provides useful guidelines for planning care. Necessary procedures can be spaced to avoid a cumulative impact on intracranial pressure, which might occur if too much activity is induced at any one time. (For a review of appropriate suctioning technique, see Table 32–4.)

**Hyperventilation Therapy.** Controlled hyperventilation is prescribed to achieve and maintain a $PaCO_2$ between 25–30 mmHg and a $PaO_2$ greater than 80 mmHg. This therapeutic approach is usually effective for approximately 72 hours. To control arterial carbon dioxide and oxygen tensions precisely within these parameters, it is usually necessary to intubate the patient and provide continuous mechanical ventilation. If necessary, pancuronium bromide (Pavulon) may be prescribed to control respiratory rate and tidal volume and to keep the patient in phase with the ventilator.

Continuous monitoring of the patient's status is essential. Continuous intracranial pressure monitoring is mandatory. Serial arterial blood gases reflect the patient's response to controlled hyperventilation and indicate that the arterial carbon dioxide and oxygen values are within the desired range. A $PaCO_2$ less than 20 mmHg may cause excessive cerebral vasoconstriction potentially predisposing to a reduction in cerebral blood flow and cerebral ischemia. Cerebral $PaO_2$ values less than 50 mmHg will result in increased blood flow (vasodilation of cerebral vasculature) to counteract hypoxia, regardless of the $PaCO_2$.

Mechanical ventilatory settings (e.g., rate, tidal volume, vital capacity, percent oxygen in inspired air) need to be assessed in conjunction with arterial blood gas values. Usually a slow rate (10–12 breaths/minute) and a high tidal volume (15 ml/kg body weight) are prescribed to attain the desired carbon dioxide and oxygen tensions. (For a discussion of nursing care of the mechanically ventilated patient, see Tables 32-6 through 32-9.)

**Use of Positive End-Expiratory Pressure (PEEP): Acute Neurogenic Pulmonary edema.** Acute neurogenic pulmonary edema (i.e., adult respiratory distress syndrome of neurogenic origin, for example, acute head injury or subarachnoid hemorrhage) is a critical complication of neurologic dysfunction.[2,3] Its development may result from an extremely rapid outpouring of nerve impulses from the injured brain, which disrupts vascular permeability and precipitates pulmonary edema.

Positive end-expiratory pressure (PEEP) is often used in the treatment of adult respiratory distress syndrome of neurogenic origin. The extra positive pressure provided within the lungs and thorax helps to control hypoxemia by preventing atelectasis (i.e., collapse of alveoli) and by decreasing transudation of fluids from the intravascular space into the pulmonary extracellular space (interstitium) and the alveoli (see Fig. 34-1).

Use of positive end-expiratory pressure in excess of "physiologic" PEEP (i.e., in amounts >3-5 cm of PEEP) presents special problems for the patient with unstable intracranial pressure. Increasing intrathoracic pressures impede venous return from the intracranial venous sinuses via the internal jugular veins and superior vena cava. This interruption of venous outflow from the brain causes intracranial volume to increase, predisposing to an increase in intracranial pressure. Increased intrathoracic pressures also retard venous return to the heart from the systemic circulation. This causes a consequent decrease in cardiac output and systemic arterial blood pressure, which, in turn, may reduce cerebral perfusion pressure.

Patients with unstable intracranial pressure should have concomitant intracranial and hemodynamic pressure monitoring so that the interaction of these physiologic phenomena can be assessed on a continuous basis. The arterial pressure monitoring line also serves as an access for obtaining blood samples for monitoring arterial blood gases.

### *Maintenance of Optimal Patient Positioning*

The position a patient assumes or is passively placed in by the critical care nurse is crucial to the maintenance of effective ventilatory function, baseline intracranial pressure, cerebral blood flow, and tissue perfusion. The patient should be placed in a semi-Fowler's position with the head of the bed elevated 30-45 degrees. This position assists drainage of blood and cerebrospinal fluid from the cranial vault via gravity; it allows maximum unimpeded chest excursion and lung expansion, facilitating ventilation and oxygenation and preventing atelectasis; and it minimizes the danger of aspiration in patients with compromised protective reflexes (cough, gag, and epiglottal closure).

The patient's body should be aligned in a midline position and the head maintained in a neutral position with the use of sandbags. If needed, a towel roll can be placed under the patient's shoulders. The use of pillows should be avoided. Neck flexion and head rotation should also be avoided because these positions may impair free circulation and outflow of blood and cerebrospinal fluid from the cranial vault. Hip flexion and flexion of the knees may increase intra-abdominal and intrathoracic pressures, which may impede free flow of blood from the cerebral circulation via the internal jugular veins and vena cavae.

Proper body alignment facilitates flow of cerebrospinal fluid from the brain into the central canal and subarachnoid space of the spinal cord. Because venous sinuses have no valves, these measures also facilitate venous return from the brain via the internal jugular veins. This unobstructed flow of cerebrospinal fluid and blood enables the autoregulatory and compensatory mechanisms to adjust intracranial volume and pressure on a moment-to-moment basis; when such controls are impaired, maintaining free flow of cerebrospinal fluid and blood from the brain may help to minimize changes in intracranial volume and corresponding intracranial pressure.

Placement of the patient in a prone position is contraindicated because compression of the abdomen interferes with venous circulation in the great veins, and the accompanying rotation of the head directly compresses the jugular vein. Together, these positions decrease venous blood and cerebrospinal fluid outflow from the cranium, and as intracranial volume increases, intracranial pressure rises accordingly.

The patient should be turned with great care so that proper body alignment is maintained during the turning and positioning procedure. These activities are essential to mobilize pulmonary secretions and to prevent pooling. The electrified rocking or kinetic bed (e.g., Rotorest bed) may be especially helpful in this regard. Turning and positioning also help to maximize tissue perfusion, thus promoting and maintaining skin integrity during the acute stage.

Proper positioning of the patient can also prevent thrombus formation with potential pulmonary embolism. Avoid crossing the patient's legs or placing a pillow under the knees. The knee gatch should remain flat. Antiembolic stockings should be applied, with removal once each shift for 20-30 minutes. Passive exercises should be performed at regular intervals guided by intracranial pressure monitoring. Athrombic pumps or venodynes, if available, are especially effective in this regard. All of these measures reduce the risk of compromising blood flow and prevent pooling of blood in the extremities.

### *Avoidance of Valsalva-Type Maneuvers*

The responsive patient at risk of developing intracranial hypertension presents a special kind of problem—how to assist the patient to avoid Valsalva-type activities, which can precipitate a rise in intracranial pressure. Valsalva's maneuver involves a forced exhalation against a closed glottis. It increases central venous and intrathoracic pressures, which impede outflow of venous return from the brain, resulting in an increase in intracranial pressure.

Patient teaching is critical if Valsalva-type maneuvers are to be avoided. The patient must be instructed to allow himself/herself to be moved passively in bed. Nurses should *lift* the patient to prevent a rise in intrathoracic pressure. The patient should be taught to exhale or to blow out through the mouth when moving, turning, or defecating. Exhaling requires an open glottis and, thus, prevents initiation of Valsalva's maneuver.

Passive range-of-motion exercises should be performed by the nurse or physical therapist. Isometric exercises, such as bracing oneself to sit up or pushing against the bed frame or side rails, need to be discouraged. Use of footboards should be avoided entirely. Isometric muscle contractions increase muscle tension, which may increase intracranial pressure. Coughing and sneezing increase intrathoracic and intra-abdominal pressures, which, in turn, are transmitted through blood vessels and subarachnoid space of the spinal cord to the brain. The end result can be an increase in intracranial pressure, and, therefore, these activities must be discouraged. Emotional stimuli and environmental noise should be kept at a minimum to foster relaxation. The patient's condition should not be discussed at the bedside or within the patient's hearing because this may cause an increase in intracranial pressure. Undisturbed rest periods must be provided for the patient.

**Muscle Relaxation: Drug Therapy.** Moving the unresponsive, intubated patient may precipitate posturing (i.e., abnormal flexor [decorticate], abnormal extensor [decerebrate], or a combination of both responses). In patients manifesting these abnormal motor responses, muscle relaxation therapy may be indicated. Such therapy can also be used to keep the patient in phase with the ventilator.

Pancuronium bromide (Pavulon) and diazepam (Valium) are frequently prescribed for the ventilated patient to provide muscle relaxation (Table 9-2). Pavulon causes skeletal muscle paralysis, requiring continuous mechanical ventilation. Respiratory muscle paralysis occurs within 2 to 3 minutes of an intravenous dose. The effects of the drug begin to subside within 35-45 minutes. If necessary, these effects can be reversed by neostigmine or pyridostigmine.

TABLE 9-2
**Pharmacologic Therapy in the Management of Intracranial Hypertension**

The following is a list of drugs commonly used in the treatment of increased intracranial pressure. For specific details on drugs used to treat the critical phase of illness including dose, mode of administration, adverse reactions, and nursing implications, see Appendix A.

Diuretics
1. Osmotic diuretic—mannitol (Osmitrol)
2. Loop diuretic—furosemide (Lasix)
—ethacrynic acid (Edecrin)
3. Thiazide diuretic—chlorothiazide (Diuril)

Corticosteroids
1. Dexamethasone (Decadron)
2. Hydrocortisone (Solu-Cortef)
3. Methylprednisolone (Solu-Medrol)

Anticonvulsants
1. Diazepam (Valium)
2. Phenobarbital (Luminal)
3. Phenytoin (Dilantin)

Muscle Relaxant
1. Pancuronium bromide (Pavulon)

Sedatives
1. Morphine sulfate
2. Pentobarbital (Nembutal)

Gastrointestinal
1. Histamine$_2$ antagonists—ranitidine (Zantac)
2. Antacids—Maalox, others

Miscellaneous
1. Calcium antagonist—verapamil (Calan, Isoptin)
2. Antipyretic—acetaminophen (Tylenol)
3. Antihypertensive—nitroprusside (Nipride), hydralazine, diazoxide, trimethaphan, nifedipine, others

Responsive and alert patients receiving Pavulon require constant teaching and reassurance that their needs will be anticipated and met. A system of communication should be established, if possible, before the drug is administered. Loss of motor control may cause anxiety and apprehension, which can themselves cause an increase in intracranial pressure.

Morphine sulfate is prescribed frequently in conjunction with Pavulon therapy because it exerts a sedative effect. The loss of control of all skeletal muscle function in the responsive patient can be a frightening experience, and sedation is a necessary adjunct to Pavulon therapy. Morphine should be used judiciously because it depresses the level of consciousness and respirations, and it alters pupillary size and reactivity. Ongoing neurologic assessment requires a consideration of drug-related responses, which may mask underlying signs and symptoms. All drugs mentioned require that equipment be available for resuscitation, particularly with parenteral administration (as in the case of diazepam). (For information related to dose, administration, adverse reactions, and nursing implications of these drugs, see Appendix A.)

### *Maintenance of Cerebral Perfusion Pressure and Cerebral Blood Flow*

**Hemodynamic Considerations.** Cerebral perfusion pressure depends largely on: (1) mean systemic arterial blood pressure, (2) level of intracranial pressure, and (3) autoregulatory mechanisms within the brain that serve to maintain cerebral perfusion pressure in the face of wide fluctuations in systemic arterial blood pressure (60–150 mmHg). When intracranial pressure increases beyond the autoregulatory capabilities of the brain, intracranial blood volume and cerebral blood flow become *passively* controlled by the systemic arterial blood pressure. Thus, a rise in systemic blood pressure increases intracranial blood volume and cerebral blood flow, causing intracranial pressure to rise; a fall in systemic blood pressure reduces cerebral blood volume and cerebral blood flow, predisposing to cerebral ischemia. The concomitant reduction in brain compliance associated with intracranial hypertension further complicates the patient's status because very small increases in intracranial volume precipitate large increases in intracranial pressure (see Fig. 8–1).

To reduce and/or maintain intracranial pressure within acceptable physiologic limits (<20 to 25 mmHg) in the patient with compromised autoregulatory and compensatory mechanisms, it is necessary to: (1) promote cerebral venous outflow (using methods discussed above), (2) minimize fluctuations in systemic arterial blood pressure, and (3) maintain the *mean* systolic pressure between 80–100 mmHg.

Patients experiencing an insult to the brain often become hypertensive as the autoregulatory/compensatory mechanisms within the brain attempt to preserve cerebral perfusion pressure in the face of cerebral ischemia, cellular hypoxia, cerebral edema, and rising intracranial pressure. It may be necessary to administer antihypertensive drug therapy if systemic blood pressure cannot be controlled by other means (e.g., fluid restriction, use of diuretics). Antihypertensive agents (e.g., nitroprusside) to reduce high blood pressure must be administered carefully in patients with increased intracranial pressure because a reduction in systemic arterial blood pressure may further reduce cerebral perfusion pressure and cerebral blood flow. Antihypertensive drugs may themselves increase intracranial pressure, and their administration requires close, ongoing scrutiny of the patient's status.

The presence of systemic hypotension needs to be assessed carefully to determine its underlying cause. Insults to the head rarely precipitate a hypotensive state unless there is a severe laceration of the scalp or damage to vital vasomotor centers in the brain.

**Fluid Management.** Careful management of fluid intake is necessary to maintain intravascular volume while concomitantly allowing the patient to be slightly dehydrated. The premise here is that limiting fluid intake will help to decrease extracellular fluid in all tissues, including the brain. To be meaningful and useful, documented fluid intake should reflect *all* fluids taken, including that in the diet, intravenous therapy (including that used to "piggyback" the administration of medications), enteral or parenteral feedings, and fluids taken to swallow medications or flush a nasogastric tube.

Fluid intake data are only significant when assessed in terms of fluid output. Urine output; fluid losses from vomiting, diarrhea, and gastric suctioning; iatrogenic losses; and an estimate of *insensible* losses (i.e., fluid loss via skin, wound drainage, and lungs) need to be documented carefully. Daily weight is the best indicator of fluid status. It should be initiated as soon as the patient's condition warrants it. Hydration status is assessed by monitoring trends in hemodynamic parameters (e.g., central venous pressure) and serum BUN, as well as by observing clinical signs of dehydration (e.g., sunken eyeballs, poor skin turgor over forehead or sternum, decreased blood pressure, thready pulse, thirst, listlessness) and overhydration (e.g., increased weight, peripheral edema, elevated blood pressure, bounding pulse).

The approach to fluid management in the patient with, or at risk of developing, intracranial hypertension is to *restrict* fluid intake usually to 1200 to 1500 ml/day. The rationale underlying fluid restriction is that a decrease in extracellular fluid volume may minimize or prevent cerebral edema formation. When initiated in conjunction with pharmacologic therapy (e.g., hyperosmolar agents, diuretics, and corticosteroids), fluid restriction can be very effective in this regard. (Specific pharmacologic therapy in the treatment of intracranial hypertension is discussed below. Also, see Table 9–2.)

***Monitoring Serum Electrolytes.*** In addition to monitoring serum BUN, it is essential to monitor serum electrolytes daily or more frequently if the patient's condition warrants it. For patients on fluid restriction who are receiving diuretic therapy (e.g., furosemide), serum sodium and potassium levels need to be evaluated very carefully. Electrolyte imbalances, including hypernatremia, hypokalemia, and hypochloremia, frequently occur. The patient's electrocardiogram should be evaluated for changes reflective of electrolyte imbalance (see Fig. 23–2; Figs. 40–51 through 40–54).

***Monitoring Serum Osmolality and Urine Specific Gravity.*** Manipulation of the serum osmolality is particularly important in caring for patients who have sustained craniocerebral insults resulting in cerebral edema formation. Osmolality is the amount of osmotic pressure exerted by particles dissolved in solution. It can be calculated from the following formula:

$$\text{Serum Osmolality} = 2\begin{pmatrix}\text{serum sodium}\\\text{concentration}\end{pmatrix} + \frac{\text{blood urea nitrogen concentration}}{2.8} + \frac{\text{serum glucose concentration}}{18}$$

(For further discussion, see Chapter 16.)

Hyperosmolar agents, corticosteroids, and diuretics are commonly administered to reduce and/or minimize cerebral edema. Hyperosmolar agents act to increase serum osmolality to create an osmotic gradient favoring movement of fluid from brain interstitium into the intravascular compartment. The desired effect is a reduction in the cerebral edema associated with the craniocerebral insult. The hyperglycemic effect of corticosteroids increases serum osmolality, favoring a water diuresis. This, in conjunction with the anti-inflammatory effects and membrane stabilization activities of steroids, further reduces cerebral edema. Diuretics (e.g., furosemide) reduce extracellular fluid volume by decreasing the reabsorption of chloride and sodium ions in the renal tubules, thereby increasing fluid excretion and increasing serum osmolality. Measurement of serum osmolality assists in evaluating the patient's status and response to therapy (see section entitled "Pharmacologic Therapy in the Treatment of Intracranial Hypertension" below).

Monitoring of urine specific gravity assists in distinguishing an *induced* diuresis from that of diabetes insipidus, a potential complication of head injury. While the urine specific gravity is low in both instances (as low as 1.005), induced diuresis directly follows the administration of hyperosmotic agents; the diuresis of diabetes insipidus occurs in the absence of osmotherapy (see Table 16–2).

Monitoring of urine specific gravity is also helpful in distinguishing between an induced diuresis and the syndrome of inappropriate secretion of antidiuretic hormone (SIADH). In both instances serum osmolality is low (<280 mOsm/kg). However, urine specific gravity is increased in SIADH and decreased in induced diuresis.[4] (For a review of clinical manifestations and treatment of fluid and electrolyte imbalances, see Chapter 23.)

### Maintenance of Normothermia

Temperature control is an important goal of patient management. Elevated temperatures increase cerebral metabolism; and the metabolic end-products, carbon dioxide and lactic acid, are both potent vasodilators of the cerebral vasculature. The consequent increase in cerebral blood volume and cerebral blood flow, in turn, increases intracranial pressure.

An oral temperature greater than 37.5°C (99.5°F) or a rectal temperature above 38°C (100.5°F) indicates fever. Fever may be associated with infection, seizure activity, or hypothalamic dysfunction. It is frequently accompanied by a rapid pulse (>100 beats/minute), tachypnea (>25 to 30 breaths/minute), restlessness, irritability, warm dry skin, flushed face, and chills. In the neurologically compromised patient experiencing an increase in intracranial pressure, an elevated temperature may be accompanied by such findings as bradycardia, changes in the level of consciousness with associated irritability and restlessness, and changes in respiratory pattern or rhythm. The respiratory rate may remain within a normal range (i.e., <20 breaths/minute).

Hyperthermia is reflected by a body temperature above 41.1°C (105°F). In the neurologic patient, hyperthermia may result from pathophysiology involving the temperature-regulating center in the hypothalamus (see Fig. 6–12). Fever associated with pathology to the anterior portion of the hypothalamus may be accompanied by profuse diaphoresis and vasodilation of blood vessels in the skin; involvement of the lateral portion of the hypothalamus is associated frequently with shivering and vasoconstriction.[5]

Efforts to control body temperature and achieve normothermia (i.e., normal range: 36.5°C to 38.0°C; 97.7°F to 100.4°F) include treatment with antipyretic medication (e.g., acetaminophen). The patient's room should be kept cool, and a minimum of bed coverings should be used. Patients with hyperthermia associated with hypothalamic involvement may not respond well to antipyretic therapy. If conservative measures to reduce body temperature are unsuccessful, or if the body temperature is greater than 41.0°C (105°F), use of the hyperthermia blanket may be indicated.

**Hypothermia Therapy.** Hypothermia therapy is the intentional reduction of body temperature to between 30°C and 32°C (86°F and 89.6°F) for the purpose of controlling intracranial pressure by reducing cerebral metabolic oxygen demands. The desired effect of hypothermia therapy in the patient with a craniocerebral insult is to reduce the risk of cerebral ischemia. It usually requires that efforts be employed to prevent shivering especially during initial cooling and rewarming phases, because this will increase oxygen consumption by muscles. The enhanced metabolic activity increases body temperature and circulation and may cause a corresponding increase in intracranial pressure. Chlorpromazine may be prescribed to prevent shivering. This drug must be used with caution in patients with liver dysfunction because it is metabolized primarily in the liver. Side effects of chlorpromazine are not uncommon and may include tachycardia, hypotension, and electrocardiographic changes with nonspecific and reversible Q wave and T wave changes. In addition, chlorpromazine may alter metabolism of other drugs such as phenytoin, predisposing to phenytoin toxicity; the drug can also prolong and intensify the action of central nervous system depressants such as narcotics and barbiturates.

In general, hypothermia therapy has not been consistently proven to be of therapeutic value in preventing and/or treating secondary effects of craniocerebral insults (e.g., cerebral ischemia, injury and infarction, cerebral edema). Currently, the goal is to achieve normothermia via use of conservative methods and antipyretic therapy.

### *Pharmacologic Therapy in the Treatment of Intracranial Hypertension*

Drug therapy can be used as a primary mode of treatment in the patient with increased intracranial pressure (e.g., cerebral edema) or as a temporary measure to reduce intracranial volume until surgery can be performed (expanding space-occupying lesion). Major categories of drugs used include hyperosmolar agents, diuretics, corticosteroids, anticonvulsants, and barbiturates (see Table 9-2). (For information related to the dose, route of administration, adverse reactions, and nursing implications for specific drugs, see Appendix A.)

**Hyperosmolar Agents (Osmotherapy).** Hyperosmolar agents are also called *osmotic* diuretics, of which mannitol is the prototype. Their therapeutic effect depends on establishing an osmotic (concentration) gradient across the blood-brain barrier (i.e., between the circulating blood in the intravascular compartment and the extracellular, or interstitial, compartment of brain tissue). By increasing the osmolality of circulating blood, these agents cause fluid to move down its concentration gradient from the brain interstitium into the intravascular compartment. The initial diuresis is usually profound, and bladder catheterization is necessary. The reduction in intracranial volume results in a corresponding decrease in intracranial pressure.

To be effective osmotic diuretics require an intact blood-brain barrier (see Fig. 6-11). A disrupted blood-brain barrier allows entry of the drug into the brain interstitium, eliminating the osmotic gradient. As the osmolality of the blood, brain, and cerebrospinal fluid equilibrate, drug action ceases.

Often, even when the blood-brain barrier is intact, patients will experience a "rebound" increase in intracranial pressure as much as 12 hours after the osmotic diuretic has been administered. Mannitol's effectiveness as a diuretic agent is attributed directly to the size of its molecule, which is for the most part too large to easily traverse the blood-brain barrier. Thus, the osmotic concentration gradient that underlies mannitol's action as a diuretic is established.

However, over time, and in the presence of an impaired or leaky blood-brain barrier associated with cerebral ischemia or edema, a sufficient number of mannitol molecules do move into the brain interstitium, compromising the effectiveness of the osmotic concentration gradient. Eventually, water is drawn back into the brain interstitium from the intravascular space, thus accounting for the "rebound" effect.

Mannitol is the most common osmotic diuretic in use, although urea is sometimes used in this regard. Mannitol's peak effect occurs within the first 3 hours after administration. A reduction in intracranial pressure should be observed within 15 minutes after starting the infusion. Its diuretic effect may last for up to 9 hours. In addition to its action as an osmotic diuretic, mannitol may also decrease formation of cerebrospinal fluid. Specific nursing implications related to administration of mannitol are listed in Table 9-3.

**Diuretic Therapy.** *Furosemide (Lasix)* acts to dehydrate the entire body. Its effectiveness in reducing cerebral edema is increasingly making it the first drug of choice in the treatment of head-injured patients. The site of action of furosemide is the kidney tubules where it inhibits the reabsorption of chloride and sodium. A direct reduction of sodium transport in brain tissue is also attributed to the action of furosemide. It may be the drug of choice in patients who have developed adult respiratory distress syndrome of neurogenic origin.

Nursing implications related to the use of furosemide involve the potency of its diuretic effect. Its peak diuretic effect occurs within 30 minutes of intravenous administration and is gone within 8 hours. A profound depletion of water and electrolytes can occur. The patient's hydration status, vital signs, intake and output, daily weight (unless contraindicated), and laboratory data (serum electrolytes, BUN, creatinine) must be regularly evaluated. Serum potassium should be particularly closely monitored if the patient is also receiving digitalis preparations. Continuous cardiac monitoring is essential. Intravenous doses of furosemide should be administered slowly over a period of at least 2 minutes to minimize risk of ototoxicity. (See Appendix A for additional nursing implications.)

**Corticosteroid Therapy.** While corticosteroid therapy has not been shown to be effective in the initial treatment of patients who have sustained a craniocerebral insult (e.g., head injury), corticosteroids continue to receive wide usage particularly in patients with cerebral edema. Dexamethasone (Decadron) and methylprednisolone (Solu-Medrol) are the two types of glucocorticosteroids most frequently used. The precise mechanism of action remains unknown. It has been suggested that the anti-inflammatory effects of corticosteroids may help to relieve cerebral edema. The mechanism involved may be the capacity to stabilize cell membranes, thus preventing the activation of noxious lysosomal enzymes. Steroids may help to re-establish and maintain the integrity of the blood-brain barrier. The patient's hydration and electrolyte

TABLE 9-3
### Administration of Mannitol: Nursing Implications

Important nursing implications related to the administration of mannitol (osmotic diuretic):

1. Mannitol needs to be warmed prior to administration if crystals are present; otherwise, use filter as prescribed.
2. An intravenous filter should be used for administration of the drug.
3. Rapid infusion of large doses of mannitol may expand the blood volume over and above the capacity of kidneys to clear the additional fluid. The consequent circulatory overload increases cerebral blood flow, predisposing to an increase in intracranial pressure.
   A. The patient should be closely monitored for signs of increasing intracranial pressure and circulatory overload. Cardiac dysrhythmias associated with circulatory overload may occur.
   B. Renal function should be closely monitored, including hourly fluid intake and output, daily weight (unless contraindicated), and laboratory data (serum BUN and creatinine).
4. Loss of electrolytes in conjunction with the diuresis may cause an electrolyte imbalance.
   A. Serum electrolytes and serum osmolality must be monitored closely.
   B. Serum potassium should be monitored regularly, particularly in patients receiving digitalis preparations. A potassium supplement may be required.
5. When using mannitol, it is necessary to monitor intracranial pressure very carefully because initially the vasodilating effect of the drug on cerebral blood vessels may aggravate an already elevated intracranial pressure, prior to the onset of its diuretic effect.
6. "Rebound" effect, an increase in intracranial pressure, can occur as much as 12 hours after the administration of mannitol. Normally, molecules of mannitol are too large to traverse the blood–brain barrier easily. Over time and/or in the presence of impaired or leaky cellular membranes, mannitol molecules move into the brain interstitium and eventually establish an osmotic concentration gradient. This draws fluid from the intravascular space back into the brain interstitium. The resultant increase in cerebral edema is an effect opposite to the desired effect of reducing cerebral edema. (For additional information, see Appendix A.)

status must be monitored closely because steroids promote water and electrolyte excretion.

Serum glucose must also be monitored closely because the hyperglycemia induced by corticosteroid therapy may be difficult to control. When administered intravenously, corticosteroids should be given slowly over at least 1 minute. High doses given for over 5 days suppress the hypothalamic–pituitary–adrenal axis. Doses should be tapered slowly to prevent addisonian's crisis (i.e., acute adrenal insufficiency). Although the ulcerogenic properties of corticosteroids remain controversial, prophylactic therapy in this regard is usually initiated (see next section). Vigilant nursing care is required, especially with patients having invasive procedures, because corticosteroids depress the immune response and may mask signs of infection, including fever.

**Gastric Ulceration: "Prophylactic" Therapy.** While there is no firm evidence that histamine$_2$ antagonists or antacids have prophylactic properties, such therapy is usually initiated in patients who have sustained a major craniocerebral insult and for whom corticosteroid therapy has been prescribed. Ranitidine (Zantac) is the drug currently prescribed to prevent and/or reduce the risk of gastric ulceration. The action of ranitidine is localized to histamine$_2$ receptors within the gastric mucosa, where the drug acts to reduce acid secretion, increase gastric pH, and reduce the activity of the enzyme, pepsin. Antacids may also be prescribed to neutralize gastric acid in the presence of gastric or duodenal ulceration and/or to prevent stress ulceration.

In patients with a nasogastric tube, gastric pH should be monitored each shift, or more frequently if there is a problem maintaining gastric pH greater than 4.5. Nasogastric drainage and stools should also be monitored for occult blood.

**Anticonvulsant Therapy.** Drugs commonly used for the treatment and/or prevention of seizure activity include diazepam, phenytoin (Dilantin), and phenobarbital. In patients receiving diazepam, intravenous doses should be administered at a rate not to exceed 5 mg/minute. The patient should be assessed for signs of respiratory depression. The anticonvulsant activity of diazepam diminishes within 15–30 minutes after an intravenous dose. Cimetidine, another histamine$_2$ antagonist, inhibits metabolism of diazepam, and its use is contraindicated.

Intravenous doses of phenytoin should be administered at a rate not to exceed 50 mg/minute to prevent hypotension and cardiovascular collapse. Vital signs and cardiac rhythm should be monitored continuously. Phenytoin has many drug interactions and adverse reactions (see Appendix A).

**Barbiturate Coma Therapy.** Barbiturate coma therapy is sometimes instituted to reduce uncontrolled intracranial hypertension refractory to conventional therapeutic modalities. Uncontrolled intracranial pressure is loosely defined as intracranial pressure greater than 25–30 mmHg for periods of time exceeding 20–30 minutes.

The mode of action is unclear, but several physiologic effects of barbiturates may account for their efficacy in reducing intracranial hypertension. Barbiturates cause cerebral vasoconstriction, reducing the blood volume within the cerebral vasculature. There is a concomitant decrease in systemic blood pressure, which is reflected as a lowered hydrostatic pressure within the cerebral circulation. The reduction in cerebral blood pressure may help to decrease cerebral edema. There is a reduced responsiveness to stimuli with a consequent decrease in the cerebral metabolic demands for oxygen and glucose. Suppression of seizure activity also reduces the cellular demand for these metabolic substrates.

***Nursing Management of the Patient in Barbiturate Coma.*** Nursing management of the patient in barbiturate coma is a challenging and demanding undertaking in which complete, supportive care for this essentially anesthetized patient must be provided. All vital physiologic functions must be monitored and, if necessary, supported by artificial means. Because of respiratory depression the patient is unable to breathe spontaneously and requires continuous, controlled mechanical ventilation. The adequacy of ventilation is evaluated by regular arterial blood gas studies. Loss of protective reflexes (cough, gag, epiglottal closure) necessitates timely suctioning of nasopharyngeal and tracheobronchial secretions to ensure a patent airway and safeguard against aspiration.

Continuous intracranial pressure monitoring is absolutely essential because the dosage of barbiturate (usually 3–5 mg/dl) is titrated according to intracranial pressure measurements. The usual neurologic assessment parameters (e.g., level of consciousness, respiratory pattern, pupillary and motor responses) are obliterated once coma is established, and intracranial pressure monitoring is the only reliable way to evaluate the patient's response to therapy.

Continuous arterial pressure monitoring is essential to determine cerebral perfusion pressure and to evaluate hemodynamic function. High doses of barbiturates (usually pentobarbital) can cause significant systemic hypotension, which may require vasopressors (e.g., dopamine) to maintain systolic blood pressure at 90 mmHg. At lower blood pressures, cerebral and renal perfusion may be compromised. Insertion of a pulmonary artery flotation catheter (e.g., Swan-Ganz catheter) permits evaluation of left ventricular function and the patient's hemodynamic status. Drug-induced myocardial depression can precipitate left ventricular insufficiency with a reduced cardiac output, and elevation in pulmonary capillary wedge pressures. Monitoring pulmonary blood pressures is invaluable in evaluating heart function and fluid replacement therapy. Continuous cardiac monitoring is essential to determine presence of dysrhythmias.

Restriction of fluid intake, use of diuretics, and continuous gastrointestinal decompression may potentially alter fluid and electrolyte balance. In addition to continuous systemic and pulmonary artery pressure monitoring, serial laboratory data, including serum electrolytes, BUN and creatinine, hematology profile, and serum osmolality, must be evaluated. The patient should be assessed for clinical signs of dehydration, and fluid intake and output should be monitored hourly.

Usually a nasogastric tube is inserted to maintain gastric decompression, which prevents vomiting and aspiration and compromise of diaphragmatic excursion; to evaluate and monitor pH of gastric secretions; and to assess for gastrointestinal bleeding. The abdomen should be assessed for distention in the presence of paralytic ileus; for bowel sounds on auscultation; and for possible fecal impaction.

Nursing measures should be implemented to safeguard against infection. Invasive monitoring techniques, immobility, and inadequate nutrition place the patient at increased risk of developing an infection.

A major aspect of patient care involves an assessment of the emotional needs of the patient's family and/or significant others. Frequent explanations regarding the patient's status and his/her response to therapy should be provided. Explanations may need to be reiterated and clarified because stress may alter comprehension by family members. Family members should be encouraged to ask questions. The nurse should remain accessible to the patient's family, listen to their feelings and concerns, and identify coping mechanisms to assist them in this time of crisis. Referral of family members to a psychiatric liaison nurse, social worker, and/or chaplain may be helpful.

## REFERENCES


1. Arsenault, L: Selected postoperative complications of cranial surgery. Journal of Neurological Nursing 17(3):155–163, 1985.
2. Littleton, M: Complications of multiple trauma. Critical Care Nursing Clinics of North America 1(1):75, March 1989.
3. Muwaswes, M: Increased intracranial pressure and its systemic effects. Journal of Neurosurgical Nursing 17(4):242, 1985.
4. Manifold, SL: Craniocerebral trauma: A review of primary and secondary injury and therapeutic modalities. Focus on Critical Care 13(2):33, 1986.
5. Snyder, M: A Guide to Neurological and Neurosurgical Nursing. John Wiley & Sons, New York, 1983, pp 515–516.

CHAPTER 10

# Nursing Management of the Patient with Acute Head Injury

## CHAPTER OUTLINE



## LEARNING OBJECTIVES

**At the end of this chapter you should be able to:**

1. Describe mechanisms of craniocerebral injury.
2. Report on the significance of skull fractures in terms of nursing care.
3. Differentiate specific types of primary head injuries and their significance in terms of neurologic dysfunction and therapeutic management.
4. List types of secondary injury and implications for medical and nursing management.
5. Implement the nursing process in the management of the patient with acute head injury:
   - Assessment
   - Nursing diagnosis
   - Planning: Desired patient outcomes
     - Nursing interventions

## CLASSIFICATION OF HEAD INJURY

This chapter will examine pathophysiology underlying acute head injury and the nursing management of the patient who sustains such injury. Head injury can be classified as primary or secondary. *Primary* head injury encompasses the actual brain damage resulting from the initial force or impact of the injury; *secondary* injury reflects the pathophysiologic consequences of the initial damage as the body responds to the injury. An increase in intracranial pressure, a decrease in cerebral perfusion pressure, cellular hypoxia, cerebral edema, and intracranial bleeding are common sequelae of acute head injury. Without timely and aggressive management, such sequelae may cause more damage than the initial insult.

The type of injury sustained can be classified as open, or penetrating, injury or closed, or nonpenetrating, injury. Open injuries disrupt the integrity of the skull and dura exposing the intracranial contents to the external environment; closed injuries do not disrupt this barrier, and the skull and its intracranial contents remain intact.

### Mechanisms of Head Injury

When the head impacts on an object, or vice versa, kinetic energy is absorbed by the scalp, skull, and meninges. The remaining energy becomes dissipated within the contents of the cranial vault. Usually, most of this energy is absorbed effectively by the protective layers of hair, scalp, bony skull, and the meninges. Very often the scalp enables an energy force to glance off the head rather than causing the head to absorb the full energy of impact directly. With especially violent trauma, however, these protective layers may not be able to absorb all of the forces of impact, and the remaining energy is transmitted to the brain causing damage and disruption of these delicate tissues.

The degree of structural and/or functional disruption of neuronal activity that occurs relates directly to the magnitutde of the force applied and the time span over which it is applied. Basically, the greater the force applied and the shorter the time of impact, the greater the likelihood of neurologic damage. The protection afforded by the scalp and skull should not be underestimated. The very fact that a skull fracture occurs may be a protective mechanism that dissipates the energy of impact before it affects the fragile brain tissues. Clinically, patients are occasionally seen with very severe scalp lacerations accompanied by large, open skull fractures, who are awake and alert soon after the injury, and whose cerebral functions remain intact. On the other hand, patients who have sustained no skull fracture, but in whom significant forces impacted directly on the brainstem, may exhibit signs and symptoms characteristic of severe neurologic disruption.

Acceleration-deceleration forces cause injuries classified as *coup* and *contrecoup*. Coup injuries occur directly beneath the site of impact; contrecoup injuries occur opposite to the site of impact. Take, for example, a passenger riding in a car that suddenly comes to a complete stop. As the forehead of the passenger hits the dashboard, a coup injury to the underlying tissues of the frontal lobe is sustained; as the brain rebounds within the skull, a contrecoup injury involving brain tissues opposite to the site of impact occurs, which in this instance is the occipital lobe.

Because of their different inertias, the skull and brain move at different velocities. In the presence of the protective cerebrospinal fluid cushion, such differences account for the acceleration, deceleration, and rotational shearing motions that can occur with head injury. The consequent intracranial stress precipitated by such forces may cause fragile brain tissue and blood vessels to be compressed, pulled, or torn apart. Shearing-type injuries to the brain can also occur when upon impact the base of the brain is thrown up against the sharpened edges of the basal bones at the base of the cranial vault (see Fig. 6-5).

## SKULL FRACTURES: IMPLICATIONS FOR NURSING CARE

The type of skull fracture sustained in head injury depends on the velocity and mass of the object, its direction, and its force of impact. Skull fractures are usually classified as linear (simple), comminuted (fragmentation of bone into pieces), depressed (interruption of contour of skull by inward displacement of bony fragments), and compound (perforated fracture that usually involves a scalp laceration creating an external pathway or openings; the dura may or may not be involved).

Of the bones comprising the cranial vault, the squamous portion of the temporal bone is the thinnest, and, thus, very vulnerable to injury. The clinical significance of a fracture of this bone is discussed in the section entitled "Epidural Hematoma" (below).

### Basilar Skull Fractures

Basilar fracture involves disruption of bones in the base of the cranial vault, especially in the area of the anterior and middle fossae (see Fig. 6-5). The petrous process of the temporal bone is commonly involved, as are the fragile bones comprising the paranasal sinuses (frontal, maxillary, ethmoid). Of additional consequence is the intimate attachment of the dura to these bones.

Disruption of the dura, which often accompanies a basilar fracture, accounts for leakage of cerebrospinal fluid via the nose or ear. Rhinorrhea defines drainage of cerebrospinal fluid and blood via the nose, otorrhea defines similar drainage from the ear. The significance of these signs is that dural tears or disruptions become pathways for infection (e.g., meningitis). The *halo* sign is occasionally noticed on dressing or linen. It consists of dark or bloody drainage encircled by a yellow halolike stain. It is highly suggestive of a cerebrospinal fluid leak. Testing the drainage with a Dextrostix is more definitive. If the stick is positive, the drainage contains cerebrospinal fluid; cerebrospinal fluid contains glucose whereas mucus is glucose-free.

Basilar skull fractures may cause injury to the cavernous sinus at the base of the brain (see Fig. 6-10); fracture of the petrous bone may cause damage to the transverse sinus, which runs in a groove adjacent to the petrous bone. Disruption of these sinuses predisposes to the spread of infection via the orbit or the ear, respectively.

Additional signs of possible basilar skull fracture

reflect bleeding into bone. Ecchymosis over the mastoid process of the temporal bone (Battle's sign) becomes evident approximately 30 hours after injury; bilateral ecchymosis of medial or circumscribed orbital areas is termed "raccoon eyes."

Any patient sustaining a skull fracture should be suspected of having an associated injury to the cervical spine. Complete caution must be used in supporting the patient until fracture of the cervical spine has been ruled out. Any patient sustaining a skull fracture should be suspected of having underlying trauma to brain tissue. Therefore, management of such fractures requires ongoing neurologic assessment with early recognition of clues suggestive of secondary injury (e.g., increase in intracranial pressure, cerebral edema, infection).

In patients with possible basilar skull fracture, assessment of vital parameters is important because of the proximity of vital centers along the brainstem to the base of the skull. Patients with possible basilar skull fracture should never be suctioned, unless intubated; alert, responsive patients should be cautioned *not* to blow their noses. A nasogastric tube should not be passed in patients suspected of having a dural tear and leaking cerebrospinal fluid. In both of these instances the concern is the introduction of infection. The patient with a basilar skull fracture is usually kept flat on complete bedrest to decrease the amount of cerebrospinal fluid that is draining. This position may facilitate spontaneous closure of the dural tear.

## PRIMARY HEAD INJURY

When an acute blow to the head causes unconsciousness, the question to be asked is what effect did this injury have on the underlying brain? Is there a possibility of intracranial bleeding? Physiologically, loss of consciousness, whether for minutes or hours, suggests that the patient has sustained widespread dysfunction of the cerebral hemispheres and/or brainstem. On initial assessment it is usually not possible to determine how long the state of unconsciousness will last. Assessment of the other variables—respiratory status, pupillary size and reactivity, extraocular movement and motor responses—helps determine the severity of the injury.

Primary head injuries include concussion, cerebral contusion, cerebral laceration, and intracranial hemorrhage with hematoma formation.

### Concussion

A concussion is a transient period of unconsciousness in response to head trauma, from which the patient recovers in minutes to hours without any definitive sequelae other than transient post-traumatic amnesia (i.e., the inability to recall events that occur after the injury) and/or retrograde amnesia (i.e., the inability to recall events that occurred prior to the injury).

The mechanism of injury may involve a rapid acceleration-deceleration type injury, or one causing deformation of the skull without fracture. In both cases pathology seems related to a sudden rise in pressure, which impacts on nerve pathways critical to consciousness (see Chap. 6). Disruption of axons in the white matter of the cerebral hemispheres via shearing forces may also be a pathogenic mechanism.

The clinical post-trauma presentation is an immediate, transient loss of consciousness usually lasting a matter of minutes; reflexes and vital signs may be depressed (e.g., decreased blood pressure and bradycardia); residual amnesia or memory loss may be evident. Recovery is usually prompt, although patients sustaining a more severe concussion may experience amnesia for several weeks or up to several months.

The duration of the unconsciousness may be used to determine if hospitalization is necessary. Such patients must be observed for up to 24 hours to detect any signs of focal or progressive neurologic changes (e.g., degree of alertness; orientation to person, place, time; and response to stimuli). The patient is discharged provided that a family member is available to arouse the patient hourly, and that person is instructed to seek medical assistance immediately if the patient becomes difficult to arouse.

### Cerebral Contusion

A cerebral contusion is an actual bruising of the brain with edema formation and capillary hemorrhages in the affected area(s) of the brain. It is considered much more serious than a concussion.

In assessing the patient it is important to establish the mechanism of injury. In acceleration-deceleration type injuries, for example, injury to the side of the head opposite to that sustaining the initial impact (i.e., contrecoup) must always be considered a possibility and assessed for accordingly.

Clinically, the patient's behavior may range from an altered state of consciousness (e.g., confusion, restlessness, agitation, or combativeness) to a state of coma in which the patient is unresponsive to stimuli. The loss of consciousness caused by a contusion can last for hours, days, and even weeks.

Contusions of the brain are significant because of the degree of secondary injury caused by cerebral edema and/or bleeding. The consequent increase in intracranial pressure is reflected by alterations in neurologic function (e.g., level of consciousness, breathing pattern, pupillary size and reactivity, motor function).

## Cerebral Laceration

A cerebral laceration is an actual tear in brain tissue associated with shearing forces, which cause the brain to strike irregular, rigid surfaces, particularly at the base of the cranial vault (see Fig. 6–5). A concomitant break in the integrity of the meningeal layers usually occurs. A laceration is a severe head injury with more extensive neurologic dysfunction than that associated with concussion.

In general, differentiation of concussion, contusion, and laceration may be difficult to establish. Each patient who sustains a head injury must be evaluated and treated on an individual basis. The initial neurologic examination should establish baseline cerebral function to which subsequent assessments can be compared to determine which way the pathologic process is moving and the response to therapy. (For details on the neurologic assessment, see Chap. 7.)

## Intracranial Hemorrhage: Hematoma Formation

A major complication of acute head injury is intracranial hemorrhage. Regardless of the severity of trauma sustained to the head, the possibility of intracranial bleeding is a major consideration and warrants ongoing neurologic assessment so that should bleeding occur, it will be diagnosed *early* in its development and treated accordingly.

Because of the structural arrangement of the meningeal layers surrounding, supporting, and protecting the brain (see Fig. 6–6), intracranial bleeding may be limited to the spaces between these membranes. Such bleeding, which is relatively or completely confined to such spaces, is referred to as a *hematoma*. Thus, bleeding into the potential space between the periosteal dural sheath and the skull is called epidural (extra dural) hematoma; bleeding within the subdural space between the dural and arachnoid membranes is called a subdural hematoma; and bleeding into the parenchyma of the brain itself is called an intracerebral hematoma.

### *Epidural Hematoma*

An epidural hematoma is a collection of blood within the potential space between the periosteal dura and the skull (see Fig. 8–7). Distinguishing features of an epidural hematoma include temporal bone fracture, rapid deterioration in the level of consciousness, and signs of uncal herniation. An epidural hematoma is a rare but extreme surgical emergency.

The squamous portion of the temporal bone is the thinnest bone of the skull, and blows to the head frequently result in a linear fracture of this bone. Such a fracture can result in a laceration of the middle meningeal artery or one of its many branches, which occupy grooves within the inner table of the bone. The consequent hemorrhage is *arterial* in origin and rapidly expands under the high pressure system. The increased pressure strips the periosteal dura from the inner table of the skull creating a space within which a rapidly expanding mass develops.

The classic clinical history of an epidural hematoma is a blow to the head in the temporal-parietal area following which the patient becomes momentarily unconscious. This is followed by a wakeful, lucid period lasting for an hour to several hours. But as the hematoma expands, the patient's condition deteriorates. There may be complaints of headache and noticeable changes in the level of consciousness. The rapidity of deterioration depends on how quickly the mass expands. Once clouding of consciousness develops, abnormal pupillary signs and hemiparesis rapidly ensue, accompanied by a deepening coma. An epidural hematoma occurs as a unilateral expanding lesion and eventually develops into a supratentorial herniation syndrome, most commonly that of *uncal herniation* with lateral brainstem compression. (For a discussion of uncal herniation, see Chap. 8.)

Dignosis of epidural hematoma is based on: (1) the patient's clinical history regarding the mechanism of head injury, and the events following the injury; (2) clinical manifestations; and (3) computed axial tomography (CAT) scan. Treatment is surgical evacuation of the hematoma, which, if performed early enough, may allow for full recovery.

### *Subdural Hematoma*

A subdural hematoma evolves from bleeding within the space between the dura and arachnoid membrane (see Fig. 8–6). It is one of the more common sequelae of head injury and largely results from disruption of small veins that bridge the subdural space. Contusion or laceration of the brain may also cause subdural hemorrhage. Clinically, the onset of symptoms is relatively slower than that of an epidural hemorrhage because venous blood pressure is considerably lower than that of the arterial system.

Subdural hematomas have been classified as acute, subacute, and chronic. This classification is based largely on the clinical manifestations exhibited by the patient and the time interval between the occurrence of the head injury and the onset of symptoms.

**Acute Subdural Hematoma.** Acute subdural hematoma is associated with severe head injury with the onset of symptoms within the first 24–48 hours. The skull may remain intact; rather, pathology is related to contusion and/or laceration of underlying brain tissue. Signs and symptoms may initially present as headache with progression to an altered state of consciousness. Rapid deterioration of consciousness may be accompanied by abnormal changes in respiratory rate and rhythm, pupillary dysfunction, dysconjugate eye movements, and abnormal motor responses.

Signs and symptoms of subdural hematoma frequently fluctuate from hour to hour or even day to day. Plum and Posner[1] suggest that many types of expanding lesions produce fluctuations in their clinical manifestations once the stage is reached where "intracranial structures can barely compensate for the expanding mass" and the consequent increase in intracranial pressure.

The subdural hematoma usually involves the accumulation of blood throughout the entire frontotemporoparietal area, which acts as a generalized expanding mass supratentorial lesion. In contrast to the epidural hematoma, the downward rostral to caudal (head to toe) deterioration of an acute subdural hematoma may occur without substantial associated focal signs of a hemispheric mass lesion. Rather, its pathologic course more closely reflects that of the *central syndrome* of rostral to caudal brain herniation (see Chap. 8). An acute subdural hematoma requires early diagnosis and surgical evacuation of the clot to prevent secondary injury and permanent sequelae.

**Subacute Subdural Hematoma.** Subacute subdural hematomas are also associated with contusions to underlying brain, the symptoms of which begin to appear between 2 days and 2 weeks after injury. Brain damage is usually less severe, affording a better prognosis. Subacute subdural hematomas are often associated with intracerebral bleeding. These hematomas are commonly located over the hemispheric areas. They may cause progressive changes in the level of consciousness with irritability and confusion; ipsilateral pupillary changes may become evident along with ophthalmoplegia; and hemiparesis may occur along with the Babinski's response. Seizure activity may become evident.

The diagnosis of subacute subdural hematoma depends on the patient's initial signs and symptoms and findings on CAT scan. Surgery may be deferred if no midline shift of cerebral structures is observed on CAT scan, and if the patient remains neurologically stable. Recovery may be possible without surgical intervention.

**Chronic Subdural Hematoma.** Chronic subdural hematomas evolve very slowly over several weeks or months. By the time changes are observed in the patient's behavior, the initial injury may have been forgotten. This type of hematoma is especially prevalent in the elderly. The patient may be unable to remember the circumstances of the initial trauma, and the presence of vague symptoms (e.g., headache, lethargy, slowed mentation, mood or personality changes) may be attributed to the aging process, cerebral atrophy, or the misdiagnosis of Alzheimer's disease. Elderly patients who present to the Emergency Room with a Colles' (wrist) fracture should be assessed for possible head injury.

As the blood clot resolves, dark blood spreads diffusely over the brain within the subdural space, congeals, and becomes walled off. The resultant viscous, highly concentrated jellylike substance draws fluid from the surrounding tissue, and gradually the fluid mass expands. Onset of symptoms by this expanding lesion includes headache, which gets progressively worse; behavioral changes (e.g., giddiness, drowsiness, confusion, slow cerebration); pupillary changes; hemiparesis; and seizures. With progressive enlargement, the encapsulated mass may cause further bleeding by tearing surrounding tissue, membrane, or blood vessels.

Diagnosis of a chronic subdural hematoma is based on the patient's age and clinical history and is confirmed by CAT scan. Treatment involves surgical aspiration of the clot via burr holes or craniotomy. If symptomatology is minimal, surgery may be deferred and the clot is allowed to resolve over time.

### *Intracerebral Hematoma*

*Intracerebral* hematoma (see Fig. 8-5) refers to bleeding into the brain parenchyma often associated with injury to small blood vessels in response to rotational or shearing forces. These hematomas may occur singularly or as multiple lesions. They are found most frequently in the frontal and temporal lobes and are frequently accompanied by serious contusions and laceration of brain tissue. Because intracerebral hematomas are not compartmentalized by the meninges as are epidural and subdural hematomas, they can cause more direct brain damage and be more difficult to evacuate surgically.

The clinical course of a serious intracerebral bleed is characterized by rapidly developing coma, a contralateral hemiplegia, and dilatation of the ipsilateral pupil. As intracranial pressure increases, evidence of developing supratentorial herniation becomes apparent, and the prognosis is very grave. CAT scan and angiography studies may help to diagnose the condition, but surgical intervention has met with limited success. Mortality rates are high.

## SECONDARY HEAD INJURY

Secondary head injury occurs as a consequence of the primary injury as the body responds physiologically to the actual insult. Examples of secondary injury include cerebral edema, increasing intracranial pressure with a consequent reduction in cerebral perfusion pressure and cerebral blood flow, cerebral ischemia, and cellular hypoxia. If unrelieved, the increasing intracranial pressure can precipitate brain herniation (see Fig. 8–4).

The major goal in the management of the patient who has sustained an acute head injury is to control and/or prevent secondary injury to optimize the patient's neurologic recovery. Therapeutic interventions are concerned with minimizing cerebral edema and reducing and/or maintaining intracranial pressure within the acceptable physiologic range (i.e., 0–15 mmHg). (For an indepth discussion of increased intracranial pressure, its consequences and nursing management, see Chapter 8; specific therapeutic approaches used in the treatment of intracranial hypertension are discussed in Chapter 9.)

# MANAGEMENT OF THE PATIENT WITH ACUTE HEAD INJURY

## Medical Management (See Chapters 8 and 9.)

Medical management is concerned with sustaining life and minimizing brain damage. An attempt is made to diagnose the type of underlying lesion (e.g., epidural versus subdural hematoma); to localize the level of brain function (e.g., hemispheric, diencephalic, midbrain, or lower brainstem); and to prescribe the appropriate course of treatment (e.g., medical and/or surgical intervention).

### *Intracranial Pressure Monitoring*

Intracranial pressure monitoring (ICPM) is initiated and maintained to monitor the high-risk patient's status, to evaluate the patient's response to therapy, and to serve as a guideline for the patient's overall care. Drainage of cerebrospinal fluid via an intraventricular catheter rapidly reduces intracranial pressure.

### *Ventilatory Support*

Ventilatory management is concerned with the prevention of hypercapnia and hypoxemia. A patent airway is established and maintained. With severe head injury the patient is intubated, and mechanical ventilation is initiated. Hyperventilation therapy is usually prescribed to maintain the $PaCO_2$ 25–30 mmHg, and the $PaO_2$ >80 mmHg. In the presence of unstable intracranial hypertension (i.e., increasing intracranial pressure), pancuronium bromide (Pavulon) may be prescribed to keep the patient in sync with the ventilator. Arterial blood gases are obtained periodically to evaluate the effectiveness of the ventilatory therapy.

### *Circulatory Support*

Effective circulatory management requires close, ongoing scrutiny for changes in vital signs (including blood pressure, pulse pressure, heart rate, pulmonary artery pressure, and cardiac output), which may herald significant changes in the patient's physiologic status, and his/her response to therapy.

An arterial pressure line is inserted to monitor and evaluate the patient's systemic blood pressure and pulse pressure. In conjunction with intracranial pressure monitoring, it facilitates close monitoring of cerebral perfusion pressure; it assists in evaluating the close interaction between intracranial and hemodynamic pressure phenomena. In the intubated patient an arterial line affords an access for arterial blood gas monitoring.

A pulmonary artery catheter (e.g., Swan-Ganz catheter) is inserted to assess and maintain the patient's fluid state. In the presence of cerebral edema, a slightly dehydrated state is desired. A Foley catheter is usually inserted to facilitate accurate documentation of fluid output, and to prevent bladder distention in the setting of aggressive diuretic treatment of cerebral edema.

### *Pharmacologic Support*

Pharmacologic therapy in the treatment of intracranial hypertension is discussed in detail in Chapter 9. Such therapy includes the use of hyperosmolar agents, diuretics, corticosteroids, anticonvulsants, "prophylactic" therapy to prevent gastric ulceration, and barbiturate coma therapy.

## Surgical Intervention

Surgical intervention is employed in emergent situations to stop intracranial hemorrhage, evacuate clots, and prevent an increase in intracranial pressure that may precipitate brain herniation. Techniques include craniotomy (i.e., surgical opening of the skull), craniectomy (i.e., surgical excision of part of skull), and cranioplasty (i.e., repair of defect in the skull).

## Nursing Management

### *Therapeutic Goals*

The major therapeutic goal in the initial nursing care of the patient with acute head injury is to control and/or prevent episodes of intracranial hypertension, which can predispose to *secondary* injury (e.g., reduction in cerebral perfusion pressure and cerebral blood flow, cerebral ischemia, cellular hypoxia, and cerebral edema). Such injury, if allowed to occur, can be life-threatening. At the very least, such injury can predispose to devastating neurologic deficits, seriously compromising the quality of life for the patient, family, and/or significant others. The potential for rapid and precipitous deterioration in body functions and associated irreversible brain damage makes the survival of the individual and the quality of life post-recovery especially dependent on timely, appropriate, and skilled nursing care.

Implementation of nursing process in the care of the patient with acute head injury revolves around the following therapeutic goals:

1. Perform a thorough ongoing neurologic assessment comparing physical findings and trends with established baseline data.
2. Establish and/or maintain a patent airway.
3. Implement prescribed hyperventilation therapy, carefully monitoring the patient's clinical status and arterial blood gas values.
4. Provide hemodynamic support necessary to stabilize mean arterial pressure at a value sufficient to maintain cerebral perfusion pressure >60 mmHg.
5. Maintain fluid and electrolyte balance to sustain the patient in a slightly dehydrated state.
6. Maintain acid–base balance.
7. Minimize anxiety and discomfort, and promote rest and relaxation.
8. Provide nutritional support.
9. Maintain urinary and bowel elimination.
10. Prevent infection.[2]
11. Prevent gastrointestinal complications associated with stress.
12. Prevent complications associated with physical immobility.
13. Maintain skin integrity and musculoskeletal function.
14. Establish a working rapport with patient, family, and/or significant others.
15. Provide emotional and psychologic support to patient, family, and/or significant others.

### *Nursing Diagnoses, Desired Patient Outcomes, and Nursing Interventions*

Pertinent nursing diagnoses, desired patient outcomes, and nursing interventions in the care of the patient with acute head injury are presented in Table 10–1. (See also the case study of the patient with closed head injury in Chap. 3, and Table 3–3.)

## CASE STUDY WITH SAMPLE CARE PLAN:* ACUTE HEAD INJURY

T.N., a 19-year-old with no previous medical history, was accidentally struck in the head by a baseball bat during a softball game. He was unconscious momentarily (his friends said about 5 seconds), then awakened and was alert and responsive. T. returned home complaining to his mother of a "splitting" headache and some nausea. An icepack was applied to the injury site, and T. fell asleep for the night.

When T. awoke the next morning, the headache had increased in severity and T. vomited several times. As the day wore on, T. became increasingly drowsy and lethargic, and his mother had difficulty in waking him. His mother also noted that T. seemed very confused. She immediately brought him to the local hospital emergency department.

Within the treatment area, T.'s condition was stable. A cervical spine film was taken to rule out cervical injury, and it was negative. On assessment, T. was noted to have an altered state of consciousness; he was confused and became combative when aroused. T.'s respiratory pattern was eupneic, with occasional sighs and yawns. His pupils were 2 mm bilaterally and reacted sluggishly to light. Eye movements were slightly divergent; oculocephalic reflexes were intact. There appeared to be some weakness in T.'s left arm and leg; a Babinski's response was noted bilaterally.

As T. was prepared to have a CAT scan of his head, his condition appeared to deteriorate. His verbal responses became inappropriate, spontaneous eye opening occurred only to speech or when prodded, and there was a gross withdrawal response of the right arm to a painful stimulus (pressure applied over a nailbed).

The results of the CAT scan revealed a large subdural hematoma on the right side of the brain, with a shift of the falx cerebri and lateral ventricle to the left. Upon consultation with the neurosurgeon, the decision was made to evacuate the hematoma surgically, and T. was prepared for surgery.

### Initial Nursing Diagnoses

1. Alteration in cerebral perfusion pressure, related to a large, right-sided acute subdural hematoma, and potential cerebral edema formation.
2. Ineffective breathing pattern, related to an expanding right-sided acute subdural hematoma with consequent brainstem compression.
3. Ineffective airway clearance, related to compromised protective reflexes (e.g., cough, gag reflex), and an altered state of consciousness.
4. Impaired gas exchange, related to widespread atelectasis, and potential neurogenic pulmonary edema.
5. Potential for injury: Seizures, related to cerebral hypoxia associated with an increase in intracranial pressure with a consequent decrease in cerebral perfusion pressure;

*Sample Care Plan appears on p. 168.

(*continues on p. 172*)

## TABLE 10-1. CARE PLAN FOR THE PATIENT WITH ACUTE HEAD INJURY

| Nursing Diagnoses | Desired Patient Outcomes | Nursing Interventions | Rationales |
|---|---|---|---|
| ***Nursing Diagnosis #1*** Alteration in cerebral perfusion pressure, related to:<br>1. Cerebral edema.<br>2. Potential intracranial bleeding and hematoma formation. | Patient will:<br>1. Maintain:<br>• Cerebral perfusion pressure > 60 mmHg.<br>• Intracranial pressure < 15 mmHg.<br>• Mean arterial blood pressure ~ 80 mmHg.<br>2. Exhibit intact level of consciousness and mentation.<br>• Oriented to person, place, time.<br>• Memory intact.<br>3. Demonstrate intact sensorimotor function.<br>• Distinguish pinprick from crude pressure.<br>• Purposeful response to painful stimuli. | • Refer to Table 8-2 for presentation of the following nursing interventions/rationales:<br>○ Monitor for signs and symptoms of increasing intracranial pressure.<br>○ Maintain the integrity of the intracranial pressure monitoring system.[3]<br>○ Implement measures to prevent and/or reduce intracranial pressure:<br>– Maintain optimal positioning.<br>– Prevent increase in cerebral blood flow.<br>– Limit or decrease cerebral edema.<br>– Minimize cellular metabolism.<br>– Plan nursing care activities to prevent cumulative increase in intracranial pressure.[4] | |
| ***Nursing Diagnosis #2*** Breathing pattern ineffective, related to:<br>1. Brainstem compression associated with:<br>a. Cerebral edema.<br>b. Rapidly expanding mass lesion (e.g., subdural hematoma). | Patient will demonstrate effective breathing pattern:<br>1. Respiratory rate < 25/min.<br>2. Rhythm and depth of spontaneous breathing—eupneic.<br>• Tidal volume > 7-10 ml/kg.<br>• Vital capacity > 12-15 ml/kg.<br>3. Adequate alveolar ventilation:<br>• $PaCO_2$ < 30-35 mmHg.<br>• $PaO_2$ > 80 mmHg.<br>• pH 7.35-7.45. | • Refer to Table 9-1, Nursing Diagnosis #2, for specific nursing interventions/rationales including:<br>○ Assess airway patency and spontaneous ventilatory effort.<br>○ Implement measures to maintain airway patency.<br>○ Implement measures to improve breathing pattern. | |

| | | | |
|---|---|---|---|
| ***Nursing Diagnosis #3***<br>Airway clearance ineffective, related to:<br>1. Compromised cough.<br>2. Thick tenacious secretions. | Patient will:<br>1. Maintain patent airway with normal breath sounds.<br>2. Demonstrate secretion-clearing cough (unless contraindicated by increased intracranial pressure). | • Refer to Table 9–1, Nursing Diagnosis #3, for specific nursing interventions/rationales. | |
| ***Nursing Diagnosis #4***<br>Impaired gas exchange, related to:<br>1. Neurogenic pulmonary edema (i.e., adult respiratory distress syndrome [ARDS] of neurogenic origin):<br>• Right to left shunting.<br>• Ventilation/perfusion mismatch.<br>• Diffusion defect. | Patient will:<br>1. Be alert and oriented to person, place, time.<br>2. Demonstrate appropriate behavior.<br>3. Maintain effective cardiovascular hemodynamics:<br>• Mean arterial blood pressure within ~10 mmHg of baseline.<br>• Cardiac output ~4–8 liters/min.<br>• Hematocrit >30–35%.<br>• Hemoglobin >10 g/100 ml.<br>4. Maintain optimal arterial blood gases:<br>• $PaCO_2$ ~30 mmHg.<br>• $PaO_2$ >80 mmHg.<br>• pH 7.35–7.45. | • Refer to Table 34–3, Nursing Diagnosis #1, for specific nursing care activities including:<br>○ Establish baseline assessment parameters for neurologic, respiratory, and cardiovascular function.<br>○ Administer prescribed humidified oxygen therapy.<br>• In addition:<br>• Implement positive end-expiratory pressure (PEEP) as prescribed, carefully monitoring effect on intracranial pressure.<br>○ Perform ongoing intracranial and arterial pressure monitoring.<br>○ Assess effectiveness of interaction of intracranial and hemodynamic phenomena in terms of maintaining adequate cerebral perfusion pressure (>60 mmHg; ideally 80–90 mmHg). | • Consequent increase in intrathoracic pressure impedes venous outflow from the cranial vault via the venous sinuses, internal jugular veins, and superior vena cava; the resulting increase in intracranial volume may cause a precipitous rise in intracranial pressure in patients with unstable intracranial pressure and reduced brain compliance. |
| ***Nursing Diagnosis #5***<br>Alteration in fluid and electrolyte balance:<br>1. Fluid volume excess with associated:<br>• Cerebral edema.<br>2. Fluid volume deficit, related to:<br>• Diuretic therapy.<br>• Diabetes insipidus.<br>3. Altered electrolytes, related to:<br>• Diuretic therapy. | Patient will:<br>1. Maintain effective hemodynamic function:<br>• Mean arterial blood pressure ~80 mmHg.<br>• Heart rate at baseline for patient.<br>• Cardiac rhythm regular, without dysrhythmias. | • See Chapters 23 and 30.<br>• Refer to Table 9–1, Nursing Diagnosis #5, for presentation of the following nursing interventions/rationales:<br>○ Monitor for signs and symptoms of diabetes insipidus.<br>○ Implement measures to maintain adequate fluid intake to prevent dehydration (in the scenario of diabetes insipidus).<br>○ Administer prescribed medications (to treat diabetes insipidus). | |

*(continued)*

**TABLE 10–1. CARE PLAN FOR THE PATIENT WITH ACUTE HEAD INJURY *(Continued)***

| Nursing Diagnoses | Desired Patient Outcomes | Nursing Interventions | Rationales |
|---|---|---|---|
| ***Nursing Diagnosis #5 (cont.)***<br>• Corticosteroid therapy.<br>• Acid–base imbalance. | 2. Demonstrate intact level of consciousness and mentation:<br>• Oriented to person, place, time.<br>• Memory intact.<br>• Appropriate responses to verbal commands.<br>3. Maintain balanced intake and output:<br>• Daily weight stable at patient's baseline (unless contraindicated).<br>• Urine output $>30$ ml, $<200$ ml/hr.<br>• Urine specific gravity 1.010–1.025.<br>4. Maintain laboratory parameters within acceptable range:<br>• Hematocrit, hemoglobin.<br>• Serum electrolytes, BUN, and creatinine.<br>• Serum osmolality. | | |
| ***Nursing Diagnosis #6***<br>Alteration in oral mucous membranes, related to:<br>1. Dehydration (diabetes insipidus).<br>2. Compromised nutritional intake. | Patient will maintain oral mucous membranes that are intact, moist, and free of infection. | • Assess for evidence of dehydration including the following parameters:<br>∘ Assess vital signs; intake and output; skin turgor over forehead or sternum; presence of sunken eyeballs.<br>∘ Assess mouth and oropharynx for dryness, cracking, fissures, bleeding, or other lesions.<br>• Provide supportive care:<br>∘ Maintain hydration as prescribed. | • Dry, cracking, or fissured mucous membranes reflect dehydrated state.<br>∘ Ongoing assessment assists in determining changes in the mucosa and response to fluid therapy.<br>∘ Ideally, the patient is maintained in a slightly dehdyrated state to minimize risk of cerebral edema. |

| | | | |
|---|---|---|---|
| | | ◦ Provide oral hygiene at frequent intervals. | ◦ Provides comfort, is aesthetically appealing, reduces risk of oral infection in compromised patient (e.g., *Candida albicans*). |
| | | ◦ Apply Vaseline or swabs with glycerin. | ◦ Prevents cracking and fissure formation. |
| ***Nursing Diagnosis #7***<br>Potential for injury:<br>Seizures, related to:<br>1. Cerebral hypoxia associated with:<br>• Increased intracranial pressure.<br>• Reduced cerebral perfusion pressure.<br>2. Cerebral irritation associated with:<br>• Craniocerebral trauma.<br>• Surgical manipulation of fragile brain tissue.<br>• Cerebral edema.<br>• Infection (e.g., meningitis). | Patient will:<br>1. Remain seizure-free.<br>2. Maintain effective serum levels of phenytoin (Dilantin).<br>• Usual serum levels: 10–20 $\mu$g/ml. | • Refer to Table 9–1, Nursing Diagnosis #6, for presentation of the following nursing interventions/rationales:<br>◦ Assess characteristics of seizure activity.<br>◦ Implement safety measures during *actual* seizure activity.<br>◦ Implement safety measures to prevent seizure activity.<br>– Avoid activities that increase intracranial pressure.<br>– Monitor for signs of meningeal irritation.<br>– Initiate and maintain seizure precautions.<br>– Administer prescribed anticonvulsant therapy, and monitor response to therapy. | |
| ***Nursing Diagnosis #8***<br>Potential for infection:<br>Meningitis, related to:<br>1. Open, penetrating wound/trauma with leakage of cerebrospinal fluid.<br>2. Surgical disruption of integrity of meninges.<br>3. Iatrogenic causes via invasive procedures.[2]<br>4. Compromised immune response associated with corticosteroid therapy. | Patient will:<br>1. Maintain body temperature ~98.6°C (37°C).<br>2. Remain free of signs of meningeal irritation: negative Kernig's/Brudzinski's signs.<br>3. Demonstrate normal cerebrospinal fluid analysis including WBC and protein levels.<br>4. Maintain serum WBC within normal range. | • Refer to Table 9–1, Nursing Diagnosis #7, for presentation of nursing interventions/rationales including:<br>◦ Monitor for signs and symptoms of infection (meningeal irritation).<br>◦ Assess for rhinorrhea and otorrhea.<br>◦ Assist with lumbar puncture.<br>◦ Implement measures to prevent infection.<br>◦ Administer prescribed course of antibiotics, and monitor response to therapy.<br>◦ See Table 49–7. | |

(continued)

**TABLE 10–1. CARE PLAN FOR THE PATIENT WITH ACUTE HEAD INJURY *(Continued)***

| Nursing Diagnoses | Desired Patient Outcomes | Nursing Interventions | Rationales |
|---|---|---|---|
| ***Nursing Diagnosis #9***<br>Potential for alteration in body temperature, related to:<br>1. Cerebral edema with altered hypothalamic function.<br>2. Infection. | Patient will maintain optimal body temperature ~98.6°F (37°C). | • Refer to Table 9–1, Nursing Diagnosis #8, for presentation of nursing interventions/rationales including:<br>○ Monitor body temperature.<br>○ Assess for signs and symptoms of hyperpyrexia.<br>○ Obtain specimens of body fluids and discharges for culture and sensitivity.<br>○ Inspect all invasive sites and wounds for signs/symptoms of infection.<br>○ Implement measures to reduce body temperature. | |
| ***Nursing Diagnosis #10***<br>Alteration in nutrition: Less than body requirements, related to:<br>1. Catabolic state.<br>2. Compromised nutritional intake associated with:<br>• Altered state of consciousness.<br>• Compromised protective reflexes (i.e., cough, gag, and epiglottal closure).<br>(See Chap. 53.) | Patient will:<br>1. Maintain body weight within 5% of patient's baseline.<br>2. Maintain total serum proteins: 6–8.4 g/100 ml.<br>3. Maintain laboratory data within acceptable range: BUN, serum creatinine, electrolytes, fasting serum glucose, hematology profile, total protein (albumin). | • Arrange consultation with nutritionist and collaborate to perform nutrition assessment.<br>○ Assess specific parameters: general state of health; baseline body weight.<br>– Physiologic factors: age, height, weight, triceps skin fold; mid-upper arm circumference. (See Fig. 53–3.)<br>– Caloric requirements of the critically ill patient.<br>– Laboratory data: fasting serum glucose; BUN, creatinine, serum electrolytes, total protein (serum albumin); hematology profile. | • For details regarding the nutrition assessment, see Chapter 53.<br>• Adequate nutritional intake is essential to meet the metabolic needs of the catabolic state.<br>– Nutritional deficiencies (especially in the elderly) are often associated with underlying chronic disease. |
| | | • Maintain optimal nutrition with prescribed enteral and/or parenteral feedings.<br>○ Special considerations:<br>– Methods of enteral and parenteral administration.<br>– Mechanical complications associated with enteral feeding tubes or with parenteral lines. | • See Chapter 53.<br>○ Patients receiving mechanical ventilation therapy are highly stressed and require additional nutritional supplements to meet hypermetabolic needs. |
| | | • Place patient in optimal position for enteral feedings (semi-Fowler's position).<br>○ Assess status of protective reflexes.<br>○ Assess for bowel sounds. | • Proper patient positioning and intact protective reflexes reduce risk of aspiration.<br>○ The presence of a paralytic ileus is a contraindication for enteral approach because of increased risk of aspiration; abdominal distention may compromise diaphragmatic excursion. |

| | | | |
|---|---|---|---|
| | | ○ Confirm placement of nasogastric tube in stomach before initiating enteral feedings.<br>• Provide frequent mouth care and other comfort measures.<br><br>• Monitor daily weight (unless contraindicated because of intracranial hypertension) and fluid intake and output.<br>• Assess bowel function:<br>○ Auscultate bowel sounds.<br>○ Implement prescribed bowel regimen.<br>– Gastrointestinal decompression.<br>– Adequate fluid intake.<br>– Use of stool softeners. | ○ Proper placement of nasogastric tube helps prevent aspiration.<br>• May be aesthetically pleasing to patient and family; reduces risk of oral infection (e.g., *candida albicans*) in the compromised patient; keeps mucous membranes moist and intact.<br><br>• Presence of a paralytic ileus may predispose to fecal impaction; measures need to be employed to minimize straining at stool because Valsalva's maneuver can increase intracranial pressure. |
| ***Nursing Diagnosis #11***<br>Potential for physiologic injury:<br>Acute upper gastrointestinal hemorrhage, related to:<br>1. Stress of catabolic state.<br>2. Corticosteroid therapy. | Patient will remain without gastrointestinal bleeding:<br>1. Hematology profile stable at patient's baseline.<br>2. Nasogastric drainage and stools negative for occult blood.<br>3. Nasogastric secretions: pH $>4.5$.<br>4. Vital signs stable; arterial blood pressure and heart rate at patient's baseline. | • Refer to Table 49–6 | |
| ***Nursing Diagnosis #12***<br>Alteration in comfort: Headache, related to:<br>1. Meningeal irritation.<br>2. Surgical scalp incision.<br>3. Anxiety. | Patient will:<br>1. Verbalize and/or indicate comfort.<br>2. Demonstrate relaxed facial expression and demeanor.<br>3. Maintain intracranial pressure $<15$ mmHg. | • Refer to Table 9–1, Nursing Diagnosis #4, for presentation of the following nursing interventions/rationales:<br>○ Assess patient for signs of pain and discomfort.<br>○ Implement measures to reduce discomfort.<br>– Administer analgesics and sedatives as prescribed, monitor response to therapy.<br>– Position patient to relieve muscle tension.<br>– Monitor dressing for tightness and constriction.<br>– Provide a quiet environment.<br>– Provide periods of uninterrupted sleep.<br>– Provide touch therapy; speak softly in soothing voice.<br>– Employ diversional and comfort measures. | |

(continued)

## TABLE 10-1. CARE PLAN FOR THE PATIENT WITH ACUTE HEAD INJURY *(Continued)*

| Nursing Diagnoses | Desired Patient Outcomes | Nursing Interventions | Rationales |
|---|---|---|---|
| ***Nursing Diagnosis #13***<br>Impaired physical mobility, related to:<br>1. Altered state of consciousness.<br>2. Restricted activity associated with intracranial hypertension.<br>3. Sedation.<br>4. Neuromuscular impairments (e.g., hemiparesis).<br>5. Pain. | Patient will:<br>1. Maintain full range of motion.<br>2. Remain without contractures.<br>3. Verbalize and/or indicate comfort. | • Assess neuromuscular function.<br>◦ Assess for limitations in range of motion, incoordination of movement, and presence of sensorimotor dysfunction.<br>◦ Assess for the presence of pain, fear, and anxiety.<br>• Consult with physical therapist regarding patient's neurologic and musculoskeletal status.<br>• Implement measures to improve mobility:<br>◦ Include passive range of motion exercises in planning care.<br>◦ Avoid cumulative effect of activities; too many activities within a short time span predispose to increases in intracranial pressure.<br>◦ Provide rest periods between patient care activities.<br>◦ Use hand/wrist splints as prescribed.<br>◦ Maintain optimal positioning; avoid crossing one leg over the other; avoid pillows under knees.<br>◦ Offer praise and encouragement. | • The degree of musculoskeletal activity should be guided by intracranial pressure measurements.<br>◦ Fear of precipitating pain or causing injury can significantly compromise musculoskeletal function.<br>• In the patient at risk of developing an increase in intracranial pressure, all activities should be guided by intracranial pressure monitoring measurements.<br>◦ Prevents pooling of blood in extremities.<br>◦ Exercise periods should be incorporated into daily care and planned around other patient care activities.<br>◦ Positioning is important in patients with reduced brain compliance to allow free flow of blood and cerebrospinal fluid from cranial vault.<br>◦ Minimizes risk of thrombophlebitis or thromboembolic episodes. |
| ***Nursing Diagnosis #14***<br>Potential for injury to eyes:<br>Abrasions, related to:<br>1. Inability to close eyes, or keep eyes closed, associated with:<br>• Altered state of consciousness. | Patient's eyes will remain intact without inadvertent abrasions. | • Assess patient's ability to close eyelids and keep them closed.<br>◦ Assess for corneal reflex. | • Disturbance in cranial nerve function can place eyeballs at risk of injury.<br>◦ Cranial nerve III dysfunction causes ptosis of upper eyelid on ipsilateral side.<br>◦ Cranial nerve VII dysfunction alters ability to close eyelid on ipsilateral side.<br>◦ Cranial nerve V dysfunction impairs corneal reflex. |

| | | | |
|---|---|---|---|
| • Neurologic deficit (cranial nerves).<br>• Periorbital edema. | | • Implement measures to protect eyes.<br>○ Administer lubricants for the eyes (e.g., Tearisol).<br>○ Gently tape eyes in closed position if necessary.<br>○ Cleanse around eyelids to prevent crusting of secretion. | • Help to protect eyes and minimize risk of infection. |
| ***Nursing Diagnosis #15***<br>Impairment of skin integrity:<br>Potential, related to:<br>1. Immobility associated with intracranial hypertension and altered consciousness.<br>2. Altered nutritional state.<br>3. Increased skin fragility associated with compromised health status. | Patient will:<br>1. Maintain intact skin with good turgor over forehead and sternum.<br>• Absence of lesions, irritations, pruritus, or infection.<br>• Absence of pressure (dermal) ulcer. | • Assess skin, especially reddened areas over bony prominences where skin is thin.<br>○ Assess for dependent edema associated with immobility.<br>• Implement measures to prevent skin breakdown.<br>○ Pressure relief device: air mattress, sheepskin, Clinitron bed, others.<br>○ Local skin care: Keri lotion, Granulex, Duoderm, Travase, Debrisan, others.<br>○ Turning and positioning.<br>• Assess nutritional status | • In patients with reduced brain compliance, turning, positioning, and nursing care activities should be guided by intracranial pressure measurements.<br>• Promote circulation and prevents venostasis. If reddened areas at pressure points do not blanch within less than 30 minutes, avoid using the position except for short periods at less frequent intervals.<br>○ Also assist to mobilize secretions and prevent pooling. |
| ***Nursing Diagnosis #16***<br>Alteration in thought processes, related to:<br>1. Cerebral ischemia and hypoxia.<br>2. Sedation. | Patient will:<br>1. Demonstrate improvement in thought processes.<br>• Oriented to person, place, time.<br>• Improved memory.<br>• Increased attentiveness.<br>• Improved ability to problem-solve and make decisions. | • Assess for alterations in mentation and thought processes.<br>○ Assess the following parameters:<br>– State of awareness or cognition.<br>– Behavior: restlessness, irritability, reduced attentiveness.<br>– Impaired memory, confusion.<br>– Ability to problem-solve.<br>• Confirm recent behavioral or personality changes with family members/significant others.<br>• Implement measures to assist patient in thought processes:<br>○ Reorient patient as follows:<br>– Reorient to person, place, and time.<br>– Call by name when talking with patient.<br>– Orient to immediate environment, but minimize stimuli at any given moment.<br>○ Repeat instructions and information, allowing adequate time for communication, explanations.<br>– Encourage to ask questions; use clear simple sentences. | • Disruption in thought processes suggests hemispheric lesion; alterations in arousal and cognition reflect disruption of reticular activating system.<br>• Helps to ascertain patient's baseline capabilities, and to plan care. |

*(continued)*

## TABLE 10-1. CARE PLAN FOR THE PATIENT WITH ACUTE HEAD INJURY *(Continued)*

| Nursing Diagnoses | Desired Patient Outcomes | Nursing Interventions | Rationales |
|---|---|---|---|
| ***Nursing Diagnosis #16 (cont.)*** | | | |
| | | ○ Plan patient's activities and write out schedule for patient to refer to:<br>– Involve in problem-solving. | ○ Writing out instructions or schedules reinforces verbal communication. |
| | | ○ Allow to choose between simple options (e.g., bathing and bedding change before or after meals).<br>– Monitor patient's readiness and ability to learn.<br>– Ascertain patient's comprehension. | ○ Provides patient with a sense of control of his/her body. |
| | | ○ Provide continuous encouragement and feedback, and praise positive gains made by patient.<br>○ Assist with self-care as indicated. | ○ Assists in motivating patient regarding self-care. |
| | | ○ Encourage patient to be independent, but provide close supervision.<br>○ Involve family members and/or significant others in care plan. | ○ Assists patient in gaining self-confidence regarding his/her capabilities. |
| | | ○ Offer reassurance regarding alterations in intellectual and emotional functions.<br>○ Be realistic when offering explanations and providing information. | ○ Depending on magnitude of insult and secondary injury, the patient may have memory loss and personality changes, which may persist for several months or longer. |
| ***Nursing Diagnosis #17***<br>Sensory-Perceptual alterations, related to:<br>1. Sensory deprivation:<br>• Restricted environment.<br>• Altered communication capabilities.<br>2. Sensory overload:<br>• Complexity of intensive care environment.<br>(See Chap. 3, sections entitled<br>• Needs of Critically Ill Patients<br>• Patient Stressors in the ICU.) | Patient will:<br>1. Demonstrate appropriate interactions with people and environment using sensory perceptions.<br>2. Verbalize restfulness and relaxed feeling. | • Assess patient's ability to interact with environment. | • Depending on the extent and location of insult, a disruption in sensation might be anticipated. |
| | | ○ Identify specific sensory deficits:<br>– Visual perception: need for glasses or contact lenses.<br>– Auditory perception: presence of language disorder (e.g., receptive dysphasia, expressive dysphasia), need of hearing aid. | ○ Major sensory capabilities include: visual, auditory, kinesthesia (spatial sense, perception of movement), tactile, gustatory, and olfactory. |
| | | ○ Tactile perception: hyperesthesia, hypoesthesia. | ○ *Hyperesthesia* is an overly acute sensitivity to touch, pain, temperature, or other stimuli.<br>○ *Hypoesthesia* is a diminished sensitivity to sensory stimuli. |
| | | ○ Identify previous coping abilities and influence on behavior. | |

- Provide usual necessary aids (e.g., glasses, hearing aid).

- Arrange environment to compensate for deficits:
  - ○ Reorient to environment as needed.
    - – Keep articles and equipment in the same place.
    - – Remove unnecessary materials from bedside.
    - – Use safety measures to prevent accidents.
- Implement measures to reduce sensory deprivation:
  - ○ Encourage communication by the patient as tolerated.
    - – Allow visits by family members as tolerated.
  - ○ Provide frequent, undisturbed rest periods.
  - ○ Provide occasional changes in routine and sensory stimuli.
    - – Provide soothing music/other radio programs.
    - – Provide diversional activities depending on patient's status (e.g., reading, television).
    - – Encourage conversations with the client; update patient on what's happening, and other conversational topics of interest to the patient.
- Implement measures to reduce sensory overload:
  - ○ Set priorities in care.
    - – Arrange patient care activities to allow for undisturbed rest periods.
    - – Provide periods of uninterrupted sleep with lights off and minimal noise.
    - – Alter environmental activities (e.g., avoid constant use of radio or television).
    - – Encourage verbalization regarding concerns, annoyances.
    - – Allow to decide on care activities and environmental stimuli.
- Recognize and accept patient's perception of stimuli (e.g., delusions, hallucinations).
    - – Reinforce reality.
    - – Maintain continuity of care.

- A comprehensive patient's clinical history helps to identify the patient's baseline capabilities and limitations.

- Fatigue may compromise patient's capabilities, leading to frustration, withdrawal, and depression.

  - ○ Minimizes fatigue and conserves strength.

  - ○ Ask family members about the patient's preferences, likes and dislikes. Familiar stimuli may motivate increased participation.

- Minimizing distractions enables the patient to concentrate on more pertinent stimuli. Ability to problem-solve and tolerate frustration decreases as the number of stimuli impacting on the individual increase.

## SAMPLE CARE PLAN FOR THE PATIENT WITH ACUTE HEAD INJURY

| Nursing Diagnoses | Desired Patient Outcomes | Nursing Interventions | Rationales |
|---|---|---|---|
| ***Nursing Diagnosis #1***<br>Alteration in cerebral perfusion pressure, related to:<br>1. Large, right-sided acute subdural hematoma.<br>2. Potential cerebral edema formation. | Patient will:<br>1. Maintain:<br>• Cerebral perfusion pressure > 60 mmHg.<br>• Intracranial pressure < 15 mmHg.<br>• Arterial blood pressure ~ 80 mmHg (mean).<br>2. Exhibit intact level of consciousness and mentation:<br>• Oriented to person, place.<br>• Memory intact.<br>3. Demonstrate intact sensorimotor function:<br>• Distinguish pinprick from crude pressure.<br>• Purposeful motor response to painful stimulus. | • Assess: level of consciousness, mentation, respiratory rate and pattern, pupillary size and reactivity, sensorimotor function (muscle tone, deep tendon reflexes, posturing). | • Patient responses to increases in ICP can change rapidly from moment to moment; a sustained increase in ICP (> 25–30 mmHg for greater than 15–20 minutes) can compromise cerebral perfusion pressure. |
| | | ∘ Assess vital signs: BP, pulse, body temperature. | ∘ A rise in BP, widening pulse pressure, and slow bounding pulse are *late* occurring signs of increasing ICP. |
| | | • Maintain integrity of intracranial monitoring system: scrupulous hand-washing and aseptic technique; monitor system for leaks, avoid drainage of CSF. | • ICP monitoring is a highly invasive system with a high risk of infection.<br>∘ Maintaining a closed system reduces risk of infection; ensures valid readings. |
| | | • Obtain/record pressure readings using appropriate procedure/protocol:<br>∘ Venting port of transducer at level of foramen of Monro. | ∘ For every inch that the measurement is off, approximately 2 mmHg is added or subtracted from the digital readout. |
| | | ∘ Monitor waveform configuration/digital readouts. | ∘ Monitoring *trends* provides essential information regarding status of ICP and intracranial compliance. |
| | | • Implement measures to prevent and/or reduce ICP:<br>∘ Maintain proper positioning; elevate head of bed; body in proper alignment. | ∘ Elevation of head facilitates drainage from cranium via gravity. |
| | | ∘ Maintain controlled hyperventilation and oxygenation; prevent accumulation of tracheobronchial secretions; use meticulous suctioning technique. | ∘ Hypercapnia causes cerebral vasodilation, increasing intracerebral blood flow.<br>∘ Proper suctioning technique reduces hypoxemia. |
| | | • Monitor response to prescribed therapy to reduce cerebral edema:<br>∘ Diuretic therapy/hyperosmolar therapy.<br>∘ Corticosteroid therapy.<br>∘ Strict intake and output. | ∘ Fluid restriction coupled with pharmacologic therapy helps to reduce extracellular fluid volume; a mildly dehydrated state is maintained. |
| | | ∘ Monitor laboratory data: BUN, creatinine, electrolytes, serum osmolality, urine specific gravity. | ∘ Craniocerebral insults frequently predispose to diabetes insipidus.<br>– Increased serum osmolality helps draw fluid from brain interstitium and reduce cerebral edema. |

| | | | |
|---|---|---|---|
| ***Nursing Diagnosis #2***<br>Ineffective breathing pattern, related to:<br>1. Expanding right-sided acute subdural hematoma with consequent brain-stem compression. | Patient will:<br>1. Demonstrate effective breathing pattern:<br>• Respiratory rate <25/min.<br>• Rhythm and depth eupneic.<br>2. Maintain adequate pulmonary function:<br>• Tidal volume >7–10 ml/kg.<br>• Vital capacity >12–15 ml/kg. | • Assess respiratory function hourly:<br>◦ Spontaneous breathing: rate/rhythm/depth.<br>◦ Monitor arterial blood gases (serially).<br>• Implement measures to improve breathing pattern:<br>◦ Maintain semi-Fowler's position.<br>◦ Maintain nasogastric decompression.<br>◦ Maintain mechanical ventilation and oxygenation: assess tidal volume and vital capacity at bedside. | • Maintenance of adequate ventilation/oxygenation is imperative because hypercapnia and hypoxemia cause cerebral vasodilation.<br>◦ Allows maximal chest excursion; facilitates drainage of blood and CSF from cranium.<br>◦ Prevents abdominal distention, which can compromise diaphragmatic excursion.<br>◦ See Chapter 32. |
| ***Nursing Diagnosis #3***<br>Ineffective airway clearance, related to:<br>1. Compromised protective reflexes (e.g., gag, cough, epiglottal closure).<br>2. Altered state of consciousness. | Patient will:<br>1. Maintain patent airway:<br>• Normal breath sounds.<br>• Absence of adventitious breath sounds (e.g., crackles, wheezes).<br>2. Demonstrate secretion-clearing cough (unless contraindicated by intracranial hypertension). | • Assess airway patency hourly:<br>◦ Status of protective reflexes (gag, cough).<br>◦ Auscultate breath sounds.<br>◦ Assess characteristics of sputum:<br>– Color, tenaciousness, amount, odor.<br>◦ Assess hydration status.<br>◦ Maintain hydration as prescribed.<br>– Humidify oxygen administered. | • Hypercapnia and hypoxemia increase cerebral blood flow.<br>◦ Compromised protective reflexes place patient at risk of aspiration.<br>◦ Presence of crackles, wheezes, and rhonchi suggests increased pulmonary secretions; or inability to mobilize or clear secretions.<br>◦ Dehydration causes tracheobronchial secretions to become thick, tenacious, and difficult to clear. |
| ***Nursing Diagnosis #4***<br>Impaired gas exchange, related to:<br>1. Widespread atelectasis.<br>2. Potential neurogenic pulmonary edema. | Patient will:<br>1. Be alert, oriented to person/place.<br>2. Demonstrate appropriate behavior.<br>3. Maintain optimal arterial blood gases:<br>• $PaCO_2$ ~30 mmHg<br>• $PaO_2$ >80 mmHg<br>• pH ~7.35–7.45 | • Assess cardiopulmonary function:<br>◦ Heart rate, skin color.<br>◦ Hemodynamic parameters: systemic arterial BP, PCWP, cardiac output.<br>◦ Presence of cardiac dysrhythmias.<br>• Monitor laboratory data:<br>◦ Arterial blood gases:<br>– pH.<br>– $PaO_2$, $PaCO_2$. | • Hemodynamic parameters reflect tissue perfusion. Evidence of cyanosis is a late sign of altered perfusion: >5 g hemoglobin are unsaturated.<br>◦ Hypoxemia is associated with myocardial irritability.<br>– Metabolic acidemia is associated with decreased tissue perfusion as the lack of oxygen predisposes to anaerobic metabolism with lactate production.<br>– Metabolic acidemia may depress myocardial function predisposing to dysrhythmias.<br>◦ Most closely reflect effectiveness of gas exchange. |

(continued)

## SAMPLE CARE PLAN FOR THE PATIENT WITH ACUTE HEAD INJURY *(Continued)*

| Nursing Diagnoses | Desired Patient Outcomes | Nursing Interventions | Rationales |
|---|---|---|---|
| ***Nursing Diagnosis #4 (cont.)*** | | | |
| | | • Calculate $AaDO_2$. | • Alveolar-arterial gradient <250 to 300 mmHg with an $FIO_2 \sim 60\%$ in the presence of deteriorating pulmonary function is highly suggestive of ARDS. |
| | | • Implement oxygen therapy as prescribed. | • $O_2$ concentration should maintain $PaO_2$ >60 mmHg. |
| | | • Implement positive end-expiratory pressure (PEEP) therapy as prescribed.<br>Monitor:<br>∘ ABGs, mixed venous oxygen tension ($SVO_2$).<br>∘ Lung compliance.<br>∘ Hemodynamic parameters (PCWP, PAP, CO). | • PEEP therapy maintains airway opening pressure at end-expiration above the atmospheric pressure, thus increasing the FRC (functional residual capacity), preventing airway collapse, and enhancing gas exchange and oxygen transport.<br>∘ Lung compliance is determined by dividing the peak inspiratory pressure (PIP) into the tidal volume. (See Chap. 34.) |
| | | • Monitor for complications of PEEP therapy:<br>∘ Reduction in venous return to the heart and cardiac output; reduction in cerebral perfusion; barotrauma. | ∘ Positive intrathoracic pressures generated reduce venous return via the great veins.<br>– Overdistention and rupture of alveoli are major complications of PEEP therapy. |
| ***Nursing Diagnosis #5***<br>Potential for injury: Seizures, related to:<br>1. Cerebral hypoxia associated with an increase in ICP with consequent decrease in CPP.<br>2. Cerebral irritation associated with cerebral trauma with bleeding.<br>3. Surgical manipulation of fragile brain tissue and meninges. | Patient will:<br>1. Remain seizure-free.<br>2. Maintain effective serum levels of phenytoin.<br>• Usual serum levels: ~10–20 μg/ml. | • Assess characteristics of seizure activity:<br>∘ Onset, influencing factors, duration.<br>∘ Type of movement: tonic-clonic.<br>∘ Associated changes in level of consciousness, pupillary size/reactivity.<br>∘ Vomiting, urinary/bowel incontinence.<br>• Implement measures to prevent seizure activity:<br>∘ Avoid activities that cause a substantial sustained increase in ICP (>25–30 mmHg/15 to 20 minutes).<br>∘ Monitor for signs/symptoms of meningeal irritation: nuchal rigidity, photophobia, persistent headache, positive Kernig's and/or Brudzinski's signs.<br>• Initiate and maintain seizure precautions:<br>∘ Oral airway; padded side rails and headboard, side rails in up position, bed in low position. | • Seizure activity can precipitate a significant increase in ICP; it increases cellular metabolism and the oxygen demand; it raises body temperature. |

| | | | |
|---|---|---|---|
| | | ◦ Administer prescribed anticonvulsant therapy.<br>◦ Evaluate patient's response to anticonvulsant therapy (obtain serial blood levels of phenytoin). | |
| ***Nursing Diagnosis #6***<br>Alteration in fluid and electrolyte balance (potential), related to:<br>1. Aggressive diuretic therapy and corticosteroid therapy.<br>2. Diabetes insipidus. | Patient will:<br>1. Maintain hemodynamic function:<br>• Mean systolic BP ~80 to 100 mmHg.<br>• Heart rate at patient's baseline.<br>• Regular rhythm without dysrhythmias.<br>2. Maintain balanced intake/output.<br>• Stable weight (unless contraindicated).<br>• Urine output: >30 ml, <200 ml/hr.<br>• Urine specific gravity: 1.010 to 1.025. | • Assess hydration status:<br>◦ Daily weight if not contraindicated by the presence of a labile ICP.<br>◦ Intake and output.<br>◦ Status of skin/mucous membranes; edema.<br>• Implement fluid replacement regimen as prescribed.<br>• Monitor for signs/symptoms of diabetes insipidus:<br>◦ Presence of polyuria, polydipsia.<br>◦ Urine specific gravity ~1.005.<br>◦ Presence of dehydration: poor skin turgor, sunken eyeballs.<br>• Monitor laboratory parameters: serum electrolytes, osmolality, BUN, creatinine, hematology profile. | • Patients at risk of developing cerebral edema, or an increase in ICP, are maintained in a slightly dehydrated state.<br>• Diabetes insipidus may occur secondary to craniocerebral trauma, infection. |

cerebral irritation associated with cerebral trauma with bleeding; and/or surgical manipulation of fragile brain tissue.

6. Alteration in fluid and electrolyte balance (potential), related to aggressive diuretic therapy and corticosteroid therapy; and diabetes insipidus.

These nursing diagnoses are documented on the Care Plan on p. 158. (Table 10–1.)

Additional nursing diagnoses may include:

7. Alteration in oral mucous membranes, related to dehydration (associated with diabetes insipidus), and compromised nutritional intake.
8. Potential for infection, related to craniocerebral surgery, iatrogenic causes via invasive procedures, and compromised immune response associated with aggressive corticosteroid therapy.
9. Alteration in nutrition: Less than body requirements, related to catabolic state with compromised nutrition intake associated with an altered state of consciousness and compromised protective reflexes (e.g., cough and gag reflexes).
10. Potential for physiologic injury: Gastric ulceration, related to stress, catabolic state, and corticosteroid therapy.
11. Alteration in comfort: Headache, related to meningeal irritation, anxiety, surgical scalp incision.
12. Impaired physical mobility, related to altered state of consciousness, and neurologic impairment (e.g., hemiparesis).
13. Potential for injury to eyes: Abrasions, related to altered state of consciousness; altered cranial nerve function associated with cerebral edema.
14. Potential for impairment of skin integrity, related to immobility, compromised nutritional status.
15. Sensory-perceptual alterations, related to sensory deprivation/overload.

## REFERENCES


1. Plum, F and Posner, J: The Diagnosis of Stupor and Coma, ed 3. FA Davis, Philadelphia, 1980, p 124.
2. Smith KA: Head trauma: Comparison of infection rates for different methods of intracranial pressure monitoring. Journal of Neuroscience Nursing 19(6):310–314, 1987.
3. Robinet, K: Increased intracranial pressure: Management with an intraventricular catheter. Journal of Neurological Nursing 17(2):95–104, 1985.
4. Hendrickson, S: Intracranial pressure changes and family presence. Journal of Neuroscience Nurs 19(1):14–17, 1987.

CHAPTER 11

# Nursing Management of the Patient with Cerebrovascular Disease

## CHAPTER OUTLINE



## LEARNING OBJECTIVES

**At the end of this chapter, you should be able to:**

1. Define cerebrovascular accident and discuss its significance in terms of mortality and morbidity.
2. Identify risk factors implicated in cerebrovascular disease.
3. Differentiate ischemic and hemorrhagic cerebrovascular disease in terms of underlying pathophysiology, clinical manifestations, and treatment.
4. Implement the nursing process in the management of the patient with a cerebrovascular accident:
   Assessment
   Nursing diagnosis
   Planning: Desired patient outcomes
   Nursing interventions

Cerebral vascular disease encompasses two clinical syndromes: *ischemic* cerebrovascular disease, and *hemorrhagic* cerebrovascular disease. Ischemic disease includes what is commonly referred to as a cerebrovascular accident (CVA), or stroke. The most common causes of stroke are cerebral thrombosis and cerebral embolism. Hemorrhagic disease encompasses hypertensive intracranial hemorrhage and ruptured cerebral aneurysm with subarachnoid hemorrhage.

## ISCHEMIC CEREBROVASCULAR DISEASE

### Cerebrovascular Accident (CVA), or Stroke

#### *Definition*

A cerebrovascular accident, or stroke, is characterized by the sudden onset of focal neurologic deficits in response to cerebral ischemia caused directly or indirectly by a localized disturbance or alteration in cerebral blood flow.

### Mortality and Morbidity

Stroke is the third leading cause of death in the United States, behind heart disease and cancer. The morbidity of this syndrome is reflected by the impact its consequent disabilities have on the lives of patients and their families. The effect on their personal (physical, psychologic, emotional), social (including the health-care system and the cost of health care), and economic (loss of earnings and opportunities for self-expression and creativity) well-being can be devastating. The situation is further complicated by the fact that the patient with stroke is commonly over the age of 65 and has other complicating health problems, such as diabetes mellitus, peripheral vascular disease, and heart disease.

### Risk Factors

Certain risk factors predispose an individual to stroke. These are listed in Table 11–1. Hypertension, hyperlipidemia, and age are major contributors to the pathogenesis of stroke.[1] As part of the "aging process," blood vessels throughout the body, but particularly the cerebral vasculature, become less compliant and predispose to increased vascular resistance and hypertension. There is also a greater tendency to develop degenerative diseases with increasing age, placing the older patient at still greater risk.

### Stroke and Cerebral Blood Flow: Clinical Significance

Alterations or disruptions of the cerebral circulation predispose to cerebral ischemia, injury, and neuronal death from infarction. The highly metabolically active nerve cells require a constant, copious supply of blood because their nutritive and oxygen reserves are minimal. Interruption of cerebral blood flow for even a few seconds can precipitate a loss of consciousness. The significance of a cerebrovascular accident is that it causes disruption of cerebral blood flow leading eventually to cerebral ischemia, injury, and infarction. (For a summary of factors influencing cerebral blood flow, see Table 6–7.)

### Major Cerebral Artery Syndromes: Location and Clinical Manifestations of Neurologic Deficits

Whether neurologic deficits associated with stroke and manifested clinically are temporary or permanent depends on a number of factors. These include the size of the involved blood vessel(s), the site of vessel pathology, the degree of vessel occlusion (partial or complete), and the extent of collateral circulation available to maintain adequate blood supply to the involved tissues.

In attempting to establish a correlation between symptomatology associated with specific cerebral artery disease and the actual clinical manifestations exhibited by the particular patient, much difficulty is encountered. Part of this difficulty is attributed to the variability of *collateral* circulation

TABLE 11–1
**Cerebrovascular Accident (Stroke): Risk Factors**

| | |
|---|---|
| Hypertension | A major risk factor, which, together with atherosclerosis, is highly implicated in the pathophysiologic processes underlying vascular disease. |
| Age | Incidence of stroke and deaths attributed to stroke increase with age. Individuals over 65 years of age are at great risk. |
| Diabetes mellitus | Associated metabolic disorders may contribute to atherosclerosis. *Hypercholesterolemia* and *hyperlipidemia* have been found to exist concomitantly in stroke patients and are implicated in the atherogenic process. |
| Heart disease | A major contributor to cerebral infarction.<br>• Rheumatic heart disease with valvular pathology, and subacute bacterial endocarditis are widely recognized as precursors to the development of cerebral embolism.<br>• Cardiovascular disease and hypertension predispose to left ventricular failure. |
| Use of oral contraceptives | This has been implicated in the development of stroke. The risk involves an alteration in blood clotting related to estrogen. New oral contraceptive preparations contain reduced doses of estrogen and are considered to be safer. |
| Other risk factors | Other risk factors implicated in the pathogenesis of cerebrovascular disease and stroke include:<br>cigarette smoking obesity<br>sedentary lifestyle arteritis<br>polycythemia vera congenital vessel anomalies<br>family history: genetic predisposition |

from one person to the next. While one patient may remain symptomless, another patient with similar pathology may become neurologically compromised.

Major clinical syndromes have been attributed to pathology of specific areas of the brain (Table 11-2). It is important to appreciate the variety and complexity of neurologic dysfunction, which can occur depending on the cause of the stroke, the vessel(s) impaired, and the area of the brain that is affected (i.e., the area of the brain supplied by a particular cerebral artery).

The major clinical syndromes are reflective of pathology involving the *anterior* cerebral circulation (i.e., via the internal carotid arteries) and include the internal carotid artery syndrome and the anterior and middle cerebral artery syndromes. Those involving *posterior* cerebral circulation (i.e., via the vertebral arteries) include vertebral and basilar artery syndromes and the posterior cerebral artery syndrome. The circle of Willis connects the anterior and posterior cerebral circulations and contributes to collateral circulation (see Fig. 6-9).

**Middle Cerebral Artery Syndrome.** Because the middle cerebral artery syndrome is the most common, it is useful to examine this particular clinical syndrome more closely.

The middle cerebral artery is the largest artery to arise from the internal carotid artery as it enters the base of the brain. This artery, in turn, gives rise to superficial cortical and the deeper penetrating arteries and accounts for about 80 percent of the blood supply to the cerebral hemisphere. The distribution of middle cerebral artery circulation is predominantly over the *lateral* surface of the hemisphere. It may be recalled that innervation to areas of the body concerned with intricate functions originates here. Thus, hands, fingers, thumb, face, lips, and so forth, are well represented, and they receive their blood supply via the middle cerebral artery (see Fig. 6-20).

Occlusion of the middle cerebral artery at its origin (i.e., the internal carotid artery) causes infarction of those areas of the brain concerned with motor and sensory function as represented by the somesthetic cortex. Clinically, the underlying pathology is reflected as the classic picture of: contralateral hemiplegia (i.e., paralysis of one side of the body including face, arm, and leg opposite to that of the lesion), hemianesthesia (i.e., loss of tactile sensibility), and homonymous hemianopsia (i.e., loss of sight in corresponding halves of both eyes). If the lesion occurs in the dominant hemisphere (commonly the left cerebral hemisphere), the patient may also experience aphasia (dysphasia), that is, difficulty in or impairment of the ability to communicate through speech, writing, or symbols. *Expressive* aphasia refers to an impairment in all *output* modalities (e.g., speech, gesturing, and writing). *Receptive* aphasia involves impairment of *input* modalities (e.g., auditory comprehension, reading, and thought processing speed).[2]

Patients with a nondominant hemispheric lesion (commonly the right cerebral hemisphere) may present clinically with apraxia rather than dysphasia. Apraxia refers to a disturbance in the execution of learned movements, or the manipulation of objects in space. While right hemispheric deficits are more subtle than the aphasias, they are just as integral to the performance of activities of daily living, social interactions, and work.[3] Although apraxia can result from injury to either hemisphere, the nature of the clinically manifested deficit(s) depends on which hemisphere is damaged.

Other deficits most commonly related to right hemispheric pathology, which are often not documented, include unilateral spatial and visual neglect. These deficits describe a spectrum of behavioral disorders characterized by decreased surveillance of the left side of one's body and immediate environment, and may involve visual, auditory, and tactile stimuli.[3] Thus, patients fail to look to the left side of space, fail to copy the left side of figures and diagrams, and read only the right portion of words and sentences. Patients may see only one side of their meal tray and may be unaware of anyone approaching from their left.

Anosognosia describes a lack of awareness by patients of the presence of neurologic deficits (e.g., hemiplegia). Some patients may vehemently deny that there is anything the matter with them; others may acknowledge that their limbs are weak, or that a hemiparesis is present, but exhibit little concern about the significance of the deficit and the ramifications for rehabilitation and recovery. Such lack of concern or awareness may interfere with rehabilitative efforts because patients may be less motivated to work at correcting or overcoming their deficits.

Disturbances in affect (i.e., an emotional reaction or feeling) and its communication are frequently associated with hemispheric pathology. This is especially true in patients with right frontal lobe lesions who are unable to express the desired affective tone in their speech. Pitch, rhythm, tone, accent, and emphasis all add meaning to what is spoken. Yet, when asked to say a phrase (e.g., "pick up the pencil") in an *angry* tone, these patients are unable to do so.

In contrast, patients with left hemispheric lesions, who often fail to understand language and its meaning, experience little difficulty in recognizing whether what was said was conveyed in an angry tone. It is important to appreciate that in addition to deficits in recognition and expression of feelings, patients experiencing stroke (particularly those with right cerebral hemisphere involvement) undergo a real change in affective or emotional makeup, which impacts on the rehabilitative and recovery process.

TABLE 11–2
## Major Cerebral Artery Syndromes: Location and Clinical Manifestations of Neurologic Deficits

| Syndromes: | Internal Carotid Artery | Anterior Cerebral Artery | Middle Cerebral Artery | Vertebral Artery, Basilar Artery | Posterior Cerebral and Thalmic Syndrome |
|---|---|---|---|---|---|
| Occurrence: | Common | Least common | Most common | Less common | Less common |
| Origin: | Common carotid | Internal carotid | Internal carotid | Subclavian artery | Basilar artery |
| Gives rise to: | Ophthalmic artery<br>Anterior cerebral<br>Middle cerebral | Anterior communicating | Superficial cortical and deeper penetrating arteries | Both vertebral arteries unite to form the basilar artery in the area of the pons. | Basilar artery |
| Distribution of blood supply: | Optic nerve, retina | Medical surface of frontal and parietal lobes<br>Internal capsule (major route connecting cerebral cortex with brainstem and spinal cord)<br>Corpus callosum (connects hemispheres) | Provides 80% of blood supply to cerebral hemishere, including lateral aspects of frontal, parietal, and temporal lobes | Medulla including the pyramid where decussation of nerves occurs<br>Medial lemniscus and lateral medullary area<br>Posterior, inferior portions of cerebellar hemisphere | Diencephaon (thalamus); midbrain, visual (occipital) cortex; choroid plexuses of lateral and third ventricles |
| Neurologic deficits (signs and symptoms): | • Mimics middle cerebral syndrome, the major artery arising from internal carotid as it enters the base of the brain<br>• Contralateral hemiplegia<br>• Dysphasia (aphasia)<br>• Headache<br>• Alteration in sensory function<br>• Altered state of consciousness<br>• Retinal insufficiency with monocular blindness (*amaurosis fugax*)<br>• May mimic some signs of anterior cerebral artery dysfunction because this artery also arises from internal carotid artery<br>• Possible optic nerve dysfunction. | • Motor dysfunction with hemiplegia of contralateral leg with foot-drop; impaired gait<br>• Paresis of contralateral proximal arm with damage of internal capsule<br>• Sensory dysfunction with sensory deficit over lower leg and foot on contralateral side<br>• Frontal lobe dysfunction: primitive reflexes on contralateral side (grasp and sucking reflexes)<br>• Decreased cerebration<br>• Dementia with flat affect, lack of spontaneity, confusion<br>• Urinary incontinence<br>• Abulia (inability to make decisions or to perform acts voluntarily) | Classic picture of:<br>• Contralateral hemiplegia involving face, arm, and leg<br>• Hemianesthesia (loss of tactile sensibility)<br>• Homonymous hemianopsia (loss of sight in corresponding lateral halves of both eyes)<br>• Dysphasia (aphasia) with lesion of left cerebral hemisphere (~96% of population: Broca's speech center in left hemisphere)<br>• Expressive and receptive aphasias<br>• Apraxia (right hemisphere)<br>• Unilateral spatial and visual neglect<br>• Anosognosia<br>• Disturbances in affect<br>• Communication and language deficits<br>• Altered state of consciousness, coma | *Vertebral* artery:<br>• Clinical manifestations vary considerably from one individual to the next<br>• Lateral medullary syndrome:<br>• Paresthesias with numbness, tingling, and burning sensations over face<br>• Ataxia<br>• Cranial nerve dysfunction: vertigo, nausea, vomiting (VIII)<br>• Dysphagia, hoarseness, impaired gag reflex (IX, X)<br>*Basilar* artery:<br>• Supplies pons, cerebellum, and posterior cerebral area<br>• Signs and symptoms: weakness of all extremities, paralysis with complete occlusion | Homonymous hemianopsia; visual field defects (the patient may be unaware of visual field defects and may be described as "bumping into objects"<br>*Thalamic syndrome:*<br>• Contralateral sensory diminution or loss<br>• Alterations in proprioception (position sense) and tactile sensation |

*(continued)*

TABLE 11-2
**Major Cerebral Artery Syndromes: Location and Clinical Manifestations of Neurologic Deficits *(Continued)***

| Syndromes: | Internal Carotid Artery | Anterior Cerebral Artery | Middle Cerebral Artery | Vertebral Artery, Basilar Artery | Posterior Cerebral and Thalmic Syndrome |
|---|---|---|---|---|---|
| | | | • Depending on extent and severity of cerebral infarction, alteration in neurologic function may reflect changes in: Respiratory rate and breathing pattern Pupillary size and reactivity Extraocular movements Motor function with abnormal flexor or extensor rsponses | • Visual disturbances: diplopia, various degrees of alteration in conjugate gaze; visual field defects; blindness • Vestibular and auditory disturbances (horizontal and/or vertical nystagmus, dizziness, tinnitus, and deafness) • Bilateral cerebellar ataxia; bilateral motor and sensory dysfunction | |

Finally, patients with a middle cerebral artery syndrome, who experience extensive tissue injury and infarction, will present clinically with corresponding physiologic changes, and the level of brain functioning will be reflected by changes in the level of consciousness; alterations in breathing pattern, pupillary size and reactivity, and extraocular movements; and the presence of abnormal flexor or extensor responses. (See Table 11-2 for specific information related to the major clinical syndromes.)

### *Stroke: Etiology and Pathophysiology*

The underlying etiologic mechanisms of stroke include thrombosis and embolism. The consequent interruption or impairment of blood flow to any part of the brain predisposes to tissue ischemia and, ultimately, to cerebral infarction. The duration of the ischemic episode will determine the extent of the infarction.

The occurrence of an infarction predisposes the individual to secondary injury. A disruption of the integrity of plasma membranes leads to cerebral edema. As the edema increases, capillaries become compressed and the vicious cycle of impaired cerebral circulation with consequent cerebral tissue ischemia is perpetuated. In the presence of extensive infarction with significant injury and necrosis of brain tissue, the episode may cause the patient's death (see Fig. 8-4).

**Thrombosis.** Cerebral arterial thrombosis is the most common cause of stroke, and its occurrence is thought to involve a number of pathophysiologic mechanisms.[4] These include inflammatory disease of the vessel wall associated with sepsis; connective tissue diseases such as lupus erythematosus or polyarteritis nodosa; mechanical constriction; prolonged vasospasm commonly associated with subarachnoid hemorrhage; shock states; hypercoagulability syndromes; dissecting aortic aneurysm; carotid artery trauma; and postradiation necrosis.

***Atherosclerosis.*** The most widely recognized pathophysiologic mechanism underlying arterial thrombosis is the process of atherosclerosis. Although much about the atherosclerotic process remains obscure, some possible contributors to its development have been identified. Atherosclerosis is a disease process involving the arterial wall, which may be initiated in response to vessel wall injury due to hemodynamic, mechanical, and/or chemical factors. More specifically, in its earliest stage, damage involves the endothelial lining and sublying intima of the vessel wall. Smooth muscle cells proliferate and migrate from the media layer into the evolving lesions.There is an accompanying infiltration of lipoproteins and cholesterol into these lesions, forming the atheromatous plaque.

In association with the atheromatous plaque formation, the intima becomes thin and fibrous, and there is loss of the smooth muscle cell layer (media) and disruption of the internal elastic lamina. As the pathologic changes evolve, fibroblasts infiltrate the degenerative areas, leading to progressive fibrosis (sclerosis) of the involved arteries. Calcium often precipitates together with the lipids to form calcified plaques.

As a result of this atherosclerotic process, arteries lose their distensibility and are easily ruptured. Most importantly, the atheromatous plaques, with their rough, uneven surfaces, protrude into flowing blood and provide a *nidus*, or a focal point of lodgement, for blood clots to develop. Eventually, thrombosis or embolus forms. Thrombosis occurs most readily in vessels where the atheromatous plaques have caused a narrowing of the vessel lumen.

The coagulation mechanism occurs concomitantly with the evolving plaque formation. As connective tissue is exposed from disrupted intima, platelets adhere to the roughened surfaces and release adenosine diphosphate (ADP) and enzymes, which stimulate the formation of the platelet plug and initiation of the coagulation cascades (see Chap. 61). The significance here is that a platelet plug may break off, producing an embolism, or it may remain in place and eventually cause complete occlusion of the artery secondary to thrombosis formation.

Clinically, it is difficult to separate the atheromatous process from other factors such as hypertension, diabetes mellitus, hyperlipidemia, or cardiac disease. These factors are all interrelated in the evolution of cardiovascular disease. The development of atherosclerosis in smaller cerebral blood vessels is particularly influenced by hypertension.

Vascular sites most commonly affected by the atherosclerotic process include: the site of bifurcation of the common carotid artery into the internal and external carotid arteries (carotid sinus); bifurcation of the middle cerebral artery; junction of the vertebral arteries to form the basilar artery; and specific sites in the distribution of the anterior and posterior cerebral arteries. It becomes obvious that in addition to vessel size, turbulent flow of blood occurring at bifurcations of blood vessels is a significant atherogenic factor.

The extent of neurologic impairment in the stroke patient varies depending on the location and size of the ischemic, injured, and/or infarcted area resulting from an arterial occlusion. The availability of collateral circulation has a critical role in salvaging injured tissue and limiting the size of the infarction.

In general, stroke is characteristically manifested by a sudden onset of symptoms frequently occurring at rest or during sleep. Specific signs and symptoms are assessed to determine the arterial system involved and, thus, the anticipated area of underlying pathology. For example, the presence of unilateral hemiplegia, hemianesthesia, homonymous hemianopsia, and aphasia suggests a *middle* cerebral artery syndrome involving the contralateral cerebral hemisphere; signs and symptoms reflective of bilateral disturbances in cranial nerve and cerebellar function suggest a *basilar* artery syndrome. Clinically, such syndromes are not nearly so distinct because of the variability of collateral circulation.

***Classification of Arterial Thrombosis.*** Arterial thrombosis is often classified as (1) transient ischemic attacks (TIAs); (2) reversible ischemic neurologic deficit (RIND); (3) stroke in evolution; and (4) completed stroke.

*Transient Ischemic Attacks (TIAs).* Transient ischemic attacks refer to brief, usually recurrent episodes of focal neurologic deficits caused by cerebral ischemia. The neurologic deficits are reversible and clear completely within minutes. Rarely do they last longer than 24 hours.

The significance of transient ischemic attacks is that there is a recurrence of the same signs and symptoms with each episode, suggesting involvement of the same blood vessel(s). This is an important consideration in the differential diagnosis of thrombosis. It also warns of underlying pathophysiology. Clinical manifestations due to emboli, for example, may be similar to that of a thrombosis, but it is unlikely that a consistent, repetitive pattern would be observed with each attack, simply because emboli tend to seed many different blood vessels. A thorough patient history is invaluable in this regard.

Approximately one third of patients who exhibit transient ischemic attacks will eventually sustain a cerebral infarction due to thrombosis; another third may have transient episodes without developing permanent dysfunction; while in the other third, attacks will cease spontaneously. The recurrence of transient ischemic attacks is not to be taken lightly, because their very presence suggests an alteration of cerebral circulation, which signals the potential for developing a cerebral infarction.

*Reversible Ischemic Neurologic Deficits (RIND).* The term reversible ischemic neurologic deficits is sometimes used to describe reversible focal neurologic deficits caused by cerebral ischemia that may last longer than the 24-hour period used to define transient ischemic attacks. It is assumed that the underlying pathophysiologic process is similar in each case and the neurologic deficits clear completely. Thus, the major difference between transient ischemic attacks (TIAs) and reversible ischemic neurologic deficits (RINDs) is the time it takes for the deficits to clear.

*Stroke in Evolution.* A stroke in evolution is the development of a full-blown thrombotic stroke in response to cerebral arterial occlusion. Commonly, there is but a single episode, with the entire process of a completed stroke (see below) evolving within a period of several hours.

In some instances, a stroke may progress stepwise or intermittently over a period of hours or days. An incomplete or partial stroke may be followed by a period of improvement, only to be followed by a rapid progression of permanent neurologic deficits.

*Completed Stroke.* A completed stroke usually reflects permanent neurologic dysfunction. Once a completed stroke is sustained the patient is at risk of developing another. The course of a cerebral arterial thrombosis commonly involves a progression of neurologic dysfunction. Such progression is most likely related to an increasing stenosis of the involved artery and/or extension of the thrombosis to adjacent vessels. If the patient survives the initial insult, there will be a gradual improvement in his/her condition. With a small or limited infarction, total recovery may occur within a few days; when the infarction is extensive, there may be little significant improvement in the patient's condition even after months of intensive therapy. (For specific information related to cerebral thrombosis, intracranial bleeding, and other cerebrovascular disorders, see Table 11–3.)

**Embolism.** Cerebral embolism is the second most common cause of stroke. In contrast to thrombosis, cerebral embolism can occur at any age but more frequently occurs in the younger individual. Embolization may be the underlying cause of transient ischemic attacks and reversible ischemic neurologic deficits.

The occurrence of embolic stroke may be related to several types of etiologic factors: extracranial atheromatous plaques or thrombosis occurring most frequently in the carotid, aortic, or vertebral arteries; the presence of a foreign substance, including fat (associated with long bone fracture), air, or tumor, in the circulating blood; or alterations in the coagulable state. Bacterial vegetations released from heart valves may be a source of infection (e.g., encephalitis).

Cerebral embolism is primarily a manifestation of heart disease. Embolic material breaks away from a thrombus within the heart and lodges within a cerebral blood vessel. The middle cerebral artery and its branches are the cerebral vessels most often involved because this artery is a direct continuation of the internal carotid artery as it enters the intracranial cavity at the base of the brain. Heart conditions that predispose to cerebral embolism include myocardial infarction with mural thrombosis; atrial fibrillation and other dysrhythmias associated with hypertensive, rheumatic, or congenital heart disease; and bacterial endocarditis and valvular heart disease, among others.

A cerebral embolism can strike at any time whether at rest, during sleep, or when strenuous physical exercise is involved. There is a sudden loss of function with no warning signs. The nature of the clinical picture depends on the vessels involved. In general, infarctions due to cerebral emboli tend to be more extensive than those associated with cerebral thrombosis. Thrombosis reflects a more gradual pathologic process, which allows time for development of collateral circulation. With the rapidly occurring cerebral emboli, there is very little time to enlist assistance from adjacent anastomatic vessels.

The course of the illness and its prognosis are similar to cerebral thrombosis. Some patients recover rapidly, many without neurologic sequelae; in others who, for example, have experienced a massive insult to the brainstem following occlusion of the basilar artery, the results may be catastrophic. (For additional information on cerebral embolism, see Table 11–3.)

### *Medical-Surgical Management of Ischemic Cerebrovascular Disease*

The ultimate outcome of the patient who sustains a stroke will depend on the type of care the patient receives. During the acute phase (i.e., first 48 hours after the stroke), the primary therapeutic goals include: (1) support of vital functions; (2) restoration and/or improvement of cerebral circulation; and (3) prevention of further neurologic damage.

### Medical Management

***Ventilatory Support.*** In the responsive patient the effectiveness of the spontaneous ventilatory effort is monitored by bedside tidal volume and vital capacity measurements, and by periodic arterial blood gas studies, as indicated. Supplemental humidified oxygen therapy using inspired oxygen concentrations of 24–28% via Venturi mask, or 2–3 liters via nasal canula, may be prescribed to maintain optimal arterial oxygen tensions. In the comatose patient with compromised protective reflexes (e.g., cough, gag, epiglottal closure), endotracheal intubation and mechanical ventilation therapy may be necessary. Hyperventilation therapy may be prescribed to prevent hypercapnia and hypoxemia.

***Circulatory Support.*** A major ischemic insult to the brain disrupts its autoregulatory mechanisms. In the absence of such mechanisms, the focus of circulatory support is to increase mean arterial blood pressure so as to increase cerebral perfusion pressure and relieve ischemia. Closely regulated intravenous fluid therapy and the use of vasopressors (e.g., dopamine) may assist in this regard. In patients hypertensive prior to the stroke, antihypertensives (e.g., diazoxide) may be prescribed. In some patients with long-standing hypertension, however, it may be necessary to maintain blood pressure at pre-existing levels. Cerebral vascular

TABLE 11–3
## Intracranial Bleeding—Cerebrovascular Disorders

| Characteristics | Epidural Hematoma | Subdural Hematoma | Cerebral Thrombosis | Cerebral Embolism | Subarachnoid Hemorrhage/ Aneurysm | Hypertensive Intracerebral Hemorrhage |
|---|---|---|---|---|---|---|
| Age | Any age | Any age | Mos common CVA >65 lears | Any age, frequently young | 30–65 years | 40–60 years |
| Etiology | Trauma—blunt blow to squamous portion of temporal bone, with fracture or closed head injury; laceration of middle meningeal artery | *Acute*—skull fracture; high impact closed head trauma; contusions *Subacute/ chronic*—seemingly mild head trauma; elderly; alcoholic; anti-coagulation therapy | Inflammatory artery disease; athero-sclerosis, prolonged vasospasm TIAs with gradual pathologic progression | Atherosclerosis; rheumatic heart disease; myocardial infarction Hypertensive heart disease; bacterial endocarditis | Trauma—rupture of an ancurysm | Fractured skull; penetrating skull injury; contrecoup injury; severe contusion and laceration of brain tissue |
| Location | Bleeding into potential space between periosteal dura and inner table of skull | Bleeding into space between dura and arachnoid, usually laceration of bridging veins | Occlusion of internal carotids, middle cerebral artery or its branches; basilar-vertebral system; anterior cerebral artery | Brain tissue nourished by branches of middle or anterior cerebral arteries | Bleeding into subarachnoid space between pia and arachnoid | May be widely dispersed; bleeding into brain parenchyma |
| Onset | Rapid—minutes to hours | *Subacute/ chronic*—insidious | Minutes to hours, sometimes days | Sudden | Sudden and acute | Rapid, minutes to a few hours |
| Duration | Brief period of uncon-sciousness followed by lucid period; thereafter, rapid deterioration. | *Acuter—hours Subacute/ chronic*—months | Permanent with infarction; reversible with minimal damage and collateral circulation | May improve rapidly if collateral circulation is established | Variable; reversible neurologic deficits may improve with time | Large breed = permanent damage; small bleed = reversible |
| Associated factors | Predisposition to trauma | Alcoholism Trauma | Atherosclerosis Hypertension Diabetes mellitus and other risk factors | Heart disease | Aneurysms, arteriovenous malformation, tumor, abscess, trauma | Hypertension Atherosclerosis |
| Pathology with loss of autoregulatory mechanisms | 1. Usually arterial bleed = increase in cerebral blood volume = increase in ICP = cerebral ischemia = cerebral infarction and cerebral edema = further increase in ICP, etc. 2. Displacement of intracranial structures with compression and ischemia | Venous bleeding more common 1. Usually venous bleed = increase in cerebral blood volume = increase in ICP = cerebral ischemia = cerebral infarction and cerebral edema = further increase in ICP, etc. | Formation of atheromatous plaques with progressive vessel occlusion = cerebral ischemia with infarction | Sudden occurrence—collateral circulation may be minimal = increased tissue ischemia and infarction | | Hemorrhage into brain parenchyma; expanding mass causes compression of adjacent tissues with cerebral ischemia, edema, and infarction |

*(continued)*

TABLE 11-3
**Intracranial Bleeding — Cerebrovascular Disorders *(Continued)***

| Characteristics | Epidural Hematoma | Subdural Hematoma | Cerebral Thrombosis | Cerebral Embolism | Subarachnoid Hemorrhage/ Aneurysm | Hypertensive Intracerebral Hemorrhage |
|---|---|---|---|---|---|---|
| | | 2. Displacement of intracranial structures with compression and ischemia | | | | |
| Blood vessels involved | Middle meningeal artery | Bridging blood vessels in subdural space | Internal carotids; basilar-vertebral systems; anterior and middle cerebral arteries | Middle cerebral artery | Circle of Willis | Middle cerebral artery |
| Relation to activity | Usually sudden with trauma | Depends on force of impact; may be acute | Frequently occurs at rest or sleep | Occurs at any time | May occur at any time | During activity |
| Clinical features | | | | | | |
| • Level of consciousness | After a lucid period, rapid deterioration to coma | *Acute* — rapid deterioration to coma<br>*Subacute* — confusion, disorientation, progressive to coma<br>*Chronic* — may resemble organic brain syndrome with impairment of consciousness, orientation, memory, intellect, judgment and insight; defects evolve over time (months) | Usually conscious, may be confused and disoriented<br>TIAs | Depends on the extent of damage; usually conscious; coma rare | Explosive onset of headche; coma common | Rapidly developing coma |
| • Respiratory pattern | Cheyne-Stokes initially = central neurogenic hyperventilation | → Same | Signs and symptoms depend on site and extent of infarction and collateral circulation; and the specific arterial system involved | → Same | → Same | → Same |
| • Pupillary reaction | Ipsilateral pupil dilatation; sluggish to unreactive | Depends on location of lesion; may be pinpoint to moderately dilated, sluggishly reactive | Usually equal in size and reactive | Usually equal in size and reactive depending on location of lesion | Variable response depending on location of lesion | → Same |

*(continued)*

TABLE 11-3
**Intracranial Bleeding—Cerebrovascular Disorders *(Continued)***

| Characteristics | Epidural Hematoma | Subdural Hematoma | Cerebral Thrombosis | Cerebral Embolism | Subarachnoid Hemorrhage/ Aneurysm | Hypertensive Intracerebral Hemorrhage |
|---|---|---|---|---|---|---|
| • Eye movement | Vary—conjugate to dys-conjugate; sluggish oculo-cephalic reflex | → Same | Homonymous hemianopsia | → Depends on site and extent of insult | Depends on site and extent of insult | → Same |
| • Motor response | Contralateral hemiparesis or hemiplegia; posturing | → Same | Contralateral hemiplegia | → Depends on site and extent of insult | Contralateral hemiparesis and hemiplegia | Depends on site and extent of insult |
| • Nuchal rigidity | Possible but rare | Possible but rare | Absent | Absent | Usually present | Frequent |
| CSF | Usually normal | Usually normal | Usually normal | Usually normal | Grossly bloody | Frequently bloody |
| Convulsions | Frequent | Infrequent | Infrequent | Rare | Common | Common |
| ICP | Increased—aggravated by hypercapnia and hypoxia | Probably increased | Not usually elevated | Not usually elevated | Frequently elevated | Frequently elevated |
| Complications | | | | | | |
| • Herniation | Uncal or lateral tran-stentorial | Uncal (lateral tran-stentorial) and/or central (transten-torial) | Uncommon | Uncommon | Common | Very common |
| • Cerebral ischemia | Secondary change related to initial trauma | Occurs in response to compres-sion from expanding mass with dis-placement of intracranial contents | Depends on area of brain affected and presence of collateral circulation | → Same | Secondary to vasospasm as well as primary insult | Secondary to vasospasm and primary insult |
| • Cerebral infarction | Occurs secondary to progressive ischemia | → Same | → Same | → Same | → Same | → Same |
| • Cerebral edema | Secondary to trauma, hypoxia; disruption of blood–brain barrier | → Same | → Same | → Same | → Common | → Common |
| • Infection (cerebral) | Possible with extensive scalp injury and/or lacerated dura | Increased as dura is opened or invasive ICP monitoring | Uncommon | Uncommon | More frequent with invasive procedure | Same |
| • Vasospasm | Infrequent | Infrequent | Uncommon | Uncommon | Frequently present | Usually present |

*(continued)*

TABLE 11-3
**Intracranial Bleeding — Cerebrovascular Disorders *(Continued)***

| Characteristics | Epidural Hematoma | Subdural Hematoma | Cerebral Thrombosis | Cerebral Embolism | Subarachnoid Hemorrhage/ Aneurysm | Hypertensive Intracerebral Hemorrhage |
|---|---|---|---|---|---|---|
| Recurrence | Uncommon with appropriate and timely therapy | Possible post-surgery | Common | Common | Very common | Very common |
| Mortality | 80 percent | *Acute*: high | If patient survives initial episode, there is gradual improvement | Increased mortality due to minimal collateral circulation | | |

*Key:* CSF = cerebrospinal fluid; ICP = intracranial pressure.

hemodynamics have adjusted to the hypertension over time, and a sudden reduction in blood pressure may aggravate underlying cerebral ischemia, increasing the risk of cerebral infarction.

***Pharmacologic Therapy.*** Pharmacologic therapy is focused on the following objectives: (1) restoration and maintenance of cerebral perfusion pressure and cerebral blood flow; (2) reducing and/or minimizing risk of cerebral edema; (3) reducing neuronal cellular metabolism; and (4) relieving pain.

Pharmacologic support therapy includes the following categories of drugs: vasopressors or antihypertensives (as indicated in the previous section); hyperosmolar agents (e.g., mannitol); diuretics (e.g., furosemide); corticosteroids (e.g., dexamethasone); anticonvulsant therapy if indicated (e.g., phenytoin); analgesics (e.g., codeine, acetaminophen); histamine$_2$ antagonists if indicated (e.g., ranitidine); and antacids and stool softeners when indicated. (For a discussion of these therapeutic agents, see Chap. 9.)

*Anticoagulant Therapy.* In addition to pharmacologic support therapy, the mainstay of treatment of ischemic cerebrovascular disease or stroke is anticoagulant therapy. Anticoagulants restore and/or improve cerebral circulation, and prevent further occlusion of the compromised cerebral vasculature.

Anticoagulation therapy reduces the risk of transient ischemic attacks (TIAs) and thrombotic episodes, which predispose to cerebral infarction. Such therapy has been found to be useful in treating some patients having a stroke in evolution (i.e., a progressively evolving stroke). Patients with completed strokes, however, have not been found to benefit from anticoagulant therapy. Strokes related to thromboembolic cerebral infarction are frequently treated with anticoagulant therapy to reduce the risk of recurrent embolization. Such treatment is also helpful in reducing the incidence of pulmonary embolism and infarction.

The mainstay of anticoagulant therapy during the acute phase of stroke is heparin. Heparin may be administered as a bolus followed by continuous intravenous infusion or, alternatively, via serial subcutaneous administration. Heparin is a potent anticoagulant, and as such it has important implications for nursing care. (Heparin's pharmacokinetics, actions and uses, dosage and administration, contraindications and adverse reactions, and nursing care considerations are presented in Table 35-2. For further information related to dosage and administration, adverse reactions, and nursing implications, see Appendix A.)

Protamine sulfate is a potent antidote for heparin overdose. Administered intravenously over 1-3 minutes, its actions begin to take effect within 5 minutes, and it has a duration of about 2 hours. Hypotension and anaphylaxis are significant adverse reactions associated with the use of protamine. (For details related to its dosage and administration, other adverse reactions, and implications for nursing, see Appendix A.)

Alternatively, depending on the severity of stroke and the patient's clinical status, or as a sequel to heparin therapy, oral anticoagulant therapy may be prescribed. Warfarin (Coumadin) is the mainstay of oral anticoagulation therapy. It exerts its anticoagulant effect by blocking the essential carboxylation of the vitamin K-dependent clotting factors — II, VII, IX, and X. Vitamin K is essential for the hepatic synthesis of these major clotting factors. In their absence, clotting is impaired. As is the case with heparin, warfarin can cause spontaneous bleeding and requires close monitoring and evaluation of the patient's response to anticoagulant therapy.

Antiplatelet aggregation therapy may be prescribed for the treatment of stroke. Drugs used in this regard include dipyridamole (Persantine), sulfinpyrazone (Anturane), and acetylsalicyclic acid (aspirin). Such drugs have been prescribed on a long-term basis to reduce platelet adhesiveness and possibly reduce the risk of recurrent thrombosis or emboli.

Cerebral vasodilator therapy may also be employed to increase blood flow to areas of brain compromised by occlusion or vasospasm. Papaverine (Pavabid) is often prescribed in this regard. Papaverine exerts a nonspecific direct spasmolytic effect on smooth muscles that is unrelated to innervation. However, its effectiveness in this regard has not been definitively ascertained.

***Surgical Interventions.*** Surgical intervention is directed at improving cerebral blood flow. Carotid endarterectomy has been especially effective in this regard. More recently, extracranial-intracranial bypass surgery has been employed with mixed success in patients with inaccessible stenosis and/or occlusion of the carotid, middle cerebral, or basilar arteries. The procedure usually performed involves the anastomosis of the superior temporal artery with the middle cerebral artery. (For nursing diagnoses, patient outcomes, and nursing interventions/rationales concerned with the postoperative care of the patient having craniocerebral surgery, see Table 9-1.)

## HEMORRHAGIC CEREBROVASCULAR DISEASE

Cerebral hemorrhage is considered to be the third most common cause of stroke. Based on underlying pathologic mechanisms, 2 types of cerebral hemorrhage have been identified: hypertensive cerebral hemorrhage and hemorrhage associated with a ruptured cerebral aneurysm (subarachnoid hemorrhage).

The onset of cerebral hemorrhage is sudden and explosive, and the patient becomes critically ill. A cerebral hemorrhage is differentiated from a thrombosis in that, unlike the thrombosis, which reflects a gradual progressive pathologic process accompanied by focal and replicated neurologic signs, a cerebral hemorrhage lacks any prior signs of neurologic dysfunction. The suddenness of its appearance precludes the establishment of collateral circulation, which may occur in thrombosis, and, consequently, sequelae of cerebral hemorrhage may be more extensive.

### Hypertensive Intracerebral Hemorrhage

Longstanding hypertension predisposes to alterations in the cerebral vasculature, which are characterized as degenerative changes of the vessel wall. Such changes may result in the development of aneurysms in the cerebral microcirculation. Frank, symptom-producing cerebral hemorrhage usually involves smaller cerebral arteries. It is not known precisely what vascular lesion precipitates rupture of a vessel; the cerebral vessels most often involved are the arteries that penetrate the brain parenchyma. Thus, a hypertensive cerebral hemorrhage is *intracerebral,* as opposed to hemorrhage associated with rupture of aneurysms, which usually causes a *subarachnoid* hemorrhage (see below).

Because intracerebral hemorrhage involves a high pressure system, such bleeds rarely seal off spontaneously. Rather, there is extravasation of blood into the brain parenchyma creating a mass lesion, which compresses and displaces adjacent brain tissue and thus precipitates signs of neurologic dysfunction (see Fig. 8-5). A massive intracerebral bleed can cause extensive infarction with displacement of intracranial contents, coma, herniation, and death. If the bleed is large enough, there will probably be seepage of blood into the ventricular system. Blood in the cerebrospinal fluid may be detected on lumbar puncture.

Hypertensive intracerebral hemorrhage may occur abruptly without any warning and usually while the patient is active. A thorough patient history may reveal subtle clues to the evolution of the hemorrhage. Initially, the patient may have experienced severe headaches associated with nausea and vomiting, followed at some point by focal neurologic deficits involving sensory and motor function. The earlier symptoms may reflect an increase in intracranial pressure, while later symptomatology reflects disruption of sensory and motor pathways within the involved cerebral hemisphere. Neurologic deficits attributed to cerebral hemorrhage are never as rapidly reversible as those associated with thrombotic disease largely because of lack of adequate collateral circulation.

Specific neurologic signs and symptoms exhibited by the patient depend on the location and extent of bleeding. Cerebral lesions may reflect symptomatology discussed earlier with respect to the major cerebral artery syndromes. In addition, hemorrhage may occur in subcortical areas, basal ganglia, and/or brainstem. Intracerebral hemorrhage usually causes the most extensive and permanent neurologic deficits. It usually involves the slowest recovery. (See Table 11-3.)

### Ruptured Cerebral Aneurysm— Subarachnoid Hemorrhage

An aneurysm is a thin-walled outpouching or localized dilatation of a blood vessel. The most common type of aneurysm is described as saccular, or "berry-shaped." These aneurysms usually occur at bifurcations of blood vessels; the circle of Willis is the most common site with blood extruded into the subarachnoid space (see Fig. 6–9). Cerebral hemorrhage related to a ruptured aneurysm generally occurs in individuals between 30–65 years of age who may have more than 1 aneurysm. The occurrence of such aneurysms may reflect a developmental defect or weakness in the vessel wall. Saccular aneurysms range from the size of a pinhead to as large as 2 or 3 cm.

Clinically, there is usually no evidence of an aneurysm until the initial rupture. Occasionally, recurrent unilateral migraine headache is mentioned as being a sign of aneurysm. Very large aneurysms may cause symptoms by compressing adjacent structures. Minor leakage of blood may precede actual rupture and may cause a warning headache.

Rupture of a saccular aneurysm occurs most often while the individual is engaged in vigorous activity. Hemorrhaging of blood under arterial pressure into the subarachnoid space may be accompanied by excruciating headache and may result in a loss of consciousness. There may be a sudden loss of consciousness without other signs or symptoms. Other symptoms, if present, may include vomiting, dizziness, vertigo, sweating and chills, and changes in the level of consciousness. There is a strong probability that the aneurysm will rebleed.

Blood is especially irritating to brain tissue. The patient may exhibit signs of meningeal irritation, photophobia, fever, nausea, and vomiting. Focal neurologic signs may also be observed: motor weakness, sensory deficits, visual disturbances (diplopia), and seizure activity. (See Table 11–3.)

### Vasospasm

Cerebral vasospasm is commonly associated with rupture of a cerebral aneurysm and consequent subarachnoid hemorrhage. It is the most serious complication of a subarachnoid hemorrhage contributing significantly to its mortality and morbidity. The vasospasm reflects prolonged contraction of a blood vessel(s) and most frequently occurs within 7–10 days after the initial hemorrhage. Vasospasm alters cerebral blood flow and contributes significantly to cerebral ischemia.

Initially, there is focal vasoconstriction of cerebral blood vessels adjacent to the area of insult. Eventually, vasospasm may become widespread, resulting in ischemia, injury, and infarction of brain tissue. These alterations are manifested by the appearance of focal or diffuse neurologic deficits. Depending on the extent of the insult and area of brain affected, these deficits may include an alteration in the level of consciousness, visual disturbances, hemiparesis, hemiplegia, and seizures.

The pathogenic mechanism underlying vasospasm remains undefined. One theory suggests that certain vasoactive substances (e.g., serotonin, catecholamines, and prostaglandins) are released from the degradation of platelets and other blood products, which causes a reflex spasm within cerebral arterioles. Initially, during the acute phase, the vasospasm functions therapeutically to reduce cerebral blood flow and thus limits bleeding and/or prevents rebleeding. Vasospasm, which persists for several days or even weeks (i.e., chronic phase), largely accounts for the neurologic deficits and seriously compromises the patient's clinical course and rehabilitation.

A major consequence of vasospasm is the impairment or loss of cerebral autoregulation. The inability of the cerebral vasculature to regulate cerebral perfusion causes cerebral blood flow to fluctuate with mean arterial blood pressure. Such fluctuations compromise cerebral blood flow and predispose to cerebral ischemia. The associated cerebral acidemia alters the integrity of the cerebral microcirculation, leading to vasogenic edema and an increase in intracranial pressure (see Chap. 8). Without intervention, the progressive increase in intracranial pressure leads eventually to cerebral infarction and death.

The treatment of vasospasm has been approached on several fronts. Cerebral vasodilation has been attempted with the use of papaverine, a spasmolytic agent, which acts directly on vascular smooth muscle to relax the muscle layer and thereby cause vasodilation. Isoproterenol, a beta-adrenergic agonist, in combination with aminophylline, a smooth muscle relaxant, has been used to treat vasospasm. Use of a serotonin antagonist (e.g., reserpine) has met with some success. Reserpine interferes with binding of 5-hydroxytryptamine (serotonin) at receptor sites. Currently, use of calcium blocking agents (e.g., nimodepine) to treat vasospasm is under investigation.

### Rebleeding

In terms of prognosis, rebleeding is considered to be the most frequent cause of mortality in patients with ruptured aneurysms. Rebleeding may occur as early as 24 hours post hemorrhage; or it may occur within 7 days of the initial bleed in conjunction with the natural fibrinolytic process. As the clot, which formed initially to seal the rupture site, undergoes normal lysis or dissolution, the risk of bleeding increases.

To prevent rebleeding, some institutions use aminocaproic acid (Amicar), an antifibrinolytic agent. However, the effectiveness of this drug in this regard has not been clearly established. Probably the most effective measure to prevent rebleeding from cerebral aneurysm(s) is surgical intervention. If surgery is not indicated, conservative treatment, directed toward controlling intracranial pressure and providing support for vital functions, is implemented.

## Medical-Surgical Management of Hemorrhagic Cerebrovascular Disease

The major therapeutic goals in the initial treatment of hemorrhagic cerebrovascular disease are to stabilize and support intracranial hemodynamics and to reduce the risk of and/or prevent rebleeding. Rebleeding is the major cause of death in patients who have sustained a ruptured aneurysm.

### Medical Management

Initial support therapy includes measures to reduce intracranial pressure and to maintain effective cerebral perfusion pressure. With a massive, rapidly expanding intracerebral or subarachnoid hemorrhage, extensive infarction and displacement of intracranial contents predispose to coma, brain herniation, and death.

Measures employed in the management of acute intracranial hemorrhage may involve the use of intracranial pressure monitoring, ventilatory and circulatory support measures, and pharmacologic therapy. (These modalities are discussed in detail in Chap. 9.)

**Specific Pharmacologic Support Therapy.** Measures employed to reduce the risk of rebleeding include sedation of the patient and use of analgesics to relieve pain. Headaches and meningeal irritation associated with intracranial hemorrhage can be especially distressing to the patient. Analgesics prescribed (e.g., codeine and acetaminophen) are usually those least likely to alter neurologic function so as not to mask the actual clinical picture. Drugs that sedate the patient or alter the state of consciousness (e.g., morphine) may mask the patient's actual status. Changes in respiratory pattern or pupillary reaction can likewise be altered by such drugs, and their use should be avoided if possible. Establishing a baseline as to the patient's actual functioning is essential.

Antihypertensive therapy is indicated in hypertensive intracerebral hemorrhage. Drugs used include diazoxide (Hyperstat), methyldopa (Aldomet), and hydralazine hydrochloride (Apresoline), among others. Stool softeners (e.g., diotyl sodium sulfosuccinate [docusate, Colace]) are prescribed for the alert, responsive patient to prevent constipation with consequent straining or Valsalva's maneuver. Antipyretic agents (e.g., acetaminophen) may be prescribed to treat an increase in body temperature, which commonly accompanies a subarachnoid bleed. Use of acetylsalicylic acid (aspirin) is avoided because of its antiplatelet aggregation effect.

### Surgical Intervention

Use of surgery in the treatment of intracranial hemorrhage may be indicated in the following instances: (1) to evacuate a large intracerebral mass formed as a result of an intracranial hemorrhage, which is large enough to cause brain compression and an increase in ICP; and (2) to ligate or remove the source of bleeding to prevent its recurrence. The decision to operate depends on several factors: (1) the cause of the bleeding—hypertensive vascular disease, ruptured aneurysm or arteriovenous malformations (AVM), as determined by angiography studies; (2) the clinical status of the patient, including level of consciousness and severity of neurologic dysfunction; (3) the accessibility of the lesion to surgical intervention; and (4) the presence and extent of vasospasm.

Surgical procedures used to treat cerebral aneurysms include direct clipping or ligation of the neck of the aneurysms to enable circulation to bypass the pathology. Inoperable cerebral aneurysms may be reinforced by applying to the aneurysmal sac such materials as acrylic resins or other plastics. The gradual tightening or constricting of a vessel via the use of a clamp (e.g., carotid artery clamp) is sometimes employed to allow for growth of collateral circulation. Establishing collateral circulation helps to reduce blood pressures and blood flow within the aneurysm. (See Table 9-1 for pertinent nursing diagnoses, desired patient outcomes, and nursing interventions/rationales in the care of the patient having craniocerebral surgery.)

## CEREBRAL VENOUS THROMBOSIS

Thrombosis involving the deep cerebral venous sinuses (see Fig. 6-10) is significant because of the paucity of collateral circulation. Infection is the most common cause of deep venous thrombosis. Infections of the eye, mouth, and nasal sinuses may predispose to cavernous sinus thrombosis; infections of the ear and mastoid area may precipitate thrombosis of the transverse venous sinus. The potential for extension or spread of such infections to the venous sinuses is the fundamental reason why patients with possible basal fractures and possible leakage of cerebrospinal fluid are cautioned not to sniff or blow their noses. Drainage from the nose or ear is allowed to drain freely onto a sterile gauze pad.

Clinical manifestations of cavernous venous thrombosis may include periorbital edema, exophthalmos and pain in the eye, and photophobia. Systemic signs and symptoms related to cerebral venous thrombosis include fever, headache, general malaise, and elevated white blood count; focal seizures may also occur. The headaches may be bifrontal or generalized, and usually develop early. Nausea and vomiting may be associated with the headache. The patient may initially be irritable, followed by drowsiness, delirium, and coma if left untreated. It is important to be mindful that signs and symptoms of cerebral venous thrombosis are often diffuse and nonlocalizing.

Other important etiologies of deep cerebral venous sinus thrombosis include pregnancy and the postpartum period, ingestion of oral contraceptive pills, cancer (lymphoma), and inflammatory bowel disease.

## NURSING MANAGEMENT OF THE PATIENT WITH CEREBRAL VASCULAR DISEASE

Consistent with the therapeutic goals of medical and/or surgical management, nursing management of the patient with an acute ischemic or hemorrhagic cerebrovascular insult is focused on: (1) support of vital functions; (2) restoration and maintenance of effective cerebral circulation and cerebral perfusion pressure; (3) prevention of further neurologic damage; (4) maintenance of total body functioning; and (5) initiation of some early overtures concerned with the patient's rehabilitation and discharge planning.

The rationales underlying nursing interventions can be approached from the perspective of conserving or "keeping together" the patient's biological, personal, and social integrity in the face of catastrophic illness.[5,6] Thus, interventions can be implemented to assist the individual/family in: (1) conserving energy to prevent further damage and promote recovery; (2) conserving the structural integrity of the individual by maintaining normal physiologic function and preventing and/or minimizing further disruption in neurologic and total body function; and (3) conserving the personal integrity of the stroke patient who already may experience dysfunction in such areas as cognition, perception, feeling, sensation, and language. The sudden dependence on others for activities of daily living may predispose to a loss of self-esteem, an altered body image, hopelessness, and loneliness; (4) conserving social integrity of the individual so that, on admission, the rehabilitative process is initiated to assist the individual to return to family and community functioning at his/her utmost level or potential.[6]

The quality of life subsequently experienced by the patient who sustains a cerebrovascular accident depends in large measure on the timeliness, appropriateness, and expedience of care provided during the acute phase. In the patient experiencing a cerebral ischemic episode, the rendering of such care may minimize the extensiveness of the ischemia and consequent infarction, and, thus, preserve neurologic function. In the setting of a major intracranial hemorrhage, such care may mean the difference between the patient's survival or ultimate demise.

The nursing care of the patient with a cerebral thrombosis or embolism is especially challenging, because in spite of the magnitude of the neurologic damage the patient is usually wakeful or arousable. Because a stroke commonly involves only one cerebral hemisphere, the patient is not only arousable but, in many instances, is usually aware of at least some of the consequent neurologic deficits sustained (e.g., a hemiparesis or hemiplegia, or the inability to communicate verbally).

The patient's clinical course is further complicated by psychologic and emotional repercussions associated with cerebral vascular disease. Preconceived ideas the patient and family may have as to the ramifications of stroke and its impact on personal, social, and economic resources may also complicate rehabilitation. A major aspect of nursing care is to provide emotional and psychologic support for the patient and family members, to keep them informed regarding the patient's clinical status, and to clarify any misconceptions.

While coma is a rare occurrence in ischemic cerebrovascular disease, its presence is highly suggestive of a massive intracerebral hemorrhage. Lesions involving the brainstem may also predispose to coma. Assessment of the patient's clinical status requires that the nurse be cognizant of the potential for an alteration in consciousness. Altered states of consciousness may interfere with establishing the patient's true baseline function. Speech, memory, and visual deficits (e.g., visual field deficits, diplopia), if present, further complicate the assessment of the patient's clinical status. The expression of behavior and personality by the patient may require corroboration with family members and/or significant others.

It is essential to differentiate between ischemia with cerebral infarction and intracranial hemorrhage, because while they both are considered to be major etiologies of a cerebrovascular accident, the approach to treatment is definitively different. In the setting of cerebral ischemia and infarction, therapy is directed toward increasing cerebral perfusion pressure and cerebral blood flow and preventing intravascular clot formation. Such therapy is contraindicated in the treatment of intracranial hemorrhage. Rather, efforts are focused on minimizing the initial bleed and preventing rebleeding and vasospasm. Rebleeding and vasospasm are the two major complications of intracranial hemorrhage, regardless of its underlying etiology.

### Therapeutic Goals

Nursing care of the patient with a cerebrovascular accident (CVA) during the acute phase is focused on the following therapeutic goals:

1. Stabilize ventilatory function with prevention of hypercapnia, hypoxia, and aspiration of nasogastric secretions.
2. Stabilize cardiovascular and cerebrovascular dynamics:
   A. Ischemic cerebrovascular disease—restore/maintain cerebral perfusion pressure and cerebral blood flow.
   B. Hemorrhagic cerebrovascular disease—minimize bleeding, prevent rebleeding and vasospasm.
   C. Monitor cardiac status for dysrhythmias.
3. Establish patient's baseline neurologic function, including prior behavior and personality considerations.
4. Stabilize and maintain fluid and electrolyte balance.
5. Maintain urinary and bowel function.
6. Minimize pain: headaches, muscular aches, anxiety.
7. Monitor and/or prevent seizures.
8. Prevent physiologic injury associated with:
   A. Disruption of musculoskeletal and skin integrity.
   B. Aspiration.
   C. Ulcerogenic gastrointestinal bleeding.
9. Initiate and establish a meaningful and trusting rapport with patient and family and/or significant others.
10. Establish a system of communication in patients with dysphasia.
11. Maintain an anabolic nutritional state.
12. Identify family and individual coping strengths; reassure family that stroke is often accompanied by changes in emotional behavior.
13. Assist patient/family to identify family and community resources especially if the patient's condition requires long-term rehabilitation.

## Nursing Diagnoses, Desired Patient Outcomes, and Nursing Interventions/Rationales

For specific nursing diagnoses, desired patient outcomes, and nursing interventions that provide the basis for nursing care of the patient with a cerebrovascular accident, see Table 11-4.

## CASE STUDY WITH SAMPLE CARE PLAN: PATIENT WITH A CAROTID ARTERY ANEURYSM AND MIDDLE CEREBRAL ARTERY SYNDROME

Mrs. M., a 37-year-old mother of 3 children ages 5, 7, and 9, presented in the emergency room at University Hospital with a right hemiplegia and dysphasia. Although unable to speak, Mrs. M. appeared to be aware of her surroundings. The patient's family stated that she was well and in good health until 2 weeks ago when she started to complain of headaches. The headaches persisted over the ensuing 2 weeks, and the family reported that Mrs. M. had several episodes when she "seemed to lose her voice."

On physical examination the patient was noted to open her eyes and interact with the examiner spontaneously. She was able to vocalize but could not verbalize. A right-sided hemiplegia was noted; a Babinski's sign was present on the right; a plantar reflex was intact on the left foot. Pupils were reactive, about 5-6 mm in size, with the right pupil slightly larger than the left. The right corner of the mouth drooped; no lid lag was noted. The patient had a weak gag reflex.

Examination of the skin and integument revealed good turgor, without lesions or rashes. The chest was clear on auscultation. The heart rate was 72, rhythm regular sinus. Abdomen was soft and nontender; bowel sounds were present in all four quadrants.

Arteriogram revealed a left internal carotid aneurysm, with poor filling of the left middle cerebral artery and anterior communicating artery. The patient was admitted with a diagnosis of right hemiplegia secondary to cerebral infarction associated with carotid artery aneurysm, and subarachnoid hemorrhage. Initial therapy included Decadron, 4 mg every 6 hours; antihypertensives to maintain systolic BP less than 180 mmHg; hold the medication for BP less than 140 mmHg. Loading dose of Dilantin (phenytoin) was initiated.

A subsequent arteriogram performed 24 hours after admission revealed a large lobulated aneurysm of the left carotid (internal) artery. The treatment plan included a left pterional craniotomy with microsurgical dissection of basal cisterns.

Postoperatively, the treatment plan included: hyperventilatory therapy via mechanical ventilation. The patient was pavulonized and sedated with morphine to keep stimuli to a minimum. Vital signs were monitored closely, with the systolic blood pressure allowed to find its own level within the range of 110-190 mmHg. The patient was monitored continuously for any increase in intracranial pressure. For ICP greater than 25 mmHg, mannitol was administered intravenously. Serum osmolality was closely monitored. A cooling blanket was prescribed to maintain the afebrile state.

The patient responded well to therapy. On the third postop day, the subarachnoid bolt was removed without difficulty, and the patient was weaned off the ventilator. On the fourth postop day, the patient was extubated successfully. Nutritional support was initiated. On overall assessment, the patient appeared to be regaining preop status. Through discussions with family members, the patient's usual behavior and personality were ascer-

**TABLE 11-4. CARE PLAN FOR THE PATIENT WITH A CEREBROVASCULAR ACCIDENT (STROKE)**

| Nursing Diagnoses | Desired Patient Outcomes | Nursing Interventions / Rationales |
|---|---|---|
| ***Nursing Diagnosis #1*** Alteration in cerebral perfusion pressure, related to:<br>1. Cerebral ischemia.<br>2. Cerebral edema.<br>3. Intracranial hemorrhage.<br>4. Vasospasm. | Patient will:<br>1. Maintain: cerebral perfusion pressure >60 mmHg.<br>• Intracranial pressure <15 mmHg.<br>• Mean arterial blood pressure ~80 mmHg.<br>• Heart rate ~72/min; no dysrhythmias.<br>2. Exhibit intact level of consciousness and mentation:<br>• Oriented to person, place, time.<br>• Memory intact.<br>3. Demonstrate neurologic function:<br>• Pupils equal and reactive.<br>• Sensorimotor functions intact (e.g., can discriminate between fine and crude touch; exhibits purposeful movement). | • Refer to Table 8-2 for information on the following nursing interventions/rationales:<br>○ Monitor for signs and symptoms of increasing intracranial pressure.<br>○ Maintain integrity of intracranial pressure monitoring system.<br>○ Implement measures to prevent and/or reduce intracranial pressure.<br>–Maintain optimal positioning.<br>–Prevent increase in cerebral blood flow.<br>–Limit or decrease cerebral edema.<br>–Minimize cerebral cellular metabolism.<br>–Plan nursing care activities to prevent cumulative increase in intracranial pressure.<br>• Additional nursing considerations:<br>○ Therapeutic approaches used to minimize risk of increased intracranial pressure are likewise implemented to prevent rebleeding in patients who have sustained an intracranial hemorrhage. |
| ***Nursing Diagnosis #2*** *(cont)* Breathing pattern ineffective, related to:<br>1. Brainstem compression associated with hemorrhage or cerebral edema.<br>2. Impaired chest excursion associated with hemiparesis. | Patient will demonstrate effective breathing pattern:<br>1. Respiratory rate <25/min<br>2. Rhythm and depth eupneic:<br>• Tidal volume >7-10 ml/kg.<br>• Vital capacity >12-15 ml/kg. | • Refer to Table 9-1, Nursing Diagnoses #2 for information on the following nursing interventions/rationales:<br>○ Assess respiratory function.<br>○ Implement measures to maintain airway patency.<br>○ Implement measures to improve breathing pattern.<br>○ Plan patient care activities to minimize a cumulative increase in intracranial pressure or increase risk of rebleeding.<br>• Additional nursing considerations:<br>○ Hyperventilation therapy has not been found to be overly effective in the treatment of the stroke patient probably because there is loss of autoregulatory mechanisms. |

*(continued)*

**TABLE 11–4. CARE PLAN FOR THE PATIENT WITH A CEREBROVASCULAR ACCIDENT (STROKE) *(Continued)***

| Nursing Diagnoses | Desired Patient Outcomes | Nursing Interventions | Rationales |
|---|---|---|---|
| ***Nursing Diagnosis #2 (cont.)*** | 3. Alveolar ventilation and gas exchange adequate.<br>• $PaCO_2$ <30–35 mmHg.<br>• $PaO_2$ >80 mmHg.<br>• pH 7.35–7.45. | | |
| ***Nursing Diagnosis #3***<br>Airway clearance ineffective, related to:<br>1. Compromised cough.<br>2. Inability to handle tracheobronchial secretions.<br>3. Ineffective chewing/swallowing. | Patient will:<br>1. Maintain patent airway with normal breath sounds.<br>2. Demonstrate secretion-clearing cough (unless contraindicated by risk of increased intracranial pressure or rebleeding). | • Refer to Table 9–1, Nursing Diagnosis #3, for nursing interventions/rationales regarding assessment of respiratory function, and implementation of measures to maintain airway patency.<br>∘ Pneumonia is a frequent complication of stroke and usually develops on the paralyzed side, probably because of decreased thoracic excursion and altered pulmonary hemodynamics. To prevent pooling of secretions, it is recommended that the patient be repositioned hourly (unless contraindicated because of the risk of intracranial hypertension or rebleeding).<br>–Side-lying position allows drainage of secretions from mouth and prevents aspiration.<br>–Alternate positioning facilitates drainage of secretions from lung segments.<br>–Positioning of patient should allow for maximum chest excursion. | |
| ***Nursing Diagnosis #4***<br>Alteration in comfort: Headache, related to:<br>1. Meningeal irritation.<br>2. Surgical scalp incision. | Patient will:<br>1. Verbalize and/or indicate comfort.<br>2. Demonstrate relaxed facial expression and demeanor.<br>3. Maintain intracranial pressure <15 mmHg. | • Refer to Table 9–1, Nursing Diagnosis #4, for information on the following nursing interventions/rationales:<br>∘ Assess patient for signs/symptoms of pain and discomfort.<br>∘ Implement measures to reduce discomfort.<br>∘ Monitor head dressing for tightness or constriction.<br>∘ Provide quiet environment.<br>∘ Provide periods of uninterrupted sleep.<br>∘ Provide touch therapy; speak in a soft, soothing voice.<br>∘ Employ diversional measures. | |
| ***Nursing Diagnosis #5***<br>Anxiety related to:<br>1. Fear of dying.<br>2. Potential sequelae associated with ischemic or hemorrhagic cerebrovascular disease. | Patient will:<br>1. Verbalize feeling less anxious.<br>2. Demonstrate a relaxed demeanor.<br>3. Perform relaxation techniques. | • Refer to Table 35–3, Nursing Diagnosis #1, for information on the following nursing interventions/rationales:<br>∘ Assess for signs/symptoms of anxiety.<br>∘ Examine circumstances underlying anxiety.<br>∘ Assess patient/family coping behaviors and their effectiveness.<br>∘ Initiate interventions to reduce anxiety. | |

| | | | |
|---|---|---|---|
| 3. Intensive care setting. | 4. Verbalize familiarity with ICU routines and protocols. | | |
| ***Nursing Diagnosis #6***<br>Alteration in fluid and electrolyte balance:<br>1. Fluid volume excess with associated<br>• Cerebral edema.<br>2. Fluid volume deficit, related to:<br>• Diuretic therapy.<br>• Diabetes insipidus.<br>3. Altered electrolytes, related to:<br>• Diuretic therapy.<br>• Corticosteroid therapy.<br>• Acid–base balance. | Patient will:<br>1. Maintain hemodynamic function:<br>• Mean arterial blood pressure ~80 mmHg.<br>• Heart rate at patient's baseline; rhythm regular; no dysrhythmias.<br>2. Demonstrate intact level of consciousness and mentation:<br>• Oriented to person, place, time.<br>• Appropriate response to verbal commands.<br>3. Maintain balanced intake and output:<br>• Stable baseline daily weight.<br>• Urine output >30 ml <200 ml/min.<br>• Urine specific gravity 1.010 to 1.025.<br>4. Demonstrate good skin turgor and moist mucous membranes.<br>5. Maintain laboratory parameters within acceptable physiologic range. | • Refer to Chapters 23 and 30.<br>• Additional nursing considerations.<br>• Prevent and/or minimize cerebral edema.<br>∘ Restrict fluids as prescribed.<br>∘ Monitor intake and output; body weight, urine specific gravity, and other laboratory parameters (e.g., serum electrolytes, osmolality, total protein, BUN, and creatinine).<br>∘ Administer prescribed medication regimen and monitor response to therapy.<br>–Hyperosmolar agents, diuretics.<br>–Corticosteroids.<br>• Assess for signs of fluid overload or deficits. | • Hydration therapy is coupled with pharmacologic therapy to maintain the patient in a slightly dehydrated state to minimize cerebral edema formation. |
| ***Nursing Diagnosis #7***<br>Potential for injury: physiologic, related to:<br>1. Diabetes insipidus associated with craniocerebral insult.<br>• Hypothalamic/pituitary dysfunction. | Patient will:<br>1. Maintain vital signs at baseline values.<br>2. Maintain desired hydration status:<br>• Urine output >30 ml <200 ml/hr. | • Assess for signs and symptoms of diabetes insipidus.<br>∘ Primary findings include:<br>–Polyuria, polydipsia, dehydration, weight loss.<br>–Urine specific gravity <1.010. | • Diabetes insipidus is a frequent secondary complication of craniocerebral insult.<br>–Cerebral edema and/or intracranial hemorrhage may temporarily impair synthesis and release of antidiuretic hormone by the hypothalamus during the initial 48 hours post-insult. |

*(continued)*

**TABLE 11–4. CARE PLAN FOR THE PATIENT WITH A CEREBROVASCULAR ACCIDENT (STROKE) *(Continued)***

| Nursing Diagnoses | Desired Patient Outcomes | Nursing Interventions | Rationales |
|---|---|---|---|
| ***Nursing Diagnosis #7 (cont.)*** | • Urine specific gravity 1.010–1.025.<br>3. Remain without clinical signs of dehydration.<br>4. Maintain acceptable laboratory profile:<br>• Serum electrolytes, BUN, creatinine.<br>• Serum osmolality, serum proteins.<br>• Hematology profile. | ○ Neurologic status: level of consciousness, mentation, cranial nerve and sensorimotor function and deep tendon reflexes.<br>○ Hydration status: strict hourly fluid intake/output, body weight, urine specific gravity; signs/symptoms of fluid overload or dehydration; laboratory data: serum electrolytes, serum osmolality; hematology profile (i.e., hematocrit, hemoglobin).<br>○ Cardiopulmonary status: blood pressure, pulse, cardiac rate and rhythm.<br>–Presence of adventitious sounds.<br>–Ability to handle respiratory secretions; characteristics of sputum (e.g., thick tenacious). | ○ Patient with diabetes insipidus can quickly become dehydrated. |
| | | • Identify patients at risk. | • Clinical manifestations of diabetes insipidus post-insult may be delayed because of limited endogenous stores of antidiuretic hormone. |
| | | • Implement measures to maintain desired fluid status. | • Patient is usually maintained in a slightly dehydrated state to minimize risk of cerebral edema and reduce blood pressure. |
| | | ○ Administer prescribed medication regimen: vasopressin replacement therapy (e.g., vasopressin; desmopressin acetate); chlorpropamide, clofibrate, carbamazepine; and corticosteroid therapy. | ○ These drugs may be prescribed to heighten the efficacy of antidiuretic hormone.<br>○ Antiinflammatory effect of steroid therapy may help to minimize cerebral edema. |
| | | ○ Administer prescribed fluid regimen.<br>• Monitor effectiveness of overall thereapeutic regimen.<br>• For additional information on diabetes insipidus see Tables 16–2 and 16–3. | |
| ***Nursing Diagnosis #8***<br>Potential for injury: seizures, related to:<br>1. Intracranial hemorrhage. | Patient will:<br>1. Remain without seizure activity. | • Refer to Table 9–1, Nursing Diagnosis #6, for information on the following nursing interventions/rationales:<br>○ Assess characteristics of seizure activity.<br>○ Implement measures to protect patient during seizure activity. | |

| | | | |
|---|---|---|---|
| 2. Cerebral ischemia.<br>3. Cerebral edema. | | ○ Implement measures to prevent seizure activity. | |
| ***Nursing Diagnosis #9***<br>Potential for alteration in body temperature, related to:<br>1. Intracranial hemorrhage (subarachnoid hemorrhage).<br>2. Infection. | Patient will:<br>1. Maintain optimal body temperature ~98.6°F (37°C). | • Refer to Table 9–1, Nursing Diagnosis #8, for information on the following nursing interventions/rationales:<br>○ Monitor body temperature.<br>○ Assess for signs and symptoms of hyperpyrexia.<br>○ Obtain specimens of body fluids for culture and sensitivity.<br>○ Inspect all invasive sites.<br>○ Implement measures to reduce body temperature.<br>○ Offer reassurance to patient and family. | ○ Blood is very irritating to fragile brain tissue and predisposes to hyperpyrexia. |
| ***Nursing Diagnosis #10***<br>Potential for infection, related to:<br>1. Meningeal irritation; surgical manipulation.<br>2. Iatrogenic (e.g., invasive lines/procedures).<br>3. Pneumonia and urinary complications associated with immobility, catabolic state.<br>4. Compromised immune response possibly associated with corticosteroid therapy. | Patient will:<br>1. Maintain body temperature ~98.6°F (37°C).<br>2. Remain free of signs of meningeal irritation.<br>3. Demonstrate normal cerebrospinal fluid analysis.<br>4. Maintain serum WBC within acceptable range.<br>5. Have normal breath sounds.<br>6. Urine clear, free of microorganisms on culture. | • Refer to Table 9–1, Nursing Diagnosis #7, for information on the following nursing interventions/rationales:<br>○ Monitor for signs and symptoms of infection.<br>○ Implement measures to prevent infection.<br>○ Administer prescribed course of antibiotics.<br>○ Provide reassurance to patient and family<br>• Additional nursing considerations:<br>• Identify patients at high risk of developing an infection. | • Patients with strokes are especially at high risk; many are elderly with underlying chronic and degenerative diseases. |
| | | • Obtain baseline cultures of body secretions and drainage. | • In patients who are intubated, a baseline sputum specimen should be obtained for culture and sensitivity. Use of artificial airway and tracheobronchial suctioning contaminate the tracheo-bronchial tree, which is considered to be sterile below the level of the larynx. |
| | | • Monitor for the following parameters:<br>○ Body temperature.<br>○ Hematology profile—evidence of leukocytosis.<br>○ Sputum for changes in color, quantity, consistency, odor, and ability of patient to handle tracheobronchial secretions.<br>○ Chest x-rays for pulmonary infiltrates.<br>○ Urinary retention/distention; urinary incontinence. | • Early diagnosis with institution of timely therapy (including antibiotics) may help to prevent or minimize impact of infectious process on total body function.<br>○ Patients with stroke are at high risk of developing a pneumonia because of compro-<br>○ mised protective reflexes, altered sensorium, and immobility.<br>○ Altered state of consciousness and sensorimotor impairment may predispose to urinary retention with consequent infection. |

*(continued)*

**TABLE 11–4. CARE PLAN FOR THE PATIENT WITH A CEREBROVASCULAR ACCIDENT (STROKE) *(Continued)***

| Nursing Diagnoses | Desired Patient Outcomes | Nursing Interventions | Rationales |
|---|---|---|---|
| ***Nursing Diagnosis #10 (cont.)*** | | • Institute chest physiotherapy and bronchial hygiene (unless contraindicated by risk of intracranial hypertension or rebleeding).<br>∘ Implement turning and positioning schedule. | • Secretion removal improves ventilation and reduces pooling of secretions, which may act as foci of infection.<br>∘ Positioning and turning help to mobilize secretions; positions used should protect the compromised patient from aspiration. |
| | | • Use aseptic technique for patient care: tracheobronchial suctioning, urinary catheterization, and Foley catheter care.<br>• Maintain nutrition (anabolic state). | |
| ***Nursing Diagnosis #11***<br>Nutrition, alteration in: Less than body requirements related to:<br>1. Catabolic state.<br>2. Compromised nutritional intake associated with:<br>• Altered state of consciousness.<br>• Compromised protective reflexes.<br>• Ineffective chewing/ swallowing.<br>• Fatigue.<br>• Depression. | Patient will:<br>1. Maintain body weight within 5% of baseline.<br>2. Maintain total serum proteins 6.0–8.4 g/100 ml. | • Refer to Table 9–1, Nursing Diagnosis #10, for information on the following nursing interventions/rationales:<br>∘ Arrange consultation with nutritionist and collaborate to perform nutritional assessment.<br>∘ Maintain optimal nutrition with prescribed nutrition regimen (e.g., oral, enteral, parenteral).<br>–Maintain patient in optimal position for specific mode of nutrition intake (e.g, semi-Fowler's position in patients receiving enteral feedings).<br>–Confirm placement of nasogastric tube in stomach before initiating feedings.<br>∘ Provide frequent mouth care and other comfort measures.<br>∘ Monitor daily weight (unless contraindicated by risk of increased intracranial pressure and/or rebleeding).<br>∘ Assess bowel function; implement prescribed bowel regimen. | |
| ***Nursing Diagnosis #12***<br>Impaired physical mobility, related to:<br>1. Comatose state.<br>2. Restricted activity associated with risk of intracranial pressure or rebleeding. | Patient will:<br>1. Maintain full range of motion.<br>2. Remain without contractures.<br>3. Remain without incidence of thrombophlebitis. | • Consult with physician and physical therapist to assess neurologic and musculoskeletal status. | • The risk of intracranial hypertension and rebleeding must guide the type and extent of an activity program. A major objective is to maintain optimal function as dictated by patient's overall condition. |

| | | | |
|---|---|---|---|
| 3. Hemostasis and/or dependent edema associated with immobility; neuromuscular impairment (e.g., hemiparesis). | | • Plan and implement activity regimen:<br>○ Initiate schedule of range-of-motion exercises. | ○ Exercise maintains muscle tone and prevents atrophy; stimulates circulation and prevents hemostasis. |
| | | ○ Passive/active exercises should be performed as patient's condition warrants. | ○ Immobility associated with hemiparesis predisposes to thrombophlebitis. |
| | | ○ Allow rest periods prior to and after exercise routines. | ○ Helps to conserve patient's energy and prevent feelings of frustration associated with inability to perform daily self-care. |
| | | ○ Maintain optimal body alignment.<br>–Use hand/wrist splints as prescribed.<br>–Support affected extremities in functional position. | ○ Proper alignment is essential to prevent development of contractures and dependent edema (sacral area, buttocks, extremities). |
| | | ○ Use trochanter roll on outer aspects of thigh. | ○ Prevents external rotation. |
| | | ○ Initiate turning and positioning schedule.<br>–Encourage patient to deep breathe and cough (unless contraindicated). | ○ Turning, positioning, and deep breathing facilitate chest and lung expansion; mobilize oral and pulmonary secretions; prevent atelectasis. |
| ***Nursing Diagnosis #13***<br>Skin integrity, impairment of, related to:<br>1. Immobility.<br>2. Catabolic state.<br>3. Altered sensation.<br>4. Incontinence. | Patient's skin will remain intact:<br>• All reddened areas will blanch within 20–30 minutes of a position change. | • Implement skin care regimen.<br>○ Inspect skin and all pressure point areas for compromised perfusion.<br>○ Provide special skin care to back and joints and all pressure points.<br>○ Provide pressure relief device (e.g., air mattress, sheepskin).<br>○ Initiate pressure ulcer protocol if indicated: treat local skin areas with prescribed treatment (e.g., Skin Prep, Granulex, Duoderm, wet-to-dry dressings, other therapies). | • Maintain circulation to all areas; it is essential to prevent skin breakdown because the compromised patient is at high risk of developing an infection. |
| ***Nursing Diagnosis #14***<br>Potential for physiologic injury: thrombophlebitis, related to:<br>1. Hemostasis associated with immobility. | Patient will:<br>1. Verbalize absence of calf tenderness.<br>2. Exhibit adequate peripheral circulation:<br>• Usual skin color; no cyanosis.<br>• Extremities warm to touch.<br>• Palpable pulses: pedal, popliteal, radial. | • Assess for signs/symptoms of venous thrombosis.<br>○ Tenderness, pain, warmth, and peripheral pitting edema.<br>○ Measure circumference of thighs and calves at designated points. | • Deep venous thrombosis places patient at risk of pulmonary embolism.<br>○ Edema is a characteristic manifestation of altered venous circulation.<br>○ Evidence of edema is best assessed and monitored by determining the circumference of calves and thighs at designated points (use tape measure). |
| | | ○ Skin color and temperature.<br>–Observe extremities in both dependent and elevated positions. | ○ With altered venous circulation a bluish-red color of skin may be observed. |

*(continued)*

**TABLE 11–4. CARE PLAN FOR THE PATIENT WITH A CEREBROVASCULAR ACCIDENT (STROKE) *(Continued)***

| Nursing Diagnoses | Desired Patient Outcomes | Nursing Interventions | Rationales |
|---|---|---|---|
| ***Nursing Diagnosis #14 (cont.)*** | | • Implement measures to minimize risk of thrombophlebitis/deep venous thrombosis.<br>○ Maintain desired hydration state. | ○ Temperature of skin is assessed by touch; unusually warm temperature in the lower extremities is commonly associated with venous thrombosis.<br>○ While the patient with a cerebrovascular insult is usually maintained in a slightly dehydrated state, dehydration is to be avoided because it increases blood viscosity. |
| | | ○ Apply antiembolic hose to both extremities; remove hose once per shift.<br>○ Assist patient to perform range-of motion exercises as appropriate. | ○ Exercise enhances "skeletal-muscular" pump, which functions to prevent pooling of blood in lower extremities (venous stasis), and increases venous return to heart. |
| | | ○ Instruct responsive patient to avoid positions that compromise blood flow in the extremities (e.g., crossing of legs, prolonged sitting in one position, pillow under knees, or use of knee gatch). | ○ Positions that compromise blood flow can cause circulatory stasis. |
| ***Nursing Diagnosis #15***<br>Alteration in self-concept, related to:<br>1. Changes in body image associated with neurologic deficits.<br>2. Low self-esteem (i.e., dependence on others to achieve activities of daily living).<br>3. Alteration in role and personal identity. | Patient will:<br>1. Verbalize feelings about self.<br>2. Maintain interpersonal relationships with family members and significant others.<br>3. Participate in decision-making.<br>4. Initiate activities of self-care. | • Refer to Table 9–1, Nursing Diagnosis #11, for information on the following nursing interventions/rationales:<br>○ Encourage verbalization regarding patient's perceptions of changes in appearance and body function.<br>○ Assist patient/family to identify coping patterns/strengths and weaknesses.<br>○ Assess patient/family's readiness to participate in decision-making regarding care.<br>○ Involve patient in making choices and decisions regarding self-care.<br>○ Assist patient/family in initial goal-setting. | |
| ***Nursing Diagnosis #16***<br>Thought processes, alteration in, related to:<br>1. Cerebral ischemia and hypoxia.<br>2. Comatose state.<br>3. Sedation. | Patient will:<br>1. Demonstrate improvement in thought processes:<br>• Oriented to person, place, time. | • Refer to Table 10-1, Nursing Diagnosis #16, for information on the following nursing interventions/rationales:<br>○ Assess for alteration in mentation and thought processes.<br>○ Confirm recent behavioral or personality changes.<br>○ Implement measures to assist patient in thought processes. | |

| | | | |
|---|---|---|---|
| | • Improved memory.<br>• Increased attentiveness.<br>• Improved ability to solve problems and make decisions. | | |
| ***Nursing Diagnosis #17***<br>Sensory-perceptual alterations, related to:<br>1. Sensory deprivation.<br>2. Sensory overload. | Patient will:<br>1. Demonstrate appropriate interactions with people and environment using sensory perception (e.g., converses with visitors).<br>2. Verbalize restfulness and relaxed feelings.<br>3. Demonstrate relaxed facies and body demeanor. | • Refer to Table 10–1, Nursing Diagnosis #17, for information on the following nursing interventions/rationales:<br>∘ Assess patient's ability to interact with environment.<br>∘ Provide usual necessary aids (e.g., eyeglasses).<br>∘ Arrange environment to compensate for neurologic deficits.<br>∘ Implement measures to reduce sensory deprivation.<br>∘ Implement measures to reduce sensory overload.<br>∘ Recognize and accept patient's perceptions of stimuli (reinforce reality). | ∘ See Chapter 3, sections entitled "Needs of Critically Ill Patients" and "Patient Stressors in the ICU." |
| ***Nursing Diagnosis #18***<br>Communication impaired, related to:<br>1. Aphasia (dysphasia).<br>2. Dysarthria (i.e., disturbance in articulation) (left cerebral hemisphere involvement). | Patient will:<br>1. Use language to verbalize or communicate needs or answer questions. | • Assess for difficulty in using language to verbalize needs and answer questions.<br>∘ Consult with speech pathologist, if possible, to assess patient's clinical status and design a care plan. | • Primary speech center (Broca's) is predominantly in frontal lobe of left cerebral hemisphere. Cerebrovascular insult to this area can result in languge deficits. |
| | | • Implement measures that enhance communication:<br>∘ Speak slowly, using simple sentences.<br>∘ Repeat questions or directions.<br>∘ Use supplemental gestures or pictures; blackboard or slate board.<br>∘ Face the patient directly when speaking.<br>∘ Avoid speaking too loudly.<br>∘ Encourage patient to express his/her thoughts; avoid rushing the patient.<br>∘ Minimize distractions.<br>∘ Offer encouragement; praise the patient for his/her accomplishments.<br>• Anticipate patient's needs. | • Directives here suggest some of the ways communication can be facilitated. In the clinical setting, ideally, speech therapy is conducted in collaboration with a speech pathologist so that specific communication problems can be addressed appropriately.<br>∘ A language problem doesn't mean the patient can't hear.<br>∘ Assist the patient to concentrate on communicating.<br>∘ Assist the patient in gaining self-confidence.<br>• May help to allay concerns regarding dependency on others. |

*(continued)*

**TABLE 11–4. CARE PLAN FOR THE PATIENT WITH A CEREBROVASCULAR ACCIDENT (STROKE) *(Continued)***

| Nursing Diagnoses | Desired Patient Outcomes | Nursing Interventions | Rationales |
|---|---|---|---|
| ***Nursing Diagnosis #19***<br>Coping, alteration in: Patient and family, related to:<br>1. Situational crisis.<br>2. Temporary family disorganization.<br>3. Inability to problem-solve.<br>4. Altered thought processes.<br>5. Catastrophic illness with long-term effects. | Patient/family will:<br>1. Identify useful coping mechanisms.<br>2. Demonstrate ability to assess, problem-solve, and make decisions.<br>3. Express realistic expectations of each other. | • Establish a rapport and trusting relationship with patient and family.<br>◦ Observe family dynamics and interactions.<br>–Assess family relationships and communication pattern: usual coping mechanisms, usual decision-making process, especially during stressful or crisis situations.<br>–Assess response of patient/family to stressful situations: identify strengths/weaknesses. | • These observations may help to identify strengths and weaknesses, and effective coping capabilities. Assisting patient/family to acknowledge their own strengths may help them cope more effectively. |
| | | • Implement measures to assist in coping:<br>◦ Provide opportunity for patient and family members to express feelings and emotions:<br>–Encourage honest communication among family members. | ◦ Recognizing feelings and emotions helps one to deal with them. |
| | | ◦ Assist patient to prioritize daily activities. | ◦ Reduction in level of stress assists in coping. |
| | | ◦ Encourage patient/family to assist in decision-making process regarding care:<br>–Assist in identifying options and their consequences. | ◦ Assists patient/family to be responsible for self-care, and level of health desired. |
| | | ◦ Advise patient/family regarding community resources. | ◦ Sequelae from cerebrovascular disease can be catastrophic; it is essential for the patient/family to identify family and community resources. |
| ***Nursing Diagnosis #20***<br>Unilateral neglect, related to:<br>1. Altered sensorimotor function associated with cerebrovascular accident.<br>2. Alterations in thought processes: perceptual. | Patient will:<br>1. Demonstrate awareness as to position or placement of all four extremities.<br>2. Demonstrate awareness of looking toward affected side in terms of:<br>• Self-care (personal hygiene, grooming, dressing).<br>• Safety measures.<br>• Eating habits. | • Assess sensorimotor function related to:<br>◦ Special senses: visual field defects, dysphasia (aphasia).<br>◦ General senses: pain and temperature, tactile sensations. | • It is essential to determine what deficits exist so that an appropriate approach to therapy can be individualized for the patient.<br>◦ Often sensory deficits are permanent, necessitating that the patient learn what his/her deficits are, and how to accommodate actions and behaviors accordingly. |

| | | | |
|---|---|---|---|
| ***Nursing Diagnosis #21***<br>Self-care deficits, related to:<br>1. Neuromuscular impairments (e.g., paresis, apraxia, visual/sensory defects, anosognosia) (right cerebral hemisphere involvement).<br>2. Reduced attention span. | Patient will identify:<br>1. Activities of daily living for which the patient requires some assistance.<br>Patient will verbalize:<br>1. Feelings regarding dependency.<br>Patient will:<br>1. Determine priorities.<br>2. Plan activities of daily living, leaving ample time to accomplish tasks. | • Implement measures to assist patient to learn what types of sensorimotor deficits exist, and the extent of the deficits in terms of self-care.<br>○ Visual field deficits:<br>–Teach patient to scan immediate environment and note the placement of objects and equipment.<br>–Approach patient from intact side. | • It is important to involve patient and family members in patient care.<br>○ Frequent praise encourages and motivates patient and family. |
| ***Nursing Diagnosis #22***<br>Potential for injury: (Safety), related to:<br>1. Altered sensory/perceptual function.<br>2. Altered musculoskeletal function. | Patient will remain free from falls or other injury. | –Position bed so that the intact side can fully visualize the doorway.<br>–Keep bedside uncluttered. | –Prevents possible injury. |
| | | ○ Dysphasia:<br>○ Attempt to evaluate type of dysphasia.<br>○ Enlist the assistance of speech pathologist, if available, to establish program for patient, family members, and health-care professionals working with patient, designed to facilitate communication.<br>○ Helpful measures may include:<br>–Speak slowly and face the patient.<br>–Use short, simple sentences.<br>–Repeat directions or explanations as necessary.<br>–Use gestures to further clarify what is being said. | ○ Dysphasia (aphasia) is particularly associated with dominant cerebral hemisphere lesion (usually the left hemisphere). |
| | | ○ General sensorimotor functions:<br>–Dressing and grooming:<br>–Teach patient to care for affected side first when bathing or dressing; and to undress the affected side last.<br>–Use sensory stimuli to help patient become aware of affected part of body.<br>–Use exercises that enable affected side to cross midline. | ○ Apraxia, unilateral spatial and visual neglect, and anosognosia are neurologic deficits associated with nondominant cerebral hemisphere involvement (usually the right hemisphere involvement). |
| | | ○ Reassure patient and family regarding progress:<br>–Praise positive responses and activities. | ○ The patient's rehabilitation should begin during the acute phase; activities initiated during this period lay the foundation for patient/family participation in self-care. |

## SAMPLE CARE PLAN FOR THE PATIENT WITH A CAROTID ARTERY ANEURYSM AND MIDDLE CEREBRAL ARTERY SYNDROME

| Nursing Diagnoses | Desired Patient Outcomes | Nursing Interventions | Rationales |
|---|---|---|---|
| ***Nursing Diagnosis #1***<br>Alteration in cerebral perfusion, related to:<br>1. Cerebral infarction with consequent cerebral edema.<br>2. Vasospasm associated with subarachnoid bleeding. | Patient will:<br>1. Maintain cerebral perfusion pressure >60 mmHg; ICP <15 mmHg; mean arterial blood pressure ~80 mmHg.<br>2. Remain without cardiac dysrhythmias.<br>3. Exhibit intact level of consciousness and mentation:<br>• Oriented to person/place.<br>• Memory intact. | • Monitor for signs/symptoms of increasing ICP:<br>○ Establish baseline parameters for level of consciousness, mentation, respiratory rate and pattern, pupillary reactions, and sensorimotor function. | • Initial treatment is focused on stabilizing and supporting intracranial dynamics, and reducing and/or preventing rebleeding.<br>○ Baseline measurements are used to compare subsequent responses. |
| | | • Maintain the integrity of the ICP monitoring system:<br>○ Check for leaks, air; stopcocks in appropriate positions.<br>–Perform insertion site care as per protocol. | • ICP monitoring is a highly invasive technique, which places the patient at considerable risk of infection.<br>○ Inadvertent loss of CSF in the presence of increased ICP can alter intracranial hemodynamics and precipitate herniation. |
| | | • Obtain and record accurate pressure measurements:<br>○ Confirm accurate placement of transducer at level of foramen of Monro. | ○ Venting port of transducer should always be at pressure source (i.e., the foramen of Monro). For every inch above or below the pressure source, the pressure reading may be as much as 2 mmHg off. |
| | | ○ Analyze waveforms and pressure readings and identify trends.<br>○ Calculate and record cerebral perfusion pressure hourly. | ○ Trends are more significant in determining status of ICP and intracranial compliance. |
| | | • Implement measures to prevent and/or reduce ICP:<br>○ Maintain proper positioning and body alignment; elevate head of bed; avoid head rotation or flexion on chest. | ○ Allows for optimal venous drainage from cranium via gravity. Prevents jugular vein compression or obstruction. |
| | | • Prevent increase in cerebral blood flow:<br>○ Initiate and maintain hyperventilation via mechanical ventilation to maintain $PaCO_2$ at 25–35 mmHg; $PaO_2$ >80 mmHg. | • Hypercapnia and hypoxemia predispose to cerebral vasodilation and increased cerebral blood flow. |
| ***Nursing Diagnosis #2***<br>Alteration in comfort: Headache, related to:<br>1. Meningeal irritation.<br>2. Surgical incision. | Patient will:<br>1. Verbalize feeling relieved of pain.<br>2. Demonstrate a relaxed demeanor. | •Assess for signs/symptoms of menigeal irritation:<br>○ Nuchal rigidity, photophobia, headache, positive Kernig's and Brudzinski's signs. | • Intracranial bleeding is highly irritating to meningeal and brain tissues. |

| | | | |
|---|---|---|---|
| | | • Implement nursing measures to reduce headache and prevent bleeding:<br>∘ Move patient carefully, minimizing head movement or sudden jarring of patient or bed; turn q2h.<br>∘ Dim the patient's bedside light, and maintain a quiet environment with minimal stimuli.<br>–Handle patient gently when providing care.<br>–Caution patient not to cough, sneeze, or strain.<br>• Administer analgesics as prescribed, and monitor effectivness of medication in relieving pain and relaxing the patient. | ∘ Turning helps to mobilize tracheobronchial secretions and redistribute pressure points to maximize circulation.<br>∘ Dimming the lights helps reduce the discomfort of photophobia.<br>∘ These activities cause an increase in ICP.<br>• Headaches can be excruciating. |
| ***Nursing Diagnosis #3***<br>Potential for injury: Seizures, related to:<br>1. Cranial cerebral insult (cerebral infarction and edema; intracranial bleeding). | Patient will:<br>1. Remain seizure free.<br>2. Maintain serum levels of phenytoin within the acceptable therapeutic range. | • Assess/monitor for seizure activity, documenting characteristics: onset, location, type of movement, associated changes in body function.<br>• Maintain seizure precautions as per protocol.<br>• Administer prescribed anticonvulsants.<br>∘ Monitor serum levels of phenytoin (Dilantin) (serial) | • Craniocerebral insults place the patient at risk of having seizures; anticonvulsant medications are usually prescribed prophylactically. |
| ***Nursing Diagnosis #4***<br>Nutrition, alteration in, less than body requirements, related to:<br>1. Altered state of consciousness.<br>2. Compromised protective reflexes.<br>3. Ineffective chewing or swallowing.<br>4. Fatigue.<br>5. Depression. | 1. Patient will maintain an anabolic state:<br>• Body weight within 5% of baseline.<br>• Total serum proteins within the acceptable range: albumin 3.5–5.0 g/100 ml.<br>2. Patient will verbalize having an appetite. | • Consult with nutritionist to determine caloric and nutritional needs.<br>• Initiate prescribed nutritional regimen:<br>∘ Hyperalimentation; fluid restriction.<br>• Monitor response to hyperalimentation:<br>∘ Intake and output.<br>∘ Laboratory parameters: BUN, creatinine, total protein, and albumin.<br>∘ Daily weight when patient's condition permits.<br>• Maintain the integrity of the hyperalimentation system as per unit protocol. | • Critical illness increases nutritional needs; these patients can rapidly experience a catabolic state when maintained on intravenous fluid replacement therapy. (One liter of dextrose and water contains 600 calories.) |

**SAMPLE CARE PLAN FOR THE PATIENT WITH A CAROTID ARTERY ANEURYSM AND MIDDLE CEREBRAL ARTERY SYNDROME *(Continued)***

| Nursing Diagnoses | Desired Patient Outcomes | Nursing Interventions | Rationales |
|---|---|---|---|
| ***Nursing Diagnosis #5***<br>Airway clearance, ineffective, related to:<br>1. Compromised cough.<br>2. Need for minimizing activity of any kind during the acute phase.<br>3. Limited mobility. | Patient's airway will remain patent; breath sounds will be normal, without adventitious sounds (e.g., crackles, wheezes, rhonchi). | • Assess breath sounds/adventitious sounds. | • Abnormal breath sounds or the presence of adventitious sounds suggests accumulation and pooling of secretions. |
| | | • Suction patient *only* when absolutely necessary, using meticulous technique.<br>○ Limit each pass to 10 seconds.<br>○ Prevent accumulation of secretions. | • Suctioning may increase intracranial pressure.<br>○ Pneumonia is a frequent complication and usually develops on the paralyzed side (in this case, the right upper and lower lobes). A decrease in thoracic excursion and altered pulmonary hemodynamics are contributory factors. |
| | | • Maintain ventilation and oxygenation as prescribed. | |
| ***Nursing Diagnosis #6***<br>Communication impaired, related to:<br>1. Dysphasia and dysarthria. | Patient will:<br>• Demonstrate use of alternative means of communication (e.g., nodding the head, pointing the finger, writing on a tablet, slate board).<br>• Demonstrate ease and comfort when groping for words. | • Assess the patient's communication status:<br>○ Ask simple questions and determine patient's ability to answer.<br>○ Evaluate appropriateness of the answer, and the use of words, grammar, and syntax.<br>○ Evalute the patient's understanding of the spoken word by asking the patient to follow simple instructions. | • Assessment identifies the skills that remain intact.<br>• Lesions of the left cerebral hemisphere frequently disturb Broca's area, resulting in an expressive aphasia. |
| | | • Loss of the ability to communicate can be devastating. A calm, reassuring approach and supportive manner are essential. | • Develop a system of communication that facilitates understanding, taking into consideration the patient's deficits. |

| | | | |
|---|---|---|---|
| ○ Assure patient that speech will improve over time and with rehabilitation. | | • Encourage and reassure patient; anticipate needs; verbalize fears, frustrations for patient.<br>○ Convey acceptance of the patient's behavior.<br>• Approach to the patient:<br>○ Encourage verbalization.<br>○ Spend time with patient. | ○ Feeling unhurried may be reassuring as the patient searches for words to express herself. |
| ***Nursing Diagnosis #7***<br>Anxiety, related to:<br>1. Fear of dying.<br>2. Potential sequelae related to neurologic deficits. | 1. Patient will write out needs and concerns on a slate board or tablet.<br>2. Demonstrate relaxed demeanor and perform relaxation techniques as condition permits. | • Assess for signs/symptoms of anxiety:<br>○ Wide-eyed look, clenched fists, increased heart rate.<br>○ Identify cause, if possible, and treat.<br>• Initiate interventions to reduce anxiety: stay with patient to reassure; verbalize fears/frustrations the patient may be experiencing; indicate acceptance of the patient. | • Severe anxiety can aggravate the patient's overall condition. Because Mrs. M. is unable to communicate verbally, her anxiety level may be especially high. |

tained. They were pleased with the way Mrs. M. "was coming around."

On physical examination, the eyes opened spontaneously; the patient was able to smile spontaneously with evident right facial palsy; the patient moved her left arm purposely, wiggled her fingers, and gripped the examiner's hand; movement of the left leg was also evident. A right hemiplegia with dysphasia persisted.

On the fourth postop day, the patient was alert, vocalizing, and had regained preop level of motor and psychic activity; she was tolerating clear fluids. Hyperalimentation was continued. The dressing site over the left carotid artery was clean and dry with no exudate. Physical therapy program was initiated.

The patient was very concerned about her children. Her mother was caring for the family since the hospitalization. A social service consult was requested to evaluate the home situation and to plan for eventual placement of the patient in a rehabilitation center.

## Initial Nursing Diagnoses

1. Alteration in cerebral perfusion pressure, related to cerebral infarction associated with carotid aneurysm and consequent cerebral edema; vasospasm associated with subarachnoid bleeding.
2. Alteration in comfort: Headache, related to meningeal irritation and surgical incision.
3. Potential for injury: Seizures, related to cerebral edema, intracranial bleeding.
4. Nutrition, alteration in, less than body requirements, related to altered state of consciousness, compromised protective reflexes (e.g., gag and cough); ineffective chewing or swallowing; fatigue and depression.
5. Airway clearance, ineffective, related to compromised cough, need for minimizing activity of any kind during the acute phase; and limited mobility due to neurologic deficits.
6. Communication impaired, related to dysphasia and dysarthria.
7. Anxiety, related to fear of dying, potential sequelae, related to neurologic deficits.

These nursing diagnoses are documented in the Sample Nursing Care Plan that follows. Additional nursing diagnoses may include:

8. Coping, alteration in: Individual and family, related to situational crisis, temporary family disorganization; catastrophic illness with long-term effects on lifestyle.
9. Unilateral neglect, related to altered sensorimotor function associated with cerebral insult.
10. Self-care deficits, related to sensorimotor deficits.
11. Thought processes, alteration in, related to cerebral ischemia, altered level of consciousness, and sedation.
12. Impaired physical mobility, related to altered state of consciousness; restricted activity associated with risk of bleeding (surgical site).
13. Skin integrity, impairment of: (Potential) related to sensorimotor deficits, immobility, and altered nutrition.
14. Potential for infection, related to craniocerebral surgery and invasive monitoring.
15. Anxiety, related to fear of dying; Potential sequelae associated with the cerebrovascular insult.

## REFERENCES


1. Wald, ME: Cerebral thrombosis: Assessment and nursing management of the acute phase. J Neurosci Nurs 18(1):36, 1986
2. Yarnell, P: Stroke rehabilitation. Current Concepts of Cerebrovascular Disease Stroke XXI(3):9–12, 1986
3. Stein, R, Hier, D, and Caplan, L: Cognitive and behavioral deficits after right hemisphere stroke. Current Concepts of Cerebrovascular Disease Stroke XX(1):1–5, 1985.
4. Rudy, E: Advanced Neurological and Neurosurgical Nursing. CV Mosby, St Louis, 1984, p 204.
5. Taylor, JW: Nursing management of Stroke: Acute care—Part I. Cardiovascular Nursing 21(1):1–5, 1985.
6. Taylor, JW: Nursing management of stroke: Acute care—Part II. Cardiovascular Nursing 21(2):7–12, 1985.

CHAPTER 12

# Nursing Management of the Patient with Spinal Cord Injury

## CHAPTER OUTLINE



## LEARNING OBJECTIVES

**At the end of this chapter, you should be able to:**

1. Define spinal cord injury and terminology used to indicate extent of injury and related sequelae.
2. Differentiate mechanisms of vertebral and spinal cord injuries.
3. Define spinal shock and its clinical significance.
4. Differentiate incomplete spinal cord syndromes in terms of pathophysiology and clinical presentation.
5. List nursing considerations in the patient experiencing autonomic dysreflexia.
6. Delineate the priorities of nursing care in the acute management of the spinal cord-injured patient including:
   A. Respiratory function
   B. Cardiovascular function
   C. Musculoskeletal integrity
   D. Body temperature instability
   E. Gastrointestinal function
   F. Renal function
   G. Skin integrity
   H. Nutritional status
   I. Rehabilitation
7. Implement the nursing process in the management of the patient with acute spinal cord injury:
   Assessment
   Nursing diagnosis
   Planning: Desired patient outcomes
   Nursing interventions

## SPINAL CORD INJURY: INTRODUCTION

Spinal cord injury is a catastrophic event having far-reaching and devastating consequences for the victim, family, the community, and today's society as a whole. Nearly 10,000 Americans sustain a traumatic spinal cord injury each year. Of this number approximately 80% are under the age of 40, the majority between 15–25 years of age, and predominantly male.

Motor vehicle accidents (MVAs) account for 50% of the total number of traumatic spinal cord injuries occurring each year, followed by falls (predominantly in the over-65 age group), sports accidents (i.e., contact sports and diving accidents), and violent trauma (e.g., use of guns). Strict enforcement of laws requiring use of seatbelts and use of car seats for young children has helped to reduce the risk and/or extent of injury sustained in a motor vehicle accident. Persons driving while impaired or intoxicated are one of the major contributing factors to the incidence of motor vehicle accidents and associated spinal cord injury.

Although the yearly incidence of spinal cord injury may be low, the cost of treating and maintaining the spinal cord-injured individual is phenomenal. Changes occur in virtually all body functions. The individual is subjected to a tremendous amount of stress—physically, emotionally, and psychologically as he/she strives to survive the insult, eventually to adjust to and cope with a changed lifestyle, an altered body image and self-concept, and a low self-esteem.

The challenge to critical care nurses caring for the spinal cord-injured patient is formidable as an effort is made early on to sustain life, prevent further neurologic damage, and assist the individual in restoring life processes to a new state of dynamic equilibrium. Care of the spinal cord-injured patient requires a collaborative, interdisciplinary approach to provide effective, quality care and management from acute care through the ongoing rehabilitative process.

## Spinal Cord Injury: Defined

Spinal cord injury refers to an acute pathologic insult to the spinal cord that interrupts sensory and motor communication within the central nervous system (CNS), and between the CNS and the peripheral nervous system (PNS). Depending on whether the lesion is complete or incomplete the individual will experience a wide range of impairments to all life processes. Physiologically, all major organ systems are involved. Psychologically, sequelae emerge that are associated with lengthy and difficult adjustments and rehabilitation necessitated by physiologic dysfunction. The social, economic, and emotional ramifications of spinal cord injury are indeterminable.

### Definition of Terms

**Quadriplegia (Tetraplegia).** Quadriplegia (tetraplegia) refers to paralysis involving all four extremities and the trunk. It results from injury to thoracic cord segment $T_1$ or above. Lesions at these levels impair autonomic nervous system function, especially that of the sympathetic (thoracolumbar) system. Such dysfunction places the paralyzed individual at risk of developing postural (or orthostatic) hypotension and autonomic dysreflexia. Respiratory insufficiency is a significant concern (Table 12-1).

***Complete Quadriplegia and Incomplete Quadriplegia.*** Complete quadriplegia describes loss of cord function above $C_6$ cord segment. It leaves the individual with minimal or no potential for independence. An intact cord segment at $C_6$ is sometimes referred to as the line of demarcation between complete dependence and the potential for independence. Incomplete quadriplegia describes loss of neurologic function below the $C_6$ spinal cord segment.

**Respiratory Quadriplegia (Pentaplegia).** Respiratory quadriplegia (pentaplegia) refers to lesions of the spinal cord involving the upper cervical cord segments $C_1$ through $C_4$. Such patients experience acute respiratory insufficiency characterized by possible lack of spontaneous respirations (associated with paralysis of diaphragm), reduced lung volumes and capacities, poor gas exchange with retention of carbon dioxide, progressive decline in lung and thoracic compliance, and a loss of or severely weakened cough with inability to handle pulmonary secretions. Mechanical ventilatory support may be required during the acute stage, and the patient may remain ventilator-dependent with a permanent tracheostomy.

**Paraplegia.** Paraplegia refers to paralysis of the lower half of the body, which includes both lower extremities and may involve the trunk. Paraplegia occurs with injury to the second thoracic cord segment ($T_2$) or below. Lesions at this level enable upper body strength and full use of upper extremities to be preserved. Functionally, the paraplegic individual has the potential of becoming independent in all aspects of daily living (ADL) with wheelchair mobility (Table 12-2).

## Mechanisms of Spinal Injury

### Mechanisms of Vertebral Injury

The vertebral column functions to support the skull and to provide protection for the spinal cord and spinal nerves. The relationship between the spinal cord and vertebral column is so intricate and unique that pathology to the vertebral column may have far-reaching implications on spinal cord function, and on the functioning of the body as a whole.

Injury to the spinal cord occurs most frequently as a result of trauma to the vertebral column and/or ligaments. The irregular bony structure and intervertebral articulations (see Fig. 6-15) cause the vertebral column to be vulnerable to flexion, extension, and rotational forces and are easily fractured. The degree, direction, and type of force exerted on the vertebral column at the moment of impact determines the extent of injury. Injury, when it does occur, most often involves those sections of the vertebral column that have the greatest mobility, namely, cervical levels C-4 to C-7, and the thoracolumbar junction, T-11, T-12, L-1. The

TABLE 12–1
**Spinal Cord Injury—Functional Status of Quadriplegia**

| Level of Injury: *Vertebral* | Level of Injury: *Cord Segment** | Motor Function | Sensory Function, Light/Deep Touch, Pain—Pinprick | Respiratory Function | Bladder and Bowel Function | Assessment—Movements Requested of Patient | Potential Outcomes |
|---|---|---|---|---|---|---|---|
| C–1 to 3 | $C_{1-3}$ | • Partial function of accessory muscles of breathing; limited movement of head and neck<br>• $C_{2-7}$ innervate: sternocleido-mastoid, scalenus muscles<br>• Cranial nerve XI also innervates sterno-cleidomastoid muscles<br>• Respiratory quadriplegia | • Full sensation to head and upper neck | • Respiratory quadriplegia<br>• Lack of spontaneous respirations<br>• Ventilator dependent | • Loss of bowel and bladder control<br>• Dependent on assistance<br>• At risk for urinary tract infection | • $C_{2-5}$ nerve roots form phrenic nerve, which innervates diaphragm. Loss of this innervation results in respiratory paralysis<br>• Loss of intercostal muscle function<br>• Tracheostomy<br>• Mechanical ventilation<br>• Maintain patent airway—removal of secretions | • Balance head, which assists in maintaining upright position in wheelchair; allows mouth stick activities<br>• With development of accessory muscles, potential to remain off respirator for brief periods<br>• Completely dependent for ADL<br>• Reduced respiratory reserve; at risk for respiratory infection<br>• Postural hypotension<br>• At risk for autonomic dysreflexia |
| C–4 | $C_4$ | • Muscle function of head and neck as above<br>• Some shoulder movement<br>• Some diaphragm control | • As above<br>• Shoulder tops ($C_{3-4}$) | • As above<br>• Compromised respiratory status | • As above | • As above<br>• Shrug shoulders | • As above<br>• Dependence for ADL and transfers |
| C–4 to 5 | $C_5$ | • Complete control of head, neck, and shoulders<br>• Elbow flexion<br>• Trapezius muscle intact<br>• Quadriplegia complete | • Full sensation to head, neck, and shoulder tops<br>• Upper anterior chest and upper back<br>• Lateral aspect of upper arms | • Phrenic nerve intact<br>• No intercostal muscle function<br>• Independent respiratory function but poor pulmonary capacity and reserve (tidal volume ~300 ml) | • Some independence with adaptive equipment and raised toilet seat | • As above<br>• Request patient to take a deep breath; diaphragm should descend causing bulging of abdomen; upper chest does not move due to loss of innervation to intercostal muscles<br>• Bend elbow | • As above<br>• Independence with electric wheelchair and use of adaptive equipment to feed and groom self |

*(continued)*

TABLE 12-1
**Spinal Cord Injury—Functional Status of Quadriplegia *(Continued)***

| Level of Injury *Vertebral* | *Cord Segment** | Motor Function | Sensory Function, Light/Deep Touch, Pain—Pinprick | Respiratory Function | Bladder and Bowel Function | Assessment—Movements Requested of Patient | Potential Outcomes |
|---|---|---|---|---|---|---|---|
| C-5 to 6 | $C_6$ | • Full elbow flexion<br>• Some wrist extension<br>• Possible incomplete quadriplegia | • As above<br>• Thumb and index finger | • As above | • Independent with adaptive equipment | • Bend wrist up | • Independence in use of manual wheelchair<br>• Independence in feeding and grooming using adaptive devices<br>• Helps to dress self<br>• Dependent for transfers |
| C-6 to 7 | $C_7$ | • As above, with elbow extension, some finger control<br>• Quadriplegia incomplete | • As above<br>• Middle finger<br>• Part of ring finger | • As above | • As above | • Make a fist<br>• Opposite thumb to each fingertip | • Independence in ADL<br>• Use of wrist extensor splint to induce finger flexion<br>• Some assistance in transfers<br>• May be able to drive |
| C-7 to T-1 | $C_8$-$T_1$ | • As above<br>• Moderate to full control of arm, wrist, and fingers | • Full sensation to entire hand and medial aspects of upper and lower arm | • As above | • As above | • As above | • Independent in transfers with adaptive equipment<br>• Can grasp and release hands voluntarily<br>• Independent in ADL |

**Terminology*: The cord segment level reflects the lowest cord level at which neurologic function is intact. Example: A $C_5$ quadriplegia means that the $C_5$ cord segment and roots are intact while $C_6$ is not.

thoracic region is less vulnerable to injury as the articulating rib cage imparts a rigidity and stability to this area.

Major mechanisms of vertebral injuries include hyperextension, hyperflexion, vertical compression, and/or rotation of the vertebral column.

**Hyperextension-Hyperflexion Injuries.** Hyperextension-hyperflexion injuries result when strong forces impact on the body causing the unsupported head first to rapidly hyperextend, and then hyperflex on the neck. The *acceleration* forces of a rear-end collision cause *hyperextension*-hyperflexion injuries.

Hyperextension injuries are seen in elderly persons who frequently have degenerative changes of the vertebral column and are prone to falls. Damage results when the force of the fall impacts on the chin and snaps the head backwards. Elderly patients seen in the emergency department for the treatment of a Colles' (wrist) fracture warrant a thorough history and physical examination to rule out head and/or spinal injuries associated with the fall. In *hyperextension* injuries the greatest stress point is at cervical vertebral levels C-4 and C-5.

**Hyperflexion-Hyperextension Injuries.** The *deceleration* forces of a head-on collision result in *hyperflexion*-hyperextension injuries. On impact the head and body continue to move forward until they contact the dashboard or windshield. Forceful hyperflexion of the head on the neck occurs, followed by a forceful hyperextension as the head snaps backwards. Diving accidents or blows impacting on the back of the head frequently result in cervical injury due to hyperflexion. In *hyperflexion* injuries the greatest stress points are cervical vertebral levels C-5 and C-6.

TABLE 12-2
**Spinal Cord Injury—Functional Status of Paraplegia**

| Level of Injury: *Vertebral* | Level of Injury: *Cord Segment** | Motor Function | Sensory Function, Light/Deep Touch, Pain—Pinprick | Respiratory Function | Bladder and Bowel Function | Assessment—Movements Requested of Patient | Potential Outcomes |
|---|---|---|---|---|---|---|---|
| T-2 | $T_3$<br>$T_4$ (nipple line) | • Full control of upper extremities<br>• Some intercostal function | • Sensation intact to midchest including upper extremities ($T_{1-2}$) and to nipple line ($T_4$) | • Some control of intercostal muscles<br>• Pulmonary capacities within physiologic limits (tidal volume—500–700 ml) | • Independent with adaptive devices | | • Completely independent in wheelchair and ADL<br>• Potential for full-time employment<br>• At risk for postural hypotension and autonomic dysreflexia |
| T-8 to 9<br><br>T-11 to 12<br>T-12<br>L-1 | $T_{10}$ (umbilicus)<br><br>$T_{12}$<br>$T_{12}$ | • Full control of abdominal and trunk muscles<br>• Hip rotation and some hip flexion ($L_{1-3}$) | • Sensation intact below waist: $T_{10}$ supplies umbilicus, $T_{12}$ supplies groin area, $L_1$ pubis, $L_2$ hips.<br>• Some sensation to anterior and medial thigh | • Full control of intercostals<br>• No interference with respiratory function | • As above | • Tighten abdomen<br>• Flex hip | • As above with complete abdominal, back, and respiratory control<br>• Participation in athletic activities |
| L-1 | $L_3$–$S_1$ | • As above<br>• Knee extension ($L_{3-4}$)<br>• Dorsiflexion of ankle ($L_{4-5}$–$S_1$)<br>• Foot movement ($L_{4-5}$–$S_1$)<br>• Knee flexion ($L_4$–$S_1$)<br>• Plantar flexion ($S_{1-2}$) | • Sensation to upper legs ($L_{1-3}$)<br>• Anterior/posterior and lateral surfaces of lower leg and dorsum of foot ($L_{4-5}$) | • As above | • Independent with or without adaptive devices | • Flex hip<br>• Straighten (extend) leg<br>• Bend and straighten toes | • As above<br>• Optimal use of long leg braces<br>• Note: Sympathetic innervation largely intact |
| L-1 to 2 | $S_{2-4}$ | • As above; some foot control; reflex centers for bowel, bladder, and sexual function | • Note: *Lumbar* nerves innervate part of lower legs and feet<br>• *Sacral* nerves innervate lower legs, feet, and perineum | • As above | • As above | • Tighten anal sphincter around examining finger<br>• Sensorimotor assessment of perineal area is critical to determine extent of function | • Independent with or without short leg braces<br>• Involvement of $S_{2-4}$ can cause considerable disability related to bowel, bladder, and sexual dysfunction |

*Terminology: The cord segment level reflects the lowest cord level of which neurologic function is intact. Example: A $T_{12}$ paraplegia means that the $T_{12}$ cord segment and roots are intact while $L_1$ is not.

Hyperflexion injuries may also occur to the thoracolumbar junction (T-11, T-12, L-1). This region of the vertebral column has considerable mobility and, like the cervical area, is vulnerable to forces impacting on this area. A classification of vertebral injuries is presented in Table 12-3.

### *Mechanisms of Spinal Cord Injury*

Mechanisms of spinal cord injuries include concussion, compression, contusion, laceration, partial section, or transection. As with injuries to the vertebral column, the extent and permanency of spinal cord dysfunction depend on the degree, direction, and type of injury. A classification of spinal cord injuries is presented in Table 12-4.

## Spinal Cord Injury: Pathophysiology

### *Localized Edema Formation: Impact on Spinal Cord Function*

Most insults to the spinal cord predispose to edema formation. This is due largely to a localized inflammatory response wherein changes in the permeability of tissue capillaries cause a disruption of osmotic gradients, enabling fluid to move from the intravascular to the interstitial spaces. The edema so formed impairs circulation of blood to parenchymal tissues and may cause inhibition of spinal cord function. In some cases, as the edema resolves, such function may be restored with a minimum of permanent sequelae.

The significance of edema formation involving the spinal cord becomes critical when the cervical region is affected. Edema may involve several cord segments above and below the level of the lesion. In the case of injury to cord segment $C_5$, for example, edema formation may advance to $C_{3-4}$ levels where it may impair phrenic nerve function and precipitate respiratory insufficiency and/or arrest. Likewise, edema occurring at the $C_{1-2}$ levels may progress upward to the medulla and impair other vital functions.

It is essential for the critical care nurse to establish *baseline* assessment data as to the level of cord function so that changes in function reflective of advancing edema formation can be readily identified and appropriate intervention can be initiated. Changes in breathing pattern, mental status, sensorimotor function, and reflex responses may pro-

TABLE 12-3
**Classification of Vertebral Injuries**

Vertebral injuries may be classified as follows:

A. *Simple fracture*—involves spinous or transverse processes; vertebral body rarely affected; ligaments and spinal cord usually intact.
B. *Compression fracture (wedged fracture)*—involves compression of vertebral body anteriorally as occurs in hyperflexion injuries; intraspinous ligaments may be stretched but spinal cord usually remains intact.
C. *Comminuted fracture (burst fracture)*—involves an actual shattering of a vertebral body into many pieces; the spinal cord may sustain severe injury if bony fragments are driven into it.
D. *Dislocation*—disruption of vertebral alignment may result in injury to supporting ligaments. With impairment of ligaments the vertebral column becomes unstable, placing the cord at risk for injury. A partial dislocation is termed a *subluxation*.
E. *Sacral-coccygeal fractures*—these fractures are usually associated with falls onto the buttocks. Associated injury to the cord in this area is significant because the reflex centers for bowel, bladder, and sexual function occur in the spinal cord segments $L_2-S_5$.

TABLE 12-4
**Classification of Spinal Cord Injuries**

Spinal cord injuries may be classified as follows:

A. *Cord concussion*—defined as a momentary disturbance of cord function usually of a short duration without evidence of residual functional loss.[1]
B. *Compression*—associated with vertebral injury; may require surgery to relieve pressure on the cord; if relieved promptly before permanent cord damage is sustained, full function should be preserved. Underlying pathophysiology involves edema and/or direct pressure from malaligned or partially dislocated vertebrae; associated vascular injury can predispose to tissue ischemia/injury.
C. *Contusion*—associated with injury to vertebrae and/or disruption of ligaments resulting in an unstable vertebral column; major pathophysiologic concern is the possible impairment of collateral circulation predisposing to local cord ischemia.
   The blood supply to the vertebral column and spinal cord is not extensive; if the blood supply remains adequate, no major functional losses become apparent; poor collateral circulation may result in tissue injury and necrosis with permanent damage. The contused area reflects localized edema with microscopic hemorrhages and degenerative and demyelinated changes in spinal cord parenchymal tissue.
D. *Laceration (partial section)*, associated with fracture—dislocations of the vertebral column with severance or sectioning of spinal tracts resulting in a permanent loss of function as nerves within the CNS do not regenerate. As the section of the cord is only partial, varying degrees of function are preserved.
E. *Transection*—involves severance of spinal cord with loss of neurologic function below the level of the lesion. (The cord segment identified reflects the lowest cord level at which neurologic function is intact. Thus, a C5 quadriplegia means that the $C_5$ cord segment and roots are intact, while $C_6$ is not.)
   1. *Complete transaction*—reflects a complete loss of neurologic function below the level of the lesion.
   2. *Incomplete transection*—reflects varying degrees of neurologic function or dysfunction below the level of the lesion depending on the severity of cord damage. (See laceration, above.)
F. *Hematomyela*—hemorrhage of blood into the spinal cord. Usually occurs as a post-traumatic lesion.

vide clues to underlying pathophysiology and its progression. The nurse must be able to recognize changes indicative of deteriorating cord function. In the case of injury to $C_5$ for example, it may be important to intubate the patient prophylactically to ensure adequate respiratory function should further deterioration of spinal cord function occur.

### *Spinal Shock*

A sudden complete transection of the spinal cord causes immediate loss of all neurologic function below the level of the lesion, and an interruption of tonic impulses from the higher centers. A state of spinal shock ensues. There is complete cessation of motor, sensory, reflex, and autonomic function below the level of the lesion. Spinal shock may also occur in an incomplete transection of the cord resulting in variable neurologic dysfunction. Spinal shock usually ensues within 30–60 minutes following cord injury.

Clinically the phenomenon of spinal shock has been well documented, yet it remains little understood. Guyton explains[2] that normally, the resting state of excitability of cord neurons depends on a constant flow of tonic impulses from higher centers via descending pathways (e.g., corticospinal and reticular spinal tracts). Sudden interruption of this continuous flow of impulses from the brain causes abrupt changes in these neurons, greatly diminishing their resting excitability and resulting in a transient inability of the cord to respond.

#### Clinical Presentation

***Motor Function.*** Flaccid, total paralysis of all skeletal muscles below the level of injury reflects interruption of descending pathways including the upper and lower motor neurons of the corticospinal tracts (see Fig. 6–19). Loss of low motor neuron (LMN) function is reflected by the absence of all skeletal muscle reflexes integrated within the cord (e.g., deep tendon reflexes).

***Sensory Function.*** Interruption of ascending pathways (e.g., dorsal columns, spinothalamic tracts, etc.) is reflected by the loss of all sensation below the injury including tactile sensation, vibration, proprioception, pain, and temperature. There is an absence of somatic and visceral sensation below the level of the lesion.

***Autonomic Function.*** Loss of sympathetic tone results in a lowered and unstable arterial blood pressure. There is an inability to perspire below the level of injury. The presence of a paralytic ileus and an absence of visceral sensations largely reflect loss of parasympathetic tone. Bowel and bladder dysfunction and loss of sexual reflexes reflect the total loss of autonomic function.

The duration of spinal shock varies with each individual and may extend from days to weeks and even months. The average duration of spinal shock is 1–6 weeks. Recovery from shock may result in a state of hyperactivity. This is demonstrated by the *spastic* paralysis associated with loss of upper motor neuron (UMN) function. In the case of lower motor neuron (LMN) function, reflexes remain hypoactive or absent with *flaccid* paralysis (Table 12–5).

TABLE 12–5
**Clinical Manifestations of Upper and Lower Motor Neuron Dysfunction**

| | Upper Motor Neuron | Lower Motor Neuron |
|---|---|---|
| Muscle tone (Major effect) | Spasticity<br>Spastic paralysis<br>Contracture development | Flaccidity<br>Flaccid paralysis |
| Reflexes | Hyper-reflexia<br>Babinski's sign | Hyporeflexia or areflexia<br>No Babinski's sign |
| Fasciculations | Absent | Present |
| Muscle bulk | Slight atrophy (disuse) or no atrophy | Marked atrophy |
| Distribution of dysfunction | Decussation at medulla:<br>Damage above—contralateral<br>Damage below—ipsilateral | Specific muscles supplied by damaged nerve usually ipsilateral |

## Spinal Cord Syndromes: Pathophysiology and Clinical Manifestations

In *incomplete* spinal cord syndromes there is partial preservation of neurologic function depending on the extent and severity of cord damage. This includes varying degrees of motor, sensory, and autonomic function. The significance of incomplete cord syndromes is that there is the potential for recovery. Symptoms of spinal shock may occur in regions of the cord that have not been severed but have sustained injury by another mechanism such as contusion, compression, hemorrhage, or altered blood supply.

Incomplete spinal cord injuries having distinct patterns of neurologic dysfunction have been defined. It is unusual to see these syndromes in pure form. Rather, there are characteristics of one or more in the patient with an incomplete lesion.

### *Anterior Cord Syndrome*

The anterior cord syndrome is associated with flexion and dislocation injuries to the cervical region. Pathology, whether due to direct injury, compres-

TABLE 12–6
**Spinal Cord Syndromes**

| Syndrome | Mechanism of Vertebral Injury | Mechanism of Spinal Cord Injury | Motor/Sensory Pathways Disrupted | Clinical Manifestations |
|---|---|---|---|---|
| Anterior cord syndrome 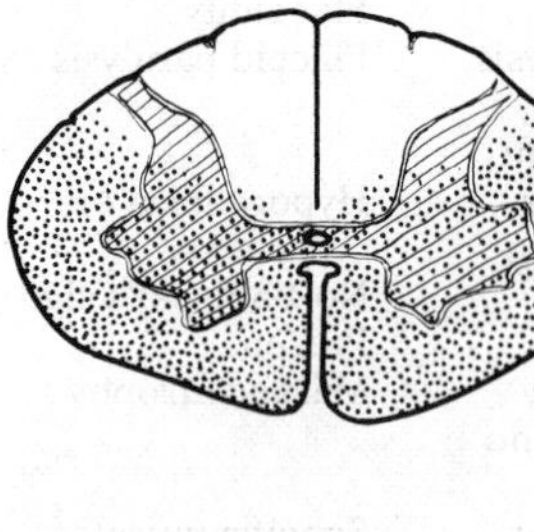 | • Flexion and dislocation injuries to cervical cord | • Direct injury; compression or vessel occlusion; infarction<br>• Compromised anterior spinal artery | • Ventral and lateral corticospinal motor tracts<br>• Ventral and lateral spinothalamic sensory tracts; spinal cerebellar tract<br>• Pathways intact: dorsal columns | • Loss of all motor function below lesion; upper motor neuron disruption: positive bilateral Babinski's signs; spastic paralysis<br>• Loss of pain and temperature sensation below lesion<br>• Sensation intact: light touch, proprioception, vibration |
| Central cord syndrome 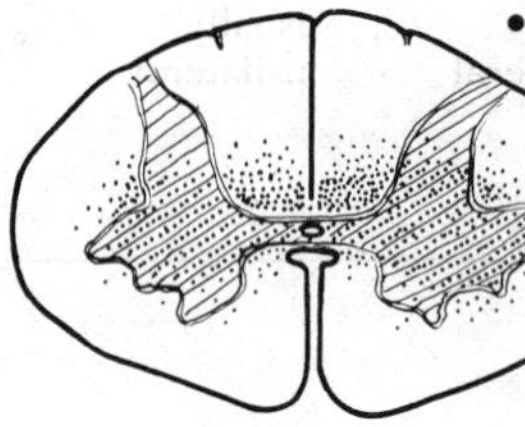 | • Severe hyperextension injury to cervical cord<br>• Spinal cord tumor | • Compression of cord between degenerated intervertebral disks<br>• Centralized cord edema | • Centrally located nerve tracts, which innervate upper extremities, are disrupted | • Greater neurologic (motor/sensory) deficits in upper extremities than in legs<br>• Varying degrees of bladder dysfunction may be seen<br>• Occurs more often in elderly |
| Brown-Sequard syndrome (hemisection of spinal cord) 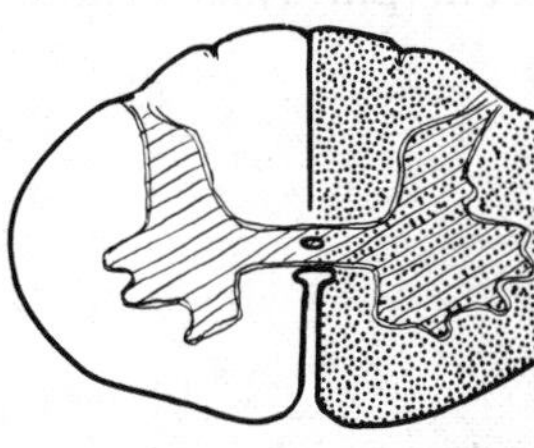 | • Direct pentrating injury such as stab wound or gunshots | • Laceration and hemisection of spinal cord | • Lateral and ventral corticospinal tracts (ipsilateral side)<br>• Ipsilateral dorsal columns | • Paresis or paralysis on ipsilateral side<br>• Loss of tactile sensation, proprioception, and vibratory sense on ipsilateral side<br>• Loss of pain and temperature on contralateral side |
| Conus medullaris cauda equina injury 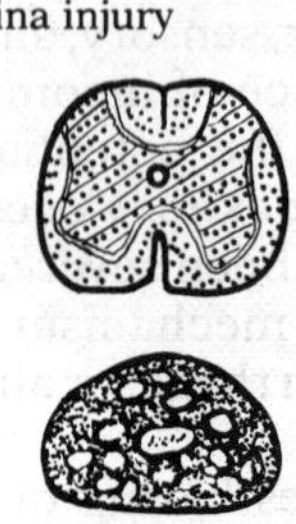 | • Fracture dislocation | • Compression, contusion, or laceration of conus and sacral spinal nerve roots | • Spinal nerve segments $S_2$–$S_4$, which house the reflex centers for bowel, bladder, and sexual functions<br>• Lower motor neuron disruption | • Neurologic deficits are variable<br>• Nerve root injury commonly causes loss of both motor and sensory functions either unilaterally or bilaterally<br>• Disruption of lower motor neuron causes loss of bowel, bladder, and sexual reflexes |
| Sacral sparing 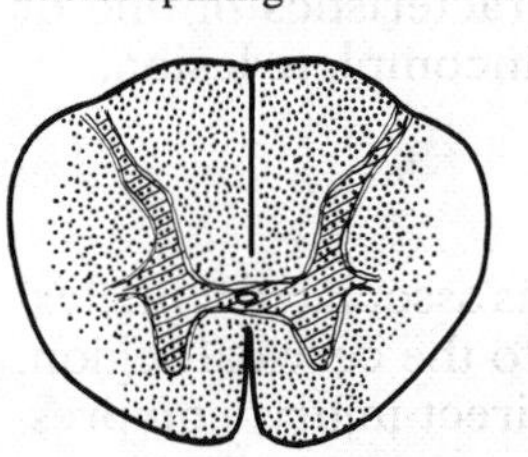 | | • Direct trauma to major portion of cord<br>• Spinal cord ischemia or infarction caused by disruption of spinal cord circulation<br>• Radicular arteries remain intact | • Peripheral rim of cord tissue is preserved, which includes innervation to sacral area | • Sensation to sacral area is preserved in an otherwise completely paralyzed patient with loss of sensation below the level of the lesion |

sion, or vessel occlusion (infarction), compromises the anterior spinal artery, which supplies blood to the anterior (ventral) two thirds of the cord. Only the posterior (dorsal) third of the cord, which encompasses the dorsal columns, remains unaffected (Table 12-6).

Clinically, there is loss of function below the level of the lesion of that portion of the cord, which contains major motor pathways including ventral and lateral corticospinal tracts, and major sensory pathways including primarily, ventral, and lateral spinothalamic tracts, and ventral spinocerebellar tracts.

In assessing signs and symptoms, it is important to recall the circuitry of the major motor and sensory tracts and that portion of the spinal cord (white matter) in which these tracts are contained (see Fig. 6-19). Thus, disruption of corticospinal tracts causes immediate loss of motor function below the lesion; disruption of ventral and lateral spinothalamic tracts results in loss of pain and temperature sensation below the injury. The presence of bilateral Babinski's signs reflects upper motor neuron (UMN) involvement, and a spastic paralysis may evolve postspinal shock.

Sensations that remain intact include light touch, proprioception, and vibration, all of which are conducted via the intact dorsal columns.

### *Central Cord Syndrome*

The central cord syndrome is associated with hyperextension injuries to the cervical region, which results in cellular damage to the central portion of the cord only (see Table 12-6). It occurs more frequently in elderly persons who are at greater risk due to arthritic and degenerative changes of the vertebral column. Pathology is characterized by central edema and compression of the cord between degenerated intervertebral disks.

Clinically, there are greater neurologic deficits in the upper extremities as nerve tracts to these areas are more centrally located than those for the lower extremities. Thus, motor and sensory function in the arms may be lost while that to the legs may remain completely intact. Varying degrees of bladder dysfunction may also be seen.

### *Brown-Sequard's Syndrome (Hemisection of Spinal Cord)*

The Brown-Sequard's spinal cord syndrome results when only one side of the cord is damaged following penetrating injuries such as stab wounds or gunshot wounds (see Table 12-6). In practice, such definitive cord injury is rarely seen. Its significance here demonstrates that although only one side of the cord is damaged, clinically the patient experiences neurologic deficits on both sides of the body.

Recall the circuitry of the major nerve tracts (see Fig. 6-19). Most nerve fibers of the corticospinal tracts cross at the medulla, as do fibers of the dorsal columns. Fibers of the lateral spinothalamic tracts, however, cross at the level of entry into the spinal cord and ascend directly to the thalamus.

Thus, the clinical presentation includes: an ipsilateral (same side as lesion) paresis or paralysis; an ipsilateral loss of light touch, pressure, proprioception, and vibration sensations; and a contralateral (opposite side) loss of pain and temperature sensation.

### *Conus and Cauda Equina Injuries*

Injury to the conus medullaris and spinal nerve roots comprising the cauda equina result from direct trauma with fracture dislocation. Clinically, neurologic deficits are variable. In nerve root injury there is commonly a loss of both motor and sensory function, and this may occur unilaterally or bilaterally. Of clinical significance are the spinal nerve segments $S_{2-4}$, which house the reflex centers for bowel, bladder, and sexual functions. Lower motor neuron involvement causes bowel, bladder, and sexual dysfunction (see Table 12-6).

### *Sacral Sparing*

Sacral sparing occurs when a major portion of the cord is traumatized or its circulation is impaired. The peripheral rim of spinal cord tissue is spared, however, because circulation to this area via the radicular arteries remains intact (see Table 12-6). Clinically, sensation to the sacral area is preserved in an otherwise completely paralyzed patient with loss of sensation below the level of the lesion.

## PRIORITIES OF NURSING CARE IN THE EARLY MANAGEMENT OF THE SPINAL CORD-INJURED PATIENT (CERVICAL CORD INJURY)

Management of the patient who has sustained a spinal cord injury begins with the stabilization of the patient at the scene of the accident. Goals of emergency care include prevention of death from asphyxia and/or mass hemorrhage, and prevention of further neurologic damage. Admission to the intensive care setting starts the patient's long-term rehabilitative process, one that requires sophisticated nursing interventions to restore life processes to equilibrium.

Nursing assumes a major responsibility for the care of the patient throughout the rehabilitative process. If this process is to be successful, it is essential that nurses have an understanding of the underlying principles and strategies involved in the patient's care. Critical care nurses caring for the spinal-cord injured patient during the acute phase must be cognizant that events occurring early on in the care of the patient and his/her family, be they physiologic, psychologic, and/or sociologic, may have considerable impact over the long term.

## Therapeutic Goals

1. Stabilize cardiopulmonary function.
2. Prevent further neurologic injury to the spinal cord.
3. Determine extent of injury.
4. Establish baseline assessment data.
5. Reduce spinal cord edema.
6. Maintain renal function and fluid/electrolyte balance.
7. Prevent complications of gastrointestinal function.
8. Initiate and establish a meaningful and trusting rapport with patient, family, and/or significant others.
9. Maintain skin integrity.
10. Maintain anabolic nutritional state.

## Nursing Diagnoses, Patient Outcomes, and Nursing Interventions

For specific nursing diagnoses, desired patient outcomes, and nursing interventions related to the spinal cord-injured patient, see Table 12-7. (Refer also to Case Study with Sample Care Plan on Patient With Spinal Cord Injury in Chap. 2.)

### *Respiratory Function in the Spinal Cord-Injured Patient*

**Initial Airway Assessment and Management.** It is essential to maintain adequate tissue perfusion to protect the fragile, highly sensitive nerve tissue from ischemia, injury, or infarction. Airway obstruction is a frequent occurrence in cervical injury particularly when head and face trauma have also been sustained. Resuscitation efforts must avoid unnecessary manipulation of the fractured neck to prevent extension and/or compromise of blood supply to the cord.

To re-establish and maintain airway patency, the neck should be straightened without hyperextension, and an oral airway should be inserted. Ventilation via bag-mask resuscitator should be initiated with oxygen concentrations of 8–12 liters/minute. To ensure effectiveness of the spontaneous ventilatory effort, arterial blood gases should be obtained. The patient should be allowed to breathe room air for about 3 minutes prior to obtaining the arterial blood gas sample. If the $PaO_2$ is less than 80 mmHg, the $PaCO_2$ is greater than 45 mmHg, and/or if the patient has a compromised ventilatory effort, intubation with mechanical ventilatory support may be indicated.

Intubation requires use of special techniques, such as the jaw-thrust maneuver, to prevent hyperextension of the neck. Use of a nasotracheal tube may be preferred, or a tracheostomy may be performed. Early tracheostomy facilitates secretion clearance and is the primary choice when long-term use of an artificial airway is anticipated. Hyperventilation therapy is usually initiated to maintain $PaCO_2$ at 30–35 mmHg.

Nasotracheal suctioning should be performed as necessary to maintain a patent airway. Management of pulmonary secretions is especially important if the patient has a weakened or absent cough reflex. Hypoxemia in the spinal cord-injured patient is most commonly caused by retained secretions. Humidified oxygen should be provided to keep secretions loose and to ensure adequate oxygenation.

**Assessment and Promotion of Ventilatory Effort.** The effectiveness of the patient's ventilatory effort needs to be carefully assessed and evaluated. Cervical cord transection at $C_8$–$T_1$ and above causes paralysis of intercostal and abdominal muscles and results in "paradoxical respiration." Clinically, the thoracic rib cage is observed to collapse passively on inspiration while the diaphragm descends, and to expand on expiration as the diaphragm ascends. This is a reversal of normal ventilatory mechanics and reflects intercostal muscle paralysis.

Paralysis of intercostal muscles ($T_2$–$L_1$) prevents adequate expansion of the rib cage and decreases effective alveolar ventilation by as much as 60%. Increased rapid shallow respirations frequently reflect a deterioration in respiratory function in the spinal cord-injured patient. The abdominal muscles ($T_{7-12}$) assist primarily with expiration and effective coughing.

The ability to cough requires the actions of intercostal and abdominal muscles, which build up pressure in the thorax and abdomen, allowing air to be vigorously forced through the closed larynx. With loss of function of these muscles, the patient is unable to cough up secretions and becomes susceptible to pulmonary complications. A moist-sounding but unproductive cough signals retention and pooling of pulmonary secretions.

*Quad-assist coughing* is a technique used to simulate the natural cough reflex. This method incorporates a Heimlich-type maneuver wherein the nurse places a fist or the palm of his/her hand between the xiphoid process and umbilicus and vigorously applies a thrust during the coughing effort. This technique can be very effective in raising pulmonary secretions when performed in conjunction with chest physiotherapy and nasotracheal suctioning.

**TABLE 12-7. CARE PLAN FOR THE INITIAL MANAGEMENT OF THE SPINAL CORD-INJURED PATIENT (CERVICAL CORD INJURY)**

| Nursing Diagnoses | Desired Patient Outcomes | Nursing Interventions | Rationales |
|---|---|---|---|
| ***Nursing Diagnosis #1***<br>Breathing pattern, ineffective, related to:<br>1. Altered ventilatory mechanics associated with paralysis of intercostal and abdominal muscles.<br>2. Limited diaphragmatic excursion associated with paralytic ileus (abdominal distention).<br>3. Immobility. | Patient will:<br>1. Demonstrate effective minute ventilation with trend of improving:<br>• Tidal volume >7–10 ml/kg.<br>• Respiratory rate <25/min.<br>2. Achieve a vital capacity >15–20 ml/kg.<br>3. Verbalize ease of breathing. | • Perform a comprehensive respiratory assessment.<br>○ Airway patency.<br>○ Rate, rhythm, depth of breathing.<br>○ Chest and diaphragmatic excursion.<br>○ Use of accessory muscles. | • Major goal of airway management is to establish and/or maintain adequate alveolar ventilation.<br>○ Baseline data are essential to evaluate effectiveness of therapeutic interventions and to follow trends.<br>○ Increased rapid, shallow respirations may signal deterioration of respiratory function.<br>○ $C_{3-5}$ cervical cord injury may disrupt innervation of diaphragm; paralysis results in respiratory arrest. |
| ***Nursing Diagnosis #2***<br>Airway clearance, ineffective, related to:<br>1. Ineffective cough associated with paralysis of intercostal and abdominal muscles.<br>2. Immobility. | Patient will:<br>1. Demonstrate clear breath sound on auscultation.<br>2. Demonstrate a secretion-clearing cough.<br>3. Maintain arterial blood gas values:<br>• $PaO_2$ > 80 mmHg.<br>• $PaCO_2$ 35–45 mmHg, if no head injury (<30 mmHg with injury).<br>• pH 7.35–7.45. | ○ Auscultation of breath sounds.<br>○ Monitor arterial blood gases (ABGs).<br>• Assess ability to cough and clear secretions.<br>○ Status of protective reflexes: cough, gag, and epiglottal closure. | ○ May detect evidence of secretion accumulation; airway obstruction.<br>○ Determine baseline respiratory function and monitor adequacy of ventilation/oxygenation.<br>○ Hypoxemia in the spinal cord-injured patient is most commonly caused by retained secretions.<br>• Loss of intercostal and abdominal muscles compromise the patient's ability to cough effectively.<br>○ Loss of protective reflexes places patient at risk of developing aspiration pneumonia; a moist-sounding, unproductive cough signals retention and pooling of pulmonary secretions. |

*(continued)*

## TABLE 12–7. CARE PLAN FOR THE INITIAL MANAGEMENT OF THE SPINAL CORD–INJURED PATIENT (CERVICAL CORD INJURY) *(Continued)*

| Nursing Diagnoses | Desired Patient Outcomes | Nursing Interventions | Rationales |
|---|---|---|---|
| ***Nursing Diagnosis #2 (cont.)*** | | | |
| | | ◦ Monitor quality, quantity, color, and consistency of sputum.<br>– Obtain sputum for culture and sensitivity. | ◦ Baseline data enable changes in sputum production and characteristics to be identified. Infection or other pulmonary insult may increase quality and quantity of sputum; a pulmonary embolism may cause *hemoptysis.* |
| | | ◦ Assess secretions for state of hydration or need for mucolytic therapy. | ◦ Thinning of secretions facilities mobilization and clearance of secretions. |
| | | • Monitor serial pulmonary function tests:<br>◦ Tidal volume.<br>◦ Vital capacity. | • Serial monitoring enables trends to be identified; progressive decline in pulmonary function may signal need for elective intubation and mechanical ventilation. |
| | | • Assess neurologic status:<br>◦ Level of consciousness; mentation. | • Hypoxia may be reflected by changes in patient's mental status or behavior (e.g., restlessness, irritability). |
| | | • Implement measures to ensure adequate respiratory function:<br>◦ Establish and maintain airway patency. | ◦ Airway obstruction frequently occurs with spinal cord injury or injuries involving head and neck. |
| | | ◦ Maintain head and neck in straight alignment without hyperflexion or hyperextension. | ◦ Reduces risk of further neurologic damage; allows for unimpeded flow of blood and cerebrospinal fluid from cranial vault; head injury often accompanies traumatic cord injuries. |
| | | ◦ Implement intubation and mechanical ventilation as per unit protocol. | ◦ Elective intubation and mechanical ventilation are often performed with cervical injury $C_{5-6}$ and above. |
| | | (For details related to the care of the intubated, mechanically ventilated patient, see Chap. 32.) | |
| | | ◦ Initiate oxygen therapy to maintain arterial blood gases within physiologically acceptable range.<br>◦ Initiate measures to clear secretions.<br>–Provide humidified oxygen.<br>–Maintain hydration. | |
| | | ◦ Implement nasotracheal suctioning as necessary to maintain airway patency. | ◦ Vagal stimulation may cause severe bradycardia in the spinal cord-injured patient who is already bradycardic. |

| | | | |
|---|---|---|---|
| | | ◦ Initiate chest physiotherapy techniques as tolerated.<br>–Postural drainage.<br>–Percussion and vibration | ◦ Loosens and dislodges secretions and enhances movement toward trachea from where they are accessible to removal by coughing and/or suctioning.<br>◦ Quad-assist coughing method may be helpful in patients with weakened cough (see text for details). |
| | | ◦ Encourage deep breathing and coughing.<br>◦ Instruct patient in use of incentive spirometry (see Table 32–2). | ◦ Increases vital capacity; helps to more evenly match ventilation with perfusion.<br>◦ Use of incentive spirometry encourages deep breathing, reducing risk of atelectasis. |
| | | ◦ Ensure hydration status.<br>–Monitor intake and output, daily weight.<br>◦ Insert nasogastric tube. | ◦ Adequate hydration moistens, loosens, and liquefies secretions.<br>◦ To decompress stomach: Helps to prevent aspiration and allows for full diaphragmatic excursion. |
| | | ◦ Use a calm, reassuring approach.<br>–Anticipate needs.<br>–Be accessible; offer explanations. | ◦ Anxiety is a major problem in the spinal cord-injured patient who may be fearful of dying. |
| ***Nursing Diagnosis #3***<br>Cardiac output, alteration in:<br>Decreased, related to:<br>1. Decreased venous return associated with spinal shock (pooling of blood in dilated vasculature).<br>2. Orthostatic hypotension.<br>3. Bradycardia. | Patient will:<br>1. Maintain stable hemodynamics:<br>• Blood pressure within 10 mmHg of baseline.<br>• Heart rate >60 <100/min.<br>• Cardiac output ~4–8 liters/min.<br>• Central venous pressure 0–8 mmHg.<br>• Pulmonary capillary wedge pressure 8–12 mmHg. | • Assess for presence of neurogenic or spinal shock: Blood pressure, pulse, body temperature, skin; orthostatic hypotension. | • Complete transection of spinal cord at $T_{4-6}$ and above precipitates spinal shock with loss of sympathetic autonomic reflex activity.<br>◦ Hypotension occurs due to loss of sympathetic vasomotor tone with resultant vasodilation of systemic vasculature.<br>◦ Bradycardia occurs due to unopposed parasympathetic (vagal) tone to the heart. |
| | | • Rule out concomitant hemorrhagic, hypovolemic shock:<br>◦ Neurogenic shock: Hypotension, bradycardia, warm dry skin.<br>◦ Hemorrhagic shock: Hypotension, tachycardia, thready pulse, cool clammy skin.<br>–Assess for signs of bleeding in spinal cord-injured patient who is tachycardic. | • Infrequently, spinal cord trauma may be accompanied by internal injuries with possible bleeding.<br>◦ Presence of internal bleeding may be difficult to detect in the insensate patient; a high degree of suspicion and meticulous assessment are essential. |

*(continued)*

**TABLE 12–7. CARE PLAN FOR THE INITIAL MANAGEMENT OF THE SPINAL CORD-INJURED PATIENT (CERVICAL CORD INJURY) *(Continued)***

| Nursing Diagnoses | Desired Patient Outcomes | Nursing Interventions | Rationales |
|---|---|---|---|
| ***Nursing Diagnosis #3 (cont.)*** | | | |
| | | • Perform ongoing cardiovascular assessment: | |
| | | ◦ Continuous cardiac monitoring. | ◦ Cardiac and cerebral tissue hypoxia can occur with hypoxemia precipitating dysrhythmias. |
| | | ◦ Continuous hemodynamic monitoring. | ◦ Offers significant data regarding cardiopulmonary function; access for serial blood gas measurements. |
| | | ◦ Arterial, central venous pressure (CVP) and pulmonary capillary wedge pressure (PCWP). | ◦ PCWP assists in determining hydration status; the patient in neurogenic or spinal shock is *not* hypovolemic and should not receive large amounts of fluids; overhydration may increase edema formation at site of injury. |
| | | ◦ Cardiac output. | ◦ Positive pressure mechanical ventilation increases intrathoracic pressures, which impedes venous return and reduces cardiac output. |
| | | • Implement measures to stabilize cardiopulmonary function:<br>◦ Initiate prescribed intravenous fluid therapy ~75–100 ml/hr to maintain systolic blood pressure ~100 mmHg. | • CVP and PCWP should be monitored to determine trends and to evaluate patient's response to hydration therapy. |
| | | ◦ Monitor fluid intake and output. | ◦ Intact mental status, and acceptable urine outputs ensure adequate tissue perfusion. |
| | | ◦ Initiate activities to minimize orthostatic hypotension:<br>–Apply antiembolic stockings:<br>–Abdominal binder.<br>–Gradual increase to vertical position (sitting up at 90°) as tolerated. | ◦ Orthostatic hypotension results from venous stasis associated with impaired vasomotor tone and skeletal muscle paralysis.<br>◦ Observe patient carefully when sitting up; syncopal episodes secondary to hypotension may occur. |
| ***Nursing Diagnosis #4***<br>Injury, potential for, related to:<br>1. Vertebral instability.<br>2. Spinal cord edema. | Patient will:<br>1. Maintain immobilization of head, neck, and back. | • Determine extent of injury and baseline assessment data.<br>• Patient history: | |

| | | | |
|---|---|---|---|
| 3. Stress. | 2. Maintain and/or improve neurologic function.<br>3. Demonstrate effective ventilatory effort. | ○ Obtain information regarding circumstances of injury/accident: Mechanism of injury? Neurologic status post-injury? | ○ Knowledge of mechanism/location of spinal cord injury assists in determining type and extent of spinal injury and the presence of other injuries. |
| | | ○ Did the patient lose consciousness? If so, for how long? Was there seizure activity? Was the patient incontinent—bowel? bladder? | ○ Concomitant head injury is always a possibility especially with cervical cord injury. |
| | | ○ Type of treatment administered at scene of injury: Medications? Fluids?<br>–Mode of transportation to the hospital? How long a delay between occurrence of injury and admission to emergency department?<br>–Patient's status on arrival to the hospital? | ○ Interview EMTs, and family member if present, about the circumstances of the injury. |
| | | ○ Obtain pertinent information regarding the patient's past history: Pre-existing disease: Pulmonary, cardiac, renal, endocrine, neurologic, mental/emotional/ psychologic; known allergies?<br>○ Use of medications? | ○ A thorough assessment and database assist in developing a treatment plan and individualizing care. |
| | | • Physical examination:<br>○ Estimate extent of cord involvement. Level and areas of neurologic deficits can be delineated by checking sensation, muscular strength, and reflexes. | ○ Knowledge regarding level of cord injury assists in determining level of function and in anticipating problems. *Example*: Impending danger of phrenic nerve dysfunction with cord injury at $C_{3-5}$ or above. Documentation of this information is critical to the continuity of patient care. |
| | | ○ Grade muscle strength with scale of 0–5.<br>0 = no movement.<br>5 = movement against reflexes. | ○ Organized approach ensures thoroughness of testing all major muscle groups. |
| | | ○ Test for sensory function using touch and pinprick as stimuli. | ○ To assist in demarcating areas of function from areas of altered sensation progress from area of neurologic deficit to area where sensation is intact. |
| | | ○ Assess patient's neurologic status every 1 to 2 hr during initial 48–72 hr post injury. | ○ Neurologic deterioration with additional loss of function may be caused by spinal cord edema, hemorrhage, compromised blood supply, and tissue ischemia. |
| | | ○ Examine patient thoroughly to determine if other injury has been sustained. | ○ The neurologically compromised patient may not be able to tell you that other problems exist. |
| | | ○ Look for signs of internal and/or external bleeding if tachycardia is present. | ○ Thoracolumbar injury is frequently associated with internal abdominal complications caused by sheer violent force of such injuries. |

*(continued)*

**TABLE 12–7. CARE PLAN FOR THE INITIAL MANAGEMENT OF THE SPINAL CORD–INJURED PATIENT (CERVICAL CORD INJURY) *(Continued)***

| Nursing Diagnoses | Desired Patient Outcomes | Nursing Interventions | Rationales |
|---|---|---|---|
| ***Nursing Diagnosis #4 (cont.)*** | | | |
| | | • Establish baseline laboratory and other diagnostic studies: serum glucose, electrolytes, BUN, creatine; CBC with differential, hemoglobin, hematocrit; type and crossmatch, coagulation studies; baseline urinalysis, hematuria. | • To be used for comparison in evaluating patient's status and response to therapy. |
| | | • Obtain pertinent x-rays. | • Patient should not be moved until cervical spine x-rays have been carefully evaluated and the patient's status has been determined. Cervical vertebrae: All seven must be definitively viewed. |
| | | *Note*: Once the patient's condition is stabilized, a more extensive history in terms of the patient's functional health patterns should be obtained. | |
| | | • Implement measures to stabilize cervical spine. | • To prevent further neurologic damage. |
| | | ◦ Use principles underlying traction:<br>–Weights are never removed, but must be allowed to hang freely at all times. | |
| | | ◦ When turning, positioning, or moving patient, obtain adequate assistance; patient should be lifted using a sheet. | ◦ Skeletal traction must be in effect at all times. |
| | | ◦ Implement nursing measures in caring for the patient with a halo immobilization brace. | ◦ For details regarding the care of the patient with a halo brace see Table 12–9. |
| | | • Monitor for neurologic changes associated with spinal cord edema.<br>◦ Assess respiratory function: rate, rhythm, depth, and pattern of breathing; arterial blood gas studies. | • In cervical spinal cord injury, ascending edema may compromise phrenic nerve innervation to diaphragm, precipitating respiratory arrest. It may be necessary to intubate patient and initiate mechanical ventilation. |
| | | ◦ Monitor response of patient to corticosteroids. | ◦ Steroids have been found to be efficacious in incomplete cord transections. May reduce inflammation and edema. |
| | | ◦ Perform serial neurologic assessments comparing sensory and motor function with the baseline data. | |
| | | • Monitor gastrointestinal function.<br>◦ Monitor pH of gastric solutions.<br>◦ Monitor response to antacids.<br>◦ Monitor hematest gastric secretions.<br>◦ Monitor stool for guaiac. | ◦ Steroids predispose to stress ulcer development. Exogenous steroids may potentiate effect of endogenous steroids in this regard. (Actual role played by steroids in this regard remains controversial.) |

| | | | |
|---|---|---|---|
| ***Nursing Diagnosis #5***<br>Anxiety, related to:<br>1. Loss of sensorimotor function below level of lesion.<br>2. Immobilization.<br>3. Impact of lifestyle. | Patient will:<br>1. Verbalize feeling less anxious.<br>2. Demonstrate a relaxed demeanor.<br>3. Verbalize familiarity with ICU routines and protocols.<br>4. Initiate attempts to discuss magnitude of this catastrophe and what it means to the patient. | • Refer to Nursing Diagnosis #1 in Table 35–3 for information concerning the following nursing activities:<br>○ Assess for signs and symptoms of anxiety.<br>○ Examine the circumstances underlying anxiety.<br>○ Assess patient/family coping.<br>○ Initiate interventions to reduce anxiety. | |
| ***Nursing Diagnosis #6***<br>Ineffective thermoregulation associated with autonomic dysfunction.<br>***Nursing Diagnosis #7***<br>Potential alteration in body temperature. | Patient will:<br>1. Maintain body temperature ~98.6°F (37.0°C).<br>2. Verbalize comfort and absence of chilling or diaphoresis above level of lesion. | • Monitor body temperature and complaints of chilliness or sweating.<br>• Maintain a constant room temperature.<br>○ Use of extra blankets should be guided by patient's temperature.<br>○ Avoid drafts.<br>–Avoid use of excessive bedding. | • Impaired homeothermia causes the patient's body to assume environmental temperature.<br>• This is the most effective way of controlling patient's temperature.<br>○ Drafts can precipitate an episode of autonomic dysreflexia in patients with spinal cord injury above $C_7$–$T_1$. |
| ***Nursing Diagnosis #8***<br>Urinary retention, related to atonic bladder associated with spinal shock.<br>***Nursing Diagnosis #9***<br>Urinary elimination, alteration in. | Patient will:<br>1. Have a urine volume of <400–450 ml on intermittent catheterization program.<br>2. Demonstrate absence of suprapubic distention.<br>3. Balance intake with output. | • Monitor urinary function.<br>○ Assess for bladder distention hourly.<br>○ Insert Foley catheter if prescribed.<br>–Avoid overdistended bladder.<br>○ Provide meticulous aseptic catheter care.<br>○ Minimize duration of use of indwelling catheter.<br>• Initiate intermittent catheterization program as early as possible.<br>○ Establish necessary criteria: fluid intake <2000 ml/24 hr; absence of urinary infection on culture and sensitivity.<br>○ Monitor fluid intake.<br>–Limit fluid intake after the evening meal.<br>–Avoid beverages that have a diuretic effect (e.g., caffeinated colas, tea, coffee). | • Urinary retention predisposes to complications of infection and autonomic dysreflexia.<br>○ During spinal shock, atonic bladder predisposes to urinary retention and urinary tract infection.<br>○ Indwelling Foley catheters place patient at high risk of infection.<br>○ Prolonged use of indwelling catheter may contribute to bladder atony, compromising efforts to train bladder for reflex emptying.<br>• Minimizes renal/urinary complications associated with infection.<br>○ Intermittent catheterization program should be initiated as early as possible, even during acute state if feasible. This simulates normal bladder filling and emptying and facilitates bladder training.<br>○ Efforts to establish effective urinary management require a collaborative approach involving patient, family and/or significant others, and health-care providers. |

*(continued)*

**TABLE 12–7. CARE PLAN FOR THE INITIAL MANAGEMENT OF THE SPINAL CORD–INJURED PATIENT (CERVICAL CORD INJURY) *(Continued)***

| Nursing Diagnoses | Desired Patient Outcomes | Nursing Interventions | Rationales |
|---|---|---|---|
| ***Nursing Diagnosis #10***<br>Alteration in fluid and electrolytes: Fluid volume deficit, related to nothing-by-mouth (NPO) status associated with weakened protective reflexes and paralytic ileus. | Patient will:<br>1. Maintain baseline body weight.<br>2. Balance fluid intake with output.<br>3. Have stable vital signs, clear breath sounds, absence of peripheral or dependent edema.<br>4. Maintain laboratory studies (e.g., electrolytes, BUN, creatinine, total protein, hematology profile) within acceptable physiologic range. | • See Chapter 23.<br>• Additional nursing considerations:<br>• Maintain fluid and electrolyte balance.<br>○ Monitor intravascular fluid volume to maintain systemic blood pressure (systolic). | ○ Adequate renal perfusion maintains glomerular filtration and renal function. |
| | | ○ Assess for fluid volume *deficit*. Signs and symptoms include:<br>–Weakness, listlessness; diminished urinary output; decreased central venous pressure.<br>–Hypotension, rapid thready pulse, increased heart rate, respiratory rate.<br>–Poor skin turgor over sternum and forehead; sunken eyeballs.<br>–Weight loss. | ○ Hemoconcentration may predispose to electrolyte imbalance, increased viscosity of blood, thromboembolic complications. |
| | | ○ Assess for fluid volume *overload*: Signs and symptoms include:<br>–Confusion, dilutional hyponatremia, elevated central venous pressure.<br>–Neck vein distention in upright position (45°).<br>–Shortness of breath, rales, hypertension, bounding pulse, dependent edema, weight gain. | ○ Fluid volume overload increases risk of pulmonary congestive heart failure.<br>○ Hemodilution may predispose to electrolyte imbalance.<br>○ Can potentiate cord edema. |
| | | • Prevent fluid and electrolyte imbalance.<br>○ Administer fluids based on fluid losses (include insensible losses) and state of hydration.<br>○ Administer electrolytes as indicated by clinical and laboratory status. | • *Note:* Disruption of sympathetic vasomotor tone precipitates a hypotensive state, which triggers an increased secretion of aldosterone, with sodium retention.<br>○ Nasogastric decompression results in loss of hydrogen and chloride ions; hypokalemia may occur because the kidneys retain hydrogen ions while excreting potassium ions. |

| | | | |
|---|---|---|---|
| | | ○ Signs/symptoms of hypokalemia: Weakness, paralysis, respiratory arrest, mental status disturbances, paralytic ileus, coma; arrhythmias; ECG changes. | ○ May be difficult to differentiate some symptomatology in the spinal cord-injured patient.<br>○ An inability to perspire due to disruption of sympathetic innervation contributes to fluid and electrolyte imbalance. |
| ***Nursing Diagnosis #11***<br>Bowel elimination, alteration in:<br>Constipation, related to atonic bowel (paralytic ileus) associated with spinal shock. | Patient will:<br>1. Remain without constipation and fecal impaction.<br>2. Establish regular bowel elimination management regimen. | • Prevent complications of gastrointestinal function. | • Level of cord injury determines the extent of gastrointestinal and bowel dysfunction.<br>○ Entire gastrointestinal tract becomes atonic with onset of spinal shock 24 to 48 hr post injury. |
| | | ○ Insert nasogastric tube to decompress gastrointestinal tract.<br>–Relieve distention associated with paralytic ileus.<br>–Prevent vomiting/aspiration. | ○ Prevents aspiration of gastric contents. Abdominal distention may limit diaphragmatic excursion. |
| | | ○ Assess patient with high degree of suspicion.<br>–Measure abdominal girth.<br>–Be alert for signs/complaints of "referred" pain.<br>–Auscultate in all quadrants.<br>○ Assess for signs of constipation: Dull sound over descending colon on percussion; palpation of hard, rigid stool over areas of bowel. | ○ With loss of sensation, patient may be unaware of signs of bleeding, ileus, impaction. |
| | | ○ Be suspicious of diarrhea.<br>–Hematest gastric secretions, stool for guaiac. | ○ It may signal presence of fecal impaction. |
| | | • Initiate bowel continence program post spinal shock and resolution of paralytic ileus:<br>○ Establish regular routine: Dulcolax suppository inserted, digital examination.<br>○ Same hour of day, usually after breakfast.<br>–Maintain appropriate diet. | • Critical care nurse can be instrumental in initiating and maintaining bowel and bladder program.<br>○ Takes advantage of peristalsis initiated by eating. |
| ***Nursing Diagnosis #12***<br>Skin integrity, impairment of:<br>Potential, related to:<br>1. Immobility.<br>2. Urinary and bowel incontinence.<br>3. Catabolic state. | Patient's skin will remain intact. | • Assess for alteration in skin integrity.<br>○ Identify areas at risk (weight-bearing bony prominences depending on position assumed) (i.e., supine, prone, and so forth). | • Loss of mobility and sensation, impaired circulation, and inadequate nutrition predispose to skin breakdown.<br>○ Pressure develops when there is lack of continuous movement and distribution of weight. |

(continued)

## TABLE 12–7. CARE PLAN FOR THE INITIAL MANAGEMENT OF THE SPINAL CORD–INJURED PATIENT (CERVICAL CORD INJURY) *(Continued)*

| Nursing Diagnoses | Desired Patient Outcomes | Nursing Interventions | Rationales |
|---|---|---|---|
| ***Nursing Diagnosis #12 (cont.)*** | | | ○ Pressure most concentrated between bone and skin surfaces that support body weight. |
| | | ○ Inspect skin after each position change. | ○ Reddened areas should blanch within 20–30 minutes after a position change. |
| | | ○ Inspect for open or ulcerated areas and localized edema (dependent/orthostatic edema). | ○ Dependent edema is incriminated in the pathophysiology of skin breakdown; it interferes with cellular nutrition and increases susceptibility of tissues to the effects of pressure. Susceptibility increased during period of spinal shock. |
| | | • Implement measures to promote tissue perfusion. | • Meticulous systematic surveillance of all pressure points from body position, bed, or traction equipment, is the key to maintaining intact skin integrity. |
| | | ○ Provide therapeutics:<br>○ Turning and positioning at least every 2 hr.<br>–Document rotation of positions. | ○ Prevents stasis and tissue ischemia. |
| | | ○ Maintain proper alignment.<br>–Passive range-of-motion exercises with dorsiflexion of feet. | ○ Prevents further neurologic damage, contractures, frozen joints. |
| | | ○ Use footboard—splints. | ○ Prevents foot drop. |
| | | ○ Provide pressure relief device: Air mattress, sheepskin, and so forth. | ○ Helps to displace weight more evenly and soften surfaces in contact with pressure points. |
| | | ○ Administer lotion to bony and reddened areas. | ○ Stimulates circulation. |
| | | • Monitor and evaluate response to therapy; monitor nutritional intake. | • Anticipate and prevent problems; intervene early on. |
| ***Nursing Diagnosis #13***<br>Potential for physiologic injury: Deep venous thrombosis; related to:<br>1. Hemostasis associated with immobility;<br>2. Loss of skeletal muscle pump; | Patient will:<br>1. Exhibit adequate peripheral circulation:<br>• Usual skin color; no cyanosis.<br>• Extremities warm to touch.<br>2. Maintain consistent calf and thigh | • Monitor for signs and symptoms of deep venous thrombosis. | • Venous stasis, skeletal muscle paralysis, and immobilization place patient at risk of developing deep venous thrombosis and pulmonary embolism. |
| | | ○ Assess skin color and temperature. | ○ Assessment for deep venous thrombosis is difficult because of sensorimotor deficits in spinal cord-injured patient. |
| | | ○ Assess calf and thigh circumference. | ○ A slowly increasing circumference suggests a possible underlying thrombosis. |

| | | | |
|---|---|---|---|
| 3. Pooling of blood in dilated capacitance vessels (e.g., absence of vasomotor tone during spinal shock). | circumference measurements.<br>3. Maintain effective respiratory function.<br>4. Maintain stable vital signs. | • Monitor for signs and symptoms of pulmonary embolism.<br>○ Assess sudden onset of respiratory difficulties (e.g., tachypnea, dyspnea, cough with hemoptysis); altered pulmonary function tests: tidal volume, vital capacity; neurologic findings: restlessness, lethargy.<br>• Implement measures to minimize risk of deep venous thrombosis and pulmonary embolism.<br>○ Maintain desired hydration.<br>–Monitor intake and output.<br>–Monitor daily weight.<br>–Hematology profile.<br>○ Apply antiembolic stocking to both lower extremities.<br>○ Institute exercise program.<br>–Passive range-of-motion exercises with dorsiflexion of feet.<br>–Maintenance of proper body alignment.<br>–Use splints as directed.<br>–Avoid crossing legs, using knee gatch, or pillow under knees.<br>–Avoid prolonged sitting or lying in one position.<br>○ Administer prophylactic heparin therapy as prescribed. | ○ Prevents increase in blood viscosity, which predisposes to a hypercoagulable state. |
| ***Nursing Diagnosis #14***<br>Alteration in nutrition: Less than body requirements, related to:<br>1. Nothing-by-mouth (NPO) status during spinal shock associated with paralytic ileus.<br>2. Weakened or absent protective reflexes (e.g., cough, gag, epiglottal closure).<br>3. Anorexia associated with depression, or inability to self-feed. | Patient will:<br>1. Maintain baseline body weight within 5% of baseline.<br>2. Maintain triceps skinfold measurements within baseline range.<br>3. Maintain laboratory parameters within acceptable physiologic range:<br>• BUN, creatinine.<br>• Total protein, albumin.<br>• Hematology profile.<br>4. Verbalize increase in appetite.<br>5. Remain free of infection. | • Obtain a complete nutritional assessment within 24–48 hr of admission.<br>○ Baseline nutritional status.<br>○ Nutritional requirements of the compromised state.<br>○ Blood chemistry and hematology.<br>○ Height and weight.<br>○ Pre-injury nutritional status: dietary habits, likes, and dislikes.<br>• Consult with nutritionist. Determine anthropometric data.<br>• Establish and maintain a balanced nutritional state—positive nitrogen balance.<br>○ Administer nutritional supplements: (as per unit protocol); parenteral nutrition (TPN and PPN) during period of spinal shock and paralytic ileus. | • Baseline nutritional needs must be identified to ensure adequate nutritional intake; individualized care.<br>○ Stress increases energy needs by 50%.<br>○ Baseline data assist in planning a nutrition program specific to the needs and desires of patient.<br>• Balanced nutritional intake promotes wound healing and prevents complications.<br>○ See Chapter 53. |

*(continued)*

**TABLE 12–7. CARE PLAN FOR THE INITIAL MANAGEMENT OF THE SPINAL CORD-INJURED PATIENT (CERVICAL CORD INJURY) *(Continued)***

| Nursing Diagnoses | Desired Patient Outcomes | Nursing Interventions | Rationales |
|---|---|---|---|
| ***Nursing Diagnosis #14 (cont.)*** | | | |
| | | ○ Initiate nasogastric tube feedings when paralytic ileus subsides but protective reflexes are still compromised.<br>–Assess location/patency of nasogastric tube prior to each feeding.<br>○ Evaluate patient's response to therapy; emphasis placed on prevention of complications.<br>○ Document daily caloric intake, fluid intake and output, daily weight, vital signs including temperature.<br>○ Assess blood chemistry and hematology.<br>○ Assess wound healing, skin integrity.<br>○ Assess patient's overall physical, mental, emotional state. | ○ Depression can cause anorexia. |
| ***Nursing Diagnosis #15***<br>Potential for physiologic injury: Episode of autonomic dysreflexia, related to noxious stimuli (e.g., distended bladder or rectum, others; see text, Table 12–8). | Patient will not experience an episode of autonomic dysreflexia.<br>• Stable vital signs; without pounding headache and profuse diaphoresis. | • Assess for presence of signs and symptoms of autonomic dysreflexia: Classic manifestations include: paroxysmal elevation in systolic blood pressure (>240–300 mmHg); pounding headache with blurred vision; anxiety, fright, nausea; profuse diaphoresis. | • Vasomotor tone to areas *above* cord lesion can receive signals from higher brain centers. When blood pressure rises, the sympathetic tone is reduced and vasodilation of these vessels occurs. This accounts for the profuse diaphoresis, headache, and flushing *above* lesion.<br>○ *Below* the lesion, an intense sympathetic response remains as inhibition from higher brain centers is blocked. Blood vessels, therefore, remain severely constricted, resulting in skin pallor and coolness, pilomotor erection (i.e., goose bumps), and paralytic ileus. |
| | | • Implement emergent measures to treat autonomic dysreflexia.<br>○ Follow protocols.<br>○ Place patient in upright position.<br>–Monitor blood pressure and heart rate. | ○ Helps to lower blood pressure. |
| | | ○ Notify physician. | ○ Physician should be notified if blood pressure is severely elevated (>240 mmHg) and/or unresponsive to therapy. |
| | | ○ Identify underlying cause and remove if possible. | ○ This is best treatment for autonomic dysreflexia. |

| | | | |
|---|---|---|---|
| | | ○ Administer prescribed antihypertensive drug therapy.<br>○ Stay with patient, provide reassurance and emotional support. | ○ Anxiety and fright increase catecholamine secretion, potentiating massive sympathetic response. |
| | | ○ Monitor blood pressure every 4 hr post crisis and for 24 hr thereafter.<br>• Implement preventive nursing interventions. | • See Table 12–7. |
| ***Nursing Diagnosis #16***<br>Sensory-perceptual alteration: Visual, tactile, related to:<br>1. Immobilization.<br>2. Sensory deficits associated with disruption of ascending nerve pathways at level of cord lesion. | Patient will:<br>1. Verbalize comfort in visualizing people and objects within immediate visual field.<br>2. Verbalize areas where tactile sensation is perceived. | • Assess underlying reason for alteration in sensory perception.<br>• Assess patient's view of immediate environment.<br>○ Consider type of spinal stabilization and use of specialized bed (e.g., Roto-Rest, Clinitron bed).<br>–Skeletal traction.<br>○ Halo immobilization brace. | • Viewing immediate environment from patient's perspective assists in arranging environment so desired materials are accessible to patient.<br>○ See Table 12–9. Nurses caring for the patient with a halo should receive continuing education regarding how to maximize effectiveness of brace and prevent complications. |
| | | • Implement measures to make immediate environment accessible to patient's field of vision.<br>○ Arrange desired objects as patient requests.<br>○ Position mirrors to enhance patient's view.<br>○ Place self within patient's field of vision when speaking to patient. Direct others to do same. | ○ Helps to provide increased visualization and stimulation.<br>○ Reduces sensory deprivation. |
| | | • Assess patient's tactile and pain sensation.<br>○ Use touch and pinprick stimuli:<br>–Test for sensory perception progressing from area of deficit to area of intact function.<br>–Frequently touch patient in areas demarcated as having sensory perception intact.<br>–Touch patient with different textured objects. | • Touching patient in areas of intact sensation helps to provide stimulation. |
| | | • Implement measures to reduce sensory overload.<br>○ Set priorities in care. | • Minimizing distraction helps patient to concentrate on more pertinent stimuli, and on how best to perceive environment from a new vantage point. |

*(continued)*

**TABLE 12–7. CARE PLAN FOR THE INITIAL MANAGEMENT OF THE SPINAL CORD–INJURED PATIENT (CERVICAL CORD INJURY) *(Continued)***

| Nursing Diagnoses | Desired Patient Outcomes | Nursing Interventions | Rationales |
|---|---|---|---|
| ***Nursing Diagnosis #16 (cont.)*** | | | |
| | | ○ Allow patient choices and options. | ○ Helps to give patient a feeling of some self-control. |
| | | ○ Encourage verbalization; carefully observe facial expression; provide a listening ear. | ○ What is not verbalized may be reflected in patient's facial expression. |
| ***Nursing Diagnosis #17***<br>Coping, alteration in: Patient and family, related to:<br>1. Situational crisis.<br>2. Temporary family disorganization. | Patient/family will:<br>1. Identify useful coping mechanisms.<br>2. Demonstrate ability to assess, problem-solve, and make decisions.<br>3. Express realistic expectations of each other. | • Establish a rapport and trusting relationship with patient and family. | |
| | | • Observe patient/family dynamics and interactions. | • These observations may help to identify strengths, weaknesses, and effective coping capabilities. |
| | | ○ Assess family resources; usual coping mechanisms. | ○ Long-term rehabilitation places tremendous burden on family resources. |
| | | • Implement measures to assist in coping: | |
| | | ○ Provide opportunity for patient and family members to express feelings and emotions.<br>–Encourage honest communication. | ○ Recognizing feelings and emotions is the first step in dealing with them. |
| | | ○ Provide emotional support and relieve anxieties by making appropriate explanations. | ○ Support and reassurance assist patient/family to cope with catastrophic event. |
| | | ○ Keep patient and family informed:<br>–Be honest and realistic.<br>–Be accessible to patient/family.<br>–Allow time for questions to be asked and feelings vented. | |
| | | ○ Increasingly include patient/family in decision-making process as they demonstrate a readiness to do so (e.g., the ability to verbalize and discuss feelings). | ○ Enables patient to feel useful, to have some control.<br>○ Promotes involvement in the rehabilitation process. |

| | | | |
|---|---|---|---|
| ***Nursing Diagnosis #18***<br>Social isolation, related to:<br>1. Immobility.<br>2. Prolonged hospitalization.<br>3. Depression. | Patient will:<br>1. Demonstrate desire to interact and maintain relationships.<br>2. Verbalize feelings of isolation.<br>3. Participate in diversional activities. | • Assess patient's usual degree of social interaction.<br>• Assess for signs/symptoms suggestive of social isolation.<br>∘ Specific signs/symptoms might include: Expression of loneliness or feelings of rejection; flat affect; depression; uncommunicative; withdrawn, preoccupied. | |
| | | • Encourage verbalization regarding patient's sense of isolation.<br>∘ Assess patient's feelings about self: Sense of being "out of control"; hopelessness. | • It is important to establish a therapeutic nurse/patient relationship, one in which the patient is able to comfortably air thoughts and concerns. |
| | | • Develop a plan of action to decrease feelings of social isolation.<br>∘ Provide effective alternative method of communication.<br>∘ Encourage interactions with significant others. | ∘ Helps to reassure that his/her needs are being met, and they have not been forgotten. |
| | | ∘ Assist patient to set up visiting schedule with family/friends.<br>∘ Encourage participation in diversional activities.<br>∘ Initiate referrals to appropriate resources (e.g., occupational, recreational therapist when feasible). | ∘ Knowing when to expect a visit or call can be reassuring. |

The phrenic nerve, which innervates the diaphragm, arises from cord segments $C_{3-5}$. Injury to the cervical cord places the patient at risk of developing respiratory insufficiency or respiratory arrest. Interruption of phrenic innervation causes paralysis of the diaphragm, and apnea results. The occurrence of ascending edema may cause a temporary paralysis of the diaphragm. Patients with cervical injuries ($C_5$–$C_6$) frequently require mechanical ventilatory assistance until the edema resolves and the cord stabilizes. At this point, the patient can be weaned from the ventilator.

**Prevention of Pulmonary Complications.** Pulmonary complications are the major cause of death during the acute phase following spinal cord injury. The critical care nurse has a primary responsibility to identify patients at risk of developing pulmonary complications, and to continuously assess respiratory function. Early changes in mental status may reflect hypoxia, manifested clinically as restlessness, fatigue, confusion, headache, and lethargy. Skin color (ashen) and cyanosis of lips, nailbeds, and earlobes reflect hypoxia and/or hypercapnia. Respiratory rate and pattern need to be monitored closely. Use of accessory muscles (e.g., sternocleidomastoid, scapular elevators, and anterior serrati [$C_{5-6}$], and scalene muscles [$C_{6-8}$]), considerably increases the work of breathing, depleting energy stores and fatiguing the patient.

Vital capacity is a useful measurement of the effectiveness of the patient's ventilatory effort. It is measured easily at the bedside using a spirometer. A lowered vital capacity (e.g., a trend leading to a vital capacity of <15–20 ml/kg), together with abnormal changes in the other assessment parameters, may signal the need for mechanical ventilatory support. Abnormal or absent breath sounds may be observed. Arterial blood gases (room air) also serve as a measurement as to the effectiveness of the ventilatory effort.

The nurse is concerned with maintaining a patent airway, preventing pooling of secretions, ensuring adequate chest expansion, and preventing or recognizing, early on, major pulmonary complications including atelectasis, hypostatic/aspiration pneumonia, pulmonary edema, or pulmonary emboli. A nasogastric tube is usually inserted to prevent aspiration of vomitus associated with paralytic ileus and/or swallowed blood from facial injuries. Preventive nursing measures include frequent turning and positioning, humidification and adequate hydration to keep secretions moist, chest physiotherapy, intermittent positive pressure breathing, and teaching the patient breathing exercises in the post-acute phase. The nurse needs to work closely with the physical therapist to initiate a program designed to facilitate these measures, and to establish an exercise regimen to promote and maintain optimal cardiopulmonary function.

**Weaning the Spinal Cord-Injured Patient: Nursing Considerations.** For patients requiring mechanical ventilatory assistance ($C_{4-6}$), weaning can be an arduous process requiring a collaborative effort on the part of the patient's nurse, physician, respiratory therapist, and physical therapist. An individualized weaning program is initiated, and its effectiveness is evaluated based on trends in the patient's respiratory parameters. These include tidal volume, vital capacity, peak inspiratory pressure, respiratory rate, and arterial blood gas values.

Intermittent mandatory ventilation (IMV), or a T-piece, may be used to accomplish weaning. The concept underlying the T-piece method is that the diaphragm, as a muscle, requires exercise periods to increase muscle tone, build up endurance, and minimize fatigue.[3] Use of the T-piece allows patients to breathe spontaneously, thus using their respiratory muscles including the diaphragm, while at the same time maintaining desired oxygen concentrations. The T-piece consists of a T-shaped tube, with one end connected to the patient's endotracheal tube or tracheostomy, one end connected to the oxygen source (inhalation end), and the third end acting as a gas reservoir (exhalation end). On inhalation, the patient draws gas with the desired oxygen concentration in from the system (i.e., inhalation end); on exhalation, the presence of an additional length of tubing (i.e., the gas reservoir) prevents the oxygen concentration of the inhaled gas to be diluted significantly by drawing in room air.

For details regarding oxygen therapy, endotracheal suctioning, and mechanical ventilation, see Chapter 32. See Table 12–7 for nursing diagnoses, patient outcomes, and nursing interventions related to respiratory function in the patient with cervical cord injury.

### *Cardiovascular Function in the Spinal Cord-Injured Patient*

Alterations in the cardiovascular status of the spinal cord-injured patient are largely attributed to autonomic dysfunction and include spinal shock, postural (orthostatic) hypotension, and autonomic dysreflexia.

**Neurogenic Shock (Spinal Shock).** Neurogenic shock, or spinal shock, is a consequence of the interruption of all neurologic function below the level of the lesion in patients with spinal cord injury at the level of $T_{4-6}$ and above. Specifically, autonomic dysfunction is characterized by loss of sympathetic vasomotor tone and vasomotor reflex activity below the level of the lesion. This results in the syndrome of spinal shock manifested clinically by hypotension, bradycardia, warm dry skin, and lowered body temperature.

Loss of vasomotor tone, which results in vasodilation of the systemic vasculature, accounts for the hypotension. There is pooling of blood in the capacitive blood vessels of the lower extremities and splanchnic circulation, decreasing venous return to the heart and resulting in a low cardiac output and reduced tissue perfusion. Venous blood pooling is particularly significant in that the patient becomes at increased risk of developing a deep venous thrombosis (see below). Vasodilation also accounts for the warm, dry skin and lowered body temperature, as body heat is lost via the dilated peripheral blood vessels.

The bradycardia characteristic of spinal shock occurs as a result of *unopposed* parasympathetic innervation to the heart via the vagus nerve. Heart rate in the spinal cord-injured patient who is hypotensive may help to distinguish two types of shock sometimes encountered in cervical cord trauma (i.e., neurogenic or spinal shock, and hemorrhagic and/or hypovolemic shock, see below).

Spinal shock is best treated by elevation of the lower extremities and application of antiembolic stockings to decrease venous pooling and increase venous return to the heart. The patient is *not* hypovolemic and should not receive large amounts of fluid because this may aggravate edema formation at the site of injury. This type of shock is usually responsive to vasoconstrictor drug therapy. The heart rate remains bradycardic, and the quality of the pulse is slow and bounding. The skin remains warm and dry.

**Hemorrhagic (Hypovolemic) Shock.** Patients sustaining a spinal cord injury infrequently experience hemorrhagic or hypovolemic shock as a result of trauma and internal injuries. Hemorrhagic or hypovolemic shock is characterized by hypotension, tachycardia, and cool clammy skin (see Chap. 46). The pulse in this case is weak, rapid, and thready, and the skin is pale, cool, and moist. The hypotension is caused by a decrease in intravascular fluid volume commonly due to extensive hemorrhaging (>1000 ml). The heart rate increases as the compensatory mechanisms within the body respond to the hypotensive state.

In the patient with hypovolemic shock without spinal cord injury, there is also a concomitant compensatory vasoconstriction of the systemic vasculature as sympathetic innervation is intact. Therapy in this type of shock involves administration of large amounts of fluid, plasma expanders and blood, to replenish the intravascular volume. Vasopressors may also be administered.

In the patient with suspected spinal cord injury who is hypotensive and tachycardic, the patient should be examined carefully for signs of bleeding. Internal injuries may accompany spinal cord injuries, yet because of loss of sensation below the level of the cord, the patient may not experience pain.

Loss of sympathetic innervation below the cord lesion also predisposes the patient to additional bodily dysfunction. Cardiac dysrhythmias frequently occur, especially in older patients, and ongoing cardiac monitoring is required.

**Postural or Orthostatic Hypotension.** Postural or orthostatic hypotension is an especially serious problem in terms of mobilizing the patient. It results from the pooling of blood in the systemic vasculature associated with loss of vasomotor tone. A program of gradual increases in sitting the patient up is implemented. Usually the patient must be able to tolerate the head of the bed at a 90-degree angle before an attempt is made to sit the patient in a chair. Antiembolic stockings and an abdominal binder are employed to enhance venous return. A CircO-lectric bed is sometimes used to assist the patient to gradually tolerate the upright position. If the patient experiences a syncopal episode, the bed is easily tilted back to a position tolerated by the patient.

**Deep Venous Thrombosis-Pulmonary Embolism.** The combination of vasomotor paralysis with pooling and stasis of blood, skeletal muscle paralysis, and immobilization places the patient at risk of developing deep venous thrombosis and thromboembolic disease. Assessment and diagnosis of deep venous thrombosis in the spinal cord-injured patient are especially difficult because the patient is unaware of pain and tenderness, which might otherwise suggest the presence of deep venous thrombosis.

Consequently, it is necessary for the nurse to maintain a high degree of suspicion in this regard, and to regularly assess for signs of venous thrombosis. Skin color and temperature of lower extremities should be assessed. A bluish-red color of the skin on inspection and an unusually warm temperature on palpation suggest a possible venous thrombosis. Circumference of thighs and calves should be measured at designated points daily. A slowly increasing circumference suggests a possible underlying venous thrombosis.

The patient should be monitored for signs and symptoms of pulmonary embolism. The sudden onset of respiratory difficulties (e.g., tachypnea, dyspnea, cough with hemoptysis), alterations in cardiopulmonary function (e.g., tachycardia, hypotension, cyanosis), and neurologic findings (e.g., restlessness, lethargy, confusion), all suggest a pulmonary embolism. (For the diagnostic evaluation of pulmonary embolism, see Table 35-1.)

Deep venous thrombosis prophylactic therapy includes measures to reduce the risk of venous stasis and to stimulate venous return to the heart. Application of antiembolic stockings to lower extremities, passive range-of-motion exercises including dorsiflexion of each foot, and maintenance of proper body alignment at all times assist in minimizing the risk of deep venous thrombosis. Other measures include avoiding positions that compromise blood flow, such as a pillow under the knees or use of knee gatch, crossing of legs, or prolonged sitting in one position. The patient breathing spontaneously should be encouraged to breathe deeply each hour to expand the lungs and prevent atelectasis. Low-dose heparin may also be initiated prophylactically to prevent thromboembolic formation and clot dispersion.

**Autonomic Dysreflexia (Autonomic Hyperreflexia).** Autonomic dysreflexia (autonomic hyper-reflexia) is defined as a clinical emergency characterized by an exaggerated sympathetic response occurring below the level of the spinal cord lesion and resulting in an uncontrolled paroxysmal hypertension (as high as 240–300 mmHg/150 mmHg). The consequences can be life-threatening, and there is the potential for a fatal stroke, subarachnoid hemorrhage, and seizures.[4]

Autonomic dysreflexia occurs in spinal cord-injured patients with lesions at the $T_{4-6}$ level or above. In patients with lesions at this level or lower, enough sympathetic nervous system function under the control of vasomotor centers in the brain is preserved to avoid this exaggerated abnormal response.

Approximately 80% of individuals with spinal cord lesions above the $T_{4-6}$ level experience autonomic dysreflexia within the first year after injury after spinal shock has resolved. It may occur spontaneously several years (~6 years) after injury even if the person has never experienced a prior episode.

***Pathogenesis.*** Under normal physiologic conditions the central nervous system (CNS) exerts its influence on autonomic function via reflex centers in the frontal cortex, limbic system, hypothalamus, brainstem, and spinal cord. When spinal cord injury occurs, this tonic, inhibitory outflow of impulses from the higher centers is blocked, enabling sympathetic reflex activity below the level of the lesion to continue unabated.

The sequence of events in the pathogenesis of autonomic dysreflexia is as follows:

1. Constant, intense local stimuli, as for example, a distended bladder, cause impulses to be initiated and conducted into the spinal cord, where they ascend to the level of the lesion. It is at this point that communication is interrupted and the sensation of a "full bladder" is never perceived. Instead, these impulses stimulate sympathetic reflex centers in the intermediolateral gray horn of the thoracolumbar cord, which, uninhibited by impulses from above, precipitate an enormous sympathetic response.
2. There occurs a reflex arteriolar spasm throughout the extensive vasculature of abdominal and pelvic organs and the skin. The result is severe, sudden hypertension.
3. Baroreceptors in the carotid sinus, aortic arch, and cerebral vessels detect the elevated blood pressure, and compensatory activities occur immediately to reduce the pressure. Parasympathetic innervation via the vagus (cranial nerve X) slows the heart rate and attempts to stimulate vasodilation of blood vessels in the splanchnic viscera and the skin. However, the parasympathetic vasodilatory effect on these blood vessels is minimal at best. In response to the hypertensive crisis, reflex centers in the brain signal a reduction in sympathetic tone. However, this inhibitory influence of higher brain centers on sympathetic reflexes within the cord is blocked at the level of the lesion, and the overwhelming sympathetic vasoconstrictor response continues unabated.

***Clinical Presentation.*** The classic clinical manifestations that occur *above* the level of the cord lesion reflect the effects of the body's compensatory mechanisms triggered in response to the hypertension. These include profuse diaphoresis, flushing (i.e., superficial or cutaneous vasodilation), and a pounding, throbbing headache. Other signs and symptoms may include blurred vision, nasal congestion, nausea, anxiety, and fright. Bradycardia persists owing to vagal stimulation.

Symptomatology occurring *below* the cord lesion reflects the effects of the exaggerated sympathetic response and consequent severe vasoconstriction, and includes skin pallor, chills, paralytic ileus, and pilomotor erections (i.e., goose bumps). The severe vasoconstriction of splanchnic vessels and those in the skin underlies the hypertension.

***Causes of Autonomic Dysreflexia.*** Causes of autonomic dysreflexia are linked intimately with nursing interventions and preventive aspects of the rehabilitative process. They include a variety of abnormal stimuli arising from localized areas below the cord lesion primarily in the abdominopelvic region:

*Urinary*

- Distended bladder due to urinary retention
- Kinking or plugging of catheter, if in place
- Genitourinary infection
- Calculi formation
- Pressure on genitals (testicles)
- Genitourinary procedures (e.g., cystoscopy)

*Bowel*

- Distended rectum
- Fecal impaction
- Digital examination

*Skin*

- Decubitus ulcer
- Sharp object pressing into skin
- Wind drafts in room

*Pain receptors*
- Ingrown toenails
- Pressure on glans penis
- Inguinal rash

*Abdominal problems*
- Internal bleeding post-instrumentation

*Pregnancy*
- Uterine contractions during labor

***Emergent Nursing Interventions.*** When an episode of autonomic dysreflexia is triggered, emergent treatment includes the following:

1. Place patient in an upright position to lower blood pressure (i.e., postural hypotension).
2. Monitor blood pressure and heart rate.
3. Notify physician if indicated (e.g., a severely elevated systolic blood pressure ~240 mmHg and/or unresponsive to interventions).
4. Identify underlying cause and remove if possible.
5. Administer drug therapy as per unit protocol for persistent hypertension after removal of the triggering stimulus; or if the stimulus cannot be identified. *Drugs of choice:* diazoxide (Hyperstat) and hydralazine (Apresoline). (See Appendix A for information regarding these drugs and others used to treat a hypertensive crisis.)
6. Stay with patient; provide reassurance, psychologic and emotional support; recognize that anxiety and fright increase catecholamine secretions potentiating the mass sympathetic response.
7. Monitor patient's blood pressure every 4 hours for 24 hours after the crisis; should hypertension persist, an oral antihypertensive drug may be prescribed.

***Preventive Nursing Interventions.*** The best treatment of autonomic dysreflexia is *prevention*. The nurse plays a pivotal role in preventing the occurrence of this complication and in teaching patient, family, and/or significant others about how to prevent it and what to do if it should occur. Specific preventive nursing interventions are listed in Table 12–8.

### Body Temperature Instability

Disruption of sympathetic innervation following high cord injury also impairs regulation of body temperature. An inability to perspire in areas of the body below the lesion prevents normal loss of body heat when body temperature is elevated, while the vasodilation of peripheral blood vessels causes an increased heat loss. In effect, the body's temperature fluctuates with that of room temperature. Early management of the spinal cord-injured patient requires an ongoing assessment of the patient's temperature (every 2–4 hours), as well as that of the environment. Actions should be taken to

TABLE 12–8
**Autonomic Dysreflexia: Preventive Nursing Interventions**

1. Identify patients at risk of developing autonomic dysreflexia, including patients with spinal cord lesions at $T_{4-6}$ or above, and especially quadriplegics ($C_{6-7}$ and above).
2. Avoid abnormal stimuli having the potential of triggering a mass sympathetic discharge.
   A. Avoid urinary retention and bladder distention.
      1) Monitor intake and output carefully.
      2) Avoid overhydration (increases risk of bladder distention/overdistention).
      3) Teach patient to avoid drinking large amount of fluid at any one time.
      4) Maintain patency of indwelling catheter.
      5) Observe for bladder spasms.
   B. Avoid bowel retention or fecal impaction.
      1) Strict adherence to bowel regimen.
      2) Use dibucaine ointment (Nupercainal) for digital exam or removal of fecal impaction.
      3) Appropriate diet and fluid intake.
   C. Examine skin for pressure areas and impaired integrity.
      1) Special examination of sensitive perineal, perianal, and genital regions for pressure areas, excoriations, or rashes. Ascertain spontaneous body response to inadvertent sexual stimulation.
      2) Pressure areas of the skin require regular, consistent monitoring with appropriate position changes. Patients at risk of developing autonomic dysreflexia should not be placed in a flat, lying-down position because this might provide a triggering stimulus in the sensitive patient. Sitting positions lower blood pressure.
   D. Avoid wind drafts in room.
3. Recognize clinical manifestations.
   A. Specific signs and symptoms (*above* cord lesion)
      1) Sudden elevation in systolic blood pressure.
      2) Pounding headache, often associated with blurred vision.
      3) Profuse diaphoresis.
      4) Flushing above level of lesion.
      5) Nasal congestion.
      6) Nausea.
      7) Anxiety, fear.
      8) Bradycardia.
   B. Specific signs and symptoms (*below* cord lesion):
      1) Skin pallor, cold to touch.
      2) Chills, pilomotor erections (goose bumps).
      3) Intestinal relaxation (i.e., paralytic ileus).
4. Provide patient and family with education regarding autonomic dysreflexia, what it is, what triggers it, signs and symptoms, and treatment.
   A. Stress importance of reporting signs and symptoms.
   B. Assist patient/family to identify the triggering stimulus so that efforts can be made to avoid it.
   C. Recommend to patients prone to developing autonomic dysreflexia the importance of carrying identification cards that stipulate course of action for emergency care:
      1) Place in upright position.
      2) Monitor blood pressure, heart rate, pulse.
      3) Identify underlying cause and/or triggering stimulus.
      4) Remove triggering stimulus and/or correct underlying cause.
      5) Seek emergency medical assistance.
      6) Administer drug therapy for an episode of autonomic dysreflexia as prescribed.
      7) Stay with patient; offer reassurance; relieve anxiety.

minimize fluctuations of body and room temperature. For example, if the room is cool, an extra blanket may be placed over the patient to prevent heat loss if his/her body temperature is normal.

In general, the quadriplegic patient ($T_1$ and above) presents with hypotension (90–100/60 mmHg), bradycardia (~60 beats/minute), and hypothermia (i.e., body heat loss attributed to vasodilation of peripheral vasculature). Paraplegics with a high thoracic lesion ($T_{1-6}$) may experience these signs to a lesser extent, while others with a lower thoracolumbar lesion ($T_{11}$–$L_1$) may not manifest any of these signs because sympathetic innervation remains intact.

### Musculoskeletal Integrity

To prevent further neurologic damage, a major goal in the initial treatment of the patient with spinal cord injury is to immobilize the head, neck, and back. Transfer of the patient is avoided until the patient's condition is assessed (including cervical spine x-rays in which all seven cervical vertebrae are definitely viewed) and stabilized. If transfer or movement of the patient is necessary, a 4-man lift technique should be used with 1 team member maintaining manual cervical traction, alignment, and immobilization.

**Surgical Stabilization.** After initial treatment to stabilize the patient's vital functions, the extent and exact location of the vertebral and/or spinal injuries are assessed. Whether medical or surgical treatment is to be instituted remains a controversial issue. Rudy[5] summarizes indications for surgical intervention as: (1) unstable injuries especially if cord transection is incomplete; (2) open injuries of the cord; and (3) evidence of progressive neurologic dysfunction. Surgical stabilization can be accomplished in several ways: (1) surgical wiring; (2) placement of Harrington rod; (3) laminectomy with fusion; and (4) anterior fusion wherein the integrity of the laminae is not interrupted. If necessary, postsurgical nursing care is facilitated by using a specialized kinetic bed (e.g., Rotorest or Clinitron bed).

### Nonsurgical Stabilization

***Therapeutic Goals.*** Techniques of nonsurgical stabilization and immobilization are employed to: (1) prevent further neurologic damage and facilitate return of potential neurologic function; (2) maintain correct body alignment while ensuring necessary position changes to prevent skin breakdown, muscle fatigue, and contractures; (3) facilitate return of weakened musculature while promoting maximum function of unaffected muscles; and (4) minimize muscle spasms and promote patient comfort.

Cervical immobilization and continuous traction may be achieved via the use of skull tongs (e.g., *Gardner-Wells*, and to a lesser extent, *Crutchfield* tongs). Skeletal traction can achieve both reduction and immobilization of the fracture/dislocation.

*Halo Immobilization Brace.* An alternative and increasingly used method of achieving cervical immobilization, as well as traction, positioning, and alignment, is the application of the halo immobilization brace. It consists of a metal halo-ring attached to the skull via screws and to a metal frame of adjustable, interlocking metallic bars. These bars connect the ring to a rigid plastic vestlike jacket with a soft liner. It provides complete external immobilization for cervical instability, without flexion, extension, or rotational movements of the head.

The use of the halo brace has several advantages for the spinal cord-injured patient:[6] (1) early application (can be placed on the patient in the emergency room if necessary) for prompt cervical reduction and alignment; (2) easy and safe patient transport; (3) timely institution of vigorous pulmonary hygiene and physiotherapy; (4) pain reduction; (5) early mobilization and ambulation, reducing risk of such complications as pulmonary compromise (e.g., atelectasis, hypostatic pneumonia associated with pooling of pulmonary secretions), impaired skin integrity, occurrence of deep venous thrombosis and pulmonary embolism, and sensory deprivation, among others; (6) easy removal of anterior and posterior chest plates allows for careful inspection of skin and implementation of necessary skin care protocols; (7) decreased length of hospital stay (acute phase) and earlier, active participation of the patient in the rehabilitation process.

When caring for a patient with a halo immobilization brace the nurse should be cognizant of ongoing nursing care management considerations including those listed in Table 12–9. In general, in clinical settings where the halo brace is employed nursing personnel are taught to maximize the effectiveness of this treatment and prevent any complications.[6]

Initially, the patient and family may be frightened because the halo brace is unsightly. The weight of the brace may make the patient feel "top heavy" and awkward, and the patient may experience lightheadedness and nausea commonly associated with postural hypotension. As the patient progresses from intensive to convalescent phase, a program of gradual ambulation can be implemented.

### Gastrointestinal Function

The level of the spinal cord lesion largely determines the extent of gastrointestinal and bowel dysfunction. Immediately after spinal cord injury when spinal shock ensues, the entire gastrointesti-

TABLE 12–9
**Nursing Management Considerations for the Patient with a Halo Immobilization Brace[6]**

1. Avoid using the metal frame as a handle to turn, lift, or position the patient; avoid hitting the metal frame because bone conduction of the sound may be annoying to the patient.
2. Move the patient and halo immobilization brace as a unit to avoid undue stress on any one part.
3. Check pins and screws daily to ensure proper tightness.
4. Clean pin site areas twice daily with normal saline and hydrogen peroxide followed by an application of povidone-iodine ointment.
5. Examine pin sites for any evidence of inflammation—pain, redness, swelling, drainage, increased body temperature, or headache, and report findings to patient's physician.
6. Examine skin under vest every 8 hours for pressure points and skin integrity. If possible, place patient in prone position to facilitate skin inspection and relieve pressure on scapulae and shoulders. Pressure points often occur over spinous processes T-1 to T-3. Be alert for unusual odors, which might indicate skin breakdown. Identify patients at risk for developing skin breakdown as, for example, the patient with diabetes mellitus or the severely debilitated patient. The paralyzed patient is unable to feel pain and requires diligent inspection and assessment after each position change.
7. Turn patient regularly to prevent skin breakdown and undue pressure on pin sites.
8. Maintain cleanliness with daily washing. Vest liners can be changed, and sheepskin padding can be applied to pressure areas.
9. All nurses caring for a patient with a halo brace should know how to remove the anterior section of the brace in the event that cardiopulmonary resuscitation is needed. A wrench must be available at bedside to unlock the bolts that attach the anterior bars to the vest.
10. When the condition of the patient with a halo brace is stabilized, he/she may gradually be assisted into a sitting position, and eventually into a wheelchair. The transition to a sitting position is gradual to prevent postural hypotension.
11. When patient ambulates, caution patient to examine heights of doorways prior to entering them.

nal tract becomes atonic. There is a loss of sensation, which complicates assessment of the patient. The patient does not experience pain nor is there abdominal guarding in response to palpation of a tender area if present. A high degree of suspicion is necessary to thoroughly assess the patient. Be especially alert for the presence of *referred* pain; auscultate the abdomen in all four quadrants for the presence or absence of bowel sounds. Measure abdominal girth at the level of the umbilicus every 8 hours. Maintain baseline function.

**Paralytic Ileus.** Paralytic ileus commonly occurs in the patient with spinal cord injury. It is defined as a state of complete atony of the small bowel with an absence of peristalsis. Although the cause is unknown, paralytic ileus is related to a sudden, abrupt interruption of autonomic innervation. Its onset varies depending on the level of the lesion or insult. In thoracolumbar cord injuries the onset may occur within the first 24 hours post injury; in lesions involving the cervical cord its onset may initially be delayed for the first 48 hours.

Associated with paralytic ileus is the danger of aspiration of vomitus due to acute gastric dilatation. Abdominal distention may limit diaphragmatic excursion and in this way predispose to respiratory complications including poor ventilatory effort with reduced vital capacity, and hypostatic and/or aspiration pneumonia. Initial management involves insertion of a nasogastric tube to decompress the stomach and minimize abdominal distention. Zejdlik[7] reports that unrecognized paralytic ileus coupled with a weak or ineffective coughing capability is the most common cause of sudden death within the first 48 hours post injury in a quadriplegic patient.

**Gastric Ulceration.** Development of acute peptic ulcer is always a potential complication in the spinal cord-injured patient, particularly during the first week post injury. The patient is at risk for developing an acute gastrointestinal bleed. Such pathology in response to trauma and stress is thought to be associated with endogenous release of corticosteroids and an increased gastric secretion of hydrochloric acid resulting from unopposed vagal stimulation. Administration of exogenous corticosteroids may potentiate this pathologic process, but clinical evidence in this regard remains controversial.

The nurse must constantly be alert for signs of gastrointestinal bleeding. Gastric contents should be tested for presence of blood (hematemesis), and the stool should be tested for guaiac. Vital signs should be monitored for any drop in blood pressure or increase in heart rate. Daily blood work should include hematocrit and hemaglobin levels. Antacid and ranitidine therapy may be prescribed to minimize the irritating effects of steroids and increased hydrochloric acid secretions.

**Bowel Management.** Early management of bowel function is concerned with prevention of bowel distention and fecal impaction. The rectum should be checked for stool, which, if present, should gently be removed with a well-lubricated gloved finger. A lidocaine jelly should be used to minimize a noxious stimulus. The nurse must be alert for signs of constipation, which might include a dull sound over the descending colon on percussion, and/or palpation of hard, rigid stool over different areas of bowel. A well-lubricated rectal tube may be placed for limited periods of time (<30 minutes) to help relieve flatus. A rectal tube should not be used for longer periods of time because of the danger of injuring the delicate bowel lining. Enemas are *not* given because fluid will accumulate in the atonic bowel, causing distention.

A major long-term goal of health care of the spinal cord-injured patient is to assist the patient to establish an effective bowel management program to ensure adequate elimination and maintain gastrointestinal function. During the acute phase of illness, critical care nurses monitor bowel status and prevent complications (e.g., constipation, diarrhea, intestinal obstruction). Through interactions with patient, family, and/or significant others, critical care nurses initiate efforts to establish and nurture a trusting relationship, and to assess and collect data of importance to the implementation of a bowel regimen. Information regarding the patient's pre-injury status, including diet, personal habits, and attitudes regarding bowel control, can be helpful in establishing an effective bowel management program.

***Defecation Reflexes.*** The act of defecation involves the combined activity of innervation at three levels.[8] At the local level, the *intrinsic* defecation reflex innervates the bowel via the myenteric plexuses located within the bowel wall. Very weak peristaltic waves are initiated in response to distention of the bowel by the presence of feces. These weak peristaltic waves are greatly intensified by innervation via the parasympathetic defecation reflex center located in the spinal cord at sacral segments $S_{2-4}$. Parasympathetic innervation enhances peristalsis and bowel motility, stimulates secretions, and relaxes sphincter activity. Its activity is largely responsible for large bowel movements. Sympathetic activity is antagonistic to that of the parasympathetic system and causes decreased peristalsis and bowel motility, inhibition of secretions, and contraction of sphincters.

The act of defecation is controlled at the level of the brain by innervation to the external anal sphincter. This sphincter reflexly relaxes when stool is propelled toward the anus. The conscious mind assumes voluntary control of this skeletal muscle sphincter, increasing its tone if the time for defecation is inconvenient or inappropriate, or relaxing the sphincter to allow defecation to occur if the moment is acceptable. Voluntary suppression of the defecation reflexes may be effective for several hours before another urge to defecate is experienced. The actual process of defecation is enhanced by straining the abdominal muscles and bearing down. This Valsalva's maneuver involves taking a deep breath and attempting to exhale against a closed glottis while tightening the abdominal muscles. The increased intrathoracic and intraabdominal pressures assist in expelling stool. Stimulation of abdominal muscles requires an intact thoracic cord, $T_{6-12}$.

The level of spinal cord injury largely determines the extent of bowel control. Spinal cord injury above the conus medullaris, which contains the spinal defecation reflex center, $S_{2-4}$, interrupts activity of the upper motor neurons (UMN) (Fig. 12-1). The result is loss of ability to voluntarily control the activity of the external anal sphincter. Depending on the level of the injury, there may also be an inability to contract abdominal muscles. Ascending sensory information is also interrupted, resulting in the inability to feel fullness in the lower bowel and the urge to defecate.

The significance of an upper motor neuron (UMN) lesion is that the spinal defecation reflex center remains intact and continues to exert a tone on bowel and sphincters. This results in *spastic* bowel dysfunction.[9] Bowel training in this instance is directed toward using the intact defecation reflexes to evacuate the bowel on a regular basis.

Injury to lower motor neurons (LMN), either directly to the defecation reflex center within the conus medullaris or to the sacral nerve roots in the cauda equina (see Table 12-6), results in *flaccid* bowel dysfunction (see Fig. 12-1). In this instance the reflex center and/or final pathways are destroyed and no tonic activity exists. The presence of a flaccid sphincter means incontinence can occur at any time without rectal or anal stimulation provided stool is present in the rectum. In the case of an upper motor neuron lesion, defecation can be initiated at a convenient time enabling bowel evacuation to be planned and incontinence prevented. Characteristics of these two neurogenic bowel dysfunction syndromes and implications for care are listed in Table 12-10.

### *Renal Function*

**Urinary Bladder Management.** Micturition, or the act of emptying the bladder, becomes disrupted when injury to the spinal cord occurs. The significance of micturition is reflected by the fact that renal dysfunction ranks high as a major cause of death in patients with spinal cord injuries. The critical care nurse plays a pivotal role in caring for the spinal cord-injured patient during the acute post-injury phase in: (1) maintaining adequate renal/urinary function; (2) preventing complications of acute urinary retention with bladder overdistention and overflow incontinence; (3) preventing infection related to stasis of urine, use of indwelling catheter, or urethral reflux of urine to upper urinary tracts and kidneys; (4) establishing and nurturing a trusting relationship with the patient and his family; (5) initiating assessment and data collection related to the patient's pre-injury status, including diet, personal habits, knowledge and attitude regarding urinary control, prior coping capabilities, and family resources.

Micturition involves a cyclic sequence of events initiated by stretch receptors in the bladder wall in response to the bladder filling with urine. Sensory impulses thus generated activate the micturition or voiding reflex center located within cord segments

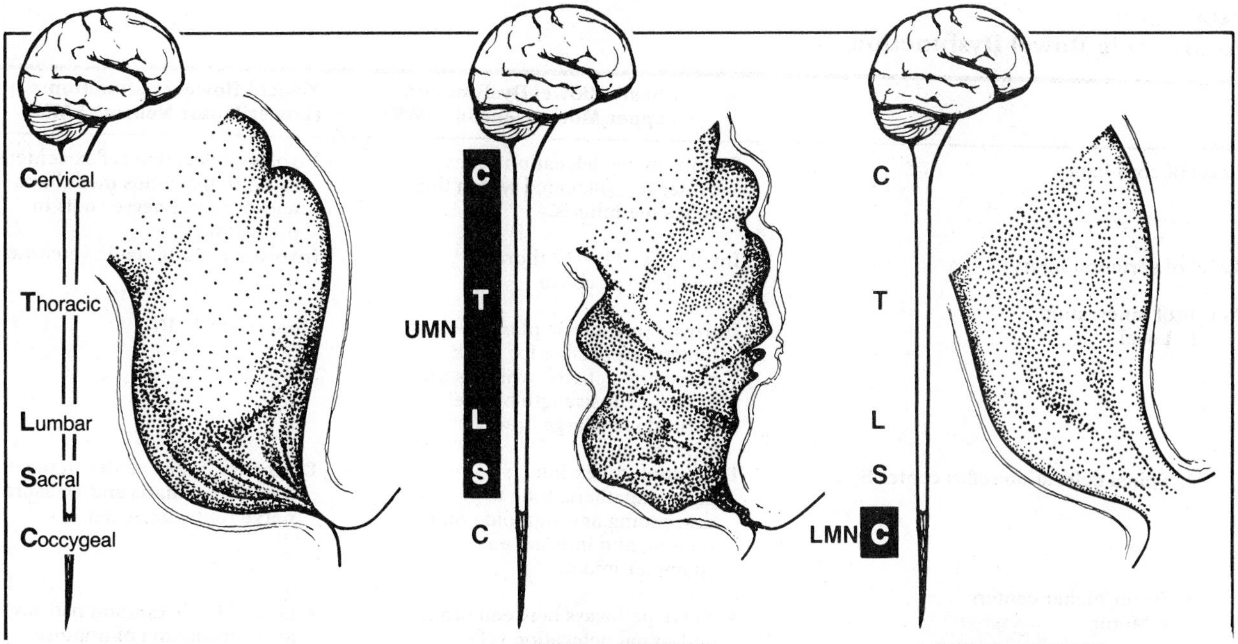

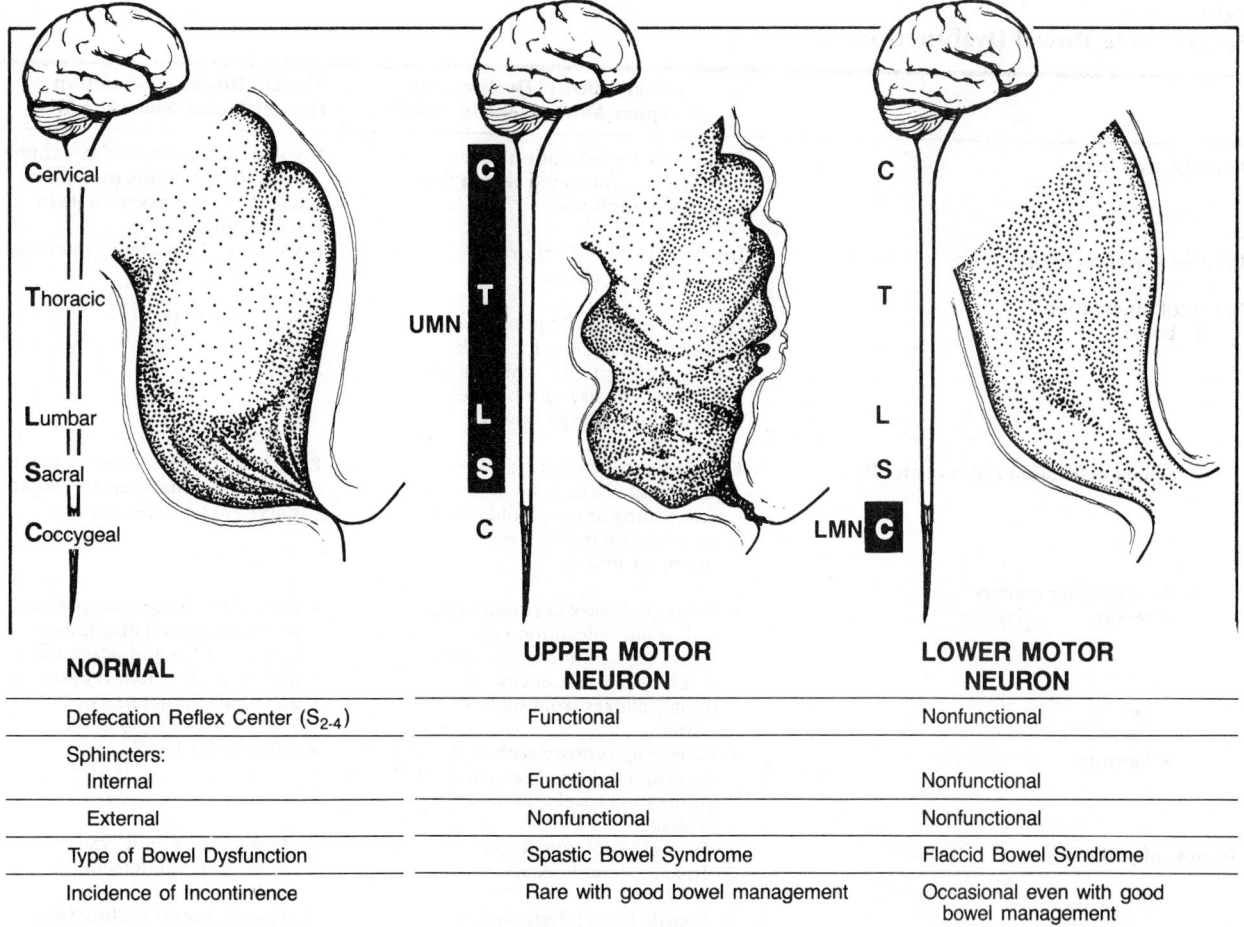

| NORMAL | UPPER MOTOR NEURON | LOWER MOTOR NEURON |
|---|---|---|
| Defecation Reflex Center ($S_{2-4}$) | Functional | Nonfunctional |
| Sphincters: Internal | Functional | Nonfunctional |
| External | Nonfunctional | Nonfunctional |
| Type of Bowel Dysfunction | Spastic Bowel Syndrome | Flaccid Bowel Syndrome |
| Incidence of Incontinence | Rare with good bowel management | Occasional even with good bowel management |

**Figure 12-1.** Innervation underlying bowel function and dysfunction, and potential for achievable bowel management. The level of spinal cord injury largely determines the extent of achievable bowel control. Interruption of UMN innervation results in the loss of voluntary control of the activity of the external anal sphincter, which becomes completely dysfunctional, and an interruption of ascending sensory information resulting in the inability of the individual to feel fullness in the rectum or the urge to defecate. The spinal defecation reflex center ($S_{2-4}$) remains functional and continues to exert a tone on the bowel and internal anal sphincter. This results in a *spastic* bowel syndrome, and bowel training is focused on using the intact defecation reflexes to evacuate the bowel on a regular basis (usually every other day). Prognosis for good bowel management with but rare episodes of incontinence is excellent.

Interruption of LMN innervation to the bowel and internal anal sphincter results in an atonic or *flaccid* bowel syndrome. Prognosis for good bowel management in this instance is less favorable because in the presence of a nonfunctional spinal defecation reflex center and internal anal sphincter, incontinence can occur at any time that stool enters the rectum. Because innervation between the higher centers and external anal sphincter is also interrupted, the external anal sphincter is also nonfunctional. Even with good bowel management, incontinence can occur.

$S_{2-4}$, resulting in reflex bladder contractions and relaxation of the internal sphincter. A complete cycle consists of a progressive increase of pressure within the bladder as it fills with urine, which increases sensory input into the micturition reflex center within the sacral cord. Efferent output from the reflex center produces a progressive increase in and strengthening of bladder contractions. This process is intensified as the volume of urine within the bladder increases and contractions of the detrusor muscle within the bladder become more powerful.

Eventually the micturition reflex becomes powerful enough to force open the bladder neck (internal sphincter). Stretch of the bladder neck stimulates still another reflex, which inhibits the well-defined, skeletal muscle external sphincter. If this inhibition is more powerful than the cerebral influence, the external sphincter reflexly relaxes and voiding occurs.

Neural control of micturition includes both autonomic and voluntary control. Nerve fibers of the parasympathetic nerve system arise within the micturition reflex center within the cord and stimulate

TABLE 12–10
**Neurogenic Bowel Dysfunction**

| | Spastic Bowel Dysfunction (Upper Motor Neuron; UMN) | Flaccid Bowel Dysfunction (Lower Motor Neuron; LMN) |
|---|---|---|
| Level of cord injury | Occurs above defecation reflex center ($S_{2-4}$) located within the conus medullaris. | Involves defecation reflex center ($S_{2-4}$) in the conus medullaris and/or sacral nerve roots in the equina. |
| Level of vertebral injury | Involves T-11—12 thoracic vertebrae or above. | Involves T-12 thoracic vetebrae or below. |
| Levels of innervation: | | |
| 1. Local | Intrinsic (myenteric plexus) intact; responsible for weak peristaltic activity, which is not of sufficient strength by itself to produce a large bowel movement. | Same as for UMN. |
| 2. Spinal defecation reflex center $S_{2-4}$ | Defecation reflex intact; parasympathetic tone to descending and sigmoid colon, rectum, and internal anal sphincter intact. | Defecation reflex center in the conus medullaris and/or sacral nerve roots destroyed. |
| 3. Brain/higher centers | | |
| • Motor | • Nerve pathways between brain and spinal defecation reflex center ($S_{2-4}$) interrupted: loss of inhibitory influences on spinal reflexes from higher centers. | • Loss of final common pathway for transmission of impulses between CNS and descending and sigmoid colon, rectum, and anal sphincters. |
| • Sensory | • Ascending sensory pathways interrupted: loss of sensation of fullness in bowel and urge to defecate. | • Same as for UMN. |
| Results of pathology | 1. Loss of UMN innervation. 2. Intact spinal defecation reflexes. 3. Spastic bowel dysfunction with spastic contraction of bowel and anal sphincters. | 1. Loss of LMN innervation. 2. Loss of spinal defecation reflexes. 3. Flaccid bowel dysfunction. |
| Prognosis for bowel control* | With intact defecation reflexes, bowel training is aimed at using these reflexes to evacuate the bowel. Bowel and anal sphincters respond to rectal/anal stimulation, enabling a planned bowel regimen, which empties the rectum and prevents incontinence. Prognosis is excellent for good bowel control. | With loss of spinal defecation reflex activity and LMN innervation, the bowel and anal sphincters are flaccid. They do not respond to planned rectal or anal stimulation. Arrival of feces in the rectum results in incontinence. Bowel training is deployed to evacuate stool from rectum. Presence of stool in rectum precipitates incontinence. Prognosis is favorable for bowel control providing a routine of regular bowel evacuation removes the stimulus for bowel emptying, preventing incontinence. |
| Occurrence of bowel incontinence | Rarely with good bowel management due to spastic contraction. Diet is a significant factor in effective bowel management. | Occasionally even with good bowel management due to flaccid sphincters. As with spastic bowel dysfunction, diet is a significant factor in effective bowel management. |
| Bowel training program | Regularly scheduled evacuation usually every other day. | Evacuation necessary on a daily basis to keep rectum clear of feces and prevent incontinence. |

TABLE 12-10
**Neurogenic Bowel Dysfunction *(Continued)***

| | Spastic Bowel Dysfunction (Upper Motor Neuron; UMN) | Flaccid Bowel Dysfunction (Lower Motor Neuron; LMN) |
|---|---|---|
| Use of medications including: Suppositories Laxatives | Responsive to a combination of laxatives (milk of magnesia), stool softener (dioctyl sodium sulfosuccinate [docusate, Colace]), and suppositories (Dulcolax). | Response to medications less effective than with spastic bowel dysfunction. |
| Digital stimulation | Used to initiate a planned reflex bowel evacuation. | Nonresponsive to digital stimulation; manual removal of stool from rectum may be required. |

*Successful bowel training depends on many factors, including level of injury, prior bowel habits, patient/family motivation, teamwork, among others.

contraction of the detrusor muscle of the bladder wall and relaxation of the internal sphincter of the bladder neck (trigone). Nerve fibers of the sympathetic nervous system arise from cord segments $T_{11}$ to $L_2$ and may play a role in the contraction of the internal bladder neck/sphincter.

Although the micturition reflex is a completely autonomic cord reflex, it can be stimulated or inhibited by higher centers within the central nervous system. Guyton[10] identifies two probable centers, including strong facilitatory and inhibitory centers in the brainstem (pons) and several cortical areas which are mainly inhibitory. Specific effects of higher centers on the micturition act include: (1) keeping the micturition reflex partially inhibited until it is desirable to void; (2) preventing micturition even in the presence of a powerful micturition reflex, by contraction of the external urinary sphincter; and (3) facilitating the micturition reflex center to initiate micturition while inhibiting contraction of the external sphincter so that urination can occur.

The level of spinal cord injury largely determines the extent of urinary control.[11] Spinal cord injury above the micturition reflex center ($S_{2-4}$), located within the conus medullaris, interrupts ascending sensory pathways and upper motor neurons (UMN) (Fig. 12-2). Interruption of upper motor neurons causes a loss of voluntary, coordinated control over the micturition reflex center in the cord. The reflex center itself remains intact so that a *spastic* automatic bladder results and can be identified after spinal shock. Patients with a spastic bladder are unable to sense bladder fullness or the urge to void due to interruption of ascending sensory pathways. As the bladder fills with urine, the micturition reflex is triggered, resulting in incontinence. The patient needs to be assessed frequently for overdistention of the bladder, which can occur if there is spasm of the bladder sphincters.

Injury to the lower motor neutrons (LMN) (see Fig. 12-2), either directly to the micturition reflex center in the conus medullaris or to sacral nerve roots in the cauda equina, causes a *flaccid* autonomous bladder. In this instance, the reflex center and/or final pathways are destroyed and no tonic activity exists. As is the case with upper motor neuron paralysis, the patient is unaware of bladder distention and the need to void due to interruption of ascending pathways. A primary concern is bladder overdistention.

Injury occurring to nerve roots at the junction of the conus medullaris and cauda equina can result in mixed bladder dysfunction as, for example, a flaccid bladder with a spastic external sphincter. It is important to diagnose the type of sphincteric damage because this will influence treatment and prognosis. Characteristics of these two neurogenic bladder dysfunction syndromes are listed in Table 12-11.

### *Skin Integrity*

Loss of mobility and sensation, impaired circulation, and inadequate nutrition predispose patients with spinal cord injury to skin breakdown. The primary factor involved in the disruption of skin integrity is excessive pressure. Pressure develops when there is a lack of continuous movement and distribution of body weight. It is most concentrated between bone and skin surfaces that support body weight. When unrelieved, pressure causes a "sustained ischemia," which disrupts cellular metabolism and leads to varying degrees of tissue injury and necrosis.

There is a definite relationship between the amount and duration of pressure and the development of a pressure sore or decubitus ulcer. Weight-bearing bony prominences must be identified as the patient is placed in different positions (prone, su-

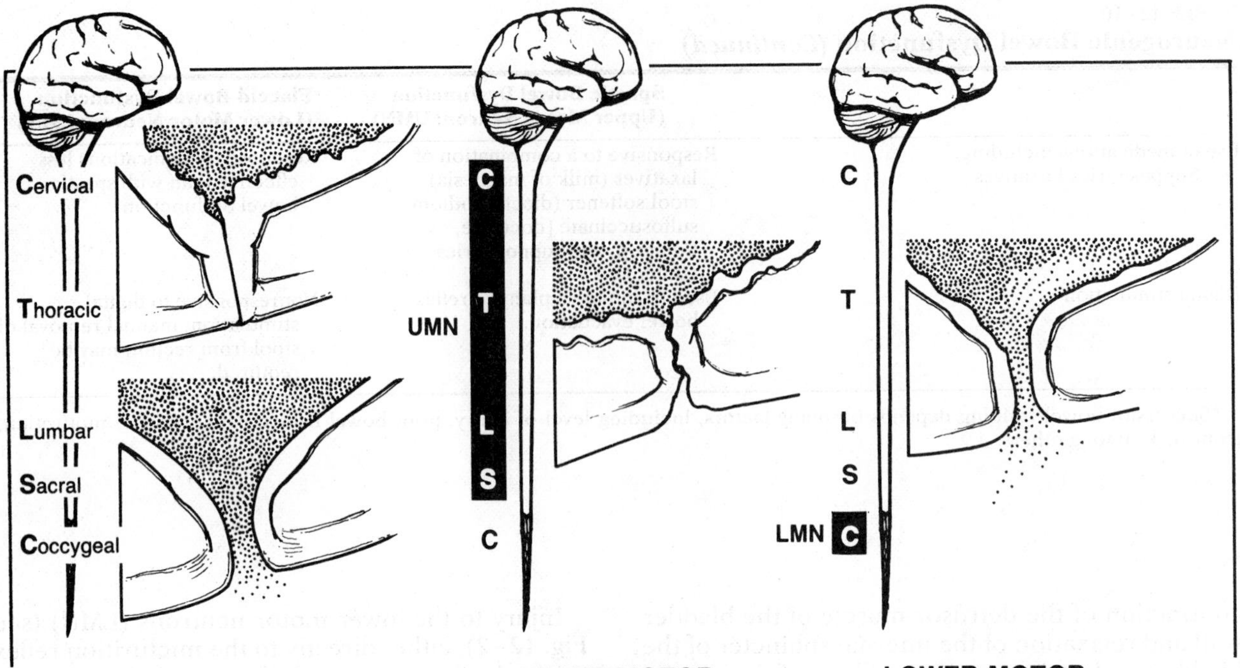


| NORMAL | UPPER MOTOR NEURON | LOWER MOTOR NEURON |
|---|---|---|
| Micturition Reflex Center ($S_{2-4}$) | Functional | Nonfunctional |
| Sphincters: Internal (Not a well-defined sphincter) | Functional | Nonfunctional |
| External | Nonfunctional | Nonfunctional |
| Type of Bladder Dysfunction | Spastic (automatic) Bladder | Flaccid (autonomous) Bladder |
| Prognosis for Planned Reflex Voiding | Favorable | Unfavorable Intermittent bladder catheterization program may be best approach |

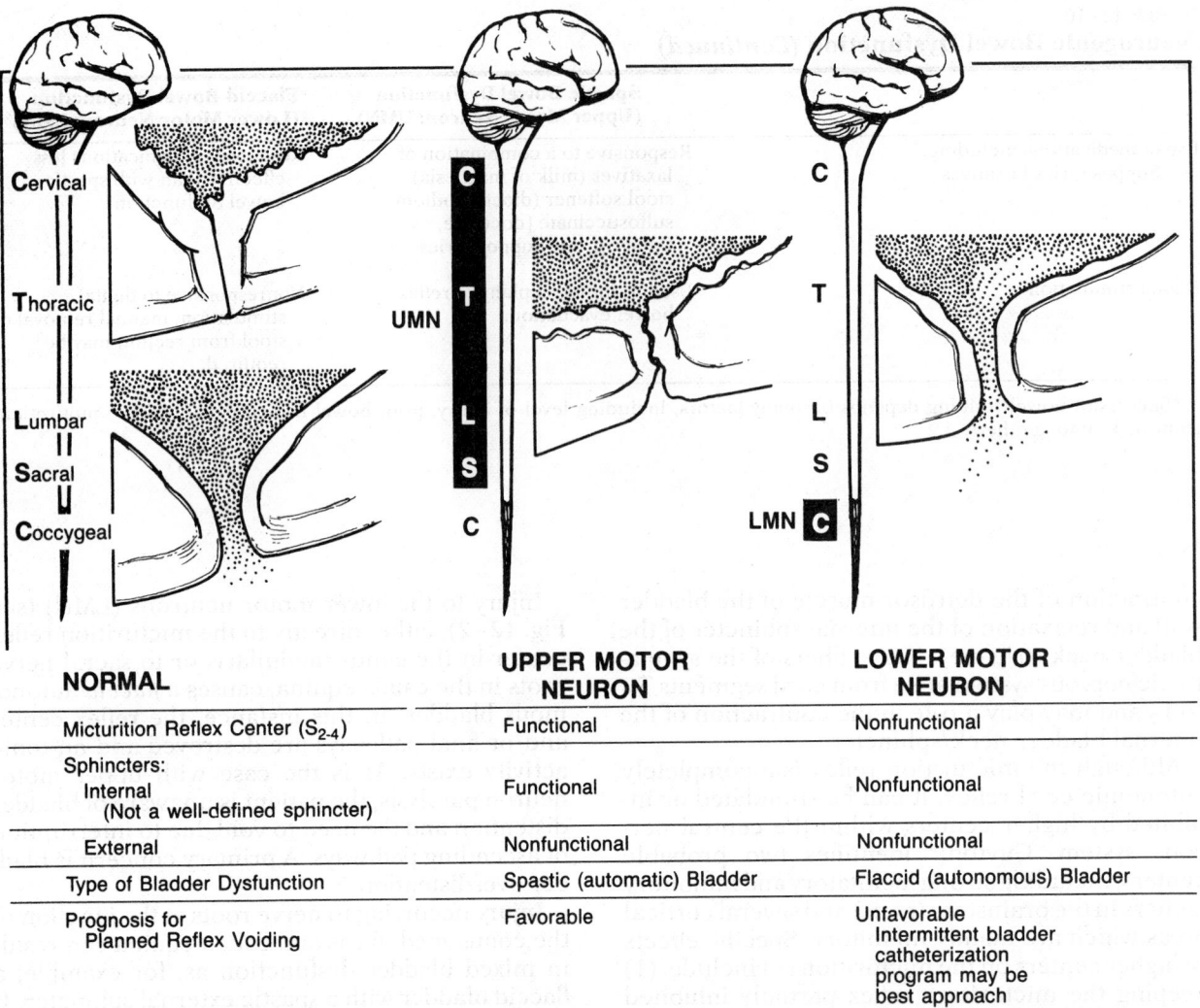

**Figure 12-2.** Innervation underlying bladder function and dysfunction, and potential for achievable bladder management. The level of spinal cord injury largely determines the extent of achievable urinary bladder control. Interruption of UMN innervation results in loss of voluntary, coordinated control of the external sphincter, which becomes completely nonfunctional, and an interruption of ascending sensory information resulting in the inability of the individual to feel bladder fullness or the urge to urinate. The micturition reflex center ($S_{2-4}$) remains functional and continues to exert a tone on the bladder and internal sphincter, thereby resulting in a *spastic* bladder syndrome. In this instance, bladder training is focused on using the intact micturition reflexes to establish some regularity to bladder emptying resulting in a favorable prognosis for planned reflex voiding.

Injury sustained to LMN innervation causes complete interruption of LMN innervation to the bladder and internal sphincter, resulting in an atonic or *flaccid* bladder. The bladder should be assessed on a regular basis to determine bladder overdistention. Prognosis for planned reflex voiding in this instance is unfavorable. Intermittent bladder catheterization may be the best approach.

pine, side-lying, sitting). With each position change the skin must be scrutinized carefully for any disruption of its integrity. Reddened areas that do not blanch or fade within 20–30 minutes after a position change suggest that other positions be assumed and the duration of time spent in a given position be decreased. Pressure that is unrelieved at least every 2 hours places the patient at risk for decubitus ulcer formation.

The skin should also be inspected for open or ulcerated areas and localized edema. Dependent or orthostatic edema is incriminated in the pathophysiology of skin breakdown. It occurs as a result of decreased vasomotor tone and the immobility of paralyzed muscles. Venous return to the heart becomes sluggish, and blood pools in dependent areas: lower extremities when sitting, sacral area in the supine position. The resulting edema interferes with cellular nutrition and increases susceptibility of these tissues to the effects of pressure. Such susceptibility is heightened especially during spinal shock. Frequent position changes are essential to

TABLE 12–11
**Neurogenic Urinary Dysfunction**

| | Spastic (Automatic) Urinary Dysfunction (Upper Motor Neuron; UMN) | Flaccid (Autonomous) Urinary Dysfunction (Lower Motor Neuron; LMN) |
|---|---|---|
| Level of cord injury | Occurs above micturition reflex center ($S_{2-4}$) located within the conus medullaris. | Involves micturition reflex center ($S_{2-4}$) in the conus medullaris and/or sacral nerve roots in the cauda equina. |
| Level of Innervation: | | |
| 1. Local | Stretch receptors in bladder wall and afferent neuron intact. | Same as for UMN. |
| 2. Spinal micturition reflex ($S_{2-4}$) | Micturition reflex intact. Parasympathetic innervation to detrusor muscle and bladder neck sphincter (internal) intact. | Micturition reflex center in conus medullaris and/or sacral nerve roots destroyed. |
| 3. Sympathetic innervation cord segments $T_{11-12}$ | Reflexes may be intact depending on level of cord injury. | Same as for UMN. |
| 4. Brain/higher center | | |
| • Motor | • Nerve pathways between brain and spinal micturition reflex center ($S_{2-4}$) interrupted; loss of inhibiting influences on spinal reflexes from higher centers. | • Loss of final common pathway for transmission of impulses between CNS and detrusor muscle and bladder sphincters (internal and external). |
| • Sensory | • Ascending sensory pathways interrupted; loss of sensation of bladder distention and urge to urinate. | • Same as for UMN. |
| Results of pathology | 1. Loss of UMN innervation. 2. Intact micturition reflexes. 3. Spastic bladder dysfunction. | 1. Loss of LMN innervation. 2. Loss of micturition reflexes. 3. Flaccid bladder dysfunction. |
| Prognosis for bladder control* | Bladder training is aimed at using micturition reflexes and "trigger" stimulus to establish planned reflex voiding. | Unable to establish reflex voiding; intermittent bladder catheterization may be best method for bladder management. |

*Bladder training depends on many factors including level of injury, prior bladder habits, patient/family motivation, and teamwork, among others.

stimulate circulation and prevent tissue edema associated with venous pooling. The skin should be kept clean and dry.

### Nutritional Status

Stress increases energy needs by as much as 50%. Glycogen stores within the body provide an immediate source of energy, but these stores are quickly used up (within 24 hours or less). Once carbohydrate stores are depleted, the body draws on its stores of fats and proteins to provide a source of energy. Gluconeogenesis is the process of breaking down proteins into glucose to be used to meet energy requirements. This catabolism of protein prevents its use for tissue building and repairs. There is an increased loss of nitrogen in the urine, and a negative nitrogen balance ensues. A nitrogen imbalance predisposes the spinal cord-injured patient to massive tissue wasting, severe weight loss, fluid and electrolyte imbalances, infections, and disruption of other body systems.

In the patient with spinal cord injury it is essential to maintain nutritional balance to promote wound healing and prevent complications. Neurologic changes, including spinal shock, paralytic ileus, and immobility, impact virtually on every body system, placing the patient at risk of developing secondary, often life-threatening complications. Malnutrition is a potential complication.

Early on in the acute phase after spinal cord injury, the patient may be hemodynamically unstable with compromised respiratory function. The danger of aspiration pneumonia dictates that the patient receive no oral intake. Presence of a paralytic ileus precludes the use of nasogastric or tube feedings, which could cause gastric dilatation. Bowel distention and dilatation prevent respiratory excursion, further compromising respiratory function. Intravenous fluid therapy alone is inadequate to meet the nutritional requirements of the spinal cord-injured patient. A liter of dextrose 5%/water, for example, provides only 600 calories. The patient becomes at risk to develop a state of malnutrition in 3–5 days.

Total parenteral nutrition (TPN) has become an essential therapeutic modality in treating the patient with spinal cord injury. It provides a source of essential amino acids, glucose, and additives, including electrolytes, vitamins, and minerals, and is administered via a central line. Although not without its potential complications, including, among others, pneumothorax on insertion of the central line and infection that can rapidly progress to septicemia, TPN is nevertheless being used more and more in the treatment of the severely compromised patient.

Administration of TPN requires careful, sophisticated patient care in initiating, maintaining, and monitoring the system. Very strict aseptic technique must be adhered to to prevent sepsis, and the patient must be evaluated daily to determine the response to therapy. A complete nutritional assessment should be obtained within the first 24 hours post injury to determine the patient's baseline nutritional status, to appraise the patient's current nutritional requirement, and to determine how these needs can best be met.

The critical care nurse needs to appreciate those criteria that best reflect progress toward, and maintenance of, a balanced nutritional state. Ongoing evaluation of the patient's response to therapy includes: daily caloric and fluid intake and output; daily weight; vital signs, including body temperature; close monitoring of blood chemistry and hematology data; wound healing; skin integrity; and the patient's overall physical, mental, and emotional state. (For specific details related to nutrition see Chap. 53.)

## Rehabilitation: Ultimate Goal

Rehabilitation is broadly defined as a "dynamic process in which a disabled person is aided in achieving optimum physical, emotional, psychological, social or vocational potential in order to maintain dignity and be as self-fulfilling as possible."[12]

The ultimate goal of rehabilitation of the spinal cord-injured individual is to help him/her to achieve the highest level of personal independence possible within the restrictions and limitations imposed by the injury. The concept of rehabilitation begins at the moment of injury, continues throughout the critical phase, and remains as a progressive, ongoing, dynamic, and lifelong process.

Meticulous and diligent nursing care can make a difference in the quality of life experienced by the patient, his/her family, and significant others. Largely dependent on nursing interventions during the critical phase after spinal cord injury, is the stabilization and maintenance of cardiopulmonary function. Maintenance of a patent airway with effective alveolar ventilation (either spontaneous or via ventilator support) prevents hypercapnia and hypoxemia and protects fragile and highly sensitive nerve tissue from further ischemia, injury, and infarction. Pulmonary complications as, for example, hypostatic pneumonia, which can be life-threatening in the spinal cord-injured patient, are prevented.

During the period of spinal shock (i.e., neurogenic shock), nursing interventions are directed toward maintaining an effective cardiac output and systemic blood pressure to ensure adequate tissue perfusion. Nursing measures (e.g., application of antiembolic stockings to the lower extremities, passive range-of-motion exercises, maintenance of proper body alignment, and diligent and astute ongoing assessments) are instituted to prevent such complications as deep venous thrombosis and pulmonary embolism, which are associated with venous blood pooling, skeletal muscle paralysis, and immobilization.

Nurses must recognize and prevent autonomic dysreflexia, a clinical emergency in spinal cord-injured patients with lesions above the $T_{4-6}$ level. They must minimize those stimuli (e.g., distended bladder with urinary retention, kinking or plugging of a urinary catheter, fecal impaction, wind drafts in the patient's room, and many others) that can precipitate this abnormal sympathetic response. Patient/family education concerned with the recognition and treatment of this phenomenon is a nursing responsibility.

Maintenance of musculoskeletal integrity and prevention of further neurologic damage are major nursing concerns. Cervical immobilization (e.g., via skull tongs, halo apparatus, other) and maintenance of correct body alignment while implementing necessary position changes to prevent pooling of pulmonary secretions, impairment of skin integrity, muscle fatigue, and contractures are vital to the recovery of the patient.

The effectiveness of bowel and urinary management in the spinal cord-injured patient over the long term depends in part on nursing interventions initiated during the critical phase. Ascertaining pre-injury personal habits, diet, and attitudes regarding bowel and urinary control is very important. Early implementation of bowel and urinary control (training) programs and prevention of complications (e.g., constipation, fecal impaction, urinary retention with bladder distention, urinary tract infection) are major patient care considerations.

The critical care nurse must assist the patient/family to stabilize life processes and to begin the rehabilitative process. Assessment of patient and family attitudes, coping and adjustment capabilities, familial resources, and psychosocial, cultural, and economic concerns is initiated during the critical phase. Such data assist in: evaluating the impact of the disability on the patient and family; identifying the need for additional professional assistance; providing a basis for patient/family education; and initiating plans for the patient's eventual discharge to a rehabilitation center and/or home environment.

In a collaborative effort with other members of the interdisciplinary health team the nurse functions to prevent physical and psychologic deterioration, to minimize suffering, and to engage the patient/family as integral, active participants on the health team.[13] Such teamwork begins the moment the patient/family enter the health-care system and enables all aspects of patient care to be approached collectively and simultaneously. Rehabilitation must *not* be viewed as something that begins *after* the acute phase, but rather, the critical care nurse and colleagues in health care must learn to "think rehab" on initial patient contact, and incorporate this concept into their daily practice.

## REFERENCES

1. Hickey, JV: The Clinical Practice of Neurological and Neurosurgical Nursing, ed 2. JB Lippincott, Philadelphia, 1986, p 385.
2. Guyton, AC: Textbook of Medical Physiology, ed 7. WB Saunders, Philadelphia, 1986, p 617.
3. Richmond, TS: A critical care challenge, the patient with a cervical spinal cord injury. Focus on Critical Care 12(2):26, 1985.
4. Bell, J and Hannon, K: Pathophysiology involved in autonomic dysreflexia. J Neurosci Nurs 18(2):86, 1986.
5. Rudy, EB: Advanced Neurological and Neurosurgical Nursing. CV Mosby, St Louis, 1984, p 403.
6. Browner, C, et al: Halo immobilization brace care: An innovative approach. J Neurosci Nurs 19(1):24, 1987.
7. Zejdlik, C: Management of Spinal Cord Injury. Wadsworth Health Sciences Division, Monterey, CA, 1983, p 255.
8. Guyton, AC: Textbook of Medical Physiology, ed 7. WB Saunders, Philadelphia, 1986, p 768.
9. Zejdlik, C: Management of Spinal Cord Injury. Wadsworth Health Sciences Division, Monterey, CA, 1983, p 337.
10. Guyton, AC: Textbook of Medical Physiology, ed 7. WB Saunders, Philadelphia, 1986, p 461.
11. Zejdlik, C: Management of Spinal Cord Injury. Wadsworth Health Sciences Division, Monterey, CA, 1983, p 275.
12. Hickey, JV: The Clinical Practice of Neurological and Neurosurgical Nursing, ed 2. JB Lippincott, Philadelphia, 1986, p 179.
13. Zejdlik, C: Management of Spinal Cord Injury. Wadsworth Health Sciences Division, Monterey, CA, 1983, p 44.

CHAPTER 13

# Nursing Management of the Patient with Neurologic Dysfunction: Meningitis, Seizures, Guillain-Barré Syndrome, Myasthenia Gravis, and Amyotrophic Lateral Sclerosis

## CHAPTER OUTLINE



## LEARNING OBJECTIVES

**At the end of this chapter, you should be able to:**

1. State the significance of an infectious disease of the central nervous system in terms of its underlying pathophysiology, clinical course, and potential for complete recovery.
2. Identify data obtained from the patient's clinical history and physical examination that is supportive of a diagnosis of meningitis.

## LEARNING OBJECTIVES—*CONTINUED*

3. Delineate tentative nursing diagnoses that provide the basis for the nursing management of the patient with meningitis.
4. Define seizure and status epilepticus.
5. Specify major classifications of seizures and etiologic considerations.
6. Describe four phases of a generalized tonic-clonic seizure and clinical manifestations.
7. State approach to drug therapy in the emergent treatment of status epilepticus, and implications for nursing care.
8. List tentative nursing diagnoses that provide the basis for nursing management of the patient with status epilepticus.
9. Report on Guillain-Barré syndrome, its etiology and pathophysiology.
10. Identify the key clinical manifestations of Guillain-Barré syndrome, its clinical course and potential life-threatening complications.
11. Delineate tentative nursing diagnoses that provide the basis for the nursing management of the patient with Guillain-Barré syndrome.
12. Report on myasthenia gravis, its pathophysiology and clinical presentation.
13. Differentiate myasthenic crisis from cholinergic crisis.
14. Identify tentative nursing diagnoses that provide the basis for nursing management of the patient in myasthenic crisis.
15. Describe pathophysiology underlying the clinical presentation of amyotrophic lateral sclerosis.
16. Identify tentative nursing diagnoses that provide the basis for the nursing management of the patient with amyotrophic lateral sclerosis during the acute phase.

## MENINGITIS

Meningitis is an infectious process causing acute inflammation of the meningeal coverings of the brain and spinal cord. Once having gained access to the subarachnoid space and the cerebrospinal fluid contained therein, the infectious process can extend and spread throughout the subarachnoid space to reach the ventricles of the brain. Meningitis is an extremely serious infection requiring prompt recognition and treatment if neurologic sequelae are to be prevented or minimized.

### Pathogenesis

Infections of the meninges can be caused by bacteria, viruses, parasites, or fungi. Most commonly, bacteria are implicated in the pathogenesis of meningitis. *Neisseria meningitidis* (meningococcal meningitis) and *Streptococcus pneumoniae* (pneumococcal meningitis) are strains frequently associated with meningitis in adults; *Hemophilus influenzae* (haemophilus meningitis) is the most common strain occurring in children.

Viral meningitis, when it does occur, is frequently a sequela of an antecedent viral infection, most commonly mumps. Viruses have also been implicated in a possible mechanism underlying autoimmunity (see Chap. 54).

#### *Mechanisms of Pathogenesis*

Meningitis may occur as a primary focal infection of the meninges or as a secondary infection following hematogenous dissemination of bacterial emboli or infectious thrombi from a primary focal infection occurring elsewhere in the body.

Meningitis may occur secondarily to infections involving other cranial structures such as the ears (e.g., otitis media, mastoiditis), the orbits, or nasal sinuses (e.g., sinusitis); it may follow disruption of the blood-brain barrier (see Fig. 6-11); or it may occur as a result of craniocerebral trauma in which the integrity of the meninges has been impaired.

Less commonly, meningitis can result from the erosion or rupture of a brain abscess into the subarachnoid space. A small number of cases of meningitis have been attributed to iatrogenic causes associated, for example, with lumbar puncture or craniotomy procedures.

### Pathophysiology

Clinically, two types of meningitis have been identified based largely on examination of cerebrospinal fluid: suppurative and nonsuppurative.[1] In suppurative meningitis the cerebrospinal fluid is characteristically turbid in appearance; it has a high leukocytosis with neutrophils as the predominant cell type; it has an increased protein and a low to normal glucose content. In nonsuppurative meningitis the cerebrospinal fluid is characteristically clear; the leukocyte count is low with a predominance of lymphocytes; the protein is increased, but the glucose is within normal limits.

Suppurative meningitis is associated with infections of bacterial origin, primarily those previously mentioned (i.e., meningococcal, pneumococcal, and hemophilus), and usually occurs subsequent to an upper respiratory infection. This antecedent infection may be subclinical (meningococcal) or symptomatic (pneumococcal and hemophilus), and the causative organisms are usually disseminated via the bloodstream to the meninges. Nonsuppurative or aseptic meningitis is primarily viral in origin; its clinical presentation is less severe; and it is usually self-limiting with complete recovery.

Bacterial invasion of the meninges initiates an inflammatory response (Table 13–1), the consequence of which is the production of a suppurative exudate within the subarachnoid space. The presence of this exudate accounts for the characteristic findings in the cerebrospinal fluid (as described above). The exudate is especially irritating to the many blood vessels traversing the subarachnoid space and some of these blood vessels subsequently become engorged, rupture, and/or thrombose. The infection may spread into the brain parenchyma via perivascular spaces that penetrate the pia mater to supply the underlying tissue; or it may involve cranial and spinal nerves. The exudate in the cerebrospinal fluid may interfere with its circulation and reabsorption and predisposes to obstructive hydrocephalus and an increase in intracranial pressure.

TABLE 13–1
**Phases of the Inflammatory Response**

*"Rubor et tumor cum calore et dolore"* by Cornelius Celsus, Roman writer, First Century AD.

In response to trauma, infection, or other insult, a complex of sequential changes occurs at the site of tissue damage, which constitute the inflammatory process. Briefly, these changes include:

A. The release by injured cells of enhanced amounts of chemical substances including histamine, bradykinin, and serotonin; proteolytic enzymes.

B. The occurrence of a vascular response mediated by these chemical substances and characterized by:
- A transient vasodilation increasing local blood flow to the injured tissues (*rubor*—erythemia) (*calore*—heat or warmth)
- An immediate increase in vascular permeability resulting in transudative extravasation of fluid from intravascular to interstitial space (*tumor*—swelling or edema) (*dolore*—pain).

C. The occurrence of a cellular response facilitated by the vascular changes and characterized by:
- Migration of leukocytes (initially neutrophils followed by monocytes, and later by lymphocytes) from the circulation into the area of damaged tissues where they trigger several important processes:
  - *Chemotaxis*: Force of attraction on circulating leukocytes facilitating their movement to area of tissue injury.
  - *Phagocytosis*: Force exerted by neutrophils involving destruction of pathologic antigen via engulfment and/or intracellular killing, or force exerted by neutrophils and macrophages wherein the pathologic antigen is captured for presentation to lymphocytes with triggering of the
  - *Immune response*: Via cell-mediated or humoral (antibodies) mechanisms.
  - *Complement System*: Potent mediator of inflammatory response, triggered by antibody and nonantibody dependent events.

D. The occurrence of wound healing by:
- Tissue regeneration: Replacement of lost cells with similar cell types.
- Tissue repair: Replacement of lost cells with connective tissue usually with scar formation.

## Clinical Presentation

Clinically, the early signs and symptoms of meningitis reflect meningeal irritation and include severe headache, photophobia, nuchal rigidity, seizures, and the classic Kernig's and Brudzinski's signs (see Chap. 7). The patient may complain of general malaise and may appear to be lethargic with a shortened attention span.

As the patient becomes septic with hematogenous dissemination of the infectious organism(s), toxic manifestations appear and include hyperpyrexia, shaking chills, hypotension, and rapid, shallow breathing. Alterations in the level of consciousness and mentation commonly occur. A skin rash (meningococcal meningitis) may also be observed.

Progressive accumulation of exudate and cerebrospinal fluid (with obstructive hydrocephalus) in the subarachnoid space is accompanied by a consequent increase in intracranial pressure. Clinically, the patient experiences an altered level of consciousness; rapid shallow breathing may give way to a Cheyne-Stokes respiratory pattern; and papilledema may be observed on fundoscopy. Vomiting frequently occurs, placing the patient at risk of aspiration. Blood pressure may become elevated.

## Diagnosis

The diagnosis of meningitis is suspected based on the patient's clinical history and physical examination; it is confirmed by laboratory examination and culture of cerebrospinal fluid.

Components of the clinical history are examined in detail in Chapter 7. In patients with possible meningitis, it is also important to elicit information concerned with the following: Has the patient had any recent upper respiratory infections, sinusitis, tonsilitis, mastoiditis, or otitis media? Has the patient had, or been exposed to, mumps, herpes simplex, mononucleosis, meningitis, other viral infections?

Has the patient sustained a recent head injury or trauma? Has there been recent exposure to, or ingestion of, toxic chemicals or poisons? What drugs does the patient take and why? Is there an allergic hypersensitivity to any drug? If so, what kind of reaction is experienced? Has the patient had seizures observed by family and/or significant others? How are they described? Focal? Generalized tonic-clonic? Opisthotonos (i.e., a form of spasm in which head and heels are bent backward and body bowed forward; in meningitis, the patient's neck is rigid)? Has there been a recent change in the patient's behavior or personality? If so, in what way?

It is also important to establish if the patient has had any illness or condition involving the immune system. Has the patient experienced frequent bacterial infections, altered serum immunoglobulin levels? Or is there a history of recurrent viral or fungal infections? Has the patient been exposed to acquired immune deficiency syndrome (AIDS)? Has the patient received any recent immunizations? Or traveled recently? Is the patient receiving long-term corticosteroid therapy? If so, why? Is the patient receiving chemotherapy? Radiation therapy? Is the patient receiving parenteral nutritional therapy? If so, for how long? Why?

In the physical examination the patient is assessed for signs of meningeal irritation; fever, malaise, presence of sore throat, nausea, vomiting; photophobia, diplopia, nystagmus, or pain with ocular movements. It is also important to assess for a rash reflective of petechial or purpural skin lesions. Endothelial fragility may occur in response to the infectious process precipitating capillary disruption and bleeding.

## Management of the Patient with Meningitis

### *Medical Interventions*

The mainstay of medical intervention is the administration of antibiotic therapy. Initial therapy may include a combination of penicillins (e.g., ampicillin) and an aminoglycoside (e.g., gentamicin) until the causative organism(s) is definitely established. Chloramphenicol is frequently prescribed because it penetrates the blood–brain barrier exceedingly well. While these drugs are especially effective for treating bacterial meningitis they are not without adverse reactions. (For nursing implications related to drug therapy, see Appendix A.)

Institution of supportive therapeutic modalities depends on the severity of the patient's clinical status. Analgesics (usually non-narcotic) are prescribed for headache and pain relief; an antipyretic is prescribed for control of fever. In patients at risk of developing an increase in intracranial pressure, intubation and mechanical ventilatory therapy may be initiated. Intravenous fluid and vasopressor therapies are instituted to treat septic shock; cardiac status is monitored continuously for significant dysrhythmias.

### *Nursing Management*

In caring for the patient with meningitis, an infectious disease, isolation precautions may be instituted and enforced as per hospital protocol. Antibiotics are administered as prescribed, and the patient's condition is monitored closely for the response to therapy and for possible adverse drug reactions. The patient's temperature is also monitored closely, with antipyretic medication administered as necessary. Tepid sponge baths or hypothermia therapy may be instituted for exceedingly high body temperatures (i.e., >103°F; 39.5°C).

To make the patient as comfortable as possible, environmental stimuli should be reduced, and the patient's room should be kept dark and quiet as much as possible. Nursing care activities should be planned to enable the patient to have long rest periods. Seizure precautions should be in effect.

Seizure precautions are focused on protecting the patient from seizure-related injury. Side rails may be padded and kept in the up position; the bed is placed in the low position. An oral airway is placed conspicuously at the patient's bedside, and suction equipment is available and ready to use. In patients at risk of having seizures, a laryngoscope and resuscitative equipment should be placed nearby and ready to use. (For other nursing care considerations related to seizure activity, actual or potential, see the section below entitled "Seizures" and Table 13–4.)

Any infection involving the nervous system can be distressing to patient, family, and/or significant others. The presence of neurologic deficits can be especially frightening, raising the concern of permanent neurologic sequelae and even death. It is important to keep patient and/or family members informed as to the patient's status and to give them the opportunity to ask questions, discuss their perceptions of the situation, and to vent fears, anger, and concerns.

It is essential to establish a rapport and to help the patient/family better understand the patient's underlying problem, current status, response to therapy, and overall prognosis. Misinformation can be corrected, and anxiety levels can be reduced. Stressors can be identified, and methods of coping can be explored. It is important to include patient/family in decision-making regarding care, and in assessing the need for patient/family education.

Often the patient's nurse helps to coordinate the various therapies administered to the patient, and to act as a liaison between the patient, family, and other health-care providers. The patient/family coping mechanisms need to be assessed, identified, and reinforced. The nurse needs to be emotionally supportive, to be accessible, and to take the time to listen. Assistance should be provided to help the patient and/or family members to communicate, to recognize their strengths individually and collectively, and to identify other family and community resources.

**Tentative Nursing Diagnoses: Basis for Treating Patient with Meningitis.** Specific nursing diagnoses, patient outcomes, and nursing interventions in the management of the patient with increased intracranial pressure are included in Table 8–2. Other tentative nursing diagnoses that provide the basis for the nursing treatment of the patient with meningitis include:

1. Alteration in comfort: Severe headache, photophobia, related to:
   A. Meningeal irritation.
   B. Increase in intracranial pressure associated with accumulation of exudate in the subarachnoid space; and/or consequent obstructive hydrocephalus.
2. Anxiety, related to:
   A. Presence of neurologic deficits.
   B. Fear of permanent neurologic sequelae.
   C. Fear of dying.
3. Potential for physiologic injury associated with seizures, related to:
   A. Meningeal irritation (see Table 8–2).
4. Thought processes, alteration in, related to:
   A. Altered level of consciousness and mentation.
5. Fluid and electrolyte balance, alteration in, related to:
   A. Nothing-by-mouth (NPO) status.
   B. Gastric decompression (see Table 8–2).
6. Knowledge deficit: Meningitis—implications for recovery.

## SEIZURES

A seizure is a spontaneous paroxysmal episode of abnormal neuronal activity, which interrupts the ongoing mental and behavioral activities of the individual. This abnormal neuronal activity may be characterized as excessive and disorganized electrical discharges from neurons within the brain, and it is manifested clinically by transient alterations in the level of consciousness, impairment of mentation, and disturbances of sensorimotor function.

### Pathophysiology

The mechanism underlying seizure activity remains undefined. It may involve an autonomous paroxysmal discharge of electrical activity that can be enhanced or minimized depending on the neurotransmitter that is active on the postsynaptic membrane.[2] Such activity, originating in one epileptic focus, may induce similar activity in synaptically related areas. The electrical discharges reflect rapid, repetitive depolarization of the involved cells. An intracellular accumulation of sodium, with a concomitant depletion of intracellular potassium, may underlie the continuous hyperexcited state. Cessation of seizure activity is associated with a period of hyperpolarization during which there is a reversal of polarity. (For further details related to electrophysiology, see Chap. 6.)

During a seizure, the cerebral oxygen consumption increases by as much as 60%. To meet the enhanced metabolic demands there is a substantial increase in cerebral blood flow. This increase in cerebral blood flow can respond to the metabolic demands associated with seizure activity providing that hypoxemia and hypoglycemia do not develop. In the scenario of repeated seizures (as in status epilepticus), oxygen and glucose consumption by skeletal muscle contraction, in conjunction with periods of apnea, rapidly depletes oxygen and nutritive stores, leading to hypoxemia, hypercapnia, and hypoglycemia. The increase in cellular lactate associated with anaerobic metabolism further complicates the pathophysiologic state. The end result is an energy debt, which rapidly leads to cellular exhaustion.

The hyperactivity of an epileptogenic focus can result in partial and generalized seizure activity. *Partial* seizures may be caused by a localized hyperexcited focus, which eventually ceases; or the hyperactivity may spread to synaptically related areas, but does not involve the entire brain. Enough resistance is offered by adjacent cells so that impulse firing stops. When the rapid, repetitive electrical discharges spread throughout the central nervous system, the resulting seizure is described as a *generalized* seizure.

### Classification of Seizures

The classification system most frequently cited in the literature is that of the International Classification of Epileptic Seizures, which is based on the clinical nature of the onset of the seizure. The two major classes are partial and generalized seizures.

#### Partial Seizures

Partial seizures are usually unilateral, involving a localized or focal area of the brain. These seizures occur without loss of consciousness and involve one category of symptoms, sensory or motor. The *jacksonian* seizure is an example of a partial seizure. It is characterized by a focal onset, as, for example, a twitching of the fingers, and progressively increases in a step-wise fashion. The seizure is said to "march along" as the successive parts of the body become involved, and this activity is reflective of the spread of seizure activity within the brain.

#### Generalized Seizures

Generalized seizures reflect involvement of the entire brain and are characterized at the onset by a sudden loss of consciousness and immediate bilateral symmetric motor activity. Two of the more frequently occurring types of generalized seizures include the petit mal and tonic-clonic seizures.

**Absence (Petit Mal) Seizures.** An absence, or petit mal, seizure is characterized by short lapses of consciousness lasting but a few seconds. There may be a vacant stare, a brief pause in conversation, or rapid eye-blinking. This type of generalized seizure occurs most frequently in young children and may disappear completely after puberty.

**Tonic-Clonic Seizures.** The tonic-clonic (grand mal) seizure is the classic epileptic seizure and is seen frequently in the critical care setting and in the scenario of status epilepticus. It may begin with an aura (i.e., a sensory and/or emotional phenomenon such as a momentary visual or auditory sensation, dizziness, a taste or smell, or a peculiar abdominal sensation). The seizure begins with a sudden loss of consciousness and is characterized by an opisthotonus posturing (i.e., a stiffening of the body in an arched position), tonic followed by clonic movements, and autonomic nervous system dysfunction such as bladder and/or bowel incontinence.

## Etiologic Considerations

Although most seizures are idiopathic (i.e., of unknown cause), seizures occurring in critically ill patients are often symptomatic of an underlying disease (e.g., hepatic or renal failure, cerebrovascular disease). The *major* immediate cause of seizures is patient noncompliance with prescribed anticonvulsant therapy. Head trauma (e.g., epidural, subdural, or intracellular hematomas; brain laceration) is a common cause of generalized seizures. Such seizures may result from actual or structural damage to the skull and/or brain, or they may occur secondary to the metabolic derangements caused by cerebral ischemia, cerebral edema, and/or infarction.

Metabolic alterations, including hypoxemia, hypercapnia, acid–base and electrolyte imbalances, and hypoglycemia, have all been implicated in neuronal dysfunction predisposing to seizure activity. Hypoxemia and hypoglycemia result in a depletion of energy stores so vital for the maintenance of ionic gradients and the resting membrane potential; electrolyte imbalance disrupts the integrity of the cell membrane and its permeability to diffusion of ions into or out of the cell. As mentioned previously in the discussion of pathophysiology, an intracellular accumulation of sodium and a depletion of intracellular potassium ions may be involved in the mechanism(s) underlying seizure activity.

Decreased serum levels of ionized calcium are known to increase neuromuscular irritability and may precipitate tetany; prolonged or severe depression of serum calcium levels can alter myocardial function.

Other altered states of metabolism known to precipitate seizures in critically ill patients include hepatic coma, uremic encephalopathy, hyperglycemic, hyperosmolar nonketotic coma (HHNK), and chronic alcohol withdrawal.

Focal or generalized seizures may accompany a variety of disorders associated with cerebrovascular disease, including cerebral thrombosis or embolism, subarachnoid hemorrhage with vasospasm, and hypertensive encephalopathy. Local tissue injury associated with cerebral hemorrhage is known to give rise to focal or generalized seizure activity.

Infectious processes, such as meningitis, encephalitis, brain abscess, and high fever, are known to predispose to seizure activity. Likewise, brain tumors and metastatic lesions to the brain may directly irritate brain tissue, setting up an epileptogenic focus.

## Tonic-Clonic Seizures: Phases and Clinical Manifestations

The tonic-clonic seizure involves major motor activity accompanied by a loss of consciousness. Four phases have been identified:

1. *Pre-ictal or aura phase*—The primary manifestation of this phase is the occurrence of an aura or prodrome. Most patients probably have no definitive warning of an impending seizure. More often, vague signs and symptoms occur, suggesting possible signs of an aura. These include restlessness, irritability, a sense of uneasiness, confusion, nausea, and visual disturbances, among others. If a definitive aura does occur, it may provide clues as to the origin of the seizure. This prodromal period may precede the actual tonic-clonic seizure by several hours or days.
2. *Tonic phase*—This phase is characterized by a sudden loss of consciousness (the suddenness may result in injury due to falling), accompanied by generalized contraction of muscles throughout the body (tonic convulsion). This phase may be heralded by a shrill cry due to the forced exhalation of air through closed vocal cords as the muscles of the trunk become contracted. The body stiffens in the opisthotonus position, the jaw snaps shut, and the tongue may be bitten. Respirations cease during this phase, which may last as long as a minute; cyanosis may become apparent. The pupils dilate and remain fixed in response to severe hypoxia. The heart rate slows in response to vagal stimulation; bladder and possibly bowel incontinence may occur. This phase lasts approximately 15 seconds and terminates abruptly as the clonic phase begins.
3. *Clonic phase*—This phase is characterized by

violent, rhythmic jerking movements accompanied by strenuous and loud hyperventilation (stertorous respirations). The face is contorted, the eyes roll back, and there is excessive salivation with frothing from the mouth. Profuse sweating and tachycardia may be evident. The clonic jerking movements, the result of simultaneous contraction and relaxation of opposing muscle groups, eventually subside.

4. *Postictal phase*—The clonic jerking and increased muscle tone are gradually replaced by flaccidity. The patient may experience a period of unconsciousness lasting from a few minutes to one-half hour. Upon regaining consciousness, the patient may appear drowsy or confused, complain of headache and muscle aches, and may need to sleep for several hours after the seizure because of neuromuscular exhaustion attributed to hypoxemia and hypoglycemia. There is usually no recollection of the seizure.

### *Seizure Activity: Assessment Considerations*

In assessing the patient with seizures, an initial consideration is to determine whether the signs and symptoms are, in fact, seizures or a disorder that mimics seizures. Table 13–2 lists major factors to be considered when assessing seizure activity. A thorough history obtained from the patient, family, and/or significant others will best characterize the seizure type, cause, duration, prior treatment, and current status.

As information regarding seizure activity is examined, it is important to appreciate that seizures are dynamic and changing. Information derived from one seizure episode may not apply to succeeding episodes. Furthermore, depending on the underlying cause of the seizure activity, such responses may be associated at different times with a variety of disease processes. The occurrence of a seizure may be an early symptom of an occult pathologic process, which otherwise might not be apparent.

In addition to eliciting a careful history, the physical examination may reveal neurologic defects associated with recent or remote neurologic lesions (e.g., prior trauma, cranial surgery, cerebrovascular accident, infection, or longstanding seizure disorder). The presence of a systemic infection or infection involving cranial structures, such as the ears, nasal sinuses, or the orbits, increases the possibility of intracranial infection.

Laboratory studies assist in delineating metabolic disturbances that may underlie seizure activity. Examples of such disorders include hypoglycemia, fluid and electrolyte disturbances (e.g., water intoxication), renal dysfunction, hepatic encephalopathy, and anemia. Patients on long-term anticonvulsant therapy should have appropriate blood level assays for the drugs in question.

TABLE 13–2
**Assessing Seizure Activity: Major Considerations**

Major factors to be considered when assessing seizure activity include the following:

1. The time of day the seizure(s) occurred and the frequency of occurrence.
2. The activity the patient was involved in when the seizure occurred.
3. The precipitating event/other precipitating factors.
4. A description of any warning signs or aura experienced by the patient.
5. A detailed description of the onset of the seizure:
   A. Was there a shrill cry?
   B. Was there loss of consciousness? Did the patient fall?
   C. In what part of the body did seizure activity begin? How did it proceed?
   D. What type of movement occurred?
6. A description of the phases of the seizure and the progression from one phase to another.
7. Notation of any changes in the size and reactivity of the pupils; evidence of dysconjugate or deviant gaze.
8. Presence of urinary or bowel incontinence.
9. The duration of the apneic period if present; evidence of cyanosis of lips, mucous membranes, and nailbeds.
10. The duration of the entire seizure, as well as that of each specific phase.
11. Evidence of altered level of consciousness; or state of unconsciousness throughout the entire seizure.
12. Notation of patient's behavior after seizure:
    A. Alert, drowsy, confused?
    B. Evidence of weakness or paralysis—unilateral or bilateral?
    C. Fatigue, muscle aching?
    D. Length of sleep after seizure?

## Status Epilepticus

Status epilepticus is a state of recurrent, successive, and/or prolonged seizure activity or convulsions without intervening periods of physiologic recovery by the patient. The patient experiences successive tonic-clonic seizures with each succeeding seizure occurring before the postictal phase of the preceding seizure has ended. Because of the potential for developing anoxia, cardiac dysrhythmias, and acidosis, the occurrence of status epilepticus is a life-threatening medical emergency. The mortality can be as high as 10–12% in cases of status epilepticus unrelieved within 1–2 hours, and there is a substantial risk of permanent neurologic sequelae.[3]

### *Management of Status Epilepticus*

**Drug Therapy.** The drug of choice in the emergent treatment of status epilepticus is diazepam (Valium). Because diazepam is short acting it is usually administered with phenytoin or phenobarbital. Dosages, adverse reactions, and nursing implications related to these drugs are presented in Table 13–3. (See Appendix A.)

A major concern in treating status epilepticus is respiratory depression and laryngospasm. Conse-

TABLE 13-3
## Drugs Used to Treat Status Epilepticus*

| Drug | Description | Use | Dosage and Administration | Adverse Reactions | Nursing Implications |
|---|---|---|---|---|---|
| Diazepam (Valium) | Drug of choice in treatment of status epilepticus. A short acting anticonvulsant; seizures may recur within 30 min. Frequently given in conjunction with phenytoin for treatment of status epilepticus. | Functions to interrupt seizure activity; it cannot prevent further seizures. | Intravenous administration. *Dose Range*: 5-10 mg IV. Rate of administration. *IV push*: 10 mg. *IV drip*: 2-5 mg/min to maximum of 20 mg/24 hr. | Respiratory: Depression and possible respiratory arrest. Cardiovascular: Hypertension, tachycardia. Eyes: Blurred vision, diplopia, nystagmus. Renal: Urinary retention. CNS: Drowsiness, fatigue, headache, slurred speech. | Do not mix or dilute with other drugs or solutions. Do not add to IV fluids. Resuscitative equipment in readiness. |
| Phenytoin (Dilantin) | Formerly, diphenyl-hydantoin. Often used in conjunction with phenobarbital. | Tonic-clonic (grand mal) generalized seizures. Status epilepticus. Effective in prevention of seizure activity or transmission of seizures. | Initial dose: ~500 mg IV at 50 mg/min, slow intravenous infusion. Maintenance dose: 3-7 mg/kg/day PO, IV, or IM in 1 to 3 individual doses. Use IV line containing normal saline; phenytoin precipitates in dextrose solutions. | Cardiovascular: Potential for dys-rhythmias-brady-cardia, heart block, and ventricular fibrillation. • ECG continuous monitoring. • Blood pressure. • Hypertension. Respiratory depression. CNS: Nystagmus, diplopia, drowsiness, lethargy. Hypersensitivity: Pruritus, fever. | For parenteral administration use only special diluent. Margin between therapeutic and toxic doses is very small. Solubility of phenytoin is pH dependent; avoid mixing with other drugs or solutions. Filter within IV line should be used. |
| Phenobarbital (Luminal) Phenobarbital sodium (Luminal Sodium) | Used to control status epilepticus when diazepam and phenytoin have failed. Most widely used anticonvulsant. Often given in conjunction with phenytoin. | Used in management of tonic-clonic (grand mal) generalized seizures. Status epilepticus. Other seizures states. | Intravenous administration for management of acute seizures: *Dose*: 200-600 mg IV push. IV doses should be administered at a rate not to exceed 60 mg/min. | Respiratory depression. Barbiturates induce hepatic microsomal enzyme activity and may decrease effects of other drugs. Overdosage: Respiratory depression, pupillary constriction, oliguria, circulatory collapse, pulmonary edema. Associated with IV use: Coughing, hiccoughing, laryngospasm. Contraindications: Sensitivity to barbiturates, severe respiratory disease. | Monitor respiratory rate and rhythm. Solutions for injections should not be used if a precipitate is present or if the solution is not clear. Constantly assess patient during IV use, resuscitation equipment available. Increased secretions, may need suctioning. |

*(continued)*

TABLE 13–3
**Drugs Used to Treat Status Epilepticus***

| Drug | Description | Use | Dosage and Administration | Adverse Reactions | Nursing Implications |
|---|---|---|---|---|---|
| Pentobarbital (Nembutal) | A rapidly acting barbiturate. | Use in the emergency treatment of status epilepticus when diazepam and phenytoin have failed. | Dose in treatment of seizures: 100–500 mg by slow IV push not to exceed 50 mg/min. | Doses that exceed 50 mg/min can precipitate laryngospasm, respiratory depression, and hypotension.<br>This drug has additive effects when given with other central nervous system depressants. | Pentobarbital is highly alkaline; extravasation may cause local tissue injury.<br>Prepare solutions for IV infusion in $D_5W$.<br>Patient must be mechanically ventilated. |

*General anesthesia considered if anticonvulsant therapy is unsuccessful.

quently, these patients are usually intubated, and mechanical ventilation is initiated. If seizures persist, general anesthesia is considered because the seizures must be *stopped if the patient is to survive.* Pentobarbital (Nembutal) is usually the drug of choice in this event. If the patient becomes hypotensive, hydration and vasopressor (e.g., dopamine) therapy may be indicated.

Controlling seizure activity requires that the underlying cause and precipitating factors be determined and appropriate treatment implemented. In the critical care setting, this may mean diagnosis and treatment of secondary metabolic disturbances associated with head trauma, intracranial surgery, drug overdose, or toxicity related to anticonvulsant therapy. Therapy is focused on treating underlying respiratory, cardiovascular, renal, and liver dysfunction.

### *Nursing Management*

Therapeutic goals of nursing treatment of the patient with status epilepticus are focused on sustaining vital functions, including maintaining respiration and oxygenation, controlling seizures, protecting the patient from injury, and preventing complications.

**Airway Management.** Maintenance of patent airway is of primary concern because *hypoxemia* predisposes to brain damage. During a seizure, support the head in a manner that allows secretions to drain out of the mouth rather than down into the pharynx. This reduces risk of aspiration. If possible, remove dentures, food, or other substances from the mouth and insert an oral airway. *Do not try to force* any objects into the patient's mouth during a seizure. *Do not try to pry* the mouth open when the teeth are clenched. *Do not insert* fingers into the patient's mouth.

Loosen any constricting clothing from neck and chest to allow for respiratory excursion and observation. Assess breathing pattern, length of apneic period, cyanosis, labored breathing. If necessary, use suction to help maintain airway patency; ventilate and oxygenate with a hand resuscitator. Anticipate endotracheal intubation and initiation of mechanical ventilation. Appropriate equipment for these modalities should be available at the patient's bedside. Obtain sample for arterial blood gas analysis.

**Seizure Precautions — Patient Safety.** There is always the potential for patient injury related to seizure activity. A major nursing responsibility is to protect the patient from possible injury. Factors concerned with seizure precautions and patient safety are listed in Table 13–4. Neurologic assessment and observation for seizure activity should be ongoing, and findings should be documented accordingly.

**Maintenance of Cardiovascular Function.** Continuous cardiac monitoring is essential because of possible cardiac dysrhythmias associated with hypoxemia and administration of phenytoin. Phenytoin has a narrow therapeutic index, and elevated levels of the drug can predispose to serious cardiac dysrhythmias. It is essential that serial levels of phenytoin be ascertained and monitored. Vital signs should also be monitored closely. Drugs used to treat seizures can have a hypotensive effect. Adequate hydration is essential. Urine output should be closely monitored to ensure adequate renal perfusion.

TABLE 13–4
**Seizure Precautions: Patient Safety**

Nursing care considerations concerned with seizure precautions and patient safety include:

1. Side rails padded and kept in up position. (Patients with a seizure disorder may request not to have their bed rails padded due to the stigma often associated with seizure disorder.)
2. Bed placed in low position.
3. Oral airway conspicuously placed at head of bed.
4. Laryngoscope and resuscitative equipment available nearby.
5. Suction equipment available and ready for use.
6. Drugs used for treatment of seizures immediately available.
7. Oxygen source available and ready for use.
8. Use of rectal rather than oral thermometer.
9. Removal of all potentially harmful objects and unnecessary furniture from bedside.
10. No smoking allowed by patient and/or visitors.

**Maintenance of Metabolic Functions.** Metabolic activity associated with seizures include acid–base and electrolyte disturbances. The sustained contractions of skeletal muscle and cessation of respirations associated with the tonic phase of grand mal seizures place the patient at risk of developing acidemia. Laboratory and clinical parameters reflective of the patient's acid–base and electrolytes status must be meticulously monitored. Intake and output should be closely monitored in conjunction with serum electrolyte levels.

Serial serum glucose levels also need to be monitored. Motor activity associated with seizure activity can be very energy consuming. Hypoglycemia needs to be avoided because it can predispose to altered neurologic function and seizure activity.

**Maintenance of Psychologic and Emotional Integrity.** The occurrence of seizures can be a frightening experience for patient and family. The nurse plays an especially important role in helping the patient and family to understand the underlying disease, its clinical course, and expectations of full recovery. Timely and appropriate explanations help to dispel fears and misconceptions, while reassuring patient and family that they are active participants in the health-care process.

**Tentative Nursing Diagnoses: Basis for Treating Patient with Status Epilepticus.** Tentative nursing diagnoses that provide the basis for the nursing treatment of the patient with status epilepticus include:

1. Breathing pattern, ineffective, related to:
   A. Altered respiratory mechanics associated with tonic phase of grand mal seizure.
2. Airway clearance, ineffective, related to:
   A. Inability to handle secretions during seizure.
3. Potential for self injury, related to:
   A. Seizure activity.
   B. Aspiration.
4. Knowledge deficit, related to:
   A. Understanding of seizure activity.
   B. Medication regimen and follow-up care.
5. Communication, impaired, related to:
   A. Seizure activity and altered state of consciousness.
6. Coping, ineffective: Individual and family, related to:
   A. Misconceptions regarding seizure disorder.

## GUILLAIN-BARRÉ SYNDROME

Guillain-Barré syndrome (GBS), also referred to as polyradiculoneuritis and acute idiopathic polyradiculopathy, is a rapidly developing, progressive, and self-limiting condition distinguished by an inflammatory process involving the peripheral nervous system (PNS). The condition may evolve clinically with severe paralysis and respiratory arrest. It is characterized by a demyelination and degeneration of the myelin sheath of peripheral nerves, including cranial and spinal nerves, dorsal root ganglia, and the ventral and dorsal spinal roots (see Chap. 6). The pathology of GBS is usually reversible with good potential for complete recovery within weeks to months in most cases. Mortality, when it does occur, is usually associated with respiratory complications.

Guillain-Barré syndrome can produce total body paralysis while mental processes remain completely intact. For the afflicted individual and family, the experience can be devastating as the integrity of the individual's life processes becomes disrupted and function is compromised. Treatment requires supportive care to maintain vital functions and prevent complications until such time as the pathophysiologic processes reverse themselves.

### Etiology

The precise etiology of Guillain-Barré syndrome remains unknown, but an infectious process and/or autoimmune phenomenon has been implicated in its causation. Its association with illnesses of viral origin is well documented. The onset of Guillain-Barré syndrome is most commonly preceded by a febrile illness of probable viral origin, occurring approximately 1–3 weeks prior to the onset of neurologic symptoms. This prodromal illness can be as undefined as a head cold, sore throat, or gastrointestinal upset, or it may be specific, as in the case of viral hepatitis or infectious mononucleosis. Eliciting a careful patient history is especially important in the diagnosis of Guillain-Barré syndrome.

## Pathophysiology

Many neurons throughout the nervous system have axons that are myelinated, that is, they have a lipid-protein substance, myelin, which is deposited along the axons so as to form a myelin sheath (see Fig. 6–1). The myelin sheath is separated or interrupted at regular intervals called nodes of Ranvier. The significance of the myelin sheath and the presence of such nodes is that they facilitate rapid impulse transmission via saltatory conduction (see Fig. 6–3). In this type of impulse conduction, the action potential jumps from one node to the next as it propagates along the axon, thus increasing the speed of impulse conduction.

Conduction of nerve impulses requires that the integrity of the myelin sheath be intact. The Schwann cell synthesizes myelin and maintains the myelin sheath in peripheral nerves and spinal roots. In Guillain-Barré syndrome there is a disruption of Schwann cells and destruction of myelin, which envelops peripheral nerves. This demyelination process affects both motor and sensory neurons, with sensory neurons affected to a lesser degree. Loss of myelin abolishes the transmission of nerve impulses by saltatory conduction. The resultant slowing of conduction and/or conduction blockage explain the muscle weakness and paralysis caused by Guillain-Barré syndrome.

An altered immune response may underlie the pathophysiology of Guillain-Barré syndrome. For example, new antigens expressed on virus-infected cells may induce immune responses, which cross-react with antigens expressed on normal cells of the same type. Thus, both the normal and abnormal cells could be destroyed. This is an example of an autoimmune response, that is, a breakdown in the natural immunologic tolerance to self-antigens, in this case, possibly induced by a viral infection (see Chap. 54).

Whether caused by an infectious process and/or an altered immune response, an inflammatory response ensues (see Table 13–1). It is characterized by a perivascular infiltration of lymphocytes and macrophages (phagocytes) responsible for phagocytosis of myelin. There is consequent exudate formation and edema. The result is segmental demyelination and degeneration of the myelin sheath and the nerve itself. Edema may be severe enough to compress the nerve and, in this way, block conduction.

Demyelination classically begins in distal nerves and ascends in a symmetric manner causing an ascending muscle weakness/paralysis and accompanying sensory deficits. The process may arrest at any point along the way or progress rostrally to involve cranial nerves and cause a bulbar paralysis. Remyelination occurs gradually in a descending manner with restoration of function to proximal areas occurring first and then proceeding distally. Complete recovery occurs in the majority of cases. In cases where residual problems persist, there is commonly motor weakness and an absence of tendon reflexes.

## Clinical Presentation

The clinical presentation of Guillain-Barré syndrome is variable with the full extent of neurologic impairment depending on the intensity of its underlying pathophysiologic processes. Characteristically, its onset is abrupt and usually follows an antecedent event within 1–3 weeks. Signs and symptoms reflect motor and sensory impairment, including cranial nerve dysfunction, and disruption of autonomic innervation.

The syndrome usually evolves in three phases: the *acute* phase reflects the sudden impairment and deterioration of neurologic function; the *plateau* phase embodies a cessation of the progressive loss of function, with those deficits that have occurred remaining static; and the *recovery* phase involves the remyelination and axonal regeneration process resulting in a reversal of neurologic deficits with a gradual return of function.

The initial complaint of a patient with Guillain-Barré syndrome is commonly muscle weakness occurring bilaterally, usually in the lower extremities, accompanied by difficult walking. It ascends symmetrically to involve the trunk, upper extremities, and cranial nerve distribution. Deterioration of function can occur at any level. Muscle weakness may evolve into a full-blown flaccid paralysis within 48–72 hours, or more slowly over several days to weeks. Deep tendon reflexes may be depressed or absent.

The appearance of sensory deficits may occur prior to, concurrently with, or subsequent to the appearance of motor dysfunction. Initial sensory disturbances reflect a hypersensitivity of the skin with paresthesias, for example, numbness, tingling, prickling, or burning sensations of the extremities occurring in a distal to proximal distribution, and often in a "glove and stocking" distribution. There may be complaints of severe headache, stiff neck, or photophobia. Upon neurologic examination, a decreased position (i.e., proprioception) and vibratory sense may be detected.

Pain is one of the most significant complaints made by the patient with Guillain-Barré syndrome; most patients with pain progress to have severe paralysis.[4] When experienced, the pain is usually severe enough to be recalled spontaneously upon questioning. It has been described as muscle tenderness, backache, or "charley-horse." Other descriptive phrases include: "chest feels bound up tightly with adhesive tape"; "a deep, steady ache like a toothache in the back of my legs"; "bandages wrapped as tight as you could"; "a deep aching and burning"; "shock-like deep muscle pain."

Pain usually occurs in the most profoundly weak muscles. It may be intensified at night. Some patients do not experience pain in the early stages of their illness. In patients who develop pain late in the course, the pain may be more severe, relentless, and unbearable, requiring narcotics for relief.

Cranial nerve dysfunction is commonly involved in the pathophysiology of Guillain-Barré syndrome. The facial (VII), glossopharyngeal (IX), and vagus (X) nerves are most commonly involved, and pathology is usually bilateral. Facial nerve involvement is reflected by the inability of the patient to wrinkle his/her forehead, close eyelids, and use facial muscles of expression (i.e., smile, frown, and so forth). Weakness/paralysis of cranial nerves IX, X, XII may impair speaking, swallowing, and mastication functions. The rare involvement of cranial nerves III, IV, VI will weaken extraocular movements (EOM), causing diplopia and dysconjugate eye movements. Assessment of these parameters is discussed in detail in Chapter 7.

Potential life-threatening complications can occur when motor paralysis ascends to involve the muscles of respiration. The function of abdominal and intercostal muscles may become compromised with involvement of the thoracic nerve roots. The patient's respiratory effort may become impaired, and respiratory insufficiency may occur. This is especially so in the patient who is fatigued. As the paralysis ascends to include the cervical nerve roots and lower brainstem (i.e., bulbar paralysis), all innervation to the diaphragm via the phrenic nerves ceases, and respiratory arrest ensues.

It is of critical importance that the patient be assessed continuously for signs of impending respiratory failure. Subtle changes may initially be observed, including shortness of breath while the patient is at rest, rapid shallow respirations, and a change in the respiratory pattern to one that is irregular and ineffective. A tidal volume (TV) of less than 5 ml/kg and a vital capacity (VC) of less than 12–15 ml/kg signal the onset of respiratory failure. Perhaps the *earliest* sign of impending respiratory failure is restlessness. Changes in the patient's level of consciousness and mental status, along with arterial blood gas results, may corroborate this suspicion.

The critical care nurse needs to develop a high degree of suspicion in assessing the patient with Guillain-Barré syndrome in order to anticipate complications before they occur and to keep the patient informed as to expectations of the course of the disease. Serial neurologic and respiratory assessments are imperative.

In spite of the severity of the illness and the extent of paralysis, the patient with Guillain-Barré syndrome is fully *conscious* and experiences all the pain, fear, and devastation associated with this syndrome. The level of consciousness, pupillary signs, and cerebral functions remain intact. Vision and hearing usually remain unaffected. The difficulty of adjusting from total independence to total dependence is profound whether it entails scratching one's nose or maintaining life support systems. The emotional and mental anguish is inestimable and presents the nurse with an unparalleled challenge.

Autonomic nervous system dysfunction, characterized by a variety of signs and symptoms reflective to a large extent of the reciprocal activity of the sympathetic versus the parasympathetic systems, also complicates the course of illness. The exact mechanism or trigger underlying this dysfunction remains unknown, but it is manifested by either an excessive or inadequate amount of autonomic activity. Signs and symptoms may range from brief duration and mild extent to a severe circulatory collapse. Wide fluctuations in blood pressure may occur. Hypertension during the acute phase may reflect release of catecholamines. The consequent vasoconstriction of the peripheral vasculature underlies the hypertension. Disruption of autonomic reflexes (e.g., baroreceptors), which control blood pressure and circulation, may predispose to hypotension. Use of vasopressors (e.g., dopamine) may be necessary to maintain adequate perfusion to vital organs.

Cardiac dysrhythmias including sinus tachycardia and atrioventricular blocks are not uncommon. The danger of asystole has occurred in some instances requiring insertion of a temporary pacemaker.[5] Autonomic function may become so labile that suctioning can precipitate an episode of bradycardia or asystole via vagal stimulation. Other signs and symptoms of autonomic disturbances include postural hypotension, facial flushing, diaphoresis, and urinary retention, among others. Death can occur from respiratory or cardiac failure, or from complications associated with immobility. Other complications may include hypostatic/aspiration pneumonia, paralytic ileus, thromboembolic disease, nosocomial infections, and impairment of skin integrity.

Maximum paralysis commonly peaks approximately 3 weeks post-onset, followed by a short plateau period in which there is neither improvement nor deterioration in function. This is followed by the recovery phase, which may take months when nerve regeneration becomes necessary.

## Diagnosis

The diagnosis of Guillain-Barré syndrome is based primarily on its distinct clinical history, clinical presentation, and clinical course (e.g., the progression of signs and symptoms). In the early phase, diagnosis may be difficult because vague complaints of muscle weakness, muscle aching, and paresthesias can easily be mistaken as resulting from the "flu" or other ailments.

In the majority of patients, the health history reveals the occurrence of a preceding event usually 2–3 weeks prior to the onset of neurologic symptoms. Following the onset of symptomatology, which is characteristically sudden and acute, there is an advancing, symmetric, nearly predictable progression of the disease ranging from minimal muscle weakness in the extremities to full-blown paralysis including acute respiratory dysfunction. Accompanying the alteration in motor function is a whole range of sensory deficits.

Neurologic assessment reveals a level of consciousness and mental status that are *intact*. Frequently there is alteration in cranial nerve function, especially cranial nerves VII, IX, and X. Sensory deficits related to fine touch, proprioception, and vibratory sense may be detected, and may correlate with segmental levels reflecting motor dysfunction. Deep tendon reflexes may be diminished or absent.

The clinical course of Guillain-Barré syndrome, although variable, reflects a period of acute disease progression, followed by an interim period when no definitive changes occur, and, finally, by the recovery period. There is no cure for this illness; it simply must run its course.

## Nursing Management

The primary treatment prescribed for the patient with Guillain-Barré syndrome is comprehensive and skilled nursing care. Major goals of treatment include supportive care, management of symptoms, and prevention of complications. A critical concern during the acute phase is maintenance of adequate respiratory function in the presence of rapidly advancing paralysis. Use of mechanical ventilation is frequently necessary during the acute phase of this illness.

Autonomic dysfunction can cause wide fluctuations in vital parameters, which need to be carefully monitored. It may be necessary to use vasopressors in order to maintain blood pressure or a temporary pacemaker to ensure adequate cardiac output.[5]

Use of corticosteroids to decrease the inflammatory process is controversial. To date there has been no definitive evidence presented that indicates steroids are efficacious in the treatment of Guillain-Barré syndrome. Some health-care providers reason that the potential complications of steroid use far outweigh their questionable therapeutic benefits.

Plasmapheresis, or plasma exchange,[6] has been instituted in certain instances, particularly in patients with extensive paralysis and respiratory dysfunction requiring long-term mechanical ventilation. The efficacy of this therapeutic modality remains questionable in the treatment of Guillain-Barré syndrome.

Thromboembolic complications in the patient with Guillain-Barré syndrome are a major concern, and use of prophylactic anticoagulation may be prescribed in certain instances. Pain control may require the use of narcotics or other analgesics. Morphine, for example, may be prescribed for the ventilated patient. The respiratory depressant effects of the drug are negated by the mechanical ventilation therapy; the sedative and analgesic effects of the drug can be very effective in making the patient feel comfortable physically, emotionally, and psychologically.

Nutritional support is a major aspect of treatment in the patient who is immobilized. It is not unusual for the patient with Guillain-Barré syndrome to lose upwards to one half of his/her total body weight during the course of prolonged paralysis. Supplemental feedings may be indicated to maintain sufficient caloric intake for energy, a positive nitrogen balance, and a balance of fluids and electrolytes. Nasogastric feedings may be instituted for the patient experiencing dysphagia. In the presence of paralytic ileus, total parenteral nutrition (TPN) may be the therapy of choice to provide adequate nutritional support. Prophylactic antibiotics are sometimes prescribed for the patient with multisystem problems.

Throughout the course of the illness, it is necessary to keep the patient and family updated regarding what Guillain-Barré syndrome is and the expectations and impact of its clinical course. A supportive environment needs to be provided. This will motivate the patient and assist in transfer from a totally independent to dependent role. The underlying goal of therapy is to assist the patient to maximize his/her capabilities and maintain a perspective regarding the ultimate goal.

### *Therapeutic Goals*

The ultimate goal of nursing care in treating the patient with Guillain-Barré syndrome is to assist the individual to restore his/her life processes to an equilibrated state. An apparently healthy, independent individual is suddenly rendered immobile and completely dependent, within hours or a few days, by an illness that is at once overwhelming, life-threatening, and devastating. Distorted sensations and disrupted motor function cause the individual to feel frightened, helpless, and alone. Although the patient may be completely paralyzed, he/she can think, feel, and perceive, and remains completely conscious throughout the course of the illness.

During the acute phase of the illness, nursing care is directed toward maintaining life-support systems, preventing complications, providing comfort measures, and initiating a system of communication with patient and family, keeping them informed as to what they can expect over the course of the illness and assisting them to keep the goal of eventual recovery in proper perspective.

Major nursing interventions in the early management of the patient with Guillain-Barré syndrome are related to the following therapeutic goals:

1. Maintain adequate respiratory function.
2. Assess and establish levels of neurologic function.
3. Establish an efficient means of communication.
4. Troubleshoot for signs of autonomic dysfunction.
5. Maintain fluid and electrolyte balance.
6. Maintain anabolic nutritional state.
7. Maintain integrity of gastrointestinal function.
8. Prevent complications of immobility:
   A. Peripheral vascular-thromboembolic disorder.
   B. Impairment of skin integrity.
   C. Musculoskeletal impairment: contractures, foot/wrist drop.
9. Maintain the integrity of psychologic and emotional processes.

### *Tentative Nursing Diagnoses: Basis for Treating Patient with Guillain-Barré Syndrome*

Tentative nursing diagnoses that provide the basis for treating the patient with Guillain-Barré syndrome include:

1. Breathing pattern, ineffective, related to:
   A. Compromised function of respiratory musculature and reduced diaphragmatic excursion.
   B. Anxiety.
2. Airway clearance, ineffective, related to:
   A. Compromised protective reflexes (e.g., cough, gag, epiglottal closure).
3. Cardiac output, alteration in: Decreased, related to:
   A. Compromised autonomic function
   B. Bradycardia and cardiac dysrhythmias.
   C. Reduced venous return (compromised vasomotor tone).
4. Anxiety, related to:
   A. Loss of sensorimotor function.
   B. Lack of knowledge regarding underlying disease and follow-up care.
   C. Change in lifestyle.
   D. Change in self-concept/body image.
5. Alteration in nutrition: Less than body requirements, related to:
   A. Nothing by mouth status.
   B. Catabolic state.
6. Skin integrity, impairment of, related to:
   A. Immobility with venous stasis.
   B. Altered nutritional status.
7. Urinary elimination, alteration in pattern of, related to:
   A. Urinary retention.
   B. Incontinence.
8. Bowel elimination, alteration in pattern of, related to:
   A. Paralytic ileus.
   B. Constipation.
9. Social isolation, related to:
   A. Immobilization.
   B. Prolonged hospitalization.
10. Knowledge deficit, related to:
    A. Underlying disease process and its clinical course.
    B. Follow-up care and expectations regarding recovery.
11. Self-care deficit, related to:
    A. Compromised sensorimotor function.
12. Self-concept, disturbance in, related to:
    A. Dependent status necessitated by compromised sensorimotor function.
13. Injury, potential for: Physiologic, related to:
    A. Musculoskeletal impairment.
    B. Compromised sensorimotor function.
    C. Aspiration pneumonia.
    D. Thromboembolic disorder.
    E. Gastrointestinal ulceration (stress related).
14. Potential for infection, related to:
    A. Compromised respiratory function.
    B. Invasive procedures.
    C. Catabolic state.

## MYASTHENIA GRAVIS

Myasthenia gravis is a chronic, progressive neuromuscular disease associated with an autoimmune phenomenon involving the neuromuscular junction and characterized by weakness of skeletal (voluntary) muscles. The muscle groups involved and the degree of severity differ in each patient. Commonly involved are muscles of chewing, swallowing, and speaking; facial muscles; and muscles of extraocular movement.

In some patients with myasthenia gravis, a sudden, severe increase of overall muscle weakness, termed myasthenic crisis, may occur, requiring hospitalization and intensive care to prevent life-threatening complications associated with respiratory insufficiency.

### Etiology

The etiology of myasthenia gravis remains unknown. In patients who have myasthenia gravis, it is necessary to be aware of those factors that can precipitate a myasthenic crisis. Such factors include, among others, inadequate anticholinesterase drug levels, infection (e.g., influenza, other viral infection), emotional stress and anxiety, certain drugs (e.g., phenothiazines, barbiturates, tranquilizers, narcotics, quinidine, and certain -mycin antibiotics), and fatigue. The characteristic weakness of myasthenia gravis is greater after periods of activity and improves with periods of rest.

## Pathophysiology

The pathophysiology underlying myasthenia gravis is now known to involve an autoimmune response, which occurs at neuromuscular junctions, specifically, on the postsynaptic membrane of skeletal muscle fibers. It is here that antibodies (AChR-Ab) destroy acetylcholine receptor sites (AChR), thereby reducing the number of receptors available for interaction with the neurotransmitter, acetylcholine (ACh). The overall decrease in available acetylcholine receptor sites diminishes and/or blocks neuromuscular transmission, predisposing to the skeletal muscle weakness characteristic of myasthenia gravis. (See the section entitled "Neuromuscular Junction" in Chap. 6.)

An autoimmune response ensues when the natural immunologic tolerance to self antigens breaks down. Why antigens associated with the acetylcholine receptor sites (AChR) are no longer recognized as self is unclear. What is clear is that serum antibodies, directed against acetylcholine receptors, are found in the majority of patients with myasthenia gravis. Plasmapheresis (i.e., plasma exchange), which removes circulating autoantibodies from the blood, has been found to produce temporary improvement in most patients with myasthenia gravis.

A significant incidence of thymoma and thymic hyperplasia (i.e., an excessive proliferation of normal cells within the thymus) is associated with myasthenia gravis. The thymus is the site for the transformation and proliferation of T-lymphocytes. An autoimmune response may develop if there is a change in the population of immunologically tolerant lymphocytes so that they lose their tolerant state. Immunologic tolerance is a state of immunologic *in*activity or diminution, so that an antigen that would ordinarily induce an immune response does not.

An additional consideration supportive of the autoimmune theory is that myasthenia gravis is frequently associated with other autoimmune diseases, for example, systemic lupus erythematosus. (For further discussion of the autoimmune phenomenon, see Chap. 54.)

## Clinical Presentation

The primary symptom of myasthenia gravis is skeletal (voluntary) muscle weakness. The weakness may be restricted to specific muscle groups or may be generalized. It may involve symmetric or asymmetric muscle groups. There are no sensory deficits, and the patient's state of consciousness remains intact; autonomic innervation (which involves smooth or involuntary muscle) also remains intact.

The muscle weakness of myasthenia gravis is distinct. It is not the same weakness or fatigue one experiences after a full day's work; nor can it be overcome by will or determination. Muscle groups affected tend to be weaker after use or in the evening when the individual is fatigued. The weakness is exacerbated by exercise and temporarily relieved by rest. With progression of the disease, weakness occurs with less exertion and increasingly earlier in the course of the day's activities.

Characteristically, muscles of the eyes are affected initially, resulting in ptosis, diplopia, and ocular palsy (i.e., loss of ability to move or to control movement). The ptosis is intensified when the patient tries to look up. Pupillary reaction to light and accommodation remains intact because it involves muscles (involuntary) innervated by the autonomic nervous system.

Involvement of the facial nerve (cranial nerve VII) results in difficulty in closing the eyelids. There is a characteristic, almost expressionless face. Dysphagia, accompanied by the inability to handle saliva or to close the jaw, reflects involvement of muscles of chewing and swallowing. The patient becomes at risk of aspiration. Muscles involved in speaking may be affected. The voice becomes high-pitched with a nasal quality; it may become weak and fades with conversation.

Weakness of neck muscles may cause the head to fall forward; involvement of muscles of the shoulder girdle prevents the individual from raising the arms over the head. If the hands are involved, the individual may be unable to perform intricate movements as, for example, eating, typing, writing, or playing a musical instrument. In some patients, the hips and lower extremities may be afflicted.

The most life-threatening aspect of myasthenia gravis, and the underlying reason for admission to the intensive care unit, is weakness of the muscles of respiration leading to respiratory insufficiency. The earliest sign of respiratory involvement is breathlessness or dyspnea at rest.

### *Myasthenic Crisis and Cholinergic Crisis*

In patients with myasthenia gravis who are receiving anticholinesterase therapy, a sudden increase in the severity of muscle weakness may signal the onset of a cholinergic crisis. Because myasthenic crisis and cholinergic crisis present clinically with a similar picture, edrophonium chloride (Tensilon), a short-acting anticholinesterase agent, may be given to differentiate the two: If muscle weakness decreases upon receiving the drug, the patient

TABLE 13–5
**Myasthenic Crisis Versus Cholinergic Crisis[11] During Administration of Anticholinesterase Therapy**

| | Myasthenic (Not Enough Medication) | Cholinergic (Too Much Medication) |
|---|---|---|
| Ocular symptoms | Ptosis<br>Diplopia | None |
| Bulbar symptoms | Dyspnea<br>Dysarthria<br>Dysphagia<br>Dysphonia<br>Difficulty chewing | "Thick tongue"<br>Dysarthria<br>Dysphagia<br>Difficulting chewing<br>Dyspnea |
| GI symptoms | None | Salivation<br>Anorexia<br>Nausea<br>Burping<br>Vomiting<br>Abdominal cramps<br>Diarrhea |
| General muscle symptoms | Generalized weakness<br>Dyspnea | Muscle fasciculations<br>Generalized weakness |
| Miscellaneous symptoms | None | Increased bronchial secretions<br>Lacrimation<br>Perspiration<br>Miosis, blurred vision |
| Psychic symptoms | Anxiety<br>Psychomotor restlessness | Irritability<br>Restlessness<br>Anxiety |
| Management | Administer additional cholinergic medications | Administer anticholinergic drugs |

is in myasthenic crisis; if symptoms worsen, the patient is in cholinergic crisis. Table 13–5 provides a comparison of these two clinical states.

## Diagnosis

The diagnosis of myasthenia gravis is based on the patient's history, physical examination, and selected diagnostic studies. It is absolutely essential to establish the patient's baseline level of functioning, because this serves as a measure for evaluating the patient's status and response to therapy. The patient may present with complaints of feeling especially tired and weak after a day's work; characteristically, muscle strength and recovery from fatigue occur with rest. Weakness of specific muscle groups may be associated with repetitive use.

On physical examination, asking the patient to perform repetitive actions using involved muscle groups assists in assessing for fatigability. Other physical signs may vary depending on the type and number of muscle groups afflicted and the severity of the consequent weakness.

Diagnostic studies include determining the presence of serum antibodies (AChR-Ab) directed against acetylcholine receptors (AChR). The anticholinesterase test using Tensilon (as described above) assists in differentiating myasthenic crisis and cholinergic crisis in the critical care setting. If results of this test are inconclusive using Tensilon, neostigmine may be used instead.

## Treatment

There is no known cure for myasthenia gravis, but symptoms may be minimized and, in some cases, relieved by various treatments or combination of treatments. The overall goal of treatment is to enhance or intensify transmission of nerve impulses at the neuromuscular junction. Drug therapy is the most widely used approach to treatment. Anticholinesterase drugs relieve muscle weakness by blocking the breakdown of acetylcholine at the neuromuscular junction. This is accomplished by interrupting the action of the enzyme, acetylcholinesterase. Ambenonium chloride (Mylelase), pyridostigmine bromide (Mestinon), and neostigmine bromide (Prostigmin) are oral preparations available. Ephedrine sulfate, an adrenergic agonist, may also be prescribed because it enhances the therapeutic response to anticholinesterase therapy.

Immunosuppressive drugs are prescribed to minimize the autoimmune response. Prednisone is the most widely used drug in this regard. It is frequently administered in combination with anticholinesterase therapy.

Plasmapheresis is used most commonly during myasthenic crisis to remove circulating acetylcholine receptor antibodies. Immunosuppressive therapy (e.g., prednisone or azathioprine [Imuran]) is frequently prescribed in conjunction with plasmapheresis therapy to prevent an increase in synthesis of the antibodies in question. In patients whose thymus scan reveals thymoma or thymic hyperplasia, or whose chest x-ray reveals thymic abnormality, thymectomy may be performed.

## Nursing Management

During the acute phase of myasthenic crisis, nursing care of the patient is focused on maintaining life-support systems, preventing complications, initiating a system of communication with the patient and family/significant others, establishing a trusting rapport, keeping patient and family/significant others informed as to the expectations of the illness, and educating the patient and family/significant others to maximize the quality of living within the limitations of the disease.

### *Maintenance of Respiratory Function*

The overriding concern in the treatment of the patient in myasthenic crisis is the maintenance of a patent airway with adequate alveolar ventilation, and the prevention of life-threatening complications, such as respiratory failure. As muscle weakness worsens, ventilatory capacity is diminished leading to ventilation/perfusion mismatch, and right to left shunting associated with atelectasis. Tidal volume (TV) and vital capacity (VC) decrease, and the inadequacy of alveolar ventilation and alveolar–capillary gas exchange is reflected in deteriorating arterial blood gas values.

During the acute phase, meticulous assessment of pulmonary function on an hourly basis is essential so that subtle signs of deterioration in pulmonary function may be detected before life-threatening respiratory failure ensues. Patients must be observed closely because impending muscle weakness leading to respiratory insufficiency can occur with alarming speed. Assessments of respiratory rate, breathing pattern and depth of breathing, breath sounds, and pulmonary function tests (e.g., tidal volume, vital capacity, and inspiratory forces) are necessary prerequisites to the detection of pulmonary complications. Breathlessness and dyspnea at rest are perhaps the earliest signs of impending compromise of pulmonary function.

The presence of abnormal breath sounds or adventitious sounds suggests a build-up of pulmonary secretions, which commonly occurs in patients in myasthenic crisis. This is particularly so in patients who are receiving anticholinesterase drug therapy because these drugs induce an increase in pulmonary secretions by the respiratory epithelium, which, in addition, is especially sensitive to irritants and foreign matter in the respiratory tract.

The ability of the patient to handle pulmonary secretions is further compromised by a weakened cough reflex. The weakness of the respiratory musculature compromises the ability of the myasthenic patient to take the necessary deep breath to execute the coughing mechanism. The inability to generate an intensified contraction of muscles involved in epiglottal closure further compromises the coughing mechanism. The patient is at increased risk of aspiration as well. A special effort is necessary to encourage the patient at regular intervals, preferably after periods of rest or after administration of an anticholinesterase drug, to try to breathe as deeply as possible. Chest physiotherapy, postural drainage, and nasotracheal suctioning of pulmonary secretions are an integral aspect of the patient's ongoing care.

Nasotracheal suctioning is a critical nursing measure and one that, if not performed appropriately, could compromise the patient's respiratory status. This is especially so in the ventilated patient who may be unable to move air effectively when removed from the mechanical ventilator. Consequently, hand ventilation and oxygenation should be performed prior to and after each suctioning pass. Each pass should be limited to 10 seconds so as not to unduly compromise the ventilatory status. Suctioning may be especially therapeutic when performed approximately 1 hour after a dose of anticholinesterase drug is administered. (For key features regarding appropriate suctioning technique, see Table 32–4).

In patients with impending respiratory failure, mechanical ventilation is instituted, usually in the assist-control mode. Use of this mode is preferred over the intermittent mechanical ventilation (IMV) mode in patients with myasthenia gravis because of difficulties that may be encountered by the patient in overcoming the present resistance offered by the ventilator. The patient may become frightened if he/she experiences an insufficient exchange of air. Nurses caring for these patients must be especially sensitive to the concerns of patients and their ventilatory needs, and must make this known to the patients. Patients must be reassured at frequent intervals that they need not panic.

A major nursing responsibility in caring for patients with myasthenia gravis who are receiving anticholinesterase drug therapy is that these drugs *must be given on time.*[7] A delay in administration of even a few minutes may cause a sufficient decrease in plasma levels of the drug to result in a marked increase in muscle weakness, thus compounding the already existing problems. Close monitoring of pulmonary function parameters is essential to accurately evaluate the patient's response to therapy.

### *Potential for Infection: Reducing the Risk*

Infection is a major complication in the patient with myasthenia gravis. Compromised pulmonary function and immunosuppressive therapy place these patients at great risk of developing a nosocomial infection. Concurrent plasmapheresis treatment may increase the possibility of infection. Thorough handwashing, use of aseptic technique in suctioning, and performing invasive procedures may help to minimize the risk of infection (see Table 49–7).

### *Maintenance of Adequate Nutrition—Preventing Complications*

Involvement of muscles of mastication and swallowing can present major concerns in the care of the patient with myasthenia gravis. Compromised swallowing leads to the accumulation of foods and secretions in the pharynx, which can be aspirated, predisposing to aspiration pneumonia. The inability to chew and swallow may also reduce the overall nutritional state to one that is less than body requirements.

Measures to assist the patient to chew and to

swallow are focused on conserving muscle strength and avoiding fatigue. A rest period one-half hour prior to eating may enhance muscle strength. The patient should be encouraged to chew slowly and to rest in between bites. It may be helpful to provide the main meal earlier in the day because weakness and fatigue are increased as the day moves along. Soft foods may reduce the need to chew, thus conserving strength. Swallowing liquids may be especially difficult; using a cup instead of a straw may be helpful because the patient's facial muscles may not be sufficiently strong to use the straw. Placing the patient in a high Fowler's position (at 60–90 degrees) should facilitate swallowing. Milk should be avoided because it stimulates formation of secretions.

#### *Communication: Basis for Effective Nursing Care*

Weakening of muscles of speech may seriously compromise the patient's ability to communicate. The inability to generate strong contractions of muscles of phonation and articulation (e.g., lips, mouth, tongue, larynx) results in speech that is soft, high-pitched, nasal in quality, and barely perceptible. Subtle changes in the patient's ability to speak may signal deterioration in the patient's condition and need to be monitored closely.

A system of communicating with the patient should be established. This is essential to the development of a trusting nurse–patient relationship; ventilation by the patient of feelings of frustration, fear, and panic; and evaluation of the patient's overall status. Attentive listening and allowing time for the patient to speak, however slowly that may be, are essential aspects of patient care. Some patients may find the experience of speaking even a few words tiring and fatiguing. In the course of communicating, it is important to validate and clarify information to ensure that communication is accurate.

Communication may be facilitated by using a blackboard or writing slate. For patients unable to use their hands, eye blinking may be used to reflect a "yes" or "no," until muscles involved become too weak. A wiggle of a finger or nodding of the head may be helpful. Once a successful means of communicating is established, it should be shared with all members of the health team caring for the patient, as well as with family members and significant others.

#### *Tentative Nursing Diagnoses: Basis for Treating the Patient in Myasthenic Crisis*

Tentative nursing diagnoses that provide the basis for treating the patient in myasthenic crisis include:

1. Breathing pattern, ineffective, related to:
   A. Weakness of muscles of respiration.
2. Airway clearance, ineffective, related to:
   A. Weakness of muscles of respiration.
   B. Weakened cough reflex.
   C. Increased pulmonary secretions associated with anticholinesterase drug therapy.
3. Gas exchange impaired, related to:
   A. Atelectasis with ventilation/perfusion mismatch and right to left shunting (see Chap. 28).
4. Communication, impaired, related to:
   A. Weakened respiratory musculature and muscles of speech.
5. Activity intolerance, related to:
   A. Altered neural transmission at the neuromuscular junction resulting in consequent muscle weakness.
6. Nutrition, alteration in: Less than body requirements, related to:
   A. Weakness of muscles of chewing and swallowing.
7. Swallowing, impaired, related to:
   A. Weakness of muscles of swallowing.
8. Injury, potential for: Physiologic (aspiration pneumonia), related to:
   A. Compromised protective reflexes (cough, gag, and swallowing).
9. Infection, potential, related to:
   A. Compromised pulmonary status.
   B. Immunosuppressive therapy.
10. Fear (panic), related to:
    A. Inability to breathe, air hunger.
11. Self-concept, disturbance in: Body image, self-esteem, related to:
    A. Progressive weakness and inability to carry out activities of daily living and usual lifestyle.
12. Coping, ineffective individual/family, related to:
    A. Chronic, progressively degenerating disease.
13. Self-care deficit, related to:
    A. Generalized weakened state.

## AMYOTROPHIC LATERAL SCLEROSIS

Amyotrophic lateral sclerosis (ALS) is a motor neuron disease involving the degeneration of upper and lower motor neurons of the spinal cord, brainstem (bulbar region), and cortex. It is manifested clinically by marked muscle weakness and atrophy. *Amyotrophic* means marked wasting and malnutrition of involved muscles; *sclerosis* refers to the degenerative hardening of nervous elements (e.g., myelin sheath) involving the lateral and anterior regions of the spinal cord. Its onset is insidious, its course is progressive, and its cause is unknown. It is now believed that ALS may represent a variety of motor neuron diseases. It is generally a disease of middle life with the mean age at onset being the mid-50s. Symptoms of the disease have been manifest as early as the teen years, and as late as the 80s.

Because ALS is a disease of *motor* neurons, the presenting symptom is usually weakness. Commonly the lower extremities are involved initially, followed by the upper extremities and bulbar region (i.e., the area of the medulla oblongata). Cranial nerve involvement in ALS is usually confined to the motor nuclei in the lower brainstem; hence, the term *bulbar symptoms* is used to reflect cranial nerve dysfunction.

ALS is generally felt to be a relentlessly progressive disease. Recovery from ALS is rare. Survival after onset is usually 3–5 years. Patients exhibiting a bulbar onset may have a shorter survival. Survival progressively decreases with increasing age at onset. Men generally have shorter survival than women.

Deaths from ALS are attributed largely to pulmonary complications. Upper respiratory infection and pneumonia are associated with pooling or aspiration of pulmonary secretions. Cardiopulmonary arrest is also implicated as a cause of death; hypoxic deaths and/or cardiac dysrhythmias have been identified as causes of death in patients with ALS.[8,9]

## Pathophysiology

The degenerative process reflective of ALS initially involves the cell bodies of the upper and lower motor neurons and the motor nuclei of cranial nerves in the bulbar region of the lower brainstem. (For a cross-sectional view of the spinal cord, see Fig. 6–16; for the pathway of upper motor neurons, see Fig. 6–19.) It may be recalled (see Chap. 6) that it is within the anterior gray horns of the spinal cord where the axonal nerve endings of the upper motor neurons synapse with the lower motor neuron, the final common pathway for innervation of skeletal muscle.

As the degenerative process progresses, it proceeds along the length of the axon to its termination. With involvement of lower motor neurons, there is a consequent interruption of the electrochemical stimulation of the muscle fiber, which, in turn, atrophies and becomes nonfunctional (i.e., flaccid paralysis). Hyper-reflexia and spasticity occur when upper motor neuron degeneration has occurred but the lower motor neuron remains intact. In this circumstance, spinal cord reflex arcs maintain some stimulation of muscle fibers, and spasticity may be observed clinically. The spasticity results as the modulating influence of the upper motor neuron is interrupted. Ultimately, progressive lower motor neuron degeneration results in the weakness, paralysis, and muscle atrophy characteristic of ALS. (See Table 12–5 for a comparison of clinical manifestations of upper and lower motor neuron involvement.)

## Clinical Presentation

The major symptom of ALS is muscle weakness, usually accompanied by muscle atrophy and fasciculations (i.e., involuntary muscle contraction or twitching of muscle fibers). The initial onset of symptoms will depend on the area of the body involved. Commonly, patients notice an asymmetric weakness or fatigue of one muscle group, which progresses to involve other muscles in the same extremity. Following involvement of one extremity the same muscle groups in the other extremity may be afflicted. The presence of a Babinski's sign reflects upper motor neuron involvement (see Fig. 7–1).

If the initial onset of symptoms involves the hand, the individual will experience difficulty in performing intricate maneuvers such as writing or typing. Bulbar symptoms are manifested by weakness of muscles of chewing, swallowing, and speaking. Tongue weakness and fasciculations may be apparent. The patient may experience dysarthria (i.e., difficult or defective speech due to impairment of the tongue muscles and other muscles essential for speech). Facial weakness, unlike that involving the extremities, is usually bilateral and symmetric.

Loss of inhibition of complex motor reflex acts concerned with laughter and crying results in a characteristic emotional lability. The presence of a hyperactive gag reflex and jaw jerk reflects upper motor neuron involvement of corticobulbar nerve tracts.

Although muscle weakness and atrophy in the upper and lower extremities lead to severe impairment, it is the weakness of the muscles of respiration that leads to the severest morbidity, and it is the cause of death in most cases. The effect on respiratory function presents clinically in several ways:[10] (1) weakness of the diaphragm and external intercostals leads to decreased inspiratory pressures, low lung volumes, and impaired gas exchange; (2) debility of the external intercostals and abdominal muscles results in an ineffective cough and the inability to clear secretions adequately; and (3) compromise of the gag reflex and muscles of the pharynx leads to the failure to protect the airway, predisposing to aspiration pneumonia.

Respiratory failure is the most important factor leading to morbidity and death in patients with ALS. It is almost always a result of aspiration pneumonia or occurs secondary to weakened respiratory musculature. There is a reduced rate of survival when the bulbar area of the central nervous system is affected initially. This is associated with the inability to protect the airways.

## Diagnosis

With involvement of the lower extremities, the patient may describe difficulty in picking up his/her feet in walking or climbing. With bulbar involvement, a history of increasing difficulty in chewing and swallowing, inability to handle secretions (e.g., drooling), and difficulties in speaking may be elicited. Family members may describe episodes of inappropriate laughter or crying. The patient's mental status remains intact.

On physical examination there are atrophy and weakness of normal muscle mass for an individual of a given age. Distal extremities are usually involved initially, followed by proximal muscle groups. Fasciculations may be observed in some muscle groups. Atrophy of muscle mass of the neck, shoulders, and chest warrants a close examination of pulmonary function. Gait abnormalities are related to weakness in the extremities because cerebellum function remains intact. There is no involvement of autonomic nervous system function.

Diagnostic tests include electromyography (EMG) and muscle biopsy. Pulmonary function tests are performed early to establish the presence and degree of respiratory system involvement including the status of the respiratory musculature and the possibility of respiratory insufficiency. These tests are also useful in following the progression of the disease.

Pulmonary function tests commonly performed include measurement of lung volumes, airflow, and arterial blood gases, in addition to an assessment of the status of muscles of respiration. A decrease in lung volumes is associated with a decrease in inspiratory muscle strength.

The maximal voluntary ventilation (MVV) provides an important measure of pulmonary function in patients with ALS. Although airway obstruction can lead to a reduced MVV, individuals with a normal forced expiratory volume/forced vital capacity ($FEV_1/FVC$) ratio also have a reduced MVV in the face of respiratory muscle weakness.[10]

Another pulmonary function test of special diagnostic value in diseases involving neuromuscular dysfunction measures pressures produced at the mouth. The specific tests performed measure the maximal inspiratory pressure ($P_I$ max) and maximal expiratory pressure ($P_E$ max) produced at the mouth. This study has demonstrated the ability to differentiate between parenchymal and neuromuscular disease, and should be followed on a regular basis in patients with ALS. Very importantly, such studies enable changes in pulmonary function to be observed over time.

The basic abnormalities in pulmonary function in the patient with ALS occur as a result of weakness of the respiratory musculature. There is an increase in the residual volume (RV) secondary to weakened expiratory muscles. The increase in RV associated with ALS needs to be differentiated from the increased RV seen in emphysema, which occurs secondary to air trapping from airway collapse (see Chap. 33). There is a reduction in vital capacity (VC) associated with both inspiratory and expiratory muscle weakness. As respiratory muscle function continues to deteriorate, there is a progressive drop in total lung capacity (TLC), vital capacity, and expiratory reserve volume, and a larger than expected increase in RV. (For a review of lung volumes and capacities, see Chap. 28.)

The reduction in maximal voluntary ventilation seen in ALS reflects the inability of the weakened respiratory muscles to move air in and out rapidly. Weakness of both inspiratory and expiratory muscles is implicated. Arterial blood gas values indicate that a mild hypoxemia exists over the course of ALS, and the $PaO_2$ (i.e., partial pressure of oxygen in arterial blood) is well preserved until the later stages of the disease. Hypercapnia (i.e., carbon dioxide retention), when recognized, is usually a poor prognostic sign, more commonly seen in cases presenting in respiratory failure.

## Treatment

Management of respiratory failure in the patient with ALS presents the patient, family, and health-care providers with major problems—medical, social, economic, and ethical. The decision to intubate these patients must be undertaken with the full realization that, although some ALS patients have been successfully weaned, ultimately the patient becomes completely and permanently ventilator dependent.

When the presence of ALS is suspected, patients are hospitalized briefly for diagnostic testing and an evaluation of the patient's overall body function, including the status of respiratory function. Thereafter, because of the risk of nosocomial infections, patients are only hospitalized when medically indicated.

## Nursing Management

In caring for the patient during the acute phase, it is essential to obtain as much information as possible about the patient's status from the patient, family, and/or significant others. Commonly, patients with ALS and families of these patients who require intensive nursing care have probably lived with the disease for a period of time and may have developed their own system of communication and routines of daily living. Every effort must be made to continue to maintain the patient at his/her optimal functioning within the limits imposed by the disease process.

A complete and candid discussion of the impending respiratory problems should be conducted early in the course of the disease. The patient and family should understand the options available to them. It is essential that the responsibility involved in the care of the paralyzed, ventilator-dependent patient be made perfectly clear. Caring for the ALS patient in the home can be draining on the family's emotional and financial resources.

For patients with ALS who are hospitalized because the need for mechanical ventilation is imminent, it is important to discuss with the patient and family/significant others what their feelings are regarding the use of life-support systems and the issue of "do not resuscitate" if it applies. When the respiratory musculature can no longer sustain adequate alveolar ventilation, it is the patient/family's decision as to whether ventilatory therapy is initiated or not. The task of deciding which option to pursue can be difficult. Family counseling should be available to support the patient and family in this decision-making process.

If chronic ventilator dependence is accepted as an alternative, there are reasonable approaches to accommodate the ventilated patient in the home environment. The support systems available for the care of the ventilator-dependent patient in the home continue to expand. Home ventilators that are safe, relatively inexpensive, and easy to operate are now available. Service contracts and regular home visits by a respiratory therapist can now be arranged.

Family education and training in the care of the ventilator-dependent patient is extensive and should be initiated in the hospital setting and continued in the home environment. Supportive and dependable follow-up care can usually be provided through the well-coordinated efforts of the health-care team and a reputable and responsible medical and/or respiratory care service.

If a long-range goal is to accommodate the ventilated patient in the home setting, it is essential to have a stable home environment. Adequate support systems are absolutely necessary. Utilization of qualified health-care aides is strongly recommended. Such support assists family members in providing day-to-day care and provides a means of relieving family members of the responsibility for care of the patient on a continuous basis. Such assistance is crucial to the prevention of "family burnout." The local ALS community support group may be invaluable in this regard. Hospitalization of patients with ALS should only continue until such time that the patient's condition is stabilized and he/she can be discharged to home or nursing care facility.

For patients with ALS, there eventually comes the time when death is near. Supporting the patient and family/significant others in working through the grieving process, the denial, the anger, the hopes, and the fears, entails that every effort be made to assist the individual and family to experience dignity in dying and peace in death.

### *Tentative Nursing Diagnoses: Basis for Treating the Patient with ALS During the Acute Phase*

Tentative nursing diagnoses that provide the basis for treating the patient with ALS include:

1. Anxiety, related to:
   A. Altered respiratory function.
   B. Lack of understanding of the underlying disease process and expectations.
2. Nutrition, alteration in: Less than body requirements, related to:
   A. Dysphagia, inability to chew.
   B. Loss of protective reflexes (e.g., gag reflex, epiglottal closure).
   C. Inability to feed self.
3. Impaired verbal communication, related to:
   A. Weakness of muscles involved in speaking.
4. Skin integrity, impairment of (potential), related to:
   A. Immobility.
5. Physical mobility, impairment of, related to:
   A. Weakness/paralysis of skeletal muscles.
6. Self-care deficit, related to:
   A. Progressive weakness.
7. Injury, physiologic (pneumonia), related to:
   A. Compromised respiratory function.
   B. Inability to mobilize and raise pulmonary secretions.
   C. Compromised cough reflex.
   D. Dysphagia.
8. Self-concept, disturbance in, related to:
   A. Dependence on others.
9. Coping, ineffective, individual/family, related to:
   A. Progressive compromise of ability to carry out activities of daily living.
   B. Poor prognosis and limited survival.
10. Knowledge deficit, related to:
    A. Lack of understanding of underlying disease process, and expectations of the progression of the disease.
11. Breathing pattern, alteration in, related to:
    A. Weakened respiratory musculature.
12. Airway clearance, ineffective, related to:
    A. Weakened to absent cough.
    B. Weakened muscles of respiration; weakened abdominal muscles.
13. Gas exchange, impaired, related to:
    A. Atelectasis with ventilation/perfusion mismatch, and right to left shunting (see Chap. 28).
14. Infection, potential, related to:
    A. Compromised pulmonary status.

## CASE STUDY WITH SAMPLE CARE PLAN: PATIENT WITH GUILLAIN-BARRÉ SYNDROME*

Mr. L.L., a well-nourished, 21-year-old white male, arrived at the emergency room of University Hospital with a chief complaint of progressive weakness of all extremities (lower extremities weaker than upper) and difficulty speaking and swallowing. Further history revealed that the patient had "the flu" approximately 4 weeks prior to this admission with symptoms of malaise, frontal headache, and a cough productive of greenish sputum. He visited his private physician 1 week ago, who treated him with amoxicillin without improvement. When he began to feel tingling in his fingers and toes, accompanied by progressive weakness, he decided to be examined in the hospital emergency room.

On physical examination, Mr. L. was seen to be awake, alert, and oriented, with intact but depressed cranial nerve function; motor strength in the lower extremity was rated 3/5; the upper extremity was rated 4/5. Sensation to light touch was intact. Deep tendon reflexes (DTR) were 1+ in lower extremities, 2+ in upper. Lumbar puncture revealed normal pressure, with a protein of 55 (mildly elevated). While in the emergency room, the patient complained of becoming short of breath and was having difficulty speaking because of this. Mr. L. was admitted to the medical ICU with a probable diagnosis of Guillain-Barré syndrome.

On the first day of admission Mr. L.'s condition deteriorated rapidly. He experienced increasing shortness of breath and fatigue. Arterial blood gases revealed a progressive hypercapnia and hypoxemia, and his vital capacity was 600 ml. The patient was intubated and mechanical ventilation initiated with an $FIO_2$ of 30%, on assist/control rate of 12/min, and a tidal volume of 700 ml. Motor strength in the lower extremities was 2/5; in the upper 3/5; there was increased numbness in the lower extremities to the waistline, and decreased sensation below T-12 level; deep tendon reflexes were absent in the lower extremities, and 1+ in the upper. A repeat lumbar tap revealed a protein level of 152, and a cytomegalovirus titer of 1:64.

An examination of the cranial nerves on the second day after admission revealed cranial nerves III, IV, and VI grossly intact with the patient able to look up and down and to shut his eyes tightly (cranial nerve VII). He experienced decreased sensation over the maxillary and mandibular distribution of cranial nerve V, bilaterally; there was decreased facial tone symmetrically, and the patient was unable to show his teeth. Cranial nerve VIII was intact; IX and X were not examined (patient was intubated); motor function of muscles innervated by cranial nerve XI was 5/5; examination of XII revealed weakened motor activity of tongue. Nerve conduction studies done at this time revealed severe demyelinating neuropathy. A Keofeed tube was placed, and enteral feedings were started at this time.

On the third day of hospitalization, Mr. L. was able to move his hands and arms slightly and to shrug his shoulders. There was slight movement of the toes; the legs were flaccid bilaterally. The patient was able to move his head side to side. Mr. L. was placed on a kinetic bed. He also complained of abdominal cramping, and his tube feedings were slowed.

On the fourth day of hospitalization, laboratory data revealed a serum albumin of 2.9, which was felt to be due to the interrupted Keofeed feedings because of abdominal cramping. ABGs were as follows: pH 7.39, $PaCO_2$ 42, $PaO_2$ 64, and percent hemoglobin saturation 93%. An increase in the $FIO_2$ from 30% to 40% produced ABGs as follows: pH 7.41, $PaCO_2$ 42, $PaO_2$ 106. The patient was incontinent of urine, and a Foley catheter was inserted. Physical therapy/occupational therapy program was initiated.

The patient's mother and father were with the patient almost 24 hours/day, and both the patient and family were becoming increasingly anxious and frightened. Referral was made to the psychiatric clinical nurse specialist who became involved with the patient and family at this time.

The patient's motor function continued to deteriorate over the next several days. The vital capacity was 200 ml; the negative inspiratory force (NIF) generated was a −8. Enteral feedings were increased to 1800 calories/day, but remained far short of the 2900 calories/day required because of persistent abdominal cramping.

On the eighth hospital day the patient was found to have a vital capacity of 140 ml, and a tracheostomy was placed. Serum albumin stabilized at 3.7. The patient was very depressed, tearful, and constantly ringing the bell, afraid to be alone. An effort was made to expand the family support system by arranging for visits by the hospital chaplain, volunteers; a schedule of visitors was set up to enable someone to be with the patient for the better part of the 24-hour day. A former patient with Guillain-Barré was invited to speak with the patient and family, an interaction that seemed to brighten and reassure both patient and family.

On the 10th day through the 18th day after admission, the patient experienced his most compromised level of function. His vital capacity was 60 ml; he was unable to close his eyes completely and developed diplopia. An eye patch was placed over one eye to decrease the diplopia during wakeful periods. Pupils were equal in size and reacted to light and accommodation (PERRLA); there was a re-

*This case study was prepared by Kathleen Daley White and Margaret Connelly.

duced shoulder shrug, and motor function in all extremities was 0/5. Mr. L. had some runs of supraventricular tachycardia (SVT), which was treated with verapamil 5 mg; blood pressure became labile with a scale of 120/80 to 210/90. Cytomegalovirus titer was 1:256, suggesting an acute CMV episode.

On the 20th hospital day there appeared to be some improvement in motor function; the patient was able to close his eyes completely; and motor function in the upper extremities ranged from 1 to 2+. Vital capacity improved to 100 ml and then to 270 ml; negatively generated inspiratory force increased to a −3 to −6 mmHg. The $FIO_2$ was decreased to 30% with ABGs: pH 7.4 $PaCO_2$ 42 and $PaO_2$ 104 mmHg. The patient could move his right bicep and left little finger; there was increased facial and shoulder movement, and return of motor function continued to progress bilaterally.

Over the course of the next week the patient was able to wrinkle his forehead, squeeze his eyes shut, and smile. His dysphagia resolved, and he began to swallow clear fluids. He was now moving both hands and his right leg. Vital capacity improved to 350 ml, and the inspiratory force was measured at −8 mmHg.

By the 30th hospital day the vital capacity increased to 460 ml and the negative inspiratory force to −30 mmHg. A T-piece was placed, and the $FIO_2$ was reduced to 21%. On the 34th day after admission, the vital capacity was 800 ml, inspiratory force was −30 mmHg. An active program of weaning continued until the trach could be plugged and the patient was able to mobilize and cough up pulmonary secretions.

The continued recovery of the patient enabled the tracheostomy to be removed, and he was transferred to a medical unit, awake, alert, and oriented, and worried about the possibility of a tracheostomy scar. Cranial nerves were intact; motor strength was 2/5 in lower extremities, 3–4/5 in the upper extremities; gross incoordination persisted, and the patient was unable to perform fine motor skills.

During the sixth week of hospitalization, the patient was able to move both lower extremities side to side horizontally and to wiggle his toes. He was still unable to move legs against gravity. Patient and family were both pleased and heartened by the patient's continued progress.

Mr. L. was transferred to a progressive rehabilitation center during the seventh hospital week. After 4 months of intensive rehabilitation, the patient was able to function independently. He was discharged home with daily rehabilitation follow-up.

## Initial Nursing Diagnoses

1. Ineffective breathing pattern, related to compromised function of the respiratory musculature, reduced diaphragmatic excursion, and anxiety.
2. Ineffective airway clearance, related to compromised protective reflexes and weakness/paralysis of intercostal (internal) and abdominal muscles.
3. Alteration in comfort: Pain (deep muscle tenderness, achiness).
4. Verbal and nonverbal communication, impaired, related to intubation, weakness of muscles of speech.
5. Self-care deficit, related to dependent status necessitated by compromised sensorimotor function.

These nursing diagnoses are documented on the Nursing Care Plan that follows. Additional nursing diagnoses may include:

6. Anxiety, related to:
   A. Loss of sensorimotor function.
   B. Lack of knowledge regarding underlying disease and follow-up care.
   C. Change in lifestyle.
   D. Change in self-concept/body image.
7. Sleep deprivation, related to ICU environment and continuous monitoring.
8. Alteration in nutrition: Less than body requirements, related to nothing by mouth status and catabolic state.
9. Fear of permanent paralysis, related to the diagnosis of Guillain-Barré syndrome.
10. Bowel elimination, alteration in pattern of, related to:
    A. Paralytic ileus.
    B. Constipation.
11. Urinary elimination, alteration in pattern, related to:
    A. Urinary retention.
    B. Incontinence.
12. Potential for infection, related to:
    A. Compromised respiratory function.
    B. Invasive procedures.
    C. Catabolic state.
13. Injury, potential for physiologic: Gastrointestinal (ulcerogenic), related to stress.
14. Injury, potential for: Physiologic, related to:
    A. Musculoskeletal impairment.
    B. Compromised sensorimotor function.
    C. Aspiration pneumonia.
    D. Thromboembolic disorder.
15. Knowledge deficit, related to:
    A. Underlying disease process and its clinical course.
    B. Follow-up care and expectations regarding recovery.
16. Depression (situational), related to powerlessness and length of recovery/rehabilitation.
17. Social isolation, related to inability to verbalize, initiate conversation; immobilization and prolonged hospitalization.

## SAMPLE CARE PLAN: PATIENT WITH GUILLAIN-BARRÉ SYNDROME

| Nursing Diagnoses | Desired Patient Outcomes | Nursing Interventions | Rationales |
|---|---|---|---|
| ***Nursing Diagnosis #1***<br>Breathing pattern, ineffective, related to:<br>1. Compromised function of respiratory musculature.<br>2. Reduced diaphragmatic excursion.<br>3. Anxiety. | Patient will maintain adequate respiratory function:<br>• Respiratory rate ~14–18/min.<br>• Respiratory rhythm: Eupneic.<br>• Arterial blood gas values:<br>pH 7.35–7.45<br>$PaCO_2$ ~35–45 mmHg.<br>$PaO_2$ ~80 mmHg | • Assess respiratory function hourly.<br>◦ Specific parameters:<br>– Rate, rhythm, depth, breath sounds, dyspnea; use of accessory muscles; status of pulmonary secretions: cough with sputum production. | • Progression of the underlying pathophysiologic process of Guillain-Barré syndrome is acutely reflected by increasing respiratory insufficiency.<br>◦ Guillain-Barré syndrome is an ascending disease of motor function; it enables the patient to be intubated prophylactically, rather than to have an emergency and potentially traumatic intubation. |
| | | ◦ Vital capacity and negative inspiratory force generated. | ◦ Vital capacity and negative inspiratory force generated by the patient are especially crucial in identifying disease progression or improvement. |
| | | • Prepare patient/family for possibility of intubation and mechanical ventilation therapy.<br>◦ Answer questions, take the time to explain what is happening.<br>◦ Establish alternative means of communication: blinking eyes, wiggle of finger, use of slate board or picture cards. | • Family and patient will accept initiation of mechanical ventilation therapy as part of the overall supportive therapy for patients with this syndrome. |
| | | • Place patient on Roto-Kinetic bed. | • Use of the Roto-Kinetic bed helps to prevent pooling of tracheobronchial secretions. |
| | | • Maintain optimal body alignment:<br>◦ Position patient so that chest is not restricted (e.g., if on his side, place arm slightly in front or back of patient). | ◦ The weight of the patient's flaccid arms should be kept off his chest to allow for maximal chest wall excursion and lung expansion. |
| | | • Notify physician of any changes in above assessment and document trends. | • By documenting data, trends can be followed and the stage of the disease progression can be pinpointed, facilitating quality of care. |
| ***Nursing Diagnosis #2***<br>Airway clearance, ineffective, related to:<br>1. Compromised protective reflexes.<br>2. Weakness/paralysis of intercostal and abdominal muscles. | Patient will:<br>1. Maintain patent airway:<br>• Normal breath sounds.<br>• Absence of adventitious sounds (e.g., crackles, wheezes). | • Assess airway patency hourly:<br>◦ Status of protective reflexes (cough, gag, epiglottal closure).<br>◦ Ability to handle tracheobronchial secretions. | • Cranial nerve dysfunction is commonly involved in the pathophysiology underlying Guillain-Barré syndrome. Involvement of cranial nerves VII, IX, X, and XII predisposes to compromised chewing, swallowing, and speaking. |
| | | • Maintain hydration state as prescribed.<br>◦ Humidify oxygen administered | • Dehydration may cause tracheobronchial secretions to become inspissated. |

*(continued)*

## SAMPLE CARE PLAN: PATIENT WITH GUILLAIN-BARRÉ SYNDROME *(Continued)*

| Nursing Diagnoses | Desired Patient Outcomes | Nursing Interventions | Rationales |
|---|---|---|---|
| ***Nursing Diagnosis #2 (cont.)*** | | | |
| | 2. Demonstrate secretion-clearing cough. | | |
| ***Nursing Diagnosis #3***<br>Alteration in comfort: Pain, related to:<br>1. Sensorimotor dysfunction. | Patient will be able to verbalize relief from pain, and demonstrate a relaxed demeanor. | • Assess pain, including severity, location/radiation, and type or quality of pain. | • Pain is one of the most significant complaints made by patients with Gullain-Barré syndrome. It occurs in the most profoundly weakened muscles and is more intensified at night. |
| | | • Provide comfort measures:<br>○ Assist patient into positions of comfort and correct body alignment.<br>○ Remain with patient to reassure. | • Maintaining body in appropriate alignment may help to ease some of the ache. |
| | | ○ Work with family members to help them understand what is happening and how they may best help their loved one.<br>○ Enlist hospital volunteers/chaplain or others to spend some time with the patient. | ○ Families often feel helpless in this circumstance; allowing them to participate in the patient's care may be reassuring to both patient and family. |
| | | • Administer analgesics as prescribed; monitor effectiveness in relieving pain. | • Pain may become severe enough to require narcotics for relief. |

| | | | |
|---|---|---|---|
| ***Nursing Diagnosis #4***<br>Communication impaired, verbal/nonverbal, related to:<br>1. Intubation.<br>2. Weakened muscles of speech.<br>3. Generalized muscle weakness/paralysis. | 1. Patient will be able to demonstrate alternative means of communication.<br>2. Patient will verbalize feeling comfortable with alternative means of communication.<br>3. Patient will verbalize why alternative means of communication may be necessary. | • Assess for difficulty in speaking.<br>• Keep patient/family appraised of expectations.<br>• Constantly reassure patient that his needs will be met.<br>• Initiate alternative means of communication before dysfunction occurs. | • Cranial nerve involvement may compromise muscles of speech; eventually, the patient may not even be able to blink his eyes; yet, throughout this ordeal, the patient remains conscious and aware.<br>• Keeping patient/family abreast of what is happening may help them to adjust to dysfunctional changes more easily.<br>• Mr. L.'s constant bell ringing reflected his frustration with his dependency and his fear of not having his needs met. |
| ***Nursing Diagnosis #5***<br>Self-care deficit, related to:<br>1. Dependent status necessitated by compromised sensorimotor dysfunction. | 1. Patient will be able to verbalize feelings about being dependent on others.<br>2. Patient will identify activities requiring assistance.<br>3. Patient will set priorities as to which dependent activities will be accomplished first. | • Identify with patient/family those activities over which the patient can have control (e.g., when to bathe, when to turn, when to have visitors).<br>• Work with family to assist the patient in some of his activities of daily living; assist the family to understand why they should respect the patient's need to maintain control of some of his care activities.<br>○ Encourage family members to verbalize thoughts and concerns.<br>• Allow patient to ventilate frustrations about dependency. | • Allowing patient to make decisions over care will help the patient to maintain some control over his body.<br>• If the patient refuses to see family members or states he doesn't want them to do anything for him, the patient's family should be reassured that it's okay for the patient to do these things and they should not feel rejected.<br>○ The patient's illness places a tremendous strain on family relationships, interactions, and lifestyle. |

## REFERENCES


1. Thompson, JM, et al: Clinical Nursing. CV Mosby, St Louis, 1986, p 1561.
2. Hickey, JV: The Clinical Practice of Neurological and Neurosurgical Nursing, ed 2. JB Lippincott, Philadelphia, 1986, p 558.
3. Pitts, LH and Simon, RP: Seizures. In Hilliary, D (ed): Decision-Making in Critical Care. CV Mosby, St Louis, 1985, p 8.
4. Ropper, AH and Shahani, B: Pain in Guillain-Barré Syndrome. Arch Neurol 41: 511, 1984.
5. Narayan, D, Huang, M, and Mathew, PK: Bradycardia and asystole requiring permanent pacemaker in Guillain-Barré syndrome. Am Heart J 108(2):426, August 1984.
6. McCarter, KA: Plasma exchange in Guillain-Barré syndrome. Nursing Times 78:319, February 14, 1982.
7. Noroian, EL: Myasthenia gravis: A nursing perspective. J Neurosci Nurs 18(2):74, April 1986.
8. Stone, N: Amyotrophic lateral sclerosis: A challenge for constant adaptation. J Neurosci Nurs 19(3):166, 1987.
9. Caroscio, JT, et al: Amyotrophic lateral sclerosis: Its natural history. Neurol Clin 5(1):1, 1987.
10. Braun, SR: Respiratory system in amyotrophic lateral sclerosis. Neurol Clin 5(1):9, 1987.
11. Mathewson, MK: Pharmacotherapeutics: A Nursing Process Approach. FA Davis, Philadelphia, 1986, p 354.

# UNIT TWO

# Bibliography

Arsenault, L: Selected postoperative complications of cranial surgery. J Neuro Nurs 17(3):155, June 1985.
Ayres, SM, Schlichtig, R, and Sterling, M: Care of the Critically Ill, ed 3. Year Book Medical Publishers, Chicago, 1988.
Barnes, PH: Guillain-Barré syndrome. Crit Care Nurse 4(1):68, January/February 1984.
Bell, J: Understanding and managing myasthenia gravis. Focus on Critical Care 16(1):57, February 1989.
Bell, J and Hannon, K: Pathophysiology involved in autonomic dysreflexia. J Neurosci Nurs 18(2):86, April 1986.
Boortz-Marx, R: Factors affecting intracranial pressure: A descriptive study. J Neurosurg Nurs 17(2):89, April 1985.
Braun, SR: Respiratory system in amyotrophic lateral sclerosis. Neurol Clin 5(1):9, February 1987.
Brown, JD: Acute disturbances of consciousness. In WJ Sibbald (ed): Synopsis of Critical Care, ed 3. Williams & Wilkins, Baltimore, 1988, p 163.
Brown, JD and Lindsay, RM: Acute disturbance of consciousness. In WJ Sibbald (ed): Synopsis of Critical Care, ed 2. Williams & Wilkins, Baltimore, 1984.
Browner, C, et al: Halo immobilization brace care: An innovative approach. J Neurosurg Nurs 19(1):24, February 1987.
Caroscio, JT, et al: Amyotrophic lateral sclerosis: Its natural history. Neurol Clin 5(1):1, 1987.
DeJong, RN, et al: Essentials of the Neurological Examination. Smith Kline Corporation, Philadelphia, 1979.
Epstein, F and Hamilton, G: Initial approach to the brain-injured patient. Crit Care Q 5(4):14, 1983.
Gilman, S and Winans, SS: Essentials of Clinical Neuroanatomy and Neurophysiology, ed 7. FA Davis, Philadelphia, 1987.
Hendrickson, S: Intracranial pressure changes and family presence. J Neurosci, 19(1):14, 1987.
Hickey, J: The Clinical Practice of Neurological and Neurosurgical Nursing, ed 2. JB Lippincott, Philadelphia, 1986.
Hotter, AN: The pathophysiology of shock brain. In KA Gould (ed): Critical Care Nursing Clinics of North America 1(1):123, March 1989.
Hughes, RA, et al: Immune responses to myelin antigens in Guillain-Barré syndrome. J Neuroimmunol 6(5):303, August 1984.
Jones, C: Glasgow Coma Scale. Am J Nurs 79(9):1551, September 1979.
Kirsch, JR, et al: Medical management and innovations. In KA Gould (ed): Critical Care Nursing Clinics of North America 1(1):143, March 1989.
Manifold, SL: Craniocerebral trauma: A review of primary and secondary injury and therapeutic modalities. Focus Crit Care 13(2):22, April 1986.
McCarter, KA: Plasma exchange in Guillain-Barré syndrome. Nursing Times 78:319, February 24, 1982.
Mitchell, PH, et al: Neurological Assessment for Nursing Practice. Reston Publishing, Reston, Virginia, 1984.
Morrison, CA: Brain herniation syndromes. Crit Care Nurse 7(5):34, September/October 1987.
Muir, BL: Pathophysiology: An Introduction to the Mechanisms of Disease, ed 2. John Wiley & Sons, New York, 1988.
Munaswes, M: Increased intracranial pressure and its systemic effects. J Neurosurg Nurs 17(4):238, August 1985.
Narayan, D, Huang, M, and Mathew, PK: Bradycardia and asystole requiring permanent pacemaker in Guillain-Barré syndrome. Am Heart J 108(2):426, August 1984.
Nikas, DL: Neurological assessment of altered states of consciousness. Focus Crit Care 11(1):54, February 1984.
Nikas, DL: Neurological assessment of altered states of consciousness. Focus Crit Care 10(6):10, December 1983.
Noroian, EL: Myasthenia gravis: A nursing perspective. J Neurosci Nurs 18(2):74, April 1986.
Oertel, LB: The dilemma of cerebral vasospasm treatment. J Neurosurg Nurs 17(1):7, February 1985.
Pallett, PJ and O'Biren, MT: Textbook of Neurological Nursing. Little, Brown & Co, Boston, 1985.
Passarella, P and Lewis, N: Nursing Application of Bobath principles in stroke care. J Neurosci Nurs 19(2):106, April 1987.
Pitts, LH and Simon, RP: Seizures. In D Hillary (ed): Decision-Making in Critical Care. CV Mosby, St Louis, 1985.
Plum, F and Posner, JB: The Diagnosis of Stupor and Coma, ed 3. FA Davis, Philadelphia, 1980.
Pollack-Latham, CL: Intracranial pressure monitoring: Part I. Physiologic principles. Crit Care Nurse 7(5):40, September-October 1987.
Richmond, TS: A critical care challenge: The patient with a cervical spinal cord injury. Focus Crit Care 12(2), April 1985.
Richmond, TS: Perspectives on brain resuscitation. In KA Gould (ed): Critical Care Nursing Clinics of North America 1(1):115, March 1989.
Robinet, K: Increased intracranial pressure: Management with an intraventricular catheter. J Neurol Nurs 17(2):95, April 1985.
Ropper, AH and Shahani, B: Pain in Guillain-Barré syndrome. Arch Neurol 41:511, May, 1984.
Smith, KA: Head trauma: Comparison of infection rates for different methods of intracranial pressure monitoring. J Neurosci Nurs 19(6):310, December 1987
Stein, R, Hier, D, and Caplan, L: Cognitive and behavioral deficits after right hemisphere stroke. Current Concepts of Cerebrovascular Disease (STROKE) XX(1):1, January-February 1985.
Stone, N: Amyotrophic lateral sclerosis: A challenge for constant adaptation. J Neurosci Nurs 19(3):166, June 1987.
Sullivan, J: Nursing interventions. In KA Gould (ed): Critical Care Nursing Clinics of North America 1(1):155, March 1989.
Taylor, J: Nursing management of stroke: Acute care—Part I. Cardiovascular Nursing 21(1):1, January-February 1985.
Thompson, JM, et al: Clinical Nursing. CV Mosby, St Louis, 1986.
Wald, ME: Cerebral thrombosis: Assessment and nursing management of the acute phase. J Neuroscience Nursing, 18(1):36, February 1986.
Yarnell, P: Stroke rehabilitation. Current Concepts of Cerebrovascular Disease (STROKE) XXI(3):9, May-June 1986.
Zejdlik, CP: Management of Spinal Cord Injury. Wadsworth Health Sciences Division, Monterey, California, 1983.

UNIT THREE

# Endocrine System

The functional integrity of the body as a whole and of the tissues and organs that comprise it is regulated by two major systems: the nervous system and the endocrine system. The nervous system exerts its control by initiating electrical impulses (action potentials). It uses a complex neuronal circuitry in which conduction of electrical impulses is facilitated by chemical neurotransmitters. The endocrine system exerts its control by secreting hormones, or "blood-borne chemical messengers," which affect many cellular functions throughout the body.

In Chapter 14, an effort is made to distinguish the characteristics common to all endocrine glands. In subsequent chapters, the anatomy, physiology, and pathophysiology of selected endocrine glands are closely examined and include the hypothalamic-pituitary (hypophyseal) system, thyroid and adrenal glands, and the endocrine pancreas.

Nursing process in the diagnosis and management of the patient with endocrine dysfunction is explored. Nursing care plans are based on nursing diagnoses, and include specific patient outcomes, nursing interventions and their rationales.

## UNIT OUTLINE

## UNIT OUTLINE—*CONTINUED*

CHAPTER 14

# General Features of the Endocrine System

## CHAPTER OUTLINE



## LEARNING OBJECTIVES

**At the end of this chapter, you should be able to:**

1. Explain the concepts of "control" system and "negative feedback" mechanism as they pertain to endocrine function.
2. Define endocrine gland, hormone, and characteristic features of hormones.
3. List the major endocrine glands, their specific hormones, and their major regulatory function.
4. Classify major types of hormones and their respective roles in endocrine function.
5. Discuss the significance of plasma-binding protein in terms of hormonal transport and overall hormonal activity.
6. Relate the rates of hormonal secretion, metabolism, and excretion to total plasma concentration of any hormone.
7. Describe mechanisms underlying hormonal action.
8. Identify pathophysiologic states predisposing to endocrine dysfunction.

The endocrine system is principally responsible for regulating metabolic functions. Such functions include the control of rates of biochemical reactions, the facilitation of transport of substances through the plasma membrane, growth and development, the stress response, and reproduction. The establishment and maintenance of fluid and electrolyte, acid–base, and energy balance are largely influenced by endocrine activity.

## CONCEPT OF "CONTROL" SYSTEM

A "control" system is defined as a collection of interconnected components that function to keep a physical or chemical parameter of the body relatively constant, or within a predetermined range of values.[1] A control system consists of three basic components not unlike those of the reflex arc (see Chap. 6). These include a *receptor*, which receives a stimulus or detects an alteration in environmental conditions; a *processing* or *integrating center,* the output of which reflects the net effect of the total input; and an *effector,* which results in the response or altered activity.

An example of a hormonal control system is the secretion of parathormone in response to hypocalcemia (see Chap. 24). Special cells within the parathyroid glands (receptors) continuously monitor the concentration of ionized calcium in circulating blood. If a state of hypocalcemia exists, parathormone is secreted by the parathyroid glands (processing/integrating center) directly into the bloodstream to act on distal target cells in bone, gut, and kidney (effectors). As a result of the hormonal influence, levels of ionized calcium are returned to appropriate physiologic levels, and the secretion of parathormone is reduced to shut off accordingly.

### Concept of "Negative Feedback" Mechanism

Negative feedback causes an increase in the output of the system to result in a decrease in the input. The example of an increase in parathormone secretion in response to hypocalcemia is illustrative of a negative feedback mechanism. The consequent increase in parathormone secretion results in an increase in the serum calcium level. This, in turn, feeds back on the parathyroid glands, which reduce parathormone secretion.

The negative feedback mechanism operates in other hormonal systems. An increase in serum levels of thyroid hormones (thyroxine and triiodothyronine) and cortisol, for example, causes the hypothalamus to reduce its secretion of thyrotrophic and corticotrophic releasing hormones, and the adenohypophysis (i.e., anterior pituitary gland) to decrease its secretion of thyrotropic and adrenocorticotropic stimulating hormones. The net effect of this mechanism is a reduction in the secretion of thyroid hormones and cortisol by the target glands, thyroid and adrenal cortex, respectively, with a consequent decrease in the serum levels of these hormones.[2]

The basic function of an endocrine gland is to secrete hormone, which regulates the activity of its target cells in a specific direction. To maintain function, it is essential that endocrine glands receive continuous feedback regarding the status of the cells or organ system regulated.

## ENDOCRINE GLAND AND HORMONE: DEFINED

An endocrine gland is ductless and consists of a group of specialized cells that synthesize and secrete a specific chemical mediator or hormone directly into the bloodstream. This hormone acts very specifically on target tissue in another part of the body. Endocrine glands produce and release their hormones according to the dictates of regulatory feedback mechanisms.

It is now widely recognized that synthesis and secretion of hormones are not limited to an endocrine gland per se. Rather, some hormones are formed in peripheral tissues from circulating precursors or prohormones. Examples of these hormones include angiotensin and the active metabolite of vitamin D, 1,25-dihydroxycholecalciferol. Prostaglandins are considered to be *tissue* hormones not primarily synthesized by a specific structure but by a wide variety of tissues. Prostaglandins exert variable effects. For a list of major endocrine glands, the hormones they secrete, and their major regulatory functions, see Table 14–1.

Hormones are generally secreted in very small amounts. Despite their low concentrations, they exert a marked metabolic and biochemical effect on their target tissues. Some hormonal effects occur in seconds (e.g., epinephrine); others may require hours to several days to commence action (e.g., growth hormone). Target tissue hormonal receptors are highly specific, meaning that they are responsive to a particular hormone.

## CLASSIFICATION OF HORMONES

### Releasing and Inhibiting Hormones

Functionally, hormones can be classified as releasing and inhibiting, trophic, and peripheral hormones. Releasing and inhibiting hormones are synthesized and secreted by special neurons within the hypothalamus, which function to control the secretion of anterior pituitary hormones. For each hormone secreted by the anterior pituitary gland (i.e., adenohypophysis), there is thought to exist both a releasing and inhibiting hormone secreted by the hypothalamus. These substances, in turn, stimulate and inhibit, respectively, the secretion of adenohypophyseal hormones. Specific hypothalamic releasing and inhibiting hormones and their functions are listed in Table 14–1.

### Trophic Hormones

Trophic hormones are secreted by the anterior pituitary gland. They affect growth, metabolism, nutrition, and the function of other glands (i.e., target glands such as the thyroid and adrenal glands). Trophic hormones, as well as other adenohypophyseal hormones, and their functions are listed in Table 14–1.

Synthesis and secretion of trophic hormones are

TABLE 14-1
**Major Endocrine Glands, Their Hormones, and Major Regulatory Functions**[3]

| Gland | Hormone | Major Regulatory Functions |
|---|---|---|
| Hypothalamus | Releasing hormones | Control of hormonal secretion by anterior pituitary gland: |
| | Growth hormone releasing hormone (GHRH) | Stimulates secretions of growth hormone (GH) |
| | Thyrotrophic releasing hormone (TRH) | Stimulates secretion of thyrotropic stimulating hormone (TSH) and prolactin |
| | Corticotrophic releasing hormone (CRH) | Stimulates secretion of adrenocorticotropic hormone (ACTH) |
| | Gonadotrophic releasing hormone (GnRH) | Stimulates secretion of luteinizing hormone (LH) and follicle stimulating hormone (FSH) |
| | Prolactin releasing hormone (PRH) | Stimulates secretion of prolactin |
| | Inhibiting hormones | |
| | Growth inhibiting hormone (GIH) (somatostatin) | Inhibits secretion of growth hormone and several other hormones |
| | Prolactin inhibiting hormone (PIH) | Inhibits secretion of prolactin |
| | Other hormones | |
| | Oxytocin | Milk "let-down" reflex; uterine contractility |
| | Antidiuretic hormone (ADH) (vasopressin) | Water balance; excretion of water via kidneys |
| Anterior pituitary | Growth hormone (GH) (somatotrophic hormone) | Growth, metabolism; secretion of *somatomedrin* by liver (Somatomedrin: growth promoting peptides released from liver in response to GH stimulation) (See liver, below) |
| | Thyrotropic stimulating hormone (TSH) | Thyroid hormones thyroxine ($T_4$) and triiodothyronine ($T_3$) |
| | Adrenocorticotropic hormone (ACTH) | Adrenal cortical hormones |
| | Gonadotropic hormones | Gonads—Sex hormones |
| | Luteinizing hormone (LH) | —Gamete production and maturation |
| | Follicle stimulating hormone (FSH) | |
| | Prolactin | Breast—Lactation |
| Posterior pituitary (see hypothalamus, above) | Oxytocin | Milk "let-down" reflex |
| | Antidiuretic hormone (ADH) (vasopressin) | Water regulation |
| Thyroid | Thyroid hormones: Thyroxine ($T_4$), Triiodothyronine ($T_3$) | Energy production, metabolism, and growth |
| | Calcitonin | Serum calcium |
| Parathyroids | Parathyroid hormone (parathormone) (PH) | Serum calcium and phosphate |
| Pancreas (islets of Langerhans) | Insulin, Glucagon, Somatostatin | Metabolism; serum glucose levels |
| Adrenal glands | | |
| Cortex | Cortisol | Metabolism; stress response |
| | Aldosterone | Sodium/potassium excretion via kidneys |
| | Androgens | Growth, sex drive (women) |
| Medulla | Epinephrine, Norepinephrine | Metabolism, cardiovascular function, and stress response |

(continued)

TABLE 14-1
**Major Endocrine Glands, Their Hormones, and Major Regulatory Functions[3] *(Continued)***

| Gland | Hormone | Major Regulatory Functions |
|---|---|---|
| Gonads | | |
| Female—ovaries | Estrogens<br>Progesterone | Reproduction, growth and development, secondary sex characteristics in women |
| Male—testes | Testosterone | Reproduction, growth and development, secondary sex characteristics in men |
| Other Glands | | |
| Kidneys | Renin (enzyme) angiotensin | Aldosterone secretion by adrenal cortex, blood pressure |
| | Erythropoietin | Erythrocyte production |
| | 1,25-Dihydroxycholecalciferol | Calcium balance, gastrointestinal absorption of calcium |
| Gastrointestinal tract | Gastrin<br>Secretin<br>Cholecystokinin<br>Gastric inhibitory peptide<br>Somatostatin | Gastrointestinal function: liver, pancreas, and gallbladder |
| Liver | Somatomedrin | Bone growth |
| Thymus | Thymic hormone (thymosin) | Lymphocyte development |
| Pineal | Melatonin | Circadian rhythms, sexual maturation |

controlled by two factors: the effect of releasing and inhibiting hormones secreted by the hypothalamus, and the blood level of hormones secreted by the target glands. The target hormones circulating in the blood generally exert a negative feedback control in which an increased serum level of these hormones causes a decreased secretion of trophic hormones by the anterior pituitary, and decreased releasing hormone by the hypothalamus. For example, an increase in the serum levels of the thyroid hormones ($T_3$ and $T_4$) will, in turn, diminish the secretion of thyrotropic stimulating hormone by the adenohypophysis and thyrotrophic releasing hormone by the hypothalamus.

### Peripheral Hormones

Peripheral hormones act directly upon peripheral tissues. They are gland-specific in origin, which means that they are synthesized within, and secreted by, the same gland. Examples of peripheral hormones include parathormone, which is synthesized and secreted by the parathyroid glands and exerts its effect on bone, kidney, and gut; and insulin, which is synthesized and secreted by the islets of Langerhans found within the pancreas and exerts its effect on liver, muscle, and adipose tissue.

## HORMONAL TRANSPORT AND DEGRADATION

### Transport

There are three categories of hormone structure: peptides and peptide derivatives, steroids, and amines. Hypothalamic, pituitary, thyroid, parathyroid, and pancreatic hormones are included in the first category; hormones of the adrenal cortex and gonads in the second; and hormones of the adrenal medulla in the third. This last category includes the catecholamines, epinephrine and norepinephrine.

Transport of hormones in the blood depends in part on their chemical structure. The more soluble peptides and amines are transported freely in blood; the relatively insoluble steroidal hormones and thyroid hormones are transported highly bound to specific plasma-binding proteins. The total concentration of a protein-bound hormone circulating in the blood depends on the amount of hormone available, the amount of binding protein, and the affinity or attraction of the protein for the specific hormone. The intactness of the normal feedback mechanisms ensures that the ratio of protein-bound to free or unbound hormone remains within appropriate physiologic levels.

## Degradation

The total plasma concentration of any hormone is a function of both its secretion rate and the rate at which it is metabolized and excreted. Changes in the rate of metabolism and excretion do not cause endocrine pathology as long as the feedback regulatory systems are intact. The major pathway for degradation and excretion of most hormones is via the liver and kidneys.

## MECHANISMS UNDERLYING HORMONAL ACTION

One of the distinguishing characteristics of hormones is that they are highly specific. Hormone receptors are viewed as specific molecules in the target tissue with which a particular hormone interacts to initiate its hormonal effect. This hormone-receptor interaction may occur, for example, on the cell surface or via an intracellular receptor mechanism (Fig. 14–1).

Some hormones classified as peptides, peptide derivatives, and amines exert their effect via the activation of cAMP (i.e., cyclic adenosine monophosphate). The hormone–cell surface receptor combination activates the enzyme, adenyl cyclase, which catalyzes the intracellular conversion of ATP (i.e., adenosine triphosphate) to cAMP. cAMP, also referred to as the "second messenger," triggers a cascade of intracellular events reflective of the cell's overall response to the particular hormone.

Not all peptide hormones use cAMP as their second messenger. In some instances, cyclic guanosine monophosphate (cGMP) or calcium is used as the second messenger. In still others, as for example insulin, the relevant second messenger has yet to be identified.

The intracellular receptor mechanism involves the lipid soluble steroidal hormones (e.g., adrenal cortical and gonadal hormones), which easily diffuse through the plasma membrane of their specific target cells into the cell's cytoplasm. Once within the cell, the hormone interacts with its specific protein receptor to form a hormone-receptor complex, which subsequently carries the steroid molecule into the cell's nucleus. It is within the nucleus that the hormone mediates the response characteristic of the cell.

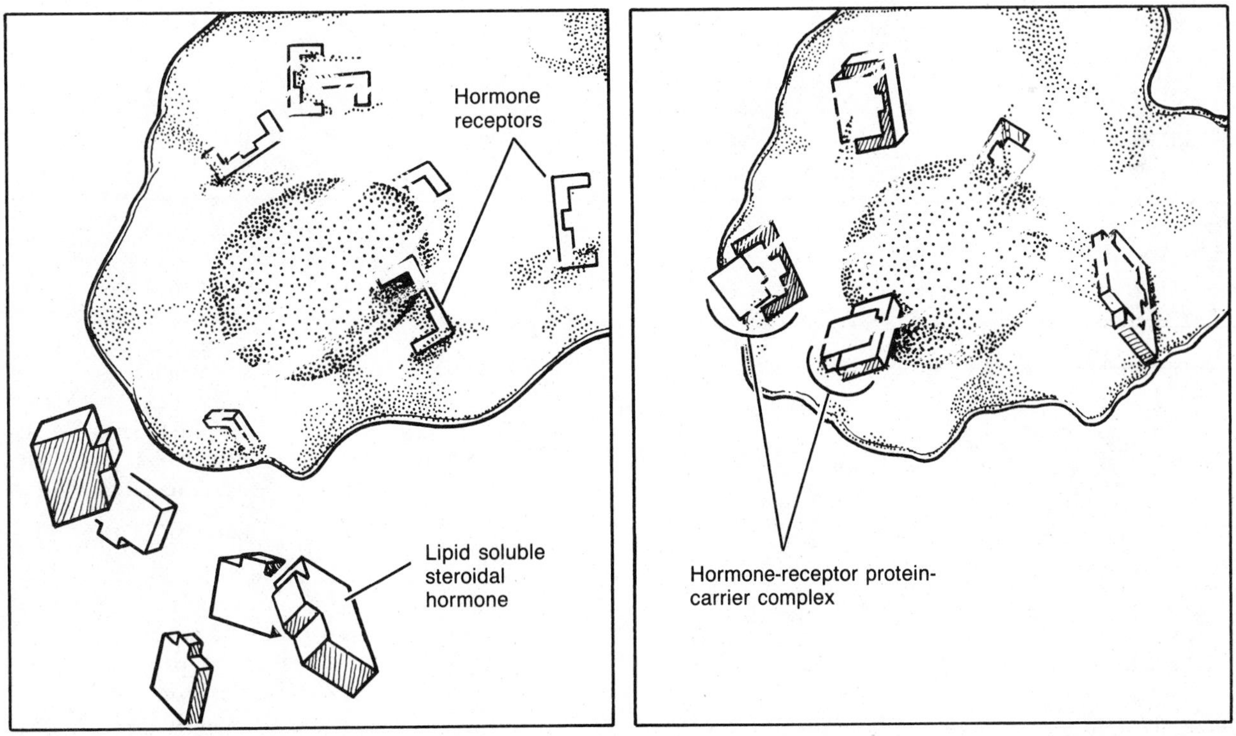


**Figure 14–1.** The interaction of a hormone with its receptor molecule is highly specific. Hormone receptors are viewed as specific and distinct molecules within the target tissue with which a particular hormone interacts to initiate its hormonal effect.

## PATHOPHYSIOLOGY: ENDOCRINOPATHIES

Endocrinopathies may be caused by hormone deficiency, hormone excess, or hormone-resistant states. In the case of hormonal resistance, primary hormone receptor abnormality and the presence of antireceptor antibody have been implicated as underlying pathophysiologic mechanisms.[4] If one considers the normal physiologic sequence of events necessary for hormonal action to occur, it is possible to identify the locus of the pathology.

## SUMMARY

For a hormone to influence its target tissue, the following mechanisms must remain intact:

The hormone must be:

1. Synthesized, unaltered and in sufficient quantity.
2. Secreted appropriately into body fluids.
3. Metabolized to its active metabolite if necessary. (Whenever metabolic activation of a hormone is required, a deficiency of the enzymes that mediate the activation process may in itself predispose to endocrine dysfunction.)
4. Transported to its target tissues.
5. Interact with its specific receptor molecule either on the cell surface or via an intracellular receptor mechanism.
6. Trigger the appropriate set of cellular reactions by virtue of the hormone–cell receptor interaction.

It is also critically important for the feedback regulatory systems to be intact.

## REFERENCES

1. Vander, A, Sherman, J, and Luciano, D: Human Physiology: The Mechanisms of Body Function, ed 4. McGraw-Hill, New York, 1985, pp 147–148.
2. Hershman, J: Endocrine Pathophysiology: A Patient-Oriented Approach, ed 3. Lea & Febiger, Philadelphia, 1988, p 2.
3. Vander, A, Sherman, J, and Luciano, D: Human Physiology: The Mechanisms of Body Function, ed 4. McGraw-Hill, New York, 1985, pp 232–233.
4. Eil, C: Hormone receptor physiology in clinical medicine. Crit Care Q 6(3):93, December 1983.

## SUGGESTED READINGS

Clark, M, et al: A user's guide to hormones. Newsweek, January 12, 1987, p 50.

CHAPTER 15

# Assessment of Endocrine Function

*Maria Elayne DeSimone*

## CHAPTER OUTLINE



## LEARNING OBJECTIVES

**At the end of this chapter, you should be able to:**

1. Describe the significance of a comprehensive database in terms of diagnosing, planning, implementing, and evaluating nursing care.
2. Identify the major components of the health history and physical examination as they pertain to endocrine function.
3. Explain the significance of functional health patterns as a basis for the nursing assessment of the patient with, or suspected of having, endocrine dysfunction.
4. Recognize clinical patterns associated with endocrine dysfunction as they emerge in the patient history and physical examination.

## ASSESSMENT OF ENDOCRINE FUNCTION

### Introduction

This chapter focuses on the data obtained by history and physical examination as they relate to endocrine dysfunction. General assessment techniques and human responses to alterations in pituitary, thyroid, adrenal, pancreatic, and parathyroid function are discussed.

Hormones affect each person's ability to interact with the environment. To assess and positively influence this interaction the nurse must take an organized, intellectual approach to the collection and documentation of data. A thorough knowledge of the pathophysiologic basis for clinical signs and symptoms, coupled with specific assessment skills, enables the nurse to formulate nursing diagnoses and to institute a plan of care. The "high level of suspicion" referred to in other chapters is not merely an intuitive process, but rather results, in this instance, from an understanding of endocrine-related symptomatology. The nurse must know what questions to ask in order to discover the etiologies that are amenable to nursing therapy.

Assessment of the endocrine system presents a formidable challenge to the critical care nurse. Due to the complexity of hormonal interactions, symptoms are often subtle and misleading. It is helpful to keep in mind that the clinical patterns seen in endocrine disorders represent the accentuation or absence of a hormone's physiologic actions. For example, blood pressure is regulated by several hormones, particularly cortisol, aldosterone, and catecholamines. Overproduction of these hormones in patients with Cushing's syndrome, primary aldosteronism, and pheochromocytoma, respectively, is associated with hypertension. On the other hand, hypotension is seen in patients with cortisol deficiency, hypoaldosteronism, or sympathetic dysfunction.[1]

Accurate nursing diagnosis begins with the recognition of clinical patterns as they emerge in the history and physical examination. When the nurse begins to recognize a pattern it must be pursued with increased specificity. For example, a patient may report polyuria for the past month. Polyuria is a symptom that occurs in several endocrine disorders, including both diabetes insipidus and diabetes mellitus. The nurse, patient, and family must explore the cluster of symptoms related to each disease process. Additional objective findings obtained from physical examination and laboratory data help establish a pattern of dysfunction.

The initial assessment of any critically ill patient is often conducted under less than optimal conditions. The need for rapid assessment and treatment of life-threatening events frequently precludes a relaxed and lengthy interview with the patient. Even so, every attempt should be made to obtain a comprehensive database. The importance of the contributions made by family and significant others cannot be overemphasized.

## Interview

Begin by introducing yourself and stating the purpose of the interview and physical examination. It should be made clear that the data gathered will remain confidential and will be used for the purposes of planning and evaluation. Maintain privacy and remain nonjudgmental. This will establish rapport and trust, essential components of any nurse–patient relationship.

Find out whether this is the first admission for this problem or an exacerbation of chronic disease. The answer to this question will vary the approach to assessment. Patients with chronic endocrine disorders are often required to alter their health practices to maintain survival. Hospitalization may represent a patient's inability for self-care. This may result from physiologic, psychologic, or environmental factors. Determining the cause of the exacerbation personalizes the plan of care.

Do not assume that length of disease bears any relationship to the degree of knowledge a patient may have. Rather, systematically establish what measures have been taken by the patient and family to maintain integrity and identify the dysfunctional health patterns specific to the patient's present state. Some of the questions to be asked in this regard are listed in Table 15–1.

TABLE 15–1
**Health Practices Assessment**

| |
|---|
| Key questions: |
| Does the patient take medication? On a daily basis? Weekly basis? (Type, dosage, route, adverse effects, efficacy?) |
| Can the patient describe symptoms of exacerbation of his/her disease? |
| Can the patient list measures to prevent complications? |
| Does the patient wear an alert bracelet or other form of identification? |
| What changes have been made in diet and activity? |
| Have there been recent hospital admissions related to this disorder? |

Throughout the interview, gather an overall impression of the patient. Does the patient seem lethargic or "jittery"? Does he/she demonstrate signs of anxiety disproportionate to the situation? Allow patients ample time to answer each question. Pay attention to both the content and manner of their responses. Note whether facial expressions, voice, and bodily movements vary appropriately with topics under discussion. Hypothyroidism often manifests itself in lethargy and slowed mentation (slowed speech pattern), whereas an overproduction of thyroid hormone will cause a patient to appear nervous and jittery.

### Chief Complaint and History of Present Illness

Determine why the patient was hospitalized. Explore thoroughly the nature of the patient's "chief complaint." A complete investigation of the present illness will reveal its onset, manner, location, duration, and severity (see Table 7–1). Ask the patient about aggravating or alleviating factors and any attempts at treatment (including home remedies).

### Past Health History

Ask about past health history. This should include the following points:

- Childhood illnesses and treatments: Common conditions such as acne were once treated with radiation. These patients may now be at risk for the development of thyroid cancer.
- History of hospitalizations, surgical procedures, chronic conditions.
- History of trauma (especially recent head trauma).
- History of allergies.
- Smoking history, use of alcohol or street drugs. Drug abuse may cause a myriad of symptoms that mimic endocrine dysfunction.
- Medication use (includes prescriptions, over-the-counter drugs, and vitamins).

### *Family History*

Complete the discussion of past history by inquiring about the health of the patient's family, both living and deceased, because many endocrine disorders have familial tendencies.

## Functional Health Pattern Assessment/Physical Examination

Document the remainder of the nursing assessment according to Gordon's functional health patterns[2] (see Appendix C). This approach will help identify actual or potential health problems amenable to nursing intervention. A discussion of some of the patterns most relevant to endocrine assessment follows. Included in the discussion of each pattern is a description of both subjective and objective data. In actual practice it is most efficient to first review each pattern verbally with the patient and family, and then perform a head to toe physical examination. The documentation is then integrated according to the nursing assessment format.

### *Health Perception–Health Management Pattern*

As stated previously, a complete discussion of health practices will help identify inadequacies in health maintenance. Alterations in this pattern may be due to a problem in one of the three domains of learning: the cognitive, psychomotor, and affective domains.

The *cognitive* domain of learning refers to the patient's ability to understand facts and concepts. Determine the patient's level of knowledge regarding pathophysiology, self-care requisites, and consequences of inadequate management. Level of education, native language, and socioeconomic status may all influence this domain.

The *psychomotor* domain encompasses the motor skills necessary to manage self-care. Does the patient have physical limitations that prevent health maintenance? An example of this is a patient who has diabetic retinopathy and is unable to draw up the correct dosage of insulin.

The *affective* domain relates to the way patients feel about their disease. Do they deny its existence? Do they believe in its seriousness? Do they believe they can influence its course? These beliefs will greatly influence the manner of health maintenance.

Finally, determine the presence of other factors that affect health management. Determine if financial restrictions preclude the purchase of necessary medications and equipment. Does lack of transportation prevent the patient from visiting the health provider or diagnostic laboratory?

### *Nutritional–Metabolic Pattern*

Endocrine disorders frequently cause significant changes in the body's ability to metabolize nutrients. Detecting an alteration in this pattern requires careful consideration of the pattern of food and fluid intake, body composition, and the characteristics of the integument (skin, hair, nails, and mucous membranes).

Ask the patient to describe what he/she ate for the last few days and determine if this is the usual pattern of food intake. Does the patient follow a restricted or special diet? If so, how does he/she tolerate it? Does the patient experience anorexia, nausea, vomiting, dysphagia, polyphagia, or excessive thirst? Any of these symptoms may indicate endocrine dysfunction.

Inquire about a recent history of infection and changes in the condition of the skin, hair, or nails. Establish a pattern of weight change with the patient and family.

**Body Composition.** Fluctuations in weight occur with several endocrine diseases. Classic examples of weight loss are seen in patients with new onset of uncontrolled diabetes mellitus and in patients with hyperthyroidism. In both cases this symptom relates to an altered metabolism and is accompanied by a voracious appetite. Weight loss coupled with anorexia is a frequent complaint of patients with adrenocortical insufficiency. In addition to weight gain, the patient with Cushing's syndrome experiences a redistribution of body fat, manifested by truncal obesity, the development of a "moon facies," and fat deposition over the cervical spine ("buffalo hump") (see Chap. 18).

Rapid fluctuations in weight most likely reflect the loss or gain of water. The complaint of rapid weight change should prompt the investigation of other symptoms related to fluid balance. These include polyuria, polydipsia, orthostatic hypotension, dizziness, excessive perspiration, dry tongue, dry skin, constipation, and the presence or absence of edema.

Dehydration is often a predominant clinical finding in diabetes insipidus, diabetic ketoacidosis, hyperosmolar coma, hypercalcemia, and adrenal crisis. This fluid volume deficit causes the skin to "tent" or temporarily lose its normal shape when gently pinched between thumb and forefinger. The best place to test for skin turgor is over the sternum, especially in the elderly patient who has lost much of the elasticity of the skin. Other clinical signs of dehydration include orthostatic hypotension, increased pulse, dry tongue and mucous membranes, concentrated urine, and changes in mental status.

Electrolyte imbalance often accompanies alterations in fluid balance. In addition to careful monitoring of laboratory results, the critical care nurse can detect such imbalances through history and physical assessment.

Signs and symptoms of potassium imbalance are often cardiac in nature and may cause irregularities in the apical and radial pulse. Signs and symptoms of sodium imbalance are, in part, neurologic and may range from mild confusion to frank coma.

Alterations in calcium levels have a profound effect on the neurologic system. The patient who is hypocalcemic will demonstrate signs of neuromuscular irritability. These include laryngeal spasm, respiratory stridor, muscular twitching, hyperactive reflexes, and possibly tetany and convulsions. Tests for Trousseau's and Chovstek's signs will be positive. In Trousseau's sign the patient's hand will spasm when pressure is applied to the arm. This is done with a blood pressure cuff inflated to 10 mmHg above the patient's systolic blood pressure. To test for Chovstek's sign, tap the facial nerve near the lower jaw. This will result in spasm of the facial muscle on the same side.

Hypercalcemia results in an opposite clinical picture. The patient is lethargic with sluggish reflexes. There is muscle weakness and lack of coordination. Additional clinical findings include hypertension, sluggish bowel sounds, and possible flank pain secondary to renal calculi.

**Integumentary Changes.** Hormonal imbalance often manifests itself in noticeable changes in the integument. Although obvious to the trained examiner, these changes may be ignored or not considered significant by the patient and family. A detailed history and careful physical examination will sort out these seemingly unrelated symptoms.

Common cutaneous effects of endocrine imbalance include infection, capillary fragility, changes in skin turgor and pigmentation, and changes in the hair and nails.

Hyperglycemia greatly increases the risk of infection. Early recognition of actual or potential infection is facilitated by questions relating to the following areas: recent injuries, areas of induration, swelling or drainage, pain or decreased sensation, condition of teeth and gums, and visits to the dentist and podiatrist.

In patients with some endocrine disorders such as Addison's disease or diabetes mellitus, infections that are not treated promptly may result in a rapid deterioration in health status. Carefully inspect all skin surfaces and mucous membranes, including the spaces between toes and folds of skin. Inspect the mouth, gums, and teeth. Auscultate the lungs for decreased breath sounds. This sign, along with dullness to percussion, may indicate consolidation secondary to pneumonia. Note that this finding may be masked in a dehydrated patient, and reevaluation may be necessary. Auscultate the abdomen for the presence and quality of bowel sounds, and palpate for tenderness. Percuss the spine for tenderness in the costovertebral angle.

The skin, hair, and nails are particularly vulnerable to alterations in the level of circulating thyroid hormone. Warm, flushed, moist skin, palmar erythema, fine silky hair, and onycholysis are hallmarks of hyperthyroidism. A lowered metabolic rate secondary to hypothyroidism results in brittle hair and nails. The skin is coarse, dry, and scaly, and often appears yellow due to increased levels of carotene.

Other changes in pigmentation include melanosis and vitiligo. The patient with adrenocortical insufficiency may report unusually persistent tanning following sun exposure or notice increased pigment over pressure points, scars, and mucous membranes. Adrenal cortex hyposecretion, diabetes mellitus, and hyperthyroidism may all cause vitiligo, which appears as irregular patchy areas of depigmentation.

To establish a history of capillary fragility, ask the patient about easy bruisability, bleeding tendencies, and the presence of ecchymosis. Patients with hypercortisolism often may complain of purple "stretch marks" on the breasts, abdomen, and hips.

### *Elimination Pattern*

Patients with endocrine dysfunction frequently experience alterations in their patterns of excretion. Questions should be directed at the excretory function of the bowel, bladder, and skin. Changes in regularity, timing, and frequency are reported more often than usual in patients with endocrine disease.

**Bowel.** Constipation results when there is significant dehydration or a decrease in gastrointestinal motility. In hypercalcemia and hyperglycemia osmotic diuresis pulls water from the gut and causes the patient to pass hard stools, often with difficulty.

The pattern of constipation seen in hypothyroidism is an example of the gastrointestinal effects of thyroid hormone. It is logical to assume, therefore, that the hyperthyroid patient will report the passage of increased stools per day.

Patients with longstanding diabetes mellitus may develop a neuropathy of the gastrointestinal tract leading to early satiety, constipation, or diarrhea, and possibly incontinence of stool at night.

**Bladder.** A change in urinary elimination is a salient feature of several endocrine disorders, particularly diabetes mellitus, diabetes insipidus, and hypercalcemia. Patients who complain of polyuria report an increased frequency and amount of voided urine. Elderly patients may describe a urinary incontinence problem. These statements should prompt the nurse to elicit more specific information regarding the color and odor of the urine as well as learn the results of related urine tests (urinalysis and culture, urine osmolality and 24-hour urine collection). Inquire about dysuria, urgency, and the presence of back pain, which may indicate the presence of a urinary tract infection.

Back pain can also be a symptom of renal calculi secondary to hyperparathyroidism.

**Skin.** Under normal temperate conditions, the skin will excrete approximately 100–500 ml of water per day. Normal skin is slightly warm and dry to the touch. Patients who are experiencing a hypermetabolic state will have warm, moist, flushed skin as a result of capillary dilatation. The complaints of heat intolerance and excessive perspiration are frequently related to states in which the metabolism is increased. Both hyperthyroidism and pheochromocytoma may cause this problem.

### *Activity–Exercise Pattern*

Detecting an alteration in activity–exercise pattern will reveal the effect of endocrine dysfunction on the cardiorespiratory and musculoskeletal system. Inquire about the ability to carry out activities of daily living. If there has been a change, document when this occurred and the patient's or family's explanation.

Intolerance to activity may take the form of fatigue, weakness, or impaired mobility. Determine if there are related symptoms to each of these complaints. Dizziness, shortness of breath, palpitations, and muscle cramps often accompany fatigue or weakness. Bone, muscle, and joint pain is often associated with impaired mobility.

Alterations in cardiac output may be perceived by the patient as fatigue or weakness. This can be secondary to diabetes, thyroid dysfunction, electrolyte imbalance resulting from adrenal insufficiency, or parathyroid disease. An examination of the cardiac and respiratory system may provide additional data to substantiate these complaints.

Determine if the patient can maintain an effective airway and breathing pattern. Patients with altered states of consciousness will require more frequent respiratory assessment. A classic example of an altered breathing pattern occurs in diabetic ketoacidosis. The respirations are rapid and deep and accompanied by a fruity odor to the breath as the lungs attempt to rid the body of excess carbon dioxide and ketones. This pattern is known as Kussmaul's breathing.

The frequent determination of blood pressure, pulse, and respirations helps to rapidly judge the integrity of the patient's cardiorespiratory system. Changes in the vital signs can reflect the body's attempt to compensate for fluid and electrolyte derangements or may result directly from hormonal imbalance.

Impaired mobility may be the result of bone loss secondary to osteoporosis. When sufficient calcium is lost, there is an increased risk of fracture. Complaints about back pain, coupled with evidence of loss of height, may indicate an episode of vertebral compression fractures. As more vertebrae become compressed, the spine develops a kyphoscoliosis, which leads to functional impairment and eventual respiratory compromise. This is commonly seen in patients with Cushing's disease.

Muscle weakness may also contribute significantly to mobility impairment. Inspect the muscles for symmetry and fasciculation, and assess strength bilaterally.

### *Cognitive Perceptual Pattern*

This pattern is designed to evaluate certain aspects of the patient's neurologic and cognitive function. Assessment of the five senses, perception of pain, and mental status is included.

The most striking examples of alterations in sensory perception are perhaps noted in the patient who has diabetes mellitus. Visual changes related to hyperglycemia include intermittent blurry vision, impaired extraocular movements, decreased peripheral vision, and retinal damage. Patients with diabetes mellitus have an increased incidence of glaucoma, cataracts, and retinal hemorrhage. Document any reported change in vision along with the frequency of visits to the ophthalmologist and therapeutic interventions (e.g., laser treatments). Include a complete evaluation of the eyes in the physical examination.

Peripheral neuropathy greatly decreases the diabetic patient's ability to perceive environmental stimuli through the skin. Reports of numbness or tingling in the extremities or observations of painless ulcers will validate an alteration in the sense of touch.

Determine if the patient is experiencing pain of any kind. Direct questions to the characteristics of pain: its onset, quality, duration, and radiation, as well as alleviating and aggravating factors. Determine what the patient and family have done to cope with this symptom.

Lastly, evaluate the patient's cognitive function. Acute and chronic changes in mental status may be secondary to an endocrine disorder such as diabetes mellitus, hypothyroidism, or pituitary disease. Components of the mental status examination are: level of consciousness, attention span, memory (recent and remote), thought process and content, and an evaluation of affect and mood (see Chap. 7).

Many tools have been developed to objectively evaluate aspects of mental status. The Glasgow Coma Scale is often used to rapidly assess level of consciousness. This scale evaluates three types of response to stimuli: verbal performance, eye opening ability, and motor ability (see Table 7–2). If a patient does not respond to a verbal stimulus, the examiner administers a painful stimulus. A score is assigned to each response and totaled at the end of the examination. The use of this scale will decrease subjectivity when examining patients with alterations in consciousness. Several brief tests have been developed to evaluate cognitive function.

Among the most useful is the Mini Mental Status Examination, a well-validated tool to screen for cognitive impairment.

In addition to completing the mental status examination, the nurse should evaluate sensory function and cranial nerves when assessing this pattern.

## SUMMARY

The remaining functional patterns, although not addressed in this chapter, will influence each patient's interaction with the environment and, therefore, must not be overlooked.

Clinical observations made by the critical care nurse often form the immediate database from which life-saving measures are implemented. The information obtained through inspection, palpation, percussion, and auscultation, when combined with the history, strengthens the foundation for the nurse's diagnosis and ongoing treatment plan. It is necessary, therefore, for the critical care nurse to master and maintain a high level of skill in assessment. The expert in critical care uses a consistent approach to the assessment and is able to adapt these techniques to rapidly changing clinical situations and patient conditions.

## REFERENCES

1. Jubitz, W: Endocrinology: A Logical Approach for Clinicians, ed 2. McGraw-Hill, New York, 1985.
2. Gordon, M: Manual of Nursing Diagnosis, ed 2. McGraw-Hill, New York, 1987.

## SUGGESTED READINGS

Abels, L: Critical Care Nursing—A Physiological Approach. CV Mosby, St Louis, 1986.

Bates, B: A Guide to Physical Examination and History Taking, ed 4. JB Lippincott, Philadelphia, 1987.

Folstein, M, Folstein, S, and McHugh, PR: Mini Mental Status—A practical method for grading the cognitive state of patients. J Psychiatr Res 12:189, 1975.

Gordon, M: Manual of Nursing Diagnosis 1986–1987. McGraw-Hill, New York, 1986.

Greenspan, F and Forsham, P: Basic and Clinical Endocrinology. Lange Medical Publications, Los Altos, CA, 1985.

Jubitz, W: Endocrinology: A logical Approach for Clinicians, ed 2. McGraw-Hill, New York, 1985.

Metz, R and Larson, E: Blue Book of Endocrinology. WB Saunders, Philadelphia, 1985.

Porter, P, et al: Diabetes Education Center Manual. Winthrop University Hospital, Mineola, NY, 1982.

Thompson, J: An Introduction to Clinical Endocrinology. Churchill Livingstone, New York, 1981.

# CHAPTER 16

# Nursing Management of the Patient with Hypothalamic-Pituitary Dysfunction

## CHAPTER OUTLINE



## LEARNING OBJECTIVES

**At the end of this chapter, you should be able to:**

1. Identify the fundamental importance of the hypothalamic-hypophyseal system.
2. Describe the pituitary gland and its structural and functional relationships.
3. Define osmolality and its significance in terms of water and electrolyte (solute) balance.
4. Describe the role of antidiuretic hormone (vasopressin) in the regulation of total body water balance.
5. State physiologic regulatory mechanisms of antidiuretic hormone secretion and water balance.
6. Describe diabetes insipidus (DI)—etiology, pathophysiology, clinical presentation, and treatment.
7. Describe syndrome of inappropriate secretion of ADH (SIADH)—etiology, pathophysiology, clinical presentation, and treatment.
8. Delineate the nursing process in the management of patients with diabetes insipidus, or syndrome of inappropriate secretion of ADH, including:
   - Assessment.
   - Nursing diagnosis.
   - Planning, including: Desired patient outcomes
     - Nursing interventions/rationales.

## INTRODUCTION

The hypothalamic-hypophyseal (pituitary) system provides for direct communication and interchange between the two major regulatory systems of bodily functions, namely, the nervous system and endocrine system. The unique relationship between the hypothalamus and pituitary enables the hypothalamus to exert a major effect on hormonal regulation. The significance of this relationship is underscored when one realizes that the hypothalamus receives signals from almost all areas within the nervous system. In essence, it is a collecting and processing center for all information and activities associated with maintaining the body in a state of dynamic equilibrium, and, accordingly, it influences bodily functions to maintain the state of well-being. While the anterior pituitary is frequently referred to as the "master" endocrine gland in the body, to be more succinct, the hypothalamus, with its many neural interconnections and glandular functions, is probably the "true" master gland.

## PITUITARY GLAND (HYPOPHYSIS): STRUCTURAL RELATIONSHIPS

The pituitary gland, or hypophysis, is a small gland that lies in the sella turcica at the base of the brain and is connected to the hypothalamus by a pituitary or *hypophyseal stalk* (Fig. 16–1). Anterior and superior to the pituitary as it sits in the sella turcica is the *optic chiasm.* This anatomic relationship is especially significant because the most common sign of extension of a pituitary tumor beyond the confines of the sella is a visual field defect. *Bitemporal hemianopsia* (i.e., blindness in the temporal half of the visual field in each eye) is the most frequently occurring disturbance caused by tumor pressing on the crossing central fibers of the chiasm while the uncrossed lateral fibers are spared.

Other significant structures lying adjacent to, and on either side of, the sella include the internal carotid arteries as they enter through the base of the skull, the cavernous sinuses, and the cranial nerves (III, IV, V, VI) that traverse the sinuses. The sphenoidal sinus occurs anterior and inferior to the sella, and it is through this sinus that a surgical transphenoidal approach to the pituitary is made.

## PITUITARY GLAND (HYPOPHYSIS): A DUAL ROLE

The pituitary gland is in actuality two distinct organs: the anterior pituitary, or *adeno*hypophysis, and the posterior pituitary, or *neuro*hypophysis. The continuity between the hypothalamus and posterior pituitary occurs via hypothalamic-neurohypophyseal *nerve* tracts wherein axons of neurons originating in the paraventricular and supraoptic nuclei travel down through the pituitary stalk to terminate in the posterior pituitary (see Fig. 16–1).

Antidiuretic hormone (ADH), also called vasopressin, and oxytocin are the two hormones synthesized by separate and distinct neurons within the hypothalamic nuclei, packaged together with carrier proteins or neurophysins, and transported down the axons to be stored in the axonal endings in the posterior pituitary.[1] These hormones are secreted directly into the blood in response to action potentials generated in the hypothalamus and conducted down the axons to the axonal endings.

In contrast to the posterior pituitary, there is no neural connection between the anterior pituitary and hypothalamus. Rather, these two organs are connected via the hypothalamic-hypophyseal *portal* system (i.e., blood vessels that connect separate and distinct capillary beds). In this circumstance, the portal vessels connect the hypothalamic capillary bed with that of the anterior pituitary (see Fig. 16–1). The anterior pituitary is a highly vascular organ with an extensive capillary network surrounding the glandular cells within it.

There are several different cell types within the anterior pituitary, with one type of cell responsible for the synthesis and secretion of each specific hormone. The one exception concerns follicle stimulating hormone (FSH) and luteinizing hormone (LH), which may be synthesized and secreted by the same cell.

Of the various hormones secreted by the anterior pituitary (see Table 14–1), which play a significant role in maintaining the life processes in a state of dynamic equilibrium, those of particular concern to critical care nursing include thyrotropic stimulating hormone (TSH) and adrenocorticotropic hormone (ACTH). (The role played by these hormones will be examined more closely in Chaps. 17 and 18, respectively.) The present discussion will focus on a close examination of the posterior pituitary hormone, antidiuretic hormone (ADH), and its role in the maintenance of fluid balance.

## SERUM OSMOLALITY: STIMULUS FOR ANTIDIURETIC HORMONE SECRETION

The composition of body fluids is largely maintained by the kidneys (see Chap. 23), which play a central role in water and electrolyte (solute) balance. Reabsorption and secretion of electrolytes must be accompanied by equivalent changes in water reabsorption and excretion if total body equilibrium is to be maintained.

The kidneys have the capacity to efficiently concentrate or dilute urine to maintain the osmolality of the extracellular fluid compartment.[2] This efficient compensatory mechanism for maintaining water balance is primarily attributed to the ability of the kidneys to excrete excess water without altering the usual excretion of salt and other molecules. This critical physiologic function, in turn, is regulated in part by antidiuretic hormone (ADH), which is secreted by the posterior pituitary in response to changes in serum osmolality.

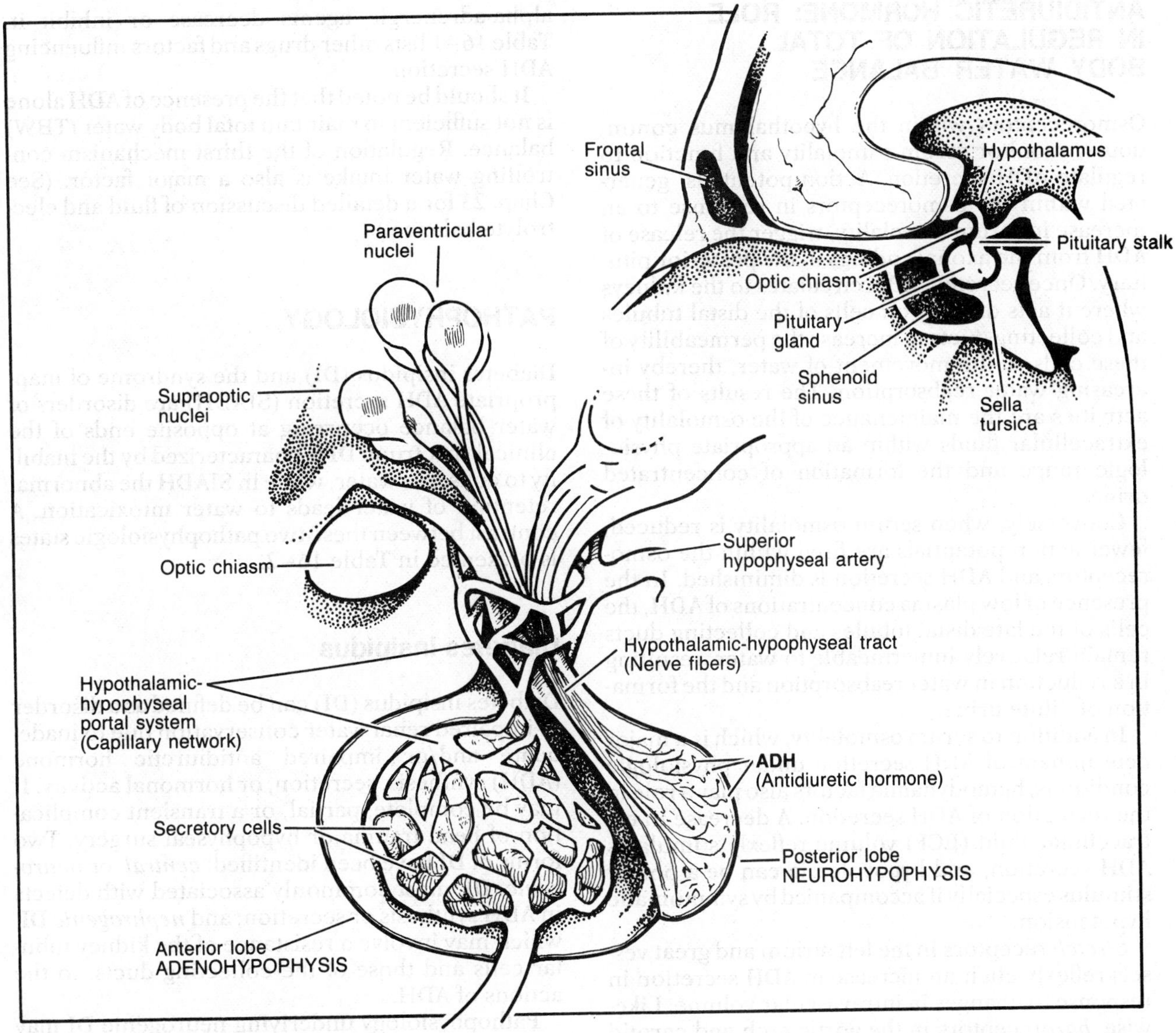


**Figure 16-1.** The pituitary gland, or hypophysis, lies within the bony sella turcica at the base of the skull. It is connected to the hypothalamus by the hypophyseal stalk. Anterior and superior to the pituitary as it sits in the sella turcica is the optic chiasm; anterior and inferior to the pituitary is the sphenoidal sinus. These structural relationships account for the visual field deficits experienced by individuals with a pituitary tumor. During pituitary-related surgery, access to the pituitary is through a transsphenoidal approach (i.e., through the sphenoid sinus into the sella turcica). Continuity between the hypothalamus and neurohypophysis occurs via hypothalamic-neurohypophyseal nerve tracts; continuity between the hypothalamus and adenohypophysis is non-neural; rather, it occurs via the hypothalamic-hypophyseal portal system.

## Osmolality: Defined

Osmolality is a measurement of the particles dissolved in the serum,[3] or the amount of osmotic pressure exerted by particles of solute per kilogram of body weight. Osmolality is affected by electrolytes (including sodium, chloride, and bicarbonate, predominantly) and inactive molecules such as glucose and urea. Serum osmolality can be calculated as follows:

$$\text{Serum Osmolality} = \left\{2 \times \text{Serum Sodium Concentration}\right\} + \frac{\text{Blood Urea Nitrogen Concentration}}{2.8} + \frac{\text{Serum Glucose Concentration}}{18}$$

Normal range: 285–295 mOsm/kg.

## ANTIDIURETIC HORMONE: ROLE IN REGULATION OF TOTAL BODY WATER BALANCE

Osmoreceptors within the hypothalamus continuously monitor serum osmolality and function to regulate ADH secretion. Action potentials, generated within the osmoreceptors in response to an increase in serum osmolality, trigger the release of ADH from the axonal endings in the posterior pituitary. Once secreted, ADH circulates to the kidneys where it acts directly on cells of the distal tubules and collecting ducts to increase the permeability of these cells to the movement of water, thereby increasing water reabsorption. The results of these activities are the maintenance of the osmolality of extracellular fluids within an appropriate physiologic range and the formation of concentrated urine.

Conversely, when serum osmolality is reduced, fewer action potentials are fired within the osmoreceptors and ADH secretion is diminished. In the presence of low plasma concentrations of ADH, the cells of the late distal tubules and collecting ducts remain relatively impermeable to water, resulting in a reduction in water reabsorption and the formation of dilute urine.

In addition to serum osmolality, which is a major determinant of ADH secretion under physiologic conditions, hemodynamic factors also play a role in the regulation of ADH secretion. A decrease in extracellular fluid (ECF) volume reflexly stimulates ADH secretion, and hypovolemia can be a potent stimulus especially if accompanied by symptomatic hypotension.

*Stretch* receptors in the left atrium and great vessels reflexly elicit an increase in ADH secretion in response to changes in intravascular volume. Likewise, *baro*receptors in the aortic arch and carotid sinuses, which monitor arterial blood pressure, also participate in the control of ADH secretion. While volume/pressure receptors are less sensitive to change in water balance than are osmoreceptors under ordinary circumstances, should hypovolemia be severe and/or arterial blood pressure decline precipitously, the magnitude of the ADH response is much greater than that seen via the osmotic stimuli (i.e., increased serum osmolality). Stretch and baroreceptors transmit information via vagal afferent fibers to the hypothalamus.

In terms of hemodynamic function, ADH exerts a potent pressor effect (i.e., constriction of peripheral arterioles), which is why it is also called vasopressin.

A number of other factors may affect ADH release. These include trauma, pain, and emotional stress, which stimulate ADH release. Many drugs may enhance or inhibit ADH secretion. Cholinergic and beta-adrenergic agents increase ADH secretion, while anticholinergics (e.g., atropine) and alpha-adrenergic agents decrease or inhibit it. Table 16-1 lists other drugs and factors influencing ADH secretion.

It should be noted that the presence of ADH alone is not sufficient to maintain total body water (TBW) balance. Regulation of the thirst mechanism controlling water intake is also a major factor. (See Chap. 23 for a detailed discussion of fluid and electrolyte balance.)

## PATHOPHYSIOLOGY

Diabetes insipidus (DI) and the syndrome of inappropriate ADH secretion (SIADH) are disorders of water balance occurring at opposite ends of the clinical spectrum. DI is characterized by the inability to conserve water, while in SIADH the abnormal retention of water leads to water intoxication. A contrast between these two pathophysiologic states is presented in Table 16-2.

### Diabetes Insipidus

Diabetes insipidus (DI) can be defined as a disorder of impaired renal water conservation due to inadequate and/or impaired antidiuretic hormone (ADH) synthesis, secretion, or hormonal activity. It may be complete, partial, or a transient complication of head trauma or hypophyseal surgery. Two forms of DI have been identified: *central,* or *neurogenic,* DI, most commonly associated with defects in ADH synthesis or secretion; and *nephrogenic* DI, which may involve a resistance of the kidney tubular cells and those of the collecting ducts, to the actions of ADH.

Pathophysiology underlying neurogenic DI may involve one or more mechanisms (see Table 16-2). Nephrogenic DI usually occurs when the kidneys fail to respond to ADH. Of the two forms of DI, nephrogenic DI rarely presents with the massive polyuria characteristic of the neurogenic form, possibly because the ability to concentrate urine is somewhat preserved in the nephrogenic form.

#### *Clinical Presentation*

The major clinical manifestations of DI include polyuria, excessive thirst, and polydipsia. In either form, neurogenic or nephrogenic, as long as the thirst mechanism remains intact and the individual is driven and able to drink adequate amounts of fluids, the effects of the underlying pathophysiology will remain obscured. Impairment of the thirst mechanism, lack of accessibility to water, or the inability to ingest large volumes of water, can, in the setting of DI, result in rapidly developing dehydration leading to circulatory collapse.

TABLE 16-1
**Factors That Affect ADH Secretion**

| Factors That Increase ADH Secretion | Factors That Decrease ADH Secretion |
|---|---|
| 1. Increased serum osmolality/decreased blood volume<br>A. Dehydration—hypovolemia<br>B. Hemorrhage<br>C. Hypotension<br>D. Decreased cardiac output<br>E. Hypernatremia<br>F. Hyperglycemia | 1. Decreased serum osmolality/increased blood volume<br>A. Overhydration—hypervolemia<br>B. Hypertension<br>C. Increased cardiac output<br>D. Hyponatremia |
| 2. Central nervous system stimulation<br>A. Trauma<br>Head injury<br>Skull fracture<br>Epidural/subdural hematoma<br>Subarachnoid hemorrhage<br>B. Pain<br>C. Nausea/vomiting—emesis<br>D. Emotional stress—fear, anxiety<br>E. Hyperthermia | 2. CNS depression<br>A. Hypothermia |
| 3. Drugs<br>A. Cholinergic—nicotine<br>B. Beta-adrenergics<br>C. Angiotensin (stimulates thirst)<br>D. General anesthetics<br>E. Morphine/barbiturates<br>F. Chlorpropamide (oral hypoglycemic)<br>G. Antineoplastic agents<br>Vincristine<br>Cyclophosphamide<br>H. Clofibrate (antilipemic)<br>I. Carbamazepine (anticonvulsant)<br>J. Chlorthiazide diuretics | 3. Drugs<br>A. Anticholinergic—atropine<br>B. Alpha-adrenergics<br>C. Ethanol<br>D. Morphine antagonist—naloxone hydrochloride<br>E. Phenytoin (diphenylhydantoin)<br>F. Clonidine hydrochloride<br>G. Reserpine<br>H. Lithium |

### *Clinical Data and Diagnostic Findings*

In considering the diagnosis of DI, any patient with an otherwise unexplained polyuria and polydipsia should be suspected of having DI. Thorough history taking is critical to the diagnosis of DI. Recent illness, trauma (e.g., head injury), surgery (e.g., transphenoidal-hypophyseal surgery), and cerebrovascular insult (e.g., intracranial bleed associated with cerebral aneurysm, cerebral vascular accident) are all implicated in DI, and their occurrence needs to be ascertained. Drug use and abuse need to be investigated. A familial history of neoplasms, metastatic carcinoma, primary renal disease, diabetes mellitus, among others, may contribute to differential diagnosis.

Physical examination usually reveals a dehydrated state. Visual field defects reflective of pressure on the optic chiasm (e.g., bitemporal hemianopsia) suggest a pituitary problem. Laboratory findings usually reflect a high serum osmolality, hypernatremia, a low urine specific gravity, and low urinary sodium. In the scenario of polyuria and polydipsia, serum/urine glucose screening is essential to rule out diabetes mellitus. The osmotic diuresis associated with an increased glucose load may manifest clinically with this symptomatology. (See Table 16-2 for specific data related to diagnostic findings and differential diagnosis.)

### *Treatment*

The treatment and management of DI largely depend on its cause and the clinical circumstances. The immediate complication is hypovolemia and dehydration with rapid progression to shock and circulatory collapse. Efforts are directed toward reestablishing and maintaining fluid and electrolyte balance and treating the underlying cause.

Antidiuretic hormone (ADH) replacement therapy may be initiated and requires special attention to the mode and technique of administration to ensure optimum dosage with the least amount of discomfort to the patient. The patient's condition needs to be monitored closely to evaluate the effectiveness of therapy and to assess for any adverse drug effects.

Other drugs in varying combinations may be used to increase release of ADH or to enhance its

TABLE 16-2

## Contrast: Diabetes Insipidus and Syndrome of Inappropriate ADH Secretion

| | Diabetes Insipidus | SIADH |
|---|---|---|
| Defined | State of decreased ADH secretion, increased water excretion, very dilute urine<br>Types: Central neurogenic and nephrogenic<br>Classification: Partial or complete; permanent or temporary | State of increased ADH secretion, increased water reabsorption, very concentrated urine |
| Pathophysiology | 1. Inability of cells in hypothalamic nuclei to synthesize/transport ADH<br>2. Failure of ADH release from axonal endings in posterior pituitary<br>3. ADH secretion in subnormal amounts<br>4. Defective osmoreceptors—altered threshold requires higher serum osmolality levels to elicit response<br>5. Presence of ADH antibiodies accelerates ADH breakdown<br>6. Resistance or unresponsiveness of cells of late distal tubule and collecting ducts to ADH (nephrogenic) | 1. Increased secretion of ADH in setting of low serum osmolality and in the absence of a physiologic stimulus such as hypovolemia, hypotension, or dehydration<br>2. Failure of negative feedback related to osmolality of ECV and fluid volume<br>3. Increase in total body water (TBW) *without* edema formation |
| Etiology | 1. 45–50% idiopathic (unknown cause)<br>2. Trauma (acute head injury most common)<br>3. Pituitary tumors<br>4. Pituitary or intracranial surgery<br>5. Cerebral edema<br>6. Infection: Meningitis, encephalitis, other<br>7. Inflammatory/degenerative processes: Tuberculosis<br>8. Cerebrovascular lesions: Aneurysms, subarachnoid hemorrhage, others<br>9. Drugs: alcohol, phenytoin, others | 1. Ectopic production of ADH via malignant tumors: Bronchogenic (oat cell) carcinoma, leukemias, Hodgkin's disease<br>2. Central nervous system (CNS) disorders: Infection—meningitis, others; Guillain-Barré syndrome; cerebrovascular disruption; seizures; head injury; tumors or metastatic lesions<br>3. Intrathoracic pathology: Pneumonia, tuberculosis, COPD, cardiac failure<br>4. Endocrine disorders: Adrenal insufficiency<br>5. Drugs:<br>Drug-related SIADH (ADH replacement therapy): Chlorpropamide, clofibrate, carbamazepine<br>Drugs that stimulate ADH release: Vincristine, cyclophosphamide<br>Drugs that potentiate action of ADH: Chlorpropamide, acetaminophen, thiazide diuretics, others |
| Clinical presentation | Onset: May be sudden<br>Signs/symptoms: Polyuria, excessive thirst (polydipsia), dehydration, weight loss | Onset: Gradual<br>Signs/symptoms related to: Water intoxication and hyponatremia<br>Mild—Headache, confusion, disorientation, lethargy, muscle cramps, anorexia, nausea, weight gain<br>Moderate—Restlessness, irritability, personality changes, nausea/vomiting/diarrhea, abdominal cramps, weakness, twitching, diminished deep tendon reflexes<br>Severe—Seizures, coma, death if untreated |
| Clinical history | Recent head trauma/surgery, cerebrovascular insult, drug usage, tumors/malignancies, renal disease, others | Malignant tumors; CNS insult—trauma, infection, cerebral hemorrhage, seizures, Guillain-Barré syndrome; pulmonary disease—tuberculosis, pneumonias<br>Drug usage—ADH replacement therapy<br>Mechanical ventilation<br>Other |
| Physical examination | Signs of dehydration: Sunken eyeballs, poor skin turgor over sternum or forehead, weight loss, weakness, listlessness<br>Visual field defects (bitemporal hemianopsia) | Personality changes, confusion, weakness, hostility<br>Fluid overload—neck vein distention, hyperpnea, rales, decreased deep tendon reflexes |
| Laboratory studies | | |
| Serum osmolality | >295 mOsm/kg | <280 mOsm/kg |
| Urine osmolality | 50–100 mOsm/kg | Equal to or greater than serum osmolality |
| Serum sodium | >148 mEq/liter | <130 mEq/liter |
| Urinary sodium | <20 mEq/liter | >180 mEq/liter |
| Urine specific gravity: | ~1.005 | >1.030 |
| Summary of serum/urine values | Increased serum osmolality<br>Decreased urine osmolality<br>Hypernatremia<br>Decreased urinary sodium | Decreased serum osmolality<br>Increased urine osmolality<br>Hyponatremia<br>Increased urinary sodium |

TABLE 16–2

**Contrast: Diabetes Insipidus and Syndrome of Inappropriate ADH Secretion *(Continued)***

| | **Diabetes Insipidus** | **SIADH** |
|---|---|---|
| | (*Urine osmolality*: A measurement of the number of particles in urine. Variable range from 50–1400 mOsm/kg, with an average of 500–800 mOsm/kg.)<br>(*Urine specific gravity*: A measurement of the degree of concentration of urine, which reflects the kidney's ability to concentrate urine. Range: 1.010–1.025.) | |
| Diagnostic studies | *Water Deprivation Test:*<br>Procedure:<br>1. Patient is deprived of water intake until urine osmolality on 3 consecutive specimens obtained 1 hr apart reflect a urine osmolality of less than 30 mOsm/kg.<br>2. Once urine osmolality is stabilized, 5 units of aqueous vasopressin or pitressin is administered subcutaneously, with urine osmolality measured 1 hr later.<br>3. Results:<br>Patients with neurogenic DI will have a greater than 9% increase in urine osmolality after vasopressin.<br>The patient requires diligent surveillance during the course of the test for signs of dehydration predisposing to hypovolemic shock. | *Water Loading Test:*<br>Procedure:<br>1. The patient is given a large fluid challenge.<br>2. Subsequent urine output is measured.<br>3. Results:<br>If less than one-half of the fluid volume is excreted, the presence of SIADH is highly suggested.<br>Urinary sodium will also be exaggerated. |
| Differential diagnosis | Diabetes mellitus<br>Psychogenic polydipsia<br>Chronic nephritis—increased BUN, albumin in urine<br>Others | Pseudohyponatremia in presence of hyperglycemia (increased serum glucose pulls fluid from the ICV to the ECV)[4]<br>True sodium depletion associated with diarrhea, diabetes mellitus, renal disease, diuretics<br>Endocrine dysfunction—Hypothyroidism, adrenal insufficiency<br>Chronic renal failure<br>Others |
| Complications | Dehydration<br>Hypovolemic shock<br>Circulatory collapse<br>Ureteral/bladder dilatation and/or hypertrophy<br>Resistance to vasopressin/pitressin therapy | Coma<br>Seizures<br>Death |
| Treatment goals | 1. Prevent dehydration.<br>2. Correct electrolyte imbalance.<br>3. Resolve underlying cause. | 1. Prevent water intoxication.<br>2. Correct electrolyte imbalance.<br>3. Resolve underlying cause. |
| Plan of care | 1. Fluid replacement<br>2. Hormonal replacement<br>3. Identification/treatment of underlying cause | 1. Strict fluid restriction<br>2. Administration of sodium chloride<br>3. Identification and treatment of underlying cause |
| Implementing care plan | 1. Fluid administration to correct dehydration and hypovolemia; hypotonic fluids recommended; oral fluid intake encouraged<br>2. ADH replacement therapy:<br>Monitor response to drug therapy; assess for allergies/side effects; assess for drug resistance; monitor all electrolytes; ongoing assessment of vital signs<br>Vasopressor properties of replacement drug may predispose to angina especially in patients with coronary artery disease<br>3. Use of thiazide diuretics may decrease urine volume output to 3–6 liters/24 hr, as opposed to 10 or more liters/24 hr<br>(See Tables 16–3 and 16–4 for pertinent nursing diagnoses, patient outcomes, and nursing interventions/rationales in the care of the patient with diabetes insipidus or syndrome of inappropriate secretion of ADH.) | 1. Fluid restriction: Fluid intake should equal urine output only until serum sodium normalizes and signs/symptoms abate.<br>As patient's status normalizes, fluid intake should equal urine output plus estimated insensible losses.<br>Hypertonic saline recommended.<br>2. Diuretic therapy<br>Furosemide (Lasix)<br>Potassium chloride supplements<br>3. Hypertonic peritoneal dialysis (4.25% dialysate solution)<br>4. Reevaluation of ADH replacement therapy (Overly vigorous ADH replacement therapy can predispose to SIADH.) |

action. These include chlorpropamide, clofibrate, and carbamazepine drug therapy. (Hypoglycemia may complicate the use of chlorpropamide.) These drugs exert an antidiuretic effect, reducing polyuria and polydipsia. They may also increase ADH secretion and potentiate its activity on the cells of the late distal tubules and collecting ducts of the nephrons. Thiazides reduce polyuria by decreasing plasma volume and depleting sodium, both of which are stimuli for renal water and sodium reabsorption.

Although some of these therapeutic approaches are more likely to be implemented in an acute care setting, the critical care nurse needs to be familiar with such regimens because of the occasional complication of SIADH precipitated by too aggressive ADH hormonal therapy. History taking in this regard is especially important.

### *Nursing Care of the Patient with Diabetes Insipidus*

**Therapeutic Goals.** Implementation of nursing process in the care of the patient with, or at risk of developing, DI revolves around the following therapeutic goals:

1. Identify patients at risk (see etiology section in Table 16–2), and establish a comprehensive database including:
   A. Clinical history (functional health patterns).
   B. Physical examination.
   C. Laboratory/diagnostic data.
2. Implement therapeutic regimen to restore fluid and electrolyte balance.
3. Promote/maintain optimal neurologic function.
4. Promote/maintain optimal cardiopulmonary function.
5. Alleviate/minimize anxiety.
6. Prevent injury related to:
   A. Altered sensorium, seizures.
   B. Altered visual fields.
   C. Infection.
   D. Untoward drug interactions or adverse effects.
   E. Iatrogenic SIADH associated with overly aggressive ADH replacement therapy.
7. Promote/maintain skin and musculoskeletal integrity.
8. Establish a working rapport with patient and family/significant others.
9. Provide emotional and psychologic support to patient and family/significant others.

**Nursing Diagnoses, Desired Patient Outcomes, and Nursing Interventions.** Pertinent nursing diagnoses, desired patient outcomes and nursing interventions/rationales in the care of the patient with DI are presented in Table 16–3.

## Syndrome of Inappropriate Secretion of ADH

The syndrome of inappropriate ADH secretion (SIADH)[5] is characterized by the inappropriate and continued secretion of ADH in a setting of low serum osmolality, and in the absence of a physiologic stimulus for ADH release such as hypovolemia, hypotension, or dehydration. The impairment in free water excretion leads to water intoxication and dilutional hyponatremia (see Chap. 23).

Failure in the negative feedback system that regulates ADH secretion results in continued reabsorption of solute-free water, which expands the extracellular fluid volume. Ordinarily, any decrease in the osmolality of extracellular fluids, or dilution and expansion of body fluids, provides the stimuli that inhibit ADH release. In the case of SIADH, the system fails to respond to decreased osmolality or increased extracellular (including intravascular and interstitial compartments) fluid volume, resulting in the continued inappropriate secretion of ADH.

### *Clinical Presentation*

Clinically, manifestations of SIADH occur secondary to two primary pathophysiologic states: water intoxication and hyponatremia (see Table 16–2). There may be an initial gradual onset of neurologic symptoms, including headache, confusion, disorientation, and weakness, together with nausea, vomiting, diarrhea, and anorexia associated with the hyponatremia. The patient may progress rapidly to muscle cramps, twitching, and seizures. These signs and symptoms are nonspecific; thus a high index of suspicion is necessary in assessing the patient. As is the case with diabetes insipidus, a thorough history is critical to help differentiate etiologic or contributing factors. For example, it is important to elicit information regarding the recent use of chlorpropamide or vasopressin preparations, because highly aggressive treatment of DI can predispose to SIADH.

Positive pressure breathing (e.g., mechanical ventilation) can predispose to an increase in ADH secretion. The underlying mechanism is associated with the reduction in venous return and cardiac output, resulting from positive pressures generated within the thorax during the inspiratory phase. The consequent reduction in cardiac output reflexly (e.g., via baroreceptors) triggers the release of ADH. Nurses caring for the ventilated patient should be especially vigilant for signs and symptoms of SIADH.

## TABLE 16–3. CARE PLAN FOR THE PATIENT WITH DIABETES INSIPIDUS

| Nursing Diagnoses | Desired Patient Outcomes | Nursing Interventions | Rationales |
|---|---|---|---|
| ***Nursing Diagnosis #1***<br>Fluid volume deficit: Actual, related to:<br>1. Decreased ADH synthesis and/or secretion.<br>2. Defective osmoreceptors.<br>3. Altered immunologic function (presence of ADH antibodies).<br>4. Unresponsiveness of cells in the late distal tubules and collecting ducts to action of ADH (nephrogenic DI).<br>(See Nursing Diagnosis #1 in Table 23–3.) | Patient will maintain stable:<br>1. Hydration status:<br>• Body weight within 5% of baseline.<br>• Balanced intake and output.<br>*Laboratory studies:*<br>• Serum osmolality: ~285–295 mOsm/kg.<br>• Urine specific gravity: ~1.010–1.025.<br>2. Neurologic status:<br>• Alert, oriented to person, place, and date.<br>• Visual fields at baseline for patients.<br>• Motor function: Muscle tone and strength intact; absence of twitching or seizure activity.<br>• Deep tendon reflexes brisk. | (For a detailed presentation of the nursing interventions and their rationales related to fluid volume deficit, see Table 23–3, Nursing Diagnoses #1 #2, #3; Table 23–7, Nursing Diagnosis #1.)<br>In addition, consider the following:<br>• Assess for signs and symptoms of DI:<br>○ Specific symptomatology includes:<br>–Polyuria (urine output: 4–6 liters/24 hr or more).<br>–Polydipsia (fluid intake: 4–6 liters/24 hr or more).<br>–Weight loss.<br>–Signs of dehydration: Sunken eyeballs, poor skin turgor, dry mucous membranes, hypotension, rapid pulse. | • DI is a state of reduced ADH synthesis and/or secretion, or diminished response of cells of the distal tubules and collecting ducts of kidneys to the actions of ADH. Osmoreceptors may be impaired.<br>○ Loss or absence of ADH compromises water reabsorption, resulting in excretion of large volumes of water despite a high serum osmolality (e.g., >295 mOsm/kg). |
| | | ○ Laboratory findings:<br>–Serum osmolality: >295 mOsm/kg.<br>–Serum sodium: >148 mEq/liter.<br>–Urinary sodium: <20 mEq/liter.<br>–Urine specific gravity: ~1.005. | ○ Excretion of water without concomitant excretion of sodium and other solute predisposes to hypernatremia and high serum osmolality. Urine excreted is, therefore, very dilute (e.g., low specific gravity), and urinary sodium is reduced as it is reabsorbed in renal tubules. |
| | | • Collaborate with other health-care providers to implement and monitor therapeutic regimen.<br>○ Monitor neurologic function: Mental status; level of consciousness; sensory/motor function; deep tendon reflexes.<br>○ Implement measures to protect patient from injury caused by altered sensorium, seizure activity.<br>–Pharyngeal airway and suction intact at bedside; padded side rails; bedside free of potential hazards (unnecessary equipment/furniture, electrical appliances, and so forth). | ○ DI may result in total body water deficit. Alterations in cerebral function may reflect cerebral intracellular dehydration with cell shrinkage (crenation). |

*(continued)*

**TABLE 16–3. CARE PLAN FOR THE PATIENT WITH DIABETES INSIPIDUS *(Continued)***

| Nursing Diagnoses | Desired Patient Outcomes | Nursing Interventions | Rationales |
|---|---|---|---|
| ***Nursing Diagnosis #2***<br>Cardiac output, alteration in: decreased, related to:<br>1. Severely contracted intravascular volume. | 3. Hemodynamic status:<br>• Blood pressure within 10 mmHg of baseline.<br>• Pulse strong; rate >60, <100 beats/min.<br>• Hemodynamic parameters:<br>CVP—mean 0–8 mmHg<br>PCWP—mean 8–12 mmHg.<br>CO—4–8 liter/min. | • Monitor hemodynamic status:<br>○ Vital signs: Heart rate, peripheral pulses, arterial blood pressure.<br>○ Hemodynamic parameters: CVP, PCWP, and CO.<br>○ Hydration status: Hourly fluid intake and output; daily weight; urine specific gravity. | • Severe dehydration reduces circulating intravascular blood volume, diminishing venous return to the heart and compromising cardiac output.<br>○ Progression of hypovolemic state to hypotensive shock and circulatory collapse can occur rapidly in the setting of DI. |
| ***Nursing Diagnosis #3***<br>Electrolyte imbalance, related to:<br>1. Excess water loss with hypernatremia (see Table 23–7, Nursing Diagnosis #1). | 4. Renal status:<br>• Hourly urine outputs: >30, <200 ml/hr.<br>*Laboratory studies:*<br>• BUN and creatinine at baseline for patient.<br>• Serum sodium: 135–148 mEq/liter.<br>• Urinary sodium: 80–180 mEq/liter.<br>• Other electrolytes within acceptable range for patient.<br>• Serum glucose: 70–110 mg/100 ml.<br>• Hematology profile within acceptable range (hematocrit, hemoglobin). | • Implement fluid replacement regimen<br>○ Administer hypotonic fluids initially.<br>○ Monitor all vital parameters during fluid replacement therapy.<br>○ Monitor serial laboratory studies: serum electrolytes, osmolality, BUN and creatinine, hematology profile; urinary sodium and osmolality.<br>○ Monitor cardiac status: Cardiac output, peripheral pulses (quality, amplitude, contour); neck vein distention.<br>–Overhydration: Full, bounding pulse; neck vein distention.<br>–Dehydration: Weak, thready pulse; flat neck veins.<br>• Administer ADH replacement therapy as prescribed; monitor response to therapy.<br>○ Pharmacologic preparations include vasopressin (Pitressin), vasopressin tannate, lypressin (Diapid), and desmopressin acetate (DDAVP). | • Major goal of therapy in treating DI is to prevent hypovolemia and dehydration.<br>• Fluid therapy is prescribed to correct hypovolemia and dehydration.<br>○ Hypotonic fluids initially allow for more vigorous treatment of hyperosmolar state; provide patient with access to copious amounts of fluid because of intense thirst.<br>○ Aggressive fluid replacement therapy can predispose to fluid overload; elderly patients (>65 years) are more susceptible to fluid overload because their total body water (TBW) is lower than in young persons.<br>○ Overhydration can precipitate congestive heart failure and pulmonary edema.<br>○ Vasopressin drug therapy should be accompanied by water ingestion to minimize side effects of nausea and abdominal cramps. |

| | | | |
|---|---|---|---|
| | | ○ Monitor for side effects:<br>–Vasopressin may cause diaphoresis, tremor, pounding headache; nausea, abdominal/uterine cramps, diarrhea; hypertension, angina, water intoxication. | ○ Vasopressin preparations in oil base require warming the ampule and shaking vigorously to disperse medication evenly in the oil medium.<br>○ Subcutaneous and intramuscular injections may be painful; a large needle is recommended. |
| | | –Rhinorrhea, nasal congestion, headache, increased blood pressure, flushing of skin, and abdominal cramps may accompany use of lypressin and desmopressin. | –Lypressin and desmopressin acetate are administered intranasally. These drugs should not be inhaled; keep refrigerated. |
| | 5. Respiratory status:<br>• Respiratory rate <25–30 breaths/min.<br>• Rhythm: Eupneic.<br>• Breath sounds: Clear to auscultation.<br>• Absence of adventitious sounds. | • Administer prescribed thiazide diuretic therapy. | • Antidiuretic response may be potentiated by concomitant administration of chlorpropamide, clofibrate, or carbamazepine.<br>○ Thiazides promote sodium excretion, which may help to prevent hypernatremia in the face of excessive water loss.<br>○ Thiazides may be prescribed in nephrogenic DI to promote water reabsorption via mechanisms independent of ADH effect. |
| | | • Monitor respiratory function: presence of tachypnea, dyspnea.<br>○ Presence of adventitious breath sounds —crackles (rales), wheezes. | ○ Presence of crackles/rales may suggest pulmonary congestion associated with overly aggressive fluid replacement. |
| | | ○ Presence of cough, productive or nonproductive? | ○ Overhydration: Thin, copious secretions. Dehydration: Thick, tenacious secretions. |
| | | • Establish regimen for positioning, turning, deep breathing, and coughing; chest physiotherapy and bronchial hygiene. | • These activities as tolerated by the patient assist in mobilizing and removing secretions by coughing and/or suctioning. |
| ***Nursing Diagnosis #4***<br>Oral mucous membranes, alteration in, related to:<br>1. Dehydration state. | Mucous membranes will remain clean, moist, and without cracking or fissures. | • Monitor integumentary status:<br>○ Assess skin/mucous membranes. | ○ Patients with DI are at great risk of becoming dehydrated when they are no longer able to maintain fluid intake to match fluid loss. |
| | | ○ Initiate oral hygiene regimen. | ○ Severely dehydrated patient is at increased risk of infection; wound healing may be compromised. |

*(continued)*

**TABLE 16–3. CARE PLAN FOR THE PATIENT WITH DIABETES INSIPIDUS *(Continued)***

| Nursing Diagnoses | Desired Patient Outcomes | Nursing Interventions | Rationales |
|---|---|---|---|
| ***Nursing Diagnosis #5***<br>Skin integrity, impairment: potential, related to:<br>1. Dehydration, diarrhea. | Skin warm and dry; turgor over sternum or forehead, elastic; skin intact. | ○ Initiate skin care regimen:<br>–Frequent turning and positioning.<br>–Active/passive ROM exercises.<br>–Initiate pressure relief device (air mattress, sheepskin, other).<br>○ Monitor nutritional intake. | ○ Maximizes tissue perfusion, prevents stasis of blood and decubitus ulcer formation. |
| ***Nursing Diagnosis #6***<br>Bowel elimination, alteration in, related to:<br>1. Diarrhea (possible side effect of vasopressin therapy). | Patient will establish and maintain effective bowel function:<br>1. Bowel pattern to return to patient's baseline.<br>• Stool formed and soft.<br>• Absence of diarrhea and abdominal cramping.<br>2. Bowel sounds appropriate throughout all quadrants. | • Assess gastrointestinal function:<br>○ Specific symptomatology includes:<br>–Anorexia, nausea, vomiting, abdominal cramping and distention; and diarrhea.<br>–Increased bowel sounds associated with increased peristalsis.<br>• Implement measures to maintain optimal gastrointestinal function with least discomfort.<br>○ Provide copious amounts of fluid at patient's disposal.<br>–Monitor strict intake and output.<br>–Monitor electrolytes. | ○ Abdominal cramping, increased gastrointestinal mobility, and diarrhea are associated with large doses of vasopressin.<br>○ Gastrointestinal symptomatology may be associated with hypernatremic state.<br>○ Severe thirst requires large fluid intake to prevent dehydration.<br>○ Water taken in conjunction with ADH replacement therapy may help to minimize side effects of abdominal cramping. |
| ***Nursing Diagnosis #7***<br>Sensory-perceptual alteration: visual, related to:<br>1. Pressure on optic chiasm associated with pituitary tumor; edema as occurs with head injury or hypophysectomy. | Patient will:<br>1. Demonstrate awareness of visual field defect if present.<br>2. Demonstrate maneuvers in activities of daily living to compensate for defect.<br>3. Verbalize improvement in vision. | • Assess visual function:<br>○ Specific parameters include:<br>–Visual acuity.<br>–Extraocular movement.<br>○ Visual fields.<br>–Direct consensual light reflex.<br>–Pupil shape, size, reactivity, and accommodation.<br>• Implement measures to minimize risk of injury due to visual field defect.<br>○ Teach patient to become aware as to where "blind spots" are in the overall field of vi- | • It is important to establish baseline function to measure patient's response to therapy.<br>○ Bitemporal hemianopsia: Blindness in temporal half of the visual field in each eye. This is a most frequently occurring disturbance in patients with pituitary pathology because of structural contiguity between optic chiasm and sella tursica and its contents (i.e., pituitary gland). |

| | | | |
|---|---|---|---|
| | | sion, and how to compensate for defect by turning the head.<br>∘ Keep patient's immediate environment uncluttered, free of unnecessary equipment, furniture, and so forth.<br>∘ Teach patient to place personal articles within reach.<br>∘ Assist patient with activities of daily living. | |
| ***Nursing Diagnosis #8***<br>Nutrition, alteration in: Less than body requirements, related to:<br>1. Anorexia, nausea associated with hypernatremic state.<br>2. Abdominal cramping associated with ADH replacement therapy.<br>3. Fatigue associated with excessive thirst and fluid intake. | Patient will:<br>1. Maintain body weight between 2% and 5% of patient's baseline.<br>2. Maintain serum electrolytes within acceptable range:<br>• Sodium: 135–148 mEq/liter.<br>3. Maintain serum proteins within acceptable range:<br>• Total protein: 6–8.4 g/100 ml.<br>4. Verbalize dietary restrictions:<br>• Low sodium diet. | • Collaborate with nutritionist to perform comprehensive nutritional assessment.<br>• Implement nutritional regimen as prescribed:<br>∘ Monitor parameters reflective of nutritional status.<br>– Weigh daily under same conditions.<br>– Monitor intake and output.<br>– Monitor serum electrolytes, plasma proteins, and serum osmolality.<br>• Provide comfort measures:<br>– Assist with frequent oral hygiene.<br>∘ Encourage family to bring patient's favorite foods, if possible.<br>– Offer a variety of fluids.<br>∘ Provide frequent rest periods.<br>• Initiate patient/family education regarding nutritional requirements and dietary limitations.<br>∘ Limit salt intake. | • Provides baseline for planning nutrition.<br>• Major objectives of nutritional therapy:<br>1. Provide sufficient calories to prevent protein catabolism.<br>2. Provide sufficient protein to ensure tissue healing and to prevent breakdown.<br>3. Limit salt intake until fluid and sodium balance stabilizes.<br>• May assist in improving appetite.<br>∘ Home cooked food, coupled with company at mealtime, may improve nutritional intake.<br>∘ Fluid intake of 4–6 or more liters/24 hr may be fatiguing.<br>∘ Hypernatremia associated with excess water loss can be significant. Efforts need to be directed toward limiting sodium intake until fluid and electrolyte balance is reestablished. |
| ***Nursing Diagnosis #9***<br>Injury, potential for physiological: Thrombophlebitis, deep venous thrombosis, pulmonary embolism, related to:<br>1. Immobility.<br>2. Hemoconcentration associated with severe water deficit and dehydration.<br>(See Table 35–3, Nursing Diagnosis #6.) | Patient will remain without thromboembolic complications:<br>1. Absence of calf pain, tenderness, swelling.<br>2. Peripheral pulses palpable.<br>3. Usual skin color and temperature in extremities. | • Assess for signs/symptoms of venous thrombosis:<br>∘ Symptomatology may include:<br>∘ Tenderness, warmth, pain.<br>– Changes in skin color and temperature.<br>– Increase in mid-thigh or mid-calf circumference.<br>• Implement measures to reduce risk of thromboembolic disease:<br>∘ Encourage position changes at frequent intervals.<br>∘ Avoid positions that compromise blood flow (e.g., crossing legs, use of knee gatch or pillow under knees). | ∘ Positive Homan's sign reflects pain in calf when the knee is placed in a flexed position and the examiner abruptly dorsiflexes the ankle. This maneuver will elicit pain in some patients with deep venous thrombosis (DVT). However, absence of calf pain does not rule out DVT; the presence of pain may also occur with herniated lower intervertebral disks or lumbosacral problems. |

*(continued)*

**TABLE 16–3. CARE PLAN FOR THE PATIENT WITH DIABETES INSIPIDUS *(Continued)***

| Nursing Diagnoses | Desired Patient Outcomes | Nursing Interventions | Rationales |
|---|---|---|---|
| ***Nursing Diagnosis #9 (cont.)*** | | ◦ Assist with ROM exercises for 5–10 min every 1–2 hr.<br>◦ Apply antiembolic stockings if appropriate.<br>◦ Monitor hematology profile. | ◦ Venous stasis coupled with hemoconcentration increases the risk of thromboembolic disease. Exercise increases venous return and reduces risk of pooling of blood in the extremities.<br>◦ Serial hematocrit/hemoglobin studies help to evaluate fluid status. |
| ***Nursing Diagnosis #10***<br>Coping, ineffective, individual, related to:<br>1. Excessive thirst and the need to drink large volumes of fluid. | Patient will:<br>1. Verbalize feelings regarding thirst and fluid status.<br>2. Identify approach to fluid intake: When, how much, how often, and what kinds of fluids. | • Collaborate with patient and family/significant others to define the magnitude of the water imbalance and to explore how the problem can best be addressed.<br>◦ Specific measures:<br>–Discuss the importance of balancing intake with output.<br>–Teach patient/family how to record intake and output accurately.<br>–Emphasize importance of daily weight.<br>–Identify fluids and other sources of water (e.g., watermelon) that appeal to patient.<br>◦ Encourage participation in decisions regarding care (e.g., what to drink or eat, how much, how often). | • Hypovolemic and dehydration can progress rapidly to hypovolemic shock and circulatory collapse.<br>◦ Involving patient and family/significant others in decision-making process regarding care enables the patient to assume responsibility for self-care and may increase compliance with prescribed therapeutic regimen. |
| ***Nursing Diagnosis #11***<br>Anxiety, related to:<br>1. Excessive thirst and its underlying cause. | (See Table 35–3, Nursing Diagnosis #1.) | (For pertinent nursing interventions and their rationales in the care of the patient exhibiting anxiety, the reader is referred to Table 35–3, Nursing Diagnosis #1.) | |

**TABLE 16–4. CARE PLAN FOR THE PATIENT WITH INAPPROPRIATE SECRETION OF ANTIDIURETIC HORMONE (SIADH)**

| Nursing Diagnoses | Desired Patient Outcomes | Nursing Interventions | Rationales |
|---|---|---|---|
| ***Nursing Diagnosis #1*** Fluid volume, alteration in: Excess, related to:<br>1. Increased secretion of ADH in presence of low serum osmolality.<br>(See Tables 23–4 and 23–5.) | Patient will maintain stable:<br>1. Neurologic status:<br>• Mental status—alert, oriented to person, place, and date.<br>• Appropriate behavior.<br>• Without seizure activity, tremors, weakness.<br>• Deep tendon reflexes brisk. | (For a detailed presentation of pertinent nursing interventions and their rationales related to fluid volume excess, See Table 23–4, and Table 23–5, Nursing Diagnosis #1; and Table 23–7, Nursing Diagnosis #2.)<br>In addition, consider the following:<br>• Assess for signs and symptoms of SIADH:<br>∘ Specific symptomatology reflects alterations in cerebral function:<br>∘ Assess for confusion, disorientation, irritability, restlessness, lethargy; tremors, seizure activity, hyperreflexia. | • Excess water of SIADH is distributed almost entirely to *intra*cellular compartment; clinically, the patient presents with CNS manifestations reflective of cerebral swelling.<br>• Hyperosmolality of intracellular compartment creates osmotic gradient for free water to flow from ECF to ICF space. |
| ***Nursing Diagnosis #2*** Electrolyte imbalance, related to:<br>1. Hyponatremia (dilutional).<br>2. Water intoxication.<br>(See Tables 23–6 and 23–7.) | 2. Hemodynamic status:<br>• Weight within 2–5% of baseline.<br>• BP within 10 mmHg of baseline.<br>• Pulse strong. >60 <100 beats/min.<br>• Hemodynamic parameters:<br>CVP—$\overline{\text{mean}}$ 0–8 mmHg.<br>PCWP—$\overline{\text{mean}}$ 8–12 mmHg.<br>CO—4–8 liters/min.<br>3. Renal status:<br>• Hourly urine output >30 ml/hr.<br>• Laboratory studies:<br>∘ BUN and creatinine at baseline<br>∘ Serum osmolality—285–295 mOsm/kg.<br>∘ Serum sodium—135–148 mEq/liter. | ∘ Hemodynamic status: Vital signs—arterial blood pressure, peripheral pulses, heart rate and rhythm; respiratory rate and pattern; body temperature.<br>–Body weight.<br>–Signs of fluid overload.<br>∘ Laboratory parameters:<br>–Serum osmolality: <280 mOsm/kg.<br>–Serum sodium: <130 mEq/liter.<br>∘ Urine osmolality: ~ to serum osmolality.<br>∘ Urine sodium: >180 mEq/liter.<br>–Urine specific gravity: ~1.030.<br>–Other serum electrolytes: Potassium and chloride. | ∘ Water intoxication of SIADH is largely distributed to cells (intracellular); in extracellular compartments (i.e., interstitium, intravascular space), fluid volume is diminished. Therefore, classic signs/symptoms of fluid overload may not be observed (e.g., pulmonary congestion, congestive heart failure, neck vein distention, pitting edema, hypertension, bounding pulse, and so forth) at least initially.<br>∘ Early signs and symptoms of SIADH are highly nonspecific; therefore, a high index of suspicion is necessary in assessing patient's overall status. A gradual onset may progress rapidly to muscle cramps, twitches, and seizures.<br>∘ Hallmarks of SIADH: Production of concentrated urine in the presence of low serum osmolality; dilutional hyponatremia.<br>∘ Urine osmolality equal to or greater than serum osmolality is classic finding highly suggestive of SIADH.<br>∘ Continued elevation in urinary sodium, if present, assists in differential diagnosis. |

*(continued)*

**TABLE 16–4. CARE PLAN FOR THE PATIENT WITH INAPPROPRIATE SECRETION OF ANTIDIURETIC HORMONE (SIADH) *(Continued)***

| Nursing Diagnoses | Desired Patient Outcomes | Nursing Interventions | Rationales |
|---|---|---|---|
| ***Nursing Diagnosis #4 (cont.)*** | | | |
| | ∘ Serum potassium — 3.5–5.5 mEq/liter.<br>∘ Serum chlorides — 100–106 mEq/liter.<br>∘ Urine specific gravity — 1.010–1.025.<br>∘ Urine sodium — 80–180 mEq/liter.<br>∘ Serum glucose — 70–110 mg/100 ml.<br>∘ Hematology profile: Hematocrit, hemoglobin. | • Implement therapeutic regimen:<br>∘ Fluid intake:<br>– Initial intake limited to urine output/24 hr.<br>– As serum sodium level normalizes and CNS symptoms abate, additional fluid is given equal to that of estimated insensible losses (i.e., fluid lost via skin, lungs). | • Approach to therapy is guided by CNS symptomatology and hyponatremia status: initial goal is to relieve CNS dysfunction. |
| | | ∘ Aggressive fluid therapy: | ∘ Aggressive fluid therapy may be necessary in the face of severe CNS symptomatology: Seizures, coma, serious cardiac dysrhythmias. |
| | | ∘ Administration (IV) of 3% hypertonic saline. | ∘ Hypertonic saline will reverse hyponatremia quickly as fluid is drawn into intravascular space; overly rapid correction can precipitate congestive heart failure; continuous cardiac monitoring is essential. |
| | | ∘ Administer/monitor diuretic therapy:<br>∘ Furosemide therapy in conjunction with prescribed fluid replacement therapy. | ∘ Furosemide therapy is accompanied by rapid losses of sodium and potassium and requires close monitoring of serum electrolytes.<br>∘ Correction of serum sodium to levels that relieve CNS symptomatology is primary goal of therapy; serum sodium need not be totally corrected. |
| | | ∘ Hypertonic peritoneal dialysis may be considered to relieve fluid excess. | ∘ Use of hyperosmolar glucose dialysate solutions functions osmotically to pull fluid into the peritoneal cavity. From these it can be drained from the body. |
| | | ∘ Close ongoing monitoring of the following is necessary to evaluate effectiveness of therapy:<br>– CNS function.<br>– Intake/output and body weight.<br>– Cardiac status, cardiopulmonary function: Dyspnea, tachypnea, productive cough with pink-tinged sputum, presence of adventitious breath sounds — crackles, wheezes.<br>– Laboratory parameters (as above). | |

| | | | |
|---|---|---|---|
| ***Nursing Diagnosis #3***<br>Thought processes, alteration in, related to:<br>1. Hyponatremia (dilutional) and water intoxication. | Patient will:<br>1. Demonstrate improved neurologic status:<br>• Alert, oriented to person, place, date.<br>• Longer attention span.<br>• Improved memory; speech intact.<br>• Relaxed demeanor | • Assess thought/behavioral processes.<br>○ Specific neurologic parameters:<br>–General cerebral functions: Consciousness and mentation.<br>–Immediate memory—ask patient to repeat a series of numbers, then have patient repeat another series of numbers backwards; ability to calculate; abstract reasoning.<br>–Thought content: Spontaneous, logical; flight of ideas, inappropriate recurrent thoughts, or excessive repetition of thoughts. | • See Chapter 7 for a detailed description of assessment parameters. |
| | | ○ Inquire of family/significant others as to recent change in behavior or personality. Have such changes occurred suddenly or gradually? Are the changes in behavior/response associated with some event? | ○ Ascertaining usual behavior of patient assists in establishing baseline data with which to evaluate subsequent responses. |
| | | • Implement measures to foster optimal thinking and expression of thoughts:<br>○ Specific considerations:<br>–Provide quiet environment with minimal distractions.<br>–Allow adequate time for communication; be accessible to patient/family.<br>–Provide explanations in clear, concise terms; repeat questions or directions to the patient's understanding.<br>○ Involve patient and family/significant others in decision-making regarding care and activities. | ○ Involvement in decision-making regarding care raises awareness and consciousness in self-care; participation in self-care increases interest in what is happening and stimulates thinking processes. |
| ***Nursing Diagnosis #4***<br>Coping, ineffective, individual/family, related to:<br>1. Strict fluid restrictions. | Patient/family will be able to:<br>1. Explain need for fluid restriction.<br>2. Develop schedule for fluid intake.<br>3. Decide on nutritional fluids for intake. | • Collaborate with patient and family/significant others to develop/implement prescribed therapeutic regimen:<br>○ Fluid restrictions:<br>–Discuss reasons for strict fluid intake, balanced with output.<br>–Encourage patient/family to ask questions and express concerns.<br>–Assist patient/family to develop plan as to when and how much fluid will be ingested per 24-hr schedule.<br>–Teach patient/family how to record intake and output accurately. | ○ The significance of fluid restriction therapy in SIADH cannot be overestimated. If patient's neurologic status is unstable, the family can be involved in assisting with implementation of fluid restriction. |

*(continued)*

**TABLE 16–4. CARE PLAN FOR THE PATIENT WITH INAPPROPRIATE SECRETION OF ANTIDIURETIC HORMONE (SIADH) *(Continued)***

| Nursing Diagnoses | Desired Patient Outcomes | Nursing Interventions | Rationales |
|---|---|---|---|
| ***Nursing Diagnosis #4 (cont.)*** | | | |
| | | ○ Emphasize importance of daily weight.<br>–Identify fluids especially enjoyed by patient. | ○ Body weight, taken daily, is best indicator of fluid status. |
| | | ○ Offer praise for accomplishments in implementing fluid restriction.<br>–Remain accessible to patient/family.<br>–Lend a listening and concerned ear. | ○ It is very difficult for family/significant others to cope when their loved one is limited to an intake of 500 ml of fluid/24 hr. Reassurance and encouragement may be helpful. Family members can often be a positive influence on the patient's compliance with therapeutic regimen. |
| ***Nursing Diagnosis #5***<br>Nutrition, alteration in: Less than body requirements, related to:<br>1. Reduced oral and nutritional intake. | Patient will:<br>1. Maintain body weight between 2% and 5% of patient's baseline.<br>2. Maintain serum electrolytes within acceptable range:<br>• Sodium >135 mEq/liter.<br>• Potassium 3.5–5.5 mEq/liter. | • Consult with nutritionist to perform comprehensive nutritional assessment. | |
| | | • Implement fluid restriction on nutritional regimen as prescribed.<br>○ Explain therapeutic regimen to patient/family. | • Fluid restriction prevents further fluid intake retention. |
| | | ○ Encourage fluids/foods with high sodium content. | ○ Hyponatremia underlies CNS symptomatology; when hyponatremia is corrected, CNS dysfunction will abate. |

| | | | |
|---|---|---|---|
| | 3. Verbalize why it is necessary to restrict fluid intake.<br>4. Develop schedule of fluid intake for each 24-hr period including amount and types of foods taken. | | |
| ***Nursing Diagnosis #6***<br>Injury, potential for, related to:<br>1. Seizures/convulsions. | Patient will remain injury-free. | • Perform assessment of patient's immediate environment for potentially injurious equipment or materials.<br>• Minimize neurologic/neuromuscular stimulation.<br>• Institute seizure precautions: Bed in low position, side rails padded; pharyngeal airway and suction equipment at bedside. | • Assessment of patient's immediate bedside environment helps to reduce risk of injury by removal of potentially hazardous objects.<br>• CNS dysfunction associated with hyponatremia may include seizures and altered state of consciousness. |

### *Clinical Data and Diagnostic Findings*

In addition to a thorough clinical history, physical examination may reveal cerebral alterations such as confusion, weakness, and diminished reflexes; blurring of vision may be present; signs of fluid overload may become evident including neck vein distention, rapid and deep breathing (hyperpnea), and adventitious sounds (e.g., crackles, wheezes). Peripheral edema is not a usual occurrence despite the degree of water overload, which suggests an *intra*cellular fluid excess; edema is usually associated with extracellular fluid excess.

Laboratory findings reflect decreased serum sodium and osmolality; urine sodium, on the other hand, is elevated. The reason for this is twofold: there is decreased reabsorption of sodium in the renal tubules, and an increased excretion of sodium occurs as a result of the expanded plasma volume, which increases the glomerular filtration rate. The result is a severely reduced serum osmolality coupled with urine hyperosmolality.

### *Treatment*

Treatment of SIADH involves strict fluid restriction with administration of sodium chloride, ongoing assessment of neurologic and hydration status, and identification and treatment of the underlying cause. Usual fluid administration guidelines include: (1) water intake not to exceed urine output until serum sodium normalizes and symptoms abate; (2) fluid intake is then given to equal urine output plus insensible fluid loss; and (3) continued careful laboratory monitoring and patient assessment to determine effectiveness of therapy.

In addition to fluid restriction and sodium chloride administration, treatment of the underlying cause is indicated. This might include surgical removal of a bronchogenic carcinoma or discontinuance of drug therapy.

### *Nursing Care of the Patient with Syndrome of Inappropriate Secretion of ADH*

**Therapeutic Goals.** Implementation of nursing process in the care of the patient with SIADH revolves around the following therapeutic goals:

1. Identify patients at risk (see Etiology section in Table 16–2), and establish a comprehensive database including:
   A. Clinical history (functional health patterns)
   B. Physical examination
   C. Laboratory/diagnostic data.
2. Implement therapeutic regimen to restore fluid and electrolyte balance.
3. Promote/maintain optimal neurologic function.
4. Promote/maintain optimal cardiopulmonary function.
5. Establish a working rapport with patient and family/significant others.
6. Provide emotional and psychologic support to patient and family/significant others.

**Nursing Diagnoses, Desired Patient Outcomes, and Nursing Interventions.** Pertinent nursing diagnoses, desired patient outcomes and nursing interventions/rationales in the care of the patient with SIADH are presented in Table 16–4.

## REFERENCES

1. Rabin, D and McKenna, TJ: Clinical Endocrinology and Metabolism Principles and Practice. Grune & Stratton, New York, 1982, pp 89–90.
2. Hershman, JM: Endocrine Pathophysiology: A Patient-Oriented Approach, ed 3. Lea & Febiger, Philadelphia, 1988, p 310.
3. Widmann, FK: Clinical Interpretation of Laboratory Tests, ed 9. FA Davis, Philadelphia, 1983, p 271.
4. Rice, V: Problems of water regulation, diabetes insipidus and syndrome of inappropriate antidiuretic hormone. Crit Care Nurse 3(1):79, January/February 1983.
5. Johndrow, P and Thornton, S: Syndrome of inappropriate antidiuretic hormone, a growing concern. Focus on Critical Care 12(5):29, October 1985.

CHAPTER 17

# Nursing Management of the Patient with Thyroid Gland Dysfunction

## CHAPTER OUTLINE



## LEARNING OBJECTIVES

**At the end of this chapter, you should be able to:**

1. Describe structure and function of the thyroid gland.
2. Define the regulation of thyroid hormone synthesis and secretion.
3. State the major functions of thyroid hormones and their effects on specific body mechanisms.
4. Differentiate tests of thyroid function and discuss patient care considerations.
5. Describe the clinical presentation of hyperthyroidism and hypothyroidism.
6. Describe pathophysiology, etiology, clinical presentation, and treatment of hyperthyroid crisis and myxedema coma.
7. Delineate the nursing process in caring for patients with hyperthyroid crisis:
   Assessment.
   Nursing diagnosis.
   Planning: Desired patient outcomes
   Nursing interventions/rationales.

## THYROID GLAND: STRUCTURE AND FUNCTION

The thyroid gland lies in the neck anterior to, and on either side of, the trachea (Fig. 17–1). It consists of two lateral "butterfly-shaped" lobes connected by a narrow *isthmus* that crosses the trachea just below the cricoid cartilage. In about one third of the population an additional pyramidal lobe is present and extends upward from the isthmus near the left lobe.

The function of the thyroid gland is to synthesize, store, and release hormones (thyroxine and triiodothyronine) concerned with regulation of cellular

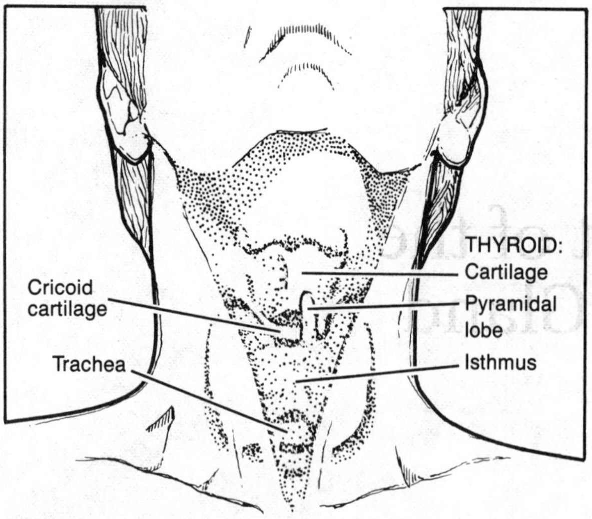


**Figure 17-1.** The thyroid gland lies in the neck, anterior to and on either side of the trachea. It consists of two lateral "butterfly-shaped" lobes connected by a narrow isthmus, which crosses the trachea just below the cricoid cartilage. In approximately one third of the population, an additional pyramidal lobe is present and extends upward from the isthmus usually from the left lobe. In the individual with a normal thyroid gland, the thyroid gland is largely nonpalpable. An enlarged thyroid gland may be visible on inspection and palpable; the presence of palpable nodules should be ruled out on physical examination. Because the thyroid is a highly vascularized organ, a thrill, or vibration, may be detected on palpation; auscultation over the lobes of the thyroid gland may reveal the presence of a bruit (i.e., a blowing type sound similar to that of a murmur).

metabolism, and with maintenance of serum calcium levels within the physiologic range (thyrocalcitonin). The hormones thyroxine and triiodothyronine are collectively referred to as the *thyroid hormones.*

Microscopically, the thyroid gland consists of two types of cells. Follicular epithelial cells, the principal cells within the thyroid gland, are responsible for the synthesis, storage, and secretion of thyroid hormones. A smaller population of cells, called parafollicular cells, or C cells, function in the regulation of calcium metabolism by secreting the hormone, thyrocalcitonin. (The role of thyrocalcitonin in calcium metabolism is discussed in Chap. 24.)

The thyroid gland differs from other endocrine glands in that it has a unique and highly developed mechanism for the *extra*cellular storage of the synthesized thyroid hormones. In contrast, other endocrine glands are limited to *intra*cellular storage of synthesized hormone. This unique extracellular storage capacity within the lumen of thyroid follicles accounts in part for the continued release of thyroid hormone for several weeks to 2 to 3 months after synthesis of the hormones has ceased.

The thyroid gland is a highly engorged organ with a close-meshed plexus of capillaries surrounding each follicle. Because of its high vascularity, structural abnormalities within the thyroid gland can often be detected by palpating for a thrill (i.e., vibration) or auscultating for a bruit (i.e., blowing type sound similar to that of a murmur) over the thyroid area. Between the dense network of capillaries of adjacent follicles lie the blind terminations, or end-points, of numerous lymphatic vessels. The lymphatics are significant pathways for the transport of hormone to the circulating blood.

Innervation of the thyroid gland occurs via numerous nerve fibers that accompany the capillaries as they ramify (branch) among the follicles. Sympathetic innervation to the thyroid occurs via postganglionic fibers originating in the middle and superior cervical ganglia. Innervation to the thyroid is presumed to be mainly vasomotor. An intact nerve supply may not be necessary for hormonal secretion.

## Thyroid Hormones: Synthesis, Release, and Transport

### *Synthesis*

The biosynthesis of thyroid hormones, thyroxine ($T_4$) and triiodothyronine ($T_3$), requires two basic ingredients: iodine and the nonessential amino acid, tyrosine.[1] Iodine is ingested orally in the diet or via medications and absorbed via the gastrointestinal tract into the blood in its iodide form. Approximately one third of the circulating iodide is taken up immediately by the thyroid gland; the remaining two thirds are excreted via the urine. Tyrosine amino acids are incorporated into the large glycoprotein molecule, *thyroglobulin,* which is synthesized within the follicular epithelial cells and stored within the follicular lumen. In addition to supplying necessary tyrosine molecules, it is within the thyroglobulin that the synthesized thyroid hormones are stored.

### *Release*

Small portions of thyroglobulin are reabsorbed from the follicular lumen into the cytoplasm of the epithelial cells by the process of *pinocytosis* (i.e., the cellular process of engulfing liquid). Here, the thyroglobulin molecule is hydrolyzed (i.e., addition of water) liberating the thyroid hormones, $T_3$ and $T_4$. These hormones diffuse through the cell membrane and are finally secreted into circulating blood.

### *Transport*

The thyroid hormones ($T_3$ and $T_4$) are transported in the blood highly bound to plasma proteins. These plasma proteins include thyroxine-binding globulin (TBG), thyroxine-binding prealbumin, and al-

TABLE 17-1
**Factors that Alter the Level of Thyroid-Binding Globulin (TBG)[2]**

| Increased TBG | Decreased TBG |
|---|---|
| Drugs: | Drugs: |
| Estrogen therapy | Glucocorticoids |
| Oral contraceptives | Anabolic steroids |
| Phenytoin—impairs binding of thyroid hormone to TBG | Diseased states: |
| Pregnancy—newborn | Nephrotic syndrome |
| Diseased states: | Chronic liver disease |
| Acute hepatitis | Systemic illness (severe) |
| Chronic liver disease | Genetically determined |
| Inborn errors in metabolism: | |
| Acute intermittent porphyria | |
| Genetically determined | |

bumin. (Table 17-1 lists factors that alter levels of thyroid-binding globulin.) The amount of thyroxine ($T_4$) circulating in the blood far exceeds that of triiodothyronine ($T_3$). This fact assumes greater significance when one considers that concentrations of the more physiologically active $T_3$ are largely derived from conversion of $T_4$ in the circulating blood.

The active, unbound form of the thyroid hormones present in miniscule amounts is in constant equilibrium with the protein-bound fraction. It is the free, unbound hormone that exerts the physiologic effects. A reduction in total plasma proteins, for whatever reason, may have a direct effect on the availability of the free, unbound fraction of the thyroid hormones in circulating blood. Distinguishing features of thyroid hormones are listed in Table 17-2.

## Regulation of Thyroid Hormone Synthesis and Secretion

Maintenance of basal metabolic rate requires that precisely the right amount of thyroid hormone be secreted at all times. To maintain this physiologic balance the activity of the thyroid gland is regulated closely by multilevel feedback control mechanisms involving higher brain centers, the hypothalamus, adenohypophysis (anterior pituitary), and the thyroid gland.

Thyrotropic-releasing hormone (TRH) is the major hypothalamic hormone triggering secretion of thyrotropic-stimulating hormone (TSH) by the adenohypophysis. Neural input to the hypothalamus, although undefined, is responsible for alterations in the secretion of TRH, which impacts on TSH secretion.

TSH, in turn, stimulates synthesis and release of thyroid hormone from the thyroid gland (i.e., its target gland). In addition, TSH stimulation causes an increase in the size and number of thyroid follicular epithelial cells (i.e., thyroid hypertrophy and hyperplasia) and their secretory activity.

Thyroid hormones ($T_3$ and $T_4$) exert a feedback inhibition on the hypothalamic-pituitary axis. They indirectly inhibit secretion of TRH by the hypothalamus by possibly decreasing the sensitivity of TSH-secreting cells in the adenohypophysis to the stimulation of TRH.[4] Levels of thyroid hormone in the blood exert a direct effect on TSH-secreting cells—lowered serum levels of thyroid hormone stimulate secretion of TSH, while excess circulating thyroid hormone depresses TSH secretion.

## Thyroid Hormones: Major Functions

The thyroid hormones have two major overall effects on bodily processes: (1) they increase metabolic rate, and (2) they stimulate body growth. Specific effects of thyroid hormone on physiologic mechanisms and functions are presented in Table 17-3.

## Diagnostic Tests of Thyroid Function[6]

When assessing thyroid function it is important to be cognizant of the ubiquitous effects thyroid hormones have on overall body function. Therefore, all organ systems of the body must be considered in the assessment. History-taking must be thorough; physical examination must be meticulous and comprehensive. (See Chap. 15 for specific assessment considerations.)

In addition, when thyroid dysfunction is present or suspected, a variety of diagnostic tests of thyroid function are available and may assist in confirming and/or differentiating the clinical diagnosis. Table 17-4 lists diagnostic tests of thyroid function currently available. Normal values and results differentiating hyperthyroidism and hypothyroidism are included.

Initial determinations usually obtained in a case of suspected thyroid dysfunction are total serum thyroxine ($T_4$) levels and triiodothyronine uptake ($RT_3U$). A good rule of thumb when interpreting these test results is that: (1) when *both* the $T_4$ and $RT_3U$ are *high*, the patient is hyperthyroid; (2) when both results are *low*, the patient is hypothyroid; and (3) when one is high and the other is low, the problem is usually an abnormality of protein binding rather than of thyroid function.[7] Inconsistencies do occur in tests of thyroid function. Therefore, one cannot rely exclusively on the results of any one test. Thorough history-taking and physical examination are essential in evaluating the patient's overall status.

In addition to thyroid function tests listed in

TABLE 17-2
## Distinguishing Features of Thyroid Hormones

| | Thyroxine, $T_4$ | Triiodothyronine, $T_3$ |
|---|---|---|
| Thyroid hormonogenesis (hormone formation) | Principal secretory product of thyroid gland<br>May act primarily as a biologically active *pro*hormone giving rise to $T_3$ in circulating blood | Most $T_3$ retained and recycled within thyroid gland<br>In disorders of thyroid gland, $T_3$ may be released in increased amounts<br>Most circulating $T_3$ is derived from circulating $T_4$<br>$T_3$ is produced by the monodeiodination of $T_4$ in blood and peripheral tissues[3] |
| Concentrations in circulating blood: | | |
| Total | 4–12 ng/100 ml | 70–190 ng/100 ml |
| Free | 1–4 ng/100 mg | 0.2–0.4 ng/100 mg |
| Affinity for plasma-binding proteins: | High affinity | Less affinity but still highly bound |
| Thyroid-binding globulin (TBG) | $T_4$ predominantly bound to TBG and TBPA | Minimal binding to TBG |
| Thyroid-binding prealbumin (TBPA) | | Slightly more binding to other plasma proteins |
| Of the total amount of thyroid hormone bound to plasma proteins, $T_4$ exceeds $T_3$ by at least 20 times in the healthy adult. | | |
| Factors influencing serum levels of $T_3$ and $T_4$: | | |
| Age | $T_4$ levels do not decline with age | $T_3$ levels decreased in fetus; rise shortly after birth.<br>$T_3$ levels decline slightly with advancing age—after age 70 in men; and age 80 in women |
| Exposure to cold, drop in body temperature | $T_4$ secretion increased via neural input to hypothalamus | $T_3$ secretion increased via neural input to hypothalamus |
| Stress, acute illness (e.g., pneumonia, myocardial infarction); chronic illness (e.g., liver disease, renal dysfunction); and malnutrition | Conversion of $T_4$ to $T_3$ impaired | Conversion from $T_4$ impaired |
| Drugs: glucocorticoids, beta-blockers, propylthiouracil, and radiopaque dyes | Conversion of $T_4$ to $T_3$ impaired | Conversion from $T_4$ impaired |
| Hormones (catecholamines and ADH) | Direct stimulatory effect on thyroid gland, which increases level of $T_4$ in blood | Direct stimulatory effect on thyroid gland, which increases level of $T_3$ in blood |
| *Note:* A synergistic relationship exists between catecholamines (e.g., epinephrine, norepinephrine, dopamine) and the thyroid hormones. Thyroid hormones potentiate the catecholamine effect possibly by stimulating synthesis of beta-adrenergic receptors. Antidiuretic hormone (ADH) also exerts a direct stimulating effect on the thyroid, which results in an increase in $T_4$ and $T_3$ levels in the circulation. | | |
| Target tissues | Most cells in the body (exceptions are brain, retina, lungs, and spleen) | Most cells in the body |
| Release to tissues | Very slowly released | Rapidly released; readily transferred to target tissues as a result of its decreased affinity for plasma proteins |
| Potency | Much less than $T_3$ | Potency of $T_3$ is more than 10 times the potency of $T_4$<br>$T_3$ is considered to be the most important thyroid hormone regulating activities of target tissues |
| Elimination | | |
| Liver metabolism (bile) | 10–20% of free $T_3$ and $T_4$ excreted in feces as glucuronide | Same |
| Renal excretion | Some free $T_3$ and $T_4$ cleared via the kidneys | Same |

TABLE 17-3
## Effects of Thyroid Hormones on Specific Body Mechanisms

| Body Mechanism/Function | Effects of Thyroid Hormones[5] |
|---|---|
| Carbohydrate metabolism | An increase occurs in:<br>1. Rate of absorption of glucose via gastrointestinal tract<br>2. Glucose uptake by cells—synergistic effect between thyroid hormones and insulin; increase in insulin secretion<br>3. Glycolysis<br>4. Gluconeogenesis (especially in the presence of excess thyroid hormone secretion) |
| Fat metabolism | All aspects of fat metabolism are enhanced. An increase occurs in:<br>1. Mobilization of lipids from fatty tissue stores<br>2. Serum concentrations of free fatty acids<br>3. Oxidation of free fatty acids by the cells (major source of long-term energy supplies) |
| Serum concentration of:<br>Cholesterol<br>Phospholipids<br>Triglycerides | Serum levels of thyroid hormones:<br>*Increased levels* / *Decreased levels*<br>Decreased / Increased<br>Decreased / Increased<br>Decreased / Increased<br>Severe arteriosclerosis is often associated with a large increase in serum lipids in the patient with prolonged hypothyroidism. |
| Vitamin metabolism | Vitamins function as coenzymes in many biochemical reactions. The increase in cellular metabolism in the presence of thyroid hormones may predispose to vitamin deficiency. |
| Basal metabolic rate (BMR) | Thyroid hormones increase cellular metabolism and thereby increase the BMR. |
| Body weight | Serum levels of thyroid hormone:<br>*Increased*—Usually associated with weight loss<br>*Decreased*—Usually associated with weight gain<br>Weight loss may be masked by increased appetite, which is also stimulated by increased levels of thyroid hormones. |
| Cardiovascular function:<br>Cardiac output | Increased cellular metabolism in response to thyroid hormonal stimulation results in an increased oxygen utilization and consumption, and an increase in metabolic waste products.<br>Vasodilatation with increased blood flow occurs to provide oxygen and nutrients to the cells while removing waste products of metabolism.<br>Blood flow to the skin is increased to dissipate body heat generated by increased cellular metabolism.<br>Cardiac output is increased to maintain adequate blood flow. |
| Heart rate | Thyroid hormones may have a direct effect on the excitability of the heart, resulting in an increased heart rate.<br>Heart rate is a very sensitive index for determining whether the patient has excessive or diminished thyroid hormone production. |
| Contractility | The presence of excessive amounts of thyroid hormones markedly depresses heart muscle strength and contractility, probably secondary to the increased protein catabolism within the heart. Cardiac decompensation is a serious concern in the patient with thyrotoxicosis. |
| Blood volume | Vasodilatation, which may occur in response to increased cellular metabolism, may account for increased blood volume in the intravascular space. |
| Arterial blood pressure | Arterial blood pressure remains largely unchanged as increased cardiac output in response to increased thyroid hormone is probably offset by dilatation of peripheral vasculature due to local hormonal effects and hyperthermia.<br>Pulse pressure may increase secondary to increased run-off of blood through dilated peripheral blood vessels. |
| Respiratory function:<br>Cellular Level | Thyroid hormones stimulate energy-producing electron transfer processes in the cytochrome chains within cell mitochondria. |
| Respiratory Rate and Pattern | Increased oxygen utilization and consumption increase the concentration of carbon dioxide in extracellular and intravascular fluid compartments.<br>Carbon dioxide is a potent respiratory stimulus. Increased levels of $CO_2$ stimulate an increase in rate and depth of respirations. |
| Gastrointestinal function:<br>Appetite<br>Digestive juices<br>GI tract motility | Thyroid hormones increase appetite and food intake and rate of secretion of digestive juices.<br>Diarrhea is associated with increased thyroid hormones.<br>Constipation may occur in the presence of reduced levels of thyroid hormone. |

*(continued)*

TABLE 17–3
**Effects of Thyroid Hormones on Specific Body Mechanisms *(Continued)***

| Body Mechanism/Function | Effects of Thyroid Hormones[5] |
|---|---|
| Central nervous system function | Thyroid hormones play a significant role in development of the nervous system. Hypothyroid infants (cretins) are mentally retarded, a defect associated with decreased thyroid hormones. Early initiation of thyroid hormone replacement therapy may prevent mental retardation. |
| Beta-adrenergic receptors | Thyroid hormones stimulate synthesis of beta-adrenergic receptors. This stimulation may be the basis of their beta-adrenergic sympathomimetic effect. |
| | Increased secretion of thyroid hormones may predispose to extreme nervousness, psychoneurotic tendencies (anxiety, paranoias), and may potentiate the "fight or flight" sympathetic response. |
| | Thyroid hormones regulate the reaction of reflexes in peripheral nerves. |
| Skeletal muscular function | |
| Muscle weakness | Exceedingly large increases in levels of thyroid hormones may predispose to muscle weakness related to excessive protein catabolism. |
| Muscle tremor | A fine muscle tremor is characteristic of excessive levels of thyroid hormones. |
| Effect on sleep | The exhausting effect of thyroid hormones on CNS and musculoskeletal function predisposes to extreme fatigue; yet, the excitable effects of excess thyroid hormones on synapses make sleeping difficult. |
| Effect on other endocrine glands | Thyroid hormones increase:<br>1. Rates of secretion of most other hormones<br>2. Demand and sensitivity of the tissues for other hormones<br>*Examples:*<br>1. Increase in glucose metabolism in response to thyroid hormonal stimulation creates a corresponding need for increased insulin secretion by the endocrine pancreas.<br>2. Increase in metabolic activities associated with bone formation and calcium metabolism causes the need for increase in parathormone secretion.<br>3. Thyroid hormone increases the rate of inactivation of glucocorticoids by the liver. This initiates the negative feedback system wherein the decreased level of circulating glucocorticoids stimulates an increase in ACTH release by the adenohypophysis; an increased secretion of ACTH, in turn, stimulates glucocorticoid secretion of the adrenal cortices. |
| Effect on sexual function | Excess thyroid hormone frequently causes impotence in the male and oligomenorrhea (reduced menstrual bleeding) or amenorrhea in females. Deficit of thyroid hormone may cause loss of libido in females; menorrhagia and excessive menstrual bleeding may also occur in females. |

Table 17–4, a number of other diagnostic studies are available.

*Thyroid scanning* is useful in determining the overall size of the thyroid gland and in detecting presence of nodules. The accumulation of technetium 99m or radioactive iodine (RAI) in the thyroid tissue enables critical characteristics of the thyroid to be discerned. Areas of decreased function appear as "cold" spots, while areas of increased function occur as "hot" spots. A palpable nodule appearing as a "cold" spot is highly suggestive of malignancy.

*Ultrasonography* allows the thyroid gland to be visualized by variable reflectance of high-frequency sound waves.[8] The test is used primarily to distinguish cyst from thyroid tumors.

*Thyroid antibodies* to various thyroid-related antigens have been found to accompany such disease states as thyroiditis, hyperthyroidism (Graves' disease), hypothyroidism, or thyroid carcinoma. Thyroglobulin is frequently implicated as a thyroid-related antigen, and autoantibodies (i.e., antibodies directed against self tissue) directed against thyroglobulin are frequently measured in the serum of patients with thyroid dysfunction.[9] Similarly, autoantibodies directed against the microsomal antigen of thyroid follicular epithelial cells are frequently encountered in patients with thyroiditis. High titers of thyroglobulin and microsomal antibodies strongly reflect the presence of autoimmune thyroiditis.[10] A family history of thyroid dysfunction, pernicious anemia, adrenal or parathyroid dysfunction, nonviral or nontoxic liver disease, or renal dysfunction should arouse suspicion of possible autoimmune disease.

### Diagnostic Tests of Thyroid Function: Nursing Care Considerations

Many diagnostic tests of thyroid function (e.g., radioactive iodine uptake—RAIU) may be affected by total-body stores of iodine. Patients need to be questioned regarding use of exogenous sources of iodine including many over-the-counter self-medication preparations (e.g., cough syrup, suntan lotion, vaginal suppositories). Recent radiography involving use of contrast dyes is especially important information because of the prolonged effect of certain contrast media (several weeks to months or even years). Information regarding recent intravenous pyelogram, gallbladder studies, and the like,

TABLE 17–4
**Diagnostic Tests of Thyroid Function**

| Tests | Normal Values | Hyperthyroidism | Hypothyroidism |
|---|---|---|---|
| Total serum thyroxine concentration (serum $T_4$) | 4–12 ng/100 ml | Total and free $T_4$ are measured: Increased | Decreased |
| Resin $T_3$ uptake ($RT_3U$) | Normally 25% to 35% of radioactive $T_3$ binds to resin. | Detects changes in serum thyroid-binding proteins: Increased | Decreased |
| Free thyroxine index ($FT_4I$) | Calculated from serum $T_4$ and $RT_3U$ values | Distinguishes whether a change in total serum concentration of thyroid hormones is due to increased production and release of hormone or to a change in hormone binding with plasma proteins. | |
| Radioactive iodine uptake (RAIU) | Radioactive iodine accumulation in thyroid: After 2 hr—1%–13% After 6 hr—2%–25% After 24 hr—15%–45% | Elevation indicative of thyroid hyperfunction, but levels are not always elevated in hyperthyroidism | Not reliable |
| Total serum $T_3$ concentration ($T_3RIA$) | 70–190 ng/100 ml (varies with age) | Elevated in thyrotoxicosis; $T_3$ levels frequently increased to a greater extent than serum $T_4$ levels | Not reliable; may be within "normal" physiologic range |
| Thyrotropic hormone stimulation test (TSH) | 0.5–3.5 $\mu$U/ml | Less than 0.1 $\mu$U/ml No response | Elevated levels are indicative of hypothyroidism; more frequently serum TSH levels are used instead. |
| Thyrotropic-releasing hormone stimulation test (TRH) | After administration of TRH, levels of TSH occur as follows: 15–30 min—TSH rises by a factor of 2.5 to 4. 2–4 hr—TSH levels return to baseline. | Hyperthyroid patients have no rise in TSH after injection of TRH. | Primary hypothyroidism may reflect an elevated baseline TSH and an exaggerated response to an intravenous bolus of TRH. |
| Thyroid-circulating antibodies: | | High titers: Hashimoto's thyroiditis | |
| Antithyroglobulin | Titer: <1:20 | Low titers: Thyroid dysfunction | |
| Antimicrosomal | Titer: <1:100 | Pernicious anemia, Myasthenia gravis, Myxedema | |

should be ascertained, including date, place, and nature of tests performed. Such exogenous sources of iodine can interfere with test results and their interpretation.

A major nursing responsibility is the coordination of patient care activities to successfully complete the diagnostic workup. Nurses need to know the underlying basis for prescribed tests and the procedures necessary for their successful implementation. The patient's condition needs to be monitored closely throughout the diagnostic workup to evaluate the patient's tolerance of testing procedures, to obtain feedback, and to expand the patient's overall assessment database. A comprehensive diagnostic workup is critical to the successful management of the patient with an endocrine disorder.

## PATHOPHYSIOLOGY: HYPERTHYROIDISM AND HYPOTHYROIDISM

### Terminology

The terminology of thyroid disorders is frequently confusing. For example, hyperthyroidism is synonymous with thyrotoxicosis, and its most common form is also called Graves' disease. Hyperthyroid crisis is frequently referred to as "thyroid storm," or thyrotoxic crisis. In the discussion to follow, the terms hyperthyroidism and hypothyroidism will be used to reflect the disorders of too much or too little thyroid activity, respectively; the terms hyperthyroid crisis and myxedema coma, respectively, will be used to reflect the toxic, life-threatening forms of thyroid dysfunction.

### Hyperthyroidism

Hyperthyroidism is a condition characterized by excessive secretion of the thyroid hormones, thyroxine ($T_4$) and triiodothyronine ($T_3$). The cause of this hyperactivity of the thyroid gland is largely unknown. It occurs in women more frequently than in men. Its onset is insidious, usually during the third and fourth decades of life.

### Hypothyroidism

Hypothyroidism is a clinical disorder resulting from decreased circulating levels of free thyroid hormones or from resistance of target cells to the action of thyroid hormones. While it is one of the more common endocrinopathies occurring in adults, some cases of hypothyroidism can exist without recognizable symptomatology; it is frequently overlooked.

#### *Clinical Presentation*

Clinical manifestation of hyperthyroidism and hypothyroidism is related primarily to the metabolic effects of too much or too little thyroid hormonal activity, respectively. Clinical manifestation of hyperthyroidism is also associated with enhanced sympathetic nervous system activity. Commonly, the signs and symptoms of these disorders are nonspecific and lack a recognizable pattern. No one clinical feature will assist in diagnosing the disease, but taken together, clinical findings may make the diagnosis unmistakable. As a review, features of the clinical presentation of hyperthyroidism and hypothyroidism, including the clinical history, physical examination, and pertinent laboratory data, are presented in Table 17-5.

## PATHOPHYSIOLOGY: HYPERTHYROID CRISIS AND MYXEDEMA COMA

### Hyperthyroid Crisis

Hyperthyroid crisis (Table 17-6), or thyroid storm, is a rare but acute medical emergency involving multisystem dysfunction accompanied by hyperpyrexia (i.e., extremely high fever). The pathophysiology underlying this syndrome remains obscure. While its clinical manifestations reflect an exaggeration of the usual signs and symptoms of hyperthyroidism (see Table 17-5), levels of thyroid hormones during the crisis are not appreciably more elevated than those found in the hyperthyroid state. Thus, clearly the cause of hyperthyroid crisis cannot be attributed to the levels of thyroid hormones alone.

Because hyperthyroid crisis seems always to be precipitated by a stressful event, the synergism of the thyroid hormone-catecholamine interaction may be implicated as a pathophysiologic mechanism underlying the crisis. Another consideration as to the pathophysiology underlying hyperthyroid crisis involves an alteration in the serum levels of thyroid-binding proteins. A decrease in total serum proteins, for whatever reason, may directly affect the levels of the free, active, unbound fraction of thyroid hormones circulating in the blood. As the availability of free thyroid hormone increases, there is a consequent increase in the rate of metabolic reactions and a potentiation of sympathetic activity.

The etiology of hyperthyroid crisis remains largely undefined. It can occur spontaneously, but it is usually associated with a stressful event in patients with preexisting hyperthyroidism. The patient with inadequately controlled hyperthyroidism is at increased risk of developing hyperthyroid crisis. The difference between a severe hyperthyroid state and hyperthyroid crisis remains unclear. Other potential causes of hyperthyroid crisis are included in Table 17-6.

#### *Clinical Presentation*

Patients in full-blown hyperthyroid crisis present a dramatic picture reflective of multisystem disturbance. The physiologic effects of thyroid hormones (see Table 17-3) are intensified, and there is a heightened exaggeration of the symptomatology of preexisting hyperthyroidism. Hyperpyrexia (body temperature elevation as high as 41 °C [106 °F]) is a classic clinical finding as the body literally "burns up" with unusable energy. It is accompanied by tachycardia, dysrhythmias, tachypnea, and profuse diaphoresis. (See Table 17-6 for specific symptomatology reflective of multisystem disturbances. Pertinent laboratory findings are also listed.)

#### *Treatment*

Appropriate treatment of hyperthyroid crisis depends primarily on early diagnosis.[12] Once the diagnosis is suspected, treatment cannot be delayed to await laboratory confirmation. Hyperthyroid crisis requires rapid, timely, and aggressive management. A delay in diagnosis and treatment

TABLE 17–5
## Clinical Presentation of Hyperthyroidism and Hypothroidism

| | Hyperthyroidism | Hypothyroidism |
|---|---|---|
| Onset | Usually gradual and insiduous; occasionally abrupt | Usually insidious; may be difficult to detect in early stages unless the patient has preexisting hypothyroidism |
| Clinical history | Nervousness, fine tremors, irritability; agitation, shortened attention span<br>Wide mood swings: mild exhiliration to depression and apathy<br>Emotional lability, behavior problems<br>Intense fear, paranoia, other psychiatric symptoms<br>Proximal muscle weakness<br>Easy fatigability; dyspnea on exertion; decreased exercise tolerance<br>Heat intolerance; fever; excessive sweating<br>Palpitations<br>Nausea, vomiting, diarrhea<br>Weight loss despite good appetite<br>Nails: "Dirt under nails difficult to clean"<br>Hair: "Won't hold a perm!"<br>Menstrual irregularity: Oligomenorrhea or amenorrhea; decreased libido; impotence in men | Lethargy, weakness; fatigue, memory impairment, slowed speech; slowing of mental functions<br>Depression; somnolence; apathy<br>Coarsening or hoarseness of voice related to myxedematous infiltration of tongue and larynx<br>Paranoia, agitation, other psychiatric reactions<br>Arthralgia, paresthesias, muscle cramps<br>Dyspnea on exertion; diminished respiratory effort (hypoventilation)<br>Cold intolerance, decreased sweating; decreased body temperature, swelling of face and extremities (peripheral edema)<br>Constipation<br>Modest weight gain with anorexia<br>Coarse, dry skin, brittle hair, and loss of hair<br>Menorrhagia, other menstrual irregularities; decreased libido; infertility in females; impotence in men |
| Physical examination | Resting tachycardia; widened pulse pressure<br>Prominent third heart sound; systolic murmur heard best over aortic and pulmonic area<br>Angina pectoris<br>Premature ventricular contractions<br>Supraventricular tachyarrhythmias:<br>Atrial fibrillation<br>Paroxysmal atrial tachycardia<br>Congestive heart failure (elderly)<br>Skin—Flushed, warm, smooth, moist; palmar erythema; spider angiomata; hyperpigmentation; exacerbation of eczematous dermatitis; pretibial edema<br>Hair—Fine, soft, silky, easily broken; increased hair loss<br>Nails—onycholysis<br>Fine tremors of hands and tongue<br>Muscle weakness, wasting; proximal myopathy<br>Thyromegaly; palpable thrill and audible bruit over thyroid; thyroid gland usually palpable<br>Prominent adominal findings in critically ill hyperthyroid patient: Abdominal pain; vomiting, diarrhea, liver failure with severe jaundice and pruritus; constipation in elderly<br>Gynecomastia in men<br>Diffuse lymphadenopathy and splenomegaly<br>Ophthalmopathy (Graves' disease):<br>Characteristic stare; periorbital edema; lid lag; decreased blinking; ophthalmoplegia, diplopia; exophthalmos; corneal ulceration<br>Dermopathy (Graves' disease):<br>Pretibial edema<br>Hyperpigmentation; pruritus | Bradycardia and diminished pulse pressure related to decreased cardiac contractility and cardiac output<br>Pleural and pericardial effusions; congestive heart failure<br>Hypertension may develop<br>Poor wound healing due to impaired protein synthesis<br>Thickened, dry skin with pallor or yellow tint (Thyroid hormones promote synthesis of vitamin A from carotene. In thyroid hormone deficiency, levels of carotene increase, causing the yellowing of skin.)<br>*Myxedema:* Reflective of advanced stage of hypothyroidism, and characterized by accumulation of mucopolysaccharide in subcutaneous and other tissues; periorbital edema, and puffy coarsened facial features are characteristic. Bruising may occur due to increased capillary fragility<br>A chronic deficiency of thyroid stimulation may result in atrophy and scarring of the thyroid gland over time; iodine deficiency may cause thyroid hypertrophy or goiter<br>Peripheral neuropathy—numbness; carpal tunnel syndrome may occur as a result of nerve entrapment in myxedematous thickening; hypoactive deep tendon reflexes |
| Laboratory data | Increased levels of serum $T_4$, $RT_3U$, $T_3$ RIA, RAIU<br>No significant TSH response to TRH<br>Blood chemistries—often abnormal:<br>Elevated serum alkaline phosphatase<br>Elevated bilirubin, SGOT<br>Lowered cholesterol levels | Free $T_4$ index is usually decreased.<br>Elevated TSH level is a sensitive index of hypothyroid function.<br>Hyponatremia; decreased red blood cell mass with normochromic anemia<br>Elevated serum cholesterol and triglyceride levels; increased tendency toward atherosclerosis and coronary artery disease<br>Elevated serum levels of CPK, SGOT, and LDH |

TABLE 17-6
## Contrast: Hyperthyroid Crisis and Myxedema Coma

| | Hyperthyroid Crisis | Myxedema Coma |
|---|---|---|
| Definition | Hyperthyroid crisis: An acute, life-threatening exacerbation of all the signs/symptoms of hyperthyroidism (see Table 17-5). It involves multisystem failure accompanied by hyperpyrexia. | Myxedema coma: An acute life-threatening complication of untreated hypothyroidism characterized by an exaggeration of the signs and symptoms of hypothyroidism (see Table 17-5). |
| Pathophysiology | 1. Thyroid hormone-catecholamine synergistic interactions:<br>• Thyroid hormones stimulate synthesis of beta-receptors and may increase the sensitivity of these receptors to catecholamines (epinephrine and norepinephrine).<br>• Enhanced sympathetic response coupled with the metabolic effects of increased levels of circulating thyroid hormone may account in part for hyperthyroid crisis.<br>2. Reduction in total serum thyroid-binding protein:<br>• Reduction in serum proteins may increase availability of free, circulating thyroid hormones.<br>• Excess free thyroid hormone reacts with tissues, increasing rates of metabolic reactions and potentiating the sympathetic effect. | 1. Thyroid hormone insufficiency may be related to decreased circulating levels of thyroid hormones, or to a resistance of target cells to the action of thyroid hormones.<br>2. Myxedema coma may be associated with destruction of the thyroid gland itself (primary) or with a disturbance in the hypothalamic-anterior pituitary-thyroid axis (secondary). Destruction of the thyroid gland is most commonly attributed to an autoimmune inflammatory process; inadequate secretion of thyrotropic-releasing hormone (TRH) by the hypothalamus may predispose to diminished TSH secretion.<br>3. Iodine deficiency predisposes to thyroid gland hypertrophy.<br>4. All clinical manifestations are directly related to the hypometabolic effect of too little thyroid hormone.<br>5. Myxedematous state involves the interstitial accumulation of mucopolysaccharides, which attract water, causing the nonpitting type of edema over the face and peripheral areas of the body. |
| Etiology | 1. Stressful event in the patient with preexisting hyperthyroidism:<br>• Trauma, acute infection (especially pulmonary)<br>• Surgery, vigorous manipulation of thyroid gland<br>• Uncontrolled diabetes mellitus, diabetic ketoacidosis, insulin-induced hypoglycemia<br>• Toxemia of pregnancy, parturition<br>• Myocardial infarction, pulmonary embolus<br>• Radioactive iodine therapy, severe drug reaction<br>• Severe fright or emotional upheaval<br>2. Increased risk in patient with hyperthyroidism that is inadequately controlled<br>3. Insufficient antithyroid therapy in the hyperthyroid patient; noncompliance with drug regimen<br>4. Excessive administration of exogenous thyroid hormone to the patient with hypothyroidism<br>5. X-ray contrast studies | Myxedema coma is preceded by a long period of hypothyroidism (usually of several years' duration).<br>1. Stressful events in the patient with preexisting hypothyroidism include trauma, infection or intercurrent illness, surgery (thyroidal), exposure to cold, sedative-type drugs, psychotropic drugs, other physical stress.<br>2. Insufficient exogenous thyroid hormone replacement therapy, most characteristically in the patient who stops taking prescribed thyroid hormone medications.<br>3. Post-subtotal thyroidectomy, less common today<br>4. Post-radioactive iodine therapy, a more frequent occurrence due to difficulty in determining the dosage desired for adequate irradiation |
| Clinical presentation | 1. Intensification of the physiologic effects of thyroid hormones (see Table 17-3)<br>2. Heightened exaggeration of signs/symptoms of hyperthyroidism (see Table 17-5) | 1. Diminution of the physiologic effects of thyroid hormones (see Table 17-3); a severe thyroid hormone deficiency state characterized by greatly depressed metabolic activity and central nervous system function, hypothermia, and hypoventilation |
| | 3. Hyperpyrexia—38-41°C; profuse sweating | • Hypothermia requires that the rectal thermometer be shaken down to lowest point to ensure accurate assessment of body temperature. |
| | 4. Multisystem disturbances:<br>• Cardiovascular: Resting tachycardia; premature ventricular contractions; supraventricular tachyarrhythmias; atrial fibrillation, paroxysmal atrial tachycardia; dyspnea; congestive heart failure, pulmonary edema, cardiogenic shock; hypotension, circulatory collapse<br>• Gastrointestinal: Nausea/vomiting; diarrhea and severe abdominal pain; liver failure, jaundice, hepatomegaly; abnormal liver function tests; weight loss | • Cardiovascular disturbances usually occur, including hypotension and bradycardia; hypercapnia due to hypoventilation |

TABLE 17–6
## Contrast: Hyperthyroid Crisis and Myxedema Coma *(Continued)*

| | Hyperthyroid Crisis | Myxedema Coma |
|---|---|---|
| | • Central nervous system: Restlessness, agitation, disorientation; delirium, frank psychosis; convulsions, tremors, muscle weakness; coma | • Depressed level of consciousness, seizure activity, and coma reflect central nervous system depression. Most frequently, patients arrive at the emergency room in coma. |
| Laboratory data | Elevated serum levels of: $T_4$, $RT_3U$, $T_3RIA$<br>Abnormal liver function tests: Serum alkaline phosphatase, bilirubin, SGOT<br>• The elevation of thyroid hormone levels provides no definitive distinction between the uncomplicated hyperthyroid state and hyperthyroid crisis.<br>• The thyrotropic-releasing hormone (TRH) stimulation test is considered by some to distinguish the critically ill patient with possible hyperthyroid crisis from one who is euthyroid.[11] | Decreased levels of: $RT_3U$, $T_3RIA$, $T_4$<br>• Increased TSH levels (primary hypothyroidism); decreased TSH levels in secondary hypothyroidism (dysfunction of hypothalamic–anterior pituitary–thyroid axis)<br>• Hypoglycemia, dilutional hyponatremia, decreased serum osmolality<br>• Increased serum cholesterol and triglycerides |
| Other studies | ECG monitoring: Resting sinus tachycardia; atrial fibrillation; premature atrial and ventricular contractions | ECG monitoring; sinus bradycardia; Q-T interval prolongation, low voltage |
| Treatment | 1. Emergency treatment of hyperthyroid crisis includes:<br>A. Inhibition of thyroid hormone synthesis<br>• Propylthiouracil (PTU) 900–1200 mg PO<br>B. Blockade of thyroid hormone release:<br>• Sodium iodide solution 1 g tid IV<br>Iodide therapy is initiated 1 to 2 hr after the administration of antithyroid agent (PTU).<br>• Oral preparations: Lugol's solution 10 g++ tid PO | 1. Measures to support body temperature, circulation, ventilation, fluid and electrolytes, and thyroid hormone replacement therapy are the foundations of treatment of myxedema coma.<br>A. Thyroid hormone replacement therapy is critical. Drug of choice is L-thyroxine: Initial stat dose 300–400 μg slowly intravenously. Daily doses are 50–100 μg per day. Intravenous administration of thyroid hormone therapy is necessary, initially because of risk of aspiration and uncertain gastrointestinal absorption. As the patient's condition stabilizes, the drug may be administered orally. Improvement in body temperature and overall clinical status should become apparent within 6–12 hr following initial dose of thyroxine. |
| | 2. Antagonism of peripheral effects of thyroid hormone:<br>• Propranolol 1–3 mg q 3–4 hr IV, 20–80 mg q 4–6 hr PO | 2. Cardiovascular function: Hypotension is treated by volume expansion with isotonic saline; alpha-adrenergic agents are avoided because the peripheral vasculature is already constricted in profound myxedema.<br>• Associated hyponatremia responds best to thyroid hormone replacement therapy; hypertonic saline is not administered except in profound hyponatremia. |
| | 3. Glucocorticoid therapy:<br>• Hydrocortisone sodium succinate (Solu-Cortef) 300 mg/day IV | 3. Glucocorticoid therapy is initiated because of the blunting of adrenal response to stress caused by the effects of long-standing hypothyroidism. |
| | 4. Supportive therapy:<br>A. Reduction of fever via use of cooling blanket; use of nonsalicylate antipyretics—acetaminophen 600 mg PO<br>B. Administration of fluids/electrolytes<br>C. Maintenance of physiologic acid–base balance<br>D. Supplemental oxygen<br>E. Treatment of cardiovascular dysfunction: Congestive heart failure—digitalis, diuretics; supraventricular tachyarrhythmias; hypotension<br>• Use of invasive monitoring techniques as the patient's condition warrants<br>F. Sedation as required<br>G. High-calorie, high-protein diet with supplemental multivitamins and trace elements | 4. Hypothermia: Therapy should not be implemented to raise body temperature because this serves to increase metabolic demands for oxygen; efforts should be made to minimize heat loss by using multiple blankets. |
| | 5. Therapy for extreme cases of hyperthyroid crisis: Removal of excessive circulating thyroxine<br>A. Exchange transfusion—Plasmapheresis<br>B. Peritoneal dialysis | 5. Cardiopulmonary function: Hypoxemia and hypercarbia ($PaO_2 < 60$ mmHg, $PaCO_2 > 45-50$ mmHg), associated with airway obstruction (enlarged tongue), and hypoventilation, may need to be treated by immediate placement of an endotracheal tube and assisted mechanical ventilation. |

Drug dosages adapted from Mathewson, MK: Pharmacotherapeutics: A Nursing Process Approach. FA Davis, Philadelphia, 1986, p 1354.

will increase mortality and morbidity. Even with the best treatment, mortality of patients with hyperthyroid crisis is about 15–20%.

Emergency treatment of hyperthyroid crisis includes the following: (1) inhibition of thyroid hormone synthesis; (2) blockage of thyroid hormone release; (3) antagonism of peripheral effects of thyroid hormone; (4) establishment of adequate supportive care; (5) identification and treatment of precipitating cause(s). Optimal treatment lies in identifying the circumstances that predispose to hyperthyroid crisis and in adequately treating the underlying hyperthyroidism. It is essential that treatment of the precipitating illness occurs in conjunction with the overall treatment of hyperthyroid crisis, because the causative illness may have triggered the crisis, or this illness may be exacerbated by the crisis. Specific drug and supportive therapies are presented in Table 17–6.

### *Nursing Care of the Patient in Hyperthyroid Crisis*

Hyperthyroidism, a common, seemingly benign illness frequently found in young, previously healthy women (predominantly), is characterized by fluctuations in severity. Such fluctuations, attributed to the potent systemic effects of abnormally elevated amounts of circulating thyroid hormones and to an associated overwhelming adrenergic response, may signal the onset of potentially life-threatening complications in a manner so rapid and dramatic that it takes the patient and health-care provider by surprise.

Nursing care of the patient in hyperthyroid crisis presents a unique and formidable challenge to the critical care nurse. While the patient may be faced with a life-threatening situation, the manifestations of the crisis may not be readily apparent clinically. In fact, some of the patient's signs and symptoms may actually be misleading, as in the case of the patient who presents with severe abdominal pain. This chief complaint may actually direct the attention of the undiscerning practitioner away from the possible hyperthyroid crisis. Likewise, in the patient who presents with nonspecific behavioral problems (restlessness, agitation, hyperactivity) and/or emotional lability (depression, apathy), it may be easy to conclude naively that the patient is a "psych" case.

Each of these situations reflects symptomatology characteristic of hyperthyroid crisis, yet, by themselves, these clinical findings may not assist in recognizing its presence. No specific clinical patterns or tests can be used readily to diagnose hyperthyroid crisis (except in those patients with Graves' disease who exhibit established signs of ophthalmopathy and dermopathy). The challenge to the critical care nurse lies in knowing what questions to ask and what signs to look for, so that significant relationships that exist between diverse signs and symptoms and that herald the onset of hyperthyroid crisis can be identified.

The life-threatening nature of hyperthyroid crisis requires timely, rapid, and aggressive management. Therapy cannot be delayed to await laboratory confirmation. Rather, such therapy is often initiated based solely on corroborating clinical findings and keen clinical instincts.

Once initiated, the appropriateness and effectiveness of ongoing treatment depend on the moment-to-moment monitoring and assessment of the patient's response to therapy, a responsibility largely assumed by the critical care nurse in collaboration with the patient's physicians. Treatment is modified continually to meet the changing needs of the patient.

During the crisis phase of hyperthyroidism, nursing care is directed toward identifying the individual at risk, preventing life-threatening events, assisting the individual to restore life processes to a state of dynamic equilibrium, and working with the individual and family to help them understand the nature of the disease and its overall impact on the lifestyle and integrity of each individual.

**Therapeutic Goals.** Implementation of nursing process in the care of the patient in hyperthyroid crisis revolves around the following therapeutic goals:

1. Establish a thorough and comprehensive database including:
   A. Clinical history (functional health patterns).
   B. Physical examination.
   C. Laboratory/diagnostic studies.
2. Implement prescribed drug regimen to reduce thyroid hormone synthesis and release, and inhibit adrenergic hyperactivity.
3. Institute measures to reduce hyperpyrexia.
4. Maintain effective cardiopulmonary function.
5. Maintain fluid and electrolyte balance.
6. Maintain adequate nutrition to meet tissue requirements of the hypermetabolic state.
7. Maintain the integrity of neurologic and psychologic processes.
8. Provide emotional and psychologic support to patient/family.
9. Initiate patient/family education to assist in developing and implementing prophylactic health-care practices.

**Nursing Diagnoses, Desired Patient Outcomes, and Nursing Interventions/Rationales.** Pertinent nursing diagnoses, desired patient outcomes, and nursing interventions/rationales in the care of the patient in hyperthyroid crisis are presented in the care plan in Table 17–7.

## TABLE 17–7. CARE PLAN FOR THE PATIENT WITH HYPERTHYROID CRISIS

| Nursing Diagnoses | Desired Patient Outcomes | Nursing Interventions | Rationales |
|---|---|---|---|
| ***Nursing Diagnosis #1***<br>Cardiac output, alteration in: Decreased, related to:<br>1. High output cardiac failure associated with increased metabolic demand, and exaggerated adrenergic effect.<br>2. Cardiac dysrhythmias.<br>3. Reduced circulating blood volume associated with excessive diaphoresis vomiting, diarrhea. | Patient will maintain:<br>1. Usual mental status: Alert, oriented to person, place, date; deep tendon reflexes brisk.<br>2. Adequate cardiovascular function:<br>• Cardiac rate and rhythm—heart rate $>60$, $<100$ beats/min; rhythm—regular sinus, without symptomatic dysrhythmias.<br>Hemodynamic status:<br>• CVP: 0–8 mmHg ($\overline{\text{mean}}$)<br>• PCWP: 8–12 mmHg ($\overline{\text{mean}}$)<br>• CO: 4–8 liters/min<br>• Arterial blood pressure within 10 mmHg of baseline supine and upright.<br>3. Renal status:<br>• Urine output $>30$ ml/hr<br>4. Respiratory status:<br>• Respiratory rate and breathing pattern: $<25$–30 breaths/min; eupnea | • Maintain adequate cardiovascular function.<br>∘ Assess the effect of hypermetabolic state on cardiovascular function: cardiac rate and rhythm; occurrence of chest pain and/or palpitations.<br>∘ Assess changes in heart sounds, extra heart sounds ($S_3$ and $S_4$), murmurs. | • Hypermetabolic state increases myocardial oxygen consumption predisposing to ischemia; cardia ischema may precipitate cardiac dysrhythmias and/or anginal pain.<br>∘ Reflect increased force of myocardial contraction; may be associated with cardiac dysrhythmias. |
| | | ∘ Breath sounds: abnormal, or adventitious breath sounds (e.g., crackles, wheezes).<br>∘ Assess hemodynamic parameters: Arterial blood pressure (supine/upright); widened pulse pressure; CVP, PCWP, CO, systemic vascular resistance (SVR). | ∘ Increased risk of developing hypovolemic shock due to dehydrated state.<br>∘ Widening pulse pressure reflects increase in stroke volume and decrease in systemic vascular resistance.<br>∘ Hemodynamic parameters reflect cardiac status; assist in evaluating fluid state and response to overall therapy. |
| | | ∘ Assess predisposition to congestive heart failure, pulmonary edema. | ∘ Related to cardiac oxygen demand in excess of adequate supply, with tissue ischemia and injury; high-output cardiac failure related to hypermetabolic demands. |
| | | ∘ Monitor for symptomatic cardiac dysrhythmias, which can predispose to cardiogenic shock:<br>– Supraventricular tachyarrhythmias: Paroxysmal atrial tachycardia; atrial tachycardia with rapid ventricular response.<br>∘ Symptomatic bradycardia, heart block, and conduction disturbances.<br>– Ventricular dysrhythmias: Premature ventricular contractions, ventricular tachycardia, ventricular fibrillation. | ∘ Conduction disturbances and bradycardia may be associated with propranolol therapy. |
| | | ∘ Anticipate the occurrence of potential lethal dysrhythmias. The following equipment should be available at bedside:<br>– Antiarrhythmia drugs.<br>– Pacemaker and insertion equipment.<br>– Equipment for cardioversion/defibrillation.<br>∘ Monitor cardiac rate and rhythm continuously. | ∘ Patients in hyperthyroid crisis are at increased risk of catastrophic events related to potential lethal dysrhythmias. |

## TABLE 17–7. CARE PLAN FOR THE PATIENT WITH HYPERTHYROID CRISIS *(Continued)*

| Nursing Diagnoses | Desired Patient Outcomes | Nursing Interventions | Rationales |
|---|---|---|---|
| ***Nursing Diagnosis #1 (cont.)*** | | | |
| | | • Implement prescribed drug regimen to reduce thyroid hormone synthesis and release, and to inhibit adrenergic hyperactivity. | |
| | | ◦ Administer therapy to block thyroid hormone synthesis:<br>– Propylthiouracil (PTU). | ◦ PTU functions to reduce circulating levels of thyroid hormone over days to weeks by blocking a strategic step in the synthesis of thyroid hormones. |
| | | ◦ Administer via nasogastric tube if patient is unable to swallow or to cooperate. | ◦ PTU is not available in parenteral form. |
| | | ◦ Assess the patient for adverse drug reactions. | ◦ Patients can develop minor side effects such as urticaria, epigastric distress, granulocytopenia, and, over the long term, lupus-like syndrome. Hepatitis has been known to occur.<br>– Abrupt withdrawal can precipitate thyroid crisis. |
| | | ◦ Administer antithyroid drug of choice, which acts to block thyroid secretion:<br>◦ Sodium iodide. | ◦ Iodides have an immediate effect in reducing serum levels of thyroid hormone; full therapeutic effect takes 10–14 days. |
| | | ◦ Establish any prior incidence of allergy to iodine preparations; contrast dye. | ◦ Presence of allergy to iodine may require an alternative approach to therapy. |
| | | ◦ Assess the patient for adverse drug reactions. | ◦ Patient can develop minor side effects—urticaria or other skin lesions. |
| | | ◦ Administer $beta_2$-adrenergic blocker to inhibit adrenergic overactivity.<br>– Propranolol is the drug of choice. | ◦ Propranolol markedly reduces the effects of excessive thyroid hormone on cardiovascular function by competing with epinephrine and norepinephrine for $beta_2$-adrenergic receptors.<br>◦ Propranolol is available in oral and parenteral preparations; this drug may be lifesaving because its therapeutic effects, via intravenous use, are achieved rapidly.<br>◦ Intravenous propranolol warrants thorough and continuous monitoring of vital signs and cardiac rhythm.<br>◦ Propranolol acts to reduce heart rate, cardiac contractility, and oxygen consumption; it reduces myocardial irritability and associated supraventricular tachyarrhythmias; it ameliorates clinical manifestations |

| | |
|---|---|
| | of adrenergic overactivity including palpitations associated with forceful heart contractions, nervousness, tremors, profuse diaphoresis, and heat intolerance. |
| ○ Establish baseline vital sign parameters; closely monitor heart rate, rhythm, blood pressure, apical and peripheral pulses, respiratory rate and pattern. Observe for desired and adverse effects. | ○ Untoward reactions to $beta_2$-adrenergic blockage may include a symptomatic bradycardia, heart block, heart failure, and respiratory insufficiency. |
| ○ Be cognizant of contraindications to the use of propranolol. | ○ Contraindications to the use of propranolol include: Asthma, chronic obstructive pulmonary disease; nonhyperthyroidal heart failure; symptomatic sinus bradycardia; atrioventricular heart block.<br>○ $Beta_2$-adrenergic blockade causes bronchiole constriction.<br>○ Tachyarrhythmias may remain refractory to therapy until the underlying hyperthyroidism is under control.<br>○ Intravenous propranolol can have sudden adverse effects: Sudden bradycardia; hypotension (orthostatic); syncope; evidence of congestive heart failure, dyspnea, respiratory compromise, and cardiac arrest. |
| ○ Maintain the following drugs within easy access:<br>– Atropine for symptomatic bradycardia.<br>– Vasopressors (e.g., dopamine) for hypotension.<br>– Isoproterenol (positive inotropic effect).<br>– Aminophylline for bronchospasm.<br>– Digoxin for heart failure.<br>– Furosemide (diuretic). | |
| ○ Monitor serum glucose (serially). | ○ Propranolol may mask signs of insulin overdosage in patients receiving insulin therapy and may prolong hypoglycemic effects. |
| ○ Administer other prescribed medications if use of propranolol is contraindicated: | |
| ○ Reserpine. | ○ Reserpine reduces synthesis of norepinephrine, and competitively inhibits its reuptake in storage granules. |
| ○ Guanethidine. | ○ Guanethidine acts to displace stored norepinephrine from storage granules; acts as a "false neurotransmitter" that effectively blocks adrenergic actions of norepinephrine. |

*(continued)*

**TABLE 17–7. CARE PLAN FOR THE PATIENT WITH HYPERTHYROID CRISIS *(Continued)***

| Nursing Diagnoses | Desired Patient Outcomes | Nursing Interventions | Rationales |
|---|---|---|---|
| ***Nursing Diagnosis #1 (cont.)*** | | | |
| | | ○ Administer prescribed glucocorticosteroid therapy. | ○ Potential accelerated turnover and degradation of glucocorticosteroids in hyperthyroid crisis warrants the administration of "stress-dose" replacement therapy. |
| | | ○ Dexamethasone.<br>– Hydrocortisone sodium succinate (Solu-Cortef). | ○ Dexamethasone also inhibits peripheral conversion of $T_4$ to $T_3$. |
| | | ○ Evaluate effectiveness of antithyroid hormone therapy:<br>– Improvements in clinical signs: Temperature reduction; clearing of mental status; reduced heart rate; stable blood pressure, pulse, respiratory rate and rhythm; reduction in palpitations, tremors, nervousness, profuse diaphoresis. | ○ The effects of antithyroid therapy and diminished adrenergic response should become clinically obvious within 6–12 hr after initiation of therapy. |
| | | ○ Improvement in laboratory studies:<br>– Serum $T_4$, $T_3$RIA, $RT_3$U. | ○ Serum levels of thyroid hormone do not significantly drop for several days after initiation of therapy; initial improvement in clinical status is probably due to the diminished adrenergic response. |
| | | ○ Improvement in liver function and other studies. | ○ Overall treatment plan may need to be modified continuously to meet the changing needs of the patient. |
| | | ○ Absence of adverse reactions to therapy. | ○ In evaluating laboratory data, it must be remembered that serum tests are measurements of thyroid hormone levels at only one point in time. It is possible for an isolated thyroid hormone value to reflect intake of exogenous iodine whether in diet or medications. It is important to question the patient regarding the intake of exogenous iodine because this may be reflected in the laboratory results. |
| | | ○ Note if the patient has any allergies to iodine-containing substances. | |
| | | ○ Assess if established protocols for specific tests are followed. | ○ It is important to follow established protocols for testing to ensure that test results are valid. |

| | | | |
|---|---|---|---|
| ***Nursing Diagnosis #2***<br>Fluid volume deficit: Actual, related to:<br>1. Hypermetabolic state with hyperpyrexia associated with profuse diaphoresis. (See Table 23–3, Nursing Diagnosis #1.)<br>***Nursing Diagnosis #3***<br>Electrolyte imbalance, related to:<br>1. Severe dehydration.<br>2. Hemoconcentration with hypernatremia. (See Table 23–7, Nursing Diagnosis #1.) | Patient will maintain effective fluid and electrolyte balance:<br>1. Neurologic status: Alert, oriented to person, date, place; deep tendon reflexes brisk.<br>2. Hemodynamic status: (As in Nursing Diagnosis #1 above).<br>3. Body weight will stabilize within 5% of patient's baseline.<br>4. Renal status: urine output >30 ml/hr.<br>5. Gastrointestinal status: Absence of anorexia, nausea, vomiting and diarrhea.<br>6. Laboratory data:<br>• Serum osmolality: ~285–295 mOsm/kg.<br>• Serum sodium: >135 <148 mEq/liter.<br>• Serum potassium: >3.5 <5.5 mEq/liter.<br>• Serum glucose, BUN, creatinine, and hematology profile at optimal levels for patient. | For pertinent nursing interventions and their rationales in the care of the patient in hyperthyroid crisis who is experiencing hyperpyrexia accompanied by fluid and electrolyte imbalance, see the following:<br>Table 23–3, Nursing Diagnoses #1, #2, and #3<br>Table 23–7, Nursing Diagnosis #1<br>Table 23–9, Nursing Diagnosis #1<br>Table 24–3, Nursing Diagnosis #1.<br>In addition, consider the following nursing interventions/rationales:<br>• Maintain fluid and electrolyte balance.<br>○ Assess the effect of hypermetabolic state on body fluid balance: | ○ The hypermetabolic state may predispose to widely fluctuating imbalance in total body fluids. |
| | | ○ Assess for signs/symptoms of fluid volume deficit: Nonproductive cough; flat neck veins, dry, parched mucous membranes. | ○ Depleted fluid state, dehydration may be due to profuse diaphoresis associated with hyperpyrexia, and to disturbances in gastrointestinal function—vomiting, and/or diarrhea. |
| | | ○ Assess for signs/symptoms of fluid volume excess:<br>– Auscultate breath sounds (crackles).<br>– Productive cough, frothy, pink-tinged sputum; neck vein distention. | ○ Fluid volume overload increases the risk of congestive heart failure and pulmonary edema.<br>○ Overly aggressive fluid replacement therapy can predispose to fluid volume excess. |
| | | ○ Monitor intake and output, urine specific gravity; serial weights. | ○ Body weight is a good indicator of insensible fluid loss. |
| | | ○ Prevent fluid imbalance.<br>○ Administer fluids based on fluid losses (include insensible losses), overall state of hydration, and serum electrolyte values.<br>– Continue to monitor closely intake and output, daily weight, vital signs, serum electrolytes, urine output and other parameters reflective of fluid state. | ○ Hemoconcentration or hemodilution can predispose to electrolyte imbalance. |
| | | ○ Consider the effects of hypermetabolic state on serum electrolytes.<br>○ Monitor for hypokalemia:<br>○ Assess signs/symptoms: General malaise, fatigue, anorexia, nausea and vomiting, diarrhea, abdominal cramps; muscle weakness, hyporeflexia; hypotension, dysrhythmias; presence of U wave on 12-lead electrocardiogram; apathy, restlessness, irritability.<br>– Monitor serial serum potassium levels. | ○ Gastrointestinal symptoms of vomiting and diarrhea, and excessive administration of diuretics to the patient with fluid overload are largely responsible for the occurrence of hypokalemia.<br>(See Table 23–8 for a contrast between hyperkalemia and hypokalemia.) |
| | | ○ Administer potassium supplements and assess clinical response. | ○ Intravenous potassium must be administered slowly to avoid lethal cardiac dysrhythmias or standstill; oral potassium supplements can cause gastrointestinal irritation. |

*(continued)*

**TABLE 17–7. CARE PLAN FOR THE PATIENT WITH HYPERTHYROID CRISIS** *(Continued)*

| Nursing Diagnoses | Desired Patient Outcomes | Nursing Interventions | Rationales |
|---|---|---|---|
| ***Nursing Diagnosis #3 (cont.)*** | | | |
| | | ○ Monitor for hyponatremia:<br>– Assess for signs/symptoms of dilutional state such as: Headache, faintness, muscle cramps; mental confusion; seizures, convulsions, coma.<br>– Monitor intake and output; serial electrolyte and osmolality levels.<br>– Restrict fluids as per medical therapeutic plan and monitor response. | ○ Hyponatremia is usually dilutional in origin, occurring due to excess in body fluid volume or hypo-osmolar state (water intoxication). *Dilutional hyponatremia:* Due to water excess.<br>(See Table 23–6 for a contrast between hyper- and hyponatremia including dilutional and depletional hyponatremia.)<br>○ Depletional hyponatremia may occur in hyperthyroid crisis because of profuse diaphoresis associated with hyperpyrexia. *Depletional hyponatremia:* Due to sodium loss. |
| | | ○ Monitor for hypercalcemia:<br>– Assess signs/symptoms including: Drowsiness, fatigue, anorexia, thirst, nausea, vomiting, constipation; neuromuscular changes are reflected in hypotonicity of muscles, with weakness; deep bone pain; central nervous system depression may be reflected by depression, lethargy, psychosis, and coma. | ○ Hypercalcemia is related to increased activity of osteoclasts causing bone resorption and demineralization.<br>○ Constipation is related to depressed tone of smooth muscles within the bowel; reduced peristalsis may progress to paralytic ileus.<br>(See Table 24–3 for a contrast between hypercalcemia and hypocalcemia.) |
| | | ○ Monitor serial serum calcium levels; observe for ECG changes reflected by a shortened Q-T interval, and dysrhythmias; maintain strict intake and output. | ○ Large amounts of calcium may be lost in urine and stool; long-term effect often involves pathologic fractures due to demineralization of bone; and renal calculi. |
| | | • Implement prescribed therapeutic plan and monitor patient's response to therapy:<br>○ Intravenous saline and diuretics. | ○ Sodium diuresis promotes renal excretion of calcium. |
| | | ○ Administration of intravenous or oral phosphates.<br>○ Administration of glucocorticoids. | ○ Phosphates induce calcium excretion, and together with glucocorticoids, inhibit calcium absorption. |
| | | ○ Administration of sodium bicarbonate. | ○ Increases fraction of calcium that is protein bound. |
| | | ○ Dialysis.<br>○ Initiate range-of-motion exercises as condition stabilizes. | ○ Inactivity contributes to bone resorption. |

| | | | |
|---|---|---|---|
| ***Nursing Diagnosis #4***<br>Hyperthermia, related to:<br>1. Hypermetabolic rate.<br>2. Enhanced adrenergic activity. | Patient's body temperature will stabilize at ~37°C (98.6°F). | • Evaluate status of body temperature.<br>∘ Assess the effect of hypermetabolic state on body functions: signs/symptoms may include the following:<br>∘ Fever as high as 106°F (41°C).<br>– Resting tachycardia; supraventricular tachyarrhythmias; congestive heart failure; hypovolemic shock.<br>– Nausea/vomiting, diarrhea; liver failure —abnormal liver function tests.<br>– State of physical, mental, emotional exhaustion.<br>– Coma. | ∘ Hyperpyrexia develops when the compensatory mechanisms of peripheral vasodilation, diaphoresis, and polyuria are no longer able to dissipate excessive heat production of the hypermetabolic state.<br>– Excessive heat production (thermal energy) largely results from exceedingly enhanced lipolysis and oxidation of fatty acids stimulated by increased circulating thyroid hormone.<br>– Body temperature may fluctuate rapidly; sudden increases or fall in body temperature stresses cardiovascular function, causing cardiac irritability and serious ventricular dysrhythmias.<br>– Untreated hyperthyroid crisis can cause death from excessive fever, cardiac and/or liver failure; exhaustion—cellular "burn out." |
| | | ∘ Monitor rectal temperature hourly or continuously if rectal probe available.<br>∘ Assess the state of hydration: Body weight, urine specific gravity; hourly intake and output; extent of diaphoresis. | ∘ Assists in evaluating trends in body temperature and response to therapy. (See Nursing Diagnosis #2 above.) |
| | | • Institute fever-reducing therapy.<br>∘ Administer antipyretic agents (acetaminophen is drug of choice). | ∘ Aspirin (acetylsalicylic acid) worsens hyperthyroid crisis by displacing thyroid hormones from serum protein thyroid hormone-binding receptors, resulting in an increase in free circulating thyroid hormone. |
| | | • Implement body surface-cooling measures (for temperature 38°C, 102°F).<br>∘ Hypothermia blanket.<br>∘ Ice packs to axilla and groin area. | • When body temperature exceeds 38°C in a patient with preexisting hyperthyroidism, it may signal that a state of physiologic decompensation and disequilibrium is in the process of evolving. |
| | | ∘ Cool environment with minimal bed covers.<br>∘ Use fans, if available, to circulate air. | ∘ Lowered body temperature decreases metabolic needs. |
| | | • Administer oxygen therapy if necessary. | • Hypermetabolic state causes increased oxygen demand and consumption. |

*(continued)*

**TABLE 17-7. CARE PLAN FOR THE PATIENT WITH HYPERTHYROID CRISIS *(Continued)***

| Nursing Diagnoses | Desired Patient Outcomes | Nursing Interventions | Rationales |
|---|---|---|---|
| ***Nursing Diagnosis #4 (cont.)*** | | • Provide supportive nursing measures: | |
| | | ◦ Scrupulous skin care with frequent tepid sponge baths and adequate skin drying. | ◦ Potential for impairment of skin integrity is increased by the catabolic state; skin is thin, friable, and easily injured. |
| | | ◦ Frequent turning and changes in position. | ◦ Increases circulation to prominent bony areas and pressure points. |
| | | ◦ Assess for shivering; muscle relaxants and/ or sedation may be necessary. | ◦ Shivering increases metabolic needs. |
| ***Nursing Diagnosis #5*** Oral mucous membranes, alteration in. (See Table 23-3, Nursing Diagnosis #2.) | Patient's mucous membranes will remain: 1. Clean, moist and without cracking or fissuring. | • Assess status of oral mucous membranes and skin integrity. | • The high metabolic state can deplete body fluid rapidly, leading to an alteration in mucous membranes with fissuring and cracking; skin becomes fragile especially over pressure points. |
| ***Nursing Diagnosis #6*** Skin integrity, impairment: Potential for. | Patient's skin will remain warm and dry; good turgor over forehead or sternum. | • Implement measures to maintain the intactness of mucous membranes and skin: | • Scrupulous skin care should be provided with frequent tepid sponging and drying. |
| | | ◦ Provide frequent mouth care; prevent encrustation; keep lips moist. | |
| | | ◦ Initiate pressure relief device (e.g., air mattress, sheepskin, egg crate mattress). | ◦ Helps to maximize perfusion. Catabolic state predisposes to thin, friable, and easily injured skin and mucous membranes. |
| | | ◦ Execute plan for turning/positioning every 2 hr. | |
| | | ◦ Monitor nutritional status. | |
| ***Nursing Diagnosis #7*** Breathing pattern, alteration in, related to: 1. Weakness of pulmonary musculature, and fatigue. | 1. Patient will maintain arterial blood gas parameters as follows: • pH: 7.35-7.45 (room air) • $PaCO_2$: 35-45 mmHg • $HCO_3$: 22-26 mEq/liter • $PaO_2$: >60 mmHg 2. Patient will verbalize ease of breathing. | • Maintain effective respiratory function. | |
| | | ◦ Assess the effects of hypermetabolic state on respiratory function: | |
| | | ◦ Respiratory rate and rhythm. – Tachypnea, dyspnea. – Use of accessory muscles of respiration. | ◦ Ineffective breathing pattern may be associated with muscle weakness and exhaustion due to hypermetabolic state. |
| | | ◦ Pulmonary function parameters: – Tidal volume, vital capacity | |
| | | ◦ Auscultation of breath sounds. | ◦ Pulmonary congestion/edema is associated with high cardiac output congestive heart failure. |
| | | ◦ Evidence of cyanosis. | |

| | | | |
|---|---|---|---|
| | | ◦ Arterial blood gas—trend. | ◦ Extreme vasodilation in response to hypermetabolic state causes skin to be flushed and warm; presence of cyanosis in lips, mucous membranes, earlobes, and nailbeds suggests decreased oxygenation related to hypoventilation and/or impaired gas exchange.<br>◦ A change in the patient's breathing pattern from hyperventilatory to hypoventilatory, coupled with a rising $PaCO_2$ (from <35 mmHg to >45 mmHg) strongly suggests that the patient is decompensating. |
| | | ◦ Obtain specimen of sputum for culture and sensitivity. | ◦ Pulmonary infection is a frequent precipitating factor in the occurrence of hyperthyroid crisis. |
| | | • Provide supportive therapy.<br>◦ Administer oxygen therapy. | ◦ Oxygen therapy will assist in meeting the increased demand for oxygen caused by the hypermetabolic state; it may help to relieve dyspnea. |
| | | ◦ Assist patient to assume a position that facilitates breathing.<br>◦ Provide a quiet environment with frequent rest periods.<br>◦ Provide explanation and feedback regarding progress of course. | ◦ All efforts are directed toward assisting the patient to conserve strength and prevent a state of exhaustion. |
| | | • Initiate antibiotic therapy to treat suspected and/or diagnosed infection. | • Infection may be an underlying cause of hyperthyroid crisis. |
| ***Nursing Diagnosis #8***<br>Nutrition, alteration in: Less than body requirements, related to:<br>1. Hypermetabolic state | 1. Patient's body weight will stabilize within 5% of baseline.<br>2. Serum proteins will be maintained within acceptable physiologic range: ~6.0 to 8.4 g/100 ml.<br>3. Serum glucose: 70–110 mg/100 ml.<br>4. Urine negative for glucose and acetone. | • Maintain adequate nutrition to meet tissue requirements of the hypermetabolic state.<br>◦ Consult with nutritionist regarding alterations in nutrition caused by hypermetabolic state.<br>◦ Assess overall nutritional status and potential alterations associated with hypermetabolic state.<br>◦ Assess for hyperglycemia: | ◦ Elevated circulating levels of thyroid hormone greatly enhance glycogenolysis and reduce serum insulin levels; increased adrenergic activity can impair insulin secretion and/or diminish tissue reponse to the effects of insulin. |

*(continued)*

**TABLE 17-7. CARE PLAN FOR THE PATIENT WITH HYPERTHYROID CRISIS** *(Continued)*

| Nursing Diagnoses | Desired Patient Outcomes | Nursing Interventions | Rationales |
|---|---|---|---|
| ***Nursing Diagnosis #8 (cont.)*** | | | |
| | | ◦ Signs and symptoms include: Polydipsia, glycosuria, polyuria, nocturia, weakness, fatigue; vision disturbances (diplopia); muscle cramping; irritability; lethargy, depression. | ◦ Polydipsia, glycosuria, and polyuria are related to the osmotic diuretic effect of elevated serum glucose. |
| | | ◦ Monitor serum glucose levels; urine for sugar and acetone. | ◦ Glycosuria may be the only symptom of altered glucose metabolism. |
| | | ◦ Administer prescribed insulin/glucose:<br>– Glucose with insulin in small amounts to control hyperglycemia. | ◦ This therapy provides an essential nutrient and ensures its use by cells—insulin is necessary for absorption and utilization of glucose by liver, muscle, and adipose tissues; the availability of glucose diminishes the occurrence of a catabolic state due to gluconeogenesis. |
| | | ◦ Maintain prescribed caloric intake. | |
| | | ◦ Provide necessary electrolytes and soluble vitamin B complex and vitamin C supplements. | ◦ Hypermetabolic rates rapidly deplete stores of vitamins and trace metals, which are vital coenzymes in many biochemical interactions. |
| | | ◦ Maintain prescribed lipid intake. | ◦ Excessive lipolysis and oxidation of free fatty acids largely account for hyperpyrexia due to inability of body to dissipate excessive heat generation. |
| | | ◦ Maintain positive nitrogen balance:<br>– Monitor BUN, creatinine. | ◦ Protein catabolism occurs at greater rate than protein synthesis. Goal of therapy is to prevent negative protein balance.<br>◦ Enhanced gluconeogenesis contributes largely to negative nitrogen balance. |
| | | ◦ Assess signs/symptoms including: Weakness, fatigue, weight loss, muscle wasting and hypoalbuminemia. | ◦ Continued weight loss may indicate inadequacy of treatment in meeting energy needs of hypermetabolic state. |
| | | ◦ Monitor body weight and serial serum protein levels. | ◦ Reduced levels of serum proteins exacerbate effect of excessive thyroid hormones due to additional free, unbound quantities of thyroid hormone. |
| | | ◦ Provide adequate nutritive intake to meet needs of hypermetabolic state.<br>– Essential amino acids and trace metals in addition to caloric intake. | ◦ Complete nutritional and supportive therapy must be provided simultaneously with therapeutic modalities to decrease serum levels of thyroid hormone. |

| | | | |
|---|---|---|---|
| | | ○ Minimize energy expenditure by coordinating overall patient care activities and allowing for uninterrupted rest periods.<br>• Assess effects of hypermetabolic state on gastrointestinal function:<br>○ Assess for signs/symptoms such as nausea, vomiting, diarrhea, abdominal pain, hepatomegaly.<br>○ Monitor mental status and presence of protective reflexes (cough and gag).<br>○ Provide frequent, small feedings. | ○ Protein catabolism, produces weakness in all muscle groups. Fatigue increases stress.<br>○ Intravenous therapy may be indicated if there is risk of aspiration.<br>○ Frequent small feedings may help to diminish epigastric distress. |
| ***Nursing Diagnosis #9***<br>Injury, potential for, related to:<br>1. Altered neurologic function associated with hypermetabolic state.<br>2. Exophthalmopathy. | Patient will:<br>1. Demonstrate usual mental status:<br>• Alert, oriented to person, place.<br>• Increased attentiveness.<br>2. Remain injury free:<br>• Without seizure activity.<br>• Corneas intact, without erosions or ulcerations. | • Maintain integrity of neurologic, physical, and psychologic processes.<br>○ Assess effect of hypermetabolic state on neurologic function.<br>○ Perform neurologic assessment every 1–2 hr during acute phase of illness. Signs/symptoms may include:<br>– Mental status: Blunted level of consciousness; disorientation, confusion, agitation, restlessness, irritability, coma.<br>– Cranial nerves: Sluggish pupillary response; impaired protective reflexes (cough, gag).<br>– Motor function: Hypokinesis, easy fatigability, muscle weakness; seizure activity.<br>– Hyperreflexia.<br>○ Employ safety measures to prevent injury:<br>○ Seizure precautions: Padded bed rails; oral airway and suction at bedside; bed in low position; soft protective restraints.<br>○ Orient to person, date, and place; provide clock and calendar in patient's room; confirm reality.<br>○ Maintain cool, quiet environment with occasional soft, soothing music.<br>○ Allow for frequent undisturbed rest periods.<br>○ Avoid sensory overload. | ○ Symptomatology related to central nervous system function is attributed largely to the hypermetabolic activity within neurons.<br>○ Rapid fluctuations in neurologic status can occur; changes in neurologic status may reflect patient's response to therapy.<br>○ Seizure activity may reflect deterioration in the patient's condition.<br>○ Goal of therapy is to maximize the resting state to minimize cellular metabolic needs.<br>○ A reduction in stimuli diminishes state of hyperactivity and cellular metabolism. |

*(continued)*

**TABLE 17–7. CARE PLAN FOR THE PATIENT WITH HYPERTHYROID CRISIS *(Continued)***

| Nursing Diagnoses | Desired Patient Outcomes | Nursing Interventions | Rationales |
|---|---|---|---|
| ***Nursing Diagnosis #9 (cont.)*** | | | |
| | | ○ Administer prescribed sedation, and monitor patient's response to therapy. | ○ Hyperactivity needs to be reduced because it exacerbates the hypermetabolic state.<br>○ Use of sedatives is avoided if possible, because they can mask changes in the patient's neurologic status. |
| | | • Assess status of exophthalmopathy.<br>○ Protect exposed corneas:<br>– Administer prescribed methylcellulose eyedrops.<br>– Tape eyes shut if necessary while patient sleeps. | • Exophthalmopathy associated with long-standing hyperthyroidism may prevent patient from closing eyelids completely. |
| | | ○ Encourage verbalization of fears and concerns regarding injury to eyes and overall appearance | ○ Verbalization of feelings and concerns may assist the patient in coping with what might be a chronic problem. |
| ***Nursing Diagnoses #10 and #11***<br>Rest-activity pattern, ineffective.<br>Sleep-pattern disturbance, related to:<br>1. Hyperactive state associated with increased metabolic rate. | Patient will:<br>1. Demonstrate performance of activities of daily living without fatigue.<br>2. Verbalize ability to sleep and feelings of rest and relaxation | • Examine nursing care considerations concerned with fostering rest and relaxation:<br>○ Identify factors that contribute to fatigue and assist patient to cope within his/her limitations.<br>– Help patient/family to identify signs of fatigue, and those activities that are especially tiring to the patient.<br>– Help to plan rest periods between patient activities to minimize fatigue. | |
| | | ○ Provide diversional activities. | ○ Such activities help to channel some of the otherwise unusable energy associated with overwhelming adrenergic response and the direct effect of thyroid hormonal action on overall metabolic rate. |
| | | ○ Initiate relaxation exercises when patient's condition stabilizes. | ○ Hyperthyroidism is often a long-term chronic illness; relaxation techniques may assist in coping. |
| | | ○ Ascertain patient's usual sleep habits:<br>– Identify disruptions in usual sleep pattern caused by illness and hospitalization. | ○ Enhance adrenergic response predisposes to restlessness, agitation, irritability. |
| | | ○ Encourage patient to verbalize feelings about sleeping capability, and ways to improve sleeping. | ○ It may also be helpful to verbalize the patient's feelings of frustration; the patient may be reassured that he/she is not all |

| Nursing Diagnosis | Desired Patient Outcomes | Nursing Interventions | Rationale |
|---|---|---|---|
| | | ○ Plan for quiet, restful period prior to sleeping.<br>– Promote a quiet, cool, and soothing atmosphere at sleep time.<br>– Allow for flexibility in the patient's daily routine.<br>○ Administer prescribed sedative if necessary; monitor effectiveness of therapy in relaxing patient and facilitating sleepfulness. | alone; that others understand and care.<br>○ Involving the patient in planning for sleep enables the patient to exert some control over his/her status. Patients sometime describe that they can't sit still; that their mind/body seems to be racing. |
| ***Nursing Diagnosis #12***<br>Thought processes, alteration in, related to:<br>1. Enhanced adrenergic activity. | Patient will:<br>1. Maintain baseline mental status:<br>• Alert, oriented.<br>• Mentation: Memory intact; able to concentrate.<br>• Behavior appropriate.<br>• Usual personality (as per family or significant others). | • Assess effect of hypermetabolic state on psychologic status:<br>○ Assess for signs/symptoms including: Insomnia, fear, anxiety, emotional lability; apathy, depression, personality changes; psychosis.<br>○ Elicit information from family members regarding patient's usual personality and behavior.<br>○ Monitor neurologic and psychologic status hourly.<br>• Implement therapeutic measures:<br>○ Explain all ongoing procedures and reasons underlying therapy (e.g., use of hypothermia blanket). Explanations should be brief and repeated as necessary.<br>○ Encourage verbalization of fears, questions, concerns; take the time to listen. | • Severe hypermetabolic state coupled with excessive adrenergic activity may predispose to psychosis and coma.<br>○ Eliciting history from family members or significant others assists in determining patient's baseline status including behavioral and personality characteristics.<br>○ Monitoring of patient's status at regular intervals assists in determining the effectiveness of therapy; enables the patient to be appraised of progress.<br>○ Appropriate explanations may help to alleviate heightened anxiety. |
| ***Nursing Diagnosis #13***<br>Knowledge deficit regarding underlying disease process, and factors that may trigger an exacerbation of the illness. | Patient/family will:<br>1. Demonstrate a readiness to learn:<br>• Interest and willingness to examine optimal level of health desired.<br>2. Verbalize details of plan of care including need for diligent follow-up care. | • Provide patient/family education to assist in developing and implementing prophylactic health-care practices.<br>○ Assess patient/family knowledge regarding disease process and therapy.<br>○ Assess readiness to learn.<br>○ Implement teaching program to include the following topics:<br>– Pertinent anatomy and physiology of thyroid gland. | ○ Understanding of underlying disease processes assists the patient/family to cope wth, and to adjust to, the limitations imposed by the disease.<br>○ Hyperthyroidism has an impact on all members of the family; interested and supportive family members should be included in the educational processes. |

*(continued)*

**TABLE 17–7. CARE PLAN FOR THE PATIENT WITH HYPERTHYROID CRISIS *(Continued)***

| Nursing Diagnoses | Desired Patient Outcomes | Nursing Interventions | Rationales |
|---|---|---|---|
| ***Nursing Diagnosis #13 (cont.)*** | | | |
| | | – Underlying pathophysiology of thyroid disease as it pertains to the patient's status.<br>– Identification of stressors that precipitate or predispose to hyperthyroid crisis in the patient with hyperthyroidism (see Table 17–6).<br>○ Identification of stressors that precipitate or predispose to hyperthyroid crisis in the patient with hyperthyroidism (see Table 17–6). | |
| | | ○ Recognition of signs and symptoms of hyperthyroid crisis (see Table 17–6) | ○ Patient/family must appreciate the importance of seeking timely medical assistance when a stressful event occurs, or with the first sign/symptom of hyperthyroid crisis. |
| | | ○ Understanding of medication regimen:<br>– Indications for antithyroid and antiadrenergic medications.<br>– Dosage and administration.<br>– Adverse side effects. | |
| | | ○ Understanding of importance of continuous medical follow-up with appropriate periodic blood testing.<br>– Initiation of self-care practices to prevent recurring crisis.<br>– Usefulness of behavioral modifications and/or relaxation techniques. | ○ The importance of maintaining therapeutic blood levels must be stressed; noncompliance with drug regimen can predispose to hyperthyroid crisis. |

| | | | |
|---|---|---|---|
| ***Nursing Diagnosis #14*** Self-concept, disturbance in: Body image, related to:<br>1. Exophthalmopathy.<br>2. Other changes in physical appearance:<br>• Hyperpigmentation.<br>• Pretibial edema.<br>• Muscle weakness/wasting.<br>• Menstrual irregularities, decreased libido in women.<br>• Impotence in men.<br>• Emotional lability. | Patient will:<br>1. Be able to verbalize feelings regarding body changes.<br>2. Be able to explore feelings associated with self-perception.<br>3. Identify own strengths/weaknesses.<br>4. Identify coping options. | • Assist patient/family to examine their values and expectations; and the desired level of health. | • Hyperthyroidism is an especially compromising condition because often it becomes chronic, and patients often become noncompliant with prescribed therapeutic regimen. |
| | | ◦ Encourage patient to identify and verbalize feelings regarding self (capabilities).<br>◦ Assist patient/family to identify coping strengths and weaknesses. | ◦ Helps patient to begin to examine self, and to begin self-acceptance. |
| | | ◦ Assess support system within family and friends/neighbors/significant others. | ◦ Patient's family and significant others can be helpful by accepting the patient as he/she is; positive support reinforces the patient's self-esteem. |
| | | ◦ Be accessible to patient/family:<br>– Provide a listening ear.<br>– Praise accomplishments.<br>– Assist in realistic goal-setting. | |
| | | ◦ Encourage expression of honest feelings about self.<br>– Be nonjudgmental; accept patient as he/she is. | ◦ Being honest with oneself helps to promote relationships with others.<br>◦ Verbalizing feelings of self increases self-awareness. |
| | | ◦ Involve in diversional activities as condition permits. | ◦ Helps the patient to avoid dwelling on self-limitations and inadequacies. |

## Myxedema Coma

Myxedema coma is the most severe clinical manifestation of hypothyroidism. (For a review of hypothyroidism, see Table 17–5.) It is a state of greatly depressed metabolic activity characterized by hypotension, bradycardia, and hypoventilation with severe carbon dioxide retention, which contributes to narcosis, altered state of consciousness, hyponatremia, and convulsions.[13] The hallmark of myxedema coma is severe hypothermia, the extent of which is often unrecognized because the thermometer used is not shaken down sufficiently or does not register temperatures low enough. Signs of severe myxedema (i.e., a relatively hard edema of subcutaneous tissues) reflect the chronic nature of underlying long-standing hypothyroidism. Specific details concerned with pathophysiology, etiology, and clinical presentation of myxedema coma are presented in Table 17–6.

### *Treatment*

When myxedema coma is suspected based on clinical presentation, appropriate blood samples should be obtained for thyroid hormone measurement, and treatment should commence immediately. The approach to therapy includes the maintenance of vital functions, replacement of thyroid hormone, and treatment of precipitating factor(s). (See Table 17–6 for further discussion of treatment of myxedema coma.)

### *Nursing Care of the Patient with Myxedema Coma*

**Therapeutic Goals.** Implementation of nursing process in the care of the patient with myxedema coma revolves around the following therapeutic goals:

1. Identify patients at risk.
2. Establish a comprehensive database including:
   A. Clinical history (functional health patterns).
   B. Physical examination.
   C. Laboratory/diagnostic data.
3. Implement measures to promote and maintain effective ventilation.
4. Implement measures to establish and maintain cardiovascular function.
5. Implement measures to promote fluid and electrolyte balance.
6. Implement measures to stabilize body temperature.
7. Maintain adequate nutrition.
8. Maintain effective bowel elimination.
9. Promote optimal musculoskeletal function.
10. Provide emotional and psychologic support to patient/family.
11. Initiate patient/family education to assist in developing and implementing prophylactic health-care practices.

**Nursing Diagnoses.** Tentative nursing diagnoses in the care of the patient with myxedema coma may include the following:

1. Cardiac output, alteration in: Decreased, related to decreased heart rate and stroke volume, and decreased contractility, associated with reduced levels of thyroid hormone.
2. Fluid volume, alteration in, related to extracellular edema associated with increased capillary permeability, and mucinosis (i.e., a condition in which mucin is present in the skin in excessive amounts).
3. Hypothermia, related to depressed cellular metabolism associated with decreased thyroid hormonal activity.
4. Breathing pattern, alteration in: Hypoventilation, related to weakness of pulmonary musculature, and transudation of mucinous material into pleural space causing pleural effusion.
5. Nutrition, alteration in, less than body requirements, related to altered digestive and absorptive processes within the gastrointestinal tract associated with reduced cellular metabolism.
6. Bowel elimination, alteration in: Constipation associated with diminished gastrointestinal motility.
7. Skin integrity, impairment of, related to tissue fragility.
8. Thought processes, impairment of, related to diminished cerebral blood flow and interstitial edema.

## REFERENCES

1. Green, W: The Thyroid. Elsevier, New York, 1987, p 9.
2. Griffin, JE: Manual of Clinical Endocrinology and Metabolism. McGraw-Hill, New York, 1982, p 53.
3. Griffin, JE: Manual of Clinical Endocrinology and Metabolism. McGraw-Hill, New York, 1982, p 49.
4. Vander, A, Sherman, J, and Luciano, D: Human Physiology: The Mechanisms of Body Function, ed 4. McGraw-Hill, New York, 1985, p 252.
5. Guyton, A: Textbook of Medical Physiology, ed 7. WB Saunders, Philadelphia, 1986, pp 900–901.
6. Hershman, JM: Endocrine Pathophysiology: A Patient-Oriented Approach, ed 3. Lea & Febiger, Philadelphia, 1988, p 43.
7. Metz, R and Larson, EB: Blue Book of Endocrinology. WB Saunders, Philadelphia, 1985, p 21.
8. Nurses Clinical Library, "Endocrine Disorders," Nursing '84 Book, Springhouse Corporation, Springhouse, PA, 1984, p 36.
9. Green, W. The Thyroid. Elsevier, New York, 1987, p 54.
10. Widmann, FK: Clinical Interpretation of Laboratory Tests, ed 9. FA Davis, Philadelphia, 1983, p 435.
11. Burman, K: Interpretation of thyroid function tests in critically ill patients. Crit Care Q 6(3):6, 1983.
12. O'Neil, JR: Thyroid crisis ACTION STAT. Nursing '87 17(11):33, 1987.
13. Payne, NR: Emergency care of the patient with myxedema coma. J Emerg Nurs 12(6):343, 1986.

CHAPTER 18

# Nursing Management of the Patient with Adrenal Dysfunction

## CHAPTER OUTLINE



## LEARNING OBJECTIVES

**At the end of this chapter, you should be able to:**

1. Describe the structure and function of the adrenal glands.
2. State the effect of the catecholamines, epinephrine and norepinephrine, on total body function.
3. Describe the underlying pathophysiology, clinical presentation, diagnosis, and treatment of the patient with pheochromocytoma.
4. List tentative nursing diagnoses underlying the nursing care of the patient with pheochromocytoma.
5. Distinguish the major functions of mineralocorticoids: Aldosterone.
6. Describe the regulation of aldosterone secretion.
7. List the major functions of glucocorticoids: Cortisol.
8. Describe the regulation of cortisol secretion.
9. Define adrenal insufficiency, and examine its pertinent pathophysiology, etiology, clinical presentation, and treatment.
10. Contrast adrenal insufficiency and Cushing's syndrome.
11. Define adrenal crisis (addisonian crisis), and examine its pertinent pathophysiology, etiology, clinical presentation, and treatment.
12. Delineate the nursing process in caring for patients in adrenal crisis including:
    Assessment.
    Nursing diagnoses.
    Planning: Desired patient outcomes
    Nursing interventions/rationales.

The adrenal glands are paired organs located at the upper pole of each kidney in the retroperitoneal space. Each individual gland is composed of two separate endocrine tissues derived from different embryologic origins and having distinctly different secretory products. They include the inner medulla, which is derived from neural crest cells and secretes catecholamines, and the outer cortex, which is derived from mesoderm and secretes steroids (Fig. 18–1).

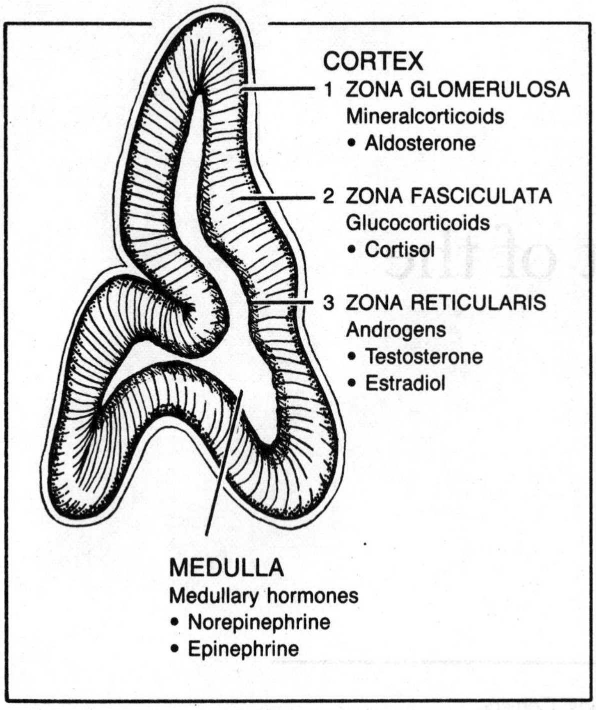


**Figure 18-1.** Each adrenal gland is composed of two separate and distinct tissues: The adrenal medulla, which forms the inner core of the gland; and the adrenal cortex, which comprises the peripheral structure of the adrenal gland. The adrenal cortex is divided structurally and functionally into three layers or zones: The outermost layer, the zona glomerulosa, secretes the mineralocorticoid, aldosterone; the middle and innermost layers, the zona fasciculata and zona reticularis, respectively, secrete the glucocorticoids (e.g., cortisol) and androgens.

Its neural origin explains the unique function of the adrenal medulla in that its specialized cells secrete the hormones, epinephrine and norepinephrine (both are catecholamines), in response to direct sympathetic outflow. These hormones, in turn, exert a sympathomimetic effect on all parts of the body. These medullary hormones are the first line of defense against stress. In response to stressful stimuli, they exert their major effect on cardiovascular function by stimulation of alpha, $beta_1$, and $beta_2$ receptors. Catecholamine-producing tumors, or pheochromocytomas, derived from adrenal medullary chromaffin cells, account for approximately 0.5% of patients with hypertension (see below).

Steroidal hormones secreted by the outer cortex are an entirely different group of hormones structurally and functionally. These corticosteroids are all synthesized from the steroid, cholesterol, and they include mineralocorticoids, glucocorticoids, and androgens. Mineralocorticoids regulate electrolytes in the extracellular fluid. Glucocorticoids regulate intermediate metabolism including carbohydrates, protein, and fats. Adrenal androgens contribute significantly to circulating levels of testosterone in women and estradiol in men.

## ADRENAL MEDULLA: SECRETION OF CATECHOLAMINES, EPINEPHRINE, AND NOREPINEPHRINE

By virtue of its neural origin, the adrenal medulla functions as part of an autonomic reflex arc. (See section entitled "Innervation of the Adrenal Medulla" in Chap. 6.) Its major secretory products resulting from its interaction with sympathetic preganglionic fibers include epinephrine and norepinephrine. Approximately 80% of the adrenal medullary secretions is epinephrine: the remainder is largely norepinephrine. Norepinephrine, the neurotransmitter secreted at adrenergic synapses, is inactivated for the most part by reuptake into the presynaptic axonal terminals (i.e., synaptic knob) (see Fig. 6-4) and via associated metabolic inactivation. In contrast, the norepinephrine and epinephrine secreted as hormones directly into the systemic circulation are able to exert a variety of physiologic effects widely dispersed throughout the body.

Sympatheticoadrenal activity has long been known to underlie the "fight or flight" response. The physiologic effects of epinephrine and norepinephrine in this regard are the maintenance of blood flow to vital organs (i.e., brain and heart); the maintenance of vasomotor tone of the systemic vasculature so as to prevent sudden changes in blood pressure; and the vasodilation of the skeletal muscle vasculature at the expense of other organs (i.e., catecholamine-related vasoconstriction of subcutaneous, mucosal, splanchnic, and renal beds). (See Tables 6-10 and 6-11 for specific responses of effector organs to adrenergic activity.)

### Pheochromocytomas

Pheochromocytomas are catecholamine-producing tumors derived largely from adrenal medullary chromaffin cells, which produce excessive amounts of epinephrine and norepinephrine. The incidence of pheochromocytomas is rare, and over 90% of tumors diagnosed are benign. The diagnosis of pheochromocytoma should be entertained in all patients presenting with signs and symptoms secondary to hypertension without any other distinguishing characteristics. There is a strong familial tendency, and the disease may be inherited as an autosomal-dominant trait. The tumors may occur at any time from infancy to old age; its greatest incidence is during the fourth and fifth decades.

The importance of pheochromocytomas is that, if untreated, these tumors are almost inevitably associated with a fatal outcome; properly handled, there is the potential for complete cure.

### Clinical Presentation

Pheochromocytomas may release hormones intermittently or continuously; symptoms occur paroxysmally or are sustained. The clinical presentation of these tumors is related to the rate of production and pattern of catecholamine secretion. Most tumors produce a combination of norepinephrine and epinephrine. Patients with tumors that secrete excessive amounts of norepinephrine usually present with hypertension as the primary finding. This is a consequence of the alpha-adrenergic sympathomimetic effect of norepinephrine on the systemic vasculature. Patients with a predominant secretion of epinephrine characteristically present with signs and symptoms reflective of largely excessive beta-adrenergic activity. Signs and symptoms may include anxiety, tremor, diaphoresis, tachycardia, palpitations, weakness, pain (anginal, abdominal), and, often, unexplained cardiac dysrhythmias.

Clinically, pheochromocytoma is characterized by the triad of hypertension, headache, and hypermetabolism. Of patients diagnosed as having a pheochromocytoma, about 90% display hypertension. Of this number, about one half demonstrate sustained elevations in blood pressure, while the remainder experience paroxysms of hypertension. Characteristically, there are very wide fluctuations in blood pressure with increases in both systolic and diastolic pressures. Blood pressures have been reported to be as high as 300/240 mmHg during an attack.

The headache associated with pheochromocytomas is prominent and may be accompanied by a pounding in the chest described as "like a sledgehammer." The patient may express nervousness, apprehension, and a sense of impending doom.

Catecholamine-initiated hypermetabolism may underlie complaints of warmth, heat intolerance, and tremulousness. These patients may display a weight loss associated with diabetes mellitus or glucose intolerance. The hallmark of diabetes in the scenario of pheochromocytoma is a weight loss disproportionate to the degree of hyperglycemia. Gastrointestinal signs and symptoms, such as nausea, vomiting, and abdominal pain, are all associated with the hypermetabolic state.

Acute episodes of hypertension may trigger visual disturbances associated with spasm of retinal arterioles. Similarly, spasm of cerebral arteries may predispose to seizures. Severe systemic vasoconstriction may underlie complaints of paresthesias, including numbness and tingling. Raynaud's phenomenon (i.e., intermittent attacks of pallor followed by cyanosis, then redness of digits, before return to normal) has been observed.

Paroxysmal (i.e., sudden and explosive) attacks may be triggered by a variety of stimuli. Some of these include an emotional event, physical upsets such as overeating with gastric/abdominal distention, full bladder, or straining at stool. Attacks may be provoked by smoking or drinking alcoholic beverages (e.g., beer, wines). In patients with coronary artery disease, anginal pain can be precipitated; catecholamine-induced dysrhythmias with congestive heart failure have been reported. Angiography, endotracheal intubation, anesthesia, and a variety of drugs are known to provoke attacks in patients with pheochromocytoma.

### Diagnosis

The cornerstone of the diagnosis of pheochromocytoma is the demonstration of excess excretion of catecholamine and catecholamine metabolites in the urine.[1] Commonly, a measure of total metanephrine (i.e., catecholamine derivatives) in the urine is used as a screening test. Because metanephrine excretion is relatively constant, a single voided (spot) urine can be used for initial screening. This test may be useful in monitoring urine catecholamines during and after the episode. When there is a high index of suspicion, 24-hour urine samples for total free catecholamines, total metanephrine, and vanillylmandelic acid (VMA; a metabolite of epinephrine) should be collected.

If the existence of a catecholamine-secreting tumor remains unproven, hormone release can be stimulated by pharmacologic manipulation. Provocative testing using intravenous histamine or phentolamine can be performed. These tests are not without hazards; continuous cardiac monitoring should be performed, and antihypertensive and antiarrhythmia drugs should be on hand. False-positive tests frequently occur. Test results can reflect the residual effects of antihypertensive drugs, and these drugs should be discontinued for 3 weeks prior to testing.

Many drugs affect urinary catecholamine measurements. Part of the nurse's responsibility in the diagnostic process is to elicit a thorough drug history from patient/family. Drugs implicated as artifacts in catecholamine testing include caffeine, MAO inhibitors, alpha-methyldopa, dopamine, chlorpromazine, clofibrate, quinidine, and isoproterenol. The presence of any recent stressors in the patient's life may alter catecholamine findings. The patient's baseline condition must be considered when evaluating urine and plasma findings. Foods, such as nuts and bananas, can also alter tests results, and a nutritional history may be pertinent.

Finally, all testing must be performed according

to standard protocol. For example, 24-hour urine specimen for catecholamine evaluation should be acidified to a pH of between 2 and 3. This is accomplished by adding 12–15 ml of concentrated hydrochloric acid to the empty collecting jar. All urine voided during the specific 24-hour period must be collected. Inattention to such details is not only costly, but may cause significant delay in determining the patient's underlying problem.

Differential diagnosis includes a variety of pathologic and physiologic conditions. Renal artery disease provoking hypertension may be associated with paroxysms of acute hypertensive episodes resembling those of pheochromocytoma. Anginal pain reflective of coronary insufficiency can precipitate marked elevation in blood pressure accompanied by diaphoresis, tachycardia, apprehension, and other signs also associated with the hypertension of pheochromocytoma. Important in the differential diagnosis is the observation that the hypertension of pheochromocytoma *precedes* pain rather than being precipitated by pain. Furthermore, agents such as nitroglycerin, narcotics, and sedatives, which relieve anginal pain and decrease blood pressure, can actually precipitate a hypertensive crisis in patients wth pheochromocytoma.

Other disorders most likely to be confused with pheochromocytomas include transient ischemic attacks, essential hypertension, hyperthyroidism, angina pectoris, or anxiety reaction. Additional diagnostic studies that may assist in localizing the tumor(s) include angiography, intravenous pyelogram (IVP), and CAT scan.

### *Treatment*

The treatment of choice in pheochromocytoma is surgical removal, with a success rate in about 90% of cases. As part of the surgical protocol to prevent perioperative and postoperative complications, operative candidates usually undergo pharmacologic stabilization of their symptoms for 1–3 weeks prior to surgery. Alpha-adrenergic blocking agents such as phenoxybenzamine, which inhibit the systemic effects of catecholamines, are usually administered. Once alpha blockade has been established, beta-adrenergic blockade, using drugs such as propranolol (a nonselective beta antagonist) and labetalol (an alpha- and beta-adrenergic blocking agent), is also achieved. (See section on sympatholytics in Appendix A.)

Perioperatively, phentolamine, an alpha antagonist, may be infused intravenously to prevent extremely high pressures, which may be triggered by anesthesia or by manipulation of the tumor. Nitroprusside, a potent vasodilator, has also been used in this regard.

For patients who are not operative candidates, or in whom surgery has not been successful, medical management involves long-term control using alpha- and beta-adrenergic antagonist therapy.

### *Nursing Care of the Patient with Pheochromocytoma*

**Therapeutic Goals.** Nursing care of the patient with pheochromocytoma is focused on the following therapeutic goals:

1. Stabilization of hemodynamic function with avoidance/prevention of paroxysmal episodes of severely high blood pressures.
2. Prevention of catecholamine-induced complications such as stroke, associated with cerebral vasospasm and resulting in neurologic impairments; or cardiac insufficiency, associated with myocarditis and cardiac dysrhythmias.
3. Assessment of patient including a thorough history as to the overall state of health, onset of symptoms and precipitating and/or predisposing cause or event surrounding the onset, types of drugs taken and why, and a nutritional history as indicated.
4. Identification/avoidance of stimuli that provoke catecholamine secretion and trigger a hypertensive episode, as, for example, an emotional upset, physical exertion, overeating, cold, bladder distention, or Valsalva's maneuver, among others.
5. Implementation of diagnostic studies following directions explicitly so as to ensure reliable results.
6. Promotion of comfort, rest, and relaxation through such measures as headache and pain relief; a quiet, warm environment free from drafts; and a calm, soothing demeanor when implementing care.
7. Maintenance of prescribed nutritional regimen with control of sodium intake, maintenance of stable body weight, and avoidance of catecholamine-potentiating foods and beverages.
8. Maintenance of adequate bladder and bowel elimination including prevention of bladder distention and constipation.
9. Education regarding the patient's underlying disease and treatment regimen including compliance with medications prescribed, precautions to be taken to reduce risk of subsequent hypertensive attacks, and follow-up care.

### *Tentative Nursing Diagnoses in the Care of the Patient with Pheochromocytoma*

Tentative nursing diagnoses in the care of the patient with pheochromocytoma include:

1. Tissue perfusion, alteration in, related to:
   A. Catecholamine-precipitated hypertensive crisis and unstable hemodynamics.
   B. Catecholamine-induced vasoconstriction of subcutaneous, mucosal, splanchnic, and renal beds.

2. Injury, potential for: Physiologic (stroke, visual impairment, seizures), related to catecholamine-induced vasospasm of retinal and cerebral vasculature.
3. Comfort, alteration in: Headache, angina, abdominal pain, tremulousness, related to hypertensive episode, tachycardia, palpitations, and cardiac dysrhythmias.
4. Nutrition, alteration in, related to hypermetabolic state.
5. Activity intolerance, related to weakness associated with a hypermetabolic state.
6. Sleep pattern disturbance, related to catecholamine-induced anxiety, apprehension, and tremor.
7. Coping, ineffective, related to:
   A. Fear of dying.
   B. Impact on individual and family lifestyle.
8. Knowledge deficit regarding underlying illness, treatment regimen, and follow-up care.

#### *Nursing Care of the Adrenalectomy Patient*

Surgery in the patient with pheochromocytoma has greater risk than most other operative procedures because manipulation of the adrenal glands and tumor can precipitate an excessive release of both adrenal medullary (i.e., catecholamines) and adrenal cortical (i.e., glucocorticoids and mineralocorticoids) hormones into the systemic circulation. Preoperative measures are focused on promoting optimal physical and emotional stamina to assist the patient to withstand the rigors of surgery and to facilitate healing postoperatively.

Because glucocorticoid excess predisposes to a catabolic state, the patient's preoperative diet is high in proteins, vitamins, and other essential nutrients. The potassium-wasting effects of increased mineralocorticoid secretion are anticipated and the patient is given foods rich in potassium and/or potassium supplements.

Following a bilateral adrenalectomy with sudden cessation of adrenal medullary and cortical hormones, the patient is treated as any individual with adrenal insufficiency, and is at risk of adrenal crisis. For nursing diagnoses, patient outcomes, and nursing interventions in the care of the patient in adrenal crisis, see Table 18–3.

## ADRENAL CORTEX: MINERALOCORTICOIDS AND GLUCOCORTICOIDS

### Mineralocorticoids: Aldosterone

Mineralocorticoids are considered to be the "life-saving" hormones secreted by a layer of tissue within the adrenal cortex, called the zona glomerulosa (see Fig. 18–1). In the absence of mineralocorticoids a major disruption of fluid and electrolyte equilibrium occurs within the body, characterized by a marked elevation in potassium ion concentration and a decrease in extracellular fluid and blood volume. If allowed to persist untreated, cardiac output diminishes progressively, predisposing to hypovolemic shock and death within several days to about 2 weeks.

Aldosterone is the major mineralocorticoid secreted by the adrenal cortex exerting at least 95% of the mineralocorticoid activity within the body. Other mineralocorticoids secreted in smaller amounts include corticosterone and desoxycorticosterone. Cortisol, the major glucocorticoid secreted by the adrenal cortex within the zonae fasciculata and reticularis, also exerts a small mineralocorticoid effect. This accounts for the fact that in acute clinical situations, use of cortisol therapy alone provides sufficient mineralocorticoid activity in addition to its glucocorticoid effects, making it unnecessary to use a separate mineralocorticoid during the acute phase.

#### *Aldosterone: Major Functions*

There are several major functions performed by aldosterone within the body. One important function is the regulation of extracellular fluid volume. Aldosterone acts on the renal epithelial cells of the distal tubules and collecting ducts (see Fig. 21–4) to promote the reabsorption of sodium and the excretion of potassium. The reabsorption of sodium ions creates an osmotic gradient between the kidney tubules and the peritubular interstitial fluid, which, in the presence of antidiuretic hormone (ADH), allows water to "follow" the movement of sodium. The net result is the reabsorption of a nearly isotonic fluid. In this way, aldosterone-induced reabsorption of sodium ions and the concomitant reabsorption of water preserve the extracellular fluid volume.

Aldosterone plays a major role in the renal regulation of potassium. It facilitates an exchange transport of sodium and potassium ions, and to a lesser extent, hydrogen ions, through the renal epithelial cells of the distal tubules and collecting ducts. For each sodium ion reabsorbed, there is a simultaneous excretion of a potassium ion (or a hydrogen ion in the presence of acidemia). The net result: sodium is conserved in the extracellular fluid while potassium ion (or hydrogen ion) is excreted in the urine. Table 18–1 lists distinguishing features and functions of aldosterone.

#### *Regulation of Aldosterone Secretion*

Guyton[2] identifies four different factors presently known to play a significant role in the regulation of aldosterone secretion. These include the potassium ion concentration in extracellular fluid; renin–

TABLE 18-1
## Distinguishing Features and Functions of Aldosterone and Cortisol

| | Aldosterone | Cortisol |
|---|---|---|
| Origin of hormone synthesis and release | Zona glomerulosa | Zona fasciculata<br>Zona reticularis |
| Daily secretion | 100–150 μg/day under conditions of adequate sodium intake | 15–20 mg/day in adults—reflected in diurnal secretory pattern:<br>Peak elevation 8:00 a.m.<br>Lowest concentration 12 midnight<br>Upper secretory limit in presence of stress: 250 mg/day |
| Peripheral blood concentration | 1–8 ng/100 ml | 12 μg/100 ml |
| Transport in blood | 50% loosely bound to plasma proteins<br>50% circulates in free form<br>In bound and free form aldosterone and cortisol are transported throughout the extracellular fluid space.<br>Synthetic compounds of corticosteroids are less well bound to plasma proteins, leaving a greater percentage of hormone in the free metabolically active state. | 90% transported in bound form: Most bound to corticosteroid-binding globulin; some loosely bound to albumin<br>< 10% circulates in free form |
| Target tissues | Renal tubular cells: Distal tubules and collecting ducts<br>Epithelial cells of sweat and salivary glands, and the intestines | Almost all cells |
| Mechanism of action | Mineralocorticoids act on cells via intracellular hormone-protein receptor mechanism. They stimulate generation of new messenger-RNA within the cell nucleus, which mediates synthesis of specific proteins necessary for expression of the mineralocorticoid effect. | Intracellular receptor mechanism: Corticosteroids act by controlling rate of intracellular protein synthesis. They stimulate generation of new messenger-RNA, which mediates synthesis of specific proteins. |
| Length of time before hormonal effect is realized | Hormonal fixation and effect in target tissues occurs within approximately 30–40 min. | Hormonal fixation and effect in target tissues occur within approximately 1–2 hr. |
| Metabolism/elimination | Metabolism and deactivation of adrenal corticol hormones occurs mainly in the liver via conjugation reactions to form glucuronides and to a lesser extent sulfates and phosphates.<br>Approximately 75% of these hormones are excreted via the urine in the form of 17-hydroxycorticosteroids; the remaining 25% is excreted via bile and feces. | |
| Major functions | Primary function: Maintain extracellular fluid volume<br>Facilitates conservation of sodium with excretion of potassium and hydrogen ions<br>Conserves sodium and chloride in sweat and salivary secretions<br>Increases absorption of sodium and chloride from intestinal tract | Primary function: Major body mechanism to cope with stress<br>Gluconeogenesis<br>Mobilization of body fat and protein<br>Insulin antagonist<br>Anti-inflammatory effect<br>Immune system depression<br>"Permissive effects" on other body hormones:<br>Glucagon<br>Epinephrine and norepinephrine<br>Antidiuretic hormone |
| Regulation of secretion | Potassium ion concentration in extracellular fluid (major factor)<br>Renin–angiotensin system<br>Decrease in total body protein<br>"Permissive effect" of ACTH<br>Sympathetic reflex input based on extracellular fluid volume and arterial blood pressure<br>Intrarenal reflex pathways: Renin-secreting cells sensitive to pressure; possibly serum sodium concentrations | Central key: Wide variety of stressors that impact on central nervous system and hypothalamus<br>Hypothalamus–adenohypophysis–adrenal cortex axis: CRH → ACTH → cortisol<br>Negative feedback mechanism of cortisol on hypothalamus and adenohypophysis<br>Possible negative feedback of ACTH on hypothalamus |
| Effect of exogenous cortisol therapy | Very minimal effect | Maximum suppression of ACTH; gradual tapering of exogenous doses of cortisol is essential to avoid adrenal insufficiency |

angiotensin system; total body sodium concentration; and the "permissive effect" of adrenocorticotropic hormone (ACTH).

The direct effect of potassium ions on the cells of the zona glomerulosa within the adrenal cortex may be the most potent factor controlling aldosterone secretion. This effect is thought to occur via a feedback mechanism: an increase in potassium ion concentration in extracellular fluid causes an increase in the secretion of aldosterone; aldosterone, in turn, enhances the excretion of potassium via the urine; as potassium levels return to normal, aldosterone secretion is reduced accordingly.

The renin-angiotensin mechanism plays an important role in regulating aldosterone secretion via another mechanism. In response to extracellular fluid depletion and decreased arterial blood pressure, sympathetic nervous system input and reflexes involving the kidneys themselves initiate a series of events that impact with considerable potency on aldosterone secretion. Specialized cells of the juxtaglomerular apparatus (see Fig. 21-8) are thus stimulated to synthesize and secrete renin, a proteolytic enzyme that catalyzes the hydrolysis of the circulating globulin, angiotensinogen, to form angiotensin I. Angiotensin I is further hydrolyzed to angiotensin II by converting enzyme found in very high concentrations within capillary endothelium primarily in the lungs. Angiotensin II is a potent stimulator of aldosterone secretion and comprises a major input to the adrenal cortex controlling synthesis and secretion of this hormone (see Fig. 21-9).

A depleted extracellular fluid volume and an elevation in potassium ion concentration are closely associated with a diminished sodium ion concentration, and probably stimulate aldosterone secretion by the mechanism discussed above. A diminished sodium concentration may directly influence the zona glomerulosa cells to increase aldosterone secretion, but this mechanism remains undefined. An increase in sodium ion concentration and/or extracellular fluid volume would have an inhibitory effect on aldosterone secretion.

The "permissive effect" of ACTH suggests that ACTH must be available in minimal amounts to maintain a functional zona glomerulosa. This layer of cells partially atrophies in the absence of ACTH with a consequent reduction in, or cessation of, aldosterone synthesis and secretion.

## Glucocorticoids: Cortisol

Glucocorticoids are the major regulators of intermediary metabolism. While the name glucocorticoid reflects the important hyperglycemic effect exhibited by these hormones, they have additional effects on protein and fat metabolism, and on a variety of other bodily functions, which, although not life-saving as in the case of mineralocorticoids, are nevertheless essential to the well-being of the individual. Over 30 glucocorticoids have been isolated, but the major glucocorticoid is cortisol (hydrocortisone). It exerts at least 95% of the overall glucocorticoid activity in the body. Small amounts of glucocorticoid activity are also provided by corticosterone and cortisone.

### *Cortisol: Major Functions*

There are several significant functions performed by cortisol within the body. These include its effect on intermediary metabolism and response to stress, its anti-inflammatory activity, its effect on the immune response, and its role in calcium/bone metabolism.

The most potent physiologic action of cortisol is on intermediary metabolism.[3] Cortisol stimulates the conversion of noncarbohydrates, such as amino acids and fatty acids, into glucose via a process termed *gluconeogenesis*. It also stimulates an increased production of liver enzymes necessary for gluconeogenesis. Cortisol functions as an insulin-antagonist, decreasing utilization of glucose by the liver, adipose, and muscle cells. The net effect of these activities is hyperglycemia; this effect distinguishes cortisol as a *gluco*corticoid.

The effect of cortisol on protein metabolism is to promote mobilization of amino acids from skin, muscle, bone, and connective tissues. This results in a reduction of protein stores in all cells except the liver. There is decreased protein synthesis and increased catabolism of protein to provide necessary amino acids for gluconeogenesis activity in the liver.

The principal effect of cortisol on fat metabolism is to promote mobilization of fatty acids from adipose tissue. This effect, coupled with the increased oxidation of fatty acids for energy (recall cortisol's insulin-antagonistic activity in the above), largely accounts for the shift in cells from utilization of glucose for energy, to utilization of fatty acids instead.

Almost any type of stress or insult to the body triggers an immediate and marked increase in ACTH secretion, followed in minutes by a greatly enhanced secretion of cortisol. When the effects of cortisol on intermediary metabolism are reviewed, it would seem that cortisol is especially well-suited to cope with stress. In a stressful situation, one often foregoes eating, yet cortisol maintains a hyperglycemic state (via gluconeogenesis), ensuring ample glucose substrate for brain cell activity; liberation of amino acids via catabolism of body protein not only provides a source of this substrate for gluconeogenesis in the liver, but also provides a potential source of amino acids, which may be necessary for repair of tissues damaged by the stressful event.

As part of its anti-inflammatory effect, cortisol functions to block the early stages of inflammation, or if the process has been initiated, it acts to resolve the inflammation and to facilitate rapid healing. Thus, cortisol decreases the permeability of capillaries and reduces loss of plasma and migration of anti-inflammatory cells (e.g., leukocytes) into the damaged site; it stabilizes lysosomal membranes reducing release of proteolytic enzymes; it depresses phagocytic activity of leukocytes; and it suppresses the immune response.

In its role in calcium/bone metabolism, cortisol reduces intestinal calcium absorption, increases excretion of calcium via the kidneys, and catabolizes bone protein. See Table 18–1, which lists some of the distinguishing features of cortisol functions.

#### Regulation of Cortisol Secretion

Regulation of cortisol secretion involves a multilevel feedback control mechanism involving higher brain centers, the hypothalamus, anterior pituitary, and the adrenal cortex. Different types of stressors impact on the hypothalamus, which responds by making appropriate adjustments in the secretory rates of the individual hypothalamic-releasing hormones over and above their basal values. In this way, the hypothalamus, using specific neuronal pathways, modulates the secretion of corticotropic-releasing hormone (CRH). Upon secretion from the hypothalamus, CRH stimulates the anterior pituitary to secrete ACTH, which, in turn, directly stimulates the adrenal cortex to secrete cortisol.

Cortisol, as the final hormone in this sequence, feeds back on the hypothalamus to reduce secretion of CRH, and, in addition, cortisol acts directly on the anterior pituitary to reduce the sensitivity of ACTH-secreting cells to the effect of CRH.[4] It is also possible that ACTH exerts a negative feedback on the hypothalamus to reduce secretion of CRH.

## PATHOPHYSIOLOGY: ADRENAL INSUFFICIENCY, HYPERACTIVITY, AND CRISIS

### Terminology

Primary adrenal insufficiency was first described in 1855 by an English physician, Thomas Addison. The term Addison's disease is frequently used to describe both acute and chronic adrenal insufficiency, and this has at times led to some confusion. Adrenal cortical insufficiency, or hypofunction, is classified as primary or secondary. *Primary* adrenal insufficiency, also called Addison's disease, is a relatively uncommon form of adrenal cortical insufficiency that results from failure of the adrenal cortex to synthesize and secrete adequate amounts of adrenal cortical hormones. This disorder results in both glucocorticoid and mineralocorticoid deficiencies.

*Secondary* adrenal insufficiency involves a failure of the hypothalamic–pituitary axis, wherein the anterior pituitary is unable to synthesize and secrete adequate amounts of ACTH. This disorder is associated with glucocorticoid deficiency only.

Cortisol excess (or adrenal hypersecretion) is referred to as Cushing's syndrome, or Cushing's disease. By convention, Cushing's *syndrome* is usually applied to clinical situations in which there is an excess of cortisol; Cushing's *disease* is usually applied to the clinical circumstance in which there is an overproduction/oversecretion of ACTH usually associated with a pituitary tumor.

The following discussion will focus on the clinically significant aspects of adrenal insufficiency, or Addison's disease. To appreciate the scope of cortisol activity within the body, a contrast of adrenal insufficiency (i.e., Addison's disease) and adrenal hyperfunction (i.e., Cushing's syndrome) is presented in Table 18–2.

### Adrenal Insufficiency (Addison's Disease)

The adrenal cortices normally have an enormous functional reserve. Clinically significant manifestations of adrenal insufficiency usually do not become obvious until greater than 90% destruction of the adrenal gland has occurred. Often the borderline patient with a slowly progressive decrease in adrenal function may live for a long time with sufficient hormonal secretion to meet everyday requirements (i.e., latent form of disease). It is only when faced with a significant stressor (e.g., surgery, trauma, infection, emotional upset) that adrenal secretion becomes inadequate to meet the body's needs and the patient develops a full-blown acute adrenal insufficiency.

Approximately 85% of all cases of adrenal insufficiency are diagnosed as idiopathic adrenal insufficiency, and most clinicians feel the underlying pathophysiology is attributed to autoimmune destruction of the adrenal cortex. Adrenal antibodies have been found in high titers in some patients with Addison's disease. The antigen–antibody reaction in adrenal corticol tissues may account for the inflammatory reaction that ultimately causes destructive adrenal atrophy. See Table 18–2 for specific pathophysiologic and etiologic factors underlying adrenal insufficiency.

#### Clinical Presentation

Most abnormalities associated with Addison's disease are ascribed to mineralocorticoid and glucocorticoid hormonal deficiencies. A lack of the min-

TABLE 18–2
## Contrast: Addison's Disease and Cushing's Syndrome

| | Addison's Disease, Primary Adrenal Cortical Insufficiency | Cushing's Syndrome, Adrenal Cortical Hypersecretion |
|---|---|---|
| Definition | Adrenal cortical *hypo*function<br>*Primary* adrenal insufficiency (Addison's disease) results from failure of adrenal cortex to synthesize and secrete adequate amounts of hormones.<br>*Secondary* adrenal insufficiency results from failure of the anterior pituitary to synthesize and secrete ACTH. This form of the disease is most frequently associated with iatrogenic causes such as too rapid withdrawal of exogenous glucocorticoid following a long course (>10–14 days) of therapy. | Adrenal cortical *hyper*function<br>*Cushing's syndrome* reflects those clinical situations characterized by an excess of cortisol.<br>*Cushing's disease* results primarily from overproduction of ACTH from a pituitary tumor. |
| Pathophysiology | Autoimmune phenomenon: Mutation of immune response gene located on chromosome six associated with malfunction of thymus-dependent suppressor lymphocytes, which ordinarily keep a check on autoimmune tendencies (see Chap. 54).<br>High adrenal antibody titers have been found in some patients with Addison's disease. The inflammatory reaction associated with the antigen–antibody response may predispose to destructive adrenal atrophy.<br>Mineralocorticoid-aldosterone deficiency: Disrupts fluid and electrolyte balance—↓ $Na^+$, ↑ $K^+$, ↓ extracellular fluid balance.<br>Glucocorticoid-cortisol deficiency: Predisposes to hypoglycemia, a decreased mobilization of fats and proteins, and a sluggish energy-generating state.<br>Melanocyte-stimulating hormone (MSH): Increased secretions of MSH coupled with melanocyte stimulatory effects of ACTH contribute to abnormal deposition of melanin pigment in skin and mucous membranes.<br>Diminished androgen secretion results in growth of hair (hirsutism) strikingly apparent in women. | Most abnormalities are ascribed to abnormal hypersecretion of cortisol, but an increased secretion of androgens from the zonae fasciculata and reticularis is also significant.<br>Hyperglycemia (>200 mg% post-meals) is related to enhanced gluconeogenesis.<br>*"Adrenal diabetes"* occurs because of a persistent hyperglycemia coupled with "insulin-antagonistic" effects of cortisol. Insulin is continuously secreted in response to hyperglycemia, but cell membranes are insensitive to its action. The net effect: Burn out of islets of Langerhans with permanent diabetes mellitus.<br>Protein catabolism: Greatly reduced tissue proteins except for liver and serum proteins. Loss of protein in muscle predisposes to severe weakness.<br>Loss of protein synthesis in lymphoid tissue diminishes the immune response.<br>Reduced collagen fibers in subcutaneous tissues; tissues tear easily (purple striae formation).<br>Diminished protein deposition in bone with consequent osteoporosis. |
| Etiology | Autoimmune phenomena<br>Iatrogenic causes, as for example the too rapid withdrawal of exogenous glucocorticoid therapy*<br>Adrenal hemorrhage associated with trauma, sepsis, or anticoagulant therapy<br>Metastatic tumors<br>Adrenalectomy as therapy for the treatment of metastatic breast cancer<br>Fungal diseases<br>Amyloidosis, histoplasmosis | Pituitary adenoma (microadenomas)<br>Overproduction of corticotropic-releasing hormone (CRH) by hypothalamus<br>Ectopic ACTH production, frequently associated with oat cell carcinoma of the lungs; abdominal carcinoma<br>Primary adrenal neoplasms (adenoma or carcinoma)<br>Hyperplasia of adrenal cortices caused by overactivity of the hypothalamic–pituitary axis |
| Diagnostic findings, history | Very important clues to pursue:<br>Prior state of health? Onset of Addison's disease may be gradual and insidious; can the patient recall when symptoms first developed? Has there been recent stress, trauma, infection?<br>Has the patient become unexpectantly ill without obvious cause? Is there a history of slow recovery from previous illnesses, surgery? The patient may be unable to cope with a stressful event due to diminished adrenal reserve.<br>Is there unusual fatigue, weakness? Does the patient tire easily? Muscle weakness occurs due to catabolism of body proteins.<br>Does the patient experience diaphoresis, faintness, or dizziness between meals or when a meal is skipped? Hypoglycemia may be due to decreased gluconeogenesis and depleted liver glycogen stores.<br>Are there gastrointestinal disturbances? Nausea, vomiting, anorexia, diarrhea? Has there been a recent weight loss?<br>Has the patient experienced mood changes, depression, confusion? Have there been any personality changes such as listlessness, apathy, paranoia, negativism? Has the patient experienced headaches, insomnia, neuralgias?<br>What medications does the patient take? Is the patient cortisone-dependent?<br>Does the patient use steroids currently? In the past? Why?<br>Is there a history of ulcerative colitis, collagen disease, or other disease treated with exogenous steroids? | |

*(continued)*

TABLE 18–2
## Contrast: Addison's Disease and Cushing's Syndrome *(Continued)*

| | Addison's Disease, Primary Adrenal Cortical Insufficiency | Cushing's Syndrome, Adrenal Cortical Hypersecretion |
|---|---|---|
| | Does the patient have an unusual sensitivity to drugs such as morphine or codeine? *Beta-endorphin*, a powerful morphinelike endogenous substance, is derived from the same precursor molecule (pro-opimelanocortin) within the anterior pituitary as is ACTH.[4] In the presence of pituitary hypofunction a decrease in the secretion of $\beta$-endorphin may account for this increased sensitivity to exogenous morphinelike sources such as morphine and codeine. There may be less competition between endogenous and exogenous morphinelike substances for the available receptor sites.<br>*Past medical history:* Have there been previous episodes of endocrine dysfunction?<br>*Family History:* Is there a familial predisposition to endocrine disorders?<br>Autoimmune-associated endocrine disorders can coexist. | |
| Physical examination | Vital sign assessment? Hypotension is characteristic of Addison's disease; hypertension is associated with Cushing's syndrome and reflects the slight mineralocorticoid effects of cortisol.<br>Examine for evidence of disease or illness in which use of steroids is suspected; scars indicating mastectomy, abdominal surgery, adrenalectomy?<br>Assessment of skin, evidence of pigmentation? Carefully question regarding the time and course of its development? Note its distribution. Did the patient notice a better suntan than usual, or one that was more prolonged? Pigmentation changes may precede the appearance of other signs and symptoms. Is there vitiligo-patchy areas of depigmentation? Inconsistent pigment alteration is attributed to an autoimmune phenomenon observed primarily in idiopathic adrenal insufficiency.<br>Is there evidence of ecchymosis or petechiae?<br>Does presence of purple striae reflect loss of collagen support?<br>Is there evidence of hirsutism? Changes in secondary sex characteristics associated with increased androgen secretion? Is gynecomastia present in a male?<br>Examine for evidence of endocrine derangement. Are there changes in the appearance of the thyroid gland? Are there complaints of vision abnormalities (homonymous hemianopsia) associated with possible pituitary pathology?<br>Observe distribution of weight. Mobilization of fat from lower part of body accompanied by extra fat deposition in thorax and upper abdomen gives rise to so-called "buffalo" torso; excess secretion of steroids leads to edematous appearance of face, the so-called moon face appearance. Both of these characteristics reflect Cushing's syndrome. In addition, acne and hirsutism may be present. | |
| Laboratory tests/diagnostic studies | Serum electrolytes: Hyponatremia, hyperkalemia, hypercalcemia (related to lack of cortisol to counteract intestinal calcium absorption).<br>Blood urea nitrogen and serum osmolality elevated due to hypovolemia.<br>Hypoglycemia; elevated eosinophil count.<br>Plasma cortisol levels:†<br>Cortisol $<10$ $\mu$g/100 ml at 8 a.m.<br>$<5$ $\mu$g/100 ml at 4 p.m.‡<br>Short ACTH stimulation test: Normal response—baseline cortisol $>5$ $\mu$g/100 ml; increment $>7$ $\mu$g/100 ml; peak $>18$ $\mu$g/100 ml.<br>Long ACTH stimulation test: Normal response—plasma cortisol $>20$–$40$ $\mu$g/100 ml after last dose, usually a 3-day period.<br>Plasma ACTH immunoassay: A baseline cortisol value of $<10\mu$g/100 ml coupled with an ACTH $>250$ $\mu$g/ml is diagnostic of primary adrenal insufficiency.<br>Urine tests: Decreased levels of 17-ketosteroids and 17-hydroxysteroids occur in adrenal insufficiency due to lack of cortisol secretion.<br>Metyrapone test: Used to determine presence of secondary adrenal insufficiency. | ACTH immunoassay: Persistently high ACTH levels coupled with high cortisol levels suggest pituitary overactivity or ectopic ACTH production.<br>Urine tests for steroids: Both 17-keto-steroids and 17-hydroxysteroids are increased when ACTH stimulation is excessive.<br>Overnight dexamethasone suppression test: Normal results—plasma cortisol $<5$ $\mu$g/100 ml.<br>Prolonged dexamethasone suppression test is a definitive test to determine the presence of Cushing's syndrome and its differential diagnosis.<br><br>*Note:* Special care is necessary in conducting laboratory testing for anterior pituitary–adrenal dysfunction. Meticulous adherence to schedules for administration of tests, medications, and collection of blood and urine specimens is essential if test results are to be reliable. |
| Other studies | X-rays and CAT scans, among others | |
| | ***Cortisol Deficiency*** | ***Cortisol Excess*** |
| Clinical presentation | Central nervous/mental status may reflect headache, vertigo, tinnitus, insomnia, confusion, listlessness, apathy, depression, irritability, and paranoia progressing to psychosis; may be labeled as psychoneurotic. | Central nervous/mental status may reflect emotional upset and personality changes including depression, anxiety, irritability, apathy.<br>Cardiovascular status almost always reflects hypertension, congestive heart failure, plethora, erythrocytosis. |

TABLE 18–2
**Contrast: Addison's Disease and Cushing's Syndrome *(Continued)***

| | **Addison's Disease,<br>Primary Adrenal Cortical Insufficiency** | **Cushing's Syndrome,<br>Adrenal Cortical Hypersecretion** |
|---|---|---|
| | Cardiovascular status usually reflects hypotension due to decrease in intravascular blood volume; orthostatic hypotension; tachycardia; there may be impaired cellular response to catecholamines due to deficient cortisol levels ("permissive effect" of cortisol).<br>Renal status may reflect impaired "free water" clearance associated with decreased glomerular filtration and hyponatremia.<br>Gastrointestinal dysfunction usually includes anorexia, nausea, vomiting, diarrhea, abdominal pain, weight loss, disruption of tastes. (Gastrointestinal symptomatology is related to a decreased secretion of digestive enzymes, and dehydration.)<br>Integumentary impairment is characterized by increased pigmentation due to increased secretions of ACTH and MSH (hyperpigmentation distributed to palmar creases, sun-exposed area, mucous membranes; areas of friction; and nipples and external genitalia). Muscular weakness and asthenia present.<br>Reproductive changes associated with diminished androgen secretion may include a decreased libido; changes in secondary sex characteristics with hirsutism and masculinization in women.<br>Reduced energy level is associated with reduced gluconeogenesis, reduced liver glycogen stores, hypoglycemia, inability to tolerate fasting, and reduced mobilization of fats and proteins. | Gastrointestinal disorders may include peptic ulcer disease due to increased gastric pepsin and hydrochloric acid secretion.<br>Weight gain associated with accumulation of adipose tissue particularly centripetal (face, neck, trunk); heavy trunk; thin extremities all reflected in "buffalo hump" and "moon face" appearance.<br>Protein catabolism reflected in muscle wasting and weakness, thin skin with formation of purple striae; ecchymosis reflective of capillary fragility; poor wound healing; osteoporosis associated with hypercalciuria.<br>Depressed immune response with increased susceptibility to infections.<br>Carbohydrate metabolism reflects poor glucose utilization and insulin resistance resulting in hyperglycemia. |
| | ***Aldosterone Deficiency*[5]**<br>Inability to reabsorb and conserve sodium results in:<br>Decreased extracellular and intravascular fluid volumes<br>Decreased cardiac output with hypotension and postural syncope<br>Hypovolemic shock<br>Prerenal azotemia<br>Weakness, weight loss<br>Increased renin production<br>Impaired renal secretion of potassium and hydrogen ions:<br>Hyperkalemia<br>Acidemia | ***Mineralocorticoid Effect of Cortisol***<br>Hypokalemia<br>Hypertension |
| Treatment | *Goals*<br>1. Replacement of cortical hormones<br>2. Correction of fluid and electrolyte disturbances<br>3. Correction of hypoglycemia<br>4. Treat precipitating event or underlying cause (e.g., antibiotic therapy for infection).<br>5. Drug regimen (hormone replacement therapy):<br>A. Cortisone is used to replace glucocorticoids.<br>B. Fludrocortisone is used to replace mineralocorticoids. | *Goal:* reduce ACTH secretion.<br>1. Surgery<br>Excision of pituitary tumor<br>Excision of adrenal tumor<br>Bilateral total or partial adrenalectomy followed by replacement steroids<br>2. Irradiation<br>3. Suppressive drug therapy |

(Implications for nursing care and patient education are discussed in Table 18–3.)

* Suppression of ACTH secretion as a consequence of chronic glucocorticoid therapy is the most common cause of secondary adrenal insufficiency.

† Normal values and diurnal rhythm do not disprove that the pituitary–adrenal axis is intact because total adrenal reserve may still be reduced. This point is of extreme importance in the patient's capacity to cope with stress.

‡ Suggest adrenal insufficiency.

eralocorticoid, aldosterone, seriously disrupts sodium reabsorption and potassium secretion in the distal renal tubules and collecting ducts. The net effect is hyponatremia, hyperkalemia, and a greatly contracted extracellular fluid volume.

Glucocorticoid (cortisol) deficiency predisposes to hypoglycemia as the individual is unable to maintain adequate serum glucose concentrations between meals and during the fasting state. There is reduced gluconeogenesis and a decreased mobilization of fats and proteins. Generation of energy becomes very sluggish and compromises the capability of the individual to withstand stress. Even a mild respiratory infection can sometimes cause death in the compromised individual.

An increase in melanin deposition in the skin and mucous membrane causes a characteristic pigmentation of the skin in the patient with primary adrenal insufficiency. An increased ACTH secretion by the anterior pituitary occurs in response to decreased serum cortisol levels. Abnormally high concentrations of ACTH exert a direct, stimulatory effect on melanocytes in the skin, predisposing to an increased deposition of the pigment. In addition, there may be an associated rise in the secretion of melanocyte-stimulating hormone (MSH) from the pituitary, which contributes further to an increased deposition of pigment. The presence of pigmentation assists in differentiating primary from secondary adrenal insufficiency. In the latter there is a complete absence of any skin pigmentation simply because there is a decreased secretion of anterior pituitary hormones, ACTH and MSH.

As a review, features of the clinical presentation of both hypersecretion and hyposecretion of adrenal cortical hormones are presented in Table 18–2. In addition, data related to the assessment and diagnostic workup of the patient with adrenal cortical dysfunction, including history, physical examination, and laboratory data, are also presented in Table 18–2.

#### Treatment

Treatment of adrenal insufficiency revolves around replacement of cortical hormones, correction of the fluid and electrolyte disturbances, and treatment of hypoglycemia. Specific treatment considerations are listed in Table 18–2.

## Adrenal Crisis (Addisonian Crisis)

Adrenal crisis, also called addisonian crisis, is the acute form of adrenal insufficiency characterized by severe prostration, weakness, dehydration, hypotension progressing to shock, and coma. It is a true medical emergency, a potentially catastrophic condition that arises when the body's requirements for adrenal cortical hormones greatly exceed the available supply. The major precipitating factor is stress. During stress the glucocorticoid requirements increase dramatically. In the well, unaffected individual the body has the capacity to increase adrenal cortical hormone secretion 10-fold. In the individual with adrenal cortical dysfunction there is an inability to respond to the stressful event.

Adrenal crisis occurs most often in individuals with preexisting undiagnosed (latent) adrenal insufficiency or in patients receiving replacement hormones for diagnosed adrenal insufficiency who fail to increase their hormone intake during a stressful period. Equally important is the occurrence of adrenal crisis after sudden withdrawal of adrenal cortical hormone therapy in the patient with chronic adrenal insufficiency. Adrenal crisis may also be precipitated by a sudden, spontaneous progression of the chronic form of the disease due to unusually rapid destruction of the adrenal glands. A thorough, comprehensive patient history assists in differential diagnosis (see Table 18–2).

Other potential causes of adrenal crisis include surgical removal of both adrenal glands or excision of a hyperfunctioning adrenal tumor in one adrenal gland that has suppressed the other. Sudden pituitary apoplexy with pituitary destruction, and injury to both adrenal glands by trauma, hemorrhage, infarction, infection, malignancy, or anticoagulation therapy have been documented as etiologic factors in adrenal dysfunction. A rare occurrence is the precipitation of adrenal crisis due to meningococcal septicemia (Waterhouse-Friderichsen syndrome).

The onset of adrenal crisis may be gradual, occurring over a period of a few days in a patient not too severely distressed; or it can appear abruptly as in patients with previously undiagnosed disease, who suffer trauma or are subjected to the stress of surgery.

#### Clinical Presentation

Clinical manifestations are nonspecific but often include fatigue, weakness, headache, nausea and vomiting, diarrhea, abdominal pain, postural hypotension, and weight loss. A high-grade fever (39°C) is common. Confusion and coma may also be present. The presence of hyperpigmentation and/or vitiligo assists in differential diagnosis; unexplained hypotension suggests the possibility of adrenal insufficiency. Other physical findings may include cyanosis, ecchymosis and petechiae, dehydration, and lymphadenopathy. Costovertebral angle tenderness may be observed in adrenal hemorrhage.

Laboratory studies reflect hyponatremia, hyperkalemia, hypoglycemia, and elevated BUN levels. Hypercalcemia is frequently present. A normal or high eosinophil count in the presence of stress strongly suggests adrenal insufficiency. Low urinary and serum cortisol levels in the setting of stress are diagnostic of adrenal insufficiency. Diagnosis is confirmed by ACTH stimulation test wherein serum cortisol levels fail to increase above 18 $\mu$g/dl 1 hour after injection of cosyntropin (Cortrosyn) 0.25 mg. Reduced cortisol levels in the presence of increased plasma ACTH levels suggests primary adrenal insufficiency or Addison's disease.

### *Treatment*

In treating the patient with adrenal crisis, corticosteroid replacement therapy is initiated after blood samples are obtained. Such therapy is usually instituted without waiting for laboratory confirmation. Initial emergency treatment includes administering any available glucocorticoid (e.g., hydrocortisone sodium succinate [Solu-Cortef] 100 mg bolus IV), administering volume expanders, controlling infection, and supporting cardiopulmonary function.

When the diagnosis has been confirmed (e.g., via ACTH stimulation test), the treatment regimen usually includes the following:

1. Hydrocortisone sodium succinate (Solu-Cortef) 100 mg intravenously, every 8 hours for 24 hours; then 50 mg intravenously, every 6 hours for the next 24 hours. (Hydocortisone sodium succinate is the drug of choice because of its mineralocorticoid effect.)
2. Rapid intravenous infusion with 5% dextrose in saline to correct hyponatremia and hyperkalemia and to expand extracellular fluid volume.
   A. From 3–5 liters of intravenous saline may be required (within 24 hours) depending on fluid and electrolyte status, cardiovascular response, and urinary output.
      - Hyperkalemia usually responds well to cortisol-saline therapy. Enhanced reabsorption of sodium increases secretion/excretion of potassium in distal tubules.
      - Use of insulin/glucose therapy to reduce serum potassium is contraindicated because it may predispose to profound hyperglycemia.
      - Use of ion-exchange resins are also contraindicated because this therapy may precipitate hypokalemia.
      - If hyperkalemia persists in spite of the above therapy, it may be necessary to institute mineralocorticoid therapy.
3. Infection, which commonly accompanies this syndrome, is treated with appropriate broad-spectrum antibiotics once cultures have been obtained.
4. Diagnosis and treatment of other precipitating events.

The response to therapy is usually rapid, with improvement seen within the first 12 hours. With continued improvement steroidal doses are tapered gradually to 30 mg/day by the fifth day. There is usually no need to give a supplemental pure mineralocorticoid as long as the patient is receiving greater than 150 mg cortisol/day. As the glucocorticosteroid is reduced further fludrocortisone (Florinef) may be required at daily oral doses of 0.05–0.20 mg.

Once the patient's adrenal crisis has resolved, diagnostic studies to pinpoint the patient's underlying condition are implemented, and an appropriate maintenance treatment regimen is initiated as necessary. Post-crisis care includes patient education for the cortisone-dependent patient and family/significant others.

### *Nursing Care of the Patient in Adrenal Crisis (Addisonian Crisis)*

In treating the patient in adrenal crisis, nursing care is directed toward identifying the individual at risk, preventing life-threatening events, and working with the individual and family/significant others to help them understand the nature of the disease and its impact on the lifestyle and integrity of each individual.

**Therapeutic Goals.** Implementation of nursing process in the care of the patient in adrenal crisis revolves around the following therapeutic goals:

1. Establish a thorough and comprehensive database including:
   A. Clinical history (functional health patterns).
   B. Physical examination.
   C. Laboratory/diagnostic studies.
2. Implement prescribed corticosteroid replacement therapy.
3. Establish and maintain effective cardiovascular function.
4. Establish and maintain fluid and electrolyte balance.
5. Maintain the integrity of neurologic and psychologic processes.
6. Maintain adequate nutrition to meet the demands of the catabolic state.
7. Provide supportive care and reduce risk of infection.
8. Provide emotional and psychologic support to patient and family/significant others.
9. Initiate patient/family education to assist in developing and implementing prophylactic health-care practices.

**Nursing Diagnoses, Desired Patient Outcomes, and Nursing Interventions.** Pertinent nursing diagnoses, desired patient outcomes, and nursing interventions/rationales in the care of the patient in adrenal crisis are presented in the Care Plan in Table 18–3.

**TABLE 18–3. CARE PLAN FOR THE PATIENT IN ADRENAL CRISIS (ADDISONIAN CRISIS)**

| Nursing Diagnoses | Desired Patient Outcomes | Nursing Interventions | Rationales |
|---|---|---|---|
| ***Nursing Diagnosis #1***<br>Cardiac output, alteration in: Decreased, related to:<br>1. Reduced circulating blood volume and decreased venous return.<br>2. Dysrhythmias associated with hyperkalemia. | Patient will maintain:<br>1. Usual mental status:<br>• Alert, oriented to person, place, date.<br>• Behavior appropriate.<br>• Usual personality (as per family/significant others). | • Establish and maintain effective cardiovascular function.<br>∘ Establish assessment data of overall body function. | • A brief but highly scrutinized assessment of the patient and family facilitates early diagnosis with institution of timely and effective therapy; once the patient's condition is stabilized, a comprehensive investigation of the patient and patient/family–environment interaction should be performed. A thorough database facilitates treatment and rehabilitation. |
| | 2. Effective cardiovascular function:<br>• Heart rate >60, <100 beats/min.<br>• Cardiac rhythm: Regular sinus, without symptomatic dysrhythmias. | • Examine for presence of Medic-Alert identification tag or bracelet.<br>• Thoroughly document all findings. | • Such identification facilitates immediate diagnosis and treatment.<br>• Provides basis for comparison; assists in evaluating response to therapy; steroid therapy may precipitate dysrhythmias because of sudden shifts in electrolytes. |
| | Hemodynamic parameters:<br>• CVP: 0–8 mmHg.<br>• PCWP: 8–12 mmHg.<br>• CO: 4–8 liters/min.<br>• Arterial BP within 10 mmHg of baseline. | • Maintain continuous assessment of vital parameters:<br>∘ Cardiac rate and rhythm.<br>–Apical/radial pulse deficit.<br>∘ Hemodynamic parameters: Central venous pressure; pulmonary artery pressure; pulmonary capillary wedge pressure; arterial pressure; cardiac output; orthostatic hypotension. | • Sudden shifts in fluid and electrolytes may precipitate cardiovascular collapse.<br>∘ Hyperkalemia may precipitate serious dysrhythmias.<br>∘ Assists in determining fluid status; prevents overhydration from too aggressive fluid replacement therapy; hypertension, congestive heart failure with pulmonary edema are potential complications of hypervolemia. |
| | 3. Renal status:<br>• Urine output: >30 ml/hr. | ∘ Arterial blood gases. | ∘ Assists in evaluating adequacy of alveolar ventilation and gas exchange. |
| | 4. Respiratory status:<br>• Respiratory rate: <25–30 breaths/min.<br>• Breathing pattern: Eupnea. | ∘ Serum electrolytes. | ∘ Diminished aldosterone secretion predisposes to hyponatremia, hyperkalemia, and extracellular fluid volume deficit. |
| | | • Institute prescribed fluid replacement: Dextrose 5% in saline; plasma expanders. | • Prevents hypovolemic shock; the amount of fluid administered is guided by hemodynamic parameters. |
| | | • Administer vasopressors (dopamine); maintain resuscitation equipment at bedside. | • Administered to relieve severe hypotension and hypovolemic shock. |
| | | • Institute immediate corticosteroid therapy. | • Immediate administration of corticosteroids may prevent cardiovascular collapse. |
| | | ∘ Administer drug regimen in highly individualized manner.<br>∘ Consider underlying pathophysiology:<br>∘ Pulmonary disease; heart disease; diabetes mellitus. | ∘ Goal of corticosteroid replacement therapy is to maximize efficacy while minimizing adverse effects.<br>∘ Minimize mineralocorticoid activity; major concern is fluid overload with concomitant risk of congestive heart failure and pulmonary edema. |

| | |
|---|---|
| ◦ Hepatic disease or hepatic dysfunction with an associated endocrine disorder (e.g., diabetes mellitus; hypothyroidism). | ◦ Liver may be unable to completely activate enterally administered exogenous steroids.<br>◦ Liver disease may impair ability to clear or metabolize exogenous steroids.<br>◦ The presence of other endocrine disorders may exaggerate response to steroids by alteration in steroid metabolism. |
| • Review mode of corticosteriod administration: | ◦ All corticosteroids can be given parenterally except prednisone, which is available only in oral form. |
| ◦ Intravenous cortisol should be given very slowly (e.g., 100 mg IV over 10–20 minutes) | ◦ Rarely, rapid infusion can result in shock and anaphylaxis in patients with acute bronchospasms. |
| ◦ Continuous monitoring of cardiac and hemodynamic parameters is absolutely essential with intravenous administration of large dosage of steroids.<br>◦ Continuous monitoring of serum electrolytes and serum glucose is absolutely essential. | ◦ Dysrhythmias may be precipitated by sudden electrolyte shifts induced by steroids; fluid overload may be precipitated by increased levels of mineralocorticoid activity. |
| ◦ Ongoing monitoring of serum proteins. | ◦ Steroids are >90% protein-bound; serum proteins should be closely monitored. |
| • Assess prescribed drug regimen and risk of adverse drug interactions. | • To prevent undesired complications, it is essential to determine the presence of incompatibility of therapeutic measures or potential alterations in physiologic processes. |
| • Monitor potassium level carefully in patient receiving furosemide or other diuretics. | • The enhanced secretion of potassium caused by these drugs, coupled with the potassium-wasting effects of steroids, may predispose to hypokalemia; major concern with digoxin use. |
| • Monitor for masked infections when administering broad-spectrum antibiotics (e.g., tetracycline). | • Antibiotic administration can predispose to opportunistic infections, the signs of which can be masked by steroids. |
| • Carefully monitor the therapeutic effects of steroids in patients receiving medications such as barbiturates, phenytoin, isoniazid, rifampin. | • Such drugs diminish the efficacy of steroids by stimulating increased hepatic microsomal enzymatic activity, which metabolizes steroids to inactive compounds. |
| • Monitor ongoing administration of steroids for associated complications. These may include:<br>◦ Metabolic: Metabolic alkalosis, potassium depletion, sodium retention, glucose intolerance, adrenal suppression.<br>◦ Cardiovascular: Edema, hypertension.<br>◦ Neurologic: Insomnia, euphoria, muscle weakness, irritability, depression, personality changes. | • Despite careful administration, steroids always have the potential of causing complications. |

*(continued)*

## TABLE 18–3. CARE PLAN FOR THE PATIENT IN ADRENAL CRISIS (ADDISONIAN CRISIS) *(Continued)*

| Nursing Diagnoses | Desired Patient Outcomes | Nursing Interventions | Rationales |
|---|---|---|---|
| ***Nursing Diagnosis #1 (cont.)*** | | ○ Gastrointestinal: Peptic ulcer disease, gastritis, hemorrhage.<br>○ Other: Impaired wound healing, increased vulnerability to infection, depressed WBC, osteoporosis, muscle wasting, glaucoma/cataracts, moon face, abdominal fat pad. | |
| ***Nursing Diagnosis #2***<br>Fluid volume deficit: Actual, related to:<br>1. Hyponatremia associated with hyposecretion of aldosterone. (See Table 23–3, Nursing Diagnosis #1.)<br>***Nursing Diagnosis #3***<br>Electrolyte imbalance, related to:<br>1. Hyponatremia and hyperkalemia associated with hyposecretion of mineralocorticoids (e.g., aldosterone) and glucocorticoids (e.g., cortisol).<br>(See Table 23–7, Nursing Diagnosis #2, and Table 23–9, Nursing Diagnosis #1.) | Patient will maintain effective fluid and electrolyte balance:<br>1. Neurologic status:<br>• Alert, oriented to person, place, date.<br>• Behavior appropriate.<br>• Usual personality (as per family).<br>• Deep tendon reflexes brisk.<br>2. Hemodynamic status:<br>• See Nursing Diagnosis #1, above.<br>3. Renal status:<br>• Urine output (hourly) $>30$ ml/hr.<br>4. Respiratory status:<br>• Respiratory rate: $<25-30$ breaths/min.<br>• Breathing pattern: Eupnea.<br>• Breath sounds clear; absence of adventitious sounds (e.g., crackles, wheezes).<br>5. Gastrointestinal status:<br>• Absence of anorexia, nausea, vomiting, diarrhea, bleeding. | For pertinent nursing interventions and their rationales related to fluid and electrolyte balance, see:<br>Table 23–3, Nursing Diagnoses #1, #2, and #3.<br>Table 23–7, Nursing Diagnosis #2.<br>Table 23–9, Nursing Diagnosis #1.<br>Table 24–3, Nursing Diagnosis #1.<br>In addition, consider the following:<br>• Maintain fluid and electrolyte balance.<br>○ Assess for signs and symptoms of hyperkalemia $>6.0$ mEq/liter.<br>– Signs and symptoms related to neuromuscular function: Muscle weakness, paralysis, paresthesias, twitching, hyperreflexia, bradycardia proceeding to cardiac arrest, ventricular fibrillation, oliguria. | • Hyperkalemia may precipitate serious dysrhythmias; a decreased serum mineralocorticoid level predisposes to hyperkalemia due to increased reabsorption of potassium via the kidney tubules in the presence of hyponatremia. |
| | | • Monitor serial electrolytes. | • Patients taking digitalis are at high risk of lethal dysrhythmias in the presence of hyperkalemia. |
| | | • Monitor for hypoglycemia. | • Fluid volume deficit can decrease cerebral perfusion, which together with hypoglycemia can predispose to coma. |
| | | • Assess for fluid volume deficit:<br>○ Cardiovascular: Decreased hemodynamic pressures, hypotension, tachycardia, tachypnea, hemoconcentration.<br>○ Neuromuscular: Paresthesias, weakness, listlessness.<br>○ Renal: Decreased urine output.<br>○ General: Poor skin turgor over sternum or forehead, sunken eyeballs, weight loss. | • Patients with underlying cardiac or renal disease are especially at high risk to develop complications associated with fluid deficit or excess. |
| | | • Assess for fluid volume excess: | • May occur with overly aggressive fluid replacement; hemodynamic parameters should be monitored very closely. |

| | | | |
|---|---|---|---|
| | 6. Laboratory data:<br>• Serum<br>Osmolality: 285–295 mOsm/kg.<br>Sodium: >135, <148 mEq/liter.<br>Potassium: 3.5–5.5 mEq/liter.<br>Glucose: 70–110 mg/100 ml.<br>Hematology profile.<br>• Urine.<br>Specific gravity: 1.010–1.025. | ∘ Cardiovascular: Elevated hemodynamic values, neck vein distention in upright position (45°), hypertension, bounding pulse, dependent edema.<br>∘ Neurologic: Confusion associated with dilutional hyponatremia.<br>∘ Pulmonary: Dyspnea, rales.<br>∘ General: Weight gain.<br>• Monitor intake and output (hourly); daily weight<br>∘ Include all gastrointestinal fluid losses.<br>∘ Insensible losses, especially in presence of fever. | • Assists in evaluating fluid status; body weight is an excellent guide to fluid state. |
| ***Nursing Diagnosis #4***<br>Tissue perfusion, alteration in: Cerebral, related to:<br>1. Fluid volume deficit.<br>2. Electrolyte disturbance:<br>• Hyponatremia.<br>• Hyperkalemia. | Patient will:<br>1. Exhibit intact level of consciousness and mentation.<br>• Alert, oriented to person, place, date.<br>• Memory intact.<br>2. Demonstrates intact sensorimotor function.<br>3. Deep tendon reflexes brisk.<br>4. Respiratory rate: <25–30 breaths/min.<br>• Breathing pattern: Eupnea. | • Maintain integrity of neurologic and psychologic processes.<br>∘ Establish baseline neurologic function:<br>– Mental status: Changes in level of consciousness, disorientation, confusion, agitation, irritability, coma.<br>∘ Sensory function: Presence of paresthesias.<br>∘ Motor function: Muscle weakness, paralysis, hyperreflexia.<br>• Establish baseline psychologic function of both patient and family.<br>∘ Assess level of anxiety.<br>∘ Assess level of knowledge regarding disease.<br>∘ Estimate developmental level.<br>∘ Record emotional/personality changes; speak with family regarding such changes in the patient:<br>– Specific changes; when did they begin to appear? Were they associated with specific stressor or stressful event?<br>∘ Assess coping capabilities: Role of patient in family nucleus: Independent? Dependent? Active, decision-maker? Passive personality? | ∘ Symptomatology is related to hypoglycemia, and decreased cerebral perfusion is due to cardiovascular instability<br>∘ May be difficult to differentiate signs and symptoms of alterations in neurologic function associated with hypoglycemia and decreased cerebral perfusion from those associated with hyperkalemia.<br>∘ Provides a base to build on because anxiety can be used constructively in certain situations.<br>∘ Age and developmental level may not necessarily be the same.<br>∘ Role of patient in family nucleus will influence rehabilitative process for all members. |

*(continued)*

**TABLE 18–3. CARE PLAN FOR THE PATIENT IN ADRENAL CRISIS (ADDISONIAN CRISIS)** ***(Continued)***

| Nursing Diagnoses | Desired Patient Outcomes | Nursing Interventions | Rationales |
|---|---|---|---|
| ***Nursing Diagnosis #4 (cont.)*** | | ∘ Identify family resources and significant others. | ∘ Observation of interactions between patient and family/significant others may provide valuable clues as to how they are coping, which may impact on the rehabilitative process. |
| | | ∘ Assess readiness to learn. | ∘ Teaching can be geared to level at which patient and family can best learn. |
| | | • Therapeutic considerations:<br>∘ Minimize stressors.<br>– Quiet, comfortable environment.<br>– Anticipate needs.<br>– Relaxed atmosphere. | ∘ A minimum of stimuli reduces risk of aggravating underlying pathophysiology. |
| | | ∘ Conserve energy.<br>– Maintain bedrest; avoid activities that may precipitate orthostatic hypotension.<br>– Frequent rest periods. | ∘ Conservation of energy helps to lessen demands of an already high catabolic state with diminished stores of muscle and liver glycogen. |
| | | ∘ Encourage verbalization of fears and concerns. | ∘ It may help to identify underlying problems or areas of particular concerns. |
| | | ∘ Observe for nonverbal communication: Eye contact, posture, movements, touch. | ∘ Nonverbal communication is especially helpful in assessing patient/family interactions. |
| | | ∘ Provide information in manageable amounts; provide opportunity for discussion and feedback. | ∘ Patient may feel overwhelmed with too much information raising anxiety levels.<br>∘ Feedback is important to enable clarification and verification of what has been said.<br>∘ Consensual validation assists in minimizing inaccurate assumptions. |
| | | ∘ Remain accessible to family members or significant others should they request to speak alone with the health-care provider.<br>∘ Enlist assistance of social worker or psychiatric liaison should such services be indicated or requested by patient, family, or significant others. | |
| | | ∘ Explain all ongoing procedures and reasons underlying therapy.<br>∘ Applaud patient/family efforts to cope. | ∘ Appropriate explanations may help to alleviate heightened anxiety. |

| | | | |
|---|---|---|---|
| ***Nursing Diagnosis #5***<br>Nutrition, alteration in: Less than body requirements, related to:<br>1. Catabolic state.<br>(See Chapter 53, Nutritional Support of the Critically Ill Patient.) | 1. Patient's body weight will stabilize within 5% of baseline.<br>2. Serum proteins will be maintained within acceptable physiologic range: 6.0–8.4 g/100 ml.<br>• Serum albumin: 3.5–5.0 mg/100 ml.<br>3. Serum glucose: 70–110 mg/100 ml.<br>4. Urine negative for glucose and acetone. | • Maintain adequate nutrition to meet the demands of the catabolic state.<br>∘ Consult with nutritionist and physician to determine nutritional needs of catabolic state:<br>– Baseline nutritional status.<br>– Nutritional requirements of compromised state.<br>∘ High carbohydrate.<br>– High protein.<br>∘ Liberal salt intake.<br>∘ Serum electrolytes, glucose, and total body proteins must be monitored on a regular basis; hematology studies are necessary.<br>∘ Intake and output; daily weight.<br>• Note therapeutic considerations when the patient can tolerate dietary intake:<br>∘ Establish which foods are best tolerated; offer nourishment between meals and at bedtime.<br>∘ Create environment conducive to eating.<br>∘ Avoid fasting or meal delays. | ∘ Baseline nutritional needs must be identified to ensure adequate nutritional intake, prevent hypoglycemic episodes, and reduce risk of infection.<br>∘ Patient is prone to hypoglycemia; it is important to establish positive nitrogen balance and decrease muscle wasting.<br>∘ Liberal salt intake offsets loss of sodium via kidneys.<br>∘ These data assist in monitoring response to therapy.<br>∘ Valuable parameters for determining fluid status.<br>∘ Foods appealing to patient may help to increase intake; smaller, more frequent meals may be better tolerated; hypoglycemic reactions may be avoided.<br>∘ Activities that promote nutritional intake should be encouraged; food brought from home may help to ensure necessary nutritional intake.<br>∘ A severe hypoglycemia reaction may be triggered by extending the fasting state or delaying meals; an increased sensitivity to insulin coupled with a low serum glucose may precipitate a hypoglycemic reaction. |
| ***Nursing Diagnosis #6***<br>Potential for infection, related to:<br>1. Catabolic state.<br>2. Compromised immune response.<br>(See Table 49–7, Potential for Infection, Nursing Care Considerations.) | Patient will:<br>1. Maintain body temperature within acceptable range: ~98.6°F (37°C).<br>2. Maintain white blood count: ~5000–10,000/mm³.<br>3. Remain without signs/symptoms of infection: Pain, redness, swelling, suppuration. | • Provide supportive measures to reduce risk of infection.<br>∘ Assess for signs of infection.<br>∘ Vigilant assessment of all invasive lines is critical.<br>– Observe for redness, pain, swelling at all invasive sites; dressing changes of invasive lines should occur every 48 hr or according to unit protocol.<br>– Culture catheter tips. | ∘ Infection presents a serious stressor capable of inducing circulatory collapse if untreated.<br>∘ Steroids suppress the immune response and place patient at greater risk of developing infection; the anti-inflammatory effects of steroids may mask signs of infection by decreasing pain, swelling, redness, and other signs of infection. |

*(continued)*

**TABLE 18–3. CARE PLAN FOR THE PATIENT IN ADRENAL CRISIS (ADDISONIAN CRISIS) *(Continued)***

| Nursing Diagnoses | Desired Patient Outcomes | Nursing Interventions | Rationales |
|---|---|---|---|
| ***Nursing Diagnosis #6 (cont.)*** | | | |
| | 4. Lungs clear to auscultation; chest x-ray without infiltrates.<br>5. Cultures negative: Blood, urine, sputum, wound, intravenous access sites. | | ○ Temperature may be low grade or normal and may not reflect an underlying infectious process. Antipyretic agents may be prescribed. |
| ***Nursing Diagnosis #7***<br>Oral mucous membranes, alteration, related to:<br>1. Dehydrated state. (See Table 23–3, Nursing Diagnosis #2.) | Mucous membranes will remain moist and intact. | • Provide comfort measures.<br>○ Assist in personal hygiene. | • Measures need to be implemented to maximize circulatory and pulmonary functions while conserving energy; such measures may help to reduce risk of infection. |

*(continued)*

| | | | |
|---|---|---|---|
| ***Nursing Diagnosis #8***<br>Skin integrity, impairment: Potential.<br>(See Table 23–3, Nursing Diagnosis #3.) | Skin will remain intact with good turgor. | ∘ Assess integrity of skin for pressure areas, swelling, ecchymosis.<br>– Apply lotion.<br>∘ Assist with turning and positioning; apply antiembolic stockings.<br>∘ Encourage deep breathing.<br>∘ Passive range-of-motion exercises.<br>∘ Provide frequent rest periods. | ∘ Increase in capillary fragility is associated with protein wasting.<br>∘ Frequent turning and deep breathing assist in mobilizing pulmonary secretions and preventing atelectasis; these activities are helpful in preventing pulmonary complications including pneumonia or pulmonary embolism.<br>∘ Limited musculoskeletal activities maintain muscle tone and decrease resorption of bone calcium; such activities improve circulation and increase venous return. |
| ***Nursing Diagnosis #9***<br>Self-concept, alteration in: Body image, related to:<br>1. Increased pigmentation.<br>2. Hirsutism.<br>3. Fat distribution: "moon face," "buffalo hump," masculinizing (women), gynecomastia (men). | Patient will verbalize concerns/feelings regarding body changes. | • Encourage verbalization of fears and concerns regarding body changes.<br>• Exhibit acceptance of patient as individual.<br>• Offer reassurance; be accessible. | • It may help identify problems or areas of concern.<br>• Encourages patient to talk about self. |

## REFERENCES

1. Hershman, JM: Endocrine Pathophysiology: A Patient-Oriented Approach, ed 2. Lea & Febiger, Philadelphia, 1988, p 115.
2. Guyton, A: Textbook of Medical Physiology, ed 7. WB Saunders, Philadelphia, 1986, p 913.
3. Martin, CR: Endocrine Physiology. Oxford University Press, New York, 1985, p 216.
4. Vander, A, Sherman, J, and Luciano, D: Human Physiology: The Mechanisms of Body Function, ed 4. McGraw-Hill, New York, 1985, pp 217, 245, 249.
5. Metz, R and Larson, EB: Blue Book of Endocrinology. WB Saunders, Philadelphia, 1985, p 53.

CHAPTER 19

# Nursing Management of the Patient with Endocrine Pancreas Dysfunction: Diabetic Ketoacidosis and Hyperglycemic, Hyperosmolar, Nonketotic Coma

## CHAPTER OUTLINE



## LEARNING OBJECTIVES

**At the end of this chapter, you should be able to:**

1. Describe the pancreas and its structure and function.
2. Define the metabolic states: Absorptive and postabsorptive.
3. Describe the regulation and control of body metabolism and energy utilization.
4. List the major functions of insulin and its effects on specific body mechanisms.
5. Describe the regulation of insulin secretion.
6. Distinguish the major function of glucagon and its effects on specific body mechanisms.
7. Describe the regulation of glucagon secretion.
8. Define diabetic ketoacidosis and examine its pathophysiology, etiology, clinical presentation, and treatment.
9. Define hyperglycemic, hyperosmolar, nonketotic coma, and examine its pathophysiology, etiology, clinical presentation, and treatment.
10. Delineate the nursing process in caring for the patient with diabetic ketoacidosis including:
    Assessment.
    Nursing diagnosis.
    Planning: Desired patient outcomes
    Nursing interventions/rationales.

## BODY METABOLISM AND ENERGY UTILIZATION

Energy within the body and between the body and the environment is maintained in a dynamic equilibrium. Intake of energy in the form of food must be sufficient to replace the energy expended by the various physiologic activities. Energy expenditure includes, for example, the utilization of ATP (adenosine triphosphate) to perform work, the dissipation of energy as heat, and net molecular synthesis with energy storage.

Metabolism reflects the ability of the body to capture and store the energy derived from foods and to make that energy available in the appropriate form when needed. Through metabolic processes the chemical energy in foodstuffs is transformed into other forms of energy necessary for physiologic activities. These forms of energy include mechanical (e.g., muscle contraction, active transport), electrical (e.g., action potential initiation and transmission), and chemical (e.g., synthetic reactions).

Metabolism encompasses the total collection of chemical reactions in the body. *Anabolic* reactions occur during the absorptive state (i.e., food ingestion) and involve a net synthesis of the major endogenous (i.e., within the body) energy sources, including glycogen, body protein, and triglycerides; *catabolic* reactions occur during the postabsorptive state (i.e., fasting state, as, for example, between meals) and involve a net breakdown of these sources with release of energy.

Efficient management of energy resources requires a precise control and integration of these metabolic processes. The endocrine pancreas, through its synthesis and secretion of the hormones, insulin and glucagon, plays a major role in regulating metabolic processes and utilizing energy.

## PANCREAS: STRUCTURE AND FUNCTION

The pancreas serves two functions: digestive and hormonal. Its digestive function is served by the *exocrine* portion of the gland within which digestive juices and enzymes are elaborated and carried via ducts to the duodenum (see Unit Seven); its hormonal function is carried on by the *endocrine* (ductless) portion, the secretions of which play a significant role in the control of carbohydrate metabolism in the body.

The pancreas is comprised of two major tissue types. *Acinar* tissue (exocrine function) is composed of many lobules bound together by loose connective tissue through which pass blood vessels, nerves, lymphatics, and the excretory ductal system, which carries digestive secretions to the duodenum; and the *islets of Langerhans* (endocrine function), well-defined and richly vascularized small clusters of endocrine cells scattered throughout the exocrine portion of the pancreas. These cells are responsible for synthesizing and secreting the hormones, insulin, glucagon, and somatostatin, directly into the blood. These hormones function to regulate activities of the absorptive and postabsorptive metabolic states.

The islets of Langerhans contain distinct cell types. The A (alpha) cells are the source of glucagon; the B (beta) cells are the source of insulin; and the D (delta) cells are the source of somatostatin.

In addition to being a highly vascular organ, the pancreas has a diffuse lymphatic system with direct drainage of lymph between the duodenum and pancreas. This continuity between the duodenum and pancreas via the lymphatic system explains the frequent involvement of both organs in carcinoma.

The pancreas receives dual innervation via the autonomic nervous system. The parasympathetic branch innervates the smooth muscles of the pancreatic ducts, facilitating passage of digestive juices and enzymes into the duodenum in response to eating. The sympathetic branch innervates the pancreatic acini and islets of Langerhans. Sympathetic innervation, together with circulating epinephrine from the adrenal medulla, stimulates glucagon secretion by alpha cells, while inhibiting the secretion of insulin by the beta cells. These systems together with the hormones, insulin, glucagon, and somatostatin, play a significant role in the regulation of body metabolism and energy utilization. (For additional discussion of pancreatic structure and function, see Chap. 47. Also see Fig. 47–8.)

## METABOLIC STATES: ABSORPTIVE AND POSTABSORPTIVE STATES

The absorptive and postabsorptive states are the two functional states that encompass the mechanisms involved in overall body metabolism. The absorptive or "eating" state reflects the digestive period during which nutrients are ingested, digested, and absorbed from the gastrointestinal tract into the blood. The postabsorptive or "fasting" state reflects the nondigestive period occurring between meals, during which the gastrointestinal tract is empty and energy must be supplied by the body's endogenous stores.[1]

During the absorptive state endogenous energy stores are revitalized with the resynthesis of body proteins and structural fats. Glucose is the major energy provider during this period with only a very small fraction of ingested amino acids and fats used for this purpose. Most amino acids and fats, as well as carbohydrates not used for energy, are converted to fat and stored in adipose tissue for use as the major energy source during the postabsorptive state.

In contrast to the absorptive state, the postabsorptive state is characterized by a net breakdown or catabolism of body protein and structural fat. The oxidation of endogenous fat stores provides the major source of energy, whereas the use of carbohydrates for this purpose is greatly reduced.

The major consideration during the postabsorptive state is the fact that neural and retinal tissues, for the most part, use only glucose as their main source of energy. Therefore, it is during this state that physiologic processes, including the endocrine and neural regulation of body metabolism, have as their top priority the maintenance of serum glucose at concentrations sufficient to meet the nutritive needs of vital tissues.

During the postabsorptive, or fasting, state, activities that function in this capacity include the mobilization of endogenous stores of glucose and glucose-sparing by the utilization of fat for energy.[2] Endogenous sources of glucose include glycogen stores in liver and muscle, and catabolism of triglyceride stores into glycerol and fatty acids. Once liberated from adipose tissue, glycerol circulates to the liver, which converts it into glucose with subsequent release into the blood.

During prolonged fasting, the major endogenous source of glucose is body protein. Via the process of gluconeogenesis in the liver, glucose is synthesized from amino acids liberated by the proteolysis (i.e., breakdown) of body protein. Glucose derived in this manner is then released into the blood by the liver. The catabolism of body protein and its utilization as the major substrate for glucose synthesis during the prolonged fasting state largely account for the muscle wasting and weakness associated with this state.

### Glucose-Sparing by Fat Utilization

The utilization of fat as the primary energy source with concomitant sparing of glucose stores is an essential modification that takes place in the transition from the absorptive to postabsorptive state. While nerve tissue continues to use glucose, nearly all other tissues significantly reduce their use of this major energy source. Thus, serum glucose concentrations are preserved as glucose derived via gluconeogenesis and released into the blood becomes available to meet the nearly exclusive continuous energy needs of neural tissue alone. (The exceptions are retinal and germinal tissues, and red blood cells, which also use glucose as their major energy source.)

### Metabolism of Triglycerides with Ketone Body Formation

Fatty acids, liberated along with glycerol in the catabolism of triglycerides in adipose tissue, are taken up by nearly all tissues (except neural tissue), which metabolize these fatty acids to carbon dioxide and water with the release of energy. The liver also metabolizes fatty acids as its energy source.

In addition, hepatic ketogenic pathways are activated wherein fatty acids are oxidized to form *ketone bodies.* These include beta-hydroxybutyric acid, acetoacetic acid, and acetone. In the presence of insulin, ketone bodies circulating in the blood provide an important energy source for many of the body's peripheral tissues during the fasting state.

When a deficiency or lack of insulin exists, peripheral metabolism of ketones is impaired, and these organic acids accumulate in unusually large quantities in blood and body fluids, a condition called *ketosis.* This impaired ketone metabolism associated with an insulin lack, coupled with the continued production and release of ketone bodies by the liver, exhausts the compensatory capabilities of body buffers, and a severe metabolic acidosis evolves. If untreated, it can lead to coma and death. These events underlie the pathogenesis of diabetic ketoacidosis (see below).

## REGULATION AND CONTROL OF BODY METABOLISM AND ENERGY UTILIZATION

The transition from absorptive to postabsorptive states, the shift from glucose utilization to fat utilization, the determination as to whether nutrients are stored, oxidized, or converted to another form, are all largely controlled by the actions of the pancreatic hormones, insulin and glucagon.

As an anabolic hormone, insulin functions to increase body energy stores through synthesis of glycogen, body proteins, and triglycerides. Glucagon, a catabolic hormone, mobilizes energy from these stores to fuel vital physiologic activities. At any given moment, the overall status of energy stores in the body is reflected by the ratio of these two hormones. The storage tendency and positive nitrogen balance of the body in the healthy individual suggests that this ratio favors to a greater extent the anabolic effects of insulin.[3]

Other hormones within the body also influence metabolism. Thyroid hormones, glucocorticoids (adrenal cortex), and growth hormone (anterior pituitary) exert a regulatory effect on metabolic processes. Thyroid hormones function to control the metabolic rates of anabolism and catabolism, and the transformation of energy into its various forms for cellular utilization. Glucocorticoids regulate intermediary metabolism and maintain serum glucose at concentrations necessary to meet metabolic needs. Growth hormone exerts a hyperglycemic effect, increasing serum glucose levels.

The hormone somatostatin, secreted by the delta cells within the islets of Langerhans, is also secreted along with insulin during the absorptive state. It functions to constrain rates of digestion and absorption in the gastrointestinal tract to prevent delivery of excessive loads of nutrients into the blood. It also has the capacity to inhibit secretions of both insulin and glucagon. Somatostatin is analogous to growth hormone-inhibiting hormone (GHIH) secreted by the hypothalamus (see Table 14-1).

Other factors influencing metabolism include epinephrine, secreted by the adrenal medulla, and sympathetic innervation to the pancreas, liver, and adipose tissue. The sympathetic influence is to inhibit insulin secretion during periods of exercise or stress.

## Insulin: Major Functions

Insulin acts directly or indirectly on most cells of the body with the exception of neural tissue. Two general categories of change attributed to the actions of insulin include alterations in membrane transport and in enzymatic activities. Insulin stimulates the *facilitated diffusion* of glucose into most cells of the body, particularly cells of muscle and adipose tissue (notable exceptions include the brain and liver). It also stimulates the active transport of amino acids into most cells, increasing the availability of these nutrients for protein synthesis. As a result of the enhanced membrane transport induced by insulin, glucose is used as the major energy source, and a net synthesis of glycogen, body protein, and triglycerides ensues.

This absorptive-state pattern is duplicated by the effects of insulin on enzymatic activities. Insulin modifies the activities and/or concentrations of many intracellular enzymes involved in anabolic and catabolic reactions. Among these are glucokinase, phosphofructokinase, and glycogen synthetase, all of which function in glycogenesis (i.e., formation of glycogen from glucose). Concomitantly, insulin inhibits the enzyme, phosphorylase, which catalyzes glycogenolysis (i.e., the breakdown of glycogen). In this way, insulin helps to maintain glycogen stores.

Insulin stimulates protein synthesis by enhancing uptake of amino acids by most cells and stimulating the activity of ribosomal enzymes, which increases the translation of messenger-RNA necessary for protein synthesis. Concomitantly, insulin inhibits almost all the critical enzymes that catalyze gluconeogenesis (i.e., formation of glycogen from noncarbohydrate sources such as amino acids and fatty acids). This maintains body protein stores because amino acids are the substrate most often used for synthesis of glucose. It is important to note that, unlike glucose (glycogen) and fatty acids (triglycerides), there is no storage form of protein. Thus, excess protein is used to synthesize glucose or is converted to triglycerides, the storage form of fat.

Similarly, insulin acts to enhance body stores of fat in the form of triglycerides, while inhibiting enzymes (e.g., lipase) that might function otherwise to break down fat stores.

Insulin has little to no direct effect on uptake and utilization of glucose by brain tissue. Brain cells are permeable to glucose without any mediation by insulin; they rely primarily on the concentration of glucose in the blood. Therefore, a certain minimal serum glucose level must be maintained at all times. The hypoglycemic effects of insulin may indirectly impact on brain function. An excess of insulin may precipitate hypoglycemic shock (see Chap. 20). The clinical manifestations of hypoglycemic shock include progressive irritability, fainting, seizure activity, and coma, all of which are reflective of the consequent alteration in brain function.

## Regulation of Insulin Secretion

Direct and precise regulation of insulin secretion involves the serum glucose concentration flowing through the pancreas. Changes in serum glucose levels are sensed very quickly as entry into beta cells of the islets of Langerhans is unaffected by insulin. It involves a simple negative feedback mechanism wherein an increase in serum glucose concentration stimulates insulin secretion; insulin reduces serum glucose levels by stimulating rapid entry of glucose into cells and decreasing the glucose output by the liver. These activities, in turn, reduce the serum glucose concentration and thereby remove the stimulus for insulin secretion, which returns to normal.

An elevation in serum levels of certain amino acids causes an enhanced secretion of insulin. Insulin promotes membrane transport of amino acids into cells and also stimulates intracellular protein synthesis.

Other factors influencing insulin secretion include the activity of thyroid, growth, and gastrointestinal hormones, and autonomic nervous system innervation. (For additional information about the distinguishing features of insulin, its physiologic activity, and the regulation of that activity, see Table 19-1.)

### Serum Glucose Levels

The physiologic effects of insulin and regulation of its secretion are so finely tuned that the serum glucose concentration is maintained within very narrow limits: 70-110 mg/100 ml (fasting). Precise control of insulin secretion and serum glucose levels is necessary for adequate brain function. A serum glucose level less than 70 mg/100 ml can cause changes in the level of consciousness; at levels less than 20 mg/100 ml, coma ensues.

### Renal Handling of Glucose

Glucose is filtered by the renal glomerulus and almost completely reabsorbed in the proximal tubule providing its serum concentrations do not exceed

TABLE 19–1
## Distinguishing Features and Functions of Insulin and Glucagon

| | Insulin | Glucagon |
|---|---|---|
| Origin of hormone: Synthesis/secretion | Beta cells within the islets of Langerhans (pancreas) | Alpha cells within the islets of Langerhans (pancreas) |
| Overall effect on target tissues | Anabolic hormone functions to decrease serum glucose and fatty acid concentrations<br>Net increase in glycogen, body protein, and triglyceride stores<br>Promotes absorptive state | Catabolic hormone functions to increase serum glucose and fatty acid concentrations<br>Net decrease in glycogen, body protein, and triglyceride stores<br>Promotes postabsorptive state |
| Major stimulus for hormone release | Elevated serum glucose concentrations as occurs during eating or absorptive state<br>Amino acids | Reduced serum glucose concentrations as occurs in fasting or postabsorptive state<br>Ingestion of amino acids: Arginine, alanine<br>Hormones: Pancreozymin, epinephrine |
| Major inhibition of hormone release | Fasting or postabsorptive state; hypoglycemia | Eating or absorptive state; hyperglycemia and increased free fatty acid levels<br>Hormones: somatostatin and insulin |
| Other factors affecting hormone secretion<br>Serum amino acid levels | Elevated serum levels increase insulin secretion | Elevated serum levels of amino acids strongly stimulate glucagon secretion. (This is of major adaptive value because the hyperglycemic effects of glucagon offset potential hypoglycemic effects of insulin.) |
| Autonomic nervous system:<br>Parasympathetic | Stimulates insulin secretion during eating or absorptive state | |
| Sympathetic | Inhibits insulin secretion | Stimulates glucagon secretion into bloodstream |
| Hormonal influence:<br>Epinephrine (adrenal medulla) | Inhibits insulin secretion during exercise or "stress" | Stimulates glucagon secretion during exercise, "stress," or postabsorptive state via its hyperglycemic effects:<br>Increased glycogenolysis in liver<br>Increased gluconeogenesis in liver<br>Increased lipolysis in adipose tissue<br>Enhanced utilization of fatty acids for energy by most cells |
| Cortisol (adrenal cortex) | Exerts a hyperglycemic effect via increased gluconeogenesis in liver; insulin antagonist | |
| Thyroid and growth hormones | Insulin acts in a synergistic capacity with these hormones to increase uptake of amino acids to promote growth | |
| Gastrointestinal hormones:<br>Gastrin<br>Cholecystokinin<br>Gastric inhibitory peptide | Increased secretion of these hormones in response to eating and absorptive state stimulates insulin secretion | Gastrointestinal factors whose release is triggered by protein ingestion increase glucagon secretion |
| Target cells | Most cells, but primarily liver, muscle, and adipose tissue; major exceptions include neural tissue, retina, and germinal tissue | Target cells include liver and adipose tissue |
| Mechanism of action | Basically unknown; it is known that insulin binds to its specific receptor-protein on the surface of plasma membranes; the insulin-receptor complex triggers a sequence of intracellular events, which ultimately reflect insulin's effect on membrane transport and enzymatic activity | Thought to involve activation of adenyl cyclase with generation of cyclic AMP as the "second messenger." Glucagon interacts with a specific receptor on the plasma membrane, which triggers the activation of adenyl cyclase with a rise in intracellular cyclic AMP. Through a cascade system, cAMP activates protein kinase and phosphorylase, which break down liver glycogen stores. |

*(continued)*

TABLE 19-1
**Distinguishing Features and Functions of Insulin and Glucagon *(Continued)***

| | Insulin | Glucagon |
|---|---|---|
| Metabolism | Insulin is rapidly (within minutes) removed from blood and degraded by the liver | Glucagon is metabolized primarily by the liver |
| Serum glucose levels | Normal fasting: 70–110 mg/100 ml<br>Hyperglycemia: >110 mg/100 ml<br>Hypoglycemia: 40–70 mg/100 ml | |
| Renal threshold for glucose | Normal threshold: ~160–180 mg/100 ml<br>Serum glucose: >180 mg/100 ml results in glycosuria | |
| Major actions | Significant physiologic effects:<br>A. Enhanced membrane transport of glucose and amino acids into most cells via facilitated diffusion and active transport, respectively<br>B. Duplication of absorptive state pattern via effects on enzymatic activities<br>C. Specific actions:<br>1. *Glycogen synthesis:*<br>• Stimulates glucose uptake and utilization via the enzymes:<br>Glucokinase<br>Phosphofructokinase<br>Glycogen synthetase<br>• Inhibits phosphorylase, the enzyme that catalyzes glycogenolysis<br>2. *Protein synthesis:*<br>• Enhances amino acid uptake by most cells, increasing activity of ribosomal enzymes necessary for protein synthesis; inhibits enzymes that catalyze gluconeogenesis in liver<br>3. *Triglyceride synthesis* (storage form of fat):<br>• Enhances uptake of glucose by adipose tissue; insulin acts as a "fat-sparer" by increasing cellular utilization of glucose for energy<br>*Note:* These actions of insulin occur within minutes of tissue exposure to insulin. | Significant physiologic effects:<br>A. Glucagon exerts its hyperglycemia effect by:<br>1. Increasing glycogenolysis in the liver by activating the enzyme phosphorylase<br>2. Stimulating hepatic gluconeogenesis and ketogenesis<br>B. Glucagon stimulates increased lipolysis in adipose tissue releasing:<br>1. Glycerol—A subtrate for gluconeogenesis in the liver<br>2. Fatty acids—A major energy source for most cells<br>C. Additional effects of glucagon (if present in increased amounts) include:<br>• Enhanced myocardial strength<br>• Increased bile secretion<br>• Increased secretion of calcitonin<br>• Inhibition of gastric acid secretion<br>D. Glucagon is a major insulin antagonist; insulin, on the other hand, inhibits glucagon release |
| Major control mechanisms of hormonal secretion: | Negative feedback mechanism: | Negative feedback mechanism: |
| Serum glucose levels | "Reflex" pathway wherein beta cells in the islets of Langerhans monitor serum glucose levels of blood perfusing the pancreas:<br>↑ serum glucose = ↑ insulin release<br>↓ serum glucose = ↓ insulin release | "Reflex" pathway wherein alpha cells in the islets Langerhans monitor serum glucose levels of blood perfusing the pancreas:<br>↑ serum glucose = ↓ glucagon release<br>↓ serum glucose = ↑ glucagon release |
| Serum amino acid levels | An increase in amino acid serum concentration stimulates insulin release with increased amino acid uptake by most cells:<br>↑ amino acids in serum = ↑ insulin secretion | Similar effect to that with insulin; glucagon secretion is strongly stimulated by a rise in serum amino acid concentration:<br>↑ amino acids in serum = ↑ glucagon secretion |
| Gastrointestinal hormones | In the presence of food these hormones stimulate insulin release—an "anticipatory" component of glucose regulation, which serves to ensure sufficient and timely availability of insulin | |
| Other hormones:<br>Cortisol<br>Thyroid hormones<br>Growth hormone | Effects on glucose metabolism and insulin secretion are listed above | |

*(continued)*

TABLE 19-1
**Distinguishing Features and Functions of Insulin and Glucagon *(Continued)***

| | Insulin | Glucagon |
|---|---|---|
| Neural control: | | |
| Parasympathetic | This innervation is activated during eating and stimulates insulin secretion. It constitutes another type of "anticipatory" regulation | |
| Sympathetic and epinephrine effects | Inhibits insulin secretion during exercise or stress | Stimulates glucagon secretion during exercise or stress |
| Insulin/glucagon ratio[4] | The insulin/glucagon (I/G) ratio reflects the overall status of energy stores in the body at any given time.<br>1. Under normal physiologic conditions the I/G ratio is 2.3/1. This ratio reflects the absorptive, anabolic state with a net storage tendency and a positive nitrogen balance.<br>2. Elevation of the I/G ratio reflects an increased anabolic state with weight gain. Secretion of insulin is enhanced by the "overfed" state.<br>3. A reduction in the I/G ratio reflects a catabolic state with weight loss. Secretion of glucagon is enhanced by fasting or "underfed" state. | |

180 mg/100 ml. The normal renal threshold for glucose is defined by a serum glucose concentration of 160–180 mg/100 ml. When the serum glucose concentration rises above the critical level, glycosuria occurs. The excretion of excess glucose load is accompanied by the excretion of water (i.e., osmotic diuresis) and electrolytes. These mechanisms figure very strongly in the pathophysiology underlying diabetic ketoacidosis and hyperglycemic, hyperosmolar, nonketotic coma (see below).

## Glucagon: Major Functions

The major effects of glucagon on body metabolism are opposite to those of insulin. Glucagon's overall effect is to increase serum glucose and fatty acid concentrations, and in this regard it is a critically important hormone secreted during the postabsorptive state.

As a catabolic hormone, glucagon exerts its hyperglycemic effect via two mechanisms: one, glucagon increases serum glucose levels via breakdown of liver glycogen (glycogenolysis); and two, glucagon largely stimulates glucose synthesis in the liver via gluconeogenesis. Glucagon also stimulates breakdown of triglyceride stores in adipose tissue (lipolysis), releasing glycerol (substrate for gluconeogenesis) and fatty acids (energy substrate for cellular utilization).

## Regulation of Glucagon Secretion

The major stimulus for glucagon secretion is a decreasing serum glucose concentration. This induces increased secretion of glucagon, which by its catabolic effects on glycogen and triglycerides serves to restore serum glucose levels while also supplying cells with fatty acids to meet their energy needs. Glucagon secretion, like that of insulin, is also strongly stimulated by an increase in the serum amino acid concentration. In this regard, the activity of glucagon is *identical* rather than opposite to that of insulin. The adaptive value and clinical significance of this relationship between serum amino acid levels and glucagon become apparent when one considers dietary intake.

During absorption of a high-carbohydrate, low-protein meal, insulin secretion alone increases in response to the rise in serum glucose. Conversely, during absorption of a low-carbohydrate, high-protein meal, secretion of glucagon, in addition to insulin, also occurs in response to the increased amino acid load. The increase in insulin secretion in the presence of a limited amount of absorbed carbohydrate could cause a marked and sudden drop in serum glucose, placing the individual at risk of developing a hypoglycemic reaction. In the presence of increased glucagon secretion this does not occur because the hyperglycemic effects of glucagon offset the hypoglycemic effects of insulin, and the net result is a stable serum glucose level. Thus, glucagon helps to protect against hypoglycemia.

In addition to low serum glucose levels (<70 mg/100 ml) and high serum concentrations of amino acids, the secretion of glucagon, like that of insulin, is controlled by autonomic nervous system innervation. Contrary to its effect on insulin, sympathetic activation stimulates glucagon secretion, an effect of considerable adaptive importance for exercise and stress. (For additional information about the distinguishing features of glucagon, and a contrast between insulin and glucagon, see Table 19-1.)

## PATHOPHYSIOLOGY: DIABETIC KETOACIDOSIS AND HYPERGLYCEMIC, HYPEROSMOLAR, NONKETOTIC COMA

### Diabetic Ketoacidosis (DKA)

Diabetic ketoacidosis (DKA) is an acute metabolic disorder in which the underlying pathophysiologic processes are attributed to an absolute or relative lack of insulin. It usually requires emergency treatment with insulin, intravenous fluids, electrolyte replacement, and other support measures. The hallmarks of diabetic ketoacidosis include hyperglycemia, glycosuria, uncontrolled lipolysis, ketogenesis, and unrestrained gluconeogenesis with loss of nitrogen and potassium. Details of these pathophysiologic mechanisms and the underlying hormonal alterations are presented in Table 19–2.

As a result of the altered metabolism associated with insulin insufficiency, profound changes occur in fluid, electrolyte, and acid–base balance. Hyperglycemia predisposes to intracellular and extracellular dehydration. Initially, the extracellular fluid volume is maintained at the expense of intracellular fluid volume because the hyperosmolality of the extracellular fluid causes a shift of intracellular fluid into the extracellular compartment. When the degree of hyperglycemia causes the filtered load to exceed a critical level (i.e., the renal threshold; serum glucose levels > 180 mg/100 ml), glycosuria occurs, accompanied by fluid loss and extracellular dehydration.

The pivotal factor, therefore, predisposing to total body dehydration is the renal handling of glucose excretion. Under normal physiologic conditions with adequate intravascular volume and an appropriate glucose load, all glucose filtered is reabsorbed from the renal tubules back into the blood. If, however, the glucose load exceeds the reabsorptive capacity (renal threshold) of the renal tubules, the excess glucose is excreted in the urine along with profound water and sodium losses (i.e., an osmotic diuresis).

Uncontrolled lipolysis with a consequent excessive ketogenesis further aggravates hyponatremia and induces a marked acidemia. Production of ketone bodies, acetoacetic acid, beta-hydroxybutyric acid, and acetone increases the hydrogen ion concentration in the blood, causing the pH to decrease markedly.

The kidneys initially attempt to conserve sodium and to correct the acidemia by increasing sodium available for hydrogen-ion exchange in the distal tubules and by excreting the ammonium salts of ketoacids. In the presence of severe osmotic diuresis, however, these renal compensatory mechanisms are inadequate and a profound acidemia ensues. Hypovolemia and associated pre-renal azotemia also ensue. Hypovolemic shock reduces tissue perfusion, causing severe tissue hypoxia. The hypoxic state necessitates that cells shift to anaerobic glycolysis with consequent lactate formation. This further aggravates the underlying metabolic acidemia and acidosis.

Etiologic factors and circumstances in which DKA is likely to occur are listed in Table 19–3. Also included in this table are clinical data related to the assessment and diagnostic workup of the patient with DKA, including the patient's clinical history, physical examination, laboratory data, and differential diagnosis.

#### *Clinical Presentation*

DKA can be classified as mild, moderate, or severe (Table 19–4). Specific clinical manifestations reflective of underlying pathophysiologic mechanisms are also considered in Table 19–3.

#### *Treatment*

Prevention is the best treatment for DKA. The key to prevention is patient/family education about the underlying disease process and the antidiabetic therapy regimen instituted. Appropriate education helps to prevent ketoacidosis and/or ensures that its symptomatology will be recognized early and treatment instituted before serious complications occur. In the acute setting, therapy is focused on the following goals:

1. Restore fluid balance.
2. Restore effective carbohydrate, fat, and protein metabolism using insulin therapy.
3. Restore electrolyte and acid–base balance.
4. Diagnose and treat underlying cause.
5. Maintain function of related systems and prevent complications.
6. Assess patient/family knowledge of diabetes mellitus and its management. Initiate and implement appropriate self-care educational programs. (Specific treatment considerations are listed in Table 19–3.)

#### *Nursing Care of the Patient with Diabetic Ketoacidosis (DKA)*

Full-blown DKA is an acute medical emergency requiring expedient, skillful, and meticulous bedside care if the patient is to survive.

**Therapeutic Goals.** Implementation of nursing process in the care of the patient with DKA revolves around the following therapeutic goals:

1. Identify the patient at risk of developing DKA.
2. Establish a thorough and comprehensive data base including:
   A. Clinical history (functional health patterns).
   B. Physical examination.

TABLE 19–2
## Hallmarks of Diabetic Ketoacidosis (DKA)

| Hallmarks of DKA | Underlying Pathophysiologic Mechanisms | Underlying Hormonal Activity (Normal) Effects of Insulin Lack |
|---|---|---|
| Hyperglycemia | Increased hepatic glucose production via:<br>Enhanced glycogenolysis<br>Enhanced gluconeogenesis<br>Reduced peripheral uptake of glucose particularly in muscle and adipose tissue | Insulin effect: Inhibits net release of glucose by the liver<br>Insulin lack: Results in increased hepatic glucose production and release into bloodstream<br>Excess catabolic hormones (glucagon, epinephrine, cortisol) catalyze gluconeogenesis |
| Glycosuria | Glucose load exceeds renal threshold resulting in osmotic diuresis | |
| Uncontrolled lipolysis (i.e., the decomposition of fat) | Enhanced lipolysis of stored triglycerides catalyzed by hormone-dependent enzyme, lipase<br>Excessive free fatty acid mobilization and release from peripheral adipose tissue stores | Insulin effect: Lipogenic; inhibits lipolytic effect of lipase<br>Insulin lack: Increased lipase activity<br>Excess catabolic hormones stimulate lipase activity |
| Ketogenesis (i.e., production of ketone bodies) | Suppression of fatty acid synthesis greatly enhances hepatic fatty acid oxidation and the generation of acetyl-CoA<br>Excess acetyl-CoA is converted to ketone bodies: acetoacetic acid, beta-hydroxybutyric acid, acetone | Insulin effect: Stimulates incorporation of fatty acids into triglycerides for storage in adipose tissue<br>Insulin lack coupled with excess glucagon: Inhibition of long chain fatty acid synthesis |
| Ketonemia (i.e., acetone bodies in blood) | Enhanced availability of free fatty acids in blood<br>Decreased utilization of ketones by peripheral tissues<br>Inability of peripheral tissues to use the by-products of fat catabolism at a rate equal to their production leads to accumulation of ketones[5] and diabetic ketoacidosis | Insulin lack: Peripheral tissues unable to use excess ketones |
| Negative nitrogen balance; hypokalemia[6] | Loss of anabolic effect of insulin with greatly reduced protein synthesis<br>Increased proteolysis with greatly enhanced release of amino acids and potassium from muscle cells into blood<br>Enhanced gluconeogenesis in liver<br>*Initial* hypokalemia as kidneys excrete excess potassium lost from muscle | Under basal absorptive circumstances there is always a net leakage or efflux of amino acids and potassium from skeletal muscle<br>Insulin effect: Exerts a "tonic-restraining" effect, which minimizes the extent of this leakage<br>Insulin lack: Intracellular protein synthesis curtailed; increased proteolysis<br>Excess glucagon stimulates gluconeogenesis in liver cells |
| Hyperkalemia | *Later,* associated reduction in plasma volume reduces renal blood flow and glomerular filtration, resulting in impaired potassium excretion and hyperkalemia<br>There is a shift of potassium out of cells into extracellular fluid in the presence of acidemia<br>Total body potassium deficit exists even in presence of hyperkalemia<br>Increased aldosterone levels associated with activation of the renin–angiotensin system in response to volume deficit causes further loss of potassium | |

TABLE 19–3

**Contrast: Diabetic Ketoacidosis (DKA) and Hyperglycemic, Hyperosmolar, Nonketotic Coma (HHNK)**

| | **Diabetic Ketoacidosis** | **Hyperglycemic, Hyperosmolar, Nonketotic Coma** |
|---|---|---|
| *Definition* | DKA is an acute metabolic disorder in which the major underlying hormonal abnormality is an absolute or relative insulin deficiency. DKA is a syndrome associated with severe, uncontrolled diabetes and characterized by hyperglycemia, ketonemia, fluid and electrolyte imbalance, and a negative nitrogen balance. | HHNK is a syndrome associated with a relative insulin deficit and characterized by marked hyperglycemia and minimal to absent ketonemia. The patient has sufficient insulin to prevent fatty acid breakdown but inadequate amounts for carbohydrate metabolism. Thus, this syndrome is characterized by severe hyperglycemia and hyperosmolality without significant ketoacidosis. |
| *Clinical setting/epidemiology* | DKA occurs most frequently in patients with type I insulin-dependent diabetes (IDDM). | HHNK occurs most frequently in patients with type II non-insulin-dependent diabetes (NIDDM). |
| Age | Young population | Middle-aged or elderly |
| Onset | Sudden or gradual | Gradual, several days to weeks |
| Previous history of diabetes | 85% | 60% |
| Drug history | Usually take insulin | Use of oral hypoglycemics; insulin usually not necessary. Other drugs taken for associated or chronic illness: Thiazide diuretics, furosemide, glucocorticoids, propranolol, cimetidine, or ranitidine |
| Frequency of occurrence | DKA six times more common than HHNK | |
| Precipitating illness | Usually a factor | Usually a factor |
| Mortality | 15% annually; directly linked to degree of metabolic derangement | 40–70% annually |
| *Pathogenesis* | Pathogenesis of DKA is largely attributed to insulin lack, and an alteration in the balance between anabolic and catabolic hormonal influences.<br>Major pathophysiologic consequences:<br>Hyperglycemia, glucosuria<br>Excessive lipolysis<br>Ketogenesis<br>Unrestrained gluconeogenesis with loss of nitrogen and potassium<br>Fluid and electrolyte disturbances<br>Metabolic ketoacidosis<br>The underlying mechanism of these hallmarks of DKA is presented in Table 19–2. | Sequence of events in pathogenesis of HHNK:<br>Stressful event with release of stress hormones, glucagon, epinephrine, and cortisol. These hormones function to increase serum glucose levels.<br>Insulin deficiency diminishes transport of glucose into cells and hyperglycemia results.<br>Hyperglycemia causes (1) extreme hyperosmolality with fluid shifts from intra- to extracellular fluid compartments; (2) osmotic diuresis with fluid loss from extracellular compartments and a concomitant loss of serum electrolytes.<br>Dehydration and hypovolemic state reduce glomerular filtration rate and renal excretion of glucose load.<br>The result: Severe hyperglycemia, hyperosmolar, dehydrated state with associated electrolyte imbalance. |
| *Etiology* | DKA occurs most commonly as:<br>A. Initial presentation of a previously undiagnosed patient with diabetes mellitus<br>B. In the type I insulin-dependent (IDDM) patient who:<br>1. Omits an insulin dose or decreases the dose<br>2. Has uncontrolled diabetes with inadequate insulin coverage<br>3. Experiences a severe stress without appropriate adjustment in insulin coverage: | Precipitating causes of HHNK:<br>• Acute illness: Infection (e.g., pneumonia, sepsis, gastroenteritis), pancreatitis, cerebrovascular insult<br>• Chronic illness: Renal disease, compromised cardiovascular function<br>• Drugs: Thiazide, furosemide, Dilantin (phenytoin), propranolol, steroids (cortisol), diazoxide<br>• Procedures:<br>• Peritoneal dialysis with hypertonic glucose solution<br>• Hemodialysis |

*(continued)*

TABLE 19-3
**Contrast: Diabetic Ketoacidosis (DKA) and Hyperglycemic, Hyperosmolar, Nonketotic Coma (HHNK) *(Continued)***

| | Diabetic Ketoacidosis | Hyperglycemic, Hyperosmolar, Nonketotic Coma |
|---|---|---|
| | • Infection: Respiratory, urinary tract<br>• Gastrointestinal illness with nausea/vomiting and diarrhea<br>• Trauma, surgery, pregnancy<br>DKA occurs less commonly in the patient with type I insulin-dependent diabetes who:<br>A. Takes medications that can impair glucose metabolism:<br>1. Diuretics and antihypertensive agents<br>• Thiazides suppress insulin secretion.<br>• Furosemide may cause hyperglycemia by reducing serum potassium, which is necessary for glucose uptake by cells.<br>2. Glucagon and glucocorticoids have a catabolic effect and cause hyperglycemia via gluconeogenesis in the liver.<br>3. Catecholamines: Epinephrine, isoproterenol stimulate glycogenolysis and inhibit insulin secretion.<br>4. Psychotropic drugs: Haloperidol, tricyclic antidepressants, phenothiazines, lithium carbonate<br>5. Analgesics, anti-inflammatory agents:<br>• Aspirin, acetaminophen<br>• Indomethacin<br>6. Anticonvulsants: Phenytoin suppresses insulin secretion; patients with diabetes mellitus should be carefully monitored for hyperglycemia.<br>7. Beta-adrenergic blocker, propranolol, may mask signs of insulin overdosage.<br>B. Has other illnesses (e.g., Addison's disease with corticosteroid replacement; acute pancreatitis; thyroid crisis<br>Other causes of DKA:<br>A. Salicylate intoxication<br>B. Alcohol intoxication<br>C. Total parenteral nutrition | • Total parenteral nutrition (TPN)<br>• Intravenous glucose in patient with severe burns<br>• General anesthesia<br>• Hypothermia<br>• Associated endocrinopathies:<br>• Cushing's syndrome<br>• Acromegaly<br>• Thyrotoxicosis |
| *Clinical Assessment:*<br>Clinical history | • Establish chief complaint. Frequently one of the classic symptoms of diabetes mellitus is mentioned: Polyuria, polydipsia, nausea/vomiting/diarrhea, epigastric discomfort, abdominal pain, leg cramps, weakness, weight loss?<br>• Determine state of prior health. Preexisting, previously diagnosed diabetes? Type I insulin-dependent (IDDM) or type II non-insulin-dependent (NIDDM)?<br>Number of years a known diabetic?<br>Therapeutic regimen: Daily insulin dosage? Oral hypoglycemic?<br>Diet? Exercise?<br>Medic-Alert bracelet or wallet card?<br>• In undiagnosed but suspected diabetes—Ascertain onset of illness. Acute, abrupt, of recent onset (type I presentation)? Vague, gradual course? Diagnosis made during treatment of unrelated illness (type II presentation)?<br>• Recent illness, trauma, or other stressor? Emotional or psychologic?<br>• Any associated illnesses—Renal disease, cardiac disease? Hypertension, obesity, other endocrine disorders—Addison's disease with glucocorticoid replacement therapy? Thyroid crisis? Acute pancreatitis? Hepatitis? | |

*(continued)*

TABLE 19–3
**Contrast: Diabetic Ketoacidosis (DKA) and Hyperglycemic, Hyperosmolar, Nonketotic Coma (HHNK) *(Continued)***

| | Diabetic Ketoacidosis | Hyperglycemic, Hyperosmolar, Nonketotic Coma |
|---|---|---|
| | • Medications other than insulin or oral hypoglycemics? Prescribed drugs—Diuretics, antihypertensives? Other? Over-the-counter drugs? Recreational drugs—Marijuana?<br>• Personal: Ascertain personal habits: Cigarette smoking—packs per day, for how long? Alcohol intake—What kind, how much, over how long a period of time? Sleep habits? Occupation, type of work? Stressors? Personality type: Role in family nucleus—dependent; decision-maker? Family resources? Coping capabilities? Health-care management?<br>• Determine family history: Diabetes mellitus, hypertension, obesity? Renal disease, coronary artery disease, hypertriglyceridemia, hypercholesterolemia?<br>• Knowledge of patient and family regarding disease? Its underlying pathophysiology, signs and symptoms, complications? Self-care—Self-administration of insulin, oral hypoglycemic, or other medication? Foot care? Skin care? Overall treatment regimen? Continued medical follow-up? | |
| Physical examination | • Neurologic status: Altered level of consciousness, lethargy, drowsiness, progressing to coma? Headache, visual disturbances, transient hemiparesis, diminished deep tendon reflexes, presence of Babinski's response? Anxiety?<br>• Cardiovascular status: Hypovolemic shock with hypotension, tachycardia, decreased cardiac output, postural hypotension? Decreased central venous (CVP), pulmonary artery (PAP), and pulmonary capillary wedge (PCWP) pressures? Reduced tissue perfusion? Hypoxia? Flushed skin (related to vasodilation caused by ketones)? Cardiac dysrhythmias?<br>• Signs of dehydration: Weakness, prostration? Hypothermia, gram-negative sepsis? Hyperthermia? Dry, crusty mucous membranes? Poor skin turgor over forehead or sternum? Soft or sunken eyeballs? Thready, weak pulses?<br>• Respiratory status: Air hunger, vigorous and rapid respirations (Kussmaul breathing) associated with pH <7.20? Presence of fruity odor of acetone to breath?<br>• Renal status: Presence of glycosuria with osmotic diuresis—Polyuria, oliguria, altered specific gravity? Odorous, cloudy urine? | |
| *Laboratory Data* | | |
| Serum tests: | | |
| Glucose | | |
| Range | 300–1200 mg/100 ml | 400–4000 mg/100 ml |
| Mean | 400–600 mg/100 ml | 800–1200 mg/ml |
| Fluid volume deficit: | | |
| Mild | 1–2 liters | Usually severe: Between 15% and 25% of total body water volume. |
| Moderate | 3–4 liters | |
| Severe | 5–8 liters | |
| Electrolytes | | |
| Potassium | Early hypo- to normokalemia not uncommon; later, hyperkalemia; total body deficit always present | Usually normal to slightly elevated initially; then hypokalemia with total body deficit |
| Sodium | Initial hypernatremia, but more commonly hyponatremia as sodium is lost in the osmotic diuresis | May be elevated, normal or low initially; then total body sodium deficit |
| Mild | >135 mEq/liter | Similar to values for DKA |
| Moderate | ~130 mEq/liter | |
| Severe | <130 mEq/liter | |
| Phosphorus | Hypophosphatemia <1.0 mg/100 ml | Hypophosphatemia |
| Magnesium | Initial hypermagnesemia, then hypomagnesemia | Similar to values for DKA |
| Calcium | Usually within normal physiologic range; with severe hypophosphatemia, hypercalcemia may occur. | Similar to values for DKA |
| BUN | Elevated with severe dehydration | Often markedly elevated: >80 mg/100 ml BUN/creatinine ratio >1:10 |
| Osmolality | <330 mOsm/kg | >330 mOsm/kg; mean ~405 mOsm/kg |
| Hematocrit | Elevated | Elevated |
| WBCs | Elevated | Elevated |
| Fatty acids | Markedly elevated | Minimally elevated |
| Arterial blood gases | pH <7.20; mean 7.07; $HCO_3^-$ <10 mEq/liter; markedly lowered in severe DKA | pH >7.20; mean 7.25; $HCO_3^-$ >10 mEq/liter; normal to moderately lowered |
| Anion gap | >15 mmol/liter | <15 mmol/liter |
| Ketonemia | Markedly elevated; acetone strongly positive | Usually normal |

*(continued)*

TABLE 19–3
**Contrast: Diabetic Ketoacidosis (DKA) and Hyperglycemic, Hyperosmolar, Nonketotic Coma (HHNK) *(Continued)***

| | **Diabetic Ketoacidosis** | **Hyperglycemic, Hyperosmolar, Nonketotic Coma** |
|---|---|---|
| Urine Studies | Glycosuria | Glycosuria |
| Ketonuria | Acetone elevated | Acetone normal |
| Proteinuria | Trace | Trace |
| Sodium | Decreased | Decreased |
| Chloride | Decreased | Decreased |
| Specific gravity | Elevated, > 1.025 | Elevated, > 1.025 |
| Cultures | As indicated (throat, sputum, blood, urine, stool, invasive sites) | Similar to DKA |
| ECG (12-lead) | S-T segment and T-wave abnormalities; cardiac dysrhythmias | Similar to DKA |
| *Differential diagnosis* | In the presence of altered level of consciousness or coma, consideration must be given to other etiologies including: Hypoglycemia, cerebrovascular accident, drug intoxication, uremia, hepatic coma, hypertensive encephalopathy, head trauma, other CNS lesions, sepsis, severe lactic acidosis.<br>If patient has abdominal pain an acute or "surgical" abdomen must be ruled out; respiratory or urinary infection may also need to be ruled out. The presence of hyperpyrexia or hypopyrexia is variable and cannot be relied on exclusively as to the presence or absence of infection. | |
| *Treatment*<br>Restoration of fluid balance | Aggressive fluid therapy with isotonic saline:<br>A. 1–2 liters 0.9 N saline over first hour<br>B. 500–1000 ml over each subsequent hour until hypotension is corrected and urine output is stable at 1–2 ml/min<br>C. 0.45 N saline substituted for (0.9 N saline) when blood pressure is stabilized<br>D. Dextrose 5%/0.45 N saline substituted for 0.45 N saline when serum glucose falls to 250 mg/dl<br>E. Blood or plasma expanders (albumin) may be necessary for hypotension unresponsive to therapy<br>▪ Close monitoring of vital parameters to evaluate response to therapy and to prevent fluid overload (pulmonary edema)<br>▪ Rule out silent myocardial infarction and/or attendant dysrhythmias if hypotension persists.<br>▪ Closely monitor for the following symptomatology: | Initial treatment similar to DKA. Fluid deficit may average 8–12 liters.<br>A. Administration of isotonic saline (0.9 N saline) 1–3 liters over first hour; protocol similar to that for DKA<br>B. Plasma expanders may be required in the presence of hypovolemic shock<br>C. Guideline: One-half of estimated fluid deficit is replaced within first 12 hr, with remaining fluid deficit replaced over subsequent 24 hr<br>D. Cardiac status must be assessed upon initiation of therapy and throughout its course; ECG and hemodynamic parameters should be assessed frequently to assess response to therapy and prevent fluid overload. |

| | Respiratory | Cardiovascular | Central Nervous | Musculoskeletal | Gastrointestinal |
|---|---|---|---|---|---|
| Hypoglycemia | Air hunger | Pallor, diaphoresis, tachycardia | Headache, blurred vision, confusion, coma, convulsions | Weakness; muscle twitching | |
| Hypokalemia | Respiratory muscle weakness proceeding to paralysis; cyanosis, respiratory arrest | Hypotension, dysrhythmias, cardiac arrest | Confusion, lethargy, irritability, paresthesias, coma | Weakness, muscle cramps, hyporeflexia | Anorexia, nausea/vomiting, abdominal pain; paralytic ileus |
| Cerebral edema | Changes in respiratory pattern | | Confusion, lethargy, somnolence progressing to coma | | |

*(continued)*

TABLE 19-3
**Contrast: Diabetic Ketoacidosis (DKA) and Hyperglycemic, Hyperosmolar, Nonketotic Coma (HHNK) *(Continued)***

| | **Diabetic Ketoacidosis** | **Hyperglycemic, Hyperosmolar, Nonketotic Coma** |
|---|---|---|
| Insulin therapy | *Goal:* To ensure a sustained, progressive reduction in serum glucose levels | |
| | Low-dose regular insulin regimens favored:<br>A. Intravenous approach (example):<br>1. Intravenous loading dose 0.3 U/kg regular insulin. (Flush IV line with 5-10 U regular insulin in 100 ml 0.9 N saline, prior to infusion into patient.) (All insulin therapy regimens must be individualized for each patient.)<br>2. Initiate continuous infusion at 0.1 U/kg/hr and titrate dose so as to reduce serum glucose to approximately 250 mg/100 ml over a period of 6-12 hr.<br>3. When 250 mg/100 ml is attained, insulin infusion rate is reduced. Intramuscular or subcutaneous insulin therapy can be initiated at this time with subsequent termination of IV insulin therapy. At this stage intravenous solution is switched from N saline to dextrose 5% in water or saline. This reduces risk of hypoglycemia. | Insulin therapy is usually necessary in HHNK but must be employed cautiously because these patients are often unusually sensitive to exogenous insulin.<br>• Recommended approach: 5 units regular insulin, intravenously. If necessary, this dose may be repeated hourly in conjunction with serum glucose studies.<br>Commonly, <40 U regular insulin is administered over the initial 24-hr period. |
| | Insulin therapy requires that serum glucose be monitored at frequent intervals. | |
| Electrolyte replacement therapy | Electrolyte replacement therapy includes restoration and maintenance of the following major electrolytes: Sodium, potassium, chloride, phosphorus, calcium, magnesium, and bicarbonate. Refer to Table 19-5, Nursing Diagnoses #1 and #2, for nursing considerations in administering and monitoring electrolytes. | |
| Glucose therapy | Glucose therapy is initiated when serum glucose levels reach 250 mg/dl.<br>*Approach:* Administration of dextrose 5%/0.45 N saline; monitor serum glucose levels very carefully; anticipate the occurrence of hypoglycemia. | Similar to DKA |
| Identification/treatment of underlying cause | Diligent and careful search may be necessary to identify underlying cause of DKA.<br>Thorough patient/family assessment including health history and physical examination of patient is crucial to the diagnostic process.<br>Patient should be carefully evaluated for the presence of intercurrent illness; upper respiratory infection, pneumonia, bronchitis, urinary tract infection, or other illness that may not readily be apparent. | Similar to DKA |

C. Laboratory/diagnostic studies.
3. Implement measures to restore and maintain fluid and electrolyte balance.
4. Implement measures to restore and maintain effective cardiovascular function.
5. Implement measures to restore and maintain acid-base balance.
6. Implement prescribed insulin therapy regimen.
7. Maintain adequate nutrition in conjunction with insulin therapy.
8. Maintain effective respiratory function.
9. Maintain integrity of neurologic and psychologic processes.
10. Provide supportive care to reduce the risk of complications: Fluid overload, infection, deep venous thrombosis, pulmonary embolism.

TABLE 19-4
**Diabetic Ketoacidosis: Clinical Classifications**

| | Mild | Moderate | Severe |
|---|---|---|---|
| History | Increasing polyuria with excessive thirst<br>Weakness, fatigue, lassitude<br>Weight loss (recent) | "Can't catch breath," air hunger with marked hyperventilatory effort<br>Marked weakness, unable to cope with physical exertion<br>Excessive thirst; marked polyuria<br>Nausea, vomiting, epigastric discomfort<br>Somnolence, lethargy | Marked drowsiness and lethargy progressing to coma<br>Deep and rapid Kussmaul breathing via an open mouth |
| Physical examination | Skin flushed<br>Tachycardia<br>Hyperventilation: Increased rate and depth of respirations<br>Possible slight odor of acetone (fruity smell) to breath | Drowsy, weak?<br>Respirations more vigorous; use of accessory muscles<br>Signs of dehydration: Dry mucous membranes, poor skin turgor (forehead or sternum), soft eyeballs, dry mouth (mouth breathing)<br>Hypovolemia: Narrowed pulse pressure<br>Noticeable acetone breath | Severe dehydration with hypovolemic shock: Hypotension tachycardia, reduced cardiac output<br>Air hunger<br>Lethargy<br>Coma<br>Temperature:<br>Subnormal—sepsis?<br>Vasomotor collapse?<br>Elevated—infection? |

11. Provide emotional and psychologic support to patient/family.
12. Initiate patient/family education to assist in developing and implementing prophylactic health-care practices.

**Nursing Diagnoses, Desired Patient Outcomes, and Nursing Interventions/Rationales.** Pertinent nursing diagnoses, desired patient outcomes, and nursing interventions/rationales in the care of the patient with DKA are presented in the Care Plan in Table 19–5.

## Hyperglycemic, Hyperosmolar, Nonketotic Coma (HHNK)

Hyperglycemic, hyperosmolar, nonketotic coma (HHNK) is a syndrome associated with a relative insulin deficit that occurs most commonly in patients with non-insulin-dependent diabetes mellitus (NIDDM).[12] The hallmarks of this disorder include a severe hyperglycemia and consequent hyperosmolality, with minimal to absent ketonemia. The patient has sufficient insulin to prevent lipolysis (i.e., fatty acid breakdown) but inadequate amounts for carbohydrate metabolism.

In addition to hyperglycemia and hyperosmolality, other prominent features of the syndrome include glycosuria, severe hypovolemia, and dehydration with associated alterations in the state of consciousness. Additionally, there is a wide spectrum of disturbances in fluid and electrolyte balance. The primary difference between HHNK and DKA is that in the former, there are sufficient levels of circulating insulin to inhibit lipolysis and ketogenesis.

The pathogenesis of HHNK is presented in Table 19–3. The major precipitating factor is usually a stressful event (e.g., infection, acute illness, surgery, or procedures such as hyperalimentation, tube feedings without sufficient free water, dialysis, or drugs such as mannitol, corticosteroids, and diuretics, among others). Other etiologic factors are listed in Table 19–3. In addition, details related to the assessment and diagnostic workup of a patient with a metabolic disorder, including the patient's history, physical examination, and laboratory findings, which are presented in Table 19–3, largely apply to both DKA and HHNK. (Also see Chap. 15.)

Patients with HHNK usually have laboratory values similar to those of patients with DKA (see Table 19–3 for contrast between DKA and HHNK). The exceptions include a more severe hyperglycemia and hyperosmolality, and the absence of a severe ketoacidemia. Frequently, renal function studies (e.g., BUN, creatinine) reveal some impairment in renal function, which is not surprising because HHNK most commonly occurs in the older population. Total body fluid deficits may be greater in HHNK as a consequence of the more severe hyperglycemia, hyperosmolality, and longer clinical course, which may span several weeks in certain instances.

### *Clinical Presentation*

A subacute course of HHNK is common, with a subtle polyuria and polydipsia. There may be an

## TABLE 19–5. CARE PLAN FOR THE PATIENT WITH DIABETIC KETOACIDOSIS (DKA)

| Nursing Diagnoses | Desired Patient Outcomes | Nursing Interventions | Rationales |
|---|---|---|---|
| ***Nursing Diagnosis #1***<br>Fluid volume deficit: Actual (total body dehydration), related to:<br>1. Osmotic diuresis caused by extreme glycosuria associated with hyperglycemic state.<br>2. Ketosis and ketonemia associated with enhanced lipolysis caused by insulin insufficiency.<br>(See Table 23–3, Nursing Diagnosis #1.)<br>***Nursing Diagnosis #2***<br>Electrolyte imbalance, related to:<br>1. Profound osmotic diuresis caused by extreme glycosuria.<br>2. Acidemia and ketonemia associated with enhanced lipolysis; and lactic acidosis associated with tissue hypoxia.<br>3. Profound dehydration and hypovolemia.<br>4. Nasogastric suctioning.<br>5. Profuse diaphoresis.<br>(See Tables 23–6, 23–7, 23–8, 23–9, 23–10, 24–3, and 24–5.) | Patient will maintain stable:<br>1. Neurologic status:<br>• Alert, oriented to person, place, and date.<br>• Appropriate behavior.<br>• Usual personality (per family).<br>• Sensorimotor function intact.<br>• Deep tendon reflexes brisk.<br>2. Hemodynamic status:<br>• BP within 10 mmHg of baseline.<br>•Heart rate >60, <100 beats/min.<br>•Cardiac rhythm: Regular sinus.<br>Hemodynamic parameters:<br>•CVP $\overline{\text{mean}}$ 0–8 mmHg.<br>•PCWP $\overline{\text{mean}}$ 8–12 mmHg.<br>•Cardiac output: 4–8 liters/min.<br>3. Renal status:<br>• Body weight within 5% of baseline.<br>• Urine output >30 ml/hr.<br>4. Laboratory status:<br>*Serum:*<br>• Osmolality: 285–295 mOsm/kg.<br>• Sodium: 135–148 mEq/liter.<br>• Potassium: 3.5–5.5 mEq/liter. | For pertinent nursing interventions and their rationales related to fluid volume deficit and electrolyte imbalance, see:<br>Table 23–3, Nursing Diagnosis #1.<br>Table 23–7, Nursing Diagnosis #1.<br>Table 23–9, Nursing Diagnosis #1.<br>Table 24–3, Nursing Diagnosis #1.<br>Table 24–5, Nursing Diagnosis #1.<br>In addition, consider the following:<br>• Assess impact of osmotic diuresis on total body fluid and electrolyte status. | • Extreme glycosuria related to hyperglycemic state precipitates profound fluid loss via a glucose osmotic diuresis.<br>○ As an osmotically active molecule, the presence of glucose in the glomerular filtrate after the renal tubules have reabsorbed the maximum amount possible requires an obligate loss of water. |
| | | ○ Assess neurologic status:<br>– Mental status, level of consciousness.<br>– Behavior and personality.<br>– Sensorimotor function.<br>– Deep tendon reflexes. | ○ Severe hyperosmolality related to hyperglycemia can predispose to alterations in neurologic function. |
| | | ○ Assess fluid status:<br>– Body weight, vital signs.<br>– Intake and output.<br>– Skin turgor, signs of dehydration: Dry, parched skin and mucous membranes; sunken eyeballs.<br>– Gastrointestinal fluid losses; nasogastric suctioning; diarrhea.<br>– Insensible fluid losses via lungs and skin (excessive ventilatory effort of Kussmaul respirations can lead to considerable fluid loss).<br>– Stress, fever, excessive diaphoresis. | ○ Hypovolemic state is reflected by decreased arterial and venous blood pressures; pulse may be rapid and thready; potential risk of hypovolemic shock must be anticipated and carefully assessed for.<br>○ Severe dehydration further exacerbates the hyperglycemic state by increasing secretions of stress hormones (e.g., glucagon, cortisol, and epinephrine), which function to increase tissue resistance to the action of insulin. |
| | | ○ Laboratory tests: Serum osmolality; electrolytes; serum glucose, phosphorus and calcium. | ○ Laboratory values may appear elevated due to hemoconcentration (i.e., severe volume contraction related to total body dehydration). |
| | | ○ BUN and creatinine.<br>– Hematology profile: Hematocrit, hemoglobin.<br>– Total protein (blood).<br>– Urine specific gravity. | ○ Decreased renal perfusion diminishes the glomerular filtration rate, predisposing to oliguria and placing the severely dehydrated patient at risk of developing acute renal failure. |

- Chloride: 100–106 mEq/liter.
- Calcium: 8.5–10.5 mg/100 ml.
- Phosphorus: 3.0–4.5 mg/100 ml.
- Glucose: 70–110 mg/100 ml.
- Hematology profile, total protein.

*Urine*:
- Sodium: 80–180 mEq/liter.
- Specific gravity: 1.010–1.025.
- Negative for glucose and acetone.

– Urine glucose and acetone.

○ Assess sources of electrolyte loss:
  – Profound osmotic diuresis with sodium loss.

○ Loss of sodium contributes to hyperkalemia because there is a decrease in potassium secretion in the distal renal tubules in the absence of sodium reabsorption.
○ In the presence of acidemia, there is a shift of potassium ions from the intra- to extracellular space in exchange for hydrogen ions.
○ Shift of potassium ions from the intra- to extracellular compartment in exchange for hydrogen ions contributes significantly to hyperkalemia.
○ It is estimated that for every 0.1 decrease in pH, the serum potassium concentration increases by 0.6 mEq/liter.
○ While hyperkalemia might be anticipated in the initial clinical presentation of ketoacidemia, normokalemia is equally as common and hypokalemia is not uncommon.

○ Losses of sodium and chloride occur with vomiting and nasogastric suctioning.

○ Serum electrolytes must be evaluated in terms of total body water status because such values, if assessed separately, may not reflect the true electrolyte status. For example, while hypernatremia might be anticipated in the face of a significant osmotic diuresis, the osmotic effect of the glucose load within the *extra*cellular fluid compartment causes water to be extracted from the *intra*cellular compartment, expanding the extracellular fluid volume. Thus, in actuality, a dilutional hyponatremia may occur.

*(continued)*

**TABLE 19–5. CARE PLAN FOR THE PATIENT WITH DIABETIC KETOACIDOSIS (DKA) *(Continued)***

| Nursing Diagnoses | Desired Patient Outcomes | Nursing Interventions | Rationales |
|---|---|---|---|
| ***Nursing Diagnosis #2 (cont.)*** | | | |
| | | | – A formula developed to compensate for this dilutional hyponatremia secondary to the osmotic effect of glucose in the ECF compartment may be a helpful assessment tool. A 1.6–3.0 mEq/liter reduction in serum sodium occurs per every 100 mg elevation of serum glucose.[7] |
| | | ○ In the presence of severe ketoacidemia, a concomitant increase in the urinary excretion of phosphates may predispose to hypophosphatemia. | ○ Phosphorus is a major constituent of ATP. Excessive deficit of phosphorus reduces ATP energy stores and predisposes to alterations in cellular metabolism. At serum phosphorus levels less than 1.0 mg/100 ml, muscle weakness may become sufficiently profound to depress myocardial contractility or produce respiratory arrest.<br>– Reduction in stores of 2,3-diphosphoglycerate (DPG) within red blood cells compromises oxygen delivery to tissues. In the absence of 2,3-DPG, hemoglobin unloads very little oxygen at the tissue level contributing to tissue hypoxia. A decrease in 2,3-DPG stores causes the oxyhemoglobin-dissociation curve to shift to the left (see Fig. 28–15). |
| | | • Implement prescribed fluid replacement regimen: | • Rapid rehydration with isotonic saline (0.9 N saline) is the treatment of choice; use of hypotonic saline (0.45 N saline) may produce a precipitous fall in extracellular fluid osmolality generating rapid intracellular fluid shifts and cerebral edema. |
| | | ○ Administer aggressive fluid therapy (see Table 19–3, under Treatment for specific considerations).<br>– Overall goal of fluid restoration is the rapid and effective correction of the fluid volume deficit. | ○ Because patients with DKA manifest varying degrees of fluid and electrolyte imbalance, fluid and electrolyte replacement therapy must be individualized and guided by continuous monitoring and assessment. |

| | |
|---|---|
| ∘ Monitor for signs/symptoms of fluid excess: Cardiac rate and rhythm; hemodynamic parameters—CVP, PCWP, CO.<br>– Physical signs: Extra heart sounds (gallop rhythm); full bounding pulse; neck vein distention at 45° (upright position); dependent edema. | ∘ Rapid fluid replacement necessitates close monitoring of vital signs and hemodynamic function to avert overhydration with its attendant danger of CHF and pulmonary edema. Patients with compromised cardiac and/or renal function are especially at high risk.<br>∘ See Table 19–3, Treatment: Restoration of Fluid Balance, for specific symptomatology related to hypoglycemia, hypokalemia, and cerebral edema. |
| ∘ Closely monitor for hypoglycemia, hypokalemia, and cerebral edema.<br>– Serial serum glucose studies. | ∘ When serum glucose levels approach 250 mg/100 ml, dextrose 5% in 0.45 N saline is substituted for normal saline to avoid precipitating a hypoglycemic reaction. |
| ∘ Insert Foley catheter during the acute phase to more closely monitor urine output. | ∘ Accurate assessment of urinary output is essential to assess renal function and to determine fluid and electrolyte therapy.<br>∘ Precise documentation of fluid intake and output is necessary to determine fluid replacement therapy and the patient's response to such therapy. |
| • Restore and maintain electrolyte balance.<br>∘ Implement electrolyte replacement therapy.<br>∘ Administer prescribed saline therapy. | • Serum sodium and potassium concentrations are variable, but total body concentrations are severely depleted.<br>∘ Provides necessary sodium and water replacement. (See Table 19–3, Treatment, for specific details related to fluid and saline therapy.) |
| ∘ Assess for signs and symptoms of *hyper*kalemia (see Tables 23–8 and 23–9).<br>– Monitor ECG for peaked T-wave and S-T segment changes.<br>– Monitor serum electrolytes and pH. | ∘ Hyperkalemia is associated with profound osmotic diuresis with hemoconcentration; shifting of potassium ions from intra- to extracellular space due to ketoacidemia; and retention of potassium ions in intravascular compartment in the absence of insulin.[6] |
| ∘ Assess for signs and symptoms of *hypo*kalemia (see Tables 23–8 and 23–9).<br>– Monitor ECG for inverted or flattened T wave; appearance of U wave; prolonged Q-T interval.<br>– Monitor serum electrolytes and pH. | ∘ Hypokalemia becomes manifest within 2–4 hr of initiation of insulin, fluid, and electrolyte replacement therapies. Physiology underlying the total body potassium deficit: Dilutional factor with rehydration; reduction in ketoacidemia related to insulin therapy—shift from fatty acid to glucose metabolism; movement of potassium ions into cells with glucose in the presence of insulin; increase in renal perfusion with consequent fluid and electrolyte loss. |
| ∘ Administer potassium replacement therapy as prescribed. One approach is the following: | ∘ Goal is to restore and maintain normal extracellular potassium concentrations during the acute period. |

*(continued)*

**TABLE 19–5. CARE PLAN FOR THE PATIENT WITH DIABETIC KETOACIDOSIS (DKA) *(Continued)***

| Nursing Diagnoses | Desired Patient Outcomes | Nursing Interventions | Rationales |
|---|---|---|---|
| ***Nursing Diagnosis #2 (cont.)*** | | | |
| | | – *Hyper*kalemia: Withhold initial potassium therapy until serum potassium level returns to within normal physiologic range.<br>– *Normo*kalemia: Potassium chloride 10–20 mEq/hr is added to intravenous replacement fluids.<br>– *Hypo*kalemia: Initial potassium replacement therapy is more aggressive: 20–40 mEq/hr administered with intravenous approach.<br>– In the absence of cardiac dysrhythmias and with good renal perfusion, potassium replacement therapy may be safely initiated even before the serum potassium is known. Recommended dose: 10–15 mEq/hr. | – Severely dehydrated patients who present with oliguria upon admission should be observed for underlying renal disease.<br>– In patients who remain oliguric despite sodium repletion, a trial with furosemide should be attempted. If oliguria persists, intrinsic renal disease becomes highly suspect and further fluid and electrolyte replacement therapy must be administered cautiously. |
| | | ○ Continuous monitoring of ECG and serial serum potassium levels is critical. | ○ Close monitoring of serum potassium and ECG changes is essential because alterations in serum potassium can precipitate serious/lethal dysrhythmias. |
| | | ○ Administer phosphate replacement therapy usually in conjunction with potassium therapy. | ○ Total body phosphate depletion is usually associated with severe DKA.<br>– Initial hyperphosphatemia followed by precipitious fall with hypophosphatemia post-implementation of fluid and insulin therapy.<br>– Overly aggressive phosphate replacement therapy unnecessary.<br>– Phosphates given in conjunction with potassium replacement therapy: Potassium chloride is alternated with potassium phosphate during the initial phase of therapy.<br>– There are no definitive consequences of hypophosphatemia.<br>– Caution must be taken to prevent hyperphosphatemia (overshoot) because this in turn may predispose to hypocalcemia and hypomagnesemia. |

| | | | |
|---|---|---|---|
| | | • Implement prescribed insulin replacement therapy.<br>○ Low-dose regular insulin regimens are usually prescribed. (See Table 19–3, Treatment, for specific dose schedules.) | • Goal is to ensure a sustained, progressive reduction in serum glucose levels.<br>○ Insulin therapy requires that serum glucose be monitored at frequent intervals. In DKA, prolonged insulin therapy is required after serum glucose levels reach 250 mg/100 ml, because correction of ketoacidemia takes longer to resolve. |
| ***Nursing Diagnosis #3***<br>Acid–base balance, alteration in, related to:<br>1. Ketoacidosis associated with insulin insufficiency.<br>2. Enhanced lipolysis.<br>3. Lactic acidemia associated with reduced tissue perfusion and tissue hypoxia. | 1. Patient's arterial blood gases will normalize as follows:<br>• pH: 7.35–7.45.<br>• $PaCO_2$: 35–45 mmHg, or optimal for patient.<br>2. Anions will stabilize as follows:<br>• $HCO_3^-$: 22–26 mEq/liter.<br>• Chloride: 100–106 mEq/liter.<br>• Anion gap: <12–15 mEq/liter. | • Implement measures to restore and maintain acid-base balance.<br>○ Monitor acid-base balance:<br>– Serial arterial blood gases.<br>– Serial electrolytes.<br>– Calculation of anion gap: The major two anions are chloride ($Cl^-$) and bicarbonate ($HCO_3^-$). They account for all but 10–15 mmol/liter of the total anion charge in the body.[8] To calculate: Anion gap = $Na^+ - (Cl^- + HCO_3^-)$<br>○ Normal anion gap: <15 mmol/liter.<br>○ If pH is <7.0, bicarbonate therapy may be prescribed. Approach to therapy:<br>– Administer 1 ampule of sodium bicarbonate (44.6 mEq/liter) at a time; follow blood study results carefully. When pH is >7.0, discontinue bicarbonate therapy.<br>○ Monitor ketoacidotic state:<br>– Presence of prominent gastrointestinal symptomatology: Epigastric distress, nausea, vomiting; abdominal pain, distention, ileus.<br>– Heavy, labored breathing (Kussmaul).<br>– Flushed skin; fruity odor to breath. | • Ketoacidemia is a major distinctive finding in DKA with marked depression of the arterial pH (<7.20) due largely to ketosis.[9]<br>○ Serum and urine are highly positive for acetoacetic acid, beta-hydroxybutyric acid, and acetone. *Note:* Ketostix test for acetoacetic acid and acetone does *not* test for beta-hydroxybutyric acid. Thus, in the patient with predominantly elevated levels of this latter ketone, a severe ketoacidemia may exist without a positive serum acetone.<br>— An anion gap greater than 15 mmol/liter indicates existence of another anion(s). In DKA, the source of these additional anions are the ketones, acetoacetic and beta-hydroxybutyric acids, and acetone.<br>○ If bicarbonate therapy is initiated (for pH <7), caution must be taken to avoid too rapid restoration of pH; this may predispose to alterations in cerebral functions due to paradoxical cerebrospinal fluid (CSF) acidosis. *Remember:* Carbon dioxide penetrates the blood–brain barrier much more easily than the bicarbonate ion ($HCO_3^-$) does. |

*(continued)*

**TABLE 19–5. CARE PLAN FOR THE PATIENT WITH DIABETIC KETOACIDOSIS (DKA)** ***(Continued)***

| Nursing Diagnoses | Desired Patient Outcomes | Nursing Interventions | Rationales |
|---|---|---|---|
| ***Nursing Diagnosis #4*** Cardiac output, alteration in: Decreased, related to:<br>1. Severe volume depletion with reduced venous return.<br>2. Cardiac dysrhythmias. | | • Restore and maintain effective cardiovascular, neurologic, and renal function. | • Of immeidate concern in the clinical setting of severe DDA with intra- and extracellular fluid volume depletion is the impact on cardiovascular and renal function. |
| | | ○ Establish baseline data reflective of cardiovascular/renal function: Cardiac rate and rhythm; hemodynamic parameters—arterial BP, CVP, PCWP, cardiac output, peripheral pulses. | ○ Baseline assessment data provide a basis for comparison and assist in evaluating the patient's response to therapy. |
| ***Nursing Diagnosis #5*** Tissue perfusion, alteration in cerebral, peripheral, related to:<br>1. Hypovolemic state, severe dehydration.<br>2. Extreme hyperosmolality with hemoconcentration. | | ○ Urine output: Hourly measurement of urine output; specific gravity; fluid intake; body weight (daily).<br>○ Establish baseline data reflective of neurologic function: Mental status, state of consciousness; behavior/personality; sensorimotor function; deep tendon reflexes. | |
| | Patient will maintain stable:<br>1. Neurologic status.<br>2. Hemodynamic status.<br>3. Renal status.<br>4. Laboratory parameters.<br>(For specific patient outcomes, see Nursing Diagnosis #1 above.) | ○ Assess cardiovascular function for signs/symptoms of fluid overload (see Tables 23–4 and 23–5). | ○ Sudden shifts in fluid and electrolytes may precipitate fluid excess; careful ongoing assessment (following trends) helps to obviate overhydration from too aggressive fluid replacement therapy; hypertension, congestive heart failure with pulmonary edema are potential complications of hypervolemia. |
| | | ○ Assess for evidence of hypovolemic shock:<br>– Hemodynamic: Hypotension, tachycardia (weak, thready peripheral pulses), decreased hemodynamic pressures.<br>– Neurologic: Altered state of consciousness, weakness, paresthesias.<br>– Renal: ↓ hourly urine output.<br>– Skin: Cool, clammy, mottled. | ○ Plasma expanders and vasopressors (dopamine) in addition to isotonic saline therapy may be necessary to maintain perfusion to vital tissue during hypovolemic shock state. |
| | | ○ Administer fluids, volume expanders (e.g., dextrose, blood, plasma, albumin), vasopressors (as prescribed). | ○ Very careful, ongoing assessment of vital parameters forms the basis for fluid and pharmacologic resuscitation. |

| | | | |
|---|---|---|---|
| ***Nursing Diagnosis #6***<br>Skin integrity, impairment of, related to:<br>1. Compromised peripheral perfusion associated with volume depletion and reduced cardiac output.<br>2. Immobility.<br>3. Catabolic state. | Patient's skin will remain:<br>1. Dry and warm to touch.<br>2. Without cyanosis or mottling.<br>3. With peripheral pulses palpable and full.<br>4. Intact, without evidence of pressure areas or skin breakdown.<br>5. With capillary refill spontaneous.<br>6. With minimal or absent pain of diabetic neuropathy.<br>7. Without edema. | • Maintain integrity of skin and mucous membranes.<br>○ Inspect skin and mucous membranes.<br>– Establish state of turgor, moisture, edema (pitting, dependent), pressure areas, cracking, fissuring, lesions.<br>– Monitor circulation to extremities.<br>– Peripheral pulses, capillary refill. | • Vascular insufficiency associated with diabetes increases risk of injury to skin especially in lower extremities.<br>○ Sensory/motor deficits due to peripheral vascular disease increase risk of injury. |
| ***Nursing Diagnosis #7***<br>Oral mucous membranes, alterations in, related to:<br>1. Severe dehydrated state.<br>2. Catabolic state. | Patient's mucous membranes will remain clean, moist, and without cracking or fissuring. | ○ Apply therapeutic measures:<br>○ Lubricate skin.<br>– Keep skin clean and dry.<br>○ Use egg-crate mattress or sheepskin.<br>○ Avoid very hot water when bathing. | ○ Lubricating skin helps to improve circulation and protects from infection.<br>○ Pressure relief devices.<br>○ Scalding can easily occur in presence of sensory deficits often experienced by patients with diabetes. |
| | | ○ Provide supportive care and comfort measures: Assist in personal hygiene; in turning and positioning; encourage deep breathing<br>○ Apply antiembolic stockings.<br>– Active/passive range-of-motion exercises as tolerated; early ambulation.<br>– Provide for frequent rest periods in a quiet milieu.<br>– Encourage gradual increase in self-care. | ○ Supportive and comfort measures need to be implemented to maximize circulatory and pulmonary function and reduce risk of infection.<br>○ Venous thrombosis and disseminated intravascular coagulation (DIC) are serious complications associated with DKA. Major contributing factors:<br>– Dehydrated state with hemoconcentration, and elevated serum protein with consequent increase in blood viscosity.<br>– Altered hemodynamics associated with peripheral vascular disease and venous stasis.<br>– Altered platelet adhesiveness and aggregation.<br>– Alteration in levels of clotting factors. |
| | | ○ Minimize pain associated with diabetic neuropathy: Aching and burning sensation in extremities especially at night.<br>○ Encourage walking (if possible) to relieve pain; use of foot cradle.<br>○ Maintenance of serum glucose within therapeutic range. | ○ Prevents contact of extremities with bed clothes.<br>○ Neuropathic pain is most often associated with increased serum glucose levels. |

(continued)

**TABLE 19–5. CARE PLAN FOR THE PATIENT WITH DIABETIC KETOACIDOSIS (DKA) *(Continued)***

| Nursing Diagnoses | Desired Patient Outcomes | Nursing Interventions | Rationales |
|---|---|---|---|
| ***Nursing Diagnosis #8*** Breathing pattern, ineffective: Hyperventilation (Kussmaul breathing), related to:<br>1. Severe ketonemia and acidemia associated with excessive lipolysis in the absence of insulin (pH <7.20).<br>2. Tissue hypoxia associated with impaired perfusion. | Patient will:<br>1. Maintain ventilatory effort as follows:<br>• Respiratory rate: <25–30 breaths/min.<br>• Tidal volume (TV): >5–7 ml/kg.<br>• Vital capacity (VC): >15 ml/kg.<br>2. Demonstrate eupnea, without use of accessory muscles of breathing.<br>3. Avoid fatigue with reduced work of breathing. | • Establish baseline assessment database:<br>○ Assess pertinent parameters of respiratory function:<br>○ Respiratory rate, rhythm, and pattern of breathing.<br>○ Hyperventilation (Kussmaul).<br>– Tachypnea, dyspnea.<br>○ Use of accessory muscles of respiration.<br>○ Pleuritic pain.<br>○ Pulmonary function parameters:<br>– Tidal volume.<br>– Vital capacity.<br>○ Auscultation of breath sounds. | • Goal of therapy is to maintain effective respiratory function as guided by arterial blood gas, tidal volume, vital capacity, and neurologic function.<br>○ Ineffective breathing pattern often associated with muscle weakness caused by hypokalemia; patient is at great risk of developing respiratory arrest.<br>○ Kussmaul breathing associated with severe ketoacidemia; it is a compensatory response of the body to blow off excess $CO_2$ and thereby increase arterial pH.<br>○ Use of accessory muscles may cause undue fatigue.<br>○ Severely dehydrated state may predispose to pleuritic friction rub. |
| ***Nursing Diagnosis #9*** Gas exchange, impaired, related to:<br>1. Tissue hypoxia associated with decreased tissue perfusion.<br>2. Increase in ventilation/perfusion mismatch.<br>3. Diffusion defect. | The patient's parameters will stabilize as follows:<br>1. Arterial blood gases:<br>• pH >7.35.<br>• $PaO_2$ >80 mmHg.<br>• $PaCO_2$ return to baseline (normally 35–45 mmHg).<br>Hemoglobin oxygen saturation: >95%.<br>2. Neurologic status: Oriented to person, place, date; protective reflexes (cough, swallowing) intact.<br>3. Skin and mucous membranes—No cyanosis. | ○ Arterial blood gases: Trends.<br>○ Cyanosis of lips, mucous membranes, and nailbeds.<br>○ Acetone odor to breath.<br>○ Neurologic status.<br>• Provide supportive therapy.<br>○ Administer humidified oxygen.<br>○ Assist patient to assume a position that facilitates breathing. | ○ Adventitious sounds (rales, rhonchi, wheezes) may signal pulmonary congestion progressing to pulmonary edema; wheezing reflects congested airways due in part to inability of patient to handle secretions.<br>○ A rising $PaCO_2$ suggests decreasing ventilatory capability.<br>– A $PaO_2$ <60 mmHg predisposes to tissue hypoxia.<br>○ Cyanosis reflects decreased tissue oxygenation related to altered ventilation.<br>○ Reflects ketogenesis.<br>○ Ongoing neurologic assessment is essential to detect alterations in cerebral function due to paradoxic CSF acidosis.<br>○ May assist in relieving tissue hypoxia; prevents thick tenacious secretions of dehydrated state.<br>○ Efforts must be directed toward assisting patient to conserve strength. |

| | | | |
|---|---|---|---|
| | | | ◦ Insertion of nasogastric tube may be necessary to prevent gastric dilation, which limits diaphragmatic excursion and increases the risk of aspiration with consequent aspiration pneumonia. |
| | | ◦ Encourage deep breathing. | ◦ Deep breathing minimizes atelectasis.<br>◦ Position changes minimize pooling of secretions. |
| | | ◦ Initiate ventilatory assistance if indicated (respiratory arrest). | ◦ Ventilatory support may be needed in presence of altered state of consciousness, ineffective breathing pattern, inability to handle secretions. |
| ***Nursing Diagnosis #10***<br>Anxiety, related to:<br>1. Fear of dying.<br>2. ICU setting.<br>3. Seriousness of compromised health state.<br>4. Personal and social responsibilities (e.g., effect of illness on job). | 1. Patient and family will be able to verbalize fears and concerns regarding current illness, diabetes mellitus, and its complications.<br>2. Patient and family's behavior will demonstrate less apprehension or withdrawal; increased interest in learning about illness state. | • Maintain integrity of neurologic and psychologic process.<br>◦ Establish baseline neurologic function:<br>– Mental status: Changes in level of consciousness, disorientation, confusion, agitation, irritability, coma.<br>– Cranial nerve function.<br>– Sensory function: Paresthesias.<br>– Motor function: Muscle weakness, paralysis, hyperreflexia.<br>– Seizure activity. | ◦ Alterations in neurologic function related to hyperglycemia with extreme hyperosmolality, and severe acidemia.<br>◦ It is essential to appreciate that the patient with DKA can shift from a coma state to hypoglycemia shock *without regaining consciousness.* Neurologic status must be carefully evaluated in conjunction with cardiovascular function and serum glucose levels. |
| | | ◦ Establish baseline psychologic function including patient and family:<br>– Assess level of anxiety, apprehension. Does behavior reflect withdrawal, disinterest, apathy? | |
| ***Nursing Diagnosis #11***<br>Communication, impaired: Verbal, related to:<br>1. Altered state of consciousness associated with severe dehydration and acidotic state. | 1. Patient will remain alert and oriented to person, place, date.<br>2. Patient will verbalize needs and whether they have been met. | ◦ Estimate developmental level.<br>◦ Assess coping capabilities: Role of patient in family nucleus: Dependent, independent? Decision-maker?<br>– Identify family resources and significant others. | ◦ Age and developmental level may not necessarily be the same.<br>◦ Role of patient in family nucleus will influence rehabilitative process for all members. |
| ***Nursing Diagnosis #12***<br>Thought processes, alteration in, related to:<br>1. Altered state of consciousness related to severe hyperosmolality (hyperglycemia); severe volume depletion. | 1. Patient will exhibit appropriate behavior; thought processes intact.<br>2. Patient will demonstrate the ability to think and make decisions regarding care, likes and dislikes. | ◦ Assess readiness to learn.<br>◦ Consider the following when providing care:<br>– Be an attentive, interested, caring listener. | ◦ Teaching can be geared to level at which patient and family can best learn. Observation of interactions between patient and family may provide valuable clues as to how they are coping, which could be an important consideration in the rehabilitative process. |

*(continued)*

## TABLE 19-5. CARE PLAN FOR THE PATIENT WITH DIABETIC KETOACIDOSIS (DKA) *(Continued)*

| Nursing Diagnoses | Desired Patient Outcomes | Nursing Interventions | Rationales |
|---|---|---|---|
| ***Nursing Diagnosis #13***<br>Self-concept, disturbance in: Body image, self-esteem, related to:<br>1. Chronic illness. | Patient will feel comfortable talking about what diabetes means and how it will affect lifestyle and optimal level of health desired. | ○ Encourage verbalization of fears and concerns.<br>○ Explain all ongoing procedures.<br>○ Involve patient/family in decision-making process.<br>– Support patient/family efforts in coping.<br>– Remain accessible to patient and family.<br>– Provide emotional support to patient and family. | ○ It may help to identify problems or areas of concern.<br>○ Appropriate explanations may help to alleviate heightened anxiety.<br>○ Management of diabetes, a chronic disease syndrome, requires self-care health practices by patient and family; their active involvement is essential if they are to evolve a meaningful life within the constraints of the disease. |
| ***Nursing Diagnosis #14***<br>Nutrition, alteration in: Less than body requirements, related to:<br>1. Catabolic state.<br>2. Insulin lack. | Patient's condition will stabilize as follows:<br>1. Body weight will stabilize within appropriate range.<br>2. Positive nitrogen balance will be maintained.<br>3. Combination of insulin, diet, and exercise therapies will maintain serum glucose levels within optimal range.<br>4. Abdominal discomfort will be minimized; gastric aspiration will be averted. | • Implement prescribed nutritional regimen.<br>○ Perform an abdominal assessment:<br>– Subjective: Anorexia, nausea, vomiting, epigastric discomfort, abdominal pain.<br>– Objective: Tender, distended abdomen, absence of bowel sounds, paralytic ileus; limitation of diaphragmatic excursion.<br>○ Insert nasogastric tube.<br>○ Monitor serum glucose, ketones, electrolyte levels, and arterial blood gases.<br>○ Monitor intake, output; daily weight.<br>○ Initiate dextrose 5% in 0.45 N saline infusion when serum glucose drops to 250 mg/dl in the presence of insulin therapy.<br>○ Consult with nutritionist, physician, patient, and family to determine specific nutritional needs. | ○ Alterations in serum potassium and severe acidemia predispose to impaired gastric motility and abdominal discomforts and symptomatology.<br>○ Limitations of diaphragmatic excursion may compromise ventilatory effort, increasing risk of atelectasis.<br>○ Gastric decompensation reduces abdominal discomfort and risk of aspiration.<br>○ With initiation of insulin therapy, metabolism shifts from fatty acids to glucose with a resultant drop in serum glucose and ketones.<br>○ Overall goals of nutritional therapy:<br>1. Meet the basic nutritional requirements. |

| | | | |
|---|---|---|---|
| ***Nursing Diagnosis #15***<br>Knowledge deficit: Nutritional/insulin therapy regimen. | Patient and family will:<br>1. Discuss underlying principles of diabetic diet therapy.<br>2. Specify dietary restrictions and their significance.<br>3. Relate how diet therapy coincides with insulin and exercise regimens.<br>4. Demonstrate proficiency in performing and interpreting tests for serum glucose.<br>5. Identify action to be taken in the event of gastrointestinal disorder or significant stressor.<br>6. Verbalize concerns regarding the disease syndrome and overall anti-diabetes therapy regimen. | ○ Baseline nutritional needs.<br>• Initiate teaching program regarding dietary therapy for the diabetic patient.<br>○ Involve patient/family in diet planning and decision-making.<br>– Provide booklets and pamphlets to reinforce teaching.<br>– Stress importance of regularity of diet and exercise; rest, sleep, and relaxation.[10]<br>– Encourage verbalization of feelings regarding impact of diabetes on family lifestyle and the integrity of each individual.<br>• Teach the importance of, and how to document, significant data, including:[11]<br>– Insulin dosage, time.<br>– Site of injection.<br>– Serum glucose (glucometer or Dextrostix).<br>– Urinary sugar and acetone.<br>– Diet.<br>– Exercise.<br>– Stressors. | 2. Attain and/or maintain ideal body weight.<br>3. Prevent complications (e.g., hypoglycemia).<br>○ Therapeutic anti-diabetes treatment regimen requires that diet therapy coincide with insulin and exercise regimen.<br>○ Ideal body weight should be established and maintained.<br>○ Diet therapy is an essential aspect of anti-diabetes therapy.<br>○ Self-care is an absolute requirement for successful management of diabetes. Participation in decision-making and planning increases motivation and compliance.<br>○ Data assist in evaluating response to therapy so that appropriate adjustments can be made as necessary. |
| ***Nursing Diagnosis #16***<br>Injury, physiologic, potential for: Hypoglycemia, related to:<br>1. Ineffective dietary/insulin regimen.<br>2. Noncompliance with therapeutic regimen.<br>3. Stressful event.<br>(See Chap. 20.) | 1. Patient will maintain optimal serum glucose levels:<br>• Fasting serum glucose: 70–110 mg/100 ml<br>• 1–2 hr postprandial: <160–180 mg/100 ml<br>2. Patient will be able to verbalize signs and symptoms of hypoglycemic and hyperglycemic states. | | |

*(continued)*

**TABLE 19–5. CARE PLAN FOR THE PATIENT WITH DIABETIC KETOACIDOSIS (DKA) *(Continued)***

| Nursing Diagnoses | Desired Patient Outcomes | Nursing Interventions | Rationales |
|---|---|---|---|
| ***Nursing Diagnosis #17***<br>Potential for infection, related to:<br>1. Catabolic state associated with insulin insufficiency.<br>(See Table 49–7.) | Patient will:<br>1. Remain nonfebrile.<br>2. Keep white blood count within acceptable physiologic range.<br>3. Verbalize a general feeling of well-being.<br>4. Remain without signs/symptoms of infection: Pain, redness, swelling, suppuration.<br>5. Have lungs clear on auscultation.<br>6. Have negative cultures: Blood, urine, sputum, wound, intravenous access sites. | • Implement activities to reduce the risk of infection.<br>○ Assess for signs of infection.<br>– Vigilant assessment of all invasive lines is critical.<br>– Observe for redness, pain, swelling at all invasive sites; dressing changes should occur every 48 hr or according to unit protocol.<br>– Culture catheter tip.<br>– Assess lungs for adventitious sounds of pulmonary congestion or increased secretions.<br>– Examine urine for cloudiness or unusual odor.<br>– Assess body temperature.<br>– Monitor white blood count.<br>– Culture all body fluids/secretions in presence of increased body temperature.<br>– Blood, sputum, urine, wounds.<br>– Administer antibiotic therapy as prescribed; assess for response to therapy. | ○ Infection is a serious stressor, which can disrupt diabetic control and precipitate DKA. |

associated marked increase in food intake and sugar-containing beverages. While the patient can drink fluids, the dehydration may not be severe. Elderly persons frequently have an inadequate fluid intake due to debility or a nonrecognition of thirst. A thorough patient history, including events surrounding the dysfunction, should be obtained.

Specific clinical manifestations of HHNK reflective of underlying pathophysiologic mechanisms are similar to those of DKA, with the major exception being those clinical findings associated with ketonemia. As mentioned previously, the patient with HHNK usually has sufficient insulin secretion to prevent lipolysis, but not sufficient to prevent hyperglycemia. Consequently, the respirations in HHNK are not of the Kussmaul's type, and the breath lacks the characteristic acetone or fruity odor. With hypovolemia caused by excessive sodium and fluid losses, the triad of hypotension, tachycardia, and oliguria is manifested.

### Treatment

The overall goal of treatment is a *gradual* correction of the hyperglycemia, hyperosmolality, and hypovolemia. Too rapid correction of hyperosmolality may precipitate cerebral edema; too rapid reduction in serum glucose can precipitate hypoglycemic/hypovolemic shock. Specific details regarding the therapeutic regimen are included in Table 19–3.

### Nursing Care of the Patient with Hyperglycemic, Hyperosmolar, Nonketotic Coma

**Therapeutic Goals.** Implementation of nursing process in the care of the patient with hyperglycemic, hyperosmolar, nonketotic coma revolves around the following therapeutic goals:

1. Identify patients at risk.
2. Establish a comprehensive database including:
   A. Clinical history (functional health patterns).
   B. Physical examination.
   C. Laboratory/diagnostic findings.
3. Implement measures to restore and maintain effective cardiovascular function.
4. Implement measures to restore and maintain effective fluid and electrolyte balance.
5. Implement measures to restore and maintain effective acid–base balance.
6. Prevent complications:
   A. Respiratory dysfunction associated with overly vigorous fluid replacement therapy; pulmonary embolism; pneumonia.
   B. Fluid overload: Congestive heart failure, pulmonary edema.
   C. Hypoglycemic shock associated with overly aggressive insulin therapy.
   D. Sepsis.
7. Maintain adequate nutrition.
8. Maintain effective bowel elimination.
9. Provide emotional and psychologic support to patient/family.
10. Initiate patient/family education to assist in developing and implementing prophylactic health-care practices.

**Nursing Diagnoses.** Tentative nursing diagnoses in the care of the patient with HHNK may include the following:

1. Fluid volume deficit, actual, related to hyperglycemia with glycosuria.
2. Cardiac output, alteration in: Decreased, related to severe dehydration with decreased venous return.
3. Electrolyte imbalance, related to osmotic diuresis associated with glycosuria.
4. Tissue perfusion, alteration in: Cerebral, related to hyperosmolality and severe dehydration (hypovolemia).
5. Oral mucous membranes, alteration in, related to severe dehydration.
6. Skin integrity, impairment: Potential, related to severe dehydration, catabolic state, and limited mobility associated with weakened state.
7. Nutrition, alteration in: Less than body requirements, related to catabolic state and inadequate nutritional and fluid intake.
8. Sensory-perceptual alteration: Potential, related to cerebral dysfunction associated with severe fluid depletion.
9. Knowledge deficit regarding underlying disease process, and factors that trigger an exacerbation of the illness.

(Specific nursing diagnoses, desired patient outcomes, and nursing interventions for the patient with diabetic ketoacidosis, listed in Table 19–5, likewise apply to the nursing care of the patient with HHNK.)

## REFERENCES


1. Vander, A, Sherman, J, and Luciano, D: Human Physiology: The Mechanisms of Body Function, ed 4. McGraw-Hill, New York, 1985, p 506.
2. Vander, A, Sherman, J, and Luciano, D: Human Physiology: The Mechanisms of Body Function, ed 4. McGraw-Hill, New York, 1985, p 511.
3. Hershman, JM: Endocrine Pathophysiology: A Patient-Oriented Approach. Lea & Febiger, Philadelphia, 1988, p 205.
4. Muir, BL: Pathophysiology: An Introduction to the Mechanisms of Disease, ed 2. John Wiley & Sons, New York, 1988, p 232.

5. Roberts, SL: Physiological Concepts and the Critically Ill Patient. Prentice-Hall, Englewood Cliffs, NJ, 1985, p 288.
6. Metheny, NM: Fluid and Electrolyte Balance: Nursing Considerations. JB Lippincott, Philadelphia, 1987, p 274.
7. Boehm, TM: Hyperglycemia in critical care medicine. Crit Care Q 6(3):51, 1983.
8. Rabin, D and McKenna, TJ: Clinical Endocrinology and Metabolism: Principles and Practice. Grune & Stratton, New York, 1982, p 165.
9. Hershman, JM: Endocrine Pathophysiology: A Patient-Oriented Approach. Lea & Febiger, Philadelphia, 1988, p 229.
10. Gavin, JR: Diabetes and exercise. Am J Nurs 88(2):178, 1988.
11. Callahan, M and Bradley, D: Why you should teach your diabetic patients to chart. Nursing '88, 18(3):48, 1988.
12. Hershman, JM: Endocrine Pathophysiology: A Patient-Oriented Approach. Lea & Febiger, Philadelphia, 1988, p 233.

CHAPTER 20

# Nursing Management of the Patient with Hypoglycemia (Hypoglycemic Shock)

## CHAPTER OUTLINE



## LEARNING OBJECTIVES

**At the end of this chapter, you should be able to:**

1. Define *hypoglycemia* and examine its pathogenesis, etiology, diagnostic findings, clinical presentation, and treatment.
2. Delineate the nursing process in the care of the patient with hypoglycemia including the following:
   Assessment.
   Nursing diagnosis.
   Planning: Desired patient outcomes
   Nursing interventions/rationales.

## HYPOGLYCEMIA

Hypoglycemia is a symptom complex initiated by alteration in glucose homeostasis wherein serum glucose concentrations decline to levels insufficient to meet the metabolic demands of the nervous system. The diagnosis of hypoglycemia requires an abnormally depressed serum glucose level (usually below 55 mg/100 ml) and a distinct clinical presentation.[1]

### Pathogenesis

Glucose homeostasis reflects the balance between glucose entry into and removal from the bloodstream. Glucose input into the circulation occurs via (1) absorption of exogenous glucose (food intake); (2) hepatic glycogenolysis (glycogen breakdown); and (3) hepatic gluconeogenesis (formation of new glucose from lactate, pyruvate, amino acids, and glycerol). Removal of glucose or its uptake from the circulation takes place in virtually all tissues within the body and predominantly in nerve tissue and muscle.

Hypoglycemia ensues: (1) when glucose uptake and utilization are too rapid; (2) when glucose release and availability are inadequate to meet tissue demands; or (3) when excessive insulin is released into the bloodstream.

### Classification and Etiology

Hypoglycemia can be classified based on underlying pathophysiologic mechanisms. Thus, hypoglycemia may be caused by: (1) excess antidiabetic medication including insulin or oral hypoglycemic therapy; (2) underproduction of glucose by the liver during the postabsorptive (fasting) state; and (3) a too rapid glucose uptake and utilization.

#### *Excess Antidiabetic Medication*

By far, the most common and most easily recognized cause of hypoglycemia is antidiabetic medication, which includes insulin as well as oral hypoglycemic agents. For patients with diabetes who are taking insulin or oral hypoglycemics (sulfonylureas; e.g., chlorpropamide, acetohexamide, glyburide), hypoglycemia is an ever-present risk. This risk increases with concomitant administration of other medications, including, for example, propranolol and oxytetracycline. Such drugs may prolong and potentiate the action of antidiabetic medications. Propranolol is thought to induce hypoglycemia by inhibiting glycogenolysis. As a beta-blocker, propranolol may also mask signs of hypoglycemia because it blocks adrenergic activity.

Patients with chronic renal disease who receive insulin are especially susceptible to hypoglycemia, perhaps due in part to impaired inactivation of insulin by the kidneys. Endogenous production of insulin may be increased in the presence of tumors or primary liver disease. Islet cell tumors (insulinomas), for example, secrete excessive amounts of insulin, which inhibit hepatic glucose production. Liver disease (hepatitis, cancer, cirrhosis) alters the ability of the liver to store and release glucose.

More recently, hypoglycemia associated with insulin-binding autoimmune antibodies has been recognized.[2,3] While the underlying mechanism by which insulin antibodies produce hypoglycemia is uncertain, possible explanations include the liberation of excessive amounts of insulin from a large pool of bound insulin during the fasting state, or potentiation of insulin effect by antibody aggregation.

Factitious hypoglycemia may arise from surreptitious use of insulin or other hypoglycemic agents. Autoimmune hypoglycemia may be very difficult to distinguish from surreptitious insulin administration. In the latter case patients are often psychiatrically disturbed, and a high degree of suspicion coupled with a thorough, astute assessment is necessary to identify the underlying cause.

Elderly patients with mild diabetes (NIDDM), receiving long-acting sulfonylureas, frequently develop hypoglycemia. Sulfonylureas sensitize islet cells and directly stimulate insulin secretion from the pancreas. See Table 20–1 for a list of etiologic/precipitating factors of hypoglycemia.

#### *Underproduction of Glucose*

Heavy alcohol consumption superimposed on an inadequate dietary intake may precipitate hypoglycemia. Ethanol directly blocks several steps in hepatic gluconeogenesis and in this way reduces glucose availability during the postabsorptive state. Additional drugs incriminated as causative factors of hypoglycemia include acetylsalicylic acid (aspirin), disopyramide (Norpace), haloperiodol, propoxyphine (Darvon), phenylbutazone, dicumoral, and others.

Underproduction of glucose by the liver during the postabsorptive state may be attributed to a variety of other causes. Insufficient dietary intake associated with missed or delayed meals or snacks, or an overall deficient nutritional status, decreases availability of necessary substrates for hepatic gluconeogenesis. Decreased requirements for exogenous insulin may be associated with recovery from a stressful episode or insult (e.g., infection, surgery, trauma). In this setting hypoglycemia may be precipitated if appropriate and timely readjustments in insulin and diet are not made. Strenuous physical exercise or severe stress without a compensatory increase in food intake or decrease in insulin dosage may precipitate a hypoglycemic episode.

Primary hormonal causes of hypoglycemia include reduced levels of cortisol associated with Addison's disease, or hypopituitarism. Cortisol, like glucagon, epinephrine, and growth hormone, is an insulin counter-regulatory hormone that stimulates hepatic gluconeogenesis during the fasting state. Reduced levels of cortisol compromise gluconeogenic activity within the liver. Hypopituitarism may predispose to hypoglycemia by decreasing levels of growth hormone and adrenocorticotropic (ACTH) hormone. A decrease in ACTH, in turn, reduces levels of cortisol secretion by the adrenal cortices. Hypoglycemia may be caused by specific enzymatic deficits leading to impaired glycogenolysis or gluconeogenesis. Such defects are usually associated with infants and children. See Table 20–1 for additional factors responsible for the underproduction of glucose.

#### *Too-Rapid Glucose Uptake and Utilization*

Too-rapid glucose uptake and utilization have been associated with gastrointestinal disease frequently requiring surgical intervention (e.g., subtotal gastrectomy, vagotomy, pyloroplasty, gastroenterostomy). Extrapancreatic tumors can also cause hypoglycemia by increasing glucose utilization and inhibiting glucose release.

TABLE 20-1
**Etiologic/Precipitating Factors of Hypoglycemia**

| Excess Insulin or Oral Hypoglycemic Agents | Underproduction of Glucose | Too-Rapid Glucose Uptake and Utilization |
|---|---|---|
| Antidiabetic medication:<br>Insulin<br>Oral hypoglycemics<br>(Sulfonylureas)<br>Acetohexamide<br>Chlorpropamide<br>Tolazamide<br>Drugs that potentiate action of antidiabetic medications: Propranolol, oxytetracycline, others<br>Surreptitious use of insulin or oral hypoglycemic agents<br>Islet cell tumor (insulinomas)<br>Pancreatic islet cell disease with inappropriate insulin output<br>Renal disease: Impaired inactivation of insulin<br>Presence of circulating insulin-like factors associated with:<br>Adrenal tumor<br>Mesothelioma<br>Retroperitoneal fibrosarcoma<br>Autoimmune phenomenon | Heavy ethanol consumption<br>Other drugs:<br>Acetylsalicylic acid<br>Disopyramide (Norpace)<br>Haloperidol (Haldol)<br>Propoxyphene HCl (Darvon)<br>Phenylbutazone<br>Dicumarol<br>Others<br>Insufficient food intake:<br>Missed or delayed meals and snacks<br>Overall deficient nutritional state—negative nitrogen balance<br>Strenuous physical exercise or stress without compensatory increase in food intake or decrease in insulin dose<br>Primary liver disease—hepatitis, cancer, cirrhosis<br>Secondary liver disease associated with right-sided congestive heart failure<br>Primary endocrine deficiency:<br>Addison's disease—reduced levels of cortisol<br>Hypopituitarism—reduced levels of ACTH and cortisol<br>Enzyme deficiency (e.g., galactosemia) | Post gastrointestinal surgery<br>Extrapancreatic tumors |

## Diagnosis

The diagnosis of hypoglycemia is determined based on a thorough patient history including an assessment of the patient's functional health patterns, and a meticulous physical examination. Diagnosis is corroborated by serum glucose values usually below 55 mg/100 ml. Details related to the patient's history and physical examination are included in Table 20-2. See also Chapter 15.

## Differential Diagnosis

When hypoglycemia is suspected, it is important initially to rule out the following potential causes: drugs, alcohol, surreptitious self-administration of insulin or sulfonylureas, hepatic or renal disease, endocrine disorders including adrenal or pituitary insufficiency, and the occurrence of insulinemia due to tumors particularly in the thorax, liver, abdomen, retroperitoneal space, and pelvis.

## Clinical Presentation

The clinical manifestations of hypoglycemia comprise two major categories: (1) symptoms reflective of autonomic nervous system stimulation; and (2) symptoms related to an inadequate glucose supply to neural tissues (i.e., neuroglucopenia).

With a rapid decline in serum glucose levels there is a compensatory activation of the sympathetic nervous system with a concomitant release of epinephrine from the adrenal medulla. Consequently symptomatology includes feelings of nervousness, marked apprehension, hunger accompanied by headache, and general weakness; palpitations, tremulousness, and circumoral numbness may also be experienced. Patients complain of fatigue, nausea, and vomiting; and typically, the symptoms of the "fight or flight" sympathetic reaction are observed, including dilated pupils, pallor, tachycardia, and profuse diaphoresis.

When the decline in serum glucose is slower, severe, and more prolonged, symptomatology reflects central nervous system manifestations including headache and restlessness, which may be accompanied by difficulty in thinking and speaking. The patient may present with visual disturbances, hemiplegia, paraplegia, convulsions, and loss of consciousness. Family members may report on personality changes; emotional instability; aggressive, maniacal behavior; catatonia; or acute paranoia. Hypothermia in the presence of coma presents a significant clue to the underlying presence of hypoglycemia.

TABLE 20-2
**Diagnostic Considerations in Assessing the Patient with Hypoglycemia**

**Clinical History**

A thorough detailed history is essential to the diagnosis of endocrinopathies, and hypoglycemia is no exception. If the patient presents with an altered level of consciousness, as much information as possible should be obtained from family or significant others. If the patient can respond, it is essential to focus on the following information, which will assist in diagnosis and treatment over the acute phase of illness, and provide the basis for planning and implementing care over the long term.

It is necessary to establish the chief complaint by asking the patient to describe his/her problems or symptoms. Manifestations of hypoglycemia can be very subtle, so it is important to encourage the patient and family to talk about their perceptions of what is happening. Has it happened before? When? The patient may complain of having "spells" brought on by missing a meal or by exercise, and relieved with food. Try to establish the onset of symptoms: What kind of symptoms, when, and over how long a period of time? What was happening to the patient at that time? Try to establish the precipitating factor(s). If the patient is an established diabetic, try to determine the relationship between the onset of symptoms, food intake, and insulin/oral hypoglycemic therapy. What has been the course since onset? Have the symptoms recurred? If so, under what circumstances?

Ascertain the existence of any unusual stressor(s) that may have precipitated the symptoms. Did the stressor(s) necessitate a change in the patient's usual routines and activities of daily living? In the established diabetic, what are the usual symptoms related to a hypoglycemic state? What are the precipitating factor(s)?

***Functional Health Patterns***

*Health Perception–Health Management*

What was the patient's prior health? Is there preexisting diagnosed diabetes? If so, what type? For how long? What is the treatment regimen—antidiabetic medication, diet, exercise? How knowledgeable is the patient and family regarding the diabetic syndrome, its treatment and long-term ramifications?

Has the patient experienced recent illness, trauma, surgery (e.g., gastrointestinal), or other stressor? Emotional or psychologic? Be especially cognizant of complaints of depression, fatigue, apathy, which are attributed to hypoglycemia.

Are there associated illnesses—hypertension, obesity? Cardiovascular or renal disease? Other endocrine disorders—Addison's disease with glucocorticoid replacement therapy? Glucocorticoids can cause drug-induced hypoglycemia. Thyroid disorder? Is there a history of liver disease—hepatitis, cirrhosis, cancer? Is there a family history of any of these disorders?

Is the patient currently taking medications other than insulin or oral hypoglycemics? If so, what kind, for what reason, in what dosage, for how long? Are over-the-counter drugs used? Abused? Does the patient drink alcohol—what kind, how much, how often, over how long a period of time? Is there a history of alcoholism, emotional or mental illness in the family? Does the patient have any allergies? Autoimmune disease?

*Sleep–Rest Pattern*

What are the patient's personal habits—sleep, work, leisure, recreation, smoking, diet? What is the patient's occupation? Has having diabetes impacted on his/her livelihood? How? What does the patient do to "unwind"? Diversional activities?

*Role–Relationship Pattern*

How does the patient perceive his/her role in the family nucleus? Is he/she dependent, independent, the decision-maker? What are the family resources and key family interrelationships? Financial resources?

*Coping—Stress Tolerance*

How is stress handled? What are the coping capabilities? Patterns of behavior? Attitudes toward health and disease? If the patient has diabetes, how is it perceived by the individual? By family members?

**Physical Examination**

Closely observe the patient's behavior for signs reflective of adrenergic activity (e.g., anxiety, nervousness, apprehension, diaphoresis, tremors, complaints of hunger, weakness). Vital signs should be assessed and evaluated at specific intervals.

A baseline neurologic assessment must be established as a basis for comparison of subsequent assessments. A thorough neurologic assessment is especially important in the patient experiencing hypoglycemia. Repeated hypoglycemic insults can predispose to permanent neurologic sequelae.

Have there been any changes in the level of consciousness? Cerebral function, intellectual capacities? Personality changes? The patient's family may be helpful in establishing a baseline in this regard. Is cranial nerve and brainstem function intact? Is there seizure activity? Focal? General? Under what circumstances do seizures occur?

Specific neuroglycopenic symptoms are addressed in the section on Clinical Presentation (see text). (See Chap. 7 for details.)

### Somogyi Phenomenon

Somogyi phenomenon refers to a rebound hyperglycemia provoked by secretion of insulin counterregulatory hormones, glucagon and epinephrine, in response to hypoglycemia.[4] Patients with unexplained wide fluctuations in serum glucose, from too low to very high, should be suspected of having the Somogyi reaction.

The mechanism underlying this phenomenon is largely unknown, but it involves the following: To control rising serum glucose levels, the insulin dose is usually increased. As the glucose level falls in response to insulin, this, in turn, stimulates secretion of epinephrine, glucagon, corticosteroids, and growth hormone, all of which oppose the excessive insulin activity. Epinephrine triggers glycogenolysis in the liver; the corticosteroids stimulate gluconeogenesis. The result of these activities is a rebound *hyper*glycemia. Should this be perceived as a deterioration in the underlying diabetes prompting an increase in the insulin dose, such ac-

## TABLE 20–3. CARE PLAN FOR THE PATIENT WITH HYPOGLYCEMIA (HYPOGLYCEMIC SHOCK)

| Nursing Diagnoses | Desired Patient Outcomes | Nursing Interventions | Rationales |
|---|---|---|---|
| ***Nursing Diagnosis #1***<br>Cerebral function, alteration in, related to:<br>1. Hypoglycemia | Patient's condition will stabilize:<br>1. Neurologic status:<br>• Mental status: Oriented to person, place, date.<br>• Level of consciousness: Arousal and awareness intact.<br>• Cranial nerve function intact.<br>• Cerebellar function intact.<br>• Sensorimotor function intact.<br>• Deep tendon reflexes brisk.<br>2. Vital signs:<br>• Arterial blood pressure within 10 mmHg of patient's baseline.<br>• Heart rate: >60, <100 beats/min.<br>• Cardiac rhythm: Regular sinus.<br>• Respirations: <25–30 breaths/min.<br>• Breathing pattern: Eupnea.<br>3. Serum glucose: Stable at 70–110 mg/100 ml. | • Implement patient care to stabilize glucose metabolism. | |
| | | ○ Establish baseline neurologic function: Neuroglycopenia.<br>– Mental status: Changes in level of consciousness, disorientation, confusion; headache, lightheadedness, visual disturbances, irritability, lethargy; inappropriate behavior, convulsions, paralysis, coma. | ○ Primary energy substrate for the brain is glucose. Serum glucose levels <55 mg/100 ml can produce alterations in cerebral functions; appropriate and timely treatment is necessary to avert permanent neurologic damage. |
| | | ○ Cranial nerve function.<br>○ Cerebellar function. | ○ Appropriate cranial nerve and cerebellar functions reflect an intact brainstem. |
| | | – Sensory/motor function: Paresthesias, hemiparesis, paralysis, seizures, convulsions.<br>– Deep tendon reflexes. | |
| | | ○ Establish baseline adrenergic function: Vital signs—Blood pressure, heart rate, pulses, respiration, temperature. | ○ Adrenergic stimulation is a compensatory reaction by the body in response to hypoglycemia; it is largely responsible for symptomatology that occurs early in the course of hypoglycemia. |
| | | ○ Administer 50 ml of 50% dextrose in water intravenously as prescribed.<br>– If venous access not available, administer glucagon 1 mg, intramuscularly.<br>– Infusion of 10% dextrose should be initiated to maintain serum glucose levels between 100 and 200 mg/100 ml; and until the patient can safely ingest oral intake. | ○ Draw blood sample prior to administration of glucose for retrospective diagnosis.<br>○ A rapid and dramatic response should be expected upon glucose administration; if coma persists in spite of therapy, suspect cerebral edema.<br>○ Establish that protective reflexes—gag, swallowing, cough—are intact before offering food/drink for oral consumption, to prevent aspiration. |
| | | ○ Keep emergency dose of glucose at bedside. | ○ Wide fluctuations in serum glucose can occur rapidly. |
| | | ○ Monitor all vital signs and ECG throughout acute phase. | ○ Assists in evaluating response to therapy. |
| | | ○ Carefully monitor serum glucose levels. | |

*(continued)*

**TABLE 20–3. CARE PLAN FOR THE PATIENT WITH HYPOGLYCEMIA (HYPOGLYCEMIC SHOCK) *(Continued)***

| Nursing Diagnoses | Desired Patient Outcomes | Nursing Interventions | Rationales |
|---|---|---|---|
| ***Nursing Diagnosis #2***<br>Injury, potential for: Seizures, related to:<br>1. Altered neuronal cellular metabolism associated with hypoglycemia. | Patient will remain seizure-free and without injury. | • Implement measures to protect patient from potential injury associated with seizure activity and neuroglucopenia.<br>∘ Identify patient at risk of developing seizures.<br>∘ Assess for seizure activity:<br>– Patient's activity at time of seizure.<br>– Precipitating event.<br>– Description of onset and progression. Note any changes in pupil size and reactivity; urinary or bowel incontinence.<br>– Duration of apneic periods if generalized seizure.<br>– Duration of seizure activity.<br>– Patient's post-seizure behavior.<br>∘ Institute seizure precautions:<br>– Side rails padded and kept in up position.<br>– Bed placed in low position if possible.<br>– Oral airway conspicuously placed at head of bed.<br>– Suction equipment available for emergency care.<br>– Available oxygen source.<br>– Removal of potentially harmful objects from bedside. | ∘ Precautions can be taken to avert seizure activity and to protect the patient from injury.<br>∘ An alteration in the level of consciousness may occur due to a variety of circumstances. Careful assessment and description of seizure activity may be helpful in diagnosing and treating the underlying problem. |
| ***Nursing Diagnosis #3***<br>Nutrition, alteration in: Less than body requirements, related to:<br>1. Altered glucose metabolism. | Patient'ss condition will stabilize:<br>1. Serum glucose levels maintained within normal physiologic range: 70–110 mg/100 ml.<br>2. Body weight will stabilize within appropriate range; positive nitrogen balance will be maintained. | • Implement patient care activities to assist patient/family to understand and execute prescribed nutritional regimen.<br>∘ Assess patient for the following:<br>– Anorexia, nausea, vomiting, diarrhea, hunger, weakness, diaphoresis, tremors.<br>∘ Inquire of patient and/or family if this adrenergic symptomatology occurred at home and under what circumstances.<br>∘ Consult with nutritionist, physician, patient, and family to determine nutritional needs: | ∘ Hypoglycemia stimulates sympathetic nervous system activity; such symptomatology suggests a low serum glucose.<br>∘ It is essential to identify the precipitating cause of hypoglycemic episodes in order to determine how they can be prevented. |

| | | | |
|---|---|---|---|
| | 3. Patient will verbalize an increase in strength and improved appetite.<br>4. Patient will verbalize the effects of alcohol on glucose metabolism. | ○ Baseline nutritional status.<br>– Must include patient/family past eating habits, food preferences, and preparation. | ○ Baseline nutritional needs must be identified to ensure adequate nutritional intake with: (1) maintenance of glucose homeostasis; (2) prevention of recurring hypoglycemic episodes; (3) and reduction of risk of infection or other stressor. |
| | | ○ Involve patient and family in planning immediate and long-term treatment regimen. | ○ In the presence of diabetes, nutritional regimen must coincide with insulin or oral hypoglycemic therapy and exercise regimen.<br>○ Involving patient and family in decision-making process fosters compliance. |
| | | ○ Consider 6 small meals per day plan. | ○ Helps to maintain serum glucose within acceptable range; prevents wide fluctuations with periods of hypoglycemia alternating with hyperglycemia. |
| | | ○ Use of anticholinergic therapy. | ○ Used in conjunction with small meals, anticholinergic therapy can reduce rapid gastric emptying.<br>○ Rapid gastric emptying and accelerated intestinal glucose absorption can provoke hypoglycemia in some patients. While the underlying mechanism is unclear, gastrointestinal hormones may contribute to an exaggerated glucose-initiated insulin release. The triad of gastrointestinal disease, early onset of hypoglycemia after eating (within 1–3 hr), and the excessive discharge of insulin characterizes the syndrome of alimentary or "intestinal-hurry" hypoglycemia. |
| | | ○ Encourage patient and family to verbalize feelings regarding alcohol consumption.<br>– Discuss use of alcohol and impact on patient's overall status. | ○ Alcohol interferes with hepatic gluconeogenesis, decreasing availability of glucose during the postabsorptive state. |
| ***Nursing Diagnosis #4***<br>Knowledge deficit regarding underlying disease, and overall therapeutic regimen: Nutritional/insulin or hypoglycemic therapy/exercise.<br>***Nursing Diagnosis #5***<br>Health maintenance, alteration in. | Patient will be able to:<br>1. Relate hypoglycemia with level of health desired.<br>2. Specify major underlying principles regarding therapeutic regimen: Diet, insulin or oral hypoglycemics, and exercise. | • Determine the presence of knowledge deficit regarding overall treatment regimen, and diet in particular.<br>• Initiate teaching program regarding diet therapy with emphasis on self-care.<br>○ Patient/family should become familiar with signs of hypoglycemia and institute treatment immediately on their appearance. | • Knowledge of overall therapeutic regimen will facilitate self-care and health management; complications will be minimized.<br>○ Patient should verbalize the need to carry a rapid-acting sugar source on his or her person at all times; a Medic-Alert bracelet or wallet card is important to have at all times. |

*(continued)*

**TABLE 20–3. CARE PLAN FOR THE PATIENT WITH HYPOGLYCEMIA (HYPOGLYCEMIC SHOCK) *(Continued)***

| Nursing Diagnoses | Desired Patient Outcomes | Nursing Interventions | Rationales |
|---|---|---|---|
| ***Nursing Diagnosis #5 (cont.)*** | | | |
| | 3. Explain why it is necessary to carry a rapid-acting sugar source, and usefulness of wearing a Medic-Alert tag.<br>4. State the early signs and symptoms of hypoglycemia and actions to be taken.<br>5. Demonstrate self-care activities: Monitoring blood/urine; self-medication. | • Assess patient/family knowledge regarding disease syndrome and its essential long-term therapy.<br>○ Assess readiness to learn.<br>• Implement teaching program on self-care health-care practices. | • Understanding of underlying disease processes assists patient and family to cope with, and to adjust to, the limitations imposed by the illness. |
| ***Nursing Diagnosis #6***<br>Noncompliance: Denial. | Patient will be able to:<br>1. Admit he/she has diabetes mellitus or a hypoglycemic disorder.<br>2. Ask pertinent questions regarding care.<br>3. Actively plan necessary changes in lifestyle to include self-care of underlying illness.<br>4. Verbalize need for continued and regular follow-up care.<br>5. Report on available resources within the family and community setting. | • Assess patient's attitude regarding chronic illness.<br>• Allow patient and family to verbalize fears and concerns regarding underlying disease.<br>• Encourage patient to make decisions regarding care.<br>○ Have patient/family explain the significance of continued follow-up care. | • Fostering a positive attitude helps to ensure compliance.<br>• Verbalization assists in identifying misconceptions and unwarranted fears; patient and family attitudes regarding the health state desired can be ascertained.<br>• When patient feels in control, he/she may readily assume responsibility for self-care. |

tion would merely serve to perpetuate the vicious cycle of hypoglycemia–hyperglycemia characteristic of the Somogyi phenomenon. The appropriate therapy in this circumstance is to *lower* the insulin dose and allow the diabetes to stabilize.

It is important to identify the patient at risk of developing the Somogyi reaction and to anticipate its occurrence. A definitive diagnosis requires the presence of adrenergic and central nervous system alterations (i.e., neuroglycopenia) in the presence of serum glucose levels less than 55 mg/100 ml (symptomatic hypoglycemia).

## Treatment

Once hypoglycemia is suspected, blood should be drawn for retrospective diagnosis followed by the immediate administration of glucose. Initial treatment of serious hypoglycemia with altered consciousness is the intravenous administration of 50 ml of 50% dextrose in water. A continuous infusion of glucose should be initiated to prevent hypoglycemia until the patient is alert and able to ingest food safely. While oral glucose intake is critical to restoration of hepatic glycogen stores, patients with depressed levels of consciousness should not be given oral glucose because of the risk of aspiration. Additionally, oral glucose is not as reliable and does not act as rapidly as intravenous glucose.

If a venous access is not immediately available, glucagon (0.5 to 1 mg or more) intramuscularly will usually correct hypoglycemia induced by insulin or sulfonylureas. Alcohol-induced hypoglycemia is less responsive to such therapy, and it, as well as sulfonylurea-induced hypoglycemia, tends to be more profound and long-lasting. When chlorpropamide is the sulfonylurea involved, hypoglycemia is more likely to last for several days. If hypoglycemia recurs, an infusion of 10% dextrose should be initiated and maintained at a rate sufficient to maintain serum glucose levels between 100 and 200 mg/100 ml.

Once the patient's condition is stabilized, the circumstances surrounding the occurrence of drug-induced hypoglycemia need to be investigated.

## Nursing Care of the Patient with Hypoglycemia (Hypoglycemic Shock)

While hypoglycemia is most closely identified as a major complication in the patient with diabetes, it can occur as a separate and distinct endocrinopathy. Thus, in treating the patient with hypoglycemia, nursing care is directed toward identifying the individual at risk, preventing life-threatening complications, and assisting the individual and family/significant others to understand the nature of the illness, necessary prophylactic measures, and its impact on the lifestyle and integrity of each individual.

### *Therapeutic Goals*

Implementation of nursing process in the care of the patient with hypoglycemia (hypoglycemic shock) revolves around the following therapeutic goals:

1. Identify the patient at risk.
2. Establish a thorough and comprehensive database including:
   A. Clinical history (functional health patterns).
   B. Physical examination.
   C. Laboratory/diagnostic studies.
3. Stabilize glucose metabolism with serum glucose within acceptable physiologic range.
4. Protect patient from potential injury associated with seizure activity (neuroglucopenia).
5. Assist patient to implement prescribed nutritional/hypoglycemic/exercise regimen.
6. Initiate patient/family self-care educational program to assist in health-care management and implementation of prophylactic health-care practices.

### *Nursing Diagnoses, Desired Patient Outcomes, and Nursing Interventions*

Pertinent nursing diagnoses, desired patient outcomes, and nursing interventions/rationales in the care of the patient with hypoglycemia are presented in the care plan in Table 20–3. See also Table 19–5 for additional pertinent nursing diagnoses.

## REFERENCES

1. Hershman, JM: Endocrine Pathophysiology: A Patient-Oriented Approach. Lea & Febiger, Philadelphia, 1988, p 289.
2. Metz, R and Larsen, E: Blue Book of Endocrinology. WB Saunders, Philadelphia, 1985, p 289.
3. Muir, BL: Pathophysiology: An Introduction to the Mechanisms of Disease, ed 10. John Wiley & Sons, New York, 1988, p 241.
4. Ramsey, PW: Hyperglycemia at dawn. Am J Nurs 87:1424, November 1987.

# UNIT THREE

# Bibliography


Bates, S and Ahern, J: Tight control: What does it mean (diabetes mellitus). Am J Nurs, November 1986.

Boehm, TM: Hyperglycemia in critical care medicine. Crit Care Q 6(3), December 1983.

Burman, KD: Interpretation of thyroid function tests in critically ill patients. Crit Care Q 6(3), December 1983.

Callahan, M and Bradley, D: Why you should teach your diabetic patients to chart. Nursing '88 18(3), March 1988.

Christman, C and Bennett, J: Diabetes: New names, new test, new diet. Nursing '87, 17(1), January 1987.

Cooper, KL: Making the diabetes connection. Am J Nurs, September 1986.

Coralli, C, Raisz, L, and Wood, C: Osteoporosis: Significance, risk factors and treatment. Nurse Practitioner 11(9), September 1986.

Duffens, K and Marx, JA: Alcoholic ketoacidosis—A review. J Emerg Med 5(5), September/October 1987.

Dumont, JE, Roger, PP, and Ludgate, M: Assays for thyroid growth immunoglobulins and their clinical implications: Methods, concepts, and misconceptions. Endocrine Rev: 8(4), November 1987.

Evangelisti, J and Thorpe, C: Thyroid storm: A nursing crisis. Heart Lung 12(2), March 1983.

Felig, P, Baxter, J, and Frohman, L: Endocrinology and Metabolism, ed 2. McGraw-Hill, New York, 1987.

Flavin, K and Haire-Joshu, D: Drugs for diabetes: The pharmacologic repertoire. Am J Nurs, November 1986.

Gavin, JR: Diabetes and exercise. Am J Nurs 88(2), February 1988.

Greenspan, F and Forsham, P: Basic and Clinical Endocrinology. Lange Medical Publications, Los Altos, CA, 1985.

Griffin, JE: Manual of Clinical Endocrinology and Metabolism. McGraw-Hill, New York, 1982.

Haire-Joshu, D: Contrasting type I and type II diabetes. Am J Nurs, September 1986.

Hershman, J: Endocrine Pathophysiology: A Patient-Oriented Approach, ed 3. Lea & Febiger, Philadelphia, 1988.

Johndrow, P and Thornton, S: Syndrome of inappropriate antidiuretic hormone. Focus Crit Care 12(5), October 1985.

Martin, CR: Endocrine Physiology. Oxford University Press, New York, 1985.

Metheny, NM: Fluid and Electrolyte Balance, Nursing Considerations. JB Lippincott, Philadelphia, 1987.

Metz, R and Larson, E: Blue Book of Endocrinology. WB Saunders, Philadelphia, 1985.

Muir, BL: Pathophysiology: An introduction to the mechanisms of disease, ed 2. John Wiley & Sons, New York, 1988.

O'Neil, JR: Thyroid crisis, action STAT. Nursing '87, November 1987.

Payne, NR: Emergency care of the patient with myxedema coma. J Emerg Nurs 12(6), November/December 1986.

Poole, D: Type II diabetes mellitus update: Diagnosis and management. Nurse Practitioner, 11(8), August 1986.

Rabin, D and McKenna TJ: Clinical Endocrinology and Metabolism: Principles and Practice. Grune & Stratton, New York, 1982.

Ramsey, PR: Hyperglycemia at dawn. Am J Nurs 87:1424, November 1987.

Rice, V: Problems of water regulation, diabetes insipidus and syndrome of inappropriate antidiuretic hormone. Crit Care Nurse, January/February 1983.

Roberts, SL: Physiological Concepts and the Critically Ill Patient. Prentice-Hall, Englewood Cliffs, NJ, 1985.

Skelly, A and Van Son, A: Insulin allergy in clinical practice. Nurse Practitioner 12(4), April 1987.

Widmann, FK: Clinical Interpretation of Laboratory Tests. FA Davis, Philadelphia, 1983.

UNIT FOUR

# The Renal/Urinary System

Maintenance of a stable internal environment is essential to the life processes of each individual. Concentrations of such important substances as water, sodium, potassium, calcium, and hydrogen ions must be maintained in a state of dynamic equilibrium if optimal cellular function is to be achieved.

While the nervous system and endocrine system are responsible for coordinating the numerous physiologic and metabolic phenomena occurring within cells, it is the renal/urinary system that is largely responsible for the existence of stable ionic conditions in the extracellular fluid, which bathes each cell and within which these phenomena occur. Total body water balance is achieved by mechanisms occurring within the kidneys. The physiologic balance of electrolyte concentrations within the body is maintained within very narrow limits by the kidneys precisely by selective excretion or retention of substances. Excretory functions of the kidneys include the elimination of metabolic waste products including urea, creatinine, and uric acid. The kidneys also eliminate foreign chemicals from the body such as drugs, poisons, and food additives, among others. The kidneys also contribute to the regulation of serum osmolality, and they play a major regulatory role in acid–base balance (see Chap. 30).

Finally, in addition to regulatory and excretory functions, the kidneys function as endocrine glands secreting hormones—renin, the active metabolite of vitamin D (1,25-dihydroxycholecalciferol); erythropoietin factor; and renal prostaglandins. Thus, the kidneys also play a vital role in the regulation of blood pressure, calcium metabolism, and red blood cell synthesis and maturation.

In the chapters to follow, an effort is made to distinguish these vital activities of the renal/urinary system, and to appreciate the unique relationship between structure and function. Emphasis will be placed on the kidney's role in maintaining fluid and electrolyte balance. Nursing process in the diagnosis and management of the patient with renal dysfunction is explored, including the care of patients with acute renal failure, end-stage renal disease, and renal transplantation. Discussions of renal assessment, fluid and electrolyte balance, and calcium metabolism are also included. Nursing care plans are based on nursing diagnoses and include specific patient outcomes, nursing interventions, and their rationales.

## UNIT OUTLINE

CHAPTER 21

# Anatomy and Physiology of the Renal/Urinary System

## CHAPTER OUTLINE



## LEARNING OBJECTIVES

**At the end of this chapter, you should be able to:**

1. Describe the gross anatomical structures of the kidney and urinary system.
2. Describe the microanatomy of the kidney and urinary system.
3. Relate the unique anatomical features of the renal blood supply to renal physiology.
4. Describe the renal processes of glomerular filtration and tubular reabsorption and secretion.
5. Define renal clearance and its significance.
6. Describe the renal processes for sodium, chloride, and water.
7. Review the regulatory role of renin and angiotensin.
8. Describe renal regulation of potassium balance.
9. Define the renal contribution to calcium homeostasis.
10. Explain why individuals with chronic renal failure develop anemia.
11. Summarize the major functions of the kidney.

## ANATOMICAL STRUCTURE OF THE KIDNEYS AND URINARY SYSTEM

Knowledge of renal anatomy is essential to the understanding of the mechanisms of urine formation. The renal/urinary system includes the kidneys, ureters, urinary bladder, and urethra. Urine formed within the kidneys collects in the renal pelvis and then flows through the ureters into the bladder from which it is eliminated from the body by the urethra.

### General Features

The bean-shaped kidneys are paired organs located in the retroperitoneal space on either side of the vertebral column, T-12 to L-3. The kidneys are somewhat protected by adjacent organs including the overlying peritoneum and intestines anteriorly, and the lower two ribs and hefty musculature posteriorly.

Blood vessels and ureters enter the kidney by way of the renal hilus (Fig. 21-1). Located within the hilus is the renal pelvis, which expands into 3 or more major calyces. The major calyces are supplied by a variable number of minor calyces (12-18). Each minor calyx, in turn, is supplied by 1 or 2 renal papillae from which urine, formed within the kidney, is emptied into the minor and major calyces and collected in the renal pelvis.

The inner gross structure of the renal parenchyma shows regional differences, which reflect the structure and location of the nephrons. The cortex comprises the outer parenchymal layer and has a granular appearance because it contains all the glomerular components of the nephrons. The medulla makes up the inner parenchymal layer and contains the renal pyramids. These are triangular-shaped structures (usually 8-18 in number) with a striated appearance reflective of the tubular components of the nephrons. The base of the renal pyramids faces the cortex, while the apices (renal papillae) face the kidney hilus and extend into the minor calyces (see Fig. 21-1).

The walls of the renal calyces, pelvis, the ureters, and bladder contain smooth muscle, which contracts rhythmically and helps to propel urine along its course by peristalsis. The transitional cells lining these structures are unique in that they can accommodate a large degree of stretch in response to varying volumes of urine.

## Microanatomy of the Nephron — Functional Unit of the Kidney

Each kidney is composed of approximately a million nephrons. As the structural and functional unit of the kidney, the nephron consists of a "filtering component," called the *glomerulus*, and a *tubule* extending out from the glomerulus.[1] The glomerulus functions to filter solute and water from the

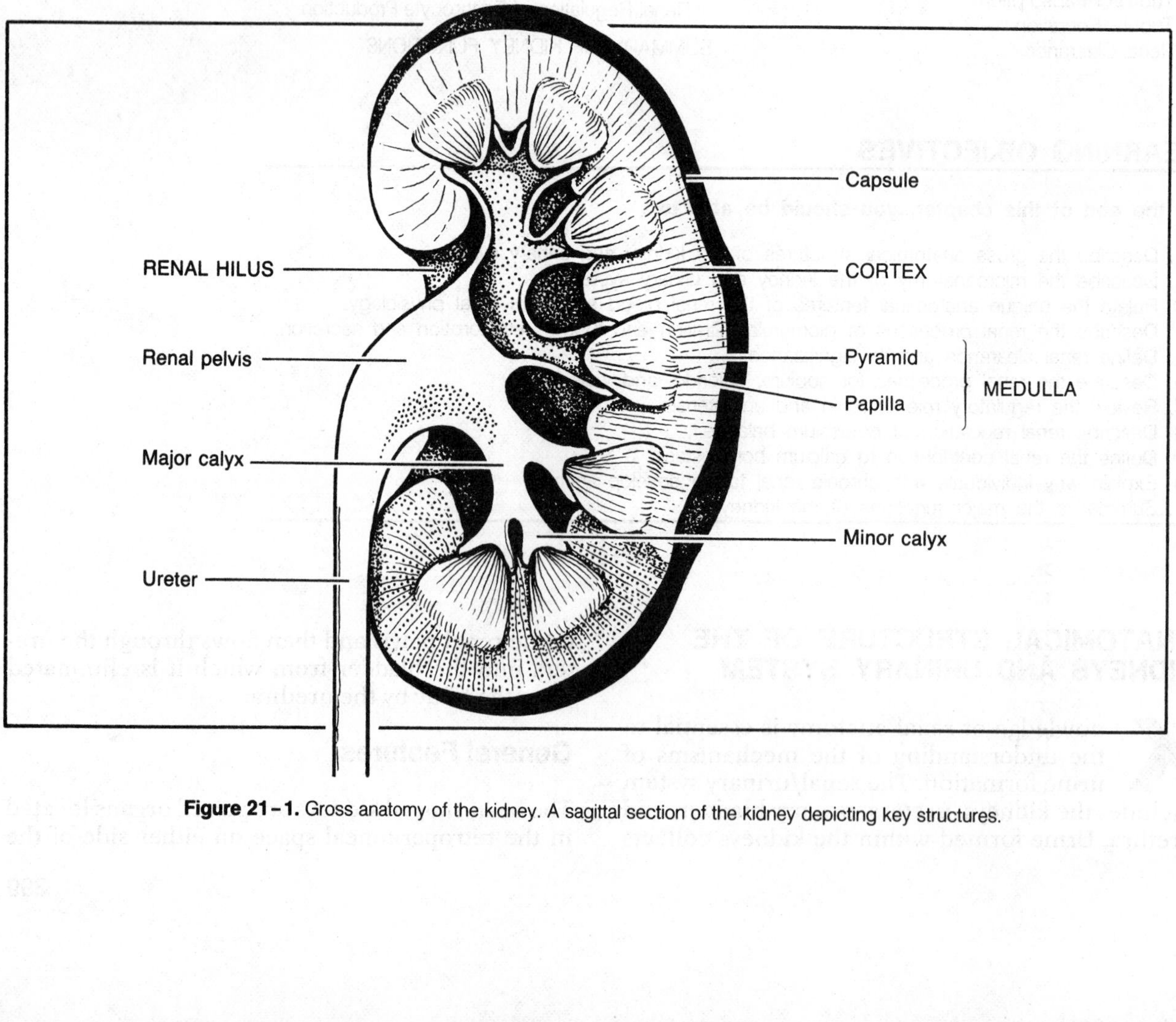


**Figure 21-1.** Gross anatomy of the kidney. A sagittal section of the kidney depicting key structures.

blood; and the tubule functions to reabsorb essential substances from the filtrate, to secrete unessential substances, and to permit these substances and metabolic waste products to flow into the calyces and renal pelvis as urine.

There are 2 types of nephrons in the kidney named according to their overall location: cortical nephrons and juxtamedullary nephrons (Fig. 21–2). Approximately 85% of all nephrons are of the cortical type, and about 15% are of the juxtamedullary type. Cortical nephrons are located almost entirely within the cortex, with but a small portion of the loop of Henle dipping down into the medulla. The bulk of renal regulatory, excretory, and secretory functions is performed by the cortical nephrons.

The juxtamedullary nephrons have glomeruli, which lie adjacent to the cortical–medullary interface, and tubular systems, which have an extended thin segment of the loop of Henle that penetrates deeply into the medulla, within the renal pyramids. The primary function of juxtamedullary nephrons is to establish and maintain the osmolality of the medullary interstitium, creating osmotic gradients necessary for the concentration of urine (see below).

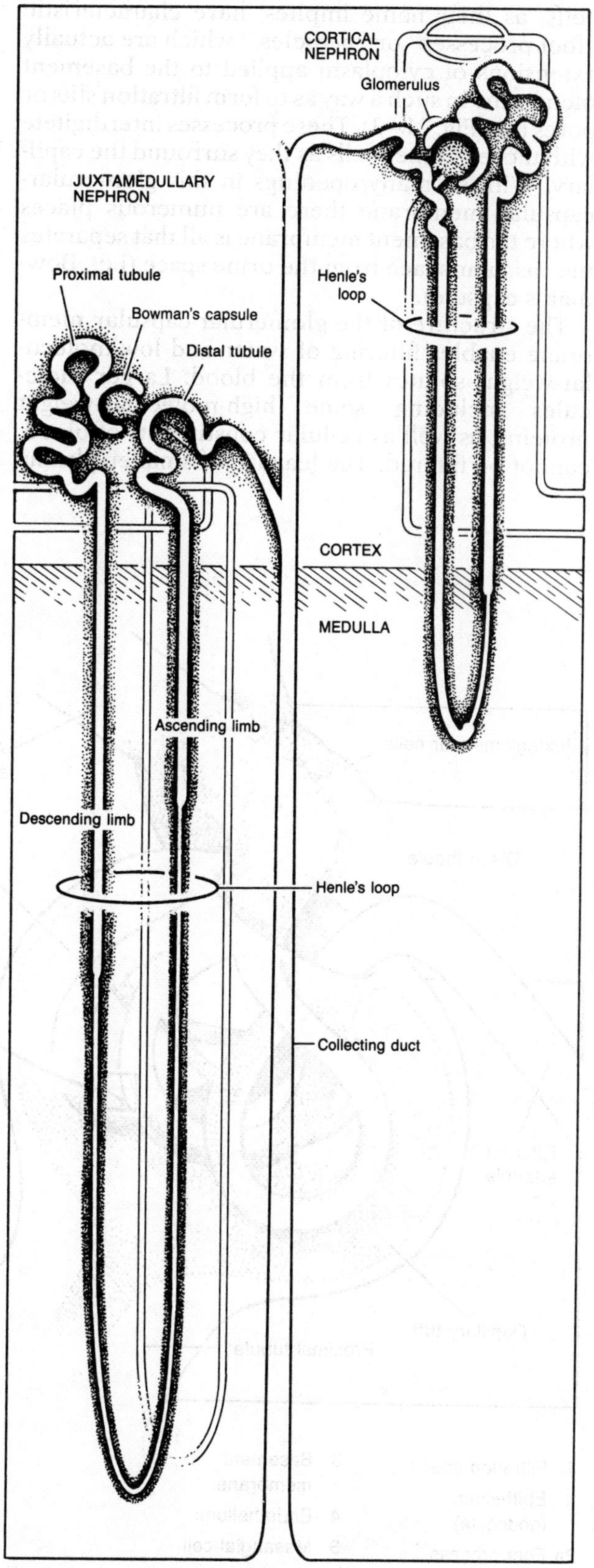


**Figure 21–2.** The nephron, the structural and functional unit of the kidney. Two types of nephrons, the cortical nephrons and juxtamedullary nephrons, are depicted.

### *Glomerulus*

The glomerulus consists of a tuft of capillaries (glomerular capillaries) and a balloonlike hollow capsule (Bowman's capsule) into which the capillary tuft protrudes. These glomerular capillaries, which form the "vascular" space, are derived from the afferent arteriole entering the glomerulus; they eventually converge to form the efferent arteriole, which leaves the glomerulus and, in turn, subdivides into a second set of capillaries (see section entitled "Renal Blood Supply" below). The "urine" space is provided by Bowman's capsule, which communicates and is continuous with the proximal convoluted tubule (Fig. 21–3).

**Glomerular-Capsular Membrane.** The primary function of the glomerular-capsular membrane is to filter water and solutes in the blood. It consists of (1) endothelial cells, which line the capillary lumen; (2) epithelial cells or podocytes, which line that portion of Bowman's capsule that is aligned with the endothelium; and (3) a basement membrane, which separates these 2 layers (see Fig. 21–3).

The endothelial cells comprising the glomerular-capsular membrane are distinctive. Unlike capillaries elsewhere in the body, these cells are characterized by having many openings or fenestrations ("Swiss cheese" appearance), which facilitate the filtration process. The podocytes likewise are adapted to facilitate the filtration process. These cells, as their name implies, have characteristic "foot processes" or "pedicles," which are actually extensions of cytoplasm applied to the basement membrane in such a way as to form filtration slits or pores (see Fig. 21–3). These processes interdigitate with those of other cells as they surround the capillary. With so many openings in this glomerular-capsular membrane there are numerous places where the basement membrane is all that separates the vascular space from the urine space (i.e., Bowman's capsule).

The structure of the glomerular-capsular membrane enables filtering of water and low-molecular-weight solutes from the blood. Larger molecules including some high-molecular-weight proteins, as well as cellular constituents of blood, cannot be filtered. The leakage of smaller plasma proteins, such as albumin, does occur and can be significant. However, most proteins that are filtered are largely reabsorbed in the proximal convoluted tubule. Consequently, proteinuria and hematuria are distinct abnormalities. Substances that have been filtered pass into Bowman's capsule and flow as the "filtrate" into the proximal tubule.

**Mesangial (Intercapillary) Cells.** Mesangial or intercapillary cells are also found within the glomerulus (see Fig. 21–3). These cells do not communicate directly with either the vascular or urine spaces. They constitute 35%–40% of all cells within the glomerulus and are thought to provide a specialized form of connective tissue support. They may also assist in preserving the integrity of the glomerular-capsular membrane by their phagocytic activity.

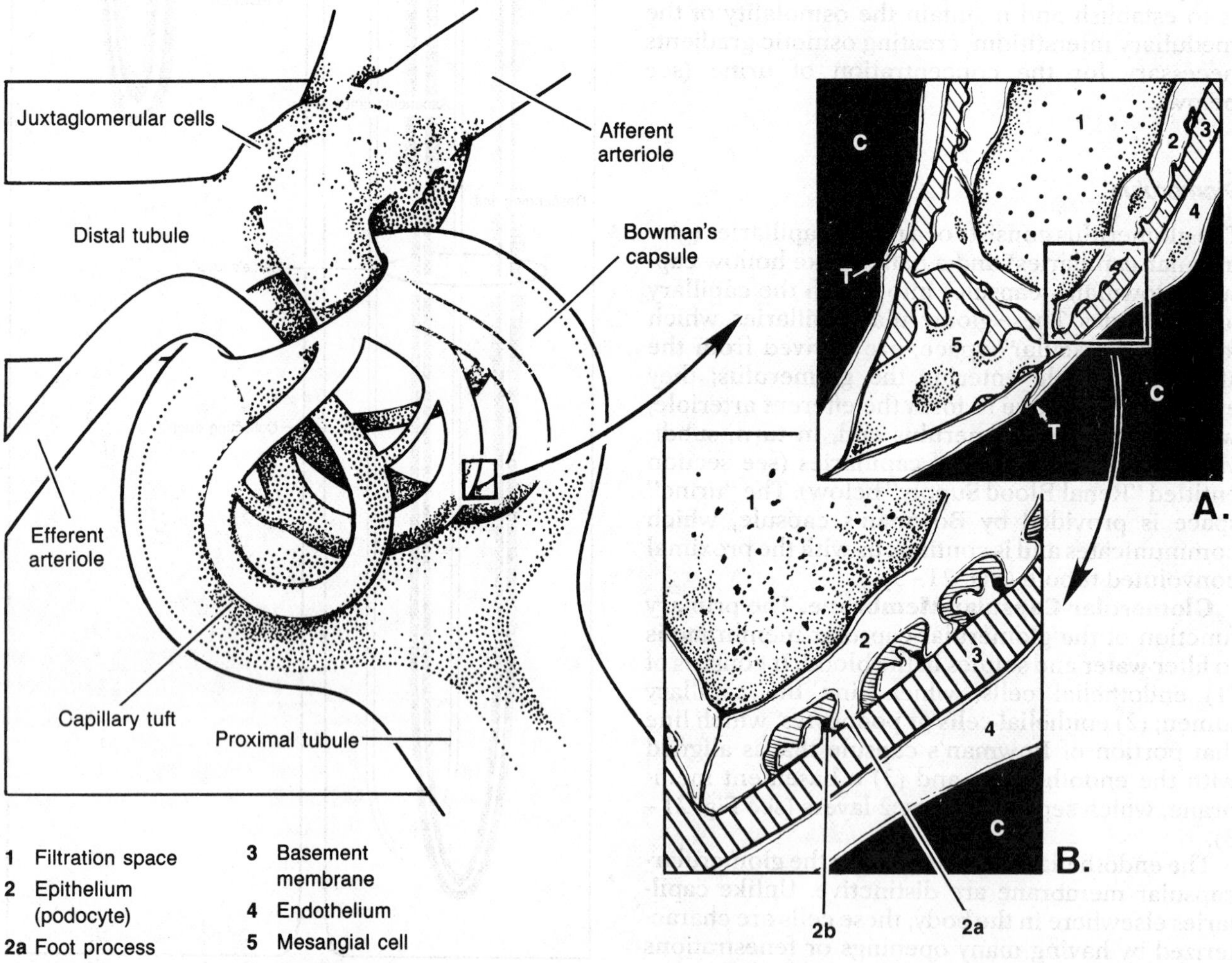


1 Filtration space
2 Epithelium (podocyte)
2a Foot process
2b Slit pore
3 Basement membrane
4 Endothelium
5 Mesangial cell
C Capillary
T Tight junction

**Figure 21–3.** The glomerulus and glomerular-capsular membrane. The glomerulus consists of a "vascular" space, the capillary tuft, surrounded by a "urine" space formed by Bowman's capsule. Key microscopic structures comprising the glomerular-capsular membrane are depicted. The unique relationship of these structures to each other facilitates filtration.

### *Tubular System*

The renal tubular system consists of the proximal convoluted tubule, the loop of Henle, distal convoluted tubule, and the collecting ducts. The structure of each portion of the tubular system differs reflecting their differing functions (Fig. 21–4).

**Proximal Convoluted Tubule.** The proximal convoluted tubule (PCT) comprises the bulk of the tubular system within each nephron. It originates at Bowman's capsule and occurs largely within the renal cortex. It is concerned primarily with the reabsorption of substances from the filtrate. Numerous microvilli on the luminal (tubular) border of these cells greatly increase the surface area for reabsorption. The presence of many mitochondria provides energy for the active transport of many of these substances.

**Loop of Henle.** The loop of Henle is a continuation of the PCT and commonly consists of a descending limb, a thin segment, and an ascending limb. Cells lining this portion of the tubules are flat with a paucity of microvilli and mitochondria, suggesting that very little reabsorption occurs here. In the juxtamedullary nephrons, this portion of the tubules is concerned primarily with the maintenance of the osmolality of the medullary interstitium, which is critical to the formation of concentrated urine (see Fig. 21–4).

**Distal Convoluted Tubule.** The distal convoluted tubule (DCT), like the PCT, occurs largely within the cortex of the kidney with a portion of it approximating the glomerular hilus, that is, the juxtaglomerular apparatus (see below). The occurrence of some microvilli and an abundance of mitochondria facilitate the reabsorption and secretion processes that occur here (see Fig. 21–4).

**Collecting Ducts.** The collecting ducts receive the distal tubules of several nephrons within the cortex and pass down through the medullary pyramids where they merge to form the major collecting ducts that open into the minor calyces in the tip (apex) of each renal papilla. It is across the membrane lining the collecting ducts that the bulk of the urine concentrating process occurs (see Fig. 21–4).

### Renal Blood Supply

Blood enters the kidney by the renal artery, which arises from the aorta at a right angle and subdivides into progressively smaller branches including interlobar, arcuate, and interlobular arteries. At the level of the glomeruli, the interlobular arteries give rise to *af*ferent arterioles (i.e., those arterioles that carry blood *to* the glomeruli). These afferent arterioles, in turn, give rise to the tufts of glomerular capillaries. These capillaries converge to form the *ef*ferent arterioles (i.e., those arterioles that carry blood *away* from the glomeruli).

Each efferent arteriole, in turn, gives rise to a second bed of capillaries. The cortical capillary plexus surrounds the tubular system of cortical nephrons; the peritubular capillary bed, or vasa recta, surrounds the tubular system of juxtamedullary nephrons. The capillaries of the vasa recta are unique in that they form an intimate and extensive network surrounding the juxtamedullary tubular system progressing into hairpin-loop vessels that run parallel to the loop of Henle and the collecting ducts (Fig. 21–5). This anatomical relationship is critical to the maintenance of the hyperosmolality of the medullary interstitium, essential for the concentration of urine (see below).

## BASIC RENAL PHYSIOLOGY

The kidneys function to maintain the composition and volume of extracellular fluid by urine formation. Urine formation begins with the filtration of essentially protein-free plasma across the glomerular-capsular membrane into Bowman's capsule. The final urine that enters the renal pelvis is considerably different from the glomerular filtrate because as the filtered fluid flows through the various portions of the tubular system its composition is altered significantly. The processes of tubular reabsorption and tubular secretion (see below) are largely responsible for this change. The intimate relationship of the tubules and peritubular capillaries permits transfer of solutes and water between the peritubular plasma and the tubular lumen, thereby facilitating these processes.

### Glomerular Filtration

Glomerular filtration is a passive process in which a portion of the blood plasma flowing through the glomerulus is transferred from the capillaries (vascular space) across the glomerular-capsular membrane into Bowman's capsule (urine space). The energy required for glomerular filtration is derived from the hydrostatic blood pressure generated by each contraction of the heart muscle. Pressure gradients between the blood flowing through the glomerular capillaries and the filtrate in Bowman's capsule provide the driving force that facilitates the passive movement of solutes and fluid across the porous glomerular-capsular membrane.

The special features of the glomerular-capsular membrane (see Fig. 21–3) facilitate selective filtration of water, crystalloids, and other low-molecular-weight solutes while impeding movement of large proteins and colloids, protein-bound substances, and other macromolecules. The glomerular-capsular membrane presents an enormous surface area through which constituents of blood can be filtered selectively. The filtrate that flows into the

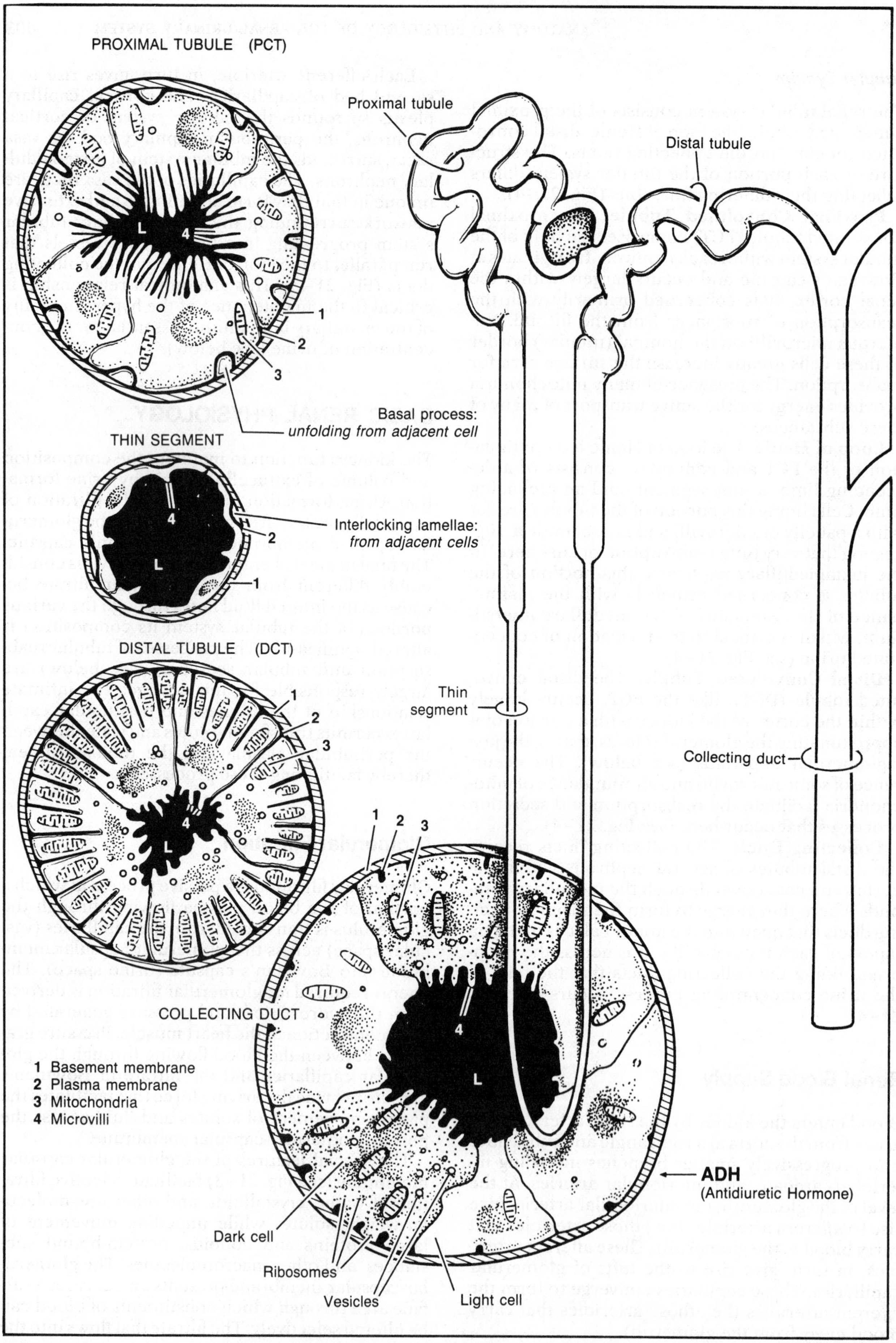


**Figure 21–4.** Microanatomy of the renal tubular system, which consists of the proximal convoluted tubule (PCT), the loop of Henle, distal convoluted tubule (DCT), and the collecting duct. The structures of these various components, which underlie their unique functions, are depicted in cross-section.

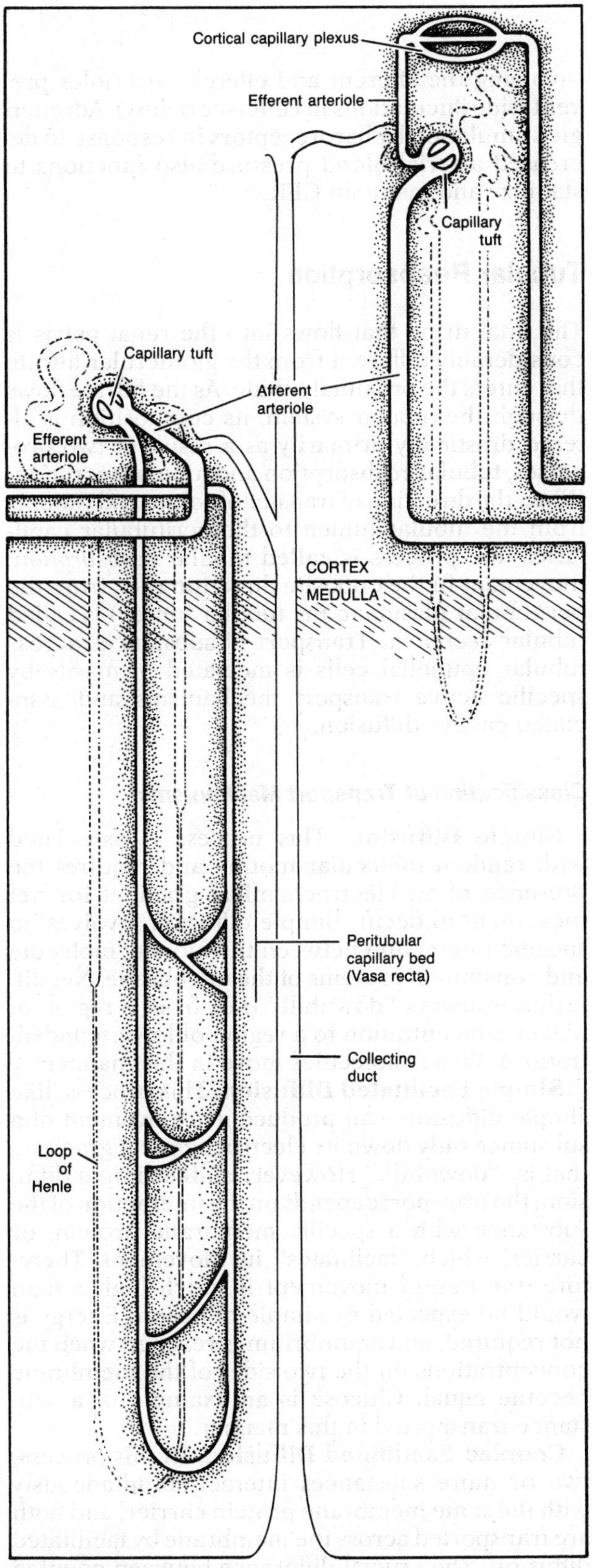


**Figure 21–5.** Vascular component of the nephrons. Blood supply to the cortical and juxtamedullary nephrons is differentiated. In each case, afferent arterioles carry blood *to* the glomeruli where they give rise to the capillary tuft; these capillaries converge to form the efferent arterioles, which carry blood *away* from the glomeruli. Each efferent arteriole, in turn, gives rise to a second bed of capillaries, the cortical capillary plexus, and the vasa recta, or peritubular capillaries. (See also Fig. 21–2 to appreciate the intimate relationship between the tubular system and vascular supply.)

proximal convoluted tubule from Bowman's capsule is nearly isotonic with blood plasma except for a reduced concentration of protein and the nearly complete absence of RBCs.

### Net Filtration Pressure

The existing pressure gradients within the glomerulus are favorable for filtration. The net filtration pressure (NFP) reflects the sum of the opposing hydrostatic blood pressure minus the colloid osmotic pressures acting across the capillary. The hydrostatic blood pressure at the afferent end of the glomerular capillaries is greater than the colloid osmotic pressure, thus favoring filtration (Fig. 21–6). As blood flows through the glomerular capillary bed, this NFP is gradually reduced and net filtration may actually cease as blood flow approaches the efferent end of the capillary bed.

These changes in the magnitude of the filtration force are explained by two factors: (1) as blood flows through the capillary bed, hydrostatic blood pressure is somewhat reduced owing to the resistance to flow offered by the capillaries; (2) because the filtration process removes water but very little protein from the plasma, the concentration of plasma proteins is increased as blood flow approaches the efferent end of the capillary bed. When the consequent rise in colloid osmotic pressure becomes high enough to counteract the blood hydrostatic pressure, net filtration ceases.[2] Glomerular filtration is a critically important process because it provides the filtrate on which the rest of the tubules act. If there is no filtrate, there can be no urine formation.

### Glomerular Filtration Rate

Nearly 25% of the total cardiac output flows through the kidneys each minute. Of this amount of blood plasma entering the glomerular capillaries by the afferent arterioles, about 20% is filtered and becomes the glomerular filtrate; the remaining 80% remains in the blood and passes into the peritubular capillary bed.

The glomerular filtration rate (GFR) is the rate at which the glomerular filtrate is formed. Normally, it amounts to approximately 125 ml/minute, or the enormous amount of 180 liters/24 hours. Because less than 1.8 liters of urine are formed and excreted, over 99% of the filtrate is reabsorbed. This ability of the kidney to filter and process such an enormous volume of plasma largely accounts for its excretion of large quantities of metabolic waste products and its precise regulation of the constituents of the internal environment.

The magnitude of the glomerular filtration rate is determined simply by the algebraic sum of forces favoring filtration (i.e., glomerular hydrostatic

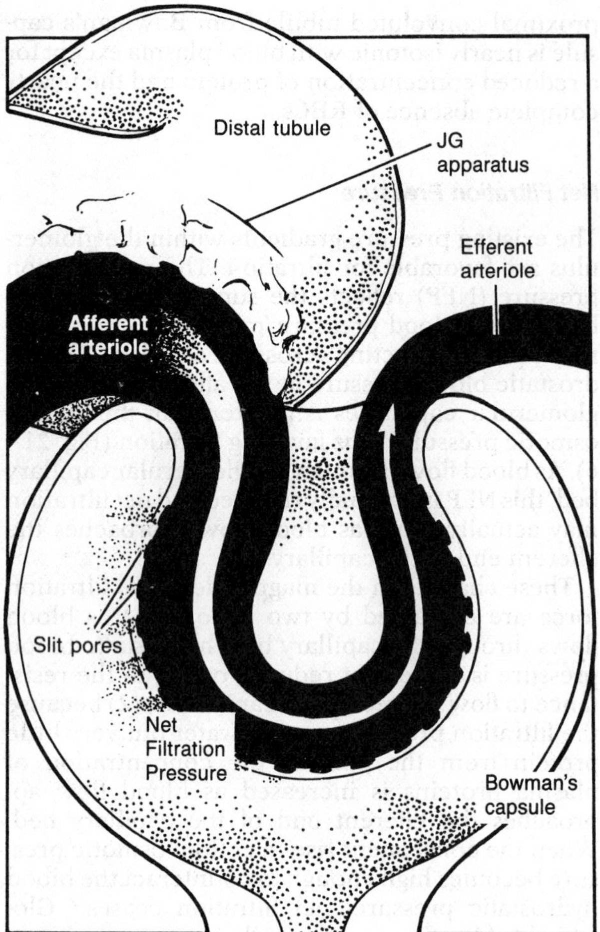


**Figure 21-6.** The existing pressure gradients within the glomerulus are favorable for filtration. The net filtration pressure (NFP) reflects the sum of the opposing hydrostatic blood pressure minus the colloidal osmotic pressure acting across the glomerular-capsular membrane. As blood flows toward the efferent arteriole, hydrostatic pressure diminishes and net filtration eventually ceases.

blood pressure) and those opposing filtration (i.e., hydrostatic pressure exerted by the filtrate in Bowman's capsule and the colloid osmotic pressure of the plasma). Accordingly, any change either in the hydrostatic pressures within the glomerular capillaries or Bowman's capsule, or in the osmotic pressure of the plasma, can alter the net glomerular filtration rate. For example, a drop in systemic arterial pressure associated with hypovolemia, or with left ventricular failure, will decrease the GFR; a drop in colloid osmotic pressure associated with hypoproteinemia will increase the GFR; a ureteral obstruction might eventually decrease GFR by increasing capsular hydrostatic pressure. These examples illustrate how changes in pressures favoring or opposing filtration can alter the GFR. Fortunately, intrinsic autoregulatory mechanisms involving the afferent and efferent arterioles prevent wide fluctuations in GFR (see below). Adrenergic stimulation by baroreceptors in response to decreased arterial blood pressure also functions to stabilize and maintain GFR.

## Tubular Reabsorption

The final urine that flows into the renal pelvis is considerably different from the glomerular filtrate that enters the proximal tubule. As the filtrate flows through the tubular system, its composition is altered drastically primarily as a result of two processes, tubular reabsorption and tubular secretion. When the direction of transfer of solute and water is from the tubular lumen to the peritubular capillaries, the process is called tubular *reabsorption*; movement in the opposite direction (i.e., from the peritubular plasma to the tubular lumen) is called tubular *secretion*. Transport of substances across tubular epithelial cells is mediated primarily by specific active transport mechanisms and associated passive diffusion.

### *Classification of Transport Mechanisms*[3]

**Simple Diffusion.** This process is associated with random molecular motion and requires the presence of an electrochemical gradient for net movement to occur. Simple diffusion involves no specific interaction between the moving molecule and constituent proteins of the membrane. Net diffusion is always "downhill" (i.e., from a region of higher concentration to a region of lower concentration). Water molecules move in this manner.

**Simple Facilitated Diffusion.** This process, like simple diffusion, can produce net movement of a substance only down its electrochemical gradient, that is, "downhill." However, unlike simple diffusion, the transport depends on the interaction of the substance with a specific membrane protein, or carrier, which "facilitates" its movement. Therefore, the rate of movement is much higher than would be expected by simple diffusion. Energy is not required, and equilibrium is reached when the concentrations on the two sides of the membrane become equal. Glucose is an example of a substance transported in this manner.

**Coupled Facilitated Diffusion.** In this process, two or more substances interact simultaneously with the same membrane protein carrier, and both are transported across the membrane by facilitated diffusion. The crucial difference between coupled and simple facilitated diffusion is that movement of one of the co-transported substances is "uphill" (i.e., against its electrochemical gradient). The net uphill transport uses energy liberated by the simultaneous downhill diffusion of the other co-transported substances. Thus, as one of the substances moves with its electrochemical gradient, the energy released somehow is able to drive the other substance uphill against its electrochemical gradient. Sodium is frequently the substance moving downhill in coupled facilitated diffusion systems, and the co-transported substance being simultaneously moved uphill is said to undergo *secondary active transport.*

**Primary Active Transport.** In this process the transported molecule also interacts with a membrane protein carrier and is moved across a membrane against an electrochemical gradient (i.e., "uphill"). The energy for this net uphill "active" transport comes directly from the splitting of ATP. Thus, "primary" active transport specifically denotes that chemical energy is the direct source of energy for this process. In this way, primary active transport differs from the secondary active transport mechanism described above.

**Passive Transport.** Passive transport occurs as a result of electrochemical gradients created by active transport reabsorption of specific substances along the tubular system, and by osmotic gradients associated with the relative increased protein content of blood in the peritubular capillaries. About 80% of the total water filtered is passively reabsorbed in the PCT in association with active reabsorption of sodium and glucose. Chloride and bicarbonate ions are reabsorbed passively due to the electrical gradient created by active sodium reabsorption.

Urea reabsorption is an example of a passive process that is completely dependent on the reabsorption of water. Because urea is not reabsorbed from the PCT at the same rate as water, its intratubular concentration eventually exceeds the peritubular plasma urea concentration. Accordingly, urea diffuses down its concentration gradient from the tubular lumen into the peritubular capillaries.

### Transport Mechanisms in Tubular Reabsorption

Most substances reabsorbed in the renal tubules must cross *two* membranes in their journey from tubular lumen through the tubular epithelial cell to the interstitial fluid. These include the *luminal* membrane, which separates the luminal filtrate from the cell cytoplasm, and the *basolateral* membrane, which separates the cell cytoplasm from the interstitial fluid. Thus, in order to fully characterize the overall reabsorption of a substance across the tubular epithelium it is important to appreciate what transport characteristics exist for each of these membranes.

### Sodium Tubular Reabsorption

In the tubular reabsorption of sodium, for example, two types of transport mechanisms are involved, namely, simple facilitated diffusion and primary active transport. Movement of sodium ions across the luminal membrane into the cell cytoplasm occurs mainly by simple facilitated diffusion. Transport of sodium ions across the basolateral membrane into the interstitial fluid occurs by an active transport mechanism involving a Na/K-dependent ATPase "pump" found only in the basolateral membrane (Fig. 21–7). Finally, once within the interstitial fluid, sodium and water move into the peritubular capillaries by bulk flow. Bulk flow or simple diffusion into peritubular capillaries is the final step in the reabsorption of all substances.

The unidirectional reabsorptive movement of sodium ions is facilitated by the "asymmetry" of the luminal and basolateral membrane transport processes. The continued net movement of sodium ions across the luminal membrane depends on the electrochemical gradient created and maintained by the basolateral membrane Na/K-dependent ATPase pump. By keeping the cytoplasmic sodium concentration low and the cell interior negatively charged, this pump facilitates sodium tubular reabsorption.

### Glucose Tubular Reabsorption[4]

The types of transport mechanisms involved in the reabsorption of glucose include coupled facilitated diffusion (with sodium) and simple facilitated diffusion. Glucose is an example of "uphill" transport characteristic of coupled facilitated diffusion. The energy used to drive the uphill movement of glucose from the tubular lumen through the luminal membrane and into the cell cytoplasm is derived from the simultaneous downhill movement of sodium. This mechanism is so efficient that glucose is virtually completely reabsorbed. Upon entry into the cell, the glucose exits across the basolateral membrane by simple facilitated diffusion, this downhill movement being driven by the high intracellular concentration of glucose achieved in the cell by the action of luminal transport processes. What is fundamental to appreciate is that the entire process of glucose reabsorption depends ultimately on the primary active Na/K-dependent ATPase pump in the basolateral membrane. This pump maintains the electrochemical gradient for net sodium diffusion across the luminal membrane, and this downhill process provides the energy for the simultaneous uphill movement of glucose (see Fig. 21–7). In addition to glucose, other substances as, for example, amino acids and phosphates, are reabsorbed by this mechanism.

### Maximal Tubular Capacity ($T_m$)

The maximal tubular capacity ($T_m$) is defined as the maximal rate of mediated transport of a substance across the luminal or basolateral membrane. Most, if not all of the active reabsorptive systems in the

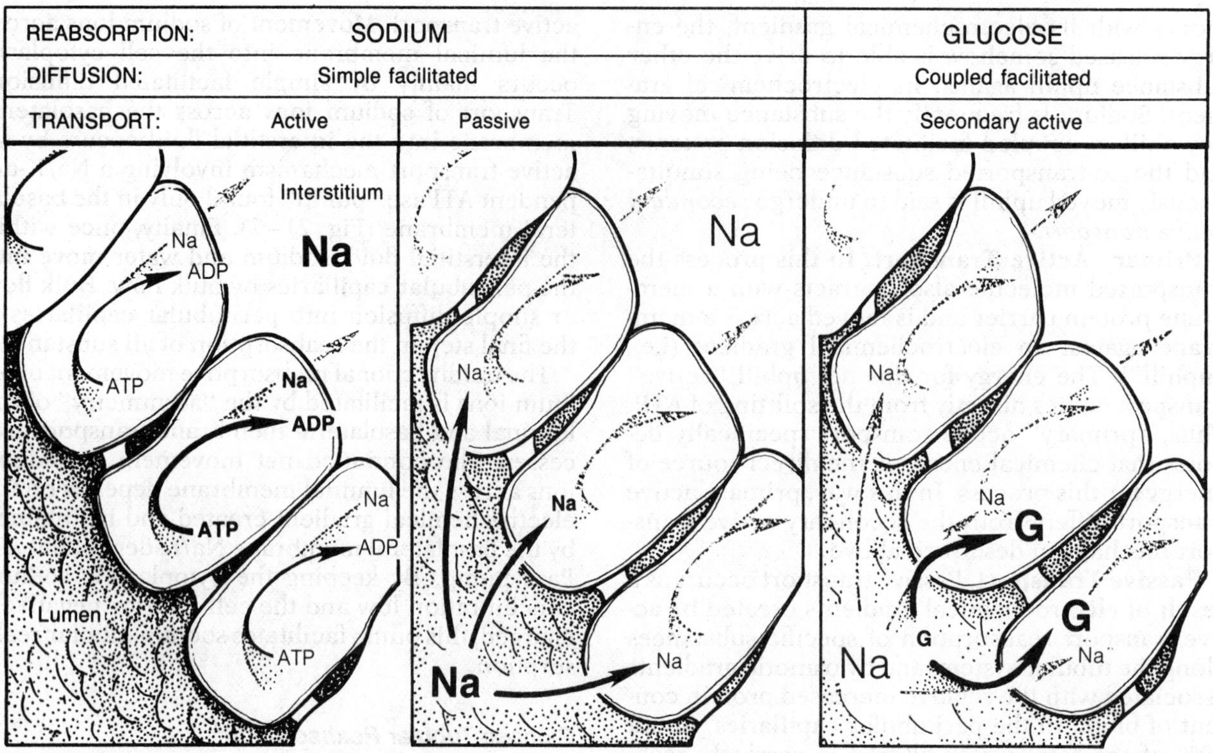


**Figure 21-7.** Tubular reabsorption of sodium and glucose. The primary active transport of sodium through the basolateral membrane of the peritubular cell into the interstitium establishes the appropriate electrochemical gradient, resulting in the net facilitated diffusion of sodium into the cell at its luminal surface. Reabsorption of glucose (G) occurs by coupled facilitated diffusion. The coupled facilitated transport of glucose "uphill" is driven by the "downhill" movement of sodium, which moves down the electrochemical gradient fueled by the primary active Na/K-dependent ATPase pump in the basolateral membrane.

renal tubules have a limit as to the amounts of substrate (e.g., glucose) they can transport per unit time. The reason for this is that each membrane protein carrier has a finite number of receptor sites for the specific substrate. Once these receptor sites have been filled, or saturated, no further transport can take place regardless of the amount of substrate available. In other words, the maximal tubular capacity of $T_m$ for the substance has been reached.

The classic example is the transport process for glucose in the proximal tubule. Normally, glucose is not excreted in the urine because its tubular reabsorption is virtually complete. But should the plasma glucose and filtered glucose load continue to rise (as, for example, in the patient with uncontrolled diabetes mellitus), a point is reached where glucose finally appears in the urine (i.e., the $T_m$ for glucose has been reached). From this point on, any further increase in plasma glucose is accompanied by an increase in excreted glucose because the $T_m$ has been reached. The tubules are reabsorbing the maximum amount of glucose possible, and any amount of glucose filtered in excess of this quantity cannot be reabsorbed and so appears in the urine. The plasma level at which a substance begins to appear in the urine is known as its *threshold.*

## Tubular Secretion

The mechanism of tubular secretion is similar to that of reabsorption except that it transfers substances *out* of the blood in the peritubular capillaries and *into* the tubules. The types of transport mechanisms that achieve tubular secretion, as, for example, simple and coupled facilitated diffusion, and primary active transport, are the same as previously described for tubular reabsorption.

Among the most important secretory processes are those involved in the secretion of hydrogen and potassium ions in the distal tubules (see below). These processes are crucial to the maintenance of acid–base and electrolyte balance. There are a variety of other low-specificity secretory systems that secrete a variety of normally occurring foreign organic substances. The fact that these secretory systems are relatively nondiscriminating makes them especially important for the elimination of drugs and other chemicals from the body.

In addition, substances metabolized within the tubular epithelial cells are added to the luminal fluid and excreted in the urine. Ammonia, for example, is synthesized by luminal cells and secreted into the tubular lumen where it binds with hydrogen ions and is excreted as the ammonium ion ($NH_4^+$) (see Fig. 30-1). This mechanism plays an essential role in the maintenance of acid-base balance (see Chap. 30).

## Renal Clearance

The clearance of a substance is the volume of plasma from which that substance is completely "cleared" by the kidneys per unit time. As the filtrate moves through the tubules, a large number of substances are not reabsorbed but, rather, they are removed (cleared) from the blood and eliminated in the urine. Every substance in the blood has its own distinct clearance values, and the units are always in volume of plasma per time.

Inulin is an excellent example for determining renal clearance. Inulin is only filtered and neither reabsorbed nor secreted. Because all inulin that is excreted must come from the plasma, it follows that a certain volume of plasma loses its inulin while flowing through the kidney (i.e., a certain volume of plasma has been "cleared" of inulin). Because inulin is neither reabsorbed nor secreted, the volume of blood completely cleared of inulin is equal to the GFR. This volume is termed the inulin clearance. The basic clearance formula for inulin and other substances is

$$C_x = \frac{\text{Mass of x excreted/time}}{P_x} =$$

$$C_x = \frac{U_x V}{P_x}$$

where:
$C_x$ = the clearance of substance x (e.g., inulin),
$U_x$ = urine concentration of x,
V = urine volume per time, and
$P_x$ = plasma concentration of x.

In general, whenever the clearance of a freely filterable substance is less than the inulin clearance, tubular reabsorption of that substance must have occurred; conversely, whenever the clearance of a substance is greater than the inulin clearance, tubular secretion of that substance must have occurred. Glucose, for example, is freely filtered, but usually completely reabsorbed (i.e., it is completely returned to the blood). The net renal clearance of glucose is, therefore, zero. Urea clearance is lower than that of inulin; because of the amount of urea filtered, approximately 50% is reabsorbed.

Creatinine is an example of a substance that is freely filtered, but not reabsorbed. In addition, a small amount of creatinine is secreted by the tubular epithelial cells. Thus, renal clearance of creatinine is higher than that of inulin. Clinically, because the creatinine clearance is a close approximation of the GFR, it may be used to determine the GFR. More commonly, a measure of the plasma creatinine alone can be a useful indicator of GFR.

## Renal Hemodynamics

### *Autoregulation*

The renal circulation receives 25% of the total cardiac output each minute. A unique feature of the renal vascular network is its inherent autoregulation wherein the afferent and efferent arterioles have the capacity to alter their renal vascular resistance independently of external neural or hormonal influences. As a result of autoregulation, the rate of blood flow through the kidney is relatively constant in the face of wide changes in mean arterial blood pressure, which may range between 80 and 180 mmHg. The net result is that the GFR shows only small changes in the face of large changes in mean arterial pressure, thereby preventing large changes in solute and water excretion that could otherwise occur.

The major site of renal autoregulatory resistance changes in the face of changes in arterial pressure is within the afferent arterioles. A rise in arterial pressure, for example, triggers enhanced contraction of afferent arteriolar smooth muscle resulting in vasoconstriction. This increases the pressure drop between the arteries and glomerular capillaries preventing the transmission of the increased arterial pressure to the glomerulus. Conversely, a fall in arterial pressure elicits a relaxation of afferent arteriolar smooth muscle resulting in vasodilation and an increase in renal blood flow. Thus, autoregulation functions to minimize changes in GFR in the face of significant changes in arterial pressure.[5] Should mean arterial pressure fall below 70 mmHg, however, autoregulation becomes virtually absent.

### *Neural Control of Renal Hemodynamics*

Renal autoregulatory changes may be overcome by sympathetic innervation reflexly mediated by the baroreceptors in the carotid sinus and aortic arch, and increased levels of circulating epinephrine. Sympathetic stimulation increases both afferent and efferent arteriolar vasoconstriction causing a decrease in renal blood flow and GFR. However, the GFR tends not to decrease as much as the renal blood flow because the increased resistance offered by the efferent arterioles that lie beyond the glomerular capillaries raises glomerular-capillary pressure.

## Other Factors Influencing Renal Hemodynamics

### *Angiotensin*

In addition to inherent renal autoregulation and the effects of epinephrine and norepinephrine, angiotensin is a powerful vasoconstrictor to which renal arterioles are quite sensitive. Whenever renin secretion is elevated significantly, angiotensin-induced renal vasoconstriction occurs. (The renin–angiotensin–aldosterone system is discussed below.) (See also Fig. 21–9.)

### *Renal Prostaglandin Production*

Prostaglandins are a group of extremely active biologic substances derived from fatty acids (arachidonic acid) and present in many tissues throughout the body including the kidneys. Renal production of prostaglandins includes the vasodilator, prostaglandin $E_2$ ($PGE_2$), which is produced by medullary interstitial cells. Its concentration parallels that of renin and may partially counteract the vasoconstriction associated with enhanced sympathetic activity and angiotensin II.[6] Secretion of $PGE_2$ functions to appropriately minimize any rise in blood pressure. Renal vasoconstriction with consequent increase in blood pressure has been associated with a reduction in $PGE_2$ release. It is estimated that one third of patients with essential hypertension (i.e., hypertension with no observable or obvious external cause) may have reduced levels of urinary $PGE_2$.[7] Prostaglandin $I_2$ (prostacyclin) is produced by the vascular bed and also increases renal blood flow.

The kidneys also produce a prostaglandin with vasoconstriction activity, called thromboxane $A_2$. Renal production of thromboxane $A_2$ is increased in severe stress and acts to decrease renal perfusion.

## Renal Processes for Handling Sodium, Chloride, and Water

Sodium, chloride, and water are all freely filtered at the glomerulus and undergo significant tubular reabsorption so that normally less than 1% is excreted in the urine. Control of the renal excretion of sodium, chloride, and water constitutes the most important mechanism for the regulation of these ions and water. The kidney can readily alter its excretion of salt and water over a wide variable range depending on salt ingestion and overall hydration status.

Approximately 65% of filtered sodium, chloride, and water are reabsorbed in the PCT, which is highly permeable to water. The tubular mechanisms for the reabsorption of these substances involve the active tubular reabsorption of sodium, which provides the primary force, resulting in the reabsorption of chloride and water as well. The reabsorption of chloride is coupled to the active reabsorption of sodium; the reabsorption of water occurs by simple diffusion and depends primarily on the reabsorption of sodium and chloride.

### *Control of Sodium Excretion*

Because sodium is freely filtered at the glomerulus and actively reabsorbed but *not* secreted by the renal tubules, the amount of sodium excreted in the urine reflects the net effect of these two processes (i.e., glomerular filtration and renal tubular reabsorption). Sodium excretion can, therefore, be adjusted by controlling either or both of these two variables. For example, if the amount of sodium filtered increases but the rate of reabsorption remains unchanged, sodium excretion increases. If the amount of sodium reabsorbed is decreased but the GFR remains constant, sodium excretion is similarly increased. Sodium excretion can be increased by increasing the GFR while also reducing sodium reabsorption. Conversely, sodium excretion can be decreased by lowering the GFR or raising sodium reabsorption, or both.

Three important factors are involved in the control of sodium excretion—the GFR, aldosterone, and third factors (e.g., natriuretic factor). As discussed previously, GFR is determined by glomerular capillary hydrostatic blood pressure, the hydrostatic pressure exerted by the filtrate in Bowman's capsule, and the plasma osmotic pressure. Anything that alters the magnitude of these factors can be expected to change GFR. Thus, a fall in arterial blood pressure decreases GFR by lowering the glomerular capillary hydrostatic pressure; conversely, an increase in arterial blood pressure has just the opposite effect (i.e., an increase in GFR). Increased sympathetic activity or circulating epinephrine causes renal vasoconstriction, which reduces glomerular capillary hydrostatic pressure with a consequent decrease in GFR. Sympathetic innervation and increased amounts of circulating catecholamines also enhance sodium tubular reabsorption. Enhanced sodium reabsorption is also triggered by baroreceptors in response to pressure changes associated with a decrease in intravascular volume.

Changes in osmotic pressure exerted by plasma proteins also impact on overall GFR. An increase in plasma osmotic pressure, which occurs, for example, in severe dehydration, will decrease net filtration. Any decrease in the net filtration rate, for whatever reason, will, in turn, decrease the amount of sodium and other substances filtered (see Fig. 21–6).

### *Regulatory Role of Renin and Angiotensin*

While the sympathetic nervous system largely controls GFR, the renin–angiotensin–aldosterone system is the major regulatory pathway concerned with sodium tubular reabsorption.

**Juxtaglomerular Apparatus.** The juxtaglomerular apparatus (JGA) is the functional unit involved in the secretion of renin that initiates a sequence of reactions leading to the secretion of aldosterone. Anatomically, the JGA is localized at the glomerular hilus (Fig. 21–8) and consists of three cell types: (1) specialized granular cells, or juxtaglomerular cells, of the afferent arterioles; (2) mesangial cells, which have an uncertain origin and function; and (3) macula densa cells.

The juxtaglomerular cells of the afferent arteriole synthesize and secrete renin, a proteolytic enzyme (cleaves peptides) that triggers the pivotal events of the renin–angiotensin–aldosterone system. Thus, renin proteolyzes the large protein angiotensinogen (synthesized in liver and circulated in blood) to form angiotensin I; angiotensin I is further proteolyzed by converting enzyme (within lung capillary endothelium) to form angiotensin II. Angiotensin II is a major stimulator of aldosterone secretion by the zona glomerulosa cells of the adrenal glands. Aldosterone stimulates the active tubular reabsorption of sodium in the distal tubules and collecting ducts (Fig. 21–9).

**Control of Aldosterone Secretion.** The control of aldosterone secretion involves several mechanisms. Angiotensin II is a most important regulator of aldosterone secretion, and its serum concentration is determined mainly by the rate of renin secretion. The rate of renin secretion, in turn, is controlled by neural and hormonal mechanisms, and by inherent renal reflexes. Systemic baroreceptors (carotid sinus and aortic arch) initiate sympathetic innervation to the vascular and tubular components of the JGA. Juxtaglomerular cells may themselves act as baroreceptors monitoring pressure/distention within the afferent arteriole and accordingly varying their secretion of renin. Renal sympathetic innervation and circulating levels of epinephrine stimulate renin secretion by constriction of afferent arterioles. Cells of the macula densa, which lie in intimate contact with juxtaglomerular cells in the afferent arteriole (see Fig. 21–8), may stimulate secretion of renin by these latter cells in response to the composition of fluid in the distal tubule, particularly the sodium concentration.

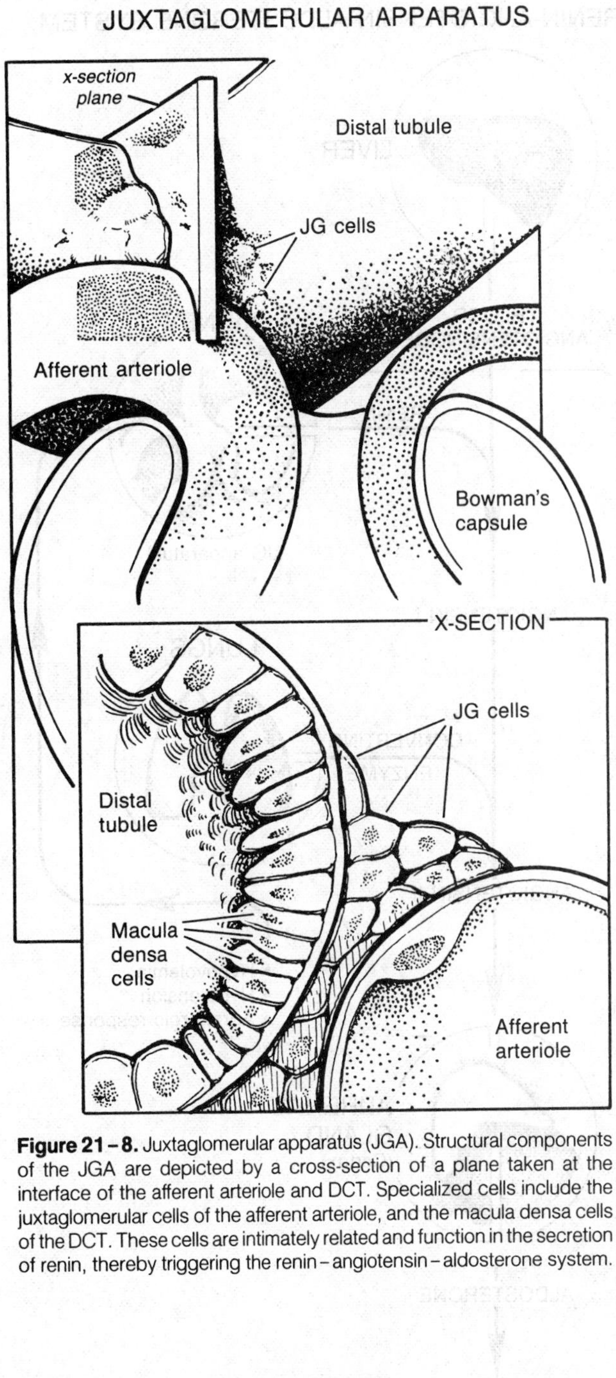


**Figure 21–8.** Juxtaglomerular apparatus (JGA). Structural components of the JGA are depicted by a cross-section of a plane taken at the interface of the afferent arteriole and DCT. Specialized cells include the juxtaglomerular cells of the afferent arteriole, and the macula densa cells of the DCT. These cells are intimately related and function in the secretion of renin, thereby triggering the renin–angiotensin–aldosterone system.

### *Natriuretic Factor (Atriopeptin)*

Atriopeptin[8] is a recently discovered hormone secreted within the atria of the heart. Its major actions are to promote loss of fluid and electrolytes and to decrease vascular tone. It causes both renal vasodilation and an increase in sodium excretion. The increase in GFR attributed to this factor accounts in part for the increased excretion of sodium as well as calcium, magnesium, and phosphate; it has no known effect on potassium.

The mechanism(s) by which atriopeptin exerts its effect on the kidney is unknown. It does play a role inhibiting aldosterone secretion, thereby reducing sodium reabsorption in the distal tubules and collecting ducts. Some atriopeptin circulates in the blood at all times, but secretion of atriopeptin is increased in response to an increase in blood volume (hypervolemia) and to an increase in central venous and right atrial pressures. Fluid volume

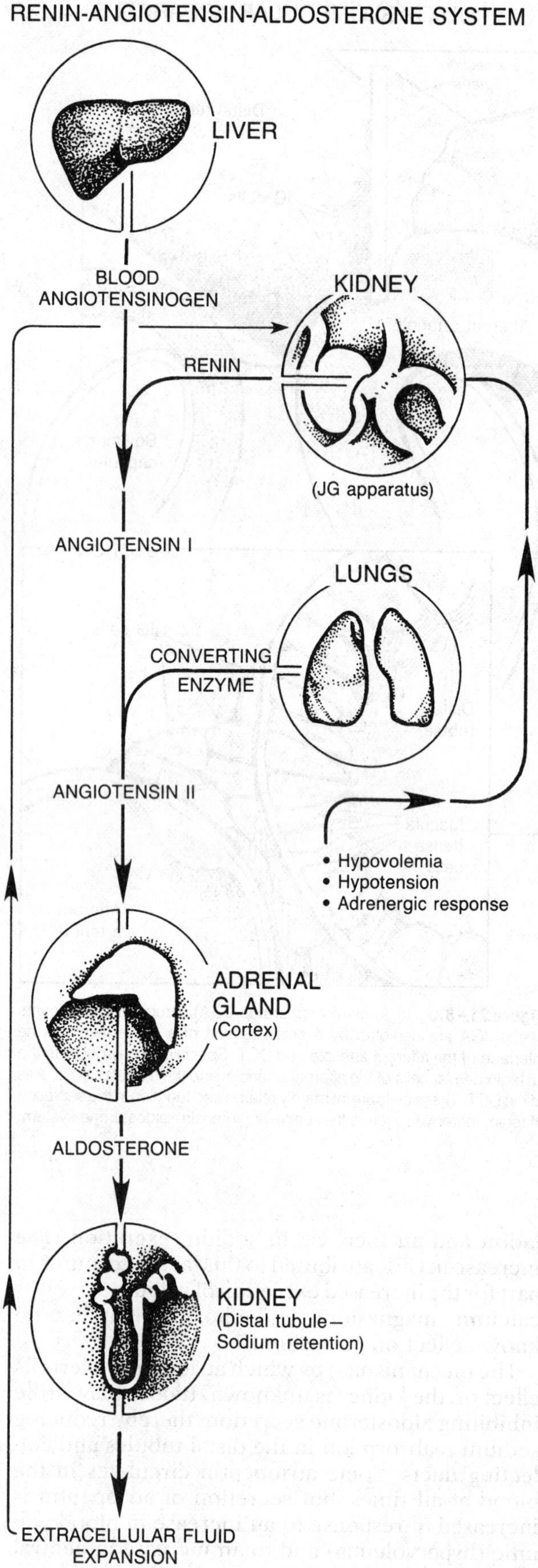


overload associated with congestive heart failure or renal failure results in elevated circulating levels of atriopeptin. Levels of atriopeptin are also elevated in the scenario of atrial tachycardia or in other cardiac dysrhythmias that predispose to an increase in right atrial pressures.

## Renal Regulation of Extracellular Osmolality

Approximately 600 mOsm/day of metabolic waste products (e.g., urea, uric acid, creatinine, sulfates, phosphates, and other nonessential substances) must be excreted, requiring a minimal obligatory water loss of 0.4 liters/day at a maximal urine concentration of 1400 mOsm/liter. The ability to concentrate urine requires a complex interplay of events involving the collecting ducts, juxtamedullary nephrons, and the vasa recta. This interplay of events constitutes the medullary countercurrent system, the purpose of which is to establish and maintain a hyperosmotic medullary interstitium. A hyperosmotic medullary interstitium provides the driving force for water movement and urine concentration or dilution.

As previously discussed, the initial step in urine formation involves glomerular filtration of water and solutes from the blood into Bowman's capsule. The glomerular filtrate has essentially the same composition as plasma except it contains little protein. As the filtrate passes through the tubular system, changes occur in its composition that are reflective of the physiologic processes acting on it. Such processes function to maintain the body's fluid, electrolyte, and acid–base balance.

### *Proximal Convoluted Tubule*

As the filtrate flows through the proximal tubule, approximately 65% of filtered sodium, chloride, and water and virtually all glucose and proteins are reabsorbed. Because the PCT is highly permeable to water, electrochemical gradients established by the active transport of solutes facilitate the passive diffusion of water down its concentration gradient from the tubular lumen, into the tubular epithelial cells, and then into the renal interstitium. Specifically, the active reabsorption of sodium is accompanied by the reabsorption of water, which occurs at a rate that maintains the osmolality of the filtrate at the end of the proximal tubule *iso*-osmotic to that of plasma. The volume of fluid entering the loop of Henle is about 25% of the original filtrate.

**Figure 21–9.** The renin–angiotensin–aldosterone system is depicted, including the roles played by the liver, kidneys, lungs, and adrenal glands, which culminate in the secretion of aldosterone.

### Loop of Henle

Approximately 25% of filtered sodium and chloride, and about 15% of water are reabsorbed in the loop. While the descending limb is highly permeable to water, the ascending limb is nearly completely impermeable to water (Fig. 21–10). In contrast to the PCT, in the ascending loop of Henle chloride is the ion *actively* reabsorbed, establishing an electrochemical gradient that secondarily induces the passive reabsorption of sodium. With the reabsorption of much more solute (i.e., sodium chloride) than water, the osmolality of the filtrate reaching the distal tubule is *hypo*-osmotic to that of plasma. The volume of filtrate entering the DCT is reduced further by about 5%.

### Distal Convoluted Tubule (Early)

Most of the remaining sodium and chloride is reabsorbed along the distal tubule and collecting ducts so that the final urine contains less than 1% of the

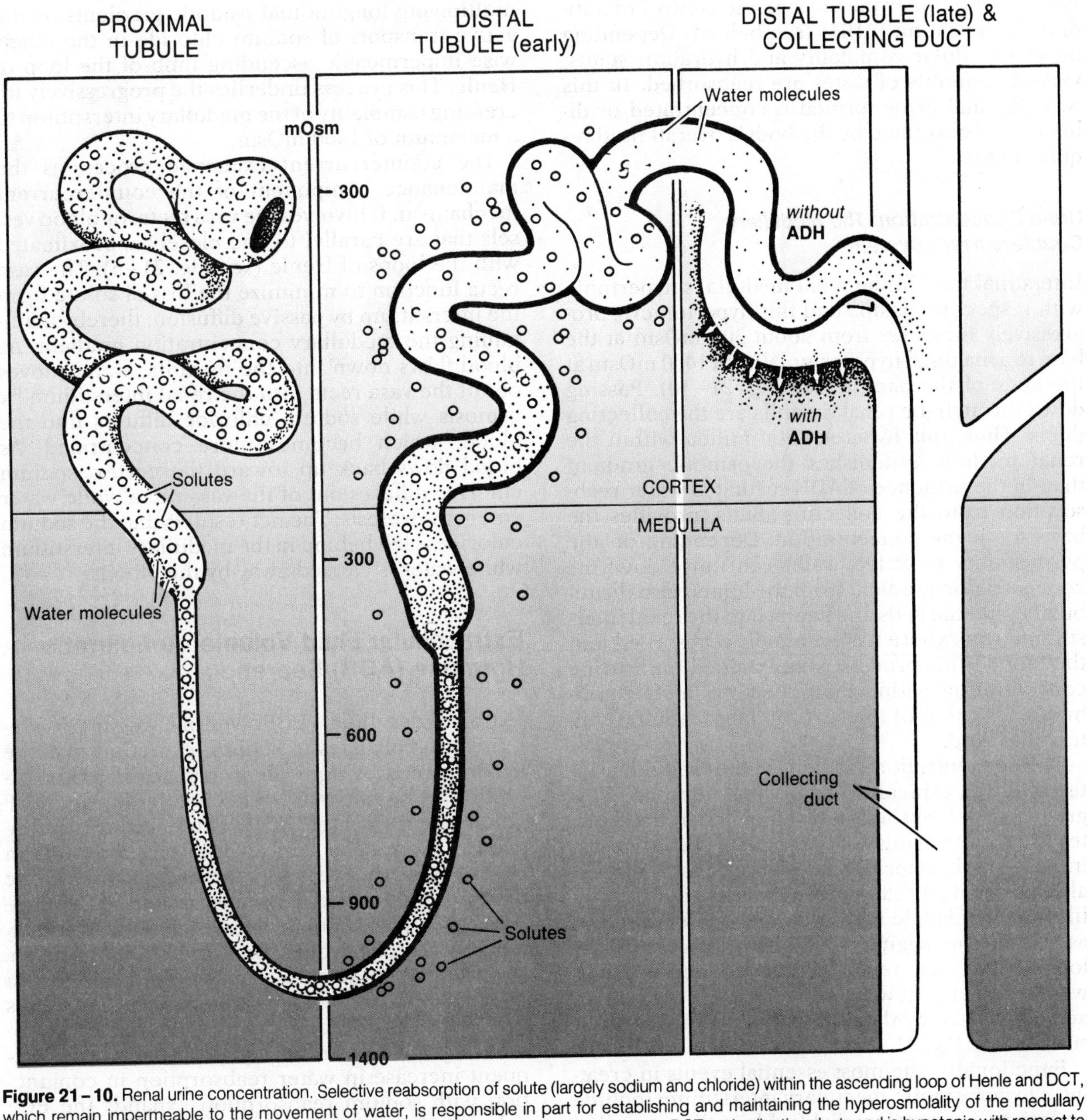


**Figure 21–10.** Renal urine concentration. Selective reabsorption of solute (largely sodium and chloride) within the ascending loop of Henle and DCT, which remain impermeable to the movement of water, is responsible in part for establishing and maintaining the hyperosmolality of the medullary interstitum. The reabsorption of solute in excess of water creates a filtrate that flows into the DCT and collecting ducts and is hypotonic with respect to blood and the surrounding medullary interstitium. In the presence of ADH, cells of the distal tubule and collecting ducts become permeable to water, which, owing to the large osmotic pressure gradient, is passively reabsorbed. A concentrated urine is thus formed. In the absence of ADH, these cells remain impermeable to water, and a dilute urine is excreted.

total sodium and chloride filtered. The permeability of the early distal tubule to water continues to be extremely low and relatively constant so that, despite the large osmotic gradient, virtually very little water is reabsorbed. Filtrate flowing into the late distal tubule is *hypo*-osmotic with respect to plasma.

### Distal Convoluted Tubule (Late) and Collecting Ducts

In contrast to the early DCT, the permeability of the late distal tubules and collecting ducts to water is *variable* and under the physiologic control of antidiuretic hormone (ADH) (see below). Depending on extracellular osmolality and hydration status, varying amounts of water are reabsorbed. In this way the final urine formed is concentrated or diluted as necessitated by the body's overall fluid requirements.

### Urine Concentration: The Medullary Countercurrent System

Interstitial fluid in the renal medulla is hypertonic with respect to plasma and this hypertonicity progressively increases from about 300 mOsm at the base to a maximal hyperosmolality of 1400 mOsm at the apex of the papilla (see Fig. 21–10). Passing down through the renal medulla are the collecting ducts. Thus, this hyperosmotic milieu within the renal medulla establishes the osmotic gradient that, in the presence of ADH-mediated water reabsorption from the collecting ducts, provides the basis for urine concentration. Depending on the permeability to water, water can move down its concentration gradient from the lumen into the tubular epithelial cells and finally into the renal interstitium from where it is eventually reabsorbed into the blood. This process is maintained until urine concentration within the collecting ducts equilibrates with that of the surrounding medullary interstitial fluid.

The concentration gradient in the medullary interstitium is critical to urine concentration. This gradient is established and maintained by the countercurrent mechanisms. Essential to the processes involved in this mechanism is the intimate and parallel anatomical relationship between the hairpinlike loops of Henle with extended descending and ascending thin segments; the hairpinlike capillary loops of the vasa recta; and the collecting ducts, which descend down through the renal medulla and are bathed by the fluid of the medullary interstitium (see Fig. 21–5).

Functionally, the most essential events in creating a hyperosmotic medullary interstitium include an active reabsorption of chloride in the ascending limb coupled with the passive reabsorption of sodium; an ascending limb that is always impermeable to water; and a descending limb that does not actively transport either sodium or chloride but is highly permeable to water.

The operation of the countercurrent mechanism involves two processes: countercurrent multiplication and countercurrent exchange. The countercurrent multiplication process occurs within the loops of Henle of the juxtamedullary nephrons. Fluid moves through the loop in such a way that the flow (i.e., current) in the ascending limb is in the opposite direction (i.e., counter) to the flow in the descending limb. The creation of a hypertonic interstitial fluid results from the generation of multiplying longitudinal osmotic gradients by the active transport of sodium chloride in the otherwise impermeable ascending limb of the loop of Henle. This process underlies the progressively increasing osmolality of the medullary interstitium to a maximum of 1400 mOsm.

The countercurrent exchange process is the maintenance component of the countercurrent mechanism. It involves the vasa recta, or blood vessels that are parallel to and closely approximated with the loops of Henle (see Fig. 21–5). The vasa recta function to minimize the loss of solute from the interstitium by passive diffusion, thereby maintaining the medullary concentration gradient. As blood flows down into the medulla, water moves out of the vasa recta into the renal interstitium by osmosis while sodium chloride diffuses into the blood, which becomes more concentrated. As blood flows back up toward the cortex, sodium chloride diffuses out of the vasa recta while water enters by osmosis. The net result is that the sodium chloride is left behind in the medullary interstitium while water is carried away by the blood.

## Extracellular Fluid Volume: Antidiuretic Hormone (ADH) Secretion

Extracellular fluid (ECF) volume regulation requires that changes in sodium excretion must be accompanied by equivalent changes in water excretion to be maximally effective in altering ECF volume. A decreased ECT volume reflexly stimulates an increase in aldosterone secretion (sodium reabsorption), as well as an increase in antidiuretic (ADH) secretion (water reabsorption). ADH, synthesized by a group of neurons within the hypothalamus, is secreted from axonal endings in the posterior pituitary in response to an increase in serum osmolality. This hormone acts specifically on cells lining the distal tubules and collecting ducts, increasing their permeability to water. The consequent increase in water reabsorption in conjunction with sodium reabsorption expands the ECF volume. (For a detailed discussion regarding ADH and its mechanism of action and control, see Chap. 16.)

## Renal Regulation of Potassium

Serum levels of potassium are regulated within a very narrow range (3.5–5.5 mEq/liter), which is of critical importance primarily because of the role played by potassium in the excitability of nerve and muscle. The ratio of extra- and intracellular potassium concentration largely accounts for the resting membrane potentials (RMP) of these tissues. An increase in extracellular potassium concentration lowers the RMP, causing slow response action potentials to be fired, which depress cellular excitability; a decrease in extracellular potassium concentration hyperpolarizes the cell membrane, stimulating fast response action potentials (at least initially) and increasing cellular excitability.[9]

Like sodium, potassium is freely filterable at the glomerulus. Approximately 90% of the filtered potassium is reabsorbed actively by the tubular system by the time the filtrate reaches the distal tubule. About 65% of the filtered potassium is reabsorbed actively in the proximal tubule, and another 20–25% is reabsorbed in the ascending loop of Henle. This reabsorption apparently occurs irrespective of changes in body potassium. Consequently, it is the late distal tubules and early collecting ducts that are primarily involved in achieving potassium homeostasis.

The mechanism of potassium secretion involves two critical steps: (1) active potassium transport (active potassium pump) from the interstitium into the tubular epithelial cell; and (2) passive potassium diffusion from the epithelial cell into the lumen. This latter step is driven by the large concentration gradient created by a high concentration of intracellular potassium, which, in turn, results from the active transport of potassium.

### Control of Potassium Secretion

Control of potassium secretion involves several mechanisms. An increase in serum potassium itself enhances active uptake of potassium by the tubular cell and thus raises potassium excretion. In addition, aldosterone-secreting cells of the zona glomerulosa monitor serum potassium levels. Any increase in the extracellular concentration of this ion directly stimulates aldosterone synthesis and secretion by the adrenal cortex, which, in turn, increase potassium secretion by the distal tubules and early collecting duct. The net result is an increased potassium excretion.

Renal mechanisms for handling potassium are related intimately to those for sodium and hydrogen ions. The presence of alkalemia or acidemia in some way alters the critical mechanism (i.e., active potassium transport and/or passive diffusion) involved in the renal handling of potassium. Thus, in the presence of alkalemia (i.e., reduced hydrogen-ion concentration), an increase in potassium secretion and excretion occurs; in the presence of acidemia (i.e., increased hydrogen-ion concentration), there is a decrease in potassium secretion and excretion.

## Renal Contribution to Calcium Homeostasis

Calcium plays an essential role in a variety of physiologic processes including, in particular, its profound effect on neuromuscular excitability. Hypocalcemia, if severe, can precipitate hypocalcemic tetany, whereas hypercalcemia can depress neuromuscular activity and cause cardiac dysrhythmias or cardiac arrest. Consequently, it is critical for extracellular calcium concentrations to be maintained within very narrow limits.

In contrast to sodium and water homeostasis where the kidneys exert the major homeostatic control, renal handling of calcium is but one of three major effector sites for calcium homeostasis including bone and the gastrointestinal tract as well. (While Chap. 24 discusses calcium metabolism in depth, it is useful here to review the role of the kidney.)

It is important to recall that approximately 40%–50% of serum calcium is protein-bound. The remaining serum calcium is freely ionized, and this fraction exerts the physiologic effects of calcium. Because of the protein-bound fraction, only about 55%–60% of serum calcium is filterable at the glomerulus, all of which is actively reabsorbed except for about 1%.

The serum pH level exerts an important effect on serum calcium levels. Alkalemia increases the protein-bound fraction, decreasing the free, ionized fraction; acidemia decreases the protein-bound fraction, thus increasing the concentration of freely ionized calcium.

Sodium reabsorption exerts the most important influence on calcium reabsorption probably by some type of coupling mechanism that facilitates sodium and calcium reabsorption in the proximal tubule and loop of Henle. In the distal tubule, however, the reabsorption of these ions becomes dissociated due to the specificity of their major hormonal controls—aldosterone (sodium) and parathyroid hormone (calcium).

Parathyroid hormone, vitamin D, and calcitonin are the major regulatory hormones of calcium homeostasis. While calcitonin functions to promote deposition of calcium in the bones and thereby decrease calcium concentration in the extracellular fluid, parathyroid hormone and vitamin D influence all three effector sites, kidney, gastrointestinal tract, as well as bone.[10]

Parathyroid hormone directly influences the role of the kidney in calcium homeostasis by increasing tubular reabsorption of calcium in the distal tubule while inhibiting the reabsorption of phosphate. In addition, this hormone inhibits hydrogen-ion secretion in the proximal tubule, thereby facilitating bicarbonate reabsorption. The resultant increase in extracellular hydrogen-ion concentration thus increases the freely ionized calcium fraction in the blood by the mechanism described above.

The kidneys play a critical role in calcium metabolism. In the kidneys vitamin D is converted to its most biologically active form, 1,25-dihydroxycholecalciferol. In this form, vitamin D stimulates active calcium (and phosphate) absorption by the intestines, its major action. Vitamin D also stimulates renal tubular reabsorption of calcium and phosphate, but this role may not be physiologically significant.

## Renal Regulation of Erythrocyte Production

In addition to renin and the active metabolite of vitamin D, the kidneys secrete an additional hormone, renal erythropoietic factor (REF). Upon secretion, this factor enzymatically proteolyzes a serum globulin (synthesized and secreted by the liver) with the resultant formation of erythropoietin. Erythropoietin stimulates an increased production of erythrocytes by the bone marrow. Secretion of REF may be diminished in renal disease and may account in part for the occurrence of anemia in chronic renal disease.

## SUMMARY OF KIDNEY FUNCTIONS

| | |
|---|---|
| Excretory: | Elimination of urea (protein metabolism). |
| | Elimination of creatinine (muscle). |
| | Elimination of uric acid (DNA and RNA metabolism). |
| Regulatory: | Regulation of extracellular fluid volume (Chap. 23). |
| | Osmolality of body fluids (Chap. 16). |
| | Electrolyte balance (Chap. 23). |
| | Acid–base balance (Chap. 30). |
| Secretory: | Secretion of renin. |
| | Secretion of erythropoietin. |
| | Secretion of prostaglandins. |
| | Secretion of active metabolite of vitamin D (Chap. 24). |

## REFERENCES

1. Vander, AJ: Renal Physiology, ed 3. McGraw-Hill, New York, 1985, p 7.
2. Vander, AJ: Renal Physiology, ed 3. McGraw-Hill, New York, 1985, p 22.
3. Vander, AJ: Renal Physiology, ed 3. McGraw-Hill, New York, 1985, p 30.
4. Vander, AJ: Renal Physiology, ed 3. McGraw-Hill, New York, 1985, p 32.
5. Ayres, S, Schlictig, R, and Sterling, M: Care of the Critically Ill. Year Book Medical Publishers, Chicago, 1988, p 268.
6. Ayres, S, Schlictig, R, and Sterling, M: Care of the Critically Ill. Year Book Medical Publishers, Chicago, 1988, p 269.
7. Rose, B: Pathophysiology of Renal Disease, ed 2. McGraw-Hill, New York, 1987, p 482.
8. Muir, BL: Pathophysiology: An Introduction to the Mechanisms of Disease, ed 2. John Wiley & Sons, New York, 1988, p 299.
9. Sweetwood, HM: Clinical Electrocardiography for Nurses. Aspen, Rockville, Maryland, 1983, pp 15–85.
10. Guyton, AC: Textbook of Medical Physiology, ed 7. WB Saunders, Philadelphia, 1986, pp 946–948.

CHAPTER 22

# Renal/Urinary Assessment

## CHAPTER OUTLINE



## LEARNING OBJECTIVES

**At the end of this chapter, you should be able to:**

1. Describe essential aspects of the clinical history as they pertain to renal function and dysfunction.
2. List the cardinal symptoms of renal/urinary dysfunction.
3. Elicit assessment data based on knowledge of functional health patterns.
4. Describe techniques/procedures used in the physical examination of the renal/urinary system.
5. Delineate key diagnostic tests and procedures for evaluating renal/urinary disorders.
6. Identify key nursing considerations in the diagnostic workup of renal/urinary disorders.

## INTRODUCTION

The renal system plays a pivotal role in maintaining relatively constant the composition of the internal environment (i.e., the cells and the fluid that surrounds them). Renal disease induces abnormalities in the composition and regulation of body fluids and, consequently, such disease may predispose to alterations in other organ systems, the signs and symptoms of which may not be immediately evident. The variable clinical presentation of renal disease requires a sophisticated clinical evaluation to diagnose and manage not only the primary renal disease, but also the secondary derangements that may result in other organ systems.

The initial step in the assessment of the patient with actual or suspected renal disease must be to take a comprehensive health history and perform a thorough physical examination. The pathophysiology underlying renal disease often follows a gradually evolving course from a completely asymptomatic state to the terminal phase of advanced uremia.

Patients may or may not feel ill. In fact, patients who have diminished renal reserve, as for example, the reduction of the glomerular filtration rate (GFR) to approximately 50%–90% of normal, may remain completely asymptomatic with blood urea nitrogen (BUN) and serum creatinine levels within the normal range. The hypertrophy of existing functioning nephrons often meets the demand for effective renal function. Clinical manifestations of renal disease in these patients may only become apparent after the individual has sustained a bodily injury or insult as, for example, infection, or exposure to a nephrotoxin, such as an aminoglycoside, or contrast media.

Patients who develop renal insufficiency (i.e., destruction of up to 75% of the nephrons and a reduction in GFR to 20%–50% of normal) may also remain relatively asymptomatic. They may look and feel well. Often, the existence of renal disease in these patients becomes evident on a routine health examination. BUN and serum creatinine are usually elevated, and the patient may report subtle changes in urinary elimination as, for example, the occurrence of nocturia (see below). More often than not, the existence of renal disease becomes apparent when the patient seeks treatment for an extrarenal manifestation such as pneumonia or anemia.

In patients with a GFR of 5%–10% of normal, the kidneys lose the ability to regulate the internal environment. These patients become symptomatic, reflecting alterations in other body systems. The patient may complain of headache; fluid retention with edema, shortness of breath, anorexia, nausea, and vomiting; and changes in mental status, behavior, and personality. The BUN and serum creatinine in these patients are elevated and rising; examination of urine may reveal hematuria and proteinuria. This scenario is highly suggestive of end-stage renal disease.

To perform a thorough comprehensive assessment of renal function, the nurse must be cognizant of a wide variety of symptomatology reflective of actual renal disease and the impact of such disease on total body function. Furthermore, the variability of the clinical presentations of renal disease requires that the nephrologic history and physical examination be adapted to meet the specific needs and problems of each individual and the stage of the disease process.

The critical-care nurse is in a pivotal position to assist in the diagnostic and therapeutic processes through history-taking, physical examination, implementation and evaluation of diagnostic studies, and the overall ongoing patient–family–nurse interaction. The critical-care nurse needs to be familiar with the cardinal signs and symptoms of prerenal (hypotensive hypovolemia or cardiac insufficiency), intrarenal (ischemic or vascular nephropathy, nephrotoxicity), and postrenal (obstructive uropathy) azotemia. The stages of the disease process, including diminished renal reserve, renal insufficiency, and end-stage renal disease must also be known. Knowledge of pertinent clinical data and laboratory indices is essential to differential diagnosis.

An ongoing evaluation is necessary to determine the disease course and the patient's response to therapeutic measures. With this knowledge the nurse can identify patients at high risk of developing renal disease and be aware of those situations in which it is likely to occur.

## CLINICAL HISTORY

In initiating the assessment of the patient's health status, the nurse must consider the patient's immediate status and whether the patient is experiencing distress. The extent and comprehensiveness of the initial history and examination should be modified accordingly.

### Components of the Clinical History

#### Chief Complaint

The chief complaint is the major reason the patient has sought health care at this point in time. Complaints associated with renal dysfunction commonly reflect an alteration in urination and may include frequency, urgency, hesitancy of urination, burning on urination, pyuria (cloudiness), dysuria, or hematuria. Complaints of polydipsia with polyuria, or oliguria with weight gain and edema, are frequently encountered. The problem of incontinence sometimes prompts patients and families to seek health care. The patient may complain of tenderness in the costovertebral angle area, the flank, or groin. Occasionally, as is the case in some patients with renal calculi, patients may arrive at the emergency room with severe, unbearable, colicky pain.

Less well-defined complaints may include fever, anorexia, nausea and vomiting, weakness or fatigue, weight gain with edema or weight loss with muscle wasting, hypertension, a bleeding tendency, or changes in mental status, behavior, and personality as confirmed by the patient's family and/or significant others.

#### History of Present Illness

The history of the present illness serves to elaborate the details surrounding the chief complaint and should include its *onset*, the *course since onset*, and *current* status. Use of the "SLIDT" tool (Table 7–1) assists in eliciting specific information about the nature of the complaint.

When eliciting the history of the present illness it is important to determine if the patient has experienced recent trauma, surgery, hemorrhage, sepsis, severe dehydration as in acute gastroenteritis, or cardiac insufficiency as in myocardial infarction. Hypotension associated with such insults may compromise renal perfusion and places the patient at risk of developing prerenal azotemia (see Chap. 25 for details regarding pre-, intra-, and postrenal azotemia).

Establishing an early and accurate diagnosis is essential because once the underlying cause has been identified, expedient and appropriate interventions can be initiated. Implementation of timely therapy may prevent the usually reversible pathology of *pre*renal azotemia from progressing to a hypotensive acute tubular necrosis with irreversible *intra*renal pathology.

The presence of an intrarenal azotemia may be related to recent or current exposure to nephrotoxic drugs or combinations of drugs (e.g., aminoglycoside plus cephalosporin), radiographic contrast media, or occupational exposure to heavy metals or toxic industrial solvents.

Eliciting the medication history is essential in the patient with possible renal disease. Has the patient been taking any medications? If so, are they physician-prescribed, or over-the-counter? Determine the name, dosage, mode of administration, and the reason for usage. How long has the patient been taking the medication? Has it been effective in relieving the underlying problem? Were there any untoward effects? Is the patient allergic to any drugs, whether prescribed or over-the-counter? Has the patient had any recent diagnostic procedures in which a contrast medium was used? Were there any untoward effects? Acute renal failure (ARF) may occur in response to the effects of nephrotoxic drugs, and it has been associated with untoward reactions to contrast media, especially iodinated agents. Contrast media may also potentiate nephrotoxicity in patients with multiple myeloma. However, the development of ARF in this setting is more likely related to prior dehydration.[1]

History of recent infection and/or immunologic disorder is especially important where renal function is concerned. Beta-hemolytic streptoccocal upper respiratory infection, for example, has been identified as a causative factor in acute glomerulonephritis. Excess immune complexes formed as a result of antigen (*Streptococcus*)–antibody reactions are deposited within the glomerular-capsular membrane, precipitating an inflammatory reaction that causes structural changes and disrupts glomerular filtration. Autoimmune diseases, such as systemic lupus erythematosus, in which the immune system produces antibodies against the patient's own renal tissue (basement membrane of glomerular-capsular membrane) can eventually lead to irreversible renal damage. (See Chap. 54 for a detailed discussion of immune mechanisms and the autoimmune phenomenon.)

The presence of a *post*renal azotemia should be ruled out in all cases of acute renal failure. An oliguria that progresses to total anuria (urine output less than 50 ml/24 hours) suggests the possible presence of obstructive uropathy. Other pertinent historical data of potential significance in postrenal azotemia include, among others, the presence of prostatic disease, bladder malignancy, recent pelvic surgery, and history of renal calculi. A familial history of renal calculi is particularly significant because there is a tendency for such disorders to recur in some families. A history of episodic, often unbearable, flank pain is highly suggestive of renal calculus disease.

Patients with symptomatic renal insufficiency or end-stage renal disease frequently present with symptomatology involving other organ systems of the body. Hypertension, reflective of altered cardiovascular function, is commonly encountered. The hypertension is related to sodium and fluid retention, and possibly to an impairment of the renin–angiotensin–aldosterone system. Dysrhythmias may occur in response to electrolyte imbalance, metabolic acidosis, or fluid volume overload, or they may be dialysis-related. Commonly, anemia is present and may be attributed to a diminished renal secretion of renal erythropoietic factor (REF) (see Chap. 21). Frequently, the patient complains of a pleuritic-type pain. Pleuritis and pericarditis are associated with elevated BUN and serum creatinine levels.

Disturbances in neurologic function include peripheral neuropathies (e.g., restless leg or burning feet syndrome) and encephalopathy. Patients may complain of headache, insomnia, restlessness, or irritability. Psychological problems are associated with bodily changes, and the patient may experience disturbances in self-image, self-concept, and self-esteem.

Gastrointestinal complaints are common. They may include changes in taste and smell, anorexia, nausea, vomiting, and thirst. Hiccups are associated with the uremic state, as is the presence of uremic fetor (i.e., a urinelike odor to the patient's breath). Constipation is a common problem associated with decreased fluid intake, use of phosphate binders, and diet restrictions.

Patients with chronic renal failure sometimes present with a bleeding tendency. Uremia interferes with the release of platelet factor III by platelets (see Chap. 61). Thus, while the platelet count is numerically within the normal range, functionally these platelets are ineffective, predisposing to bleeding.

**Cardinal Symptoms of Renal Dysfunction.** Cardinal symptoms of renal dysfunction include lower urinary tract symptoms including frequency, urgency, nocturia, dysuria, and incontinence; hematuria; pain including renal colic or renal parenchymal pain; and edema.

### *Lower Urinary Tract Symptomatology*

*Patterns of Urination.* Micturition, or the passage of urine from the urinary bladder, may occur in various patterns, which may or may not be of significance in terms of underlying renal and urinary function, and thus require closer scrutiny. *Frequency* is defined as micturition or voiding at short intervals. It may be associated with increased urine formation, high residual volume or reduced bladder capacity, or an irritable or inflamed bladder (e.g., cystitis). While frequency is variable and often poorly defined by patients, *nocturia* (i.e., urinating at night) may have greater significance in terms of underlying renal pathology. When not associated with large fluid volume intake prior to sleeping or the use of diuretics late in the day or at night, nocturia may reflect primary renal disease in which the kidneys lose the ability to concentrate urine. Nocturia is sometimes associated with prostatic hypertrophy, congestive heart failure with edema, or inflammation of the bladder or urethral mucosa.

Nocturia should be distinguished from *polyuria* (i.e., excessive micturition), which is commonly associated with use of diuretics; osmotic diuresis as occurs, for example, in diabetes mellitus; renal parenchymal disease causing a urine concentrating defect; or with polydipsia (i.e., extreme thirst).

*Urgency*, or the inability to wait to void, is usually associated with urinary tract infections. *Dysuria*, described as difficulty or pain in urination, is likewise associated with urinary tract infection (e.g., cystitis, urethritis, or prostatitis).

Urinary *incontinence* (i.e., the inability to prevent discharge or dribbling of urine) may be a significant finding in a previously continent patient. It has been associated with urinary tract infections, prostatic hypertrophy, or with neurogenic bladder (see Fig. 12–2). Patients with advanced diabetes may present with neurogenic incontinence, and a thorough history regarding the diabetes should be obtained.

*Hematuria.* Hematuria, or blood in the urine, is frequently a presenting symptom that requires thorough assessment to determine its origin and significance. The color and appearance of the urine should be carefully described. Urine that appears grossly red or red-brown in color suggests the presence of red blood cells, hemoglobin, or myoglobin; dark yellow or amber (concentrated) urine is associated with a febrile, dehydrated state; straw-colored (dilute) urine suggests overhydration or an underlying clinical disorder (e.g., diabetes mellitus or diabetes insipidus); cloudy urine may reflect the presence of a variety of substances including, among others, bacteria, epithelial cells, blood cells, pus, protein, or fat. Certain drugs may also result in color changes of urine, and the patient's medication history should be obtained. Hematuria is a common complication of anticoagulant therapy, and the patient should be asked about bleeding elsewhere.

Other details regarding hematuria should be ascertained. For example, pure blood at the beginning or end of micturition suggests a lower urinary tract origin either in the bladder or urethra. Bleeding in this circumstance may be accompanied by a burning pain on micturition. The presence of flank pain or a ureteric colic suggests a renal origin for the bleeding.

*Proteinuria.* Proteins are filtered from the blood only to a limited degree. Those filtered are usually of low molecular weight and consist largely of small amounts of albumin. Filtered proteins are usually reabsorbed within the proximal convoluted tubule so that only a trace (40–80 mg) to no protein is excreted in the urine. This lack of protein (albumin) filtration is physiologically important because it prevents loss in the urine, thereby preserving the plasma colloidal osmotic pressure.

*Glomerular* proteinuria is associated with increased glomerular-capsular permeability. It is characterized primarily by albuminuria, although globulin excretion may also be increased. *Tubular* proteinuria occurs when there is enhanced excretion of the normally low-molecular-weight proteins such as immunoglobulins. Tubular proteinuria occurs when there is impairment of proximal tubular reabsorption, or when production and subsequent filtration of low molecular weight proteins are increased to a level that exceeds the tubular reabsorptive capacity. The latter is often seen in multiple myeloma with immunoglobulin light chains (see Fig. 54–4) being excreted in the urine.[2]

The presence of protein in the urine may be determined by the use of a dipstick (e.g., Albustix). The dipstick is especially sensitive to albumin but may not detect low-molecular-weight proteins. An accurate assessment of protein excretion is best achieved with a 24-hour urine collection.

***Pain of Renal Origin.*** Pain may arise anywhere along the urinary tract from the kidney to the urethra. Of major concern is "true" renal pain, which may be of two types: pain arising from the renal capsule and surrounding tissues, and pain that is characteristically ureteric colic. Any condition that produces distention of the renal capsule (e.g., acute infection, nephrolithiasis, or renal vein thrombosis) may cause pain usually described as dull, aching, and vaguely localized at the costovertebral angle (see Fig. 22–1).

The pain of ureteric colic is classic. It is commonly caused by renal calculi (nephrolithiasis), and less frequently by blood clot and/or infarction of renal parenchyma. It is described as very severe and colicky in nature, occurring in waves and superimposed upon a continuous persistent underlying dull background of pain. The pain, which may originate anteriorly or posteriorly over the kidney, usually radiates to the groin and may extend to the scrotum or labia. Some patients initially suspected of having pain of renal origin may, in fact, have an underlying musculoskeletal problem. A thorough history and clinical evaluation assist in differential diagnosis.

***Edema.*** With advanced renal disease the kidneys lose the ability to maintain and regulate the composition of body fluids. A consequence of this is fluid retention, resulting in edema. Hypoproteinemia and proteinuria are major factors contributing to edema formation associated with underlying renal disease.

It is important to distinguish between edema associated with cardiac dysfunction and that of renal origin. Differential diagnosis can usually be made based on the clinical history. For example, orthopnea and paroxysmal nocturnal dyspnea (PND) characteristic of cardiac dysfunction are usually not features of renal dysfunction. Periorbital edema is commonly observed in renal failure. Fluid pools in the lower extremities during daytime activities and then becomes redistributed overnight, giving rise to facial edema.

An effort should be made to determine sodium intake, including a review of the patient's diet and eating habits, and any drugs the patient is taking. Many drugs, including some antihypertensives and steroids, predispose to edema formation and should be identified.

**Functional Health Patterns.** Assessment of the patient's functional health patterns is essential to elaborate on the chief complaint and to elicit pertinent assessment data, which form the basis for diagnosing, planning, implementing, and evaluating nursing care. Such information assists in providing appropriate patient/family education, and in discharge planning.

***Health Perceptions—Health Management.*** It is essential to determine what the patient's overall health status has been and whether there have been any significant changes in health or lifestyle. Does the patient appear healthy or ill? Is the patient emaciated with muscle wasting? Muscle wasting associated with renal dysfunction can result in hypoalbuminenia and reduction in total body protein. Does the patient appear to be the stated age? Commonly, adults with renal disease may look older than their actual age.

Is the patient alert and oriented to person, place, and time? Is the patient able to concentrate? Is the ability to remember intact? An assessment of the patient's mental status is important because patients with severe azotemia or uremia may experience impairment of mental functions and encephalopathy. (See Chap. 7 for details related to the neurologic assessment.)

Details regarding the patient's usual lifestyle should be elicited. Does the patient smoke? How many packs of cigarettes per day for how long a period of time? Cigarette smoking has been associated with cancer of the bladder in women. What are the patient's usual drinking habits, including the amount, frequency, and type of fluid? Excessive alcohol intake has been implicated in hepatorenal syndrome (see Chap. 50).

What type of work does the patient do? Is it satisfying? How has the current illness impacted on the patient's working abilities? What might the impact of an extended illness be on the patient's job and the family's overall economy?

***Nutritional–Metabolic.*** What are the usual dietary and eating habits of the patient/family? What foods are eaten, and who prepares the food? How much does the patient eat, and how often? Does the patient use table salt? Does the patient frequent fast-food establishments? Fast-food diets are frequently high in salt. A daily food intake high in sodium predisposes to fluid retention and edema.

Are there any allergies to specific foods? If so, have the patient describe the reaction that usually occurs. What quantity of beverages high in caffeine are consumed? High caffeine intake may be irritating to the bladder.

***Elimination Pattern.*** See the sections entitled "History of Present Illness" and "Cardinal Symptoms of Renal/Urinary Dysfunction."

***Sleep–Rest Pattern.*** Has the patient experienced a recent change in sleeping habits? Is there an associated nocturia? What amount of food or fluid does the patient consume prior to bedtime? Does the patient take diuretics? If so, what type of diuretic? What is the reason for using diuretics? What is the dose, frequency, and time of day taken? Does the urge to urinate awaken the patient from sleep? How often? What volume of urine is eliminated with each voiding?

***Coping–Stress–Tolerance.*** Throughout the clinical assessment it is essential to evaluate the patient's emotional and mental status. Has the illness occurred suddenly, or has there been a gradual, progressive disease process? Does the patient appear anxious or distraught regarding the illness and its impact on personal and family lifestyle?

What role does the patient assume in familial interactions? Who is the decision-maker? What resources are available to the patient and family? Ask the patient/family to identify coping mechanisms that have been effective in previous stressful events. What resources are available to patient/family?

### *Past Medical History*

What previous illnesses, operations, or injuries has the patient experienced? Is there a history of urinary tract infections, diabetes mellitus, hypertension, tuberculosis, or nephrolithiasis? Has the patient experienced a recent streptoccocal infection? Is there a history of immune-related diseases such as systemic lupus erythematosus?

What is the patient's past and present drug history? (See section entitled "History of Present Illness.") Kidney failure has been associated with chronic self-medication frequently involving salicylates (e.g., aspirin), nonsteroidal anti-inflammatory agents (e.g., indomethacin), and antibiotics (e.g., aminoglycosides).

#### Family History

Is there a family history of chronic renal disease, renal calculi, diabetes mellitus, hypertension, polycystic kidney disease, Goodpasture's syndrome, or renal tubule acidosis? The patient's racial and cultural background should be noted. Race may be an important factor in the incidence of some renal diseases. For example, malignant hypertension, which may predispose to nephrosclerosis and renal failure if untreated, is more common among blacks.

## PHYSICAL EXAMINATION

The kidneys maintain and regulate the composition of all body fluids, intracellular and extracellular. Consequently, to assess renal/urinary function it is necessary to assess *all* organ systems, including cardiovascular, respiratory, renal/urinary, gastrointestinal, hematologic, musculoskeletal, neurologic, and integumentary systems. Psychological function is also evaluated.

### Cardiovascular

#### Vital Signs

An assessment of vital signs should include: the blood pressure taken in each arm with the patient sitting (if possible), and supine; cardiac rate and rhythm, peripheral pulses; respiratory rate and rhythm, use of accessory muscles; body temperature; and body weight. In the intensive care setting, monitoring hemodynamic parameters (e.g., central venous pressure, pulmonary artery and pulmonary capillary wedge pressures, and cardiac output) may be indicated.

A differential drop in blood pressure greater than 10 mmHg and a concomitant increase in the pulse with position changes suggest postural (orthostatic) hypotension, which is associated with fluid volume deficit. Irregularities in apical and peripheral pulses may reflect fluid and electrolyte imbalance. A full bounding pulse suggests fluid volume overload; a thready pulse reflects dehydration.

Alterations in cardiovascular function are by far the most serious sequelae associated with acute and chronic renal disease. Hypertension is almost always present and largely associated with sodium and fluid retention. Dependent edema and distended neck veins (with patient sitting at 45 degrees) reflect fluid overload.

On auscultation, the presence of a gallop rhythm suggests fluid volume excess and may be associated with congestive heart failure. A systolic murmur may reflect anemia. Detection of a pericardial friction rub is not uncommon, especially in the scenario of uremia.

Electrolyte and acid–base imbalances commonly occur in patients with renal disease, and result in disturbances in cardiac rate and rhythm. Hyperkalemia is especially alarming because it predisposes to profound conduction disorders and cardiac dysrhythmias. Continuous cardiac monitoring is essential, and periodic assessment of the 12-lead ECG is indicated. (For a discussion of potassium imbalance and associated 12-lead ECG changes, see Chap. 23.)

### Respiratory

An assessment of respiratory function should include respiratory rate and rhythm, symmetry of chest expansion, nasal flaring, and use of accessory muscles to aid in breathing. Pleuritic pain and pleural effusion are not uncommon in patients with uremia and may predispose to atelectasis and pneumonia.

Lung fields should be auscultated for normal and adventitious breath sounds. The presence of crackles suggests fluid overload and, possibly, pulmonary edema, a major complication of renal failure. Rhonchi and wheezes reflect partially obstructed airways, which may be associated with an underlying infection (e.g., pneumonia, uremic pneumonitis). The presence of a cough, productive or nonproductive, should be noted. Patients with uremia are especially susceptible to infection because uremic toxins impair white blood cell function and may depress the cough reflex. A rapid, deep breathing pattern (Kussmaul) may be observed in metabolic acidemia (pH less than 7.2).

### Renal/Urinary

An assessment of the kidneys is performed during the abdominal examination. The abdomen is assessed for asymmetry, fullness, distention, and the presence of tenderness or masses. The palpable and tender liver may be associated with hepatorenal disease. Diminished peristalsis and hypoactive bowel sounds often occur with uremia. Abdominal distention may reflect accumulated feces in the intestinal tract; constipation is a common problem in patients with renal disease. A full bladder may also underlie abdominal distention.

Dullness elicited on percussion of the flanks suggests the presence of ascites. The *fluid-wave* test is a maneuver used to detect ascites. With another person pressing down with the palm of the hand on the abdomen, in the midline, the examiner places one palm on one of the patient's flanks and sharply taps the opposite flank. If a fluid wave is felt in the resting palm, fluid is present.

A bimanual technique is used for deep palpation to feel the kidney. One technique is to place the patient in a supine position with pillows placed under the head and knees. This helps to relax the abdominal musculature. To palpate the right kidney, the right hand is placed midway between the costal margin and the iliac crest anteriorly, with fingers pointing toward the umbilicus; the examiner's left hand is placed under the right flank and aligned with the right hand. With the patient breathing normally, the examiner presses the hands together during each inhalation, progressively increasing the pressure until a maximum palpation depth is achieved. The patient is then asked to take a deep breath during which time the examiner feels for the lower pole of the kidney as it moves down between the palpating hands. The contour and size of the kidney should be noted. The area is also assessed for nodules, masses, and/or tenderness. The procedure is repeated with the left kidney. (See Chap. 48 for discussion of techniques used in abdominal assessment.)

Kidneys are usually unpalpable except in very thin patients, or in cases where the kidney is enlarged. Normal kidneys, if palpable, feel firm and smooth (in adults) and are of similar size. Enlarged kidneys suggest tumor, polycystic kidney disease, or hydronephrosis.

Tenderness associated with renal pathology may be elicited by delivering a blunt blow to the area over the costovertebral angle posteriorly. With the patient in a sitting or side-lying position, the examiner places the palm of one hand over the costovertebral angle and firmly strikes the back of that hand with the ulnar surface of the other fist. If tenderness is elicited, one can suspect acute inflammation (Fig. 22-1).

The urinary bladder should also be assessed during the abdominal examination. A normal empty bladder is not palpable, and a tympanic sound elicited on percussion indicates an empty bladder. If retained urine is suspected (>150 ml of urine), the bladder may be palpable just above the symphysis pubis. A bladder that feels smooth and firm indicates the presence of urine. A dull sound is elicited on percussion over the urine-containing bladder. Excessive urine retention may cause abdominal distention. An atonic or flaccid bladder may not be palpable even when grossly distended with urine.

Auscultation for bruits is an important part of the physical examination. Bruits are sounds of vascular origin described as blowing or swishing sounds. Auscultation for bruits should include areas over the abdominal aorta and renal arteries, the iliac and femoral arteries. Bruits detected over renal arteries suggest renal stenosis.

(Further discussion of the techniques used to assess the kidneys, bladder, and genitalia is beyond the scope of this text, and the reader is referred to an appropriate text.)

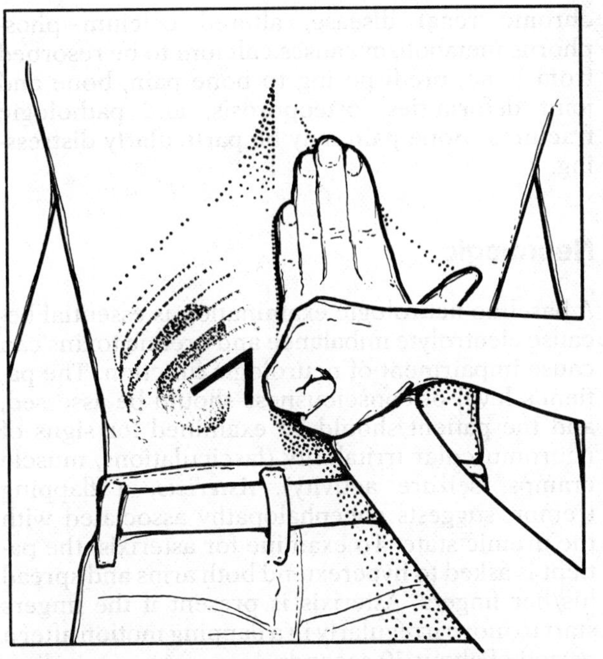

**Figure 22-1.** Costovertebral angle. A blunt blow delivered over the costovertebral angle, as indicated, may elicit tenderness associated with underlying renal pathology. The examiner places the palm of one hand over the costovertebral angle and firmly strikes the back of the hand with the ulnar surface of the other fist. If tenderness is elicited, an acute inflammation should be suspected.

## Gastrointestinal

Patients with uremia may experience uremic fetor (i.e., urine-smelling breath) and hiccuping. Gastrointestinal drainage, vomitus, and stool should be examined for occult blood. (For indepth discussion of the assessment of gastrointestinal function, see Chap. 48.)

## Hematologic

Patients with renal disease are at risk of developing alterations in hematologic function, which may be observed on physical examination. A skin pallor associated with anemia was mentioned earlier. Alterations in platelet function predispose to petechiae and ecchymosis. Altered white blood cell function increases the risk of infection in these patients. Body temperature and other vital signs (e.g., blood pressure and pulses) should be assessed at regular intervals.

## Musculoskeletal

Muscle weakness and easy fatigability are commonly observed in patients with renal disease. In chronic renal disease, altered calcium–phosphorus metabolism causes calcium to be resorbed from bone, predisposing to bone pain, bone and joint deformities, osteoporosis, and pathologic fractures. Bone pain may be particularly distressing.

### Neurologic

A baseline neurologic examination is essential because electrolyte imbalance and uremic toxins can cause impairment of neurologic function. The patient's level of consciousness should be assessed, and the patient should be examined for signs of neuromuscular irritability (fasciculations, muscle cramps, seizure activity). *Asterixis*, a flapping tremor, suggests encephalopathy associated with the uremic state. To examine for asterixis, the patient is asked to hyperextend both arms and spread his/her fingers. Asterixis is present if the fingers start to move irregularly in a flapping motion after a period of about 30 seconds.

Patients with end-stage renal disease frequently experience peripheral neuropathy. An early sign that may be observed is the "restless leg" syndrome. The patient experiences "pins and needles" or prickling sensations in the lower extremities, which are relieved by movement.

### Integumentary

Alterations in the integumentary system involve the skin, hair, and nails, and are most commonly seen in patients with chronic renal disease. The skin should be carefully examined. A yellow-tan, sallow appearance may be evident. This results from retained pigments (e.g., urochrome) normally excreted by kidneys. A pallor associated with anemia, or compromised respiratory function (e.g., altered breathing pattern, dyspnea, or fatigue) may also contribute to overall skin coloring.

Fluid volume overload may be reflected by the presence of edema over the sacral area, ankles, and feet; periorbital edema may also be observed, especially upon rising from a night's sleep. Fluid volume deficit may be reflected by poor skin turgor; flattened neck veins; rapid, thready pulse; and hypotension.

The presence of petechiae (platelet dysfunction) and areas of ecchymosis suggests a bleeding disorder or coagulopathy, which is frequently associated with renal/urinary dysfunction. Patients may report that they bruise easily. Epistaxis may also be encountered.

Atrophy of sebaceous and sweat glands underlies a change in skin texture, which becomes dry, scaly, and rough. Skin irritation from repeated scratching may also be evident.

Deposition of calcium–phosphorus crystals in the skin predisposes to pruritus. Areas of excoriation resulting from scratching may be observed. Subcutaneous nodules of deposited calcium–phosphorus may be palpable on physical examination.

### Psychological

Major psychological sequelae of longstanding renal disease are related to the morbidity of its end-stage, in which patients must rely on dialysis therapy unless a compatible donor is found and the patient can withstand the rigors of transplantation surgery and its after-care. Many patients become depressed. They despair and lose hope. Others may appear to be anxious, questioning, and in need of frequent reassurance. Changes in body appearance disrupt the individual's view of self, and these patients commonly experience a low self-esteem.

## RENAL/URINARY DIAGNOSTIC WORKUP

### Laboratory Evaluation: Urine and Blood Analysis

Laboratory data provide strategic information regarding the patient's general health status and contribute conclusively to the differential diagnosis of renal/urinary disease. Analysis of urine and blood may indicate the presence of renal/urinary dysfunction.

Urine tests assist in assessing the diluting and concentrating capacities of the renal tubules; serum electrolytes, BUN, and serum creatinine level assist in evaluating the ability of the kidneys to regulate the composition of the internal environment. Such tests reflect the ability of the kidneys to eliminate waste products, as well as their overall glomerular and tubular function.

Nurses play a key role in the diagnostic workup to ensure that prescribed tests/procedures are executed as designed. This ensures the validity of test results. Patients should understand the reasons/rationales for specific diagnostic studies and what is entailed in effectively implementing them, including what is expected of them. Preparation of the patient is largely within the domain of nursing.

Diligent implementation of diagnostic tests/procedures ensures reliable results. For example, data gleaned from a simple, inexpensive urinalysis are most pertinent when a clean midstream ("clean catch") urine specimen is obtained, followed by *prompt* laboratory analysis. Many tests of renal function (e.g., urea clearance tests performed to estimate glomerular filtration) require collection of a 24-hour urine specimen. Depending on the na-

**TABLE 22-1**
## Urine Analysis: Constituents and Characteristics of Significance in Renal Function

| Constituent Characteristics | Values/Volume/ Descriptions | Clinical Significance |
|---|---|---|
| Volume (per 24 hr) | 1200–1800 ml/day | |
| | Polyuria > 1800 ml/day | Excess fluid intake; osmotic diuresis; diuretic phase of ARF; early chronic renal failure (CRF). |
| | Oliguria < 400 ml/day | Severe dehydration; acute renal failure (e.g., acute glomerulonephritis) |
| | Anuria < 50 ml/day | Obstructive uropathy; oliguric ARF (rarely) |
| Gross characteristics: | | |
| Color | Clear, amber | Reflects osmolality, degree of concentration; color changes—may be diet/drug-related |
| Clarity | Clear | Cloudy urine may reflect infection; foamy, if albumin is present |
| Odor | Mildly fragrant or aromatic (fresh specimen) | Pungent on standing, in dehydration, drug-related, or urinary tract infection |
| pH | Range: 4.4–8.0 | Usually slightly acidic due to excretion of acid by-products of metabolism. Decreased glomerular filtration reduces excretion of acid load<br>Alkaline: Urinary tract infection; diet-related; respiratory/metabolic alkalemia, other<br>Acidic; high-protein diet, pyrexia, respiratory/metabolic acidemia, other |
| Specific gravity[3] | • Range: 1.005–1.035 | Higher in dehydration or when the kidneys conserve water (concentrated urine)<br>>1.030: Proteinuria, glycosuria; x-ray contrast media, severe dehydration<br>Lower in fluid volume excess or when kidneys excrete water (dilute urine)<br><1.010: Diabetes insipidus; overhydration<br>Fixed: In severe renal disease, urine specific gravity becomes fixed at ~ 1.010, the same as the glomerular filtrate prior to tubular activity. |
| Osmolality | • Range: 270–900 mOsm/kg; mean ~550 mOsm/kg | Depends on serum osmolality and overall hydration status<br>Severe renal disease causes urine osmolality to be fixed, or the same as the glomerular filtrate prior to tubular activity. |
| Urine chemistry: | | |
| 1. Electrolytes | | Electrolytes in urine occur as a result of selective tubular reabsorption and secretion. |
| Sodium | • Range: 43–217 mEq/liter/24 hr | |
| Potassium | 27–123 mEq/liter/24 hr | In renal failure, renal tubular regulation of electrolytes becomes compromised, altering electrolyte excretion. |
| Chlorides | 170–250 mEq/liter/24 hr | |
| Calcium | 50–300 mg/24 hr | Calcium excretion decreases because of reduced synthesis and secretion of activated vitamin D metabolite. |
| Phosphorus | Varies with intake ~ 1 g/day | |
| Magnesium | <150 mg/24 hr | Analysis for electrolytes requires 24-hr urine specimens. |
| 2. Glucose | Negative | Filtered glucose is normally totally reabsorbed in tubules.<br>Glucose appears in urine when renal threshold is exceeded. |
| 3. Acetone | Negative | Frequently seen in urine during starvation states and diabetic ketoacidosis (DKA)<br>A false-positive result occurs in patients taking salicylates. |
| 4. Protein | Negative to trace, <10 mg/100 ml | Protein molecules are usually too large to be filtered. All filtered protein is normally reabsorbed in tubules.<br>Heavy proteinuria is usually associated with altered glomerular function (e.g., glomerulonephritis) and/or renal tubule pathology.<br>A 24-hr urine specimen is required. |
| 5. Creatinine | 15–25 mg/kg/day | Concentration in urine decreases in renal disease. |

*(Continued)*

TABLE 22-1
## Urine Analysis: Constituents and Characteristics of Significance in Renal Function *(Continued)*

| Constituent Characteristics | Values/Volume/ Descriptions | Clinical Significance |
|---|---|---|
| Microscopic elements: | | |
| 1. Red blood cells | None to very minimal cell count | Hematuria indicates renal and/or urinary tract pathology (e.g., renal disease, tumor, ureteral calculi, infection, other). |
| 2. White blood cells | None to minimal cell count | Elevated WBC count suggests renal/urinary infection. |
| 3. Crystals: Urates (acidic urine) Phosphates (alkaline urine) | Usually none | Seen in nephrolithiasis or following certain intoxications (e.g., oxalate calculi of ethylene glycol) Composition of crystals may provide clue as to calculus formation. |
| 4. Casts: | | |
| Hyaline | Few (<5000) | Casts are precipitates of proteinaceous material formed in the tubules and collecting ducts by agglutination of protein, cells, or cellular debri, and flushed loose by flow of urine. |
| RBC casts | None | Present in glomerular disease (e.g., glomerulonephritis) |
| WBC casts | Few | Reflect infection or inflammation (e.g., pyelonephritis) |
| 5. Bacteria: | | |
| Culture and sensitivity | >100,000 organisms/ml | Indicates renal and/or urinary infection |
| Creatinine clearance | 104–125 ml/min<br>150–180 liters/day | This test is used to determine presence or progression of renal disease and to estimate percentage of functioning nephrons.<br>Equation: $\frac{Ucr \times V}{Pcr} = Ccr$<br>where:<br>Ucr = amount of urinary creatinine excreted<br>V = urine volume/min<br>Pcr = plasma creatinine level |

TABLE 22-2
## Blood Analysis: Parameters of Significance in Renal Function

| Constituents/ Characteristics | Values/Volume/ Descriptions | Clinical Significance |
|---|---|---|
| Hematology Profile | | |
| 1. Complete blood count: | | |
| Red blood cells | Range: 4.2–5.9 million/mm³ | In chronic renal disease, diminished secretion of renal erythropoietic factor reduces level of erythropoietin necessary for production, maturation, and release of RBCs from bone marrow and blood-forming tissues. |
| White blood cells (leukocyte) | 4300–10,800/mm³ | Elevation indicates infection. |
| Hematocrit | 37–52% | Alterations in Hct and Hbg may reflect hydration status. |
| Hemoglobin | 12–18 g/100 ml | |
| Platelet count | 150,000–350,000/mm³ | Patients with chronic renal disease develop bleeding tendencies despite platelet counts within the acceptable range; uremia impairs release of platelet factor III by platelets. |
| 2. Coagulation screening tests: | | |
| Bleeding time | Range: 3–9 minutes | Reflects platelet function/dysfunction |
| Prothrombin time | <2-second deviation from control | Uremic toxins cause alterations in coagulation factors predisposing to bleeding. |
| Partial thrombo-plastin time | 25–37 seconds | |
| Blood Chemistry | | |
| 1. Electrolytes | Range: | Because the kidneys are concerned with regulating the composition of body fluids, any alteration in renal function predisposes to fluid and electrolyte imbalance. |
| Sodium | 135–145 mEq/liter | Sodium levels are evaluated in terms of hydration status. In renal failure, sodium renal reabsorption becomes impaired: during polyuric stage, serum sodium levels may be low; during oliguric stage hypernatremia may become evident. |

TABLE 22-2
## Blood Analysis: Parameters of Significance in Renal Function *(Continued)*

| Constituents/ Characteristics | Values/Volume/ Descriptions | Clinical Significance |
|---|---|---|
| | | In advanced renal disease, fluid retention may have a dilutional effect on serum sodium levels; dietary sodium restriction may also contribute to hyponatremic state. |
| Potassium | 3.5–5.5 mEq/liter | Potassium levels are a function of variations in aldosterone secretion, pH, and serum sodium and glucose levels.<br>In renal failure, kidneys lose the ability to regulate potassium reabsorption and secretion. |
| Chloride | 100–106 mEq/liter | Major extracellular anion, which interacts with sodium to maintain osmotic gradients<br>Serum chloride levels are related to $HCO_3^-$ levels and, thus, reflect acid–base status.<br>Hyperchloremia is associated with metabolic acidemia because the kidneys conserve chloride ions to replace base. |
| Calcium<br>Phosphorus inorganic) | 8.5–10.5 mg/100 ml<br>3.0–4.5 mg/100 ml | A reciprocal relationship exists between calcium and phosphorus. Under the influence of parathyroid hormone, the kidneys selectively reabsorb or excrete phosphorus to maintain calcium/phosphorus balance.<br>Chronic renal disease impairs conversion of vitamin D to its active metabolite; calcium reabsorption from the gut becomes impaired.<br>Diminished renal excretion of phosphorus predisposes to hyperphosphatemia. |
| 2. Total protein<br>Albumin<br>Globulin | 6.0–8.4 g/100 ml<br>3.5–5.0 g/100 ml<br>2.3–3.5 g/100 ml | Serum proteins function to maintain osmotic pressure gradients within the blood necessary for normal distribution of water in the intracellular and extracellular (interstitium and intravascular) compartments.<br>Hypoalbuminemia predisposes to edema and anasarca. |
| 3. Blood urea nitrogen | 8–25 mg/100 ml | Elevated BUN level reflects an increase in nitrogenous waste products derived from protein metabolism. Urea is synthesized in the liver from $NH_3$ and excreted by the kidneys.<br>BUN level should be assessed in terms of other renal function tests and the clinical status.<br>BUN-to-creatinine ratio: 10 to 1 = normal. >20 to 1 = extra-renal problem (e.g., dehydration, catabolic state).<br>Elevation in both BUN and creatinine results from a decrease in GFR associated with renal disease. |
| 4. Creatinine | 0.6–1.5 mg/100 ml | Most closely reflects changes in GFR. A proportional relationship exists between creatinine excretion and production. An elevated serum creatinine reflects serious renal disease. |
| 5. Glucose | 70–110 mg/100 ml (fasting) | Normally all glucose filtered at the glomerulus is reabsorbed in the proximal tubule.<br>In renal dysfunction, elevated glucose levels or glucose intolerance may be associated with altered insulin synthesis and degradation, and with tissue insensitivity to action of insulin. |
| 6. Uric acid | 3.0–7.0 mg/100 ml | In renal disease, decreased renal clearance and tubular secretion of uric acid predisposes to elevated serum levels of uric acid. |
| Serum osmolality | 285–295 mOsm/kg | Serum osmolality regulates ADH release; simultaneous serum and urine osmolality determinations assist in evaluating responsiveness of distal tubules and collecting ducts to the effects of circulating ADH. |
| Arterial blood gas analysis:<br>pH<br>$PaCO_2$<br>$HCO_3^-$ | <br>7.35–7.45<br>35–45 mmHg<br>22–26 mEq/liter | Arterial blood gas analysis assists in evaluating acid–base status. $PaCO_2$ reflects integrity of the respiratory component; $HCO_3^-$ reflects the integrity of the metabolic (renal) component. pH reflects the hydrogen-ion concentration.<br>In renal dysfunction, inability to excrete hydrogen ions leads to progressive fall in pH. |

TABLE 22–3
**Diagnostic Studies and Procedures for Evaluating Renal Dysfunction**

| Test/Study | Description | Clinical Significance and Nursing Implications |
|---|---|---|
| Radiography:<br>KUB | Flat plate x-ray of kidneys, ureters, and bladder | Reveals kidney position, size, and structure; gross malformations, renal calculi.<br>No special preparation and follow-up care required. |
| Excretory urography (intravenous pyelography) (IVP) | A series of radiographs taken following intravenous administration of contrast media; and before and after voiding | Allows visualization of renal parenchyma, major and minor calcyces, renal pelvis, ureters, bladder, and urethra.<br>Reveals altered renal anatomy; renal calculi; post-voiding residual urine.<br>Procedure:<br>1. Rule out iodine sensitivity.<br>2. NPO or clear liquids 12 hr prior to test unless contraindicated.<br>3. Evacuate bowel.<br>4. Obtain informed consent.<br>5. Following procedure, encourage fluids and monitor for dehydration and signs of delayed sensitivity to contrast media. |
| Retrograde pyelography | Series of radiographs taken following injection of contrast media by cystoscope | Allows visualization of renal collecting system including calyces, pelvis, and ureter.<br>May reveal obstruction to flow of urine in collecting system caused by calculi, neoplasms, blood clot, stricture, or adhesions.<br>Procedure: (see cystoscopy below)<br>1. Determine iodine sensitivity. |
| Renal angiography | Series of radiographs taken after injection of contrast media into renal vasculature during phases of arterial, nephrographic, and venous filling<br>Vascular access: Femoral artery is most commonly used. | Delineates renal vasculature and may reveal renal tumors, renal cysts, renal artery stenosis, aneurysm or fistula; renal abscess; or trauma.<br>Procedure: (see excretory uropathy above).<br>Follow-up care:<br>1. Bedrest for several hours.<br>2. Observe venipuncture site for evidence of bleeding (hematoma formation); puncturing of peripheral artery with consequent hematoma, embolism, and thrombosis are serious complications.<br>3. Monitor peripheral pulses.<br>4. Monitor for delayed reaction to contrast media. |
| Intravenous digital subtraction angiogram (DSA) | Allows visualization of main renal arteries | Less invasive than renal arteriography, but false-negative rate is about 10%–12%. |
| Voiding cystogram (cystourethrography) | Instillation of contrast media through a catheter introduced through the urethra and into the bladder; fluoroscopic films and overhead radiographs demonstrate bladder filling and emptying as patient voids. | May reveal urinary tract abnormalities, such as ureteral stricture or stenosis; ureteral reflux; measurement of post-voiding residual urine volume.<br>Procedure:<br>1. Rule out iodine sensitivity.<br>2.Establish baseline vital parameters (e.g., blood pressure, heart rate, respiratory rate, temperature). |
| Retrograde cystography | Radiographic examination follows instillation of contrast media into bladder. | Assists in diagnosing bladder rupture; presence of neurogenic bladder; residual urine volume; suspected vesicoureteral reflex; tumors; other.<br>Procedure: (see voiding cystogram above). |
| Retrograde urethrography | | Provides information about status of urethra and visualization of membranes, bulbar and penile portions in males. |
| Cystoscopy | Passage of rigid flexible cystoscope into bladder and ureters under local or general anesthesia, and under strict aseptic techniques | Facilitates calculi removal.<br>Procedure:<br>1. NPO.<br>2. Evacuate bowel<br>3. Obtain informed consent.<br>4. Sedation as prescribed.<br>Follow-up care:<br>1. Encourage fluids.<br>2. Monitor fluid intake and urine output.<br>3. Monitor for urine retention, bleeding, infection. |

(*Continued*)

TABLE 22–3
**Diagnostic Studies and Procedures for Evaluating Renal Dysfunction *(Continued)***

| Test/Study | Description | Clinical Significance and Nursing Implications |
|---|---|---|
| Renal computerized tomography scan | A series of tomograms, or cross-sectional slices, are translated by a computer and displayed on an oscilloscope screen.<br>The density of the image reflects the amount of radiation absorbed by renal tissue.<br>Renal CT scan may be performed after administration of contrast media, which accentuates the density of the renal parenchyma and assists in differentiating renal masses. | Permits identification of masses and other lesions of different densities, as, for example, renal cysts, renal tumors; and other abnormalities (e.g., polycystic kidney disease, congenital anomalies, calculi and other obstructions).<br><br>Procedure:<br>1. Determine sensitivity to contrast media. |
| Nuclear magnetic resonance (NMR) | | Provides same information as CT scan but has the advantage of not using x-rays. |
| Renal scan (radionuclide imaging) | Injection of nuclide is followed by scintiphotography. | Allows identification of structure of kidneys and can demonstrate lesions, intrarenal masses, and traumatic injury.<br>Dynamic scans assist in evaluating renal perfusion and can identify compromised circulation in patients with renovascular hypertension and abdominal aortic pathology.<br>Abnormalities of the collecting system (e.g., ureteral obstruction) can be detected.<br>Follow-up care: Handle urine with gloves for 24 hr post-procedure; encourage fluid intake. |
| Renal ultrasonography | High-frequency sound waves are transmitted from a transducer through the kidneys and surrounding structures.<br>The resulting echoes are amplified and converged into electrical impulses and displayed on an oscilloscope screen as anatomical images. | Differentiates between solid and cystic structures and localized fluid collections.<br>Assists in visualizing renal anatomy; structure of perirenal tissues; location of urinary obstruction; abnormal accumulation of fluid; and in assessing and diagnosing complications post-renal transplantation.<br>Noninvasive; no special preparation or after-care is required. |
| Renal biopsy | With visualization of kidney by fluoroscopy or ultrasound, an insertion of biopsy needle is performed percutaneously or by open incision. | Highly invasive procedure.<br>Assists in diagnosis of renal disease that cannot be definitively determined by other methods.<br>Procedure:<br>1. NPO for 6–8 hr prior to procedure.<br>2. Maintain patent intravenous access.<br>3. Obtain informed consent.<br>4. Sedation as prescribed.<br>5. Assess for hypertension, bleeding, or coagulation disorders.<br>Follow-up care:<br>1. Serial vital signs until stable.<br>2. Monitor for complaints of pain and hematoma formation.<br>3. Monitor hematocrit.<br>4. Bed rest for 24 hr.<br>5. Encourage fluids; monitor hourly urine output; observe for hematuria.<br>6. Chest x-ray as prescribed to rule out iatrogenic pneumothorax.<br>For open biopsy, follow unit post-operative protocols. |

ture of the test, urine collected may require preservation, either by chemical means or by refrigeration. Appropriate patient preparation, including the patient's role in properly performing the test(s), facilitates the diagnostic process. Table 22–1 lists some important data that can be obtained by urinalysis, normal range of values, and clinical significance in terms of renal function.

Use of a variety of dipsticks (e.g., Diastix, N-Multistix) affords rapid bedside screening. Nurses need to understand the importance of data obtained in this manner and be able to evaluate its significance in terms of the patient's overall condition. Table 22–2 lists specific blood parameters of significance in evaluating renal/urinary function.

## Diagnostic Tests/Procedures: Nursing Implications

Results of urine and blood analyses frequently reveal abnormal findings that suggest the presence of underlying renal disease, which mandate further diagnostic study. Such radiologic examination tests include excretory urography (formerly intravenous pyelography), retrograde pyelography and urethrography, cystoscopy, radionuclide imaging, renal ultrasonography, and renal biopsy, among others. Table 22–3 lists specific tests/studies available for the diagnostic workup of suspected renal/urinary dysfunction, a description of each study, its clinical significance in terms of renal/urinary function, and implications for nursing care.

## REFERENCES


1. Rose, BD: Pathophysiology of Renal Disease, ed 2. McGraw-Hill, New York, 1987, p 91.
2. Rose, BD: Pathophysiology of Renal Disease, ed 2. McGraw-Hill, New York, 1987, p 14.
3. Whittaker, AA: Acute renal dysfunction: Assessment of patients at risk. Focus Crit Care 12(3):12, 1985.

CHAPTER 23

# Fluid and Electrolyte Physiology and Pathophysiology

## CHAPTER OUTLINE



## LEARNING OBJECTIVES

**At the end of this chapter, you should be able to:**

1. Describe the overall fluid and electrolyte composition of extracellular and intracellular body compartments.
2. Define "third spacing," and delineate examples of this phenomenon.
3. List physiologic factors influencing total body water balance.
4. Contrast extracellular and intracellular fluid disorders including etiology, clinical manifestations, laboratory data, and treatment.
5. Contrast electrolyte disorders including etiology, clinical manifestations, laboratory data, and treatment for the following:
   - Hypernatremia—Hyponatremia
   - Hyperkalemia—Hypokalemia
   - Hyperchloremia—Hypochloremia
   - Hypermagnesemia—Hypomagnesemia
6. Delineate the nursing process in caring for the patient with fluid and electrolyte imbalance including:
   - Assessment
   - Nursing diagnosis.
   - Planning: Desired patient outcomes
     - Nursing interventions/rationales.

Fluid, electrolyte, and acid–base disturbances are common occurrences encountered in the care of the critically ill patient. An understanding of the pathophysiology underlying these abnormalities helps the critical care nurse recognize their clinical manifestations, anticipate those situations in which they are likely to occur, and assist in the implementation of appropriate and timely treatment when they do occur. Many of the symptoms of fluid and electrolyte disturbances are nonspecific and require a high index of suspicion if they are to be recognized and/or prevented. Simple treatment can reverse the vast majority of these conditions, yet, failure to recognize them may lead to needless deleterious consequences.

## BODY COMPOSITION

A major function of the kidney is the maintenance of the integrity of the internal environment. To accomplish this task, the kidney regulates the volume and composition of extracellular fluid, specifically, by controlling the amounts of water and electrolytes reabsorbed or excreted from the blood.

### Total Body Water and the Fluid Compartments

Depending on age, sex, skeletal muscle mass, and fat content, approximately 60%–70% of body weight is water. In terms of volume, the total body water (TBW) amounts to about 40 liters, for example, in an adult male who weighs about 62 kg. The distribution of TBW is of major importance in regulating fluid and electrolyte balance. TBW is compartmentalized into two major spaces: about two thirds, or 25 liters, is located within the intracellular fluid (ICF) space; and the remaining one third, or 15 liters, is confined to the extracellular (ECF) space. The plasma cell membrane separates the fluid in these two compartments.

The extracellular fluid (ECF) itself is subdivided into the intravascular space (about 3 liters) and the interstitial fluid (about 12 liters). Also included as part of the ECF volume are the *transcellular* fluid spaces. These spaces are relatively small and are separated from the interstitial fluid by a layer of epithelium. Transcellular fluid includes cerebrospinal fluid; intraocular fluid; fluid within the pleural, pericardial, and peritoneal cavities; joint fluid; and the gastrointestinal secretions. Transcellular fluid volume becomes a significant factor when an abnormal fluid accumulation occurs in a transcellular space, as for example, the occurrence of *ascites*. Ascites occurs when there is an abnormal intra-abdominal fluid accumulation. Because fluid shifts between the transcellular spaces and interstitium occur very slowly, fluid is "confined" to these spaces, a condition often referred to as "*third-spacing.*"

Third-spacing, a commonly occurring phenomenon in critically ill patients, reflects a shift of fluid from the intravascular space into the transcellular space. While no actual decrease in total body fluid volume (no weight loss) occurs, the intravascular plasma volume becomes contracted, resulting in a decrease in the circulating blood volume. Examples of third-spacing include[1]: ascites, a serous accumulation in the peritoneal cavity related to portal hypertension (cirrhosis); intestinal obstruction, with fluid accumulation in the intestines proximal to the obstruction (fluid accumulation accounts for the abdominal distention often seen in this disorder); peritonitis, with fluid accumulation in the peritoneal cavity associated with infection or inflammation; continuous ambulatory peritoneal dialysis (CAPD), a frequent cause of peritonitis in patients with renal disease; acute pancreatitis in which the inflammatory response is associated with the loss of digestive juices into surrounding tissues; fistulous drainage; and burns. Ascites is not always considered as third-spacing because it can be removed by paracentesis.

As part of the ECF compartment, the plasma within the intravascular space is distinguished by its high protein concentration. The distribution of serum proteins in the body is limited almost exclusively to the intravascular space. These proteins, particularly albumin, function primarily to maintain the volume of the small but vital intravascular space. They exert a colloidal osmotic pressure, which attracts fluid into this space and keeps it there. Thus, while comprising but a small fraction of ECF volume, the plasma volume remains constant even in the face of severe contraction of the interstitial fluid volume.

Rapid changes of water balance usually affect the intravascular volume first, with the interstitial fluid functioning as an immediate buffer. As fluid is lost from the intravascular space, hemoconcentration occurs within this space, creating an osmotic force that draws water from the interstitium. This serves to maintain the critical volume of fluid within the intravascular space.

Similarly, the interstitial fluid volume acts as a reservoir for intracellular fluid needs, providing water to the cells when needed, or accepting it from the cells when fluid is in excess. It is the volume of fluid in the interstitium that is assessed clinically when the patient is examined to determine the overall fluid status. The interstitial fluid volume serves to minimize the effects of changes in TBW on intravascular and intracellular fluid volumes. A contrast between extracellular and intracellular fluid is presented in Table 23–1.

#### *Physiologic Factors Influencing Water Balance*

**Osmolality of Body Fluids.** Regulation of water balance occurs largely in conjunction with electrolyte balance, and its distribution within the ICF and ECF compartments is influenced directly by the osmolality of the fluids within these compartments. Osmotic gradients are established and maintained by solutes, which, unlike the freely penetrating water molecule, are largely confined to their respective compartments. Potassium, magnesium, phosphates, sulfates, and proteins are the major *in-*

TABLE 23–1
**Contrast: Extracellular and Intracellular Fluids[2]**

| | Extracellular | Intracellular |
|---|---|---|
| Type of fluid | "Saline" solution reflects high sodium and chloride content of ECF compartment. | "Potassium" solution because this ion is primarily intracellular; this solution is isotonic with the extracellular fluid. |
| Distribution | 20% of total body weight; one third of total body fluid; approximately 12–15 liters<br>Depends on age, sex, skeletal muscle mass and fat content | 40% of total body weight; two thirds of total body fluid; approximately 25–30 liters; depends on age, sex, skeletal muscle mass, and fat content |
| Area | Interstitial and intravascular | Intracellular |
| Excess | Compartment expanded, reflects edema | Solute diluted (hyponatremia) |
| Deficit | Compartment contracted | Solute concentrated (hypernatremia) |
| Fluid movement | Saline solution taken into the body remains in ECF compartment.<br>Saline losses are from ECF compartment. | Water taken into the body is distributed: one third goes into ECF compartment; two thirds goes into ICF compartment<br>Water losses are from both compartments in proportions stated above |
| Major electrolytes | Sodium ($Na^+$)<br>Chloride ($Cl^-$)<br>Bicarbonate ($HCO_3^-$)<br>Proteins | Potassium ($K^+$)<br>Magnesium ($Mg^{2+}$)<br>Phosphate ($HPO_4^{2-}$)<br>Proteins |
| Sensible loss (perceptible) and insensible loss (imperceptible) | Immediate loss from the ECF compartment | Eventual loss from the ICF compartment |

*tra*cellular osmotic solutes, while sodium and its accompanying anions, chloride and bicarbonate ($HCO_3^-$), comprise the major *extra*cellular solutes.

The osmolality of the intravascular fluid (plasma) is a critical value because it influences the volume and composition of fluids within the other compartments. One can appreciate, therefore, why the renal regulation of the reabsorption and secretion of the constituents of plasma constitutes the most important mechanism for maintaining bodily processes in an equilibrated state.

Various physiologic processes influence fluid and electrolyte balance. Finely regulated control of serum osmolality occurs with regulation of water intake by the thirst mechanism, and its reabsorption or excretion in response to antidiuretic hormonal secretion. These two mechanisms are concerned largely with control of intracellular fluid (ICF) volume. When volume is restored and serum osmolality returns to within physiologic range, these mechanisms are shut off.

**Aldosterone Secretion.** Aldosterone secretion by the adrenal cortex plays an important role in the regulation of ECF volume by increasing sodium reabsorption in the distal tubule. Accompanying the reabsorption of sodium is an obligatory retention of water, which functions to expand the ECF volume and decrease serum osmolality. Major stimuli of aldosterone secretion include potassium-ion concentration of ECF, renin–angiotensin system, decrease in total body sodium concentration, and the "permissive effect" of ACTH (see Chap. 18). As fluid volume and electrolyte concentrations are stabilized, these stimuli are diminished and the secretion of aldosterone is turned off by negative feedback mechanisms.

**Baroreceptors.** Baroreceptors located in the carotid sinus and aortic arch respond to the degree of stretch of the vessel wall generated by the volume of blood flowing through it. In response to a drop in arterial blood pressure, these receptors generate fewer impulses, which reflexly excite the sympathetic vasomotor center in the medulla resulting in an accelerated heart rate, and an increase in blood pressure by peripheral vasoconstriction (increased peripheral vascular resistance). Concomitantly, sympathetic innervation of afferent and efferent arterioles at the glomerulus reduces glomerular filtration, resulting in a decrease in urine formation and excretion. These mechanisms thus function to maintain a stable intravascular fluid volume, and, in turn, the ECF compartment fluid volume.

**Intravascular Proteins.** Maintenance of intravascular volume also depends on the osmotic (colloidal) pressure exerted by the serum proteins. Depletion of proteins results in a contraction of intravascular volume.

***Fluid Intake and Output***

To maintain an equilibrated state between fluid compartments, the body's daily fluid intake must equal its output. The average healthy adult requires about 2000–2800 ml/day. Of this about 1000–1500 ml is consumed in liquid form; another 800–1000 ml is ingested in foods; and the oxidation of foodstuffs in body tissues accounts for an additional 200–300 ml.

Fluid loss in the average healthy adult from all sources usually amounts to about 2500 ml/day. Of this amount about 1500 ml occurs as urine; up to 200 ml is excreted in feces; and the remainder is lost through the lungs and skin (insensible losses).

The occurrence of an illness state can quickly and radically change the equilibrium between fluid intake and output. Fever and hyperventilation can cause an increase in fluid losses by perspiration and the lungs, respectively. Patients on mechanical ventilators or another source of humidified oxygen can *absorb* up to an additional 1000 ml of fluid daily, while unhumidified oxygen therapy can result in a net *loss* of fluid. Altered gastrointestinal function such as occurs with vomiting, diarrhea, and gastric suctioning can significantly reduce fluid intake, while dramatically increasing fluid loss. Overzealous use of diuretics can quickly deplete body fluids and electrolytes. Wound drainage offers another source of significant fluid loss.

## Assessment of the Fluid State

The clinical assessment of total body water (TBW) is very inaccurate at best. More than 10% of TBW may be lost before evidence of hypovolemia appears. The thirst mechanism is activated when the decrease in TBW reaches about 2%. Serial assessment of body weight is probably the most reliable parameter, especially because water makes up such a large proportion of total body weight. As a general rule, each kilogram (2.2 lb) of body weight is equal to approximately 1 liter of fluid.

Intravascular (plasma) volume is assessed by evaluating the effectiveness of the circulation in meeting tissue needs. Key factors that must be considered include the effectiveness of the heart as a pump (cardiac output) and the peripheral vascular resistance to blood flow offered by the systemic vasculature.

Important assessment considerations include: mental status; temperature and skin color (mottling or cyanosis?) of peripheral parts of the body; heart rate and blood pressure (lying, and sitting or standing); central venous pressure reflected in the degree of neck vein distention; shortness of breath or dyspnea; and urinary output.

Laboratory studies having diagnostic value in evaluating fluid status include: serum electrolytes, serum osmolality, hematocrit, blood urea nitrogen (BUN), and urine specific gravity. Serum sodium is the best indicator of intracellular fluid disorders. The hematocrit reflects the proportion of blood plasma to red blood cells. Fluid loss causes hemoconcentration; fluid gain causes hemodilution. Serum osmolality reflects the actual number of osmotically active particles in blood. Fluid loss increases serum osmolality because particles become more concentrated; fluid excess decreases serum osmolality because particles become diluted. A rise in BUN frequently reflects a fluid deficient state: a fluid deficit causes urine to be concentrated (specific gravity $>1.030$); a fluid excess dilutes urine (specific gravity $<1.010$).

# FLUID IMBALANCES

Fluid imbalances may reflect a significant increase or decrease in total body fluid, or an altered distribution of body fluid as occurs for example in third-spacing (see Table 23-2). These conditions are especially challenging to the critical care nurse because there are no definitive laboratory tests that are pathognomonic of these disorders. Rather, their recognition and/or prevention require astute observation and assessment skills (history-taking and physical examination), coupled with a sound understanding of the principles underlying fluid and electrolyte physiology. The critical care nurse must be able to recognize signs and symptoms suggestive of fluid imbalance, and to integrate these data with the patient's overall clinical status to determine their significance and treatment.

## Extracellular Fluid Volume Deficit

Extracellular fluid (ECF) volume deficit (Table 23–2) reflects a severely contracted ECF compartment attributed to a significant extracellular fluid loss and/or accumulation of fluid in transcellular spaces (third-spacing.) Because extracellular fluid consists predominantly of sodium and chloride ions, both of which tend to attract water, disorders of the ECF compartment are often referred to as "saline" disorders (see Table 23–1). Gastrointestinal dysfunction is most commonly identified as the underlying cause of ECF volume deficit. Other etiologies include renal dysfunction, profuse diaphoresis associated with high fever, serum hypoproteinemia, and hemorrhage.

Clinically, ECF volume deficit is characterized by an acute weight loss of greater than 0.5 kg/day. Altered cardiovascular function largely reflects the underlying ECF volume deficit. Symptoms may include: changes in heart rate; postural hypotension (i.e., a decrease of 10 mmHg or more on sitting or standing, than while lying supine); dizziness, ver-

TABLE 23–2
**Contrast: Extracellular and Intracellular Fluid Deficit Disorders**

| | Extracellular Fluid Volume Deficit | Intracellular Fluid Volume Deficit |
|---|---|---|
| Definition | *Hypovolemia:* Contracted ECF compartment, ECF volume deficit | Total body water (TBW) deficit; *hypernatremia* |
| Etiology | General dysfunction: Fever with profuse diaphoresis<br>Gastrointestinal dysfunction (most common):<br>Fluid and electrolyte loss: Anorexia; reduced oral intake; vomiting with loss of $H^+$ ion; sodium and chloride<br>Diarrhea: Increased peristalsis preventing adequate resorption of fluid and electrolytes; loss of $HCO_3^-$; fistula or wound drainage; continuous gastrointestinal suction<br>Overdose of cathartics; excessive tap water enemas; Hypotonic solution causes electrolyte shift into intestinal lumen from whence they are lost in feces.<br>Renal dysfunction:<br>Renal disease—Tubular damage causes loss of sodium and serum proteins.<br>Overzealous use of diuretics causes excessive loss of sodium, chloride, and water.<br>Neurologic dysfunction:<br>Mental status changes, lethargy, coma<br>Endocrine dysfunction: Diabetes insipidus<br>Other fluid losses: Hypoproteinemia, hemorrhage, tachypnea<br>*Third-spacing*—Shift of fluid into transcellular spaces where it becomes inaccessible. Shift occurs from intravascular space into transcellular space. While no actual decrease in total fluid volume (no weight loss) occurs, the intravascular plasma volume becomes contracted. | Insufficient water intake: Inability to respond to thirst stimulus: Comatose patient; organic brain syndrome; inability to swallow<br>Excessive water loss. Extensive insensible (skin, lungs) fluid losses: Profuse diaphoresis associated with hyperpyrexia; hyperventilation<br>Diabetes insipidus<br>Osmotic diuresis: Diabetes mellitus; iatrogenic via administration of osmotic diuretics (mannitol, hypertonic dextrose, radiopaque dyes)<br>(*Note:* Patients having special procedures requiring the use of contrast media are often further dehydrated by being NPO [nothing by mouth] for several hours prior to the procedure. Intravenous fluid replacement must be provided during this interim.) |
| Clinical presentation | *Acute weight loss:* > 0.5 kg/day<br>*Neurologic:* Changes in mental status; disorientation, agitation; lethargy, loss of consciousness; convulsions, muscle cramps<br>*Cardiovascular:* Hypovolemic shock; postural hypotension; blood pressure decrease > 10 mmHg on sitting or standing than while lying down; dizziness, vertigo, syncope; tachycardia—Pulse weak and thready; absence of neck vein distention; decreased CVP; decreased pulmonary artery pressures; decreased cardiac output<br>*Gastrointestinal:* Nausea, vomiting, anorexia<br>*Fluid intake vs. output:* increased thirst with increase in fluid intake if patient is conscious; coupled with a decreased urine output < 200 ml/8 hr; poor skin turgor over sternum or forehead; dry skin and mucous membranes, but skin may become cold, clammy, and cyanotic in presence of shock state; sunken eyeballs; hyperthermia associated with diaphoresis and loss of salt (with dehydrated state there is less water available for cooling) | Intracellular fluid volume deficit is reflected predominantly by alterations in central nervous system function.<br>*Neurologic:* Changes in level of consciousness and mental status; restlessness or agitation; lethargy and listlessness. Muscle weakness may occur, and seizure activity is not uncommon.<br>*Respiratory:* Disruptions in respiratory rate and rhythm may occur followed by respiratory arrest.<br>*Renal:* Oliguria (< 30 ml/hr)<br>*Skin:* Warm and flushed; hyperpyrexia is common. |
| Laboratory data | No electrolyte parameter (by itself) is indicative of an *extra*cellular fluid deficit. Contributing data: Reflective of hemoconcentration. | Serum sodium is an excellent indicator of ICF volume deficit:<br>Serum sodium level > 148 mEq/liter (hypernatremia) strongly suggests ICF volume deficit.<br>Low or normal serum sodium with elevated serum glucose is associated with ICF volume deficit. |
| Hematocrit | Increased | Normal to increased |
| Hemoglobin | Increased | Normal to increased |

*(Continued)*

TABLE 23–2
**Contrast: Extracellular and Intracellular Fluid Deficit Disorders *(Continued)***

| | Extracellular Fluid Volume Deficit | Intracellular Fluid Volume Deficit |
|---|---|---|
| Serum: | | |
| Proteins | Increased | Increased |
| Osmolality | Normal (285–295 mOsm/kg) | >310 mOsm/kg |
| BUN | >20 mg/100 ml | >20 mg/100 ml |
| Urine: | | |
| Sodium | <50 mEq/liter | Measurable amount |
| Osmolality | >500 mOsm/kg | >500 mOsm/kg |
| Specific gravity | >1.030 | >1.030 |
| Treatment | 1. Restore fluid and electrolyte balance using intravenous isotonic saline until oliguria is relieved, hemodynamic parameters stabilize, and neurologic status is intact. Extreme caution is required to prevent fluid overload (with congestive heart failure and cerebral edema).<br>2. Treat underlying cause. | 1. Aggressive fluid replacement usually with 5% dextrose/water. Vital parameters need to be monitored closely to prevent fluid overload.<br>2. Treat underlying cause. |

tigo, syncope; tachycardia (in hypovolemic shock, the pulse may feel weak and thready); and a decrease in venous return to the heart as reflected by flat neck veins, lowered central venous pressure, and reduced pulmonary artery pressures. Frequently there are complaints of nausea with vomiting. A cough, productive of thick tenacious mucus (dehydrated mucous glands) may be evident. Symptomatology reflective of the dehydrated state may be apparent: changes in mental status, muscle cramps, sunken eyeballs, and poor skin turgor over the forehead and sternum. Oliguria (<30 ml/hour) occurs in severely dehydrated states.

Laboratory tests provide data supportive of the diagnosis of ECF volume deficit. A reduction in plasma volume causes an increase in hematocrit and serum proteins (hemoconcentration); serum sodium levels are nonspecific in the diagnosis of extracellular fluid volume disorders and may be high, low, or normal.

Treatment of ECF volume deficit entails judicious fluid replacement (isotonic saline) orally and/or intravenously, until oliguria is relieved, hemodynamic parameters stabilize, and neurologic status is normal. Extreme caution needs to be exercised in fluid replacement therapy to avoid fluid overload. Continuous monitoring of vital parameters, intake and output, and daily weight is essential.

Nursing care considerations are focused on reestablishing and maintaining fluid and electrolyte balance. Nursing diagnosis, interventions, and rationales in the care of the patient with a fluid and/or electrolyte imbalance are presented in the Care Plan in Table 23–3.

## Intracellular Fluid Volume Deficit

A decrease in the volume of fluid distributed intracellularly constitutes an intracellular fluid (ICF) volume deficit (see Table 23–2). In contrast to the ECF (saline) compartment, disorders of the ICF compartment are primarily considered to be "water" disorders because of the miniscule concentration of sodium and chloride intracellularly. These disorders reflect a problem with the concentration and dilution of intracellular solute, which is specifically reflected by the concentration of sodium. When there is an excess of total body water (TBW), sodium concentration is diluted, resulting in *hypo*natremia; when a TBW deficit exists, sodium becomes concentrated and *hyper*natremia occurs.

ICF volume deficit is caused by either an insufficient water intake or an excessive water loss. The patient who is comatose and unable to respond to the thirst stimulus, or the patient who is unable to swallow, is at high risk of developing ICF volume deficit unless fluid is replaced in some way. ICF volume deficit may occur in the presence of extensive insensible (by skin or lungs) fluid losses. A high fever with profuse diaphoresis, and hyperventilation are two mechanisms that can cause considerable fluid losses. Diabetes insipidus (see Chap. 16) predisposes one to significant fluid losses either because there is a decreased secretion of antidiuretic hormone (ADH) and/or because cells in the distal tubule and collecting ducts are unresponsive to this hormone. The osmotic diuresis often associated with diabetes mellitus causes fluid loss.

Clinically, ICF volume deficit is reflected by alter-

## TABLE 23-3. CARE PLAN FOR THE PATIENT WITH FLUID AND ELECTROLYTE IMBALANCES: FLUID VOLUME DEFICIT

| Nursing Diagnoses | Desired Patient Outcomes | Nursing Interventions | Rationales |
|---|---|---|---|
| ***Nursing Diagnosis #1***<br>Fluid volume deficit:<br>Actual, related to:<br>1. Extracellular dehydration (hypovolemia).<br>2. Intracellular dehydration (hypernatremia). | Patient's condition will stabilize:<br>1. Neurologic status: Oriented to person, place, date; deep tendon reflexes brisk.<br>2. Hemodynamic status will stabilize as follows:<br>• Heart rate >60 <100 beats/min.<br>• Arterial BP within 10 mmHg of baseline.<br>• CVP mean 0–8 mmHg.<br>• PAP <25 mmHg (systolic).<br>• PCWP mean 8–12 mmHg.<br>• CO 4–8 liters/min.<br>3. Body temperature ~98.6°F (37.0°C).<br>4. Body weight will stabilize within 5% of baseline.<br>5. Serum osmolality will stabilize at 285–295 mOsm/kg.<br>6. Serum sodium; >135 <148 mEq/liter.<br>7. Serum glucose; BUN, creatinine, hematocrit stabilized at optimum levels for patient.<br>8. Hourly urine output: >30 ml/hr. | • Assess impact of fluid volume deficit on body processes. | • Decreased intravascular volume triggers three compensatory mechanisms:<br>○ Renin–angiotensin–aldosterone system.<br>○ Thirst mechanism.<br>○ Antidiuretic hormone secretion in response to serum hyperosmolality. |
| | | • Assess neurologic status.<br>○ Level of consciousness.<br>○ Behavioral changes: Irritability, restlessness, listlessness, lethargy. | • Hyperosmolar state associated with severe dehydration usually reflects intracellular fluid deficit as well as contraction of the ECF volume; alterations in neurologic status primarily reflect *ICF* volume deficit (see below). |
| | | • Assess status of hemodynamic function. | • Alterations in hemodynamic function primarily reflect *ECF* volume deficit. |
| | | ○ Heart rate; peripheral pulses (quality—weak, thready).<br>○ Tachypnea, "air hunger." | ○ Hypovolemia causes tachycardia (heart rate >100); the increase in heart rate is a compensatory mechanism to maintain cerebral and renal perfusion in the presence of a depleted intravascular blood volume. |
| | | ○ Postural (orthostatic) hypotention. | ○ A drop in systolic pressure >10 mmHg from supine to upright position signals compromised hemodynamics. |
| | | ○ CVP reduced: <1 mmHg. | ○ Reduced CVP reflects decreased venous return to heart caused by hypovolemia. |
| | | ○ PCWP reduced: <4 mmHg. | ○ PCWP reflects status of left ventricular function and ECF volume. |
| | | • Monitor body temperature: Fever | • Profuse diaphoresis associated with fever aggravates underlying dehydrated state; dehydration decreases the amount of body water available for cooling, and, thus, body temperature rises. |
| | | • Assess renal function. | • Reduced renal perfusion associated with hypovolemia may compromise renal function; reduced glomerular filtration rate predisposes to oliguria. |
| | | ○ Blood urea nitrogen (BUN), serum creatinine, serum osmolality, BUN/creatinine ratio.<br>○ Urine output—decreased; specific gravity—increased (>1.030). | ○ When BUN/creatinine ratio increases in favor of BUN (i.e., >10 : 1), conditions such as hypovolemia or reduced renal perfusion may be present. |

*(continued)*

**TABLE 23–3. CARE PLAN FOR THE PATIENT WITH FLUID AND ELECTROLYTE IMBALANCES: FLUID VOLUME DEFICIT *(Continued)***

| Nursing Diagnoses | Desired Patient Outcomes | Nursing Interventions | Rationales |
|---|---|---|---|
| ***Nursing Diagnosis #1 (cont.)*** | | | |
| | | ◦ Total fluid intake and output including urine output; insensible losses by lungs and skin; gastric suctioning; gastrointestinal losses by vomiting, diarrhea; wound drainage; iatrogenic losses (blood sampling). | |
| | | • Assess gastrointestinal function: Anorexia, nausea, vomiting, abdominal cramps and distention; diarrhea or constipation. | |
| | | • Assess body weight (daily). | • Change in body weight is best indicator of fluid state; weight should be measured daily under the same conditions. |
| | | • Monitor laboratory values. | • These values may be elevated due in part to severe volume contraction with intravascular hemoconcentration. |
| | | ◦ Total serum protein. | ◦ Hypoproteinemia may require replacement if protein loss is from the intravascular space; colloidal intravascular osmotic pressure is essential for maintaining intravascular volume. |
| | | ◦ Hematocrit, hemoglobin, and serum electrolytes. | |
| | | • Monitor other parameters. | |
| | | ◦ Mucous membranes. | ◦ Dry mucous membranes reflect dehydrated state. |
| | | ◦ Skin turgor over sternum and forehead; sunken eyeballs. | ◦ Loss of interstitial (ECF) fluid reduces elasticity of skin. |
| | | ◦ Third-spacing, fluid accumulation. | ◦ Fluid accumulation in third spaces is lost to body use; a tape measure can be used to determine expansion of body parts due to progressive fluid accumulation as, for example, abdominal girth (ascites). Mark areas clearly, and measure at the same point using same tape measure. |
| | | • Collaborate with physician to correct underlying cause of fluid imbalance (see Table 23–2). | • Correction of the underlying cause contributing to the fluid loss is essential if hypovolemia is to be successfully treated and normovolemia restored. |
| | | ◦ Causes of ECF volume deficit: | |
| | | – Infection with hyperpyrexia and diaphoresis. | |
| | | ◦ Renal: Overly aggressive diuretic therapy. | ◦ Results in excessive loss of Na, Cl and $H_2O$. |
| | | ◦ Gastrointestinal dysfunction. | ◦ GI secretions contain large amounts of Na, Cl, and $H_2O$. |
| | | – Third-spacing fluid accumulation. | |

| | |
|---|---|
| ◦ Causes of ICF volume deficit:<br>◦ Insufficient water intake (comatose patient; postoperative patient).<br>◦ Excessive water loss (fever with profuse diaphoresis; gastroenteritis with diarrhea; diabetes mellitus—diabetic ketoacidosis; diabetes insipidus). (See Chapters 19 and 16 respectively.) | ◦ Unable to respond to thirst stimulus; NPO without adequate intravenous replacement. |
| • Implement fluid replacement regimen.<br>◦ Extracellular fluid deficit: Saline deficit | • Goal of fluid replacement therapy is to restore volume without rapid fluid shifts or alteration in electrolyte concentrations. |
| ◦ Implement prescribed treatment: Saline fluid replacement orally or intravenously until oliguria is relieved, hemodynamic parameters stabilize, and neurologic status is intact. | ◦ Rapid rehydration with isotonic saline is treatment of choice in fluid volume deficit due to *extra*cellular fluid imbalance.<br>◦ Guideline: One half of estimated fluid deficit is replaced within first 12 hr; remaining fluid deficit replaced over subsequent 24 hr.<br>◦ Fluid volume and rate of administration will depend on severity of dehydration and effectiveness in relieving underlying cause. Isotonic saline (0.9N saline) or lactated Ringer's solution is usually prescribed. |
| ◦ Monitor rehydration closely: Careful documentation of all fluid intake and losses; fluid losses include urinary output, gastric suctioning, insensible losses by lungs and skin, iatrogenic losses.<br>◦ Insert Foley catheter to monitor urine output closely.<br>– Monitor for signs of fluid excess: Elevated hemodynamic parameter; neck vein distention in upright position (45 degrees); dependent and/or pitting edema. | ◦ Overly aggressive fluid replacement therapy may precipitate fluid excess, with its attendant danger of congestive heart failure/pulmonary edema, and cerebral edema.<br>◦ Accurate assessment of urinary output is essential to assess renal function and to determine fluid and electrolyte therapy.<br>◦ Edema reflects an extracellular imbalance. |
| ◦ Intracellular fluid deficit: Water deficit (hypernatremia).<br>– Assess neurologic function: Weakness, restlessness, irritability; hyperpnea with danger of sudden respiratory arrest; tetany.<br>◦ Implement: Water replacement orally or intravenously with 5% dextrose in water IV, and avoid further water loss: keep patient and environment cool; use of antipyretics may be indicated for fever. | ◦ Loss of *intra*cellular fluid (as opposed to extracellular fluid loss discussed above) causes a shrinkage in cell size due to loss of water; shrinkage of brain cells in this manner underlies the symptomatology associated with intracellular fluid loss.<br>◦ Rapid rehydration with 5% dextrose in water is treatment of choice in fluid volume deficit due to intracellular fluid imbalance. |
| ◦ Monitor serum sodium levels, serum proteins, urinary sodium, and urine specific gravity. | ◦ A sodium level > 148 mEq/liter indicates intracellular fluid deficit. Urinary sodium may be detectable in measurable amounts; urine specific gravity is elevated. |

(continued)

## TABLE 23-3. CARE PLAN FOR THE PATIENT WITH FLUID AND ELECTROLYTE IMBALANCES: FLUID VOLUME DEFICIT *(Continued)*

| Nursing Diagnoses | Desired Patient Outcomes | Nursing Interventions | Rationales |
|---|---|---|---|
| ***Nursing Diagnosis #2*** Oral mucous membranes, alteration in. | 1. Mucous membranes will remain clean, moist, and without cracking or fissures. | • Implement supportive nursing care measures<br>○ Assist with oral hygiene.<br>○ Maintain hydration as prescribed.<br>○ Assess mouth and pharynx for lesions, fissures, bleeding.<br>○ Apply Vaseline or swabs with glycerin.<br>–Offer fluids as indicated/tolerated. | ○ Keeps mucous membranes moist.<br>○ Assists in determining changes in the mucosa and the effectiveness of therapy.<br>○ Prevents cracking and fissure formation. |
| ***Nursing Diagnosis #3*** Skin integrity, impairment: Potential. | 1. Skin warm and dry; turgor over forehead and sternum elastic. | ○ Maintain skin integrity.<br>○ Assess skin for edema, breakdown, dryness.<br>○ Provide comfort measures: Massaging, turning, positioning, protecting bony prominences.<br>○ Involve patient/family in daily care when appropriate.<br>○ Prescribe appropriate level of activity:<br>– Bedrest while orthostatic (postural) hypotension and heart rate changes are significant; progressive activity as tolerated. | ○ Daily inspection helps in recognizing potential problem area enabling timely intervention to prevent complications.<br>○ In illness, tissues are more easily impaired.<br>○ Participation in self-care enables patient/family to assume responsibility for their health.<br>○ Progressive increase in activity as tolerated promotes general well-being and reduces risk of complications associated with immobility (e.g., impairment of skin integrity thromboembolic complications). |

Arterial BP = systolic/diastolic; CVP = central venous pressure; PAP = pulmonary artery pressure; PCWP = pulmonary capillary wedge pressure; CO = cardiac output.

ations in central nervous system function. Changes in level of consciousness and mental status may occur. The patient may exhibit restlessness, agitation, lethargy, and listlessness. Muscle weakness may occur, and seizure activity is not uncommon. Disruptions in the respiratory rate and rhythm may occur, followed by respiratory arrest. In contrast to ECF volume deficit, the skin of the patient with ICF volume deficit is warm and flushed, often with a concomitant fever. Oliguria may be severe.

The serum sodium test is a diagnostic indicator for intracellular fluid disturbances. A serum sodium level greater than 148 mEq/liter reflects the presence of an intracellular fluid volume deficit (hypernatremia). An intracellular fluid deficit may also occur in the presence of elevated serum glucose levels, while serum sodium levels remain within the normal range. Serum protein levels may also be elevated.

Treatment of ICF volume deficit (hypernatremia) involves fluid replacement usually with 5% dextrose in water. (For nursing care considerations, see the Care Plan in Table 23–3, Nursing Diagnosis #1B).

## Extracellular Fluid Volume Excess

An increase in extracellular fluid (ECF) volume (Table 23–4) causes an expansion of the ECF compartment. Primary causes of ECF excess include cardiovascular dysfunction as, for example, congestive heart failure with pulmonary edema. Overhydration by too rapid administration of intravenous saline may be a contributing factor in this instance. Primary renal disease with reduced glomerular filtration rate (GFR) and altered tubular reabsorption and secretion causes increasingly larger amounts of fluid to be held in the circulation. Reduced renal perfusion (hypotensive state) decreases GFR; this reduces the volume of filtrate presented to the tubular system for excretion. The net effect is expansion of ECF compartment. Hyperaldosteronism causes an increase in ECF volume by the enhanced reabsorption of sodium by the kidney tubules, with an obligatory retention of water.

Clinically, there are distinct signs and symptoms of ECF volume excess. A weight gain in excess of 5% of total body weight (>0.5 kg/day) reflects an ECF volume excess. Classically, ECF volume excess is reflected by alterations in cardiovascular function. Edema reflects an expansion of the interstitial fluid; *pitting* edema always indicates an ECF volume excess. Hypertension, tachycardia progressing to bradycardia, neck vein distention, and elevated central venous and pulmonary artery pressures all reflect expansion of ECF volume. Associated respiratory dysfunction may include shortness of breath, dyspnea, cough, and adventitious breath sounds (rales or crackles).

Laboratory data supportive of the diagnosis of ECF volume excess are largely nonspecific. There is no specific electrolyte test of diagnostic value. The hematocrit is usually reduced because red blood cells find themselves in an increased intravascular volume. Urinary sodium may be decreased due to sodium reabsorption.

Treatment of ECF volume excess is directed toward sodium (saline) and fluid restriction, administration of diuretics, and treatment of the underlying cause. Hypertonic intravenous solutions (e.g. mannitol, 10% and 50% dextrose in water) are commonly used for their osmotic diuretic effect. Diuretic therapy is prescribed to increase excretion of the extracellular fluid load. Nursing diagnosis, desired patient outcomes, and nursing interventions in the care of the patient with extracellular fluid volume excess are presented in the Care Plan in Table 23–5.

## Intracellular Fluid Volume Excess

An increase in the volume of fluid distributed *intracellularly* constitutes an ICF volume excess (see Table 23–4). The major cause of ICF volume excess is renal disease. The syndrome of inappropriate secretion of antidiuretic hormone (SIADH) causes water excess (water intoxication). An excessive oral and/or intravenous water intake has also been associated with ICF volume excess.

Clinical manifestations of ICF volume excess are classically exhibited by central nervous dysfunction. The underlying pathophysiology involves swelling of brain cells, which predisposes to an increase in intracranial pressure (ICP). Specific symptomatology includes changes in level of consciousness and mental status; headaches frequently occuring along with nausea and vomiting; and weakness, muscle cramps, muscle twitchings, and seizure activity, progressing to convulsions and coma.

The major laboratory indicator of ICF volume excess is the serum sodium concentration. Sodium levels less than 130 mEq/liter strongly indicate an ICF volume excess. In contrast to ECF volume excess in which the hematocrit falls, in ICF volume excess the hematocrit usually remains within the normal physiologic range because the red blood cells swell in proportion to the increase in plasma volume.

Treatment of ICF volume excess involves fluid restriction. Initially, fluid replacement is limited to the urine output volume only; as serum sodium rises and symptoms abate, the volume of fluid administered is increased to equal the fluid volume losses by urine and the insensible fluid losses (skin and lungs); continuous assessment of patient's con-

TABLE 23-4
## Contrast: Extracellular and Intracellular Fluid Excess Disorders

| | Extracellular Fluid Volume Excess | Intracellular Fluid Volume Excess |
|---|---|---|
| Definition | *Hypervolemia:* Expanded ECF compartment, ECF volume excess | Total body water (TBW) excess; *hyponatremia* |
| Etiology | Cardiovascular dysfunction: Congestive heart failure with pulmonary edema may result in reduced renal perfusion with decreased glomerular filtration and increased retention of fluid in intravascular space.<br>Too rapid administration of intravenous saline (overhydration) may precipitate congestive heart failure.<br>Renal dysfunction: Primary renal disease; renal failure: Reduced renal filtration, reabsorption, and secretion cause increasingly larger amounts of fluid to be held in circulation.<br>Serum protein depletion and hyponatremia cause ECF volume to become hypotonic to ICF; fluid shifts to intracellular compartment.<br>Cirrhosis with ascites and portal hypertension—alters renal blood flow; increased capillary fragility<br>Endocrine dysfunction: Hyperaldosteronism | Renal dysfunction: Renal disease is major cause of ICF volume excess; renal parenchymal damage disrupts renal handling of water, resulting in fluid overload.<br>Syndrome of inappropriate secretion of antidiuretic hormone (SIADH)<br>Excessive oral and/or intravenous intake |
| Clinical presentation | *Weight gain:* In excess of 5% of total body weight or >0.5 kg/day<br>*Neurologic:* Changes in mental status and level of consciousness; seizures, paralysis<br>*Cardiovascular:* Hypertension, tachycardia with bounding pulse initially, possibly progressing to bradycardia if treatment is delayed; neck vein distention; increased CVP and pulmonary pressures (associated with increased intravascular volume)<br>*Edema:* Reflects expansion of interstitial ECF volume; periorbital, presacral, extremities, *true pitting edema indicates ECF excess;* skin—taut and shiny<br>*Respiratory:* Shortness of breath, tachypnea, dyspnea, cough; rales, pulmonary edema<br>*Renal:* Urine output is disproportionately less than fluid intake. | Classic manifestations of ICF volume excess reflect central nervous system dysfunction. Increase in intracranial pressure associated with swelling of brain cells accounts for the following symptomatology:<br>*Neurologic:* Changes in level of consciousness, mental status; headache; weakness, muscle cramps, muscle twitchings; seizure activity; nausea and vomiting frequently accompanying the headache |
| Laboratory data | No electrolyte parameter (by itself) is indicative of an extracellular fluid disorder. Contributing data are reflective of hemodilution. | • Serum sodium is an excellent indicator of ICF volume deficit: Serum sodium level <130 mEq/liter (hyponatremia) strongly suggests ICF volume excess. |
| Serum: | | |
| Hematocrit | Normal to low | • Normal |
| Hemoglobin | Normal to low | • Normal |
| Proteins | Normal to low | • Normal to low |
| Osmolality | ~285–295 mOsm/kg | • <285 mOsm/kg |
| BUN | Normal to low | • Normal to low |
| Urine: | | |
| Sodium | Reduced | • Reduced |
| Osmolality | <500 mOsm/kg | • <500 mOsm/kg |
| Specific gravity | <1.010 | • <1.010 |
| Treatment | 1. Reduce fluid retention by salt and fluid restriction.<br>2. Diuretics to increase fluid excretion:<br>• Osmotic diuretics<br>• Salt-poor albumin<br>3. Treat underlying cause. | 1. Reduce total body water (TBW) by strict fluid restriction:<br>• Initially fluid replacement is equal to urine output only.<br>• As symptoms abate and sodium returns to within normal limits, fluid replacement therapy is increased to include insensible losses in addition to urine output.<br>2. Treat underlying cause. |
| | Continuous assessment of patient's condition and response to therapy, and evaluation of laboratory data are essential to prevent fluid deficit and hypovolemic shock. | |

## TABLE 23–5. CARE PLAN FOR THE PATIENT WITH FLUID AND ELECTROLYTE IMBALANCE: FLUID VOLUME EXCESS

| Nursing Diagnoses | Desired Patient Outcomes | Nursing Interventions | Rationales |
|---|---|---|---|
| ***Nursing Diagnosis #1***<br>Fluid volume, alteration in: Excess, related to:<br>1. Extracellular overhydration (hypervolemia) (circulatory overload).<br>2. Intracellular overhydration (hyponatremia). | Patient's condition will stabilize:<br>1. Neurologic status:<br>• Oriented to person, place, time; deep tendon reflexes brisk.<br>2. Hemodynamic status will stabilize as follows:<br>• Heart rate >60 <100 beats/min.<br>• Arterial BP within 10 mmHg of baseline.<br>• CVP mean 0–8 mmHg.<br>• PAP <25 mmHg (systolic).<br>• PCWP mean 8–12 mmHg.<br>• CO 4–8 liters/min.<br>3. Body temperature ~98.6°F (37°C).<br>4. Body weight will stabilize within 5% of baseline.<br>5. Serum osmolality will stabilize at ~285–295 mOsm/kg.<br>6. Serum sodium: >135 <148 mEq/liter.<br>7. Serum glucose, BUN and creatinine, hematocrit stabilized at optimum for patient.<br>8. Hourly urine output: >30 ml/hr.<br>9. Respiratory status:<br>• Lung fields resonant and without rales (crackles). | • Assess impact of fluid volume excess on body processes.<br>○ Assess neurologic status: Level of consciousness; mental status changes: confusion, lethargy; behavioral changes: irritability, restlessness, listlessness; headache; weakness; muscle twitchings, convulsions, coma. | ○ Hypo-osmolar state (excess of water or sodium depletion) usually reflects intracellular fluid volume excess, which is characterized by alterations in neurologic function.<br>○ An increase in intracranial pressure is related to swelling of brain cells from water excess. |
| | | ○ Assess status of hemodynamic function: Pitting and/or dependent edema reflect expansion of interstitial fluid volume; skin pale, moist, and cool to touch in edematous areas; heart rate: tachycardia; peripheral pulses: bounding quality; elevated systolic blood pressure. | ○ Alterations in hemodynamic function primarily reflect extracellular fluid volume excess.<br>○ Elderly patients may develop dependent edema with relatively little fluid excess (e.g., mild congestive heart failure). |
| | | ○ CVP increases >6–8 mmHg. | ○ Increased CVP reflects the increased venous return caused by hypervolemia. |
| | | ○ PCWP increases >15 mmHg.<br>– Neck vein distention in upright position (45 degrees). | ○ PCWP reflects left ventricular function and its effectiveness in handling increased fluid volume. |
| | | ○ Heart sounds: An $S_3$ and $S_4$ frequently occur in the setting of fluid overload with congestive heart failure.<br>○ Assess pulmonary function: Tachypnea, dyspnea, increased respiratory rate, moist rales, productive cough.<br>○ Assess gastrointestinal function: Anorexia, nausea, vomiting, constipation. | ○ Congestive heart failure with pulmonary edema may be precipitated when the increased fluid volume is in excess of the amount of fluid the heart can effectively pump. |
| | | ○ Assess renal function: Oliguria, periorbital edema, blood urea nitrogen, serum creatinine, urine output, urine specific gravity. | ○ ECF volume excess is commonly associated with primary renal disease, or with conditions that reduce renal perfusion (e.g., congestive heart failure, liver disease). |
| | | ○ Assess body weight (daily); weight gain >5% of baseline weight is significant. | ○ Body weight measurement is an excellent indicator of total body water. Rule: 1 kg (2.2 lb) equals 1 liter fluid; weight should be measured daily under same conditions. |
| | | ○ Monitor laboratory data:<br>○ Serum sodium <135 mEq/liter.<br>– Serum proteins, albumin decreased. | ○ Reduced serum sodium is the best indicator of ICF volume excess. |

*(continued)*

**TABLE 23-5. CARE PLAN FOR THE PATIENT WITH FLUID AND ELECTROLYTE IMBALANCES: FLUID VOLUME DEFICIT *(Continued)***

| Nursing Diagnoses | Desired Patient Outcomes | Nursing Interventions | Rationales |
|---|---|---|---|
| ***Nursing Diagnosis #1 (cont.)*** | | | |
| | | ◦ Hematocrit: Low in ECF volume excess; normal in ICF volume excess. | ◦ Number and size of red blood cells remain unchanged in increased plasma volume. |
| | | • Collaborate with physician to correct underlying cause of the fluid imbalance.<br>◦ Causes of ECF volume excess: | ◦ Correction of underlying cause contributing to fluid gain is essential if the hypervolemia is to be successfully treated and normovolemia restored. |
| | | ◦ Cardiac insufficiency, congestive heart failure.<br>– Cirrhosis, hepatic insufficiency; hypoproteinemia; overly aggressive intravenous fluid therapy. | ◦ Decreased renal perfusion with decreased glomerular filtration rate predisposes to oliguria. |
| | | ◦ Causes of ICF volume excess:<br>◦ Parenchymal renal disease most common cause; iatrogenic (e.g. excessive administration of hypotonic fluid); syndrome of inappropriate antidiuretic hormone secretion. | ◦ Diseased kidneys unable to excrete water load. |
| | | • Implement treatment for *ECF* volume excess.<br>◦ Implement prescribed treatment of sodium (saline) and fluid restriction. | • Goal of therapy is to reduce fluid volume without rapid fluid shifts or alteration in electrolyte balance. |
| | | ◦ Intravenous therapy is usually prescribed in amounts to cover sensible (urine) and insensible (skin and lungs) fluid losses only (initially). | ◦ Goal of fluid restriction is the loss of approximately 0.5 kg of body weight/day. |
| | | ◦ Hypertonic intravenous solutions may be used:<br>– Osmotic diuretic agents include mannitol, 10% and 50% dextrose in water, and urea preparations. | ◦ Hypertonic solutions increase osmotic gradient favoring the movement of fluid from interstitial to intravascular space; excess fluid is excreted by the kidneys. |
| | | ◦ Oral fluid intake and/or intravenous therapy must be monitored very carefully to ensure an overall decrease in extracellular fluid volume. | ◦ Diligent monitoring of fluid intake and output must continue until the body has compensated for the fluid imbalance, and body weight again approaches the ideal value for the patient. |
| | | ◦ Implement prescribed diuretic therapy. | ◦ Diuretics are prescribed to increase excretion of extra fluid. |

| | |
|---|---|
| ◦ Monitor the following:<br>◦ Serum potassium; metabolic alkalosis. | ◦ Most diuretics cause an increased excretion of potassium; a concomitant metabolic alkalosis can predispose to hypokalemia and hypochloremia. |
| ◦ Elevation of blood urea nitrogen (BUN); ECF volume depletion. | ◦ Overly aggressive diuretic therapy may predispose to fluid volume deficit. |
| ◦ ECG. | ◦ Changes in electrolyte concentrations can predispose to altered ECG. |
| • Implement major nursing interventions.<br>◦ Measure and carefully document:<br>◦ Fluid intake: Oral, intravenous; piggyback administration of medications; ice chips.<br>– Fluid output: Urine, gastrointestinal losses by vomiting, gastric suctioning, diarrhea; wound or fistula drainage; insensible losses by skin and lungs; iatrogenic losses (blood sampling).<br>– Daily body weight. | ◦ Accurate intake and output is essential to determine fluid therapy and the effectiveness of therapy.<br>◦ Avoid overly rapid infusions of intravenous fluids. |
| ◦ Assess for signs of fluid overload:<br>– Neurologic: confusion.<br>– Cardiovascular: Tachycardia, bounding pulse; elevated blood pressure and hemodynamic parameters; neck vein distention in upright position (45 degrees).<br>◦ Edema (pitting/dependent).<br>– Respiratory: Dyspnea, tachypnea; productive cough; rhonchi and rales. | ◦ Dependent edema may result in unobservable fluid retention (e.g., as much as 4–8 liters of fluid can be retained in a supine position without detectable edema).<br>◦ See Table 23–3, Nursing Diagnosis #1. |
| ◦ Assess for signs of fluid volume deficit associated with over-zealous fluid restriction and diuretic therapy. | |
| • Implement treatment regimen for *ICF* volume excess.<br>◦ Restrict water intake as prescribed:<br>– Administration of oral and/or intravenous fluid therapy should be planned for each 12–24-hr period.<br>– Rate of administration of intravenous fluids should be carefully regulated to avoid too rapid, or too slow administration. | ◦ Initially, fluid replacement is restricted to the amount of urine output and insensible losses; as patient outcomes are achieved and fluid state approaches normalcy, adjustments can be made in fluid intake. |
| ◦ Assess neurologic status frequently for changes in sensorium and level of consciousness. | ◦ Neurologic findings reflect intracellular fluid excess. |
| ◦ Monitor serum sodium carefully. | ◦ A serum sodium <130 mEq/liter is diagnostic of ICF volume excess. |

(continued)

## TABLE 23–5. CARE PLAN FOR THE PATIENT WITH FLUID AND ELECTROLYTE IMBALANCES: FLUID VOLUME DEFICIT *(Continued)*

| Nursing Diagnoses | Desired Patient Outcomes | Nursing Interventions | Rationales |
|---|---|---|---|
| ***Nursing Diagnosis #1 (cont.)*** | | | |
| | | ◦ Implement nursing actions. | |
| | | ◦ Offer explanations to patient and family regarding the significance of fluid restriction.<br>– Fluid restrictions that may be as low as 500 ml/24 hr require cooperation of patient and family. Constant reassurance is important; offer praise for each accomplishment. | ◦ An understanding of the reasons for strict fluid restriction may assist patient and family to comply with treatment regimen. |
| | | ◦ Prescribe appropriate level of activity as tolerated by patient. | ◦ Progressive increase in activity as tolerated promotes general well-being and reduces risk of complications associated with fragile, edematous tissues, and immobility (e.g., impaired skin integrity). |

Arterial BP = systolic/diastolic; CVP = central venous pressure; PAP = pulmonary artery pressure; PCWP = pulmonary capillary wedge pressure; CO = cardiac output.

dition and response to therapy, and evaluation of laboratory data are essential. Treatment of the underlying cause is imperative. (See the Care Plan in Table 23–5 for nursing diagnosis, desired patient outcomes, and nursing interventions in the care of the patient with fluid volume excess.)

Often there is a combination of fluid imbalances as, for example, a concomitant ECF deficit and an ICF excess. The ECF deficit may reflect fluid loss by profuse diaphoresis, gastrointestinal losses, or overzealous diuretic use. When the extracellular losses become severe, oliguria develops due to a reduced renal blood flow caused by the hypovolemic state. Associated with the hypovolemia is an increase in serum osmolality, which stimulates ADH secretion causing an increase in free water reabsorption by the kidneys. When the increase in free water intake becomes greater than obligatory fluid losses, an ICF excess develops.

The combination of extracellular and intracellular fluid excess is another example of a combined problem. In the patient with ECF saline excess, an excessive concentration of sodium in the ECF compartment will attract an increased amount of free water of which one third will distribute to the ECF compartment, and two thirds will distribute to the ICF compartment. Such combined disorders need to be recognized and treated separately. It is essential to identify and treat the underlying cause.

# ELECTROLYTES

Electrolytes comprise a major portion of solute within each fluid compartment. Potassium and phosphates are the major intracellular electrolytes, while sodium, chloride, and bicarbonate constitute the major extracellular electrolytes. Although concentrations of electrolytes differ, their combined electrical activity establishes an essentially electrically neutral milieu.

Electrolytes are largely involved in the maintenance of the osmolality of body fluids. They function to establish and maintain transmembrane potentials and, thus, are instrumental in the transmission of electrochemical impulses at synapses and neuromuscular junctions. Electrolytes contribute to acid–base balance, and they participate in cellular metabolism.

Concentration of electrolytes is measured in milliequivalents per liter (mEq/liter), which reflects the chemical activity of the electrolyte (i.e., its ability to combine to form compounds) in solution. Concentrations of electrolytes in the body are well defined in both the ECF and ICF compartments. The concentration of an electrolyte is a function of its intake and excretion. A change in intake without a proportional change in output will alter the electrolyte concentration in the body disrupting electrochemical events and predisposing to illness. In particular, serum concentration of electrolytes is maintained within narrow limits (see Table 22–2).

Electrolytes to be discussed in this section include sodium, potassium, chloride, and magnesium. (See Chap. 24 for an indepth discussion of calcium.)

## Sodium

### *Distribution in the Body*

The concentration of serum sodium is regulated within a narrow range: 135–148 mEq/liter. Sodium is the primary cation in extracellular fluid contributing about 90% of the total cation content. This accounts in part for the dominant role played by sodium in the regulation of total body water. The average adult usually consumes more than the minimum daily requirement for sodium, which is about 2 g. Sodium is actively absorbed by the intestines and excreted by the kidneys and skin.

### *Physiologic Activity*

Because sodium is the most abundant cation in extracellular fluid, it exerts the predominant effect on controlling ECF volume. Its ability to attract water enables sodium to influence intracellular (water) volume as well.

In conjunction with potassium, sodium largely influences the excitability of nerves and muscles. It is a critically essential factor in the generation and synaptic transmission of action potentials. Sodium also functions in the conduction of electrical impulses to muscle fibers via the neuromuscular junction.

Sodium is a key factor in acid–base balance. Renal reabsorption of sodium can occur in three ways: it may be accompanied by the reabsorption of either chloride ($Cl^-$) or bicarbonate ($HCO_3^-$), both negatively charged ions (anions); or in exchange for potassium ($K^+$) or hydrogen ($H^+$) ions. A hyponatremia accompanied by a hypochloremia is often associated with a metabolic alkalosis. The stimulus for sodium reabsorption in this setting is potent. However, due to the chloride depletion, an increased amount of sodium is reabsorbed, with bicarbonate contributing to a metabolic alkalosis. Furthermore, because a greater percentage of sodium is reabsorbed in exchange for potassium or hydrogen ions, hypokalemia occurs as the supply of potassium ions is depleted; and the alkalosis is worsened by the secretion of hydrogen ions.

### *Sodium Regulation*

Regulation of sodium concentration is primarily determined by the volume needs of the ECF compartment. Water intake is adjusted by variations in the thirst mechanism; water excretion depends on release of antidiuretic hormone (ADH) by the hypothalamic-neurohypophyseal system, and an intact intrarenal mechanism capable of responding to ADH.

Aldosterone is a potent stimulator of sodium reabsorption. However, despite the increase in sodium reabsorption triggered by the action of aldosterone on cells of the distal tubules, little change (<3%) occurs in the overall sodium concentration because of the obligatory reabsorption of water along with the sodium.

### *Pathophysiology*

A decrease in ECF volume for whatever reason triggers two regulatory mechanisms that function to restore ECF volume (Fig. 23-1). The first mechanism occurs in response to the slight increase in serum osmolality that accompanies the loss of extracellular fluid, and involves the thirst-ADH mechanism described above. The increase in water ingestion coupled with the increase in free water reabsorption from the distal tubule and collecting ducts in response to ADH secretion operate to prevent further water loss and to restore the ECF volume to its physiologic norm.

The second mechanism involves the renin-angiotensin-aldosterone system. A reduction in ECF volume (intravascular volume) reduces renal blood flow and glomerular filtration rate, which stimulates renin secretion. The result of this series of reactions is an enhanced secretion of aldosterone. This hormone stimulates sodium reabsorption in the distal tubules and it operates to restore the ECF volume because of the water that is passively reabsorbed with the sodium.

Another factor that operates in restoring sodium and water balance is an increase in arterial pressure, which, by increasing the glomerular filtration rate (GFR), increases sodium loss by the kidney. (The increase in GFR increases the amount of filtrate presented to the renal tubules for processing and, therefore, the likelihood of an increase in the amount of sodium excreted in the urine.) In contrast, an increase in venous pressure reduces sodium loss. These factors are especially important in congestive heart failure in which arterial pressure is reduced while venous pressure is increased.[3]

**Hypernatremia (Dehydration).** Serum sodium levels greater than 148 mEq/liter constitute hypernatremia and are usually due to the effect of water loss (predominantly) or sodium excess. Most commonly hypernatremia is observed in conditions in which both water and sodium losses occur, but the water loss is quantitatively greater than the sodium loss. Dehydration hypernatremia is commonly the result of water loss due either to an inadequate intake and/or excessive loss by kidneys and skin.

Reduction of water in the extracellular fluid pro-

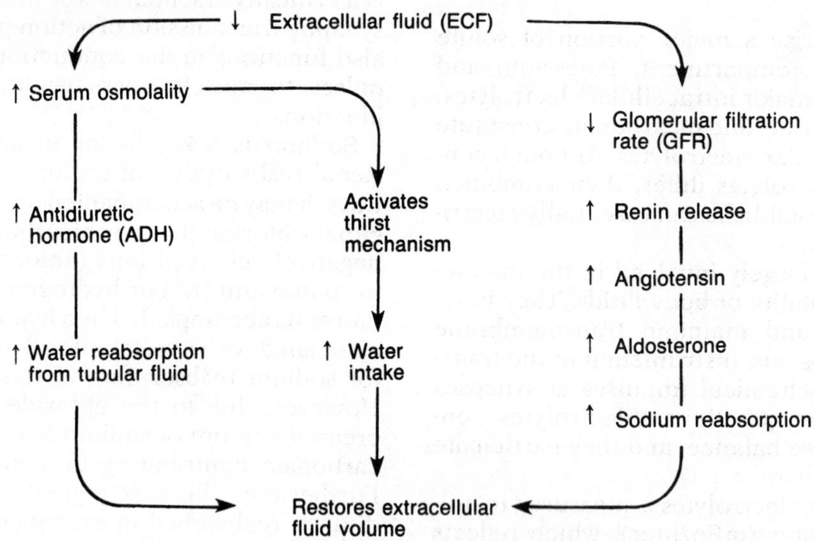


**Figure 23-1.** Sodium and water balance mechanism. A reduction in extracellular fluid (ECF) volume for any reason activates two mechanisms that function to restore ECF volume: the thirst mechanism and enhanced secretion of antidiuretic hormone (ADH); and the initiation of the renin-angiotensin-aldosterone system (see Fig. 21-9).

An increase in serum osmolality associated with water loss activates the thirst mechanism, which promotes water ingestion. Slight increases in serum osmolality also stimulate the production/secretion of ADH. ADH acts on the cells of the distal tubules and collecting ducts to permit an increase in free water reabsorption (see Fig. 21-10).

A reduction in ECF volume also reduces GFR, which triggers an increase in renin production/secretion. Renin acts to increase serum levels of angiotensin, which, in turn, acts to stimulate aldosterone secretion by the adrenal cortex. Aldosterone stimulates sodium reabsorption in the distal tubules, which is accompanied by an obligatory reabsorption of water. (Adapted from Sibbald, WJ: Synopsis of Critical Care. ed 3. Williams & Wilkins, Baltimore, 1988, p. 135, with permission.)

duces a rise in serum osmolality.[3] This, in turn, draws water from the intracellular space. Loss of fluid from the ICF compartment stimulates (by osmoreceptors) the antidiuretic (ADH) mechanism with a consequent conservation of body water by a reduction in urine volume. The thirst mechanism is also stimulated, promoting water ingestion.

Hypernatremia from a sodium excess is much less common and reflects the ingestion or retention of sodium in excess of water. As the sodium concentration in extracellular fluid rises, water is drawn out of cells. The result is a combination of ECF volume excess and ICF volume deficit. Table 23-6 details characteristics of hypernatremia, including etiology, clinical presentation, diagnosis, and treatment. Nursing diagnoses, patient outcomes, and nursing interventions in the care of the patient with hypernatremia are presented in the Care Plan in Table 23-7. The overall therapeutic approach depends on the underlying pathophysiologic mechanisms.

**Hyponatremia.** Serum sodium levels less than 134 mEq/liter constitute hyponatremia, which may result from two main mechanisms: sodium loss or water excess. Hyponatremia associated with sodium loss is called *depletional* hyponatremia; that due to water excess is termed *dilutional* hyponatremia or *water intoxication*. The clinical presentation of depletional hyponatremia is characterized by *contraction* of the ECF compartment; dilutional hyponatremia is characterized by an *expansion* of the ECF compartment. Distinguishing between these two disorders is essential to determine appropriate therapy. A reduction in serum sodium levels occurs, for example, when elevated serum glucose levels increase serum osmolality, thus enhancing a shift of water from the ICF to the ECF compartment. The combination of elevated glucose and low sodium concentrations is often seen in the ICU setting and needs to be recognized by the critical care nurse.

The mechanism of depletional hyponatremia[4] involves the occurrence of a sodium deficit, whether due to an excessive loss or reduced sodium intake, which leads to a decrease in the osmolality of extracellular fluids. A reduced serum osmolality suppresses ADH secretion, thus contributing to an increased water excretion (polyuria). At the same time, a reduced osmolality of interstitial fluid causes water to shift from the ECF to ICF compartment.

These mechanism succeed (at least initially) in maintaining serum sodium levels but at the expense of ECF volume contraction. With further reduction in ECF volume, two additional events are triggered, both of which lead to oliguria. There is a reduction in glomerular filtration rate and eventually, stimulation of ADH secretion.

Depletional hyponatremia warrants particular concern because the body's initial response to the loss of sodium is to maintain serum sodium levels at the expense of ECF contraction. Serum electrolytes at this stage may not reveal much early decrease in the sodium level, and the patient's complaints are usually nonspecific—headache, nausea, vomiting, lethargy, cramps. As the condition progresses, signs of altered cerebral function are reflected by delirium, asterixis, seizures, and coma. Serum sodium levels that approach 100 mEq/liter are associated with a greater than 50% mortality.

Characteristics of depletional and dilutional hyponatremia, including etiology, clinical manifestations, and treatment, are presented in Table 23-6. Depletional hyponatremia is characterized by a sodium deficit, a contracted ECF volume, and dehydration. Dilutional hyponatremia is characterized by water excess with expansion of both ECF and ICF volumes. Both disorders may present with signs of altered cerebral function. Syndrome of inappropriate secretion of ADH is characterized by an increase in volume but without edema formation. There is an absence of postural hypotension, and the jugular venous pressure is usually normal. (SIADH is examined in detail in Chap. 16) Nursing diagnoses, patient outcomes, and nursing interventions concerned with the care of the patient with a sodium imbalance are presented in the Care Plan in Table 23-7.

## Potassium

### *Distribution in the Body*

The concentration of serum potassium is regulated within a very narrow range: 3.5-5.5 mEq/liter. While this small extracellular concentration of potassium does not accurately reflect total body potassium, even the slightest fluctuations beyond this narrow range can have deleterious effects on body function. Potassium is predominantly an *intra*cellular cation.

The daily dietary requirement for potassium is about 40/mEq. Potassium is absorbed from the gastrointestinal tract and is freely filterable at the glomerulus. About 80% of ingested potassium is excreted in the urine, and approximately 20% is excreted in feces and by the skin each day. Potassium balance is regulated by the kidney, which excretes excess amounts of potassium when concentrations are high, but is unable to conserve potassium when levels are low. Tubular cells of the distal tubule and collecting ducts have the capacity to both secrete and reabsorb potassium, and the rate at which these processes occur is variable. It is now clear that the majority of urinary potassium is derived from potassium secretion in the distal tubules. The final contribution can be either a net reabsorption or a net secretion of potassium.

TABLE 23-6
## Contrast: Hypernatremia and Hyponatremia

| | Hypernatremia | Hyponatremia |
|---|---|---|
| Definition | Serum sodium levels > 148 mEq/liter | Serum sodium levels < 134 mEq/liter |
| Pathophysiologic mechanisms[6] | Water loss in excess of sodium loss: dehydration (most common) may occur as a combined ECF and ICF volume deficit.<br>Sodium excess without proportional increase in water intake | Sodium loss (depletional): Characterized by contraction of the ECF volume<br>Water excess (dilutional, water intoxication): Characterized by an ECF volume excess and an ICF volume excess |
| Etiology | Inadequate fluid intake—Elderly or postoperative patient whose water intake is not perceived to be insufficient<br>Water loss in excess of sodium: Diabetes mellitus—water loss by high serum glucose osmotic diuresis<br>Chronic renal failure—Inability of kidneys to respond to volume contraction by reducing urine volume<br>Diaphoresis—Fluid lost in sweat is relatively hypotonic to serum.<br>Gastrointestinal losses—Diarrhea<br>Diabetes insipidus<br>Sodium excess:<br>Salt craving—High sodium intake without water supplement<br>Hyperaldosteronism<br>Cushing's syndrome, Excessive steroid administration } Excessive sodium reabsorption in excess of water | *Depletional:* (Sodium deficit)<br>Diuretics<br>Salt-poor diet<br>Excessive gastrointestinal losses: Severe vomiting, nasogastric suctioning, diarrhea<br>Renal disease with impaired ability to conserve salt when necessary<br>Adrenal insufficiency with altered aldosterone secretion<br>Use of water only to replace sodium and water losses associated with sweating, blood loss, or by transudation of fluid into transcellular spaces (e.g., pleural or peritoneal cavities)<br>*Dilutional:* Water excess commonly seen in cardiac failure, hepatic insufficiency, and nephrotic syndrome (inability to excrete free water)<br>Excessive water ingestion or administration of hypotonic electrolyte-free intravenous solutions; excessive tap water enemas and gastric irrigations in which water is used rather than a saline solution<br>Syndrome of inappropriate secretion of ADH (see Tables 16-2 and 16-4) |
| Clinical presentation | Specific symptomatology depends on underlying mechanisms:<br>Water loss in excess of sodium: A state of dehydration (refer to symptomatology of fluid deficit presented in Table 23-2)<br>Alterations in neurologic function associated with increased neuronal excitability due to increased sodium concentrations: Changes in mental status, restlessness, irritability, agitation, lethargy, confusion, coma, tremors, seizures<br>Sodium excess: Sodium gain in excess of water (when both are increased) constitutes an extracellular fluid excess (refer to symptomatology of extracellular fluid excess presented in Table 23-4). | Specific symptomatology depends on underlying mechanism:<br>*Depletional* (sodium deficit):<br>Contracted ECF volume with dehydration; (refer to symptomatology of fluid deficit presented in Table 23-2)<br>Altered cerebral function: mental status changes; headache; lethargy, confusion, seizures, coma<br>Cardiovascular: Hypotension, postural hypotension; reduced jugular venous pressure<br>*Dilutional* (water excess):<br>Cardiac, hepatic and/or renal disease (non-SIADH):<br>Expansion of ECF and ICF volumes (refer to symptomatology of fluid excess presented in Table 23-4)<br>Cardiovascular: No postural hypotension; possible increased jugular venous pressure<br>SIADH: There is an increase in fluid volume but an absence of edema formation; there is no postural hypotension and jugular venous pressure is usually normal.<br>Neurologic/cerebral functions are altered by dilutional hyponatremia. |
| Laboratory data | Hemoconcentration:<br>Hematocrit: Increased<br>Hemoglobin: Increased<br>Serum osmolality > 295 mOsm/kg<br>Serum sodium > 148 mEq/liter | *Depletional vs. Dilutional*<br>Serum sodium < 134 mEq/liter. Serum sodium levels should be scrutinized carefully in determining type and severity of hyponatremia. |

TABLE 23-6
**Contrast: Hypernatremia and Hyponatremia *(Continued)***

| | Hypernatremia | Hyponatremia |
|---|---|---|
| | Urine:<br>Urinary sodium <20 mEq/liter<br>Urine osmolality >500 mOsm/kg<br>Urine specific gravity >1.015 | In depletional hyponatremia, serum sodium falls very slowly until the condition becomes severe; in dilutional states the fall in serum sodium is more rapid.<br>Serum osmolality <285 mOsm/kg<br>Depletional—delayed fall<br>Dilutional—markedly reduced from onset<br>Urine sodium<br>Depletional <20 mEq/liter (excludes depletion due to primary sodium loss)<br>Dilutional >30 mEq/liter<br>SIADH<br>Serum sodium <134 mEq/liter<br>Serum osmolality <285 mOsm/kg<br>Urine sodium >20 mEq/liter<br>Urine osmolality >500 mOsm/kg<br>Note that urine sodium and urine osmolality are inappropriately high despite a reduced serum sodium and serum osmolality. |
| Treatment | Therapeutic approach depends on the underlying pathophysiologic mechanisms: | |
| | *Hypernatremia/dehydration* (water loss in excess of sodium loss):<br>Fluid replacement therapy usually with an isotonic or hypotonic intravenous solution. 5% dextrose solution is commonly given over first 48 hr depending on severity of dehydration (cerebral edema may occur if hypernatremia is corrected too rapidly).<br>Electrolyte replacement therapy should begin as fluid loss is corrected.<br>*Sodium excess:*<br>Sodium and fluid restriction<br>Administration of hypotonic intravenous fluids<br>Diuretics | *Depletional* (sodium loss):<br>Fluid and sodium replacement therapy using intravenous normal saline (avoid undue haste to correct the abnormality)<br>*Dilutional* (water excess) (excluding SIADH):<br>Diuretics (furosemide)<br>Treat underlying cause: Cardiac, hepatic or renal disease.<br>Spironolactone may be given to reverse secondary hyperaldosteronism.<br>*Dilutional SIADH*<br>Fluid restriction<br>Diuretics (furosemide); demeclocycline to block action of ADH<br>Urinary fluid losses replaced with normal saline |

### *Physiologic Activity*

As the major intracellular cation, potassium functions to maintain intracellular osmolality and electrical neutrality. It is a dynamically active ion constantly moving into and out of the cell, and its movements, like those of sodium, are regulated by the sodium–potassium pump. Potassium contributes to the resting membrane potential, and, along with sodium, it is essential for the generation and transmission of action potentials. It plays a significant role in neuromuscular excitation and transmission, especially in cardiac muscle, skeletal muscle (70% of total body potassium occurs in skeletal muscle), and the smooth musculature of the gastrointestinal tract. Alterations in serum potassium can have a significant impact on neuromuscular function. The heart is especially sensitive to serum potassium levels, and small changes can precipitate serious dysrhythmias.

In conjunction with its influence on neuromuscular activity, potassium is involved in the glucose–insulin mechanism, which functions to supply muscle with ample amounts of glucose necessary for energy metabolism. Insulin causes glucose uptake by cells and stimulates the sodium–potassium pump, which moves sodium out of the cells and potassium in. As potassium moves into the cell and sodium moves out, the electrical neutrality within the cell is maintained. Often, in patients with hyperkalemia, intravenous glucose/insulin therapy is provided to move potassium out of the extracellular space and into the cells, thus reducing the serum potassium levels.

Potassium also plays a key role in acid–base balance. Acidemia is often associated with hyperkalemia, and alkalemia with hypokalemia. One of the mechanisms accounting for this relationship is that $H^+$ ions and $K^+$ ions freely exchange across plasma cell membranes. In acidemia, excess $H^+$ ions are buffered by moving into cells in exchange for $K^+$

## TABLE 23–7. CARE PLAN FOR THE PATIENT WITH A SODIUM IMBALANCE

| Nursing Diagnoses | Desired Patient Outcomes | Nursing Interventions | Rationales |
|---|---|---|---|
| ***Nursing Diagnosis #1***<br>Electrolyte imbalance, related to:<br>1. Hypernatremia.<br>2. Water deficit.<br>(See Table 23–3, Nursing Diagnoses #1, #2, and #3.) | Patient's condition will stabilize:<br>1. Neurologic status: Alert, oriented to person, place, date; absence of: headache, muscle cramps, convulsions, coma.<br>2. Hemodynamic status will stabilize as follows:<br>• Heart rate >60 <100 beats/min.<br>• Arterial BP = within 10 mmHg of baseline.<br>• CVP $\overline{\text{mean}}$ 0–8 mmHg.<br>• PAP <25 mmHg (systolic).<br>• PCWP $\overline{\text{mean}}$ 8–12 mmHg.<br>• CO 4–8 liters/min.<br>3. Body weight will stabilize within 5% of patient's baseline.<br>4. Serum studies will stabilize as follows:<br>• Osmolality 285–295 mOsm/kg.<br>• Sodium >135 to <148 mEq/liter.<br>• Potassium 3.5–5.5 mEq/liter.<br>• Chloride >100 to <106 mEq/liter.<br>• Proteins, glucose, BUN, creatinine, hematocrit, and osmolality will stabilize at optimum levels. | • Assess impact of hypernatremia and hyperosmotic state on body processes. (See Table 23–3, Nursing Diagnosis #1.) | • Hyperosmolar state associated with severe dehydration reflects primarily an ICF volume deficit.<br>○ Hypernatremia is usually caused by a water deficiency rather than an actual increase in sodium concentration. |
| | | ○ Assess neurologic status:<br>– Level of consciousness, mental status.<br>– Behavioral changes: Irritability, restlessness, listlessness, lethargy.<br>– Deep tendon reflex. | ○ Alterations in neurologic function reflect an intracellular fluid volume deficit. |
| | | ○ Assess hemodynamic function:<br>○ Heart rate increased.<br>– Pulses, weak and thready. | ○ Hypovolemia causes tachycardia (heart rate ≥100/min), a compensatory measure to maintain cerebral and renal perfusion. |
| | | ○ Postural hypotension. | ○ A drop in systolic BP >10 mmHg from supine to upright position signals compromised hemodynamics. |
| | | ○ All hemodynamic parameters are reduced including: CVP <1 mmHg; PCWP <4 mmHg. | ○ These parameters reflect diminished venous return to heart and left ventricular function. |
| | | ○ Monitor body temperature. | ○ Fever and associated diaphoresis contribute to the dehydrated state. |
| | | ○ Assess renal function:<br>– Urine output: <400 ml/24 hr suggests acute renal failure.<br>– Urine specific gravity >1.030. | ○ A reduction in renal perfusion and glomerular filtration rate predisposes to oliguria. |
| | | ○ BUN, serum creatinine, and osmolality all elevated.<br>– Total intake and output. | ○ Hemoconcentration related to hypovolemic state. |
| | | ○ Assess gastrointestinal function:<br>– Anorexia, nausea, vomiting, abdominal distention, diarrhea, constipation. | |
| | | ○ Assess body weight. | ○ Body weight most closely reflects fluid changes; weight should be measured daily under the same conditions. |
| | | ○ Monitor laboratory studies:<br>○ Serum sodium >148 mEq/liter. | ○ Serum sodium most closely reflects intracellular fluid volume deficit. |
| | | – Serum protein.<br>– Hematocrit/hemoglobin. | – Serum parameters may expect to be elevated due to hemoconcentration associated with hypovolemic state. |

| | | |
|---|---|---|
| 5. Urine studies:<br>• Urine output > 30 ml/hr.<br>• Specific gravity 1.010–1.025.<br>• Sodium 50–130 mEq/liter.<br>• Osmolality 500–800 mOsm/kg. | ○ Monitor other parameters.<br>– Mucous membranes.<br>– Skin turgor.<br>– Third-spacing. | |
| | • Collaborate with physician to correct underlying cause of hypernatremia.<br>○ Fluid volume deficit.<br>○ Sodium excess. | ○ See Table 23–3, Nursing Diagnosis #1. |
| | ○ Implement treatment program as prescribed:<br>○ Treatment of hypernatremia and dehydration (water loss) involves water replacement therapy:<br>○ Hypotonic or isotonic solutions are administered intravenously. 5% dextrose in water is frequently the solution prescribed. | ○ Therapeutic approach depends on underlying pathophysiologic mechanisms (e.g., water loss in excess of sodium, or excess sodium intake without supplemental water intake).<br>○ Hypotonic or isotonic solutions serve to reverse hypertonicity of body fluids.<br>– A hypotonic sodium solution is considered safer because it allows a gradual reduction in the serum sodium levels and reduces risk of cerebral edema.[6] |
| | ○ Oral fluids are administered as tolerated using salt-free fluids. | ○ Avoid offering salty fluids such as bouillon, tomato or V-8 juices, cocoa beverages, among others. |
| | ○ Treatment of hypernatremia (sodium excess) involves salt restriction.<br>– Hypotonic intravenous solutions and salt-free oral fluids are administered as described above. | |
| | • Nursing care considerations:<br>○ Implement nursing treatments in caring for the patient with ICF volume deficit and sodium excess:<br>○ Establish baseline data (e.g., vital signs, laboratory data). | ○ Such data provide a framework for evaluating effectiveness of therapy. |
| | ○ Document fluid intake and output from all sources: Fluid intake including oral and intravenous fluids; intravenous piggyback medications; irrigation of gastric tube; saline used for endotracheal suctioning; humidifed oxygen therapy; enemas. | ○ These measurements provide a basis for prescribing therapy. |
| | ○ Fluid output including urine; gastrointestinal losses—vomiting, diarrhea, gastric suctioning; wound, fistula or ostomy drainage; iatrogenic losses (blood sampling); insensible losses by lungs and skin; third-spacing. | ○ A considerable amount of body fluid can be lost due to iatrogenic causes, including blood samples for electrolyte assessment and arterial blood gases. |

(continued)

## TABLE 23-7. CARE PLAN FOR THE PATIENT WITH A SODIUM IMBALANCE *(Continued)*

| Nursing Diagnoses | Desired Patient Outcomes | Nursing Interventions | Rationales |
|---|---|---|---|
| ***Nursing Diagnosis #1 (cont.)*** | | | |
| | | ○ Estimates of third-spacing are critical; Careful measurements of abdominal girth or diameter of thighs should be performed; appropriate markings and the use of the same tape measure contribute to consistency, accuracy, and usefulness of the data. | ○ Fluid accumulation in third-spaces is unavailable for body use and thus contributes to fluid deficit. |
| | | ○ Assess weight daily. | ○ For accuracy, the same scale and conditions should be used with each measurement. |
| | | ○ Monitor serum sodium (>148 mEq/liter indicates hypernatremia). | |
| | | ○ Monitor neurologic, cardiovascular, and respiratory parameters at regular intervals. | ○ Overly aggressive fluid replacement therapy can predispose to fluid overload.<br>– Cerebral edema, congestive heart failure, and pulmonary edema are associated with fluid overload. |
| | | ○ Patient, family interaction:<br>– Offer appropriate explanations regarding therapy and course of the illness.<br>– Elicit expectations of underlying illness and its impact on family lifestyle.<br>– Involve in decision-making process. | ○ Insight and understanding breeds cooperation and compliance. |
| | | ○ Supportive care:<br>– Oral hygiene.<br>– Skin integrity. | |
| ***Nursing Diagnosis #2***<br>Electrolyte imbalance, related to<br>1. Hyponatremia. (Depletional hyponatremia = sodium deficit. Dilutional hyponatremia = water excess. [See Table 23-5, Nursing Diagnosis #1].) | Patient's condition will stabilize:<br>1. Neurologic status: Alert, oriented to person, place, and time; deep tendon reflexes brisk; seizure-free.<br>2. Hemodynamic status will stabilize within patient's baseline values.<br>3. Body weight will stabilize within 5% of patient's baseline. | Hyponatremia occurs in two forms: Depletional and dilutional. *Depletional* hyponatremia is characterized by a sodium loss with contraction of ECF volume (dehydration); *dilutional* hyponatremia is characterized by a water excess (water intoxication). | |
| | | • Assess impact of hyponatremia on body processes: | • For assessment and management, see Table 23-3, Nursing Diagnosis #1 (depletional); and Table 23-5, Nursing Diagnosis #1 (dilutional). |
| | | ○ Neurologic status. | ○ Altered fluid states associated with sodium imbalances predispose to neurologic dysfunction. |
| | | ○ Hemodynamic status. | ○ Major concern is to provide appropriate fluid therapy to maintain cerebral, renal, and peripheral perfusion without precipitating fluid volume overload. |

| | | |
|---|---|---|
| 4. Serum and urine parameters will stabilize at optimum levels for patient. (See Nursing Diagnosis #1, above, for specific hemodynamic and laboratory parameters.) | ○ CVP, PCWP. | ○ Monitoring of these parameters guides fluid and electrolyte replacement therapy. |
| | ○ Respiratory function: Respiratory rate and pattern; evidence of adventitious breath sounds. | ○ Continuous assessment of cardiopulmonary status helps to prevent complications (e.g., fluid overload with congestive heart failure and pulmonary edema). |
| | ○ Renal status.<br>– Urine output and specific gravity. | ○ A reduction in renal perfusion and glomerular filtration rate (depletional) predisposes to oliguria and acute renal failure. |
| | ○ Body weight.<br>– Fluid accumulation in third-spaces. | ○ Most closely reflects hydration status. |
| | ○ Monitor laboratory data:<br>○ Serum sodium. | ○ Serum sodium levels should be scrutinized carefully to determine type and severity of hyponatremia. |
| | ○ Serum osmolality.<br>– Urine sodium, osmolality. | ○ Monitoring of laboratory data assists in evaluating response to fluid and electrolyte therapy. |
| | • Collaborate with physician to correct underlying cause of hyponatremia. (See Table 23–6 for possible etiology.) | • Therapeutic approach depends on underlying pathophysiologic mechanism. |
| | ○ Implement treatment program as prescribed and monitor response to therapy.<br>○ Treatment of *depletional* hyponatremia (sodium loss) involves fluid and sodium replacement therapy. Intravenous isotonic saline is commonly prescribed. An increase in dietary sodium may also be prescribed if tolerated. | ○ See Table 23–3, Nursing Diagnosis #1.<br>– Intravenous normal saline replaces sodium as well as water. Avoid undue haste to correct the abnormality to prevent fluid overload. |
| | ○ Treatment of *dilutional* hyponatremia (water excess) involves modalities to reduce water concentration; diuretic therapy (furosemide); and treatment of underlying cause. | ○ Dilutional hyponatremia has a higher incidence than the depletional form.<br>– See Table 23–5, Nursing Diagnosis #1.<br>– Underlying cardiac, hepatic, or renal disease may require aggressive therapeutics. |
| | • Nursing care implications: See Nursing Diagnosis #1, above):<br>○ Document and interpret baseline data: Intake and output, daily weight. | ○ Provide a basis on which to determine fluid therapy and to evaluate the effectiveness of therapy. |
| | ○ Implement measures to reduce water intake in treatment of dilutional hyponatremia:<br>○ Avoid excessive water intake: Tap water orally, or by enema; electrolyte-poor intravenous fluid; or irrigation of gastric tube with distilled water. | ○ Excessive water intake by these routes will further complicate the fluid excess associated with dilutional hyponatremia or water intoxication state. |

*(continued)*

## TABLE 23-7. CARE PLAN FOR THE PATIENT WITH A SODIUM IMBALANCE *(Continued)*

| Nursing Diagnoses | Desired Patient Outcomes | Nursing Interventions | Rationales |
|---|---|---|---|
| ***Nursing Diagnosis #2 (cont.)*** | | | |
| | | ○ Monitor neurologic status closely:<br>– General cerebral function, mental status, level of consciousness, cranial nerve function, deep tendon reflexes, sensorimotor function. | ○ Close monitoring of the neurologic status is essential to prevent complications associated with fluid dehydration/overhydration states depending on whether the underlying cause is depletional versus dilutional hyponatremia, respectively. |
| | | ○ Monitor cardiovascular function:<br>– Hemodynamic parameters: CVP, PCWP.<br>– Heart rate and rhythm; presence of neck vein distention, quality of peripheral pulses (bounding, or weak and thready on palpation). | ○ Data provided by hemodynamic parameters and meticulous serial assessments assist in determining the status of venous return to the heart and left ventricular function. |
| | | ○ Assess respiratory function: Rate, rhythm, effort, presence of adventitious breath sounds. | ○ In the setting of fluid overload, especially due to chronic cardiac, hepatic, or renal disease, it is critical to perform ongoing assessment of neurologic and cardiopulmonary function to prevent and/or recognize signs of impending cardiac failure. |
| | | • Initiate efforts to obtain a comprehensive patient/family history including the functional health patterns. | • Family history may assist in assessing potential problems, including coping capabilities and stress tolerance. |
| | | ○ How does patient/family perceive the impact of the illness on individual and family lifestyles? Coping capabilities? Stress tolerance?<br>○ Can the patient/family identify family support systems? | ○ Fluid and electrolyte imbalances are often the result of serious underlying cardiac, hepatic, or renal disease requiring intensive care and follow-up. Knowing how to cope, and how to assume responsibility for self-care may assist in minimizing impact of illness on individual and family lifestyles. |
| | | ○ Teach patient/family the importance of maintaining prescribed fluid intake/restriction. Enlist their assistance in keeping a meticulous intake and output. Encourage to participate in decision-making regarding care. | ○ In patients on strict fluid intake (e.g., 500 ml/24 hr), it is essential to assist patient/family to adjust to this critical limitation. Decisions regarding when to drink may be left for the patient/family to decide. Such participation may ensure better compliance with the therapeutic regimen. (See Table 16-4, Nursing Diagnosis #4.) |

ions, which move into the plasma. In this way acidemia can cause hyperkalemia.

Hyperkalemia may develop in acute acidemia as a result of the ion-exchange mechanism in the distal tubule. Normally sodium reabsorption in the distal tubule and early collecting ducts occurs in exchange for $H^+$ ions or $K^+$ ions, which are secreted into a tubular lumen and excreted in the urine. In acidemia $H^+$ ions are plentiful; the kidney tends to secrete these ions while retaining $K^+$ ions. The net result is hyperkalemia.

As might be expected, in alkalemia these activities are reversed. $H^+$ ions move out of cells while $K^+$ ions move in; and sodium reabsorption in the distal tubule is coupled with the secretion of potassium, which is excreted in the urine. The net result is hypokalemia.

Contrary to the above situations in which the primary problem is an acid–base imbalance predisposing secondarily to a potassium imbalance, the reverse is also true (i.e., the primary problem may be a potassium imbalance, which secondarily causes an acid–base imbalance). Thus, in hyperkalemia more $K^+$ ions move into the cells displacing $H^+$ ions into the serum; and the reabsorption of sodium in the distal tubule is coupled with the secretion of potassium while $H^+$ ions are retained. The net result is acidemia.

Likewise, in hypokalemia, $K^+$ ions shift from the cells into the serum causing $H^+$ ions to be shifted into cells; and in the distal tubule, with fewer $K^+$ ions available for exchange with sodium, there is an increase in $H^+$ ion excretion. The net result is alkalemia.

### *Potassium Regulation*

Several mechanisms are involved in serum potassium regulation. An increase in serum potassium concentration itself enhances active uptake of potassium by tubular epithelial cells. This increased amount of potassium within the distal tubular cells is available for secretion in exchange for sodium reabsorption. Aldosterone acts to facilitate the reabsorption of sodium in exchange for potassium secretion. Aldosterone-secreting cells of the zona glomerulosa in the adrenal cortex monitor serum potassium levels and influence the reabsorption or secretion of potassium by cells in the distal tubule and early collecting ducts. This mechanism functions to maintain serum potassium levels within a very narrow therapeutic range.

In general, renal potassium excretion is increased by an increase in dietary intake, aldosterone, alkalemia, and diuretics; it is decreased by sodium deficiency (hyponatremia), acidemia, and spironolactone. The point to be remembered is that it is the plasma concentration of potassium that influences cardiac conduction and the occurrence of dysrhythmias. These are the most serious effects of all alterations in potassium metabolism.

### *Pathophysiology*

**Hyperkalemia.** A serum potassium level greater than 5.5 mEq/liter constitutes hyperkalemia. The major cause of hyperkalemia is renal disease including the oliguric phase of acute renal failure or the later stage of chronic renal failure. The key here is oliguria, because in the patient with an adequate urine output it is almost impossible to develop hyperkalemia. Because potassium is principally an intracellular ion, any disruption of cellular integrity will cause a loss of potassium into the ECF compartment (e.g., crushing injuries, extensive tissue injury, or burns).

Administration of potassium-sparing diuretics (e.g., spironolactone or triamterene) may predispose to hyperkalemia. A deficiency of aldosterone contributes to hyperkalemia as potassium secretion coupled with sodium reabsorption is reduced. It is important to be aware that overly aggressive potassium replacement therapy for hypokalemia (especially by the intravenous route) can produce serious hyperkalemia. Specific features of hyperkalemia are presented in Table 23–8.

The signs and symptoms of hyperkalemia are nonspecific, and diagnosis in high-risk patients depends on a high index of suspicion and frequent measurements of serum potassium levels. Hyperkalemia may be the most dangerous of the electrolyte disorders. Once the serum potassium level reaches 7.0 mEq/liter, serious cardiac dysrhythmias and/or cardiac arrest are imminent.

Hyperkalemia directly impacts on the excitability of cardiac cells. Elevated levels of serum potassium cause hypopolarization (a decrease in negativity within the cell) of the cardiac cell resting membrane potential (RMP). As the RMP moves closer to threshold, slow response (calcium channel) action potentials are triggered, producing a depressed or diminished response. This results in serious conduction delays and blocks within the heart, and can predispose to ventricular standstill or ventricular fibrillation (Fig. 23–2.)

The treatment of hyperkalemia will vary with the severity of the problem. Serum potassium levels less than 6.5 mEq/liter may be adequately managed with sodium polystyrene sulfonate (Kayexalate). If serum potassium levels exceed 6.5 mEq/liter and/or there is severely impaired renal function, emergency measures may need to be employed. Calcium gluconate infusion is usually prescribed to relieve the cardiotoxic effects of hyperkalemia. Continuous cardiac monitoring is essential.

In addition, because calcium does not lower the serum potassium level, other therapies need to be introduced. These include: 500 ml 10% glucose with 10 units regular insulin infused over 30 minutes. Hypertonic glucose and insulin therapy help to drive potassium into cells, thus reducing serum levels. Sodium bicarbonate therapy is given to treat the acidemia. As the pH rises, potassium moves into

TABLE 23-8
## Contrast: Hyperkalemia and Hypokalemia

| | Hyperkalemia | Hypokalemia |
|---|---|---|
| Definition | Serum potassium levels > 5.5 mEq/liter | Serum potassium levels < 3.5 mEq/liter |
| Etiology | Acute renal failure, oliguric phase; chronic renal failure, later stage<br>Disruption of cellular integrity: Crushing injury, trauma, burns<br>Potassium-sparing diuretics: spironolactone, triamterene<br>Acidosis<br>Aldosterone deficiency (Addison's disease)<br>Overly aggressive potassium replacement therapy (iatrogenic)<br>Factitious hyperkalemia: Hemolysis of RBCs in blood sample; thrombocytosis; hemoconcentration; use of tight tourniquet when drawing blood<br>Medications high in potassium (e.g., penicillin) | Inadequate dietary intake: Contributory<br>Gastrointestinal disorders: Persistent vomiting contributes to hypokalemia by loss of potassium-containing secretions or marked urinary loss of potassium due to metabolic alkalosis.<br>• Persistent diarrhea contributes to hypokalemia by direct loss of potassium or reduced gastrointestinal absorption of potassium due to increased peristalsis.<br>Renal losses:<br>• Diuretics<br>• Hyperaldosteronism: Hormonal imbalance causes reabsorption of sodium and enhanced secretion of potassium.<br>• Renal tubular disorder: Tubular dysfunction causes loss of fluid and electrolytes.<br>Resistance to ADH<br>Drugs: Gentamicin and carbenicillin cause increased urinary excretion of potassium. |
| Clinical presentation | Signs and symptoms highly nonspecific<br>Neuromuscular irritability; weakness; cramps, progressing to an ascending flaccid paralysis; paresthesias of face, tongue, extremities; symptoms of hyperkalemia often similar to those of hypokalemia<br>*Gastrointestinal*, *Neurologic*, *Respiratory* } See hypokalemia<br>*Cardiovascular:* Hypotension, dysrhythmias<br>*ECG changes:* Tented, symmetric T waves (shortened repolarization); widened QRS, reduced R wave amplitude, depressed ST segment; prolonged PR interval; flattening to absent P waves (see Fig. 23-2)<br>• Heart block<br>• Cardiac arrest | Signs and symptoms highly nonspecific<br>Reduction in overall muscle tone<br>*Skeletal muscles:* Fatigue, weakness, hyporeflexia, flaccid paralysis<br>*Gastrointestinal:* Anorexia, nausea, vomiting, constipation, abdominal distention, paralytic ileus<br>*Neurologic:* Apathy, depression, irritability, drowsiness, lethargy, paresthesias<br>*Respiratory:* Respiratory muscle weakness, compromised respiratory excursion, respiratory muscle paralysis, respiratory arrest with anoxia leading to cardiac arrest<br>*Cardiovascular:* Hypotension, dysrhythmias; digitalis toxicity—interplay between digoxin, diuretics and hypokalemia, a potentially dangerous combination<br>*ECG changes:* Peaked P wave, prolonged PR interval; flattened T wave; depressed ST segment, and elevated U wave (see Fig. 23-2)<br>Evidence of digitalis toxicity: Paroxysmal atrial tachycardia with Wenckebach (digitalis creates entrance block at AV node slowng ventricular response in atrial fibrillation); AV nodal block may result in junctional escape rhythms; exit block to His-Purkinje system; ventricular tachycardia |
| Treatment | Therapeutic goals: 1. Correct underlying cause<br>2. Avoid overly aggressive or too rapid correction of the potassium imbalance | |
| | Treatment will vary with the severity of the imbalance.<br>Serum $K^+$ level 5.5-6.5 mEq/liter with adequate renal function: Sodium polystyrene sulfonate (Kayexalate) 15-30 g orally or by enema, two to three times/daily<br>Serum $K^+$ level > 6.5 mEq/liter and/or severely impaired renal function:<br>• Emergency measures: 10% calcium gluconate is usually administered with continuous cardiac monitoring<br>• 500 ml 10% glucose with 10 units regular insulin, IV over 30 min<br>• Sodium bicarbonate 2-3 amps, in 500 ml glucose, IV over 1-2 hr or as prescribed | Potassium replacement therapy dictated by severity of deficit and presence of dysrhythmias:<br>Serum levels 2.5-3.5 mEq/liter: Oral potassium therapy; increased dietary potassium; oral potassium supplements. Relief of gastrointestinal disturbances (nausea/vomiting) may be necessary<br>Serum levels < 2.5 mEq/liter coupled with cardiac dysrhythmias may require more aggressive potassium replacement therapy: Intravenous KCl at concentrations not exceeding 40 mEq/liters, at a rate not exceeding 40 mEq/hr. If fluids need to be restricted: Intravenous KCl 10-20 mEq via buretrol over 1 hr or as prescribed |

TABLE 23–8
**Contrast: Hypernatremia and Hypokalemia *(Continued)***

| Hyperkalemia | Hypokalemia |
|---|---|
| • Kayexalate (as above)<br>• Diuretics (furosemide)<br>• Hemodialysis, especially in cases of impaired renal function | Additional considerations:<br>• Correct alkalosis and/or prevent its occurrence<br>• Monitor serum potassium closely<br>• Monitor renal function: urine output >30 ml/hr<br>• Monitor ECG continuously<br>• Patients allowed nothing by mouth (NPO) (e.g., post-surgery) should receive minimal potassium maintenance dosage in intravenous fluids<br>• A burning sensation at IV site may indicate that the KCl concentration is overly toxic and the rate should be slowed and/or the dosage decreased |

the cells. Kayexalate therapy may also be initiated at this time. Finally, diuretics may enhance urinary excretion of potassium. Nursing diagnoses, patient outcomes, and nursing interventions in the care of the patient with a potassium imbalance are presented in the Care Plan in Table 23–9.

**Hypokalemia.** A serum potassium level less than 3.5 mEq/liter constitutes hypokalemia, and a potassium deficit is probably the most common electrolyte imbalance. Common causes of hypokalemia are listed in Table 23–8. It is important to appreciate the effect of gastrointestinal and renal dysfunction on serum potassium levels. Hypokalemia is a serious disorder requiring a high index of suspicion and an awareness of those situations in which potassium loss is likely to occur.

Because potassium is distributed largely to muscles (skeletal, cardiac, and smooth), it is not surprising that the principal manifestation of an evolving hypokalemia is a reduction in muscle tone. Of particular concern is the effect of hypokalemia on cardiac muscle and the muscles of respiration. Hypokalemia may cause weakness of respiratory muscles, progressing to paralysis and respiratory arrest; anoxia may cause dysrhythmias, leading to cardiac arrest.

Hypokalemia impacts on cardiac cell excitability by causing hyperpolarization (increased negativity within the cardiac cell) of the resting membrane potential (RMP). As the RMP moves further away from threshold, fast response (sodium channel) action potentials are triggered, leading to an irritable ventricular response with the danger of serious/lethal dysrhythmias (see Fig. 23–2.)

The combination of digoxin, diuretic therapy, and hypokalemia requires special mention. Patients with hypokalemia are especially sensitive to the digitalis effect and are at high risk of developing digitalis toxicity. The potassium-wasting effects of diuretics (furosemide) may potentiate the digitalis toxicity. Patients who are at risk of developing hypokalemia should be identified, and special care should be taken to prevent the hypokalemic state from occurring. Serum potassium levels should be monitored closely, with potassium therapy provided as indicated, in conjunction with continuous cardiac monitoring. Nursing diagnoses, patient outcomes, and nursing interventions in the care of the patient with a potassium imbalance are presented in the Care Plan in Table 23–9.

## Chloride

### *Distribution in the Body*

The concentration of serum chloride in the extracellular fluid ranges between 100 and 106 mEq/liter. It is the major anion (negatively charged ion) in the extracellular fluid. Together with sodium, chlorides make up the "saline" milieu of the ECF compartment. Both of these ions have the capacity to "attract" water molecules. The concentration of chloride varies according to the changes in the quantity of extracellular fluid. Its concentration is also a function of chloride intake (largely sodium chloride or table salt) and its urinary excretion. Chlorides are distributed in the interstitial and lymph fluids; they are also found in specialized cells as, for example, nerve cells.

### *Physiologic Activity and Regulation*

Chloride, along with sodium, functions to maintain blood volume by influencing osmotic pressures within the intravascular and interstitial spaces. Chloride regulation is linked closely to sodium regulation. For each sodium ion reabsorbed in the

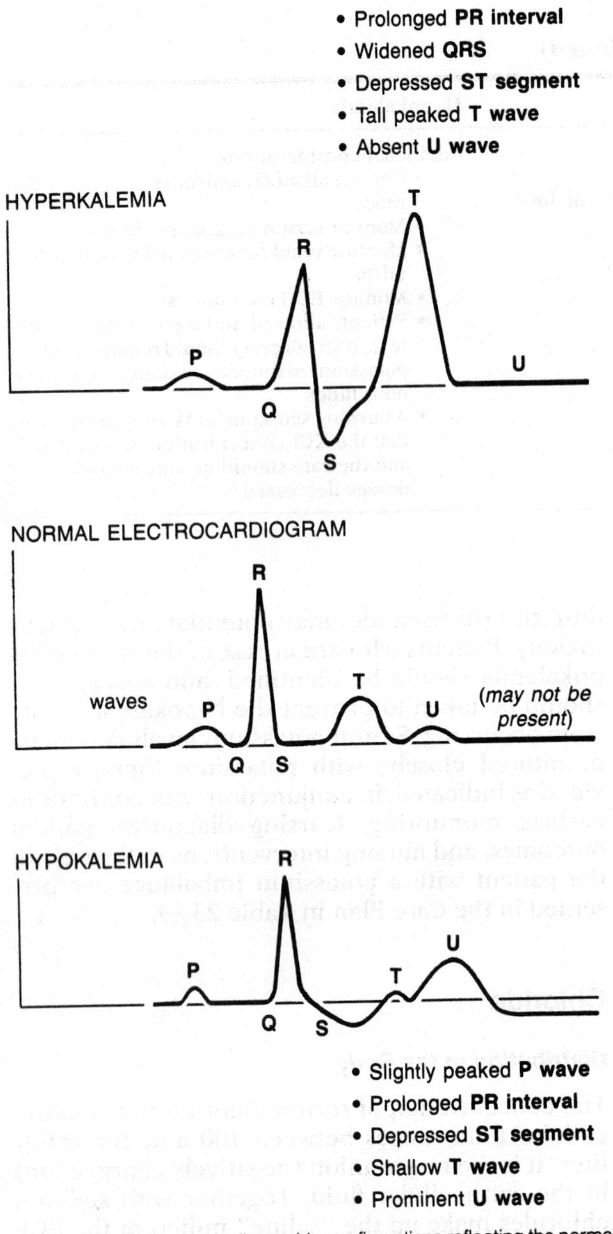


**Figure 23-2.** Electrocardiographic configurations reflecting the normal circumstance and changes from normal that occur in the presence of hyperkalemia and hypokalemia.

renal tubules, a chloride or bicarbonate ion is also reabsorbed. The acid-base status within the body determines which of these two anions is reabsorbed with sodium. Aldosterone indirectly controls chloride levels because as it stimulates sodium reabsorption in the distal tubule, chloride reabsorption also occurs.

### *Pathophysiology*

To preserve the acid-base status of extracellular fluid, the total number of anions (chloride and bicarbonate ions) must equal the total number of cations (sodium). Normally an inverse relationship exists between chloride and bicarbonate ($HCO_3^-$) ions. The significance of this inverse relationship is demonstrated in metabolic alkalemia associated with sodium chloride and ECF volume depletion. In this situation the readily reabsorbable chloride anion is not made available to the renal tubule in amounts sufficient to allow the kidney to reject the excess filtered $HCO_3^-$ load, despite the fact that the accompanying ECF volume depletion is a potent stimulus for sodium reabsorption. The continued enhanced reabsorption of $HCO_3^-$ ion accompanying sodium reabsorption suggests that the priority here is the restoration of ECF volume rather than the correction of the *hypochloremic* metabolic alkalemia.

**Hyperchloremia.** Hyperchloremia is a major consideration in the differential diagnosis of metabolic acidemia. In this instance, the state of the unmeasured anion gap is used to differentiate causes of metabolic acidemia into two groups: *normal anion gap* or *hyperchloremic* metabolic acidemia; and *increased anion gap* metabolic acidemia. The normal physiologic anion gap is expressed as follows: (normal range: ~10-14 mMol/liter

$$\text{Anion gap} = Na^+ - (Cl^- + HCO_3^-)$$

The "normal" physiologic anion gap reflects unmeasurable anions, including proteinates, phosphates, and sulfates; measurable anions include chloride and bicarbonate ions. (For further discussion of the anion gap and its clinical significance, see the section entitled "Anions and the Anion Gap," in Chap. 30.)

States of metabolic acidemia with a normal anion gap are usually due to losses of $HCO_3^-$ by the gastrointestinal or renal routes. While the level of $HCO_3^-$ ion is decreased, the level of choride ion is increased and, thus, the accompanying hyperchloremia. Metabolic acidemia with an increased anion gap is usually associated with the addition of acids to body fluids at a rate in excess of renal ability to excrete them (see Table 30-3). The characteristic features of hyper- and hypochloremia, including etiology, clinical presentation, and treatment, are listed in Table 23-10.

## Magnesium

### *Distribution in the Body*

The serum magnesium concentration is regulated within a very narrow range: 1.5-2.5 mEq/liter. Magnesium is the second most prevalent *intra*cellular cation. The body requires a daily intake of magnesium, which is absorbed by the intestines. It is reabsorbed or excreted by the kidney depending on serum concentration. Of the total body magnesium, approximately one half is found in bone, and the rest is found in muscle and other soft tissues.

## TABLE 23–9. CARE PLAN FOR THE PATIENT WITH A POTASSIUM IMBALANCE

| Nursing Diagnoses | Desired Patient Outcomes | Nursing Interventions | Rationales |
|---|---|---|---|
| ***Nursing Diagnosis #1***<br>Cardiac output, alteration in: Decreased, related to dysrhythmias associated with *hyper*kalemia (>5.5 mEq/liter). | Patient's status will stabilize as follows:<br>1. Neuromuscular status: Muscle strength intact; absence of muscle twitching or seizures; deep tendon reflexes brisk.<br>2. Cardiovascular status:<br>• Heart rate >60, <100 beats/min.<br>• Arterial BP = within 10 mmHg of patient's baseline.<br>• CVP = 0–8 mmHg.<br>• PCWP = 8–12 mmHg.<br>• CO = 4–8 liters/min.<br>3. ECG: Regular sinus rhythm.<br>• Rounded P wave.<br>• PR interval 0.12–0.20 seconds.<br>• QRS duration 0.06–0.12 seconds.<br>• ST segment = isoelectric.<br>• Rounded, asymmetric T wave.<br>4. Serum potassium 3.5–5.5 mEq/liter.<br>5. Arterial blood gases:<br>• pH = 7.35–7.45.<br>• $PCO_2$ = 35–45 mmHg.<br>• $HCO_3^-$ = 22–26 mEq/liter.<br>6. Respiratory status: Lung fields resonant; no rales (crackles).<br>7. Gastrointestinal function intact. | • Assess impact of hyperkalemia on physiologic processes: | • Assists in differential diagnosis of underlying pathophysiology; altered cardiopulmonary dynamics may reflect a compensatory response to some other primary diagnosis. |
| | | ◦ Elicit comprehensive patient history:<br>– Current cardiopulmonary status.<br>– Past medical history: Hypertension; coronary artery disease; angina; myocardial infarction; medications.<br>– Family history: Obesity; diabetes mellitus; hypertension; coronary artery disease; renal disease. | ◦ May help to identify patient at risk of developing a potassium imbalance. |
| | | ◦ Assess neuromuscular status: Evidence of twitching or seizure activity; muscle strength; deep tendon reflexes. | ◦ Potassium is intricately involved in establishing and maintaining cellular excitability; alterations in serum potassium are reflected by signs and symptoms of neuromuscular irritability. |
| | | ◦ Assess cardiopulmonary dynamics:<br>– Heart rate; peripheral pulses.<br>– Arterial blood pressure.<br>◦ CVP.<br>◦ PCWP. | ◦ Establishment of baseline data provides a basis for comparison and evaluation of effectiveness of therapy.<br>◦ Reflects volume of venous return.<br>◦ PCWP reflects the effectiveness of left ventricle in handling the volume of venous return to the heart; dysrhythmias associated with potassium imbalance decrease cardiac output. |
| | | ◦ Respiratory rate and pattern; breath sounds: Adventitious (rales or crackles). | ◦ The occurrence of rales may reflect left heart failure. |
| | | ◦ Fluid volume intake-output. | ◦ Fluid overload may cause cardiac failure in compromised heart. |
| | | ◦ Neck vein distention (45 degrees). | ◦ Neck vein distention reflects high central venous pressures associated with fluid overload and/or congestive heart failure. |
| | | ◦ Assess renal function.<br>– Urine output/hr. | ◦ Reduced renal perfusion related to decreased cardiac output may predispose to oliguria and fluid overload. |
| | | ◦ Assess gastrointestinal function: Abdominal distention, paralytic ileus. | ◦ Altered serum potassium disrupts smooth muscle excitability in gastrointestinal tract. |
| | | ◦ Evaluate arterial blood gases: pH, $PaCO_2$, $HCO_3^-$. | ◦ Metabolic acidosis drives hydrogen ions into cells in exchange for potassium ions; the result is hyperkalemia. |

*(continued)*

**TABLE 23–9. CARE PLAN FOR THE PATIENT WITH A POTASSIUM IMBALANCE *(Continued)***

| Nursing Diagnoses | Desired Patient Outcomes | Nursing Interventions | Rationales |
|---|---|---|---|
| ***Nursing Diagnosis #1 (cont.)*** | | | |
| | 8. Renal function: Urine output > 30 ml/hr. | • Collaborate with physician to correct underlying cause of hyperkalemia (see Table 23–8, Etiology).<br>– Metabolic acidosis. | • Correction of the underlying cause is essential to establish potassium homeostasis. |
| | | ◦ Implement treatment regimen (see Table 23–8, Treatment):<br>◦ Emergency measures: Serum potassium > 6.5 mEq/liter and/or severely impaired renal function: | ◦ Treatment will vary with the severity of electrolyte imbalance. |
| | | ◦ 10% calcium gluconate, as prescribed, with continuous cardiac monitoring. | ◦ Calcium is given to stimulate the heart; it should not be administered to patients taking digitalis preparations because the combined treatment may precipitate dysrhythmias. |
| | | ◦ 500 ml 10% glucose (hypertonic) with 10 units regular insulin IV over 30 min. | ◦ Potassium is driven into cells along with insulin-facilitated movement of glucose intracellularly (by K/Na pump). |
| | | ◦ Sodium bicarbonate, 2–3 amps in 500 ml glucose IV, or as prescribed. | ◦ Bicarbonate therapy relieves acidemia, causing potassium to move into cells in exchange for hydrogen ions; overall result is a decrease in serum potassium levels. |
| | | ◦ Additional therapy to correct hyperkalemia:<br>◦ Sodium polystyrene sulfonate (Kayexalate) 15–30 g orally or by enema, 2–3 times daily. | ◦ Kayexalate functions as an exchange resin absorbing potassium in the gastrointestinal tract and eliminating it in the feces. |
| | | • Nursing implications in hyperkalemia:<br>◦ Monitor cardiac function continuously.<br>◦ Electrical activity (ECG) (see Table 23–8 for list of specific ECG changes associated with hyperkalemia; see Fig. 23–2). | ◦ Potassium is the primary intracellular ion; alterations in potassium concentration predispose to neuromuscular irritability and dysrhythmias. |
| | | ◦ Mechanical activity (cardiac contractility) as reflected by: Arterial blood pressure, pulmonary pressures, cardiac output. | ◦ Electrical-mechanical asynchronization leads to reduced cardiac output, reduced arterial blood pressure, and reduced tissue perfusion. |
| | | ◦ Monitor arterial blood gases: pH, $PaCO_2$, $HCO_3^-$, $PaO_2$, $O_2$ saturation of hemoglobin. | ◦ Acidemia predisposes to hyperkalemia as hydrogen ions move into cells in exchange for potassium.<br>◦ $O_2$ administration may be indicated if $PaO_{PaCO_2}$ > 45 mmHg; an increase in carbon dioxide further contributes to acidemia. |

| | | | |
|---|---|---|---|
| | | ○ Monitor serum electrolytes: Notify physician of significant changes in serum electrolytes; serum potassium.<br>○ Decreased serum sodium. | ○ It is important to follow trends in arterial blood gases and serum electrolytes to evaluate effectiveness of therapy.<br>○ May also contribute to hyperkalemia. |
| | | ○ Monitor renal function:<br>– Urine output > 30 ml/hr.<br>○ Accurate documentation of intake and output.<br>– Daily weight. | ○ Potassium should not be administered in the presence of oliguria.<br>○ Fluid restriction may be necessary in presence of compromised cardiac function. |
| | | ○ Auscultate lung fields.<br>– Maximize ventilatory effort: semi-Fowler's position reduces pressure on diaphragm.<br>○ Comfort measures: Provide frequent rest periods; provide reassurance to patient and family; keep them informed.<br>○ Monitor effectiveness of prescribed medications and potential drug interactions: | ○ Presence of rales may suggest congestive heart failure. |
| | | ○ Diuretics (furosemide). | ○ Reduces intravascular volume and increases potassium excretion. |
| | | ○ Digitalis preparation. | ○ Stimulates contractility, slows heart rate, and increases cardiac output. |
| | | ○ Morphine. | ○ Alleviates anxiety, decreases venous return to the heart by decreasing peripheral vascular resistance |
| ***Nursing Diagnosis #2***<br>Cardiac output, alteration in: Decreased, related to dysrhythmias associated with *hyper*kalemia (>3.5 mEq/liter). | Patient's condition will stabilize as follows:<br>1. Neurologic status: Alert, oriented to person, place, date.<br>2. Neuromuscular status: Muscle strength intact; deep tendon reflexes brisk.<br>3. Respiratory function: Respiratory rate and pattern maintain arterial blood gases within acceptable physiologic limits:<br>• pH 7.35–7.45.<br>• $PaCO_2$ 35–45 mmHg.<br>• $HCO_3^-$ 22–26 mEq/liter. | • Assess impact of hypokalemia on physiologic processes (see Nursing Interventions for Nursing Diagnosis #1, above). Additionally:<br>○ Evaluate arterial blood gases: pH, $PaCO_2$, $HCO_3^-$. | ○ Metabolic alkalemia contributes to hypokalemia by driving potassium into cells in exchange for hydrogen ions. |
| | | • Collaborate with physician to correct underlying cause of hypokalemia (see etiologies listed in Table 23–8). | • Correction of the underlying cause is essential to establish potassium homeostasis. |
| | | ○ Metabolic alkalemia. | ○ Shift of potassium into cells in exchange for hydrogen may contribute to hypokalemia. |
| | | ○ Metabolic acidemia. | ○ A normal serum potassium in the presence of an acidemia indicates a potassium deficit. |
| | | ○ Implement treatment regimen (see Treatment in Table 23–8). Additionally:<br>– Identify patient at risk. | ○ Treatment will vary with the severity of electrolyte imbalance. |
| | | ○ Prevent conditions that may contribute to hypokalemia. For example, diuretic abuse (e.g., furosemide, thiazides). | ○ Serum potassium should be closely monitored because these diuretics increase potassium excretion. |

*(continued)*

## TABLE 23–9. CARE PLAN FOR THE PATIENT WITH A POTASSIUM IMBALANCE *(Continued)*

| Nursing Diagnoses | Desired Patient Outcomes | Nursing Interventions | Rationales |
|---|---|---|---|
| ***Nursing Diagnosis #2 (cont.)*** | | | |
| | • $PaO_2 > 60$ mmHg.<br>• $O_2$ Sat > 90%.<br>4. Cardiovascular function and ECG (see Patient Outcomes for Nursing Diagnosis #1, above). | – Minimal maintenance dose should be prescribed for patients with restricted oral intake of potassium:<br>○ NPO preoperative; diagnostic studies.<br>– NPO postoperative.<br>– Nasogastric suctioning. | – Additional losses of potassium associated with tissue injury, vomiting, and diarrhea, for example, should be replaced.<br>○ When potassium losses cannot be prevented, it is critical that they be replaced. |
| | 5. Serum electrolytes maintained as follows:<br>• Potassium 3.5–5.5 mEq/liter.<br>• Sodium 135–148 mEq/liter.<br>• Chloride 100–106 mEq/liter.<br>• Bicarbonate (as above). | ○ Administer potassium replacement therapy as prescribed: 40 mEq/liter KCl in 1000 ml of 5% dextrose/water.<br>○ A variety of potassium supplements are available for oral use.<br>– The occurrence of gastrointestinal symptomatology (nausea, vomiting, abdominal pain, distention, or bleeding) signals that oral potassium should be discontinued. | ○ Oral potassium supplements must be administered cautiously as these preparations cause gastric irritation; oral preparations should be administered completely dissolved to prevent gastrointestinal irritation.<br>– Serum potassium must be monitored closely to prevent hyperkalemia. |
| | 6. Renal function: Urine output > 30 ml/hr.<br>7. Gastrointestinal function intact. | ○ Potassium therapy should not begin until renal function has been evaluated.<br>– Intravenous potassium administration requires continuous cardiac monitoring. | ○ The kidneys are the major potassium-excreting organs. |
| | | • Other nursing considerations:<br>○ Maintain accurate intake/output.<br>○ Evaluate neuromuscular status hourly during acute phase of illness. | ○ Urine output should be maintained at > 30 ml/hr. |

| | | |
|---|---|---|
| | ○ Monitor cardiac status continuously (see Clinical Manifestations listed in Table 23–8 for specific ECG changes associated with hypokalemia; see Fig. 23–2). | |
| | ○ Monitor serum electrolytes and arterial blood gases:<br>○ Metabolic alkalemia, symptomatology: Nausea, vomiting, diarrhea, shallow breathing. | ○ Alkalemia predisposes to hypokalemia as potassium moves into cells in exchange for $H^+$ ions.<br>– Shallow breathing is a compensatory mechanism to increase carbon dioxide retention so as to help relieve alkalemic state. |
| | ○ Anticipate potential cardiac dysrhythmias in patients receiving digitalis and diuretics.<br>○ Assess patient for digitalis toxicity; Anorexia, nausea, vomiting, diarrhea; all types of dysrhythmias—paroxysmal atrial tachycardia, multifocal premature ventricular beats; atrioventricular conduction blocks, ventricular dysrhythmias. | ○ Digoxin normally slows conduction through atrioventricular node (junction); potential digitalis toxicity results in heart blocks. |

Arterial BP = systolic/diastolic; CVP = central venous pressure; PAP = pulmonary artery pressure; PCWP = pulmonary capillary wedge pressure; CO = cardiac output.

TABLE 23-10
**Contrast: Hyperchloremia and Hypochloremia**

| | Hyperchloremia | Hypochloremia |
|---|---|---|
| Definition | Serum chloride level > 106 mEq/liter | Serum chloride level <96 mEq/liter |
| Etiology | Metabolic acidemia associated with normal anion gap (hyperchloremic)<br>• Gastrointestinal loss of $HCO_3^-$: Diarrhea, small-bowel, biliary, or pancreatic drainage/fistula; ureterosigmoidostomy<br>• Renal loss of $HCO_3^-$: Carbonic anhydrase inhibitors (acetazolamide); renal tubular acidosis<br>Other | Metabolic alkalemia associated with:<br>• Direct chloride ion loss ($HCO_3^-$ is reabsorbed with chloride depletion)<br>• Direct hydrogen ion loss<br>• Gastrointestinal: Vomiting, gastric drainage, villous adenoma of colon<br>Diuretic therapy: Conditions that increase sodium loss with chloride following:<br>• Osmotic diuresis<br>• Excessive diaphoresis<br>• Other |
| Clinical presentation | Symptomatology largely reflects that of metabolic acidemia (see Table 30-3).<br>*Neurologic:* Drowsiness, lethargy, headache, weakness, tremors<br>*Cardiovascular:* Dysrhythmias<br>*Respiratory:* Tachypnea, dyspnea, Kussmaul's breathing with pH <7.20, hyperventilation | Symptomatology nonspecific; largely reflects that of metabolic alkalemia (see Table 30-3)<br>*Neuromuscular:* Irritability, muscle cramps, weakness, hyperactive deep tendon reflexes, tetany-alkalemia decreases freely ionized serum calcium.<br>*Cardiovascular:* Dysrhythmias associated with hypokalemia<br>*Respiratory:* Depressed function |
| Treatment | Therapeutic goals:<br>1. Treat the underlying cause<br>2. Restore fluid and electrolyte balance<br>Treat underlying cause of metabolic acidemia.<br>Emergency treatment: Intravenous administration of bicarbonate to increase pH<br>Intravenous fluid therapy with Ringer's lactate—liver converts lactate to bicarbonate, further increasing base and pH. | Treat underlying cause of metabolic alkalemia.<br>Intravenous fluid replacement therapy with sodium chloride and potassium chloride |

#### *Physiologic Activity*

The actual role of magnesium within the body is not yet clearly understood, but some activities and relationships of clinical importance should be mentioned. Magnesium has been identified as an essential coenzyme in numerous metabolic reactions including, for example, the kinase enzymatic systems involved in carbohydrate metabolism, and key reactions of the citric (Krebs') cycle. Magnesium is recognized as an essential component in the transmission of neuromuscular impulses. Magnesium may be involved in bone metabolism. As mentioned, approximately one half of total body magnesium occurs within bone. Parathyroid hormone regulates the renal reabsorption of magnesium in much the same way it affects that of calcium.

#### *Pathophysiology: Hypomagnesemia*

Hypomagnesemia[5] is relatively common in critically ill patients because of dietary deficiencies, increased gastrointestinal losses, and an impairment of renal reabsorption of magnesium. Medication (e.g., diuretics, aminoglycosides, and digoxin) may also contribute to hypomagnesemia. Magnesium levels below 1.5 mEq/liter may precipitate signs of neuromuscular irritability similar to those found with hypocalcemia, including convulsions. Cardiac dysrhythmias, ECG changes (e.g., flattened T waves, prolonged QT and PR intervals, and ST depression) may also be observed. Decreased intracellular levels of magnesium inhibit the sodium–potassium ATPase pump, which produces electrophysiologic abnormalities similar to those seen with hypokalemia.

Hypomagnesemia is treated with 1-2g 10-20% solutions of magnesium sulfate not to exceed 1.5 ml/minute. A deficiency of magnesium can be prevented by the administration of about 10 mEq/day.

#### *Pathophysiology: Hypermagnesemia*

Hypermagnesemia is an uncommon disorder usually associated with the use of magnesium-containing medications. Clinically, hypermagnesemia depresses central nervous system function. Muscle weakness and hyporeflexia appear at plasma levels around 6 mEq/liter. At levels of 10 mEq/liter, hypermagnesemia causes hypotension and dysrhythmias. This condition is treated by eliminating the causative medications. Transiently, the administration of intravenous calcium may ameliorate the imbalance. Features of hypomagnesemia and hypermagnesemia, including etiology, clinical presentation, and treatment, are presented in Table 23-11.

TABLE 23-11
**Contrast: Hypermagnesemia and Hypomagnesemia**

| | Hypermagnesemia | Hypomagnesemia |
|---|---|---|
| Definition | Serum magnesium levels > 2.5 mEq/liter | Serum magnesium levels < 1.5 mEq/liter |
| Etiology | Renal failure, oliguric phase, resulting in decreased urinary excretion of magnesium<br>Excessive use of magnesium-containing compounds: Laxatives—Milk of magnesia; antacids—Gelusil, magnesium oxide; Epsom salts<br>Overdose of magnesium replacement therapy; excessive parenteral administration<br>Hemoconcentration (dehydration) | Gastrointestinal losses: Malabsorption syndrome: Severe diarrhea, steatorrhea; long-term gastrointestinal suctioning; intestinal fistula; malnutrition; pancreatitis secondary to alcoholism<br>Renal disorders: Renal failure—diuretic phase; post-diuretic administration (e.g., furosemide)<br>Hyperaldosteronism<br>Hyperparathyroidism, thyrotoxicosis<br>Toxemia of pregnancy<br>Chronic alcoholism (increased urinary loss and probably decreased intake)<br>Post-drug use: Aminoglycosides, cisplatin, digoxin, ethyl alcohol |
| Clinical presentation | Symptomatology reflects CNS depression with coma, lethargy, decreased respiratory rate, and bradycardia, which can progress to cardiac arrest.<br>There is depressed neuronal activity and transmission of neuromuscular impulses. Muscle weakness and an ascending flaccid paralysis may occur.<br>Hypotension frequently occurs.<br>ECG changes similar to those occurring in hyperkalemia (e.g., peaked T wave) may become evident. | Symptomatology reflects increased neuromuscular excitation characterized by muscle weakness, tremors, muscle spasms.<br>Severe hypomagnesemia may present with generalized tetany, and seizures.<br>Other signs and symptoms may include: Confusion, coma, dizziness, gastrointestinal symptoms including anorexia and nausea.<br>ECG changes: Flat or inverted T wave; possible ST segment depression; prolonged QT interval |
| Treatment | Therapeutic goals:<br>1. Correct underlying disorder.<br>2. Restore and maintain fluid and electrolyte balance.<br>3. Identify high-risk patients.<br>In renal failure dialysis may be indicated: Hemodialysis or peritoneal dialysis.<br>Calcium gluconate may be administered to antagonize the effects of hypermagnesemia.<br>Observe for respiratory distress while efforts are made to reduce the magnesium levels.<br>Monitor continuous ECG, and magnesium levels. | Emergency treatment:<br>• Magnesium sulfate 1-2 g 10-20% solution IV not to exceed 1.5 ml/minute; kidney function should be assessed.<br>• Observe patient for signs of magnesium toxicity: Flushing due to peripheral vasodilation, hypotension, weakness, diminished to absent deep tendon reflexes, drowsiness, lethargy.<br>Magnesium toxicity can be treated with calcium gluconate, diuretics; tapering of magnesium-containing drugs; and by dialysis.<br>Maintenance magnesium dosage: 10 mEq/day.<br>Establish seizure precautions.<br>Note that hypomagnesemia will enhance digitalis effect predisposing to digitalis toxicity. Monitor ECG. |

## REFERENCES


1. Metheny, N: Fluid and Electrolyte Balance: Nursing Considerations. JB Lippincott, Philadelphia, 1987, p 45.
2. Stroot, V, Lee, C, and Barrett, C: Fluid and Electrolytes, A Practical Approach. FA Davis, Philadelphia, 1984, p 45.
3. Linton, A: Electrolyte disturbances. In Sibbald, WJ (ed): Synopsis of Critical Care, ed 3. Williams & Wilkins, Baltimore, 1988, p 134.
4. Linton, A: Electrolyte disturbances. In Sibbald, WJ (ed): Synopsis of Critical Care, ed 3. Williams & Wilkins, Baltimore, 1988, p 137.
5. Ayres, SM, Schlichtig, R, and Sterling, M: Care of the Critically Ill, ed 3. Year Book Medical Publishers, Chicago, 1988, p 307.
6. Metheny, N: Fluid and Electrolyte Balance: Nursing Considerations. JB Lippincott, Philadelphia, 1987, p 57.
7. Johnson, D: Nephrotic syndrome: A nursing care plan based on current pathophysiologic concepts. Heart and Lung 18(1):85, January 1989.

CHAPTER 24

# Nursing Management of the Patient with Altered Calcium Metabolism

## CHAPTER OUTLINE



## LEARNING OBJECTIVES

**At the end of this chapter, you should be able to:**

1. Describe the role of calcium in physiologic processes.
2. Specify factors involved in the maintenance of physiologic levels of serum calcium and phosphorus.
3. Specify the distribution of calcium in blood.
4. Distinguish the functions of parathyroid hormone in the regulation of calcium metabolism.
5. Identify the functions of vitamin D in the regulation of calcium metabolism.
6. State the functions of calcitonin (thyrocalcitonin) in the regulation of calcium metabolism.
7. Describe feedback mechanisms essential to the control of calcium metabolism.
8. Differentiate hypercalcemia and hypocalcemia in terms of pathophysiology, etiology, diagnostic findings, clinical manifestations, and treatment.
9. Delineate the nursing process in the care of the patient with a calcium disorder:
   Assessment.
   Nursing diagnosis.
   Planning: Desired patient outcomes
   Nursing interventions/rationales.

## CALCIUM: PHYSIOLOGIC FUNCTIONS

Calcium plays an essential role in physiologic processes, including its effect on biologic membranes, neural and neuromuscular activity, cardiac action potential and contractility, endocrine glands and other secretory apparatus, blood coagulation, activation of complement, and regulation of many enzyme systems. It is the major constituent of bone, teeth, and nails.

### Effect on Biologic Membranes

As an important constituent of biologic membranes, calcium functions to help maintain the permeability and electrical properties of cellular membranes. Intracellular concentration of calcium is usually extremely low in virtually all cells because of active transport of calcium out of the cell into the extracellular space. Thus, there exists a large gradient for diffusion of calcium. When cell membrane calcium channels open up, an influx of calcium into the cells occurs, with a consequent lowering of calcium concentration in interstitial and intravascular spaces. This difference in calcium concentration gradients underlies, in part, the increase in excitability of cellular membranes. Clinically, this change is reflected in the serum calcium. A decrease in serum calcium causes an increase in permeability and excitability of biologic membranes.

### Effect on Neural and Neuromuscular Activity

Calcium influences neuronal transmission and acts to link the excitation-contraction mechanism in muscle. Depolarization of the sarcolemma releases calcium from the sarcoplasmic reticulum, which initiates contraction by binding to troponin. Calcium binding to troponin produces conformational changes in tropomyosin, which cause tropomyosin to shift out of the way so that actin and myosin bridges can form, resulting in muscle contraction (see Figs. 37–11 and 37–17). Calcium also activates ATPase, which hydrolyzes ATP to ADP with the release of energy. When energy is released, muscle contraction occurs.

Calcium is an important component in neurotransmission. It is considered to be the link between depolarization of the presynaptic membrane by an arriving action potential and the neurotransmitter release (e.g., acetylcholine at cholinergic synapses; see Fig. 6–4). Clinically, a decrease in serum calcium concentration increases excitability of nerve tissues and neuromuscular activity, and predisposes to hypocalcemic tetany. An excessive elevation of serum calcium causes cardiac dysrhythmias and depresses neuromuscular excitability.

### Effect on Cardiac Action Potential and Contractility

The initial sodium-dependent depolarization of the cardiac muscle cell opens calcium channels within the cell membrane. Influx of calcium by way of the cell membrane causes intracellular stores of calcium in the sarcoplasmic reticulum to be mobilized. This calcium plays a pivotal role in: (1) prolonging the cardiac action potential in a depolarized state (i.e., absolute refractory period); (2) facilitating cardiac electrical-mechanical synchronization; and (3) preventing cardiac muscle tetany. (See sections on Myocardial Mechanical and Electrochemical Physiology in Chap. 37.)

Changes in extracellular and cytoplasmic calcium concentrations can cause alterations in the cardiac action potential and cardiac muscle contractility. Clinically, hypercalcemia shortens the duration of the cardiac action potential, and on ECG, it produces a shortening of the QT interval. Calcium exerts a positive inotropic effect on cardiac contractility; in excessive amounts it may cause cardiac irritability reflected by the occurrence of premature contractions and dysryhthmias.

Hypocalcemia prolongs the duration of the cardiac action potential, and on ECG, it produces a prolongation of the QT interval. A low serum calcium decreases myocardial contractility, predisposing to cardiac arrest.

### Effect on Endocrine Glands and Other Secretory Apparatus

Calcium, controlled by a variety of inputs, acts as a "second messenger" (the "first messenger" being the original stimulating hormone) or intracellular hormonal mediator in a variety of cells including muscle, nerve, and gland cells. Its role as a second messenger is frequently termed "coupler" in that it relays the message between the membrane event and the secretory or contractile apparatus. For example, calcium ions, in association with the calcium-binding protein, calmodulin, function as a "second messenger" system. Upon entry into the cell, whether stimulated by electrical phenomena that open calcium channels or by hormones interacting with membrane receptors that similarly open calcium channels, calcium ions bind with calmodulin. Calcium binding activates calmodulin, which, in turn, activates many intracellular enzymatic systems as, for example, myosin kinase, which acts directly on the myosin of smooth muscle to cause smooth muscle contraction.[1]

## Effect on Blood Coagulation

Calcium is necessary for blood coagulation because it is an essential cofactor in many of the clotting-sequence reactions in the blood clotting pathways. (See Chap. 61.) A recently discovered calcium-activated phospholipid-dependent enzyme, protein kinase C, has been found to be responsible for the activation of a variety of receptors including those for thrombin, platelet-activating factor, metabolites of arachidonic acid (e.g., prostaglandins and leukotrienes), insulin, and interleukin-2 (see Chap. 54), among others.[2] As part of the calcium messenger system, protein kinase C and calmodulin-dependent kinase (see above) work together with cyclic adenosine monophosphate (cAMP) to regulate cellular functions.

## Effect on Activation of the Complement System

Calcium is an important component in the activation of the complement system. The complement system involves a group of plasma proteins, which, when activated, participate in type II, cytotoxic immunologic responses, resulting in destruction of bacteria or other causative organisms. These activated plasma proteins also facilitate the inflammatory response. (Complement is discussed in Chap. 54; see Fig. 54–13.)

# MAINTENANCE OF CALCIUM/PHOSPHORUS HOMEOSTASIS

Maintenance of calcium homeostasis is required to preserve bone structure and function, and to facilitate other calcium-dependent reactions within the body. The major effector sites for calcium homeostasis include the gastrointestinal tract, bone, and kidney. Maintenance of calcium homeostasis depends on the balance between calcium input and output, and on the extracellular and serum concentrations of phosphorus. The two major sources of serum calcium input are the diet and bone with its large pool of calcium salts. Output of calcium involves deposition in bone or excretion by urine, feces, and skin.

Absorption of calcium from the intestinal lumen into the blood requires an active transport system. A considerable amount of dietary calcium is not absorbed from the intestines, and simply leaves by way of the feces. Absorption of calcium from the intestinal lumen is hindered because many of its salts are insoluble. Many variables reduce calcium absorption from the gastrointestinal tract. Among these are stress, including elevated levels of cortisol and thyroid hormones; alterations in intestinal motility (e.g., rapid peristalsis), immobilization, and aging. Diminished renal conversion of vitamin D to its active metabolite, 1,25-dihydroxycholecalciferol, is a major factor in reducing calcium absorption from the gastrointestinal tract.

Bone provides a large reservoir of calcium consisting of approximately 99% of total body calcium, much of it bound to phosphorus in the form of calcium phosphate crystalline salts called hydroxyapatites. The remaining 1% of total body calcium is found in extracellular fluid, including the blood.

The kidneys can selectively control reabsorption and excretion of calcium, depending on the calcium-ion concentration in the blood. Calcium is excreted by urine, feces, and, in the presence of a hyperthyroid state or extremely elevated temperature, by the skin.

The metabolism of calcium and phosphorus is closely and reciprocally related. Calcium and phosphorus are found in many of the same foods. While calcium is poorly absorbed from the gastrointestinal tract, phosphorus is absorbed exceedingly well, except when dietary intake of calcium is elevated. In this instance, calcium and phosphorus combine to form calcium phosphate, an insoluble salt, which is excreted in feces. Like calcium, phosphorus is deposited in bone or excreted by urine and feces.

Phosphorus plays a major regulatory role in body metabolism. It is present in extracellular fluid as inorganic phosphate ($PO_4$) and exists within cells primarily as phosphorylated organic compounds. A number of these compounds, for example, adenosine triphosphate (ATP), are critically important to energy metabolism. Additionally, the phosphorylation (that is, the addition of a phosphate group to an organic molecule) and dephosphorylation of various enzymes play a major role in the regulation of their metabolic activity. Approximately 85% of total body phosphate is contained in bone as calcium phosphate; about 1% is in extracellular fluid, with the remainder in the intracellular fluid compartment.

Renal handling of phosphorus plays an important role in regulating levels of extracellular and serum calcium. About 80%–90% of phosphate filtered at the glomerulus is reabsorbed by the renal tubules. Thus, the kidney plays a major role in regulating total body phosphate. When dietary phosphate intake increases, the rise in serum phosphate causes a reciprocal lowering of serum calcium, which stimulates secretion of parathyroid hormone. Parathyroid hormone acts to decrease renal tubular reabsorption of phosphate, while increasing calcium reabsorption, thereby restoring serum levels of these minerals toward normal. When the intake of phosphates is reduced, renal tubular reabsorption increases so that urinary loss of phosphates is minimal. In general, phosphate excretion is increased by parathyroid hormone, expansion of ECF volume, and to a lesser extent by calcitonin.

There is a narrow concentration range of ionized

calcium in extracellular fluid and blood that is required for intracellular biochemical reactions. Maintenance of this range within narrow limits is critical to provide sufficient ionized calcium for physiologic activities, while preventing life-threatening complications such as tetany or cardiac dysrhythmias, which are associated with hypo- and hypercalcemia, respectively. Maintenance and regulation of this narrow range largely depend on the hormonal activity of parathyroid hormone, vitamin D, and calcitonin, on the intestines, bone, and kidneys.

## Distribution of Calcium in Blood

Approximately 99% of total body calcium is localized in bone, teeth, and nails. The 1% remaining resides in extracellular fluid and predominantly in the blood. Calcium in blood is present in three different forms:

- Protein-bound, nondiffusible 41%
- Free, ionized, readily diffusible 50%
- Bound to organic substances in plasma (e.g., citrate, phosphate, sulfur, bicarbonate) 9%

The free, ionized fraction of serum calcium is the biologically active form, and this form is tightly regulated. The nurse must be cognizant of the relationship between protein-bound and free, ionized fraction of calcium in the blood. In evaluating the serum concentration of free, ionized fraction of calcium, it is important to consider that this value will be influenced by the amount of protein-bound calcium. Thus, a low serum albumin may result in a lower total serum calcium value in the presence of a normal ionized fraction of calcium. It is essential to assess total serum protein in conjunction with total serum calcium.

The normal range of serum calcium varies with the laboratory, but it is usually as follows:

- Normal physiologic range 8.5–10.5 mg/100 ml
- Hypercalcemia >10.5 mg/100 ml
- Hypocalcemia < 8.5 mg/100 ml

## Mechanism of Bone Formation: Significance in Calcium Homeostasis

Because 99% of body calcium and 85% of body phosphate are contained in bone, it is apparent that bone has an important regulatory role in calcium and phosphate metabolism. The major cell types involved in normal bone turnover include osteoblasts, which continually form bone; osteoclasts, which resorb or dissolve bone; and osteocytes, which are trapped osteoblasts implicated in the process of bone crystallization.

The activities of osteoblasts and osteoclasts occur simultaneously and are ongoing. While one section of bone is being built up, another is being broken down. Although the activity of these cells is normally closely coupled, hormonal and local regulatory factors can rapidly alter the deposition–resorption balance. Normally, about 500 mg/day of calcium is involved in hormonally regulated bone turnover controlled by osteoblasts and osteoclasts. Another 4000 mg or so is available for ionic exchange controlled by various factors, such as pH, and serum concentrations of calcium and phosphate. The amounts of "exchangeable" free, ionized calcium are quite large in relation to the total ECF calcium pool. Thus, changes in the ECF–bone equilibrium for calcium and phosphate in response to hormonal, ionic, pH, and other factors can rapidly alter the concentrations of calcium and phosphate extracellular fluid.[3]

## Calcium Metabolism: Function of Parathyroid Glands

The major function of the parathyroid glands is to synthesize and secrete parathyroid hormone in response to changes in ionized serum calcium. The parathyroid glands are responsible for the minute-to-minute fine tuning of the serum concentration of ionized calcium. These glands respond briskly to slight changes in free, ionized calcium levels by increasing or decreasing parathyroid hormone secretion when the serum calcium rises or falls. In this way, the activities of the parathyroid glands maintain the serum calcium levels within the narrow, optimal physiologic range.

### *Parathyroid Hormone*

Parathyroid hormone (PTH) is probably the most important factor involved in the regulation of calcium metabolism, and it acts specifically to control the concentration of ionized serum calcium. It also lowers the serum phosphate levels. Its release into the bloodstream varies with the serum concentration of free, ionized calcium perfusing the parathyroid glands. PTH release occurs in response to hypocalcemia; PTH suppression occurs in response to hypercalcemia.

PTH exerts its regulatory effect on calcium metabolism by specific action on the major effector sites for calcium homeostasis—bone, kidneys, and the gastrointestinal tract. Its immediate effect on bone is to stimulate osteoclastic activity in preexisting bone cells to mobilize calcium and phosphates from the exchangeable calcium pool. Transiently, it depresses osteoblastic activity. Its long-term effect is to stimulate proliferation of new osteoclastic resorption of bone matrix in addition to resorption of calcium and phosphate salts. PTH requires the permissive influence of 1,25-dihydroxycholecalciferol to effectively act on bone.

The immediate effect of PTH on the kidney is to stimulate rapid loss of phosphate by a greatly diminished proximal tubular reabsorption of phosphate ions. Over the long term, PTH stimulates an increase in calcium reabsorption. It is essential for conversion of vitamin D to its most potent metabolite, 1,25-dihydroxycholecalciferol. In addition, PTH increases urinary excretion of sodium, potassium, and bicarbonate, while decreasing the urinary excretion of magnesium, hydrogen, and ammonium ions.

PTH enhances both calcium and phosphate ion absorption from the intestines. It potentiates the action of vitamin D on intestinal calcium absorption. Thus, by increasing synthesis of 1,25-dihydroxycholecalciferol in the kidneys, PTH directly increases intestinal absorption of calcium. Table 24–1 lists the major hormonal effects of PTH on calcium metabolism and the important influence of the hormones, vitamin D and calcitonin on PTH activity.

#### *Calcium Metabolism: Role of Vitamin D*

Vitamin D has a less pronounced effect on calcium metabolism than does parathyroid hormone (PTH), but it nevertheless plays an essential role. It occurs in more than one form but is converted to its most biologically active form, 1,25-dihydroxycholecalciferol, by the kidneys. Its primary function is to stimulate intestinal absorption of calcium, an action that is potentiated by PTH. The highly active metabolite of vitamin D may be required for mineralization of the organic matrix of bone; this form of vitamin D also helps to maintain stores of calcium in mitochondria of bone cells. A lesser metabolite of vitamin D, 25-hydroxycholecalciferol, stimulates renal tubular reabsorption of calcium and phosphate (see Table 24–1).

#### *Calcium Metabolism: Role of Calcitonin*

Calcitonin (also called thyrocalcitonin) is a hormone secreted by the thyroid gland in response to elevated levels of free, ionized calcium. Its principal effect is to decrease serum levels of ionized calcium by decreasing bone resorption, and increasing bone deposition by osteoblastic activity. Calcitonin acts on the kidneys to increase phosphate excretion. It inhibits renal conversion of vitamin D to its highly active metabolite, 1,25-dihydroxycholecalciferol. Calcitonin has no definitive action on the intestines. Other details related to calcitonin and its physiologic activities are presented in Table 24–1.

### Regulation of Calcium Metabolism

Control of calcium metabolism is extremely complex yet finely tuned. Such control is characterized by constant, transient shifts of calcium between bone, extracellular fluid, blood, the kidneys, and the gastrointestinal tract, and requires ongoing dynamic interactions and continual feedback at the hormonal and cellular levels.

The major factor in the regulation of calcium involves the actual serum concentration of free, ionized calcium, which feeds back directly on the parathyroid glands. These glands respond by adjusting their secretion of PTH so as to maintain serum calcium levels within the normal physiologic range (i.e., ~8.5–10.5 mg/100 ml). A decrease in the serum concentration of free, ionized calcium stimulates the release of PTH; conversely, an increase in serum concentration of calcium reduces PTH secretion.

There are numerous other interactions involved in the regulation of calcium metabolism, some of which are presented in Table 24–2. Reciprocal feedback effects occur between each of the hormones involved in calcium metabolism (i.e., PTH, vitamin D, and calcitonin). Such interactions demonstrate the sophistication and intricacy of activities within the body concerned with maintaining all of the life processes in a state of dynamic equilibrium.

## PATHOPHYSIOLOGY: HYPERCALCEMIA AND HYPOCALCEMIA

As a key participant in so many critical physiologic processes, any disturbance or alteration in calcium metabolism can cause profound, far-reaching, and even life-threatening effects on total body function. The occurrence of *hyper*calcemia (i.e., total serum calcium of >10.5 mg/100 ml), or *hypo*calcemia (i.e., total serum calcium of <8.5 mg/100 ml) is not uncommon in the critically ill patient, who often experiences multiorgan disease usually accompanied by a diminished nutritional state. The recognition and timely treatment of a calcium imbalance can be essential to patient survival. Yet, the early clues as to its presence may be so subtle as to go unnoticed to the unsuspecting health-care provider.

### Hypercalcemia

Hypercalcemia is defined as an increase in the free, ionized serum calcium. Because approximately one half of total serum calcium is bound to protein, when evaluating serum calcium, factors affecting

TABLE 24-1
## Hormonal Effects on Calcium Metabolism

| | Parathyroid Hormone (PTH) | Vitamin D | Calcitonin (CT) |
|---|---|---|---|
| Primary function | Regulation/maintenance of free, ionized serum calcium concentration within physiologic range. | Stimulation of intestinal calcium absorption. | Reduction in free, ionized serum calcium concentration; a weak hypocalcemic agent. |
| Prohormone (precursors) | Preproparathyroid and proparathyroid hormones. | Vitamin $D_2$ (ergocalciferol) —Dietary source, fortified milk; vitamin $D_3$ (cholecalciferol)—Skin sterols. | |
| Stimulus for hormone release | 1. Decreased free, ionized serum calcium levels.<br>2. Increase in circulating catecholamines.<br>3. Increase in circulating levels of cortisol.<br>4. Elevated serum phosphate levels: Hypophosphatemia induces increased renal synthesis of 1,25-$(OH)_2D$,* which increases the intestinal absorption of phosphate as well as calcium. | Decreased free, ionized serum calcium levels stimulate release of active metabolite. | Large increases in free, ionized serum calcium levels stimulate calcitonin release. |
| Inhibition | PTH inhibited by increased serum calcium and severely reduced serum magnesium. | | Decreases in free, ionized serum calcium levels inhibit calcitonin release. |
| Metabolites | | Highly active metabolite 1,25-$(OH)_2D$<br>Lesser metabolites: 25-(OH)D, 24,25-$(OH)_2D$ | |
| Actions | | | |
| Bone | 1. Immediate effects:<br>• Stimulates osteoclastic activity in preexisting bone cells to mobilize calcium and phosphates from exchangeable calcium pool.<br>• Transiently depresses osteoblastic activity.<br>2. Long-term effects:<br>• Stimulates proliferation of new osteoclastic resorption of bone matrix in addition to calcium and phosphate salts.<br>3. Requires permissive influence of 1,25-$(OH)_2D$ to effectively act on bone. | Highly active metabolite of vitamin D (1,25-$(OH)_2D$) may be required for mineralization of the organic matrix of bone; this form of vitamin D also helps to maintain stores of calcium in mitochondria of bone cells.<br>Lesser metabolites of vitamin D: 25-(OH)D and 24,25-$(OH)_2D$ enhance synthesis of bone matrix and its mineralization, possibly to a greater extent than does 1,25-$(OH)_2D$. | Decreases activity of osteoclasts in bone resorption.<br>Decreases formation of osteoclasts.<br>Net effect on bone:<br>Bone resorption.<br>Bone deposition by osteoblasts.<br>Hypermagnesemia = increase in release of calcitonin. |
| Kidney | 1. Immediate effect:<br>• Stimulates rapid loss of phosphate by a greatly diminished proximal tubular reabsorption of phosphate ions.<br>2. Long-term effect:<br>• Stimulates increase of calcium reabsorption. | Lesser metabolite (25-(OH)D) stimulates renal tubular reabsorption of calcium and phosphate (possibly to a greater extent than does 1,25-$(OH)_2D$). | Increases excretion of sodium, chloride, and calcium.<br>Increases phosphate excretion.<br>Inhibits renal conversion of vitamin D to its highly active metabolite, 1,25-$(OH)_2D$. |

*(continued)*

TABLE 24–1
## Hormonal Effects on Calcium Metabolism *(Continued)*

| | | | |
|---|---|---|---|
| | 3. Essential for conversion of vitamin D to its most potent metabolite, $1,25\text{-}(OH)_2D$.<br>• Increases urinary excretion of sodium, potassium, and bicarbonate.<br>• Decreases urinary excretion of magnesium, hydrogen, and ammonium ions. | | |
| Intestines | • Enhances both calcium and phosphate ion absorption from the intestines.<br>• Potentiates action of vitamin D on intestinal calcium absorption.<br>• Thus, indirectly increases calcium absorption by the intestines by increasing $1,25\text{-}(OH)_2D$ synthesis in the kidneys. | Primary function of $1,25\text{-}(OH)_2D$: Potent stimulator of intestinal calcium-ion absorption. | No definitive action on intestines. Increased levels of gastrointestinal hormones, gastrin and pancreozymin, stimulate calcitonin release. |

* Vitamin D: 1,25-dihydroxycholecalciferol ($1,25\text{-}(OH)_2D$).

TABLE 24–2
## Regulation of Calcium Metabolism

| Factors Affecting Parathyroid hormone (PTH) | Factors Affecting Vitamin D Metabolites | Factors Affecting Calcitonin (CT) |
|---|---|---|
| ***Free, Ionized Serum Calcium Levels***<br>↑ Serum calcium = ↓ PTH secretion.<br>↓ Serum calcium = ↑ PTH secretion. | | ↑ Serum calcium = ↑ CT release.<br>↓ Serum calcium = ↓ CT release. |
| ***Actions of ↑ PTH***<br>Enhances conversion of vitamin D to its highly active form ($1,25\text{-}(OH)_2D$) in the kidney.<br>PTH increases bone resorption.<br>PTH increases calcium reabsorption in distal tubules and collecting ducts within the kidneys. | ***Actions of Vitamin D***<br>$1,25\ (OH)_2D$ greatly increases calcium absorption by intestinal mucosa.<br>Active metabolites inhibit release of PTH possibly by direct stimulation of calcium uptake by cells within the parathyroid glands. Sensory receptors within these glands interpret the increased calcium uptake as an increase in serum calcium levels even though actual serum levels of free, ionized calcium may not have changed. | ***Actions of Calcitonin***<br>Calcitonin exerts an antagonistic effect on PTH.<br>Calcitonin decreases serum calcium by inhibiting calcium mobilization from bone. |
| ***Permissive Effects***<br>PTH requires permissive effect of vitamin D to exert its effect on bone resorption and maintenance of serum calcium levels within physiologic range. | PTH is required to convert vitamin D to its highly active metabolite, $1,25\text{-}(OH)_2D$. This function requires unimpaired renal integrity.<br>PTH potentiates action of vitamin D metabolite on intestinal mucosa. | |
| ***Serum Magnesium Levels***<br>Hypermagnesemia inhibits PTH release; alterations in serum magnesium may interfere with PTH secretion. | | Hypermagnesemia = ↑ CT release. |

TABLE 24–2
**Regulation of Calcium Metabolism *(Continued)***

| | | |
|---|---|---|
| ***Serum Phosphorus Levels*** | ↓ Serum phosphorus:<br>• Enhances conversion of vitamin D in kidney.<br>• Increases absorption of calcium from gut.<br>• Net effect: Increase in free, ionized serum calcium. | Calcitonin decreases phosphate levels by inhibiting bone remodeling; and possibly by increasing urinary loss of phosphates. |
| ↑ Serum phosphorus:<br>• Enhances PTH secretion. | ↑ Serum phosphorus:<br>• Decreases conversion of vitamin D in kidney.<br>• Net effect: Decrease in free, ionized serum calcium levels. | |
| ***Other Factors***<br>Catecholamines } ↑ PTH secretion<br>Cortisol | Serum levels of lesser vitamin D metabolites = decreased by barbiturates; phenytoin; chronic liver disease. | ↑ Gastrin, pancreozymin hormonal secretions in gastrointestinal tract = ↑ CT release |
| Arterial pH: Influences free, ionized calcium. | *Alkalemia:* | Calcium binding to protein increases. Free, ionized calcium decreases. |
| | *Acidemia:* | Calcium binding to protein decreases. Free, ionized calcium increases. |
| ***Effect of Anabolic Hormones***<br>• Growth hormone: Indirect involvement in bone formation; influences liver to synthesize somatomedin whose action increases cartilage growth.<br>• Thyroid hormones: Exert an anabolic effect on bone formation.<br>• Sex hormones:<br>Estrogen } promote bone growth and development.<br>Testosterone | | |
| ***Effect of Catabolic Hormones***<br>• Glucocorticoids:<br>1. Act to break down bone by removing bone matrix with secondary loss of hydroxyapatite.<br>2. Interfere with intestinal calcium absorption. | | |

the amount of protein-bound calcium must be considered. An increase in the albumin concentration in blood (e.g., as in dehydration) or an increase in abnormal binding protein (e.g., as occurs in multiple myeloma) may lead to an increase in total serum concentration but without an increase in the ionized fraction. Acidemia decreases the amount of protein-bound calcium, resulting in an increase in its free, ionized fraction; conversely, alkalemia increases the amount of calcium that is protein-bound, thus reducing the free, ionized fraction.

### Clinical Presentation

Clinical manifestations of hypercalcemia depend on the rapidity of its development and the extent and duration of the abnormality. It can vary in severity from an asymptomatic longstanding condition, detected accidentally on routine blood tests, or to an acute, life-threatening illness. Symptomatology may occur when total serum calcium levels exceed 11.0–12.0 mg/100 ml; serum calcium in excess of 15 mg/100 ml represents a medical emergency.

Renal, neurologic, and cardiovascular functions are those primarily affected by hypercalcemia. Renal manifestations are largely due to hypercalciuria caused by the increased filtered load of calcium and can vary from kidney stones to renal failure. Polyuria and nocturia may be among the earliest renal manifestations of hypercalcemia caused by the increased osmotic load of calcium and loss of ability to concentrate urine. Dehydration may rapidly ensue. With sustained hypercalcemia, glomerular filtration rate is diminished due to hypovolemia and nephrocalcinosis (i.e., calcium deposits in the renal parenchyma). There is the potential for renal calculi formation (nephrolithiasis) associated with hypercalciuria. Flank pain may occur in the presence of renal calculi.

Hypercalcemia has a depressive effect on the central nervous system, manifested as lethargy, depression, emotional lability, and personality changes depending on the duration of the disorder. Headache and fatigue are common, and generalized muscle weakness progressing to hypotonia, hyporeflexia, and paresis may occur if the hypercalcemic state remains untreated. Reduced intestinal motility can cause constipation, a subtle but frequently presenting symptom. Anorexia and nausea are common.

Calcium has a positive inotropic effect on the heart. Hypercalcemia can alter conduction within the heart predisposing to heart block. There is a shortened QT interval and shorted ST segment on ECG, and a tendency to dysrhythmias. In patients receiving digoxin, increased serum calcium can potentiate the effect and precipitate digitalis toxicity. Hypercalcemia may also be associated with hypertension. Possible underlying mechanisms include a direct increase in peripheral vascular resistance and alterations in the renin–angiotensin–aldosterone system.

There is an increased incidence of peptic ulcer disease and pancreatitis in patients with hypercalcemia. These patients may also experience deposition of calcium salts in soft tissues (especially the lungs, kidneys, blood vessels, and joints). Soft tissue deposition occurs most commonly when there is an associated elevation in phosphate as occurs in renal failure and vitamin D intoxication.

### *Treatment*

The most important initial measure in the treatment of hypercalcemia is to restore normal intravascular fluid volume by replacing sodium and water that have been lost as a result of calcium-induced osmotic diuresis. This approach increases renal blood flow and glomerular filtration rate, thus enhancing calcium excretion. In addition, because sodium and calcium compete for reabsorption in the renal tubules, administration of sodium accelerates calcium excretion. Sodium and water may be given as alternating normal (0.9%) and half-normal (0.45%) saline solution until the central venous pressure (CVP) is restored to normal. Cautious administration of a loop diuretic (e.g., furosemide) prevents fluid overload in the face of continuing saline administration. Overzealous use of diuretic can precipitate intravascular volume depletion exacerbating the hypercalcemia.

These measures should significantly reduce serum calcium levels in virtually all patients with hypercalcemia who have reasonably normal renal function. Additional therapeutic measures may include restricting calcium intake, mobilizing the patient when possible to stimulate calcium deposition in bone, and treatment of the underlying cause.

### *Nursing Care of the Patient with Hypercalcemia*

As the health-care provider most intimately involved in patient care, the critical care nurse must be cognizant of the potential risks and dangers of a calcium imbalance developing in the critically ill patient. Early detection and timely implementation of preventive measures may be necessary to maintain calcium homeostasis.

In patients with hypercalcemia, initial therapy involves aggressive fluid (saline) and diuretic (usually furosemide) therapy. Overly aggressive fluid replacement therapy can predispose to fluid overload and congestive heart failure; too rigorous antihypercalcemic therapy can precipitate hypocalcemia. Thus, it is essential for the critical care nurse to closely monitor cardiovascular function and fluid and electrolyte balance. Close monitoring of serial calcium and phosphorus levels helps to anticipate and prevent hypocalcemia. The nurse must also be alert for signs of increased neuromuscular excitability (e.g., muscle twitching, spasms, or seizure activity), which are indicative of the hypocalcemic state.

Hypercalcemia causes a decrease in smooth muscle tone of the gastrointestinal tract, resulting in an alteration in bowel elimination. Stool softeners may be prescribed to reduce problems with constipation. Laxatives should be used judiciously to avoid diarrhea with its associated disruption in fluid and electrolyte balance. Efforts may be employed to reduce gastrointestinal absorption of calcium. The patient may be placed on a calcium-restricted diet. Fruits and fiber stimulate peristalsis and decrease absorption time; efforts can be made to maximize exercise activity as tolerated because this helps to increase peristalsis and overall muscle tone. Increased muscular activity also contributes to calcium deposition in bone, reducing serum calcium levels.

Additional supportive care measures of concern to nursing include the importance of early mobilization, prevention of thrombophlebitis, maintenance of skin integrity, and patient/family education. This information is included in the Care Plan in Table 24–3. Nursing diagnoses, patient outcomes, and nursing interventions in the care of the patient with hypercalcemia are presented.

## Hypocalcemia

Hypocalcemia is characterized by a decrease in the free, ionized calcium fraction in the blood, and its occurrence is most commonly associated with a depression of parathyroid function. Severe hypomagnesemia also suppresses PTH function. Hyper-

## TABLE 24–3. CARE PLAN FOR THE PATIENT WITH HYPERCALCEMIA

| Nursing Diagnoses | Desired Patient Outcomes | Nursing Interventions | Rationales |
|---|---|---|---|
| ***Nursing Diagnosis #1***<br>Electrolyte imbalance: Hypercalcemia, related to:<br>1. Impaired renal function (renal tubular acidosis).<br>2. Alkalemia.<br>3. Prolonged immobilization.<br>4. Hypophosphatemia.<br>5. Hyperparathyroidism.<br>6. Others. | Patient's condition will stabilize as follows:<br>1. Neurologic status:<br>• Alert, oriented to person, place, and time.<br>• Absence of fatigue, mood appropriate, memory intact.<br>• Verbalizes comfort, without pain or headache.<br>2. Cardiovascular status:<br>• Heart rate >60, <100 beats/min.<br>• Arterial BP within 10 mmHg of patient's baseline.<br>• ECG: Regular sinus rhythm, ST segment isoelectric, QT interval within normal range.<br>3. Serum studies:<br>• Calcium 8.5–10.5 mg/100 ml.<br>• Phosphorus 3.0–4.5 mg/100 ml.<br>• Sodium 135–148 mEq/liter.<br>• Potassium 3.5–5.5 mEq/liter.<br>• Magnesium 1.5–2.0 mEq/liter.<br>• Proteins (total) 6.0–8.4 g/100 ml.<br>4. Renal status: Urine output >30 ml/hr (depends on status of renal function). | • Assess impact of hypercalcemia on physiologic processes.<br>○ Elicit pertinent aspects of patient/family history (see Table 24–4). | • Personal characteristics and state of health play a crucial role in determining the ability of the patient/family to cope with the stress of hypercalcemia and its underlying cause.<br>○ While many signs/symptoms may accompany hypercalcemia, they are usually nonspecific and difficult to recognize. The patient's assessment requires a high degree of suspicion and a meticulous examination of laboratory data. |
| | | ○ Perform physical examination. | ○ Establish baseline data with which subsequent assessments can be compared. |
| | | ○ Neurologic status: Mental status, level of consciousness, alertness, orientation to person, place, time. | ○ Calcium is a key factor in cellular permeability, and in the transmission of electrical impulses. |
| | | ○ Lethargy, confusion, memory status; emotional lability; personality changes (as per family/significant others); headache, pain.<br>– Cranial nerve function. | ○ Hypercalcemia causes depression and sluggishness of central and peripheral nervous systems; it alters neuromuscular responses. |
| | | ○ Neuromuscular function: Extreme fatigue; decreased muscle strength; generalized muscle weakness; muscle hypotonicity, flaccidity; muscle twitchings, spasms; neuromuscular hypoactivity; diminished deep tendon reflexes; bone pain; flank pain. | ○ Prolonged immobilization increases movement of calcium from bone into the bloodstream, contributing to hypercalcemic state. |
| | | ○ Cardiovascular status: Heart rate and rhythm; arterial blood pressure; pulmonary artery and capillary wedge pressures; cardiac output. | ○ Hypertension associated with high cardiac output and extremely enhanced cardiac contractility has been known to occur in the scenario of hypercalcemia. |
| | | ○ Assess for exaggerated, inotropic effect of increased serum calcium levels on cardiac contractility.<br>– ECG. | ○ The potent inotropic effect of elevated serum calcium predisposes to cardiac dysrhythmias, conduction delays, and cardiac arrest. There is an increased incidence of heart blocks in such clinical states. |
| | | ○ Respiratory status.<br>○ Respiratory rate and rhythm. | ○ Shortness of breath may reflect weakened state. |

*(continued)*

**TABLE 24–3. CARE PLAN FOR THE PATIENT WITH HYPERCALCEMIA *(Continued)***

| Nursing Diagnoses | Desired Patient Outcomes | Nursing Interventions | Rationales |
|---|---|---|---|
| ***Nursing Diagnosis #1 (cont.)*** | | | |
| | Serum studies:<br>• BUN 8–25 mg/100 ml<br>• Creatinine 0.6–1.5 mg/100 ml. | ∘ Hydration status: Evidence of congestive heart failure and pulmonary edema: tachypnea, dyspnea; adventitious breath sounds (crackles, rales, wheezes); cough, productive of frothy, pink-tinged sputum. | ∘ Fluid volume overload increases risk of congestive heart failure and pulmonary edema, especially in patients with prior limitations in cardiac reserve. |
| | | ∘ Acid–base status—Arterial blood gases: pH, $PaCO_2$, $HCO_3^-$. | ∘ Metabolic alkalemia increases binding of calcium to serum proteins; the net effect—hypocalcemia.<br>∘ Metabolic acidemia increases freely ionized serum calcium fraction. |
| | | ∘ Renal status and fluid and electrolyte status: | ∘ Polydipsia and polyuria are frequently associated with an increased or forced calcium excretion.<br>∘ Baseline data are essential to evaluate the patient's response to therapy. |
| | | ∘ Determine fluid intake/output.<br>– Determine body weight.<br>– Assess hematocrit/hemoglobin.<br>– Assess BUN and creatinine levels.<br>– Establish baseline electrolyte levels: | ∘ Aggressive fluid therapy can predispose to fluid overload with congestive heart failure. |
| | | ∘ Calcium. | ∘ Highly bound to serum proteins. |
| | | ∘ Sodium. | ∘ Calcium excretion is largely dependent on concomitant excretion of sodium. |
| | | ∘ Phosphorus. | ∘ Exhibits a reciprocal relationship with calcium. |
| | | ∘ Proteins (total and albumin). | ∘ Approximately one half of serum calcium is freely ionized; the remainder is bound to proteins and organic molecules. |
| | | ∘ Assess urine output for stones. | ∘ Renal calculi formation can be a major complication because of the increased excretion of high concentrations of calcium by the nephrons. |
| | | • Collaborate with other health-care providers to implement therapeutic regimen to restore serum calcium to within physiologic range.<br>∘ Initiate fluid and drug therapy to reduce serum calcium to appropriate physiologic range. (Refer to section on Treatment in Table 24–4 for specific therapies.) | ∘ Goal of fluid and drug therapy is to attain an asymptomatic serum calcium level and reverse process causing the hypercalcemia. |

| | |
|---|---|
| ◦ In addition:<br>◦ Administer prostaglandin inhibitors, as prescribed. | ◦ Prostaglandin inhibitors, as for example, indomethacin, or aspirin, may lower serum calcium when hypercalcemia is associated with prostaglandin-producing tumors. |
| ◦ Initiate efforts to determine and treat underlying cause of hypercalcemic state.<br>◦ Treatment of underlying cause should be initiated once the acute phase is under control.<br>◦ Precipitants of hypercalcemia, especially prolonged immobilization and volume depletion, should be diligently avoided. | |
| ◦ Anticipate the occurrence of hypocalcemia with too rigorous antihypercalcemic therapy.<br>– Be alert for signs of increased neuromuscular excitability: Muscle twitchings and spasms; seizure activity; tetany. | ◦ Wide fluctuations in serum calcium levels may occur and require very close monitoring. |
| ◦ Implement measures to restore and maintain fluid and electrolyte balance.<br>◦ Establish and maintain hydrated state. | ◦ Patient may be unable to conserve free water due to ADH resistance. Rehydration = dilutional effect on serum calcium. |
| ◦ Administer normal saline infusion in conjunction with administration of furosemide (diuretic therapy).<br>◦ Avoid use of thiazide diuretics. | ◦ Combination of normal saline and diuretic therapy increases glomerular filtration rate and renal excretion of calcium.<br>◦ There is a concomitant decrease in urinary calcium excretion when thiazide diuretics are administered. |
| ◦ Strain urine for stones.<br>◦ Assess for signs/symptoms associated with passage of stone: Severe colicky flank pain, hematuria.<br>◦ Consider acid-ash diet to keep urine acidic and avoid renal calculi formation. | ◦ Elevated renal excretion of calcium predisposes to renal calculi formation. |
| ◦ Correlate serum electrolytes with clinical status.<br>◦ Carefully monitor serial serum calcium and phosphorus levels. | ◦ Following the trend of serum calcium levels assists in determining the effectiveness of therapeutic regimen.<br>◦ Close monitoring of serum calcium levels helps to anticipate and prevent hypocalcemia.<br>– A reciprocal relationship between these two ions usually exists. Hypophosphatemia frequently occurs in hypercalcemia. |

*(continued)*

**TABLE 24–3. CARE PLAN FOR THE PATIENT WITH HYPERCALCEMIA *(Continued)***

| Nursing Diagnoses | Desired Patient Outcomes | Nursing Interventions | Rationales |
|---|---|---|---|
| ***Nursing Diagnosis #1 (cont.)*** | | | |
| | | ◦ Carefully monitor total serum proteins to determine state of free, ionized serum calcium.<br>– ↑ In serum proteins = ↓ in free, ionized calcium.<br>– ↓ In serum proteins = ↑ in free, ionized calcium. | ◦ Approximately 45–50% of serum calcium is protein bound. |
| | | ◦ Carefully monitor serum potassium and magnesium.<br>◦ Replace urinary losses. | ◦ Depletion of serum potassium and magnesium levels frequently occurs, and their monitoring is mandatory to prevent alterations in cardiac function.<br>– Combination of hypercalcemia and hyperkalemia causes cardiac irritability.<br>– Ultimate goal of therapy is to establish an asymptomatic serum calcium level without alterations in neuromuscular or cardiac functions. |
| | | ◦ Monitor cardiovascular function.<br>– Cardiac rate and rhythm (continuously).<br>◦ Administer digitalis carefully in patients with hypercalcemia.<br>◦ Monitor arterial and pulmonary capillary pressures. | ◦ Calcium will enhance digitalis effect and may precipitate digitalis toxicity.<br>◦ Assist in managing fluid status: fluid volume overload must be avoided because patients are at increased risk of congestive heart failure and pulmonary edema. |
| | | ◦ Implement peritoneal or hemodialysis in life-threatening situations. | ◦ Either peritoneal or hemodialysis is capable of efficiently removing calcium from blood; the mode of dialysis depends on several considerations, as for example, the acuteness of the situation, age, and clinical status of patient. |

| | | | |
|---|---|---|---|
| ***Nursing Diagnosis #2***<br>Bowel elimination, alteration in: Constipation, related to:<br>1. Smooth muscle hypotonicity with inadequate peristalsis associated with hypercalcemia. | Patient will establish and maintain effective bowel function:<br>1. Bowel pattern to return to patient's baseline.<br>• Stool soft and formed.<br>• Absence of constipation, abdominal distention, fecal impaction with diarrheal incontinence. | • Assess gastrointestinal function:<br>○ Ascertain bowel habits/pattern; establish pre-illness diet; presence of anorexia, nausea, vomiting; constipation, diarrhea.<br>○ Determine attitudes of patient/family regarding nutrition.<br>○ Perform abdominal examination: Bowel sounds; evidence of tenderness or guarding ; distention.<br>○ Determine hydration status. | • Hypercalcemia causes a decrease in smooth muscle contractility of the gastrointestinal tract; the bowel becomes hypoactive with reduced muscle tone. |
| ***Nursing Diagnosis #3***<br>Potential for injury: Peptic ulcer disease, related to:<br>1. Increased gastric acid secretion associated with elevated serum calcium levels. | 2. Bowel sounds appropriate and heard throughout all quadrants.<br>3. Absence of epigastric pain; relaxed facial expression and demeanor.<br>4. Stool/gastric secretions negative for occult blood.<br>5. Gastric pH >4.5. | ○ Assess for potential complications.<br>○ Peptic ulcer disease. | ○ Enhanced gastric secretions in the presence of hypercalcemia predispose to peptic ulcer disease. |
| | | ○ Acute pancreatitis. | ○ Associated with activation of pancreatic enzymes or plugging of pancreatic duct. |
| | | • Initiate comprehensive approach to reducing calcium absorption from the intestines.<br>○ Diet (as per nutritionist).<br>– Calcium restriction. | |
| | | ○ Fruit and fiber. | ○ Bulk stimulates peristalsis. |
| | | ○ Avoid caffeine-containing foods/fluids. | ○ Reduces hydrochloric acid secretion. |
| | | ○ Medications (as prescribed).<br>○ Stool softeners. | ○ Prevent constipation. |
| | | ○ Judicious use of laxatives. | ○ Diarrhea must be avoided because of associated fluid and electrolyte imbalance.<br>– Presence of diarrhea may suggest fecal impaction in patients with constipation. |
| | | ○ Histamine antagonists (cimetidine, ranitidine). | ○ Inhibit gastric secretions. |
| | | ○ Antacids.<br>– Administer phosphates to increase calcium excretion. | ○ Reduce gastric acidity. |
| | | ○ Maximize exercise activity as tolerated. | ○ Exercises (abdominal) assist to increase peristalsis and increase overall muscle tone. |

(continued)

**TABLE 24-3. CARE PLAN FOR THE PATIENT WITH HYPERCALCEMIA *(Continued)***

| Nursing Diagnoses | Desired Patient Outcomes | Nursing Interventions | Rationales |
|---|---|---|---|
| ***Nursing Diagnosis #4*** Mobility, impaired physical.<br>***Nursing Diagnosis #5*** Activity intolerance, potential. | Patient will:<br>1. Achieve maximum mobility without discomfort, weakness, or fatigue.<br>2. Demonstrate maximum range of motion. | • Implement therapeutic regimen to restore/maintain mobility and activity tolerance.<br>○ Maintain proper body alignment.<br>○ Establish a progressive exercise program as tolerated (as per physical therapist).<br>– Encourage range-of-motion exercises to all joints.<br>– Initiate passive exercises when appropriate, and progress to active exercises.<br>– Avoid rough handling; support joints to minimize pain and prevent trauma.<br>○ Avoid overfatigue; provide rest periods. | ○ Pathologic fractures are often associated with hypercalcemia and its underlying cause.<br>○ Exercise and mobilization reduce resorption of calcium from bone; and functions to maintain muscle strength and prevent contractures and fractures.<br>○ Providing a quiet, safe environment with frequent rest periods helps to conserve energy. |
| ***Nursing Diagnosis #6*** Skin integrity impaired, potential for, related to:<br>1. Immobilization.<br>2. Altered nutrition. | Patient will:<br>1. Maintain intact skin and mucous membranes. | • Maintain skin integrity.<br>○ Turn and position every 2 hr.<br>– Lubricate skin.<br>○ Initiate pressure relief device (e.g., air mattress).<br>○ Assess nutritional status.<br>○ Assess pressure area at planned intervals to determine status.<br>○ Perform local site care as per unit protocol and/or physician's orders. | ○ Reddened areas that do not blanch within 20–30 min of position change dictate that the position be avoided, or the duration in that position be reduced. |
| ***Nursing Diagnosis #7*** Potential for injury: Thrombophlebitis, related to:<br>1. Immobilization. | Patient will:<br>1. Remain without evidence of thrombophlebitis:<br>• Increased calf/thigh circumference.<br>• Pain upon dorsiflexion of foot.<br>• Absence of redness or swelling of extremities. | • Establish precautions related to thrombus formation and thrombophlebitis.<br>○ Apply anti-embolic stockings.<br>○ Assess for redness, pain, and swelling of calves; measure circumference of extremity.<br>○ Perform range-of-motion exercises as above. | • Immobility contributes to venous stasis and increases risk of thromboembolic disease.<br>○ Provides a measure to evaluate for presence of thrombophlebitis. |

| | | | |
|---|---|---|---|
| ***Nursing Diagnosis #8***<br>Knowledge deficit regarding followup/ preventive care. | Patient will:<br>1. Verbalize knowledge of underlying disease process and therapy.<br>2. Verbalize understanding of therapeutic regimen:<br>• Medications: Indication, dosage, administration, schedule for taking, potential side effects.<br>• Diet.<br>• Exercise. | • Assess patient/family knowledge regarding disease process and therapy.<br>○ Assess readiness to learn. | • Understanding of underlying disease processes assists the patient/family to cope with, and to adjust to, the limitations imposed by the disease.<br>○ Depending on the underlying causes, hypercalcemia may impact on all members of the family. Interested and supportive family members should be included in the educational process. |
| | | • Implement teaching program to include the following topics:<br>○ Pertinent anatomy and physiology of calcium metabolism.<br>○ Underlying pathophysiology.<br>○ Identification of precipitating stressors or other factors.<br>○ Recognition of signs and symptoms of the hypercalcemia state.<br>○ Appreciation of the importance of seeking timely assistance when the stressful event occurs, or with the first sign/ symptom of hypercalcemia.<br>○ Understanding of medication regimen for disorders underlying the occurrence of hypercalcemia.<br>– Dosage and administration.<br>– Adverse side effects.<br>○ Understanding the importance of continuous health-care followup.<br>○ Initiation of self-care, health-oriented practices to prevent recurring episodes.<br>○ Nutritional counseling. | |

phosphatemia predisposes to calcium precipitation and decreased renal vitamin D synthesis, thereby indirectly contributing to hypocalcemia.

### Clinical Presentation

The diagnosis of hypocalcemia can be made in the asymptomatic patient on inadvertent detection by routine blood testing; or the patient may demonstrate significant symptomatology. Clinical manifestations are associated with disturbances in neuromuscular function and may include the presence of paresthesias (e.g., numbness and tingling sensations of the hands, feet, tongue, and circumoral areas), which often become pronounced during periods of fatigue. The patient may become irritable and restless with a limited attention span. Enhanced motor neuron excitability underlies observable muscle spasms or twitchings involving the forearm and hand with flexion and abduction of the metacarpal-phalangeal joints across the palm; a similar pattern is demonstrated in the ankle and foot (carpopedal spasm). Tetany is manifested initially by muscle cramps and then by carpopedal spasm. Tonic-clonic seizures are not uncommon, and the occurrence of bronchospasm and laryngospasm may rapidly precipitate respiratory arrest.

Characteristic diagnostic signs of tetany may be demonstrated by Chvostek's sign, that is, a twitching of the ipsilateral facial muscles and upper lip elicited by a brisk tap over the facial nerve in front of the ear; and Trousseau's sign, which is elicited by inflating a blood pressure cuff to just above systolic pressure for a 3-minute period. A positive response consists of paresthesias followed by tetany in the occluded extremity. Cardiac dysrhythmias, decrease in cardiac contractility, and an insensitivity to beta-adrenergic agonists may occur. The ECG may be normal, or it may demonstrate a prolongation of the QT interval and ST segment. The occurrence of vomiting, diarrhea, paralytic ileus, abdominal pain, tenderness, and distention reflects the effect of the hypocalcemia on gastrointestinal function.

### Treatment

Acute symptomatic hypocalcemia (<7.0 mg/100 ml) of any cause must be treated aggressively with intravenous calcium because of the immediate danger of seizures, laryngospasm, and respiratory and cardiac arrests. Emergent treatment includes 10–20 ml of 10% calcium gluconate administered intravenously, not to exceed 0.5 ml/minute. Subsequent calcium may need to be supplied by a slow intravenous infusion while the threat of tetany remains. Oral calcium supplementation can commence as soon as necessary requirements can be tolerated. Caution must be observed in patients taking digitalis because calcium's inotropic effects can potentiate the action of digitalis and precipitate digitalis toxicity.[4]

The salient clinical features of hypercalcemia and hypocalcemia are contrasted in Table 24–4. Specifically, differences in underlying pathophysiology, etiologies, diagnostic findings, clinical presentations, and treatment are addressed.

### Nursing Care of the Patient with Hypocalcemia

The critical care nurse collaborates with other health-care providers to implement a therapeutic regimen to restore serum calcium levels to within the normal physiologic range. In patients with hypocalcemia, aggressive calcium replacement therapy is often required to attain an asymptomatic serum calcium level with absence of neuromuscular and cardiac alterations. Meticulous monitoring of cardiac rate, rhythm, and output is essential because hypocalcemia weakens myocardial contractility and can predispose to heart failure and cardiac arrest.

To prevent exacerbation of neuronal excitability and irritability associated with hypocalcemia, nursing measures should be implemented to minimize neurologic and neuromuscular stimulation. A cool, quiet environment should be maintained with limited stressors and avoidance of drafts, bright lights, and sudden noises. Seizure precautions should be initiated, and equipment necessary for insertion of an artificial airway should be available at the patient's bedside because the hypocalcemic state increases the risk of laryngo-bronchospasm. Laryngeal stridor and wheezing reflect a compromised airway (see Chap. 29). The patient's breathing pattern must be monitored closely. Hyperventilation, for example, induces an alkalemia, which, because of increased serum protein binding of calcium, may cause a further decrease in free, ionized serum calcium levels.

A major nursing concern is the monitoring and maintenance of fluid and electrolyte balance. Alterations in serum electrolytes can exacerbate neuromuscular irritability. Serum calcium and phosphorus levels are monitored closely because there is a reciprocal relationship between serum levels of these two elements. When one is elevated, the other is usually low. The presence of hypophosphatemia requires replacement therapy prior to the administration of calcium. Hypophosphatemia induces increased renal synthesis of 1,25-dihydroxycholecalciferol, which increases intestinal absorption of both calcium and phosphate. Hyperphosphatemia, attributed to phosphate therapy or reduced renal excretion, may be associated with hypocalcemia and deposition of calcium in bone and soft tissues.

In conjunction with the monitoring of serum calcium levels, it is essential to monitor total serum protein. Approximately 45–50% of serum calcium is protein-bound. An increase in serum protein re-

TABLE 24–4
**Contrast: Hypercalcemia and Hypocalcemia**

| | Hypercalcemia | Hypocalcemia |
|---|---|---|
| Definition | Hypercalcemia is defined as an increase in total serum calcium above 10.5 mg/100 ml.<br>Symptomatic hypercalcemia may occur when total serum calcium levels exceed 11.0–12.0 mg/100 ml. | Hypocalcemia is defined as a decrease in total serum calcium below 8.5 mg/100 ml.<br>Symptomatic hypocalcemia may occur when serum calcium levels drop below 7.0–7.5 mg/100 ml. |
| Major concern | Progressive suppression of cardiac function by abnormally high levels of free, ionized serum calcium. | Increased neuromuscular excitability is caused by increased neuronal membrane irritability.<br>Enhanced excitability of nerve fibers causes them to discharge spontaneously and rapidly, generating impulses that pass to neuromuscular junctions (skeletal muscle) where they elicit tetanic contractions. |
| Pathophysiology | Underlying pathophysiologic basis may reflect:<br>A. Abnormal calcium input into the circulation.<br>B. A decreased removal or output of calcium from the circulation.<br>Increased resorption of calcium from bone:<br>A. Hyperparathyroidism.<br>B. Immobilization.<br>C. Hyperthyroidism (Graves' disease).<br>Abnormally large dietary intake of calcium and/or excessive intake of vitamin D.<br>Altered renal tubular reabsorption of calcium.<br>Hypercalcemia may also reflect an increase in free, ionized calcium. Because approximately one half of total serum calcium is bound to serum proteins, factors affecting the amount of protein-bound calcium must be considered.<br>A. Dehydration increases serum protein concentration, which may reflect an increase in total serum calcium without an increase in the free, ionized fraction.<br>B. Acidemia decreases the amount of protein-bound calcium resulting in an increase in its free, ionized fraction. | Underlying pathophysiologic basis may reflect:<br>A. Inadequate calcium input into circulation<br>B. Excessive losses of calcium.<br>Excessive losses of calcium:<br>A. Gastrointestinal disorders—Diarrhea.<br>B. Secondary to diuretics.<br>C. Increased lipoprotein levels.<br>Inadequate intake:<br>A. Malabsorption syndromes—Vitamin D deficiency. |
| Etiology | Primary hyperparathyroidism associated with benign adenoma and resulting in increased tubular reabsorption of calcium.<br>Malignancy (metastatic carcinoma), which releases calcium into circulation.<br>Prolonged immobilization, resulting in increased resorption of calcium from bone, teeth.<br><br><br><br><br>Alkalemia increases calcium binding to protein, which decreases free, ionized serum levels; potent stimulus for PTH release, with resulting increase in serum calcium.<br>Excessive administration of vitamin D resulting in increased intestinal calcium absorption.<br>Hypophosphatemia.<br>Hyperthyroid crisis.<br>Longstanding thiazide diuretic therapy.<br>Renal tubular acidosis.<br>Use of sex hormonal therapy in the treatment of disseminated breast cancer is known to precipitate acute hypercalcemia.<br>Acidemia: Aggressive correction of acidemia may reveal an underlying hypocalcemia. | Most frequently encountered in patients following removal of, or damage to, parathyroid glands during neck surgery; hypoparathyroidism may occur within 2 days following surgery.<br>Malignancy:<br>A. Osteoblastic metastasis depletes calcium stores due to abnormal bone formation.<br>B. Thyroid carcinoma with abnormal secretion of calcitonin stimulates osteoblastic activity.<br>Alkalemia may independently increase neuronal excitability; patients with chronic hypocalcemia may develop tetany if they become alkalotic.<br>Alkalosis due to vomiting, alkali ingestion, or hyperventilation may precipitate asymptomatic hypocalcemia.<br>Chronic renal failure:<br>A. Hyperphosphatemia precipitates peripheral deposition of calcium phosphate salts in soft tissues.<br>B. Vitamin D resistance caused by alterations in Vitamin D—Mediated intestinal calcium absorption.<br>C. Vitamin D deficiency states resulting from inadequate metabolism of vitamin D prohormones to active metabolites due to chronic hepatic and renal failure. |

*(continued)*

TABLE 24–4

## Contrast: Hypercalcemia and Hypocalcemia *(Continued)*

| | Hypercalcemia | Hypocalcemia |
|---|---|---|
| | | Chronic malabsorption states associated with:<br>• Gastrectomy<br>• High fat diet: Fat impairs intestinal calcium absorption<br>• Small bowel disorders with inability to absorb dietary sources of vitamin D (prohormone)<br>Hypomagnesemia: Inhibits PTH secretion and use; hypomagnesemia must be corrected before normal serum calcium levels can be achieved.<br>Acute pancreatitis with precipitation of calcium in inflamed pancreas, and intra-abdominal lipids.<br>Idiopathic hypoparathyroidism. |
| Diagnostic workup/history | *What is chief complaint?*<br>*History of present illness?*<br>Onset, Course, Current status } General state of health? Easy fatigability: muscle weakness—proximal and lower extremity?<br>Neuromuscular: Headache?<br>Lethargy, drowsiness, paresthesias?<br>Emotional lability, apathy, depression, personality changes?<br>Visual disturbances or photophobia related to calcium deposits in the eye, conjunctivitis?<br>Renal status: Polyuria, kidney infections, renal calculi?<br>Abdominal status: Anorexia, thirst, nausea, vomiting, epigastric distress, abdominal discomfort, constipation?<br>*Past health history? Pertinent family history?*<br>Previous illnesses, hospitalizations? Endocrine illness, obesity? Hyperthyroidism or hypothyroidism? Bone disease? Prolonged immobilization?<br>Tumor or malignancy? Cataracts? Mental retardation?<br>Previous neck surgery and/or irradiation?<br>Previous gastrointestinal surgery: Gastrectomy, small bowel resection? Recent malabsorption syndrome?<br>Nutritional derangements; high fat or protein diets?<br>Recent massive infection?<br>Renal disease? Rickets?<br>Acute pancreatitis?<br>History of alcohol abuse? Associated hypomagnesemia?<br>Recent massive blood transfusions?<br>Current medications?<br>• Anticonvulsants? Antibiotics? Aminoglycosides?<br>• Vitamin D supplements—excessive intake?<br>• Corticosteroid therapy? Chronic thiazide diuretics?<br>• Phosphate binders?<br>• Phenobarbital? Heparin? Cimetidine?<br>• Theophylline? Cytotoxic agents?<br>*Functional health patterns?* (See Appendix C). | Neuromuscular: Tingling or twitching around mouth? Extremities? Evidence of lowered sensory/motor excitability thresholds?<br>Cramping, stiffness, clumsiness?<br>Seizure activity, convulsions?<br>Evidence of autonomic ganglia hyperirritability: Alterations in gastrointestinal functions—nausea/vomiting, diarrhea, abdominal pain? |
| Physical examination (see also section on Clinical Manifestations, below.) | *Neuromuscular status:*<br>*Skeletal:* Pathologic fractures, extraosseous calcifications in soft tissues (hyperparathyroidism).<br>*Ocular/visual status:* Metatastic calcifications with calcium deposition in cornea; band keratopathy.<br>*Cardiovascular considerations:* Increased serum calcium levels can potentiate digoxin effect and predispose to dysrhythmias and/or cardiac arrest. | *Neuromuscular status:*<br>Mild hypocalcemia: muscle spasms, tremors.<br>Severe hypocalcemia: Tetany, grand mal tonic/clonic seizures.<br>*Classic manifestations:* Tetany.<br>Overt tetany may vary from muscle cramps, abdominal cramping, and pain, to laryngospasms and bronchospasms, to grand mal tonic-clonic seizures.<br>Latent tetany detected via:<br>A. Chvostek's sign: Elicited by tapping cheek over facial nerve: observe for twitching of upper lip and facial muscles on the side stimulated. This sign is not specific for hypocalcemia. |

TABLE 24–4
**Contrast: Hypercalcemia and Hypocalcemia *(Continued)***

| | Hypercalcemia | Hypocalcemia |
|---|---|---|
| | | B. Trousseau's sign: Elicited by inflating blood pressure cuff to just above systolic pressure for 3 min. A positive response consists of paresthesias followed by tetany in the occluded extremity. |
| | | *Pulmonary status:* Compromised function related to bronchospasm and airway obstruction:<br>Labored, shallow breathing; hypoventilation; adventitious breath sounds, wheezes; limited thoracic cage movement with involvement of muscles of respiration; use of accessory muscles.<br>Neuromuscular irritability may precipitate laryngeal spasm with airway obstruction and respiratory arrest. |
| | *Gastrointestinal status:* Vomiting; predisposition to peptic ulcer disease due to increased gastric acid secretion in response to elevated calcium.<br>Smooth muscle hypotonicity with inadequate peristalsis, constipation, paralytic ileus, abdominal distention and pain.<br>*Renal status:* Renal calculi may occur with flank pain. | *Gastrointestinal status:* Vomiting, paralytic ileus; abdominal pain and tenderness, distention. |
| Diagnostic studies<br>Serum studies | Serum calcium: 8.5–10.5 mg/100 ml (normal physiologic range).<br>Serum calcium > 10.5 mg/100 ml.<br>Symptomatic > 11.0–12.0 mg/100 ml. | Serum calcium < 8.5 mg/100 ml.<br>Symptomatic < 7.0–7.5 mg/100 ml. |
| Rule-out studies | Specific laboratory tests:<br>Creatinine, BUN = renal function.<br>Liver enzymes, total protein = liver function.<br>Alkaline phosphatase: Evaluate liver and bone isoenzymes.<br>Amylase = pancreatic function.<br>Phosphorus: Hyper- or hypophosphatemia.<br>Magnesium: Hyper- or hypomagnesemia. | Parathyroid hormone (PTH)—Serum levels. This value will help to distinguish hypocalcemia due to PTH deficiency from that due to skeletal resistance. |
| Urine test | Sulkowitch's urine test for calcium | |
| X-ray studies<br>Rule-out studies | Renal calculi.<br>Nephrocalcinosis (i.e., calcium deposition in the renal parenchyma). | Skeletal bone survey to rule out:<br>• Pseudofractures.<br>• Pseudohypoparathyroidism.<br>• Osteomalacia.<br>• Osteoblastic lesions.<br>• Cancer-induced hypocalcemia. |
| ECG studies | Reveals shortened ST segment and QT interval.<br>Dysrhythmias | Reveals prolonged ST segment and QT interval; findings may reflect impaired myocardial contractility, predisposing to cardiac arrest.<br>Dysrhythmias |
| Clinical manifestations | Signs and symptoms of hypercalcemia or hypocalcemia depend on the rapidity of its development, and the extent and duration of the abnormality. Neurologic, cardiac, and renal function are those primarily affected. | |
| Neurologic function | *Mental status:* Lethargy, depression, emotional lability; poor recent memory; stupor, coma (severe).<br>Personality changes depending on duration.<br>Headache, generalized muscle weakness; fatigue; neuromuscular weakness progressing to flaccidity. | *Mental status:* Irritability, restlessness, limited attention span.<br>Acute hypocalcemia: Enhanced motor nerve excitability characterized by: Muscle twitching; neuromuscular irritability; paresthesias, numbness and tingling of extremities, lips and mouth; carpopedal spasm, stridor, seizures, and tetany; the occurrence of bronchospasm and laryngospasm may rapidly precipitate respiratory arrest. |

*(continued)*

TABLE 24–4

**Contrast: Hypercalcemia and Hypocalcemia *(Continued)***

| | Hypercalcemia | Hypocalcemia |
|---|---|---|
| | | Chronic hypocalcemia: Predisposes to changes in integumentary system with pigmented dry, scaly skin, alopecia; and psychiatric complaints ranging from mild depression to clear-cut psychosis. |
| Cardiovascular function | Increase in extracellular calcium levels predisposes to myocardial irritability, dysrhythmias with increased incidence of heart block, and cardiac arrest.<br>Increased peripheral vascular resistance; hypertension. | Major concern: Decrease in cardiac contractility predisposing to cardiac arrest. |
| Renal function | Early clinical manifestations:<br>A. Diminished ability to concentrate urine due to a form of antidiuretic hormone (ADH)-resistance.[5] This causes polydipsia, polyuria, and nocturia.<br>B. With sustained hypercalcemia, glomerular filtration rate is diminished due to hypovolemia and nephrocalcinosis (i.e., calcium deposits in renal parenchyma).<br>There is the potential for nephrolithiasis due to hypercalciuria.<br>Flank and thigh pain may be associated with the presence of calcium calculi in the urinary system. | Hypocalcemia related to PTH resistance may predispose to pathophysiologic defects in the kidney; patients with PTH resistance are believed to have impaired formation of 1,25-$(OH)_2D$. |
| Skeletal function | Deep bone pain: Pathologic fractures. | Prolonged hypocalcemia predisposes to osteoporosis. |
| Gastrointestinal function | Anorexia, weight loss, nausea.<br>Constipation due to dcreased smooth muscle contractility of intestinal wall.<br>Activation of pancreatic enzymes or plugging of pancreatic ducts may predispose to acute pancreatitis. | Diarrhea due to smooth muscle irritability. |
| Integument | Soft tissue calcification. | |
| Eyes | Band keratopathy (i.e., linear deposits of calcium in the cornea). | |
| Treatment | Acute symptomatic hypercalcemia (>12.0 mg/100 ml) requires immediate therapy to prevent life-threatening ventricular dysrhythmias and altered neural excitability and transmission, leading to coma. A combination of approaches to therapy are used and include:[6]<br>A. Forced saline diuresis: Urinary excretion of calcium is linked to that of sodium. Administration of normal saline and furosemide accelerates calcium excretion. Potassium and magnesium depletion may occur and require careful monitoring. Patients with diminished cardiac reserve require close monitoring for signs of congestive heart failure and pulmonary edema. A fluctuating fluid state may require hemodynamic pressure monitoring.<br>B. Mithramycin, a cytotoxic antibiotic, is a potent hypocalcemic agent especially indicated in the treatment of malignancy-related hypercalcemia. One dose is found to normalize the serum calcium of most patients within the first 48 hr. Its calcium-lowering activity is variable, requiring close monitoring of serum calcium levels. Rarely it is associated with toxic effects such as renal/hepatic toxicity; thrombocytopenia. | Acute symptomatic hypocalcemia (<7.0 mg/100 ml) of any cause must be treated aggressively with intravenous calcium because of the immediate danger of seizures, laryngospasm, tetany, respiratory and cardiac arrests.<br>Dosage: Urgent treatment includes:<br>A. 10–20 ml of 10% calcium gluconate intravenously, not to exceed 0.5 ml/min.<br>B. Subsequent calcium may need to be supplied by a slow intravenous infusion while the threat of tetany remains.<br>C. Oral calcium supplementation can commence as soon as necessary requirements can be tolerated.<br>Caution must be exercised in patients taking digitalis because calcium's inotropic effects can potentiate the action of digitalis and precipitate digitalis toxicity.<br>Serum magnesium should be measured and monitored because hypomagnesemia inhibits both the release and action of PTH. Correction of hypomagnesemia can be made with magnesium sulfate, which has a rapid onset of action. The dose administered is magnesium sulfate 1–2 g every 4–6 hr intramuscularly depending on the extent of hypomagnesemia and the clinical status of the patient. |

TABLE 24-4
**Contrast: Hypercalcemia and Hypocalcemia *(Continued)***

| Hypercalcemia | Hypocalcemia |
|---|---|
| C. Glucocorticoids function to decrease intestinal calcium absorption and increase renal excretion. They are especially effective in the treatment of hypercalcemia associated with malignancies and sarcoidosis, the highest success rate being observed in patients with multiple myeloma, lymphosarcoma, and breast cancer. Glucocorticoid therapy is used in conjunction with other therapeutic modalities because its maximum hypocalcemic effect may not be realized for several days.<br>D. Calcitonin therapy is administered concomitantly with glucocorticoid therapy and acts to decrease calcium release from bone while increasing its renal excretion. Its effect is rapid and without significant adverse reactions.<br>E. Phosphate administration may be prescribed for the treatment of hypercalcemia associated with a low to normal serum phosphate.<br>• Short-term glucocorticoid therapy and growth hormone administration increase renal reabsorption of phosphates.<br>• Controversy exists as to whether or not phosphate therapy is appropriate. Administration of phosphates will decrease serum calcium, but such therapy may cause extraosseus calcifications with deposition of calcium in soft tissues including kidney and lung.<br>F. Peritoneal dialysis and hemodialysis efficiently remove calcium and can be used in life-threatening situations.<br>G. Administer $K^+$ and magnesium supplements to prevent depletion of these electrolytes. | Long-term replacement therapy may include: Oral calcium and vitamin D supplements as prescribed. |

duces the free, ionized calcium fraction; a decrease in serum protein increases the free, ionized calcium. For every 1 g/100 ml change in serum albumin, there is a 0.8 mg/100 ml change in total serum calcium.[7]

Fluid and electrolyte monitoring should include serum magnesium levels. Hypomagnesemia decreases PTH release and utilization, aggravating an already hypocalcemic state. (PTH functions to raise serum calcium levels.) The presence of hyperkalemia potentiates myocardinal irritability in the presence of hypocalcemia. When obtaining blood specimens for serum calcium studies, if the tourniquet is left in place too long, the total calcium level may be falsely elevated due to hemoconcentration. Also noteworthy, transfusions of citrated blood may predispose to hypocalcemia due to chelation of circulating calcium.

Additional supportive care measures of concern to nursing in patients with hypocalcemia include nutrition, implementation of a program of progressive mobilization and ambulation, psychological support in coping with the illness, and patient/family education. This information is included in the Care Plan in Table 24-5. Nursing diagnoses, patient outcomes, and nursing interventions in the care of the patient with hypocalcemia are presented.

## TABLE 24–5. CARE PLAN FOR THE PATIENT WITH HYPOCALCEMIA

| Nursing Diagnoses | Desired Patient Outcomes | Nursing Interventions | Rationales |
|---|---|---|---|
| ***Nursing Diagnosis #1***<br>Electrolyte imbalance: Hypocalcemia, related to:<br>1. Alkalemia associated with vomiting, alkali ingestion, or hyperventilation.<br>2. Chronic renal failure with hyperphosphatemia.<br>3. Vitamin D deficiency state.<br>4. Chronic malabsorption state.<br>5. Hypomagnesemia.<br>6. Acute pancreatitis.<br>7. Idiopathic hypoparathyroidism. | Patient's condition will stabilize as follows:<br>1. Neurologic status:<br>• Alert, oriented to person, place, and time.<br>• Absence of muscle spasms or cramping, tremors, seizure activity, or tetany.<br>2. Respiratory status:<br>• Eupnea, unlabored respirations.<br>• Full chest wall excursion.<br>• Absence of adventitious breath sounds: Rales, crackles, wheezes.<br>• Absence of laryngospasm, airway obstruction (bronchospasm).<br>3. Cardiovascular status:<br>• Heart rate >60 <100 beats/min.<br>• Arterial BP within 10 mmHg of patient's baseline.<br>• ECG regular sinus rhythm:<br>ST segment isoelectric.<br>QT interval within normal range.<br>4. Renal status:<br>• Urine output >30 ml/hr (depends on status of renal function).<br>• BUN 8–25 mg/100 ml.<br>• Creatinine 0.6–1.5 mg/100 ml. | • Assess impact of hypocalcemia on physiologic processes:<br>◦ Elicit pertinent aspects of patient/family health history. (See section on Diagnostic Workup in Table 24–4). | ◦ Personal characteristics and state of health play a crucial role in determining the ability of the patient/family to cope with the stress of hypocalcemia and its underlying cause.<br>◦ Unlike *hyper*calcemia where the clinical presentation may be so nonspecific as to require laboratory confirmation, hypocalcemia is characterized by definitive diagnostic findings upon history and physical assessment.<br>◦ Based on these assessment data, a decision must be made as to whether or not the progress of the illness represents an immediate threat to life. |
| | | • Collaborate with other health-care providers to implement therapeutic regimen to restore serum calcium to within physiologic range. | • Therapeutic goal is to raise serum calcium levels to >8.5 mg/100 ml. Reduced serum calcium levels precipitate neuromuscular irritability and seizure activity. |
| | | ◦ Administer calcium replacement therapy: 10–20 ml of 10% calcium gluconate, intravenously, not to exceed 1.5 ml/min. (See section on Treatment in Table 24–4). | ◦ Goal of calcium replacement therapy is to attain an asymptomatic serum calcium level with absence of neuromuscular and cardiac alterations.<br>◦ Calcium gluconate (or calcium chloride) preparation must be administered slowly to avoid high serum calcium concentrations and associated cardiac conduction delays. |
| | | ◦ Use intracath for intravenous administration, and dilute method versus IV push. | ◦ Calcium preparations can cause vein irritation and inflammation; calcium chloride causes tissue necrosis and is associated with an increased incidence of thrombophlebitis. |
| | | ◦ Administer calcium slowly to patients receiving digitalis therapy. | ◦ In patients on digitalis therapy, a rapid infusion of calcium may potentiate digitalis effect and precipitate cardiac dysrhythmias and cardiac arrest.<br>◦ Cardiac monitoring of rate and rhythm must be continuous. |
| | | ◦ Avoid simultaneous administration of calcium and sodium bicarbonate in the same line. | ◦ Calcium will precipitate in an alkaline solution. |

| | | |
|---|---|---|
| 5. Serum studies:<br>• Calcium 8.5–10.5 mg/100 ml.<br>• Phosphorus 3.0–4.5 mg/100 ml.<br>• Sodium 135–148 mEq/liter.<br>• Potassium 3.5–5.5 mEq/liter.<br>• Magnesium 1.5–2.0 mEq/liter.<br>• Proteins (total) 6.0–8.4 g/100 ml. | ◦ Avoid use of saline for infusions. | ◦ Saline increases calcium excretion by the kidneys. |
| | ◦ Monitor serum calcium, phosphorus, and total protein. | ◦ Monitoring of serum values assists in evaluating effectiveness of therapeutic plan. (See fluid and electrolyte interventions, below.) |
| | ◦ Monitor 24-hr urine for calcium as total body calcium approaches an equilibrated physiologic state. | ◦ It is important to monitor total body calcium to prevent the occurrence of a hypercalcemic state. |
| | ◦ Administer vitamin D or its active metabolites:<br>◦ Monitor for hypercalciuria.<br>– Monitor serum calcium levels closely to prevent hypercalcemia. | ◦ Vitamin D preparations increase intestinal calcium absorption.<br>◦ Hypercalciuria and associated calculus formation may occur with doses of vitamin D sufficient to relieve tetany and normalize serum levels of calcium. |
| | ◦ Correct hypomagnesemia if present: Magnesium sulfate 1–2 g every 4–6 hr intramuscularly depending on state of hypomagnesemia. | ◦ Magnesium deficit may inhibit PTH release and utilization. |
| | ◦ Initiate efforts to determine and treat underlying cause of hypocalcemic state: | ◦ Treatment of underlying cause should be initiated once the acute phase is under control. |
| | • Consider nursing implications related to the care of the patient with hypocalcemia.<br>◦ Identify patients at risk of developing seizures.<br>◦ Assess neurologic status: Mental status and level of consciousness; status of cranial nerve function; presence of hyperreflexia. | ◦ Establish baseline data with which subsequent assessment can be compared. |
| | ◦ Presence of:<br>◦ Chvostek's sign | ◦ Chvostek's sign is not specific for evaluating the effect of the hypocalcemic state on neuromuscular function because it is present in approximately 10% of normal individuals. |
| | ◦ Trousseau's sign | ◦ Trousseau's sign can be helpful in evaluating the patient's response to therapy. |
| | ◦ Implement measures to minimize neurologic and neuromuscular stimulation:<br>◦ Maintain cool, quiet environment; limit stressors; avoid drafts, bright lights, and sudden noise or movements. | ◦ Reduction in stimuli helps to prevent exacerbation of neuromuscular hyperexcitable and hyperirritable state; reduces risk of seizure activity and tetany. |
| | ◦ Institute seizure precautions:<br>◦ Maintain at bedside: Suction, oral pharyngeal airway, oxygen source and access.<br>– Emergency drugs and equipment: Anticonvulsants; Valium. | |

(continued)

**TABLE 24–5. CARE PLAN FOR THE PATIENT WITH HYPOCALCEMIA *(Continued)***

| Nursing Diagnoses | Desired Patient Outcomes | Nursing Interventions | Rationales |
|---|---|---|---|
| ***Nursing Diagnosis #1 (cont.)*** | | | |
| | | ∘ Tracheostomy set, endotracheal airways.<br>∘ Side rails padded and maintained in up position; bed in lowest position; call light accessible to patient. | ∘ Hypocalcemic state increases risk of laryngo-bronchospasm. |
| | | ∘ Monitor (record) seizure activity: Precipitating event? How initiated? Part of body involved? Unilateral or bilateral? Level of consciousness? Pupillary size and reactivity? Urinary/bowel incontinence? | |
| | | ∘ Protect patient from injury during seizure.<br>∘ Turn on side if possible. | ∘ Reduces risk of aspiration of airway obstruction from tongue falling to back of throat. |
| | | ∘ Implement measures to maintain effective respiratory function. | |
| | | ∘ Assess for and anticipate bronchospasm: Respiratory rate, rhythm; dyspnea, tachypnea; use of accessory muscles; auscultate all lung fields. | ∘ The hypocalcemic state increases sensitivity and excitability of laryngeal and bronchial musculature placing patient at risk of developing laryngo-bronchospasms. |
| | | ∘ Assess effctiveness of cough and handling of secretions.<br>– Monitor pulmonary function: Tidal volume; vital capacity. | ∘ Laryngeal stridor and wheezing reflect a compromised airway. |
| | | ∘ Monitor for hyperventilation associated with stress. | ∘ Hyperventilation induces an alkalemia. |
| | | ∘ Evaluate arterial blood gases and implement measures to correct:<br>∘ Alkalemia (pH >7.45). | ∘ Alkalemia increases serum protein-binding of calcium, causing a further drop in free, ionized calcium levels, which may precipitate tetany. |
| | | ∘ Acidemia (pH <7.35). | ∘ Acidemia decreases serum protein-binding of calcium, causing an increase in levels of free, ionized calcium.<br>– When correcting the acidemic state, monitor for signs of hypocalcemia because as the pH rises toward alkalemia, more calcium becomes protein-bound, reducing levels of free, ionized calcium. |

| | |
|---|---|
| ○ Maintain effective cardiovascular function:<br>○ Assess the effect of heightened neuromuscular activity on cardiac function.<br>– Monitor all vital signs: Temperature, heart rate, blood pressure; hemodynamic parameters if indicated: pulmonary artery pressure (PAP); pulmonary capillary wedge pressure (PCWP); cardiac output.<br>– Continuous cardiac monitoring of rate and rhythm. | ○ Symptomatic hypocalcemia weakens myocardial contractility; impaired myocardial contractility can predispose to heart failure and cardiac arrest. |
| ○ Implement measures to maintain fluid and electrolyte balance:<br>○ Correlate serum electrolytes with clinical status:<br>○ Follow serum calcium and phosphorus. | ○ Alterations in serum electrolytes can exacerbate neuromuscular irritability.<br>○ There is a natural reciprocal relationship between serum levels of calcium and phosphorus: When one is elevated, the other is usually low.<br>– The presence of hypophosphatemia requires replacement therapy prior to administration of calcium.<br>– Hypophosphatemia induces increased renal synthesis of 1,25-$(OH)_2D$, which increases intestinal absorption of both calcium and phosphate.<br>– Hyperphosphatemia attributed to phosphate therapy or reduced renal excretion may be associated with hypocalcemia and deposition of calcium in bone and soft tissues. |
| ○ Monitor total serum protein. | ○ Approximately 45–50% of serum calcium is protein-bound. |
| ○ Monitor serum magnesium levels. | ○ Hypomagnesemia decreases PTH release and utilization, aggravating an already hypocalcemic state. (PTH functions to raise serum calcium levels.) |
| ○ Monitor serum potassium. | ○ Hyperkalemia potentiates myocardial irritability in the presence of hypocalcemia.<br>– If the tourniquet is left in place too long when obtaining blood specimens for serum calcium studies, the total calcium level may be falsely elevated due to hemoconcentration.<br>– Transfusions of citrated blood may predispose to hypocalcemia due to chelation |

**TABLE 24–5. CARE PLAN FOR THE PATIENT WITH HYPOCALCEMIA *(Continued)***

| Nursing Diagnoses | Desired Patient Outcomes | Nursing Interventions | Rationales |
|---|---|---|---|
| ***Nursing Diagnosis #1 (cont.)*** | | ◦ Assess for signs and symptoms of altered fluid state.<br>– Monitor intake and output; daily weight; serum osmolality and urine specific gravity; serum electrolytes; hematocrit and hemoglobin. | of circulating calcium.<br>◦ Dehydration may accompany disturbances in gastrointestinal function (e.g., vomiting, diarrhea); hemoconcentration or hemodilution may predispose to an electrolyte imbalance. |
| ***Nursing Diagnosis #2***<br>Injury, potential for: Trauma, related to:<br>1. Seizure activity associated with hypocalcemia. | Patient will:<br>1. Remain seizure-free and injury-free.<br>2. Maintain serum calcium levels: 8.5–10.5 mg/100 ml.<br>3. Verbalize understanding of potential for seizure activity and necessary safety precautions. | • Perform injury-potential assessment of patient's immediate environment.<br>• Minimize neurologic and neuromuscular stimulation.<br>• Institute seizure precautions.<br>• Instruct patient/family regarding potential for seizure activity and necessary precautions to be taken to prevent injury. | • Environmental assessment helps to reduce risk of injury by removal of potentially hazardous objects.<br>• Refer to nursing interventions listed under Nursing Diagnosis #1, above. |
| ***Nursing Diagnosis #3***<br>Nutrition, alteration in: Less than body requirements (calcium intake), related to:<br>1. Malabsorption syndrome (e.g., vitamin D deficiency).<br>2. Increased lipoprotein levels.<br>Nutrition, alteration in: Less than body requirements (calcium loss), related to:<br>1. Gastrointestinal disorders: diarrhea.<br>2. Secondary to diuretics. | Patient will:<br>1. Maintain adequate nutritional status:<br>• Body weight within 5% of baseline for patient.<br>• Serum proteins within acceptable range.<br>• Serum electrolytes within acceptable range.<br>• Hematology profile stable.<br>2. Demonstrate increased strength and activity tolerance.<br>3. Remain without signs of infection. | • Provide nutritional and supportive care:<br>◦ Assess nutritional needs: Dietary habits of patient/family; attitudes regarding nutrition.<br>◦ Nutritional needs of hypocalcemic state: Low-phosphorus and high-calcium diet.<br>◦ Perform an abdominal assessment: Presence of bowel signs; evidence of tenderness, abdominal distention.<br>• Collaborate with nutritionist to incorporate dietary instructions in overall patient/family education.<br>• Assist patient/family to coordinate medication around dietary intake.<br>• Establish a progressive exercise program tolerated by patient.<br>◦ Begin with passive range of motion exercises with progression in activity as tolerated. | ◦ Bowel hyperactivity associated with hypocalcemia may predispose to diarrhea; bowel hypoactivity is associated with hypercalcemic state.<br>• Oral calcium supplements should be taken to decrease gastrointestinal upsets; oral calcium supplements should not be taken with dairy products because the phosphorus content of these foods will decrease intestinal calcium absorption by causing calcium to precipitate in the intestinal tract and be excreted in the feces.<br>• Immobilization increases calcium resorption from bone.<br>◦ Gentle handling and positioning reduce muscle spasms; reassuring and relaxing approach reduces unnecessary stimuli. |

| | | | |
|---|---|---|---|
| ***Nursing Diagnosis #4***<br>Coping, ineffective: Individual. | Patient will:<br>1. Express willingness to participate in self-care activities.<br>2. Identify prior effective coping mechanisms (individual and/or familial).<br>3. Verbalize feelings of self-confidence. | • Assess psychologic status of patient/family.<br>○ Identify prior coping mechanisms; familial and community resources.<br>• Implement measures to assist patient/family in coping.<br>○ Explain all ongoing procedures and reasons for care.<br>○ Encourage verbalization of fears, questions, concerns.<br>• Be accessible to patient/family. | • Patient/family should be encouraged to participate in self-care.<br>○ Appropriate explanations may help to alleviate heightened anxiety.<br>○ The occurrence of tetany or seizures is a frightening experience for patient/family. |
| ***Nursing Diagnosis #5***<br>Knowledge deficit regarding followup/preventive care. | Patient/family will:<br>1. Verbalize knowledge of underlying disease process.<br>2. Verbalize understanding of therapeutic regimen:<br>• Medications: Indications, dosage, and administration, potential side effects.<br>• Diet.<br>• Exercise. | • Provide patient/family education to assist in developing and implementing prophylactic health-care practices.<br>○ Assess patient/family knowledge of the disease process and therapy.<br>○ Assess readiness to learn.<br>• Implement teaching program to include the following:<br>○ Pertinent anatomy and physiology of calcium metabolism.<br>○ Pertinent underlying pathophysiology.<br>○ Identification of precipitating stressors.<br>○ Recognition of signs/symptoms of hypocalcemic state (tetany).<br>○ Appreciation of the significance of seeking timely assistance when stressful event(s) occur, or with the first signs/symptoms of hypocalcemia.<br>○ Knowledge of medical regimen for the disorder underlying the hypocalcemia.<br>○ Knowledge of medication regimen: Dosage and administration; adverse side effects.<br>○ Understanding importance of continuous health-care followup.<br>○ Initiation of self-care, health-oriented practices to prevent reoccurring episodes.<br>○ Nutritional counseling. | ○ Understanding of underlying disease processes assists the patient/family to cope with, and to adjust to, the limitations imposed by the disease.<br>○ Hypocalcemia and its underlying course impact on all members of the family; interested and supportive family members should be included in the educational process. |

## REFERENCES

1. Guyton, A: Textbook of Medical Physiology, ed. 7. WB Saunders, Philadelphia, 1986, p 881.
2. Ayres, S, Schlichtig, R, and Sterling, M: Care of the Critically Ill, ed. 3. Year Book Medical Publishers, Chicago, 1988, p 17.
3. Hershman, JM: Endocrine Pathophysiology, A Patient-Oriented Approach, ed. 3. Lea & Febiger, Philadelphia, 1988.
4. Metheny, N: Fluid and Electrolyte Balance, Nursing Considertions. JB Lippincott, Philadelphia, 1987, p 80.
5. Griffin, JE: Manual of Clinical Endocrinology and Metabolism. McGraw-Hill, New York, 1982, p 178.
6. Metz, R and Larsen, E: Blue Book of Endocrinology. WB Saunders, Philadelphia, 1985, p 350.
7. Ayres, S, Schlichtig, R, and Sterling, M: Care of the Critically Ill, ed. 3. Year Book Medical Publishers, Chicago, 1988, p 306.

CHAPTER 25

# Nursing Management of the Patient with Acute Renal Failure

## CHAPTER OUTLINE



## LEARNING OBJECTIVES

**At the end of this chapter, you should be able to:**

1. Define *azotemia* and *acute renal failure*.
2. Differentiate categories of acute renal failure: prerenal, postrenal, and intrarenal failure.
3. Describe the etiologic and pathophysiologic mechanisms underlying acute renal failure.
4. Differentiate the phases of acute renal failure: Initial, oliguric, diuretic, and recovery, and their clinical presentation.
5. List specific clinical data and diagnostic findings associated with acute renal failure.
6. Specify the major complications of acute renal failure.
7. State the therapeutic interventions used in the treatment of acute renal failure: Conservative (medical) therapy, dialysis therapy (peritoneal and hemodialysis), and continuous arteriovenous hemofiltration.
8. Delineate the nursing process in the care of the patient with acute renal failure:
   Assessment.
   Nursing diagnosis.
   Planning: Desired patient outcomes
   Nursing interventions.

## INTRODUCTION

Acute renal failure (ARF) is defined as an acute deterioration in renal function characterized by a progressive retention of nitrogenous waste (azotemia), with or without oliguria. It may occur over hours, or within several days of an acute insult. The toxic condition that evolves from renal insufficiency is termed *uremia*. While the advent of dialysis has dramatically reduced the number of deaths attributed to uremia, nevertheless, this syndrome, with its multitude of devastating complications, still has a high mortality rate. Early recognition and management of ARF in the critically ill patient are of crucial importance. The severity and duration of failure and the ultimate degree of recovery depend largely on timely institution of appropriate therapy. A determination of etiology and an understanding of underlying pathophysiologic mechanisms are essential.

## CLASSIFICATION OF ACUTE RENAL FAILURE

There are three categories of ARF, based largely on etiology and pathogenesis. These include prerenal, postrenal, and intrarenal (parenchymal) azotemia. The pathophysiology of the first two involves *extra*renal mechanisms, while that of the third category involves renal parenchymal tissue or *intra*renal mechanisms.

Clinically, a continuum exists between prerenal and intrarenal pathophysiology. A prerenal azotemia caused by renal hypoperfusion may evolve into an intrarenal vascular nephropathy or ischemic acute tubular necrosis (ATN). Thus, prompt recognition and timely intervention are critical: (1) to halt the progression of a prerenal azotemia to a full-blown intrarenal insult; and (2) should this course of events occur, to minimize the severity and duration of the insult to overall renal function.

### Prerenal Azotemia

Prerenal disorders are characterized by renal hypoperfusion without renal tubular damage. Prerenal azotemia is probably the most common type of ARF. Its overall pathophysiology involves a decreased renal blood flow or renal hypoperfusion, which predisposes the patient to a decrease in the glomerular filtration rate (GFR), and ultimately, oliguria. Depending on the severity and duration of the reduced renal perfusion, the condition can rapidly progress to ischemic tubular necrosis with irreversible renal damage.

Causes of prerenal failure include hypovolemia, a severely depleted ECF volume (i.e., severe dehydration) associated with gastrointestinal fluid losses (e.g., bleeding, vomiting, diarrhea, nasogastric suctioning, or wound drainage); urinary losses, such as those related to overly aggressive diuretic therapy without adequate rehydration; fluid loss by way of the skin as in burns, or profuse diaphoresis associated with hyperpyrexia; and "third-spacing" of extracellular fluid. Sepsis may cause a relative hypovolemia as a result of its acute vasodilation of peripheral vasculature causing blood to pool in the extremities and decreasing venous return to the heart. Hypoalbuminemia, which disrupts colloidal osmotic pressure gradients between the intravascular and interstitial fluid spaces, results in loss of intravascular fluid volume (i.e., the circulating blood volume) and in edema formation.

Renal hypoperfusion may also be caused by hemorrhage associated with trauma or surgery. A mild hemorrhagic shock state occurs with a loss of 15–25% of total circulating blood volume, or ~1200 ml; a blood loss of 25–35%, or 1200–1700 ml, results in severe hemorrhagic shock.

In each of these examples cited, the major factor contributing to renal hypoperfusion is a decrease in cardiac output associated with a reduced circulating blood volume and a diminished venous return. Because renal blood flow consists of approximately 25% of the cardiac output each minute, any reduction in renal perfusion that exceeds the autoregulatory and compensatory capabilities of the kidneys results in decreased renal perfusion with a consequent fall in the GFR. (See section entitled "Renal Hemodynamics" in Chap. 21.) This leads to oliguria and a progressive increase in blood urea nitrogen (BUN) and serum creatinine.

A decrease in cardiac output underlying renal hypoperfusion can also be associated with cardiac insufficiency. Whether there is longstanding congestive heart failure, for example, or cardiogenic shock associated with myocardial infarction or cardiac surgery, the reduction in cardiac output results in renal hypoperfusion with compromise of renal function. This may be reflected clinically by sodium and water retention, with or without oliguria, and a potential progressive rise in BUN and serum creatinine.

### Postrenal Azotemia

Postrenal azotemia is most commonly associated with obstructive uropathy, that is, obstruction of the urinary collecting system at any point along its course. Blood clots, calculi, tumors, and prostatic hypertrophy are all implicated in the pathophysiology underlying postrenal azotemia. Whether the obstruction is partial or complete, the impediment to urine outflow through the urinary system results in a retrograde or "back-up" pressure involving both kidneys and predisposing to nephron dysfunction.

## Intrarenal (Parenchymal) Azotemia

Intrarenal disorders are characterized by renal parenchymal pathology involving the renal cortex and medulla. Intrarenal cortical involvement is associated with infectious, immunologic, or vascular disease processes. Acute glomerulonephritis (poststreptococcal infection) reflects glomerular pathology associated with type III immune responses. Circulating immune (antigen–antibody) complexes function to plug up the filtration slit pores within the glomerular-capsular membrane (Fig. 25–1). This precipitates an inflammatory process, which ultimately results in impairment of the glomerular filtration mechanism. (See section entitled "Effector Mechanisms" in Chap. 54.)

Profound disturbances in glomerular function are associated with other types of immune responses. Goodpasture's syndrome, for example, involves a type II cytotoxic humoral reaction wherein antibodies are directed against the glomerular-capsular basement membrane. The autoimmune phenomenon that occurs in systemic lupus erythematosus has also been implicated in the etiology of glomerulonephritis. Cortical involvement is also associated with disorders of vascular origin, including vasculitis of renal blood vessels related to Wegener's granulomatosis and postpartum cortical necrosis.[1]

Renal medullary involvement is characterized by renal tubular pathology. Acute tubular necrosis is the most common type of acute renal failure and may be the result of ischemic or nephrotoxic injury (e.g., papillary necrosis).[2]

Ischemic ARF is usually attributed to an altered hemodynamic state often associated with hypovolemic or hemorrhagic shock, septic shock, or major surgery. As many as 50% of all cases of ischemic ARF occur after high-risk surgery, as, for example, repair of abdominal aortic aneurysm, extensive bowel or biliary surgery, or open heart surgery. Hemodynamic alterations reflect preoperative hypovolemia, intraoperative fluid losses, and the effects of stress, anesthesia, and morphine on antidiuretic hormone secretion and total body water balance. An increased sensitivity to, and elevated levels of, circulating catecholamines may be an additional contributing factor in ischemic ARF.

Nephrotoxic ARF occurs after exposure to a nephrotoxic agent and is frequently exacerbated by a dehydrated state. Nephrotoxic drugs are particularly implicated in acute tubular necrosis. Certain antibiotics, including aminoglycosides, cephalosporins, and tetracyclines, are direct tubular toxins, and the toxicity is dose-related. Penicillins have been reported to cause an acute allergic interstitial nephritis and have been encountered in glomerulonephritis, nephrotic syndrome, or tubular basement membrane disease. Thiazide diuretics have also been identified with acute allergic interstitial nephritis.

Iodinated contrast media have been implicated in renal disease, both as direct tubular toxins and obstructive crystalluria. Patients with preexisting renal insufficiency, renal hypoperfusion associated with a hypovolemic state, congestive heart failure, diabetes mellitus, multiple myeloma, or patients who have had recent iodinated contrast studies, are at increased risk of developing a contrast media-induced ARF.[3] Ingestion of heavy metals, such as

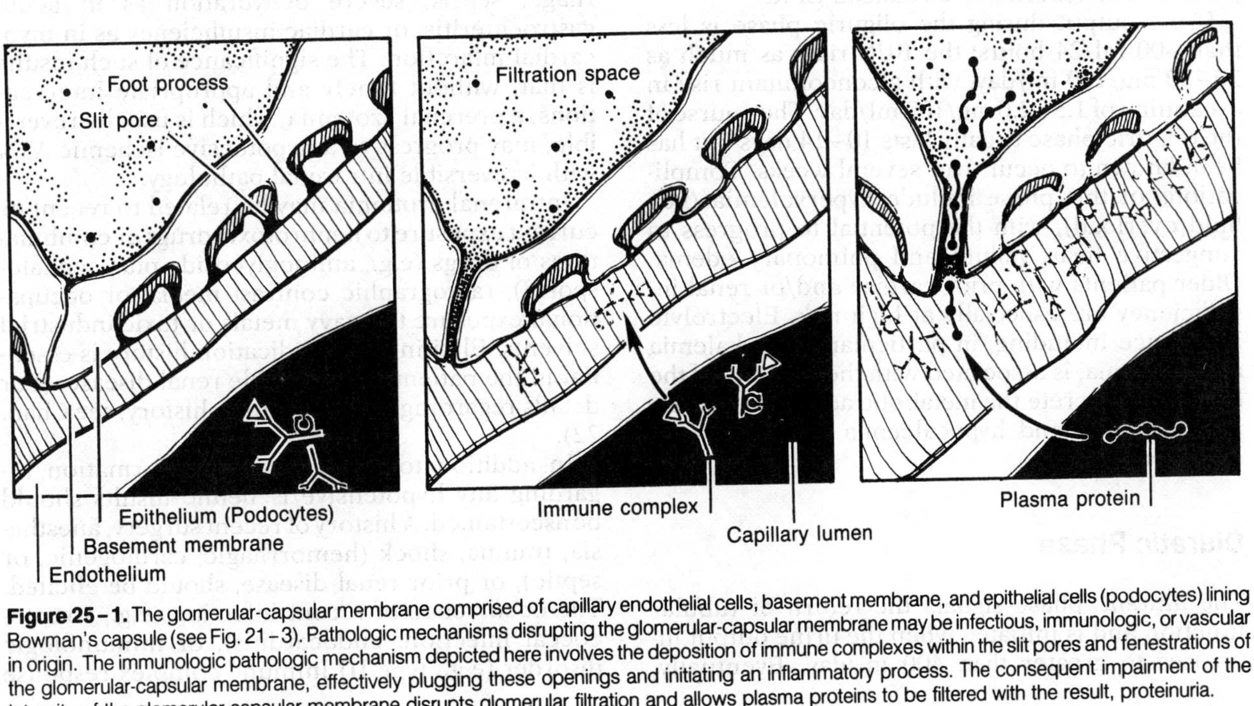


**Figure 25–1.** The glomerular-capsular membrane comprised of capillary endothelial cells, basement membrane, and epithelial cells (podocytes) lining Bowman's capsule (see Fig. 21–3). Pathologic mechanisms disrupting the glomerular-capsular membrane may be infectious, immunologic, or vascular in origin. The immunologic pathologic mechanism depicted here involves the deposition of immune complexes within the slit pores and fenestrations of the glomerular-capsular membrane, effectively plugging these openings and initiating an inflammatory process. The consequent impairment of the integrity of the glomerular-capsular membrane disrupts glomerular filtration and allows plasma proteins to be filtered with the result, proteinuria.

lead, arsenic, or mercury, or exposure to pesticides and fungicides constitute other sources of nephrotoxins. Thorough history-gathering assists in identifying patients at risk of developing nephrotoxic ARF.

## PHASES OF ACUTE RENAL FAILURE

The clinical course of oliguric ARF can be divided into four phases: onset or initial phase, oliguric, diuretic, and recovery phases.

### Initial Phase

The *initial* phase precedes the actual injury process and is associated with disruption of renal hemodynamics. A decrease in cardiac output largely accounts for the altered renal blood flow. Renal perfusion is further compromised by an increase in sympathetic nervous system activity in response to baroreceptor stimulation caused by a fall in blood pressure (systemic). The vasopressor effects of angiotensin secretion further exaggerate renal vascular resistance with a consequent reduction in overall renal perfusion.

### Oliguric Phase

The *oliguric* phase is present 24–48 hours after the initial insult, although symptoms may not be apparent for several days. A progressive azotemia accompanies the oliguria. During this phase, tubular obstruction and necrosis occur, and vasoconstriction persists, contributing to a reduced GFR.

Urine output during the oliguric phase is less than 400 ml/24 hours; the BUN rises as much as 20–30 mg/100 ml/day, with a concomitant rise in creatinine of 1.5–2.0 mg/100 ml/day. The course of the oliguric phase usually lasts 10–14 days but has been known to occur over several weeks. Complications of this phase include hypervolemia (i.e., fluid overload), with the potential to progress to congestive heart failure and pulmonary edema. Older patients with prior cardiac and/or renal insufficiency are especially at high risk. Electrolyte imbalance including, in particular, hyperkalemia and acidemia, is associated with the inability of the kidneys to excrete the metabolic acid load. Hyperphosphatemia and hypocalcemia are commonly observed.

### Diuretic Phase

The *diuretic* phase signals the return of tubular function and is initiated when the urine output increases to greater than 400 ml/day. Eventually, urine output may reach as much as 3 liters/day, or more. The physiologic mechanism underlying the high urine output involves an osmotic diuresis associated with high levels of urea and the inability of the kidneys to conserve filtered sodium and water.

During the early diuretic stage, which may last for several days, water and sodium are lost in excess of solute, causing the urine to be hypotonic. BUN and serum creatinine may continue to rise; urea clearance and excretion do not keep pace with endogenous urea production. As the diuretic phase evolves, azotemia gradually diminishes, accompanied by improvement in the overall clinical picture.

### Recovery Phase

The *recovery* phase can last from a few days up to a year. During this time, glomerular filtration and the concentrating ability of the kidneys progressively improve. While in many instances recovery of renal function is complete, permanent sequelae, most commonly a reduction in GFR, may persist.

## CLINICAL DATA AND DIAGNOSTIC FINDINGS

### Clinical History

The patient's history may provide clues as to the underlying cause of the renal dysfunction. Such clues may assist in the differential diagnosis. In the case of prerenal azotemia, it is important to determine if the patient experienced a recent *hypotensive* insult attributable to trauma, surgery, hemorrhage, sepsis, severe dehydration as in acute gastroenteritis, or cardiac insufficiency as in myocardial infarction. The significance of such insults is that, without timely and appropriate interventions, a prerenal azotemia, which is usually reversible, may progress to a hypotensive ischemic ATN with irreversible intrarenal pathology.

Intrarenal azotemia may be related to recent or current exposure to nephrotoxic drugs or combinations of drugs (e.g., aminoglycoside plus cephalosporin), radiographic contrast media, or occupational exposure to heavy metals or toxic industrial solvents. Eliciting the medication history is essential in the patient with possible renal disease. (For details regarding the medication history, see Chap. 22).

In addition to nephrotoxicity, information regarding any hypotensive/ischemic insults should be ascertained. A history of recent surgery, anesthesia, trauma, shock (hemorrhagic, cardiogenic, or septic), or prior renal disease, should be elicited. The occurrence of recent infection (e.g., streptococcal infection, endocarditis), or immunologic disorder (e.g., type III immune complex response as in acute glomerulonephritis or an autoimmune phenomenon such as systemic lupus erythematosus) is significant in patients who have, or are suspected of having, renal disease or dysfunction.

Historical data of potential significance in postrenal azotemia include, among others, the presence of prostatic disease, bladder malignancy, recent pelvic surgery, and history of renal calculi. A familial history of renal calculi is particularly significant because there is a tendency for such disorders to recur in some families. A history of episodic, often unbearable, flank pain is highly suggestive of renal calculous disease.

An oliguria that progresses to total anuria (i.e., urine output <50 ml/24 hours) suggests the possible presence of an underlying obstructive uropathy. While anuria can occur with oliguric ATN, more often, urine output in prerenal and intrarenal azotemia is characteristically between 400 and 700 ml/24 hours. However, postrenal azotemia should be ruled out in all cases of ARF. (For a detailed discussion of the components of the clinical history, including the cardinal signs/symptoms of renal/urinary dysfunction, and the functional health patterns, see Chap. 22)

## Physical Examination

Clues discovered during history-taking are followed up during the physical examination. A thorough history and meticulous physical examination are essential to differential diagnosis of renal disease. The kidneys function to maintain and regulate the composition of all body fluids; consequently, renal/urinary disease may impact on all organ systems of the body. These include cardiovascular, respiratory, renal/urinary, gastrointestinal, hematologic, musculoskeletal, neurologic, and integumentary systems. The patient's psychologic status is disrupted by renal/urinary disease. (For an indepth discussion of the assessment of function of all the major organ systems of the body, and how the impact of renal disease predisposes to dysfunction, see the section entitled "Physical Examination" in Chap. 22. Additional symptomatology reflective of renal disease is included in the section on "Clinical Presentation, below.)

## Laboratory and Diagnostic Studies

Laboratory data contribute conclusively to the differential diagnosis of ARF. When a patient develops an acute oliguria, with or without azotemia, it is imperative to determine whether the underlying insult is prerenal, intrarenal, or postrenal in origin because the treatment in each case is distinctly different. Simple measurements of serum and urine osmolality and a determination of urine sodium usually provide distinctive evidence as to renal function.

To ensure a reliable interpretation of urinary indices, samples of urine should be obtained prior to any therapeutic interventions such as diuretic administration. Establishing baseline data provides a basis for comparison of subsequent results and assists in evaluating the response to therapy. It should be noted that, because patients with ARF often have complicated and serious illnesses, the usual indices of hypovolemia (dehydration) such as hematocrit and hemoglobin levels are frequently unreliable.

In prerenal azotemia, laboratory results will be consistent with hypovolemia and reduced renal perfusion and well-preserved intrarenal function. Urine specific gravity and osmolality indices closely reflect renal tubular urinary concentrating ability. A urinary specific gravity greater than 1.020, and a urine osmolality in excess of 500 mOsm/kg, in the face of oliguria and a rising azotemia, strongly indicate that intrarenal tubular function is intact, and that the problem is very likely *pre*renal in origin (Table 25-1).

Urine sodium concentration provides additional evidence that renal tubular function is preserved in prerenal azotemia. Low urine sodium levels (<10–20 mEq/liter) indicate that the kidney can still reabsorb sodium with its obligatory water retention, in response to severe volume contraction. Thus, in the patient with oliguria and a rising BUN (azotemia), a high urine osmolality coupled with low urine sodium indicate that ARF is due to hypovolemia (prerenal causes). Upon definitive diagnosis of prerenal ARF, appropriate therapy can immediately be initiated in the form of rapid fluid repletion.

In contrast to prerenal azotemia, intrarenal pathology (e.g., ATN), reflects the inability of the kidney to reabsorb or conserve sodium and water, and thus, to concentrate urine in the setting of a severely contracted fluid volume. Consequently, laboratory indices reflect a lower specific gravity (<1.010) and urine osmolality (<400 mOsm/liter). The latter may eventually become nearly iso-osmolar with that of blood, demonstrating that renal tubular damage has impaired the urinary concentrating and diluting functions of the kidney. The presence of acute tubular damage is confirmed if the urinary sodium excretion is increased (usually >20 mEq/liter or higher).

Laboratory indices for postrenal azotemia or obstructive uropathy are less characteristic. Urinalysis may be normal in the absence of urinary tract infection. Proteinuria is usually mild or absent; sediment may reflect red cells, white cells, and granular casts. The BUN may be increased out of proportion to the serum creatinine because slowed urine flow allows increased tubular reabsorption of urea. When acute renal failure presents in the scenario of obstructive uropathy, urinary sodium and osmolal-

TABLE 25-1
**Laboratory Indices in Acute Renal Failure**

| Laboratory Indices | Prerenal Azotemia | Intrarenal Azotemia | Postrenal Azotemia |
|---|---|---|---|
| Incidence | Most common | Acute tubular necrosis (ATN) most common type of intrarenal azotemia | |
| Pathophysiologic mechanisms | Renal hypoperfusion secondary to:<br>1. Intravascular hypovolemia (hypovolemic shock)<br>• Hemorrhage<br>• Sepsis<br>• Third-spacing fluid loss<br>• Overdiuresis<br>• Gastrointestinal losses (vomiting, diarrhea, nasogastric suctioning)<br>• Hypoalbuminemia<br>2. Cardiac insufficiency<br>• Progressive rise in left ventricular end-diastolic pressure (LVEDP) with decrease in cardiac output | Renal parenchymal damage related to:<br>1. Ischemic ATN due to prolonged or severe renal hypoperfusion<br>2. Nephrotoxic drugs:<br>• Aminoglycosides<br>• Cephalosporins<br>• Diuretic abuse<br>• Iodinated contrast agent<br>3. Infection<br>4. Immunologic disorders<br>• Acute glomerulonephritis | Complete or incomplete obstruction of urinary tract along its course:<br>• Renal calculi<br>• Prostatic hypertrophy<br>• Tumors<br>• Blood clots |
| Urine studies* | | | |
| Urine output | <400-700 ml/24 hr | <400 ml/24 hr | <50 ml/24 hr |
| Specific gravity | >1.020 | <1.010 (varies) | Variable |
| Sodium | <10-20 mEq/liter<br>Low urine sodium in presence of severely contracted fluid state reflects renal reabsorptive processes remain intact. | <10 mEq/liter (cortical)<br>>20 mEq/liter (medullary) (tubular) | >20 mEq/liter |
| Urine osmolality | >500 mOsm/kg | <400 mOsm/kg | <400 mOsm/kg |
| Serum osmolality | ~285-295 mOsm/kg | ~285-295 mOsm/kg | ~285-295 mOsm/kg |
| Urine/serum osmolality ratio | >2:1 | 1:1 (urine/serum osmolalities may become equal | |
| BUN/creatinine ratio | >10:1 | <10:1 (elevated) | Elevated with complete obstructive uropathy |
| Urinalysis | Usually within normal physiologic limits<br>Urine protein, minimal to absent<br>Usual urinary sediment | More commonly abnormal:<br>1. Glomerular involvement<br>• Urine protein 3-4+<br>• Hematuria<br>• Red blood cell casts<br>2. Acute tubular necrosis<br>• Dirty brown color<br>3. Interstitial renal disease with infection<br>• Protein 1-2+<br>• Pyuria<br>4. Allergic interstitial nephritis<br>• Urinary eosinophils | Significant bacteriuria (urinary tract infection)<br>Proteinuria, mild to absent<br>Urinary sediment; red and white cell, and granular casts |

* Obtain urinary specimens prior to therapeutic intervention because results may be made uninterpretable following therapeutic measures such as mannitol or furosemide diuretic therapy. (See Tables 22-1, 22-2, and 22-3.)

ity may be variable and difficult to interpret. These urinary indices may be similar to those of acute tubular necrosis, with high sodium and decreased urine osmolality, possibly a result of chronic obstruction.

Urinalysis findings allow for further definition of the underlying etiology of ARF. Urinalysis in pre- and postrenal azotemia is characteristically within acceptable physiologic limits. The urinalysis findings in ATN may also be normal, but more commonly the urine demonstrates the presence of dirty brown epithelial cell casts, which have sloughed off within the damaged tubular system. The presence of high-grade proteinuria (3-4+) and hematuria with red blood cell casts is highly suggestive of a glomerular pathophysiologic process (see Table 25-1).

Urinalysis findings in renal interstitial disease may provide further definitive data. A low-grade proteinuria (1-2+), pyuria, and white blood cell (WBC) casts suggest an underlying infectious process; the presence of eosinophiluria raises the question of an allergic response. Urine cultures may provide evidence of infection. A renal biopsy may be necessary to definitively diagnose intrarenal pathology. (For additional information on laboratory and diagnostic studies, see Tables 22–1 and 22–2.)

### ECG Findings

Hyperkalemia is a common and major complication associated with ARF. Excretion of potassium from the body is largely controlled by the kidneys. When renal function is impaired, potassium is retained and serum potassium levels rise quickly, resulting in hyperkalemia. While only a small proportion of total body potassium is found in the intravascular space (3.5–5.5 mEq/liter), even small changes in the serum potassium concentration can have profound effects on cardiac function. Hyperkalemia (>5.5 mEq/liter) causes characteristic progressive changes in the electrical conduction within the heart, which are reflected on the electrocardiogram (ECG). These changes are presented in Figure 23–2.

## CLINICAL PRESENTATION

Specific symptomatology of ARF is related to the pathophysiologic mechanisms underlying prerenal, intrarenal, or postrenal azotemia. Because renal function impacts on nearly all body systems, it is not surprising to find that complaints related to renal dysfunction likewise reflect multisystem dysfunction.

### Prerenal Azotemia

Patients with prerenal azotemia present clinically with signs and symptoms reflective of a hypovolemic state. There may be complaints of thirst, weight loss (try to determine how much over how long a period of time), fever with diaphoresis, unexplained tiredness, and easy fatigability. Poor skin turgor over the sternum and sunken eyeballs are reflective of severe dehydration. The patient may appear listless and may lack enthusiasm and motivation. Associated gastrointestinal symptoms may include anorexia, nausea, vomiting, constipation, or diarrhea.

Cardiovascular signs may include postural (orthostatic) hypotension; tachycardia with weak, thready pulse; flattened neck veins; and reduced central venous pressure (CVP) and pulmonary capillary wedge pressures (PCWP). Dysrhythmias may become evident on cardiac monitoring. Respirations may be shallow and rapid early on, owing to anxiety and apprehension. As metabolic acidemia evolves, respirations may become deep and rapid.

Neurologically, a slowly rising BUN may underlie complaints of headaches, an inability to concentrate, or to remember; mental status changes, such as memory loss, confusion, and lethargy, may be observed.

The complaint of oliguria should be explored carefully to determine its extent. It is important to establish when the patient first became aware of the falloff in urine output. A determination of the patient's prior health may be of diagnostic assistance. Has the patient fallen ill suddenly or has there been a gradual decline in the health status? Can the patient recall when symptoms first developed? Such data are significant to differential diagnosis of pre-, intra-, or postrenal azotemia. Timely and appropriate treatment based on the underlying diagnosis is essential because the severity and duration of renal failure and the ultimate degree of recovery depend largely on the institution of such therapy.

### Postrenal Azotemia

Signs and symptoms of postrenal azotemia or obstructive uropathy include a characteristic anuria (< 50 ml/24 hours); or, should a partial obstruction exist, anuria may alternate with periods of polyuria. An oliguria that progresses to complete anuria is highly suggestive of obstructive uropathy. Additional features of postrenal azotemia may include frequency, urgency, or hesitancy of urination; suprapubic distention or pressure; pain; and hematuria.

The diagnosis of obstructive uropathy is based on history, physical examination, ultrasonography, and radiologic examination. Obvious symptomatology in the history includes difficulty with urination (see section entitled "Cardinal Symptoms of Renal/ Urinary Dysfunction" in Chap. 22), costovertebral pain or lower abdominal pain, gross hematuria, and widely varying urine output volumes.

Physical examination may reveal signs of severe dehydration due to the inability of the kidneys to conserve sodium and water (these findings are consistent with longstanding obstructive disease); less often, the clinical status may reflect fluid overload. A palpable, tender, or distended bladder may be evident; and a paralytic ileus may accompany the obstruction. Depending on the duration of the obstruction, features of chronic renal failure may be observed (see Chap. 26). Careful rectal examination should be performed; and in females, a pelvic examination is essential.

In the absence of urinary tract infection, urinalysis may be normal. Other laboratory findings are listed in Table 25–1. Ultrasonography provides the best screening for obstructive disease. More definitive evaluation consists of specific radiologic examination, including renal tomograms, excretory urography, retrograde pyelography, and voiding cystogram (cystourethrography). These and other available diagnostic studies are listed in Table 22–3.

### Intrarenal Azotemia

The clinical presentation of intrarenal azotemia, which reflects damage to the functional unit (nephron) of the kidney, is largely characterized by a state of fluid overload and electrolyte acid–base imbalance. The patient experiences a significant weight gain (>0.5 kg/day) with weakness and fatigue. Cerebral edema may be reflected by alterations in neurologic function. These may include changes in mental status and level of consciousness, shortened memory and attention span, confusion, motor dysfunction, seizure, paralysis, and/or coma.

Oliguria and the inability of the kidney to filter and selectively reabsorb solute and water predispose to fluid overload, which is reflected clinically by alterations in cardiovascular function and edema. Hypertension is characteristically present, accompanied by tachycardia with a bounding pulse, neck vein distention, and elevated CVP and PCWP. Hypertension, an associated congestive heart failure, and/or serum hypoproteinemia may alter pulmonary hemodynamics, predisposing to pulmonary edema with tachypnea; dyspnea; a cough productive of pink-tinged, frothy sputum; rhonchi; wheezes; and rales (crackles).

Hypoproteinemia results from the abnormal filtering of serum proteins (especially albumin) at the impaired glomerular-capsular membrane without subsequent tubular reabsorption. The consequent reduction in serum colloidal osmotic pressure allows fluid to leave the intravascular space to move into the interstitial space, thus contributing to edema formation. Peripheral edema may be apparent in the periorbital and presacral areas and in the extremities. (For a detailed description of clinical manifestations associated with fluid overload, see Tables 23–4 and 23–5).

## COMPLICATIONS

Because of the impact renal function has on overall body physiology, complications of ARF frequently reflect multisystem dysfunction.

### Neurologic

Alterations in neurologic function commonly involve personality/behavioral changes, headaches, asterixis, seizure activity, and peripheral neuropathies. Such abnormalities may reflect metabolic changes associated with azotemia; they may occur secondary to cerebral edema associated with fluid overload.

### Cardiovascular

Hypertension is seen commonly in patients with ARF. Its occurrence may be related to an inappropriate production and/or excessive secretion of renin by the affected kidneys in the face of adequate hydrostatic blood pressure and blood flow. Fluid overload may also be a contributing factor in the development of hypertension.

Patients with ARF may develop complications associated with specific phases of renal failure. During the oliguric phase, a fluid volume excess can predispose to congestive heart failure, pulmonary and peripheral edema, and hypoalbuminemia; while the fluid volume deficit associated with the diuretic phase can precipitate a significant drop in cardiac output, leading to hypovolemic shock. Electrolytes are also lost. Pericarditis is occasionally seen as a complication of uremia that persists into the recovery phase.

### Metabolic

Patients with ARF are especially at risk of developing fluid, electrolyte, and acid–base disturbances, and a negative nitrogen balance. The inability of the kidneys to excrete acid by-products of metabolism (organic acids, hydrogen and ammonium ions), predisposes to metabolic acidosis. The inability of the kidneys to regenerate bicarbonate further exaggerates the acidotic state. The catabolic state associated with altered nutrition and proteinuria predisposes to a negative nitrogen balance.

Hyperkalemia may occur concomitantly with metabolic acidemia in ARF. To maintain acid–base balance, the kidneys excrete hydrogen ions instead of potassium ions. Additionally, the body tries to handle the excess acid load by driving hydrogen ions into cells in exchange for potassium. The net result: hyperkalemia that may reach life-threatening proportions (>8.0 mEq/liter).

### Hematologic

Anemia and coagulopathies associated with the uremic state are frequent complications of ARF. Decreased production and secretion of erythropoietin factor by the affected kidneys reduce the number of circulating red blood cells (RBCs). This type of anemia is associated with an increase in RBC fragility and a decrease in RBC survival time. Manifestations of anemia may include pallor, weakness and fatigue, shortness of breath, and chest pain. Platelet dysfunction may predispose to blood loss within the microcirculation. Additional blood loss may occur by gastrointestinal bleeding and iatrogenically (e.g., hemodialysis).

### Infection

The debilitated state associated with ARF causes patients to be especially susceptible to infections including pneumonia, urinary tract and wound infection, and septicemia. Staphylococci and pseudomonas organisms are encountered frequently in nosocomial infections of the critically ill patient with ARF.

## TREATMENT OF ACUTE RENAL FAILURE

Therapeutic interventions are directed at the underlying pathophysiologic process and the management of potential consequences of the loss of renal function.

### Prerenal Azotemia

In prerenal azotemia, the focus of initial management is to maximize renal perfusion by repletion of intravascular volume with a consequent restoration of blood pressure. Once identified, oliguria and azotemia due to hypovolemia and renal hypoperfusion readily respond to fluid replacement therapy. Such fluid may include packed red blood cells, plasma and plasma expanders, saline, and water ($D_5W$). Furosemide may be instituted in conjunction with fluid replacement therapy.

Caution must be exercised during fluid replacement therapy to prevent fluid volume excess. Hourly assessment of mental status, vital signs, cardiovascular and pulmonary function, and total fluid intake and output, is essential to effectively monitor the patient's fluid state and to evaluate the overall response to therapy. Use of the balloon-tipped pulmonary catheter (Swan-Ganz) allows for close monitoring of cardiac output before and after a fluid challenge. The critical care nurse must be cognizant of the fact that hypovolemia and renal hypoperfusion can themselves progress to intrinsic renal disease with disruption of renal tubular function and vascular nephropathy.

### Postrenal Azotemia

Once diagnosed, the first priority in the management of obstructive uropathy with postrenal azotemia is to eliminate any life-threatening circumstance such as gram-negative septicemia or pyonephrosis. Pyelonephritis associated with partial or complete obstruction places the patient at risk of developing septicemia. The presence of pyonephrosis and/or acute papillary necrosis may require emergency surgical relief to prevent rapid destruction of renal tissue.

Renal failure may require dialysis intil definitive steps are taken to correct the obstruction. A postobstructive diuresis may occur after relief of severe obstruction leading to intravascular fluid contraction with hypotension and severe electrolyte depletion. Medical management involves fluid and electrolyte replacement therapy. Urinary tract infection with or without pyelonephritis is treated with appropriate antibiotic based on cultures and sensitivity testing. Such therapy may be continued longer than usual (3–4 weeks or more is not unusual). Antihypertensive drugs may be indicated to treat hypertension.

Once the patient's overall condition is established, steps are taken to preserve renal function and to treat the underlying cause of the obstruction. Definitive treatment of obstructive uropathy is surgical, with optimal results requiring meticulous attention to the medical aspects of therapy. Elective surgery is usually indicated for urinary retention, recurrent urinary tract infections, or evidence of progressive deterioration in renal function. Once a decision has been made for surgical intervention, the goal consists of removing the obstruction and re-establishing continuity of the urinary tract. Should the lesion not be removable, a urinary diversion may be required.[4]

### Intrarenal Azotemia: Management of Acute Tubular Necrosis

The diagnosis of acute tubular necrois (ATN) may be confirmed using the potent loop diuretic, furosemide. Following a fluid challenge (200–500 ml) in the oliguric patient, intravenous furosemide is administered as prescribed. (Note that furosemide should not be administered until the patient has been hydrated.) If the urine output does not increase to 30–40 ml/hour, within 6–8 hours of the administration of furosemide, and if the patient's clinical history, physical examination, and laboratory/diagnostic studies suggest ATN, then the diagnosis of ATN is established with reasonable certainty.[5]

In patients who respond to furosemide with an increase in urine output to within normal levels, the appropriate therapy is to continue to replace urinary and other fluid losses as tolerated in order to maintain renal perfusion. A positive response to diuretic therapy indicates that the patient may have had a *pre*renal oliguria, in which case, renal function can be expected to return to normal; or, that the oliguric ATN has been converted to a nonoliguric ATN, with the expectation that the BUN and serum creatinine levels will continue to rise, although at a slower rate.

### Fluid and Electrolyte Therapy

Specific therapy in the management of ATN is directed toward maintenance of fluid, electrolyte, and acid–base balance. The status of the ECF volume, serum electrolytes, fluid intake and output, and body weight requires close monitoring. Intravenous fluid therapy should be given in amounts that cover measured fluid losses plus an additional 600 ml/day to replace insensible losses. Sodium intake is restricted. With adequate maintenance of fluid balance, the patient with fluid retention may lose about 0.5 kg/day.

Hyperkalemia is a major concern in patients with renal failure. Emergent treatment includes administration of (1) calcium gluconate to nullify the antagonistic effects of hyperkalemia on cardiac function; (2) sodium bicarbonate to at least partially correct metabolic acidemia; and (3) hypertonic glucose and insulin therapy given intravenously as prescribed to increase movement of potassium into the cells.

Sodium polystyrene sulfonate (Kayexalete), a cation exchange resin, is usually administered to treat hyperkalemia over the long term. This drug increases potassium loss by way of the gastrointestinal tract because it actually leeches out potassium, which is then eliminated in the stool. Early and repeated hemodialysis may be necessary to treat severe hyperkalemia and to prevent its recurrence.

Metabolic acidemia is usually present in patients with renal failure because the kidneys are unable to excrete the acid by-products of ongoing cellular metabolism. Severe acidemia (pH $<$7.20, serum bicarbonate $<$12–16 mEq/liter) may require dialysis therapy. Except for emergent circumstances, sodium bicarbonate is not usually administered as part of long-term therapy. Failure of glomerular filtration predisposes to hyperphosphatemia. Treatment involves administration of phosphate-binding antacids (e.g., aluminum hydroxide), which assist in eliminating phosphates by the gastrointestinal tract. Antacids administered for this purpose may also help to decrease the risk of stress-related upper gastrointestinal bleeding.

Hypocalcemia is seen commonly in patients with renal failure but is usually asymptomatic. However, overly aggressive treatment of metabolic acidemia with sodium bicarbonate, for example, can precipitate seizure activity and tetany due to the increase in protein-binding of free, ionized calcium. In general, the metabolic acidemia and hypocalcemia seen in ARF usually require no therapy, except for close monitoring.

### Diet Therapy

In patients with established ATN, nutritional therapy is directed toward maintaining a normal calorie intake and a low protein intake that is high in essential amino acids. Such a diet, in conjunction with dialysis therapy, helps to control the azotemia. A diet of 2000–3000 calories and 1 g protein/kg of body weight is usually prescribed. Foods high in potassium are avoided. Oral high calorie supplements may be given. In patients unable to tolerate oral or enteral feedings, total parenteral nutrition may be indicated to prevent protein catabolism and to reduce susceptibility to infection. (See Chap. 53).

### Dialysis Therapy

If complications of ARF become marked (e.g., fluid volume overload with congestive heart failure, hyperkalemia [$>$6.0 mEq/liter], and severe metabolic acidemia [pH $<$7.20]), aggressive therapy with dialysis may be necessary. An indepth discussion of dialysis therapy, including hemodialysis and peritoneal dialysis, is presented in Table 25–2. (See also Chap. 26.)

### Continuous Arteriovenous Hemofiltration for Acute Renal Failure

An alternative to peritoneal and hemodialysis in the treatment of critically ill patients with renal failure and/or fluid overload is continuous arteriovenous hemofiltration (CAVH).[7] This technique uses a hemofilter that facilitates removal of water, electrolytes, and small to medium molecular weight molecules from the vascular space, while conserving the cellular and protein contents of circulating blood. The blood enters the extracorporeal circuit by an arterial access, flows through the hemofilter, and returns to the patient by way of a venous access. Blood flow is driven by the hydrostatic blood pressure; no pump is used.

The mechanism underlying hemofiltration involves the use of a transmembrane pressure gradient. This pressure gradient is achieved by the net difference between hydrostatic and osmotic pressures. The hydrostatic pressure consists of two components. These include the arterial blood pressure, which drives fluid across the semipermeable membrane into the ultrafiltrate compartment, and the pressure exerted by the fluid within the ultrafiltrate system, which drives fluid from the fibers into the ultrafiltrate. The pressure opposing the hydrostatic pressure is the colloidal osmotic pressure exerted by the plasma proteins, which do not pass through the semipermeable membrane.

The filter replacement fluid used is determined by the patient's electrolyte values, and the ultrafiltration flow rate is geared to the patient's needs. If

TABLE 25–2
## Peritoneal Dialysis Versus Hemodialysis: Nursing Implications

| Objectives | Peritoneal Dialysis | Hemodialysis |
|---|---|---|
| 1. Define peritoneal and hemodialysis. | The process of removing metabolic wastes and water from blood by use of the living semipermeable membrane, the peritoneum. | The process of removing metabolic wastes and water from blood by use of a semipermeable membrane of an artificial kidney. |
| 2. State underlying principles used in the dialysis process. | Principles used:<br>A. Osmosis—Movement of water across a semipermeable membrane from an area of lesser to one of greater concentration of solute.<br>B. Diffusion—Movement of molecules from an area of higher concentration to one of lower concentration.<br>C. Filtration—Movement of particles through a semipermeable membrane by means of hydrostatic pressure. | |
| 3. Define ultrafiltration and how it is accomplished. | The removal of fluid (water) by use of an osmotic gradient by the addition of increased concentration of dextrose to the dialysate.<br>Increased dialysis efficiency and ultrafiltration are obtained by using dextrose 4.25 g/100 ml (490–520 mOsm/kg), every sixth exchange. | The removal of fluid (water) by use of either positive or negative hydrostatic pressure or a combination of both. |
| 4. State major indications for dialysis. | Fluid overload<br>Electrolyte imbalance<br>Severe acidosis<br>Uremic symptomatology<br>Unavailable vascular access<br>Severe hemodynamic compromise<br>Severe active bleeding<br>Lack of accessible hemodialysis center | Uncontrolled hyperkalemia<br>Fluid overload<br>Peritonitis<br>Severe acidosis<br>Uremic symptomatology<br>Severe intoxication with a dialyzable substance of low volume of distribution, and low endogenous clearance (e.g., ethanol, ethylene glycol, salicylates, lithium) |
| 5. Discuss primary assessment factors indicating need for dialysis therapy in acute renal failure (ARF). | Primary indications for dialysis therapy in ARF are the presence of:<br>1. Uremic encephalopathy<br>2. Pericarditis<br>3. Bleeding<br>4. BUN $>$ 100 mg/100 ml<br>5. Creatinine $>$ 10 mg/100 ml<br>6. Potassium $>$ 6.0 mEq/liter<br>7. $HCO_3^- < 12–15$ mEq/liter<br>8. Severe fluid overload persisting despite maximum conservative therapy<br>Additional factors to be assessed include:<br>1. Relative risk of complications from dialysis therapy<br>2. Risk of hemorrhagic or infectious complications of uremia<br>3. Likelihood of prompt reversal of acute renal failure | |
| 6. Describe major contraindications for dialysis. | Peritonitis<br>Recent abdominal surgery<br>Abdominal adhesions<br>Colostomy/ileostomy | Severe hemodynamic instability (inability to tolerate rapid changes in extravascular fluid volume)<br>Active and severe bleeding<br>Intolerance to systemic heparinization |
| 7. Examine the need for anticoagulation (heparinization) in specific type of dialysis therapy. | Indicated in initial "runs" especially when fibrin clots are observed in the drainage from peritoneal cavity. Heparin is added directly to dialysate solution. | Heparinization (regional) of patient's blood is done prior to the procedure, to keep blood anticoagulated in the dialysis apparatus. *Note:* Patient must be monitored closely for signs of bleeding. |
| 8. Identify advantages of each method of dialysis treatment. | Slower process (36–48 hr)<br>Clears middle molecular weight molecules better (300–800 MW)<br>Little likelihood of disequilibrium syndrome ocurring<br>Safer, simple, less expensive<br>No need for vascular access<br>No need for dialysis technician | More efficient, faster process<br>Indicated for treatment of uncontrolled hyperkalemia<br>Clears smaller molecular weight molecules better<br>Preferred treatment for ARF due to:<br>1. Drug overdose or toxicity<br>2. Contrast-induced ARF<br>3. Nonoliguric acute tubular necrosis |
| 9. Consider disadvantages of each method of dialysis. | Risk of peritonitis<br>Does not remove potassium rapidly enough in state of uncontrolled hyperkalemia<br>Slow process (36–48 hr)<br>Loss of proteins<br>Cannot be used in presence of abdominal surgery that involves the retroperitoneum<br>Rarely, perforation of bowel or bladder | Requires trained personnel and sophisticated equipment<br>Requires heparinization, which may predispose to:<br>1. Bleeding<br>2. Retinopathy (diabetes)<br>Requires maintenance of vascular access<br>Expensive to maintain<br>May precipitate "disequilibrium syndrome" due to rapid removal of fluid |

*(continued)*

TABLE 25–2
**Peritoneal Dialysis Versus Hemodialysis: Nursing Implications *(Continued)***

| Objectives | Peritoneal Dialysis | Hemodialysis |
|---|---|---|
| 10. Distinguish major complications of dialysis therapy. | Peritonitis (most common)<br>Loss of body protein<br>Hyperglycemic, hyperosmolar, nonketotic coma<br>Pleural effusion, pneumonia<br>Electrolyte imbalance<br>Dysrhythmias | Hypotension associated with an acute decrease in serum osmolality due to:<br>1. Removal of urea<br>2. An acute decrease in intravascular volume from excessive ultrafiltration (hypovolemia)<br>3. Acetate accumulation during high clearance dialysis (treated with hypertonic mannitol or saline)<br>Hypervolemia (hypertension)<br>Electrolyte imbalance<br>Dysrhythmias<br>Dysequilibrium syndrome characterized by:<br>1. Restlessness, headache, nausea<br>2. Muscle twitching<br>3. Disorientation and seizures (severe form)<br>Prevention of dysequilibrium syndrome:<br>1. Minimize fluid/electrolyte shifts<br>2. Early and frequent dialysis<br>Hypoxemia may develop partly due to loss of $CO_2$ into dialysate with consequent reduction in minute ventilation by the patient (treated with bicarbonate solution equilibrated with $CO_2$ to a partial pressure of 35–45 mmHg, or by increasing fraction of inspired oxygen).[6]<br>Mild thrombocytopenia and leukopenia<br>Bacteremia; cellulitis<br>Thrombosis |
| 11. Describe access sites for each dialysis method. | Stiff peritoneal catheter (acute)<br>Soft Tenckhoff catheter (chronic)<br>These catheters are usually inserted percutaneously in the awake, cooperative patient. | Arteriovenous shunt<br>Arteriovenous fistula<br>Direct arterial stick: Femoral, subclavian |
| 12. Highlight major nursing process considerations in caring for the patient undergoing dialysis therapy.<br>A. Baseline assessment and patient/family preparation | 1. Body weight.<br>2. Vital signs: Blood pressure lying and sitting; apical/radial pulse; temperature; respirations: rate and rhythm.<br>3. Neurologic: Mental status; level of consciousness; cranial nerves, sensory-motor function; deep tendon reflexes<br>4. Respiratory: Breathing pattern, chest movement, use of accessory muscles; cough; breath sounds: presence of adventitious sounds; presence of pleural friction rub.<br>5. Cardiovascular: Heart sounds, extra heart sounds, murmur or pericardial friction rub; peripheral pulses; pulse—bounding or thready? Neck vein distention; interstitial edema.<br>6. Abdominal exam: Abdominal distention; bowel sounds; palpable liver border, spleen, bladder, abdominal tenderness; Last bowel movement? Costovertebral angle tenderness.<br>7. Laboratory data: Serum electrolytes, serum glucose, BUN and creatinine; calcium, phosphorus, serum albumin, total protein, CBC, hematocrit and hemoglobin; bleeding and clotting times; arterial blood gases (as indicated).<br>8. Other studies: ECG, chest x-ray.<br>9. Patient/family preparation: Patient and/or family should be able to verbalize the need/indication for dialysis therapy, duration, limitation of activity during the procedure, discomfort, risks involved, and expectations of dialysis therapy. | |
| B. Pertinent nursing diagnoses | 1. Fluid volume, alteration in: Deficit (potential).<br>2. Fluid volume, alteration in: Excess (potential).<br>3. Comfort, alteration in: Pain.<br>4. Injury, potential for: Traumatic insertion of peritoneal dialysis (PD) catheter.<br>5. Potential for infection (peritonitis).<br>6. Breathing pattern, ineffective.<br>7. Bowel elimination, alteration in: Ileus.<br>8. Skin integrity, impairment of: Potential.<br>9. Nutrition, alteration in: Less than body requirements.<br>10. Fear: Unknown procedure.<br>11. Coping, ineffective: Potential for, individual/family. | 4. Potential for injury (shunt malfunction).<br>5. Potential for infection (hepatitis).<br>6. Cardiac output, alteration in: Decreased.<br>7. Gas exchange, impaired. |

TABLE 25–2
**Peritoneal Dialysis Versus Hemodialysis: Nursing Implications *(Continued)***

<table>
<tr><th>Objectives</th><th>Peritoneal Dialysis</th><th>Hemodialysis</th></tr>
<tr><td>C. Planning:<br>1) Desired patient outcomes</td><td colspan="2">Patient will:<br>1. Remain hemodynamically stable: Blood pressure, heart rate optimal for patient; respirations—rate, rhythm, appropriate for patient; lungs clear.<br>2. Maintain body weight ideal for patient.<br>3. Maintain serum electrolytes, blood chemistries—BUN and serum creatinine, calcium and phosphorus, serum albumin and total protein, at level ideal for patient.<br>4. Maintain hematologic studies—CBC, platelets, bleeding/clotting times at level ideal for patient.<br>5. Maintain body temperature and WBC at levels ideal for patient.<br>6. Maintain nutrition state in positive nitrogen balance.<br>7. Verbalize absent to minimal discomfort.<br>8. Verbalize feelings and concerns regarding dialysis therapy and overall status of renal function.</td></tr>
<tr><td></td><td>9. Experience atraumatic insertion of PD catheter without bowel or bladder perforation.<br>10. Maintain skin integrity with absent to minimal leakage around PD catheter.</td><td>9. Experience hemodialysis therapy without hemolysis or loss of blood.<br>10. Maintain a patent shunt/fistula.</td></tr>
<tr><td>2) Nursing interventions</td><td>1. Prepare patient/family.<br>A. Explain procedure to patient and family.<br>B. Encourage patient and family to verbalize fears and concerns, and to ask questions.<br>2. Perform predialysis assessment (see Baseline assessment, above).<br>3. Assemble equipment at bedside:<br>A. Dialysate ordered (1.5%, 2.5%, or 4.25%).<br>B. Add medications to dialysate as prescribed:<br>• Heparin is added to prevent fibrin accumulation, which could cause a flap valve effect over perforated openings in PD catheter.<br>• Potassium (dialysate is potassium-free).<br>• Antibiotics.<br>• Lidocaine may be added to control local discomfort.<br>C. Provide masks, sterile gowns and gloves. Aseptic technique must be strictly maintained.<br>D. Provide additional necessary equipment—tubings, drainage bags, and so forth.<br>E. Have patient void (if producing urine) prior to procedure to reduce risk of bladder perforation.<br>F. Provide assistance with PD catheter insertion.<br>1. Assist patient during trocar insertion; document how patient tolerated the procedure.<br>2. Drain initial dialysate "run" to:<br>• Ascertain PD catheter patency.<br>• Determine how much time is needed to fill and drain the abdominal cavity (subsequently dwell period can be adjusted so that entire cycle [instill, dwell, drain] lasts 1 hr).</td><td>Shunt care:<br>1. Assess shunt patency:<br>A. Palpate for thrill.<br>B. Auscultate for bruit.<br>2. Assess for pulsations in tubing and signs of clotting: change of color of blood; separation of blood cells from serum; loss of pulsations.<br>3. Maintain sterile dressing over shunt access; change daily as per unit protocol.<br>4. Avoid use of shunt arm to:<br>A. Take blood pressure.<br>B. Perform venipuncture.<br>C. Give injections or intravenous therapy.<br>5. Instruct patient in self-care of shunt site and emergency measures should shunt separate.<br>Arteriovenous fistula care:<br>1. Assess fistula patency:<br>A. Palpate for thrill.<br>B. Auscultate for bruit.<br>2. Avoid restrictive dressing or clothing over fistula site.<br>3. Note bleeding, skin discoloration, pain, or drainage at fistula site, and report immediately.<br>4. Avoid use of arm with fistula to:<br>A. Take blood pressure.<br>B. Perform venipuncture.<br>C. Give injections or intravenous therapy.<br>Patient/family preparation:<br>1. Explain procedures to patient and family.<br>2. Encourage patient and family to verbalize fears and concerns and to ask questions.<br>Perform pre-dialysis assessment (see Baseline assessment, above).<br>Implementation: Hemodialysis requires specially trained personnel.</td></tr>
</table>

**Peritoneal Dialysis: Procedure**

*"Up-down" peritoneal dialysis:* Implementing the procedure

The first 2-liter dialysate volume may not drain completely; the missing volume is presumably in the gutters of the peritoneal cavity. Failure of the second 2-liter volume to drain completely indicates a mechanical problem. Nursing interventions in this regard include:

A. Altering the patient's position.

TABLE 25-2
## Peritoneal Dialysis Versus Hemodialysis: Nursing Implications *(Continued)*

B. Ensuring that drainage bag is below the level of the patient.
C. Establishing that there is no airlock. If these maneuvers do not solve the problem, the physician may inject Gastrografin into the PD catheter, which may reveal kinking or malplacement of the PD catheter.
D. Implementing overall procedure:
1. Subsequent "runs" include:
a. Instillation of dialysate—Inflow phase.
b. Diffusion—Dwell phase.
c. Drainage—Outflow phase.
2. Documentation:
a. Exact time the procedure started.
b. Amount/concentration of dialysate.
c. Medications added to dialysate.
d. Exact time of each phase of the "runs":
- Instillation: Time started and time completed.
- Dwell: Total time of dwell phase.
- Drainage: Time started and when instillation was completed.

e. Document color of dialysate drainage (drainage may be blood-tinged on first two or three runs).
- Dialysate drainage:
  Normal—Clear, pale yellow.
  Cloudy—Infection, peritonitis.
  Brownish—Bowel perforation.
  Amber—Bladder perforation.
  Bloody—Initial dialysate drainage may be blood-tinged; persistent bleeding suggests abdominal site or uremic coagulopathy.

f. Exact amount of total dialysate fluid drained or retained by the patient:
- Positive balance = fluid gained by patient.
- Negative balance = fluid lost by patient.

Thus, fluid retention will create a positive balance, and fluid loss will create a negative balance. The goal of therapy is a negative balance.

g. Document total intake and output. Include oral and/or intravenous intake, urine output, nasogastric drainage, emesis, diarrhea, wound drainage, and insensible losses.
- Diarrhea occurring after initial runs needs to be evaluated for significant dilution, or blood, which could indicate bowel perforation.

3. Specific nursing activities:
a. Monitor vital signs every 15 min initially and subsequently at hourly intervals.
- A drop in blood pressure or increase in heart rate warns of early shock.
- Notify physician if any signs of bleeding, severe abdominal pain, and/or respiratory distress.
- Respiratory embarrassment can occur as the peritoneal fluid volume limits diaphragmatic excursion.
- Reduction in volume of dialysate exchanges may alleviate compromised ventilatory effort.
- Pleural effusion, if present, may require thoracentesis.

b. Monitor serum electrolytes, blood chemistries, hematology studies.
- Patients receiving 2.5% or 4.25% dialysate solution should have serum glucose determinations at frequent intervals. Hyperglycemic, hyperosmolar, nonketotic (HHNK) coma is a serious complication and must be avoided.

c. Use *strict aseptic technique* with each peritoneal dialysis run to avoid peritonitis.
d. Assess patient frequently for pain/discomfort.
- Pain at catheter placement may respond to changing its position.
- Pain on initiation of peritoneal dialysis may be due to dialysate acidity and is usually relieved by adding lidocaine to the dialysate.
- Dialysate must be warmed prior to instillation for patient comfort.
- Warming also helps to dilate peritoneal blood vessels enhancing the effectiveness of the dialysis treatment.
- Pain at end of drainage phase may be due to suction of the peritoneum against the perforations in the PD catheter.
- Administer analgesic as necessary.
- Diffuse abdominal pain may herald peritonitis.

e. Assess dialysate drainage: Cloudiness suggests peritonitis.
- Obtain dialysate sample for culture; monitor body temperature.
- Initiate antibiotic therapy as prescribed. Loading dose administered orally or intravenously. Addition of antibiotic to each dialysate instillation at the concentration desired in blood. Exit wound infection may require PD catheter removal.
- Watch for fluid leakage around PD catheter; if it is observed, notify physician.

TABLE 25-2
**Peritoneal Dialysis Versus Hemodialysis: Nursing Implications *(Continued)***

| | |
|---|---|
| | f. Perform PD catheter site care *(strict aseptic technique)*.<br>• Assess site for signs/symptoms of infection: Redness, swelling, tenderness, induration, purulence.<br>• Remove dried blood and drainage: Serve as a media for bacterial growth.<br>• Examine dressings frequently; dressings should not be allowed to remain wet—contamination at PD catheter site can predispose to peritonitis.<br>g. Perform procedure for dressing change:<br>• Cleanse exit site gently with povidone-iodine solution beginning around PD catheter where it penetrates the skin and working outward.<br>• Cleanse entire circumference of catheter with povidone-iodine solution. Allow antiseptic to dry completely to allow for maximum bacteriostatic effect and to prevent gauze dressing from sticking to the skin.<br>• Secure peritoneal dialysis catheter on sterile gauze pad to avoid skin irritation and decrease risk of catheter contamination from skin.<br>• Cover site with additional sterile gauze pads and secure dressing. Allow areas of gauze to be exposed to enable skin to "breathe," thus decreasing the risk of anaerobic bacterial growth and preventing bacterial contamination. |
| Peritoneal dialysis: Major approaches in current use | Major approaches to peritoneal dialysis:<br>• "Up-down" or single bottle manual setup.<br>• "Cycler" peritoneal dialysis apparatus.<br>• Continuous ambulatory peritoneal dialysis (CAPD). |

*Note:* Major nursing care considerations related to dialysis therapy have been highlighted in this table. For an indepth discussion of this topic, which is beyond the scope of this text, see appropriate source books on this topic.

the objective is to remove extracellular fluid only, ultrafiltration is regulated at a low rate (approximately 100–300 ml/hour) without subsequent intravenous replacement; if the objective is to clear both extracellular fluid and toxic substances (e.g., urea, potassium), then high ultrafiltration rates and filter replacement fluid are used. The final composition of the ultrafiltrate might include the following: sodium 150 mEq/liter, chloride 114 mEq/liter, potassium 0, bicarbonate 37 mEq/liter, magnesium 1.6 mEq/liter, calcium 2.5 mEq/liter. Clotting of the extracorporeal circuit is prevented by the administration of low dose heparin. The dose is titrated depending on the patient's coagulation status.

Nursing care of patients undergoing continuous arteriovenous hemofiltration involves patient and equipment preparation, attachment, monitoring of patient and the hemofilter, and termination of hemofiltration. A baseline assessment, including the clinical history, physical examination, and hemodynamic profile, is essential. The hemodynamic profile includes vital signs and measurement of hemodynamic pressures (e.g., central venous, pulmonary artery, pulmonary capillary wedge pressures, and arterial pressures). The patient's weight is ascertained, and baseline laboratory data (e.g., hematology, coagulation, and chemistry profiles) are established.

An access site is established. The most commonly used sites are the femoral artery and vein; the saphenous or subclavian veins may also be used as the venous access. Scribner-type wrist shunts involving the radial or ulnar arteries and median cubital or basilic vein may also be cannulated. The hemofilter is primed, heparinized, and attached to the patient. The hemofilter must be secured carefully to the patient to prevent accidental disconnection.

Continuous monitoring of the patient's hemodynamic status is recommended and best achieved using an arterial line. Ideally, use of the pulmonary artery catheter more closely reflects the patient's fluid status. The nurse observes the flow rate every 15 minutes; outputs are recorded hourly. The goal is to remove a large amount of fluid each hour and to replace part of this volume. This results in a net loss of fluid and selected solutes (e.g., urea). The desired hourly fluid balance is specified by the physician. Laboratory values are followed closely to identify trends. It is essential to avoid fluctuations outside the normal range. *Aseptic* shunt care is imperative; monitoring of pulses distal to the access site is essential.

Patient/family education should include information about the function, purpose, and standard care of patients receiving continuous arteriovenous hemofiltration. Areas of greatest concern include the frequency of patient monitoring and the special equipment involved. The nurse should emphasize that the frequency of care is standard practice for patients receiving this form of therapy.

## TABLE 25-3. CARE PLAN FOR THE PATIENT WITH ACUTE RENAL FAILURE

| Nursing Diagnoses | Desired Patient Outcomes | Nursing Interventions | Rationales |
|---|---|---|---|
| ***Nursing Diagnosis #1***<br>Fluid volume deficit: Actual (extracellular dehydration, hypovolemia).<br>Fluid volume deficit: Actual (intracellular dehydration, hypernatremia). | (For patient outcomes, see Table 23-3.) | • For pertinent information related to total body fluid and electrolyte status, see:<br>Table 23-1. Contrast: Extracellular and Intracellular Fluids.<br>Table 23-2. Contrast: Extracellular and Intracellular Fluid Deficit Disorders.<br>Table 23-4. Contrast: Extracellular and Intracellular Fluid Excess Disorders.<br>Table 23-6. Contrast: Hypernatremia and Hyponatremia.<br>Table 23-8. Contrast: Hyperkalemia and Hypokalemia.<br>Table 23-10. Contrast: Hyperchloremia and Hypochloremia.<br>Table 23-11. Contrast: Hypermagnesemia and Hypomagnesemia.<br>• For pertinent nursing interventions and their rationales in the care of the patient with fluid deficit or excess disorders, see:<br>Table 23-3. Fluid Volume Deficit.<br>Table 23-5. Fluid Volume Excess. | |
| ***Nursing Diagnosis #2***<br>Fluid volume, alteration in: Excess (extracellular overhydration, hypervolemia circulatory overload).<br>Fluid volume, alteration in: Excess (intracellular overhydration, hyponatremia). | (For patient outcomes, see Table 23-5.) | | |
| ***Nursing Diagnosis #3***<br>Electrolyte imbalance, related to:<br>1. Water deficit.<br>2. Hypernatremia.<br>Electrolyte imbalance, related to:<br>1. Water excess.<br>2. Hyponatremia. | (For patient outcomes, see Table 23-7.) | • For pertinent nursing interventions and their rationales in the care of the patient with sodium imbalance, see:<br>Table 23-7. Patient with Sodium Imbalance. | |
| ***Nursing Diagnosis #4***<br>Cardiac output, alteration in: Decreased, related to:<br>1. Dysrhythmias associated with hyperkalemia (>5.5 mEq/liter).<br>2. Dysrhythmias associated with hypokalemia (<3.5 mEq/liter). | (For patient outcomes, see Table 23-9.) | • For pertinent nursing interventions and their rationales in the care of the patient with potassium imbalance, see:<br>Table 23-9. Patient with Potassium Imbalance. | |

| | | | |
|---|---|---|---|
| ***Nursing Diagnosis #5*** Acid–base balance, alteration in: Metabolic acidemia (acidosis). (See Tables 30–2 and 30–3.) | Patient's condition will stabilize as follows:<br>1. Arterial blood gases will normalize to baseline values:<br>• pH >7.35, <7.45.<br>• $PaCO_2$ optimal level for patient (normal range 35–45 mmHg).<br>2. Anions will stabilize as follows:<br>• Bicarbonate ($HCO_3^-$) 22–26 mEq/liter.<br>• Chloride 100–106 mEq/liter.<br>• Anion gap 12–15 mEq/liter.<br>3. Neurologic: Alert, oriented to person, time, place; deep tendon reflexes—brisk.<br>4. Serum potassium level: 3.5–5.5 mEq/liter.<br>5. Hemodynamic status will stabilize as follows:<br>• Arterial BP within 10 mmHg of baseline.<br>• CVP = $\overline{\text{mean}}$ 0–8 mmHg.<br>6. Ventilatory effort will maintain blood gas values at optimal level for patient.<br>• Respiratory rate: 12–18/min.<br>• Tidal volume: >5–7 ml/kg. | • Monitor neurologic status: Level of consciousness, mental status; cranial nerve function; deep tendon reflexes, seizure activity. | • Alterations in neurologic function are commonly associated with severe metabolic acidosis and may include confusion, headache, seizures, coma, and other manifestations. |
| | | • Monitor arterial blood gases. | • Reflect effectiveness of ventilatory effort and gas exchange; blood gas levels and pH provide essential data for assessing acid–base and electrolyte balance. |
| | | • Monitor serum potassium levels. | • Severe metabolic acidemia can predispose to hyperkalemia as excess hydrogen ions are moved into cells in exchange for potassium ions, which enter intravascular space (circulation); hyperkalemia may predispose to cardiac dysrhythmias and cardiac arrest. |
| | | • Monitor respiratory rate and rhythm. | • Hyperventilation (Kussmaul's breathing): Deep and rapid breathing—the body's compensatory response to severe acidemia (pH <7.20). |
| | | • For pertinent information related to acid–base abnormalities including definition, pathophysiology, etiology, clinical presentation, treatment, and nursing diagnoses, see:<br>Table 30–2. Respiratory Acid–Base Abnormalities: Respiratory Acidemia and Alkalemia.<br>Table 30–3. Metabolic Acid–Base Abnormalities: Metabolic Acidemia and Alkalemia. | |

*(continued)*

**TABLE 25–3. CARE PLAN FOR THE PATIENT WITH ACUTE RENAL FAILURE *(Continued)***

| Nursing Diagnoses | Desired Patient Outcomes | Nursing Interventions | Rationales |
|---|---|---|---|
| ***Nursing Diagnosis #6***<br>Nutrition, alteration in: Less than body requirements. | Patient will:<br>1. Maintain body weight between 2–5% of patient's baseline.<br>2. Maintain serum albumin within physiologic range: 3.5–5.0 g/100 ml.<br>3. Tolerate oral feedings without nausea, vomiting, diarrhea, or stomatitis. | • Collaborate with nutritionist to perform comprehensive nutritional assessment. | • Provides baseline for planning nutrition that will provide sufficient calories to prevent protein catabolism, and sufficient protein intake to meet body needs while avoiding excess production of urea nitrogen. |
| | | ○ Weigh daily under same conditions. | ○ Body weight is best indicator of fluid gain or loss. |
| | | ○ Monitor intake and output.<br>– Monitor electrolytes closely. | ○ Diligent monitoring of fluid state is essential to prevent fluid excess during oliguric phase, and fluid deficit during diuretic phase. |
| | | • Implement prescribed dietary regimen:<br>○ Caloric intake: 2000–3000 calories/24 hr. | ○ The number of calories depends on age, size, and level of activity. |
| | | ○ Low protein intake: ~1 g/kg of body weight/24 hr.<br>– Protein sources high in essential amino acids. | ○ Low protein intake helps to control azotemia associated with compromised renal excretion of nitrogenous waste. Goal of therapy: Maintain body weight and prevent protein breakdown. |
| | | ○ Avoid foods high in potassium.<br>– Offer oral high caloric supplements; vitamin and mineral supplements. | ○ Acute renal failure and associated metabolic acidemia place the patient at risk of developing hyperkalemia. |
| | | • Implement measures to enhance mealtimes:<br>○ Provide frequent oral care. | ○ Prevents stomatitis; decreases foul taste; improves appetite. |
| | | ○ Limit fluids with meals; provide more frequent small feedings. | ○ Smaller volume at mealtimes may facilitate gastric emptying and reduce gastrointestinal upsets. |
| | | ○ Encourage family to bring appropriate home-cooked foods; encourage visiting during mealtimes. | ○ Favorite foods may enhance appetite. Helps to provide a mealtime atmosphere conducive to good eating. |
| | | ○ Encourage rest periods before and after meals. | ○ Avoids undue fatigue. |
| ***Nursing Diagnosis #7***<br>Knowledge deficit: Dietary regimen in renal disease. | Patient will:<br>1. Verbalize knowledge of prescribed diet; specify dietary restrictions and their significance. | • Initiate patient/family education regarding prescribed diet and meal preparation. Stress those foods permitted versus those foods restricted. | • Compliance with long-term dietary restriction requires that patient/family understand the relationship among renal disease, diet, and medication regimen. |
| | | • Implement alternative approach to providing nutrition as dictated by patient's overall condition:<br>○ Nasogastric or enteral feedings.<br>○ Total parenteral nutrition. | • Ensures adequate intake of essential amino acids for maintaining and repairing body tissues; sufficient carbohydrate caloric source to reverse gluconeogenesis and catabolic state. |

| | | | |
|---|---|---|---|
| ***Nursing Diagnosis #8*** Infection, potential for: Depressed immunologic system. (See Table 49–7, Potential for Infection.) | Patient's condition will stabilize as follows:<br>1. Nonfebrile.<br>2. White blood count within physiologic range.<br>3. Patient will verbalize a general feeling of well-being.<br>4. Absence of infection.<br>• Negative cultures.<br>• Absence of redness, swelling, pain. | • Assess for signs of infection:<br>○ Vigilant assessment of all invasive lines and wound dressings is critical.<br>○ Observe for redness, pain, swelling at all invasive sites; dressing changes as per unit protocol.<br>○ Monitor body temperature, white blood count; obtain cultures as indicated—Sputum, blood, urine, wound.<br>○ Pulmonary function: Encourage deep breathing and coughing.<br>○ Auscultate lungs for adventitious sounds of pulmonary congestion or increased secretions; encourage frequent position changes.<br>○ Urinary function: monitor use of Foley catheter; perform perineal care and cleansing around catheter as per unit protocol; maintain the integrity of the closed drainage system; examine urine for cloudiness or unusual odor. | • Uremic state depresses the body's immunologic defenses and increases patient's susceptibility to infection.<br>○ Infection is the most common cause of death in patients with ARF.<br>○ Patient care activities are directed toward prevention of accumulation of pulmonary secretions and atelectasis.<br>○ Assists in evaluating ventilatory effort; patients with ARF are at high risk of developing pneumonia.<br>○ Use of indwelling Foley catheters in patients with ARF is associated with a high incidence of urinary tract infection (nosocomial infections). If an indwelling catheter is necessary, its insertion and ongoing care require *strict* aseptic technique.<br>○ Indwelling catheter should be removed as soon as feasible as determined by the patient's overall condition. |
| ***Nursing Diagnosis #9*** Injury, potential for: Uremia-induced gastrointestinal disorders. | Patient will:<br>1. Tolerate oral feedings.<br>2. Verbalize having an appetite.<br>3. Maintain usual bowel routine.<br>4. Nasogastric secretions and stool negative for occult blood. | • Monitor gastrointestinal function: Assess abdomen for distention, tenderness; bowel sounds in all quadrants.<br>○ Monitor for nausea, vomiting, and diarrhea; test vomitus or nasogastric aspirate and stool for occult blood.<br>○ Monitor Hct and Hgb. | • Patients with ARF are susceptible to gastrointestinal upsets, due in part to the chemical irritation caused by bacteria that hydrolyze urea to ammonia in the gut.<br>• Administration of antibiotics or other drugs alters the intestinal flora, placing the patient at increased risk of infection. |

**TABLE 25-3. CARE PLAN FOR THE PATIENT WITH ACUTE RENAL FAILURE *(Continued)***

| Nursing Diagnoses | Desired Patient Outcomes | Nursing Interventions | Rationales |
|---|---|---|---|
| ***Nursing Diagnosis #10***<br>Skin integrity, impairment of: Potential. | Patient will:<br>1. Maintain intact skin; no breaks, lesions, or infection.<br>2. Exhibit warm, dry skin, with good turgor and absence of interstitial edema.<br>3. Verbalize/demonstrate measures for optimal skin care. | • Maintain skin integrity.<br>○ Inspect skin on each shift, especially reddened areas over bony prominences where skin is thin.<br>○ Institute measures to prevent skin breakdown: frequent position changes; use of sheepskin or egg crate mattress (pressure relief device); frequent lubrication of skin; active/passive exercises as tolerated.<br>○ Teach patient/family the essentials of skin care. | • A comprehensive assessment of skin can assist in early detection of alterations in skin.<br>○ Deposition of phosphate crystals in the skin causes troublesome itching, which can lead to excoriation and infection.<br>○ Patient/family can be taught to rub a lanolin-base lotion on the skin to avoid scratching and to stimulate circulation. |
| ***Nursing Diagnosis #11***<br>Oral mucous membrane, alteration in. | Patient will:<br>1. Verbalize/demonstrate measures for optimal oral hygiene. | • Maintain integrity of oral mucous membranes: Provide oral hygiene; instruct patient/family on measures to enhance oral hygiene. | • Changes in overall health status are often reflected in the status of the oral mucous membranes and the skin. Poor oral hygiene places the patient at risk of developing stomatitis; it decreases the patient's appetite and can seriously curtail oral intake. |
| ***Nursing Diagnosis #12***<br>Comfort, alteration in: Pain (pericarditis). | Patient will:<br>1. Verbalize when in pain.<br>2. Identify appropriate pain relief measures.<br>3. Verbalize comfort.<br>4. Discuss origin of chest pain and significance in ARF. | • Evaluate pain and stress tolerance.<br>○ Assess presence of chest pain: Severity, location, duration, quality (type) of pain, influencing factors.<br>○ Assess presence of: Fever, chills, pericardial friction rub, gallop rhythm.<br>○ Administer analgesic as prescribed, and evaluate its effctiveness in relieving pain.<br>○ Instruct patient to lean forward over a pillow or bedside table.<br>○ Perform comfort measures: Repositioning; relaxation techniques.<br>○ Manipulate the environment and daily routines to provide rest periods. | • Pericarditis is frequently precipitated during the uremic state; fear of "heart attack" on the part of patient/family may complicate therapy and recovery.<br>○ Use "SLIDT" tool (Table 7-1).<br>○ Chest pain associated with pericarditis can be sudden onset, sharp and intermittent, located substernally with radiation to neck and back.<br>○ Diligent monitoring is essential because myocarditis and tamponade can lead to cardiac failure.<br>○ This positioning frequently relieves chest pain associated with pericarditis.<br>○ Comfort measures may decrease pain by promoting relaxation. |

| | | | |
|---|---|---|---|
| | | • Identify patients at risk and predisposing factors: Bacterial/viral infections associated with invasive lines, respiratory and gastrointestinal dysfunction, or wounds; poor dietary intake; depressed immunologic function. | • Prevention and/or prophylaxis is the best treatment. |
| | | ○ Assess for cardiac failure and tamponade. | ○ These complications must be anticipated and can create an acute emergency situation. The focus of diligent, ongoing assessment is to avoid these complications. |
| | | • Discuss underlying cause of pericarditis and its potential impact on patient/family lifestyle. | • An informed patient/family facilitates their participation in the care process. |
| ***Nursing Diagnosis #13***<br>Activity, alteration in: Fatigue and anemia. | Patient will:<br>1. Verbalize decrease in fatigue.<br>2. Exhibit willingness to pace activities.<br>3. Maintain Hct and Hgb within realistic range based on renal function. | • Evaluate activity tolerance — impact of anemic state: | |
| | | ○ Assess onset, time of day, and duration of fatigue, and clinical circumstances in which it occurs. | ○ Fatigue is a major clinical manifestation attributed directly to the uremic state. |
| | | ○ Monitor laboratory data to determine presence and extent of anemia: Hematocrit and hemoglobin; complete blood count (CBC), platelet count; blood urea nitrogen (BUN), serum creatinine. | ○ Anemia is often seen early in ARF and is associated with an inadequate synthesis of erythropoietin factor by the kidneys. Uremia may predispose to bleeding tendencies. |
| | | ○ Assess skin for bruising or petechiae; nasogastric aspirate and stool for occult blood. | ○ Diligent, ongoing assessment is essential to prevent anemia and/or a major bleeding disorder. |
| | | ○ Minimize iatrogenic blood loss. Draw minimal blood samples for laboratory study; handle patient carefully to prevent bleeding; avoid hypodermic injections.<br>○ Use stool softeners to prevent constipation and hemorrhoidal bleeding; use soft small-lumen nasogastric tube to minimize gastric mucosa irritation; monitor vital signs and watch carefully for signs of anemia, hemorrhage, and occult bleeding from whatever source. | ○ Efforts to minimize blood loss are essential in the presence of compromised hematologic function associated with uremia. |
| | | ○ Incorporate rest perods into daily routines. Assist patient/family to set priorities and to pace exercise and other activities alternating with timely rest periods. | ○ Conservation of strength may improve endurance. |

*(continued)*

## TABLE 25–3. CARE PLAN FOR THE PATIENT WITH ACUTE RENAL FAILURE *(Continued)*

| Nursing Diagnoses | Desired Patient Outcomes | Nursing Interventions | Rationales |
|---|---|---|---|
| ***Nursing Diagnosis #14***<br>Knowledge deficit, impact of renal disease on patient/family lifestyle when the course of ARF is extended over several weeks or months. | Patient and family will:<br>1. Verbalize understanding of acute renal failure.<br>2. Verbalize willingness to make adjustments in lifestyle as necessitated by the course of the illness. | • Knowledge deficit–health perceptions.<br>○ Assess patient/family baseline knowledge and readiness to learn.<br>○ Establish a rapport with patient and family.<br>○ Determine appropriate teaching strategies to facilitate learning:<br>– Encourage open discussions regarding renal disease: Etiology, clinical presentation, complications, treatment, and prognosis.<br>– Assist patient/family to relate dietary restrictions and exercise activities to status of renal disease.<br>– Encourage patient/family to verbalize concerns regarding renal disease and expectations of its outcome.<br>○ Reinforce learning and provide feedback for patient/family progress and achievements. | • ARF may require weeks to months for recuperation and often becomes chronic.<br>○ An informed patient/family can participate in care and make adjustments in lifestyle as necessitated by the course of the renal disease.<br>○ An environment of mutual respect and trust can enhance the learning process.<br>○ Learning should occur at a rate that is meaningful and tolerable to patient and family.<br>○ Learning is an ongoing process; praise for one's accomplishments stimulates self-motivation, and assists in determining directions for further growth. |
| ***Nursing Diagnosis #15***<br>Coping, ineffective individual/family: Potential. | Patient will:<br>1. Verbalize feelings regarding renal disease.<br>2. Identify strengths and coping capabilities.<br>3. Make decisions regarding matters of importance to the patient/family.<br>4. Identify resources available in family and community. | • Evaluate coping capabilities:<br>○ Assess patient's ability to solve problems and set priorities.<br>○ Establish a trusting and caring rapport: Patient advocacy; accessibility to patient.<br>○ Encourage verbalization of perceptions, concerns, and feelings.<br>○ Assist patient to identify past coping capabilities. Emphasize strengths; offer praise for accomplishments; encourage development of new coping mechanisms.<br>○ Assist to identify community resources and encourage patient to enlist assistance when necessary. | ○ Problem-solving capability enables patient to assume control and make decisions regarding own actions and behaviors.<br>○ A definitive, dependable support system assists the patient to assume responsibility for the level of health desired.<br>○ Unexpressed and unresolved fears and concerns may compromise ability to cope effectively.<br>○ Active participation in self-care assists the individual to gain a new sense of dignity and feelings of self-worth.<br>○ Additional resources may assist patient to gain increased awareness of self in the interaction among patient, family and environment. |

## PREVENTION OF ACUTE RENAL FAILURE

Perhaps the most efficacious treatment of ARF is *prevention*. Evidence now indicates that early and aggressive fluid and electrolyte repletion significantly reduces the incidence of intrarenal pathophysiology. Preoperative sodium-loading may have a similar effect in preventing subsequent renal damage.

Because of the drug-induced iatrogenic causes of ARF, the patient's clinical history must be scrutinized closely prior to initiation of therapy with nephrotoxic drugs administered alone or in combination with other drugs. Renal function must be monitored closely throughout the course of the therapy. Abuse of potent diuretics has also been implicated in the genesis of ARF.

## NURSING CARE OF THE PATIENT WITH ACUTE RENAL FAILURE

The kidneys play a multifaceted, complex, and intricate role in maintaining the internal environment in a state of dynamic equilibrium. Renal function impacts virtually all life processes, and any impairment in the integrity of renal function can have far-reaching effects on total body physiology and on individual-family-environment interactions.

In the event of a disruption in renal function, timely and appropriate intervention is imperative if life processes and the body as a whole are to be preserved and sustained. Nursing, as a process, has the capacity to intervene in an expedient and purposeful manner to prevent or minimize the repercussions of an actual or potential insult to renal function.

It is essential for critical care nurses to be able to identify patients at risk of developing renal failure and to be aware of those clinical circumstances within which an insult to renal function can occur. The goals of treatment are prevention and prophylaxis. Close monitoring and maintenance of total body fluid, electrolyte, and acid-base balance assist in reducing the incidence of ARF, or should it occur, in minimizing its morbidity.

Prompt recognition and timely intervention are essential to prevent progressive deterioration of renal function, and to minimize the severity and duration of the insult on overall renal, as well as total body function.

### Therapeutic Goals

The overall therapeutic goal in the care of the patient with ARF is to avoid irreversible renal parenchymal damage, and to promote recovery by meticulous attention to fluid and electrolyte balance, nutrition, prevention of infection, and emotional support to the patient and family/significant others. The therapeutic approach used will depend on the underlying insult, the stage of the disease, its duration, and the degree of disability experienced by the patient.

Should significant irreversible renal damage occur, the challenge to nursing is twofold: one, to assist the patient and family to understand the implications of renal disease in terms of their overall lifestyle; and, two, to explore with them and identify the intrafamilial and extrafamilial support systems and resources available to assist them in coping with what could eventually be the catastrophic effects of end-stage renal disease.

Implementation of nursing process in the care of the patient with ARF revolves around the following:

1. Establish a comprehensive database including:
   A. Clinical history functional health patterns.
   B. Physical examination.
   C. Laboratory/diagnostic data.
2. Promote/maintain fluid, electrolyte, and acid-base balance.
3. Promote/maintain effective cardiopulmonary function.
4. Implement prescribed nutritional regimen.
5. Prevent infection.[8]
6. Prevent impairment of integrity of skin and mucous membranes.
7. Ameliorate uremic symptomatology.
8. Provide emotional and psychologic support to patient and family/significant others.

### Nursing Diagnoses, Desired Patient Outcomes and Nursing Interventions in the Care of the Patient with Acute Renal Failure

Pertinent nursing diagnoses, desired patient outcomes, and nursing interventions/rationales are presented in the Care Plan in Table 25-3.

## REFERENCES

1. Rose, BD: Pathophysiology of Renal Disease, ed. 2. McGraw-Hill, New York, 1987, p 307.
2. Rose, BD: Pathophysiology of Renal Disease, ed. 2. McGraw-Hill, New York, 1987, p 395.
3. Cane, RD and Shapiro, B: Case Studies in Critical Care Medicine. Year Book Medical Publishers, Chicago, 1985, p 132.
4. Brogna, L and Lakaszawski, M: The continent urostomy. Am J Nurs 86(2): 160, 1986.
5. Levine, DZ: Care of the Renal Patient. WB Saunders, Philadelphia, 1983, p 177.
6. Don, H: Decision-Making in Critical Care. CV Mosby, St Louis, 1985, p 146.
7. Cotton, J, et al: Nursing management of continuous arteriovenous hemofiltration for acute renal failure. Focus Crit Care 13(5): 21, 1986.
8. Conti, M and Eutropius, L: Preventing UTIs: What works? Am J Nurs 87(3):307, 1987.

# CHAPTER 26

# Nursing Management of the Patient with End-Stage Renal Disease

*Christine M. Chmielewski*

## CHAPTER OUTLINE



## LEARNING OBJECTIVES

**At the end of this chapter, you should be able to:**

1. Define *end-stage renal disease (ESRD).*
2. Identify the etiologic and pathophysiologic mechanisms underlying end-stage renal disease.
3. Describe the stages of end-stage renal disease with respect to clinical presentation and treatment.
4. List the various body system manifestations associated with end-stage renal disease.
5. Review medications commonly used in the treatment of end-stage renal disease.
6. Describe the therapeutic interventions employed in the treatment of end-stage renal disease:
   a. Conservative management.
   b. Dialytic therapy.
7. Describe the various types of dialysis access and the basic nursing care for each.
8. Use the nursing process to organize the care of the patient with end-stage renal disease:
   Assessment
   Nursing diagnosis
   Planning: Desired patient outcomes
   Nursing interventions.

## INTRODUCTION

One needs only to review the many functions performed by the kidneys in order to fully appreciate what happens to the patient in the course of end-stage renal disease. As the excretory, regulatory, and hormonal functions of the kidneys are lost, the disease disrupts virtually every system of the body.

Decreased kidney function, appearance of uremic symptoms, and the loss of urinary output affect the renal patient physically, psychologically, and socially. These bodily changes cause the patient to experience symptoms such as nausea, weakness, fatigue, irritability, confusion, and erratic memory, among others. These symptoms, in turn, have a major impact on the patient's psychologic and social states. Difficulties and disruption occur no matter which stage of renal failure the patient is in because all affect the activities of daily living. Chronic renal disease forces a certain amount of dependency on the patient. As a result, the patient may experience an altered self-image and self-worth.

Although uremic symptoms are alleviated with dialysis and transplantation, new problems occur as a result of these treatments. The renal patient, whether controlled by diet and medications or treated by maintenance dialysis, is not well but rather is "suspended in a state of limbo between the world of the sick and the world of the well, belonging to neither yet a part of both."[1]

The focus of this chapter is on end-stage renal disease, its pathophysiology, and management. While conservative management and dialytic therapy are discussed here, renal transplantation is discussed in Chapters 27 and 57.

## END-STAGE RENAL DISEASE

Chronic renal failure (CRF) or end-stage renal disease (ESRD), as it is now more commonly called, is defined by Lancaster and Pierce as "irreversible kidney disease causing chronic abnormalities in the internal environment and necessitating treatment with dialysis or kidney transplantation for survival."[2] The patient with end-stage renal disease is faced with making the choice between life and death. Chronic maintenance dialysis and transplantation have become widely accepted as treatment modalities. Without either of these interventions, the patient will die.

Two other descriptive terms used with reference to kidney disease are azotemia and uremia. *Azotemia* pertains to the accumulation and retention of nitrogenous waste products in the blood. *Uremia*, which originally meant urine in the blood, now refers to the complex multisystem alterations that occur when the level of kidney function can no longer support the internal milieu.

Progression of renal failure occurs at a variable rate depending on such factors as etiology or additional insults to an already compromised renal status. While the patient with type I diabetes mellitus may not show evidence of clinical symptoms of renal involvement for 10 years or longer,[3,4] the patient with rapidly progressive glomerulonephritis may follow a course of renal deterioration in weeks to months.[5]

### Classification

The etiologic mechanisms underlying the development of ESRD are both numerous and varied. Yet despite this etiologic diversity, the eventual outcome is the same, though the course of the disease processes may vary.

There is no one accepted set of categories for the classification of ESRD; many exist. One such system groups the disease processes under the four major anatomical portions of the kidney, that is, the glomeruli, tubular system, vascular system, and interstitium. Differential diagnosis is often made by biopsy in order to correlate the suspected underlying etiology with morphologic and hematologic changes.

Another common approach is to classify etiology in the same manner as that used for acute renal failure, namely, prerenal (vascular), intrarenal (parenchymal), and postrenal (urologic) causes.

Descriptive categories that take into account the pathophysiologic basis for the particular disease entity include glomerular, infectious or interstitial, vascular, tubular, obstructive, collagen-related, metabolic, congenital, and nephrotoxin-induced diseases.[6,7] Again, these categories are not meant to be exclusive but rather to serve as a guide for systematic arrangement of etiologies. For the purpose of this chapter, these descriptive categories are used.

*Glomerular* diseases account for nearly half of all cases of ESRD. Although the primary defect occurs in the glomeruli, the damage eventually spreads to include the other renal structures. Glomerular changes can involve a single or a combination of histologic alterations. These include cellular proliferation, leukocyte exudation, basement membrane thickening, and sclerosis or hyalinization.[8] Each of these alterations interferes with the normal glomerular functioning and, consequently, with kidney function in general. Additionally, these changes may be described further as focal (involving only some glomeruli), segmental (involving only certain regions of the glomeruli), or diffuse (involving either the entire glomerulus or all glomeruli).

The pathogenesis of glomerular disease occurs most frequently as a result of *immunologic-mediated* processes. The presence of antigen—exogenous or endogenous—stimulates the production of antibody. The resultant effect is antigen-antibody complex deposition within the glomerulus. There are two separate mechanisms by which the immune-complex deposition takes place. First, the antigen–antibody complex circulates and becomes lodged within the glomerular capillary tuft (see Fig. 25–1). Second, as in the case of Goodpasture's syndrome, the antibody is directed against the glomerular basement membrane. (See section entitled "Effector Mechanisms" in Chap. 54 for further details regarding these immune responses.)

Glomerular damage allows passage of substances, such as red blood cells and plasma proteins, which normally cannot be filtered through the intact glomerular epithelium. Therefore, two of the major clinical manifestations of glomerular disease are *hematuria* and *proteinuria*. As proteinuria persists, hypoalbuminemia occurs. This, coupled with alterations in the sodium and water handling by the damaged kidneys, contributes to the edema seen in these patients. The renin–angiotensin-aldosterone system reacts to the physiologic cues it receives. Because the cues are released incorrectly by the damaged kidneys and because the feedback mechanisms are lost, hypertension occurs. As the number of functioning nephrons decreases, urine output falls and the oliguria is accompanied by azotemia and uremic symptoms.

*Interstitial* diseases are characterized by changes that occur primarily in the renal interstitium. Inflammation of the interstitium, often with accompanying cellular exudate, progresses on a course of renal tissue destruction. As fibrosis, hyalinization, and scarring occur, the tubular and vascular systems are affected. The most common interstitial disease category is pyelonephritis caused by the presence of longstanding, recurrent urinary tract infections. Other causes of interstitial disease are analgesic nephropathy, injury from irradiation, and certain metabolic and hereditary diseases.

The *vascular* diseases of the kidney involve changes in the renal vessels, primarily the arteries and arterioles. Narrowing results from atherosclerotic plaque formation, hyaline deposits, endothelial inflammation with scarring, or fibrous tissue formation. Occlusion can occur from emboli, thrombus formation, or simply from the progression of vessel narrowing to total occlusion.

Because of the relationship between renal blood flow and glomerular filtration rate, a compensatory mechanism exists whereby a decrease in renal perfusion activates the renin–angiotensin–aldosterone system. When this mechanism can no longer compensate or when it is beyond the scope of this mechanism to correct the decrease in renal perfusion, the decrease in blood flow leads to a concomitant drop in glomerular filtration rate.

When the major site of renal injury is found in the *tubular* system, the clinical manifestations reflect the site of tubular epithelial cell dysfunction. Those diseases that affect the proximal tubules primarily alter the reabsorptive capabilities of the kidneys, while defects in the distal tubules affect secretion and excretion. Urinary loss of electrolytes, retention of acids, and eventual inability to concentrate urine are just some of the results of tubular damage.

*Obstructions* found above the level of the bladder must be bilateral unless one kidney is already nonfunctional, congenitally absent, or surgically removed. Otherwise, the second kidney would compensate for the loss in the contralateral organ.

Obstruction of urinary outflow not only predisposes the patient to infection and, therefore, to the possibility of pyelonephritis but also causes dilation of the collecting system. This hydronephrosis translates into a back pressure that is greater than glomerular filtration pressure. Consequently, filtration ceases. Increased and prolonged pressure further compresses kidney tissues, thereby decreasing renal blood flow. Ischemic changes occur, and a multifactorial basis for irreversible kidney damage ensues.

The *collagen-related* diseases are, in themselves, multisystem diseases. Systemic lupus erythematosus (SLE), polyarteritis nodosa, and systemic sclerosis affect not only the renal system but also the cardiovascular, respiratory, musculoskeletal, and neurologic systems as well. Renal damage occurs as the result of antigen–antibody complex deposition (as in SLE) and vascular changes such as inflammation, necrosis, and narrowing of the arteries.

*Metabolic* disorders affect the kidneys in a number of ways. Changes can occur in any or all of the renal structures. Diabetes mellitus causes structural changes in the blood vessels and tubular system, while amyloidosis primarily affects the glomeruli by causing basement membrane thickening. The hallmark of *hyperoxaluria* is calcium deposition, not only in the renal tissue, but also in the blood vessels, myocardium, and other body tissues.

While some *congenital* disorders such as renal agenesis and renal aplasia are fatal, others may not cause renal dysfunction until later in life. The presence of structurally nonfunctional tissue decreases renal reserve, and altered renal status may eventually occur. Polycystic and medullary cystic diseases destroy renal tissue by displacement and compression. Infection of the fluid-filled cysts is common, and hematuria occurs secondary to the rupture of these cysts.

The final category is that of *nephrotoxin-induced* disorders. While it is possible that the patient presents with renal problems after exposure to some type of nephrotoxin, it is also possible that the patient's nephrotoxicity is iatrogenic in nature. Toxins frequently encountered outside of the hospital include heavy metals, chemicals, pesticides, and poison mushrooms. Chronic and prolonged use of phenacetin-containing analgesics is a recognized cause of renal damage.

The hospitalized patient is also exposed to a number of potentially nephrotoxic agents. These are the most preventable of causes. The most common of these agents are radiographic contrast media and the aminoglycosides. Other medications may also be implicated as causative factors especially in the patient with underlying renal impairment or other risk factors such as old age or dehydration. In addition, concomitant use of other potentially nephrotoxic agents increases the likelihood of deleterious renal effects. Some of these include amphotericin B, cephalosporins, penicillins, tetracyclines, and antineoplastic agents. Renal damage caused by these agents include glomerular, vascular, tubular, and interstitial changes. Although these changes may be acute in nature and, therefore, theoretically reversible, there may also be residual renal impairment leading to eventual ESRD.

## Stages

Patients who present with renal dysfunction may do so in a number of ways. The patient may or may not feel ill and may be seen at anytime during the course of renal disease. For instance, the patient with type I diabetes mellitus under close and continued medical supervision may be followed throughout the course of gradual but steady decline in renal function. Another patient may be seen with complaints of headache, fluid retention, shortness of breath, nausea, vomiting, and changes in mental status only to find that the patient's level of renal function is so compromised that the need for dialytic therapy is imminent. Still another patient, totally asymptomatic, may be found to have abnormal urine or serum results on a routine physical examination.

How, as in the case of the second patient, can a person live with decreasing renal function—perhaps for years—and not be aware of it until the disease reaches end-stage and uremic manifestations occur? Bricker hypothesized what is now commonly accepted as the *intact nephron theory*.[9] In essence, Bricker identified two types of nephrons in the diseased kidney: those that are affected by the disease and, therefore, rendered nonfunctional, and those that are disease-free and functionally normal. The latter group of nephrons are able to maintain homeostasis because they hypertrophy and, in doing so, are able to pick up the workload of the lost renal mass. This mechanism for maintaining the internal milieu is effective until the later stages of renal failure when the loss of functioning nephrons becomes critical and multisystem evidence of uremia appears.

This adaptive mechanism has been scrutinized by investigators studying not only the progression of renal disease, but also the effect of long-term hypertrophy in the absence of disease, as in the case of organ donors.[10] Interestingly, but not conclusively, the hypertrophy of the nephrons with its concomitant increases in glomerular capillary pressure and renal blood flow has been implicated as a causative factor in further glomerular damage. In order to reduce the high pressures and flows within the glomerulus, thereby halting progression of glomerular changes, it has been suggested that dietary protein restriction and aggressive treatment of hypertension be instituted early in the course of renal disease.

The clinical course of renal disease progresses through three stages: diminished renal reserve, renal insufficiency, and, finally, ESRD.

### *Diminished Renal Reserve*

In diminished renal reserve, the glomerular filtration rate (GFR) is approximately 50–90% of normal. Because of the hypertrophy of the functioning nephrons, homeostasis is maintained. The patient remains asymptomatic, and, for the most part, the blood urea nitrogen (BUN) and serum creatinine levels are within normal limits. At this stage of renal disease, exposure to a nephrotoxin such as contrast medium or aminoglycosides could cause an elevation in the BUN and serum creatinine. Dehydration and infection may have the same effect. No bodily signs or symptoms occur. Removal of the offending agent allows laboratory values to return to baseline.

### *Renal Insufficiency*

As GFR drops to 20–50% of normal, renal insufficiency occurs. One half to three fourths of the nephrons have been destroyed. Although the patient may still remain relatively asymptomatic, he or she now has an elevated BUN and serum creatinine. Also, changes in urine output begin at this time. The kidneys, with their increasingly small number of functioning nephrons, can no longer concentrate the urine. As a result, the patient experiences nocturia and polyuria. Urine osmolarity approaches that of the serum, and specific gravity remains fixed in the range of 1.008–1.012. Exposure to a stressful event at this stage of renal failure results in further elevation of blood values and appearance of related symptoms.

### *End-Stage Renal Disease*

With a GFR of 5–10% of normal, the kidneys lose their ability to regulate the internal environment. The BUN and serum creatinine continue to rise. The patient is symptomatic, the outcome of myriad alterations in the body systems. The patient is now in the final stage, that is, end-stage renal disease.

## Body System Manifestations

The body system alterations that occur with ESRD range from annoying to life-threatening, from easily controllable to persistently incapacitating. A brief overview of the changes the renal patient experiences is presented here. Of all of these changes, the effects of uremia on the cardiovascular and respiratory systems are, by far, the most serious encountered by the patient.

### *Cardiovascular*

Hypertension is seen in most, if not all, ESRD patients. The two major contributory factors are the retention of sodium and fluid and the inappropriate function of the renin–angiotension–aldosterone system. The presence of hypertension itself contributes to further renal damage. Congestive heart failure is seen not only in cases of fluid overload but also in some patients with a high flow vascular access used for hemodialysis. Pericardial disease, ranging from pericarditis to tamponade, appears to result most frequently in highly uremic individuals. Concurrent fluid overload has also been implicated as a causative factor in this condition.

Coronary artery disease is a condition found in many patients with renal disease. The presence of hypertension, hyperlipidemia, atherosclerosis, and lack of physical activity are each responsible, in part, for the development of heart disease. Dysrhythmias may occur for any number of reasons, for example, electrolyte imbalances, metabolic acidosis, volume overload, and dialysis-related problems. Angina may occur while the patient is receiving hemodialysis treatments. This is due not only to volume changes secondary to blood in the extracorporeal circuit but also to the anemia seen in these patients.

Lastly, but also seen more rarely these days, is arterial calcification. This results from the calcium–phosphorus imbalance. As calcium and phosphorus bind and precipitate, they form deposits in the tissues. With adequate control of dietary intake of phosphorus and the prescribed use of phosphate binders, tissue calcification is prevented.

#### Respiratory

Pulmonary edema represents an emergency, which, in many cases, may require hemodialysis therapy for fast and effective fluid removal. Altered sodium and fluid handling by the body is the precipitating factor. Noncompliance of the patient with respect to fluid and salt restrictions may be the cause, although, in the hospital, IV therapy and fluid replacement in the face of oliguria may take the blame. Pleuritis, like pericarditis, is seen in the patient with a high BUN and serum creatinine level. If left untreated, it can progress to an effusion state. Changes within the respiratory system make the lungs more susceptible to infection. Depressed cough reflex, altered white blood cell response, and sputum changes are noted. Calcifications in the lungs, as mentioned in relation to the cardiovascular system, are a rare occurrence in the individual with adequate control of calcium–phosphorus metabolism.

#### Neurologic

The neurologic complications associated with ESRD are basically categorized into two types. The first of these is peripheral neuropathy, and, in most cases, it affects the lower extremities. It tends to be bilateral and occurs as uremia worsens. The two most common neuropathies are referred to as the *restless leg* syndrome and the *burning feet* syndrome. Discomfort, burning, paresthesia, numbness, and a jumpy feeling in the legs are just some of the ways that patients describe these conditions. A notable feature is that these conditions are worse at night and interfere with the patient's comfort and rest. Both syndromes tend to improve and eventually dissipate after dialysis is instituted.

*Encephalopathy* is the second category of neurologic alteration. There are actually different types of encephalopathy recognized in ESRD. One of these is that seen in the patient whose uremia is at the stage that requires dialytic intervention. Changes in mentation and personality occur. Irritability, insomnia, and headaches are frequent complaints. If left untreated, somnolence, seizures, coma, and eventual death would ensue. For the most part, these symptoms disappear when the person is adequately dialyzed.

The *dialysis disequilibrium syndrome* may be seen with the patient who is newly started on hemodialysis. As uremic toxins are removed from the bloodstream more rapidly than across the blood–brain barrier during the course of dialysis, fluid shifts occur. Because of the principles of osmosis, fluid moves from the intravascular space into the cerebrospinal space where solute concentration is higher. The result of this fluid shift is cerebral edema. The patient may suffer from headache, nausea, and vomiting. If not corrected, seizures and coma could result. Recognition of this condition has led to some changes in how the institution of hemodialysis is carried out. Shorter dialysis time, less rapid solute removal, and use of mannitol have prevented this once common occurrence.

Another neurologic problem is a new condition referred to as *dialysis dementia*. Seen in long-term hemodialysis patients, this condition appears to be due to aluminum toxicity. The sources of this aluminum are the water source used for the dialysis treatment and the aluminum hydroxide gels used as phosphate binders. For those patients with recognized toxicity, treatment is available with a drug called desferoxamine, which is given IV during the hemodialysis treatment. It binds with the aluminum and allows for its removal during dialysis.[11]

#### Gastrointestinal

Gastrointestinal alterations occur anywhere within the entire alimentary tract. Changes in taste and smell contribute to an already decreased appetite caused by anorexia, nausea, and vomiting. Thirst may be ever present. *Uremic fetor* is the term used to describe the urinelike odor of the patient's breath. Irritation by uremic toxins causes oral, esophageal, gastric, and intestinal inflammation and ulcerations.

Hiccups may occur and are also thought to be due to the uremia. Sometimes intractable, they are difficult for the patient to tolerate, thereby increasing his or her discomfort and loss of rest. Sedatives and tranquilizers, although sometimes successful in stopping the hiccups, cause the patient to become somnolent. For the most part, hiccups disappear with the start of dialysis.

The most common GI complaint in this group of patients is constipation. Decreased fluid intake, a change in eating habits forced by diet restrictions, phosphate binders, and less physical activity all contribute to the problem.

Because the renal patient has a propensity toward bleeding and because GI irritations can add to further blood loss, it is important to check for the presence of occult blood in vomitus or stool.

### *Hematologic*

Hematologic abnormalities include anemia, bleeding tendencies, and altered white blood cell function. The etiologic mechanisms underlying the anemia associated with ESRD are many. As functional renal mass decreases with the progression of the disease, erythropoietin is affected and red blood cell (RBC) production falls. Deficiencies in body iron stores and folic acid, likewise, contribute to inadequate RBC production. Survival of circulating RBCs is affected by the presence of uremic toxins. Blood loss occurs as the result of hemodialysis where some blood remains in the dialyzer, frequent and numerous blood samples, subclinical bleeding, and damage to the RBCs from the roller pump on the hemodialysis machine. Also, the lowered hematocrit, in part, may be a reflection of volume overload and, therefore, be dilutional. Blood transfusions are not routinely given unless the patient is symptomatic, evidencing such symptoms as dyspnea, tachycardia, and fatigue. One major reason for avoiding transfusion therapy is that the increase in hematocrit secondary to the transfusion serves as a feedback mechanism to the bone marrow and RBC production is suppressed. As a result, the patient becomes transfusion dependent.

The bleeding tendency in the renal patient is due to a qualitative rather than a quantitative platelet defect. As a rule, the platelet count is normal. However, the presence of uremia seems to interfere with the release of platelet factor III, an integral component of the clotting sequence (see Chap. 61). This results in the elevated bleeding time.

Although the white blood cells (WBC) appear to be normal in number and configuration, they appear to have a slower response time in the face of uremia. Because of this, renal patients seem to be more prone to both bacterial and viral infections. Therefore, the WBC is not always the best indicator to follow to rule out the presence of infection. Also, an important piece of information to have is whether the blood specimens were obtained while the patient was on hemodialysis. Although the cause is unknown, the WBC count falls within minutes after hemodialysis is started. It is thought that there is a temporary migration of these cells to the lungs. Again, within a few hours, the count returns to its baseline. A complete blood count (CBC) drawn early in the dialysis run will provide spurious results.

### *Musculoskeletal*

Muscles, joints, and bones undergo changes in ESRD. Muscle weakness may occur secondary to electrolyte imbalances, atrophy, and uremic toxins. Joint discomfort may result from calcification from calcium–phosphorus precipitation, gout, and bone changes. Altered calcium–phosphorus metabolism is at the root of the skeletal changes. A decrease in the functional renal tissue leads to an altered and ineffective synthesis of vitamin D. Because of this, calcium cannot be absorbed as readily from the GI tract. The serum calcium level falls, and this, in turn, triggers the secretion of parathyroid hormone (PTH). PTH causes bone resorption in order to elevate the low calcium levels.

PTH, in normal conditions, also causes the kidneys to excrete the extra phosphorus. In renal failure, this cannot be accomplished. The constant effect of the low serum calcium on the parathyroid glands results in secondary hyperparathyroidism, which sometimes requires surgical intervention. If calcium continues to be extracted from the bones, renal osteodystrophy and osteoporosis occur. Bone pain, bone deformities, and pathologic fractures are all outcomes of bone resorption. Dietary phosphate restriction and phosphate binders instituted early in the course of renal failure help to stop this chain of events.

### *Integument*

Although less serious than other body system changes, the alterations in the integumentary system, nevertheless, are cause for physical and psychologic discomfort. The patient's skin, hair, and nails change in appearance. The skin takes on a tan to bronze color, the result of retained pigments in the body. Pallor from the anemia also contributes to the skin color change. The skin becomes dry and scaly as oil and sweat glands atrophy. Pruritus develops not only from the increased dryness but also from the deposition of calcium–phosphorus crystals. Excoriation and infection may result from patients scratching their skin. Ecchymotic areas appear with the most minor of trauma because of the capillary fragility. The nails and hair become dry and brittle, the result of protein wasting. Hair may fall out and, on occasion, may even change color.

### Acid-Base/Electrolyte

The acid-base disorders and electrolyte abnormalities seen in ESRD are metabolic acidosis, hyperkalemia, hypocalcemia, hyperphosphatemia, hypermagnesemia, and hyponatremia or hypernatremia. All are due to the inability of the diseased kidneys to excrete or reabsorb these substances.

### Endocrine

Finally, renal disease is responsible for a number of endocrine abnormalities, namely, thyroid dysfunction, pituitary-gonadal dysfunction, altered carbohydrate metabolism, and changes in lipid metabolism.

## Conservative Therapy

Conservative management of ESRD involves diet therapy, fluid restriction, and medications. The goals of this management are threefold, that is, preservation of renal function, alleviation of symptoms, and prevention of the multisystem complications.

### Diet Therapy

Diet therapy is employed as a mechanism to control metabolic alterations and to replace lost nutrients. Special attention is given to protein intake, caloric requirements, fluid and electrolyte restrictions, and vitamin and mineral requirements.

As the GFR approaches 10 ml/minute, protein intake and its subsequent breakdown play a major role in the accumulation of nitrogenous waste products (azotemia). At this point, a protein restriction, usually 0.5-1 g/kg of body weight/day, is instituted. This keeps the BUN and other end-products of protein metabolism at a tolerable level. This results in an overall improvement in the way the patient feels. However, an important consideration is that the patient's intake of protein, although restricted, must be adequate to prevent a negative nitrogen balance and, hence, muscle wasting. This is accomplished by the intake of high biologic value protein, which contains the essential amino acids. High biologic value foods include eggs, fish, meats and poultry, milk, and milk products.

Caloric intake should be in the range of 2000-3500 calories/day depending on the patient's age, size, and level of activity. The goals are to maintain body weight and to prevent protein breakdown. Intake of carbohydrates and fats permits this protein-sparing effect.

Control of sodium, potassium, and phosphorus intake is a necessary part of diet therapy. Sodium restriction is based on the overall evaluation of the patient's condition. As long as the kidneys are able to excrete sodium, problems are not encountered. However, certain renal conditions may cause the patient to lose excessive amounts of sodium in the urine. In these cases, hyponatremia can lead to dehydration, and sodium supplementation is a must. Later in the course of renal disease, however, sodium retention occurs, and this leads to fluid overload and its concomitant effects. Restriction at this time is imperative to prevent these complications, some of which are life-threatening.

Hyperkalemia tends to occur later in the course of renal disease, that is, when the GFR falls below 10 ml/minute. Dietary restriction poses a difficult problem because potassium is found in most foods. Even with adequate dietary control, other factors contribute to hyperkalemia and, therefore, must be carefully monitored. These include the use of salt substitutes (which contain potassium chloride), medications that contain potassium (such as potassium penicillin), metabolic acidosis, gastrointestinal bleeding and other sources of hemolysis, blood transfusions, and, finally, any catabolic state (such as trauma or infection).

With decreased renal function comes decreased excretion of phosphorus. The retention of phosphorus, coupled with the lack of vitamin D synthesis and consequent impairment of calcium absorption from the GI tract, leads to the bone disease seen in ESRD. In an effort to halt these skeletal changes, therapy has a twofold approach: first, dietary restriction of phosphorus and, second, the use of phosphate binders. Because some phosphorus will remain in the diet, these binders are taken after meals and help to prevent hyperphosphatemia.

### Fluid Restriction

Fluid intake is restricted when the kidneys can no longer maintain the body's fluid balance. Allowances range from 1000-2000 ml/24 hours. Those patients who maintain some urine output are permitted a more liberal intake and are less likely to suffer from overhydration. Thirst and habit make this restriction a difficult one for the patient to follow. It is important to keep this fact in mind, especially for the hospitalized patient whose meager oral fluid allowance is further decreased when IV therapy is instituted.

### Medication Therapy

Medications commonly used in patients with ESRD may include any or all of the following: anithypertensives, diuretics, phosphate binders, stool softeners and laxatives, antiemetics, antipruritics, cardiotonics, hormonal agents (androgen therapy), vitamins, calcium, iron, and cation exchange resins.

Fluid overload and inappropriate renin secretion both play a role in the development of the hypertension seen in ESRD. Blood pressure control can sometimes be difficult to attain, and it is not uncommon for the patient to be on more than one antihypertensive medication.

Diuretic therapy, often used in conjunction with antihypertensives, is employed in the patient who maintains a urine output. Besides ridding the body of excess fluid, some of these drugs are also able to enhance renal excretion of sodium and potassium. It must be kept in mind, however, that certain diuretics are potassium-sparing and, therefore, can lead to hyperkalemia.

Phosphate binders, or aluminum hydroxide gels, are used for prevention and treatment of the bone disease of ESRD. Taken with meals, these medications bind with the dietary intake of phosphorus, thereby preventing an increase in serum phosphorus. The major side effect noted with phosphate binders is constipation.

In addition to phosphate binders, a number of other factors contribute to the chronic constipation seen in these patients: decreased fluid and fiber intake and lack of physical activity, to name a few. Stool softeners and laxatives (usually bulk-forming) can be used, provided they do not contain magnesium or phosphorus.

As the BUN rises, GI symptoms occur. To combat the nausea and vomiting seen at this time, antiemetics can be prescribed. With the institution of dialysis, these symptoms usually subside.

Dry skin and abnormal calcium–phosphorus metabolism contribute to the pruritus experienced by patients with renal failure. When meticulous skin care and control of serum phosphorus are ineffective, the use of antipruritics becomes necessary for patient comfort.

Cardiac medications are often found in the patient's drug regimen. Atherosclerosis, coronary artery disease, hypertension, cardiac hypertrophy, congestive heart failure, and angina pectoris are some of the cardiac-related conditions associated with ESRD. Because many of these conditions contribute significantly to renal patient mortality, it is the goal of drug therapy to prevent or treat cardiac disease.

Androgen therapy is used to treat anemia that has been unresponsive to other measures, that is, diet, vitamin, and iron therapy. The medication is administered by mouth or by injection usually for a period of up to 6 months. It is not successful in all cases, and the side effects reflect the male hormone component.

Vitamin supplements consist of multivitamins, folic acid, and vitamin D. These fill the void left by inadequate intake secondary to dietary constraints. Also, once dialysis is employed, water-soluble vitamins are lost during treatment and must be replaced. An important point to remember is that serum phosphorus must be within normal limits before vitamin D is given. Otherwise, the increase in serum calcium will interact with an already elevated phosphorus, leading to potential tissue calcifications and worsening bone disease.

Oral calcium supplements are given when hypocalcemia occurs, when vitamin D has been ineffective used alone, and when serum phosphorus levels are normal. If vitamin D and calcium supplements are given concomitantly, careful monitoring of the serum calcium is necessary.

Iron supplements play a role in the correction of anemia, provided the anemia is related to depleted iron stores in the body. Usually administered in oral form, iron can be rendered inactive by phosphate binders and, therefore, should not be given at mealtime.

Use of a cation exchange resin is most commonly seen as an emergency treatment for hyperkalemia. Basically, it works by releasing sodium ions in exchange for potassium ions. The net result is a lowered serum potassium. The route of administration is by mouth or by retention enema. The dry powdered form can be mixed with either water or sorbitol, the latter being more effective in preventing constipation. Because the site of action is in the large intestine, administration by enema achieves results in approximately 30–60 minutes, whereas the oral dose can take up to 1–2 hours.

## Dialytic Therapies

As renal failure progresses to end-stage and the GFR falls below 5 ml/minute, the kidneys lose the last of their compensatory capabilities. With the loss of the excretory and regulatory functions, the kidneys cannot rid the body of metabolic waste products, acids, electrolytes, or fluid. The uremia, at this point, has affected every system of the body, and it threatens the life of the patient. Conservative therapy is no longer an effective treatment option.

The patient has one of three choices to make, that is, dialysis, transplantation, or no further treatment at all. It is not uncommon for the patient with ESRD to opt for any or all of those choices at some time. As was stated previously, it is not the intent of this chapter to cover transplantation (see Chaps. 27 and 57). Also, because refusal of or discontinuation of treatment can, in and of itself, be a lengthy topic of discussion, it will not be covered here.

There is no cure for ESRD. Although dialysis is able to sustain life, it falls short when compared to the work performed by the kidneys. While dialysis can remove some of the uremic toxins and maintain some semblance of fluid and electrolyte balance, it cannot replace the kidney's other important functions. Therefore, the patient continues to follow diet and fluid restrictions, and medications continue to play a role in the control of the disease and its manifestations.

There are two basic types of dialytic therapy: hemodialysis and peritoneal dialysis. The principles of both are the same, that is, each involves a blood compartment and a dialysate compartment separated by a semipermeable membrane. Movement of fluid and solutes across this membrane is governed by the processes of diffusion, filtration, and osmosis (see Table 25–2).

### *Hemodialysis*

Although the technical aspects of hemodialysis require the mastery of certain knowledge and skills, the process of hemodialysis is not difficult to understand. The semipermeable membrane in this case is in the dialyzer (also known as the artificial kidney). A concentration gradient exists between the blood and dialysate compartments, and solute movement occurs in both directions. For the most part, the electrolyte composition of the dialysate solution is similar to that of normal extracellular fluid. However, potassium, sodium, and calcium concentrations can vary to meet the needs of the particular patient. Acetate or bicarbonate is used to combat metabolic acidosis. Those substances, such as the metabolic waste products, that need to be removed from the patient are not found in the dialysate.

As the patient's blood is pumped through one compartment (hollow fibers or cellulose sheets, depending on the design of the dialyzer), the dialysate is pumped through the other compartment in a countercurrent direction. This flow pattern allows fresh dialysate to circulate continuously, thereby maintaining a constant concentration gradient between the two compartments.

Because blood has a tendency to clot in the extracorporeal circuit, an anticoagulant, most commonly heparin, is used. The goal of anticoagulation is to prevent clotting in the dialyzer and blood lines while, at the same time, to prevent bleeding problems in the patient. Clotting times are performed throughout the dialysis procedure to monitor the anticoagulation effects. In some patients, most notably those with decreased hematocrits, thrombocytopenia, or prolonged partial thromboplastin time (PTT), it is possible to dialyze the patient without an anticoagulant.

The major function of the dialysis machine is to allow for both a safe and effective treatment. In addition to pumping the blood and delivering the proper concentration of dialysate solution and water, it monitors a variety of factors: blood and dialysate flow rates, the temperature and conductivity of the dialysate, and arterial and venous blood line pressures. It checks for the presence of blood in the spent dialysate (which signifies a rupture in the dialyzer) and, therefore, a source of blood loss. It also monitors the blood as it returns to the patient to be sure that there is no air in the line, a potentially fatal complication.

Auditory and visual alarms alert the dialysis nurse to the presence of a potentially harmful condition or to a change in one of the parameters on the machine. Conditions that are harmful to the patient, such as air in the blood or a change in the dialysate temperature, will automatically stop the machine and, subsequently, protect the patient.

Hemodialysis requires access to the patient's vascular system. This access may be external (shunt, subclavian catheter, femoral catheter) or internal (fistula, graft). Some, as is the case with the femoral catheter, are used only as a temporary access. The need for a special vascular access is dictated by the fact that blood flow rates up to 350–400 ml/minute are required during dialysis.

The arteriovenous shunt was a major breakthrough that made chronic hemodialysis a possibility.[12] Its use today, however, is limited. It is more frequently seen in the patient with acute renal failure. An instance in which it might still be employed in ESRD is in the patient awaiting maturation of a fistula but in need of immediate dialysis.

The shunt consists of two pieces of Silastic tubing, each connected to a sturdy Teflon tip. One tip is inserted surgically into an artery, the other into a vein. A special connector holds the Silastic tubing together so that the blood flows from the artery to the vein. Placement is usually in the wrist area of the nondominant arm, with ankle placement as a second choice. Complications include infection, clotting, skin erosion, dislodgement, and hemorrhage.

Subclavian catheters are seen more frequently in the patient with acute renal failure but are used in certain instances with the ESRD patient. Indications include temporary access for short-term dialysis before a scheduled living, related donor transplant or for use until a fistula matures. Also, if a problem with a fistula or graft occurs, the catheter may be used in the interim. There is now available a permanent, surgically placed subclavian dialysis catheter, which is being used for the chronic hemodialysis patient. Complications seen with subclavian catheters are of two types: those secondary to insertion and those after the catheter has been in place. Those associated with the former include hemothorax, pneumothorax, laceration of the subclavian artery, and hematoma. The latter are clotting, emboli, subclavian vein thrombosis, and sepsis.

There are two kinds of femoral dialysis catheters. The Shaldon catheter is a single-lumen catheter that requires a second access (or a special device called a single-needle device) to avoid recirculation of the blood leading to inadequate dialysis. If two Shaldon catheters are used, they may be placed bilaterally or in the same femoral vein. The newer type of femoral catheter has a double lumen so that blood can be taken from one port and returned through the other during dialysis without any mixing of dialyzed and nondialyzed blood. The complications seen with the femoral catheters, like with the subclavians, are related to insertion and to problems afterwards. These include hematoma, retroperitoneal bleeding, and laceration of the femoral artery; infection; embolus; and femoral vein thrombosis.

With the advent of the arteriovenous (AV) fistula, another major step occurred in hemodialysis. Using the patient's own vessels, Cimino and Brescia were able to create the internal vascular access.[13] The anastomosis between the artery and vein directs arterial blood flow into the vein, resulting in venous distention. The creation of this high-flow vessel allows for direct and repeated venipunctures in the venous side of the access. The AV fistula is the most common vascular access route used. It has not only the lower incidence of complications (clotting and infection) but also the longest life span.

In some instances, it is not possible to create a fistula using the patient's own vessels. The vessels may be too small, injured, or rendered unusable by previous procedures. A graft is then used. Anastomosed between an artery and a vein, it serves as the conduit for blood flow and the site for needle placement during dialysis. Graft materials include bovine (specially treated bovine carotid artery) and polytetrafluoroethylene (PTFE). Saphenous vein grafts are rarely used today. As with the fistula, complications involve clotting and infection.

Two complications seen with the fistula and graft occur soon after surgical creation of the access. Because of their detrimental effect on the patient, these complications require immediate attention and surgical intervention. The *steal syndrome*, which is responsible for ischemic changes in the extremity distal to the access, is caused by the shunting of blood through the access and away from the distal circulation. At first, subtle changes occur in the skin temperature and sensation. Later, pain, paresthesia, swelling, and absence of pulses ensue. If allowed to continue, gangrene and limb loss are the sequelae.

*High-output cardiac failure* also results from the large volume flow through the access. In this case, increased venous return to the heart cannot be tolerated by some individuals. This leads to pulmonary congestion and heart failure. Surgical intervention includes a procedure called *banding*, in which the lumen of the high-flow vessel is narrowed.[14] If this intervention is ineffective in alleviating the problem, surgical ligation of the vessel is usually necessary.

### Peritoneal Dialysis

Peritoneal dialysis (PD), once the mainstay of acute renal failure therapy, has gained in popularity as a treatment modality for ESRD. Improvement in catheters, related supplies, and techniques has allowed peritoneal dialysis to be performed outside the hospital. When the patient enters the hospital, it is not enough for the nurse to know that the patient is on peritoneal dialysis. The nurse must be aware of which mode of dialysis the patient is on. Although each type of peritoneal dialysis accomplishes the same goal, it does so in different ways.

*Intermittent peritoneal dialysis* (*IPD*) involves 3–7 treatments per week. Because the treatment can last up to ten hours, automated equipment is used. It is often performed overnight. At the end of the treatment, the fluid is drained, and the peritoneal cavity remains empty until the next treatment.

*Continuous cyclic peritoneal dialysis* (*CCPD*), like IPD, is automated. There are two major differences between the two. First, treatments are performed every night for 8–10 hours. Second, during the last exchange, the fluid is allowed to dwell in the peritoneal cavity and remains there until the next night.

*Continuous ambulatory peritoneal dialysis* (*CAPD*), unlike the other two, does not involve automated equipment. Three to five exchanges are performed manually every day. The last exchange is performed at bedtime, and the fluid is allowed to dwell overnight.

As with hemodialysis, the process of peritoneal dialysis involves both blood and dialysate compartments separated by a semipermeable membrane, in this case, the peritoneum. Dialysate is infused by way of a special catheter into the peritoneal cavity. To maintain a concentration gradient between the two compartments, exchanges are performed every 1–6 hours, depending on the mode of the treatment.

The effectiveness of peritoneal dialysis is influenced by a number of factors, some related to the dialysate and the others to the patient. Dialysate-related factors are the amount, concentration, and temperature of the fluid, the flow rate, and the volume of dialysate in the peritoneal cavity. The other factors are blood flow to the peritoneum and effective surface area of the peritoneal membrane. The last of these can be especially influenced by the presence of peritonitis.

Access to the peritoneal cavity is achieved by means of a catheter surgically implanted when the patient is in the OR. This catheter serves as the conduit for the inflow and outflow of the dialysate. Although there are some differences in catheter design, usually involving the intraperitoneal section, each performs the same function. Care of the PD access, like the vascular access, must be meticulous. It is the patient's only means for treatment of ESRD.

Peritonitis is the most serious infectious complication associated with PD. The outcome of peritonitis ranges from quick resolution to less favorable

**TABLE 26–1 CARE PLAN FOR THE PATIENT WITH END-STAGE RENAL DISEASE**

| Nursing Diagnoses | Desired Patient Outcomes | Nursing Interventions | Rationales |
|---|---|---|---|
| ***Nursing Diagnosis #1*** Acid–base balance, alteration in: Metabolic acidosis. | Patient outcomes: See Table 25–3. | • For pertinent nursing interventions and rationales, see: Table 25–3, Nursing Diagnosis #5. | |
| ***Nursing Diagnosis #2*** Nutrition, alteration in: Less than body requirements. | See Table 25–3. | Table 25–3, Nursing Diagnosis #6. | |
| ***Nursing Diagnosis #3*** Knowledge deficit: Dietary regimen in renal disease. | See Table 25–3. | Table 25–3, Nursing Diagnosis #7. | |
| ***Nursing Diagnosis #4*** Knowledge deficit: Medications in renal disease. | Patient will:<br>1. Correctly identify medications. | • Develop teaching plan: | |
| | | ◦ Assess patient's level of understanding. | ◦ Appropriate vocabulary and teaching method are necessary for learning. |
| | 2. Verbalize understanding of the purpose and side effects. | ◦ Assess patient's level of anxiety. | ◦ Anxiety interferes with learning. |
| | | ◦ Assess patient's readiness to learn. | ◦ Patient must be ready to learn before teaching can be started. |
| | | ◦ Implement schedule that allows for short, effective teaching sessions. | ◦ Patient can become easily overwhelmed with information. |
| ***Nursing Diagnosis #5*** Infection, potential for: Depressed immunologic system. | See Tables 25–3 and 56–1. | • For pertinent nursing interventions and rationales, see: Table 25–3, Nursing Diagnosis #8. Table 56–1. | |
| ***Nursing Diagnosis #6*** Infection, potential for: Dialysis access. (See also Table 49–7.) | See Table 25–3.<br>1. Access insertion site will remain free of signs of infection. | • Shunt care:<br>◦ Change dressing prn. | ◦ Dressing routinely done by dialysis nurse. Procedure for dressing must be followed. |
| | | ◦ Assess insertion sites for redness, swelling, exudate, or other signs of infection. | ◦ Infection at insertion site can erode skin and vessel. |
| | 2. Patient on PD will remain free of peritonitis. | ◦ Use sterile gloves when handling the shunt. | ◦ Infection is major complication of shunt. |
| | | ◦ Do not disconnect shunt (e.g., to draw blood samples). | ◦ Shunt should only be used for dialysis and then only by dialysis nurse. |

| | | | |
|---|---|---|---|
| | | ◦ Monitor patient's parameters: Temperature, white blood counts, routine culture results. | ◦ Note: WBC count falls within minutes after hemodialysis is started. |
| | | ◦ Obtain cultures as necessary. | |
| | | • For pertinent nursing interventions and rationales, see Table 25–3, Nursing Diagnosis #8. | |
| | | • Subclavian catheter. | |
| | | ◦ Dressing should be sterile and occlusive. Change prn if soiled or nonocclusive. | ◦ Infection is major complication and requires removal of catheter. |
| | | ◦ Assess catheter insertion site. Note whether sutures are intact. | ◦ Sutures prevent migration of catheter. |
| | | ◦ Do not reinsert catheter if it has partially slipped out. | ◦ Introduces contaminated catheter into vessel. |
| | | ◦ Do not use the access (for blood drawing, IV route). | ◦ Access is meant only for dialysis. Heparin is used to keep catheter patent. Catheter must be aspirated to remove heparin and also to reduce risk of embolism. |
| | | • Femoral catheter (see procedure for subclavian catheter, above). | |
| | | • PD catheter (acute or newly inserted). | |
| | | ◦ Change dressing every 24–48 hr. Dressing must be sterile and occlusive. Must cover catheter insertion site. (Acute catheter dressing must cover catheter tubing junction.) | ◦ Infection can occur at insertion site or at catheter junction. |
| | | ◦ Assess site for signs of infection. | ◦ Infection can lead to catheter removal. |
| | | ◦ Use sterile gloves and masks during dressing change, when performing bag changes, or whenever system is open. | ◦ Airborne contaminants can cause infection. |
| | | ◦ Use antibacterial soap to scrub hands before disconnecting anywhere in the system. | ◦ Decreases number of microorganisms. |
| | | ◦ Check for presence of catheter clamp. Close it whenever system will be discon- | ◦ Prevents direct route into peritoneum. |
| ***Nursing Diagnosis #7*** Injury, potential for: Uremia-induced GI disorders. | See Table 25–3. | • For pertinent nursing interventions/rationales, see Table 25–3, Nursing Diagnosis #9. | |
| ***Nursing Diagnosis #8*** Skin integrity, impairment of: Potential. | See Table 25–3. | Table 25–3, Nursing Diagnosis #10. | |
| ***Nursing Diagnosis #9*** Oral mucous membrane, alteration in. | See Table 25–3. | Table 25–3, Nursing Diagnosis #11. | |
| ***Nursing Diagnosis #10*** Activity, alteration in: Fatigue, anemia. | See Table 25–3. | Table 25–3, Nursing Diagnosis #14. | |

*(continued)*

**TABLE 26-1 CARE PLAN FOR THE PATIENT WITH END-STAGE RENAL DISEASE** *(Continued)*

| Nursing Diagnoses | Desired Patient Outcomes | Nursing Interventions | Rationales |
|---|---|---|---|
| ***Nursing Diagnosis #11*** Noncompliance, potential for: Diet and fluid restrictions. | Patient will: 1. Maintain weight within 3–5 lb of dry weight. 2. Be free of signs of volume overload. 3. Have laboratory values that reflect compliance with medical regimen. | • Evaluate patient's knowledge base to rule out knowledge deficit. | • Knowledge deficit is treated differently. (See Table 25–3, Nursing Diagnosis #14.) |
| | | • Reinforce teaching of diet and fluid restrictions and medications. | • Increased understanding may lead to improved compliance. |
| | | • Allow patient to choose foods and fluids when necessary, and reinforce good choices. | • This allows patient to feel more in control of his/her situation. |
| | | • Assess patient to discover factors contributing to noncompliance. | • Anger, denial, frustration, and subconscious death wish are common factors underlying noncompliance and should be treated. |
| ***Nursing Diagnosis #12*** Bowel elimination, alteration in: Constipation. | Patient will have regular bowel pattern. | • Assess patient's usual pattern and use of aids. | • Gives baseline for comparison. |
| | | • Document bowel pattern. | • Prevents patient from developing impaction by monitoring bowel status. |
| | | • Consult with dietitian to evaluate allowable fiber and roughage in restricted renal diet. | |
| | | • Check stools for presence of blood. | • GI complications occur frequently in ESRD. Heme-positive stool may indicate subclinical to active GI bleeding. Stools will be dark if patient is on iron therapy. |

| | | | |
|---|---|---|---|
| ***Nursing Diagnosis #13***<br>Comfort, alteration in: Skeletal changes. | Patient will maintain serum calcium and phosphorus within normal limits. | • Monitor lab values.<br>• Review patient's dietary intake of phosphorus. Have dietary consult, if necessary. | |
| | | • Administer phosphate binders immediately after meals. | • Binders and food must be present in the stomach at the same time to be effective. |
| ***Nursing Diagnosis #14***<br>Coping, ineffective individual/family: Potential. | See Table 25–3. | • For pertinent nursing interventions and rationales, see: Table 25–3, Nursing Diagnosis #15. | |

outcomes including the formation of an intraperitoneal abscess, the loss of effective membrane due to scarring, the necessary removal of the catheter (usually because of unresolved peritonitis), and death of the patient. Cloudy effluent (due to the presence of white blood cells and fibrin) is the hallmark sign of peritonitis. Other signs and symptoms include abdominal pain, rebound tenderness, fever, and chills. A culture and Gram's stain of the effluent identify the causative organism(s). Antibiotics are given intraperitoneally to combat infection, and heparin is added to the dialysate to prevent catheter blockage and adhesion formation. Two other infectious complications seen with PD are subcutaneous tunnel infection and exit site infection.

The dialysate is composed of a dextrose solution with added electrolytes and minerals. The dextrose concentration is available in three standard concentrations: 1.5%, 2.5%, and 4.25% solutions. Because the dialysate is hypertonic, it removes fluid by osmotic pull. As the fluid is removed by this force, it is accompanied by small molecules. This process is called solvent drag and, in addition to diffusion, plays a role in solute removal.

Because movement occurs between both compartments, substances can be added to the dialysate that the patient will absorb. Insulin, potassium, and antibiotics are just some of the common additives. Some diabetics can even be maintained solely on intraperitoneal insulin. However, because of the high glucose load and its subsequent absorption into the bloodstream, blood sugar control may sometimes be more difficult.

There are two pieces of equipment used with peritoneal dialysis patients that the nurse may encounter. The first is the cycler. This automated machine is able to perform hourly (or longer) exchanges. By and large, it has replaced the old method of changing bags every 1-2 hours. Not only does it save time, but its major advantage is that fewer breaks occur in the system, thereby allowing fewer opportunities for contamination. Solution can be set up for up to 36 hours. The machine heats and delivers the solution; controls the inflow, dwell, and outflow cycles; and monitors the amount of fluid delivered and returned.

Because peritonitis is the major complication of CAPD (often due to touch contamination), various methods have been designed to decrease the risk of contamination. One such device is the ultraviolet light. This small, easy-to-use piece of equipment uses ultraviolet light to sterilize both the catheter spike and the outlet port of the new bag. It must be used with each CAPD exchange.

## Nursing Care of the Patient with End-Stage Renal Disease

For nursing diagnoses, desired patient outcomes, and nursing interventions in the care of the patient with end-stage renal disease, see the care plan in Table 26-1.

## REFERENCES


1. Landsman, MK: The patient with chronic renal failure: A marginal man. Ann Intern Med 82:268, 1975.
2. Lancaster, LE and Pierce, P: Total body manifestations of end stage renal disease and related medical and nursing management. In Lancaster, LE (ed): The Patient with End Stage Renal Disease. John Wiley & Sons, New York, 1979, p 4.
3. Knowles, HC: Magnitude of the renal failure problem in diabetic patients. Kidney Int 6:S2-S7, 1974.
4. D'Elia, JA, et al: Diabetic nephropathy. Comprehensive Therapy 5(9):47, 1979.
5. Leaf, A and Cotran, R: Renal Pathophysiology. Oxford University Press, New York, 1976, p 284.
6. Netter, F: Kidneys, ureters and urinary bladder. Vol. 6 in The CIBA Collection of Medical Illustrations. CIBA Medical Education Division, West Caldwell, NJ, 1974, p 113.
7. Renal and Urologic Disorders. In Nurse's Clinical Library Series. Springhouse Corporation, Springhouse, PA, 1984, p 87.
8. Leaf, A and Cotran, R: Renal Pathophysiology. Oxford University Press, New York, 1976, pp 268-269.
9. Bricker, NS, et al: The pathophysiology of renal insufficiency: On the functional transformations in the residual nephrons with advancing disease. Pediatr Clin North Am 18:595, 1971.
10. Anderson, S, Meyer, TW, and Brenner, BM: The role of hemodynamic factors in the initiation and progression of renal disease. J Urol 133:363, 1985.
11. Linamegi, E: Aluminum toxicity. NAPHT News. May 1985, p 2.
12. Quinton, W, Dillard, D, and Scribner BH: Cannulation of blood vessels for prolonged hemodialysis. Trans Am Soc Art Int Organs 6:104, 1960.
13. Cimino, JE and Brescia, MJ: Simple venipuncture for hemodialysis. N Engl J Med 267:608, 1962.
14. Krupski, WC, et al: Access for dialysis. In Cogan, MG and Garovoy, MR (eds): Introduction to Dialysis. Churchill Livingston, New York, 1985, p 66.

CHAPTER 27

# Nursing Management of the Renal Transplant Patient

*Jo-Ann Murray-Schluckebier and Christine Chmielewski*

## CHAPTER OUTLINE



## LEARNING OBJECTIVES

**At the end of this chapter, you should be able to:**

1. Identify the types of renal transplants.
2. Describe transplant donor selection.
3. Describe the care required for the cadaver donor.
4. List the components of the human immune system.
5. Identify the pathophysiologic mechanisms of transplant rejection.
6. Specify the immunosuppressants used postoperatively.
7. Describe the implications of infection in the transplanted kidney.
8. State the major complications of renal transplantation.
9. Apply the nursing process to the care of the renal transplant patient.
   Assessment.
   Nursing diagnosis.
   Planning: Desired patient outcomes
   Nursing interventions.

## INTRODUCTION

Renal transplantation is an accepted and proven method of treatment for end-stage renal disease (ESRD). Several thousand transplants are performed annually in this country alone and are available at most major medical centers. As of 1986, over 65,000 renal transplants had been performed. Significant advances in the field of immunology have been made since the first transplants between identical twins in the 1950s. The ability to better control the immune response with potent specific immunosuppressants and refinements in both surgical techniques and organ preservation have established renal transplantation as a major medical intervention.

The following multicenter data demonstrate the dramatic improvements in both patient and kidney graft survival. One-year living, related donor patient survival has increased from 84% in 1968 to 97% in the 1980s. During the same period, the

1-year survival rate for patients receiving cadaveric transplants went from 60% to 90%.[1]

Kidney transplants in which the donor is a living, genetically similar family member of the recipient have a higher rate of graft survival than do those of cadaver donors. In addition to the benefits of genetic similarities, these organs are not subjected to the ischemic changes related to prolonged preservation times. The probability for 1-year graft survival for transplants from cadaveric donors is 85% now as compared with 55% in 1968. Graft survival for living, related donor kidneys has remained over 90% throughout the years.[1]

This chapter will review several major nursing considerations in the care of the renal transplant patient. (See also Chaps. 54 and 57).

## RENAL TRANSPLANTATION

Studies of ESRD patients following transplantation often reveal successful physical and occupational rehabilitation. Transplant patients report a higher objective and subjective quality of life than did patients undergoing any form of dialysis.[2] Improvements in physical well-being following a successful renal transplant may be attributed to sufficient renal filtration and endocrine function. Fluid and dietary restrictions, with the exception of sodium, are no longer required. Normal calcium–phosphorus balance is restored, possibly halting the skeletal changes resulting from renal osteodystrophy. The anemia attributed to the lack of erythropoietin, diminished iron stores, blood loss, and the effect of uremia on red blood cell survival is reversed. Neuropathies and poor muscle tone may be restored with exercise. Impotence may improve, and women may resume ovulation and menstruation while reporting a gradual return of libido. Cardiovascular changes resulting from accelerated atherosclerosis and chronic hypervolemia may be halted. However, cardiac disease resulting from myocardial infarction or chronic congestive heart failure remains a problem despite the modality of treatment.[3]

The benefits, however, should be weighed against the risks of major surgery and the need for long-term chemical immunosuppression. Further disadvantages of transplantation include the risk of potentially overwhelming fungal, bacterial, or viral infections; aseptic necrosis of the bone; and an increased incidence of malignancies, hypertension, and ulcer disease.[4]

Few studies document the comparative morbidity rates of hemodialysis and kidney transplant patients. However, it does appear that patients with ESRD, regardless of which intervention is chosen, are at risk for developing complications of varying severity.[4]

### Donor Evaluation

Donor kidneys for transplantation come from 3 sources. The first is a living, related donor, either sibling, parent, child, or more distant relative. The determining factor of success is the selection of the most appropriate donor by matching the shared HLA antigens. The major histocompatibility complexes (MHC) on human leukocyte antigens (HLA) in humans are those genes located on the sixth chromosome that code for individual immune response. Once the donor is identified, he will undergo a series of examinations and studies ensuring that 2 normal kidneys are present and that no underlying systemic disease or infection exists. It is important for the transplant team and family to openly discuss this donation. Although it has been shown that there is little risk to the donor aside from surgery itself, nothing should be undertaken that would adversely affect the potential donor's well-being.

The second donor source is a living person, nonrelated to the recipient, usually a spouse or close friend. Although not genetically related, the donor and recipient are considered emotionally related. Very few situations would warrant this type of transplant. If a living, related donor is unavailable and a cadaver kidney is difficult to obtain, a living, nonrelated donor who is properly motivated and medically stable may be considered. The donor must be compatibly matched with the recipient.

The third and most common donor for kidney transplants is the cadaver donor. In 1985, approximately 70% of all transplants performed were from cadaver donors. Criteria for cadaveric donation customarily require that the donor be newborn to age 50; free of systemic, infectious, or metastatic disease; and brain dead. Brain death determination is made at the hospital, and requirements may vary among institutions and states. The intensive care unit nurse should be familiar with the hospital policies for brain death and potential donor referral.

Care of the donor in the intensive care unit focuses on the maintenance of cardiorespiratory and renal function. Hypoxia should be monitored by arterial blood gases and avoided. Adequate intravenous hydration prevents hypovolemia and should promote sufficient diuresis. The use of vasopressors is acceptable but should be weaned if vasoconstriction occurs with subsequent decreased renal perfusion. Laboratory studies are done routinely. Baseline serum creatinine levels are often helpful because serum creatinine elevations may result from trauma. The acceptance of brain death is extremely difficult, and support of the patient's family at this time is an integral aspect of nursing care. (For brain death criteria, see Table 57–2.) Following donor nephrectomy, the kidneys are flushed and preserved in a cold electrolyte solution. Because graft survival has been related to cold ischemic time, most institutions prefer to transplant the organ within 48 hours of the donor surgery.[5] Efforts to promote increased awareness of the need for more organ donors should further expand organ availability.

## Recipient Evaluation

The evaluation for renal transplantation is necessary to identify any potential problems resulting from preexisting conditions. It is essentially the same for all transplant recipients, regardless of the kidney donor source. Generally the evaluation includes a review of all the body systems with special attention to the cardiovascular system, as well as a psychologic and immunologic evaluation. Extensive information about transplantation, the need for long-term follow-up, and patient reliability are discussed in depth with the patient, family members, and the transplant team. A voiding cystourethrogram (VCUG) is performed to establish the existence of normal urinary tract function. Should abnormalities such as ureteral reflux be found, corrective surgery may take place prior to transplantation.

Other required studies include a chest x-ray, electrocardiogram, tuberculin skin test, urine culture, viral titers, liver function tests, a hepatitis profile, HIV, and for women a Papanicolaou smear. The presence of malignancy, coronary artery disease, active peptic ulcer disease, or infection is a contraindication to transplantation.

The benefits of blood transfusions prior to transplantation are still unclear. A 10 to 15% increase in kidney graft survival rates has been noted when 5 or more red blood cell transfusions are received by the transplant candidate prior to surgery. The blood transfusions may stimulate an immunologic enhancement, thereby diminishing the incidence and severity of rejection episodes.[6] Some patients develop cytotoxic antibodies in response to the foreign antigens received from the blood transfusions. This hypersensitivity complicates matching for a cadaver kidney and often predisposes the recipient to a long waiting period before a suitably matched donor kidney can be found.

Following the evaluation process, cadaver donor recipients are placed on a waiting list for renal transplant. Those patients who have high levels of cytotoxic antibodies, who poorly tolerate dialysis, or who have difficulty maintaining a dialysis access are considered priority patients for transplantation. Fresh recipient serum samples are obtained monthly and refrigerated. This ensures availability of recipient lymphocytes for preliminary crossmatching with all potential cadaver donors.

A potentially successful match is determined by blood group (ABO) compatibility and a negative T-cell crossmatch. The crossmatch is performed by mixing donor lymphocytes with serum from the recipient. If the recipient has preformed cytolytic antibodies to the donor, a positive crossmatch will ensue, and transplantation is contraindicated because hyperacute rejection would probably be the result.

# TRANSPLANT IMMUNOLOGY

To understand organ transplantation and consequent complications the nurse must have a basic understanding of immunology. The human immune system is responsible for recognizing and resisting foreign substances, such as bacteria, viruses, toxins, and cells unrelated to itself.[7]

Therefore, medications that suppress the immune system are required for as long as the transplanted kidney functions. Cessation of the immunosuppressive medications while the transplanted kidney is still functioning would probably cause a rejection episode that is frequently irreversible. This immunosuppression, because it interferes with the normal immune response, predisposes the patient to infections, opportunistic pathogens, and possibly malignancies. The two types of acquired immunity are cellular immunity (T-lymphocytes) and humoral immunity (B-lymphocytes or antibodies). While cell-mediated immunity is the chief mechanism whereby transplanted organs are rejected early on, humoral immune mechanisms play a role primarily in both hyperacute and chronic or long-term rejection. (See section entitled "Transplant Rejection.")

Cellular immunity involves the sensitization of the patient's T-lymphocytes to a foreign substance, for example, transplanted kidney tissue. These cells proliferate and infiltrate the kidney. The consequent inflammatory response results in tissue damage, disruption of normal renal blood flow, and rejection.

Humoral or B-cell immunity involves a series of antigen–antibody reactions. The presence of antigen or foreign tissue elicits the formation of specific antibodies, which function to attack the antigen. Such antigen–antibody reactions may account for the pathophysiology of underlying renal disease and may be encountered in hyperacute or accelerated rejection reactions (see Chap. 54).

## Transplant Rejection

Despite the advances in and availability of immunosuppressive medications, allograft rejection remains one of the most plaguing problems for transplant recipients. The majority of patients will undergo at least one acute rejection episode within the first 6 months. Rejections can be categorized as follows:

TABLE 27-1
**Symptoms of Acute Rejection**

| |
|---|
| Elevated temperature |
| General malaise |
| Tenderness over graft |
| Elevated blood pressure |
| Decreased urine output |
| Rapid weight gain |
| Peripheral edema |

*Hyperacute rejection* usually occurs within minutes to hours after the surgical anastomoses are completed. It results from the reaction of preformed cytotoxic antibodies in the recipient's body with the foreign antigen. Intrarenal vascular thrombosis results, and the kidney must be removed. Renal scans documenting poor dye uptake confirm the lack of renal function.[8]

*Accelerated rejection* can occur within the first week after transplant and is also the result of preformed antibodies. This form of rejection will not respond to immunosuppressive therapy, and the kidney will be removed.

*Acute rejection* is the most recognizable and common form of rejection. The inflammatory changes from this cellular immune response are often reversed with vigorous immunosuppression. The classic signs and symptoms of an acute rejection are a decrease in urine output, significant weight gain, peripheral edema, elevated temperature, a rise in blood pressure, and graft tenderness (Table 27-1). Patients may present with several, all, or even none of these symptoms. An elevation in the serum creatinine level is often the first indication of rejection. Differential diagnosis is facilitated by renal scans and ultrasounds, which demonstrate changes in kidney function and size. A transplant biopsy is helpful in distinguishing this cell-mediated process. Following treatment of the rejection, the patient will continue on standard immunosuppression.

*Chronic rejection* is humoral in nature and is characterized by a progressive deterioration of renal function, which may occur over a period of months to years. This form of rejection does not generally respond to treatment and is responsible for eventual failure of the graft. Changes noted on biopsy show a chronic inflammatory interstitial infiltrate and progressive fibrosis. As renal function decreases, the patient may be placed on diet restrictions and medications to control the symptoms. When graft failure occurs, dialysis or retransplantation may then take place.

## Immunosuppression

Successful renal transplantation depends on the ability to suppress the immune system judiciously. Chemical immunosuppression is achieved through various combinations of medications. During the 1970s these included prednisone, azathioprine, and antilymphocyte globulin (ALG). Since that time, more specific drugs, such as cyclosporine and monoclonal antibodies (OKT-3), have been developed. Current medication protocols stress a combination of prednisone, azathioprine, and cyclosporine for long-term management. The actions of each of these medications differ, and their simultaneous use yields a multifaceted attack on the reacting cells (Fig. 27-1).

*Cyclosporine* is a potent and specific immunosuppressant that prevents the replication of T-lymphocytes by inhibiting the production of interleu-

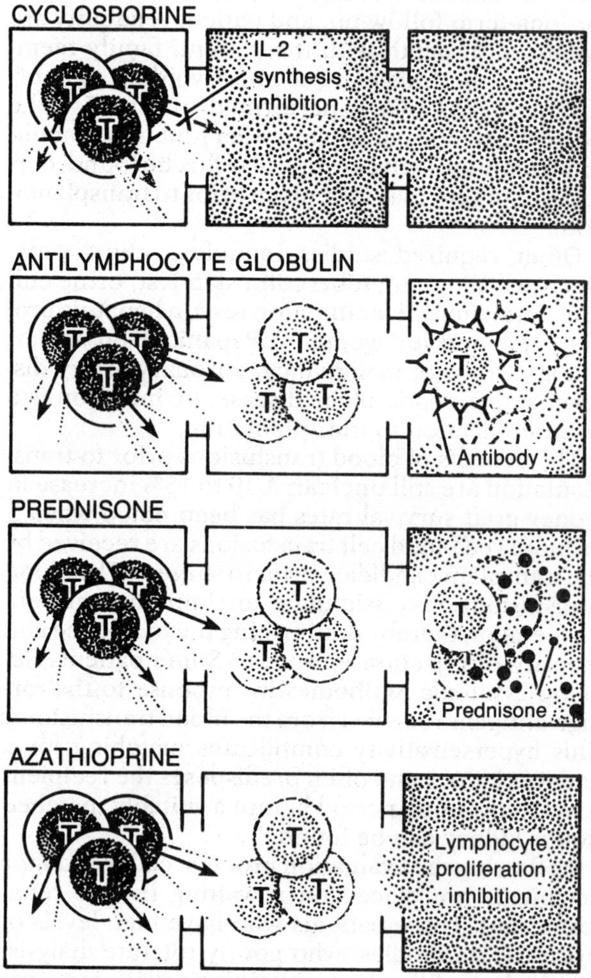


**Figure 27-1.** Pharmacologic immunosuppression in renal transplant therapy. Cyclosporine acts on T-lymphocytes inhibiting the synthesis and secretion of interleukin-2 (indicated by X in top frame), essential for the proliferation of T-lymphocytes. Hence, cyclosporine prevents lymphocytic replication. Antilymphocyte globulin (ALG) is an antiserum of lymphocytic antibodies (Y-shaped structures in frame 2) used to treat rejection by destroying circulating white blood cells. Prednisone (black dots in frame 3) acts nonspecifically as a lymphocytic agent causing the destruction of circulating lymphocytes. Azathioprine interferes with cell synthesis, thereby inhibiting lymphocyte proliferation.

kin-2 (Fig. 27–1). The recent use of cyclosporine has significantly improved cadaver graft survival rates. Nephrotoxicity can result from this medication, so it is best used after some renal function has been established in the transplanted kidney. This would be manifested by a decrease in the serum creatinine level.

*Anti-lymphocyte globulin (ALG)* is an antiserum produced by injecting human lymphocytes into horses. The lymphocytic antibodies developed in the horse are extracted from the new sera, they are purified, and they act to treat rejection by destroying the now abundant circulating white blood cells (see Fig. 27–1). ALG may be used prophylactically postoperatively until cyclosporine therapy can be initiated safely, or it may be used as treatment for acute rejection. Administration of ALG requires the use of a central line or vascular access because a high-flow vessel must be used. The nurse must monitor the patient for anaphylaxis, fever, chills, joint pain, or symptoms of infection. Symptomatic relief is achieved through administration of hydrocortisone, acetaminophen, and diphenydramine prior to injection of ALG.

*Prednisone* is a glucocorticoid whose anti-inflammatory action is cytolytic and whose immunologic action impairs the recognition and processing of foreign tissue by the immune system. Its lymphocytic action results in the destruction of circulating lymphocytes (see Fig. 27–1). The nonspecific actions of this medication yield untoward systemic effects.

*Azathioprine* acts to interfere with cell synthesis, thereby inhibiting proliferation of lymphocytes. However, its action is not specific because it also inhibits myelogenous cells, often resulting in bone marrow toxicity (see Fig. 27–1).

Administration of monoclonal antibody (OKT-3) preparations requires special precautions. Upon receiving the initial dose, the patient may experience dyspnea, wheezing, tachycardia, fever, chills, possible anaphylaxis, and bronchospasm. Pulmonary complications have been avoided by ensuring that the patient's chest x-ray is negative for infiltrates and pulmonary congestion. Nursing care focuses on assessment for fluid volume overload prior to initiation of therapy and diligent patient monitoring, and symptomatic relief.

## CLINICAL MANAGEMENT

### Preoperative Period

A fresh negative T-cell crossmatch is the final determination prior to surgery. Preparation for transplantation includes assessment of the need for dialysis prior to surgery, initiation of immunosuppressants, and cleansing of the operative site. Patient teaching and support are vital now because events take place rapidly and may be overwhelming.

### Intraoperative Period

The donor kidney is placed within the right or left iliac fossa. The donor renal vein is anastomosed to the external iliac vein. The donor renal artery is anastomosed to the hypogastric artery or to the iliac artery. The donor ureter is tunnelled into the bladder by means of a ureteroneocystotomy. Once the vascular clamps are removed, the kidney should become pink and firm, denoting adequate blood flow to the organ. It is important to avoid circulating volume deficit because hypovolemia interferes with renal function[9] (Fig. 27–2).

### Postoperative Period

In the immediate postoperative period, the patient's vital signs and hemodynamic parameters are monitored on a frequent basis. Intake and output are measured on an hourly basis to assess the patient's fluid status, and laboratory specimens are used to evaluate the patient's electrolyte and acid–base status. Complications seen in this early postoperative period include fluid volume overload or deficit, metabolic acidosis, hyperkalemia, or hypokalemia.

Fluid replacement is determined both by the patient's hourly urine output and central venous pressure (CVP) readings. Excessive diuresis may sometimes occur and with it hyponatremia and hypokalemia. This polyuria occurs secondary to diminished reabsorption in the proximal tubules. IV fluids (usually a dextrose solution with 0.45% normal saline) may contain additives to combat metabolic acidosis and/or hypokalemia.

Hyperkalemia may occur as the result of tissue trauma intraoperatively, blood transfusions administered during the surgery, or nonfunction of the transplanted kidney. Because hyperkalemia is life-threatening, emergency measures are employed to bring the serum potassium near normal until either the transplanted kidney begins to function or the need for dialysis is ascertained. These emergency measures include the IV administration of glucose and regular insulin to facilitate the movement of the potassium ions into the cells, and IV calcium chloride is given to protect the myocardium against the deleterious effects of the elevated serum potassium on the heart. Because these measures are temporary in nature (they do not lower but redistribute the potassium ions), they are followed up with the administration of Kayexalate, which may be given either by mouth or by retention enema. This medication binds with potassium and, therefore, re-

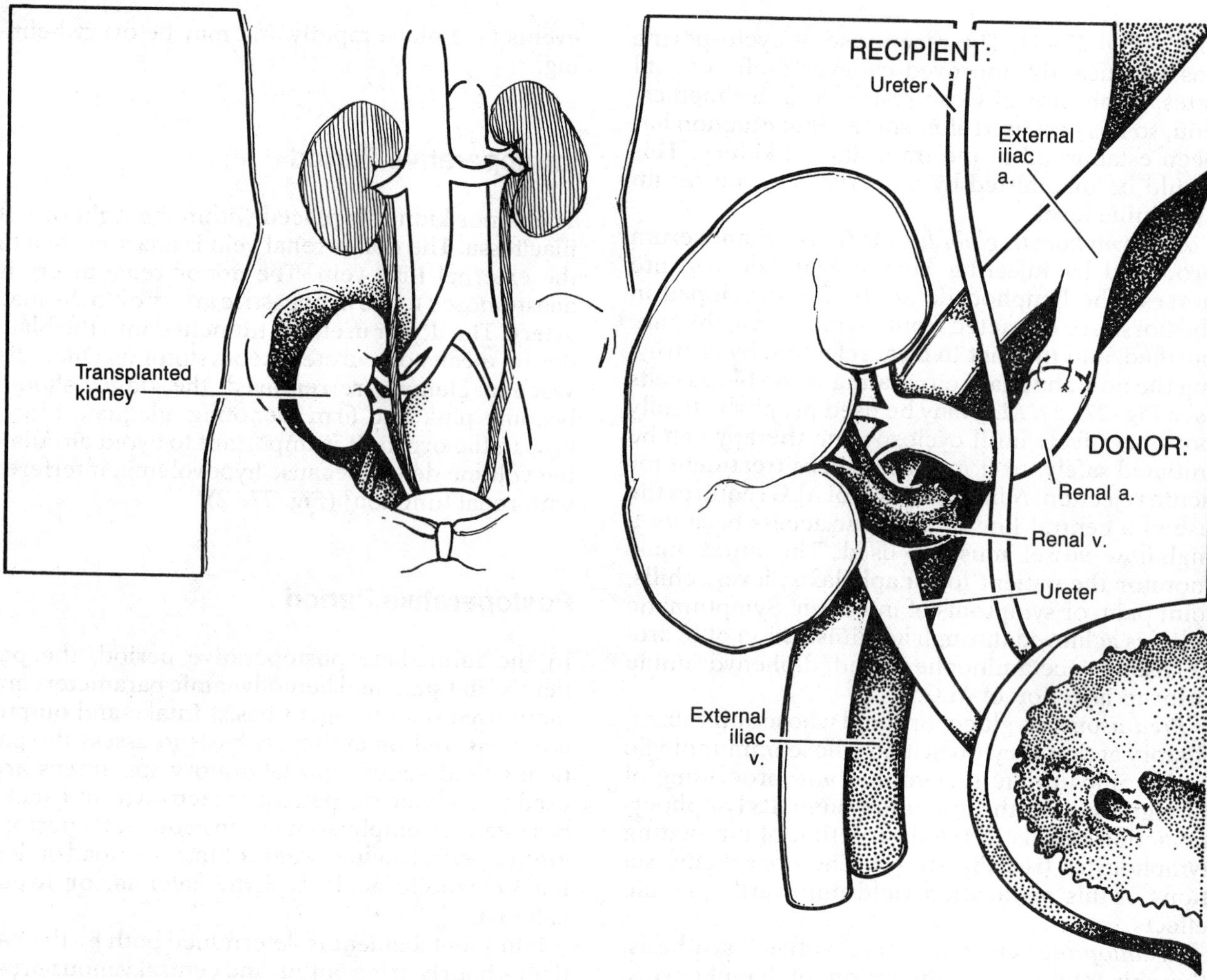


**Figure 27-2.** Surgical transplantation of donor kidney into recipient.

moves this ion from the body. Continued or recurrent hyperkalemia is an indication for dialysis.

The patient may be anuric or oliguric, the result of acute tubular necrosis (ATN) that develops from ischemic changes in the graft. ATN may never resolve or could last for as long as 6 weeks with reported full recovery of renal function.[10] The anuric patient must be supported with dialysis and monitored for infection because he/she will sometimes require increased doses of immunosuppressive medication. The patient must be given realistic encouragement. Fluid and dietary restrictions are usually required.

A sudden decrease in established urine flow indicates potential complications and mandates further assessment. The urinary catheter should be checked for patency and irrigated only under strict aseptic technique. Decreased urine flow could represent hypovolemia, ureteral leaks, or an obstruction. A vascular thrombosis (e.g., renal artery thrombosis) may cause partial or complete infarction of the transplant. Observe for abdominal distention, tenderness, or leakage from the incision. Fluid challenges with diuretics and colloids may be given. Renal scans and ultrasounds usually assist in determining the source of the problem and establishing diagnosis.

An ongoing head-to-toe assessment is performed by the nurse. Because of the propensity for infectious complications (caused by the immunosuppressive medications), the patient requires diligent monitoring for the signs and symptoms of infection. Prevention of these infectious complications is of tantamount importance and should serve as the focal point in rendering bedside care. In all other respects, the renal transplant recipient is treated as all other postoperative patients. (See the Care Plan in Table 27-2).

## TABLE 27-2. CARE PLAN FOR THE RENAL TRANSPLANT PATIENT

| Nursing Diagnoses | Desired Patient Outcomes | Nursing Interventions | Rationales |
|---|---|---|---|
| ***Nursing Diagnosis #1*** Anxiety, related to impending transplantation and uncertain outcomes. | Patient will:<br>1. Verbalize concerns.<br>2. Ask questions.<br>3. Discuss readiness for transplantation.<br>4. Use coping capabilities. | • Assess patient's knowledge of transplantation.<br>• Review teaching related to surgery, medications, possibility of a positive crossmatch, and routine hospital care.<br>• Encourage verbalization.<br>• Involve family members.<br>• Provide realistic support for patient and family. | • Despite extensive education during the transplant evaluation, many patients are still exposed to misconstrued ideas.<br>• A positive crossmatch would cancel transplant surgery. |
| ***Nursing Diagnosis #2*** Ineffective breathing pattern, related to: Anesthesia; neuromuscular weakness. | Patient will:<br>1. Maintain adequate ventilation postoperatively.<br>• Respiratory rate/rhythm/pattern at baseline.<br>• Arterial blood gases at patient's baseline. | • Assess for pulmonary edema preoperatively and postoperatively.<br>• Maintain an adequate airway.<br>• Monitor vital signs until stable.<br>• Auscultate lungs for normal/adventitious breath sounds.<br>• Encourage coughing and deep breathing. | • Pulmonary edema impairs ventilation and oxygenation.<br>• Presence of crackles on auscultation suggests fluid accumulation in alveoli indicative of pulmonary edema.<br>• Coughing and deep breathing loosen and mobilize secretions. |
| ***Nursing Diagnosis #3*** Impaired skin integrity, related to surgical procedure. | Patient will:<br>1. Experience healing of incision without complications.<br>(See Table 25–3, Nursing Diagnosis #10.) | • Inspect incision every shift for signs of redness, swelling, or drainage.<br>• Keep incision clean, dry, and well approximated.<br>• Maintain adequate nutrition. | • Immunosuppressed patients are prone to infection.<br>• Adequate intake of protein and vitamins B and C promote wound healing. |
| ***Nursing Diagnosis #4*** Potential for infection, related to a compromised immune system. | Patient will:<br>1. Remain infection free:<br>• Afebrile.<br>• Negative cultures.<br>2. Be protected from exposure to infection.<br>3. Recognize and report any signs or symptoms of infection.<br>(See Table 25–3, Nursing Diagnosis #8.) | • Obtain baseline cultures preoperatively.<br>○ Pan-culture patient if temperature increases.<br>○ Monitor bacterial, viral, and fungal cultures routinely.<br>• Review radiologic studies for fluid collections or abscesses.<br>• Administer appropriate antibiotics, follow sensitivities and response to therapy.<br>• Use strict aseptic technique. | • Chemical immunosuppression places transplant patients at high risk for infection.<br>○ Steroids may mask the symptoms of infection, so cultures are vital.<br>• Aseptic technique reduces the risk of infection. |

**TABLE 27–2. CARE PLAN FOR THE RENAL TRANSPLANT PATIENT *(Continued)***

| Nursing Diagnoses | Desired Patient Outcomes | Nursing Interventions | Rationales |
|---|---|---|---|
| ***Nursing Diagnosis #5***<br>Potential alteration in oral mucous membranes. | Patient will:<br>1. Report any breakdown or lesion immediately.<br>2. Demonstrate good personal hygiene.<br>(See Table 25–3, Nursing Diagnosis #11. | • Monitor patient for oral herpetic or fungal infections.<br>• Administer nystatin oral suspension after meals and at bedtime prophylactically. | • Immunosuppressed patients are highly susceptible to herpetic and monilial oral infections. |
| ***Nursing Diagnosis #6***<br>Potential alteration in fluid and electrolyte balance. | Patient will:<br>1. Remain normovolemic.<br>2. Maintain electrolyte balance.<br>(See Chap 23.) | • Maintain accurate intake and output and daily weights.<br>• Assess for signs and symptoms of hypovolemia or hypervolemia.<br>• Assess for signs and symptoms of hyperkalemia.<br>• Report any sudden decrease in urine output. | • These parameters are indicative of volume balance.<br>• Oliguria/anuria may result from acute tubular necrosis and may lead to hypervolemia.<br>• Serum potassium may be elevated from surgery and blood transfusions.<br>• A sudden decrease in urine flow may be related to other complications and should be followed.<br>• Diminished urine output may be a sign of acute rejection. |
| ***Nursing Diagnosis #7***<br>Potential alteration in renal function, related to rejection or obstruction. | Patient will:<br>1. Recognize and report the signs and symptoms of rejection.<br>2. Follow prescribed treatment for impaired kidney function. | • Monitor vital signs.<br>○ Assess for symptoms of rejection: elevated temperature, rapid weight gain, decreased urinary output, peripheral edema, elevated blood pressure, general malaise, tenderness over graft.<br>○ Assess for obstruction of Foley catheter. Irrigate under strict sterile technique only if clotted and absolutely necessary.<br>○ Follow daily lab results.<br>• Assess all complaints of abdominal pain, and report them promptly.<br>• Prepare patient for radiology procedures.<br>• Continue administration of immunosuppressants unless otherwise ordered. | ○ Acute rejection usually occurs during the first 3 months after transplant.<br>○ Decreased urine flow may be the result of hypovolemia, obstruction of either the catheter or ureter, or vascular thrombosis of the graft.<br>○ The serum creatinine is an indicator of renal function.<br>• Radiology may be required for diagnosis. |

| | | | |
|---|---|---|---|
| ***Nursing Diagnosis #8*** Knowledge deficit, related to recent renal transplantation. | Patient will:<br>1. Verbalize understanding of rejection, potential for infection, medications, and routine care.<br>2. Demonstrate compliance.<br>3. Report any potentially serious symptoms or changes. | • Teach patient the physiology of a transplanted kidney.<br>• Review the process of rejection and the symptoms.<br>◦ Instruct patient to monitor blood pressure, temperature, weight, and intake and output at home.<br>◦ Instruct patient to report any of the above to transplant office.<br>◦ Reinforce to the patient that acute rejection is usually promptly and effectively treated. | • While in the hospital, the patient should begin to assume responsibility for recording daily parameters and taking medications. This facilitates adjustment to home. |
| | | • Review immunosuppressant medications.<br>◦ Discuss actions and side effects. | • Medication side effects are disturbing, and the patient should be prepared for the changes in body appearance related to steroids and cyclosporine. |
| | | ◦ Instruct patient to avoid crowds or others who are ill.<br>◦ Review signs and symptoms of infections (pulmonary, urinary, operative, and so forth).<br>◦ Instruct patient to report any of above immediately to transplant office. | ◦ The transplant patient is highly susceptible to infections. |
| | | • Encourage good nutrition and daily exercise. Review patient's diet and routines. | • Assists with healing and improving muscle tone. Patients are prone to excessive weight gain with steroids. |
| | | • Instruct patient to avoid heavy lifting, and resume driving in 3–6 weeks.<br>• Enforce possible need for birth control now; sexual activity may resume when desired. | • Female patients may resume ovulation and menstruation and should avoid pregnancy the first 1–2 years following transplantations. |

## NURSING RESPONSIBILITIES

Thorough assessment and monitoring of the transplant patient cannot be overemphasized. As long as a transplanted kidney is in place, these patients will require immunosuppressants. Immunosuppressed patients with compromised cell-mediated immunity are at increased risk for developing fulminant bacterial, viral, and fungal infections. Infections are treated with antibiotics and, if the infection is life-threatening, immunosuppression may be discontinued to save the patient. Infections remain the primary cause of morbidity for this patient population.[11]

Assessment of a renal transplant recipient for either infection or rejection includes physical examination and daily laboratory work including cultures and radiographic results. Other parameters of kidney function include daily weights, intake and outputs, and vital signs.

An elevated temperature is rarely insignificant and may indicate infection or rejection. Fevers should be recorded, reported, and followed with bacterial, viral, and fungal cultures. Hepatitis profile is also to be considered. It is important to remember that large doses of steroids may mask an elevated temperature and a normal white blood cell response to an infectious process.

The surgical incision should be examined for swelling, erythema, or tenderness. Drainage should be cultured immediately and an ultrasound should be obtained. Intravenous access areas should be inspected, cleansed daily, and changed frequently. Upon removal of the IV access in the presence of fever, the catheter tips should be inspected and sent for cultures. The mouth and mucous membranes are inspected often for herpetic lesions and monilial infections. Changes in mental status, headaches, or confusion could mean central nervous system involvement and necessitate a spinal tap for cultures of cerebrospinal fluid.

The urinary catheter predisposes the transplant recipient to urinary tract infections and should be removed as soon as possible. Symptoms of a urinary tract infection warrant immediate urine cultures. Patient education on recognition of the signs and symptoms of a urinary tract infection and the principles of good hygiene is vital.

Shortness of breath, tachypnea, cough, or sputum production may reveal a pulmonary infection and should be followed with sputum cultures and chest x-rays. Viral cultures should be sent, in addition to bacterial cultures.

Hypertension is a common problem for transplant recipients, and its causes are varied. It has been correlated with higher dosages of prednisone and cyclosporine. Intrinsic changes resulting from rejection episodes or recurrence of disease lead to a renal vasculitis and diminished renal blood flow. Subsequently, there appears to be a renin–angiotensin–aldosterone component to the hypertension (see Fig. 21–9).

The forms of transplant hypertension that respond to surgical intervention are renal artery stenosis (appearing in 5%–10% of all transplant patients) and native kidney hypertension. This is induced by vasoconstrictive hormones secreted into the bloodstream. Finally, because many patients were maintained on dialysis prior to surgery there is a higher incidence of atherosclerosis.[12]

Careful monitoring of the blood pressure is required, especially if antihypertensive medications are being adjusted. Patients are taught to check their blood pressure at home and to restrict their dietary intake of sodium.

### Discharge Planning

There is a major need for education and emotional support in this particular patient population. These patients and their families must understand the full implications of a compromised immune response and the basic physiology of transplant rejection before they leave the hospital.

The nurse must serve as patient advocate and educator to ascertain that patients know how to administer their medications safely, care for themselves, and recognize potentially serious signs and symptoms, as well as understand the need for continuing medical supervision. Patients and their families will need assistance adjusting to new fears, concerns, and feelings of dependency. Increased activity and rehabilitation are encouraged.

The role of the transplant nurse is an ever-expanding one—one that changes and advances as rapidly as the progress made in the field of transplantation today.

## REFERENCES


1. Report of the Task Force on Organ Transplantation: Organ Transplantation Issues and Recommendations. US Dept. of Health and Human Services, Washington, DC, 1986, p 17.
2. Evans, R, et al: The quality of life of patients with end-stage renal disease. N Engl J Med 312(9):557, 1985.
3. Parfrey, P, Hutchinson, T, and Lowry, R: Dialysis and transplantation: Complimentary forms of treatment. In Garovoy, M and Guttman, R (eds): Renal Transplantation. Churchill Livingstone, New York, 1986, p 4.
4. Parfrey, P, Hutchinson, T, and Lowry, R: Dialysis and transplantation: Complimentary forms of treatment. In Garovoy, M and Guttman, R (eds): Renal Transplantation. Churchill Livingstone, New York, 1986, p 5.
5. Terasaki, P: Clinical Kidney Transplants 1985. The Regents of the University of California, Los Angeles, 1985, p 38.
6. Najarian, J: Immunologic aspects of transplantation. In Dixon, F, et al (eds): The Biology of Immunologic Disease. Sinauer Associates, Sunderland, MA, 1982, p 351.
7. Irwin, B: Renal transplantation: Advances in immunology —A nursing perspective. AANNT Journal 10(4):11, June 1983.
8. Simmons, RL, et al: Clinical transplantation. In Simmons,

RL and Najarian, JS (eds): Transplantation. Lea & Febiger, Philadelphia, 1972, p 474.
9. Chatterjee, S: Manual of Renal Transplantation. Springer-Verlag, New York, 1979, p 83.
10. Simmons, RL, et al: Clinical transplantation. In Simmons, RL and Najarian, JS (eds): Transplantation. Lea & Febiger, Philadelphia, 1972, p 439.
11. Irwin, B: Renal transplantation: Advances in immunology—A nursing perspective. AANNT Journal 10(4):12, June 1983.
12. Curtis, JJ: Hypertension: A common problem for kidney transplant patients. Kidney 18(2):7, 1985.

# UNIT FOUR

# Bibliography


Anderson, S, Meyer, TW, and Brenner, BM: The role of hemodynamic factors in the initiation and progression of renal disease. J Urol 133:363, 1985.

Ayres, S, Schlictig, R, and Sterling, M: Care of the Critically Ill. Year Book Medical Publishers, Chicago, 1988.

Bricker, NS, et al: The pathophysiology of renal insufficiency: On the functional transformations in the residual nephrons with advancing disease. Pediatr Clin North Am 18:595, 1971.

Brogna, L, and Lakaszawski, M: The continent urostomy. Am J Nurs 86(2):160, February 1986.

Cane, RD and Shapiro, B: Case Studies in Critical Care Medicine. Year Book Medical Publishers, Chicago, 1985.

Chatterjee, S: Manual of Renal Transplantation. Springer-Verlag, New York, 1979.

Cimino, JE, and Brescia, MJ: Simple venipuncture for hemodialysis. N Engl J Med 267:608, 1962.

Conti, M, and Eutropius, L: Preventing UTIs: What works? Am J Nurs 87(3):30, March 1987.

Cotton, J, et al: Nursing management of continuous arteriovenous hemofiltration for acute renal failure. Focus on Crit Care 13(5):21, October 1986.

Curtis, J: Hypertension: A common problem for kidney transplant patients. Kidney 18:2, 1985.

D'Elia, JA, et al: Diabetic nephropathy. Comprehensive Therapy 5(9):47, 1979.

Evans, R, et al: The quality of life of patients with end-stage renal disease. N Engl J Med 312:9, 1985.

Griffin, JE: Manual of Clinical Endocrinology and Metabolism. McGraw-Hill, New York, 1982.

Guyton, AC: Textbook of Medical Physiology, ed 7. WB Saunders, Philadelphia, 1986.

Hershman, JM: Endocrine Pathophysiology, A Patient-Oriented Approach, ed 3. Lea & Febiger, Philadelphia, 1988.

Irwin, B: Renal transplantation: Advances in immunology—A nursing perspective. AANNT Journal 10:4, June 1983.

Johnson, D: Nephrotic syndrome: A nursing care plan based on current pathophysiologic concepts. Heart & Lung 18:(1):85, January 1989.

Knowles, HC: Magnitude of the renal failure problem in diabetic patients. Kidney Int 6:S2–S7, 1974.

Krupski, WC, et al: Access for dialysis. In Cogan, MG, and Garovoy, MR: Introduction to Dialysis. Churchill Livingstone, New York, 1985.

Lancaster, LE, and Pierce, P: Total body manifestations of end-stage renal disease and related medical and nursing management. In Lancaster, LE: The Patient with Endstage Renal Disease. John Wiley & Sons, New York, 1979.

Landsman, MK: The patient with chronic renal failure: A marginal man. Ann Intern Med 82:268, 1975.

Lawyer, L and Velasco, A: Continuous arteriovenous hemodialysis in the ICU. Crit Care Nurse 9(1):29, January 1989.

Leaf, A, and Cotran, R: Renal Pathophysiology. Oxford University Press, New York, 1976.

Levine, DZ: Care of the Renal Patient. WB Saunders, Philadelphia, 1983.

Linamegi, E: Aluminum toxicity. NAPHT News, May 1985.

Lunger, D: Potassium supplementation: How and why? Focus on Crit Care 15(5):56, October 1988.

Metheny N: Fluid and Electrolyte Balance: Nursing Considerations. JB Lippincott, Philadelphia, 1987.

Metz, R, and Larsen, E: Blue Book of Endocrinology. WB Saunders, Philadelphia, 1985.

Muir, BL: Pathophysiology, An Introduction to the Mechanisms of Disease, ed 2. John Wiley & Sons, New York, 1988.

Najarian, J: Immunologic aspects of transplantation. In Dixon, F, et al: The Biology of Immunologic Disease. Sinauer Associates, Sunderland, MA, 1982.

Netter, F: Kidneys, Ureters and Urinary Bladder, Vol. 6, in The Ciba Collection of Medical Illustrations. CIBA Medical Education Division, West Caldwell, NJ, 1974.

Parfrey, P, Hutchinson, T, and Lowry, R: Dialysis and transplantation: Complimentary forms of treatment. In Garovoy, M, and Guttman, R: Renal Transplantation. Churchill Livingstone, New York, 1986.

Quinton, W, Dillard, D, and Scribner, BH: Cannulation of blood vessels for prolonged hemodialysis. Trans Am Soc Art Int Organs 6:104, 1960.

Renal and Urologic Disorders. In Nurse's Clinical Library Series, Springhouse Corporation, Springhouse, PA, 1984.

Report of the Task Force on Organ Transplantation: Organ Transplantation Issues and Recommendations. US Dept. of Health and Human Services, Washington, DC, 1986.

Rose, B: Pathophysiology of Renal Disease, ed 2. McGraw-Hill, New York, 1987.

Sawyer, D: Potential for infection: A nursing diagnosis for the patient with an indwelling catheter. Focus on Crit Care 16(1):46, February 1989.

Schumann, D: Cytomegalic virus infection in renal allograft recipients: Indicators for intervention in the SICU. Focus on Crit Care 14(3):40, June 1987.

Sibbald, WJ: Synopsis of Critical Care, ed 2. Williams & Wilkins, Baltimore, 1984.

Simmons, RL, et al: Clinical transplantation. In Simmons, RL, and Najarian, JS: Transplantation. Lea & Febiger, Philadelphia, 1972.

Stroot, V, Lee, C, and Barrett, C: Fluid and Electrolytes: A Practical Approach. FA Davis, Philadelphia, 1984.

Sweetwood, HM: Clinical Electrocardiography for Nurses. Aspen, Rockville, Maryland, 1983.

Terasaki, P: Clinical Kidney Transplants 1985. The Regents of the University of California, Los Angeles, 1985.

Vander, AJ: Renal Physiology, ed 3. McGraw-Hill, New York, 1985.

Whittaker, AA: Acute renal dysfunction, assessment of patients at risk. Focus Crit Care 12(3):12, June 1985.

# UNIT FIVE

# Respiratory System

The respiratory system plays a pivotal role in the maintenance of life processes of the individual in an equilibrated state. In conjunction with the central nervous system and cardiovascular system, the respiratory system facilitates the processes of oxygen uptake and carbon dioxide elimination by the lungs. The central nervous system provides the inherent rhythmic drive to breathe. It reflexly stimulates the diaphragm and muscular apparatus of the thorax, which together function as a "bellows" for the movement of air. The cardiovascular system provides the blood, pump, and conduits essential for gas transport between the lungs and the cells.

*Respiration* is the exchange of oxygen and carbon dioxide between the cells and the external environment. *Internal respiration* refers to the intracellular chemical reactions in which oxygen is used and carbon dioxide is produced, as the cells metabolize carbohydrates and other substances to release energy and generate adenosine triphosphate (ATP). Adequate functioning of all of these interrelated systems is essential to ensure effective respiration. A disturbance in any one of the systems can disrupt gas exchange and gas transport, and can seriously compromise these life-sustaining processes.

The chapters to follow focus on the essential elements of the respiration process. As in previous units, emphasis is placed on the relationship between structure and function. The anatomical structure of the respiratory apparatus and the physiologic phenomena associated with ventilation, gas exchange, gas transport, and the overall control of breathing are examined in detail.

The discussion of respiratory pathophysiology includes acute respiratory failure, chronic obstructive pulmonary disease (chronic bronchitis and emphysema), adult respiratory distress syndrome (noncardiogenic versus cardiogenic pulmonary edema), asthma, pulmonary embolism, pneumothroax, pleural effusion, and pneumonia.

Nursing process and the management of the patient with compromised respiratory function are explored, including pertinent nursing diagnoses. Nursing care plans are based on nursing diagnoses and include specific patient outcomes and nursing interventions.

## UNIT OUTLINE

CHAPTER 28

# Anatomy and Physiology of the Respiratory System

## CHAPTER OUTLINE



## LEARNING OBJECTIVES

**At the end of this chapter, you should be able to:**

1. Describe the functional anatomy of the respiratory system and its role in the process of respiration.
2. Identify the major features of the respiratory alveolar-pulmonary capillary membrane that facilitate its role in gas exchange.
3. Examine the unique features of the bronchopulmonary vasculature in terms of its responses to ventilation and oxygenation.
4. Describe the essential aspects of the mechanics of breathing.
5. Define compliance and its impact on the "work" of breathing.
6. Outline strategic pulmonary defense mechanisms.
7. Describe the underlying mechanisms of pulmonary ventilation.
8. Discuss the clinical significance of maximal expiratory flow studies.

## LEARNING OBJECTIVES—*CONTINUED*

9. Describe the mechanisms underlying diffusion of gases between the alveoli and pulmonary capillaries, and between the circulating blood and body tissues.
10. Examine ventilation-perfusion relationships and their clinical significance.
11. Discuss mechanisms of oxygen and carbon dioxide transport in body fluids.
12. Review the clinical significance of the oxyhemoglobin dissociation curve.
13. Describe the intricate mechanisms in the control of respiratory function.

The process of respiration involves the following physiologic activities: (1) the mechanics of pulmonary ventilation (i.e., the movement of air into and out of the lungs by bulk flow); (2) the exchange of oxygen and carbon dioxide between the alveoli and the blood by diffusion; (3) the transport of oxygen and carbon dioxide throughout the circulatory system by bulk flow; (4) the exchange of oxygen and carbon dioxide between the circulating blood and the cells by diffusion; and (5) the regulation of the activities involved in respirations. Each of these activities will be examined in this chapter. The discussion begins with a review of the overall organization of the respiratory system.

## ORGANIZATION OF THE RESPIRATORY SYSTEM

### Upper and Lower Airways of the Respiratory Tract

The entire pathway for the flow of air between the external environment and the lungs extends from the mouth or nose down to the alveolar sacs. Inhaled gas is conducted through the *upper* airways, which include the nose, nasal cavity, paranasal sinuses, mouth, oropharynx and nasopharynx, and the larynx, down through the *lower* airways, which include the tracheobronchial tree, terminal bronchioles, respiratory bronchioles, and finally ending in tiny blind sacs, the alveoli.

Throughout this system there occurs a progressive dichotomous arborization (branching) of bronchi and bronchioles. The trachea divides at the carina into right and left mainstem bronchi (Fig. 28–1), which, in turn, branch into lobar bronchi (three on the right, two on the left), segmental and subsegmental bronchi, smaller bronchi and bronchioles. In all, these conducting airways divide approximately 15 to 17 times down to the level of terminal bronchioles, which are the smallest units that do not participate in gas exchange (see Fig. 28–3).

#### *Larynx*

The larynx and pharyngeal musculature provide clinically significant protective functions essential for maintenance of normal lung physiology. The critical dividing point in separating solids and liquids from air occurs within the laryngopharynx. Here the passageway bifurcates into the larynx and esophagus, and the pharyngeal muscles function to close the glottis while initiating the *swallowing reflex*. In this way, the lungs are protected from aspiration.

**Cough Reflex.** The *cough reflex* is a major physiologic mechanism for clearing and protecting the airways. It is protective against aspiration of food or other foreign material into the airway, and assists in clearing the tracheobronchial secretions produced within the tracheobronchial tree. The cough reflex is usually initiated by stimulation of *irritant receptors* found primarily in the larynx, trachea, and major bronchi, and especially at points of bifurcation of the air passages.

#### *Trachea*

The trachea is approximately 11 to 13 cm in length and extends from the cricoid cartilage in the neck into the thorax where it branches into the right and left mainstem bronchi at a point called the *carina* (see Fig. 28–1). The carina is highly innervated and can produce severe bronchospasm and coughing when stimulated (as frequently occurs in endotracheal suctioning). The carina also serves as a strategic landmark when evaluating the placement of an endotracheal tube on a chest x-ray.

#### *Bronchi*

The right and left mainstem bronchi are anatomically asymmetric (see Fig. 28–1). The right bronchus is shorter and wider than the left and continues from the trachea in a more nearly vertical course. The left mainstem bronchus is longer and narrower and continues from the trachea at a more acute angle.

The clinical implications of these anatomical characteristics are noteworthy. Upon insertion, an endotracheal tube passed too far will enter the right mainstem bronchus. If this occurs and the cuff is inflated, the left lung will not be ventilated, a situation that can rapidly lead to atelectasis of the left lung with hypoxemia, hypoxia, and respiratory insufficiency. It is essential to observe for bilateral equal chest expansion and to auscultate both lungs immediately upon intubation. A chest x-ray should always be taken to confirm proper positioning of

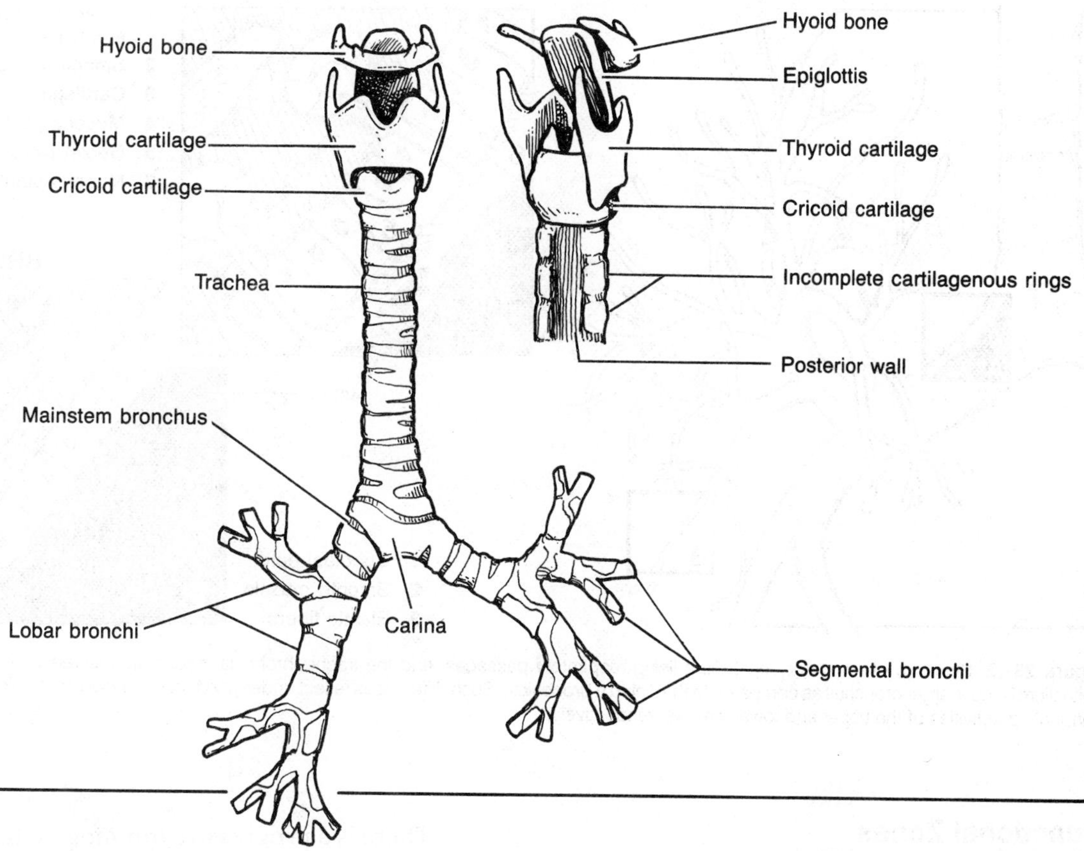


**Figure 28-1.** Structure of cartilaginous airways including the trachea and major bronchi.

the endotracheal tube, usually 1 to 2 cm above the carina.

## Respiratory Epithelium

The airways that extend from the nose down to and including the terminal bronchioles function primarily to prepare and condition the inhaled gas by filtering, warming, and humidifying it, and to facilitate its flow throughout the respiratory tract to the distal blind sacs, the alveoli.

These airways are especially well suited for these critical functions. The nose, nasal cavity, turbinates, and paranasal sinuses provide an extensive, highly vascularized surface to which inhaled gas is exposed as it flows through the respiratory tract. The luminal surface layer or mucosa of both upper and lower airways is lined with a specialized *respiratory epithelium*, or pseudostratified ciliated columnar epithelium with goblet cells (Fig. 28-2). The cilia function to protect the deeper airways by propelling tracheobronchial secretions toward the pharynx where they can be coughed up, swallowed, or expectorated.

The epithelial surface is covered by a "mucous blanket," which is secreted largely by submucosal mucous glands and, to a lesser extent, the goblet cells. Fine particles within the inhaled gas are trapped in the mucous blanket, which is continuously propelled by the cilia toward the pharynx by a process termed *mucociliary transport* or *mucociliary clearance.*

Bacteria inhaled on dust particles are similarly trapped in the mucous blanket. In this way, the mucociliary clearance mechanism contributes to the body's total defense against bacterial infection. A reduction in ciliary activity, as occurs, for example, with cigarette smoking, coupled with an increase in mucus secretion, also induced by noxious agents such as cigarette smoke, predisposes to airway congestion and obstruction caused by stationary mucus.

A rich underlying vascular network warms the gas as it flows toward the distal or peripheral areas of the tracheobronchial tree. It is largely by the "conditioning activities" of the respiratory epithelium on inhaled gas that the gas reaching the alveoli is "dust free," at body temperature, and 100% humidified.

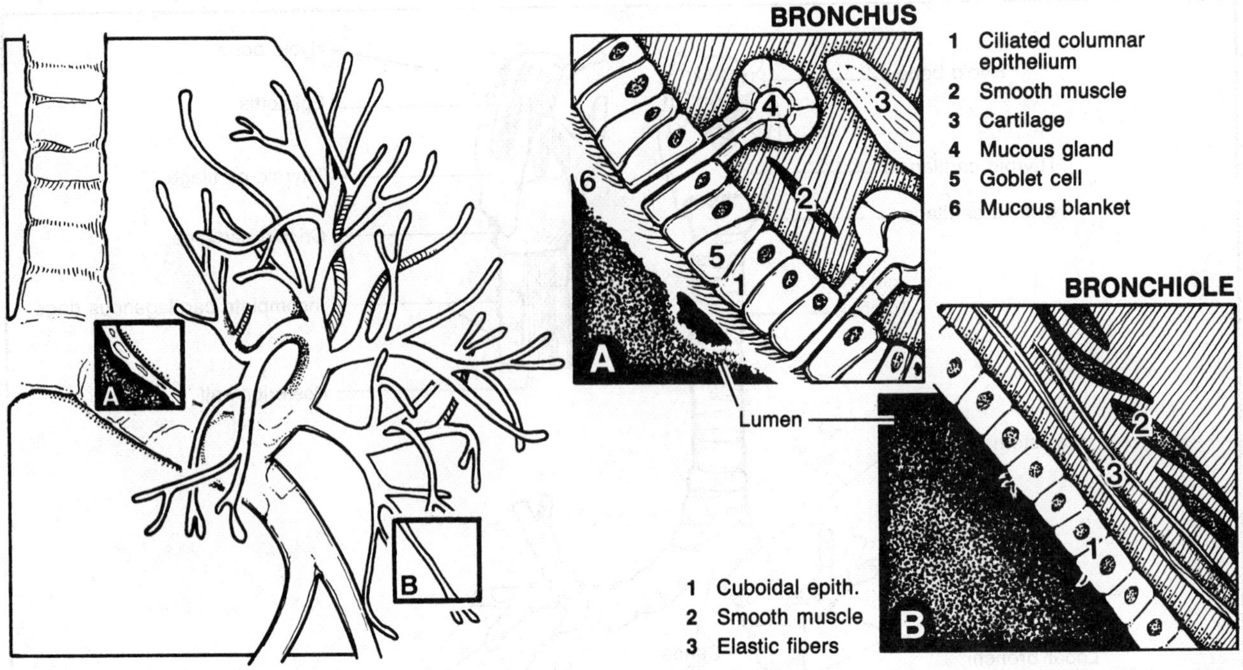


**Figure 28–2.** Structure of respiratory epithelium lining respiratory passages, and the tracheobronchial tree. Note differences in structure of the epithelium lining a larger bronchus as compared to that lining a bronchiole. Such differences reflect underlying function including the air conditioning and conducting activities of the upper and lower airways, respectively.

## Functional Zones of the Respiratory Tract

All the dichotomous subdivisions or generations of the bronchi and bronchioles, down to and including the terminal bronchioles, comprise the *conductive* zone of the respiratory tract (i.e., they are concerned with the movement of gas by bulk flow between the external environment and the respiratory zone; Fig. 28–3).

The *transitional* zone includes respiratory bronchioles, which function to transport gas distal to the terminal bronchioles into the alveolar ducts and alveoli. The appearance of alveoli in the walls of the respiratory bronchioles enables these airways to also participate in gas exchange.

The *respiratory zone*, where gas exchange takes place, is comprised of alveolar ducts and alveoli. Because the conducting airways contain no alveoli and, therefore, take no part in gas exchange, they constitute the *anatomical dead space* (see below).

### Airway Structure

Coincidental with these distinct functional zones of the respiratory tract, there occurs definitive structural changes as the airways progress distally (peripherally) in the tracheobronchial tree. These structural changes involve the respiratory epithelium, the smooth muscle layer, elastic layer, and the cartilaginous structure of the airways.

There is a progressive thinning of the respiratory epithelium as it changes from the tall, ciliated columnar cells of the conductive zone to the cuboidal, sparsely ciliated cells of the terminal bronchioles. Goblet cells, which are numerous throughout the upper airways and proximal lower airways, decrease in number until they actually disappear at the level of the terminal bronchioles (Fig. 28–4).

Significant changes in the smooth muscle layer of the airways occur at different levels of the tracheobronchial tree. In the trachea and large bronchi, the smooth muscle layer occurs as bands or a spiral network; in the small bronchi and bronchioles, the smooth muscle layer completely surrounds the airway wall. With the progressive diminution in airway size as one moves distally in the tracheobronchial tree, the smooth muscle layer is found to occupy the greater portion of the total wall thickness of these airways, becoming maximal at the level of the terminal/respiratory bronchioles.

Elastic tissue, while present in the larger airways, comprises a significant part of the walls of smaller airways and alveoli.

The cartilaginous structure of the airways also changes in configuration. In the trachea, cartilage occurs as incomplete rings, while in the larger bronchi, it occurs as sheets or plates of cartilage. These cartilaginous sheets become progressively smaller and less numerous, until, finally, they disappear completely at the level of the bronchioles.

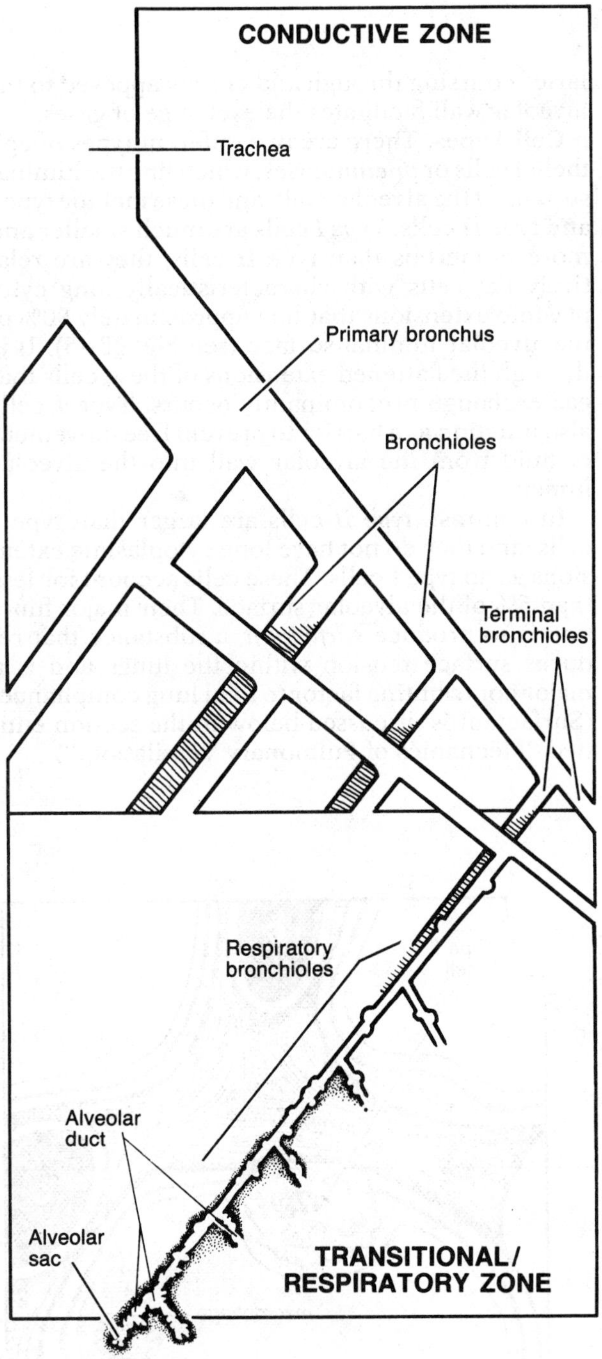


**Figure 28–3.** Functional zones of the respiratory tract. A series of dichotomous subdivisions or generations of airways and their corresponding functions, as they become progressively narrower, shorter, and more numerous, branching distally throughout the tracheobronchial tree.

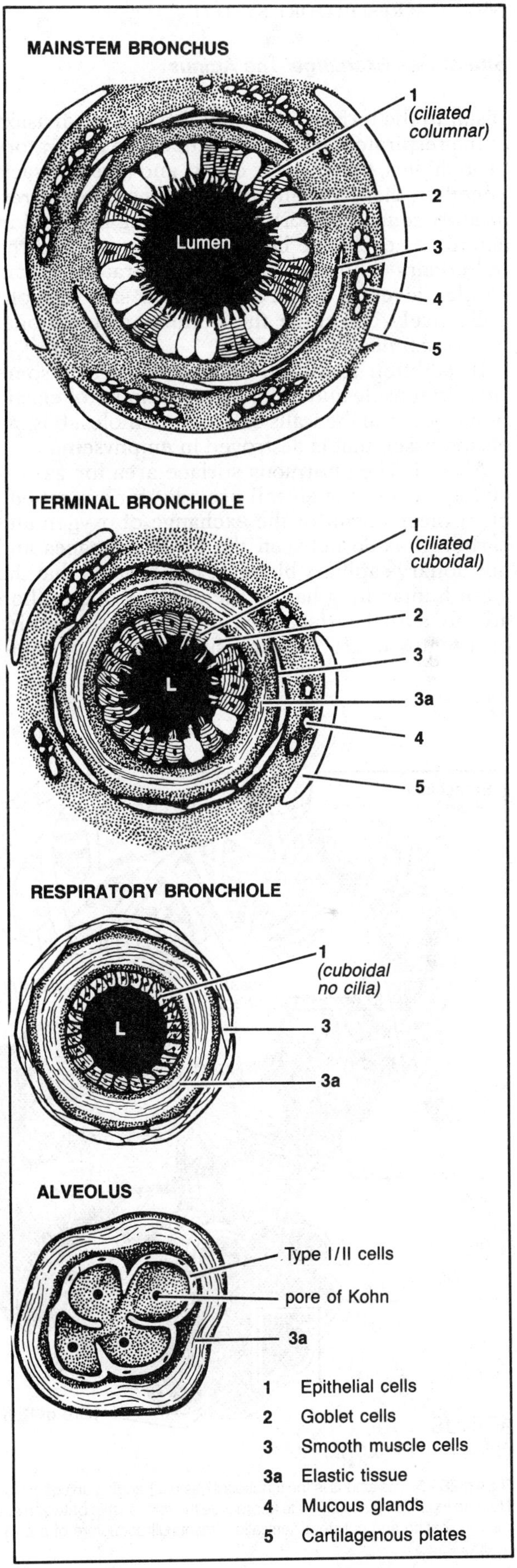


**Figure 28–4.** Microanatomy of airways in cross section, at various points within the tracheobronchial tree, including the mainstem bronchus proximally, down to the alveolus, distally. (Refer to Fig. 28–3 to appreciate the relationship between structure and function of these various airways.)

### *Site of Gas Exchange: The Acinus*

Distal to the terminal bronchioles further division of the respiratory passages includes the respiratory bronchioles, the alveolar ducts, and alveolar sacs. Together, these tiny air passages constitute the *respiratory zone*, that portion of the lung involved in actual gas exchange between the alveoli and the pulmonary capillaries. The respiratory bronchioles, alveolar ducts, and alveolar sacs (alveoli) collectively constitute the pulmonary functional unit or *acinus* (Fig. 28–5).

In addition to alveoli and alveolar sacs, some smooth muscle and a significant amount of elastic tissue occur in the walls of the bronchioles. It is the elastic tissue that is destroyed in emphysema.

**Alveoli.** The enormous surface area for gas exchange within the alveoli provides for a most efficient mechanism for the exchange of oxygen and carbon dioxide between the alveolar spaces and pulmonary capillary blood. It is estimated that the adult human lung has on the order of 300 million alveoli, a total surface area approximately the size of a tennis court. An extensive network of capillaries coursing through and closely apposed to the alveolar wall facilitates the exchange of gases.

**Cell Types.** There are two different types of epithelial cells or *pneumocytes*, which line the luminal surface of the alveolar wall, and these include type I and type II cells. *Type I* cells are much smaller and more numerous than type II cells; they are relatively flat cells with characteristically long cytoplasmic extensions that line approximately 90% of the alveolar luminal surface (see Fig. 28–5). It is through the flattened extensions of these cells that gas exchange predominantly occurs. Type I cells also function as a barrier to prevent free movement of fluid from the alveolar wall into the alveolar lumen.

In contrast, *type II* cells are larger than type I cells, and they do not have long cytoplasmic extensions as do type I cells. These cells account for less than 5% of the alveolar surface. Their major function is to produce *surfactant*, a substance that reduces surface tension within the lungs and is a major contributing factor to total lung compliance. (Surfactant is discussed below in the section entitled "Mechanics of Pulmonary Ventilation.")

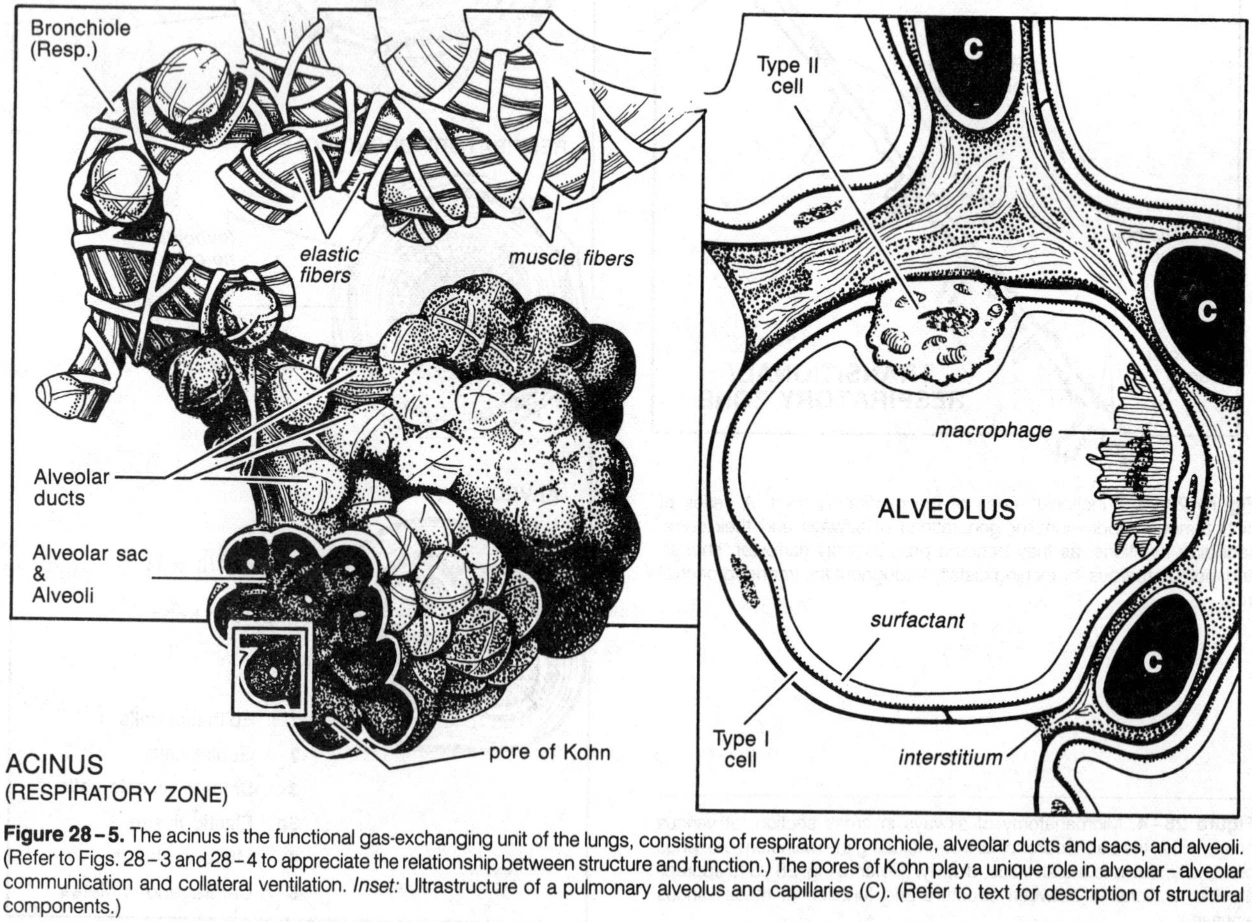


**Figure 28–5.** The acinus is the functional gas-exchanging unit of the lungs, consisting of respiratory bronchiole, alveolar ducts and sacs, and alveoli. (Refer to Figs. 28–3 and 28–4 to appreciate the relationship between structure and function.) The pores of Kohn play a unique role in alveolar–alveolar communication and collateral ventilation. *Inset:* Ultrastructure of a pulmonary alveolus and capillaries (C). (Refer to text for description of structural components.)

A third type of cell identified within the alveoli is the pulmonary alveolar *macrophage*. By the process of *phagocytosis* (engulfment/digestion of foreign material), macrophages function as a major defense against inhaled substances that have escaped the defense mechanisms of the upper and lower airways. Through their ability to process antigenic material, macrophages also play a vital role in the body's immunologic defense system (see Chap. 54).

**Pores of Kohn.** The *pores of Kohn* are alveolar-septal pores or openings within the alveolar wall that facilitate alveolar-alveolar communication and *collateral ventilation*.[1] These pores allow movement of gases between alveoli, reducing the incidence of atelectasis, and they facilitate movement of macrophages between alveoli (see Fig. 28-5).

## PULMONARY DEFENSE MECHANISMS

The process of exchanging thousands of liters of gas each day for oxygen uptake and carbon dioxide elimination, coupled with the large surface area of the lungs, which in many places is separated from circulating blood by only a thin membrane (alveolar-pulmonary capillary membrane—see below), places the pulmonary system at considerable risk to invasion by foreign substances including particulate materials, noxious chemicals, and microorganisms. Major categories of defense include the functional anatomy of the respiratory tract, presence of phagocytic and inflammatory cells to interact directly with inhaled material, and the immune system. In addition, important protective reflexes include the cough, gag, and epiglottal closure reflexes.

### Turbulent Precipitation Mechanism

The obstruction to air flow afforded by the turbinates, nasal septum, and pharyngeal wall, and the progressive dichotomous branching of the respiratory passages throughout the tracheobronchial tree down to the lung parenchyma (see Fig. 28-3) function efficiently to precipitate particulate matter at various levels depending on particle size. Each time inhaled air hits one of these obstructions, it must change its direction of flow. Particles suspended in the air, having greater mass and momentum, cannot change direction as rapidly as air, and thus precipitate out and become deposited within the respiratory epithelium. Particles deposited along the respiratory tract are transported by the mucociliary transport mechanism toward the mainstem bronchi and trachea where the cough reflex effectively clears this foreign material from the respiratory passages.

Many particles 0.1 to 0.5 micron in size (including particles in cigarette smoke) remain suspended in alveolar air and are expelled by expiration; up to one third of them do precipitate in the alveoli. Those particles entrapped in the alveoli are removed slowly by macrophages.

### Phagocytosis-Inflammatory Process

The pulmonary alveolar macrophage plays a critical role in removing foreign material that has escaped deposition in the upper airways. In addition, intracellular processing of antigenic material by macrophages is a critical preliminary step in the initiation of the immune response. (For a discussion of the role played by macrophages in the immune response, see Chap. 54.) Factors that cause macrophage dysfunction include cigarette smoke, viral respiratory tract infection, alcoholism, hypoxia, and corticosteroid therapy. (For further discussion of the macrophage, see Chap. 61.)

## PULMONARY VASCULATURE

### Bronchial and Pulmonary Circulations

All portions of the airways and the alveoli receive a rich supply of blood. The pulmonary vasculature encompasses a dual blood supply by the bronchial and pulmonary vessels. The *bronchial* circulation, which is actually part of the systemic circulation, provides nutrient blood flow to the bronchi and larger bronchioles. Distal to the terminal bronchioles including all the acini, blood in the pulmonary capillaries provides the necessary blood supply. Communication between the bronchial and pulmonary circulations occurs at the level of the terminal bronchioles, and the blood originating in the bronchial arteries returns to the heart by way of the pulmonary veins. In this instance, venous blood is returned to vessels transporting oxygenated blood to the left heart.

The *pulmonary* circulation is responsible for transporting deoxygenated blood from the right ventricle to the lungs by the pulmonary artery, and returning oxygenated blood to the left atrium by the pulmonary veins. While the pulmonary circulation handles approximately the same cardiac output from the right ventricle as does the systemic circulation from the left ventricle at a resting cardiac output (~5 liters/minute), blood supply to the lungs is uniquely different in several respects.

The pulmonary vasculature is characterized by its great distensibility, attributed largely to its thin-walled blood vessels with minimal smooth muscle. Thus, these blood vessels offer a low resistance to right ventricular ejection, reducing the work of the right ventricle.

During exercise or under conditions of increased

cardiac output, the pulmonary circulation is actually able to *decrease* its resistance so that overall, only a minimal increase in pulmonary artery pressure occurs. Mechanisms underlying this response include: (1) recruitment of blood vessels, which, under normal resting conditions, essentially receive no blood; and (2) distensibility of thin-walled pulmonary vessels, which can enlarge their diameter under increased pressure to accommodate additional blood flow (Fig. 28–6). The ability to increase the total cross-sectional area of the pulmonary vasculature on demand enables the pulmonary circulation to lower its resistance when the need for increased blood flow arises.

There is an uneven distribution of pulmonary blood flow that is strongly influenced by the low-pressure hemodynamics and the effects of gravity. In the upright position, blood flowing to the apex of each lung must flow against gravity. Under normal conditions, a mean pulmonary artery pressure of 15 mmHg is usually just sufficient to achieve adequate flow to this region.

In contrast, blood flow to the base of each lung is assisted by gravity, and, thus, there is a substantially greater blood flow to this region than to the apices. Gravity also becomes a factor with respect to blood flow to dependent areas associated with position (i.e., the supine or prone positions; see Fig. 28–13). The distribution of blood flow to the lungs has major implications for the matching of ventilation with perfusion, and local mechanisms within the lungs function to ensure optimal matching of ventilation and perfusion to individual alveoli.

One mechanism functions to adjust ventilation to perfusion by reflex changes in bronchiolar smooth muscle tone, in response to local carbon dioxide concentrations. If an alveolus is well ventilated but its blood supply is reduced, there is a consequent decrease in the alveolar carbon dioxide concentration ($PACO_2$). This reduction in $PACO_2$, in turn, causes a reflex constriction of bronchioles in the underperfused area. The end result is a decrease in ventilation to the area so as to more closely match ventilation with the available blood supply.

A second mechanism functions to adjust perfusion to ventilation by reflex changes in the smooth muscle tone of pulmonary blood vessels in response to local oxygen concentrations. A decrease in alveolar oxygen concentration (i.e., the $PAO_2$) causes nearby pulmonary blood vessels to vasoconstrict, thereby shunting blood away from alveoli with reduced ventilation. Thus, unlike blood vessels in the systemic circulation that *dilate* in the presence of hypoxemia, the pulmonary vasculature *constricts*. Pulmonary vasoconstriction in response to alveolar hypoxia is a protective mechanism designed to reduce blood flow to poorly ventilated alveoli, thereby minimizing ventilation/perfusion mismatch.

While these two mechanisms are quite effective in matching ventilation with perfusion, even in healthy individuals some ventilation/perfusion (V/Q) mismatching does exist. This largely accounts for the fact that systemic arterial gas pressures are not really exactly the same as alveolar gas pressures, that is, a gradient exists between oxygen

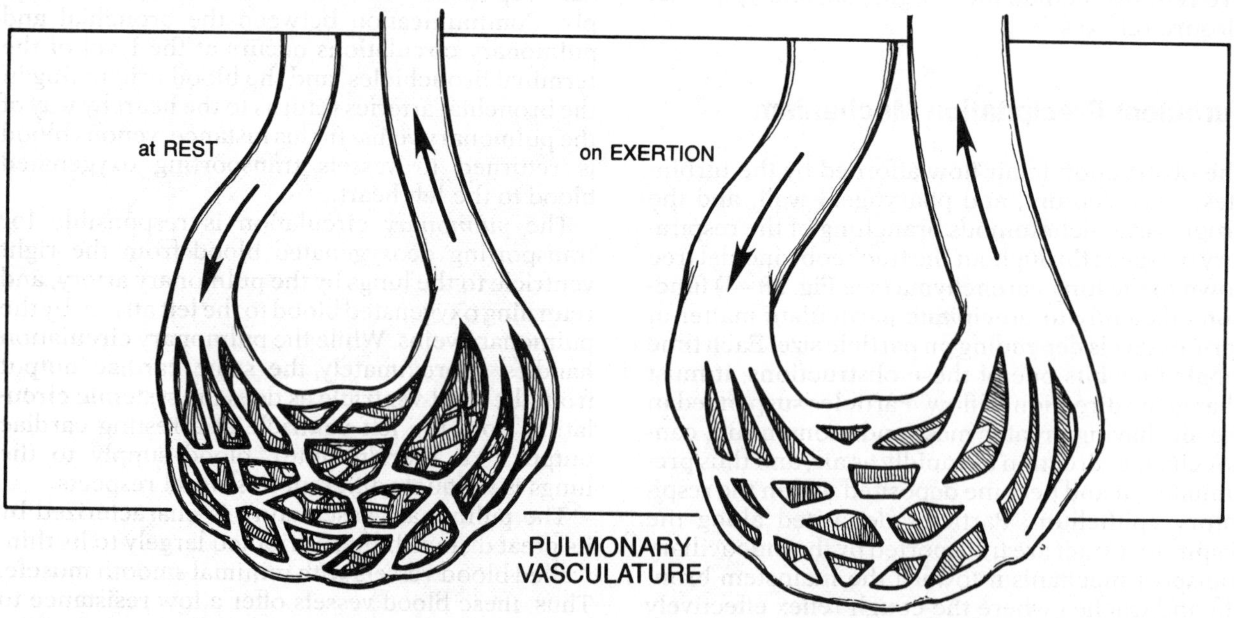


**Figure 28–6.** Effects of increases in pulmonary arterial blood pressure and blood flow (on exertion) on pulmonary vasculature resistance. Recruitment and distention of pulmonary vessels actually result in a decrease in pulmonary vascular resistance in the face of increases in pulmonary blood flow. (This is assuming that lung volumes and left atrial pressure remain constant.)

tension in alveolar air and that in arterial blood. (See section entitled "A–a Gradient" below.)

A reduction in arterial pH is also known to cause pulmonary vasoconstriction and, together with hypoxemia, may have a synergistic effect on increasing pulmonary vascular resistance. (See section entitled "Control of Respiration" below.)

The pulmonary circulation also plays an important role in the metabolism of some biologically active substances, as for example, 5-hydroxytryptamine (serotinin), bradykinin, and prostaglandins. Converting enzyme, synthesized by pulmonary vascular endothelial cells, is responsible for the proteolysis of angiotensin I to angiotensin II. Angiotensin II is a major stimulator of aldosterone synthesis and secretion by the adrenal glands. It is also a powerful vasopressor. (See Chap. 21 for further discussion regarding angiotensin and its significant metabolic role.)

## Pulmonary Lymphatic Network

An extensive network of lymphatic channels occurs within the lungs in close proximity to small pulmonary blood vessels and airways. The lymphatic system functions to return to the systemic circulation, fluid and solutes (e.g., albumin) that diffused into the interstitium from pulmonary capillaries and were not reabsorbed. In this way, the pulmonary lymphatic system helps to prevent pulmonary congestion and pulmonary edema while helping to maintain intravascular blood volume and, very importantly, serum albumin levels.

Lymphatic tissue within the respiratory system also plays a crucial role in the immune response. (This subject is discussed in Chap. 54.)

# PULMONARY VENTILATION

## Mechanics of Pulmonary Ventilation: Intrapleural and Intra-alveolar Pressures

Air, like blood or water, flows from a region of higher pressure to one of lower pressure. Inspiration occurs when alveolar pressure is less than atmospheric pressure; expiration occurs when alveolar pressure is greater than atmospheric pressure. The changes in alveolar pressure are caused by changes in the dimensions of the lungs.

### *Functional Elastic Properties of Pulmonary Structures and Intrapleural Pressure*

The lungs are highly elastic organs, open at one end to the atmosphere and enclosed within the thoracic cavity. The pleura, a thin sheet of collagen and elastic tissue, lines the thoracic cavity (parietal) and encases the lungs (visceral). A thin film of pleural fluid occurs in the intrapleural space, which allows these two surfaces to glide over each other during respiration, but prevents their separation from one another. This relationship between the thoracic wall and the lungs is analogous to two glass slides that are stuck together with water. The slides easily glide over one another, but they cannot easily be pulled apart.

While both the lungs and the thoracic wall have highly elastic properties, they act in *opposite* directions. The recoil tendency of the lungs, attributed to its elastic structure and, more importantly, to the surface tension of the fluid lining the alveoli, functions to collapse the lung and to pull it away from the chest wall; the elastic properties of the chest wall, in turn, function to expand the thoracic cavity. The consequence of these opposing recoil tendencies is the creation of a net *subatmospheric* (negative) pressure within the intrapleural space relative to atmospheric (external) pressure (Fig. 28–7). The point in the respiratory cycle at which these opposing forces are balanced, that is, pressure across the lungs and chest wall is zero (0), is the normal *resting end-expiratory phase.*

### *Mechanics of Inspiration*

At the end-expiratory position in the respiratory cycle, the intrapleural pressure is subatmospheric, the alveolar pressure is atmospheric, the respiratory muscles are relaxed, and there is no air flow. *Inspiration* is initiated by contraction of the diaphragm (predominantly) and the inspiratory musculature (external intercostals and the accessory muscles—sternocleidomastoid, scalene), which cause an increase in the size of the thoracic cavity. As the thoracic cage expands, it pulls ever so slightly away from the lung surface, causing the intrapleural pressure to become more negative. Because of the changes in intrapleural pressure, the lungs are also forced to expand. This increases the size of the alveoli, causing the pressure within them to become subatmospheric (negative). The consequent difference between atmospheric and intra-alveolar pressures causes the bulk flow of air into the lungs (see Fig. 28–7).

### *Mechanics of Expiration*

A reversal of the inspiratory process occurs on expiration when the inspiratory muscles relax and the lungs recoil. The elastic recoil of the lungs causes gas within the alveoli to become temporarily compressed. The consequent increase in intra-alveolar pressure momentarily exceeds atmospheric pressure, and air flows out of the lungs (see Fig. 28–7). In contrast to inspiration, expiration is largely a passive process.

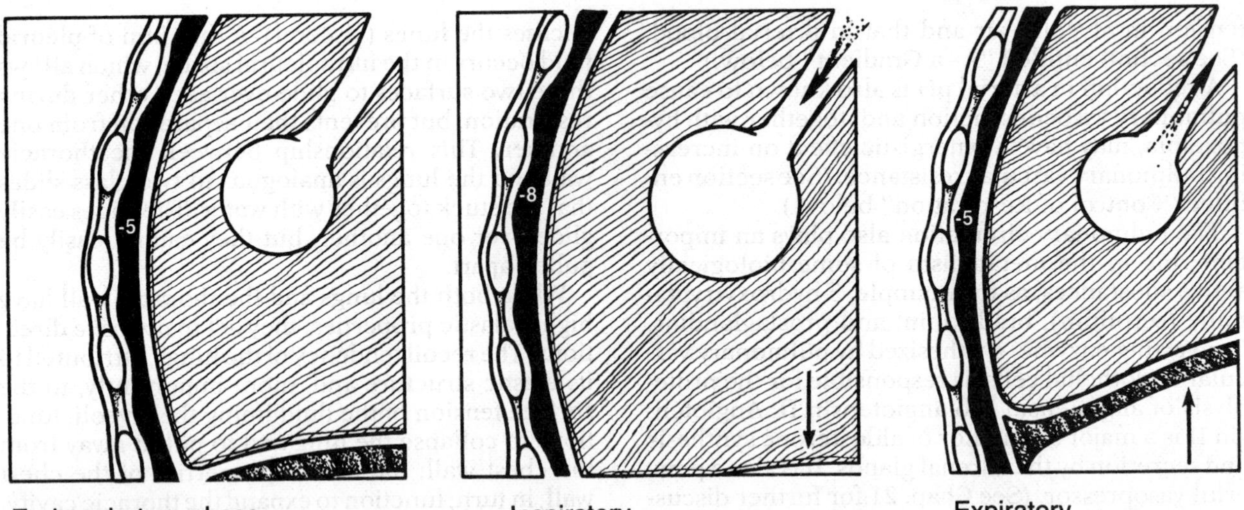


**Figure 28-7.** Pulmonary forces during quiet breathing. A schematic depiction of changes in intrapleural and intra-alveolar pressures at end-expiratory, inspiratory, and expiratory phases. A representative alveolus is depicted within the lung; lung expansion occurs as the chest cage expands and diaphragm descends (*down arrow*); lung recoil occurs as diaphragm relaxes (*up arrow*); numerical values represent change in intrapleural pressures during each phase.

*End-expiratory phase:* At end-expiration, the tendency of the lungs to recoil is balanced by the opposing recoil tendency of the chest wall to bow out, resulting in a subatmospheric intrapleural pressure (−5 mmHg). The pressure in the alveolus is atmospheric, and there is no airflow.

*Inspiratory phase:* On inspiration, contraction of inspiratory muscles (predominantly diaphragm) increases the size of the thoracic cavity, causing the intrapleural pressure to become increasingly subatmospheric (−8 mmHg) with consequent expansion of the lung. Intra-alveolar pressure becomes subatmospheric, and air flows into the lung.

Expiratory phase: On expiration, the respiratory muscles relax and the size of the thoracic cavity decreases, reducing the intrapleural pressure (−5 mmHg); the consequent recoil of the lung compresses the alveolus so that intra-alveolar pressure momentarily exceeds atmospheric pressure, and air flows out of the lung.

## Compliance and the Work of Breathing

### *Compliance*

Compliance reflects the expansibility or distensibility of the lungs and thorax and is expressed as the "volume increase in the lungs for each unit increase in alveolar pressure, or for each unit decrease in pleural pressure."[2] Compliance of the normal lungs and thorax combined is 0.13 liters/cm of water pressure. This means that every time the alveolar pressure is increased by 1 cm of water, the lung volume expands by 130 ml.

When lung compliance is diminished, the work of breathing is increased. A low compliance means that a greater pressure difference must be generated across the chest wall to produce normal lung expansion. This is accomplished by developing a greater than normal subatmospheric pressure within the intrapleural space, a feat that requires more vigorous contraction of the diaphragm and inspiratory intercostal muscles. When lung compliance is decreased, the work of breathing increases and a greater amount of energy is expended for a given amount of chest expansion.

**Surfactant.** While the elastic properties of pulmonary structures play an important role in determining lung compliance, the single most important determinant is the surface tension at air–water interfaces within the alveoli.[3] Common to all liquid–gas interfaces, surface tension reflects the attraction between molecules that tends to draw them together. Pressure within the alveoli is directly proportional to the surface tension of the alveolar wall and inversely proportional to the radius. Surfactant is a lipoprotein substance secreted by type II cells, which lines the alveolar wall and functions to reduce surface tension within the alveoli. By reducing surface tension, surfactant lowers the resistance to alveolar expansion on inspiration and the collapse of the alveoli on expiration.[4]

### *Work of Breathing*

The work or energy required to expand the lungs and thorax so as to provide for a given amount of ventilation is generated by the contraction of the inspiratory musculature, that is, the diaphragm (predominantly), intercostal muscles, and the accessory muscles (if necessary).

The actual work of breathing can be divided into three components:[5] (1) *compliance* work reflects the work required to expand the lungs against the elastic forces; (2) *tissue resistance* work is the work expenditure required to overcome the viscosity of the lungs and chest wall; and (3) *airway resistance* work reflects the work required to overcome resistance to air flow through the respiratory bronchi and bronchioles.

Clinically, the different types of work of breathing may be increased in pulmonary disease. Compliance work and tissue resistance work are frequently increased in pneumonia, pulmonary edema, adult respiratory distress syndrome (ARDS), and pulmonary fibrosis, among others. Airway resistance work is especially increased by diseases causing airway obstruction such as asthma or chronic bronchitis. Emphysema, a disease characterized by the loss of the elastic element of the lungs, has an increased lung compliance. A more detailed discussion of some of these pathologic conditions can be found in subsequent chapters within this unit.

## Atmospheric–Alveolar Pressure Gradients and Airway Resistance: Impact on Air Flow

The volume of gas that flows in or out of the alveoli per unit time is directly proportional to the pressure difference between the atmosphere and the alveoli, and inversely proportional to the airway resistance to gas flow. The magnitude of the pressure gradient is increased by increasing the forcefulness of contraction of the inspiratory musculature. The consequence of this activity is to: (1) cause a more rapid expansion of the thoracic cage, which, in turn, increases the subatmospheric intrapleural pressure and the pressure difference across the lung wall; and (2) increase lung expansion and, thus, increase the subatmospheric intra-alveolar pressure. The end result is an increased flow of gas into the lungs (see Fig. 28–7).

### *Airway Resistance*

Resistance to gas flow into the alveoli is directly proportional to the degree of interaction between the flowing gas molecules and airway length, and inversely proportional to airway radius or diameter. The radius or diameter of airways is the predominant factor determining overall airway resistance. Specifically, it is the medium to large airways rather than the more numerous small airways that provide greater resistance to air flow. The reason for this is that, despite their small diameter, the enormous number of these smaller airways comprises the greater portion of the overall cross-sectional area of the tracheobronchial tree.

Total airway resistance in the average healthy individual is so small that at rest, only a pressure of about 1 mm (1.0 mmHg) needs to be generated with each breath to move a volume of 500 ml of gas into the lungs. Airway resistance becomes a significant factor in the presence of pulmonary disease. For example, bronchospasm and the hypersecretion of bronchial mucous glands associated with asthma cause a manifold increase in airway resistance, which can seriously compromise ventilation. In patients with endotracheal tubes, airway resistance in the trachea can be increased by 50%. (For a discussion of asthma, see Chap. 36).

## Pulmonary Volumes and Capacities

Volume changes that occur with breathing do so within the boundaries of the maximum excursion of the respiratory apparatus. Four pulmonary lung volumes have been defined, which, when summed, equal the maximum volume to which the lungs can be expanded. These four volumes include the tidal volume ($V_T$), inspiratory reserve volume (IRV), expiratory reserve volume (ERV), and residual volume (RV) (Fig. 28–8).

*Tidal Volume* ($V_T$) is the volume of air inspired or expired with each normal breath. Under resting conditions in the average adult, it is ~500 ml.

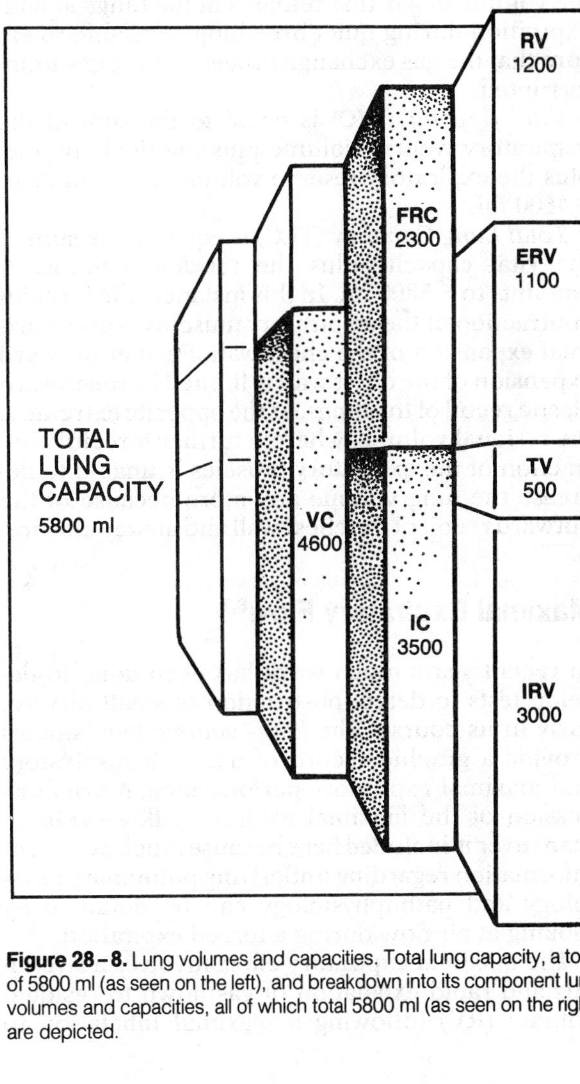


**Figure 28–8.** Lung volumes and capacities. Total lung capacity, a total of 5800 ml (as seen on the left), and breakdown into its component lung volumes and capacities, all of which total 5800 ml (as seen on the right) are depicted.

*Inspiratory Reserve Volume* (IRV) is the extra volume of air that can be inspired over and above the resting tidal volume. It amounts to ~3000 ml.

*Expiratory Reserve Volume* (ERV) is the amount of air that can still be expired by forceful contraction of the expiratory musculature after the end of a normal tidal volume expiration. It amounts to ~1100 ml.

*Residual Volume* (RV) is the volume of air still remaining in the lungs after the most forceful expiration. It amounts to ~1200 ml.

When describing events in the respiratory cycle, two or more volumes can be combined and they are called *pulmonary capacities*. They include the inspiratory capacity (IC), functional residual capacity (FRC), vital capacity (VC), and the total lung capacity (TLC; see Fig. 28–8).

*Inspiratory Capacity* (IC) is equal to the sum of the tidal volume plus the inspiratory reserve volume. It amounts to ~3500 ml.

*Functional Residual Capacity* (FRC) is equal to the sum of the expiratory reserve volume plus the residual volume. It amounts to ~2300 ml. The functional residual capacity is significant in that it is the volume of gas that remains in the lungs at end-expiration during quiet breathing, available to ensure that the gas exchange process continues uninterrupted.

*Vital Capacity* (VC) is equal to the sum of the inspiratory reserve volume plus the tidal volume, plus the expiratory reserve volume. It amounts to ~4600 ml.

*Total Lung Capacity* (TLC) is equal to the sum of the vital capacity plus the residual volume. It amounts to ~5800 ml. In this instance, the forceful contraction of the inspiratory muscles causes maximal expansion of the chest wall. Further outward expansion of the chest wall is limited by the inward elastic recoil of the lungs. At the opposite extreme is the residual volume, wherein further forceful contraction of the expiratory muscles is unable to decrease the lung volume any more because of the outward recoil of the chest wall and airway closure.

## Maximal Expiratory Flow[6,7]

In recent years much work has been done to develop tests to detect obstruction of small airways early in its course. The *flow–volume loop* studies provide a graphic record of maximal inspiratory and maximal expiratory performance. A brief discussion of the maximal expiratory flow–volume maneuver is included here because much pertinent information regarding underlying pulmonary physiology and pathophysiology can be obtained by looking at air flow during a forced expiration.

The maximal expiratory effort involves a strenuous and rapid exhalation of gas down to residual volume (RV) following a maximal inhalation to total lung capacity (TLC). In Figure 28–9, a series of expiratory curves (*A*) show the kind of flow rates generated by progressively greater expiratory efforts. In each instance, flow rises very rapidly to a high value in the initial portion of the curves but declines over the greater portion of expiration. Sig-

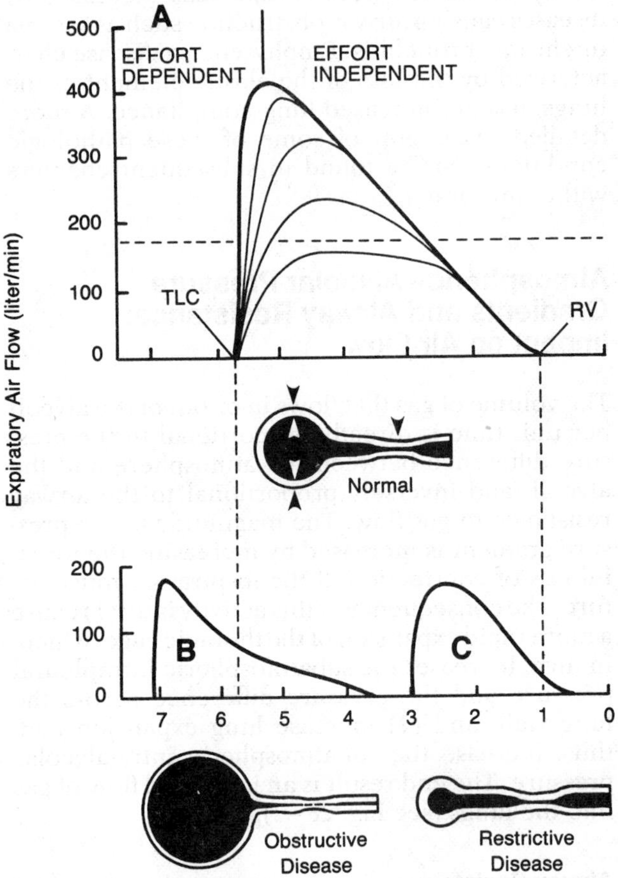


**Figure 28–9.** Maximum expiratory flow. (*A*), A series of maximal expiratory flow volume curves is depicted, reflecting increasingly greater expiratory efforts from relatively lower to a maximum effort. In each case, a maximum expiratory air flow is rapidly reached ("effort dependent"), beyond which further flow cannot be achieved, no matter what additional expiratory effort is exerted. In each instance, the descending portion of the flow–volume curves takes virtually the same path, regardless of the effort expended (i.e., "effort independent"). The major factors determining maximal expiratory flow are the external and internal pressures applied to the airways. Compression of the lungs by the intrathoracic pressure generated during expiration tends to collapse the airways. (Note the direction of arrows in the schematic airway indicating that this external pressure is applied equally to both the alveolus and bronchiole). However, this expiratory force is opposed by an increased resistance from within the airway generated by the elastic recoil of lung tissue (note direction of arrows within the airway). This internal pressure tends to keep the airway open and, thus, facilitates air flow out of the lungs until a critical point is reached. Once the bronchioles have become nearly completely collapsed, further expiratory force can still increase the alveolar pressure, but it also increases the airway resistance by an equal amount, thereby preventing any further increase in flow.[7] Thus, beyond this critical degree of expiratory force, the maximum expiratory flow has been reached.

Maximum expiratory flow volume curves are depicted for two respiratory diseases with differing pathophysiologies including: *B*, obstructive lung disease; and *C*, restrictive lung disease. Refer to text for discussion.

nificantly, the decline of each curve follows the same path regardless of the effort expended.

The initial part of the forced expiratory maneuver is termed "effort dependent" and results from an increase in intrapleural pressure associated with strenuous contraction of the expiratory musculature. In contrast, flow rates during the latter part of the maneuver are considered to be "effort independent," that is, a point is reached beyond which the expiratory flow rates decline, regardless of the effort exerted. The limiting factor to air flow during most of a forced expiration is the critical narrowing of the smaller airways or increased airway resistance.

### *Factors Determining Airway Resistance*

During a forced expiration, several factors determine airway diameter and, thus, resistance to air flow. The level at which the airway occurs in the tracheobronchial tree reflects the size of the airways and the measure of smooth muscle within the airway walls. The degree of *radial traction* exerted by surrounding lung parenchyma on airway walls is an important factor in keeping airways open during expiration. The extent of this elastic pull or "tethering" by the structural (elastic) elements of lung tissue depends to some extent on lung volumes. At greater lung volumes, this "tethering" effect contributes significantly to keeping bronchi and bronchioles open; as lung volumes diminish, this structural support also decreases and the airways collapse more easily.

### *Factors Determining Maximal Expiratory Air Flow*

Internal and external pressures are major factors involved in determining maximal expiratory flow. Figure 28-9 illustrates the even distribution of external (intrapleural) pressure on the outside of both the alveoli and bronchioles. On forced expiration such external pressures would compress the airway, preventing air flow unless counteracted by internal pressures within the airways. It is the *internal* airway pressures, largely attributed to the elastic recoil of lung tissue, that function to keep airways open in the face of strong external forces, thus facilitating air flow to the exterior. At a critical point along the airway, pressure falls sufficiently so that internal airway pressure (elastic recoil) becomes equal to pressure outside the airway (intrapleural pressure), and the maximal expiratory flow rate is reached.

Beyond this point, no matter how much additional expiratory force is applied, this is the absolute maximal expiratory flow that can be achieved. Thus, it is the *elastic recoil* pressure of the lungs (effort-independent) that is the *primary* determinant of maximal expiratory flow.

Clinically, diseases that alter the inherent elastic recoil capabilities of the lung parenchyma cause changes in the effective driving pressure for air flow, which are reflected in maximal expiratory flow rate determinations. In Figure 28-9, the normal maximum flow-volume curve is depicted together with those of two different respiratory abnormalities, *obstructive* lung disease (*B*); and *restrictive* lung disease (*C*). The normal curve indicates a total lung capacity (TLC) of nearly 6 liters and a residual volume (RV) of about 1200 ml. Maximal expiratory flow is greater than 400 ml. By comparison, there is a distinct difference between the normal curve and the two abnormal curves.

In *obstructive* lung disease (e.g., asthma, chronic bronchitis, emphysema, bronchiectasis, cystic fibrosis), maximal expiratory flow rates are significantly reduced and characteristically reflect a pattern of air flow obstruction. The actual mechanism of airway obstruction depends on the underlying pathophysiology. For example, in chronic bronchitis, maximal expiratory flow rates are reduced due to decreased airway size (increased airway resistance) associated with increased secretions of mucous glands and inflammation. In emphysema, the reduced maximal expiratory flow rates are largely caused by loss of elastic recoil due to destruction of lung tissue. There is loss of radial traction or "tethering" of airways, thus predisposing to airway collapse during expiration. Commonly, a mixture of both pathologies is present.

In general, obstructive lung disease is characterized by elevated total lung capacity (>7000 ml) and increased residual volume (3500 ml), due to air trapping within the lungs (see Fig. 28-9, *B*). The underlying airway obstruction and tendency of airways to collapse account for the greatly reduced maximal expiratory flow rates (<200 ml).

In *restrictive* lung disease including interstitial lung diseases (e.g., pulmonary fibrosis, sarcoidosis, silicosis) and thoracic cage disorders (e.g., kyphosis, scoliosis, fibrotic pleurisy), there is a reduced lung compliance and increased resistance to lung expansion. Accordingly, there is a reduced total lung capacity (about 3000 ml) and reduced residual volume (about 750 ml; see Fig. 28-9, *C*). The reduced maximal expiratory flow (<200 ml) reflects the overall reduction in lung volumes associated with restrictive lung disease, but is otherwise normal because there is no air flow obstruction.

## Alveolar Ventilation

In order to maintain arterial blood gas parameters within the normal physiologic range to ensure adequate gas exchange to the tissues, a volume of gas must be presented to the lungs that is sufficient for the necessary oxygen uptake and carbon dioxide elimination.

The average individual under resting conditions breathes about 12 to 20 times per minute and exchanges approximately 500 ml gas with each breath. The volume of gas inspired with each breath is called the *tidal volume* ($V_T$). The total volume of gas inspired each minute (i.e., respiratory rate times the tidal volume) amounts to 6 to 8 liters per minute and is called the *minute ventilation* ($\dot{V}_E$). Thus,

$$\dot{V}_E = f \times V_T$$

where f represents the respiratory rate.

Not all the gas inspired with each breath is used for gas exchange. Rather, the portion of the total minute ventilation that occupies the space within the upper airways and tracheobronchial tree, that is, the *conducting* zone, does not participate in gas exchange and constitutes the *anatomical dead space* ($V_D$; see Fig. 28–3). This "wasted" volume of gas amounts to approximately 1 ml per pound of body weight or, on the average, about 150 ml.

The portion of the tidal volume ($V_T$) that reaches the gas exchanging zones of the lungs (i.e., *transitional* and *respiratory* zones) is called the *alveolar* volume and usually amounts to ~350 ml per single normal breath. *Alveolar minute ventilation* ($\dot{V}_A$) is equal to the number of breaths per minute (i.e., the respiratory rate) times the tidal volume minus the anatomical dead space volume (i.e., the alveolar volume), thus,

$$\dot{V}_A = f \times (V_T - V_D)$$

### *Total (Physiologic) Dead Space*

The anatomical dead space is not the only type of dead space. For example, areas of the lung that normally participate in gas exchange and are fully ventilated, but do not receive adequate blood flow, contribute additional dead space volume. This volume of air is called the *alveolar* dead space. Thus, *physiologic* dead space is equal to the *anatomical* dead space plus the *alveolar* dead space.

The relationship between dead space volume and the depth and rate of breathing is clinically significant. Rapid, shallow respirations with a tidal volume of 150 ml and a respiratory rate >40 can seriously compromise alveolar ventilation because the patient is essentially only moving dead space gas, and the alveoli are not being ventilated. On the other hand, any increase in tidal volume (>500 ml), increase in depth of breathing, and reduction in the rate of breathing will enhance alveolar ventilation.

## DIFFUSION

### Behavior of Gases in Air and Body Fluids

The underlying process responsible for the net movement of oxygen and carbon dioxide between the alveoli and the blood, and between the blood and cells of the body is diffusion. Diffusion is defined as the random movement of molecules from an area of greater concentration to one of lesser concentration. The energy that fuels this process is derived from the kinetic motion of the molecules themselves. The constant impact of these molecules against a surface exerts a force or pressure, and this pressure, which is a function of the amount of the gas present, is called the *partial pressure* of the particular gas. Partial pressure is indicated by the letter P before the symbol of the gas (e.g., $PO_2$, $PCO_2$).

*Atmospheric* air at sea level is composed of approximately 79% nitrogen and 21% oxygen and exerts a total pressure of 760 mmHg (Fig. 28–10). Each of these gases contributes to the total pressure

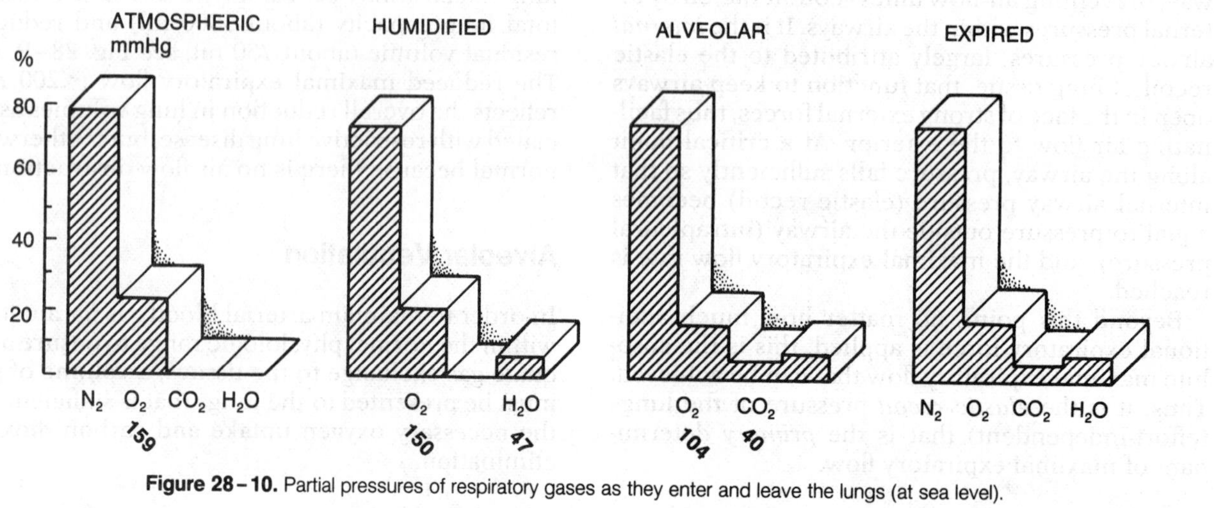


**Figure 28–10.** Partial pressures of respiratory gases as they enter and leave the lungs (at sea level).

in direct proportion to their relative concentrations or partial pressure. Nitrogen contributes 79% of the 760 mmHg or a partial pressure of 600 mmHg; oxygen contributes 21% or a partial pressure of 159 mmHg.

#### Vapor Pressure

When gas is inhaled into the respiratory tract, it is immediately conditioned by the specialized respiratory epithelium lining the respiratory passageways. This means that the inspired gas is filtered, warmed, and humidified. Humidification of gas occurs because, like other dissolved gas molecules, water molecules are continually escaping from the fluid into the gaseous state. The pressure exerted by water molecules as they escape from the water surface is called *vapor pressure.* At normal body temperature (37°C), the vapor pressure is 47 mmHg.

Humidification of atmospheric air as it flows through the upper airways means that the partial pressure exerted by water molecules becomes a definite factor in determining the composition of alveolar gases. Addition of water vapor serves to dilute all the other gases in inspired gas, and the partial pressure exerted by water molecules must always be taken into consideration when calculating the partial pressures of gases within the alveoli.

For example, inspired gas saturated with water vapor at body temperature (37°C) exerts a partial pressure of 47 mmHg. To calculate the partial pressure of nitrogen and oxygen in the humidified gas, it is necessary to subtract the partial pressure of water vapor (i.e., 47 mmHg) from the total pressure exerted by atmospheric air, which at sea level is 760 mmHg. Thus, 760 mmHg minus 47 mmHg equals 713 mmHg. Therefore, the partial pressure exerted by nitrogen in *humidified* gas is 713 mmHg times 79% (percentage of nitrogen in atmospheric air) or ~563 mmHg; the partial pressure exerted by oxygen in humidified gas is 713 mmHg times 21% (percentage of oxygen in atmospheric air) or ~150 mmHg (see Fig. 28–10).

#### Solubility of Gases

Gases dissolved in body fluids similarly exert a partial pressure because dissolved molecules move randomly and generate kinetic energy as do molecules in the gaseous state. Factors that determine the concentration of a gas in solution include the pressure exerted by the relative concentration of the gas and by its *solubility coefficient.* This latter term refers to the extent that molecules of a gas are physically or chemically attracted to water molecules. The greater the attraction, the greater the number of molecules that become dissolved. This is an important factor in determining the rate at which a gas can diffuse through the tissue. A point to remember is that carbon dioxide is 20 times more soluble than oxygen in body fluids.

### Composition of Alveolar Gas

The composition of *alveolar* gas is considerably different from that of atmospheric air (see Fig. 28–10). This difference is attributed largely to the following: (1) atmospheric air entering the respiratory tract is humidified before it reaches the alveoli (partial pressure of water vapor is 47 mmHg); (2) alveolar gases are only partially replaced by atmospheric air with each breath; (3) oxygen is constantly being absorbed from the alveoli into pulmonary capillary blood; and (4) carbon dioxide is constantly diffusing from the pulmonary blood into the alveoli. Thus, the partial pressure of oxygen in alveolar air is ~13.6% or about 104 mmHg as compared to its concentration or partial pressure in atmospheric air, which is about 21% or about 159 mmHg, respectively.

*Expired* gas reflects a combination of dead space gas and alveolar gas. Its overall composition is determined by the proportion of the expired gas that is dead space gas and the proportion that is of alveolar origin. The initial portion of this air, the dead space air, is typically humidified. Increasingly, alveolar gas becomes mixed with dead space until all the dead space gas has been expired, and only alveolar gas is exhaled at the end of expiration. The final composition of expired gas lies somewhere between humidified gas and alveolar gas (see Fig. 28–10).

### Diffusion of Gases Through the Alveolar–Capillary Membrane

Gas exchange between the alveoli and blood in the pulmonary capillaries occurs at an interface between a gas and a liquid via the alveolar–capillary membrane. The structural layers of this membrane allow for alveolar gases to be in close proximity to the blood within the capillaries, thus facilitating the rapidity of respiratory exchange of these gases.

Structurally, the layers of the respiratory membrane through which gases are exchanged include (Fig. 28–11): (1) a fluid layer lining the alveolar lumen and containing surfactant; (2) the long, narrow cytoplasmic extensions of type I alveolar epithelial cells; (3) epithelial cell basement membrane; (4) narrow interstitial space between the basement membrane of alveolar epithelial cells and that of the pulmonary endothelial cells; (5) capillary basement membrane, which commonly fuses with epithelial basement membrane, thus obliterating the interstitial space in a large portion of the alveolar–capillary interface; and (6) the capillary endothelial cell and the red blood cell.

The overall thickness of the respiratory membrane varies from 0.2 micron to an average of 0.6 micron; its total surface area approaches approximately 50 to 100 $m^2$ in the normal adult. The aver-

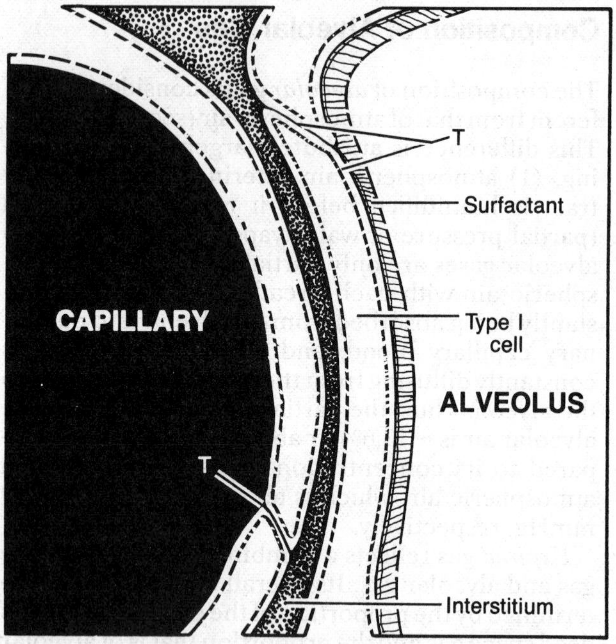


**Figure 28–11.** Ultrastructure of the alveolar–capillary membrane shown in cross section: pathway of diffusion. Diffusion of gases occurs through the various structural layers of the membrane including: the fluid surfactant layer lining the alveolus; alveolar epithelial type I cell; epithelial basement membrane; interstitial space; capillary basement membrane; capillary endothelial cell, and the red blood cell (not depicted). Tight junctions (*T*) are also depicted.

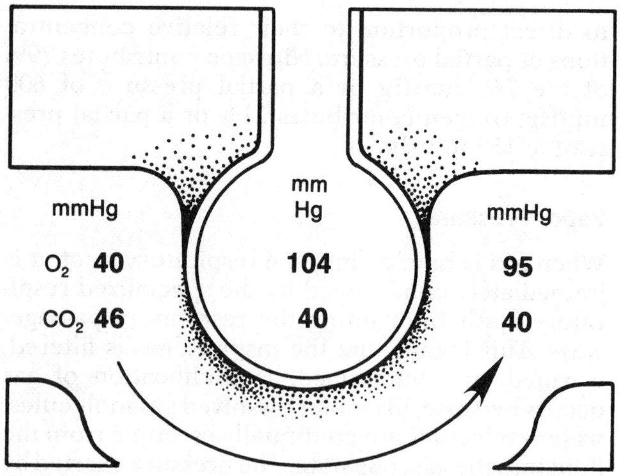


**Figure 28–12.** Transfer of oxygen and carbon dioxide between the alveolus and capillary blood. The net gradients between the partial pressure of oxygen and carbon dioxide on the two sides of the alveolar–capillary membrane provide the driving force that underlies gas exchange within the lungs. These pressure differences facilitate carbon dioxide release and oxygen uptake as blood flows through the pulmonary circulation. Following gas exchange, the partial pressures of these gases in arterial blood leaving the pulmonary circulation are 95 and 40 mmHg, respectively. The difference between the alveolar oxygen tension (104 mmHg) and that of arterial blood (95 mmHg) is largely attributed to "physiologic" dead space (i.e., the sum of anatomical and alveolar dead space). This difference is referred to as the A–a gradient.

age diameter of the pulmonary capillary is 7 to 9 microns. Because the diameter of a red blood cell (RBC) is about 7.0 micron, one can appreciate the close intimate interface that occurs between the RBC and the alveolar lumen as blood flows through the pulmonary circulation.

The usual transit time for a RBC traveling through the pulmonary capillaries is approximately 0.75 second. The diffusion of respiratory gases through the alveolar–capillary membrane is so rapid that full equilibration of partial pressures of these gases between the alveoli and pulmonary capillaries occurs within but the initial one third of the total transit time, or 0.25 second. Thus, there is a pulmonary "reserve" available for diffusion should transit time decrease, as in exercise, or should pathology alter the alveolar–capillary membrane and impair diffusion.

### Alveolar–Blood Gas Exchange

Blood entering the pulmonary capillaries by the pulmonary arterial circulation is systemic *venous* blood, and, as such, it contains a high partial pressure of carbon dioxide ($P\bar{v}CO_2$ 46 mmHg) and a low partial pressure of oxygen ($P\bar{v}O_2$ 40 mmHg) (Fig. 28–12). (The small "v" in the symbols $P\bar{v}CO_2$ and $P\bar{v}O_2$ reflects mixed venous blood.)

Normally, the partial pressures of carbon dioxide and oxygen in alveolar gas are 40 mmHg and 104 mmHg, respectively (see Fig. 28–10). The net gradient between the partial pressures of carbon dioxide and oxygen on the two sides of the alveolar–capillary membrane result in a net diffusion of carbon dioxide into the alveoli, and of oxygen into the blood.

In summary, diffusion of carbon dioxide and oxygen is influenced by the integrity of the alveolar–capillary membrane, the surface area available for gas exchange, the solubility coefficient of each gas, the net pressure gradients between the alveolar and pulmonary capillary gas pressures, the total RBC count, and the amount of hemoglobin.

## VENTILATION/PERFUSION RELATIONSHIPS

The extensive network of the pulmonary capillary bed interfacing with alveolar walls provides for an enormous surface area of intricate contact between RBCs and alveolar gas. For gas exchange to be most efficient, the appropriate amount of alveolar gas and capillary blood should be available to each alveolus, or gas-exchanging unit.

### Ventilation/Perfusion Ratio ($\dot{V}/\dot{Q}$ Ratio)

Ideally, optimal efficiency for gas exchange would be provided by an even distribution of ventilation and perfusion throughout the lung so that ventilation and perfusion are always matched. Clinically, this is not the case even in healthy individuals. Overall, alveolar ventilation is normally about 4 liters/minute and pulmonary capillary blood flow is about 5 liters/minute, making the average ratio of ventilation to blood flow 4:5, or about 0.8. This relationship is called the ventilation/perfusion ratio ($\dot{V}/\dot{Q}$ ratio).

Although the overall $\dot{V}/\dot{Q}$ ratio is about 0.8, the ratio varies remarkably throughout the lung. Because blood flow to the lungs is largely determined by hydrostatic forces (see section entitled "Pulmonary Vasculature," above), the dependent areas of each lung receive a disproportionately larger share of the perfusion while areas in the apices of the lungs are relatively underperfused. In the normal person in the upright position, the alveoli in the apices of the lungs receive a moderate amount of ventilation but little blood flow. As a result, the $\dot{V}/\dot{Q}$ ratio in the upper regions of the lungs is greater than 0.8.

Gradations of ventilation occur throughout each lung, with a greater portion going to dependent lung areas. However, ventilation and perfusion are not matched in the dependent areas because the gradient is more marked for perfusion than for ventilation. As a result, the $\dot{V}/\dot{Q}$ ratio is lower than 0.8 in the lower lung regions. Thus, gas exchange throughout the lung is not uniform but varies according to the ratio of ventilation ($\dot{V}$) to perfusion ($\dot{Q}$) in each region. Clinically, the position assumed (e.g., supine, prone, side-lying) is an important factor to be considered in terms of ventilation and perfusion to dependent areas as patients are turned and positioned (Fig. 28–13).

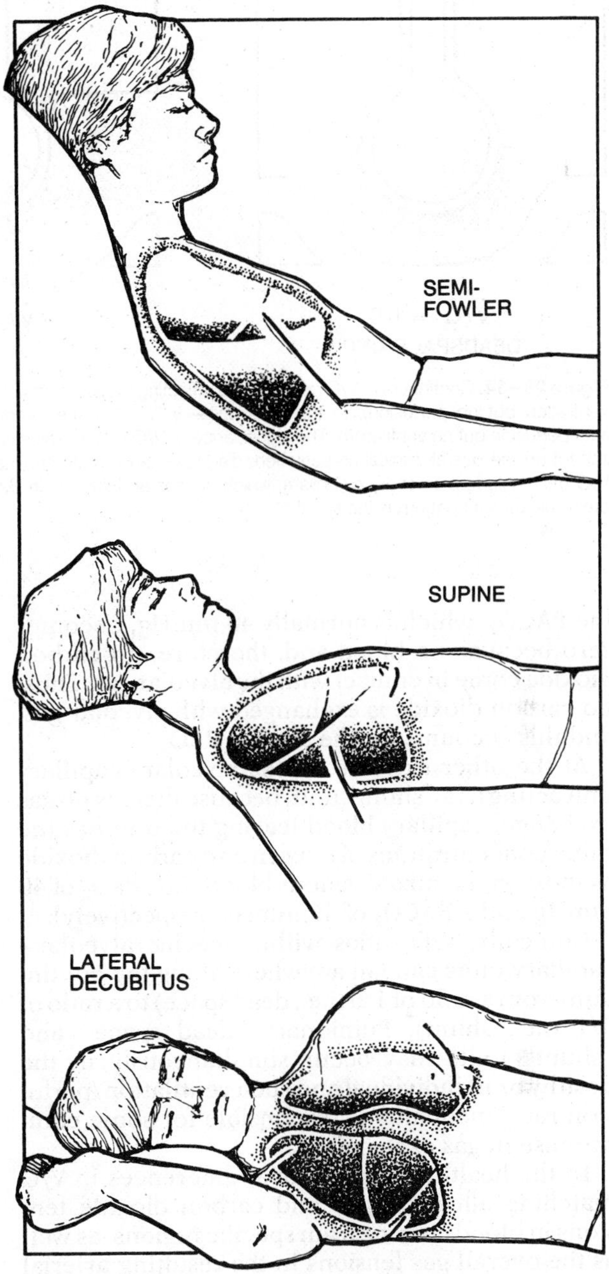


**Figure 28–13.** The effect of various position changes on the ratio of ventilation to perfusion throughout regions of the lungs. In the uppermost lung regions, the $\dot{V}/\dot{Q}$ ratio is greater than in dependent lung regions. In general, ventilation and perfusion are more closely matched in dependent lung areas, a factor that may be of significance when turning and positioning patients.

### *"Dead Space" Versus "Shunt" Units*

To better understand the effects of alterations in the ventilation/perfusion $\dot{V}/\dot{Q}$ ratio on gas exchange, it is useful to consider the dynamics of a single alveolar–capillary unit. In such a unit, a continuum of possible $\dot{V}/\dot{Q}$ relationships exists (Fig. 28–14). As discussed, in the normal situation the ventilation and perfusion are well matched and the $\dot{V}/\dot{Q}$ ratio is ideally 0.8 (or rounded off to 1/1, for this discussion). At one extreme of the continuum, ventilation is maintained but perfusion approaches zero. The $\dot{V}/\dot{Q}$ ratio in this instance approaches infinity (1/0). Insofar as gas exchange is concerned, because the alveolus is not perfused, the ventilation is "wasted" and the alveolus becomes part of the "dead space" ventilation.

At the opposite extreme of the continuum, ventilation approaches zero, while perfusion is preserved. The $\dot{V}/\dot{Q}$ ratio in this instance approaches zero (0/1). When there is no ventilation ($\dot{V} = 0$), a "shunt" exists, and oxygenation does not take place during the transit of the blood through the pulmonary circulation.

The $\dot{V}/\dot{Q}$ ratio can have profound effects on the composition of alveolar air, which reflects the altered gas exchange. In the alveolar–capillary unit acting as a "dead space" unit, the $PAO_2$ is equal to, or approaches *150* mmHg, which takes into account the normal humidification of inspired air (i.e., water vapor pressure of 47 mmHg). Normally, the $PAO_2$ is about *104* mmHg (see Fig. 28–10). The key consideration in the "dead space" unit is that

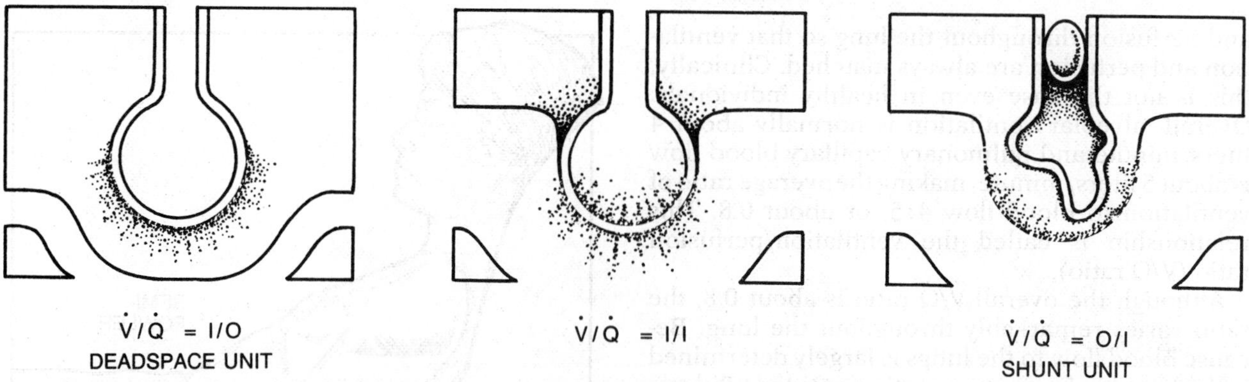


**Figure 28-14.** Continuum of V̇/Q̇ relationships reflecting the extremes of ventilation-perfusion matching: From the dead space unit—V̇/Q̇ = 1/0 (i.e., ventilation but no perfusion); to the ideal unit—V̇/Q̇ = 1/1 (i.e., ventilation and perfusion optimally matched); to the shunt unit—V̇/Q̇ = 0/1 (i.e., perfusion but no ventilation). The significance of V̇/Q̇ relationships is that each pulmonary disease state has a distinctive V̇/Q̇ pattern, which may impact on the overall clinical presentation, diagnosis, and treatment/management. Two examples of respiratory disorders and their effect on the V̇/Q̇ ratio include pulmonary embolism, which causes an increase in dead space ventilation; and adult respiratory distress syndrome in which the predominant V̇/Q̇ pattern is the shunt.[12]

the $PACO_2$, which is normally 40 mmHg, becomes zero because no blood and, therefore, no carbon dioxide come in contact with the alveolar gas. Thus, no carbon dioxide is exchanged with alveolar gas, and this accounts for the altered $PAO_2$.

At the other extreme, in the alveolar-capillary unit acting as a "shunt" unit, because there is no gas exchange, capillary blood leaving the unit has the same concentrations of oxygen and carbon dioxide as those in the mixed venous blood (i.e., $PaO_2$ of 40 mmHg and a $PACO_2$ of 46 mmHg, respectively).

Clinically, V̇/Q̇ ratios within specific alveolar-capillary units can fall anywhere along the continuum from a ratio of 1/0 (i.e., dead space) to a ratio of 0/1 (i.e., shunt). Pulmonary "dead space" and "shunt" units may occur simultaneously in the healthy or ill individual and such ventilation/perfusion ratio inequality is responsible for some compromise in gas exchange.

In the healthy lung, regional differences in V̇/Q̇ matching affect oxygen and carbon dioxide tensions in blood coming from specific regions, as well as the overall gas tensions in the resulting arterial blood returning to the left ventricle. For example, at the apex of each lung where the V̇/Q̇ ratio approaches 3.3, the $PaO_2$ is ~132 mmHg and the $PaCO_2$ is ~28 mmHg. At the bases, where the V̇/Q̇ ratio approaches 0.63, the $PaO_2$ is ~89 mmHg and the $PaCO_2$ is ~42 mmHg. The net $PaO_2$ and $PaCO_2$ of the combined blood returning from the apices, the bases, and areas in between is a function of the relative amounts of blood from each of these areas and the gas tensions of each.[8]

In respiratory disease, the V̇/Q̇ ratio is always altered, resulting in clinically significant gas exchange abnormalities. For example, in disorders that reduce alveolar ventilation, the affected lung areas receive little to no ventilation in relation to blood flow, causing the V̇/Q̇ ratio to decrease. Consequently, blood coming from these areas has a low oxygen content and saturation, which cannot be compensated for by blood from relatively preserved regions of the lung. Respiratory disorders that decrease the V̇/Q̇ ratio include hypoventilation from any cause, obstructive lung disease (e.g., asthma, emphysema, chronic bronchitis), and restrictive lung disease (e.g., pneumonia, adult respiratory distress syndrome).

In respiratory disorders that reduce pulmonary perfusion, the affected lung area receives little to no blood flow in relation to ventilation, causing the V̇/Q̇ ratio to increase. Consequently, a larger portion of the alveolar ventilation will constitute dead space ventilation and, therefore, decrease the alveolar ventilation to other areas of the lung carrying a disproportionate share of the perfusion. When the V̇/Q̇ ratio increases, the $PAO_2$ also increases while the $PACO_2$ decreases. Respiratory disorders that increase the V̇/Q̇ ratio include pulmonary embolism with partial or complete occlusion of the pulmonary artery or one of its branches; altered pulmonary vascular dynamics associated with pneumothorax or hydrothorax, and tumors; and actual destruction of pulmonary blood vessels as occurs, for example, in emphysema.

## Alveolar-Arterial Oxygen Difference (A-a Gradient)

Theoretically, under normal physiologic conditions the $PaO_2$ of blood leaving the pulmonary capillary bed should be in equilibrium with the $PAO_2$ within the alveoli. Physiologically, this is not the case because the $PAO_2$ (alveolar oxygen tension) is greater than $PaO_2$ (arterial oxygen tension) in the healthy individual, or about 104 mmHg to 95 mmHg, respectively. The difference between the alveolar and arterial oxygen tensions is called the alveolar–arterial oxygen difference, or the A–a gradient ($AaDO_2$).

The existence this gradient is attributed to the presence of normal physiologic shunts. These include the exiting of blood from lung regions with low V/Q ratios (i.e., alveoli that are underventilated in proportion to the pulmonary blood flow); drainage of venous blood from the bronchial circulation into the pulmonary veins; and drainage of coronary venous blood directly into the left atrium by the thebesian veins.

Normally, the A–a gradient is less than 15 mmHg. An $AaDO_2$ greater than 15 mmHg reflects an underlying hypoxemia-producing process. There are several reasons for an elevated $AaDO_2$ in disease. These include intrapulmonary shunts as occur in atrial or ventricular septal defects (right to left shunt), pulmonary arteriovenous malformations, or pulmonary disease wherein the alveoli are filled with fluid and/or exudate (e.g., pulmonary edema, adult respiratory distress syndrome), or there is complete alveolar collapse (e.g., pneumothorax).

Ventilation–perfusion mismatch may also cause the $AaDO_2$ to be elevated. Even when total ventilation and perfusion to both lungs are normal, if some areas receive less ventilation and more perfusion (low $\dot{V}/\dot{Q}$ ratio) while others receive more ventilation with less perfusion (high $\dot{V}/\dot{Q}$ ratio), the end result is an increase in the $AaDO_2$ with hypoxemia.

The physiologic mechanism underlying this phenomenon is that areas with a low $\dot{V}/\dot{Q}$ ratio provide relatively desaturated blood with a low oxygen content; blood coming from regions of high $\dot{V}/\dot{Q}$ ratio cannot compensate for the alteration because the hemoglobin is already fully saturated and cannot increase its oxygen content further by increased ventilation.

### Calculation of Arterial/Alveolar Ratio (a/A Ratio) and Alveolar–Arterial Gradient ($AaDO_2$)

The calculation of the arterial/alveolar ratio (a/A ratio) and/or the alveolar–arterial gradient ($AaDO_2$) can be extremely helpful in the clinical setting, particularly when one is trying to determine the reason why a patient is hypoxemic. Both these calculations are relatively simple to determine and require but two parameters to do so: arterial oxygen pressure (i.e., $PaO_2$) value obtained from an arterial blood sample and the alveolar oxygen pressure (i.e., $PAO_2$), which can be determined using the alveolar gas equation:[12]

$$PAO_2 = FIO_2\,(P_B - PH_2O) \times \frac{PaCO_2}{RQ}$$

where $FIO_2$ is the fraction of inspired oxygen; $P_B$ is the barometric pressure (assumed to be 760 mmHg at sea level); $PH_2O$ is the vapor pressure of water in the alveoli (assumed to be 47 mmHg); $PaCO_2$ is the partial pressure of carbon dioxide in arterial blood as determined on blood gas analysis; and RQ is the respiratory quotient, which reflects carbon dioxide production divided by oxygen consumption, usually a factor of about 0.8. Accordingly, the *a/A ratio* can be calculated as follows:

$$\text{a/A ratio} = \frac{PaO_2}{PAO_2}$$

The *A–a gradient* can be calculated as follows:

$$AaDO_2 = PAO_2 - PaO_2$$

### Venous Admixture and Pulmonary Shunting

Limitations in the use of the a/A ratio and $AaDO_2$ calculations occur in the scenario of venous admixture (i.e, the mixing of shunted non-reoxygenated blood with reoxygenated blood distal to the alveoli) and in the presence of intrapulmonary shunt. Venous admixture and pulmonary shunting commonly occur as complications of respiratory disorders. To determine the degree of shunting, the *classic shunt equation* is used.

$$\frac{\dot{Q}_s}{\dot{Q}_T} = \frac{CcO_2 - CaO_2}{CcO_2 - C\bar{v}O_2}$$

where $\dot{Q}_s$ is cardiac output that is shunted, $\dot{Q}_T$ is total cardiac output, $CcO_2$ is oxygen content of capillary blood, $CaO_2$ is oxygen content of arterial blood, and $C\bar{v}O_2$ is oxygen content of mixed venous blood.

In order to obtain the data necessary to calculate the degree of pulmonary shunting, the following information must be obtained: $P_B$ (barometric pressure); $PaO_2$ (partial pressure of arterial oxygen); $PaCO_2$ (partial pressure of arterial carbon dioxide); Hgb (hemoglobin concentration); $PAO_2$ (partial pressure of alveolar oxygen); $FIO_2$ (fraction of inspired oxygen); and $P\bar{v}O_2$ (partial pressure of mixed venous oxygen).[9]

In general, pulmonary shunting below 10% reflects normal lung status; a shunt between 10% and 20% is indicative of an intrapulmonary abnormality; while shunting between 20% and 30% denotes significant intrapulmonary disease and may be life-threatening in patients with compromised cardiovascular and central nervous system function. In patients with questionable perfusion status, reduced myocardial reserve, or unstable oxygen consumption/demand, calculating the degree of shunting is unreliable because these conditions directly affect oxygen content of capillary arterial ($CaO_2$) and mixed venous ($C\bar{v}O_2$) blood.

## TRANSPORT OF OXYGEN

Oxygen is transported in the blood in two distinct ways: dissolved in blood, and bound to hemoglobin within the red blood cells. Under normal physiologic conditions approximately 97% of oxygen is transported from the lungs to the tissues in chemical combination with hemoglobin. The remainder is dissolved in blood, the amount dissolved being directly proportional to its partial pressure ($PaO_2$). Because oxygen is relatively insoluble in plasma, only about 3% of total oxygen is transported in this manner.

The underlying basis for transport of oxygen from the lungs to the tissues is that the oxygen molecule binds loosely and reversibly with hemoglobin. When the $PaO_2$ is high as in the pulmonary capillaries, oxygen readily binds with hemoglobin; when the $PaO_2$ is low as in tissue capillaries, oxygen is released from hemoglobin.

Hemoglobin consists of four polypeptide chains, each containing a heme group. Oxygen specifically binds to the iron atom found within each of the four heme groups. Thus, each hemoglobin molecule can combine with four molecules of oxygen. When all four iron atoms (i.e., binding sites for oxygen) in each molecule of hemoglobin are bound with oxygen, the hemoglobin molecule is said to be fully saturated. *Saturation* is defined as the degree to which binding sites are occupied by a particular molecule, in this case, oxygen. Hemoglobin bound with oxygen is called *oxy*hemoglobin; when not in combination with oxygen, the hemoglobin is called *deoxy*hemoglobin, or *reduced* hemoglobin.

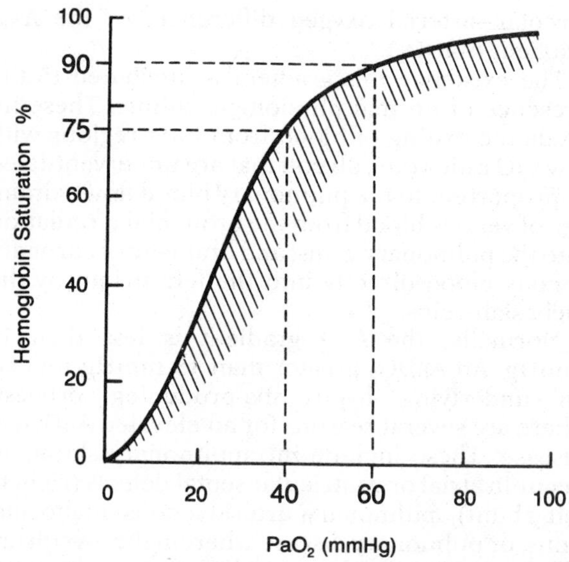


**Figure 28–15.** Oxyhemoglobin dissociation curve, relating the percent hemoglobin saturation and the partial pressure of oxygen ($PO_2$). The unique structure of the hemoglobin molecule accounts for the unusual affinity this molecule has for oxygen. When the $PO_2$ is high as in the lungs (plateau portion), oxygen readily binds with hemoglobin; when the $PO_2$ is low as in the tissue (steep portion), oxygen is readily released. Note that at a $PaO_2$ of 60, approximately 90% of the hemoglobin is saturated. Thus, clinically, oxygen therapy is often instituted to maintain a $PaO_2$ of 60 minimally, in the patient with compromised pulmonary function. Oxygen unloading at the cellular level is enhanced when the oxyhemoglobin dissociation curve is shifted to the right (*striped area*). The presence of acidemia (i.e., an increase in hydrogen-ion concentration), increase in body temperature, and increased levels of 2,3-DPG, all function to shift the curve to the right. Alkalemia, hypothermia, and reduced levels of 2,3-DPG function to shift the curve in the opposite direction, thereby reducing the release of oxygen at the cellular level.

## Oxyhemoglobin Dissociation Curve

The amount of oxygen bound to hemoglobin is a function of the partial pressure of oxygen. The quantitative relationship between oxygen bound and the partial pressure of the gas is characterized by the *oxyhemoglobin dissociation curve* (Fig. 28–15). This curve is S-shaped with a steep slope between a $PaO_2$ of 10 to 60 mmHg, and a plateau portion between a $PaO_2$ of 70 to 100 mmHg. The cooperative binding that occurs between the heme groups in a given hemoglobin molecule accounts for its sequential increase in oxygen affinity as reflected by the sigmoidal-shaped curve. As oxygen binds to one heme group, this facilitates the rapid binding of oxygen with the remaining heme groups within the same hemoglobin molecule. Thus, at the lower $PaO_2$, the extent to which hemoglobin combines with oxygen increases very rapidly from 10 to 60 mmHg, so that at a $PaO_2$ of 60 mmHg, 90% of the total hemoglobin is bound to oxygen.

At the higher $PaO_2$, the oxyhemoglobin dissociation curve reaches a plateau, which reflects that hemoglobin can only bind to so much oxygen before the binding sites become fully saturated. In general, as the partial pressure of oxygen ($PaO_2$) increases, there is a progressive increase in the percentage of hemoglobin bound with oxygen. This is called the *percent saturation of hemoglobin* ($SaO_2$). The usual saturation of arterial blood is about 97% in ambient air (at sea level); in the venous blood returning from the tissues the $PaO_2$ is about 40 mmHg with saturation of hemoglobin still about 75%. Thus, a reserve of oxygen is available on demand.

To appreciate the importance of the pivotal role played by hemoglobin in transport of oxygen, it is useful to examine mechanisms at work in the pulmonary capillaries where oxygen loading takes place, and at the tissue level where oxygen unloading occurs.

Venous blood returning to the lungs has a $P\bar{v}O_2$ of 40 mmHg, and the hemoglobin is about 75% saturated. The net pressure gradient between the alveoli ($PaO_2$ of 104 mmHg) and pulmonary capillary blood ($PaO_2$ of 40 mmHg) provides the driving force for diffusion of oxygen from the alveoli, into the blood, and subsequently, into the red blood cells where it binds to hemoglobin (see Fig. 28–12). At the tissue level, the process is reversed. The plasma $PaO_2$ (~95 mmHg) is greater than that of interstitial fluid (~40 mmHg), thus providing the driving force underlying the net diffusion of oxygen from the blood and into the interstitium. As oxygen diffuses out of the capillary, the $PaO_2$ of the plasma is reduced, thus favoring the diffusion of oxygen out of the red blood cell into the plasma. The decrease of oxygen tension within the red blood cell causes the dissociation of oxyhemoglobin, thereby liberating oxygen. Oxygen within the interstitium, in turn, moves into the cells along the concentration gradient generated by cellular utilization of oxygen.

The significance of the "oxygen reserve" alluded to earlier (i.e., hemoglobin that is still 75% upon leaving the tissues under resting conditions) is that it provides a mechanism by which cells can extract oxygen whenever they increase their metabolism. An exercising muscle, for example, uses more oxygen, thereby lowering tissue oxygen tensions; this increases the overall oxygen pressure gradient from blood to cell; oxygen diffuses out of the blood, which, in turn, reduces the oxygen tension within the red blood cells. The end result is an additional dissociation of hemoglobin and oxygen. All of these activities take place within the steep portion of the oxyhemoglobin dissociation curve (see Fig. 28–15).

It is important to appreciate that while *mixed venous* blood ($P\bar{v}O_2$) returning to the lungs may have a $PO_2$ of 40 mmHg and a hemoglobin saturation of 75%, this does not necessarily reflect the total extraction of oxygen from circulating blood by specific tissues. For example, the heart and brain extract a far greater percentage of oxygen from the circulating blood; thus, the $P\bar{v}O_2$ is much lower than 40 mmHg. The same is true of the exercising muscle.

On the contrary, tissues such as the skin and kidney, which extract much less oxygen from the blood, may have a $P\bar{v}O_2$ that is much higher than 40 mmHg. Should mixed venous blood reflect a $PO_2$ of less than 40 mmHg, or an $O_2$ saturation of hemoglobin ($S\bar{v}O_2$) that is less than 75%, these findings could indicate that the oxygen reserve is being depleted, and the compensatory mechanisms that maintain oxygen supply are being compromised.

## Effect of Hydrogen-Ion Concentration on Hemoglobin Saturation

*Acidemia* (i.e., an increase in hydrogen-ion concentration of the blood [pH $<$7.35]) can cause a shift of the entire oxyhemoglobin dissociation curve to the *right*. While the percent oxygen saturation of hemoglobin is still primarily determined by the $PaO_2$, an increase in hydrogen-ion concentration can significantly affect oxygen transport. A shift of the curve to the right means that, at any given $PaO_2$, hemoglobin has a decreased affinity for oxygen. This decreased affinity for oxygen results from an alteration in the conformation of the hemoglobin molecule by the hydrogen ion when it combines with hemoglobin.

Clinically, the more metabolically active a tissue is (e.g., heart, nerves, or an exercising muscle), the greater is its production of hydrogen ions and carbon dioxide. As the blood concentrations of these substances increase, a shift of the oxyhemoglobin dissociation curve to the right occurs. Essentially, in the tissues, the high concentrations of hydrogen ions and carbon dioxide enhance oxygen unloading; in the pulmonary capillaries, the high concentration of oxygen enhances the unloading of hydrogen ions and carbon dioxide. This is called the *Haldane effect.*

## Effect of Temperature on Hemoglobin Saturation

The effect of an increase in body temperature resembles that of increased acidity (i.e., the oxyhemoglobin curve shifts to the right; see Fig. 28–15). Clinically, this suggests that an actively metabolizing tissue (e.g., an exercising muscle) has a consequent elevation in temperature, which facilitates the release of oxygen from hemoglobin as blood flows through the tissue capillaries.

## Effect of 2,3-Diphosphoglycerate on Hemoglobin Saturation

2,3-Diphosphoglycerate (DPG) is produced by red blood cells during glycolysis. This molecule binds reversibly with hemoglobin and causes it to have a reduced affinity for oxygen. Thus, as was the case with increased hydrogen-ion concentration and temperature elevation, DPG likewise shifts the oxyhemoglobin dissociation curve to the right (see Fig. 28–15).

Clinically, tissues experiencing ischemia or reduced supply of oxygen necessitating anaerobic glycolysis generate an increased supply of DPG. The increase in DPG, in turn, causes the enhanced unloading of oxygen as blood passes through the tissue capillaries. In this way, additional oxygen is made available to the tissues.

A shift of the oxyhemoglobin dissociation curve to the *left* means that, at any given $PaO_2$, hemoglobin has an increased affinity for oxygen. The result is a significant reduction in the amount of oxygen released to the tissues. Conditions such as hypocapnia, alkalemia, and hypothermia may cause a shift of the curve to the left.

## Factors Determining Tissue Oxygen Delivery

The percent saturation of hemoglobin is most predominantly a function of the partial pressure of oxygen ($PaO_2$). Additional factors concerned with oxygen delivery to the tissues include the hemoglobin level and the cardiac output.

Reductions in the hemoglobin level can seriously compromise oxygen delivery to the tissues. In anemia, for example, with the reduction in hemoglobin levels there is a concomitant reduction in the number of oxygen binding sites, with a consequent decrease in the total oxygen content of the blood delivered to the tissues. In this circumstance, oxygen tissue delivery capability may be reduced, even though $PaO_2$ remains within acceptable physiologic range (>60 mmHg). Because oxygen delivery to the tissues depends on blood flow, any alteration in cardiac output can compromise oxygenation at the tissue level.

## TRANSPORT OF CARBON DIOXIDE

Carbon dioxide is transported in the circulation in three different forms: (1) as bicarbonate ion ($HCO_3^-$); (2) as dissolved carbon dioxide; and (3) bound to hemoglobin (*carbamino*hemoglobin). Bicarbonate is quantitatively the largest fraction and results from the combination of $CO_2$ and $H_2O$ in a reaction catalyzed by the enzyme, *carbonic anhydrase*:

$$CO_2 + H_2O \overset{\text{carbonic anhydrase}}{\rightleftharpoons} H_2CO_3 \rightleftharpoons H^+ + HCO_3^-$$

This reaction takes place within the red blood cell. $HCO_3^-$ then diffuses into the plasma in exchange for chloride ($Cl^-$) (called *chloride shift*).

While $CO_2$ is approximately 20 times more soluble than oxygen, dissolved $CO_2$ comprises only a small portion of the total $CO_2$ transported. Carbaminohemoglobin is formed from the combination of $CO_2$ and hemoglobin and depends, to a large extent, on the oxygenation status of hemoglobin (i.e., deoxyhemoglobin has a greater affinity for carbon dioxide). In the pulmonary capillary bed, the oxygenation of hemoglobin decreases its ability to bind $CO_2$ and, therefore, facilitates elimination of $CO_2$ by ventilation. As mentioned previously, these reactions reflect the Haldane effect.

## CONTROL OF RESPIRATION

### Central Neuronal Control

Alveolar ventilation (i.e., the movement of gases into and out of the lungs [alveoli]) requires a rhythmic, coordinated sequence of events involving the activity of the respiratory muscles ("respiratory pump"), under the control of the central nervous system (CNS). There is no single "respiratory center" that controls breathing. Rather, there are several neuronal networks, which are definitively involved in coordinating the respiratory effort. Breathing depends on the cyclic innervation of the inspiratory musculature (diaphragm and intercostal muscles) by neurons from these networks.

Major neuronal networks that have been identified include:[10] (1) dorsal and ventral respiratory neuronal networks located within the medulla; (2) the *pneumotaxic* center located in the superior pons; and (3) a less well-defined *apneustic* center located in the lower pons (Fig. 28-16).

The basic rhythm of breathing is generated within the medullary groups of neurons. Innervation of the inspiratory musculature occurs characteristically by alternating cycles of neuronal firing and quiescence. At the end of expiration, there is some degree of muscle tone involving the diaphragm and intercostal muscles, but not of the magnitude to move the chest wall.

Inspiration is initiated by an increased firing of impulses to the motor units, which begin to contract more forcefully. The inspiratory force increases as it proceeds, until there is an abrupt cessation of impulse firing and the inspiratory muscles relax. At this point, expiration begins. Expiration is largely a passive process, and all that is required for expiration to occur is a cessation of inspiratory neuronal activity. Expiration may be facilitated by contraction of expiratory muscles, which previously remained quiescent during inspiration.

The pneumotaxic center in the pons functions primarily to limit inspiration. Because limiting the inspiratory phase also shortens the entire period of the respiratory cycle, there is a secondary effect on the respiratory rate.

The apneustic center in the pons may signal the dorsal medullary network so as to prevent a "switch off" of inspiratory effort. The function of the apneustic center may be to provide extra drive to in-

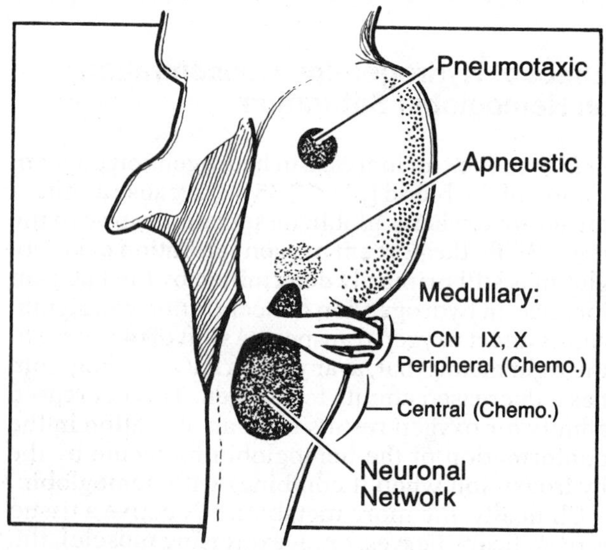


**Figure 28-16.** Regulation of respiration: central neuronal networks.

spiration, but this effect is overridden by impulses from the pneumotaxic center.

In summary, central ventilatory control is distinguished by two important features: (1) the degree of inspiratory activity (inspiratory drive), which, in turn, regulates the inspiratory gas flow rate; and (2) the timing mechanism or rhythmicity of respiration, which controls the termination of inspiration. These factors function conjointly to set the respiratory rate and tidal volume, minute ventilation, and the overall pattern of respiration.

Control of respiration by the major neuronal networks in the medulla and pons requires an intricate feedback system in order to "fine tune" the neural output of the CNS to the pulmonary musculature. In this way, the CNS is able to respond to the varied needs of the individual by appropriately increasing ventilation as, for example, during exercise or strenuous activity, while maintaining arterial blood gases within the acceptable physiologic range.

## Autonomic Nervous System Control

Regulation of respiratory function is largely under autonomic nervous system control including parasympathetic and sympathetic innervation. Specific effects of autonomic innervation on respiratory physiology include the following:

| | *Parasympathetic* | *Sympathetic* |
|---|---|---|
| Bronchiolar smooth muscle | Contraction | Relaxation |
| Pulmonary vasculature smooth muscle | Vasodilation | Vasoconstriction |
| Mucous/serous glandular secretion | Stimulation | Inhibition |

## Chemical Control of Respiration

The major neuronal networks are concerned with the mechanisms that generate spontaneity and rhythmicity of breathing. These networks in turn, receive afferent inputs from a variety of sources. The most important of these inputs concerned with the involuntary control of ventilatory volume include *peripheral chemoreceptors*, which monitor arterial oxygen ($PaO_2$), carbon dioxide ($PaCO_2$), and hydrogen-ion concentrations; and *central chemoreceptors*, which monitor the hydrogen-ion concentration of the brain's interstitial fluid. Respiratory control is designed to maintain arterial blood gas parameters within the acceptable physiologic range: $PaO_2 > 60$ mmHg; $PaCO_2$ 35 to 45 mmHg, and a pH 7.35 to 7.45.

### *Control of Ventilation by Oxygen ($PaO_2$)*

Large decreases in $PaO_2$ (e.g., $< 60$ mmHg) act as a stimulus to reflexly increase ventilation. Because the oxygen content of arterial blood is not really compromised at a $PaO_2$ above 60 mmHg (e.g., percent oxygen saturation of hemoglobin is 90), it is usually when the $PaO_2$ falls below 60 mmHg that a significant increase in ventilation occurs.

Peripheral chemoreceptors that respond to changes in the $PaO_2$ include the *carotid* and *aortic bodies*. The chemoreceptors sense the $PaO_2$ and respond specifically to dissolved oxygen and not to oxyhemoglobin (i.e., oxygen bound to hemoglobin). Afferent nerve fibers arising from these chemoreceptors pass to the medulla by way of the vagus and glossopharyngeal nerves, and stimulate the medullary inspiratory neuronal network. A compensatory increase in ventilation occurs to return the $PAO_2$ and $PaO_2$ toward normal.

### *Control of Ventilation by Carbon Dioxide and Hydrogen-Ion Concentration*

A decrease in alveolar ventilation raises the $PACO_2$, and, accordingly, an elevation in $PaCO_2$ occurs. Unlike the $PaO_2$ wherein a large decrease in $PaO_2$ ($< 60$ mmHg) must occur before the chemoreceptors respond, an increase in $PaCO_2$ of but 2 to 5 mmHg can cause a 100% increase in ventilation.[11] The slightest change in $PaCO_2$ is associated with a significant reflex change in rate and depth of ventilation. The increased ventilatory effort promotes elimination of carbon dioxide by the lungs, thus returning the $PaCO_2$ toward normal.

Conversely, a decrease in $PaCO_2$ below normal reflexly reduces the ventilatory stimulus, enabling metabolically produced carbon dioxide to accumulate. In this way, the $PaCO_2$ is returned toward normal (i.e., $> 35$ mmHg).

There are no definitive receptors for carbon dioxide per se. Rather, the impact of changes in $PaCO_2$ on the ventilatory effort are mainly due to the consequent increase in hydrogen-ion concentration that occurs with an increase in carbon dioxide concentration. Consider the following equation:

$$CO_2 + H_2O \underset{}{\overset{\text{carbonic anhydrase}}{\rightleftharpoons}} H_2CO_3 \rightleftharpoons H^+ + HCO_3^-$$

According to the law of mass action, an increase in $PaCO_2$ drives this reaction to the right, thereby increasing the hydrogen ion concentration.

Hydrogen-ion receptors include the peripheral chemoreceptors, the carotid bodies. Thus, these receptors are triggered by either a low $PaO_2$ or a high hydrogen-ion concentration in arterial blood.

The major hydrogen-ion reflex involves the *central* chemoreceptors located in the medulla. Carbon dioxide, a nonpolar substance, diffuses rapidly across the blood–brain barrier (see Fig. 6–11). Thus, any increase in $PaCO_2$ causes a rapid, similar increase in the $PCO_2$ of the brain's interstitial fluid. Accordingly, by the law of mass action (see equation above), there is a consequent increase in the hydrogen-ion concentration of the brain's interstitial fluid.

The increase in hydrogen-ion concentration stimulates the central chemoreceptors in the medulla, which, in turn, stimulate the inspiratory neuronal networks to enhance the ventilatory effort. The end result is a closely regulated hydrogen-ion concentration within the normal range. The normal pH of cerebrospinal fluid (CSF) ranges between 7.32 and 7.35.

In addition to carbon dioxide–induced changes in hydrogen-ion concentrations, peripheral chemoreceptors are also responsive to changes in arterial hydrogen-ion concentration associated with conditions other than an elevated $PaCO_2$ (i.e., hypercapnia). For example, metabolically induced increases in arterial hydrogen-ion concentration associated with increased lactic acid production can precipitate hyperventilation. *Kussmaul's* breathing (i.e., rapid, deep breathing) associated with diabetic ketoacidosis is an example of how an increase in arterial hydrogen-ion concentration can alter the ventilatory response.

In these instances, central chemoreceptors do not respond to increases in systemic arterial hydrogen-ion concentrations because, unlike carbon dioxide, the charged hydrogen ion does not easily penetrate the blood–brain barrier. Therefore, the hydrogen concentration of the brain's interstitial fluid is not appreciably increased, at least initially.

Clinically, reflex hyperventilation associated with an increase in hydrogen-ion concentration functions effectively to restore arterial pH toward normal (i.e., 7.35 to 7.45). Hyperventilation decreases the carbon dioxide concentration, which, by the law of mass action (see equation, above), lowers the hydrogen-ion concentration.

While the *stimulatory* effects of carbon dioxide on ventilation have been discussed, it is essential to appreciate that very high levels of carbon dioxide may have just the opposite effect, that is, a *depressant* effect on the CNS, including the various neuronal networks concerned with respiration. In addition, if hypercapnia and hypoxia are present simultaneously, they function synergistically to effect an enhanced ventilatory response.

## Other Controls of Ventilation

Pulmonary stretch receptors, which lie in the airway smooth muscle layer, are activated by expansion of the lung on inspiration and may provide an important "cut-off" signal for inspiration. These receptors are activated when very large tidal volumes (>1 liter) are exchanged, as for example, during exercise.

*Irritant* reflexes are elicited by stimulation of irritant receptors located within the luminal lining of the airways. Cough, bronchospasm, and tachypnea may occur in response to a noxious stimulus such as inhaled dust, chemicals, or cigarette smoke. Tachypnea may also occur in response to stimulation of *juxtacapillary* or *J receptors*, found within the pulmonary interstitium in response to an inflammatory process, or the presence of fluid and congestion in the interstitial compartment. These receptors are thought to be the source of dyspnea that occurs with pulmonary edema.

## REFERENCES


1. Des Jardins, TR: Cardiopulmonary Anatomy & Physiology: Essentials for Respiratory Care. Delmar Publishers, New York, 1988, p 28.
2. Guyton, AC: Textbook of Medical Physiology, ed 7. WB Saunders, Philadelphia, 1986, p 468.
3. Des Jardins, TR: Cardiopulmonary Anatomy & Physiology: Essentials for Respiratory Care. Delmar Publishers, New York, 1988, p 58.
4. Des Jardins, TR: Cardiopulmonary Anatomy & Physiology: Essentials for Respiratory Care. Delmar Publishers, New York, 1988, p 64.
5. Guyton, AC; Textbook of Medical Physiology, ed 7. WB Saunders, Philadelphia, 1986, p 469.
6. Weinberger, SE: Principles of Pulmonary Medicine. WB Saunders, Philadelphia, 1986, pp 69–71.
7. Guyton, AC; Textbook of Medical Physiology, ed 7. WB Saunders, Philadelphia, 1986, p 476.
8. Weinberger, SE: Principles of Pulmonary Medicine. WB Saunders, Philadelphia, 1986, p 16.
9. Des Jardins, TR: Cardiopulmonary Anatomy & Physiology: Essentials for Respiratory Care. Delmar Publishers, New York, 1988, p 177.
10. Guyton, AC; Textbook of Medical Physiology, ed 7. WB Saunders, Philadelphia, 1986, p 504.
11. Vander, A, Sherman, J, and Luciano, D: Human Physiology: The Mechanisms of Body Function, ed 4. McGraw-Hill, New York, 1985, p 412.
12. King, G: Respiratory failure in the critically ill. In Sibbald, WJ (ed): Synopsis of Critical Care, ed 3. Williams & Wilkins, Baltimore, 1988, p 55.
13. Ahrens, T, and Rutherford, K: The new pulmonary math applying the a/A ratio. Am J Nurs 87(3):337, March 1987.

CHAPTER 29

# Respiratory Assessment: Clinical History and Physical Examination

## CHAPTER OUTLINE



## LEARNING OBJECTIVES

**At the end of this chapter, you should be able to:**

1. Outline essential aspects of the clinical history as they pertain to respiratory function and dysfunction.
2. List the cardinal signs and symptoms and extrapulmonary findings of respiratory disease.
3. Identify assessment data based on knowledge of underlying patterns of restrictive and obstructive pulmonary disease.
4. Identify assessment data based on knowledge of functional health patterns.
5. Locate and describe specific anatomical landmarks and imaginary lines of the anterior, posterior, and lateral thorax.
6. List the four techniques used in the physical examination of the lungs and thorax, and the order in which they are performed.
7. Describe essential information to be obtained on inspection of the lungs and thorax.
8. Describe the key aspects of the palpatory examination of the lungs and thorax.
9. Discuss the significance of percussion in assessing for underlying pathophysiology of the lungs and thorax.
10. Describe normal breath sounds and locate the area of the chest wall where they are normally heard.
11. Define *adventitious breath sounds* and discuss possible underlying pathophysiology that they may reflect.

The major components of the patient's assessment include significant clinical history, physical examination, arterial blood gas studies, pulmonary function tests, x-rays, and other studies. In this chapter, emphasis is placed on the clinical history and on the physical examination of the lungs and thorax.

The most important factor in appraising clinical status is a carefully elicited and comprehensive history. The history provides data for developing a differential diagnosis; it establishes a baseline with which to evaluate the patient's clinical course and responsiveness to therapy.

The chronic nature of many respiratory diseases

has further implications for ongoing history-gathering: What is the nature, status, and prognosis of the patient's underlying pulmonary disease? What is the patient/family's understanding of the disease and its impact on their lifestyles? What has been their prior involvement and experience in coping with a chronic disease? What family/community resources are available? What are the patient/family's goals as to level of health desired? Are they motivated and willing to work diligently with each other and with health-care providers to achieve and maintain an optimal level of health? What do they perceive this to be?

So much of a productive longstanding relationship between patient, family, and health-care providers depends on establishing a rapport with open communication for joint caring, sharing, and learning. A thorough, ongoing history offers the information and clues upon which to develop a working relationship, one that assists each participant to more fully realize his or her potential.

## CLINICAL HISTORY

In initiating the respiratory assessment, it is essential to determine the patient's immediate status to ascertain if the patient is experiencing respiratory or other distress. The extent and thoroughness of the initial history and examination should be modified accordingly. In assessing the symptomatology, including the cardinal signs and symptoms of respiratory disease, it is important to establish the onset, progression, and current status of the illness. This is followed by a careful examination of the severity, frequency, and duration of symptoms, as well as their precipitating, aggravating, and alleviating factors. (See SLIDT tool, Table 7-1.)

### Cardinal Respiratory Signs and Symptoms

Four commonly occurring respiratory-related complaints are: dyspnea, cough, hemoptysis, and chest pain.

#### *Dyspnea*

Dyspnea reflects an uncomfortable awareness of one's own sensation of breathlessness or difficulty breathing. The patient may complain of "shortness of breath," or "difficulty catching my breath." In assessing dyspnea, it is important to ascertain the stimulus or cause of the problem, the amount of activity that precipitated it, and any associated signs or symptoms, such as cough (productive or nonproductive) and wheezing.

Dyspnea needs to be distinguished from other signs and symptoms that may have a somewhat different clinical significance. *Tachypnea*, for example, refers to a rapid respiratory rate with or without dyspnea. *Orthopnea* is described as shortness of breath upon reclining. It is often quantitated by the number of pillows needed to relieve or prevent the sensation. Underlying physiology involves an increase in venous return to the heart upon assuming the recumbent position. While often associated with left heart decompensation, it may accompany pulmonary disease, especially in patients who have a significant amount of secretions and who demonstrate difficulty in clearing secretions by coughing or other bronchial hygiene measures (e.g., deep breathing, postural drainage).

**Paroxysmal Nocturnal Dyspnea (PND).** Although very similar to orthopnea, paroxysmal nocturnal dyspnea differs in that it is not precipitated soon after the patient lies down. Rather, it occurs at some point after the patient has been asleep—he/she awakens from sleep "gasping for breath." PND is commonly associated with cardiac disease but may occur in response to the slow mobilization of body fluids as, for example, from peripheral or dependent edema.

In general, the underlying cause of dyspnea remains undefined. It may reflect an imbalance between ventilatory neural output and the "work of breathing." Virtually all disorders that affect pulmonary function may present as "shortness of breath." Differential diagnosis of dyspnea includes obstructive airway disease (e.g., asthma, chronic obstructive pulmonary disease); parenchymal lung disease (e.g., pneumonia, interstitial or fibrotic processes, adult respiratory distress syndrome); disorders of the pleura (e.g, pleural effusion, pneumothorax); and pulmonary vascular disorders (e.g., pulmonary embolism, pulmonary hypertension). Cardiovascular disorders commonly associated with dyspnea include left heart failure with a consequent increase in pulmonary pressures (as in pulmonary edema), and severe anemia. Dyspnea may also be anxiety-related.

#### *Cough*

The *cough reflex* is an inherent protective reflex against food or other substances entering the respiratory tract. In conjunction with the intrinsic mucociliary clearance mechanism of the respiratory epithelium (see Fig. 28-2), coughing functions to clear secretions produced within the tracheobronchial tree. The cough reflex is commonly stimulated by inhalation of irritant substances, such as cigarette smoke, noxious fumes, and dust. It is triggered by aspirated substances, whether oral pharyngeal secretions, gastric contents, or a foreign body. Coughing may also accompany congestive heart failure.

To generate a cough, a volume of about 2.5 liters of air is inhaled, followed by closure of the epiglottis and vocal cords. This entraps air within the lungs. The abdominal muscles contract forcefully pushing against the diaphragm, while expiratory muscles (e.g., internal intercostals) also contract.

As a result of the forceful contraction against the closed epiglottis and vocal cords, pressure within the thorax increases precipitously (as high as 100 mmHg or more). Finally, the epiglottis and vocal cords suddenly open, allowing the air, under pressure within the lungs, to be exhaled explosively. Any disruption in the ability of the patient to perform these activities can compromise the effectiveness of coughing. Knowledge of the mechanism underlying the cough maneuver can assist in determining why a patient may be unable to cough effectively, and how assistance can be offered in this regard.

When assessing a cough, it is important to identify the circumstances in which it occurs. Is it appropriate? Is it disease-related? Acute or chronic? What are its characteristics or frequency? When does the cough occur—in the morning upon arising (smoker's cough); during the day (irritant substances, possibly work-related); or in the evening (chronic postnasal drip, sinusitis)? How does it sound—dry (of cardiac origin, fibrotic lung disease), barking (croup), hacking (atypical pneumonia), or congested (upper respiratory infection, bronchitis)? Is the cough seasonal (chronic bronchitis, asthma)? Is the cough accompanied by wheezing, chest pain, or hemoptysis? Is it associated with drug usage (e.g., the beta-blocking effects of propranolol = bronchial constriction)?

Of clinical significance is whether the cough is productive or nonproductive. Is the sputum production scanty or copious? Is the amount increasing or decreasing? What is the color of the sputum? Yellow-green sputum reflects presence of anti-inflammatory cells—especially leukocytes, associated with bacterial infection; a tenacious mucoid purulent sputum, laden with neutrophils and eosinophils, is seen in acute asthma; blood-tinged or rust-colored sputum may be associated with trauma caused by coughing, as well as underlying pathology (pulmonary infarction, pneumonia); and pink, frothy sputum may be encountered in advanced pulmonary edema.

#### *Hemoptysis*

*Hemoptysis* is defined as coughing up of blood originating within the airways or the lung parenchyma itself. The origin of the bleeding is not always apparent. It must be distinguished from that originating in the nasopharynx (e.g., common nosebleed), mouth (e.g., lip or tongue-biting), or the upper gastrointestinal tract (e.g., esophagus, stomach, or duodenum). It may be confused with *hematemesis* (vomiting of blood) or associated with aspiration.

In differential diagnosis, hematemesis is acidic, usually dark red or "coffee-ground," and often contains food particles. Hemoptysis is usually frothy and alkaline and is frequently accompanied by sputum. Thin, frothy, pink-tinged sputum in the scenario of left heart decompensation is highly suggestive of pulmonary edema.

In terms of etiology, airway disease is the most common cause of hemoptysis. Heading the list are acute or chronic bronchitis, bronchogenic carcinoma, and bronchiectasis. Lesions of the pulmonary vasculature, including pulmonary embolism, or elevated pulmonary pressures associated with left ventricular failure are also high up on the list. Neoplasms should be suspected if hemoptysis occurs in a patient without any prior respiratory problems. Parenchymal hemorrhage has been associated with lung abscess, tuberculosis, pneumonia, vasculitis, and localized fungal infection (e.g., *Aspergillus*). Hemoptysis can also be caused by cystic fibrosis and pulmonary endometriosis (i.e., ectopic occurrence of uterine endometrium, innermost lining).

#### *Chest Pain*

Chest pain usually originates in the cardiovascular, pulmonary, or gastroesophageal system.[1] Chest pain reflective of pulmonary disease does not originate in the lung itself because this organ is free of sensory (afferent) pain fibers, as is the pleura. However, there are pain receptors so close to the parietal pleura that it is considered to be sensitive to pain. Chest pain arises in the intercostal muscles, ribs and overlying skin, the diaphragm, or the mediastinum, each of which is highly innervated by sensory nerve fibers specific for pain.

An inflammatory process of the parietal pleura or the diaphragm commonly produces pain. When the diaphragm is involved, the pain is *referred* to the ipsilateral shoulder (reflective of phrenic nerve distribution). Parietal pleural pain is usually well localized over the involved site; the pain is characteristically sharp, and worsened on inspiration or with coughing.

Inflammation of parietal pleura, which is pain-producing, occurs after pulmonary infarction, or with pneumonia when there is involvement of the pleural lining. Viral (coxsackie) infections affecting the pleura produce pain, as do some diseases of the connective tissue (e.g., systemic lupus erythematosus). Pneumothorax may result in the onset of pleuritic pain. Mediastinal masses have been implicated in the causation of pain.

## Extrapulmonary Findings

#### *Clubbing*

*Clubbing* is a change in the shape and configuration of the nails and the distal phalanx of fingers and toes. These changes are characterized by a loss of the normal angle between the nails and skin with an increase in the curvature of the nail; an increased

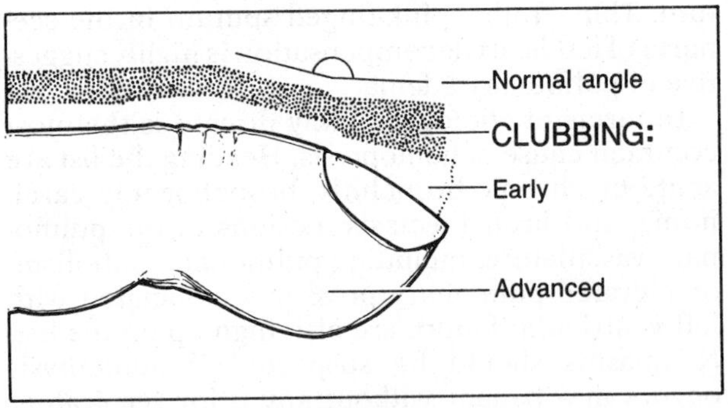


Figure 29-1.

sponginess of the tissue beneath the proximal part of the nail; and a bulbous appearance of the fingertip, with a flaring or widening of the terminal phalanx (Fig. 29-1).

Clubbing is observed most commonly in longstanding respiratory disease including, especially, bronchogenic carcinoma, chronic lung infection (bronchiectasis and lung abscess), and interstitial lung disease. Carcinoma of the lung parenchyma or pleura is the single most common cause of clubbing.

Nonpulmonary causes of clubbing include cardiovascular disease (subacute bacterial endocarditis, congenital intracardiac disease with right to left shunt), and chronic diseases of gastrointestinal system (chronic liver disease or inflammatory bowel disease). Clubbing may also be associated with hypertrophic pulmonary osteoarthropathy, which is characterized by subperiosteal bone deposition especially in long bones. This disorder causes arthralgias and arthritis. The pathophysiologic mechanism underlying clubbing remains undefined.

#### Cyanosis

*Cyanosis* is a bluish discoloration of skin, nailbeds, earlobes, and mucous membranes, associated with an increased level of deoxygenated or reduced hemoglobin. *Central* or generalized cyanosis is linked to a low $PaO_2$, resulting in insufficient oxygenation of hemoglobin in the lungs. It may also occur when systemic blood flow is reduced with a consequent increased extraction of oxygen from the blood by peripheral tissues. *Peripheral* or localized cyanosis is attributed to this latter mechanism. A reduction in venous oxygen saturation accounts for the bluish discoloration.

The percentage of the total hemoglobin that is reduced must be considered. In an individual with a serum hemoglobin of 15 g/100 ml, cyanosis may not be observed until one third or about 5 g of that amount of hemoglobin is reduced.

In anemia, if the total quantity of reduced hemoglobin is less than the amount required to produce the bluish discoloration, even a large decrease in the $PaO_2$ (<60 mmHg) may not be associated with cyanosis. In contrast, only a small decrease in $PaO_2$ (e.g., ~80 mmHg) is necessary to produce sufficient amounts of reduced hemoglobin to cause cyanosis in the patient with increased amounts of hemoglobin (e.g., polycythemia vera).

## Past Medical History

Eliciting the patient's past medical history may provide valuable information regarding the underlying etiology and pathophysiology of respiratory disease. When eliciting history, it is helpful to think in terms of restrictive or obstructive patterns of respiratory disease.

#### Patterns of Restrictive Lung Disease

Restrictive ventilatory disorders are characterized by decreased lung volumes without obstruction to air flow. Such disorders predispose to alveolar hypoventilation with compromise of normal gas exchange. A wide variety of disorders demonstrate a restrictive ventilatory pattern.

*Interstitial* lung disease, for example, causes scarring and fibrosis of the lung parenchyma, resulting in decreased lung compliance with reduction in lung volumes. Example of such disorders include (1) disorders associated with inhaled inorganic dusts (e.g., silicosis, asbestosis), (2) disorders involving an immunologic response to an inhaled antigen (e.g., hypersensitivity pneumonitis), (3) drug-induced lung disease frequently associated with the use of chemotherapeutic and cytotoxic agents, and (4) radiation-induced lung disease, a potential complication of radiation treatment for tumors within or in close proximity to the thorax (e.g., lymphoma, carcinoma of breast and/or lungs).

Idiopathic (cause unknown) pulmonary fibrosis, frequently associated with connective tissue diseases (e.g., rheumatoid arthritis, systemic lupus erythematosus, progressive systemic sclerosis or scleroderma), may present clinically with a restrictive ventilatory pattern.

A detailed history should explore the patient's past medical history, including drug sensitivities, connective tissue disease including those mentioned above and neoplastic disease involving the lungs or thorax, especially if treated with radiation and/or chemotherapeutic therapy. The patient's occupation should be determined, especially if the patient handles noxious gases or fumes, poisonous chemicals, sprays, or disinfectants currently, or whether he/she previously worked with such substances or in areas where such substances were present. Asbestosis, for example, is highly implicated in lung disease characterized by a restrictive ventilatory effort.[2]

*Chestcage deformities* (e.g., kyphoscoliosis, congenital/trauma-related deformities) may limit expansion of the thoracic cage and, in this way, cause a reduction in lung volumes. The history may provide information and clues in this regard, which may be followed up in the physical examination. *Neuromuscular* disorders (e.g., myasthenia gravis, muscular dystrophy, amyotrophic lateral sclerosis) may likewise limit chestcage expansion because of muscle weakness, fatigue, or paralysis, or uncoordinated muscles of respiration (e.g., diaphragm, external intercostals).

*Pleural* disorders may restrict lung expansion because of pleuritic pain and/or compression forces of a large pleural effusion. Atelectasis, or lung consolidation (e.g., pneumonia), can reduce lung volumes by reducing lung compliance.

Central nervous system disorders may cause a restrictive ventilatory effort associated with alveolar hypoventilation without affecting lung compliance. Drug overdose may depress central control of respirations predisposing to alveolar hypoventilation. A careful drug history should be obtained; recent behavioral or personality changes may suggest suicide tendency and need to be considered in the scenario of compromised respiratory function.

#### Patterns of Obstructive Lung Disease

Obstructive ventilatory disorders are characterized by an increased resistance to air flow whether within the airways (e.g., chronic bronchitis) or within the lung parenchyma (e.g., emphysema). Chronic bronchitis, emphysema, and asthma are the three disease entities identified in obstructive airway disease. A detailed history may be helpful in differential diagnosis. For example, a diagnosis of chronic bronchitis is based on chronic cough and sputum production on most days of 3 consecutive months for not less than 2 consecutive years. In emphysema, the clinical presentation is not nearly so distinct.

Clinically, it is useful to distinguish two types of chronic obstructive pulmonary disease: type A ("pink puffer") and type B ("blue bloater") (see Chap. 33). The former is associated with emphysema (i.e, destruction of airways distal to the terminal bronchioles) wherein the patient complains of dyspnea and must work increasingly harder (with use of accessory muscles) to expire gas from within the lung (increase in lung compliance); the latter reflects more closely the presentation of chronic bronchitis mentioned above. More often, there is a mixture of both types.

Knowledge regarding the underlying etiology and pathophysiology of these obstructive ventilatory disorders determines what information to elicit on interview. For example, cigarette smoking is highly implicated as an etiologic agent in both types, so the patient's smoking history is vital. If cigarettes are smoked, determine the number of packs smoked per day times how many years. If the patient has stopped smoking, inquire as to how long ago, the reason for stopping, and how many packs per day were smoked prior to stopping. Exacerbations of these conditions often develop after viral infection or upper respiratory infection, so information regarding a recent cold or infection may be important.

Asthma is more easily separated from chronic bronchitis and emphysema based on a history of paroxysmal attacks of wheezing. These attacks are associated with hyperreactivity of the airways accompanied by reversible episodes of bronchoconstriction (bronchospasm). While the relationship between allergies and asthma is not clear, it is nevertheless important to elicit a thorough history regarding allergic reactions of any kind, childhood through the present day. If specific allergies cannot be identified, inquire about other factors that can trigger an attack, such as, for example, exercise, infections, or stress.

#### Patterns of Cardiopulmonary Function

Clinical history related to cardiovascular function should be ascertained because of the close relationship between cardiovascular and pulmonary function. Evidence of hypertension, myocardial infarction, congestive heart failure, anemia, and hypoproteinemia should be carefully documented. If the patient has had recent chest x-ray, pulmonary function tests, arterial blood gas analysis, sputum culture, or skin tests (tuberculosis), it is important to elicit: what the underlying problem was, who treated it, how was it treated, was hospitalization necessary, how did the problem respond to therapeutic intervention, and were there any complications? Recent chest or lung-related surgery or other procedures (bronchoscopy, thoracentesis) should likewise be noted.

#### Drug and Immunization History

It is essential to obtain the patient's drug and immunization history. What drugs is the patient taking, and what is it that they were prescribed to treat? Has the patient taken the drugs as instructed? Have the drugs been effective in resolving the problem? Has the patient ever had an allergic reaction to drugs, food, or other substances? Document the patient's response on exposure to the allergen(s) in question. Note whether the patient has been immunized against pneumococcal pneumonia or influenza.

## Family History

It is important to determine the family incidence of asthma, cystic fibrosis, and emphysema (*alpha-1-*

*protease inhibitor deficiency*), because these disorders may be genetically transmitted. Similarly, it is necessary to inquire as to the occurrence of other significant diseases within the family constellation, including, among others, chronic allergies, lung cancer, tuberculosis, neuromuscular dysfunction, disorders of the thoracic cage (kyphosis, scoliosis, extreme obesity as in pickwickian syndrome, others), diabetes or other endocrine dysfunctions, renal disease, and cardiopulmonary dysfunction.

## Functional Health Patterns[3]

(Refer to Appendix C)

**Health Perception — Health Management.** Determine the patient's overall state of health, and the patient/family's perception as to what they feel is optimal health with respect to themselves. What are patient/family attitudes regarding smoking, drugs (self-medication, use of over-the-counter drugs), and alcohol consumption? Elicit patient/family perceptions as to how they feel the present illness will impact on their individual and collective lifestyles?

**Nutritional - Metabolic Patterns.** Ascertain the patient/family nutritional attitudes and eating patterns. In the patient with chronic obstructive pulmonary disease, assess how disease-related symptomatology affects appetite and actual food consumption. In the patient with emphysema, the "work of breathing" may become so energy-consuming as to leave little strength for eating. Severe dyspnea may directly compromise eating. Copious sputum production in the patient with chronic bronchitis may cause anorexia.

**Activity - Exercise Patterns.** Inquire as to how compromised ventilatory effort has affected the patient's ability to participate in daily living, recreational, and work-related activities.

**Sleep - Rest Pattern.** How does compromised ventilatory effort affect sleep? What are the patient's sleeping patterns? How many hours per day? How many pillows? Does the patient pace his/her activities so as not to become overfatigued?

**Cognitive - Perceptual Pattern.** Inquire as to patient's/family's knowledge of underlying respiratory disease, including prognosis, anticipated disease course, prescribed medications, assistance with activity of daily living? What is the patient's/family's readiness to learn?

**Self-Perception - Self-Concept.** How does the patient feel about this illness and its impact on lifestyle? Is there anger, denial, depression?

**Role - Relationship Pattern.** How does the patient view family dynamics? Is his/her role dependent, independent, interdependent? Who makes the decisions?

**Coping - Stress Pattern.** Inquire as to patient's/family's prior patterns in coping with stress. Who takes charge? How do family members react? Is there withdrawal, or denial as to the existence of a problem? What are the family resources? Identify strengths and weaknesses?

**Value - Belief Pattern.** What are patient's short- and long-term goals? Does the patient feel these goals are compromised by the illness? What plans have been made to accommodate the illness in future goal-setting? For example, has the patient's occupational history contributed to the illness (e.g., exposure to pollutants or irritants)? Is a change in occupation necessary to avert exacerbation of illness? How does patient/family respond to this reality?

# PHYSICAL EXAMINATION*

## Thoracic Landmarks — Location of Underlying Lung Lobes

To localize and describe findings on examination of the lungs and thorax, it is important to be familiar with the anatomical surface landmarks and imaginary lines drawn on the anterior and posterior thorax.

**Sternal Angle (Angle of Louis).** To be able to number the ribs accurately on the anterior chest, the sternal angle, or angle of Louis, is the best guide. The sternal angle is the horizontal bony ridge that joins the manubrium to the body of the sternum (Fig. 29–2). Lateral to this ridge occurs the second rib and costal cartilage. The intercostal space immediately below is the second intercostal space. Beneath this intercostal space is the third rib, as one counts downward along the anterior chest. Always start from the sternal angle and second rib when locating ribs or interspaces in the anterior thorax.

**Imaginary Lines of Anterior Thorax.** When inspecting the anterior thorax, there are three imaginary lines with which one needs to be familiar. These include the midsternal line, midclavicular line (a vertical line from the midpoint of the clavicle), and the anterior axillary line (a vertical line from the anterior axillary fold; see Fig. 29–2).

**Anatomical Landmarks Posterior Thorax.** When inspecting the posterior thorax, the scapulae provide an anatomical landmark in that the inferior angle (pole) of each scapula lies approximately at the level of the seventh rib or intercostal space (Fig. 29–3).

Findings may also be localized according to their relationship to the spinous processes. Upon flexion

---

* Only selected aspects of the physical examination of the lungs and thorax are presented here. For an indepth study of techniques and procedure of physical examination, see the bibliography at the end of Unit V.

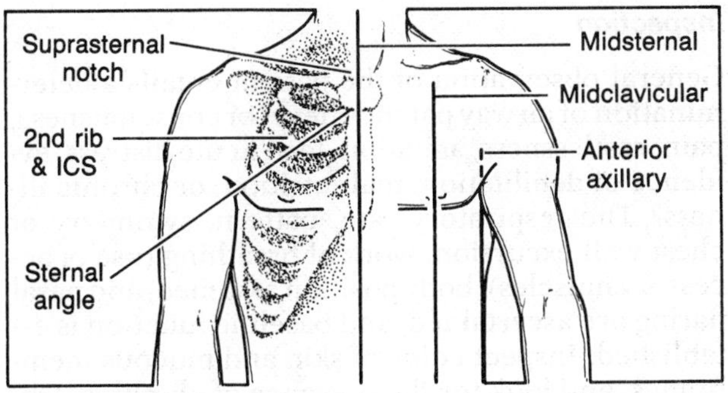


Figure 29-2.

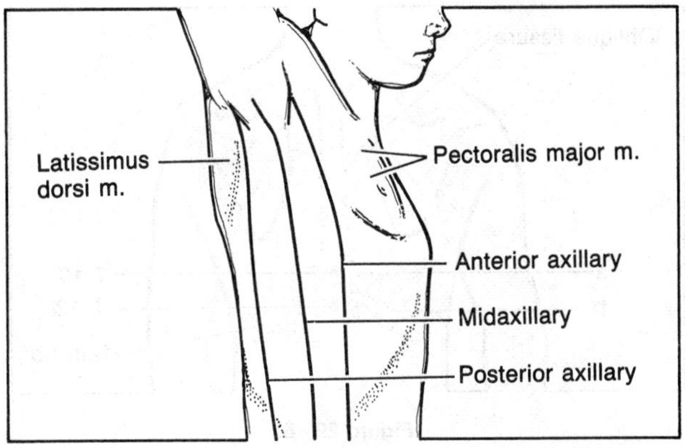


Figure 29-4.

of the head on the chest, the most prominent spinous process is usually that of the seventh cervical or first thoracic vertebrae. The spinous processes below this level can often be felt and numbered, especially when the spine is flexed. The spinous processes of thoracic vertebrae four through twelve angle obliquely downward so that each overlies the body of the vertebra below it. For example, the spinous process of thoracic vertebra six overlies the seventh thoracic vertebra, and is adjacent to the seventh rib.

**Imaginary Lines of Posterior Thorax.** The posterior thorax has two imaginary lines: the vertebral line, which occurs along the spinous processes, and the scapular line, which is vertical from the inferior angle of the scapula (see Fig. 29-3).

**Imaginary Lines—Lateral Thorax.** The imaginary lines in the lateral view include the anterior axillary line, midaxillary line (a vertical line from the apex of the axilla), and the posterior axillary line (a vertical line from the posterior axillary fold; Fig. 29-4).

**Lung Borders.** When examining the lungs and thorax, it is important to consider the location of the underlying lungs and their lobes with respect to anterior anatomical landmarks and imaginary lines. In the anterior view (Fig. 29-5), the apex of each lung rises above the medial aspect of each clavicle; the inferior border of each lung crosses the sixth rib at the midclavicular line, and the eighth rib at the midaxillary line. Posteriorly, the lower border of each lung occurs at the level of the tenth thoracic vertebra and may descend to the twelfth process with full inspiration (Fig. 29-6).

**Lung Fissures.** An oblique fissure divides each lung into upper (anterior) and lower (posterior) lobes (Fig. 29-7). The apex of each lung is actually the superior projection of the upper lobes. The lower lobes project anteriorly and laterally. The right lung is further divided by a horizontal fissure, which delineates the right middle lobe (see Fig. 29-5).

The anatomical position of each lobe of the lungs within the thorax has implications for the actual examination of the lungs. A complete examination of the apex of each lung, for example, requires both anterior and posterior examination. Anteriorly, palpation, percussion, and auscultation of the supraclavicular space are required; posteriorly, the examination should begin across the top of each shoulder.

To examine the right middle lobe (RML) appropriately, visualize its position in the right chest in the area circumscribed by the fourth rib superiorly, the sixth rib inferiorly, and laterally to the midclavicular line (see Figs. 29-5 and 29-7). This is espe-

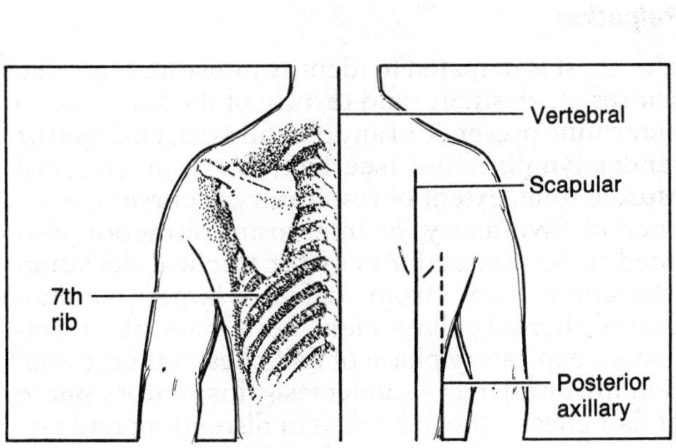


Figure 29-3.

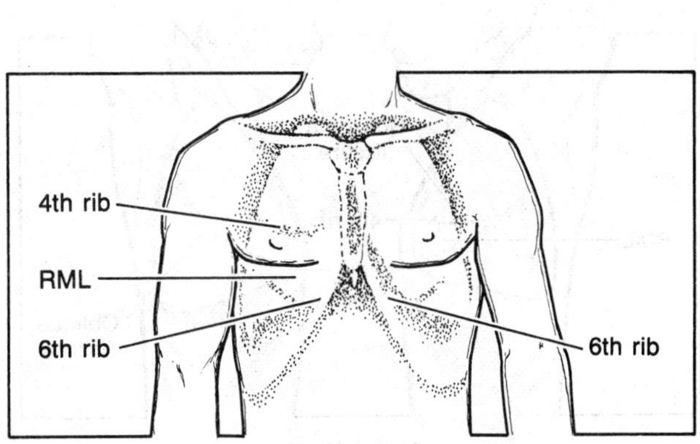


Figure 29-5.

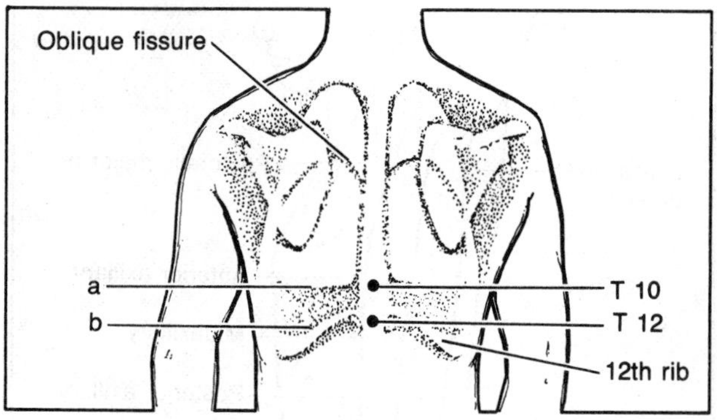


Figure 29-6.

cially important because the RML is implicated frequently in aspiration pneumonia. The more vertical course of the right mainstem bronchus from the bifurcation of the trachea makes the RML especially vulnerable to aspiration (see Fig. 28-1).

Lastly, appreciate the anterior and lateral projections of the lower lobe of each lung. Appropriate technique requires a careful examination of the lateral chest (see Fig. 29-7).

## Techniques of Physical Examination

Four methods are used in the physical examination of the lungs and thorax. These include inspection, palpation, percussion, and auscultation, *in that order*. The examination should be organized and systematic. The extent of the initial examination will depend on the patient's condition. It is important to compare one side with the other whenever symmetry of structure allows. A comparison of one side with the other allows the patient to serve as his/her own control. Throughout the examination, try to visualize underlying tissues, including the location of lobes of the lungs with respect to surface landmarks.

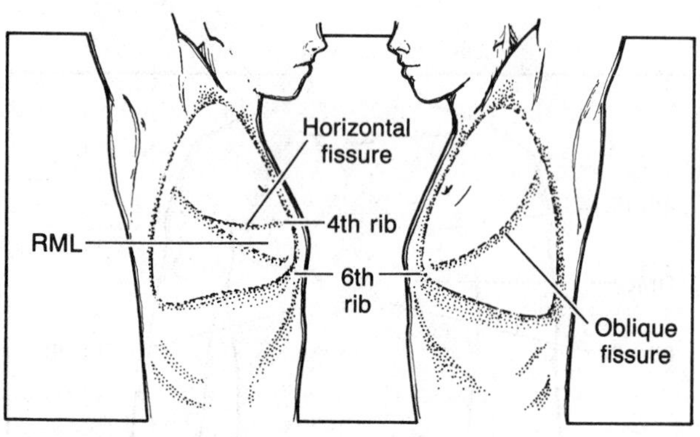


Figure 29-7.

### Inspection

General observation of the patient entails a determination of airway patency, level of consciousness, pain, restlessness, agitation, fear, acute distress; evidence of debilitation, malnutrition, or chronic illness? The respiratory rate, pattern, symmetry of chest wall excursion, work of breathing (use of accessory muscles), body position assumed, and nasal flaring are ascertained, and baseline function is established. Inspect color of skin and mucous membranes, and look for the presence of clubbing. Observe the ease with which the patient speaks and eats.

The shape and contour of the thoracic cage should be observed for deformities. A "barrel chest" suggests advanced chronic obstructive pulmonary disease. Deformities of the chestcage contours may also include kyphosis and/or scoliosis, "funnel chest" (pectus excavatum), or pigeon or chicken breast. The latter deformity involves an increase in the AP (anterior/posterior) diameter, a narrowed transverse diameter, and the presence of vertical grooves along the line of the costochondral junctions.

Respiratory motion should be observed during quiet breathing and then during deep inspiration. A respiratory cycle should have a longer inspiratory phase and a shorter expiratory phase.

The presence of "paradoxical respirations" (i.e., a reversal of normal respiratory mechanics wherein the thoracic ribcage is observed to passively collapse on inspiration while the diaphragm descends, and to expand on expiration as the diaphragm ascends) may reflect disruption of intrapleural pressures, as occurs with thoracic trauma (e.g., multiple rib fractures, flail chest, and disruption of the costosternal cartilaginous joints), or paralysis of respiratory muscles associated with cervical spinal cord injury. Asymmetry of respiratory motion may also be observed with a large pneumothorax or tension pneumothorax. In these instances, tracheal deviation to the unaffected side may be observed as well.

### Palpation

The chest is palpated to identify moisture (e.g., diaphoresis), elasticity, and texture of the skin, and to determine presence of any painful area, enlarged or tender lymph nodes (see Fig. 48-1), or crepitus. Muscle tone, extent of respiratory excursion, presence of asymmetry, or intercostal retraction also need to be assessed. Assess for tracheal deviation (deviation *away* from defect—large pneumothorax, thyroid enlargement, neck mass, pleural effusion, expiratory phase of flail chest, other; deviation *toward* defect—atelectasis, inspiratory phase of flail chest, other); neck vein distention; and tactile fremitus (diminished fremitus—pleural effusion, pneumothorax with lung collapse, obstruction of mainstem bronchus, emphysema, others; increased fremitus—pneumonia with consolidation; lung tumors, pulmonary infarction, other). *Fremitus* refers to the palpable vibrations transmitted through the tracheobronchial tree to the chest wall when the patient speaks. Usually, the palmer surface of each hand is placed flat on the posterior chest, and the patient is asked to say "99." Liquid and solid materials transmit vibrations better than air-filled spaces.

### Percussion

In percussing, the examiner notes the quality of sound elicited by tapping the middle finger of one hand against the middle finger of the opposite hand, which is applied to the chest wall. The underlying principle is similar to that of tapping a surface and judging whether what is underneath is solid or hollow. Normally, percussion of the chest wall overlying air-containing lung produces a "resonant" sound; in contrast, percussion over a solid organ, such as the liver, produces a "dull" sound. This contrast in sounds allows the examiner to detect areas with something other than air-containing lung beneath the chest wall. For example, the sound elicited over fluid in the pleural space (pleural effusion) or airless (consolidated) lung in both cases is dull to percussion. At the other extreme, air in the pleural space (pneumothorax) or a hyperinflated lung (emphysema) may produce a hyperresonant or more "hollow" sound, approaching what one hears when percussing over a hollow viscus such as the stomach (tympany) (Table 29-1).

### Auscultation

Goals of auscultation are twofold: (1) to assess the quality of breath sounds, and (2) to detect the presence of abnormal or adventitious sounds. When the examiner places the diaphragm of the stethoscope firmly on the chest wall, the sound of air flow can be heard when the patient takes a breath that is a little deeper than normal, with the mouth open. Exactly what is heard depends on where the stethoscope is placed. Sounds heard over the trachea tend to be loud, harsh, and high-pitched, with the expiratory phase slightly longer than the inspiratory phase. In contrast, when the stethoscope is placed over peripheral lung fields, sound is heard almost exclusively during the inspiratory phase, and the quality of the sound is much softer.

When interpreting the quality of breath sounds it is important to be cognizant of two factors:[5] (1) normal transmission of sound depends on airway pa-

TABLE 29-1

**Respiratory Pathophysiology—Physical Findings[4]**

| Condition | Tactile Fremitus | Percussion | Breath Sounds | Adventitious Sounds |
|---|---|---|---|---|
| Normal | Normal | Resonant | Vesicular over peripheral lung fields; bronchovesicular over large bronchi; bronchial over trachea and sternum | Usually none; transient rales (crackles) after sleep or recumbency. |
| Atelectasis (collapsed air sacs) | Decreased to absent | Dull | Decreased vesicular to absent | None |
| Bronchitis (partial airway obstruction) | Normal | Resonant | Normal to prolonged expiratory phase | Rales (crackles); wheezes; rhonchi |
| Emphysema (hyperinflated lung) | Decreased | Hyperresonant | Decreased vesicular, frequently with prolonged expiratory phase | None unless bronchitis is also present |
| Pleural effusion or pleural thickening | Decreased to absent | Dull to flat | Decreased or absent | None unless underlying airway or lung parenchymal disease |
| Pneumothorax (air in pleural space) | Decreased to absent | Hyperresonant | Decreased to absent | None |
| Pneumonia (pulmonary consolidation) | Increased | Dull | Bronchial | Rales (crackles) |
| Pulmonary edema (left ventricular failure) | Normal | Resonant | May be prolonged on expiration | Rales (crackles) at lung bases; wheezes may be detected |

tency; and (2) the presence of air or fluid in the pleural space acts as a barrier to sound. Obstruction of relatively large bronchi decreases the transmission of sound, and, on auscultation, breath sounds over the affected areas are diminished or absent. The presence of either a pneumothorax or a pleural effusion also causes breath sounds to be diminished.

**Normal Breath Sounds.** Normal breath sounds are described as vesicular, bronchovesicular, and bronchial.

***Vesicular Sounds.*** Vesicular sounds are soft and quiet, a fine rustle or swishing sound, low-pitched, and heard primarily during the inspiratory phase and early expiratory phase. The inspiratory phase is about three times longer than the expiratory phase.

The actual sounds produced are thought to be due to distention and separation of alveoli during the inspiratory maneuver. These sounds are the predominant breath sounds, and they are heard over most lung areas. They are produced in the alveoli and fine terminal and respiratory bronchioles, which comprise the lung parenchyma.

***Bronchial Sounds.*** Bronchial sounds are normally heard over the trachea and sternum and are described as a loud "tubular" sound resembling wind blowing through a long tube. These sounds are loud and high-pitched with an expiratory phase that is longer than the inspiratory phase. There is a momentary pause between these phases during which no noise or breath sound is heard. When bronchial breath sounds are heard other than over the trachea and sternum, they may be associated with a pathologic process (e.g., in pneumonia, over a pleural effusion, or with major atelectatic).

***Bronchovesicular Sounds.*** Bronchovesicular sounds reflect a mixture of both bronchial and vesicular breath sounds. They are heard best where normal lung overlies the large mainstem bronchi at the first and second intercostal space at the left and right sternal borders, below the clavicles anteriorly, and between the scapulae posteriorly. Bronchovesicular sounds are heard about equally through the inspiratory and expiratory phases. Vesicular, bronchial, and bronchovesicular sounds are all normal breath sounds when heard in the appropriate area of the thorax.

In general, sound generated by air flow is transmitted better through consolidated than air-containing lung. Thus, a bronchial-type sound might be detected over lung tissue that is consolidated due to pneumonia. Furthermore, there is a difference not only in the quality of sound, but in its relative duration of inspiration and expiration.

**Adventitious Breath Sounds.** The second goal of auscultation is to detect adventitious or abnormal breath sounds. The major types of adventitious sounds include rales or crackles, wheezes, rhonchi, friction rubs, and stridor.

***Rales (Crackles).*** Rales (crackles) are described as a series of popping or clicking noises heard over an involved area of lung. The quality of these sounds may range from that produced by rubbing two hairs together, or resembling soda fizzing, to the sound generated by opening a Velcro fastener or crumpling a sheet of cellophane. The sounds are often referred to as "opening" sounds, reflective of the opening of small airways and alveoli that may have been atelectatic or poorly ventilated, or that may be partially filled with fluid or inflammatory exudate. These sounds are heard throughout, or at the latter part of the inspiratory phase. Rales are most commonly associated with pulmonary edema, atelectasis, pneumonia, and interstitial lung disease (idiopathic pulmonary fibrosis, fibrosis associated with collagen diseases—systemic lupus erythematosus, scleroderma, sarcoidosis, and others).

***Wheezes.*** Wheezes are high-pitched sounds, often of a "whistling" quality, that are produced by air flow through narrowed airways. Airway narrowing may be caused by bronchiole smooth muscle contraction, edema, excessive secretions, or airway collapse due to inadequate support. Under normal physiologic circumstances, the diameter of the airways is decreased during expiration, and, consequently, wheezing is more pronounced during the expiratory phase. During expiration, there is some loss of the "tethering" effect by virtue of the elastic recoil of the lung parenchymal tissue. This may account, in part, for the narrowing of airways that occurs during expiration.

It is important to note that for wheezing to occur there must be a certain minimal amount of air flow. If airway narrowing becomes sufficiently severe and ventilation is seriously compromised, wheezing may no longer be heard and the patient's condition may rapidly decompensate leading to respiratory failure (see Table 29–1).

***Rhonchi.*** Rhonchi is a term that describes sound generated by secretions within the airways. When this term is used, it usually reflects breath sounds that are lower-pitched and somewhat coarser in quality than wheezes.

When rales or rhonchi are heard, ask the patient to cough. If these sounds do not disappear, or if they become accentuated with coughing, they are usually clinically significant, reflective of fluid and secretions in the tiny airways, alveolar ducts, and alveolar sacs.

***Friction Rub.*** A friction rub is the term used to describe the sounds caused by the rubbing together of inflamed or roughened pleural surfaces. These sounds are "raspy" in quality and mimic the rubbing together of two pieces of leather. They occur continuously throughout the respiratory cycle. Pleuritic pain and splinting may accompany the friction rub. Clinically, a friction rub may be associated with a primary acute inflammatory disease of the pleura, or it may be caused by lung parenchymal pathologic processes that penetrate through to the pleural surface (e.g., pneumonia, pulmonary infarction, other).

***Stridor.*** Stridor is a high-pitched noisy respiration, like the blowing of the wind. Its presence usually reflects some type of respiratory obstruction, particularly in the trachea or larynx (i.e., the upper airways). In the acute setting, the larynx is probably the major area subject to obstruction. Infection (e.g., *Hemophilus influenzae*), thermal injury and consequent laryngeal edema from smoke inhalation, aspiration of foreign body, and laryngeal edema associated with allergic reaction (anaphylaxis) have all been implicated as causes of stridor. Eliciting a thorough history may be helpful in differential diagnosis.

## REFERENCES

1. Forshee, T: Systemic origins of chest pain. Nursing 87 17(4):30, April 1987.
2. Price, S, and Wilson, L: Pathophysiology: Clinical Concepts of Disease Processes, ed 3. McGraw-Hill, New York, 1986, p 444.
3. Gordon, M: Manual of Nursing Diagnosis. McGraw-Hill, New York, 1987, pp 16–19.
4. Bates, B: A Guide to Physical Examination, ed 4. JB Lippincott, Philadelphia 1987, p 250.
5. Weinberger, S: Principles of Pulmonary Medicine. WB Saunders, Philadelphia, 1986, p 33.

CHAPTER 30

# Acid–Base Physiology and Pathophysiology

## CHAPTER OUTLINE



## LEARNING OBJECTIVES

**At the end of this chapter, you should be able to:**

1. Explain the significance of acid–base balance in terms of overall body physiology.
2. Describe the compensatory mechanisms, including the major buffering systems, and their critical role in the maintenance of acid–base balance.
3. Describe the respiratory response to changes in hydrogen-ion concentration.
4. Identify key factors in the renal regulation of hydrogen-ion concentration.
5. Define the clinical significance of blood acid–base parameters (pH, $PaCO_2$, $HCO_3^-$, and base excess); list normal values.
6. Contrast respiratory acidemia and respiratory alkalemia.
7. Contrast metabolic acidemia and metabolic alkalemia.
8. Describe the procedure for analyzing arterial blood gases.
9. Describe procedures for obtaining an arterial blood gas sample, including implications for nursing care.

Maintenance of the internal environment in a state of dynamic equilibrium requires that the acid–base balance be maintained within the optimal physiologic range (pH 7.35–7.45). Any deviation from this range can seriously disrupt enzymatic catalysis of intracellular chemical reactions and vital electrochemical processes critical to nerve conduction—synaptic transmission and muscle contraction.

The necessity of maintaining the physiologic pH takes on added significance when one considers that the waste products of metabolism are primarily acidic. Carbon dioxide combines with water to form carbonic acid, the most ubiquitous body acid. Fat and protein metabolism contribute other acid by-products including, among others, sulfuric and phosphoric acids. Mechanisms within the body function to resist changes in the pH, which would otherwise occur in the presence of large quantities of these acid by-products. Such mechanisms facilitate the excretion of these substances at a rate that coincides with their generation.

## DEFINITION OF TERMS

### pH

The *pH* of a solution is a measure of its hydrogen-ion concentration. Specifically, pH reflects the *negative logarithm* of the hydrogen-ion concentration. For example, water, which consists of hydrogen ions ($H^+$) and hydroxyl ions ($OH^-$) has a pH of 7. Numerically, the expression pH of 7 reflects the actual concentration of hydrogen ions in water, which is 0.0000001, or the negative logarithm of $10^{-7}$.

Thus, the pH and hydrogen-ion ($H^+$) concentration are *inversely* related. As the hydrogen-ion concentration rises, pH falls; as the hydrogen-ion concentration decreases, the pH rises. A low pH indicates the solution is more *acidic*; a high pH indicates the solution is more *alkaline*. The normal pH range is 1–14, where 7 is approximately neutral (i.e., the concentrations of acid and base in the solution are about equal). In water, which has a neutral pH of 7, the concentrations of hydrogen ions ($H^+$) and hydroxyl ions ($OH^-$) are about the same.

### Acids

An *acid* is a substance that can donate or contribute hydrogen ions, or protons, to a solution (i.e., proton donor). A distinction is made between strong and weak acids. *Strong* acids have a strong tendency to discharge hydrogen ions into solution and, thus, become completely dissociated or ionized in solution. Strong acids remain completely dissociated, even in strongly acidic solutions.

*Weak* acids also donate hydrogen ions to solution, but they do so far less vigorously than do strong acids. Weak acids are only partially dissociated in acidic solutions.

### Bases

A similar distinction is made between strong and weak bases. A *base* is a substance that can accept or combine with hydrogen ions to remove these ions from solution (i.e., proton acceptor). A *strong* base reacts vigorously with hydrogen ions in solution and removes these ions from solution with much avidity. Strong bases remain dissociated even in strongly alkaline solutions.

*Weak* bases also combine with hydrogen ions in solution, but they do so much less vigorously than do strong bases. Weak bases are only partially dissociated in alkaline solutions.

In the body, most acids and bases concerned with the regulation of acid–base balance are weak acids and weak bases. As such, these substances function to prevent sudden and precipitous changes in the pH of body fluids. For example, if hydrochloric acid, a strong acid, is added to water (pH 7), the pH drops precipitously to 1. If however, sodium bicarbonate, a weak base, is added to the solution, it functions to neutralize the strong acid (i.e., the hydrochloric acid) and, in turn, produces the weak acid, carbonic acid. The weak base thus minimizes the change in pH by converting a strong acid into a weak acid solution.

The following equation expresses this reaction:

| | | | | |
|---|---|---|---|---|
| $NaHCO_3 +$ | $HCl \rightarrow$ | $H_2CO_3 +$ | $NaCl$ | |
| Weak base | Strong acid | Weak acid | Salt (Sodium chloride) | (1) |

Similarly, a weak acid, carbonic acid, functions to neutralize a strong base, sodium hydroxide. When sodium hydroxide is added to water (pH 7), the pH rises precipitously, approaching 14.0. The addition of carbonic acid to this solution produces the weak base, sodium bicarbonate , thus minimizing the change in pH. The following equation expresses this reaction:

| | | | | |
|---|---|---|---|---|
| $H_2CO_3 +$ | $NaOH \rightarrow$ | $NaHCO_3 +$ | $H_2O$ | |
| Weak acid | Strong base | Weak base | Water | (2) |

In each of these reactions, a strong acid (base) is converted to a weak acid (base), thus minimizing the consequent change in pH. In other words, the strong acid (base) has been "buffered" by the addition of a weak acid (base).

## COMPENSATORY MECHANISMS IN ACID–BASE BALANCE

Maintenance of acid–base balance in the extracellular and intracellular fluids is accomplished by the precise regulation of the free hydrogen-ion concentration. These control mechanisms are so effective that the pH is normally stabilized at 7.4 for arterial blood and 7.35 for venous blood. The lower pH of venous blood is due to an increased concentration of acid by-products of cellular metabolism. The major control mechanisms responsible for the regulation of hydrogen-ion concentration include the chemical buffers, the lungs, and the kidneys.

### Chemical Buffering Systems

*Buffering* refers to the ability of a solution that contains a buffer pair, that is, a weak acid and its conjugate base (e.g., carbonic acid and bicarbonate), to minimize or resist a change in pH when either acid or base is added to the buffered solution. By accepting a hydrogen ion the buffer prevents a change in the concentration of hydrogen ions in solution, thus preventing a significant change in its pH.

The equations above demonstrate the buffering reactions. The buffer in Equation 1 is the weak base, sodium bicarbonate; in Equation 2, the buffer is the weak acid, carbonic acid.

There are four major chemical buffers in body fluids: the carbonic acid/bicarbonate system, the hemoglobin/oxyhemoglobin system in red blood cells, the phosphate system, and the protein buffers. The significance of chemical buffers is that they react *immediately* to prevent any major, consequential changes in hydrogen-ion concentration. Coupled with the dilutional effect of circulating blood, they constitute the first line of defense in preventing immediate shifts in pH. Eventually, excess hydrogen ions are eliminated by way of the lungs (carbon dioxide) and kidneys.

#### *Carbonic Acid/Bicarbonate Buffer System*

The carbonic acid/bicarbonate buffer system contributes 53% of the total buffering capacity of whole blood, including 35% in the serum and 18% in red blood cells. Carbon dioxide and water, the end-products of energy metabolism, react to form carbonic acid; carbonic acid dissociates to form hydrogen and bicarbonate ions:

$$H^+ + HCO_3^- \rightleftharpoons H_2CO_3 \rightleftharpoons CO_2 + H_2O \qquad (3)$$

The Henderson-Hasselbalch equation describes the dissociation of the carbonic acid pool (i.e., predominantly carbon dioxide gas, and to a lesser extent, carbonic acid) and expresses the relationship between pH and the ratio of bicarbonate to carbonic acid ($PCO_2$):

$$pH = pK + Log\frac{HCO_3^-}{H_2CO_3}\ \frac{Base}{Acid} \qquad (4)$$

The pK is a constant that reflects the pH of an acid at which it is half dissociated (i.e., when half of the solution occurs as carbonic acid, and the other half is ionized as hydrogen and bicarbonate ions). The pK for carbonic acid is 6.1.

In a liter of extracellular fluid there are 24–28 mEq/liter of bicarbonate ions and 1.2–1.4 mEq/liter of carbonic acid. Thus, the base to acid ratio is 20 : 1. Because carbonic acid exists in the body predominantly as carbon dioxide gas, the value of $PCO_2$ (i.e., the partial pressure of carbon dioxide) is substituted in the denominator as follows:

$$pH = pK\ (6.1) + Log\frac{HCO_3^-}{PCO_2} = \frac{20}{1}\ Ratio \qquad (5)$$

Calculate the pH where the pK for carbonic acid is 6.1, and the log of 20 is 1.3:

$$\begin{aligned} pH &= 6.1 + 1.3 \\ pH &= 7.4\ \text{(arterial blood)} \end{aligned} \qquad (6)$$

#### *Hemoglobin/Oxyhemoglobin Buffer System*

Hemoglobin, by virtue of its high concentration and ubiquitous status, is considered to be the most effective body buffer. The reaction between hemoglobin and free hydrogen ions occurs within the red blood cells (RBCs), which are readily permeable to bicarbonate ions ($HCO_3^-$). For every free hydrogen ion bound by hemoglobin, a corresponding bicarbonate ion diffuses out of the red blood cell into the plasma. In order to maintain electrical neutrality across the RBC membrane, bicarbonate ions ($HCO_3^-$) are exchanged for chloride ions ($Cl^-$). As venous blood leaves the tissues, this exchange of bicarbonate ions for chloride ions is designated the *chloride shift*, and accounts for the greater chloride content of venous blood, which, in contrast to arterial blood, has a greater carbon dioxide tension ($PaCO_2$).

#### *Protein Buffers*

In addition to hemoglobin, other proteins act as buffers both intracellularly and extracellularly. Because proteins are largely *amphoteric* (i.e., they can behave as an acid or base depending on the pH of the solution), they are suitably adapted for their buffering effect.

#### Phosphate Buffer System

Phosphate ions exert their buffer effects primarily in the intracellular fluid compartment. Monosodium phosphate ($NaH_2PO_4$) acts as the weak acid, and disodium phosphate ($Na_2HPO_4$), as the weak base. The action of this buffer pair in intracellular fluid is analogous to that exerted by the carbonic acid/bicarbonate buffer pair in extracellular fluid.

## Respiratory Response to Changes in Hydrogen-Ion Concentration

Because carbon dioxide gas is the predominant state of the carbonic acid pool in the body (see the Henderson-Hasselbalch equations 4 and 5 above), any increase in the concentration of carbon dioxide gas in body fluids decreases the pH; any decrease in the concentration of carbon dioxide gas causes the pH to rise (assuming that the numerator remains unchanged).

#### Alveolar Ventilation ($\dot{V}_A$): Impact on Carbon Dioxide Concentrations

The major factor regulating the carbon dioxide gas concentrations in body fluids is the *rate* of alveolar ventilation ($\dot{V}_A$). An increase in alveolar ventilation (i.e., *hyper*ventilation) causes carbon dioxide gas to be blown off by way of the lungs, thus decreasing the concentration of carbon dioxide in body fluids, with a consequent increase in the pH; conversely, a decrease in alveolar ventilation (i.e., *hypo*ventilation) allows body fluid concentrations of carbon dioxide to increase, with a consequent decrease in the pH.

#### Ventilatory Response to Changes in Carbon Dioxide and Hydrogen-Ion Concentrations

The rate of alveolar ventilation ($\dot{V}_A$) can affect the hydrogen-ion concentration and, thus, the pH; in turn, changes in hydrogen-ion concentration can affect the rate of $\dot{V}_A$. The slightest change in carbon dioxide and, thus, hydrogen ion concentrations, is associated with significant reflex changes in the rate and depth of breathing.

*Peripheral* chemoreceptors (e.g., carotid and aortic bodies) respond to changes in carbon dioxide ($PaCO_2$) and the hydrogen-ion concentration of circulating blood by reflexly stimulating medullary inspiratory neuronal networks. The slightest increase in $PaCO_2$ (~ 2–5 mmHg) is associated with a significant increase in alveolar ventilation. This response is designed to promote elimination of carbon dioxide by way of the lungs, thus reducing the $PaCO_2$ and returning the hydrogen-ion concentration of circulating blood toward normal.

Conversely, a decrease in $PaCO_2$ and, thus, the hydrogen-ion concentration of circulating blood reflexly decreases alveolar ventilation. Metabolically produced carbon dioxide is allowed to accumulate until the $PaCO_2$ and hydrogen-ion concentrations of the circulating blood are returned toward normal.

*Central* chemoreceptors located in the medulla comprise a major reflex mechanism whereby the hydrogen-ion concentrations of circulating cerebral blood and the brain's interstitial fluids regulate the rate and depth of alveolar ventilation. An increase in the hydrogen-ion concentration and the corresponding drop in pH can increase the rate of alveolar ventilation several times normal, depending on the magnitude of the change; conversely, a reduction in hydrogen-ion concentration and corresponding increase in pH can decrease the rate of alveolar ventilation to only a fraction of normal.

Thus, the respiratory system acts as a *feedback* regulatory system for controlling hydrogen-ion concentration. When hydrogen-ion concentrations become high (i.e., low pH), alveolar ventilation increases. This results in a consequent decrease in the carbon dioxide concentration of body fluids and in a reduction in the hydrogen-ion concentration. Any increase in alveolar ventilation wherein carbon dioxide is eliminated by way of the lungs causes the reaction to be driven to the *right* (see Equation 3 above). The end result is a decrease in the hydrogen-ion concentration.

Conversely, when hydrogen-ion concentrations become low (i.e., high pH), alveolar ventilation becomes depressed, carbon dioxide accumulates, and the hydrogen-ion concentration rises. Any decrease in alveolar ventilation reduces the elimination of carbon dioxide by the lungs, causing the reaction to be driven to the *left* (see Equation 3). The concentration of hydrogen ions increases accordingly.

Respiratory control of the hydrogen-ion concentration is limited in that such control cannot return the hydrogen-ion concentration to its normal value reflected by a pH of 7.4. The reason for this is that, as the pH approaches normal, the stimulus for the increase or decrease in alveolar ventilation is removed. (For further discussion of the control of respiration, see Chapter 28.)

## Renal Response to Changes in Hydrogen-Ion Concentration

The renal response to changes in hydrogen-ion concentration occurs much more slowly than does the respiratory response, usually over several days. (The respiratory response occurs within minutes to several hours.) The renal system functions to maintain physiologic pH by regulating the bicarbonate-ion concentration in extracellular fluid and by ridding the body of acid by-products of metabolism that cannot be eliminated by the lungs (i.e., fixed acids).

## *Bicarbonate "Reabsorption" and Hydrogen-Ion Secretion*

Bicarbonate is freely filtered at the glomerulus. Key events involved in its reabsorption include hydrogen-ion secretion, combination of hydrogen ions with bicarbonate ions in the renal tubules, and the reabsorption of sodium in exchange for hydrogen ions (Fig. 30–1).

The process of bicarbonate reabsorption involves carbon dioxide, which either diffuses into, or is formed metabolically within, the tubular epithelial cells. Within these cells, carbon dioxide combines with water to form carbonic acid in a reaction catalyzed by the enzyme, carbonic anhydrase. The dissociation of carbonic acid into hydrogen ions ($H^+$) and bicarbonate ions ($HCO_3^-$) occurs almost immediately.

The hydrogen ions generated by this reaction are secreted into the tubular lumen in exchange for sodium by a mechanism involving a sodium/hydrogen ion ($Na^+/H^+$) carrier transport protein; bicarbonate ions are absorbed into the extracellular fluid and peritubular capillaries in combination with reabsorbed sodium ions.

Once within the tubular lumen, the secreted hydrogen ions combine with filtered bicarbonate ions to form carbonic acid, which immediately converts to carbon dioxide and water. In this manner, the

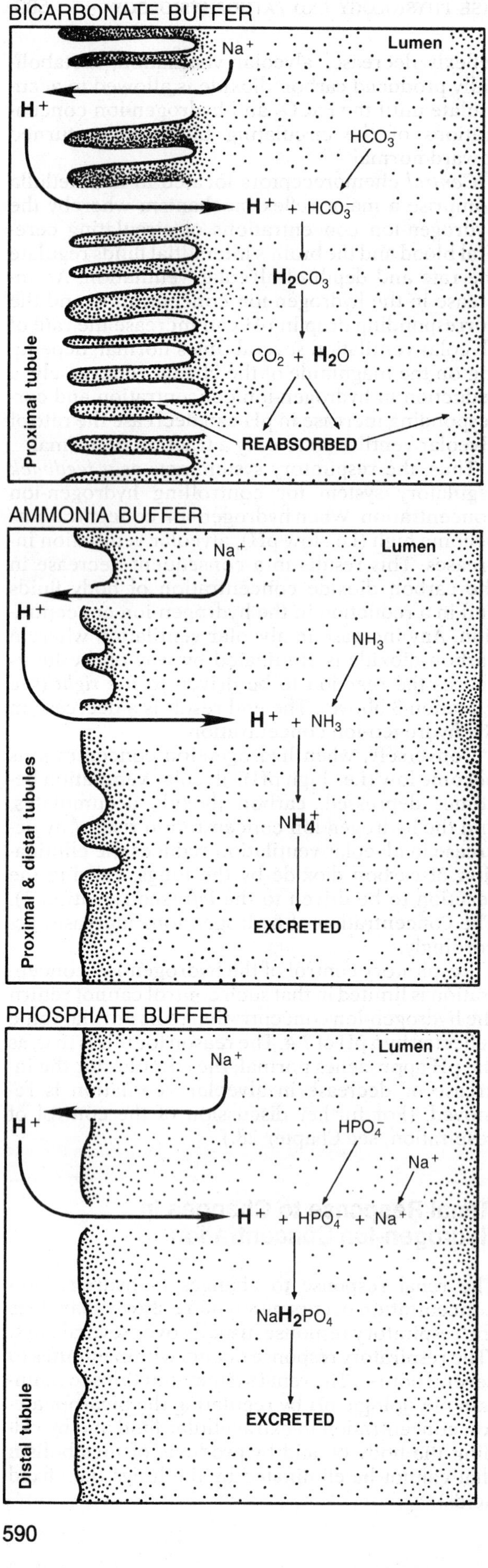


**Figure 30–1.** (*Top*) Bicarbonate "reabsorption" from the proximal tubular epithelial cell. Within the tubular cell, carbon dioxide is hydrated to form carbonic acid, a reaction catalyzed by the enzyme, carbonic anhydrase, and followed by the almost immediate dissociation of the acid into hydrogen ions and bicarbonate ions. The bicarbonate ion thus generated is "reabsorbed" by diffusing into the peritubular interstitium. The hydrogen ion formed in this reaction (as depicted) is pumped out of the cell into the tubular lumen (in exchange for sodium) where it is available to combine with filtered bicarbonate to form carbonic acid. This, in turn, is converted to carbon dioxide and water. The carbon dioxide enters the tubular cell where the entire process is again replicated. Note that the bicarbonate ion reabsorbed is not the same one filtered; note also that the hydrogen ion is not excreted but is available to be used for bicarbonate "reabsorption."

(*Middle*) Bicarbonate "regeneration" by the peritubular cell and excretion of secreted hydrogen ions with ammonia. Carbonic acid formed within the peritubular cell, as described above, dissociates into bicarbonate and hydrogen ions. The bicarbonate thus generated is absorbed into the tubular interstitium. The hydrogen ion is secreted into the tubular lumen where it reacts with ammonia ($NH_3$) formed by the tubular cells. The addition of a hydrogen ion to the ammonia forms ammonium ion ($NH_4^+$), which as a charged molecule cannot be easily reabsorbed and, thus, is excreted in the urine. This represents a net gain of bicarbonate in conjunction with the renal excretion of fixed acid.

(*Bottom*) Bicarbonate "regeneration" by the peritubular cell and excretion of secreted hydrogen ions with filtered phosphate. Carbonic acid formed within the peritubular cell, in a reaction catalyzed by carbonic anhydrase, dissociates into bicarbonate ions and hydrogen ions. The bicarbonate ion thus generated is absorbed into the tubular interstitium. The hydrogen ion is pumped out of the cell into the tubular lumen where it combines with phosphate buffer and is excreted in the urine. Thus, in this reaction, for each bicarbonate ion absorbed, a hydrogen ion is excreted. This represents a net gain of bicarbonate in conjunction with the renal excretion of fixed acids.

filtered bicarbonate is "reabsorbed." The process is again replicated as carbon dioxide diffuses into the tubular epithelial cells.

The net result of these events is that, for each hydrogen ion secreted into the tubular lumen, a bicarbonate ion is absorbed into the extracellular fluid and peritubular capillaries.

#### *Carbon Dioxide Concentration: Impact on Hydrogen-Ion Regulation*

Because carbon dioxide is involved in the reactions concerned with hydrogen-ion secretion, the greater the concentration of carbon dioxide in body fluids, the greater the rate of hydrogen-ion secretion. Thus, any factor that increases carbon dioxide tensions in body fluids (e.g., reduced alveolar ventilation, increased metabolic rate) also increases the rate of hydrogen-ion secretion. Conversely, any factor that decreases carbon dioxide tensions (e.g., hyperventilation, or decreased metabolic rate) decreases the rate of hydrogen-ion secretion.

These events of hydrogen-ion secretion and bicarbonate absorption occur throughout the renal tubular system, except for the descending loop of Henle. The proximal tubule absorbs 80-90% of the total bicarbonate filtered. The conversion of such large quantities of intraluminal carbonic acid to carbon dioxide and water in the proximal tubule is catalyzed by the enzyme, carbonic anhydrase, which resides in the microvilli of the proximal tubular epithelial cells (see Fig. 21-4).

#### *Renal Response to Acidemia*

In *acidemia* the ratio of carbon dioxide to bicarbonate ion in extracellular fluid increases (see Henderson-Hasselbalch Equation 5, above). Thus, the rate of hydrogen-ion secretion into the tubular lumen rises and exceeds the rate of glomerular filtration of the bicarbonate ion. Consequently, a great excess of hydrogen ions is secreted into the tubule, which have far too few bicarbonate ions to react with. In this instance, the excess hydrogen ions combine with urinary buffers (see below) and are excreted in the urine. Thus, the net effect of secreting excess hydrogen ions into the tubules is to increase the concentration of bicarbonate ions in the extracellular fluid, causing the pH to rise toward normal.

#### *Renal Response to Alkalemia*

In *alkalemia* the ratio of bicarbonate ions to carbon dioxide in extracellular fluid increases (see Henderson-Hasselbalch Equation 5, above). The high concentration of bicarbonate ions in the extracellular fluid increases the amount of bicarbonate filtered in excess of hydrogen ions secreted. Because it is necessary for bicarbonate ions to react with hydrogen ions in order to be "reabsorbed" (see Fig. 30-1), all the excess bicarbonate ions are excreted in the urine, usually with sodium ions. The net renal response in alkalemia is that sodium bicarbonate is removed from the extracellular fluid and the pH decreases toward normal.

#### *Elimination of Excess Hydrogen Ions: Urinary Buffer Systems*

Two major urinary buffer systems actually combine with hydrogen ions in the renal tubules and transport excess hydrogen ions into the urine: the phosphate buffer system and the ammonia buffer system.

**Phosphate Buffer System.** The *phosphate* buffer system consists of a mixture of disodium hydrogen phosphate ($Na_2HPO_4$) and monosodium dihydrogen phosphate ($NaH_2PO_4$). The phosphates are effective buffers because both forms are readily filtered, but relatively poorly reabsorbed from the renal tubules; and they become highly concentrated as water is reabsorbed from the tubules. Figure 30-1 illustrates how excess hydrogen ions are removed from the tubular fluid by the phosphate buffers. For each hydrogen ion excreted in the urine, a bicarbonate ion is absorbed from the tubular epithelial cell.

**Ammonia Buffer System.** The *ammonia* buffer system is composed of ammonia ($NH_3$) and ammonium ion ($NH_4^+$). Unlike phosphate, ammonia is not filtered but, rather, gains entry into the tubular lumen by diffusion from the tubular epithelial cells. Synthesis of ammonia occurs in all tubular cells, except those of the thin segment of the loop of Henle. The synthesis of ammonia by these cells creates a concentration gradient down which ammonia diffuses from the tubular epithelial cells into the tubular lumen. Diffusion of ammonia is facilitated by its nonionized, lipid-soluble form.

Upon combining with a hydrogen ion within the tubular lumen, the ammonium ion ($NH_4^+$) is formed. Because the luminal membrane is impermeable to the ammonium ion, it is trapped within the tubule and excreted in the urine (see Fig. 30-1).

The net effect of the reactions involving urinary buffering of excess hydrogen ions is to increase the concentration of bicarbonate in the extracellular fluid and remove the hydrogen ions associated with fixed acid production.

## ACID-BASE BALANCE: CLINICAL ABNORMALITIES

### Acid-Base Terminology

*pH* reflects the concentration of free hydrogen ions in solution. Normal physiologic pH range is 7.35-7.45.

*Acidemia* is a condition in which the hydrogen-ion concentration of the blood is elevated; the blood has an acid excess or base deficit (pH <7.35).

*Alkalemia* is a condition in which the hydrogen-ion concentration of the blood is reduced; the blood has an acid deficit or base excess (pH >7.45).

*Acidosis* is the process that causes acidemia. *Alkalosis* is the process that causes alkalemia.

## Arterial Blood Acid–Base Values

To evaluate the acid–base status, it is essential to appreciate the normal range of values for the specific blood acid–base parameters (Table 30–1). Definitive diagnosis of acid–base abnormalities depends on an evaluation of arterial blood gas values in conjunction with the patient's history, physical examination, and other diagnostic studies.

## Carbon Dioxide ($PCO_2$): Respiratory Parameter

Carbon dioxide ($CO_2$) gas is considered an *acid* substance because, when it combines with water, carbonic acid is formed; this weak acid dissociates into hydrogen and bicarbonate ions (see Equation 3).

Carbon dioxide is a major by-product of aerobic metabolism. The body eliminates carbon dioxide by way of the lungs.

There is a direct relationship between alveolar ventilation and the concentration of carbon dioxide in arterial blood ($PaCO_2$). Any alteration in the respiratory elimination of carbon dioxide out of proportion to its metabolic production can result in abnormalities of arterial $PaCO_2$ and pH.

A general rule regarding the expected change in pH resulting from changes that occur in $PaCO_2$ is:

TABLE 30–1
**Range of Physiologic Blood Acid–Base Values (at Sea Level)**

| Parameter* | Arterial Blood Values | Venous Blood Values |
|---|---|---|
| pH | 7.35–7.45 | 7.33–7.43 |
| $PaCO_2$ | 35–45 mmHg | 41–51 mmHg |
| $HCO_3^-$ | 22–26 mEq/liter | 24–28 mEq/liter |
| Base excess | −2–+2 | 0–+4 |

*These acid–base parameters apply to a person eating the average American diet. In persons eating a vegetarian diet, the bicarbonate will be elevated beyond this range.

$PaCO_2$ is the measure of the partial pressure (P) of carbon dioxide in arterial blood in millimeters of mercury (mmHg); respiratory parameter.

$HCO_3^-$ (bicarbonate ion) is a measurement of bicarbonate (base) concentration in blood; metabolic/renal parameter.

Base excess reflects the concentration of bicarbonate and other anions in the blood including serum proteins, hemoglobin, phosphates, and other metabolites. Base excess indicates the remaining base buffer after the free hydrogen ions are completely buffered. (Normal range: +2 to −2; anion excess: >2 [alkalemia]; anion deficit: <−2 [acidemia].)

pH will rise or fall 0.08 in the appropriate direction for every 10-mmHg change in $PaCO_2$. The following values loosely relate the ventilatory status to arterial carbon dioxide concentrations:

| $PaCO_2$ | Ventilatory Status |
|---|---|
| 35–45 mmHg | Effective alveolar ventilation |
| >45 mmHg | *Hypo*ventilation |
| <35 mmHg | *Hyper*ventilation |

Any factor that decreases the rate of alveolar ventilation (i.e., *hypo*ventilation), increases the concentration of dissolved carbon dioxide in the extracellular fluid ($PaCO_2$ >45 mmHg); conversely, any factor that increases the rate of alveolar ventilation (i.e., *hyper*ventilation) decreases the concentration of dissolved carbon dioxide in body fluids ($PaCO_2$ <35 mmHg).

### *Clinical Abnormalities: Respiratory Acidemia and Alkalemia*

There are two pathophysiologic conditions associated with an alteration in the ventilatory effort: respiratory acidemia and respiratory alkalemia.

**Respiratory Acidemia.** *Respiratory acidemia* is characterized by an increase in $PaCO_2$ (>45 mmHg), associated with a decreased ventilatory effort. As the concentration of carbon dioxide in the extracellular fluid increases, the reaction depicted in Equation 3 is driven to the *left* (i.e., there is an increase in the formation of carbonic acid, with a consequent increase in hydrogen-ion and bicarbonate-ion formation). Acidemia results from the increase in hydrogen-ion concentration.

As shown in the Henderson-Hasselbalch equation (Equation 5, above), as the carbon dioxide component (denominator) increases, the pH decreases. Thus, respiratory acidemia is reflected clinically by a $PaCO_2$ >45 mmHg, and a pH <7.35.

### *Respiratory Alkalemia*

*Respiratory alkalemia* is characterized by a decrease in $PaCO_2$ (<35 mmHg), associated with excessive alveolar ventilation, or hyperventilation. What occurs is a reversal of the process described for respiratory acidemia. As carbon dioxide is blown off and its concentration in extracellular fluid decreases, the reaction depicted in Equation 3 is driven to the *right* (i.e., there is a reduction in the hydrogen-ion concentration resulting in alkalemia). Referring again to the Henderson-Hasselbalch equation, as the denominator decreases, the pH will increase. Thus, respiratory alkalemia is reflected clinically, by a $PaCO_2$ <35 mmHg, and a pH >7.45.

For information related to the pathophysiology, etiology, clinical presentation, and treatment of respiratory acidemia and respiratory alkalemia, see Table 30-2.

TABLE 30-2
**Respiratory Acid-Base Abnormalities: Acidemia and Alkalemia**

| | Respiratory Acidemia | Respiratory Alkalemia |
|---|---|---|
| Definition | Respiratory acidemia is caused by a process that raises the $CO_2$ tension of blood ($PaCO_2$), increasing its hydrogen-ion concentration, with a consequent decrease in pH < 7.35.<br>Primary abnormality: elevated $PaCO_2$ (>45 mmHg). | Respiratory alkalemia is caused by a process that reduces the $CO_2$ tension of blood ($PaCO_2$), decreasing its hydrogen-ion concentration, with a consequent increase in pH > 7.45.<br>Primary abnormality: Reduced $PaCO_2$ (<35 mmHg). |
| Pathophysiology | Underlying process: Alveolar *hypo*ventilation.<br>When the lungs fail to eliminate metabolically produced $CO_2$, for whatever reason, $PaCO_2$ rises, resulting in an increase in hydrogen-ion concentration with a net decrease in pH < 7.35. This is termed *hypercapnia*. | Underlying process: Alveolar hyperventilation.<br>Hyperventilation (i.e., blowing off $CO_2$) causes a decrease in hydrogen-ion concentration, which results in an increase in pH > 7.45. This is termed *hypocapnia*. |
| Etiology | Central nervous system depression of respiratory centers in pons and medulla:<br>Drug overdose<br>Respiratory depressants<br>Neuromuscular conditions:<br>Guillain-Barré syndrome<br>Myasthenia gravis<br>Bony bellows:<br>Kyphoscoliosis<br>Massive obesity (pickwickian syndrome)<br>Airway patency:<br>Chronic obstructive pulmonary disease<br>Asthma<br>Intact alveoli:<br>Adult respiratory distress syndrome<br>Bilateral pneumonia<br>Congestive heart failure with pulmonary edema | Central nervous system dysfunction of respiratory centers in pons and medulla:<br>Fever<br>Head trauma<br>Cerebral vascular accident<br>Anxiety<br>Brain tumor<br>Salicylates<br>Alterations in pulmonary function related to:<br>Pneumonia<br>Pulmonary embolism<br>Congestive heart failure<br>Interstitial lung disease<br>Mechanical ventilation<br>Hypoxia<br>Gram-negative septicemia |
| Clinical presentation | Acute hypercapnia usually associated with hypoxemia, which dominates the clinical presentation:<br>1. Altered neurologic function: restlessness, irritability, headache (related to increase in cerebral blood flow due to vasodilatory response of cerebral vasculature to hypercapnia). Drowsiness, confusion, coma.<br>2. Cardiac dysrhythmias.<br>3. Neuromuscular status: Weakness, tremors.<br>4. Altered pulmonary function: Tachypnea, dyspnea, acute respiratory distress and insufficiency. | Acute hypocapnia is manifested by the following:<br>1. Altered neurologic function: changes in level of consciousness (hypocapnia causes cerebral vasoconstriction); coma, lightheadedness, giddiness (associated with hyperventilation). Paresthesias, weakness, muscle cramps, seizures, tetany, hyperactive deep tendon reflexes, convulsions (hypocalcemia).<br>2. Cardiac dysrhythmias. |
| Arterial blood gas values | pH < 7.35<br>$PaCO_2$ > 45 mmHg<br>$HCO_3^-$ > 26 mEq/liter<br>Serum electrolytes: Within acceptable concentrations. | pH > 7.45<br>$PaCO_2$ < 35 mmHg<br>$HCO_3^-$ < 22 mEq/liter<br>Serum electrolytes: Occasionally associated with hypokalemia and hypocalcemia. |
| Physiologic responses | Buffering: The increase in hydrogen-ion concentration is immediately buffered by noncarbonate buffers including hemoglobin and other proteins in extracellular fluid, and phosphates, proteins, and lactate in intracellular fluid. | The decrease in hydrogen-ion concentration within the extracellular fluids prompts an immediate release of hydrogen ions from the intracellular compartment, usually in exchange for potassium.<br>Cellular metabolism contributes to restoring the hydrogen-ion level by increasing production of lactate and other metabolic acids. |
| Renal compensation | The kidneys increase hydrogen-ion secretion while reabsorbing $HCO_3^-$; the increased $PaCO_2$ directly stimulates an increase in hydrogen-ion secretion, which is associated with an increased reabsorption of sodium (to maintain appropriate electrochemical balance).<br>In the setting of acute respiratory acidemia more sodium is reabsorbed in exchange for hydrogen ions, resulting in an increased chloride secretion.<br>Renal compensation also includes an increased excretion of ammonium ion ($NH_4^+$) and an increase in chloride secretion. The net result is an increase in $HCO_3^-$ concentration in extracellular fluid. | The kidneys reduce net excretion of hydrogen ions; there is a decreased reabsorption of $HCO_3^-$ in the renal tubules.<br>Because it is necessary for $HCO_3^-$ ions to react with hydrogen ions in order to be "reabsorbed," all excess bicarbonate ions are excreted in the urine, usually with sodium.<br>Net renal response: sodium bicarbonate is removed from extracellular fluid, and the pH decreases toward normal. |

TABLE 30-2
**Respiratory Acid-Base Abnormalities: Acidemia and Alkalemia *(Continued)***

| | Respiratory Acidemia | Respiratory Alkalemia |
|---|---|---|
| Correction of primary problem (pulmonary in origin) | Restoration of effective alveolar ventilation. In patients with chronic hypercapnia associated with irreversible parenchymal lung disease, a partially correct acid-base balance may only be possible. | Restoration of effective alveolar ventilation. It is necessary to alleviate hyperventilation. Hyperventilation associated with mechanical ventilation can easily be corrected; a reduction of stimulation of respiratory centers in the pons and medulla may be more difficult to achieve; if due to an irreversible pathologic process, correction may not be possible. |
| Treatment | Treatment goal: Restore and maintain effective alveolar ventilation.<br>Specific therapy may entail vigorous pulmonary toilet and/or mechanical ventilation.<br>Oxygenation as indicated by arterial oxygen tension ($PaO_2$), patient history, and physical examination.<br>Small doses of $NaCO_3$ may be prescribed in severe acidemia as a temporary measure until definitive therapy is established. The blood-brain barrier is less permeable to $HCO_3^-$ than the nonpolar $CO_2$ molecule. Consequently, correction of systemic pH may occur, while the pH of cerebral fluids may actually fall, initially.<br>Close monitoring of cardiopulmonary and neurologic function and fluid and electrolyte status is essential in acid-base imbalances. | Treatment goal: To correct or ameliorate the underlying disorder causing the hyperventilation.<br>Oxygenation to treat hypoxemia.<br>Patients on mechanical ventilation who manifest neuromuscular irritability, twitching or seizures, or cardiac dysrhythmias, may benefit from decreasing the minute ventilation and increasing dead space ventilation.<br>Occasionally, treatment with an inhaled gas mixture containing 3% carbon dioxide may be helpful when used for short periods of time.<br>Close monitoring: Same as in respiratory acidemia. |
| Nursing diagnoses | Breathing pattern, ineffective: Hypoventilation.<br>Airway clearance, ineffective.<br>Sensory-perceptual alteration: Altered level of consciousness.<br>Thought processes, alteration in.<br>Potential for injury: Cardiac dysrhythmias.<br>Electrolyte imbalance, potential for. | Anxiety.<br>Breathing pattern, ineffective: Hyperventilation.<br>Electrolyte imbalance, potential for.<br>Potential for injury: Seizure activity, tetany, cardiac dysrhythmias.<br>Sensory-perceptual alteration: Altered level of consciousness.<br>Knowledge deficit regarding role in inducing altered breathing pattern. |

## Bicarbonate Ion ($HCO_3^-$) and Base Excess (B.E.): Metabolic (Nonrespiratory) Parameters

Metabolic acid-base abnormalities include all acid-base disturbances other than those caused by excess or insufficient carbon dioxide in extracellular fluid (i.e., respiratory parameter). Two pathophysiologic conditions have been defined: metabolic acidemia and metabolic alkalemia.

### *Metabolic Acidemia*

*Metabolic acidemia* is associated with the accumulation of metabolic or fixed acid, or to a loss of bicarbonate from extracellular fluid. A distinction is made between *metabolic* or *fixed* acid, and the *respiratory* acid, carbonic acid. By convention, carbonic acid, which results from dissolved carbon dioxide, is considered as part of the *respiratory* parameter. All other acids, whether metabolically produced or ingested, comprise the *metabolic* parameter.

Clinically, metabolic acidemia is characterized by a decrease in bicarbonate-ion ($HCO_3^-$) concentration in extracellular fluid (<22 mEq/liter), by a base deficit, and by a pH <7.35 (see Table 30-1). The reduction in bicarbonate-ion concentration is associated with an increase in metabolic or fixed acid. The consequent increase in hydrogen-ion concentration necessarily uses up bicarbonate ion and other anions (see below), as part of the body's buffering response to neutralize the high acid load preventing the pH from falling too low.

**Anions and the Anion Gap.** Metabolic acidemia is commonly divided into those causes in which there is an increase in unmeasured anions and those in which bicarbonate is lost without an increase in unmeasured anions. An *anion* is a substance with a net negative charge.

The ionic composition of the major fluid compartments is such that, overall, body fluids are essentially electroneutral, that is, the number of cations (positively charged ions) match the number of anions (negatively charged ions).

Sodium accounts for 90% of the cations in extracellular fluid. The positively charged sodium ions are matched rather well by the sum of chloride and bicarbonate anions, and, to a much lesser extent, by minor anions such as sulfates, phosphates, and organic acids. Laboratory measurements of plasma concentrations of sodium, chloride, and bicarbonate ions can readily be made, and the latter, that is, chloride and bicarbonate ions, are referred to as the *measured* anions; other anions, (e.g., sulfates, phosphates, and organic acids) are difficult to assess and they are referred to as the *unmeasured* anions, or more conveniently, as the *anion gap*.

The anion gap is calculated as follows: plasma sodium concentration minus the sum of plasma chloride and bicarbonate.

$$\text{Anion gap} = Na^+ - (Cl^- + HCO_3^-)$$

Normal range: 10–14 mM/liter.

$$= 140 - (102 + 26)$$
$$= 140 - 128$$
$$\text{Anion gap} = 12 \text{ mM/liter}$$

### Metabolic Acidemia: Anion Gap > 15 mM/liter

An increase in unmeasured anions (i.e., the anion gap) is always present when a metabolic acidemia is caused by the *addition* of acid from an endogenous or exogenous source. For example, accumulations of lactic acid (anaerobic metabolism of cardiac arrest), ketoacids (diabetic ketoacidosis), or sulfates, phosphates, creatinates, and proteinates (renal failure) are *endogenous* sources of unmeasured anions. *Exogenous* sources include drug overdose/poisoning attributed, for example, to salicylates, ethylene glycol, methyl alcohol, or ingestion of other acidic substances. In each of these examples, there is an increase in the hydrogen-ion concentration of the extracellular fluids, which consumes bicarbonate ($HCO_3^-$) in the buffering process, eventually replacing the bicarbonate with an increased concentration of unmeasured anions.

### Metabolic Acidemia: Normal Anion Gap (i.e., 10–14 mM/liter)

Not all episodes of metabolic acidemia are attributed to an increase in unmeasured anions. The anion gap remains normal in acidemia associated with loss of bicarbonate ion as occurs with diarrhea and lower gastrointestinal dysfunction (e.g., fistulas, drainage of pancreatic juices, ureterosigmoidostomy), among others. Such conditions are usually associated with *hyperchloremia*. The loss of bicarbonate ion ($HCO_3^-$) in excess of a concomitant loss of chloride ions ($Cl^-$) will reduce the bicarbonate-ion level of extracellular fluid, while the chloride-ion concentration rises. See Table 30–3 and the appropriate tables on fluid/electrolytes in Chapter 23 for other details related to metabolic acidemia.

### Metabolic Alkalemia

*Metabolic alkalemia* may be associated with a net *loss* of hydrogen ions, or a net *gain* of bicarbonate ions in extracellular fluids, or a loss of chloride ions in excess of bicarbonate ions. Hydrogen-ion depletion of extracellular fluid may occur by way of the gastrointestinal tract and kidneys. Gastric losses due to vomiting or continuous nasogastric suctioning can cause a considerable loss of hydrogen ions as well as chloride ions. Serum bicarbonate levels rise if hydrogen-ion loss is greater than that gained by the diet or body metabolism.

Clinically, metabolic alkalemia is characterized by an increase in bicarbonate-ion ($HCO_3^-$) concentration in extracellular fluid (>26 mEq/liter), by a base excess, and by a pH >7.45 (see Table 30–1) (and the appropriate tables on fluid/electrolytes in Chap. 23).

**Hypochloremic, Hypokalemic Metabolic Alkalemia.** A reciprocal relationship exists between bicarbonate ($HCO_3^-$) and chloride ($Cl^-$) concentrations in metabolic alkalemia: when plasma bicarbonate concentration rises, there is a concomitant fall in the plasma chloride concentration. Chloride is the only anion, other than bicarbonate, that occurs in significant concentrations in extracellular fluid, and it is readily reabsorbed by the kidneys in conjunction with the reabsorption of sodium. Thus, any reduction in chloride levels seriously compromises bicarbonate excretion, and actually favors its reabsorption.

Hypochloremia contributes to the maintenance of metabolic alkalemia in another way. Normally reabsorption of sodium (cation) is largely accompanied by the reabsorption of chloride (anion), in order to preserve electrochemical gradients along the tubular system. Sodium is also reabsorbed by way of an exchange mechanism wherein it is reabsorbed, while another cation (e.g., potassium or hydrogen ion) is secreted. When this latter mechanism becomes predominant (as in the presence of hypochloremia), the additional loss of hydrogen ions that results contributes further to the alkalemic state.

In addition, because there is a limited concentration of potassium ions available for exchange with sodium, hypokalemia may rapidly ensue. Thus, the patient with metabolic alkalemia may ultimately experience a *hypochloremic, hypokalemic metabolic akalemia* (see Chap. 23).

TABLE 30-3

## Metabolic Acid-Base Abnormalities: Acidemia and Alkalemia

| | Metabolic Acidemia | Metabolic Alkalemia |
|---|---|---|
| Definition | Metabolic acidemia is caused by a process that increases hydrogen-ion concentration in conjunction with a decrease in bicarbonate ion ($HCO_3^-$), resulting in a decrease in pH < 7.35. | Metabolic alkalemia is caused by a process that increases bicarbonate-ion concentration (or decreases hydrogen-ion concentration), with consequent increase in pH > 7.45. |
| Pathophysiology | The bicarbonate-ion ($HCO_3^-$) concentration can be reduced in the following ways:[1]<br>1. Buffering activity: Buffering of a strong, highly dissociated acid with $HCO_3^-$.<br>2. Loss of $HCO_3^-$ from body fluids especially by way of gastrointestinal tract and kidneys.<br>3. Rapid hemodilution of fluid in extracellular space with a noncarbonate-containing fluid (e.g., isotonic saline). | The $HCO_3^-$ concentration can be elevated in the following ways:<br>1. By a net loss of hydrogen ions from extracellular fluid.<br>2. By a net addition of $HCO_3^-$ to the extracellular fluid.<br>3. Chloride loss from extracellular fluid in excess of $HCO_3^-$. |
| Etiology | Causes of metabolic acidemia:[1]<br>1. Increase in unmeasured anions (anion gap > 15 mM/liter).<br>• Diabetic ketoacidosis.<br>• Starvation ketoacidosis.<br>• Alcoholic ketoacidosis.<br>• Poisonings:<br>Salicylate<br>Ethylene glycol<br>Methyl alcohol<br>• Lactic acidosis<br>• Shock; cardiac arrest<br>• Renal failure.<br>2. Without increase in anion gap (anion gap—normal) (hyperchloremia).<br>• Diarrhea (intestinal fluids have high $HCO_3^-$ content).<br>• Drainage of pancreatic juice.<br>• Ureterosigmoidostomy.<br>• Obstructed ileal loop.<br>• Ammonium chloride therapy.<br>• Renal tubular acidosis.<br>• Dilutional acidosis.<br>• Hyperalimentation.<br>• Acetazolamide therapy* | Causes of metabolic alkalemia:<br>1. Fluid loss from upper gastrointestinal tract:<br>• Vomiting.<br>• Continuous nasogastric suctioning.<br>2. Rapid correction of chronic hypercapnia.<br>3. Diuretic therapy.<br>4. Corticosteroid therapy.<br>5. Severe hypocalemia.<br>6. Alkali administration. |
| Clinical presentation | Severe metabolic acidemia may cause the following:<br>1. Alterations in neurologic function:<br>• Headache, change in level of consciousness, drowsiness, confusion, coma.<br>2. Alteration in cardiovascular function:<br>• Depressed cardiac function, cardiac dysrhythmias.<br>• Decreased peripheral vascular resistance, with hypotension, shock, tissue hypoxia.<br>• Pulmonary edema.<br>3. Alteration of pulmonary function:<br>• Deep, rapid respirations (Kussmaul's breathing), which is especially evident when bicarbonate levels are < 15 mEq/liter.<br>4. Alterations in gastrointestinal function:<br>• Nausea, vomiting, anorexia. | A high index of suspicion is necessary in examining the patient with metabolic alkalemia because there are no specific signs and symptoms unique to this disorder.<br>A history of vomiting, diuretic usage, and complaints of weakness may provide important clues.<br>Specific considerations:<br>1. Alteration in neuromuscular function:<br>• Irritability, muscle cramps, hyperactive deep tendon reflexes, tetany. (Hypocalcemia is frequently an associated problem because levels of ionized calcium decrease as pH increases.)<br>• Muscle weakness.<br>2. Alteration in cardiovascular function:<br>• Cardiac dysrhythmias. |
| Arterial blood gas values | pH < 7.35; if severe < 7.20.<br>$PaCO_2$normal; or decreased with compensation.<br>$HCO_3^-$ < 20 mEq/liter; if severe < 15 mEq/liter.<br>Anion gap: normal or increased, depending on the underlying cause.<br>Serum electrolytes:<br>• Potassium ions: Normal or increased. (In the presence of excess hydrogen ions, these ions shift into cells in exchange with potassium ions.) | pH > 7.45<br>$PaCO_2$ normal; or increased with compensation.<br>$HCO_3^-$ > 26–30 mEq/liter.<br>Serum electrolytes:<br>• Potassium ions decreased.<br>• Chloride ions decreased. |

TABLE 30–3
**Metabolic Acid–Base Abnormalities: Acidemia and Alkalemia *(Continued)***

| | Metabolic Acidemia | Metabolic Alkalemia |
|---|---|---|
| Physiologic responses | 1. Buffering: Intracellular buffers such as hemoglobin and phosphates actively participate in the buffering process, as bicarbonate ions are used up buffering the excess hydrogen-ion concentration. | 1. Buffering: Excess bicarbonate ions are buffered primarily by hydrogen ions derived from intracellular phosphates and proteins, which shift to the extracellular fluid compartment. |
| | 2. Respiratory compensation: As the pH decreases due to a decrease in bicarbonate ions, a concomitant fall in $PaCO_2$ is essential to reestablish the 20:1 ratio (Henderson-Hasselbalch equation) and return the pH to within the normal range: 7.35–7.45.<br>• The respiratory system compensates for acidemia by increasing alveolar ventilation (e.g., Kussmaul's breathing). As the lungs "blow off" carbon dioxide, a reduction in the hydrogen-ion concentration occurs.<br>• The stimulus for the increased ventilatory effort is an increase in hydrogen-ion concentration of cerebral fluids.<br>• The respiratory response occurs quickly (within minutes) but does not reach a steady state for up to 12–24 hr. | 2. Respiratory compensation: As the pH increases due to an increase in bicarbonate ions, a concomitant increase in $PaCO_2$ is essential to reestablish the 20:1 ratio (Henderson-Hasselbalch equation), which is necessary to achieve a pH within the normal range: 7.35–7.45.<br>• Alveolar hypoventilation occurs to retain carbon dioxide and increase the $PaCO_2$. The degree of compensation is limited by the requirement to maintain $PaO_2$ at acceptable level ($PaO_2 > 60$ mmHg).<br>• Upper limits of $PaCO_2$ compensation in patients without pulmonary disease is usually about 55 mmHg, but may be higher. |
| | 3. Renal compensation: The kidney is responsible for excreting the acid load; reabsorbing and generating bicarbonate ions.<br>• A lag time of up to 24 hr occurs before the kidneys begin to impact on the acidemic state; up to 4 or 5 days may be required for maximal excretion of the acid load.<br>• The major renal mechanism for excreting excess hydrogen ions is by the urinary buffers:<br>Ammonia/ammonium ion buffer.<br>Phosphate buffer system.<br>• Because the lungs cannot excrete fixed or metabolic acid, the kidneys are ultimately responsible for correcting the acidemia and returning the pH to normal range: 7.35–7.45. | 3. Renal compensation: The kidney has the ability to rapidly excrete bicarbonate ions and restore normal levels of bicarbonate in extracellular fluid.<br>• Hypochloremia can seriously compromise renal excretion of bicarbonate, because one method of sodium reabsorption requires the concomitant reabsorption of a negatively charged ion (e.g., chloride or bicarbonate ions). In the presence of chloride-ion depletion, reabsorption of bicarbonate ion can actually be enhanced.<br>• Reabsorption of sodium in exchange for hydrogen or potassium ions further depletes $H^+$ ions. |
| Treatment | Therapeutic goal: Treat the underlying disease process responsible for the depletion of body buffers at a rate faster than the kidney can regenerate them.<br>1. Major therapeutic considerations:<br>• Severe metabolic acidemia (pH < 7.0) may require intravenous sodium bicarbonate to raise pH to > 7.20, and bicarbonate levels to > 15 mM/liter.<br>• Very rapid correction of acidemia should be avoided.<br>2. Specific therapeutic considerations when administering sodium bicarbonate:<br>• Cerebrospinal fluid acidosis may worsen initially, causing changes in the level of consciousness.<br>• Hemoglobin delivery of oxygen to the tissues may be retarded.<br>• Continuous infusion with sodium bicarbonate may compromise cardiac function; the additional sodium intake can predispose to congestive heart failure and pulmonary edema in the compromised renal and/or cardiac patient. | Therapeutic goal: Treat the underlying disease process responsible for the alkalemia, and correct factors maintaining it.<br>Specific therapeutic considerations:<br>• Correct volume depletion.<br>• Replace chloride so that kidney has the option of reabsorbing or secreting $HCO_3^-$.<br>• Sodium and potassium replacement therapy will correct volume depletion and hypokalemia.<br>• Administration of ammonium chloride ($NH_4Cl$) may be used in compromised cardiac and/or renal status.<br>• Intravenous acetazolamide may be useful because it will increase renal excretion of bicarbonate. |
| | • Close monitoring of cardiopulmonary function and fluid and electrolyte balance is essential.<br>• Close monitoring of neurologic and neuromuscular status is necessary. | • Close monitoring of cardiopulmonary function and fluid and electrolyte balance is essential. |

*(continued)*

TABLE 30-3
**Metabolic Acid-Base Abnormalities: Acidemia and Alkalemia *(Continued)***

| | Metabolic Acidemia | Metabolic Alkalemia |
|---|---|---|
| Nursing diagnoses | Thought processes, alteration in.<br>Sensory-perceptual alteration:<br>Altered level of consciousness.<br>Electrolyte imbalance, potential for.<br>Potential for infection, related to compromised protective reflexes (cough, gag, epiglottal closure).<br>Potential for injury:<br>Altered level of consciousness.<br>Cardiac dysrhythmias. | Sensory-perceptual alteration.<br>Electrolyte imbalance, potential for:<br>Hypochloremia<br>Hypokalemia<br>Hypocalcemia<br>Potential for injury:<br>Altered level of consciousness.<br>Cardiac dysrhythmias.<br>Neuromuscular irritability.<br>Seizure activity, tetany. |

*Acetazolamide inhibits intracellular and luminal (tubular) carbon anhydrase. It delays the hydrolysis of carbonic acid to carbon dioxide and water, allowing hydrogen ions to increase in the lumen, creating a gradient against hydrogen-ion secretion by tubular epithelial cells.
Intracellularly, acetazolamide inhibits hydration of carbon dioxide to carbonic acid, thus reducing the subsequent production of hydrogen and bicarbonate ions.

## Extracellular Fluid Volume Depletion: Impact on Metabolic Alkalemia

Extracellular fluid volume depletion is also instrumental in maintaining metabolic alkalemia. The kidney preserves the extracellular volume by its reabsorption of sodium, which, in turn, facilitates the reabsorption of water along osmotic gradients and in the presence of antidiuretic hormone (ADH). Volume depletion is known to increase sodium reabsorption, as well as bicarbonate reabsorption in the proximal tubule. Increased hydrogen-ion secretion is associated with the generation of bicarbonate (see Fig. 30-1). (For details regarding metabolic alkalemia, see Table 30-3; refer also to Chap. 23.)

## SUMMARY OF ACID-BASE RELATIONSHIPS: IMPACT ON pH

Referring again to the Henderson-Hasselbalch equation, the following generalities can be made:

$$pH = pK + \text{Log}\,\frac{HCO_3^-\ (\text{Base})}{PCO_2\ (\text{Acid})} = \qquad (5)$$

$$\text{Acid-Base Parameters}\quad \frac{20}{1}\ \text{Ratio}\ \frac{\text{Metabolic}}{\text{Respiratory}}$$

- Any increase in the numerator ($HCO_3^-$, other anions) without a corresponding increase in the denominator ($PCO_2$) so as to maintain the 20:1 ratio will increase pH. A pH change due primarily to alterations in bicarbonate and other anions (i.e., the numerator) is attributed to *metabolic* (nonrespiratory) causes.
- Any increase in the denominator ($PCO_2$) without a corresponding increase in the numerator ($HCO_3^-$, other anions) so as to maintain a 20:1 ratio will decrease the pH. A pH change due primarily to alterations in $PCO_2$ (i.e., the denominator) is attributed to *respiratory* causes.
- Any change in both the $HCO_3^-$ (numerator) and $PCO_2$ (denominator) that preserves the 20:1 ratio will result in a pH within the normal physiologic range (i.e., 7.35-7.45).
- Causes of acidemia and alkalemia:

| | | |
|---|---|---|
| *Acidemia — pH < 7.35* | Respiratory | $\uparrow PCO_2$ |
| | Metabolic (nonrespiratory) | $\downarrow HCO_3^-$ |
| *Alkalemia — pH > 7.45* | *Respiratory* | $\downarrow PCO_2$ |
| | Metabolic (Nonrespiratory) | $\uparrow HCO_3^-$ |

- Normal blood gas values:

| | | |
|---|---|---|
| pH | 7.4 (7.35-7.45) | |
| $PaCO_2$ | 35-45 mmHg | (Respiratory parameter) |
| $HCO_3^-$ | 22-26 mEq/liter | (Metabolic parameter) |
| Base excess | −2 to +2 | (Metabolic parameter) |

## ACID-BASE ABNORMALITIES[2]

### Acute Uncompensated

Acute or uncompensated acid-base abnormality is characterized by an abnormal pH and a change in *one* blood parameter, either the respiratory parameter ($PaCO_2$) or the metabolic parameters ($HCO_3^-$ and base excess).

## Compensated

Compensated acid–base abnormality is characterized by a change in pH, an abnormal parameter associated with the primary disorder (respiratory or metabolic), and a change in the other parameter so as to maintain a bicarbonate to carbonic acid ($HCO_3^-$) ratio of 20 : 1.

## Fully Compensated

The pH is normal. Both $HCO_3^-$ and $PaCO_2$ parameters may still be abnormal, but the ratio between them remains 20 : 1.

## Partially Compensated

The pH may have improved toward the normal range but is still slightly abnormal. In this situation, all three values—pH, $PaCO_2$, and $HCO_3^-$—are abnormal.

Compensation occurs much more slowly than the initial, immediate buffering processes, but it is much more effective in returning the pH to within the normal physiologic range. The respiratory system ($PaCO_2$) compensates for an underlying metabolic disorder; the renal system ($HCO_3^-$) compensates for an underlying respiratory disorder.

## Corrected

Corrected acid–base abnormality is characterized by all acid–base parameters (pH, $PaCO_2$, and $HCO_3^-$) returning to normal. The primary disorder is rectified: the lungs remedy the respiratory parameter while the kidneys correct the metabolic parameter.

# PROCEDURE FOR ANALYZING ARTERIAL BLOOD GASES TO DETERMINE ACID–BASE ABNORMALITIES[3]

1. Establish pH using 7.40 as a guide to acidemia or alkalemia.
2. Examine respiratory parameter, $PaCO_2$. Can it cause the change in pH?
3. Examine metabolic parameters, $HCO_3^-$ and base excess. Can these factors cause the change in pH?

# ANALYSIS AND INTERPRETATION OF ARTERIAL BLOOD GASES: CASE STUDIES

1. An 18-year old female was admitted to the hospital after taking an overdose of phenobarbital.

| *Data* | *Analysis* |
|---|---|
| pH 7.18 | (A) pH $< 7.4$, therefore underlying condition is *acidemia*. |
| $PaCO_2$ 60 mmHg | (B) Respiratory parameter elevated; *primary* cause of the acidemia. |
| $HCO_3^-$ 26 mEq/liter | (C) Metabolic parameters within normal physiologic range. |
| Base excess +1 | |

***Diagnosis.*** Acute respiratory acidemia caused by severe hypoventilation.

2. A 17-year-old, semicomatose male is seen in the Emergency Department. The patient has a fruity odor to his breath; he is an insulin-dependent diabetic.

| *Data* | *Analysis* |
|---|---|
| pH 7.20 | (A) pH $< 7.4$, therefore underlying condition is *acidemia*. |
| $PaCO_2$ 40 mmHg | (B) Respiratory parameter within normal physiologic range. |
| $HCO_3^-$ 13 mEq/liter | (C) Metabolic parameters significantly reduced; *primary* cause of the acidemia. |
| Base Excess −4 | |

***Diagnosis.*** Acute metabolic acidemia.

The anion gap in this situation would be expected to be elevated due to excess keotacids associated with diabetic ketoacidosis.

3. A 62-year-old female presents with a history of severe vomiting over the past 48 hours; she complains of severe weakness and muscle cramps.

| *Data* | *Analysis* |
|---|---|
| pH 7.56 | (A) pH $> 7.40$, therefore underlying condition is *alkalemia*. |
| $PaCO_2$ 44 mmHg | (B) Respiratory parameter within normal physiologic limits. |

| | |
|---|---|
| $HCO_3^-$ 33 mEq/liter | (C) Metabolic parameters elevated; *primary* cause of alkalemia. |

Base excess +7

***Diagnosis.*** Acute metabolic alkalemia, probably associated with hypochloremia (vomiting) and hypokalemia (weakness). Muscle cramps may be related to the effect of the alkalemic state. Alkalemia increases the protein-bound calcium, with a resultant decrease in free, ionized calcium. This patient is at risk for developing tetany. (Note: Vomiting causes loss of hydrogen ions as well as chloride.)

4. A 62-year-old male with longstanding COPD (chronic obstructive pulmonary disease) is admitted to the hospital with possible gastrointestinal bleeding.

| *Data* | *Analysis* |
|---|---|
| pH 7.34 | (A) pH borderline *acidemia.* |
| $PaCO_2$ 60 mmHg | (B) Respiratory parameter significantly elevated. |
| $HCO_3^-$ 32 mEq/liter | (C) Metabolic parameters elevated. |

Base excess +5
$PaO_2$ 75 mmHg
$O_2$ saturation 80%
Longstanding COPD suggests respiratory acidosis as the primary cause of the acidemia. The elevated base reflects renal compensation, and the nearly normal pH suggests that compensation is largely complete.

***Diagnosis.*** Compensated (fully) respiratory acidemia.

5. A 54-year-old female with longstanding pulmonary disease is admitted to the Emergency Department with severe dehydration and prostration. Her family reports that she has had the flu for the past week.

| *Data* | *Analysis* |
|---|---|
| pH 7.24 | (A) pH $< 7.35$, therefore underlying mechanism is *acidemia.* |
| $PaCO_2$ 55 mmHg | (B) Respiratory parameter elevated. |
| $HCO_3^-$ 20 mEq/liter | (C) Metabolic parameters reduced. |

Base excess −6
The elevated $PaCO_2$ and history suggest that the primary disorder is respiratory acidemia. The metabolic parameters also suggest acidemia because these values are considerably reduced. In the setting of longstanding chronic respiratory acidemia, the expectation would be for $HCO_3^-$ and base excess to be elevated (renal compensation) with a pH reflective of partial to full compensation. This is not the case here because the pH is 7.24.

***Diagnosis.*** Combined respiratory/metabolic acidemia.

## Summary

An understanding of the principles underlying acid–base physiology is essential to the care of the critically ill patient. Acid–base imbalances are constantly encountered in the critical care setting, and they impact on total body function. Coupled with clues derived from the patient's ongoing history, physical examination, and other laboratory tests and studies, information garnered from arterial blood gas analysis and interpretation assists in assessing the patient's neurologic and cardiopulmonary status, and the overall response to therapy. It is important to develop a systematic approach to analyzing and evaluating such data in terms of total body function.

TABLE 30–4
**Drawing Arterial Blood Sample from Indwelling Line**

| **Procedure** | **Rationale/Precautions** |
|---|---|
| 1. Place unheparinized syringe in 3-way stopcock nearest the patient and withdraw flush solution until blood fills the line. Discard syringe and flush solution. | Maintain sterile technique throughout procedure to decrease risk of infection. Flush solution is withdrawn so as not to dilute the sample. |
| 2. With a heparinized syringe, withdraw approximately 2 ml blood; maneuver stopcock to closed position and remove the syringe. | Stopcock should be adjusted so that it is closed to the syringe port prior to removing syringe. |
| 3. Immediately expel any air from the syringe, cap the syringe with rubber stopper or cork, immerse in ice, and deliver to laboratory. | To avoid inaccuracy in results, it is essential to prevent any air from getting into the syringe. |
| 4. Flush the stopcock used to obtain the sample, and flush the arterial line. | |
| 5. Stopcock should be returned to original position so that it is off to air and the flush solution is opened to the patient. | Assess line to make sure that no air bubbles were introduced into the system. |

TABLE 30–5

## Drawing Arterial Blood Sample by Percutaneous Puncture

| Procedure | Rationale/Precautions |
|---|---|
| 1. Select site to be used for percutaneous stick. Arterial blood can be obtained from radial, brachial, or femoral artery. Radial and brachial arteries are preferred sites. | Maintain sterile technique throughout procedure to decrease risk of infection.<br>Radial and brachial arteries have readily palpable pulses and are easily accessible. |
| 2. If radial artery is selected, collateral circulation to the hand via the ulnar artery should be determined. | Femoral artery usually used as a last resort because of higher incidence of hematoma or infection. |
| *To perform Allen's test:* | The Allen's test is performed to determine collateral circulation to the hand. |
| A. Occlude both radial and ulnar arteries while patient alternately clenches and unclenches the hand. | |
| B. When the hand blanches, release pressure on ulnar artery while maintaining pressure on the radial artery. | |
| C. If the hand quickly becomes pink, collateral circulation is good and the radial site is usable. | |
| 3. Assemble necessary equipment. Arterial blood gas sampling kit may be available. Specific equipment:<br>• 3- or 5-ml syringe.<br>• Rubber or cork cap.<br>• 1-ml ampule heparin (1000 units/ml).<br>• Povidone-iodine or alcohol swabs.<br>• 2 needles: 22 gauge, $1\frac{1}{2}$ inch<br>25 gauge, $\frac{5}{8}$ inch<br>• Gauze pads/dressing. | |
| • Appropriate laboratory request slip with necessary information. | Information on laboratory slip should include: Patient's temperature; fraction of inspired oxygen ($FIO_2$); method of oxygen delivery; ventilator settings if applicable. |
| 4. Prepare heparinized syringe by drawing up heparin from the ampule using the 22-gauge needle. Switch to 25-gauge needle, and, after rinsing syringe barrel with heparin, discard excess heparin and air from the syringe while holding the syringe with needle pointing upward. | Care should be taken to remove excess heparin and air as these may cause results to be inaccurate. |
| 5. Explain to the patient what is to be done and what the expectations might be. | Arterial stick may be uncomfortable.<br>An informed patient may be a cooperative one. |
| 6. Position the patient's wrist in hyperextension by placing a small rolled towel under it, with the palmar surface of the hand facing upward. | Proper positioning makes the artery more accessible, and it is easier to determine point of maximal impulse. |
| 7. Wash hands thoroughly and/or use sterile gloves. | Diligent handwashing helps to decrease risk of infection. |
| 8. Carefully palpate pulse, determining the approximate point for the puncture. | |
| 9. Cleanse site carefully with povidone-iodine or alcohol swab. Start at the puncture site and move outward, using circular motion. Always prep from the center outward. | Minimizes contamination of puncture site. |
| 10. Hold the syringe and needle (bevel up) directly over insertion site, while stabilizing artery with fingers of other hand. | |
| 11. Pierce the skin at approximately a 60-degree angle. As soon as the artery is punctured, blood will forcefully enter the syringe. | Once the skin is penetrated, the high blood pressure within the artery forces blood into the syringe. |
| 12. Collect approximately 2–3 ml blood and withdraw needle and syringe. | |
| 13. Apply firm pressure immediately with one hand. With the other, hold syringe with needle upright to expel any air, and promptly cork or apply a rubber stopper. Place in ice, and have specimen transported to laboratory without delay. | Firm, *continuous* pressure needs to be applied for at least 5 minutes to prevent bleeding and hematoma formation. Remember that the high pressure within the artery can easily cause bleeding at puncture site. |
| 14. After applying continuous, firm pressure to puncture site for 5 minutes, assess site for bleeding and apply pressure dressing. | |
| 15. Leave pressure dressing in place for about 30 minutes, assessing the site periodically. | |

## ARTERIAL BLOOD GASES: DRAWING THE SAMPLE

Arterial blood for blood gas analysis needs to be obtained using an appropriate technique to ensure that the integrity of the sample remains intact, and to prevent complications of bleeding and infection. For specific details related to obtaining the sample, care of the puncture site, and appropriate disposition of the sample, see Tables 30–4 and 30–5.

## REFERENCES


1. Schrier, N: Renal and Electrolyte Disorders. Little, Brown & Co., Boston, 1976, pp 83–101.
2. Broughton, J: Understanding Blood Gases. Ohio Medical Products, a Division of Airco, Inc., Wisconsin, August, 1979, p 5–9.
3. Romanski, S: Interpreting ABGs in four easy steps. Nursing 86 16(9):58, 1986.

CHAPTER 31

# Nursing Management of the Patient with Acute Respiratory Failure

## CHAPTER OUTLINE



## LEARNING OBJECTIVES

**At the end of this chapter, you should be able to:**

1. Define *acute respiratory failure (ARF).*
2. Describe the four pathophysiologic mechanisms that can impair gas exchange and cause hypoxemia:
   a. Alveolar hypoventilation.
   b. Impaired diffusion.
   c. Ventilation/perfusion mismatch.
   d. Intrapulmonary (right to left) shunt.
3. Examine the etiology and pathophysiology of the two types of acute respiratory failure:
   a. Hypercapnic/hypoxemic (alveolar hypoventilation)
   b. Hypoxemic
4. Describe the clinical presentation of acute respiratory failure.
5. Outline the treatment and management of acute respiratory failure.
6. Identify pertinent therapeutic considerations in the nursing care of the patient with acute respiratory failure.

The normal function of the respiratory system is to facilitate gas exchange. Without an adequate exchange of oxygen and carbon dioxide, the metabolic demands of the tissues would remain unfulfilled and body systems would rapidly fail. Many different types of respiratory diseases are capable of disrupting the lung's normal function as a gas-exchanging organ. Some of these cause a mild impairment of gas exchange with no, or relatively few, sequelae; in others, dysfunction is so marked as to predispose to life-threatening consequences.

When respiratory function is compromised to the degree that it can no longer maintain arterial blood gases within an acceptable range, the patient is said to be in respiratory failure. Acute respiratory failure (ARF) requires early recognition and prompt treatment to improve the patient's chances of survival. Successful management of ARF depends largely on its *anticipation* rather than treatment after the fact.

Respiratory failure can develop acutely in the patient without preexisting respiratory disease. The primary cause of the failure may be respiratory in origin, or commonly it may evolve in the patient with an acute illness involving another organ system, which is complicated by respiratory problems. The patient with advanced chronic, preexisting respiratory disease (e.g., chronic obstructive pulmonary disease [COPD]) is at high risk of developing respiratory failure. The underlying limited respiratory reserve may be further compromised by a deterioration of the preexisting pulmonary disease, or by a superimposed infection.

## RESPIRATORY FAILURE: DEFINED

Respiratory failure has been arbitrarily defined as the inability of the respiratory system to maintain adequate gas exchange as reflected by the following arterial blood gas criteria: decreasing pH $<7.25$; decreasing $PaO_2$ $<60$ mmHg; rising $PaCO_2$ $>50$ mmHg; decreasing percent saturation of hemoglobin ($SaO_2$) $<90$. These measurements are taken while the patient is spontaneously breathing ambient (room) air at sea level (760 mmHg).

In determining the acuteness of the respiratory failure, it is essential to consider the pH value, arterial blood gas values, and the patient's clinical history. Respiratory failure is considered to be "acute" if the lungs are unable to maintain adequate oxygenation in a previously healthy person, with or without an impairment of carbon dioxide elimination. The pH value in this instance is abnormal, and its cause is usually reflected (initially) by the presence of at least one grossly abnormal arterial blood gas parameter.

"Chronic" respiratory insufficiency is commonly seen in the patient with chronic obstructive pulmonary disease (COPD) and is characterized by a pH level within the normal physiologic range (7.34–7.45) despite significant abnormalities in both arterial blood gas parameters (e.g., $PaO_2$ $<60$ mmHg, $PaCO_2$ $>55$ mmHg). In the healthy person, these abnormal blood gas values would meet criteria for acute respiratory failure. In the patient with chronic lung disease, these gas parameters, together with an elevated blood bicarbonate level ($>26$ mEq/liter) and an increase in base excess ($>+2$), reflect normal renal compensation for alveolar hypoventilation and carbon dioxide retention characteristic of chronic obstructive pulmonary disease. The fact that the pH is within the normal range reflects the effectiveness of this compensatory mechanism. If there is a significant change from these usual blood gas values for this person, characterized by an abnormal pH, acute respiratory failure may have developed superimposed on the underlying pulmonary disease.

## Gas Exchange Abnormalities

Four pathophysiologic mechanisms can impair gas exchange and contribute to respiratory insufficiency and failure: alveolar hypoventilation, impaired diffusion, ventilation/perfusion mismatch, and intrapulmonary (right to left) shunt.

### *Alveolar Hypoventilation*

Alveolar ventilation ($\dot{V}_A$) is the prime determinant of $PaCO_2$, and an elevation in $PaCO_2$ signals inadequate alveolar ventilation, or alveolar *hypo*ventilation. Alveolar hypoventilation can be caused by a decrease in total minute ventilation ($\dot{V}_E$) or an increase in the proportion of total minute ventilation that is wasted or *dead space* ventilation.

It is characterized by arterial blood gas values that reflect an increase in $PaCO_2$, a decrease in $PaO_2$, and a decrease in percent saturation (oxygenation) of hemoglobin. Any change in the pattern of breathing that decreases tidal volume ($V_T$) and concomitantly increases the respiratory rate can predispose to alveolar hypoventilation.

Treatment of alveolar *hypo*ventilation is to improve alveolar ventilation. Encouraging the patient to cough and deep breathe may be helpful; chest physiotherapy and postural drainage may open up clogged airways; and the use of supplemental oxygen may minimize hypoxemia. Bronchodilators may be indicated to improve $V_A$. A review of all medications taken by the patient is essential to determine if any drug, individually or synergistically with another medication, can depress central nervous system control of ventilation, thereby contributing to alveolar hypoventilation.

### *Diffusion Impairment*

Gas exchange between the alveoli and pulmonary capillaries occurs across the alveolar–capillary membranes, which are normally thin structures, freely permeable to carbon dioxide and oxygen (see Figs. 28–11 and 28–12). Pressure gradients exist between the alveoli and the capillary blood, which provide the driving force for the diffusion of these gases. Gas exchange between the alveoli and the blood occurs very rapidly (about 0.25 second). Because it takes a red blood cell about 0.75 second to traverse the pulmonary capillary bed, there is considerable leeway (reserve) for diffusion, and equilibration of gases to take place. Consequently, only rarely does an impairment in diffusion become significant enough to alter arterial oxygenation.

When diffusion becomes impaired, a physical or anatomical alteration in the alveolar–capillary membrane is usually the cause. Such changes may increase the distance over which gas exchange occurs, or they may alter the permeability of the membrane to oxygen and carbon dioxide. The net result: it takes longer for gas exchange between the alveoli and the blood to be achieved. $PaO_2$ levels and the percent saturation of hemoglobin are mainly affected by diffusion abnormalities because oxygen diffuses about 20 times more slowly than does carbon dioxide.

Diseases implicated as causes of diffusion impairment include: interstitial lung diseases, for example, pulmonary fibrosis (increase in lung parenchymal connective tissue) and sarcoidosis (increase in alveolar wall thickness); and advanced pulmonary edema (fluid within the alveoli reduces surface area for gas exchange; see Fig. 34–1). Decreased pulmonary capillary density/blood volume can also result in diffusion defects.

Treatment of diffusion defects depends on the underlying cause. Inotropic agents (to increase cardiac output) and diuretics may be effective in treating pulmonary edema; anatomical defects associated with pulmonary fibrosis are usually permanent and treatment is supportive/preventive in nature.

#### *Ventilation/Perfusion Mismatch ("Dead Space" Units)*

Effective gas exchange depends largely on the degree to which ventilation is matched with perfusion throughout the lung. Clinically, there is an uneven distribution of ventilation and perfusion so that even when total ventilation and perfusion to each lung are normal, some areas receive more ventilation than perfusion, while others receive more perfusion than ventilation. Normally, these individual areas of the lungs balance out to maintain the overall $PaO_2$ within normal physiologic range. If, however, there is greater than normal variability in these ventilation/perfusion matchups, the overall ratio of ventilation to perfusion is disturbed and hypoxemia develops.

Lung units that are well ventilated, but that are inadequately perfused, reflect ventilation/perfusion mismatching, and such areas are referred to as "dead space" units (see Fig. 28–14). Clinically, an increase in the number of "dead space" units sufficient to cause overall ventilation/perfusion mismatching with hypoxemia can be caused by pulmonary infection, atelectasis, chronic obstructive pulmonary disease, carcinoma of the lung, pulmonary emboli, and left heart insufficiency, among others.

#### *Right-to-Left Shunting ("Shunt" Units)*

Ventilation/perfusion abnormalities may also occur in lung units that have significantly reduced to absent ventilation, but that are well perfused (see Fig. 28–14). Such "units" are termed "shunt" units because they contribute to an overall "right-to-left" intrapulmonary shunt. What this means is that blood passing by nonventilated alveoli remains unoxygenated as it returns to the left heart. The result is a decrease in $PaO_2$ over and above normal physiologic shunting.

The severity and extent of the shunt will determine, in large measure, the degree of hypoxemia. A true right-to-left shunt (i.e., mixing of unoxygenated blood with oxygenated blood upon leaving the pulmonary circulation) differs from the other causes of hypoxemia mentioned above in that even the administration of 100% oxygen concentrations ($FIO_2$) may not improve the shunting problem or relieve the hypoxemia.

Major causes of right-to-left shunting in the adult patient include adult respiratory distress syndrome, pneumonia, atelectasis, and oxygen toxicity, among others. Treatment involves administration of oxygen with ventilatory support. Positive end-expiratory pressure (PEEP) is frequently implemented. Vigorous therapy directed at correcting the underlying cause is employed.

In general, because many disease processes have several pathophysiologic abnormalities, it is not at all uncommon to see more than one of the above hypoxemia-producing mechanisms in a particular patient.

## CLASSIFICATION OF ACUTE RESPIRATORY FAILURE

Respiratory failure is broadly categorized into two types based on the pattern of blood gas abnormalities: (1) *hypercapnic/hypoxemic* (alveolar hypoventilation)—those patients in whom the $PaCO_2$ is greater than 45 mmHg, accompanied by a less than normal $PaO_2$; and (2) *hypoxemic*—those patients in whom the $PaO_2$ is less than 50 mmHg while the $PaCO_2$ is normal to low.

### Hypercapnic/Hypoxemic Respiratory Failure

In hypercapnic/hypoxemic respiratory failure, as the term reflects, hypercapnia and hypoxemia occur together. The primary mechanism causing hypercapnia is *alveolar hypoventilation*. The low $PaO_2$ is associated with an altered alveolar $PaO_2$ commensurate with the increase in $PaCO_2$. This form of respiratory failure is also characterized by an abnormal pH, which reflects the absence of or incomplete renal compensation for respiratory acidemia, which occurs secondarily to the elevated $PaCO_2$.

### Pathophysiology

The pathophysiology underlying hypercapnic/hypoxemic respiratory failure is the inability of the patient to maintain alveolar ventilation at a level sufficient to eliminate carbon dioxide while keeping the $PaO_2$ within an acceptable range ($PaO_2 > 60$ mmHg). Physiologically, effective alveolar ventilation requires an intact series of interconnected anatomical–physiologic "links." It is essential to review these links because a disturbance of more than one link in this cycle (Fig. 31–1) contributes largely to alveolar hypoventilation and hypercapnic/hypoxemic respiratory failure.

These links include: (1) the pons and medullary center; (2) the neuromuscular connections from the respiratory center to the chest cage; (3) the chest bellows or chest cage itself, and respiratory musculature; (4) patent airways; and (5) intact alveoli.

Major questions that need to be considered in hypercapnic/hypoxemic respiratory failure include: What is the total minute ventilation? What proportion of the total minute ventilation effectively eliminates carbon dioxide (alveolar ventilation)? What proportion constitutes dead space (i.e., ventilation without perfusion)? A decrease in total minute ventilation and/or a marked increase in the proportion of each breath going to dead space can seriously compromise alveolar ventilation, with a consequent fall in $PaO_2$ and rise in $PaCO_2$, despite the maintenance of seemingly adequate total minute ventilation ($\dot{V}_E$).

In addition to alveolar hypoventilation, $PaO_2$ may be further compromised in hypercapnic/hypoxemic respiratory failure by an impairment of the matchup between alveolar ventilation and capillary perfusion (i.e., ventilation/perfusion *mismatch*).

### Etiology

Drug overdose is usually considered to be the purest form of hypercapnic/hypoxemic respiratory failure. This form of failure frequently develops in patients with preexisting pulmonary disease, which compromises pulmonary function and reduces respiratory reserve. Central nervous system depres-

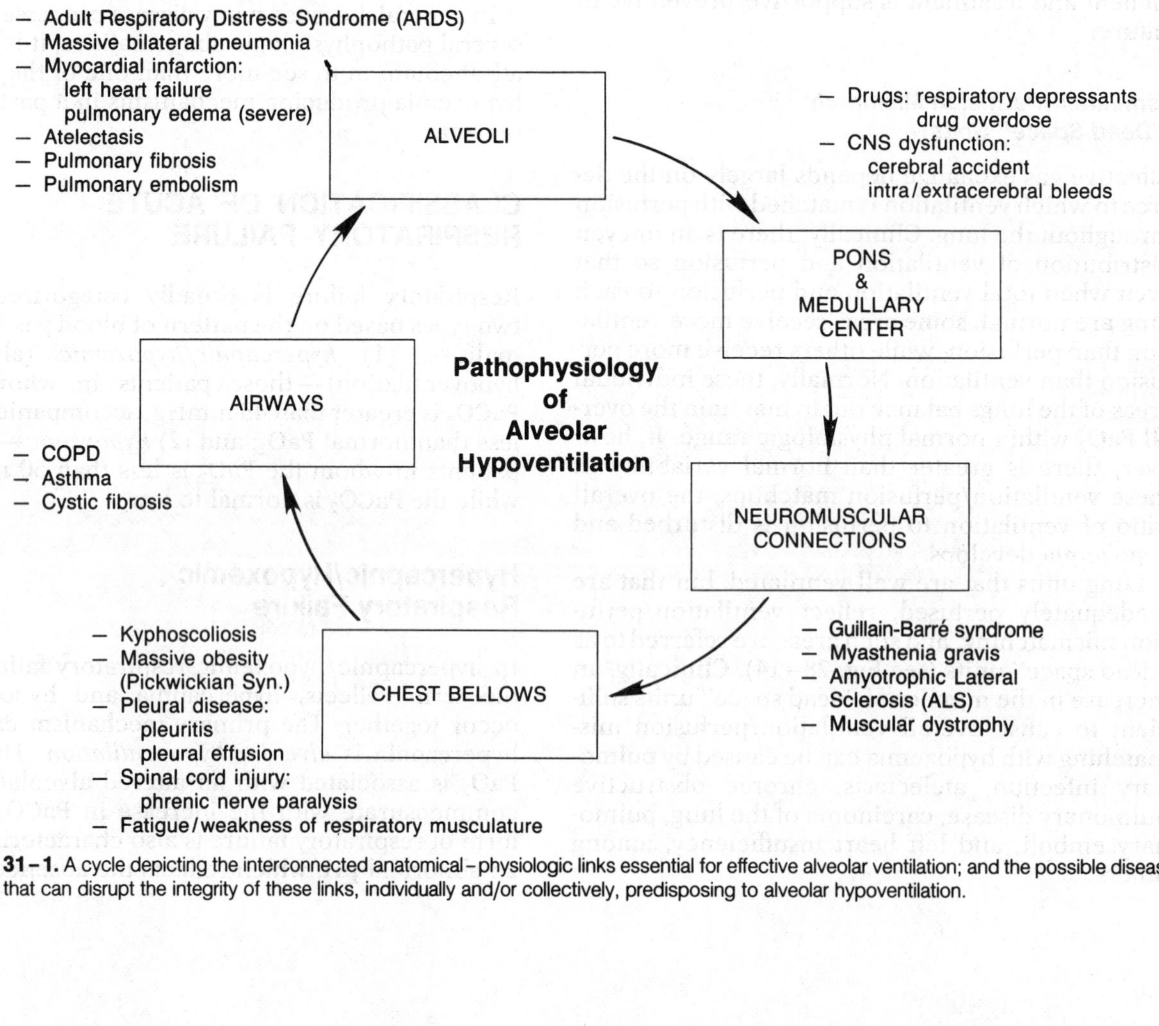


**Figure 31–1.** A cycle depicting the interconnected anatomical–physiologic links essential for effective alveolar ventilation; and the possible disease entities that can disrupt the integrity of these links, individually and/or collectively, predisposing to alveolar hypoventilation.

sion, neuromuscular disease, disorders of the chest cage (respiratory bellows), and airway disease have all been implicated in this form of respiratory failure. The patient with longstanding chronic obstructive pulmonary disease is a classic example of a person who can function well within the limitations imposed by his/her disease process, but in whom pulmonary function can rapidly deteriorate when the person develops an upper respiratory infection. This infection, superimposed on the underlying pulmonary disease, pushes the patient "over the brink," and acute respiratory failure may ultimately ensue (Table 31-1).

## Hypoxemic Respiratory Failure

*Hypoxemic* respiratory failure is characterized by an acute hypoxemia ($PaO_2$ <50-60 mmHg), with normal to low arterial carbon dioxide tension ($PaCO_2 \leq 35$ mmHg).

### Pathophysiology

The major pathophysiologic mechanisms underlying the hypoxemia usually involve a combination of *ventilation/perfusion mismatching* and *right-to-left shunting* (see Fig. 28-14). A decrease in ventilation relative to perfusion occurs, for example, in areas of the lung where alveoli are partially or completely filled with fluid or exudate (see Fig. 34-1). Ventilation may become significantly compromised or totally absent, whereas perfusion to the region remains relatively preserved. Similarly, disruption of airway patency, either by structural pathology of the airway wall or by secretions within the lumen, reduces and limits alveolar ventilation.

In other areas of the lung that have a high ventilation/perfusion ratio (ventilation in excess of perfusion), hypoxemia becomes a function of greater than normal dead space ventilation. Of particular interest is that, despite the marked derangement in oxygenation, overall carbon dioxide elimination remains adequate as reflected by normal to low $PaCO_2$.

Localized compensatory reflex responses of pulmonary tissue to alveolar carbon dioxide tension ($PaCO_2$) normally function to closely match ventilation with perfusion. A low $PaCO_2$ associated with high ventilation/low perfusion (dead space unit) causes contraction of airway smooth muscle, which increases airway resistance and, thus, decreases ventilation to the particular unit. In contrast, a high $PaCO_2$ associated with low ventilation/high perfusion (shunt unit), causes relaxation of airway smooth muscle, which decreases airway resistance and, thus, increases ventilation to the particular unit.

The response of the pulmonary vasculature to ventilation/perfusion mismatch is to constrict, thereby limiting perfusion to poorly ventilated or nonventilated areas of the lung, while shunting blood to areas of increased ventilation. When these intrapulmonary protective mechanisms are unable to compensate fully for the ventilation/perfusion mismatch, hypoxemia results. (For a review of ventilation/perfusion relationships, local and central nervous system control of ventilation, see Chap. 28).

### Etiology

Adult respiratory distress syndrome (ARDS) is a major form of hypoxemic respiratory failure. Atelectasis, pneumonia, pulmonary embolism, and chronic obstructive pulmonary disease, among

TABLE 31-1
**Comparison: Hypercapnic/Hypoxemic and Hypoxemic Respiratory Failure[1]**

| | Hypercapnic/Hypoxemic | Hypoxemic |
|---|---|---|
| Incidence | Relatively common. | Common. |
| Clinical history | Usually longstanding antecedent chronic obstructive pulmonary disease (COPD).<br>Evidence of neurologic, neuromuscular disorders; chest cage defect; impaired airway patency. | Usually normal lung function prior to acute pulmonary insult. |
| Underlying pathophysiologic mechanism | Alveolar hypoventilation.<br>Some ventilation/perfusion mismatching. | Ventilation/perfusion mismatching.<br>Right-to-left intrapulmonary shunting. |
| Typical arterial blood gas values | $\downarrow PaO_2$; $\uparrow PaCO_2$ | $\downarrow PaO_2$; $PaCO_2$ normal or $\downarrow$ |
| Resting lung volume | May be high (e.g., emphysema). | Low. |
| Lung compliance | Increased. | Decreased. |
| Alveolar ventilation ($V_A$) | Decreased. | Increased. |
| Assisted ventilation | COPD: Avoid, if titrated oxygen therapy and airway therapy effective.<br>Others: Criteria for intubation and mechanical ventilatory assistance (see Chap. 32). | Early institution. |

others, have also been implicated in this type of respiratory failure.

## Acute Respiratory Failure: Clinical Presentation

When patients develop acute respiratory failure (ARF), their symptom complex usually includes the manifestations of hypoxemia and/or hypercapnia and the specific symptomatology associated with the underlying precipitating disorder.

The signs and symptoms of hypoxemia, hypercapnia, and consequent acidemia are widespread, involving all major body systems. It is essential for the critical care nurse to appreciate the underlying etiology, pathophysiology, and clinical presentation of ARF. Patients at high risk of developing ARF can be identified, and the early, often subtle signs and symptoms of ARF can be recognized, thus preventing actual respiratory arrest. It is *anticipatory* nursing care that largely impacts on the successful management of the patient with, or at risk of developing, ARF. Pertinent signs and symptoms of hypoxemia and hypercapnia are presented in Table 31-2.

## Treatment and Management of Acute Respiratory Failure

Acute respiratory failure (ARF) reflects the inability of patients to maintain adequate gas exchange. While in some cases impairment of gas exchange is mild and responsive to "conservative" therapeutic techniques, in others it may be life-threatening, requiring emergency intervention. The survival of these patients depends on their ability to maintain adequate gas exchange over the course of the respiratory failure with the aid of timely, aggressive, and supportive forms of therapy. By supporting gas exchange for as long a period as necessary, the patient can be maintained while the underlying pathophysiologic process causing the failure is treated or allowed to resolve spontaneously.

The overall goal of treatment and management of ARF is to "normalize" the disturbed gas exchange and maintain the $PaO_2$ and pH. Normal gas exchange involves the adequate uptake of oxygen by the blood, transport of oxygen to the tissues, and the elimination of carbon dioxide. It requires a well-coordinated effort on the part of the central nervous system, which provides the rhythmic drive to breathe, and innervates the diaphragm and muscular apparatus of the chest wall to facilitate ventilation. It requires an intact cardiovascular system,

TABLE 31-2
**Hypoxemia and Hypercapnia: Effects on Bodily Functions**

| Bodily Function | Physiologic Responses |
|---|---|
| Neurologic | Mental status: Confusion, disorientation, impaired judgment, drowsiness, lethargy, eventual lapse into coma.<br>Headache (increase in cerebral blood flow associated with cerebral vasodilatation).<br>Cerebral edema with consequent increase in intracranial pressure; papilledema (profound hypercapnia). |
| Cardiovascular | Sympathetic nervous system response: Tachycardia, increase in cardiac contractility.<br>Anxiety and restlessness.<br>Peripheral vasoconstriction: increase in systolic blood pressure (early).<br>Skin cool and dry.<br>Acidemia (lactic acidemia with severe hypercapnia):<br>Depression of cardiac function—Decreased automaticity, cardiac dysrhythmias, decreased cardiac contractility; chest pain (tissue hypoxia); weakness and fatigue.<br>Later responses: Peripheral vasodilatation with hypotension, diaphoresis with cool moist skin.<br>Hypoxia (severe): Central cyanosis. |
| Respiratory | Acidemia (increase in $PaCO_2$, and hydrogen-ion concentration with stimulation of peripheral and central chemoreceptors): Increase in respiratory rate, depth and pattern of breathing. Hyperventilation may initially cause hypocapnia, tachypnea, dyspnea. (Dyspnea, when present, usually reflects the increased work of breathing; nasal flaring and use of accessory muscles of respiration may be observed.)<br>Alveolar hypoxia: Reduced alveolar ventilation is a potent stimulus for vasoconstriction of pulmonary vasculature, resulting in pulmonary hypertension over time. Right ventricular work is increased, predisposing to cor pulmonale and right heart failure. |
| Renal | Sympathetic nervous system response: Increased peripheral vasoconstriction may reduce renal perfusion and decrease urine formation.<br>Acute tubular necrosis often accompanies severe hypoxemia and hypercapnia associated with acute respiratory failure. |
| Gastrointestinal | Sympathetic nervous system response: Vasoconstriction of splanchnic circulation reduces blood flow to the gastrointestinal tract, predisposing to tissue ischemia with consequent paralytic ileus, gastric/intestinal ulceration, mesenteric infarction, and digestive disturbances. |

which functions to maintain an adequate blood flow and, therefore, effective transport of oxygen and carbon dioxide between the tissues and the lungs.

To achieve optimal oxygen transport to the tissues it is essential to maintain: arterial oxygen tension ($PaO_2$) >60 mmHg; percent oxygenation of hemoglobin ($SaO_2$) >90; an acceptable hemoglobin level within the blood (hemoglobin >12 g/100 ml; hematocrit ~37%–42%); and an adequate cardiac output (~5 liters/minute).[2]

Carbon dioxide elimination by way of the lungs is essential for maintaining acid–base balance. In managing patients with ARF who have impaired elimination of carbon dioxide, the primary goal is to achieve a pH within the acceptable physiologic range (7.35–7.45) and not necessarily a "normal" $PaCO_2$. This distinction is particularly important in patients with a hypercapnic/hypoxemic form of ARF who have a prior history of chronic respiratory disease with chronic hypercapnia ($PaCO_2$ >55 mmHg). An abrupt restoration of the $PaCO_2$ to normal ($PaCO_2$ 35–45 mmHg) in these patients can result in alkalemia and serious complications (e.g., cardiac dysrhythmias, seizures, among others).

In contrast, treatment and management of patients with the hypoxemic form of ARF who have previously healthy lungs are focused on "normalizing" the disturbed gas parameters in achieving a pH within the normal physiologic range. It is important to appreciate the principles that underlie the distinct approaches to treating each of these forms of acute respiratory failure.

In general, the treatment and management of ARF may fall into one or more of the following categories:[3] First, treatment is focused on the underlying disease or illness that is the primary cause of ARF. Examples include the use of a narcotic antagonist to treat opiate overdose; antibiotics for pneumonias or other infections; and treatment for other medical problems that may be exacerbated by co-existing ARF (e.g., cor pulmonale; fluid, electrolyte, and acid–base imbalance; or stress ulcer).

Second, if the ARF is mild (e.g., postoperatively), "conservative" techniques may be employed as the basis for therapy. These include supplemental oxygen with humidification; deep breathing with incentive spirometry, chest physiotherapy, deep coughing and nasotracheal suctioning, to mobilize and remove secretions; and use of aerosolized catecholamines (e.g., metaproterenol) and theophylline derivatives to relieve bronchospasm. Supplemental oxygen administered to patients who have ARF superimposed on an underlying chronic respiratory disease (e.g., emphysema, chronic bronchitis) must be carefully controlled to avoid suppressing the *hypoxic* drive (i.e., a decrease in the $PaO_2$ in the scenario of a chronically elevated $PaCO_2$, as the stimulus for breathing).

### Role of Oxygen Therapy

In acute respiratory failure, when the ventilation/perfusion ratio is high (i.e., ventilation exceeds perfusion, resulting in increased dead space ventilation), administration of supplemental oxygen is very effective in relieving hypoxemia. If, however, the ventilation/perfusion ratio is low (i.e., perfusion exceeds ventilation, resulting in increased right-to-left shunting), even high fractions of inspired oxygen ($FIO_2$ >60 mmHg) may be ineffective in relieving the hypoxemia. Therefore, it often becomes necessary to institute mechanical ventilation with positive end-expiratory pressure (PEEP).

The addition of positive airway pressure above that of ambient air at the end of exhalation (i.e., PEEP) functions to increase functional residual capacity (FRC). The consequent airway distention and alveolar expansion improve alveolar ventilation and help to balance the distribution of inspired gas throughout the lung, thus improving the ventilation/perfusion ratio.

For patients with acute, decompensating respiratory failure in whom gas exchange is seriously compromised ($PaO_2$ <50 mmHg; $PaCO_2$ >50 mmHg), treatment and management involve timely and aggressive respiratory support therapy. This includes oxygen therapy, chest physiotherapy, bronchial hygiene, airway management, and mechanical ventilation. These therapeutic modalities are examined more closely in Chapter 32.

## Nursing Care of the Patient with Acute Respiratory Failure

Patients with, or at risk of developing, acute respiratory failure present the critical care nurse with some of the most difficult management problems encountered in the nursing care of critically ill patients. It is here that the application of pulmonary physiologic principles to patient treatment and management is most evident and most crucial. To provide effective, intensive respiratory care, the critical care nurse must master basic concepts of pulmonary physiology, gain an indepth understanding of pulmonary disease, and appreciate the relationship between disease and its consequent impact on overall lung function.

Severe physiologic stress potentially affects all organ systems of the body, irrespective of primary etiology or pathophysiology. The lungs are especially vulnerable to such stress, which is why pulmonary dysfunction is so prevalent in critically ill patients. Pneumonia, for example, is one of the most frequently occurring *nosocomial* infections in critically ill patients, and every critically ill patient should be considered to be at high risk of developing pulmonary complications.

As the health-care providers most intimately involved in the care of the critically ill patient, the critical care nurse functions to coordinate all aspects of patient care. With a sound knowledge of the physiology of breathing and with keenly sharpened assessment skills, the nurse closely monitors the patient's responses to therapy, following trends and recognizing subtle, yet significant changes in the patient's condition.

In the patient with acute asthma, for example, the astute nurse recognizes that subtle changes in the patient's breathing pattern accompanied by diminishing breath sounds, and seemingly "normalizing" arterial blood gases may not reflect improvement in the patient's condition but rather, a progressive deterioration (see Fig. 32–4). As the work of breathing increasingly tires the patient, alveolar ventilation becomes compromised and ARF may quickly ensue. Appropriate pharmacologic management, deep breathing, chest physiotherapy, and bronchial hygiene can help to prevent the need for intubation, and can largely determine whether the patient improves or proceeds to acute respiratory failure, with the necessary institution of mechanical ventilation therapy.

Should mechanical ventilation therapy be initiated, the nurse provides meticulous, supportive care to ensure optimal benefit to the patient. Such care provides temporary support, which prevents complications, while maintaining bodily processes until the patient recovers effective, spontaneous, physiologic function. During the weaning period, the nurse plays a pivotal role in assisting patients to gain confidence in their capabilities until they are able to reestablish and maintain their respiratory function independently.

Successful management of ARF, or its prevention, requires that the critical care nurse employ an approach to patient care that is anticipatory and preventive in scope, astute in observation and recognition of significant clinical data, and timely, pertinent, and energetic in instituting therapies to alleviate and/or ameliorate dysfunction reflected by these clinical data.

The immediate therapeutic goals in the treatment and management of the patient with ARF are to relieve the hypoxemia and return the pH to within the acceptable physiologic range. Nursing care is focused on the following therapeutic considerations:

1. Thorough and meticulous ongoing assessment and monitoring the patient's overall condition.
2. Establishing and maintaining a patent airway (Chap. 32).
3. Providing appropriate ventilatory support and oxygenation to relieve the hypoxemia, hypercapnia, and consequent respiratory acidemia.
4. Providing necessary cardiovascular support to maintain cardiac output and reduce occurrence of tissue hypoxia.
5. Treating the underlying primary disease.
6. Administering prescribed drug therapy and monitoring the patient's response to therapy.
7. Maintaining hydration and nutrition.
8. Correcting and/or maintaining fluid and electrolyte balance.
9. Preventing complications related to mechanical ventilation and artificial airway management; and to hypoxemia and acid–base imbalances (e.g., confusion, tremors, seizures, cardiac dysrhythmias).
10. Preventing infection.
11. Providing emotional and psychologic support to patient and family.
12. Assisting the patient to maintain optimal physical function and performance of activities of daily living.

Details related to these therapeutic goals are examined more closely in the following chapters. Specific nursing diagnoses and care plans are included in the discussions of respiratory pathophysiology that follow.

## REFERENCES


1. King, G: Respiratory failure in the critically ill. In Sibbald, WJ (ed): Synopsis of Critical Care, ed. 3. Williams & Wilkins, Baltimore, 1988, p 53.
2. Weinberger, SE: Principles of Pulmonary Medicine. WB Saunders, Philadelphia, 1986, pp 311–312.
3. Ayres, S, Schlichtig, R, and Sterling, M: Care of the Critically Ill, ed 3. Year Book Medical Publishers, Chicago, 1988, pp 223, 243.

CHAPTER 32

# Therapeutic Modalities in the Treatment of the Patient with Acute Respiratory Dysfunction

## CHAPTER OUTLINE



## LEARNING OBJECTIVES

**At the end of this chapter, you should be able to:**

1. State the primary goal of oxygen therapy and indications for its use.
2. Describe the effectiveness of oxygen therapy in the treatment of hypercapnic/hypoxemic and hypoxemic forms of acute respiratory failure.
3. List complications of oxygen therapy.
4. Define underlying principles of oxygen therapy.
5. Describe techniques of chest physiotherapy-bronchial hygiene, and indications for their use.
6. Describe procedure for use of incentive spirometry devices.
7. Identify the major goal and risks of airway management.
8. List common causes and the clinical presentation of airway obstruction.
9. Describe types of artificial airways in current use and discuss implications for nursing care.
10. Identify primary goals of and clinical indications for mechanical ventilation therapy.
11. Describe types of mechanical ventilators in current use, modes of ventilatory assistance, ventilator controls, and guidelines for adjustment.
12. Specify complications of mechanical ventilation therapy.
13. Outline major nursing considerations in the ongoing monitoring of the patient receiving mechanical ventilation therapy.
14. Describe indications for and basic approaches to the weaning process.

A continuous supply of oxygen to the tissues is essential to sustain cellular metabolism, prevent tissue hypoxia, and maintain life processes of the person in an equilibrated state. Factors that determine the concentration of oxygen in arterial blood (i.e., $PaO_2$) include the degree of alveolar ventilation ($PAO_2$), the fraction of inspired oxygen ($FIO_2$), the percent saturation of available hemoglobin ($SaO_2$), and the distribution of ventilation and perfusion within the lungs.

*Hypoxemia,* defined as subnormal oxygenation of arterial blood with a $PaO_2$ <60 mmHg and percent saturation of hemoglobin ($SaO_2$) <90%, develops when there is a significant alteration in the physiologic status of any one or more of these factors. Hypoxemia is a feature of virtually all patients with acute respiratory failure (ARF) when they are breathing ambient air.

Regardless of its underlying cause, treatment of hypoxemia may require an increase in alveolar ventilation, an increase in the fraction of inspired oxygen, and therapy designed to reduce ventilation/perfusion (V/(Q) mismatch and intrapulmonary (right-to-left) shunting.

Treatment and management of hypoxemia involve timely and aggressive respiratory support therapy. This includes oxygen therapy, chest physiotherapy and bronchial hygiene, airway management, and mechanical ventilation. These therapeutic modalities, together with implications for nursing care, are examined more closely in the discussion that follows.

## OXYGEN THERAPY

### Therapeutic Goals

The purpose of oxygen therapy is to relieve hypoxemia and prevent tissue hypoxia. Although the basic treatment of hypoxemia is the treatment of its cause, the immediate potentially life-threatening problem may be tissue hypoxia as a consequence of the severely lowered $PaO_2$. Tissue hypoxia is assumed to be present at a $PaO_2$ <60 mmHg and a lowered $SaO_2$ <90%. Thus, regardless of the underlying cause of hypoxemia, oxygen is the initial and perhaps most important drug in its treatment.

The effectiveness of oxygen therapy in restoring a $PaO_2$ >60 mmHg depends largely on the type of ARF. For example, one type is *hypercapnic/hypoxemic* failure as seen in chronic lung disease; another is *hypoxemic* failure, commonly associated with adult respiratory distress syndrome (ARDS) (see Chap. 31). In the former, ventilation/perfusion mismatch and chronic alveolar hypoventilation are the underlying pathophysiologic mechanisms responsible for hypoxemia. Administration of supplemental oxygen in relatively low concentrations ($FIO_2$ <40%) is very effective in improving the $PaO_2$ and relieving the hypoxemia in this clinical circumstance.

In the setting of hypoxemic respiratory failure, ventilation/perfusion mismatch and right-to-left shunting are the underlying pathophysiologic mechanisms largely responsible for hypoxemia. When the fraction of the cardiac output that is "shunted" through the lungs (i.e., does not achieve oxygenation) is large, supplemental oxygen even at higher concentrations ($FIO_2$ 60%–100%) is relatively ineffective at raising the $PaO_2$ >60 mmHg. In this setting, it is often necessary to resort to mechanical ventilation with positive end-respiratory pressure (PEEP).

### Dosage and Methods of Oxygen Administration

#### Low-Flow Oxygen Systems[1]

Low-flow oxygen systems may provide either high or low $FIO_2$ at flow rates less than the patient's inspiratory demand. *Nasal catheters* and *cannulas* are the most commonly used devices for administering low-flow oxygen, and they can provide from 24 to 50% oxygen at flow rates up to 6 liters/minute. The actual $FIO_2$ delivered depends on changes in oxygen flow rate, inspiratory flow, and minute ventilation.

Simple *oxygen masks* deliver approximately 35 to 50% oxygen with flow rates of 5 liters/minute, or greater. *Masks with reservoir* (rebreathing or nonrebreathing) are capable of delivering a high $FIO_2$ >50%. A more recent method of oxygen delivery for patients requiring continuous oxygen therapy is use of the transtracheal oxygen delivery system wherein a small (16-gauge) needle is inserted percutaneously into the trachea. This method achieves higher oxygenation at lower flow rates.[2]

#### High-Flow Oxygen Systems[1]

*High-flow* oxygen systems can provide flow rates that completely satisfy the patient's inspiratory demand, either by entrainment of ambient air or by a high flow of gas. These systems can provide either high or low $FIO_2$.

*Venturi masks* are designed to deliver 24 to 28% oxygen at flow rates of 4–6 liters/minute to ensure the desired $FIO_2$. At oxygen concentrations >30%, the $FIO_2$ may not be as predictable because of inadequate and/or variable total flow rates.

*Reservoir nebulizers* and *humidifiers* with aerosol masks, face tents, CPAP masks, T-tubes, or tracheostomy collars provide both supplemental oxygen and increased water vapor or mist.

## Complications of Oxygen Therapy

It is essential for the critical care nurse to be familiar with adverse effects of oxygen therapy. Some of these include oxygen toxicity, absorption atelectasis, oxygen-induced hypoventilation, drying of respiratory mucosa, and psychologic dependence.

### *Oxygen Toxicity*

Oxygen toxicity is associated with long-term exposure to high inspired oxygen concentrations ($FIO_2$ >60% for more than 2–3 days). Topical damage to alveolar tissue may lead to the development of a thickened alveolar–capillary membrane with consequent diffusion impairment. The *free radical theory* of oxygen toxicity suggests that an increase in the rate of generation of partially reduced oxygen products (i.e., free radicals, as, for example, superoxide, hydrogen peroxide, and hydroxyl radical) within the lungs is responsible for the *cytotoxicity* of oxygen. Oxygen reduction products interact with cellular components, leading to overall structural and metabolic changes, which may eventually result in the death of the cell.

Early signs and symptoms of oxygen toxicity may include restlessness, chest pain, dyspnea, malaise, lethargy, anorexia, nausea and vomiting, and paresthesias in the extremities. Later signs and symptoms reflect progressive respiratory difficulty with dyspnea, cyanosis, and asphyxia.

The underlying pathophysiology of oxygen toxicity remains undefined. Because the therapeutic effect of oxygen entails the risk of adverse reactions, its use should be based on an assessment of the potential toxicity versus its therapeutic benefit.

### *Absorption Atelectasis*

Breathing high concentrations of oxygen increases alveolar oxygen tension ($PAO_2$), while decreasing the level of nitrogen. Unlike nitrogen, which is inert and has a slower rate of diffusion, oxygen is continuously being taken up by the blood. If an alveolus should become occluded (e.g., secretions), the oxygen within it will diffuse more rapidly than the inert nitrogen it replaced, thus leading to alveolar collapse and atelectasis.

### *Oxygen-Induced Hypoventilation*

This complication is seen in patients who develop acute respiratory failure superimposed on chronic lung disease. The increased carbon dioxide tension associated with chronic alveolar hypoventilation causes the patient's respiratory centers to become insensitive to normal fluctuations in $PaCO_2$. As a consequence, the patient's respiratory stimulus becomes a low arterial oxygen tension or *hypoxic* drive. Administration of oxygen in concentrations sufficient to obliterate this hypoxic drive may cause apnea. This is the underlying reason for administering supplemental oxygen at controlled low concentrations in patients with hypercapnic/hypoxemic respiratory failure.

### *Drying of Respiratory Mucosa*

Drying of the respiratory mucosa occurs if oxygen is administered without humidification. It results in a thickening of respiratory secretions with disruption of the integrity of the respiratory epithelium (see Fig. 28–2). Mucosal bleeding may occur, and the patient is at increased risk of developing retained secretions, leading to atelectasis or infection.

### *Psychologic Dependence*

Long-term oxygen therapy may induce psychologic dependence because patients associate oxygen gas flow with relief of their "shortness of breath."

## Principles of Oxygen Therapy

For a review of basic principles of oxygen therapy, see Table 32–1.

# CHEST PHYSIOTHERAPY–BRONCHIAL HYGIENE

## Therapeutic Goals

Retained pulmonary secretions predispose to atelectasis and infection (e.g., pneumonia) with a consequent increase in ventilation/perfusion mismatch and right-to-left shunting. The end result is hypoxemia with tissue hypoxia.

*Chest physiotherapy* is a series of manipulative assistive techniques designed to be both preventative and therapeutic. Chest physiotherapy techniques, in conjunction with bronchial hygiene (pulmonary toilet), assist in mobilizing bronchial secretions, facilitating their removal from the respiratory tract, and preventing accumulation of secretions within the tracheobronchial tree.

By eliminating potential airway obstructions, these techniques improve ventilation and its distribution within the lungs. They function to establish a more equal matching of ventilation with perfusion. Chest physiotherapy techniques assist the patient to develop more efficient use of the respiratory musculature. Respiratory exercises and overall physical conditioning improve cardiopulmonary reserve.

TABLE 32-1
**Principles of Oxygen Therapy**[3]

1. A patent airway must be maintained. Oxygen therapy is of no use without a patent airway.
2. Oxygen is a potent drug and, as such, should be administered in a prescribed dose (the $FIO_2$ is the dose) and evaluated for desired, as well as adverse effects.
3. If high concentrations are necessary, duration of administration should be kept to a minimum and reduced as soon as possible.
4. The goal is to maintain $PaO_2$ greater than 60 mmHg to produce acceptable saturation of hemoglobin ($SaO_2$ >90%) without damaging lungs or causing carbon dioxide retention.
5. Response to oxygen therapy should be evaluated in terms of its effect on tissue oxygenation rather than its effect on arterial blood gas values alone.
6. Periodic arterial blood gas monitoring is a necessary assessment parameter when oxygen concentrations above 40% are administered.
7. The pathophysiology of the patient's disease is a major determinant of the effectiveness of oxygen therapy.
8. Delivered concentrations of gas from low-flow or high-flow oxygen systems are subject to the condition of the equipment, technique of application, cooperation of the patient, and the rate, depth, and pattern of the patient's ventilations. Oxygen analyzers should be used periodically to determine actual $FIO_2$.
9. Low-flow oxygen systems do not provide the total inspired gas (patient is breathing some ambient air) and, therefore, are effective only if tidal volume is adequate, respiratory rates are not excessive, and the ventilatory pattern is stable. Variable oxygen concentrations of 21%-90+% are provided, but the $FIO_2$ varies greatly with changes in tidal volume and breathing patterns.
10. High-flow oxygen systems provide the entire inspired gas (patient is breathing only the gas supplied by the apparatus) and are adequate only if flow rates exceed inspiratory flow rate and minute ventilation. Both high and low oxygen concentrations may be delivered by high-flow systems ($FIO_2$ 24%-100%).
11. Concerns about "oxygen toxicity" should *never* prevent adequate oxygenation of the patient. While the phenomenon of oxygen toxicity is very real, hypoxemia "kills."

Techniques of chest physiotherapy include postural drainage, percussion and vibration techniques, deep breathing exercises, incentive spirometry, and intermittent positive-pressure breathing. A systematic approach to the implementation of these techniques should be used.[4,5]

### Postural Drainage

Postural drainage employs the effect of gravity to assist in drainage of secretions from the lungs. It assists in propelling mobilized secretions from the lungs toward the trachea from where they can be suctioned or coughed up, and either swallowed or expectorated.

Positions used in postural drainage are based on the segmental anatomy of each lung (see Fig. 28-1 and 28-3). Appropriate positioning of the patient to drain affected lung areas requires a familiarity with this segmental anatomy. Specific postural positions and lung areas drained are depicted in Figure 32-1.

### Percussion and Vibration Techniques

Percussion and vibration are used after the patient has been placed in a desired postural position. These techniques function to vibrate the thoracic cage and lungs, which helps to mechanically loosen and/or dislodge secretions from within the smaller airways. The increased velocity of exhalation facilitated by these vibratory techniques helps to loosen secretions and propel them toward the large bronchi and trachea from where they are accessible to coughing and/or suctioning.

### Deep Breathing Exercises

Deep breathing exercises promote maximum alveolar ventilation with increased aeration to underventilated areas of the lungs. They help to maintain functional residual capacity (FRC is the volume of gas remaining in the lungs at the end of normal expiration, i.e., the expiratory reserve plus the residual volumes) and prevent atelectasis.

Patients who have progressive chronic obstructive pulmonary disease can be taught "pursed-lip breathing." This type of breathing prevents early airway collapse and air-trapping within the lungs during exhalation. It also helps to reduce the respiratory rate.

### Incentive Spirometry

An incentive spirometry device is prescribed to encourage the patient to participate in intermittent deep breathing maneuvers.[6] A procedure for using incentive spirometry devices is included in Table 32-2.[7]

### Intermittent Positive-Pressure Breathing

Intermittent positive-pressure breathing (IPPB) is a therapeutic modality that increases the flow of gas into the lungs during inspiration by applying intermittent positive pressure (i.e., higher than atmospheric) to the airways. This technique can generate large inspiratory volumes in patients who otherwise will not or can not take deep breaths on their own. The periodic deep breath provided by IPPB therapy assists to reduce atelectasis and to achieve optimal peripheral distribution of the inspired air.

IPPB therapy is not without its disadvantages or complications. Among the complications associated with IPPB, *barotrauma* (i.e., air in extra-alveolar locations caused by positive-pressure breathing), is one of the most common. Examples of barotrauma include pneumothorax, subcutane-

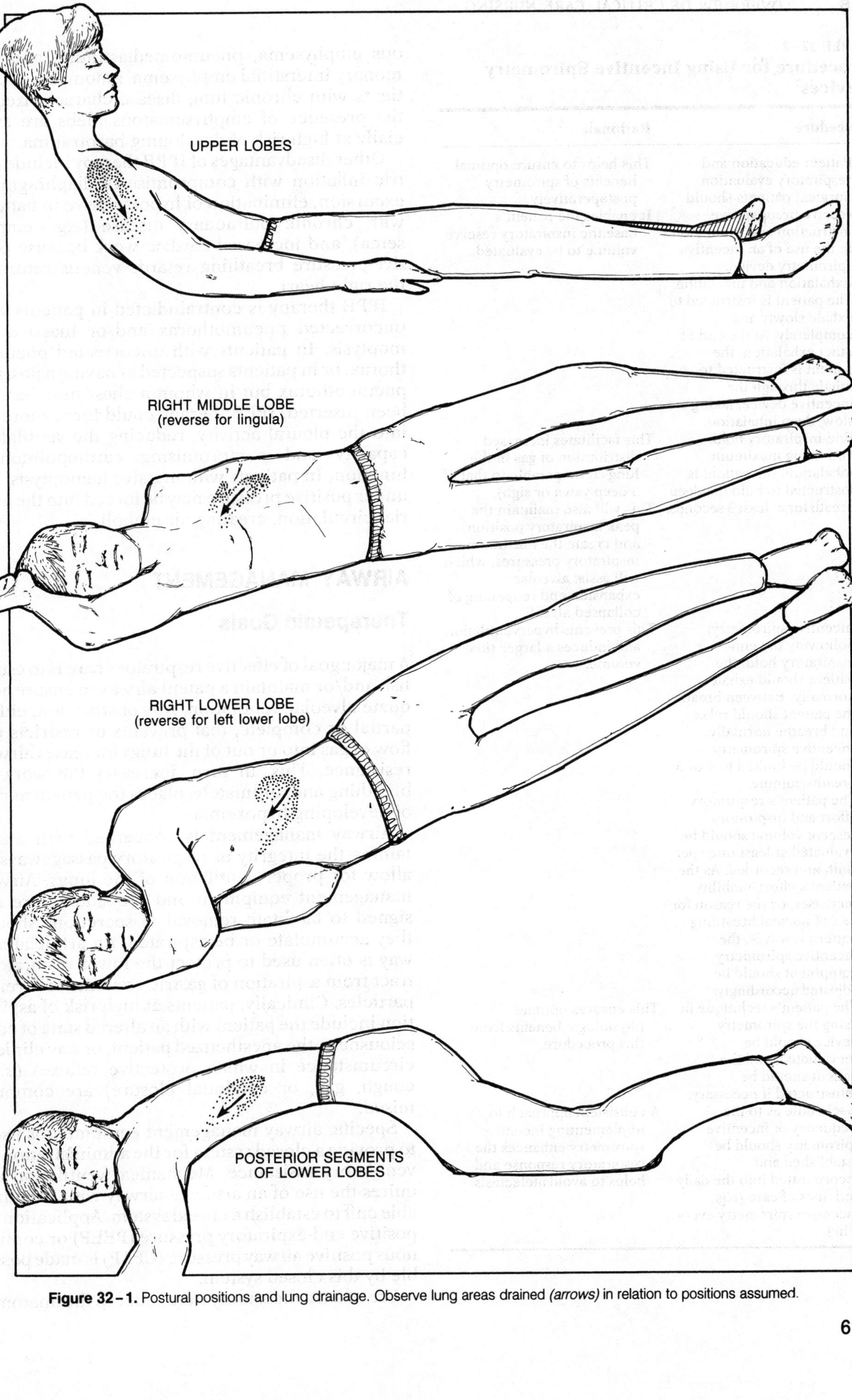


**Figure 32–1.** Postural positions and lung drainage. Observe lung areas drained *(arrows)* in relation to positions assumed.

TABLE 32-2
**Procedure for Using Incentive Spirometry Devices[7]**

| Procedure | Rationale |
|---|---|
| 1. Patient education and respiratory evaluation: Surgical patients should receive preoperative instruction and evaluation in the use of an incentive spirometry device. | This helps to ensure optimal benefits of spirometry postoperatively. It enables the patient's baseline inspiratory reserve volume to be evaluated. |
| 2. Exhalation and inhalation: The patient is instructed to exhale slowly and completely. At the end of quiet exhalation, the patient is instructed to inhale through the incentive device, taking a slow, deep inhalation. | |
| 3. End-inspiratory hold: Following maximum inhalation, the patient is instructed to hold the deep breath for at least 3 seconds. | This facilitates increased distribution of gas in the lungs (comparable to that of a deep yawn or sigh). This will also maintain the peak inspiratory position and create the maximum inspiratory pressures, which will assist alveolar expansion and reopening of collapsed alveoli. |
| 4. Incentive spirometry: Following the end-inspiratory hold, the patient should exhale normally. Between breaths, the patient should relax and breathe normally. Incentive spirometry should be limited to 4 or 5 breaths/minute. | This prevents hyperventilation and induces a larger tidal volume. |
| 5. The patient's respiratory effort and inspiratory reserve volume should be evaluated at least once per shift, and recorded. As the patient's effort/mobility increases, or the reason for loss of normal breathing pattern resolves, the incentive spirometry equipment should be adjusted accordingly. | |
| 6. The patient's technique in using the spirometry device should be reevaluated, and the patient should be reinstructed if necessary. | This ensures optimal physiologic benefits from this procedure. |
| 7. A schedule as to the frequency of incentive spirometry should be established and incorporated into the daily activities of care (e.g., incentive spirometry every 1 hr). | A consistent approach to implementing incentive spirometry enhances the respiratory response and helps to avoid atelectasis. |

ous emphysema, pneumomediastinum, and pulmonary interstitial emphysema, among others. Patients with chronic lung disease characterized by the presence of emphysematous blebs are especially at high risk of developing barotrauma.

Other disadvantages of IPPB therapy include gastric inflation with compromise of diaphragmatic excursion, elimination of hypoxic drive in patients with chronic pulmonary disease (e.g., emphysema), and increased cardiac work because positive-pressure breathing retards venous return to the right heart.

IPPB therapy is contraindicted in patients with uncorrected pneumothorax and/or massive hemoptysis. In patients with uncorrected pneumothorax, or in patients suspected of having a possible pneumothorax but in whom a chest tube has not been inserted, IPPB therapy could force more air into the pleural activity, reducing the ventilatory capacity and compromising cardiopulmonary function. In patients with massive hemoptysis, gas under positive pressure may be forced into the arterial circulation, creating air emboli.

## AIRWAY MANAGEMENT

### Therapeutic Goals

A major goal of effective respiratory care is to establish and/or maintain a patent airway to ensure adequate alveolar ventilation. Any obstruction, either partial or complete, that prevents or restricts the flow of gas into or out of the lungs increases airway resistance. This, in turn, increases the work of breathing and, ultimately, places the patient at risk of developing hypoxemia.

Airway management is concerned with maintaining the integrity of respiratory passageways to allow for proper ventilation of the lungs. Airway management equipment and procedures are designed to facilitate removal of secretions should they accumulate or be aspirated. An artificial airway is often used to protect the lower respiratory tract from aspiration of gastric contents or foreign particles. Clinically, patients at high risk of aspiration include the patient with an altered state of consciousness, the anesthetized patient, or any clinical circumstance in which protective reflexes (e.g., cough, gag, or epiglottal closure) are compromised.

Specific airway management equipment is used to provide a closed system for the administration of ventilatory assistance. Mechanical ventilation requires the use of an artificial airway with an inflatable cuff to establish a closed system. Application of positive end-expiratory pressure (PEEP) or continuous positive airway pressure (CPAP) is made possible by this closed system.

Use of a tracheostomy tube reduces the anatomical dead space within the respiratory tract by as much as 30%–50%, thus improving alveolar ventilation and facilitating a more even distribution of respiratory gases. This helps to optimize matching of ventilation with perfusion and to reduce the work of breathing.

Prevention of infection is a major goal of patient care. Activities related to airway management and total care of the patient must be implemented in a manner that reduces the risk of infection.

### Airway Obstruction

The airway may be partially or completely obstructed.[8] Partial obstruction suggests that some air movement is present, and, thus, sounds are usually audible. They may include snoring (tongue fallen back against pharyngeal wall); hoarseness (inflammation of larynx); grunting (narrowing of vocal cords); coughing (irritation of trachea and/or larger bronchi); and wheezing (narrowing or bronchospasm of bronchioles). An expiratory stridor may be present, or inspiratory squeaking together with rib retraction may be observed. The patient may experience tachypnea and tachycardia.

With complete airway obstruction, no air movement occurs. Thus, no sounds are produced. The conscious patient may experience extreme anxiety with diaphoresis and may be observed making an extreme effort to move air with deep substernal and intercostal retractions, and contraction of accessory muscles.

In general, obstruction during the inspiratory phase occurs at or above the larynx; obstruction occurring during the expiratory phase involves the airways distal to the larynx.

The *Heimlich maneuver* may be used to assist persons who are choking on foreign matter caught in the upper respiratory tract. A sudden, sharp increase in alveolar pressure caused by a forceful elevation of the diaphragm provides the basis for this maneuver. With a fist placed midway between the xiphoid process and the umbilicus, a quick upward thrust causes elevation of the diaphragm and a forceful exhalation. The foreign object is expelled from the airway as air is forced through the trachea and larynx.

*Bronchoscopy* is a technique with both diagnostic and therapeutic uses. It affords direct visualization of the trachea and tracheobronchial tree, enabling a foreign body to be visualized and identified; therapeutically, this technique may allow removal of the foreign body.

### Risks of Airway Management

The major risk encountered in airway management is a disruption of the normal integrity of the respiratory tract, with consequent contamination and potential infection of the respiratory system. The placement of artificial airways extending into the trachea bypasses the normal protective mechanisms of the upper airways involved in warming, filtering, and humidifying inhaled gases. Bypassing the upper airway defense mechanisms allows microorganisms and other foreign matter in the unfiltered inspired gas to enter the lower airways.

Under normal physiologic circumstances, the respiratory tract is considered to be sterile distal to the larynx. Consequently, all procedures involving artificial airways should be performed using *aseptic* technique. Placement of an artificial airway through the glottis interferes with or reduces the effectiveness of the coughing mechanisms, which plays a crucial role in clearing secretions from the respiratory tract.

Bypassing the humidification function of the upper airway increases the risk of dehydration of the respiratory mucosa. Consequent loss of the mucociliary transport activity of the respiratory epithelium compromises movement of secretions toward the large bronchi and trachea where they are accessible to removal by suctioning. Accumulation and pooling of secretions within the tracheobronchial tree predispose to airway obstruction and provide a milieu conducive to colonization by microorganisms. The patient is at increased risk of developing infection (pneumonia). Humidification devices are required when artificial airways are used.

Placement of most artificial airways eliminates the ability of the patient to communicate verbally. Special tubes are available that enable the patient to talk while mechanical ventilation is maintained. In patients with standard endotracheal tubes, it is imperative that some form of communication be established to enable the patient, family, and healthcare providers to understand each other more clearly.

If the patient is able to write, a writing pad should be provided. A chalkboard can be very helpful, if available. Picture cards can also be used to facilitate communication. A signal method, such as a shake of the head, blinking of the eyes, or movement of fingers, can be implemented.

Patients often become frightened when they realize that they cannot ask questions regarding their condition or care. Patients need frequent reassurance that their needs will be met and that someone is always nearby, anticipating needs or attending to problems and concerns as they arise.

## Artificial Airways

### Types of Artificial Airways

**Pharyngeal Airways.** The *naso*pharyngeal and *oro*pharyngeal airways are used for short-term airway maintenance. They function to hold the tongue away from the posterior wall of the pharynx. They are designed to allow airflow around or through them, and they easily accommodate the passage of a suction catheter into the laryngopharynx. The oropharyngeal tube may cause gagging, vomiting, or laryngospasm in the conscious or semiconscious patient (Fig. 32-2).

**Endotracheal Tubes.** Endotracheal tubes are flexible, hollow cylindrical airways designed for nasal or oral insertion (see Fig. 32-2). They come equipped with an inflatable balloon or cuff that provides a seal to prevent aspiration of oral secretions, and facilitates mechanical ventilation.

The *nasal* endotracheal tube is frequently used for long-term intubation because it is easier to stabilize, has a decreased risk of extubation, and is usually better tolerated by the conscious patient. Its major drawback is that a smaller diameter tube is required to be accommodated by the nose with a minimum of trauma (i.e., pressure exerted within the nose).

More commonly, endotracheal intubation is accomplished using the oral approach. *Oral* endotracheal tubes have a larger diameter, which lessens airway resistance and facilitates spontaneous or mechanical ventilation. These tubes are especially indicated in the clinical setting of thick, copious pulmonary secretions, which require a larger size suction catheter for effective secretion removal. Low-compliance cuffs minimize barotrauma to the trachea and larynx.

### *Intubation and Airway Placement*

**Preparation for Intubation.** Prior to intubation, competency of the cuff is established by injecting approximately 10 ml of air into the cuff, or the amount indicated on the tube. Appropriate explanations are made to the patient, and a system of communication is established, if possible. A nasogastric tube may be passed to decompress the stomach. The patient is preoxygenated with 100% oxygen for at least 1-2 minutes before intubation is initiated.

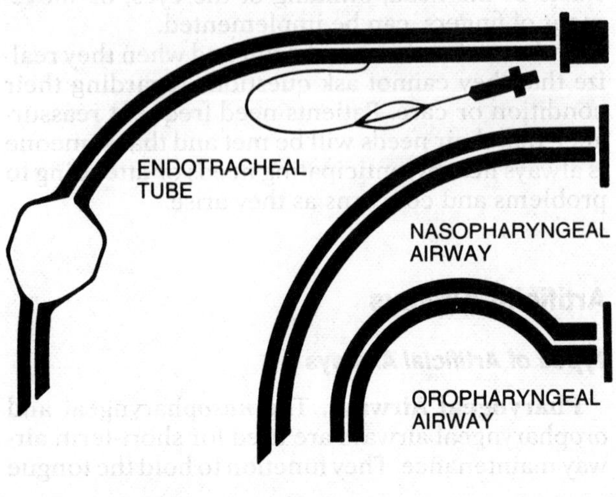


**Figure 32-2.** Artificial airways.

**Assessment for Correct Airway Placement.** Upon insertion of the airway, it is essential to assess for correct placement by: (1) feeling/listening for airflow through the tube opening; (2) observing for symmetrical bilateral chest excursion during inspiration and expiration; (3) auscultating for breath sounds over peripheral areas of the anterior and lateral chest bilaterally; and (4) obtaining an immediate chest x-ray. A sterile sputum specimen may be obtained at this time.

There is always the danger that, should the endotracheal tube be passed too far, it will enter the right mainstem bronchus, which continues from the bifurcation of the trachea in a nearly vertical course (see Fig. 28-1). Upon cuff inflation, in this event, ventilation will occur exclusively to the right lung. The unventilated left lung will develop atelectasis, and respiratory insufficiency with hypoxemia and tissue hypoxia may rapidly ensue.

Ideally, the tip of the endotracheal tube should be about 3 cm above the carina. Adequate stabilization of the airway is a major nursing concern to ensure optimal ventilation. After airway placement is confirmed, the endotracheal tube should be marked at the point at which it emerges from the mouth (gumline). The tube should be taped securely because body movements may lead to accidental extubation or endobronchial intubation. If an oral endotracheal tube is inserted, an oral airway may also be inserted to act as a "biteblock." The position of the endotracheal tube should be changed from side to side every 8 hours to relieve pressure on the lips and tongue. It is a primary nursing responsibility to secure the tube and maintain its proper placement. Frequent and aggressive oral hygiene should be provided.

**Cuff Inflation and Deflation.** Endotracheal tubes in current use have cuffs that are soft, pliable, and of low pressure if inflated properly. This has allowed endotracheal tubes to remain in place for increased periods of time. Three weeks is now considered standard. If longer-term airway management is anticipated, a tracheostomy is usually performed.

It is the responsibility of the critical care nurse to make sure that an optimal low pressure is always maintained. Cuff inflation requires only the amount of air necessary to achieve a minimal air leak. Tracheal damage occurs when the pressure exerted by the inflated cuff against the tracheal walls exceeds the tracheal capillary pressure, which is about 25 mmHg. Usually the maximum pressure exerted by an inflated cuff is approximately 15–20 mmHg. The actual pressure can be determined by connecting the balloon port to a manometer. If increasing amounts of air are needed to obtain a seal, suspect tracheal dilation or a leak in the cuff. Some patients require a *sealed* airway, and, therefore, a minimal occlusive volume (MOV) is used.

Regardless of cuff design or pressure characteristics, all cuff pressures should be evaluated every 4–8 hours. If high-quality low-pressure cuffs are used, routine deflation is unnecessary and may be of no value in minimizing tracheal damage. If deflation is to be performed, it is important to suction the oropharynx first to avoid aspiration. It may also be helpful to apply positive pressure during inspiration as the cuff is deflated. This, together with the mucociliary transport activity (if intact), establishes a retrograde flow of secretions into the oropharynx where they are removed by suctioning. The minimal air leak is then quickly re-established. In patients on continuous controlled ventilation, it is necessary to adjust the tidal volume when the cuff is deflated in order to compensate for the air leak around the deflated cuff.

**Complications of Endotracheal Intubation** (Table 32–3)[9]. Problems encountered with use of endotracheal tubes usually occur at pressure points along the respiratory tract. Nasal endotracheal tubes, for example, may cause nosebleed, sinusitis, pressure necrosis to the cartilaginous structure of the nose, or turbinate fracture. Both nasal and oral endotracheal tubes have the potential to cause

TABLE 32–3
**Complications of Endotracheal Intubation[9]**

1. Complications of laryngoscopy:
   Lip bruising and lacerations, tooth avulsion.
   Esophageal lacerations.
   Aspiration of pharyngeal and gastric contents.
2. Complications during intubation:
   Laryngospasm or bronchospasm.
   Cardiac dysrhythmias.
   Altered hemodynamics (labile blood pressure).
   Esophageal endotracheal tube placement.
   Intrabronchial-endotracheal tube placement with consequent unilateral lung expansion.
   Nasal intubation: Nosebleed, sinusitis, otitis media.
   Pressure necrosis of cartilaginous structure of the nose.
   Turbinate fracture.
   Tracheostomy: Bleeding, hematoma formation.
   Subdermal tissue dissection with consequent inability to pass tube into trachea; subcutaneous emphysema.
   Tracheostomy tube obstruction by blood, tissue, or secretions.
   Aspiration of blood and secretions into tracheobronchial tree.
   Pneumothorax, pneumomediastinum.
3. Complications post-intubation:
   Endotracheal tube kinking; obstructed with blood and secretions.
   Increased airway resistance associated with decreased endotracheal tube diameter resulting from secretion-coating within tube; increased work of breathing in patients breathing spontaneously; increased airway pressures in patients receiving mechanical ventilation; aspiration.
   Endotracheal tube cuff leak—inability to occlude air leak around the tube.
4. Complications after confirmation of correct tube placement.
   Endotracheal tube position changes with body movements.
   Neck extension causes tube to move up (cephalad). With upward movement, endotracheal tube cuff may become positioned above the vocal cords. If this occurs, an increase in cuff inflation may be necessary to maintain a seal, and the tube may be forced out of the trachea. Whenever a leak arises around the endotracheal tube cuff, the cuff should be completely deflated, the endotracheal tube repositioned, and the cuff reinflated so as to maintain a *minimal air leak*. If a *sealed* airway is desired, a *minimal occlusive volume* is used.
   Head flexion causes tube to move down into mainstem bronchus (endotracheal tube tip can move about 2 cm from a neutral position with head movement).
5. Complications post-extubation:
   Laryngospasm; glottic and subglottic edema; vocal cord edema or ulceration.
   Late complications: Vocal cord granulomas (nodular inflammatory lesion secondary to trauma); polyps, vocal cord paralysis; tracheal abnormalities—tracheitis, tracheomalacia, tracheal stenosis; tracheoesophageal fistula.

pressure-induced trauma to the glottis, the subglottic area, and the larynx. Commonly, complications involving these areas become especially significant post-extubation. With routine extubation, a sore throat and/or hoarseness is commonly experienced by patients. If, however, these symptoms persist for a week or longer, cord ulcerations, polyps, or granulomas must be suspected.

Edema of the glottis (superior opening of the larynx) is a common complication of endotracheal intubation. It is usually characterized by an *inspiratory stridor*, a high-pitched musical sound heard on inspiration as air flows through a narrowed glottic opening. If heard on extubation, stridor should be considered serious because the edema may progress over several hours.

Subglottic edema is the most serious complication occurring post-extubation.[10] It may be distinguished from glottic edema in that it does not respond to usual post-extubation therapy such as humidification, application of alpha-adrenergic medications to cause vasoconstriction and reduce edema, or the use of steroid preparations for their anti-inflammatory effect. Subglottic edema should be considered a life-threatening problem, usually requiring re-intubation.

The complications described here should establish the need for meticulous and thorough ongoing assessment. Laryngospasm and/or edema may evolve rapidly over minutes to several hours. It is important to anticipate the occurrence of these complications so that measures may be instituted to prevent and/or minimize consequent airway obstruction.

### *Tracheostomy*

Tracheostomy is the airway of choice for long-term assisted and/or controlled mechanical ventilation. It facilitates removal of thick, tenacious secretions from the tracheobronchial tree, and functions to prevent aspiration of oral or gastric secretions. A tracheostomy may be established to bypass an upper airway obstruction. It may be used to improve alveolar ventilation by decreasing dead space. A tracheostomy may be more comfortable than other airways; it allows the patient to eat, and, with some adaptations, the patient may be able to speak.

The standard tracheostomy tube (see Fig. 32–2) is designed for placement beneath the second cartilaginous ring below the cricoid cartilage (see Fig. 28–1). As a sterile procedure, it is preferable to perform a tracheostomy on an elective basis in an operating room setting. Upon insertion of the tracheostomy tube, the cuff is inflated, and the airway is assessed immediately for patency and correct placement. Auscultation for breath sounds and examination for bilateral chest wall excursion are performed. A chest x-ray is obtained to ascertain exact tube position within the trachea.

Each tracheostomy tube is packaged with a fitted obturator (Fig. 32–3). This device should be kept wrapped and in an obvious place at the tracheostomy patient's bedside where it is available if re-insertion of the tube is necessary. The obturator, with its rounded tip, eliminates the blunt edge of the tracheostomy tube and facilitates re-insertion. Another tube of the same size should be available in the event of accidental extubation and contamination.

The *fenestrated* tracheostomy tube is sometimes used to decrease airway resistance while maintaining the stoma during weaning. The fenestrated opening must be within the airway lumen and not against the tracheal wall. The cuff must be deflated when the decannulation cannula or plug is in place.

**Complications of Tracheostomy** (see Table 32–3). The most immediate complication of a tracheostomy is local wound bleeding. Aspiration of blood into the tracheobronchial tree may obstruct airways with clots, leading to atelectasis. Clotted blood also serves as an excellent culture medium for bacterial colonization with consequent infection. Inadvertent cannulation of subdermal layers

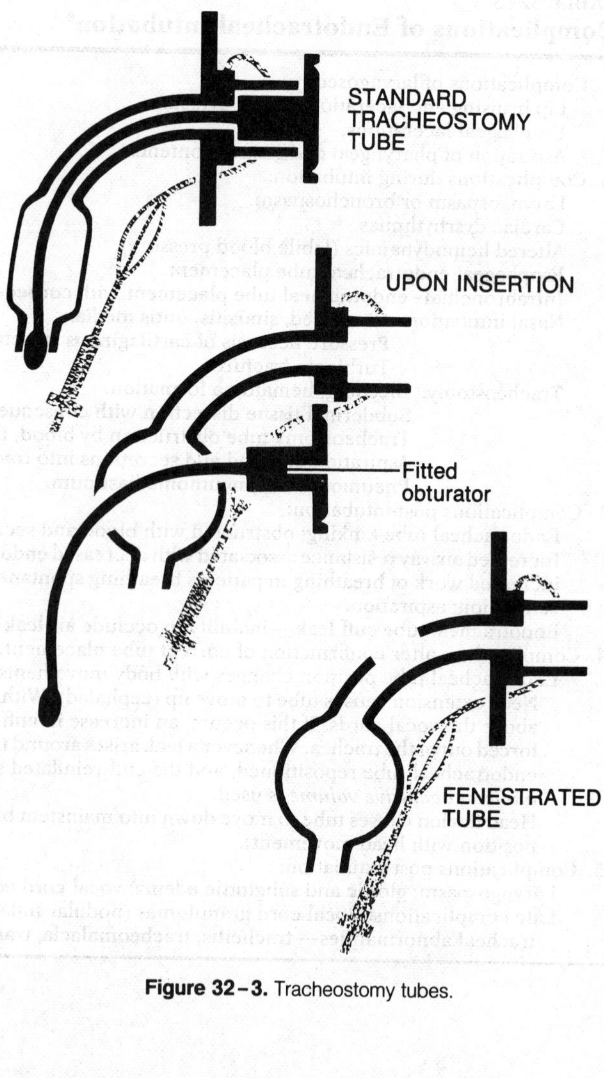


**Figure 32–3.** Tracheostomy tubes.

above the trachea may predispose to subcutaneous emphysema besides resulting in inadequate ventilation. Pneumothorax and pneumomediastinum may be caused by laceration of the pleura.

Another complication is infection, resulting from direct continuity of the trachea with the atmosphere. Bleeding, when it occurs later, is frequently associated with tracheitis; hemorrhage may occur from erosion into a large artery (e.g., innominate artery).

Complications commonly seen after removal of the tracheostomy tube include tracheomalacia (i.e., degeneration of elastic and connective tissue of the trachea) and tracheal stenosis. These complications are associated with tracheal ischemia caused by the pressure of the tracheostomy tube and its cuff (if present). Tracheostomies for long-term or permanent use in patients who are able to breathe spontaneously do not have cuffs. This alleviates tracheal damage associated with long-term use of cuffed tubes.

**Tracheostomy Care.** Tracheostomy care is performed at least every 8 hours, or more frequently if needed, to maintain airway patency, to reduce the risk of infection, and to make the tracheostomy more esthetically acceptable to patient, family, and significant others.

Stomal care should be provided using aseptic technique. A combination of hydrogen peroxide and normal saline is usually used to clean the stomal site, followed by a rinsing with normal saline and application of a dry, sterile dressing. Care should be taken not to trim or cut the gauze pads used for the dressing because the cotton filling and fibers may be aspirated or may become embedded in the surgical wound causing inflammation.

When changing tracheostomy ties, secure the tracheostomy with the clean ties before removing old ones. An untied tracheostomy tube could be accidentally extubated. When tying the tube securely in place, leave enough slack to accommodate one finger between the ties and neck.

The artificial airway should be carefully assessed for patency. Tracheal obstruction can be caused by accumulated secretions or an inflated cuff that herniates and occludes the catheter lumen. The stomal site should be inspected for signs of infection.

### *Extubation*

Tracheal extubation is appropriate when the underlying problem that necessitated placement of an artificial airway and mechanical ventilation has been resolved. In assessing the patient's readiness for extubation, the following factors need to be evaluated:

1. Level of consciousness; intact protective reflexes—cough, gag, and epiglottal closure.
2. Ability of patient to effectively remove secretions from the lungs.
3. Effectiveness of spontaneous respirations as reflected by respiratory parameters:
   - Tidal volume $\geq$ 10 ml/kg.
   - Minute volume ($V_E$) ~ 10 liters.
   - Vital capacity > 12–15 ml/kg.
   - Peak inspiratory pressure $\geq$ (−20 $cmH_2O$).
   - Respiratory rate <30–35/min.
   - Arterial blood gas values: $PaCO_2$ 35–45 mmHg (may be >45 mmHg in chronic lung disease). $PaO_2$ >60 mmHg. $SaO_2$ >90%.
4. Hemodynamic stability—vital signs (blood pressure, heart rate).
5. Cardiac status (absence of dysrhythmias).

**Extubation: Major Considerations.** In preparation for extubation, appropriate explanations are made and the patient is placed in a semi-Fowler's position. This position ensures a more open airway once the artificial airway is removed; it allows for full use of respiratory muscles; it facilitates coughing; and it minimizes risk of vomiting and consequent aspiration. The endotracheal tube should be suctioned, and, very importantly, suctioning above the endotracheal cuff should be performed. This removes pooled secretions above the cuff, which may be aspirated with cuff deflation. If tolerated, the patient should be placed in a head-down position prior to cuff deflation to promote drainage of pooled secretions that may have accumulated above the cuff and to prevent aspiration.

A resuscitator bag is attached to the endotracheal tube, and positive pressure is applied by administering maximum inflation as the tube cuff is deflated. This assists in forcing secretions toward the oropharynx where they can be swallowed or expectorated. The patient should be instructed to take deep breaths, and the endotracheal tube is removed at the point of maximal inspiration. This allows for easier and less traumtic removal with expiration.

The patient is fitted with a face mask, and the prescribed concentration of humidified oxygen is administered. The patient should be observed closely for increasing hoarseness or respiratory stridor, which warns of potential laryngeal edema or spasm. Equipment for re-intubation should be available at the bedside. The patient's tolerance to extubation should be monitored by clinical observation, ventilatory measurements, and arterial blood gas parameters.

### *Care of the Artificial Airway: Major Nursing Considerations*[11]

Use of an artificial airway bypasses the critical air-conditioning functions of the upper airways, which include filtering, warming, and humidifying inhaled gas. Consequently, in caring for the intubated patient, certain measures must be instituted routinely to ensure that adequate ventilation is maintained, and that gas reaching the tracheobronchial tree is nearly "dust-free," at body temperature, and 100% humidified. To ensure airway patency, an effort must be made to control secretions and prevent infection.

Nursing measures should include frequent mouth care to decrease pooling of secretions within the oropharynx and reduce the consequent risk of infection; it helps to relieve halitosis and induces the patient to feel more comfortable. In patients with nasopharyngeal tubes in place, the nares should be examined closely for irritation and inflammation. Exudate should be gently removed, and the mucous membranes should be kept clean and moist.

In addition to oral care, correct placement of the artificial airway should be validated. Oral endotracheal tubes should be moved from one side of the mouth to the other at least once each shift to decrease pressure necrosis to the oral mucosa. The airway should be secured carefully to prevent accidental extubation or intrabronchial intubation, and to decrease laryngotracheal trauma. Inhaled gas must be warmed and humidified to prevent dehydration of the respiratory mucosa. Without humidification, permanent damage associated with excessive mucosal drying and an increased viscosity of pulmonary secretions may occur. This increase in secretion viscosity may predispose to problems of airway secretion removal with a consequent increase in the risk of airway obstruction.

**Airway Suctioning.** Airway suctioning with secretion removal is a major goal in airway management. Suctioning should be performed on a PRN basis rather than by the clock. Signs and symptoms indicating a need for suctioning include: patient restlessness or anxiety, and diaphoresis; an increase in blood pressure and heart rate; an increase in the respiratory rate with a change in the patient's breathing pattern (e.g., dyspnea, noisy, shallow respirations); and the detection of rales (crackles) and rhonchi on auscultation. If the patient is receiving mechanical ventilation, ventilatory peak airway pressures may signal a buildup of secretions long before the problem becomes grossly evident.

Endotracheal suctioning should be an aseptic procedure, and sterile disposable catheters should be used. The bacterial flora of the upper airways may contaminate and infect the lower airways. Therefore, catheters used for suctioning the oral and nasal cavities should never be used for suctioning of the tracheobronchial tree. The procedure for endotracheal suctioning is presented in Table 32–4.[12]

***Complications of Airway Suctioning.*** Major complications of endotracheal suctioning include hypoxemia and tissue hypoxia. Significant changes in heart rate or blood pressure, or the presence of cardiac dysrhythmias suggests hypoxemia. Untoward cardiac reactions may be avoided by adequate prehyperventilatory and posthyperventilatory oxygenation and by limitations of each suctioning pass to less than 10 seconds. Vagal stimulation associated with suctioning of pharynx, larynx, and trachea may lead to bradycardia and hypotension during suctioning. This can be limited by gentle catheter insertion and limited application of intermittent suction.

Atelectasis occurs with excessive removal of residual gas volume. Use of suction catheters less than one third to one half the inner diameter of the airway may limit loss of this residual volume. Hyperinflation and preoxygenation may minimize the hazard of atelectasis.

Additional complications of endotracheal suctioning include airway trauma associated with probing and forcing the catheter on insertion, or the application of high negative pressures during suctioning. Repeated suctioning and suctioning when not necessary should be avoided because bleeding, respiratory epithelial injury, and local inflammation may occur. Such injury can be limited by gentle introduction of the catheter and by use of intermittent suctioning and a continual rotation of the catheter as it is removed.

Infection is a major complication of suctioning. Scrupulous handwashing and the stringent use of sterile equipment and aseptic technique can minimize the danger of pulmonary infection. It is important to obtain a sputum specimen before initiation of artificial airway management. This may help to establish what the baseline conditions are. Periodic laboratory testing of secretions coupled with the general monitoring of body temperature and other physiologic and laboratory parameters will assist in determining the presence of infection so that appropriate treatment can be initiated early in the course of the infection.

## MECHANICAL VENTILATION

Ventilation reflects a movement of gas into and out of the lungs. Mechanical ventilation creates a flow of gas into and out of the lungs by manipulation of airway pressures. It achieves effective ventilation by altering the relationship between intrathoracic and extrathoracic pressures. Mechanical ventilation therapy is critical to the effective management of patients in respiratory failure or at high risk of developing ARF. By supporting ventilation and, thus, gas exchange, mechanical ventilators can sustain a patient for as long a period as necessary until the acute process precipitating ARF is resolved.

### Primary Goals of Mechanical Ventilation

Mechanical ventilation is concerned with (1) maintaining alveolar ventilation (i.e., carbon dioxide elimination); (2) delivering appropriate concentra-

TABLE 32–4
**Procedure for Endotracheal Suctioning[12]**

| Procedure | Rationale |
|---|---|
| 1. Assess for signs and symptoms indicative of need for suctioning. | Unnecessary suctioning should be avoided because it is uncomfortable and may be hazardous to the patient. |
| 2. In the conscious patient the procedure should be clearly explained. Stress necessity and importance of procedure in maintaining airway patency. | This encourages patient's cooperation during the procedure. |
| 3. Position patient in semi-Fowler's sitting position at approximately 45-degree angle. | This facilitates airway alignment; straightening of trachea ensures greater patency; it allows for full use of respiratory musculature, and improves coughing. |
| 4. Wash hands. | |
| 5. Assemble sterile suctioning equipment. (A 14 Fr catheter is commonly used in adults; catheter should be less than one third the inner airway diameter.) | Catheter exceeding one third the airway diameter increases risk of suction-induced hypoxia and atelectasis. |
| 6. Pre-oxygenate and hyperventilate patient with 100% oxygen using resuscitator bag. | This helps to minimize suctioning hypoxia and atelectasis. |
| 7. Glove and maintain sterility of dominant hand; glove and maintain clean technique of nondominant hand. (Two-glove technique may be preferred.) | This decreases the incidence of contamination and infection. |
| 8. Using nondominant hand, remove ventilation tube or open suctioning port on swivel adapter. Place ventilator tubing end on sterile gauze pad or drape. | This prevents contamination of ventilator tubing. |
| 9. Using sterile gloved dominant hand, pick up catheter and connect to suction source; thumb of opposite "clean" gloved hand controls suction port. | |
| 10. Lubricate catheter with sterile saline. | Surgical lubricant is usually unnecessary and may accumulate on inner surface of endotracheal tube. |
| 11. Using sterile gloved hand, insert catheter into endotracheal tube as far as it will go. Do not force catheter. | Do not apply suction while advancing catheter because this will "steal" oxygen from within the airway. |
| 12. Withdraw catheter 1 cm to free it from respiratory mucosa; apply intermittent suction by quickly opening and closing suction thumb port. | Application of continuous suction should be avoided to prevent the catheter from "grabbing" the respiratory mucosa and causing trauma. |
| 13. Withdraw catheter using a rotating motion; entire suctioning pass should not exceed 10 seconds in duration. | Rotating motion sweeps the catheter tip against all sides of the airway as the catheter is withdrawn. |
| 14. Hyperinflate patient's lungs with 100% oxygen using resuscitator bag. | This helps to re-expand sections of the lung that may have collapsed with evacuation of air; it minimizes hypoxia due to suction-induced atelectasis. |
| 15. The above steps should be repeated each time the suction maneuver is done. | Maintain rigorous aseptic technique because impaired pulmonary defense systems place the patient at high risk of infection. |
| If the endotracheal tube cuff is to be deflated, suction above the cuff prior to deflation. | This will prevent secretions from being deposited within tracheobronchial tree. *Never* use the same catheter to suction oral and nasal cavities and then lower airways. |
| 16. Reconnect patient to ventilator or close suction port of the swivel adapter. | |
| 17. Reassess patient's airway status. | |
| **Additional tips:** | |
| 18. If secretions are thick and tenacious introduce 3–5 ml of sterile saline solution into airway and ventilate 4 or 5 times. | Introduction of saline may help mobilize secretions and aid in their removal; does not thin secretions. |
| 19. Minimize frequency and duration of suctioning when positive end-expiratory pressure (PEEP) is required. | Small suction-induced changes may have profound effects on a high-risk, refractory, hypoxemic patient. |
| 20. Patient's hydration status should be monitored closely, including daily weight and intake and output. | Hydration helps to minimize viscosity of pulmonary secretions, facilitating their removal. |
| Maintain humidification of inspired gas. | Humidification prevents drying of respiratory epithelium. |

tions of oxygen more reliably; (3) administering gas under positive pressure, which functions to increase lung volumes and reduce areas of atelectasis; (4) maintaining elective positive end-expiratory pressure (PEEP) to help prevent closure/collapse of small airways; and (5) reducing the work of breathing.

If the degree of carbon dioxide retention is increased sufficiently to cause a marked decrease in the patient's pH (<7.25), or if the patient's level of consciousness and mental status is impaired by marked hypercapnia ($PaCO_2$ >50–60 mmHg), mechanical ventilation may be indicated.

As a consequence of advanced airway obstruction, as may occur in the setting of status asthmaticus, crush injuries to the chest, or adult respiratory distress syndrome (ARDS), for example, ventilation–perfusion disturbances arise, causing major changes in blood gases and pH. The progression from normal values to severe hypoxemia, hypercapnia, and respiratory acidemia can occur with alarming rapidity in these clinical circumstances, and, therefore, it is essential to closely monitor the blood gas and pH relationships. Without early recognition and prompt intervention, these persons may be observed to pass through 3 phases: an early hyperventilatory phase, a "crossover" phase, and full-blown acute respiratory failure (Fig. 32–4).

In the early stage (hyperventilatory phase), patients can be observed using increasingly greater effort to ventilate the lungs in the face of advanced airway obstruction. There is use of accessory muscles with intercostal retraction, nasal flaring, and "pursed-lip" breathing; diaphoresis may be evident, and the patient may be tachypneic and tachycardic. Arterial blood gases, at this stage, reflect mild to severe hypoxemia ($PaO_2 \leq 60$ mmHg) and hypocapnia ($PaCO_2 < 30$ mmHg), predisposing to respiratory alkalemia with a variable degree of compensation (pH $\geq$7.50). Patients are able to maintain themselves in the face of serious underlying pathophysiology (increasing alveolar hypoventilation, ventilation/perfusion mismatch, and intrapulmonary shunting) by hyperventilating (i.e., "blowing off" carbon dioxide). But they do so at the expense of considerable energy and oxygen consumption.

As these patients become increasingly fatigued to the point of exhaustion, they eventually progress to the "crossover" phase (see Fig. 32–4). During this phase, the patient's clinical status might suggest to an unsuspecting observer that the patient's condition is actually improving. The patient appears to be breathing with less difficulty and effort; breath sounds are diminished; and arterial blood gases reflect a "normalizing" pH (~7.4) and $PaCO_2$ (~40 mmHg). Significantly, however, the hypoxemia *worsens* ($PaO_2$ <50–60 mmHg), reflecting advancing alveolar hypoventilation, serious disturbances in ventilation/perfusion matching, and significant right-to-left shunting. The diminution of breath sounds on auscultation suggests that the patient is unable to effectively move gas into or out of the lungs.

The "crossover" phase is significant because it signals the need for decisive and immediate institution of timely and aggressive therapy to treat and/or avert full-blown acute respiratory failure (pH <7.2; $PaO_2$ <50–55 mmHg; $PaCO_2$ >50 mmHg). It is absolutely essential to initiate mechanical ventilation at this time to prevent further deterioration in the patient's condition. Mechanical ventilation therapy reduces the work of breathing while maintaining adequate alveolar ventilation.

Use of positive pressure throughout the respiratory cycle (i.e., use of positive end-expiratory pressure) usually is beneficial in these patients because they experience a great deal of microatelectasis associated with fluid-filled alveoli, reduced tidal vol-

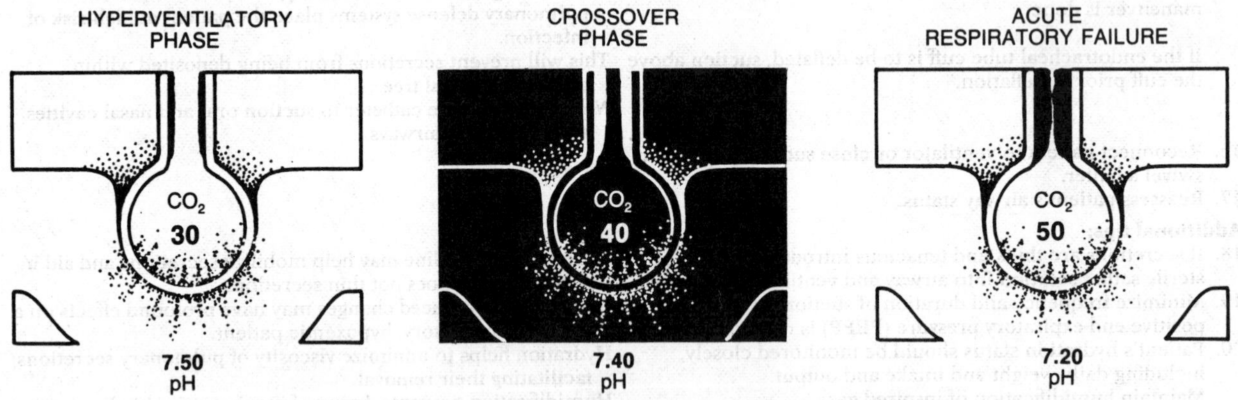


**Figure 32–4.** Blood gas and pH relationships in setting of progressive mild to severe airway obstruction. Schematically depicted are three alveoli and alveolar–capillary membranes. Numbers within the alveoli represent carbon dioxide concentrations; numbers within the capillary reflect corresponding pH.

*Hyperventilatory phase:* Characterized by hypocapnia ($PaCO_2$ ~30 mmHg) and respiratory alkalemia (pH 7.50). Mild airway obstruction predisposes to tissue hypoxia with clinical signs of anxiety, apprehension, and increased work of breathing with hyperventilation. Hyperventilation results in increased carbon dioxide elimination with consequent hypocapnia; hypocapnia underlies the respiratory alkalemia.

*"Crossover" phase:* Characterized by seemingly "normalizing" blood gas values ($PaCO_2$ ~40 mmHg, pH ~7.40). Clinically, there are diminished breath sounds and decreased work of breathing.

*Acute respiratory failure:* Characterized by hypercapnia ($PaCO_2$ >50 mmHg) and respiratory acidemia (pH <7.20). With severe airway obstruction, there is increased ventilation/perfusion mismatching, and shunting. Alveolar ventilation is significantly compromised, predisposing to the hypercapnia. Hypercapnia causes respiratory acidemia, and, if untreated, it can lead to acute respiratory failure.

The significance of the "crossover" phase is that, despite a seemingly "normalizing" clinical picture, the patient is actually in need of immediate, aggressive therapy to prevent full-blown acute respiratory failure. (Not depicted here is the $PaCO_2$, which, concomitantly, progressively worsens as the patient moves from the hyperventilatory phase, to the crossover phase, and, finally, to acute respiratory failure, if untreated.)

umes, and probable surfactant inactivation. PEEP can substantially increase the functional residual capacity (FRC) (i.e., the resting end-expiratory volume of the lungs) and helps to prevent closure of small airways and alveoli.

## Clinical Indications for Mechanical Ventilation

Indications for mechanical ventilation therapy depend largely on the degree to which a pathophysiologic process or processes impinge on cardiopulmonary reserves. This is best assessed by the patient's clinical history and physical examination, serial measurements of spontaneous ventilatory capability, and interpretation of arterial blood gases in light of minute alveolar ventilation ($V_A$).

Subjective and objective criteria for the establishment of airway access (intubation) and initiation of mechanical ventilation therapy are helpful in determining if and when such therapy is indicated. This information is presented in Table 32-5.[13] These criteria may apply to any of the following clinical situations (among others) (see Fig. 31-1):

1. Central nervous system depression with apnea due to primary causes such as drugs, cerebrovascular accidents (CVA), or increased intracranial pressure; or secondary to cerebral hypoxia caused by disturbances in cardiopulmonary function.
2. Increased intracranial pressure (ICP), which is very sensitive to changes in $PaCO_2$. In this situation, induced hypocapnia is used commonly to lower ICP.
3. Persistent hypoxemia ($PaO_2$ <60 mmHg) despite maximum $FIO_2$ by face mask and nasal prongs.
4. In the development of acute lung disease wherein initially, hypocapnia is the rule. The onset of even mild elevation of $PaCO_2$ with a consequent decrease in pH is suggestive of disease progression to a serious potentially compromising state (see Fig. 32-4).
5. Deterioration of ventilatory status of patients with neurologic and neuromuscular problems such as Guillain-Barré and myasthenia gravis, respectively.
6. Flail chest if more than 6 ribs are broken unilaterally, or 4 ribs are broken on each side, and there is evidence of respiratory compromise.
7. Post-cardiac surgery where mechanical ventilation is maintained for 11-24 hours to protect the vulnerable injured myocardium from acidemia and hypoxemia.

TABLE 32-5
**Indications for Initiation of Mechanical Ventilation Therapy*[13]**

| | |
|---|---|
| Subjective: | Is the patient awake, oriented, alert, and cooperative? |
| | Can the patient cough and deep breathe effectively? |
| | What are the secretions like and can the patient handle them effectively? |
| | Is there bronchospasm? |
| | Is there respiratory muscle discoordination (i.e., absence of synchronized movement of the diaphragm and intercostal muscles)? |
| | What is the work of breathing like? Is there impending physical and emotional exhaustion with the labored breathing? |
| | Is the patient hemodynamically stable? |
| Objective: | *Mechanics:* |
| | Tidal volume ($V_T$) <5-7 ml/kg. |
| | Vital capacity ($V_C$) <12-15 ml/kg. |
| | Peak inspiratory pressure (PIP) <20 $cmH_2O$†. |
| | Respiratory rate ("f") >30-35/min (adults). |
| | *Ventilation:* |
| | Dead space ($V_D/V_T$) <55% of $V_T$ (normal: ~25-40%). |
| | $PaO_2$ <60 mmHg; $SaO_2$ <90%. |
| | $PaCO_2$: |
| | Alveolar hypoventilation: $PaCO_2$ >45 mmHg (pH <7.25). |
| | Alveolar hyperventilation: $PaCO_2$ <35 mmHg (pH >7.45). |

*A reversal of the greater than and less than signs preceding each parameter listed above reflects criteria for *weaning* off the ventilator.

†PIP reflects the maximum inspiratory force or peak inspiratory pressure that a patient can exert against a closed system from functional residual capacity (FRC) (i.e., the end-expiratory volume).

## Types of Mechanical Ventilators[14]

Mechanical ventilators currently used for the management of ARF are positive-pressure devices (i.e., they deliver gas under positive pressure to the patient during the inspiratory phase). In contrast, negative pressures are generated during the inspiratory phase with spontaneous ventilation (Fig. 32-5). With spontaneous breathing, expansion of the chest cage and lungs creates a negative pressure within the alveoli. The resulting pressure gradient between the alveoli and the atmosphere allows air to flow into the lungs (see Fig. 28-7).

### Volume- and Pressure-Cycled Ventilators

There are two types of ventilators: *volume-cycled*, wherein each inspiration is terminated after a specified volume has been delivered by the ventilator, with expiration allowed to occur passively; and *pressure-cycled*, wherein inspiration is terminated when a specific airway pressure has been reached. Volume-cycled ventilators are most commonly used to support the critically ill patient because

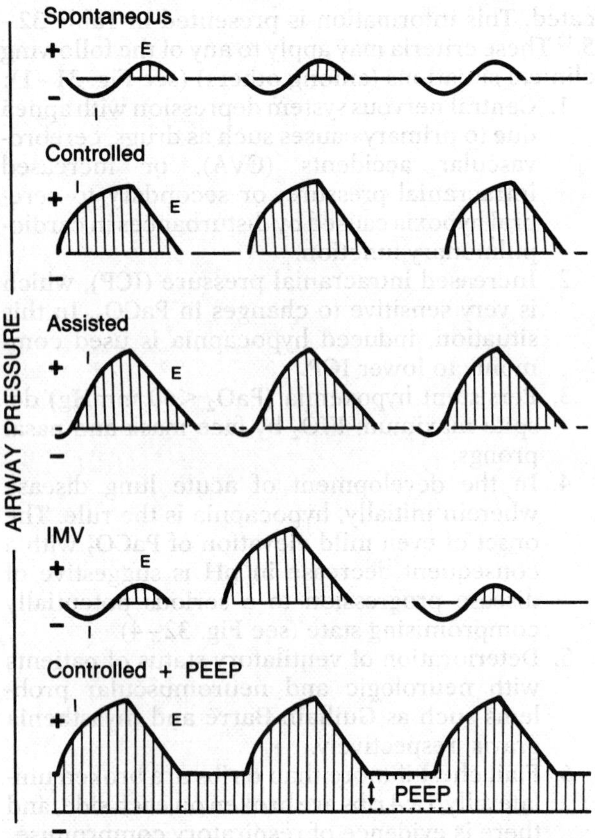


**Figure 32–5.** Airway pressures during spontaneous breathing and during mechanical ventilation with several different patterns. E = expiration; I = inspiration; IMV = intermittent mandatory ventilation; and PEEP = positive end-expiratory pressure. (Adapted from Weinberger, SE: Principles of Pulmonary Medicine. WB Saunders, Philadelphia, 1986, p 316.)

they are more reliable in delivering the volume of air desired, despite variations in airway resistance and lung compliance. They also afford better delivery of accurate oxygen concentrations and can be modified to deliver positive end-expiratory pressure (PEEP), and intermittent mandatory ventilation (IMV).

### *High-Frequency Jet Ventilation*

High-frequency jet ventilation uses a high-pressure source connected to a small-bore catheter with an interposed cycling mechanism allowing high-frequency delivery of gas. High-frequency jet ventilation, delivered at 100–150 cycles/minute, can maintain adequate gas exchange for undefined periods of time in the patient with normal lungs. This type of ventilation provides continuous ventilation in the setting of acute respiratory failure without the undesirable side effects of positive-pressure ventilation.

## Modes or Patterns of Ventilation

### *Control Mode*

In the control mode, ventilation is provided entirely by the ventilator at a respiratory rate, tidal volume, and inspired oxygen concentration prescribed by the physician. At ventilatory rates greater than 8/minute in conjunction with a tidal volume of 12–15 ml/kg, it is reasonable to assume that full alveolar ventilatory support is adequate in most instances. The use of barbiturate coma to treat head injury is an example wherein ventilation is exclusively in the control mode. However, with the availability of the assist-control and intermittent mandatory ventilation modes, which provide full ventilatory support without the inflexibility of the control mode, this mode is used infrequently.

### *Assist–Control Mode*

In the assist–control mode of ventilation, the ventilator is able to "sense" when the patient initiates inspiration, at which point the ventilator "assists" by delivering a specified tidal volume to the patient (see Fig. 32–5). The tidal volume is set by the ventilator along with at least a minimum number of breaths per minute. The respiratory rate is determined by the number of spontaneous inspirations initiated by the patient. Should the patient's spontaneous rate fall below a specified level, the ventilator supports respirations by delivering at least the minimum number of breaths for which it is set. The assist–control mode of ventilation can result in wide swings in minute ventilation if the patient's respiratory rate changes appreciably once the rate is higher than the specified minimum.

### *Intermittent Mandatory Ventilation (IMV)*

Intermittent mandatory ventilation (IMV) allows for partial ventilatory support by delivering a preset number of breaths per minute at a specified tidal volume and inspired oxygen concentration. In between the ventilator-delivered breaths, the patient is able to breathe spontaneously through the ventilator circuit without increased resistance, and at the preset inspired oxygen concentration. The ventilator does not assist the spontaneous breaths, and the tidal volume of these breaths is determined by the patient's inspiratory effort (see Fig. 32–5).

### *Synchronized Intermittent Mandatory Ventilation (SIMV)*

Most ventilators in use today have the SIMV mode. This mode allows the patient to breathe spontaneously through the ventilator circuit without increased resistance, while, at predetermined intervals, the next spontaneous breath is assisted by the machine. The ventilator and self-initiated breaths do not compete as they can with the IMV mode described above.

#### *Positive End-Expiratory Pressure (PEEP)*

When using a positive-pressure, volume-cycled ventilator, an important option available for the intubated patient with hypoxemic ARF is positive end-expiratory pressure (PEEP). PEEP refers to the existence of an airway pressure above that of ambient air at the end of exhalation. PEEP functions to increase functional residual capacity (FRC), which appears to be the primary mechanism by which alveolar ventilation and, thus, gas exchange are improved when PEEP therapy is instituted. PEEP increases FRC by distending airways and increasing alveolar size by the application of positive pressure. In fact, in ventilated patients receiving PEEP, the entire respiratory cycle is maintained under positive pressure (see Fig. 32–5).

PEEP functions to reduce the incidence of atelectasis, particularly in the scenario of altered surfactant activity. The application of PEEP therapy has been associated with an improvement in arterial oxygenation and overall lung compliance; it reduces pulmonary vascular resistance. It may be the most effective therapy in ARF where right-to-left shunting is a significant problem, because it helps to balance the distribution of the inspired volume of gas throughout the lungs.

#### *Continuous Positive Airway Pressure (CPAP)*

For patients breathing spontaneously, a variation of PEEP called continuous positive airway pressure (CPAP) is available. Principles underlying CPAP are similar to those of PEEP except that the patient is breathing spontaneously without a mechanical ventilator. Benefit is derived from the positive pressure maintained within the airways and alveoli at the end of expiration.

## Ventilator Controls: Guidelines for Adjustments

Manipulation of airway pressure is an effective approach to improving pulmonary gas exchange in acute respiratory failure. Time relationships between inspiratory and expiratory phases, respiratory rate, tidal volume, and oxygen concentration of inspired gas, all impact significantly on alveolar ventilation and, thus, gas exchange, and can be manipulated to derive the optimal benefit for the patient.

Before institution of mechanical ventilation therapy, a total clinical assessment must be performed to identify indicators for mechanical ventilation and to establish baseline data (see Table 32–5). The patient's ventilatory capacity, arterial blood gas values, and laboratory data, together with the clinical history and physical examination, all aid in the decision-making process.

A variety of control settings are available that enable mechanical ventilation to be individualized to meet the needs of each patient. Table 32–6 lists specific ventilatory controls and guidelines for usage.

## Monitoring the Ventilated Patient

General monitoring of the patient on continuous ventilatory support should include: (1) ongoing patient assessment including the status of neurologic, respiratory, cardiovascular, renal, and gastrointestinal function; (2) monitoring of ventilatory settings; (3) monitoring arterial blood gases; (4) laboratory studies; (5) pulmonary function studies; and (6) radiology studies: chest x-ray (daily).

Details related to the monitoring of the ventilated patient are included in Table 32–7.

## Complications of Mechanical Ventilation Therapy

Complications of mechanical ventilation therapy (Table 32–8) may involve problems related to the treatment of acute respiratory failure, as well as medical complications that may arise during the course of the ARF. It is important to appreciate that successful management of ARF depends on identifying high-risk patients and anticipating problems before they occur.

Intubation and mechanical ventilation therapy are not without risks or complications. The intubation procedure may trigger laryngospasms, hypoxemia, and cardiac dysrhythmias. Malposition, displacement, or kinking of the tracheal tube, or clenching of the teeth with an oral endotracheal tube in place, may increase airway resistance and compromise alveolar ventilation. Atelectasis may occur with inadvertent intrabronchial intubation.

Equipment failure or mechanical malfunction is always a potential danger of mechanical ventilation therapy. A resuscitator bag and oral airway must always be available at the bedside, and the patient should be manually ventilated until the malfunction is corrected. Inappropriate or inadequate ventilatory settings related to tidal volume, respiratory rate, and airway pressure may predispose to hypoventilation with consequent hypercapnia and respiratory acidemia. In patients with chronic pulmonary disease, excessive supplemental oxygen therapy may depress the hypoxic drive.

TABLE 32-6
## Ventilator Controls: Guidelines for Adjustments

**Minute Volume ($V_E$)**

Minute volume is a function of the tidal volume times the respiratory rate ($V_E = V_T \times$ "f"). A set tidal volume of 12–15 ml/kg body weight is usual, with a maximum of approximately 1200 ml. Use of large tidal volumes is felt to eliminate the need for an intermittent "sigh."

In patients with chronic lung disease, smaller tidal volumes (~10 ml/kg) are used to avoid gas trapping with consequent impairment of cardiac output due to high pleural pressure. Smaller volumes minimize the problem of dropping the $PaCO_2$ too rapidly.

The chest wall movements should be observed to ensure bilateral symmetry with appropriate synchronization with the phases of the respiratory cycle. In determining the tidal volume, it is important to consider that part of the gas volume delivered by the ventilator that remains within the tubing and, thus, constitutes dead space ventilation (also called *mechanical dead space*).

**Respiratory Rate ("f")**

The respiratory rate is usually set between 10 and 16 breaths/minute to achieve the required $PaCO_2$. Lower rates (<10/minute) may be used with intermittent mandatory ventilation (IMV) to maintain cardiac output and prevent hyperinflation. The *inspiratory/expiratory* ratio is usually regulated so that the inspiratory phase is shorter than the expiratory phase (usual I : E ratio is 1 : 2 or 1 : 3 in adults). The *inspiratory flow rate* can be adjusted so that the prescribed tidal volume can be completely delivered to the patient in an inspiratory time that will maintain an I : E ratio of 1 : 2 or 1 : 3.

**Fraction of Inspired Oxygen Concentration ($FIO_2$)**

Fraction of inspired oxygen concentration ($FIO_2$) can usually be dialed on most ventilator models in current use. It is usually adjusted so that the arterial oxygen tension is at an acceptable level for the patient ($PaO_2$ >60 mmHg). Use of the lowest $FIO_2$ that achieves the desired $PaO_2$ is recommended because excessively high oxygen levels (>60%) may cause oxygen toxicity. The ventilator should be checked daily with an oxygen analyzer to ensure that the desired $FIO_2$ is actually being delivered to the patient. Serial arterial blood gases should be obtained to monitor the $PaO_2$.

Continuous humidification is absolutely essential, and gas should be warmed to body temperature. Adequate humidity prevents dehydration of respiratory epithelium and thickening of tracheobronchial secretions. Ventilators also have the capacity to filter inspired air. Thus, inspired gas reaching the alveoli is warmed, humidified, and filtered by the mechanical ventilator to most closely replicate the functions of the respiratory epithelium.

**Sigh Rate**

The sigh rate can be adjusted with respect to frequency and volume of sighing. The usual sigh rate is established at a frequency of 5–10-minute intervals, usually given in multiples of 2 to 3. The volume of a sigh is approximately twice the tidal volume depending upon the patient's clinical status.

**Sensitivity Setting**

In patients receiving "assisted" ventilation, the sensitivity setting can be adjusted so that minimal patient effort (i.e., about −2 cm $H_2O$) is required to trigger the machine.

**System Pressure**

System pressure adjustments (when using the *volume*-cycle ventilator) must not be limited to a level below that necessary to deliver the preset tidal volume. Usually the pressure limit is set at 10–15 cm above the cycling pressure required to deliver the prescribed volume. If a *pressure*-cycled ventilator is used, the upper pressure limit must be set so that the prescribed tidal volume is delivered at that pressure setting. Volume is delivered only until the preset pressure is reached. Because the pressure is

TABLE 32-6
## Ventilator Controls: Guidelines for Adjustments (*Continued*)

preset and will not vary, changes in airway resistance and compliance can result in reduced volumes delivered to the patient.

PEEP can be incorporated into the mechanical ventilation system to provide positive pressure throughout the expiratory phase. The presence of positive pressures during exhalation functions to stabilize alveoli and prevent their collapse. The normal range for PEEP is usually 0–20 cm of water pressure; higher levels of PEEP can be used in specific clinical settings, as, for example, in ARDS.

**Alarm Systems**

Mechanical ventilators in current use incorporate *audible and visual alarm systems*, which act as immediate warning signals of altered ventilation. Alarms can usually be set for low and high pressures and low volume, to ensure delivery of appropriate tidal volume to the patient. Other alarms guarantee appropriate I : E ratio, appropriate concentrations of oxygen, and fail-safe alarms, which warn of disconnection or unplugging of the ventilator. Mechanical ventilators are used to support life. While alarm settings call attention to malfunction, they should not obviate the need to monitor the patient closely to assess for effectiveness of prescribed ventilation therapy.

Complications may be encountered when an endotracheal or tracheostomy tube remains in the trachea for several days to weeks. Pressure necrosis of the respiratory mucosa, submucosa, and tracheal cartilaginous rings is associated with cuff inflation and direct pressure points between the tube and airway. Consequent complications include tracheitis, tracheomalacia, tracheal stenosis, and, less commonly, tracheoesophageal fistula. Nasal stenosis may occur with use of a nasal endotracheal tube. Vocal cord ulceration and laryngeal stenosis or granulomas have been reported. Occasionally, a complication of mechanical ventilation therapy is the inability to wean the patient. This occurs more frequently in patients with preexisting chronic lung disease (e.g., chronic obstructive pulmonary disease), which severely limits reserves.

The use of positive-pressure mechanical ventilation places the patient at risk of developing barotrauma (e.g., pneumothorax or pneumomediastinum). A *tension pneumothorax* may develop, severely diminishing venous return and cardiac output. If unrecognized and untreated, a tension pneumothorax may cause lung collapse and precipitate cardiovascular collapse (see Chap. 36).

A major adverse effect of positive-pressure ventilation is a reduction in venous return to the heart. With normal spontaneous breathing, the negative intrathoracic pressure created during inspiration promotes venous return from the periphery by way of the great vessels (venae cavae). The mechanical application of positive pressure during inspiration impedes venous return and results in a reduced cardiac output. With the application of PEEP, cardiac output is further compromised. In each pa-

TABLE 32–7
## Monitoring the Ventilated Patient: Implications for Nursing Care

General monitoring of the patient on continuous ventilatory support includes:

**Patient Assessment**

A. *Neurologic status:* Level of consciousness, mental status, level of anxiety, pain? Is the patient "fighting" the ventilator? Evaluate effectiveness of nonverbal communications in meeting patient needs.

B. *Respiratory status:* Evaluate airway patency; presence of air leaks in the system. Assess respiratory rate and pattern of breathing; symmetry of chest movement. Use of positive airway pressure increases risk of barotrauma, pneumothorax.
- Evaluate breath sounds bilaterally; evidence of adventitious sounds? Diligent tracheobronchial hygiene and chest physiotherapy may be necessary on a regular basis to ensure airway patency and adequate ventilation.
- Assess body temperature.
- Frequent turning and position changes minimize pooling of secretions, provide better distribution of ventilation and perfusion, and prevent impairment of skin integrity.

C. *Cardiovascular status:* Heart rate, heart sounds, peripheral pulses, pulse pressure; neck vein distention, peripheral edema? Continuous ECG monitoring?
Hemodynamic pressure parameters:
- Arterial pressure (mean arterial pressure may drop with mechanical ventilation especially when PEEP therapy is applied as positive thoracic pressures decrease venous return).
- Pulmonary capillary wedge pressure (PCWP): Approximates left atrial pressure and can be used as a guide to blood volume, preload, and left heart function; reflects pulmonary hydrostatic pressure as a cause of pulmonary edema.
  When a patient is mechanically ventilated, the PCWP should be taken at the *end-expiratory phase* of the respiratory cycle because this most closely reflects functional residual capacity (FRC). PCWP may not reflect left atrial pressures in the presence of PEEP.
- Cardiac output measurements must be monitored carefully because venous return (preload) is compromised by positive-pressure ventilation.
- Central venous pressures reflect right heart function, blood volume (venous return), and vascular tone.

D. *Renal status:* Fluid and electrolyte balance; daily weight? Intake and output? Maintaining hydration and blood volume is essential in the mechanically ventilated patient to offset reduction of venous return in the presence of positive thoracic pressures. Careful monitoring of the fluid state is essential because the fully humidified gas supplied by the ventilator blocks otherwise insensible fluid loss by the lungs. An increase in body weight often associated with interstitial pulmonary edema is a problem frequently encountered with mechanical ventilation.

E. *Gastrointestinal status:* Nasogastric tube is commonly inserted for gastric decompression; gastric secretions are closely monitored for bleeding. Stress ulcers are commonly associated with mechanical ventilation therapy.
- Nutrition: The patient's nutritional status impacts on pulmonary function in several ways. Respiratory centers in the brain are influenced by the body's overall metabolic rate. Conditions that reduce the metabolic rate also reduce the ventilatory drive; conversely, when the metabolic rate is increased, there is a concomitant increase in the ventilatory response.
  When energy demands exceed the supply, fatigue and weakness of respiratory muscles (especially the diaphragm and intercostals) occur and may be contributing factors predisposing to respiratory failure. Vital capacity is progressively diminished with the catabolic state. A decrease in respiratory endurance has been associated with decreased arterial oxygen tensions.
  Nutritionally, the goal of treatment of the patient with ARF is to induce an *anabolic* state. It is, therefore, necessary to perform a nutritional assessment early in the course of the disease, with implementation of an appropriate nutritional regimen to meet the individual's needs.
  Information regarding the nutritional assessment, caloric and nutrient requirements, and therapeutic modalities in the treatment of the patient with altered nutritional status is presented in Chapter 53.

**Monitoring of Ventilatory Settings**

A. Minute ventilation ($V_E$) and tidal volume ($V_T$) can be measured (spirometer) directly from the artificial airway. Any drop in exhaled tidal volume may indicate a leak in the system.

B. Respiratory rate should be counted for a full minute and compared with the set ventilatory rate.

C. Oxygen concentration: The actual oxygen concentration delivered by the system should be analyzed periodically to ensure that the concentration desired reaches the patient. The lowest $FIO_2$ capable of promoting adequate arterial oxygenation should be delivered.

D. Inspiratory/expiratory ratio: Normally the I : E ratio is 1 : 2 or 1 : 3. Changes in this ratio will affect ventilation/perfusion matching.

E. Sensitivity: Reflects the amount of negative pressure the patient must generate to trigger the ventilator (assist mode).

F. Airway pressure: In volume-cycled ventilators, once the tidal volume is established, airway pressure remains relatively constant. An increase in the pressure reading on the manometer reflects an increase in the amount of pressure needed to deliver the set tidal volume to the patient's lungs. Increases in airway resistance and/or decreases in lung compliance commonly account for the increased pressure. A buildup of thick, viscous secretions, bronchospasms, atelectasis, pneumonia with consolidation, and pulmonary edema are examples of conditions that increase pressure readings; leaks in the delivery system or around the cuff of the artificial airway, or improvement in the patient's condition result in decreases in the pressure readings.

G. Deadspace measurement: Normal range of physiologic deadspace is between 25% and 40% of the tidal volume. Deadspace volume is increased by diseases that decrease pulmonary perfusion (e.g., pulmonary embolism, pulmonary hypertension). Deadspace volume ($V_D/V_T$) is easily calculated by collecting expired carbon dioxide and simultaneous $PaCO_2$.

H. Humidity and temperature.

I. Alarm system: Alarm systems should *never* be turned off.

*(continued)*

TABLE 32–7
**Monitoring the Ventilated Patient: Implications for Nursing Care (*Continued*)**

**Arterial Blood Gases**
The pH and $PaCO_2$ are correlated with minute ventilation; the $PaO_2$, $SaO_2$ (hemoglobin saturation), and arterial oxygen content ($CaO_2$) are correlated with $FIO_2$ and PEEP.[15] These measurements should be taken at least 30 minutes post change in ventilator settings, or following procedures such as suctioning, which disrupt the patency and intactness of the system.
- Alveolar–arterial gradient ($AaDO_2$): The normal $AaDO_2$ is <15 mmHg (room air). An $AaDO_2$ >15 mmHg suggests an underlying hypoxemia-producing process.

**Laboratory Studies**
A. Hematology profile: Hemoglobin, hematocrit, complete blood count.
B. Blood chemistries: Serum electrolytes, BUN, creatinine, glucose, others.

**Pulmonary Function Studies**
A. Spirometric measurements: Forced vital capacity.
Negative inspiratory force.
Maximal inspiratory pressure.
Forced expiratory volume ($FEV_1$).

**Radiologic Test**
Chest x-ray (daily).

tient, there appears to be a PEEP level at which reduction of cardiac output is of greater detriment to tissue oxygenation than the effects of improved arterial oxygen content are beneficial.[17] Usually these detrimental PEEP levels are above those that are therapeutic. Reasonable augmentation of intravascular volume must always precede the initiation of PEEP therapy.

Patients receiving prolonged mechanical ventilation are at increased risk of gastrointestinal ulceration and bleeding. Stools and nasogastric aspirate should be tested for blood. Prophylactic antacid therapy or intravenous cimetidine or ranitidine titration may be prescribed to maintain gastric pH >4.5 (based on hourly testing of gastric pH). Abdominal distention is commonly caused by increased gas in the stomach and intestines, which may be related to positive-pressure ventilation. A nasogastric tube connected to suction maintains the stomach and gut in a decompressed state, decreases risk of aspiration, and provides a source of gastric aspirate for pH testing.

Acute renal failure sometimes occurs in patients with ARF and requires careful monitoring of fluid, acid and base, and electrolyte balances. Acute renal failure frequently accompanies serious gastrointestinal bleeding.

Contamination of the respiratory system by intubation, suctioning, and other invasive procedures (e.g., fiberoptic bronchoscopy) places the patient at great risk of infection. Normal defense systems are compromised, and immunologic defenses are commonly altered in the critically ill patient. The patient is highly vulnerable to nosocomial infections and sepsis.

Lastly, psychologic depression is not uncommon in patients with ARF who are being mechanically ventilated. The inability to communicate normally can be very frightening to the patient. Occasionally, a psychologic dependence on mechanical ventilation complicates the weaning process. For details regarding complications, see Table 32–8.

## Weaning from Mechanical Ventilation Therapy[18,20]

Inherent in the decision to institute mechanical ventilation therapy is determining the factors involved in weaning the patient from it. *Weaning*, or the process of removing the patient from mechanical ventilation therapy, is affected largely by the length of time the patient has been on the mechanical ventilator; physical condition, including the tone and strength of respiratory muscles; underlying disease status; and whether or not psychologic dependence is a significant factor. It is recognized that, when patients have been maintained on mechanical ventilatory therapy, a period of gradual separation is necessary before spontaneous respirations can effectively meet ventilatory needs. Long-term mechanically ventilated patients may have their weaning complicated by infection, anemia, hemodynamic instability, nutritional and metabolic disturbances, altered elimination patterns, and sleep disturbances.

The basic guide to beginning the weaning process is to establish whether or not the indications for the implementation of mechanical ventilation have improved. Criteria for weaning are reflected in Table 32–5 simply by *reversing* the "greater than" and "less than" signs preceding each parameter.

The two basic approaches to weaning are the T-piece or nebulization trial and the intermittent mandatory ventilation (IMV) method.

TABLE 32-8
## Complications of Mechanical Ventilation Therapy

| Complication | Cause and Clinical Presentation | Management Considerations |
|---|---|---|
| ***Acid–Base Disturbances*** | | |
| 1. Post-hypercapnic alkalemia | Too rapid reduction in $PaCO_2$ by mechanical ventilation, in a patient with chronic lung disease (long standing hypercapnia with elevated serum bicarbonate—Renal compensation to maintain pH within normal limits). Reduction in $PaCO_2$ exposes underlying alkalemia. Signs/symptoms of severe alkalemia:<br>1. Depression of respiratory centers for ventilation.<br>2. Reduced serum ionized calcium level.<br>3. Increased central nervous system irritability (potential seizures); muscle weakness, ileus.<br>4. Cardiac dysrhythmias (pH >7.55). | Provide enough mechanical ventilation to reduce $PaCO_2$ only to a level that normalizes the pH.<br>Replace chloride ion to allow kidney to excrete bicarbonate ($HCO_3^-$). |
| 2. Metabolic alkalemia/alkalosis (see Table 30-3) | Associated with hypokalemia and hypochloremia related to:<br>1. Increased renal loss of potassium by diuretics, steroids, penicillins, and other drugs.<br>2. Shift of $K^+$ intracellularly in exchange with $H^+$ ion in presence of underlying alkalemia.<br>3. Inadquate intake of potassium.<br>4. Increased aldosterone secretion.<br>5. Loss of gastric acid by nasogastric drainage.<br>6. Renal retention of bicarbonate in the presence of hypercapnia. | Alkalemia may interfere with weaning.<br>Acetazolamide therapy—Renal response significantly enhanced with excretion of large urine volumes with increased bicarbonate.<br>Administration of saline or potassium chloride. |
| | Respiratory compensation for metabolic alkalemia involves alveolar hypoventilation. | Alveolar hypoventilation predisposes to atelectasis. |
| 3. Respiratory alkalemia/alkalosis (see Table 30-2) | Respiratory alkalemia can be artificially produced by overventilation of the patient.<br>Spontaneous hyperventilation may also cause respiratory alkalemia.<br>Signs/symptoms:<br>1. Reduced cardiac output.<br>2. Cardiac dysrhythmias.<br>3. Decreased lung compliance.<br>4. Increased airway resistance.<br>5. Ventilation/perfusion mismatch.<br>6. Increased right-to-left shunt.<br>7. Seizures. | Ventilatory therapy should be closely controlled to produce an acceptable pH, but not necessarily a normal $PaCO_2$.<br>Decrease alveolar ventilation:<br>• Decrease tidal volume.<br>• Decrease respiratory rate.<br>• Add mechanical deadspace.<br>Changing ventilatory mode to IMV may alleviate problem if due to patient out of sync with ventilator or assist/control.<br>Diazepam, morphine, and pancuronium may be necessary to control spontaneous hyperventilation while the patient is mechanically ventilated. |
| 4. Hypercapnic respiratory acidemia/acidosis | Inadequate alveolar ventilation or alveolar hypoventilation.<br>Retention of carbon dioxide leads to acidemia with decreased pH (pH <7.35). | Increase ($V_E$) or ($V_A$) ventilation.<br>• Larger tidal volume.<br>• Increase in respiratory rate. |
| ***Pulmonary Alterations*** | | |
| 1. Atelectasis | Collapse of alveoli associated with airway obstruction.<br>Use of low tidal volumes with mechanical ventilation therapy without a periodic "sigh."<br>Signs/symptoms:<br>1. Diminished breath sounds.<br>2. Increase in $AaDO_2$ (alveolar-arterial oxygen gradient).<br>3. Reduced lung compliance. | Institute use of "sigh" or large tidal volume.<br>Vigorous chest physiotherapy and pulmonary hygiene.<br>Increased humidification of inspired gas.<br>Vigorous tracheal suctioning. |

*(continued)*

TABLE 32–8

## Complications of Mechanical Ventilation Therapy (*Continued*)

| Complication | Cause and Clinical Presentation | Management Considerations |
|---|---|---|
| 2. Oxygen toxicity | Prolonged administration of high concentration of oxygen ($FIO_2 > 60\%$) may cause:<br>1. Absorption atelectasis (at $FIO_2$ 100%).<br>2. Impaired surfactant activity.<br>3. Pulmonary interstitial edema; fibrosis and thickening of alveolar–capillary membrane (may impair diffusion and gas exchange). | Frequent monitoring of arterial blood gases with use of $FIO_2 > 40\%$.<br>Periodic oxygen analysis to confirm that oxygen concentration reaching the patient is at the prescribed level.<br>Always use lowest possible oxygen concentration to maintain $PaO_2 > 60$ mmHg. |
| 3. Barotrauma: Pneumothorax, pneumomediastinum, subcutaneous emphysema | Associated with positive-pressure ventilation; especially with PEEP.<br>Signs/symptoms:<br>1. Restlessness; agitation.<br>2. Asymmetric chest wall excursion.<br>3. Altered breathing pattern; tachypnea.<br>4. Diminished breath sounds on affected side; hyperresonance on percussion.<br>5. Tachycardia; cyanosis. | Patients with chronic obstructive lung disease are at high risk.<br>The effects of excessive pressure and volume combined within the alveoli can lead to rupture of the membrane.<br>Possibility of tension pneumothorax must always be considered.<br>Chest x-ray. |
| 4. Inability to wean | A major problem in patients with chronic lung disease, debilitation (as in elderly), musculoskeletal disorders, cystic fibrosis. | Intubation and initiation of mechanical ventilation therapy should only be done if absolutely necessary.<br>See Chapter 33 for details related to the management of the patient with hypercapnic/hypoxemic ARF. |
| 5. Tracheal/laryngeal damage (see Table 32–3) | Pressure necrosis.<br>1. Tracheal stenosis.<br>2. Tracheomalacia.<br>3. Tracheoesophageal fistula.<br>4. Tracheoinnominate fistula. | Ongoing assessment for:<br>1. Proper placement of tube.<br>2. Maintenance of cuff pressure sufficient to achieve a minimal leak/seal.<br>3. Properly secured tube to prevent movement of the tube or accidental extubation.<br>4. Necessary humidification of inspired gas.<br>5. Airway patency: Effectiveness of secretion removal.<br>6. Use of aseptic technique in suctioning.<br>7. To minimize trauma to the airway: Alleviate clinical problems that result in disruption of tube placement (e.g., restlessness, agitation, "bucking vent," or seizure activity).<br>Support tube/tubing during patient movement to reduce traction or friction on airway. |
| 6. Pulmonary embolism (see Chap. 35) | Immobilization associated with mechanical ventilation therapy.<br>High incidence of thrombocytopenia in adult respiratory distress syndrome.[16] | Range-of-motion exercises.<br>Support stockings to lower extremities.<br>Careful assessment for calf tenderness; measure circumference of calf and thighs each shift.<br>Prophylactic heparin therapy. |
| ***Cardiovascular Alterations*** | | |
| 1. Cardiac dysrhythmias<br>a. Supraventricular<br>b. Ventricular | Hypoxemia, hypercapnia, pH changes, increased catecholamine secretion, hypokalemia, and hypocalcemia.<br>1. Disrupt depolarization and repolarization phases of action potential.<br>2. Increase automaticity.<br>3. Increase re-entry phenomenon.<br>Tracheal intubation and suctioning can stimulate vagal reflexes and predispose to dysrhythmias. | Treat hypoxemia/hypoxia.<br>Maintain continuous ECG monitoring.<br>Monitor electrolytes. |

TABLE 32–8
## Complications of Mechanical Ventilation Therapy (*Continued*)

| Complication | Cause and Clinical Presentation | Management Considerations |
|---|---|---|
| 2. Decreased cardiac output<br>a. Tachycardia<br>b. Hypotension<br>c. Tissue hypoxia | Positive intrathoracic pressures reduce preload (venous return).<br>Signs/symptoms of decreased cardiac output:<br>1. Reduced blood pressure; tachycardia.<br>2. Decreased urine output. | Maintain intravascular volume to minimize effects of changes in intrathoracic pressures on venous return to the heart.<br>Careful ongoing assessment of tidal volume, airway resistance, PEEP adjustments. |
| ***Fluid and Electrolyte Disturbances*** | | |
| 1. Water and salt retention (see appropriate tables in Chap. 23) | Controlled mechanical ventilation causes:<br>1. Alteration in renal blood flow.<br>2. Increased secretion of antidiuretic hormone (ADH) decreases urinary output.<br>3. Increase in aldosterone secretion.<br>Hypoalbuminemia and decreased colloidal oncotic pressure predispose to pulmonary interstitial edema.<br>Fluid retention due to overhydration by humidification. | Close monitoring of intake and output.<br>Daily weight.<br>Respiratory assessment every 1–2 hr for abnormal or adventitious breath sounds.<br>Monitor serum electrolytes; serum proteins.<br>Monitor arterial blood gases and $AaDO_2$.<br>Monitor vital capacity and lung compliance. |
| 2. Electrolyte imbalances<br>a. Hypokalemia<br>b. Hypochloremia (see appropriate tables in Chap. 23) | (See acid–base disturbances above.)<br>Associated with metabolic alkalemia.<br>1. Sodium renal reabsorption is associated with potassium excretion in presence of reduced hydrogen-ion concentration.<br>2. Shift of potassium intracellularly in exchange for hydrogen-ion movement into blood.<br>3. Renal reabsorption of bicarbonate in response to hypercapnia is associated with chloride excretion = hypochloremia.<br>Hypokalemia resulting from large renal losses of potassium in response to drugs:<br>1. Diuretics.<br>2. Penicillins (carbenicillin; ticarcillin, piperacillin).<br>3. Adrenocorticosteroids: Endogenous and exogenous sources.<br>Signs/symptoms:<br>1. Muscle weakness, which may interfere with weaning.<br>2. Dysrhythmias associated with or without digitalis toxicity. | Monitor as above:<br>1. Serial electrolyte, BUN, creatinine.<br>2. Review drug therapy—Avoid use of potassium-depleting medications.<br>3. Follow serum digitalis levels if the patient takes digoxin; assess for signs of digitalis toxicity.<br>CNS—Fatigue, headache, muscle weakness, mental depression, paresthesias.<br>CV—Decreased cardiac output with hypotension; dysrhythmias.<br>GI—Nausea, vomiting, diarrhea.<br>4. Continuous ECG monitoring. |
| c. Reduced ionized serum calcium (see appropriate tables in Chap. 24) | Alkalemia increases the fraction of protein-bound calcium, thus reducing available ionized calcium.<br>1. Serum calcium levels <8.0 mg/100 ml can precipitate neuromuscular irritability. | Correct hypercapnia and acidemia to reduce obligatory renal reabsorption of bicarbonate.<br>Monitor serum calcium/phosphorus levels.<br>Assess for signs of hypocalcemia. |
| ***Gastrointestinal Alterations*** | | |
| 1. Acute upper GI bleeding due to stress ulcer, peptic ulcer, gastritis<br>2. Paralytic ileus (most commonly associated with hypokalemia)<br>3. Gastric distention related to intubation and air swallowing.<br>4. Pulmonary aspiration of gastric contents. | Gastrointestinal complications frequently associated with acute respiratory failure.<br>Hypoxia enhances gastric acidity; acute increases in gastric acidity play a role in the increased incidence of peptic ulcer disease associated with chronic lung disease and acute respiratory failure. | Abdominal assessment: Bowel sounds<br>Antacid prophylaxis to keep gastric pH >4.5.<br>Cimetidine or ranitidine therapy:<br>1. Note side effects—Lethargy, confusion, depressed ventilatory drive, thrombocytopenia; cardiac dysrhythmias, GI symptoms, other.<br>Periodic testing of gastric aspirate and stools for guaiac. |
| ***Infections*** | | |
| 1. Pulmonary infections—Pneumonias<br>2. Septicemia | Debilitated and aged at increased risk.<br>Multiple invasive lines. | Obtain baseline cultures: Sputum, urine, blood. |

*(continued)*

TABLE 32-8
**Complications of Mechanical Ventilation Therapy *(Continued)***

| Complication | Cause and Clinical Presentation | Management Considerations |
|---|---|---|
| 3. Urinary tract infection | Malnutrition/protein catabolism; alteration in surfactant activity; alteration in respiratory epithelium replication invites infection and ulceration.<br>Use of antibiotics that alter normal flora.<br>Increased risk of aspiration.<br>Artificial airway and other respiratory adjuncts interfere with nonpulmonary defenses; increased risk of airway contamination.<br>Immunosuppression/decreased immunocompetence. | Monitor WBC, leukocytosis, body temperature, presence of purulent tracheobronchial secretions.<br>Pulmonary infiltrates on chest x-ray.<br>Monitor pulmonary function.<br>Vigorous chest physiotherapy (bronchial hygiene), postural drainage, percussion, regular turning/positioning.<br>Aseptic technique in suctioning, care of monitoring lines.<br>Therapeutic bronchoscopy.<br>Appropriate antibiotic therapy.<br>Nutrition maintenance. |
| ***Malnutrition*** | | |
| 1. Critical illness, increased stress cause hypermetabolic state<br>• Protein catabolism<br>2. Increased carbon dioxide production with respiratory acidosis<br>3. Energy demand greater than energy supply<br>• Fatigue and weakness of respiratory muscles | Critical illness with inadequate nutritive intake = semi-starvation.<br>Prolonged mechanical ventilation subjects respiratory muscles to passive activity, resulting in atrophy of diaphragm and respiratory muscles.<br>Excess glucose alimentation may increase carbon dioxide production and places added demands on ventilatory system. | Nutrition assessment.<br>Appropriate total parenteral nutrition.<br>Maintenance of alveolar ventilation. |
| ***Psychologic Depression*** | | |
| Anxiety: Patient and family | Inability to communicate normally during mechanical ventilation therapy.<br>Psychologic dependence on mechanical ventilation.<br>Sensory/sleep deprivation.<br>Sensory overload. | Develop system of communication patient feels comfortable with.<br>Anticipate needs.<br>Continuous monitoring.<br>Establish rapport with family. Keep patient/family informed. Involve them in care planning.<br>Offer reassurance; take time to listen and answer questions.<br>Help nurture feelings of security and human worth. |

### T-Piece or Nebulization Trial

For patients in whom there is a good potential for successful weaning, a trial of breathing humidified oxygen through a T-piece is indicated. For this method to be successful, patients should be awake, oriented, alert, and cooperative; they should be hemodynamically stable and able to take deep breaths without intercostal retraction; and they must feel confident about their ability to breathe spontaneously and effectively.

Success in using the T-piece approach is evaluated in terms of patient comfort and ease of breathing; stable hemodynamic status; respiratory rate <30/minute, tidal volume ($V_T$) >5–7 ml/kg, vital capacity >10–15 ml/kg; negative inspiratory pressure (NIP) −20–−25 cm$H_2O$; a $PaO_2$>100 mmHg on an $FIO_2$ 40%; and a $PaCO_2$ <45 mmHg. Some patients require very gradual weaning with T-piece trials, with increasing time off the ventilator.

### Intermittent Mandatory Ventilation (IMV)

The second approach to weaning involves applicatin of intermittent mandatory ventilation (IMV). The number of mechanical breaths delivered to the patient per minute is decreased to allow the patient to increasingly contribute to ventilatory demand by spontaneous breathing.

The IMV route has several advantages when properly applied. This method is safer and easier to regulate than a T-piece; the respiratory rate can be reduced according to an arbitrary time frame based on the patient's response. For example, if the initial setting was 14 breaths/minute, this rate could be decreased by 2, every 4 hours if tolerated by the patient. Some patients may require a more gradual decrease in IMV rate.

Eventually, the patient assumes complete ventilatory responsibility by spontaneous breathing. Successful weaning is evaluated using arterial

TABLE 32–9

**The Mechanically Ventilated Patient: Nursing Care Considerations***

| Nursing Interventions | Rationales |
|---|---|
| • Maintain a patent airway by proper endotracheal tube placement/taping. | • Due to anatomical structure of the mainstem bronchi, the endotracheal tube may slip into the right mainstem if positioned too low, thereby obstructing airflow to the left lung. |
| • Inflate tracheal/endotracheal tube cuff using the minimal air leak or minimal occlusive technique. | • The cuff must be adequately inflated to provide a closed system between the patient and the ventilator. Underinflation of the endotracheal tube cuff may allow aspiration of gastric contents or saliva and loss of desired tidal volume. Overinflation may cause tracheal tissue necrosis or may herniate the cuff over the tip of the tube causing partial or complete airway obstruction. |
| • Turn patient every 1–2 hours; alternate side-to-side and semi-Fowler's position. | • Both ventilation and perfusion can be preferentially delivered to the segments of the lung through positioning maneuvers that promote drainage of some segments and ventilation of others. |
| • Use nonverbal as well as verbal communication; provide slate/pencil; maintain IV in nonwriting arm. | • Intubated patients experience fear, helplessness, and despair, and communication is necessary. |
| • Evaluate respiratory status periodically noting bilateral breath sounds and symmetry of chest movement. | • Auscultation provides information regarding the flow of air through the tracheobronchial tree and the presence of fluid, mucous, or obstruction. Evaluation of symmetry with respirations provides information about air flow to lungs and may identify inadvertent right mainstem intubation. |
| • Suction airway as necessary. | • The endotracheal intubated patient usually has an ineffective cough reflex due to the interference of the tube with glottic closure. Suctioning should not be routine because unnecessary suctioning may produce excessive tracheal irritation and increase risk of infection. |
| • Hyperventilate with resuscitator bag and oxygenate pre/post-suctioning with 100% oxygen for 3-6 breaths. | • Hyperventilation minimizes atelectasis related to suctioning. High concentrations of oxygen provided prior to, and following suctioning, assist in preventing myocardial hypoxia and cardiac dysrhythmias. |
| • Monitor ECG during suctioning. | • Hypoxia is a common cause of dysrhythmias. Ventilated patients have ventilation/perfusion imbalances and often have hypoxia/hypoxemia. |
| • Maintain respiratory parameters within normal limits by frequent checks on ordered ventilatory settings: | |
| Oxygen percentage | • The lowest possible $FIO_2$ capable of promoting adequate oxygenation should be provided to the patient; lower levels (less than 50%) can be used for long periods of time without evidence of oxygen toxicity. |
| Tidal Volume | • Indicates the amount of air breathed in and out of the airway during a normal respiratory cycle; changes may indicate leakage through the machine or cuff and will affect ventilation and oxygenation. |
| Inspiratory/expiratory ratio | • Usual ratio of inspiratory phase to expiratory phase (I:E) is 1 to 2 or 1 to 3. Changes in the I:E will change the ventilatory rate and will effect ventilation/perfusion ratio. |
| Sensitivity | • Determines the amount of negative pressure that the patient must generate in the assist mode to trigger the ventilator. If the sensitivity is not adjusted, the patient can hyperventilate or at the other extreme, fight for air. |
| Airway pressure | • Once the tidal volume has been established, the airway pressure should remain relatively constant. An increase in the pressure reading on the manometer may reflect an increase in the amount of pressure needed to deliver a set volume of gas as occurs with increases in airway resistance and/or decreases in lung compliance as may occur with pneumothorax, pulmonary edema, misplacement of the ET tube. |
| Sigh (frequency and volume) | • Frequency and volume of sigh affect alveolar ventilation, promote cough, and help prevent atelectasis. |
| Humidity and temperature | • The usual warming/humidifying function of the nasopharynx has been bypassed with intubation. Humidification is necessary to maintain secretions at normal viscosity. The temperature of inspired gas should be maintained at approximately body temperature. |

*(continued)*

TABLE 32–9

**The Mechanically Ventilated Patient: Nursing Care Considerations* (*Continued*)**

| Nursing Interventions | Rationales |
|---|---|
| Rate | • Respirations should be counted for one full minute comparing the patient's respiratory rate with set ventilatory rate. Rapid respiratory rate due to the patient's triggering of the ventilator can produce abnormal blood gas values. |
| Alarm system | • Mechanical ventilators involve a series of audible and visual alarms to reflect abnormal ventilator changes and increase ventilator efficiency and patient safety, (e.g., low/high pressure alarms, I : E ratio alarms, oxygen alarms.) These alarms should never be turned off even when suctioning. |
| • Evaluate response to mechanical ventilation: level of consciousness and responsiveness; and monitor ABGs. | • Assess mental state, orientation to person, place and time; level of consciousness. Changes in arousability or behavior, or ability to follow commands, may be early indicators of hypoxia, as noted by ABGs. |
| • Patient respirations related to ventilator. | • If the patient is *bucking* or *fighting* the ventilator, it may be appropriate to sedate the patient. |
| • Constant supervision and care are required if Pavulon is used. | • Complete paralysis makes the patient totally dependent on ventilator for breathing and on nursing staff for general care. |
| • Maintenance of optimal PEEP, avoid routine suctioning. | • Each time the ventilator is disconnected, the PEEP is lost and it takes time to reestablish effective alveolar pressures again. |
| • Recognize side effects/complications: atelectasis evidenced through auscultation/palpation. | • Localized atelectasis may occur as a result of retained secretions. |
| • Decreased cardiac output evidenced by decrease in blood pressure and pulse. | • The positive pressures generated increase the intrathoracic pressure, which can potentially decrease venous return resulting in a decrease in cardiac output (especially with the use of PEEP). |
| • Monitor signs of pneumothorax (barotrauma): asymmetrical chest movements; diminished/absent breath sounds on affected side; tachycardia with weak pulse; cyanosis; decreased cardiac output with hypotension; accumulation of air under skin, crackling of skin with palpation; displacement of trachea. Note tracheal position. | • Pressures generated by the PEEP mode of ventilation may promote rupture of the alveolar walls, allowing air leaks into the pleural space, mediastinum and/or subcutaneous spaces. The patient becomes at risk of lung collapse with compromise of cardiopulmonary function.<br>• Trachea shifts away from the affected side. Depending on the size of pneumothorax and/or mediastinal or subcutaneous emphysema, chest tube insertion may be necessary. |
| • In preparation for weaning:<br>Monitor the tests related to respiratory status. | • Monitor arterial blood gases, tidal volume ($V_T$) on spontaneous breathing, vital capacity ($V_C$) >12 to 15 ml/Kg; ease of breathing. |
| Assess respirations and ventilator breaths per minute; record tidal volume for each during use of IMV for weaning. | • IMV allows the patient's own breathing pattern to be maintained with positive breaths delivered intermittently by the ventilator. |
| Monitor for signs of respiratory distress. | • Early detection and treatment of respiratory difficulty will minimize possibility of return to the ventilator. |
| **Medical Management** | |
| • Arterial line and serial ABGs. | • To assess effectiveness of ventilatory effort, gas exchange, and the weaning process. |
| • Bronchodilators | • Use may improve ventilation compromised by bronchial edema and bronchospasms. |
| • Pavulon | • Sedation or paralysis alleviates the problem of *fighting the ventilator.* Makes the patient completely dependent on mechanical ventilation. |
| • Sedatives | • The use of Pavulon does not affect the ability to think and sedation is important to reduce the unpleasant feelings that accompany the use of this drug. |
| • Addition of PEEP to ventilator regimen | • Promotes alveolar expansion and helps to prevent shunting of blood through unventilated areas of the lung thereby increasing FRC and optimizing the oxygen gradient across the alveolar/capillary membrane. |
| • IMV, SIMV, or other appropriate weaning techniques. | • Promotes use and gradual strengthening of the respiratory muscles. |

*Adapted from Doenges, ME, Jeffries, MF, Moorhouse, MF. *Nursing Care Plans: Nursing Diagnoses in Planning Patient Care,* F.A. Davis Co., Philadelphia, 1984, pp. 145–149.

See also:
TABLE 32–6. Ventilator Controls: Guidelines for Adjustments
TABLE 32–7. Monitoring the Ventilated Patient: Implications for Nursing Care
TABLE 32–8. Complications of Mechanical Ventilation Therapy

blood gas values as the parameter for determining continued decrease in the ventilatory rate. Parameters mentioned above with respect to T-piece weaning may also be used to evaluate the patient's response to the weaning process.

It is important to evaluate the patient's drug therapy. Drugs causing central nervous system depression should be discontinued (narcotics may exert an effect in some patients for up to 10 days); drugs that cause bronchoconstriction (e.g., propranolol) should also be stopped. Patients with renal or hepatic failure may have a prolonged effect with some drugs (e.g., neuromuscular blocking agents). Neuromuscular blockade has also been associated with certain antibiotics (e.g., neomycin, gentamicin, streptomycin). Aminophylline is commonly prescribed in weaning situations because it causes bronchodilatation, increases diaphragmatic contractility, increases ventricular contractility, exerts a diuretic effect, and stimulates ventilation. Electrolyte imbalance may cause muscular weakness in patients who may already have some atrophy of respiratory muscles because of prolonged mechanical ventilation.

### *Tips on Weaning*[21]

1. Never commence weaning unless you think the patient has some chance of success, that is, has met minimal criteria for weaning (see Table 32–5).
2. Always quit while you're ahead (i.e., discontinuance of the weaning routine at the earliest sign of fatigue, discomfort, or distress).
3. Develop a program with appropriate input from all staff members so that they can be consistently supportive of the approach used.
4. Keep the patient informed, and develop an incentive system.
5. The patient must be in an appropriate nutritional state and hemodynamically stable.
6. Pain must be controlled.
7. Have the patient in a position where all respiratory muscles are maximally functioning.
8. Never wean at night.

Specific nursing interventions and their rationales pertinent to the care of the patient receiving mechanical ventilation are presented in Table 32–9.

## REFERENCES


1. Fulmer, JD and Snider, GL: American College of Chest Physicians/National Heart, Lung, and Blood Institute National Conference on Oxygen Therapy. Heart Lung, 13(4):550, September 1984.
2. Clinical news, Transtracheal oxygen: The nose knows the difference. Am J Nurs 87(4):421, April 1987.
3. Alspach, J and Williams, S: Core Curriculum for Critical Care Nursing, ed 3. WB Saunders, Philadelphia, 1985, p 62.
4. Hoffman, L, Mazzocco, M, and Roth, J: Fine tuning your chest PT. Am J Nurs 87(12):1566, December 1987.
5. McHugh, J: Chest physiotherapy: Perfecting the 3 steps. Nursing '87 17(11):54, November 1987.
6. Kacmarek, R and Stoller, J: Current Respiratory Care. BC Decker, Philadelphia, 1988, p 38.
7. Rarey, KP and Youtsey, JW: Respiratory Patient Care. Prentice-Hall, Englewood Cliffs, NJ, 1981, p 145.
8. Dennison, R: Managing the patient with upper airway obstruction. Nursing '87 17(10):34, October 1987.
9. Don, H: Decision Making in Critical Care. CV Mosby, St. Louis, 1985, p 106.
10. Emanuelsen, K and Densmore, MJ: Acute Respiratory Care. Fleschner Publishing, Bethany, CT, 1981, p 155.
11. Hoffman, L and Maszkiewicz, R: Airway management, the specifics of suctioning. Am J Nurs 87(1):39, January 1987.
12. Millar, S, Sampson, L, and Soukup, SM: AACN Procedure Manual for Critical Care ed 2. WB Saunders, Philadelphia, 1985, pp 220–223.
13. King, G: Respiratory failure in the critically ill. In Sibbald, WJ (ed): Synopsis of Critical Care, ed 3. Williams and Wilkins, Baltimore, 1988, p 53.
14. Chalikian, J and Weaver, T: Mechanical ventilation: For CE credit where it's at, where it's going. Am J Nurs 84(11):1372, 1984.
15. Rarey, K and Youtsey, J: Respiratory Patient Care. Prentice-Hall, Englewood Cliffs, NJ, 1981, p 224.
16. Vincent, JE: Medical problems in the patient on a ventilator. Crit Care Q 6(2):40, September 1983.
17. Shapiro, BA: Noncardiogenic edema, adult respiratory distress syndrome and PEEP therapy. In Cane, RD and Shapiro, BA (eds): Case Studies in Critical Care Medicine. Year Book Medical Publishers, Chicago, 1985, p 184.
18. Jorgenson, S: CE weaning from the ventilator. Am J Nurs 87(9):1173–1184, September 1987.
19. Herrold, R: The drug connection. Am J Nurs 84(11):1389, November 1984.
20. Norton, LC and Neureuter, A: Weaning the long-term ventilator-dependent patient: Common problems and management. Critical Care Nurse 9(1):42–46, January 1989.
21. King, G: Respiratory failure in the critically ill. Synopsis of Critical Care, ed. 3. Williams and Wilkins, Baltimore, 1988, p 60.

CHAPTER 33

# Nursing Management of the Patient with Chronic Obstructive Pulmonary Disease in Hypercapnic/Hypoxemic Acute Respiratory Failure

## CHAPTER OUTLINE

CHRONIC OBSTRUCTIVE PULMONARY DISEASE
- Major Chronic Obstructive Pulmonary Disorders
- Pathology
- Pathophysiology
- Clinical Presentation
- Treatment

NURSING CARE OF THE PATIENT WITH CHRONIC OBSTRUCTIVE PULMONARY DISEASE IN ACUTE RESPIRATORY FAILURE
- Therapeutic Goals

*CASE STUDY WITH SAMPLE CARE PLAN: Patient with Chronic Obstructive Pulmonary Disease*

## LEARNING OBJECTIVES

**At the end of this chapter, you should be able to:**

1. Define *chronic obstructive pulmonary disease (COPD).*
2. Identify similarities and dissimilarities between chronic bronchitis and emphysema in terms of:
   a. Pathology.
   b. Pathophysiology.
   c. Clinical presentation.
3. Examine mechanisms underlying hypercapnic/hypoxemic acute respiratory failure in the patient with COPD.
4. State the therapeutic goals in the treatment and management of COPD complicated by acute respiratory failure.
5. Specify precautions to be taken when administering oxygen therapy to the patient with COPD.
6. Describe the use of respiratory support therapy, including the following therapeutic modalities:
   a. Oxygen therapy.
   b. Drug therapy.
   c. Hydration and nutritional support.
   d. Chest physiotherapy–bronchial hygiene.
   e. Intubation and mechanical ventilation.
7. Describe implications for nursing care based on nursing process:
   Assessment.
   Specific nursing diagnoses.
   Planning: Desired patient outcomes
   Nursing interventions/rationales.

# CHRONIC OBSTRUCTIVE PULMONARY DISEASE

Acute respiratory failure (ARF) is a major cause of death in patients with chronic obstructive pulmonary disease (COPD). The term chronic obstructive pulmonary disease refers to chronic respiratory disorders that disrupt airflow whether the pathologic process is predominantly within the airways or the lung parenchyma. The two major disorders within this category are chronic bronchitis and emphysema. Although the underlying pathophysiology of airflow impairment is different in these two disorders, they frequently coexist to a variable extent in different patients who present clinically with features of both.

## Major Chronic Obstructive Pulmonary Disorders

### Chronic Bronchitis

Chronic bronchitis is characterized by excessive mucous secretions in the tracheobronchial tree. Clinically, the diagnosis of chronic bronchitis is based on chronic cough and sputum production. A formal definition requires that a chronic productive cough be present on most days during at least 3 consecutive months for not less than 2 successive years. Patients with chronic bronchitis frequently have periods of exacerbation, often precipitated by an upper respiratory infection.

The symptoms of chronic bronchitis are a result of chronic bronchial irritation. Several factors have been implicated in its etiology including, among others, smoking, air pollutants, and industrial irritants. Smoking is clearly the most important, and cigarette smoking has been recognized as the major cause of chronic bronchitis. Epidemiologic studies indicate that there is a significant correlation between cigarette smoking and the symptoms of cough and sputum production.

Air pollutants and respiratory tract infections have also been implicated in the pathogenesis of chronic bronchitis. These factors are especially significant because of their potential for causing exacerbations of preexisting chronic bronchitis. Viral infection, for example, appears to be responsible for a large number of clinical exacerbations of symptoms of chronic bronchitis.

### Emphysema

Emphysema is characterized by destruction of elastic tissue within the lungs. It is associated with two main etiologic factors: cigarette smoking and a hereditary predisposition. Cigarette smoking is responsible for most cases of emphysema; a hereditary predisposition characterized by a deficiency of the protein, alpha$_1$-protease inhibitor ($A_1PI$) appears to be a causative factor in a much smaller population of persons who develop emphysema. Persons with this genetic defect have very low serum levels of this protein, and they are strongly predisposed to the premature development of emphysema, as early as the third and fourth decades of life. If the person is also a smoker, there is an even stronger likelihood of the early occurrence of emphysema.

## Pathology

### Chronic Bronchitis

The pathology of chronic bronchitis is related to excessive mucous secretion of both mucus-secreting glands and goblet cells. It is characterized by enlargement of submucosal glands and an increase in the number of goblet cells (see Figs. 28–2 and 28–4). The composition of the mucus is altered (i.e., thickened and more viscous than usual). Changes in small airways can be seen early in the disease process. Inflammation of airways with cellular infiltration can be demonstrated, and variable degrees of fibrosis may also be evident. As a result of these pathologic changes, there is a significant reduction in the diameter of small airways and bronchioles, which increases airway resistance, impairs airflow, and gives rise to the symptomatology associated with chronic bronchitis.

It is important to appreciate that these early pathologic changes involving the small airways and respiratory bronchioles occur in response to cigarette smoking and forewarn of the potential development of the more advanced lesions of chronic bronchitis and emphysema.

### Emphysema

The pathology of emphysema is characterized by destruction of alveolar walls with enlargement of respiratory airspaces distal to the terminal bronchiole. The primary defect underlying emphysema involves the proteolysis of the complex structural protein, elastin, which is found in the walls of the alveoli. The breaking down of elastin diminishes elastic recoil of the lung, which alters expiratory airflow, and reduces the respiratory epithelial surface area available for gas exchange.

Elastin is largely broken down by the enzyme elastase, which is released by two types of inflammatory cells within the lungs: alveolar macrophages and polymorphonuclear leukocytes (PMNs). If elastase, released by these cells, was allowed to exert its proteolytic effect on elastin, destruction of the alveolar wall would ensue. Such wanton destruction of the alveolar walls does not occur because normally the activity of elastase is inhibited by alpha$_1$-protease inhibitor ($A_1PI$). Current thinking suggests that there is a balance between proteolytic enzymes, such as elastase, and $A_1PI$.[1] Any disturbance in this balance associated with an increase in elastase activity or a decrease in the anti-elastase activity of $A_1PI$ can disrupt elastin and damage the alveolar wall, with the consequence of early development of emphysema.

Cigarette smoking is thought to disturb the balance between elastase and $A_1PI$. The irritating effects of smoke increase the number of inflammatory cells (especially PMNs) within the lung, thus providing a source for increased amounts of elastase. Through its direct interaction with $A_1PI$, cigarette smoke decreases the normal inhibitory activity of this molecule, which serves to limit the uncontrolled breakdown of elastin.

Two types of emphysema having distinct pathologic features dependent on the distribution of the lesions have been identified. These are panacinar (panlobular) emphysema and centriacinar (centrilobular) emphysema (Fig. 33-1).

**Panacinar Emphysema.** This is characterized by a nearly uniform enlargement and destruction of the alveoli in the pulmonary acinus. With progression of the disease, there is gradual loss of all components of the acinus until only a few strands of tissue, usually blood vessels, remain. Pathology within an involved area is relatively diffuse but may be more severe in lower lung areas. Panacinar emphysema is the usual type of emphysema described in patients who have $A_1PI$ deficiency, but it is by no means limited to this clinical circumstance.

**Centriacinar Emphysema.** This commonly occurs in cigarette smokers and is frequently accompanied by the airway changes of chronic bronchitis. Predominantly, pathologic changes are found in the proximal part of the acinus (i.e., the respiratory bronchioles). The involvement in an affected area seems to be more irregular with apparent sparing of alveolar tissue distal to the respiratory bronchioles (see Fig. 33-1).

## Pathophysiology

### *Reduced Maximal Expiratory Airflow*

The major functional abnormality found in chronic obstructive pulmonary disease is a reduction in maximal expiratory airflow.* This reduction in expiratory airflow is characteristic of both chronic bronchitis and emphysema. The mechanisms underlying flow reduction, however, are quite different in these two conditions. Measurements of lung volumes, specifically total lung capacity (TLC), functional residual capacity (FRC), and residual volume (RV), help to differentiate the effects of the underlying pathophysiology in these two obstructive disorders. It is useful to review the factors that determine these major lung volumes/capacities (see Fig. 28-9).

**Total Lung Capacity (TLC).** This reflects the point at which the maximal force generated by inspiratory muscles acting to expand the lungs is

*Review the discussion regarding the clinical significance of maximal expiratory flow studies presented in Chapter 28 before pursuing the discussion that follows.

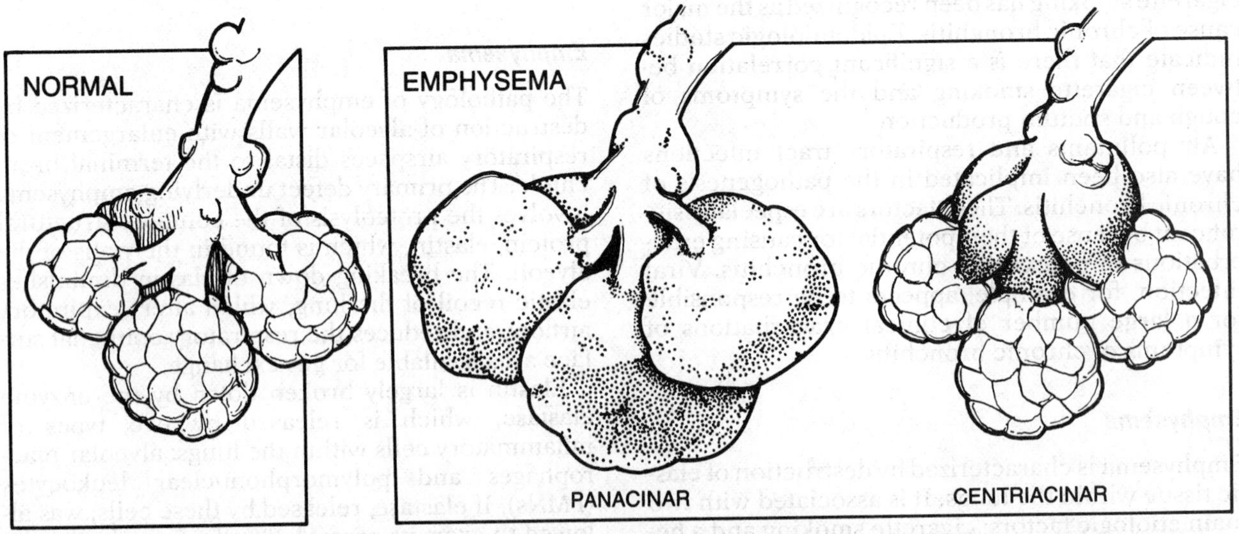


**Figure 33-1.** Schematic diagram depicting the terminal bronchiole, respiratory bronchiole, and alveoli of normal lung, and changes seen in these structures in emphysema. In panacinar type, all airways and alveoli are involved with breakdown of alveolar walls predisposing to loss of surface area for gas exchange. In centriacinar type, respiratory bronchioles are distended and communicating with one another, but distal alveoli remain intact early in the course of the disease.

equaled by the elastic recoil (mainly lung recoil) resisting expansion (see Fig. 28–8).

**Functional Residual Capacity.** This is the volume of gas remaining in the lungs after a normal expiration. It is the resting point of the respiratory system and reflects a balance between the elastic recoil of the lungs and the chest wall, which pull in opposite directions—the lungs inward and the chest wall outward.

**Residual Volume.** This is the volume of gas left within the lungs when the relatively stiff chest wall can be compressed no further by the expiratory muscles. Airway closure is an important determinant of residual volume (RV) (see Fig. 28–9).

In chronic bronchitis, maximal expiratory flow rates are reduced due to a decrease in airway size resulting from increased mucous secretions, hypertrophy and hyperplasia of mucus-secreting glands and goblet cells, and inflammatory and fibrotic changes in the airway walls. The TLC remains relatively close to normal as the elastic recoil of the lungs and strength of inspiratory muscles remain intact in chronic bronchitis. Because the recoil of both the lungs and chest cage is unchanged, the FRC also remains within normal range. FRC will increase if expiration is prolonged and the respiratory rate is rapid. In this instance, there may not be sufficient time during expiration for the patient to reach the normal resting end-expiratory point. The RV is commonly increased in chronic bronchitis due to the air trapping that occurs during expiration when small airways are narrowed or occluded.

In emphysema, the reduced maximal expiratory flow rates are largely due to loss of elastic recoil of the lungs as a consequence of the destruction of elastin. There is also loss of radial traction or "tethering" of airways. The result of these pathologic changes is a lower driving force for expiratory airflow, and an increased tendency of the airways to collapse during expiration. TLC is increased as the loss of elastic recoil reduces the force opposing that generated by the inspiratory musculature. FRC is also increased as the force generated by the outward recoil of the chest cage substantially exceeds the diminished inward recoil of the lungs. RV is also significantly increased due to early airway closure during a maximal expiration. (Study the details in Fig. 28–9 while concentrating on the material presented in this section.)

### *Abnormalities of Gas Exchange*

Characteristically in chronic obstructive pulmonary disease there is a nonuniformity of the underlying disease process. Consequently, there is a very uneven distribution of ventilation in relation to blood flow. Regions of the lung that are highly diseased receive less ventilation than less diseased areas. While compensatory mechanisms reduce blood flow to these underventilated areas, there is, nevertheless, considerable variability in ventilation/perfusion matchups. When the overall ratio of ventilation to perfusion is disrupted significantly, hypoxemia develops. Specific mechanisms underlying hypoxemia in the patient with obstructive pulmonary disease include ventilation/perfusion mismatch (most common), alveolar hypoventilation (related to increased work of breathing and an increase in dead space), and right-to-left shunting (particularly in advanced emphysematous obstructive disease).

### *Pulmonary Hypertension*

Pulmonary hypertension is a potential complication of chronic obstructive pulmonary disease. The major cause of pulmonary hypertension is hypoxia. A decrease in $PaO_2$ is a potent stimulus for constriction of pulmonary arterioles. Hypercapnia also stimulates constriction of pulmonary blood vessels, but this effect may be mediated predominantly by the consequent change in pH (respiratory acidemia).

While compensatory mechanisms within the lungs function to maintain optimal ventilation/perfusion matching in patients with chronic obstructive pulmonary disease, a point may be reached at which these compensatory mechanisms are exceeded, and acute respiratory failure with hypoxemia and tissue hypoxia develops. Pulmonary hypertension associated with longstanding hypoxemia increases the workload of the right ventricle and predisposes to right heart failure or cor pulmonale.[2]

Patients with prominent chronic bronchitis are particularly susceptible to development of pulmonary hypertension. In addition to hypoxia and respiratory acidemia, secondary polycythemia (increased blood viscosity) and destruction of pulmonary vascular bed (coexistent emphysema) also contribute to pulmonary hypertension.

## Clinical Presentation

To appreciate the clinical presentation, manifestations, and problems associated with chronic obstructive pulmonary disease, it is useful to distinguish between the two pathophysiologic types: emphysema (type A) and chronic bronchitis (type B). In practice, it is common for patients to have a combination of both types.

### *Type A—Emphysema Predominant (Pink Puffer)*

The type A patient who has a prominent emphysema and is in a more advanced stage of the disease is referred to as a "pink puffer." Dyspnea is the prominent symptom, and the patient works hard "puffing" to maintain a high minute ventilation. Arterial oxygen tensions are therefore well preserved so the patient is "pink" (not cyanotic), and carbon dioxide levels are not abnormally high. Gas exchange remains adequate in the patient with emphysema because destruction of alveolar walls involves the concomitant loss of attendant capillaries; thus, loss of ventilation and perfusion is matched. Because there is no hypoxia, pulmonary hypertension and polycythemia are not seen in this form of obstructive disease.

On physical examination, the type A patient is usually thin, underweight, and cachectic. There is an increased anteroposterior diameter (barrel-chested) indicating hyperinflation of the lungs. Supraclavicular fossae are hollowed, and the accessory muscles of respiration are hypertrophied. The patient is observed to lean forward to breathe, and "pursed-lip" breathing may also be evident. Diaphragmatic excursion is diminished. The chest is hyperresonant on percussion; breath sounds and heart sounds are distant and barely audible on auscultation. Expiration is prolonged as the patient struggles to maintain effective expiratory airflow.

#### *Type B—Chronic Bronchitis Predominant (Blue Bloater)*

The type B patient has a prominent chronic bronchitis, and chronic cough and sputum production are the major presenting symptoms. This form of obstructive disease is characterized by major gas exchange problems—hypoxemia and hypercapnia. In the more advanced stage of the disease, the patient is referred to as a "blue boater" because cyanosis is associated with significant hypoxemia and polycythemia. These patients are frequently obese and may have peripheral edema resulting from right ventricular failure (cor pulmonale). Ventilation/perfusion (V/(Q) mismatch and alveolar hypoventilation are the predominant mechanisms underlying the hypoxemia and hypercapnia. Significant hypoxia predisposes to pulmonary hypertension with eventual progression to cor pulmonale.

On physical examination the type B patient may be cyanotic, obese, and edematous. These patients appear to be in less respiratory distress than type A patients. Presence of excessive airway secretions produces wheezing and rhonchi on auscultation. In the presence of right ventricular failure, jugular venous distention and peripheral edema may be evident; and heart sounds may reflect a loud second sound ($S_2$) in the pulmonic area; extra heart sounds ($S_3$ and $S_4$) may also be heard.

There is a wide spectrum of severity in chronic obstructive pulmonary disease ranging from a mild form of the disease, in which the patient is able to pursue his/her work and lifestyle with minimal, if any, changes, to a severe stage of the disease, in which the patient experiences dyspnea even at rest. The disease course may be punctuated by periods of exacerbations usually precipitated by a respiratory tract infection. When the exacerbations are severe, the patient may experience acute respiratory failure necessitating hospitalization. Table 33-1 compares the clinical features of type A and type B obstructive pulmonary disease.

## Treatment

Acute respiratory failure (ARF) is a relatively common complication and major cause of death in patients with advanced chronic obstructive pulmonary disease (COPD). Acute respiratory failure in these patients may be precipitated by superimposed viral (commonly) or bacterial infection, or other acute respiratory insult. In patients with preexisting pulmonary disease and compromised respiratory reserve, the consequent reduction in alveolar ventilation and increase in ventilation/perfusion mismatch predispose to hypercapnic/hypoxemic or "acute on chronic" respiratory failure. Patients are diagnosed to be in ARF when they are unable to maintain a level of alveolar ventilation sufficient to eliminate carbon dioxide and maintain the pH $>7.35$; and to maintain $PaO_2 >60$ mmHg.

#### *Goals of Treatment*

The immediate therapeutic goals are to relieve hypoxemia and tissue hypoxia; to return the blood pH to within an acceptable physiologic range (pH $>7.35$) by eliminating carbon dioxide; and to reverse the precipitating cause.[3] It is important to appreciate the special problems presented by the patient with COPD because of their progressive pulmonary pathology, abnormal pulmonary mechanics, and the physiologic adaptations to these derangements.

The criteria of ARF are different in patients with COPD who often function at arterial blood gas levels ($PaO_2 <60$ mmHg, $PaCO_2 >50$ mmHg) that ordinarily define ARF in otherwise healthy persons. These patients also function on a hypoxemic (hypoxic) ventilatory stimulus, which requires low-flow supplemental oxygen. Administration of high oxygen concentrations may reverse the hypoxemia, but it may also diminish the patient's ventilatory drive, increase the $PaCO_2$ to levels causing a precipitous drop in blood pH ($<7.25$), and precipitate apnea. Improvement of the $PaO_2$ reduces tissue hypoxia and may also reverse pulmonary hypertension resulting from vasoconstriction of the pulmonary vasculature in response to hypoxia.[4]

Appropriate oxygen therapy may also minimize polycythemia vera, which is associated with long-term reduction in arterial oxygen saturation

TABLE 33-1
**Comparison: Clinical Features of Type A and Type B Obstructive Pulmonary Disease**

| Clinical Features | Type A (Emphysema) | Type B (Chronic Bronchitis) |
|---|---|---|
| Description | "Pink puffer" | "Blue bloater" |
| Pathology | Destruction of alveolar walls with dilatation of respiratory air spaces<br>Types:<br>Panacinar (panlobular)<br>Centriacinar (centrilobular) | Decreased airway size due to:<br>1. Excessive mucus production<br>2. Hypertrophy and hyperplasia of mucous glands and goblet cells<br>3. Airway inflammation and fibrosis |
| Elastic recoil of lungs | Reduced | Normal |
| Lung compliance | Increased | Normal |
| Pathophysiology | | |
| Maximal expiratory flow | Reduced | Reduced |
| Lung volumes | | |
| TLC | Increased | Normal |
| FRC | Increased | Normal |
| RV | Increased | Increased |
| Arterial blood gases | | |
| $PaO_2$ | Normal to mildly decreased | Decreased significantly |
| $PaCO_2$ | Normal to decreased | Normal to increased |
| Mechanisms of: | | |
| Hypoxemia | $\dot{V}/Q$ mismatch | $\dot{V}/Q$ mismatch |
| Hypercapnia | | Alveolar hypoventilation |
| Pulmonary hypertension | Usually absent | Usually present with advanced disease |
| Cor pulmonale | Usually absent | Usually present with advanced disease |
| Clinical presentation | | |
| History | | |
| Smoking | Usual | Usual |
| Family | $Alpha_1$-protease inhibitor deficiency | Cystic fibrosis |
| Signs and symptoms | | |
| Major symptom | Dyspnea | Chronic cough and sputum production |
| Physical examination | Thin, underweight, cachectic | Obese, edematous |
| Color | Pink | Cyanotic |
| Chest dimensions | Anteroposterior diameter increased | Within normal limits |
| Accessory muscles | Hypertrophied | Normal |
| Diaphragmatic excursion | Reduced | Usually normal |
| Breath sounds | | |
| Percussion | Hyperresonant | Usually normal |
| Auscultation | Breath sounds faint<br>Usually no adventitious sounds | Breath sound audible<br>Adventitious sounds—crackles and rhonchi |
| Expiratory rate | Increased | Increased |
| Sputum characteristics | Absent or mucoid | Copious, thick, tenacious<br>Predominantly neutrophilic |
| Laboratory | | |
| Hematocrit | Normal | Elevated (polycythemia) |
| Chest x-ray | Hyperinflation with large lung volumes<br>Flat diaphragm<br>Increased anteroposterior diameter<br>Reduced vascular markings<br>Emphysematous bullae | Normal if chronic bronchitis alone<br>Progressive disease:<br>Pulmonary hypertension<br>Cor pulmonale |

($SaO_2$). A reduced oxygen content in arterial blood stimulates erythropoiesis.

### *Treatment Modalities*

The modalities available for the treatment of chronic obstructive pulmonary disease with hypercapnic/hypoxemic respiratory failure include: (1) supplemental oxygenation and humidification; (2) bronchodilator therapy in conjunction with sympathomimetic and corticosteroid therapy; (3) antibiotic therapy; (4) mucolytic therapy; (5) chest physiotherapy; (6) phlebotomy; and (7) treatment of underlying cause.

**Supplemental Oxygen.** Supplemental oxygen with humidification is the mainstay of therapy in acute hypercapnic/hypoxemic respiratory failure. The mechanisms underlying the hypoxemia in this clinical circumstance are alveolar hypoventilation and ventilation/perfusion mismatch, both of which respond favorably to low concentrations of oxygen. Oxygen must be administered cautiously using inspired oxygen concentrations ($FIO_2$) of 24%–28% by Venturi mask, or 2–3 liters by nasal cannula.

Monitoring the patient's responses to therapy, including frequent measurements of arterial blood gases, is essential to guide treatment.

Overzealous use of high oxygen concentrations can shut off the hypoxic drive leading to alveolar hypoventilation. This results in hypercapnia with carbon dioxide narcosis and respiratory acidemia/acidosis.

The goal of oxygen therapy is to maintain the $PaO_2$ greater than 60 mmHg, because this affords near maximal saturation of hemoglobin ($SaO_2$~90%). Humidification is essential to prevent drying of respiratory mucosa and to assist in mobilization of secretions.

**Drug Therapy.**[5]. (See Appendix A for information on specific drugs.)

***Bronchodilator Therapy.*** Bronchodilator therapy is an important aspect of the treatment of patients with chronic obstructive pulmonary disease with ARF. Bronchodilators improve airflow and ventilation by decreasing bronchospasm. The most commonly used agents are aminophylline (administered intravenously in patients with acute respiratory decompensation) and sympathomimetics (e.g., beta agonists).

A steady-state concentration of theophylline and theophylline salts of 10–20 μg/ml is most efficacious, providing maximum benefit with least incidence of untoward effects. Frequent determination of theophylline levels in the critically ill is advocated because of variability of drug metabolism and clearance in these patients. Hepatic dysfunction and congestive heart failure may require dosage adjustments.

Familiarity with signs and symptoms of theophylline toxicity is essential. These may include central nervous system stimulation, nausea, diarrhea, cardiac dysrhythmias (multifocal atrial tachycardia, supraventricular ectopy), and seizures. (See Appendix A for adverse reactions and implications for nursing care.)

*Sympathomimetic* drugs complement the actions of theophylline preparations. (See specific section on sympathomimetic drugs in Appendix A.)

*Corticosteroid Therapy.* Corticosteroid therapy used in combination with bronchodilators (e.g., aminophylline, metaproterenol) has been shown to be efficacious in patients with chronic obstructive pulmonary disease (COPD). Use of steroids of low mineralocorticoid activity is preferred to prevent metabolic alkalemia (with sodium retention at the expense of hydrogen-ion excretion).

***Antibiotic Therapy.*** Antibiotic therapy is an integral part of the treatment plan because infection is the most common precipitating cause of acute respiratory failure in patients with COPD. Bacterial pneumonias are fairly common in patients with COPD; likely causative microorganisms in these circumstances are *Hemophilus influenzae* and *Streptococcus pneumoniae.*

The occurrence of fever; change in consistency, color, and amount of sputum; leukocytosis; or the appearance of new pulmonary infiltrates on chest x-ray during hospitalization requires meticulous surveillance and aggressive treatment with antibiotic therapy. Sputum cultures should be monitored at regular intervals to identify causative microorganism(s) and sensitivity to specific antibiotics. In viral pneumonias, antibiotics may be indicated to treat secondary bacterial infections superimposed on the viral infection.

*Klebsiella* and *Pseudomonas* pneumonias are gram-negative infections usually of nosocomial origin. *Klebsiella* pneumonia has a high mortality rate in patients with COPD. *Serratia,* another gram-negative organism, is a frequent contaminant of the nebulizers used in IPPB devices. A trial of therapy with the newer, safer antibiotics (e.g., cephalosporins) is usually initiated. The antibiotic therapy is provided over a 5–7 day period with close monitoring of sputum production, fever, leukocytosis, and pulmonary infiltrates on chest x-ray. (For specific antibiotics, including information related to dosage and administration, adverse reactions, and nursing care considerations, see Appendix A.)

***Antipyretic Therapy.*** Fever requires antipyretic therapy because oxygen consumption and carbon dioxide production increase approximately 10% with each degree (F) of temperature elevation.

***Mucolytic Therapy.*** Mucolytic therapy is sometimes used in conjunction with bronchodilator therapy to decrease viscosity of pulmonary secretions and facilitate secretion removal. Acetylcysteine (Mucomyst) is one mucolytic agent currently available. The benefit of hydration therapy and humidification cannot be underestimated in this regard.

**Chest Physiotherapy.** Use of chest physiotherapy to mobilize secretions is an integral aspect of the treatment of ARF in the patient with COPD. In conjunction with humidification of the tracheobronchial tree, techniques such as postural drainage, percussion and vibration, coughing and deep breathing exercises, and incentive spirometry, have been shown to improve secretion removal, ventilation, and oxygenation (see Chap. 32).

Positioning of patients can also improve arterial oxygenation. The prone position, if it can be assumed by the patient, has been shown to improve ventilation and oxygenation in patients with ARF. In unilateral lung consolidation, improved oxygenation occurs with positioning of the uneffective side down (better V/Q matching).[6] (See Fig. 28–13.)

The ability to cough is perhaps the most effective mechanism for clearing pulmonary secretions. The patient should be helped to establish and use this mechanism correctly.

**Nutritional Support Therapy.** Nutritional support therapy includes early implementation of nutritional support with enteral alimentation, supplemented with parenteral feedings to ensure sufficient nutritional intake. The semi-starvation state has been associated with a depression of the hypoxic ventilatory drive; and *hypophosphatemia* has been implicated in respiratory muscle weakness and infections in patients with COPD.[6]

A major concern in determining the nutritional regimen for patients with compromised pulmonary function is to avoid the metabolically associated increase in carbon dioxide production, which can exacerbate the worsening respiratory status. Patients with high protein intake or an overall high caloric intake may complain of dyspnea and may demonstrate an increased respiratory effort to maintain carbon dioxide at resting levels. The necessary increase in workload can further compromise lung function.

Treatment of the patient with an exacerbation of obstructive pulmonary disease is always focused on *conservative supportive therapy*. A vigorous routine of chest physiotherapy and bronchial hygiene, together with supplemental oxygen therapy, bronchodilator therapy, hydration and humidification, and nutritional support, may be sufficient to maintain the patient until the underlying insult is rectified. Through these efforts, intubation and mechanical ventilation therapy may be unnecessary.

Intubation and mechanical ventilation are generally reserved for those patients who experience fatigue, muscle weakness, and/or cardiac compromise, resulting in further deterioration in their overall conditions. The objective of mechanical ventilation in this clinical circumstance is to support the patient only for as long a period as is necessary to resolve the ARF-precipitating event.

In patients with COPD who develop ARF, mechanical ventilation therapy should be avoided, if at all possible, because of the numerous problems associated with intubation and maintenance of mechanical ventilation and the difficulty weaning these patients from the ventilator. (For an indepth examination of the essentials of airway management and mechanical ventilation, see Chap. 32.)

## NURSING CARE OF THE PATIENT WITH CHRONIC OBSTRUCTIVE PULMONARY DISEASE IN ACUTE RESPIRATORY FAILURE

The critical care nurse plays a crucial role in the assessment, diagnosis, and management of the patient with COPD who has or is at great risk of developing ARF. The nature of COPD as a chronic, usually progressive debilitating illness presents the critical care nurse with an especially challenging task of assisting the patient to prevent life-threatening complications and to regain optimal function within the limitations of the underlying obstructive disease.

The approach to nursing care must be guided by the knowledge that the patient's respiratory reserve has already been significantly compromised. It becomes necessary to manipulate and support the patient's underlying ventilatory capabilities to minimize the effects of the disease exacerbation on total body function, reduce the occurrence of potential sequelae, and afford the patient the best opportunity to resume a meaningful life for self and family.

### Therapeutic Goals

The immediate therapeutic goal of the critical care nurse is to act in an expedient and purposeful manner to relieve life-threatening hypoxemia and improve alveolar ventilation so as to reverse hypercapnia and its consequent respiratory acidemia. The critical care nurse is cognizant of the fact that a thorough ongoing assessment and evaluation of the patient's clinical status provide the basis for therapeutic intervention (see Chaps. 29 and 30).

For patients in whom gas exchange is seriously compromised, or in whom acute respiratory failure has developed, aggressive respiratory support therapy is the mainstay of treatment and management. Respiratory support therapy includes the following therapeutic modalities: oxygen therapy, drug therapy, chest physiotherapy–bronchial hygiene, airway management, and mechanical ventilation therapy. (For an indepth examination of these therapeutic modalities and the implications for nursing care see Chap. 32.)

### Nursing Diagnoses, Desired Patient Outcomes, and Nursing Interventions in the Care of the Patient with COPD in Hypercapnic/Hypoxemic Acute Respiratory Failure

Pertinent nursing diagnoses, care planning, and management of the patient with COPD who develops acute respiratory failure are related to the following therapeutic goals:

1. Establish a thorough comprehensive database (see Chaps. 29 and 30). The ongoing clinical evaluation of the patient and his/her response to therapy will consistently yield the most valuable information in terms of effective patient management.
2. Establish and maintain patent airway.
3. Provide appropriate ventilatory support and oxygenation to relieve hypoxemia, hypercapnia, and consequent respiratory acidemia (Chap. 32).
4. Provide support of cardiovascular function to maintain cardiac output and reduce tissue hypoxia.

5. Administer prescribed drug therapy, monitoring the patient's response to therapy.
6. Maintain fluid and electrolyte balance (Chap. 23).
7. Prevent complications related to hypoxemia and metabolic alkalemia.
8. Provide nutritional support without increasing the work of breathing (see Chap. 53).
9. Prevent infection.
10. Prevent impairment of skin integrity related to immobility.
11. Prevent alterations in pulmonary mechanics related to immobility and mechanical ventilation.
12. Provide emotional and psychologic support to patient and family.
13. Initiate patient/family teaching to facilitate maintenance of optimal physical functioning and performance of activities of daily living.

Specific nursing diagnoses, desired patient outcomes, and nursing interventions for the care of the patient with chronic obstructive pulmonary disease with hypercapnic/hypoxemic acute respiratory failure are detailed in the Care Plan in Table 33-2.

## CASE STUDY WITH SAMPLE CARE PLAN: PATIENT WITH CHRONIC OBSTRUCTIVE PULMONARY DISEASE*

J.D. is a 51-year-old white female with a 2-year history of COPD. She is maintained at home on nasal cannula oxygen at 2 liters, Theo-Dur 400 mg every 8 hours, Prednisone 40 mg daily, and atropine inhalers every 4 hours. For 3-4 days prior to admission she was complaining of increasing shortness of breath, cough, sputum production, and chills. On the day of admission, J.D.'s daughter found her lethargic, cyanotic, and significantly short of breath and brought her to the emergency department.

*9/30, 12:30 p.m.* On admission to the Emergency Department of University Hospital, her respiratory rate is 40/minute and labored. Arterial blood gases on nasal cannula are as follows: $PaO_2$, 40 mmHg; pH, 7.1; $PaCO_2$, 107 mmHg. She is orally intubated and then transferred to the medical intensive care unit with the diagnosis: Exacerbation of COPD due to respiratory infection.

*9/30, 1:30 p.m.* On admission to the ICU, her vital signs are: BP, 90/60 mmHg; heart rate 108/minute; sinus tachycardia, respiratory rate 16/minute, temperature 101 R.

| | |
|---|---|
| Neuro: | PERRLA. She is lethargic and difficult to arouse. |
| Cardiovascular: | Extremities are warm to touch and shaking chills noted. Peripheral pulses are weak and thready. Tissue turgor is good. |
| Respiratory: | Orally intubated and placed on a ventilator in an assist/control mode. She has no spontaneous respirations. Secretions via ETT are thick yellow in moderate amounts. Lungs reveal diminished breath sounds throughout all lung fields with scattered rhonchi and wheezing bilaterally. A chest x-ray shows bilateral infiltrates. |
| Gastrointestinal: | Abdomen is nontender with no palpable masses. Post intubation she is maintained NPO. |
| Renal/Urinary: | A Foley catheter is inserted and is draining clear amber urine. She has an IV of aminophylline running at 0.9 mg/kg hour, and 1000 ml $D_{5½}NS$ with 20 mEq/liter KCl at 100 ml/hour. |

### Initial Nursing Diagnoses

1. Ineffective airway clearance, related to thick secretions associated with respiratory infection.
2. Impaired gas exchange, related to alteration in diffusion and increased ventilation/perfusion mismatching, and respiratory infection.
3. Alteration in patterns of urinary elimination, related to altered sensorium and need for Foley catheter.
4. Potential alteration in nutrition: Less than body requirements, related to NPO status.

### Additional Nursing Diagnoses

5. Impaired communication, related to oral intubation.
6. Potential for impairment of skin integrity, related to immobility.
7. Potential for infection, related to invasive lines and procedures.
8. Anxiety, related to ICU environment and impairment in ability to communicate needs.
9. Decreased activity tolerance, related to impaired gas exchange and hypoxemia.

*By Kathleen Daley White and Margaret Connelly

## SAMPLE CARE PLAN: PATIENT WITH CHRONIC OBSTRUCTIVE PULMONARY DISEASE

| Nursing Diagnoses | Desired Patient Outcomes | Nursing Interventions | Rationales |
|---|---|---|---|
| ***Nursing Diagnosis #1*** Ineffective airway clearance, related to thick secretions associated with respiratory infection. | Patient will maintain patent airway as evidenced by:<br>1. Absent to reduced adventitious breath sounds.<br>2. Increased ease in handling secretions. | • Assess respiratory status q2h: Rate, rhythm, work of breathing; breath sounds, presence of adventitious breath sounds.<br>• Assess ability to mobilize and raise secretions.<br>• Assess sputum for changes in color, odor, amount, and consistency; obtain sputum specimen for culture/ sensitivity prior to initiating antibiotic therapy. | • Establishing a baseline as to patient's respiratory function provides a measure by which to evaluate the patient's response to therapy.<br>• Secretion removal is essential to improve alveolar ventilation.<br>• Pooling of secretions underlies airway obstruction and provides foci of infection. |
| | | • Provide humidification of inhaled gases by way of mechanical ventilator. | • Humidification and hydration therapy help to keep secretions thinned so they may be more easily mobilized and removed by suctioning. |
| | | • Administer antibiotics as prescribed; monitor response to therapy.<br>• Monitor response to bronchodilator therapy. | • Infection is the underlying cause of the exacerbation of COPD; early treatment is essential to prevent further complications. |
| | | • Initiate bronchial hygiene and chest physiotherapy as tolerated by patient.<br>○ Chest percussion and vibration.<br>○ Postural drainage. | • These procedures help mobilize secretions and relieve airway obstruction. |
| ***Nursing Diagnosis #2*** Impaired gas exchange, related to alteration in diffusion and increased ventilation/ perfusion mismatching, and respiratory infection. | Patient will maintain adequate alveolar ventilation as evidenced by:<br>1. ABGs at baseline for patient.<br>2. Usual skin color<br>3. Mental status intact; oriented to person, place, time. | • Assess arterial blood gases as ordered/indicated.<br>• Assess for cyanosis; changes in skin color. | • Arterial blood gas measurements indicate effectiveness of gas exchange at the alveolar–capillary interface; assist in evaluating ventilation/perfusion mismatching. |
| | | • Assess level of consciousness. | • Changes in mental status reflect status of hypoxemia and hypercapnia. |
| | | • Assess hematocrit/hemoglobin level. | • Reduced hemoglobin can contribute to tissue hypoxia. |
| ***Nursing Diagnosis #3*** Potential alteration in nutrition: Less than body requirements, related to NPO status. | Patient will maintain a positive nitrogen balance:<br>1. Stable body weight.<br>2. Total proteins, BUN, and creatinine within normal limits.<br>Patient will verbalize having an appetite. | • Consult with physician/nutritionist to assess dietary and nutritional needs.<br>• Provide nutritional support as prescribed: Oral, enteral, or parenteral. | • Sufficient calories and protein must be provided but without increasing obligate gain in carbon dioxide production.<br>• Semi-starvation state leads to depression of the hypoxic drive. |
| | | • Monitor daily weights. | • Daily weight provides most accurate measure of fluid status. |

*(continued)*

## SAMPLE CARE PLAN: PATIENT WITH CHRONIC OBSTRUCTIVE PULMONARY DISEASE *(Continued)*

| Nursing Diagnoses | Desired Patient Outcomes | Nursing Interventions | Rationales |
|---|---|---|---|
| ***Nursing Diagnosis #4***<br>Alteration in pattern of urinary elimination, related to altered sensorium and need for meticulous intake and output. | Patient will maintain:<br>1. Urine output greater than 50 ml/hr.<br>2. Renal function studies, electrolytes within normal range for patient. | • Monitor sensorium and mental status. | • When patient becomes alert and can request a bedpan or commode, the Foley catheter should be discontinued as it becomes another focus of infection in an already compromised patient. |
| | | • Provide perineal and Foley catheter care each shift.<br>• Monitor urine for color, cloudiness, odor. Obtain baseline culture/sensitivity.<br>• Monitor intake/output and daily weight.<br>• Monitor BUN, creatinine, and total protein and albumin, electrolytes. | • Patient is at high risk of urinary tract infection. |
| ***Nursing Diagnosis #5***<br>Impaired verbal/nonverbal communication, related to endotracheal intubation. | Patient will be able to make needs known using the approach established. | • Establish a system of communication: Current approach 2 eye blinks = yes; 1 eye blink = no; 1 finger up = yes, 1 finger down = no.<br>• Establish a trusting, reassuring rapport; anticipate needs, and follow through. | • The inability of the intubated patient to make needs known can be a frightening experience.<br>• Anticipating needs can be reassuring to the patient/family. |

## TABLE 33–2. CARE PLAN FOR THE PATIENT WITH CHRONIC OBSTRUCTIVE PULMONARY DISEASE IN ACUTE RESPIRATORY FAILURE

| Nursing Diagnoses | Desired Patient Outcomes | Nursing Interventions | Rationales |
|---|---|---|---|
| ***Nursing Diagnosis #1***<br>Airway clearance, ineffective, related to copious, thick, tenacious secretions. | Patient will:<br>1. Be alert and oriented to person, place, time.<br>2. Demonstrate deep breathing techniques and effective secretion-clearing cough.<br>3. Minimize risk of aspiration.<br>Arterial blood gases will stabilize:<br>• pH > 7.35 < 7.45.<br>• $PaO_2$ > 60 mmHg.<br>• $PaCO_2$ at level to maintain pH within acceptable range. | • Perform a comprehensive respiratory assessment including:<br>∘ Airway patency; rate, rhythm, and depth of breathing; chest and diaphragmatic excursion.<br>∘ Use of accessory muscles; presence of intercostal retraction.<br>∘ Auscultation of breath sounds. | • Major goal of airway management is to establish and/or maintain adequate alveolar ventilation.<br>∘ Baseline data are essential to evaluate effectiveness of therapeutic interventions.<br>∘ Increased work of breathing may be caused by small airway obstruction.<br>∘ May detect evidence of secretion accumulation, airway obstruction, atelectasis. |
| | | • Monitor quality, quantity, color, and consistency of sputum.<br>∘ Obtain sputum for culture and sensitivity on admission, and thereafter as dictated by patient's condition.<br>∘ Assess secretions for state of hydration or need for mucolytic therapy.<br>∘ Monitor body temperature and white blood count profile. | • Baseline data enable changes in sputum production and characteristics to be identified. Infection or other pulmonary insult may increase quantity of sputum production.<br>∘ Thinning of secretions facilitates mobilization and clearance.<br>∘ Early detection of an infectious or inflammatory process affords prompt intervention to minimize the effect of the insult on pulmonary and other body processes. |
| | | • Institute prescribed bronchodilator therapy.<br>∘ Assess pulmonary function prior to and after bronchodilator therapy.<br>∘ Assist into semi-Fowler's position.<br>∘ Monitor for signs/symptoms of bronchodilator therapy toxicity (especially when theophylline or theophylline salts are used).<br>– Monitor theophylline level. | ∘ Assists in determining effectiveness of therapy.<br>∘ Allows for best possible lung expansion.<br>∘ Theophylline and derivatives have a narrow therapeutic index. |
| | | • Initiate chest physiotherapy techniques:<br>∘ Postural drainage; percussion and vibration; deep breathing and coughing. | • Loosens and dislodges secretions and enhances movement toward trachea from where they are accessible to removal by cough and/or suctioning. |
| | | • Teach appropriate method of coughing.<br>∘ Avoid unnecessary or ineffective coughing. | • Achieve most effective cough with least amount of effort.<br>∘ May cause irritation of tracheobronchial tree. |
| | | • Institute pharyngeal and tracheobronchial suctioning as needed. | • Suctioning is not without risks (hypoxemia, atelectasis, infection); it should be performed only as indicated. |

*(continued)*

### TABLE 33–2. CARE PLAN FOR THE PATIENT WITH CHRONIC OBSTRUCTIVE PULMONARY DISEASE IN ACUTE RESPIRATORY FAILURE *(Continued)*

| Nursing Diagnoses | Desired Patient Outcomes | Nursing Interventions | Rationales |
|---|---|---|---|
| ***Nursing Diagnosis #1 (cont.)*** | | ○ Follow appropriate procedure for endotracheal suctioning (Table 32–4). | ○ Aseptic technique is essential to minimize risk of infection; oxygenation reduces risk of hypoxemia. |
| | | • Instruct patient in use of incentive spirometry (Table 32–2). | • Increases vital capacity and helps to more evenly match ventilation with perfusion. |
| | | • Provide opportunity for rest periods.<br>○ Schedule activities to avoid fatigue. | • Reduces oxygen demand; reduces fatigue. |
| | | • Assure hydration state.<br>○ Monitor intake and output; daily weight. | • Adequate hydration moistens, loosens, and liquefies secretions. |
| | | • Use a calm, reassuring approach.<br>○ Anticipate needs for emotional support.<br>○ Be accessible and offer explanations. | • Assists to reduce anxiety.<br>○ An informed patient is usually a cooperative patient. |
| | | ○ Involve in decision-making regarding care when possible. | ○ Allows patient to retain some control over his/her life. |
| ***Nursing Diagnosis #2***<br>Breathing pattern, ineffective, related to reduced maximum expiratory airflow. (See Nursing Diagnosis #11 below.) | Patient will:<br>1. Demonstrate effective minute ventilation: Tidal volume ($V_T$) >5–7 ml/kg. Respiratory rate <35/min (adult).<br>2. Achieve a vital capacity ($V_C$) >12–15 ml/kg.<br>3. Verbalize ease of breathing.<br>4. Demonstrate pursed-lip and diaphragmatic breathing.<br>5. Exhibit breath sounds: Audible throughout anterior/posterior chest. Reduced to absent adventitious sounds. | • Assess respiratory function:<br>○ Rate, rhythm, depth, and pattern of breathing. | ○ Reflect work of breathing: increased work of breathing increases oxygen consumption and results in hypercapnia and physical fatigue/exhaustion. |
| | | ○ Symmetry of chest wall and diaphragmatic excursion. | ○ Effective ventilation requires synchronous movement of chest wall, diaphragm, and abdominal wall.<br>○ Rapid, shallow respirations (tachypnea, hyperventilation) move deadspace air, significantly reducing alveolar ventilation.<br>○ Asymmetry of respiratory excursion may reflect underlying pathology (e.g., atelectasis, pneumothorax). |
| | | ○ Coordination of contraction of inspiratory and expiratory muscles.<br>○ Use of accessory muscles.<br>○ Auscultation of breath sounds. | ○ *Ventilatory dyscoordination* (a disordered sequence of the contraction of muscles of inspiration and expiration) may be an early but subtle clue as to the development of ARF. |
| | | ○ Pulmonary lung volumes: Total minute ventilation ($V_E$), tidal volume ($V_T$), respiratory rate (f), vital capacity ($V_C$). | ○ A minimal volume of ventilation is necessary to ensure adequate alveolar ventilation.<br>○ Assessment of respiratory volumes allows close evaluation of effectiveness and efficiency of respiratory effort (see Fig. 28–8). |

| | | | |
|---|---|---|---|
| | | • Assist patient into position of comfort and to allow for best lung expansion. | • Expansion of lungs facilitates more even distribution of ventilation; improves ventilation/perfusion matching. |
| | | ○ Low to semi-Fowler's position; unaffected side down in side-lying position. | ○ Reduces ventilation/perfusion mismatch. |
| | | ○ Provide table with pillow for patient to lean on. | |
| | | • Teach breathing techniques: | |
| | | ○ Pursed-lip breathing. | ○ Increases expiratory airway resistance, which functions to keep airways open longer to allow airflow and to reduce air trapping. |
| | | ○ Diaphragmatic breathing. | ○ Lifting of abdominal wall upward and outward allows for easier excursion of diaphragm by decreasing pressure within the abdomen. |
| | | ○ Avoid lying flat (supine). | ○ Causes abdominal contents to shift toward chest cavity, limiting diaphragmatic excursion; may predispose to atelectasis. |
| | | ○ Avoid hyperventilation. | ○ May predispose to metabolic alkalosis in patient with chronic lung disease. |
| | | ○ Controlled breathing: Slower, of increased depth; use abdominal muscles. | ○ Conscious control of breathing increases effectiveness of respiratory effort. |
| | | ○ Encourage hourly deep breathing in conjunction with chest physiotherapy techniques and bronchodilator therapy. | ○ Minimizes atelectasis; mobilizes secretions; improves ventilation. |
| ***Nursing Diagnosis #3***<br>Gas exchange, impaired, related to:<br>1. Alveolar hypoventilation.*<br>2. Ventilation/ perfusion mismatch.*<br>3. Diffusion impaired.†<br>4. Right-to-left shunting.† | Patient will:<br>1. Be alert and oriented to person, place, time.<br>2. Demonstrate appropriate behavior.<br>3. Maintain effective cardiovascular function:<br>• Blood pressure within 10 mmHg of baseline.<br>• Cardiac output ~5 liters/min.<br>• Without cyanosis if baseline "pink." | • Perform neurologic examination including: | • Hypercapnia may predispose to carbon dioxide narcosis with depression of central respiratory centers. |
| | | ○ Mental status; level of consciousness; appropriateness of behavior. | ○ Hypoxemia may predispose to cerebral tissue hypoxia. |
| | | ○ Deep tendon reflexes. | |
| | | ○ Complaints of headache, dizziness, nervousness, restlessness. | |
| | | • Avoid sedatives, narcotics, hypnotics, tranquilizers. | • Depress central respiratory centers predisposing to alveolar hypoventilation with hypercapnia; may mask signs of significant carbon dioxide retention. |
| | | • Monitor vital signs including: | • Circulatory impairment will interfere with adequate gas exchange within lungs and at tissue level. |
| | | ○ Blood pressure, heart rate. | |

*(continued)*

## TABLE 33–2. CARE PLAN FOR THE PATIENT WITH CHRONIC OBSTRUCTIVE PULMONARY DISEASE IN ACUTE RESPIRATORY FAILURE *(Continued)*

| Nursing Diagnoses | Desired Patient Outcomes | Nursing Interventions | Rationales |
|---|---|---|---|
| *Nursing Diagnosis #3 (cont.)* | • Lab values:<br>Hematocrit<br>Male: 45%–52%<br>Female: 37%–48%<br>Hemoglobin<br>>10–12 g/100 ml.<br>4. Maintain optimal arterial blood gases:<br>• pH 7.35–7.45.<br>• $PaO_2$ >60 mmHg.<br>• $PaCO_2$ at level to preserve normal pH.<br>5. Maintan alveolar–arterial gradient ($AaDO_2$): Within acceptable range based on $FIO_2$. | ◦ Respiratory rate; work of breathing.<br>◦ Evidence of distress; undue fatigue; secretion buildup. | ◦ Increased work of breathing increases oxygen consumption and demand; predisposes to tissue hypoxia. |
| | | • Monitor laboratory data:<br>◦ Arterial blood gases: | ◦ Most closely reflect effectiveness of gas exchange. |
| | | ◦ Calculate alveolar–arterial gradient ($AaDO_2$). | ◦ Limitation of $AaDO_2$ is that it does not look at cardiopulmonary function as a whole. |
| | | ◦ Observe for decreasing $PaO_2$ and pH, and increasing $PaCO_2$; bicarbonate ($HCO_3^-$) is elevated. | ◦ Patients with COPD will have a different range of normal than healthy individuals.<br>◦ Increased $HCO_3^-$ reflects renal compensation (i.e., reabsorption of $HCO_3^-$) in response to decreased blood pH caused by hypercapnia. |
| | | ◦ Hematology profile:<br>Hematocrit (Hct).<br>Hemoglobin (Hgb). | ◦ Sufficient red blood cells and hemoglobin are required for gas exchange to occur. In patients wth longstanding COPD, hematology should be monitored for polycythemia vera. |
| | | • Administer prescribed oxygen concentration: | • Alveolar hypoventilation and $\dot{V}/\dot{Q}$ mismatch respond favorably to low-flow supplemental oxygen therapy. |
| | | ◦ Use low-flow supplemental oxygen therapy.<br>• 24%–28% by Venturi mask.<br>• 2–3 liters/min by nasal cannula. | ◦ Overzealous oxygen therapy can wipe out hypoxic drive in patients with COPD. |
| | | ◦ Monitor arterial blood gases at regular intervals. | ◦ Reflect effectiveness of lungs in gas exchange. |
| | | ◦ Prevent complications related to precipitous decrease in $PaCO_2$. | ◦ When ventilation has been interrupted (e.g., suctioning) or the $FIO_2$ has changed, blood sample for analysis should not be obtained for at least 20 min after therapy. |
| | | • Monitor criteria for acute respiratory failure (Table 32–5).<br>◦ Additional considerations: Evidence of respiratory distress, "air hunger," secretion buildup, undue fatigue. | • Patients with COPD may experience difficult weaning from mechanical ventilatory therapy. Timely and aggressive implementation of respiratory support therapies ($O_2$ therapy, chest physiotherapy, treatment of underlying causes) may successfully prevent need for intubation and mechanical ventilation. |
| | | • Intubate and initiate mechanical ventilation therapy when criteria for acute respiratory failure have been identified. | |

| | | | |
|---|---|---|---|
| ***Nursing Diagnosis #4***<br>Cardiac output, alteration in: Decreased (diminished venous return).<br>***Nursing Diagnosis #5***<br>Tissue perfusion, alteration in: Cardiopulmonary. | Patient will:<br>1. Maintain stable hemodynamics:<br>• Blood pressure within 10 mmHg baseline.<br>• Heart rate <100 beats/min.<br>• Cardiac output ~5 liters/min.<br>• Central venous pressure (CVP) 0–8 mmHg.<br>• Pulmonary capillary wedge pressure (PCWP) 8–12 mmHg.<br>2. Remain without:<br>• Extreme weakness or fatigue.<br>• Peripheral (pedal) edema.<br>• Neck vein distention.<br>• Chest pain.<br>• Cardiac dysrhythmias.<br>3. Maintain fluid and electrolyte balance:<br>• Stable body weight.<br>• Balanced intake and output.<br>• Hourly urine output >30 ml/hr. | • Perform ongoing cardiovascular assessment:<br>◦ Continuous cardiac monitoring (establish baseline rate, rhythm, ectopy).<br>◦ Continuous hemodynamic monitoring (establish baseline): CVP, PCWP.<br>◦ Heart sounds—Loudness or intensity, splitting, extra heart sounds ($S_3$–$S_4$)?<br>◦ Breath sounds—Evidence of rales (crackles); altered pulmonary mechanics?<br>◦ Fatigue, exhaustion?<br>◦ Neck vein distention? Pedal edema?<br>◦ Serial arterial blood gases.<br>• Implement fluid replacement therapy as prescribed.<br>◦ Monitor hydration status: Daily weight, intake and output, urine specific gravity.<br>◦ Avoid fluid volume overload. | ◦ Cardiac tissue hypoxia may predispose to dysrhythmias.<br>◦ Offers significant data regarding cardiopulmonary function.<br>◦ Positive-pressure mechanical ventilation increases pressure within the thorax, which impedes venous return to the heart; decrease in venous return (preload) reduces cardiac output.<br>◦ Loud pulmonic sound or splitting is commonly seen in cor pulmonale; it is related to pulmonary hypertension due to longstanding hypoxemic state.<br>◦ In the patient with COPD, diminished breath sounds in a heretofore "noisy" chest may warn of hypoventilation with impending acute respiratory failure (see Fig. 32–4).<br>• Adequate fluid replacement therapy is essential to maintain blood volume and keep pulmonary secretions moist and easily mobilized.<br>◦ Longstanding pulmonary disease with pulmonary hypertension predisposes to right heart failure (cor pulmonale). (See Nursing Diagnosis #7, below.) |
| ***Nursing Diagnosis #6***<br>Tissue perfusion, alteration in: Cerebral. | Patient will:<br>1. Demonstrate appropriate behavior:<br>• Oriented to person, place, time. | • Assess ongoing neurologic function.<br>◦ Mental status, level of consciousness; behavior appropriate?<br>• Assess fluid and electrolyte status.<br>◦ Body weight.<br>◦ Intake and output (hourly urine output).<br>◦ Serum electrolytes, BUN, creatinine.<br>• Maintain a quiet, relaxed milieu.<br>◦ Use a calm, reassuring approach.<br>◦ Provide explanations of care. | • Compromised hemodynamics and hypoxemia predispose to cerebral hypoxia with altered cerebral function.<br>• Reduced blood volume will further compromise venous return and cardiac output; blood volume may need to be expanded to minimize this effect.<br>◦ Reduced cardiac output may diminish renal perfusion, placing patient at risk of developing acute renal failure.<br>• Minimize fear and anxiety, which increase oxygen consumption and demand. |

*(continued)*

**TABLE 33–2. CARE PLAN FOR THE PATIENT WITH CHRONIC OBSTRUCTIVE PULMONARY DISEASE IN ACUTE RESPIRATORY FAILURE *(Continued)***

| Nursing Diagnoses | Desired Patient Outcomes | Nursing Interventions | Rationales |
|---|---|---|---|
| ***Nursing Diagnosis #6 (cont.)*** | | ◦ Provide frequent periods of rest and relaxation.<br>• Monitor for effects of drugs (e.g., theophylline) on cardiopulmonary function. | ◦ The work of breathing is often taxing; it is important to conserve patient's energy.<br>• Drug toxicity may further compromise cardiopulmonary function. |
| ***Nursing Diagnosis #7***<br>Fluid and electrolyte, alterations in (see nursing diagnoses in Chap. 23 for specific fluid/electrolyte imbalances). | Patient will:<br>1. Maintain baseline body weight.<br>2. Balance fluid intake with output.<br>3. Have:<br>• Good skin turgor.<br>• Absence of peripheral edema.<br>• Absence of rales (crackles) on auscultation.<br>• Stable vital signs.<br>4. Stabilize in terms of serum electrolyte, BUN, creatinine, total protein within acceptable physiologic range. | • Monitor hydration status:<br>◦ Daily weight, intake and output, vital signs.<br>◦ Examine skin for signs of dehydration: Poor skin turgor; sunken eyeballs; dry, parched mucous membranes.<br>◦ Monitor mental status changes; lethargy; severe weakness; reduced urine output.<br>◦ Examine for signs of overhydration: Peripheral edema; hypertension; tachycardia; neck vein distention; elevated pulmonary hemodynamics; shortness of breath, dyspnea.<br>• Monitor serum electrolytes, BUN, creatinine, total protein. | • Patients receiving mechanical ventilation with humidified gas therapy are at risk to increase total body water.<br>◦ Stress increases secretion of antidiuretic hormone (ADH) by posterior pituitary gland, increasing water retention.<br>◦ Stress increases aldosterone secretion by adrenal cortex, which stimulates sodium reabsorption within the kidneys. |
| ***Nursing Diagnosis #8***<br>Acid–base balance, alteration in, related to overzealous oxygen therapy in the patient with longstanding COPD. | The patient's arterial blood gases will stabilize as follows:<br>• pH 7.35–7.45.<br>• $PaO_2 > 60$ mmHg.<br>• $PaCO_2$ sufficiently reduced to maintain pH within acceptable range for the patient. | • Administer oxygen therapy cautiously at prescribed concentration ($FIO_2$).<br>◦ Closely monitor arterial blood gas values.<br>– $PaCO_2$ must only be reduced to the level that "normalizes" pH. | • In patients with longstanding COPD with chronic hypercapnia and consequent acidemia, the kidneys respond (compensate) by reabsorbing bicarbonate ($HCO_3^-$). This buffers the excess hydrogen ions associated with the hypercapnia and stabilizes the pH.<br>◦ Overzealous administration of oxygen can cause a precipitous fall in the $PaCO_2$, reducing hydrogen-ion concentration while leaving excess bicarbonate. The result is metabolic alkalemia, which, if sufficiently severe, can lead to serious cardiac dysrhythmias and seizures. |

| | | | |
|---|---|---|---|
| ***Nursing Diagnosis #9***<br>Nutrition, alteration in: Less than body requirements. (See Chap. 53.) | Patient will:<br>1. Maintain body weight within 5% of baseline weight.<br>2. Maintain total serum proteins ~6.0–8.4 g/100 ml.<br>3. Maintain laboratory data within acceptable range: BUN, serum creatinine, electrolytes, fasting blood sugar, serum albumin, hematology profile.<br>4. Verbalize essentials of adequate diet. | • Arrange consultation with nutritionist and collaborate to perform nutrition assessment: General state of health; baseline body weight; nutritional history: Likes, dislikes, meal preparation, eating habits, cultural, religious considerations.<br>∘ Lifestyle influences.<br>∘ Physiologic factors: Height, weight, triceps skinfold, mid-upper arm circumference.<br>∘ Laboratory studies: Urinary/serum creatinine, BUN, fasting blood sugar, serum electrolytes, total protein (serum albumin), hematology profile. | • Adequate nutritional intake is necessary to meet metabolic requirements to reverse acute respiratory failure.<br>∘ Nutritional deficiencies (especially in elderly) are often associated with chronic disease. |
| | | • Maintain adequate nutrition with prescribed enteral and/or parenteral feedings.<br>∘ Special considerations. | • Clinical semi-starvation leads to depression of the hypoxic ventilatory drive.<br>∘ Patients receiving mechanical ventilation therapy are highly stressed and require nutritional supplements to meet hypermetabolic needs. |
| | | ∘ Avoid large glucose loads to meet caloric needs. | ∘ There is an obligate increase in carbon dioxide with increased glucose intake. Fat emulsions may be used to provide calories.<br>∘ In patients who are mechanically ventilated or who have reduced respiratory reserve, the increased carbon dioxide can lead to hypercapnia and may precipitate acute respiratory failure in the high-risk patient. |
| | | ∘ Avoid hypophosphatemia. | ∘ Reduced phosphate levels are associated with decreased energy levels, respiratory muscle weakness, and increased risk of infection. |
| | | ∘ Avoid high amino acid loads. | ∘ Increase $O_2$ consumption. |
| | | • Place patient in optimal position during feedings (usually semi-Fowler's position). | • Proper positioning and intact protective reflexes reduce risk of aspiration. |
| | | • Confirm placement of nasogastric tube in stomach before initiating feedings.<br>∘ Assess for protective reflexes (gag, cough, swallowing). | • Proper placement of nasogastric tube helps to prevent aspiration. |
| | | • Provide frequent mouth care and other comfort measures. | • May be aesthetically pleasing to patient/family.<br>∘ Keeps mucous membranes moist and intact. |

*(continued)*

**TABLE 33–2. CARE PLAN FOR THE PATIENT WITH CHRONIC OBSTRUCTIVE PULMONARY DISEASE IN ACUTE RESPIRATORY FAILURE *(Continued)***

| Nursing Diagnoses | Desired Patient Outcomes | Nursing Interventions | Rationales |
|---|---|---|---|
| ***Nursing Diagnosis #9 (cont.)*** | | • Monitor daily weight; fluid and intake.<br>• Assess bowel function:<br>∘ Assess bowel sounds.<br>∘ Initiate bowel regimen, if indicated. | ∘ Maintains gastrointestinal smooth muscle tone; prevents constipation or impaction. |
| ***Nursing Diagnosis #10***<br>Infection, potential for (see Table 49–7). | Patient will:<br>1. Maintain normal body temperature ~98.6°F (37°C).<br>2. Maintain white blood count at acceptable baseline level.<br>3. Remain without evidence of acute infection: Redness, swelling, pain. | • Identify patients at high risk of developing an infection: Debilitated or elderly, chronic lung disease, multiple invasive lines, semistarvation state, immunosuppressed. | • Patients with COPD are especially at high risk due to:<br>∘ Alteration in surfactant activity.<br>∘ Alterations in respiratory epithelium replication. |
| | | • Obtain baseline cultures: Sputum, urine, blood. | • Upon intubation, a baseline sputum specimen should be obtained.<br>∘ Use of artificial airway (endotracheal tube or tracheostomy) contaminates the tracheobronchial tree, which is usually considered to be sterile distal to the larynx. |
| | | • Monitor the following parameters:<br>∘ Body temperature.<br>∘ Hematology profile—Evidence of leukocytosis; eosinophilia.<br>∘ Sputum for changes in color, quantity, consistency, odor; and ability of patient to handle secretions.<br>∘ Chest x-ray for pulmonary infiltrates. | • Early diagnosis with institution of timely and vigorous therapy (antibiotic) may help to minimize the impact of the infectious process on total body function. |
| | | • Institute vigorous chest physiotherapy and bronchial hygiene. | • Secretion removal improves ventilation and reduces pooling of secretions, which may act as foci of infection. |
| | | • Use aseptic technique for patient care: Tracheobronchial suctioning, care of invasive lines.<br>• Administer prescribed antibiotic therapy.<br>∘ Monitor culture and sensitivity studies to assess response to therapy.<br>• Maintain nutrition. | • Reduces risks of infection. |

| | | | |
|---|---|---|---|
| ***Nursing Diagnosis #11***<br>Pulmonary mechanics, alteration in, related to respiratory muscle atrophy (immobility, mechanical ventilation; see Nursing Diagnosis #2 above). | Patient will:<br>1. Perform deep breathing exercises.<br>2. Achieve maximum pulmonary function:<br>• Tidal volume >7 ml/kg.<br>• Vital capacity >15 ml/kg.<br>• Maximal expiratory flow. | • Teach deep breathing exercises. | • Use of positive-pressure ventilation predisposes to atrophy of the respiratory musculature, which can present problems for weaning. |
| | | ○ Instruct regarding the importance of deep breathing exercises. | ○ Improves pulmonary ventilation, mobilizes secretions, stimulates circulation.<br>○ Teaching regarding pulmonary mechanics forms the foundation of patient's self-care after hospitalization. |
| | | ○ Allow patient to demonstrate pulmonary exercises.<br>○ Combine deep breathing therapy with other chest physiotherapy maneuvers.<br>○ Involve patient/family in decision-making (e.g., scheduling of exercise activities). | ○ Patient should be allowed to learn one task before proceeding to the next. Always establish readiness to learn on the part of patient and family.<br>○ The nature of chronic illness requires cooperation of all family members if exacerbations are to be prevented. |
| | | ○ Encourage early ambulation (e.g., sitting up in chair). | ○ Involvement in planning and decision-making enables patient/family to begin to assume responsibility for their own lives. |
| | | • Assess pulmonary volumes to determine effectiveness of therapy: Tidal volume, vital capacity. | |
| ***Nursing Diagnosis #12***<br>Skin integrity, impairment of, related to immobility, and altered nutritional status. | Patient's skin will remain intact. | • Establish routine for turning and repositioning. | • Exercise maintains muscle tone and prevents muscle atrophy. |
| | | • Assist with range-of-motion exercises to extremities. | • Exercise stimulates circulation and prevents stasis. |
| | | ○ Provide support stockings to lower extremities.<br>○ Assess extremities for calf tenderness.<br>○ Measure circumference of thighs and calves daily. | ○ Immobility predisposes to thrombophlebitis. |
| | | • Provide special skin care to back and joints, and all pressure points. | • Maintains circulation to all areas; these patients frequently have a compromised body defense system and are at high risk of infection. |
| | | ○ Establish regimen for: Skin inspection, skin care, decubitus care if necessary. | ○ It is essential to prevent skin breakdown. |
| | | ○ Provide "egg-crate" or air mattress; sheepskin; heel and ankle protectors.<br>○ Apply local skin care. | ○ Pressure relief devices. |

*(continued)*

**TABLE 33–2. CARE PLAN FOR THE PATIENT WITH CHRONIC OBSTRUCTIVE PULMONARY DISEASE IN ACUTE RESPIRATORY FAILURE *(Continued)***

| Nursing Diagnoses | Desired Patient Outcomes | Nursing Interventions | Rationales |
|---|---|---|---|
| ***Nursing Diagnosis #13***<br>Fear.<br>***Nursing Diagnosis #14***<br>Knowledge deficit regarding chronic obstructive pulmonary disease. | Patient/family will:<br>1. Be able to verbalize fears and concerns.<br>2. Identify strengths and coping capabilities.<br>3. Verbalize knowledge regarding COPD.<br>4. Verbalize intentions to make necessary adjustments in life-style.<br>5. Demonstrate ability to carry out necessary interventions.<br>6. Demonstrate self-confidence in their capabilities. | • Assess knowledge regarding COPD and expectations of the disease progression.<br>• Verbalize fears and concerns for patient and family. | • Chronic lung disease is a "family disease" impacting every member to some degree.<br>• If the patient/family are to realize optimal function within the limitations of the disease, all family members should be involved in the educating and caring processes.[7] |
| | | • Help them to recognize and to express their feelings regarding disruption in their life-style.<br>○ Encourage them to express fears regarding chronicity of disease: Necessity of oxygen therapy in the home setting; specific medication/other therapies.<br>• Assess readiness to learn (see Chap. 4).<br>○ Have patient/family assist in identifying needs and learning objectives. | |
| | | • Assist family in problem-solving techniques.<br>○ Help them identify family strengths and resources. | • Assists family in coping; increases self-confidence in their own capabilities. |
| | | ○ Initiate referral to social services for necessary support: emotional, psychologic, financial, other. | ○ It is reassuring to have specific resources available to lend assistance and support. |

* Most commonly occurring.
† Characteristic of progressive emphysematous disease.

## REFERENCES


1. Weinberger, SE: Principles of Pulmonary Medicine. WB Saunders, Philadelphia, 1986, p 90.
2. Wollschlager, C and Khan, F: Secondary pulmonary hypertension: Clinical features. Heart Lung 15(4):338, July 1986.
3. Ayres, S, Schlichtig, R, and Sterling, M: Care of the Critically Ill, ed 3. Year Book Medical Publishers, Chicago, 1988, pp 243–254.
4. Peil, M, and Rubin, L: Therapy of secondary pulmonary hypertension. Heart Lung 15(5):450, September 1986.
5. Petty, T: Drug strategies for airflow obstruction. Am J Nurs 87(2):180, February 1987.
6. Chin, R, and Pesce, R: Practical aspects in management of respiratory failure in chronic obstructive pulmonary disease. Crit Care 6(2):11, September 1983.
7. Hahn, K: Slow-teaching the COPD patient. Nursing '87 17(4):34, April 1987.

CHAPTER 34

# Nursing Management of the Patient with Adult Respiratory Distress Syndrome in Hypoxemic Acute Respiratory Failure

## CHAPTER OUTLINE



## LEARNING OBJECTIVES

**At the end of this chapter, you should be able to:**

1. Describe the adult respiratory distress syndrome (ARDS), including its clinical hallmarks.
2. List the disorders or circumstances commonly associated with the development of ARDS.
3. Define noncardiogenic pulmonary edema of ARDS and cardiogenic pulmonary edema.
4. Examine the underlying pathophysiology of ARDS.
5. Relate the clinical presentation of ARDS to its underlying pathology.
6. Outline clinical criteria diagnostic of ARDS.
7. Identify the role of mechanical ventilation and PEEP therapy in the treatment and management of ARDS.
8. Describe the nursing care of the patient with ARDS based on the nursing process:
   - Assessment
   - Diagnosis
   - Planning: Desired patient outcomes
     - Nursing interventions.

## ADULT RESPIRATORY DISTRESS SYNDROME

### Description

Adult respiratory distress syndrome (ARDS) is characterized by a rapidly progressing and fulminating form of hypoxemic respiratory failure, which often occurs in previously healthy individuals who have sustained a severe physiologic insult, pulmonary or nonpulmonary in origin. The syndrome has been associated with a variety of causes or precipitating events, including shock (whatever the origin), sepsis, diffuse pneumonias, trauma, aspiration of gastric contents, inhalation of a chemical irritant, fat embolism, and pancreatitis (Table 34–1).

Irrespective of the underlying insult, ARDS is the final common clinical and pathologic pattern predisposing to the demise of the individual. The onset of ARDS usually occurs within hours or 3–4 days after the precipitating event. Despite intensive research and advances in supportive care over the past 2 decades, the mortality rate associated with ARDS remains at approximately 50%.

### Hallmarks of ARDS

No single test is diagnostic of the syndrome; rather, its identity is based on a description of its clinical presentation. The hallmarks of ARDS include: (1) marked respiratory distress with tachypnea, use of accessory muscles, and an overall increase in the work of breathing; (2) profound hypoxemia despite ventilatory assistance with high inspired oxygen fractions ($FIO_2 > 50\%$); (3) a decrease in functional residual capacity (FRC) and lung compliance associated with interstitial and alveolar edema and alveolar atelectasis, and requiring progressively greater than normal ventilatory pressures to maintain adequate alveolar ventilation; and (4) the appearance of diffuse pulmonary infiltrates on chest x-ray, which reflect the abnormal accumulation of fluid and proteins within the lung interstitium and alveolar air spaces as a result of altered alveolar–capillary permeability.

### Pathogenesis

The pathology underlying ARDS involves an increase in the permeability of the alveolar–capillary membrane leading to pulmonary interstitial and alveolar edema, or as it is frequently termed, "noncardiogenic" pulmonary edema. It is important to distinguish between the noncardiogenic pulmonary edema of ARDS and the "cardiogenic" pulmonary edema associated with left heart failure. (Table 34–2 compares these two types of pulmonary edema.)

Under normal physiologic conditions, there is always a small net movement of fluid out of the pulmonary capillaries (intravascular space) into the lung interstitium (Fig. 34–1). An accumulation of this fluid within the interstitium does not occur because any excess fluid or protein is drained by the pulmonary lymphatic system and eventually returned to the blood.

#### *Pulmonary Edema*

Pulmonary edema occurs when there is an abnormal accumulation of fluid within the interstitial and air spaces of the lungs. The mechanisms underlying

TABLE 34–1
**Disorders Associated with ARDS**

- Shock of any etiology
- Trauma:
  - Fat embolism (long bone fracture)
  - Lung contusion
  - Nonthoracic
- Infections:
  - Gram-negative sepsis
  - Pneumonia (diffuse): Viral, Bacterial, Fungal
  - *Pneumocystis carinii*
  - Tuberculosis
- Aspiration:
  - Gastric contents
  - Fresh/salt water (near drowning)
  - Hydrocarbons
- Metabolic disorders:
  - Uremia
  - Pancreatitis
- Drug overdose:
  - Narcotics—Heroin, methadone
  - Sedatives—Barbiturates
- Inhaled toxins:
  - Oxygen toxicity
  - Smoke
  - Nitrous oxide
  - Ammonia
  - Chloride
- Neurogenic:
  - Head injury
  - Intracranial hemorrhage
  - Seizures
- Hematologic disorders:
  - Disseminated intravascular coagulation (DIC)
  - Massive transfusion/transfusion reaction

TABLE 34-2
## Cardiogenic and Noncardiogenic Pulmonary Edema: A Comparison

| | Noncardiogenic Pulmonary Edema (NCPE) | Cardiogenic Pulmonary Edema (CPE) |
|---|---|---|
| Etiology | See Table 34-1. | Occurs in the setting of left heart failure. Mitral stenosis/regurgitation can cause CPE with normal LVEDP. |
| Pathogenesis | Noncardiogenic pulmonary edema involves an increase in the permeability of the alveolar-capillary membrane, permitting the movement of fluid and protein out of the pulmonary capillary (intravascular) space into the pulmonary interstitium and alveolar air spaces. | An increase in LVEDP is reflected back to the pulmonary capillary bed increasing pulmonary intravascular hydrostatic pressure (PCWP). |
| Pulmonary capillary wedge pressure | Pulmonary hydrostatic pressures (PCWP) usually remain within normal limits, 8–12 mmHg. | An increase in PCWP forces fluid out of pulmonary capillaries into the lung interstitium, causing pulmonary congestion.<br>When the fluid in the interstitium exceeds the reabsorptive capacity of the pulmonary lymphatic system, fluid is forced into the alveoli, causing pulmonary edema. |
| Pathology | Alteration in permeability of the alveolar-capillary membrane permitting a net egress of fluid and *protein* from the pulmonary intravascular into interstitial and alveolar spaces.<br>Initial pathologic changes reflect disruption of the capillary endothelium followed by injury to types I and II pneumocytes.<br>Resulting pathology includes:<br>1. Alveolar edema, atelectasis.<br>2. Loss of type I cell elasticity.<br>3. Altered surfactant activity.<br>Underlying initiating factors predisposing to acute lung injury:[1]<br>1. Increased accumulation of polymorphonuclear neutrophilic leukocytes (PMNs) in the patient with ARDS; release of potentially toxic mediators by these cells may account for injury to, and increased permeability of, the alveolar-capillary membrane.<br>2. Activated *complement* (C5a) promotes adherence of circulating granulocytes to pulmonary capillary endothelium (*leukotaxis*); it may induce release of chemotactic factor from alveolar macrophages.<br>3. Alveolar macrophages elaborate proteases, which perpetuate the inflammatory process.<br>4. Platelets release mediators (e.g., serotonin), which cause pulmonary arterial vasoconstriction.<br>5. Mast cells trigger release of vasoactive substances.<br>The above factors may contribute to the self-destructive inflammatory response that occurs in the setting of ARDS. | In left heart failure, as cardiac output decreases, there is a "back up" of blood, which accumulates in the pulmonary capillary bed, raising pulmonary capillary hydrostatic pressure.<br>When capillary hydrostatic pressure exceeds pulmonary capillary oncotic pressure (see Fig. 34-1), fluid leaks into the pulmonary interstitium; when the reabsorptive capacity of the pulmonary lymphatic system is exceeded, fluid fills the alveoli causing pulmonary edema.<br>CPE involves the increased infiltration of a *protein-poor* fluid across the microvascular membrane. This is contrary to noncardiogenic pulmonary edema wherein the defect in endothelial permeability involves the movement of both fluid and protein.<br>Summary of pathophysiologic stages in cardiogenic pulmonary edema:[2]<br>1. *Interstitial* stage—Lung interstitium swells with fluid as lymphatics are unable to reabsorb excess fluid. Patient may become restless and anxious.<br>2. *Alveolar* stage—Alveolar flooding with significant decrease in $PaO_2$, $PaCO_2$, and a rising pH. Tachypnea increases venous return and increases the volume of blood within the pulmonary capillary bed.<br>3. *Bronchial stages*—Infiltration of fluid within air spaces alters surfactant activity with atelectasis. Frothy, tenacious, often blood-tinged sputum may become evident; there is the appearance of rales (crackles).<br>4. *Final* stage—Tissue hypoxia occurs as the patient tires; hypoventilation ensues with consequent respiratory/ acidemia (pH falls <7.35). |

TABLE 34–2
## Cardiogenic and Noncardiogenic Pulmonary Edema: A Comparison *(Continued)*

| | Noncardiogenic Pulmonary Edema (NCPE) | Cardiogenic Pulmonary Edema (CPE) |
|---|---|---|
| Pathophysiology | | |
| Arterial blood gases | ↓↓$PaO_2$ (severe hypoxemia).<br>↓To normal $PaCO_2$ (hypocapnia).<br>Respiratory alkalemia. | ↓$PaO_2$<br>↓$PaCO_2$ early stage with respiratory alkalemia. |
| Ventilation | ↑Minute alveolar ventilation ($\dot{V}_A$) (>20 liters/min).<br>↑Respiratory rate.<br>↑Deadspace ventilation ($V_D$).<br>Reduced residual volume.<br>Reduced functional residual capacity (FRC). | Hyperventilation initially.<br>Advanced stage: ↑$PaCO_2$ associated with patient exhaustion and compromised ventilatory effort.<br>↑Respiratory rate. |
| Pulmonary mechanics | ↓In lung compliance—stiffening of lung parenchyma.<br>↓Functional residual capacity (FRC).<br>↑Work of breathing and increased respiratory rate results in decreased tidal volume. | ↓In lung compliance especially with alveolar flooding; loss of surfactant activity to reduce surface tension.<br>↑Work of breathing.<br>↓Functional residual capacity. |
| Pulmonary pressures | Significantly widened alveolar–arterial oxygen tension ($AaDO_2$).<br>Significant right-to-left shunting, which causes hypoxemia to be refractory to supplemental oxygen therapy even with an $FIO_2$ >60%.<br>Ventilation/perfusion mismatching. | Widened $AaDO_2$ gradient.<br>Ventilation/perfusion mismatching.<br>Right-to-left shunting (minimal).<br>Hypoventilation ensues in later stages. |
| | Gas exchange compromised by alteration in surfactant activity.<br>Increase in pulmonary vascular resistance. | Same as for noncardiognic pulmonary edema during bronchial and final stages. |
| | Pulmonary pressures: PCWP within 8–12 mmHg. | Pulmonary pressures: PCWP >18 mmHg. |
| | Pulmonary capillary permeability: Increased.<br>Protein content of edema fluid: High. | Transudation of fluid from intravascular to interstitium and alveoli; alveolar–capillary membrane remains intact.<br>Protein content of edema fluid: Low |
| Clinical presentation | Hallmarks:<br>1. Marked respiratory distress with dyspnea and tachypnea; use of accessory muscles; increased work of breathing.<br>2. Profound hypoxemia.<br>3. Decrease in functional residual capacity and residual volume.<br>4. Decreased lung compliance.<br>5. Appearance of diffuse pulmonary infiltrates on chest x-ray.<br>6. Physical findings: Skin warm; full bounding pulses with increase in cardiac output; breath sounds reveal coarse rales. No jugular venous distention. | Left-sided heart failure:<br>1. *Initial* stage: Anxiety, restlessness, tachypnea, dyspnea, orthopnea, paroxysmal nocturnal dyspnea (PND), insomnia.<br>2. *Advanced* stage: Tachycardia; palpitation; hypotension, diaphoresis. Reduced lung compliance = ↑work of breathing. Cough productive of frothy, often blood-tinged sputum; pallor or cyanosis; cool mottled periphery. Basilar rales; bronchial wheezing. Increased jugular venous distention. Gallop rhythm (heart sounds: $S_3$, $S_4$). Chest x-ray: Initial interstitial pattern followed later by a pattern of diffuse airway disease.<br>3. *Acute* stage: Decreased level of consciousness with compromised cerebral perfusion; severely deranged gas exchange causes tissue hypoxia with shock and ventricular dysrhythmias. |
| Diagnostic criteria | 1. Precipitating factor(s) or catastrophic physiologic insult (see Table 34–1).<br>2. Physiologic parameters: $PaO_2$ <60 mmHg with an $FIO_2$ >50%. Respiratory compliance decreased.<br>3. Chest x-ray with diffuse bilateral infiltrates.<br>4. PCWP ~12 mmHg (8–12 mmHg). | In the early stages, it may be difficult to distinguish whether the pulmonary edema is cardiogenic or noncardiogenic in origin.<br>Differential diagnosis:<br>1. Presence of precipitating event.<br>2. Clinical presentation.<br>3. Chest x-ray findings. |

*(continued)*

TABLE 34-2
**Cardiogenic and Noncardiogenic Pulmonary Edema: A Comparison *(Continued)***

| | Noncardiogenic Pulmonary Edema (NCPE) | Cardiogenic Pulmonary Edema (CPE) |
|---|---|---|
| Clinical history | Commonly, the patient is essentially healthy prior to precipitating event. | Frequently the patient presents with a history of chronic congestive heart failure; or acute event preceding episode of pulmonary edema (e.g., myocardial infarction, pulmonary embolism). |
| Physical examination | Physical findings reflect high cardiac output; see clinical presentation above.<br>Lack of cardiomegaly.<br>Absence of extra heart sounds. | Physical findings reflect low cardiac output; see clinical presentation above.<br>Cardiomegaly is a frequent finding.<br>$S_3$, $S_4$ frequently present. |
| ECG findings | ECG usually normal. | ECG may reflect signs of ischemia, injury, or infarction and previous pathology. |
| Chest x-ray | Diffuse pulmonary infiltrates. | Butterfly distribution of pulmonary infiltrates. |
| Intrapulmonary shunt | Large increase is characteristic of ARDS. | Small increase |
| Hemodynamic parameters | CVP ~10 cm $H_2O$.<br>PCWP 8–12 mmHg. | CVP >20 cm $H_2O$.<br>PCWP >18 mmHg. |
| Other | | Cardiac enzyme studies may point to cardiogenic pulmonary edema in early stages. |
| Treatment (overall) | Initial treatment:<br>1. Establish and/or maintain patent aiway.<br>2. Oxygen therapy to maintain $PaO_2$ >60 mmHg.<br>3. Ventilation therapy to maintain $PaCO_2$ 35–45 mmHg.<br>4. Correct acid-base abnormalities.<br>5. Correct electrolyte abnormalities. | |
| Goals of treatment | 1. Treatment of precipitating event/disorder.<br>2. Stabilize permeability defect in alveolar-capillary membrane.<br>3. Support gas exchange until adequate pulmonary function is restored.<br>4. Prompt recognition with early institution of supportive therapy.<br>5. Prevention/decrease in risk for additional insults that further deteriorate patient's clinical status. | 1. Therapy in left ventricular failure:<br>A. Reduce PCWP.<br>B. Reduce venous return (preload).<br>C. Reduce circulating blood volume.<br>D. Reduce systemic blood pressure (afterload)<br>E. Increase cardiac contractility. |
| Specific therapeutic modalities | Mainstay of treatment:<br>Intubation with mechanical ventilation, PEEP, and oxygenation.<br>1. PEEP therapy.<br>A. Indications for PEEP therapy:[8]<br>• $PaO_2$ <60 mmHg with $FIO_2$ >50%.<br>• Diffuse lung disease bilaterally.<br>• Prophylactic use at high risk of developing ARDS.<br>B. Contraindications for PEEP therapy:<br>• Reduced extracellular fluid volume.<br>• Patchy, necrotizing pulmonary process.<br>• Unilateral lung disease.<br>C. Desired effect:<br>Recruits and maintains open lung units that are otherwise collapsed.<br>• Increases FRC.<br>• Increased tidal volumes help to prevent atelectasis.<br>• Allows for better arterial oxygenation with lower $FIO_2$. | Venodilation therapy:<br>1. A. Increases size of venous capacitance vessels enabling a larger volume of blood to pool in the venous system, thus reducing venous return to the heart.<br>B. Specific drug therapy:<br>*Morphine* is the most effective drug in emergency treatment of pulmonary edema. Its actions include: Vasodilation; sedation, which relieves anxiety and fosters muscle relaxation; it reduces myocardial oxygen demand.<br>*Diuretic therapy:* Furosemide increases venous capacitance, reducing venous return; it causes diuresis, which reduces circulatory blood volume.<br>*Vasodilator therapy:* Vasodilator agents include nitroprusside, nitroglycerin, nitropaste, others; these agents reduce vascular hydrostatic pressure and, thus, reduce PCWP; they facilitate an increase in cardiac output by decreasing left ventricular |

TABLE 34-2
## Cardiogenic and Noncardiogenic Pulmonary Edema: A Comparison *(Continued)*

| | **Noncardiogenic Pulmonary Edema (NCPE)** | **Cardiogenic Pulmonary Edema (CPE)** |
|---|---|---|
| | D. Administration of PEEP early in disease course (dose)<br>• Early 5–15 cm $H_2O$.<br>• Late 20–30 cm $H_2O$<br>PEEP level sought: Progressive increments of 3–5 cm $H_2O$ that allow maintenance of a hemoglobin-saturating $PaO_2$ with minimal compromise of cardiac output and oxygen transport.<br>E. Assessment of response to PEEP therapy:<br>• Arterial blood gases.<br>• Alveolar-arterial oxygen gradient ($AaDO_2$).<br>• PCWP and cardiac output.<br>• Mixed venous oxygen tension.<br>• Frequent determination of static compliance; large tidal volume plus PEEP allows for optimal lung compliance.<br>F. Adverse effects of PEEP:<br>• ↓Venous return = ↓cardiac output.<br>• ↑Intracranial pressure by impeding cerebral venous drainage by jugular veins.<br>• Barotrauma (pneumothorax, pneumomediastinum).<br>• Reduced bronchial blood flow to lungs.<br>• Reduced renal perfusion.<br>• During PEEP use, prostaglandins exhibit negative inotropism.<br>2. Supportive fluid therapy:<br>• Maintain PCWP between 8 and 12 mmHg to maintain cardiac output during positive-pressure and PEEP therapy.<br>3. Treatment of underlying cause or precipitating event (e.g., use of antibiotics to treat infection).<br>• Avoid prophylactic use of antibiotics.<br>4. High dose corticosteroids: Definitive benefit questionable; use in ARDS controversial.<br>5. Supportive therapy to reduce hypoxemia/hypoxia:<br>A. Increase oxygen delivery to tissues.<br>• Administration of packed red blood cells to maintain hemoglobin ~11 g/100 ml.<br>• Treatment of respiratory alkalemia and hypophosphatemia to shift oxygen-dissociation curve to right (enhances oxygen unloading at the tissue level). | end-diastolic pressure.<br>Intravenous nitroprusside and nitroglycerin decreases both preload and afterload by their vasodilating effects on systemic venous and arterial blood vessels.<br>*Aminophylline therapy:* Used in conjunction with furosemide, may induce an enhanced diuresis; it also enhances cardiac output, increasing renal perfusion; it improves the $PaO_2$ by its bronchodilator effect.<br>2. *Inotropic agents:* These agents improve cardiac output by increasing myocardial contractility; there is a concomitant reduction in left ventricular preload, which, in turn, reduces PCWP. Inotropic agents increase myocardial oxygen consumption and must be used with caution in the setting of myocardial infarction.<br>Specific agents include: Digoxin, quabain, dopamine, dobutamine.<br>3. *Antidysrhythmia therapy* (e.g., lidocaine, quinidine, procainamide, calcium-channel blockers).<br>4. Intubation and mechanical ventilation with PEEP may be instituted in pulmonary edema, which is refractory to other therapeutic modalities.<br>• Use of PEEP reduces intrapulmonary shunting; it also reduces left ventricular (LV) preload by a vasodilator effect on the venous capacitance system, and by its effects on pleural pressures; PEEP decreases left ventricular end-diastolic volume, which may improve LV ejection fraction and, thus, reduce PCWP. |

*(continued)*

TABLE 34–2
**Cardiogenic and Noncardiogenic Pulmonary Edema: A Comparison *(Continued)***

| | Noncardiogenic Pulmonary Edema (NCPE) | Cardiogenic Pulmonary Edema (CPE) |
|---|---|---|
| | B. Decrease in oxygen demand/consumption.<br>• Hypothermia: Decreases cardiac output = ↓shunt fraction; decreases oxygen demand.<br>• Cautious use of sedatives (diazepam) in restless patient to keep patent airway secure.<br>Mental status evaluation is essential to evaluate response to therapy. Use of sedation must be minimized.<br>• Muscle paralysis may be necessary in the extremely restless, hypoxic patient in whom a decrease in oxygen demand is necessary.<br>• Pancuronium bromide (Pavulon) is the drug of choice; administered with diazepam to reduce anxiety associated with muscle paralysis.<br>6. Ancillary supportive measures:<br>A. Rigorous chest physiotherapy (bronchial) hygiene.<br>B. Use of aminophylline for wheezing.<br>C. Intravenous and/or enteral nutrition. | |
| Complications | Outcome depends on nature and extent of pulmonary insult.<br>Mortality: ~50%.<br>Post-illness sequelae: Mild restrictive disease<br>Mild impairment of gas exchange: ↓$PaO_2$ especially during exercise.<br>Airflow obstruction of smaller airways. | Progressive deterioration of cardiopulmonary function:<br>Serious cardiac dysrhythmias.<br>Complications of treatment:<br>Digitalis toxicity.<br>Fluid/electrolyte imbalance.<br>Oxygen toxicity.<br>Cardiogenic shock. |

the pathogenesis of pulmonary edema may involve one or more of the following: (1) an increase in the hydrostatic pressure within the pulmonary capillaries; (2) an increase in the permeability of the alveolar–capillary membrane; and (3) an alteration in pulmonary lymphatic drainage.

**Cardiogenic (Hydrostatic) Pulmonary Edema.** Cardiogenic pulmonary edema occurs most often in the scenario of left heart failure. Its cause is essentially an imbalance between the hydrostatic and osmotic pressures that govern fluid movement within the lungs (see Fig. 34–1).

As the volume of blood in the left ventricle at the end of diastole increases, there is a consequent increase in the left ventricular end-diastolic pressure (LVEDP), which is reflected back to the pulmonary capillary bed. This increase in pulmonary intravascular hydrostatic pressure (which is represented clinically by an increase in the pulmonary capillary wedge pressure; PCWP)[3] forces fluid out of the pulmonary capillaries and into the interstitium causing pulmonary congestion. When the amount of fluid in the interstitium exceeds the drainage capacity of the pulmonary lymphatic system, or if lymphatic drainage is impeded (e.g., post-irradiation lymph fibrosis, neoplasms), fluid is forced into the alveoli causing pulmonary edema.

In this form of pulmonary edema, the permeability of the microvascular membrane remains intact limiting movement of protein out of the capillaries. (See Table 34–2 for specific details regarding underlying pathophysiologic stages.)

**Noncardiogenic Pulmonary Edema.** The mechanism leading to noncardiogenic pulmonary edema or ARDS involves an *increase* in the *permeability* of the alveolar–capillary membrane usually

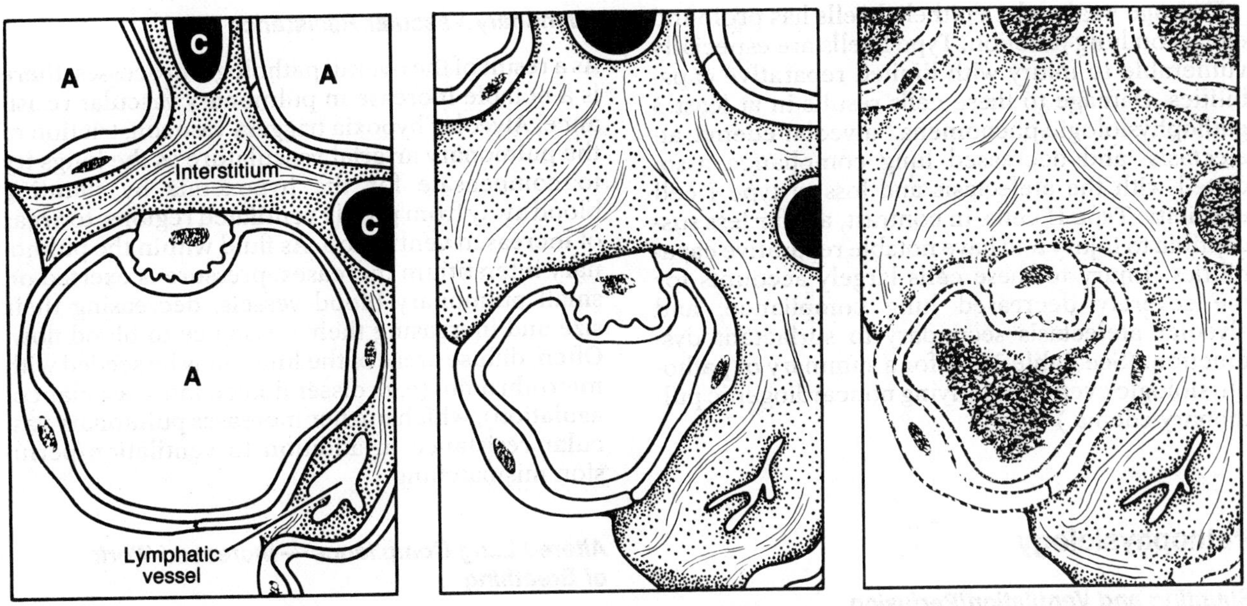


| NORMAL (mmHg) | CARDIOGENIC (mmHg) | NONCARDIOGENIC (mmHg) |
|---|---|---|
| Capillary hydrostatic pressure 8-12 | > 12 | ~ 8-12 |
| Capillary oncotic (osmotic) pressure 23-25 | ~ 23-25 | Decreased (early) <23 |
| Interstitial hydrostatic pressure −3 | Increased | Increased |
| Interstitial oncotic (osmotic) pressure 16-19 | ~ 16-19 | Increased > 19 |
| Alveolar-capillary membrane permeability | Intact | **Increased** |
| Pulmonary lymphatic drainage | Intact (early) | Intact (early) |

**Figure 34–1.** Underlying pathophysiology differentiating cardiogenic from noncardiogenic pulmonary edema. In cardiogenic edema, the alveolar–capillary membrane remains intact, but the capillary hydrostatic pressure is increased (>12 mmHg) thereby increasing movement (transudation) of fluid from the pulmonary capillary (C) (i.e., the intravascular space) into the interstitium. In noncardiogenic pulmonary edema, the capillary hydrostatic pressure remains within normal limits (~8–12 mmHg), but there is a significant drop in capillary osmotic pressure (<23 mmHg) and an increase in interstitial osmotic pressure (>19 mmHg) attributed to disruption in permeability of the alveolar–capillary membrane. This allows movement of proteins, fluid, and cells from the intravascular space (i.e., the capillary) into the interstitium and, thence, into the alveolus (A), with the consequent pressure changes.

in the presence of normal pulmonary capillary hydrostatic pressure. As a consequence of the increase in permeability, plasma proteins and red blood cells, in addition to fluid, move out of the intravascular space and into the pulmonary interstitium.

The exact cause (or causes) of the increase in membrane permeability remains undefined, but initial pathologic changes reflect disruption of the capillary endothelium, which leads to leakage of fluid, protein, and cellular material into the interstitial space. This is followed by involvement of alveolar epithelial cells including both type I cell sloughing and type II cell dysfunction.

Damage to alveolar epithelial cells has profound effects on lung function. Type I cells are especially vulnerable to injury with limited reparative capabilities. Damage to these cells results in at least 3 pathophysiologic phenomena:[4] alveolar edema, atelectasis, and decreased lung compliance associated with the atelectasis and loss of type I cell elasticity. Type II cells, in contrast, are far less susceptible to injury and have notable reparative capabilities. Injury to these cells largely accounts for the severely decreased lung compliance, and alveolar atelectasis secondary to surfactant dysfunction. (See Table 34-2 for a summary of pathophysiologic events underlying noncardiogenic pulmonary edema.)

## Pathophysiology

### *Shunting and Ventilation/Perfusion Mismatching*

Pathologic processes seen in ARDS play a major role in altering gas exchange and disrupting the mechanical properties of the lungs. Flooding of the alveoli with fluid (i.e., pulmonary edema) prevents ventilation of lung units, while perfusion may be relatively preserved. Consequently, unoxygenated blood is shunted into the pulmonary venous circulation and on into the left heart. This right-to-left shunting is a primary cause of hypoxemia in ARDS and largely accounts for the refractoriness of the hypoxemia to supplemental oxygen therapy.

In addition to areas of true shunting, there are also regions of ventilation/perfusion ($\dot{V}/\dot{Q}$) mismatching due, in part, to the uneven distribution of the pathologic processes within the lungs. Changes in blood flow do not necessarily follow those related to ventilation.

### *Ineffective Surfactant Activity*

Gas exchange is compromised due to alterations in the activity of surfactant. Surfactant is a phospholipid largely responsible for reducing surface tension within the alveoli. When fluid fills the alveoli, surfactant is inactivated and becomes ineffective as a surface tension reducer. The result is widespread alveolar collapse and atelectasis, with a consequent reduction in gas exchange and a worsening hypoxemia. Despite these alterations in gas exchange, overall ventilation in the patient with ARDS remains intact, and alveolar hypoventilation with rising carbon dioxide retention ($\uparrow PaCO_2$) usually does not occur except in the terminal stages of the disease, or when another underlying pulmonary process is present (e.g., viral pneumonia).

### *Pulmonary Vascular Resistance*

As a result of the overall pathologic processes, there is a notable increase in pulmonary vascular resistance. Alveolar hypoxia triggers vasoconstriction of the pulmonary arterial vasculature as the lungs try to compensate for the hypoxemia by shunting blood away from poorly ventilated regions, to areas of increased ventilation. As fluid within the pulmonary interstitium increases, pressure is exerted on small pulmonary blood vessels, decreasing their size and increasing their resistance to blood flow. Often, diffuse areas of the lungs may be seeded with microthrombi (e.g., disseminated intravascular coagulation), which further increases pulmonary vascular resistance in addition to ventilation/perfusion mismatching.

### *Altered Lung Compliance—Increased Work of Breathing*

Alterations in the mechanical properties of the lungs include decrease in pulmonary compliance and a decrease in functional residual capacity (FRC). The presence of increased pulmonary interstitial fluid, together with alveolar collapse, contributes to a "stiffening" of the lung parenchyma. As a result, a progressively greater effort is expended in order to expand the lungs and maintain adequate alveolar ventilation. The increased work of breathing is associated with decreased tidal volumes and an increase in respiratory rate, which increases the relative deadspace ventilation ($V_D/V_T$).

### *Reduction in Lung Volumes*

As a consequence of the increase in fluid occupying air spaces and widespread atelectasis, the volume of gas within the lungs is significantly reduced. Specifically, the FRC is significantly decreased (i.e., the volume of gas remaining within the lungs at end-expiration). Thus, not only is the work of breathing increased, but the volume of gas moved with each breath is also reduced. This rapid, shallow pattern of breathing, necessitating increased energy expenditure on the part of the patient, contributes significantly to the dyspnea so characteristic of ARDS.

## Clinical Presentation

Following the initial physiologic insult, there may be a lag of several hours to a day or more before consequences of the underlying pathologic processes become evident clinically. Dyspnea and tachypnea are usually the initial symptoms experienced by the patient. Arterial blood gases usually reflect a disturbance in oxygenation (↓$PaO_2$); carbon dioxide levels may be reduced (↓$PaCO_2$) because the patient is able to maintain adequate alveolar ventilation in the early period. An increase in the alveolar–arterial oxygen gradient ($AaDO_2$) may also become evident. Chest x-rays at this stage may be unremarkable.

With disease progression and continued leakage of fluid, protein, and blood cells from the intravascular space into interstitial and alveolar spaces, clinical findings become more definitive. The patient may become extremely dyspneic and tachypneic; breath sounds may reveal rales (crackles); hypoxemia worsens with significantly widened $AaDO_2$; and chest x-rays become grossly abnormal, revealing significant infiltrates reflective of the fluid and protein within air spaces.

The progression of ARDS is variable from patient to patient, but generally these patients become gravely ill as reflected by a mortality rate of 50%. Prior to the initial insult many of these patients have normal pulmonary function. Yet within a matter of a few days, they may progress to life-threatening respiratory failure. Those fortunate to recover may have surprisingly few sequelae with pulmonary function returning essentially to premorbid status (see Table 34–2).

## Diagnostic Considerations

The diagnosis of ARDS is based on clinical history, including the presence of precipitating factor(s); clinical findings on examination (dyspnea, tachypnea); assessment of arterial blood gases; changes in lung compliance and intrapulmonary shunt fraction; and demonstration of diffuse interstitial and alveolar infiltrates on chest x-ray.

*Hypoxemia* is the hallmark of ARDS due largely to *intrapulmonary shunting.* The hypoxemia is refractory to oxygen therapy as reflected by a $PaO_2$ less than 50–60 mmHg with an $FIO_2$ greater than 50%. Respiratory alkalemia occurs because of hyperventilation; hypercapnia is often not seen initially, and its presence early on may be an ominous sign. An A–a gradient greater than 250–300 mmHg on an $FIO_2$ of 100% is characteristic of ARDS. In terms of pulmonary function, pulmonary compliance and FRC are reduced secondary to microatelectasis and pulmonary edema.

Use of hemodynamic pressure monitoring is indicated in patients with ARDS. Monitoring of pulmonary capillary pressures helps to distinguish cardiogenic or hydrostatic pulmonary edema from the noncardiogenic pulmonary edema of ARDS. In the former, the pulmonary capillary wedge pressure (PCWP; hydrostatic pressure) is high as a result of "back-pressure" from the left heart; in the latter, the PCWP is usually normal, suggesting that the presence of interstitial and alveolar fluid is caused by an increase in alveolar–capillary permeability and not high intravascular hydrostatic pressures.

## Treatment

### *Therapeutic Goals*

Effective treatment of ARDS requires a continuous effort to diagnose and treat the underlying precipitating event, whether it involves aspiration or inhalation of chemical irritants, or occurs by way of the pulmonary circulation (sepsis, fat embolism, disseminated intravascular coagulation, and so forth; see Table 34–1). Effective treatment of the precipitating disorder, control of the permeability defect responsible for the leakage of fluid and protein, and support of gas exchange until adequate pulmonary function is reestablished are major goals in the treatment and management of ARDS.[5] As long as the underlying disorder persists, the capillary permeability defect may remain. Prompt recognition of the syndrome with early institution of supportive measures remains a fundamental goal of therapy in ARDS.

It is also essential to reduce the potential for additional insults to the respiratory system and other organ systems, which may cause further deterioration in the already severely compromised person. For example, improved survival appears to be associated with vigorous antibiotic therapy in the treatment of infection.

Maintenance of lung volumes with early intubation and controlled ventilation has been found to improve small airway function and prevents the development of interstitial and alveolar congestion and atelectasis. The mainstay of treatment is oxygenation. Because of the large shunt component characteristic of ARDS, some form of distending airway pressure becomes desirable or mandatory. Thus, intubation with mechanical ventilation is required, with subsequent application of positive end-expiratory pressure (PEEP).

### *PEEP Therapy*

Positive end-expiratory pressure (PEEP) therapy improves gas exchange and pulmonary function by maintaining a low level of positive airway pressure during the expiratory phase. This increases the FRC. Assuming that there is an upper limit to the distensibility of normal alveoli, it is within those limits that PEEP can increase FRC. PEEP reestablishes and maintains the patency of airways and alveoli, and reduces the amount of right-to-left shunting. This, in turn, allows reduction of the $FIO_2$ necessary to relieve hypoxemia, and reduces the potential for the development of oxygen toxicity associated with administration of high oxygen concentrations ($FIO_2 > 50\%$) necessitated by the refractory hypoxemia.

The goal is to achieve a PEEP level that allows maintenance of a hemoglobin-saturating $PaO_2$ without significant compromise of cardiac output and oxygen transport. Patients with an early form of noncardiogenic pulmonary edema may show significant improvement in gas exchange with a PEEP of 5–15 cm $H_2O$; severe ARDS may require as much as 15–30 cm $H_2O$ of PEEP. Subsequent increments in PEEP are based on arterial blood gas analysis ($PaO_2$), mixed venous oxygen tension ($PvO_2$), lung compliance, and status of hemodynamic parameters (e.g., PCWP and cardiac output).

**Dynamic Lung Compliance.** Dynamic lung compliance can be determined at the bedside by dividing the tidal volume ($V_T$) by the peak inspiratory pressure (PIP) minus PEEP. With initial institution of PEEP therapy, which opens up atelectic and edematous alveoli, there should be an increase in the $V_T$/PIP ratio. PEEP may be increased by increments of 3–5 cm $H_2O$ to optimize oxygen saturation of hemoglobin and delivery of oxygen to the tissues. If necessary, PEEP may be increased until the inherent stiffness of the lungs prevents further distention or expansion of air spaces. Further increase in PEEP should be avoided because the compliance may actually decrease. The goal of PEEP therapy is to achieve the maximum benefit of PEEP, or the "best PEEP" for the patient that will improve gas exchange and enable the inspired oxygenation to be adjusted so as to decrease the $FIO_2$ necessary to achieve oxygenation ($PaO_2 > 60$ mmHg).[6]

PEEP does not prevent ARDS in the clinical milieu, but rather, it is a supportive therapeutic modality that facilitates improvement in arterial oxygen tensions while reducing the necessary $FIO_2$ ($FIO_2 < 50\%$).[7]

**Complications of PEEP Therapy.** A major potential complication of PEEP therapy is a reduction in cardiac output caused by a reduced venous return to the heart. Positive intrathoracic pressure generated by PEEP is applied to the intrathoracic great veins and pulmonary vasculature and accounts for the reduction in venous return. A reduced venous return results in a decreased cardiac output. Maintaining intravascular volume is essential to minimize reduction in venous return.

PEEP may be detrimental to cerebral blood flow. By increasing pressure within the superior vena cava, cerebral venous drainage by the jugular veins may be compromised, resulting in an increase in intracranial pressure. Maintenance of head elevation at approximately 30 degrees may be sufficient to guarantee adequate cerebral venous blood flow. The patient's mental status should be closely monitored.

Barotrauma (e.g., spontaneous pneumothorax, pneumomediastinum) may occur from overdistention and rupture of alveoli. Oxygen toxicity is always a potential complication when it is necessary to administer $FIO_2$ greater than 50%. Diligent monitoring of serial arterial blood gases assists in determining the lowest $FIO_2$ that effectively treats the hypoxemia (i.e., a $PaO_2 > 60$ mmHg on an $FIO_2 < 50\%$).

**Indications for the Initiation of PEEP Therapy.** Major indications for PEEP therapy include persistent (refractory) hypoxemia ($PaO_2 < 60$ mmHg on an $FIO_2 > 50\%$); decreasing pH $< 7.25$; rising $PaCO_2 > 45$ mmHg; and diffuse lung disease. Prophylactic PEEP therapy may be used in those patients at greater risk of developing hypoxemic respiratory failure.

**Contraindications for PEEP Therapy.** While there are no absolute contraindications to the use of PEEP in patients with ARDS, the following clinical circumstances need to be assessed and evaluated: Reduced extracellular fluid volume; patchy, necrotizing nonhomogeneous lung disease; unilateral lung disease; and panlobular emphysema. The reduction in cardiac output associated with PEEP therapy may be further exaggerated by a reduced circulating blood volume. During PEEP therapy, cardiac output can be maintained by augmentation of preload by fluid therapy and pharmacologic manipulation.

### *Fluid and Electrolyte Management*

Fluid management is a major consideration in the treatment of ARDS. Overly vigorous administration of fluids may increase hydrostatic pressure within the pulmonary capillary bed and increase fluid content within the lung interstitium and air spaces. The consequence may be a larger shunt fraction contributing to hypoxemia.

On the other hand, fluid therapy may be necessary to restore and/or maintain adequate pulmonary and systemic tissue perfusion. Maintaining this delicate fluid balance requires continuous monitoring of pulmonary artery and pulmonary capillary wedge pressures, together with appropriate pharmacologic manipulation.

Skillful management of fluid status in ARDS is required because PEEP may have an adverse effect on renal perfusion. The physiologic mechanism by which PEEP alters renal perfusion may involve a direct effect on the nephron; or it may involve the indirect effect of PEEP on baroreceptors, osmoreceptors (antidiuretic hormone secretion), renin secretion, or the sympathetic nervous system.

### *Supportive Measures*

Additional measures to be considered to achieve an increase in tissue perfusion include correction of respiratory alkalemia and hypophosphatemia. These conditions cause a shift of the oxygen dissociation curve (see Fig. 28–15) to the right, increasing the concentration of oxygen released to the tissues.

Administration of blood products (e.g., packed red blood cells) may be indicated to ensure adequate oxygen transport to the tissues. However, some studies have demonstrated optimal hemoglobin for ARDS to be about 11 g/100 ml. An increase in hemoglobin levels above this level can increase blood viscosity, creating additional problems.

Methods to decrease oxygen demand and consumption may also be instituted. Careful use of sedatives (e.g., diazepam) or a muscle-paralyzing agent (e.g., pancuronium) reduces oxygen consumption by decreasing muscle tone and activity. Hypothermia also reduces oxygen demand.

Use of the various modalities may allow $FIO_2$ to be reduced to less than 50%, thus minimizing the danger of oxygen toxicity while effectively treating the hypoxemia.

Successful treatment and management of ARDS depend to a large extent on the nurse's awareness of the patient's entire clinical status in addition to the mechanical ventilatory and pharmaceutical support. Meticulous attention to the patient's responses to therapeutic modalities as well as knowledge of the adverse effects of these modalities are important considerations in the ongoing monitoring and care of the patient with ARDS.

## Nursing Care of the Patient with ARDS

Adult respiratory distress syndrome (ARDS), characterized by its sudden but commonly subtle onset frequently in previously healthy persons, and its rapidly progressive, fulminating course, which may reach catastrophic, life-threatening proportions within hours to a few days, presents health-care providers with a distinctly awesome challenge. Despite modern technologic advances in science, medicine, and health care over the past 2 decades, the mortality rate of patients with ARDS remains about 50%. And yet, those who do survive may have minimal to absent sequelae.

What does it take to get the patient through the precarious course of respiratory failure unique to ARDS with the eventual recovery of effective pulmonary function? As the health-care provider most intimately involved in patient care, the critical care nurse is especially challenged in this regard.

To effectively meet this challenge presented by ARDS, it is essential that critical care nurses have a thorough grasp of underlying cardiopulmonary physiology and an indepth understanding of this syndrome—the setting in which it occurs, its pathophysiology, clinical manifestations, and necessary therapeutic interventions. Critical care nurses must have sharp assessment skills and an instinctive and intuitive ability to perceive even the most subtle changes in the patient's condition, and to recognize their significance in terms of total body responses. For example, in the patient who is hemodynamically stabilized following a physiologic insult, a persistent but subtle hyperventilation (tachypnea) may be the only clue to the presence of respiratory insufficiency.

ARDS is not an isolated problem that can be attributed to a particular disease, trauma, or precipitating event. Frequently, precipitating factors occur in combination to initiate the underlying pathologic process. Consequently, it is necessary for critical care nurses to be able to recognize and identify possible combinations of factors that function to produce ARDS. Critical care nurses should be able to identify those disorders most commonly associated with ARDS (see Table 34–1).

What makes ARDS particularly challenging to diagnose and to treat is that, to date, no clinically valid diagnostic tests or procedures have been developed to assist in the early diagnosis of ARDS. This is regrettable because therapeutic interventions instituted early in the course of this syndrome can often mean the difference between the patient's complete recovery or ultimate demise. This fact serves to punctuate the necessity for thorough ongoing assessment and monitoring of patients who are at risk of developing ARDS.

### *Therapeutic Goals*

The overall therapeutic goal in the management of the patient in hypoxemic respiratory failure associated with ARDS is to maintain adequate gas exchange through timely, aggressive, and supportive interventions for as long a period as is necessary until the pathophysiologic process(es) underlying the failure is (are) treated or allowed to resolve spontaneously. In the previously healthy person, the focus of treatment is to "normalize" disturbed gas parameters in achieving a pH within the normal physiologic range (7.35–7.45).

Meticulous supportive nursing care is necessary to maximize the therapeutic effects and prevent complications. Nursing functions to maintain the essential bodily processes within the patient until effective spontaneous physiologic functions are restored. Patient–nurse interaction is especially significant when one considers the fact that compromised respiratory function impacts on total body function. Without adequate gas exchange, the life processes of the patient would rapidly succumb.

The critical care nurse plays a crucial role in the assessment, diagnosis, and management of the patient with ARDS who develops hypoxemic respiratory failure. The immediate therapeutic goal in the nursing care of these critically ill patients is to act in a timely and purposeful manner to relieve life-threatening hypoxemia, and to assist in re-establishing adequate gas exchange.

Current technologic sophistication in the care of

**TABLE 34–3. CARE PLAN FOR THE PATIENT WITH ADULT RESPIRATORY DISTRESS SYNDROME IN HYPOXEMIC ACUTE RESPIRATORY FAILURE**

| Nursing Diagnoses | Desired Patient Outcomes | Nursing Interventions | Rationales |
|---|---|---|---|
| ***Nursing Diagnosis #1***<br>Gas exchange, impaired, related to:<br>1. Right-to-left shunting.<br>2. Ventilation/ perfusion mismatch. | Patient will:<br>1. Be alert and oriented to person, place, time.<br>2. Demonstrate appropriate behavior.<br>3. Maintain effective cardiovascular function:<br>• Blood pressure within 10 mmHg of baseline.<br>• Cardiac ouput ~5 liters/min.<br>• Without cyanosis if preexisting pulmonary function normal<br>• Lab values:<br>Hematocrit<br>Male: 45%–52%<br>Female: 37%–48%<br>Hemoglobin<br>Male: 13–18 g/100 ml<br>Female: 12–16 g/100 ml<br>4. Maintain optimal arterial blood gases:<br>pH 7.35–7.45.<br>$PaO_2$ >60 mmHg.<br>$PaCO_2$ ~35–45 mmHg.<br>5. Alveolar–arterial oxygen gradient ($AaDO_2$): <15 mmHg on room air. | • Perform neurologic assessment:<br>∘ Mental status, level of consciousness.<br>∘ Appropriate behavior.<br>∘ Protective and deep tendon reflexes. | • Hypoxemia may predispose to cerebral tissue hypoxia. |
| | | • Monitor respiratory function:<br>∘ Respiratory rate and pattern.<br>∘ Use of accessory muscles. | ∘ Increased work of breathing fatigues the patient and predisposes to alveolar hypoventilation with hypercapnia and respiratory acidemia. |
| | | ∘ Status of weakness and fatigue.<br>∘ Degree of chest wall excursion.<br>∘ Increase in fremitus? | ∘ Consolidated lung tissue transmits vibrations better than air-filled lung spaces. |
| | | ∘ Presence of dullness on percussion? | ∘ Percussion over consolidated lung produces a "dull" sound. |
| | | ∘ Breath sounds:<br>– Abnormal breath sounds.<br>– Adventitious breath sounds. | ∘ Bronchial breath sounds are often heard in areas of the lung that normally would reflect vesicular sounds; rales (crackles) may also be heard. |
| | | • Assess cardiovascular function:<br>∘ Heart rate.<br>∘ Hemodynamic parameters:<br>– Systemic arterial pressure.<br>– Pulmonary capillary wedge pressure.<br>– Cardiac output. | • Hemodynamic parameters reflect tissue perfusion. |
| | | ∘ Evidence of cyanosis. | ∘ Late sign reflecting the desaturation of at least 5 g of hemoglobin; evidence of ventilation/perfusion mismatch and right-to-left shunt. |
| | | ∘ Cardiac dysrhythmias. | ∘ Hypoxemia is commonly associated with myocardial irritability. |
| | | ∘ Arterial blood gas values: pH. | ∘ A metabolic acidemia is often associated with decreased tissue perfusion; the consequent anaerobic metabolism causes a rise in serum lactate levels with a progressive metabolic acidosis.<br>∘ Metabolic acidosis may depress myocardial function and predispose to dysrhythmias. |

| | |
|---|---|
| • Monitor laboratory data:<br>◦ Arterial blood gases.<br>pH<br>$PaO_2$ significantly reduced <60 mmHg.<br>$PaCO_2$ reduced early <35 mmHg.<br>increased late >45 mmHg.<br>Calculate $AaDO_2$. | ◦ Most closely reflect effectiveness of gas exchange.<br>◦ Extensive right-to-left shunting causes the hypoxemia to be refractory to oxygen therapy.<br>◦ Tachypnea and dyspnea cause carbon dioxide to be eliminated, predisposing to hypocapnia.<br>◦ Alveolar–arterial gradient <250–300 mmHg with an $FIO_2$ of 100%; a classic hallmark of ARDS. |
| ◦ Hematology: Hematocrit, hemoglobin. | ◦ Maintenance of normal physiologic levels of hemoglobin ensures maximal oxygen transport and release of oxygen to the tissues. Increased hemoglobin levels increase blood viscosity. |
| • Administer prescribed humidified oxygen therapy. | • Oxygenation is the mainstay of treatment of ARDS; a large right-to-left shunt predisposes to a hypoxemia refractory to administration of even high concentrations ($FIO_2$ >50%) of oxygen.<br>◦ Oxygen is administered in conjunction with mechanical ventilation and PEEP therapy.<br>◦ Precautions associated with oxygen therapy:<br>– Oxygen is a potent drug necessitating cautious use.<br>– Oxygen concentrations should be kept to a minimum to maintain $PaO_2$ >60 mmHg.<br>– Duration of oxygen therapy should be kept to a minimum.<br>◦ Prolonged administration of high oxygen concentrations predisposes to oxygen toxicity.<br>◦ Use of an $FIO_2$ >50% over a period of 6–30 hr has been associated with oxygen toxicity.<br>◦ Maintenance of a $PaO_2$ >60 mmHg can produce a hemoglobin saturation of ~90%. |
| ◦ Monitor for signs/symptoms of oxygen toxicity: Retrosternal chest pain; paresthesias in extremities; fatigue, lethargy, malaise, restlessness; anorexia, nausea, vomiting; dyspnea, coughing. | ◦ Signs and symptoms of oxygen toxicity are often subtle and may be easily overlooked; meticulous and thorough ongoing assessment and evaluation of patient's responses to therapy assist in determining effectiveness of therapy and prevention of complications. |

*(continued)*

**TABLE 34–3. CARE PLAN FOR THE PATIENT WITH ADULT RESPIRATORY DISTRESS SYNDROME IN HYPOXEMIC ACUTE RESPIRATORY FAILURE *(Continued)***

| Nursing Diagnoses | Desired Patient Outcomes | Nursing Interventions | Rationales |
|---|---|---|---|
| ***Nursing Diagnosis #1 (cont.)*** | | | |
| | | ○ Late symptomatology: Progressive respiratory distress; dyspnea, cyanosis; asphyxia; increasing $AaDO_2$; decreased compliance and lung volumes. | |
| | | ○ Monitor serial arterial blood gas measurements. | ○ Frequent monitoring of arterial blood gases is a mandatory safety measure when an $FIO_2 > 40\%$ is used. |
| | | • Implement positive end-expiratory pressure (PEEP) therapy in conjunction with mechanical ventilatory support.<br>○ Dosage: Early noncardiogenic pulmonary edema; 5–15 cm $H_2O$ pressure; severe ARDS 15–30 cm $H_2O$ pressure. | • PEEP therapy maintains airway opening pressure at end expiration above atmospheric pressure. This distending airway pressure increases lung volumes including FRC; it prevents airway collapse; it enhances gas exchange and oxygen transport; and it functions to reduce right-to-left shunting.<br>○ Use of PEEP therapy increases $PaO_2$ without requiring an increase in $FIO_2$. |
| | | ○ Criteria used to determine effective PEEP level: Arterial blood gas analysis; mixed venous oxygen tension; lung compliance; hemodynamic parameters: pulmonary artery pressure; PCWP; cardiac output.<br>○ PEEP is usually increased in increments 3–5 cm $H_2O$ pressure until "best PEEP" is achieved. | ○ Lung compliance is determined by dividing the peak inspiratory pressure (PIP) into the tidal volume ($V_T$).<br>○ "Best PEEP" is achieved when the inherent "stiffness" of the lungs prevents further distention of air spaces; it is the level at which maximal benefit of PEEP is realized (i.e., $PaO_2 > 60$ mmHg on $FIO_2$ 50%). |
| | | ○ Monitor for complications of PEEP therapy: Reduction in venous return to the heart and cardiac output; reduction in cerebral perfusion—Assess mental status.<br>○ Barotrauma. | ○ Positive intrathoracic pressure generated by PEEP is applied to the great veins within the chest, reducing venous return to the right heart.<br>○ Overdistention and rupture of alveoli are major complications of PEEP therapy. |
| | | ○ Monitor fluid status. | ○ Overly vigorous administration of fluids may aggravate the pulmonary edema; the increased capillary hydrostatic pressure favors movement of fluid into lung interstitium.<br>○ Excessive fluid accumulation increases total lung water, causing an increase in ventilation/perfusion mismatching. |

| | | | |
|---|---|---|---|
| ***Nursing Diagnosis #2***<br>Breathing pattern, ineffective:<br>Tachypnea, hyperventilation. | Patient will:<br>1. Achieve effective minute ventilation.<br>• Tidal volume ($V_T$) >5–7 ml/kg.<br>• Respiratory rate <30/min.<br>2. Achieve a vital capacity ($V_C$) >12–15 ml/kg.<br>3. Verbalize ease of breathing.<br>• Breath sounds audible throughout anterior/posterior chest.<br>• Reduced to absent adventitious sounds. | • Assess respiratory function:<br>○ Rate, rhythm, depth, and pattern of breathing.<br>○ Symmetry of chest wall and diaphragmatic excursion: Use of accessory muscles; flaring of nares.<br>– Monitor for fatigue, exhaustion.<br>○ Lung compliance.<br>○ Pulmonary lung volumes:<br>– Total minute ventilation ($\dot{V}_E$).<br>– Tidal volume ($V_T$).<br>– Respiratory rate (f).<br>– Vital capacity ($V_C$).<br>• Assist patient into position of comfort to allow for best lung expansion.<br>• Implement mechanical ventilation (see Table 32–7 for nursing care considerations). | ○ Tachypnea is the compensatory mechanism for hypoxemia.<br>○ Hyperventilatory effort is responsible for the hypocapnia observed during the *early* course of the illness.<br>○ Accumulation of fluid, edema, and secretions within the lungs, with lung consolidation, reduces lung compliance.<br>○ Maximal respiratory effort is made to facilitate optimum ventilation.<br>○ A minimal volume of ventilation is necessary to ensure adequate alveolar ventilation; this minimal volume of gas enables gas exchange to occur during the phases of the respiratory cycle when no new gas is inspired (expiratory and end-expiratory phases).<br>• Expansion of lungs facilitates more even distribution of ventilation; increases ventilation/perfusion matching. |
| ***Nursing Diagnosis #3***<br>Airway clearance, ineffective, related to increased tracheobronchial secretions. | Patient will:<br>1. Be alert and oriented to person, place, time.<br>2. Maintain effective alveolar ventilation:<br>• Breath sounds audible throughout anterior/posterior chest.<br>• Reduced to absent adventitious sounds.<br>• Arterial blood gas values stabilized as follows:<br>pH 7.35–7.45.<br>$PaO_2$ >60 mmHg.<br>$PaCO_2$ 35–45 mmHg. | • Assess respiratory function with emphasis on status of pulmonary secretions and the patient's ability to handle secretions.<br>○ Presence of adventitious sounds.<br>– Rales (crackles) wheezes.<br>• Assess fluid status.<br>○ Intake and output; daily weight.<br>• Implement chest physiotherapy and bronchial hygiene measures. | • Patients with ARDS often have increased secretions, which impair adequate ventilation, further compromising the hypoxemia.<br>• Excessive intrapulmonary accumulation of fluid reduces compliance and further aggravates underlying right-to-left shunting and ventilation/perfusion mismatching.<br>• Pooling of secretions within the tracheobronchial tree compromises ventilation and predisposes to infection.<br>• In patients receiving PEEP therapy, an adapter should be used to maintain the positive end-expiratory pressure.<br>• Even the slightest interruption of PEEP therapy can significantly increase the hypoxemia. |

(*continued*)

**TABLE 34-3. CARE PLAN FOR THE PATIENT WITH ADULT RESPIRATORY DISTRESS SYNDROME IN HYPOXEMIC ACUTE RESPIRATORY FAILURE *(Continued)***

| Nursing Diagnoses | Desired Patient Outcomes | Nursing Interventions | Rationales |
|---|---|---|---|
| ***Nursing Diagnosis #4***<br>Cardiac output, alteration in: Decreased (diminished) venous return.<br>***Nursing Diagnosis #5***<br>Tissue perfusion, alteration in: Cardiopulmonary.<br>***Nursing Diagnosis #6***<br>Tissue perfusion, alteration in: Cerebral. | For specific patient outcomes related to these nursing diagnoses, see Table 33-2, Nursing Diagnoses #4, #5, and #6. | For specific nursing interventions and their rationales, see Table 33-2, Nursing Diagnoses #4, #5, and #6. | |
| ***Nursing Diagnosis #7***<br>Fluid and electrolytes, alteration in.<br>(See Chapter 23 for appropriate nursing diagnosis.) | For specific patient outcomes related to this nursing diagnosis, see Table 33-2, Nursing Diagnosis #7. | • Administer prescribed intravenous therapy. | • Because of the alveolar-capillary permeability defect in ARDS, the fluid of choice for intravenous administration is crystalloid rather than colloid. Colloids would leak out of intravascular space to equilibrate with interstitial fluid. |
| ***Nursing Diagnosis #8***<br>Acid-base balance, alteration in: Respiratory alkalosis (tachypnea, hyperventilation). | The patient's arterial blood gas values will stabilize as follows:<br>pH 7.35-7.45.<br>$PaO_2 > 60$ mmHg.<br>$PaCO_2$ 35-45 mmHg. | • Assess for signs and symptoms of respiratory alkalemia:<br>∘ Neurologic function: Lightheadedness, weakness, muscle cramps, twitching; paresthesias; hyperactive deep tendon reflexes, seizure activity; tetany.<br>∘ Cardiovascular function: Cardiac dysrhythmias.<br>∘ Serum calcium levels.<br>∘ Serial arterial blood gases. | • Respiratory failure in the patient with ARDS is associated with tachypnea and hyperventilation as the body tries to compensate for the severe hypoxemia.<br>∘ Hyperventilation reduces $PaCO_2$ with a consequent rise in pH.<br>∘ A rise in pH reduces the serum concentration of freely ionized calcium by causing an increase in the calcium that is protein-bound. The consequent hypocalcemia, if sufficiently severe, may predispose to neuromuscular alterations. |
| | | • Implement supportive therapy to maintain adequate ventilation and optimal gas exchange. | |

| | | | |
|---|---|---|---|
| | | ∘ Increase tidal volume.<br>∘ Decrease respiratory rate.<br>∘ If mechanically ventilated, increase dead-space ventilation; decrease minute ventilation. | ∘ Increasing tidal volume and decreasing respiratory rate decreases total minute ventilation; reduced ventilation enables the alveolar $PCO_2$ and, thus, the $PaCO_2$ to return to an acceptable physiologic range (35–45 mmHg). |
| ***Nursing Diagnosis #9***<br>Nutrition, alteration in: Less than body requirements (see Chap. 53). | For specific patient outcomes related to this nursing diagnosis, see Table 33–2, Nursing Diagnosis #9. | For specific nursing interventions and their rationales, see Table 33–2, Nursing Diagnosis #9. | |
| ***Nursing Diagnosis #10***<br>Infection, potential for (Table 49–7). | For specific patient outcomes related to this nursing diagnosis, see Table 33–2, Nursing Diagnosis #10. | For specific nursing interventions and their rationales, see Table 33–2, Nursing Diagnosis #10. | |
| ***Nursing Diagnosis #11***<br>Pulmonary mechanics, alterations in, related to respiratory muscle weakness and atrophy (immobility, mechanical ventilation). | Patient will:<br>1. Perform deep breathing exercises hourly.<br>2. Achieve maximum pulmonary function:<br>• Tidal volume >7–10 ml/kg.<br>• Vital capacity >15 ml/kg.<br>• Respiratory rate <30/min.<br>• Maximal expiratory flow. | • Teach deep breathing exercises:<br>∘ Assess emotional and physiologic readiness for such teaching.<br>∘ Allow patient to demonstrate deep breathing exercises.<br>∘ Combine deep breathing therapy with other chest physiotherapy maneuvers.<br>• Assess pulmonary volumes to determine effectiveness of therapy. | • Use of positive-pressure ventilation for a prolonged period predisposes to atrophy of the respiratory musculature.<br>∘ Breathing exercises mobilize secretions, improve ventilation, stimulate circulation, and increase muscle tone. |
| ***Nursing Diagnosis #12***<br>Skin integrity, impairment of, related to immobility. | For specific patient outcomes related to this nursing diagnosis, see Table 33–2, Nursing Diagnosis #12. | For specific nursing interventions and their rationales, see Table 33–2, Nursing Diagnosis #12. | |

(*continued*)

**TABLE 34–3. CARE PLAN FOR THE PATIENT WITH ADULT RESPIRATORY DISTRESS SYNDROME IN HYPOXEMIC ACUTE RESPIRATORY FAILURE *(Continued)***

| Nursing Diagnoses | Desired Patient Outcomes | Nursing Interventions | Rationales |
|---|---|---|---|
| ***Nursing Diagnosis #13*** Coping, ineffective individual/family. | Patient/family will:<br>1. Verbalize knowledge and understanding of the illness.<br>2. Verbalize feelings as to what this potentially life-threatening illness means to each family member, individually and collectively.<br>3. Verbalize strengths and coping capabilities.<br>4. Identify family resources.<br>5. Make decisions regarding matters of importance to patient and family. | • Assess patient/family perceptions regarding a potentially life-threatening illness. | • Knowledge of patient and family perceptions of the illness assists in identifying coping capabilities and potential coping problems. |
| | | ○ Develop a trusting relationship with patient and family. | ○ A trusting, caring, supportive relationship facilitates verbalization of concerns and fears. |
| | | ○ Establish a caring rapport: Patient advocacy; accessible to patient/family. | ○ A definitive, dependable support system assists patient/family to assume responsibility for decision-making. |
| | | ○ Encourage verbalization of perceptions, concerns, and feelings. | ○ Unexpressed and unresolved fears and concerns may compromise ability to cope effectively. |
| | | • Assist patient/family to identify past coping capabilities:<br>○ Emphasize strengths.<br>○ Assist patient/family in defining areas requiring problem-solving and decision-making.<br>– Support patient/family in this regard. | |
| | | ○ Involve in decision-making regarding care.<br>– Offer praise for accomplishments.<br>– Encourage development of new coping mechanisms.<br>– Assist patient/family to explore and identify options and the consequences of the options. Assist patient/family to implement chosen options. | ○ Active participation in self-care assists the individual/family to gain a new sense of dignity, self-worth, and self-esteem. |
| | | • Initiate referrals to intrahospital and community resources for special needs: Psychiatric social worker, family pastor, home care. | • Additional resources may assist patient/family to gain increased awareness of self in the interactions among patient, family, health-care providers, and environment. |

patients with compromised cardiopulmonary function enables these patients to be maintained with a degree of respiratory failure until the underlying problem is resolved. Through ongoing assessment and timely, appropriate interventions, the astute critical care nurse provides the quality of care necessary not only to maintain these patients over the critical course of the illness, but also to impact positively on the patient's ultimate prognosis.

Thorough ongoing assessment of the patient's responses to intensive treatment provides the basis for therapeutic interventions. (Essential details regarding the clinical history and physical examination are presented in Chap. 29; an indepth discussion of arterial blood gases and acid–base balance is presented in Chap. 30.) Aggressive respiratory support therapy remains the mainstay of treatment and management of ARDS. Therapeutic modalities include oxygen therapy, airway management, mechanical ventilation with PEEP, and chest physiotherapy–bronchial hygiene (see Chap. 32). Vigorous implementation of such therapies may help to reduce the risk of oxygen toxicity by enabling the fraction of inspired oxygen ($FIO_2$) to be decreased to a concentration less than 50%, while still relieving hypoxemia.

Implementation of nursing process in the care of the patient with ARDS and hypoxemic respiratory failure revolves around the therapeutic goals listed below.

1. Perform a thorough and meticulous ongoing assessment and monitoring of the patient's overall condition (Chaps. 29 and 30).
2. Establish and maintain a patent airway (Chap. 32).
3. Provide appropriate ventilatory support and oxygenation to relieve the severe hypoxemia associated with ARDS.
4. Provide support of cardiovascular function to maintain cardiac output and tissue perfusion to all vital organ systems (Table 33–2, Nursing Diagnoses #4, #5, and #6).
5. Maintain fluid and electrolyte balance (Chap. 23).
6. Maintain acid–base balance (Chap. 30).
7. Diagnose and treat underlying precipitating disorders, disease, or event (e.g., trauma, shock, sepsis, pneumonia with extensive lung consolidation, fat emboli, and so forth; Table 34–1).
8. Provide nutritional support (Table 33–2, Nursing Diagnosis #9, see Chap. 53).
9. Prevent infection (Table 33–2, Nursing Diagnosis #10).
10. Prevent alterations in pulmonary mechanics related to immobility and mechanical ventilation (respiratory muscle weakness and atrophy associated with positive-pressure mechanical ventilation).
11. Prevent impairment of skin integrity related to immobility.
12. Provide emotional and psychologic support to patient and family (see Chap. 3).

Pertinent nursing diagnoses, desired patient outcomes, nursing interventions and their rationales are presented in the care plan for the patient with ARDS in Table 34–3.

## REFERENCES


1. Brandstetter, RD: The adult respiratory distress syndrome—1986. Heart Lung 15(2):161, March 1986
2. Roberts, SL: Physiological Concepts and the Critically Ill Patient. Prentice-Hall, Englewood Cliffs, NJ, 1985, pp 149–150.
3. Campbell, M and Greenberg, C: Reading pulmonary artery wedge pressure at end-expiration. Focus Crit Care 15(2):60, April 1988.
4. Shapiro, BA: Noncardiogenic edema, adult respiratory distress syndrome, and PEEP therapy. In Case Studies in Critical Care Medicine. Year Book Medical Publishers, Chicago, 1985, p 178.
5. Bradley, R: Adult respiratory distress syndrome. Focus Crit Care 14(5):48, October 1987.
6. Sibbald, WJ: Pulmonary Edema. In Sibbald WJ (ed): Synopsis of Critical Care, ed 3. Williams & Wilkins, Baltimore, 1988, p 104.
7. Brandstetter, RD: The adult respiratory distress syndrome—1986. Heart Lung 15(2):156, March 1986.
8. King, E: Respiratory failure in the critically ill. In Sibbald, WJ (ed): Synopsis of Critical Care, ed 3. Williams & Wilkins, Baltimore, 1988, p 64.

CHAPTER 35

# Nursing Management of the Patient with Pulmonary Embolism

## CHAPTER OUTLINE



## LEARNING OBJECTIVES

**At the end of this chapter, you should be able to:**

1. Identify predisposing and etiologic factors associated with the pathogenesis and etiology of pulmonary embolism.
2. Describe the pathophysiology of pulmonary embolism and its impact on pulmonary and hemodynamic function.
3. Describe the clinical presentation and diagnostic evaluation of pulmonary embolism.
4. Define the therapeutic priorities in the treatment and management of pulmonary embolism.
5. Identify implications for nursing care based on nursing process:
   a. Assessment.
   b. Specific nursing diagnoses.
   c. Planning: Patient outcomes and nursing interventions/rationales.

## PULMONARY EMBOLISM

### Definition

The term pulmonary embolism refers to the movement of a blood clot (most common) or detached intravascular mass (e.g., tumor cells or fragments, fat embolism) from its site of origin (usually a systemic vein within the pelvis or lower extremities) through the right side of the heart and into the pulmonary circulation where it lodges in one or more branches of the pulmonary artery. It is estimated that 95% of all pulmonary emboli arise from thrombi in the deep veins of the lower extremities. Although these emboli commonly originate in veins of the calf, it is within the large deep veins of the thigh that emboli, sufficiently large to precipitate clinical manifestations suggestive of pulmonary embolism, are released.

Pulmonary embolism is a major cause of sudden, unexpected death in hospitalized patients. Of clinical significance is that two thirds of the cases of pulmonary embolism are misdiagnosed both in terms of overdiagnosis when not present, and underdiagnosis when present. The fact that clinical, laboratory, and roentgenographic findings of pulmonary embolism are nonspecific contributes to the overall misdiagnosis. Yet, early recognition, prompt diagnosis, and treatment of this disorder reduce mortality from as high as 40% to less than 10%. In this regard, institution of prophylactic measures (i.e., low-dose heparin, subcutaneously) has proved to be an effective therapeutic approach in certain high-risk patients (e.g., patients scheduled to undergo thoracic or abdominal surgery).

## Pathogenesis and Etiologic Factors

### *Predisposing Factors*

Three predisposing factors have been identified (Virchow's triad) in the pathogenesis of venous thrombosis. These include: (1) venous stasis; (2) endothelial injury or vessel wall abnormalities; and (3) alteration in the mechanism of blood coagulation (hypercoagulable state).

### *Etiologic Factors*

Etiologic factors contributing to the pathogenesis of venous thrombosis and consequent thromboemboli include the following: immobilization (e.g., bedrest, fractures, prolonged sitting in one position as during travel), trauma (e.g., burns, long bone fracture with fat emboli), preoperative and postoperative states (especially after hip or pelvic surgery, or surgery involving the lower extremity), underlying carcinoma, pregnancy and childbirth, and use of oral contraceptives.

Less commonly, thrombus formation occurs in the heart in association with congestive heart failure, atrial fibrillation, cardioversion, endocarditis, and infarction. The incidence of thromboembolic disease increases with age and the length of illness.

While extensive deep venous thrombosis (DVT) of the lower extremities and pelvic veins has been highly implicated in the etiology of pulmonary embolism, it may be clinically undetectable. In fact, only about 50% of all patients with pulmonary embolism manifested prior clinical signs of venous thrombosis in the lower extremities or elsewhere. This underscores the necessity to obtain a thorough clinical history and to pay close attention to subtle clinical clues and details in order to even suspect pulmonary embolism.

## Pathophysiology

Pathologically, embolic occlusion of a vessel may lead to pulmonary infarction (about 10%–15% of all pulmonary emboli); and/or congestive atelectasis of the lung parenchyma characterized by hemorrhage and edema. Often, however, neither of these pathologic changes occurs, and there may be relatively little alteration of the lung parenchyma distal to the occlusion, presumably because of incomplete occlusion or sufficient oxygen from other sources. The dual circulation (pulmonary and bronchial systems) to the lungs, for example, may provide adequate collateral circulation in these instances.

Pathophysiologic responses associated with pulmonary emboli may involve alterations in both pulmonary and hemodynamic function. Characteristically, changes in pulmonary status involve an increase in alveolar deadspace with significant ventilation/perfusion (V/Q) mismatching, bronchospasm, altered surfactant function, and pulmonary arterial hypertension associated with an increase in pulmonary vascular resistance.

### *Bronchospasm*

Bronchospasm (bronchoconstriction) of small airways may be a direct consequence of hypocapnia as the lung tries to compensate for the ventilation/perfusion mismatching by directing ventilation to perfused lung units. With the consequent increase in airway resistance, the patient experiences an increased work of breathing.

Bronchospasm is also induced by chemical mediators thought possibly to be released by the emboli themselves, although the exact source and nature of the chemical mediators are not entirely clear. Platelets that adhere to the emboli are presumably an important source of such mediators as histamine, serotonin, and prostaglandins.[1] Through their secondary effects on both airways and the pulmonary vasculature, the activity of these mediators may be an important mechanism underlying the hypoxemia in pulmonary embolism.

### *Altered Surfactant Production/Activity*

Another feature of the pathophysiology of pulmonary embolism involves a disturbance in surfactant and/or its surface tension-reducing activity in the affected areas of the lung. The absence of surfactant or its altered activity associated with pulmonary embolism contributes to alveolar collapse and atelectasis. Gas exchange may become seriously compromised due to significant ventilation/perfusion mismatching and a degree of right-to-left shunting, leading to hypoxemia. If the embolism is massive (i.e., obstruction of 50% or more of the pulmonary arterial bed), life-threatening respiratory failure and circulatory collapse may ensue.

### *Pulmonary Arterial Hypertension*

The extent and severity of the pulmonary embolism and the patient's preexisting cardiopulmonary status largely determine the overall effect on hemodynamic function. The major hemodynamic consequences of pulmonary embolism is pulmonary arterial hypertension.

Mechanical occlusion of greater than 50% of the pulmonary vascular bed increases pulmonary vascular resistance. Lesser clot burdens may increase pulmonary vascular resistance (PVR) in the presence of preexisting disease states.

Chemical mediators released in the presence of pulmonary embolism cause vasoconstriction with further compromise of the pulmonary vasculature. As the pulmonary vascular resistance increases, pulmonary artery pressure also increases, and there is a corresponding increase in the work of the right ventricle. A point may be reached when the pulmonary vascular resistance and the consequent pulmonary artery pressure may rise so high that the right ventricle may be unable to handle this acute increase in workload and right heart failure may ensue.

## Clinical Presentation

Most pulmonary emboli do not produce any significant symptoms, and the entire embolic episode may go unnoticed. When the patient becomes symptomatic, the clinical presentation may vary from mild to severe depending on the extent and severity of the pulmonary embolism. In a mild episode, the most common complaint is that of otherwise unexplained dyspnea. Only infrequently do patients present with a conclusive picture of a well-identified precipitating factor with clinically apparent deep venous thrombosis, dyspnea, pleuritic chest pain, and hemoptysis. Still another presenting pattern may reflect a massive embolism with acute cor pulmonale characterized by dyspnea, cyanosis, right heart failure, and compromising hypotension, or shock.

An abrupt onset of chest pain is thought to be associated with pulmonary infarction involving the pleura and the effects of blood clots on the pulmonary vessels. Hemoptysis may occur in the presence of pulmonary infarction and is frequently *pure* blood, which helps to differentiate an underlying pulmonary embolism from a pneumonia. In pneumonia should hemoptysis occur, the blood expectorated is usually mixed with sputum. Syncopal episodes may occur when the embolic episode causes serious disruption of cardiopulmonary dynamics with a reduction in cardiac output and a consequent decrease in cerebral blood flow.

On physical examination, dyspnea, tachypnea, and tachycardia are common findings. The chest examination may be entirely normal, or it may reveal diminished breath sounds, localized rales (crackles), or wheezing. A pulmonary infarction that extends to the pleura may produce a friction rub and a finding of pleural effusion on chest x-ray.

Evidence of acute right ventricular overload (cor pulmonale) may be revealed on cardiac examination. Fixed splitting of the second heart sound with a pronounced pulmonic component may be detected, reflecting a delay in closure of the pulmonic valve. A right-sided $S_4$ may be heard, possibly accompanied by a right ventricular heave. A murmur may also be detected over the lung field, possibly reflecting turbulent blood flow through a pulmonary blood vessel partially occluded by an obstructing embolism. Jugular venous distention may be observed, reflecting right heart insufficiency or failure.

Examination of the lower extremities may reveal changes suggestive of a venous thrombosis including tenderness, swelling, or detection of a palpable cordlike clot within a vessel. More commonly, however, there is rarely evidence of an underlying deep venous thrombosis.

Cardiac dysrhythmias, which are frequently atrial in origin, may be present; right heart strain and refractory congestive heart failure may be evident.

## Diagnostic Evaluation

As mentioned previously, a diagnosis of pulmonary embolism is often difficult to make because the clinical presentation varies depending on the size and location of the embolic episode. Many of the diagnostic studies used do not enable a definitive diagnosis of pulmonary embolism to be made but, rather, assist in differential diagnosis by ruling out other possibilities. Diagnostic tests and procedures used in the diagnostic evaluation of pulmonary embolism are listed in Table 35-1.

## Treatment and Management

### *Therapeutic Priorities*

In the setting of an acute embolic episode, the first priority may be to treat severely compromised cardiopulmonary function. Once the patient's cardiopulmonary status is stabilized, the next priority is to prevent recurrent embolization.[2]

**Cardiopulmonary Support Therapy.** The major considerations in initiating cardiopulmonary support in the scenario of acute pulmonary embolism includes the maintenance of ventilation, oxygenation, and circulation.

***Ventilatory Support.*** In patients with pulmonary embolism, the usual ventilatory consequence observed is hyperventilation with hypocapnia. In patients experiencing a massive pulmonary embolism associated with severe obtundation, hypoxemia and carbon dioxide retention with hypercapnia may occur, necessitating intubation and mechani-

TABLE 35–1
## Diagnostic Evaluation of Pulmonary Embolism

| Tests/Studies/Findings | Clinical Significance |
|---|---|
| Laboratory: | |
| • Arterial blood gases:<br>pH >7.45<br>$PaO_2$ <60 mmHg<br>$PaCO_2$ <35 mmHg | Hypocapnia with consequent respiratory alkalemia related to tachypnea and hyperventilation is a common finding when clinical manifestations of the embolic episode become evident.<br>Hypoxemia in pulmonary embolism is largely due to ventilation/perfusion mismatching. |
| • Alveolar–arterial oxygen tension gradient ($AaDO_2$) = 15 mmHg (normal = <15 mmHg) | The norm for this gradient varies with age. Patients over 60 years may have an increased $AaDO_2$. |
| • Hematology:<br>Leukocyte count <15,000/mm$^3$ | |
| • Serum enzyme studies:<br>CPK-MB<br>SGOT<br>LDH | These studies assist in differential diagnosis of myocardial infarction. |
| • Blood coagulation studies: Fibrin degradation products = increased | These studies may reflect an underlying hypercoagulable state commonly associated with thromboembolic disease and pulmonary embolism. |
| X-ray studies: | |
| • Chest x-ray: Nonspecific, frequently normal; may indicate the following findings: | |
| Hemidiaphragmatic elevation: areas of atelectasis | These findings suggest reduced lung volumes; in the presence of an embolic episode, such findings may reflect reduced ventilation associated with tachypnea, and increased airway resistance due to bronchospasm. |
| Pulmonary infiltrates | Pulmonary infiltrates may reflect a pulmonary infarction, or congestive atelectasis and hemorrhage associated with pulmonary embolism. |
| Pleural effusion, unilateral | |
| Special studies: | |
| • Perfusion lung scan:<br>Demonstrates absence of perfusion to the region of the lung supplied by the occluded blood vessel. | A major screening test for pulmonary embolism.<br>If perfusion scan is normal, pulmonary embolism is largely ruled out; abnormalities do not automatically indicate presence of embolic disease; false-positive scans are common because local decreases in blood flow may result from a preexisting lung disease. |
| • Ventilation lung scan (involves inhalation of xenon radioisotope) | Assists in differential diagnosis: If regions of decreased perfusion are secondary to airway disease, a concomitant ventilation abnormality should also be present. |
| • Pulmonary angiography (done within 2 weeks of the suspected embolic event) | The most definitive diagnostic procedure for pulmonary embolism; usually reserved to last because of the invasive nature of the procedure. |
| • Contrast venography<br>• Radionuclide venography | Highly effective for detection of occlusive venous disease proximal to the knee. |
| • Radioactive fibrinogen test | A sensitive test to detect the presence of small thrombi in the calves. |
| • Impedance phlebography | A noninvasive method for quantitating blood volume changes in the leg: obstruction of major veins in the leg decreases rate at which blood flows out of leg; reflects capacity of venous system to accommodate additional blood volume in the presence of temporary venous outflow obstruction. |
| • Impedance plethysmography $^{125}$I fibrinogen scan: Screening for deep venous thrombosis (DVT) | |
| Electrocardiogram:<br>• Findings are commonly nonspecific.<br>• The following may be evident:<br>Dysrhythmias<br>Peaked P waves<br>S wave in lead I<br>Q wave in lead III<br>An $S_1$, $Q_3$, $T_3$ togther with RBBB<br>ST segment depression<br>T wave inversion lead III | |

cal ventilation. Tidal volume and respiratory rate are adjusted to maintain the $PaCO_2$ within the range of 35–45 mmHg.

***Oxygen Therapy.*** Basic principles pertaining to the management of hypoxemia require maintenance of a patent airway with intubation and initiation of mechanical ventilation if there is need to: (1) prevent aspiration in the patient who is obtunded and in severe hypovolemic shock; or (2) administer oxygen therapy at inspired oxygen concentrations ($FIO_2$) necessary to achieve $PaO_2 > 60$ mmHg.

***Circulatory Support.*** In obstructing the pulmonary vasculature, a pulmonary embolism reduces flow of blood to the left heart, decreasing the preload, or left ventricular end-diastolic volume (LVEDV); this, in turn, results in a reduction of cardiac output and systemic arterial blood pressure.

Concurrently in response to the embolic episode, the pulmonary vasculature may itself reflexly trigger systemic peripheral arteriolar vasodilation, which likewise reduces systemic arterial blood pressure. The consequence is a "relative" volume depletion, or if severe, hypovolemic shock.

Treatment involves intravascular volume expansion to raise systemic blood pressure. Administration of intravenous fluids is best guided by hemodynamic pressure monitoring. Hypovolemic shock may require use of vasopressor therapy (e.g., dopamine).

### Prevention of Recurrent Embolization

***Anticoagulant Therapy.*** Concomitantly with the implementation of definitive therapy to maintain cardiopulmonary function until resolution of the embolic episode occurs, there is initiation of anticoagulant therapy to prevent recurrent embolization. The major goal of anticoagulant therapy is to prevent further formation of intravascular clot with embolic potential.

The mainstay of anticoagulant therapy during the acute phase is the administration of heparin. The use of heparin has several advantages. While it does not dissolve clots that have already embolized the lungs, it does prevent formation of new thrombi or propagation of old ones.

Heparin also acts to block platelet–thrombin interactions on the embolus, which might otherwise lead to release of chemical mediators (e.g., serotonin) associated with bronchospasm and hypotension.

Heparin enhances fibrinolytic activity on fresh thrombi. A major advantage of the drug is that its anticoagulant effects are promptly reversible with protamine sulfate if bleeding occurs. Heparin has an immediate onset of action.

Standard treatment for uncomplicated pulmonary embolism is anticoagulation with heparin during the acute phase followed by coumadin for 6 weeks to 6 months. Longer anticoagulant therapy is reserved for patients with conditions predisposing to recurrent emboli or who have a continuing predisposition to venous thrombosis. Because the action of coumadin is mediated through altered production of vitamin K-dependent coagulation factors in the liver (factors II, VII, IX, X), the onset of action is not immediate. Hence, the initiation of coumadin therapy should be overlapped by 2 or 3 days of heparin therapy at a slightly reduced dosage before the heparin is discontinued.

***Thrombolytic Therapy.*** Another option for treating pulmonary embolism is the use of thrombolytic agents, either streptokinase or urokinase (see Appendix A). These agents, which may actually lyse recent blood clots, must be given within the first several days of the embolic event in order to be effective. Patients with massive pulmonary embolus, or those with hemodynamic compromise as a result of vascular occlusion, are most likely to benefit from thrombolytic (fibrinolytic) therapy.

Use of thrombolytic agents is generally continued for 24–48 hours and is followed by standard anticoagulant therapy.

***Inferior Vena Caval Filter.*** Surgical intervention in the treatment of pulmonary embolism involves placement of a filtering device into the inferior vena cava. Also referred to as the "umbrella" device, the filter functions to trap thrombi originating in the deep veins of the pelvis or lower extremities, en route to the pulmonary circulation. These devices are indicated in situations where anticoagulant therapy is contraindicated (e.g., the presence of a bleeding problem) or the patient's pulmonary vascular reserve is so compromised that an additional embolus to the lungs could prove fatal.

***Prophylactic Anticoagulation.*** Prophylactic anticoagulation to prevent deep venous thrombosis in high-risk patients has proved to be an effective therapeutic approach. The most common prophylaxis is heparin administered subcutaneously in low dosage, usually 5,000 units subcutaneously, every 8–12 hours (see Appendix A). For nursing implications in heparin therapy, see Table 35–2.

## Nursing Care of the Patient with Pulmonary Embolism

The critical care nurse plays a crucial role in the prevention of pulmonary embolism in critically ill patients. Through the identification of those patients considered to be at great risk and recognition of those etiologic factors contributing to the pathogenesis of deep venous thrombosis, the critical care nurse can implement appropriate and timely interventions directed toward decreasing the risk of pul-

TABLE 35-2
## Heparin Therapy: Nursing Considerations

**Actions of Heparin**

Heparin is an anticoagulant agent that potentiates the inhibitory activity of antithrombin III on several clotting factors essential for normal blood coagulation. (See Chap. 60 for physiology underlying coagulation.)

- The key reactions that are blocked include:
  1. Conversion of prothrombin to thrombin.
  2. Conversion of fibrinogen to fibrin.
- Heparain inhibits the formation of new clots.
- Heparin may prevent extension and propagation of preexisting clots but does not facilitate lysis of these clots.

**Uses of Heparin:**

- Treatment of deep venous and arterial thrombosis, and/or pulmonary embolism.
- Prophylaxis of thromboembolic complications associated with surgery and venostasis.
- Treatment of disseminated intravascular coagulation (DIC) (rarely).

| **Dosage and Administration** | **Nursing Considerations/Rationales** |
|---|---|
| Common approaches to heparin therapy: | |
| 1. A. Use of loading dose: 5,000–15,000 IU by IV bolus followed by continuous IV heparin therapy. | A loading dose is used to achieve a therapeutic blood level rapidly. |
| B. Maintenance dose: Continuous intravenous infusion of heparin 500–3,000 IU hourly as determined by aPTT and coagulation tests. | |
| Use of continuous intravenous heparin infusion:<br>• Facilitates administration.<br>• Avoids unven anticoagulation. | During administration of heparin therapy, periodic blood samples are obtained to determine the patient's response to heparin and dosage adjustments. |
| 2. Intermittent heparin therapy:<br>A. 10,000–15,000 IU by IV bolus; followed by<br>B. Maintenance dose: 5,000–6,000 IU every 4 hr as determined by aPTT. | Activated partial thromboplastin time (aPTT) is the blood test commonly used to monitor effects of heparin therapy on blood coagulation.<br>*Goal:* To maintain aPTT 1.5–2.5 times normal baseline (usually ~65–80 sec) |
| 3. Prophylactic anticoagulation therapy.<br>A. 5,000 IU every 8–12 hr, subcutaneously. | Prophylactic approach is commonly used in patients at risk of developing deep venous thrombosis as, for example, the immobilized patient, or patients about to undergo or who have recently undergone major thoracic and abdominal surgery. |
| 4. Heparin lock flush solution to maintain patency of vascular access site.<br>• Concentrations of heparin/saline flush solution typically range from 10–1000 units/ml; and volume varies from 2–3 ml to 6–8 ml/flush procedure. The volume used should be sufficient to exceed the capacity of the heparin lock catheter. | Use of heparin flush in this instance is *not* intended for heparin therapeutic purposes. |
| • Flush heparin lock set with normal saline (1–2 ml) before and after a medication is administered. | Heparin is a highly acidic molecule; avoid mixing drugs with heparin to prevent potential drug interaction. Clinical relevance of the drug interaction is dubious. |

**Initiation of Heparin Activity**

- Intravenous route: Begins within minutes with clotting time returning to baseline within 2–6 hr after discontinuation.
- Subcutaneous route: Begins within 20–60 min; lasts for 8–12 hr, with wide variations.
- Intramuscular route: Unpredictable and unreliable.

| **Duration of Heparin Therapy** | **Nursing Considerations/Rationales** |
|---|---|
| • Course of heparin therapy is 8–10 days. | It takes 8–10 days for a clot to adhere to the vessel wall. |
| • Coumadin therapy is usually initiated during the last 2–3 days of heparin therapy. | The action of coumadin is mediated by altered production of vitamin K-dependent clotting factors and requires several days for its action to take effect. |

**Heparin Pharmacokinetics**

- 95% protein-bound.
- Small amount taken up by mast cells.
- Metabolism: Reticuloendothelial system and liver.
- Elimination by urine as partially degraded heparin; some heparin may be eliminated unchanged.

**Contraindications to Heparin Therapy**

| | |
|---|---|
| • Active bleeding; recent surgery; stroke.<br>• Hypersensitivity. | |
| *Precaution:* Advanced renal, liver, or biliary disease. | Altered metabolism may alter the action of heparin and its duration. |

*(continued)*

TABLE 35-2

## Heparin Therapy: Nursing Considerations *(Continued)*

**Adverse/Side Effects**

- Spontaneous bleeding.
- Sensitivity reaction at injection site.
- Thrombocytopenia and platelet antibodies.

**Baseline platelet count should be obtained, followed by serial platelet determinations every 3 days during heparin therapy.**
**Increased bleeding and thrombosis have been related to heparin-induced thrombocytopenia.**

**Heparin Antidote**[3]

Protamine sulfate (1% solution).

1. Onset of action of IV protamine is ~5 min with a duration of up to ~2 hr.
2. Dosage: 1 mg of protamine neutralizes the effect of 90–110 units of heparin.
3. Administration: Slow injection of the drug not to exceed 50 mg in any 10-min period.
   A. Loading dose may be given: 25–50 mg by slow injection followed by a continuous intravenous infusion.
4. Monitor vital signs.

**The strongly basic protamine combines with the highly acidic heparin to form a stable compound and, thus, nullifies the anticoagulant effect.**

**Dosage is guided by blood coagulation studies; monitor aPTT and clotting time.**

| **Nursing Interventions** | **Rationales** |
|---|---|
| • Obtain baseline studies including:<br>1. Blood.<br>A. Coagulation studies.<br>1) Activated partial thromboplastin time.<br>2) Coagulation (clotting) time.<br>B. Hematology.<br>1) Hemoglobin, hematocrit.<br>2) RBC count; platelet count. | **These tests are performed periodically throughout heparin therapy to monitor patient's response to therapy, and determine appropriate dosage adjustments.**<br>**Heparin-induced thrombocytopenia may predispose to bleeding and thrombosis.** |
| • Monitor aPTT after each dosage change, and daily once the maintenance dose is established. | **aPTT is a specific test reflecting effects of heparin therapy.** |
| • Identify patients at higher risk of developing spontaneous bleeding (e.g., patients receiving prophylactic heparin therapy post-surgery; the elderly; patients with renal, hepatic and/or biliary disease). | |
| • Assess all organ systems prior to initiation of heparin therapy to establish baseline function. | **Establishing a baseline assists in assessing patient's overall response to therapy.** |
| 1. Reassess for signs/symptoms of bleeding every 2 hr. | |
| 2. Monitor the following parameters at regular intervals:<br>A. Vital signs: Heart rate, blood pressure; respiratory rate and rhythm; body temperature. | |
| B. Neurologic status: Mental status, level of consciousness; behavioral changes; complaints of headache, dizziness. | **Changes in neurologic status may reflect intracranial bleeding.** |
| C. Petechiae: Soft palate, conjunctiva, retina.<br>D. Ecchymosis.<br>E. Hematuria.<br>F. Hematemesis; red/black stools. | **This distribution of petechiae may reflect thrombocytopenia and warrants the determination of the platelet count.** |
| 3. Continuous intravenous heparin therapy requires the following interventions:<br>A. Addition of heparin in the prescribed strength and dose, to the infusion fluid; invert 5–6 times to ensure adequate distribution of heparin. | **It is necessary to read the label carefully because heparin comes in different strengths.**<br>**It is important to prevent pooling of heparin in the solution to ensure appropriate continuous dose.** |
| B. An infusion pump should be used to deliver accurate heparin dose. | **Use of pump facilitates close monitoring.** |
| C. Examine insertion site carefully for signs of infiltration or tubing kinking. | |
| D. Inspect all invasive sites each shift for bleeding, hematoma formation, or signs of inflammation. | |
| 4. Subcutaneous administration of heparin therapy: Recommended guidelines/techniques.[4] | |
| A. Deep subcutaneous (SC) injection, preferably made to fatty layer of the abdomen, or just above iliac crest. | **Shallow SC injection should be avoided because it may be more painful, is associated with high risk of hematoma formation, and has variable duration of desired effect.** |
| B. Use tuberculin syringe, 25–26 gauge, $\frac{1}{2}$–$\frac{5}{8}$ in. needle. | **Ensures accuracy in measuring dose.** |
| C. Discard needle used to withdraw heparin from vial. | |
| D. Prepare site with alcohol sponge and allow to dry. | **Avoid massaging the injection site to avoid injury to small blood vessels.** |

TABLE 35–2
**Heparin Therapy: Nursing Considerations *(Continued)***

| | |
|---|---|
| E. Gently bunch up a defined roll of subcutaneous tissue. | Avoid pinching because this may also injure small blood vessels. |
| F. Insert needle into roll at 90-degree angle to skin surface. | |
| G. While maintaining support of tissue, slowly and steadily inject the drug. | Do not withdraw plunger to check for blood because of risk of tissue injury. |
| H. Hesitate before withdrawing needle; withdraw needle quickly in the same direction it was introduced; simultaneously, release hold of subcutaneous tissue. | This pause is to prevent trailing of drug through needle tract. |
| I. Apply gentle pressure to insertion site for approximately 1 min; do not massage the area. | |
| J. Optional application of ice to puncture site may reduce incidence of hematoma or ecchymosis. | |
| K. Keep a chart indicating rotation of injection sites. | Rotation of injection sites minimizes tissue injury and altered distribution and absorption of the drug. |
| • Patient/family education. | Critical phase of illness: Limits educational process. |
| 1. Instruct on preventive activities to reduce risk of deep venous thrombosis (DVT) and pulmonary embolism. | Stasis or stagnation of blood, and endothelial or vessel wall injury have been implicated in the pathogenesis of venous thrombosis. |
| A. Provide antiembolic stockings or support hose. | |
| B. Avoid positions that compromise blood flow (e.g., crossing legs, prolonged sitting in one position, or pillow under knees). | Instruction should involve ways to minimize stasis of blood or vessel injury and, thus, reduce risk of thrombus recurrence. |
| C. Encourage active range-of-motion exercises hourly; initiate and maintain daily exercise schedule. | Exercise of lower extremities assists the "skeletal muscle pump" to return venous blood to the heart; such exercises minimize stasis of blood in the lower extremities. Deep venous thrombosis of lower extremities has been definitively implicated as a major etiologic factor in pulmonary embolism. |
| D. Instruct patient/family regarding the following: | |
| • Avoid exposure to cold. | |
| • Stop smoking. | |
| • Maintain ideal body weight. | |
| • Maintain hydration. | Hydrated state ensures adequate blood volume; hemoconcentration associated with the dehydrated state may result in sluggish blood flow. |
| • Avoid use of oral contraceptives. | These medications are considered to increase the risk of thrombus formation. |
| • Avoid massaging any area of suspected deep venous thrombosis or thrombophlebitis. | Such activity may increase the risk of pulmonary embolism. |
| 2. Instruct regarding medication therapy including: | Following pulmonary embolism, patients are commonly maintained on long-term (6 weeks–6 months) oral anticoagulant therapy (coumarin derivative, e.g., warfarin and dicumarol). |
| A. Underlying indication/rationale. | |
| B. Dosage schedule and the importance of taking the medication as prescribed (correct dose taken at same time daily). | |
| C. Adverse/side effects. | |
| D. Necessary regular followup including periodic blood studies. | |
| E. Importance of not taking other medications including over-the-counter drugs, without first consulting with the physician. | Many over-the-counter drugs contain aspirin (salicylates), which potentiates the anticoagulant effect and may cause spontaneous bleeding. |
| F. Necessity of reporting to physician any unusual prolonged or excessive bleeding:<br>Excessive bleeding from gums, mouth; epistaxis; excessive bruising (ecchymosis); hematuria; coffee-ground hematemesis; tarry stools; excessive menses.<br>Other significant signs/symptoms:<br>Headaches, dizziness, behavioral/personality changes; sudden chest or shoulder pain; dyspnea or tachypnea; redness, swelling or pain in an extremity. | Early recognition of a bleeding problem may prevent serious complications in the patient on anticoagulant therapy. |
| G. Importance of wearing Medic-Alert band identifying the patient as being on anticoagulant therapy. | |
| 3. Instruct regarding precautions to be used in activities of daily living: | Knowledge and awareness of situations that can potentially precipitate bleeding assist in minimizing the risk of bleeding while the patient is on anticoagulant therapy. |
| A. Use of electric rather than straight-edge razor. | |
| B. Gentle flossing and brushing of teeth. | |
| C. Careful trimming of nails. | |
| D. Careful blowing of nose. | |
| E. Avoidance of straining at stool. | |
| 4. Reinforce the necessity of following prescribed care including followup visits with health-care providers. | The informed patient is more likely to exhibit compliance with prescribed treatment regimen. |
| A. Provide written instructions regarding overall plan of care. | Involvement of other family members in decision-making activities and overall treatment plan may provide the patient with additional resources and support. |
| B. Include names and telephone numbers of key health-care providers involved in patient's care. | |
| C. Allow time for questions and clarification of information provided. | |

monary embolism, preventing or eliminating those factors implicated in its pathogenesis, or, should a pulmonary embolic episode occur, preventing recurrent thrombus formation and embolization.

### Therapeutic Goals

Specific nursing interventions in the care of the patient with pulmonary embolism are related to the following therapeutic goals:

1. Relieve anxiety precipitated by a sudden (commonly) acute onset of respiratory insufficiency, possibly accompanied by chest pain and frank hemoptysis, and requiring aggressive therapy within the confines of an unfamiliar, often frightening and intimidating intensive care setting.
2. Establish and/or maintain a patent airway and initiate mechanical ventilation and oxygen therapy as determined by the patient's clinical status and arterial blood gas values.
3. Provide hemodynamic support to maintain cardiac output and tissue perfusion.
4. Prevent alterations in hemodynamic function related to immobility (e.g., venous stasis).
5. Minimize discomfort and promote rest and relaxation.
6. Initiate patient/family health education regarding thromboembolic disease including risk factors, etiology, clinical manifestations, prescribed therapy (anticoagulants), and prophylactic measures (see Table 35–2).

### Nursing Diagnoses, Desired Patient Outcomes, and Nursing Interventions

Pertinent nursing diagnoses, desired patient outcomes, and nursing interventions are presented in the care plan for the patient with pulmonary embolism in Table 35–3.

## CASE STUDY WITH SAMPLE CARE PLAN: PATIENT WITH PULMONARY EMBOLISM*

A 62-year-old obese female was admitted to the telemetry unit for monitoring of recent onset of atrial fibrillation with a ventricular rate of 80–100/min. Patient has history of an anterior myocardial infarction 6 years prior to this admission, with mild CHF controlled by no restricted diet, digoxin, and Lasix. The patient has had dyspnea on exertion over the past 2 weeks. When she went to her doctor, the atrial fibrillation was discovered. She denied having chest pain, syncope, dizziness, palpitations, and shortness of breath at rest.

On physical examination, the nurse finds decreased peripheral pulses (+1) in both extremities; pedal pulses auscultated with Doppler. Extremities cool to touch. Patient states she has never had good circulation in her legs.

*2/3, 3:00 a.m.* Patient sat up suddenly in bed complaining of dyspnea, unable to catch her breath, and rang for the nurse. Nurse notified physician and respiratory therapist immediately. Vital signs: BP 120/80, heart rate 120 (atrial fibrillation), respiratory rate at 36 and tachypneic. ABGs on room air: alkalosis/decreased $PaCO_2$, and decreased $PaO_2$.

The patient was placed on 4 liters nasal oxygen and prepared for transfer to ICU with possible diagnosis of pulmonary embolism.

*2/3, 4:00 a.m.* Admitted to MICU, where her condition continued to deteriorate. Dyspnea persisted, with cyanosis, diaphoresis, and fatigue. The patient was intubated at that time. The patient remained alert, awake, and oriented. Chest x-ray was within normal limits; ECG showed an old anterior wall MI; there was no evidence of pulmonary hypertension (no right axis shift; no peaked P wave; and no ST segment changes).

Continuous heparin therapy was started; bedside V/Q scan was positive for pulmonary embolus. Maintenance heparin was established—PT/PTT = 19.5/52.5.

*2/5* With improvement in ABGs, the patient was weaned off the ventilator using a T-piece. Heparin therapy was continued for a period of 10 days.

*2/15* Patient was discharged home with prescriptions for digoxin, quinidine, coumadin, and ASA daily, and followup visit in 1 week.

### Initial Nursing Diagnoses

1. Impaired gas exchange, related to decreased pulmonary blood flow (ventilation/perfusion mismatching).
2. Cardiac output decreased, related to decreased PA blood flow, pulmonary hypertension, right heart failure.
3. Alteration in tissue perfusion, related to: Thromboembolic disorder, deep venous thrombosis, and pulmonary embolism.
4. Potential for physiologic injury: Bleeding, related to anticoagulation therapy.

### Additional Nursing Diagnoses

5. Alteration in comfort, related to pulmonary ischemia.
6. Anxiety (patient and family), related to ICU

*By Kathleen Daley White and Margaret Connelly

## SAMPLE CARE PLAN FOR THE PATIENT WITH PULMONARY EMBOLISM

| Nursing Diagnoses | Desired Patient Outcomes | Nursing Interventions | Rationales |
|---|---|---|---|
| ***Nursing Diagnosis #1***<br>Impaired gas exchange, related to:<br>1. Altered pulmonary blood flow.<br>2. Ventilation/perfusion mismatching.<br>3. Right-to-left shunting. | Patient will maintain optimal arterial blood gas parameters:<br>• pH 7.35–7.45.<br>• $PaO_2$ >80 mmHg.<br>• $PaCO_2$ 35–45 mmHg.<br>• $HCO_3^-$ 22–26 mEq/liter. | • Assess for signs/symptoms of hypoxia, anxiety, tachypnea, dyspnea, air hunger, tachycardia, hypertension, or hypotension. | • A classic sign of a pulmonary embolism is a subtle, mild dyspnea. In the presence of pulmonary infarction associated with an embolism, sudden and severe dyspnea may reflect an underlying total or partial obstruction of pulmonary blood flow. |
| | | • Assess level of fatigue. | • The increased work of breathing may predispose to fatigue; fatigue may result in alveolar hypoventilation with worsening hypoxemia; and it predisposes to hypercapnia. |
| | | • Monitor arterial blood gas parameters. | • A metabolic acidemia is often associated with decreased tissue perfusion; the consequent anaerobic metabolism causes a rise in serum lactate levels. Arterial blood gas parameters most closely reflect effectiveness of gas exchange and pH. |
| | | • Administer prescribed humidified oxygen therapy.<br>○ Prepare for intubation. | • Oxygenation is effective in the treatment of ventilation/perfusion mismatch.<br>○ Compromised ventilatory effort, ventilation/perfusion mismatch, and right-to-left shunting may compromise gas exchange sufficiently to require mechanical ventilation. |
| ***Nursing Diagnosis #2***<br>Cardiac output, alteration in: Decreased, related to:<br>1. Pulmonary hypertension.<br>2. Right-sided heart failure.<br>3. Decrease in left ventricular end-diastolic pressure. | Patient will maintain stable hemodynamics:<br>• Heart rate <100 beats/min.<br>• CVP 0–8 mmHg.<br>• PCWP <25 mmHg.<br>• Cardiac output 4–8 liters/min. | • Assess for signs/symptoms of right-sided heart failure: Weight gain, imbalance in intake and output; hemodynamic changes—neck vein distention, tachycardia, extra heart sounds ($S_3$ and $S_4$); edematous lower extremities. | • Pulmonary hypertension is the major hemodynamic disturbance of pulmonary embolism. Hypoxemia, acidemia, and a reduced cross-sectional area of the pulmonary capillary bed contribute to the development of pulmonary hypertension. |
| | | • Administer prescribed medication regimen to treat right heart failure:<br>○ Vasopressor therapy, cardiac glycosides, morphine, diuretics, and sedatives.<br>○ Monitor response to drug therapy. | • Therapies are directed toward decreasing myocardial oxygen consumption and demand.<br>○ Morphine increases systemic venous capacitance; the reduced venous return decreases the work of the heart. |

*(continued)*

## SAMPLE CARE PLAN FOR THE PATIENT WITH PULMONARY EMBOLISM *(Continued)*

| Nursing Diagnoses | Desired Patient Outcomes | Nursing Interventions | Rationales |
|---|---|---|---|
| ***Nursing Diagnosis #3***<br>Tissue perfusion, alteration in, related to:<br>1. Thromboembolic disorder.<br>2. Deep venous thrombosis.<br>3. Pulmonary embolism. | Patient will remain without recurrent pulmonary embolism as reflected by:<br>• Absence of pain.<br>• Stable vital signs (for patient).<br>• Stable arterial blood gases. | • Assess for signs/symptoms of venous thrombosis: Tenderness, warmth, pain, and peripheral edema of lower extremities.<br>○ Measure circumference of each extremity at designated point daily.<br>○ Assess for Homans' sign each shift. | • Predominantly, pulmonary emboli arise from deep venous thrombosis. Edema is a characteristic manifestation in the presence of disruption in venous blood flow.<br>○ A positive Homans' sign occurs when pain in the calf is experienced upon dorsiflexion of the foot. It is highly suggestive of venous thrombosis. |
| | | • Apply antiembolic hose to both lower extremities; remove for 20 min/shift.<br>• Assist patient to perform active range-of-motion exercises each shift unless otherwise contraindicated. | ○ Periodic removal allows filling of superficial capillaries.<br>• Exercise enhances "skeletal-muscular pump," which functions to prevent pooling of blood in the lower extremities (venostasis) and maintains venous return to the heart. |
| | | • Instruct patient to avoid positions that compromise blood flow in the extremities.<br>• Encourage deep breathing hourly.<br>• Caution to avoid straining, breath-holding, or other Valsalva's maneuver. | • Positions that compromise blood flow can cause circulatory stasis.<br>• Expands lungs and minimizes atelectasis.<br>• Such activities increase risk of dislodging thrombi. |
| ***Nursing Diagnosis #4***<br>Potential for physiologic injury, bleeding, related to anticoagulant therapy. | Patient will experience an absence of bleeding:<br>• Stable hematocrit/hemoglobin (for patient).<br>• Stable vital signs.<br>• Absence of petechiae, ecchymosis, hematuria, occult blood in stools, or bleeding at invasive sites. | • Assess closely for signs/symptoms of bleeding. | • Anticoagulant therapy is major treatment in patients with deep venous thrombosis. Major adverse effect of heparin is the risk of bleeding. |
| | | • Teach patient to examine self for signs of bleeding: Petechiae, easy bruising, changes in color of urine or stools. | • An aware patient may afford early recognition of subtle bleeding. |
| | | • Obtain daily serum coagulation parameters (prothrombin and partial thromboplastin times); monitor closely for desired range. | • Usual PT/PTT is maintained $1\frac{1}{2}$–2 times the control. |
| | | • Monitor all invasive sites every shift.<br>• Limit puncture sites and blood drawing to only when necessary.<br>○ Use only small gauge needles when drawing blood.<br>• Teach patient to use an electric razor and to avoid vigorous toothbrushing. | • Puncture sites and invasive lines will not be able to clot as quickly during anticoagulant therapy. Large hematomas may occur without appropriate application of pressure postinjection and at puncture sites. It may be necessary to apply direct pressure to these sites for as long as 10 min, followed by application of pressure dressing. |
| | | • Maintain access to protamine sulfate for patients receiving heparin therapy. | • Protamine sulfate is the antidote for heparin and should be readily available for administration if necessary. |

## TABLE 35–3. CARE PLAN FOR THE PATIENT WITH PULMONARY EMBOLISM

| Nursing Diagnoses | Desired Patient Outcomes | Nursing Interventions | Rationales |
|---|---|---|---|
| ***Nursing Diagnosis #1***<br>Anxiety, related to:<br>1. Sudden, acute respiratory insufficiency with disruption of lifestyle.<br>2. Pain; hemoptysis.<br>3. Knowledge deficit regarding illness and its prognosis.<br>4. Intensive care setting. | Patient will:<br>1. Verbalize feeling less anxious.<br>2. Demonstrate a relaxed demeanor.<br>3. Perform relaxation techniques with assistance.<br>4. Verbalize familiarity with ICU routines and protocols. | • Assess for signs/symptoms of anxiety: Restlessness, agitation, diaphoresis; tachypnea, sighing; tachycardia, palpitations; anorexia, nausea, diarrhea; presence of anxiety-related behaviors: nailbiting, insomnia, finger tapping; uncooperative or noncompliant behaviors; verbalization of fears and concerns. | • Thorough assessment assists in discerning underlying cause of anxiety and provides a basis for intervention.<br>*Examples:* (1) Relief of pain with medication often alleviates its anxiety-related symptomatology. (2) Coping with the fear of dying with a listening ear and caring attitude may assist in reducing the patient's anxiety. |
| | | • Examine the circumstances underlying the anxiety. | • Removal of precipitating factors may reduce anxiety. |
| | | ◦ Manipulate ICU environment to provide calm, restful periods. | ◦ Reduction in stimuli is essential to assist patient/family to relax and avoid useless dissipation of compromised energy stores. |
| | | • Assess patient/family coping behaviors and their effectiveness in dealing with current stressors.<br>◦ Provide positive reinforcement when desired response is achieved. | ◦ Positive feedback nurtures self-confidence. |
| | | • Initiate interventions to reduce anxiety:<br>◦ Relieve pain or other discomfort.<br>– Medication for pain.<br>– Comfort measures: Turning, positioning, mouth care, skin care, and so forth. | ◦ Pain precipitates and/or aggravates anxiety. |
| | | ◦ Monitor effectiveness of ventilatory support and oxygen therapy if these therapies are indicated.<br>– Serial arterial blood gas values. | ◦ Inadequate gas exchange, hypoxemia, and/or hypercapnia precipitate symptomatology that contributes to the patient's "sense of doom." |
| | | ◦ Listen attentively, encourage verbalization, provide a caring touch. | ◦ These nursing activities reassure the patient that he/she is not alone. |
| | | ◦ Let patient know it's okay to feel anxious or to experience fear of dying.<br>◦ Remain with patient during periods of acute stress. | ◦ Reassurance helps patient focus on his/her feelings, work them through, and, eventually, accept them. |
| | | ◦ Assess readiness to learn and implement the following when appropriate: | ◦ Readiness to learn facilitates meaningful learning and a sense of accomplishment. |
| | | ◦ Orient to environment, ICU equipment, routines, and staff.<br>– Explain all procedures and activities involving the patient. | ◦ Knowing what to expect helps to reduce anxiety. |
| | | ◦ Involve in decision-making regarding care when possible and appropriate. | ◦ Helps patient maintain some degree of control over his/her body and health care. |

*(continued)*

**TABLE 35–3. CARE PLAN FOR THE PATIENT WITH PULMONARY EMBOLISM *(Continued)***

| Nursing Diagnoses | Desired Patient Outcomes | Nursing Interventions | Rationales |
|---|---|---|---|
| ***Nursing Diagnosis #1 (cont.)*** | | ○ Help in establishing short-term goals that can be attained.<br>○ Instruct in relaxation techniques. | ○ Builds and reinforces self-confidence.<br>○ Energy-release techniques allow an outlet for pent-up feelings; enable the patient to have some control over anxiety. |
| ***Nursing Diagnosis #2***<br>Gas exchange, impaired, related to:<br>1. Right-to-left shunting.<br>2. Ventilation/perfusion mismatch.<br>***Nursing Diagnosis #3***<br>Breathing pattern, ineffective, related to tachypnea, dyspnea. | For specific patient outcomes related to these Nursing Diagnoses, see Table 34–3. | For specific nursing interventions and their rationales, see Table 34–3.<br>For details related to the nursing care of the mechanically ventilated patient, see Table 32–7 and Table 32–9. | |
| ***Nursing Diagnosis #4***<br>Cardiac output, alteration in: decreased, related to:<br>1. Pulmonary arterial hypertension.<br>2. Right-sided congestive heart failure (cor pulmonale).<br>3. Decrease in left ventricular end-diastolic pressure (LVEDP).<br>4. Systemic arterial hypotension/hypovolemic shock. | Patient will:<br>1. Maintain stable hemodynamics:<br>• Heart rate <100 beats/min.<br>• CVP 0–8 mmHg.<br>• Pulmonary artery pressure <25 mmHg.<br>• PCWP 8–12 mmHg.<br>• Cardiac output ~5 liters/min.<br>• Systemic arterial blood pressure within 10 mmHg of baseline. | • Assess for signs/symptoms of right-sided congestive heart failure:<br>○ Weight gain; fluid intake/output.<br>○ Hemodynamic changes:<br>– Tachycardia (>100 beats/min).<br>– Jugular neck vein distention.<br>– Peripheral (dependent) edema.<br>– CVP >8–12 mmHg.<br>– Extra heart sounds; $S_3$, $S_4$; systolic murmur.<br>– Fatigue; mottled appearance of skin, cool to touch; cyanosis of nailbeds.<br>○ Breath sounds may be clear and without adventitious sounds; or breath sounds may be diminished with localized rales (crackles) or wheezing. A pleural friction rub may be detected. Breathing pattern may reflect tachypnea, dyspnea.<br>○ Hepatic involvement:<br>– Hepatomegaly, positive hepatojugular reflex; abdominal distention; ascites. | • The major hemodynamic disturbance associated with pulmonary embolism is *pulmonary arterial hypertension* (>25–30 mmHg), which may predispose to right ventricular failure.<br>○ Hypoxemia, acidemia, and a reduced cross-sectional area of the pulmonary vascular bed all contribute to the development of pulmonary hypertension.<br>○ Right ventricular failure causes alterations in systemic hemodynamics; left ventricular failure alters pulmonary hemodynamics. Commonly, failure in one ventricle causes failure of the other.<br>○ A massive pulmonary embolism with acute cor pulmonale may be characterized by dyspnea, cyanosis, and hypovolemic shock. |

| | |
|---|---|
| ◦ Gastrointestinal: Anorexia, nausea/vomiting; abdominal distention.<br>◦ Oliguria.<br>◦ Mental status changes. | |
| • Monitor diagnostic tests/studies:<br>◦ Laboratory studies: BUN, creatinine, hematocrit, serum albumin; electrolytes; arterial blood gases.<br>◦ ECG may reflect signs of ischemia; dysrhythmias (atrial).<br>◦ Chest x-rays frequently reflect cardiomegaly, pleural effusion, and possibly, pulmonary edema (left-sided heart failure). | • Serum sodium values reflect hydration status.<br>◦ Serum potassium needs to be carefully monitored especially during diuretic therapy. |
| • Administer prescribed medication regimen to treat cor pulmonale, a consequence of pulmonary hypertension. | • Therapies are directed toward decreasing myocardial oxygen consumption and demand. |
| ◦ Vasopressor therapy (e.g., dopamine in the presence of heart failure and hypovolemic shock). | ◦ A pulmonary embolic episode may reflexly trigger systemic peripheral arteriolar vasodilation with a consequent "relative" volume depletion, which, if severe, can cause hypotension or hypovolemic shock. |
| ◦ Cardiac glycosides (digoxin).<br>– Positive inotropic agent = improved contractility.<br>– Negative chronotropic agent = reduced heart rate.<br>– End result = improved cardiac output. | |
| ◦ Morphine.<br>◦ Induces systemic venous vasodilation.<br>– Reduces chest pain frequently associated with pulmonary embolism.<br>– Decreases anxiety and helps to reduce the work of breathing.<br>– Exerts a sedative effect, which assists in relaxing the patient. | ◦ Increased pooling of blood in the periphery reduces venous return to the right heart, which helps to decrease the work of the right ventricle. |
| ◦ Diuretics (e.g., furosemide). | ◦ A reduction in total blood volume reduces venous return (preload) while also reducing systemic arterial blood pressure (afterload). The end result is a decrease in myocardial work.<br>◦ Use of diuretics requires the maintenance of fluid volume. |
| ◦ Vasodilator therapy may be initiated especially in the setting of left ventricular compromise. | ◦ Vasodilators function to decrease preload and afterload and, thus, decrease the work of the heart. |
| ◦ Anticoagulant therapy.<br>– Heparin, coumadin derivatives.<br>– Aspirin (antiplatelet agent). | ◦ Major focus of therapy in the patient experiencing a pulmonary embolic episode is to *prevent* recurrent embolization; anticoagulants function effectively in this capacity. |

*(continued)*

### TABLE 35-3. CARE PLAN FOR THE PATIENT WITH PULMONARY EMBOLISM *(Continued)*

| Nursing Diagnoses | Desired Patient Outcomes | Nursing Interventions | Rationales |
|---|---|---|---|
| ***Nursing Diagnosis #5***<br>Fluid volume, alteration | Patient will:<br>1. Maintain body weight within 5% of baseline.<br>2. Balance fluid intake with output.<br>3. Have:<br>• Good skin turgor.<br>• Absence of peripheral edema.<br>• Absence of jugular vein distention.<br>• Absence of rales (crackles) on auscultation.<br>Serum electrolytes, BUN, creatinine, total protein, will stabilize within acceptable physiologic range. | • Maintain fluid and electrolyte balance.<br>◦ Administer prescribed fluid volume.<br>◦ Document intake and output, urine specific gravity.<br>◦ Record daily weight.<br>◦ Monitor electrolytes. | • Fluid therapy is directed toward reducing the work of the heart while still maintaining adequate tissue perfusion.<br>◦ Close monitoring of urine output helps to evaluate renal perfusion/function; a reduction in cardiac output may reduce renal perfusion, which is manifested clinically by a decrease in hourly urine output. |
| | | • Monitor hemodynamic parameters.<br>◦ Systemic arterial blood pressure, CVP, pulmonary artery pressure, PCWP, cardiac output. | • These measures best reflect the patient's response to therapy, and insertion of a pulmonary artery flotation catheter is commonly indicated in the setting of massive pulmonary embolism. |
| | | • Administer oxygen therapy as prescribed and monitor arterial blood gases to evaluate patient's response to therapy. | • Hypoxemia in pulmonary embolism is a consequence of ventilation/perfusion mismatching and right-to-left shunting. |
| | | • Implement nursing measures to improve and/or maintain cardiac output.<br>◦ Manipulate environment to reduce stressors and promote rest and relaxation.<br>◦ Plan frequent rest periods. | • A quiet, calm environment decreases anxiety, and reduces sympathetic nervous system stimulation. The overall net effect is to reduce the work of the heart.<br>◦ A reduction in cardiac workload reduces myocardial oxygen consumption and demand. |
| | | ◦ Maximize patient activities in accordance with the acuity of the illness. | ◦ Nursing interventions are implemented to maximize circulation, prevent pooling or stasis of blood, maintain venous return, and promote comfort. |
| | | ◦ Place in high Fowler's position.<br>◦ Assist with frequent position changes. | ◦ Facilitates ease of breathing as abdominal pressure on the diaphragm is reduced; less effort exerted = decrease in oxygen demand. |
| | | ◦ Provide special care to back and to skin over joints and pressure points.<br>◦ Assist with passive range-of-motion exercises. | ◦ Compromised circulation predisposes to tissue ischemia; stasis or pooling of blood predisposes to venous thrombosis; reduces venous return, which decreases cardiac output. |

| | | | |
|---|---|---|---|
| ***Nursing Diagnosis #6***<br>Tissue perfusion, alteration in, related to:<br>1. Thromboembolic disorder.<br>2. Deep venous thrombosis.<br>3. Pulmonary embolism. | Patient will:<br>1. Remain without recurrent pulmonary embolism as reflected by:<br>• Absence of pain.<br>• Stable vital signs (see Nursing Diagnosis #4 above).<br>• Stable arterial blood gases (within acceptable physiologic range)<br>pH 7.35–7.45.<br>$PaCO_2$ 35–45 mmHg.<br>$PaO_2$ >60 mmHg. | • Assess for signs/symptoms of venous thrombosis:<br>◦ Tenderness, warmth, pain, and peripheral (pitting) edema of lower extremities.<br>– Evidence of edema is best assessed and monitored by determining the circumference of the limb at a designated point using a tape measure. | • 95% of all pulmonary emboli arise in the deep veins of the lower extremities.<br>◦ Edema is a characteristic manifestation when alteration in tissue perfusion is due to venous interference. |
| | | ◦ Skin color and temperature.<br>– Observe extremities in both dependent and elevated positions. | ◦ In the presence of altered tissue perfusion or venous obstruction a bluish-red color of the skin may be observed.<br>◦ Temperature of skin is assessed by use of touch; usually warm temperatures in the lower extremities are commonly associated with venous thrombosis. |
| | | ◦ Bleeding/bruising tendency, petechiae, ecchymosis, hematuria, occult blood in stool. | ◦ Hypercoagulable state is often reflected by bleeding tendency. |
| | | ◦ Complaints of pain:<br>– Pain associated with deep venous thrombosis may be described as heavy, aching, or cramping.<br>– Pain associated with arterial insufficiency is characteristically sudden and sharp; the presence of cool skin temperatures suggests decreased arterial blood flow. | ◦ Pain occurs when there is an alteration in tissue perfusion. |
| | | • Monitor for signs/symptoms indicative of extended or recurrent pulmonary embolism.<br>◦ Sudden occurrence of persistent or exacerbated chest and/or shoulder pain.<br>◦ Onset of respiratory difficulties: Tachypnea, dyspnea, cough with hemoptysis.<br>◦ Alterations in cardiopulmonary function: Tachycardia, hypotension, cyanosis.<br>◦ Neurologic findings: Restlessness, lethargy, confusion. | • The presence of deep venous thrombosis places the patient at increased risk of pulmonary embolism. |
| | | • Monitor laboratory data:<br>◦ Arterial blood gas values.<br>◦ Hematologic studies: Complete blood count, hematocrit, hemoglobin.<br>◦ Coagulation studies: aPTT; prothrombin time; clotting time.<br>◦ Platelet count. | |
| | | • Implement prescribed anticoagulant therapy. | • See Table 35–2. |

*(continued)*

## TABLE 35–3. CARE PLAN FOR THE PATIENT WITH PULMONARY EMBOLISM (*Continued*)

| Nursing Diagnoses | Desired Patient Outcomes | Nursing Interventions | Rationales |
|---|---|---|---|
| ***Nursing Diagnosis #6*** | | • Implement measures to reduce the risk of recurrent pulmonary embolism.<br>○ Maintain hydrated state as prescribed. | ○ Dehydration increases blood viscosity. The consequent disturbed blood flow may predispose to endothelial injury within blood vessels, and/or a hypercoagulable state. |
| | | ○ Apply antiembolic hose to both lower extremities; remove hose once per shift.<br>○ Assist patient to perform active range-of-motion exercises; active/passive foot and leg exercises should be performed hourly unless otherwise contraindicated. | ○ Exercise enhances "skeletal-muscular pump," which functions to prevent pooling of blood in the lower extremities (venous stasis) and maintains venous return to the heart.<br>○ If a thrombosis is suspected, the involved extremity should *not* be massaged or exercised to prevent possible dislodgement of thrombi with consequent pulmonary embolism. |
| | | ○ Instruct patient to avoid positions that compromise blood flow in the extremities (e.g., gatch knees, pillow under knees, crossing of legs, prolonged sitting in one position). | ○ Positions that compromise blood flow can cause circulatory stasis. |
| | | ○ Encourage deep breathing hourly. | ○ Expands lungs and minimizes areas of atelectasis. |
| | | ○ Caution patient to avoid activities that involve a Valsalva's maneuver (e.g., straining to defecate, breath holding). | ○ Such activities increase risk of dislodging thrombi. |
| ***Nursing Diagnosis #7***<br>Comfort, alteration in: Pain associated with compromised pulmonary perfusion. (See Nursing Diagnosis #1 above.) | Patient will:<br>1. Verbalize pain relief.<br>2. Exhibit relaxed demeanor:<br>• Relaxed facial expression and body posturing.<br>• Ease of breathing. | • Determine how patient usually copes with pain.<br>○ Pain tolerance.<br>○ Willingness to discuss pain; or stoically "keeping it within" himself or herself.<br>○ Willingness to use medication for pain.<br>• Assess for nonverbal clues as to the presence of pain (e.g., restlessness, or reluctance to move; tense facial features; clenched fists; diaphoresis; rapid, shallow breathing). | |

| | | | |
|---|---|---|---|
| | | • Assess complaints of pain including severity, location/radiation; influencing factors (e.g., what precipitates, aggravates, or ameliorates the pain; and associated signs and symptoms such as diaphoresis), pain duration and the quality of pain (e.g., sharp, dull, "knifelike"). | • To assist in comprehensive assessment, see SLIDT Tool in Table 7–1. |
| | | • Implement measures to alleviate pain: | |
| | | ◦ Assist patient into comfortable position (e.g., high Fowler's). | ◦ Upright position favors better lung expansion; improves alveolar ventilation. |
| | | ◦ Encourage deep breathing hourly. | ◦ Minimizes atelectasis and improves distribution of ventilation. |
| | | ◦ Teach/assist patient to splint chest with hands or pillow when coughing, deep breathing, or repositioning. | ◦ Splinting may help to reduce discomfort. |
| | | ◦ Stay with patient until pain is relieved. | ◦ Providing support can reduce anxiety and help the patient relax. |
| | | ◦ Provide a listening ear and caring touch; encourage verbalization; explain procedures, routines, tests, and so forth. | ◦ Keeping the patient informed may help to alleviate anxieties, which may potentiate pain. |
| | | ◦ Refrain from nonessential activities. | ◦ Reducing patient's activities decreases oxygen consumption and demand. |
| | | ◦ Provide comfort measures (e.g., position change, back care, reducing environmental stimuli). | ◦ Comfort measures and touch therapy are often sufficient to alleviate pain. |
| | | • Administer analgesic medication therapy as prescribed. | |
| | | ◦ Encourage to request medication when pain is first realized rather than waiting until it gets unbearable. | ◦ Pain medication administered early on may be more effective. |
| | | ◦ Evaluate effectiveness of pain medication in relieving the patient's pain. | |
| ***Nursing Diagnosis #8***<br>Knowledge deficit, related to:<br>1. Thromboembolic disease.<br>2. Followup care.<br>3. Prevention. | Patient/family will:<br>1. Identify risk factors of significance in thromboembolic disease.<br>2. Identify activities that promote venous blood flow and reduce risks of venous thrombosis.<br>• Importance of individualized exercise program. | See Table 35–2, section on patient/family education, for information essential to the patient/family's understanding of, and compliance with, the prescribed therapeutic regimen.<br>See also Nursing Diagnoses #1 and #6 above. | |

(*continued*)

### TABLE 35–3. CARE PLAN FOR THE PATIENT WITH PULMONARY EMBOLISM *(Continued)*

| Nursing Diagnoses | Desired Patient Outcomes | Nursing Interventions | Rationales |
|---|---|---|---|
| ***Nursing Diagnosis #8 (cont.)*** | | | |
| | 3. Explain the prescribed treatment regimen and the importance of complying with it:<br>• Rationale for anticoagulant therapy.<br>• Medication routine, dosage, and side effects.<br>• Signs/symptoms to report to health-care provider.<br>• Measures to minimize risks of bleeding during anticoagulant therapy.<br>• Importance of followup care. | | |

environment, acute onset of life-threatening event.
7. Knowledge deficit, related to anticoagulation therapy.
8. Potential for drug interaction, related to anticoagulation therapy.
9. Altered home health management, related to deep venous thrombosis, anticoagulation therapy, and high-risk patient.

## REFERENCES

1. Weinberger, S: Principles of Pulmonary Medicine. WB Saunders, Philadelphia, 1986, p 163.
2. Driedger, AA and Sibbald, WJ: Acute pulmonary embolism. In Sibbald, WJ (ed): Synopsis of Critical Care, ed 3. Williams & Wilkins, Baltimore, 1988, p 107.
3. Mathewson, M: Pharmacotherapeutics, A Nursing Process Approach. FA Davis, Philadelphia, 1986, p 584.
4. Mathewson, M: Pharmacotherapeutics, A Nursing Process Approach. FA Davis, Philadelphia, 1986, p 586.

CHAPTER 36

# Nursing Management of the Patient with Respiratory Dysfunction: Asthma, Pleural Effusion, Pneumothorax, and Pneumonia

## CHAPTER OUTLINE



## LEARNING OBJECTIVES

**At the end of this chapter, you should be able to:**

1. Differentiate asthma from other forms of obstructive pulmonary disease (chronic bronchitis and emphysema) in terms of:
   a. Etiology and pathogenesis.
   b. Pathology and pathophysiology.
   c. Clinical presentation.
2. Describe the significance of the "crossover phase" in acute asthma including underlying pathophysiology and emergent therapy.
3. Identify essential factors to be considered in the diagnosis of asthma.
4. Examine therapeutic modalities in the treatment of asthma including:
   a. Supplemental oxygen therapy.
   b. Drug therapy.

## LEARNING OBJECTIVES—*CONTINUED*

c. Chest physiotherapy-bronchial hygiene.
d. Mechanical ventilation.
5. Identify pertinent nursing diagnoses, desired patient outcomes, and nursing interventions in the care of the patient with chronic obstructive pulmonary disease (Table 33-2).
6. Differentiate exudative from transudative pleural effusion.
7. List common etiologies associated with pneumothorax.
8. Describe pathophysiology of pneumothorax including its impact on intrapleural pressures, respiratory mechanics, and cardiopulmonary dynamics.
9. Outline clinical presentations of spontaneous and tension pneumothoraces.
10. List tentative nursing diagnoses related to the care of the patient with pneumothorax/pleural effusion.
11. Describe the etiology and pathogenesis of pneumonia.
12. Differentiate clinical presentation and treatment of bacterial, viral, and mycoplasmal pneumonias.
13. Define tentative nursing diagnoses related to the care of the patient with pneumonia.

## ASTHMA

Asthma is a reversible obstructive airway disorder characterized by a hyperreactivity of the airways. It affects all age groups but particularly children and young adults. Hyperreactivity of the airways (i.e., an exaggerated or increased responsiveness of the airways to a wide variety of stimuli) is the single feature that patients with asthma seem to have in common. While the stimuli triggering the event may vary from one patient to the next, the end result is usually reversible episodes of bronchoconstriction. Asthma differs from chronic obstructive pulmonary disease (COPD) in terms of its reversibility (i.e., between periods of exacerbation or asthmatic "attacks," these patients may remain relatively symptom-free); chronic, longstanding asthma, however, may cause severe debilitation from compromised respiratory function.

### Etiology and Pathogenesis

#### *Relationship to Allergy and Genetic Predisposition*

It has long been accepted that there is at least some association between asthma and allergy, but this relationship remains undefined. While a large number of asthmatics do have a history of allergies, many do not. Those included in the latter group are sometimes classified as "idiosyncratic," and their asthma is often exacerbated by upper respiratory infections. For asthmatics with a known history of allergies whose asthma is often exacerbated by exposure to substances to which they have been previously sensitized, a strong family history of asthma exists suggesting that genetic factors may play a role in its development. The specific inheritable trait is a tendency to form IgE antibodies, a trait not uncommon in other forms of allergy (e.g., eczema, allergic rhinitis).

#### *Alterations in Autonomic Nervous System Function*

Abnormalities of the autonomic nervous system may contribute to the pathogenesis of asthma by modifying the tone of airway smooth muscle. Present within the airways are adrenergic receptors, which respond largely to catecholamines (epinephrine and norepinephrine) secreted by the adrenal medulla, and, to a lesser extent, to sympathetic innervation. Cholinergic receptors are also present on airways and respond to parasympathetic innervation by the vagus nerve. Stimulation of $beta_2$-adrenergic receptors produces bronchodilation; stimulation of alpha-adrenergic and cholinergic receptors results in bronchoconstriction.

Often associated with allergic asthmatics is a decreased responsiveness or blockade of $beta_2$-receptor activity, coupled with a heightened alpha-receptor and cholinergic-receptor responsiveness. In particular, hyperresponsiveness of alpha-receptors may be a fundamental causal defect in asthma.[1]

#### *Bronchoconstriction—Common Causative Factors*

In addition to genetic factors and alterations in autonomic nervous system function, stimuli that commonly cause bronchoconstriction in the asthmatic patient include: (1) allergen(s) to which the patient is sensitized; (2) inhaled irritants (e.g., cigarette smoke); (3) emotional factors; (4) exercise; and (5) respiratory infection.

Common allergens (antigens) include dust, molds, and animal dander. As a result of prior exposure to such antigens, the patient has preformed IgE antibodies, which are bound to mast cells in the airway wall. Subsequent exposure of specific IgE-containing mast cells sensitized to the appropriate antigen initiates a series of intracellular events facilitated by the presence of calcium, which culminate with the release of chemical mediators from the mast cells. Included among these chemical mediators in asthma are: histamine, SRS-A (leukotrienes), eosinophil and neutrophil chemotactic factors of anaphylaxis, prostaglandins, bradykinin, and serotonin (see Chaps. 54 and 67).

**Chemical Mediators in Asthma.** The chemical mediators released from mast cells react in a variety of ways to exacerbate the asthma (see Fig. 54–11). Stimulation of bronchial smooth muscle causes airway constriction; alteration in vascular permeability predisposes to airway edema; and stimulation of mucosal glands and goblet cells causes airways to be filled with a characteristically thick, tenacious mucous secretion and mucous plugs. Chemotactic factors may be important in attracting inflammatory cells (polymorphonuclear neutrophils and eosinophils) into the airway wall (see Table 61–3).

Inhaled irritants (cigarette smoke, environmental dust) precipitate bronchoconstriction by reflex activity. Stimulation of irritant receptors in the large airways triggers a reflex arc with impulses traveling to the central nervous system and back to the bronchi. Efferent vagal innervation of bronchial smooth muscle completes the reflex arc, causing bronchoconstriction.

Bronchospasm has been associated with emotional upsets, which frequently involve hyperventilation with a consequent hypocapnia. Airway cooling appears to be a crucial factor in exercise-induced bronchoconstriction in the patient with asthma. At high minute ventilation, the warming and humidifying of large volumes of gas cause water to evaporate from the epithelial surface, resulting in a cooling of the respiratory epithelium. Respiratory infection (commonly viral in origin) is frequently implicated as a causative factor in asthma.

## Pathology/Pathophysiology

See the section entitled "Atopy Type I" in Chapter 54.

### *Mechanisms Underlying Increased Airway Resistance*

Pathologic changes associated with asthma include hypertrophy of the smooth muscle layer, thickening of the respiratory epithelium basement membrane, hypertrophy and hyperplasia of mucous glands, an increase in the number of goblet cells, and the presence of eosinophilic infiltrates within the bronchial wall (see Figs. 28–2 and 28–4). Consistent with these changes, the major pathophysiologic mechanisms responsible for the increased airway resistance characteristic of asthma include bronchial smooth muscle contraction (bronchospasm), mucosal edema, and accumulation of secretions.

Clinically, the effects of increased airway resistance in the asthmatic patient can be demonstrated by measuring pulmonary function. Such studies, performed during an asthmatic attack, indicate a reduction in forced expiratory flow rates as well as evidence of air trapping (see Fig. 28–9). Measurement of lung volumes in these patients confirms air trapping as reflected by the increases in functional residual capacity (FRC) and, in particular, the residual volume (RV). Such findings are consistent with those of other obstructive airway diseases, specifically, chronic bronchitis and emphysema (see Chap. 33).

### *Characteristic Pattern of Arterial Blood Gas Values in Acute Asthmatic Attack*

During an acute asthmatic attack, the disruption in airflow also disturbs gas exchange. The characteristic pattern of arterial blood gases early in the attack (hyperventilatory phase) reflects a mild to severe hypoxemia ($PaO_2$ <60 mmHg) due largely to ventilation/perfusion mismatching; hypocapnia ($PaCO_2$ <30 mmHg) caused by hyperventilation and an increased respiratory effort; and a consequent respiratory alkalemia (pH >7.50) (see Fig. 32–4). An increase in the $PaCO_2$ to normal or above, a decrease in pH, and a persistent hypoxemia often reflect a deterioration in the patient's condition, whether due to a worsening airflow obstruction or extreme fatigue, or both. The patient may be unable to maintain the hyperventilatory effort in the face of significant airflow obstruction ("crossover phase"). Without timely and aggressive therapy at this stage, the patient may eventuate into the phase of full-blown, acute respiratory failure.

## Clinical Presentation

Clinically, symptoms of asthma may range from mild complaints of unexplained cough or breathlessness on exertion, to a full-blown status asthmaticus. The term status asthmaticus is applied to asthmatic episodes that are refractory to hydration and bronchodilator therapy and may become life-threatening in severity. An asthmatic attack is characterized by restlessness, anxiety, altered mental status, dyspnea with use of accessory muscles of respiration (the patient may be too short of breath to talk or eat), a prolonged expiratory phase, wheezing on auscultation, cough productive of characteristic thick, sticky sputum with mucous plugs, chest tightness, and abnormal blood gases.

## Diagnosis

The diagnosis of asthma should include a comprehensive clinical history of any prior episodes of cough, dyspnea, and wheezing. While wheezing is often a prominent symptom in asthma, the presence of wheezing does not always indicate a diagnosis of asthma. Nor do all asthmatics wheeze. In very severe asthma, no wheeze may occur if airflow is too impaired to generate an audible wheeze or any breath sounds. When eliciting the patient's history, it is important to exclude other etiologies of wheezing (e.g., aspiration of foreign object or food).

The past medical history should be elicited to determine evidence of hay fever, allergic rhinitis, eczema, or other *atopy* (i.e., conditions characterized by a predisposition for hyperproduction of IgE antibodies). A family history of such disorders should be established.

It is essential to obtain the patient's medication history, including use of specific drugs (e.g., bronchodilators, nonsteroidal anti-inflammatory drugs, antihistamines, prescribed or over-the-counter), reasons for taking the drugs, dosages, effectiveness in relieving the symptoms, and any untoward effects.

Drug allergies must be noted, including the drug(s) involved and a description of the "allergic" response. Some asthmatics, for example, are particularly sensitive to ingestion of aspirin and may experience an exacerbation of the asthma after taking aspirin or other nonsteroidal anti-inflammatory drug. It is now known that these drugs increase production of leukotrienes, which are extraordinarily potent bronchoconstrictors.[2]

Other data of importance to the diagnosis of asthma include the clinical presentation (as discussed above) and the presence of many eosinophils on sputum smear, and an increased number in the blood. While eosinophils are usually associated with allergies, their increased presence may be demonstrated even when asthma has no clear relationship to allergies. In this instance, the underlying factor may be a genetic deficiency of the group of T cells that regulate IgE production (see section entitled "Atopy-Type I" in Chap. 54).

Demonstration of reversible airflow obstruction by pulmonary function tests (e.g., RV, FRC, TLC, $FEV_1/FVC$) is helpful in diagnosis. Commonly, the diagnosis of asthma is made based on the clinical history, findings of expiratory wheezes or rhonchi, and intercostal retractions, as well as pulmonary function studies.

## Treatment

### Goals of Treatment

The treatment of asthma is focused on correcting the abnormal gas exchange, relieving bronchospasm, and clearing airway secretions. Supplemental oxygen therapy ($FIO_2$ of 24%, 28%, or 35%) by Venturi mask or nasal cannula is usually effective in raising the $PaO_2 > 60$ mmHg. The mechanisms underlying the hypoxemia during an acute asthmatic attack include, predominantly, ventilation/perfusion mismatching and alveolar hypoventilation, both of which usually respond favorably to oxygen therapy.

If, however, there is a rise in the $PaCO_2$ with mental status changes, the patient may have reached the "crossover phase" (mentioned above), and institution of assisted ventilatory support may be indicated. Mechanical ventilation therapy is itself associated with significant complications (see Table 32–8). Therefore, such therapy should only be considered if all other measures have failed.

### Therapeutic Modalities

**Drug Therapy.** Drug therapy is a major therapeutic modality in the treatment of asthma, and consists of several categories of drugs including bronchodilators, anti-cholinergic drugs, anti-inflammatory agents, antibiotics, and drugs that inhibit the release of chemical mediators from the mast cells (Table 36–1).

The most commonly used agents are those that increase intracellular cAMP (cyclic adenosine monophosphate) levels in both bronchial smooth muscle cells and mast cells. Increased levels of cAMP in bronchial smooth muscle result in bronchodilation, while in mast cells cAMP inhibits release of chemical mediators that secondarily cause bronchoconstriction (bronchospasm). Among these mediators are histamine, leukotrienes, serotonin, bradykinin, and prostaglandins. Agents that increase intracellular levels of cAMP include the methylxanthines (theophylline and aminophylline)

TABLE 36–1
**Drug Therapy in the Treatment of Asthma***

| |
|---|
| Bronchodilators |
| Sympathomimetics |
| Epinephrine |
| Isoproterenol |
| Isoetharine |
| Metaproterenol |
| Terbutaline |
| Albuterol |
| Xanthines |
| Theophylline |
| Aminophylline |
| Anticholinergics |
| Atropine |
| Corticosteroids |
| Dexamethasone |
| Methylprednisolone |
| Antibiotics |
| Cephalosporins |
| Penicillins |
| Aminoglycosides |
| Miscellaneous antimicrobials |
| Cromolyn (disodium cromoglycate) |

*See Appendix A for information related to dosage, administration, adverse reactions, and nursing implications for specific drugs.

and sympathomimetic agents (epinephrine, isoetharine, metaproterenol, terbutaline, and albuterol).

Anticholinergic agents (e.g., atropine) also cause bronchodilation by blocking parasympathetic innervation at the cholinergic receptors on the larger airways. When used in the treatment of asthma, atropine is usually given by aerosol treatment. Newer anticholinergic drugs are currently under investigation and should be available within the next 1–2 years.

Another pharmacotherapeutic agent used in the treatment of asthma is cromolyn sodium. It stabilizes the membrane of mast cells and prevents release of chemical mediators, which cause bronchoconstriction. The drug is inhaled as a powder and, therefore, can be irritating to the airway mucosa. Consequently, it is not used to treat acute asthmatic attacks, but is generally given during periods of remission to prevent subsequent exacerbations.

Corticosteroids are also used to treat asthma. Although these agents are widely used, their mechanism of action remains undefined. During an asthmatic attack, these drugs may be started at high doses and tapered relatively quickly. Agents frequently used include dexamethasone and methylprednisolone. (For information on dosage, administration, adverse reactions, and implications for nursing care, see Appendix A.)

In the presence of infection (upper respiratory infection), antibiotic therapy is initiated. Commonly such drug therapy is initiated after specimens of sputum, blood, and urine are obtained for culture and sensitivity studies. Appropriate revisions are made based on the outcome of such studies. It is important to emphasize that antibiotic therapy is given only when the presence of infection is established.

**Chest Physiotherapy–Bronchial Hygiene.** Bronchial secretions in asthma are characteristically thick, sticky, and tenacious, with numerous mucous plugs, which may completely obstruct some of the airways. Initial therapy is focused on *hydrating* the patient by the intravenous administration of fluids, thinning secretions so that they may be more easily mobilized, and improving the effectiveness of the cough reflex in raising secretions. Body fluid balance needs to be carefully monitored to prevent overhydration, especially in elderly patients or those with compromised cardiac function.

The techniques of chest physiotherapy, including postural drainage with percussion and vibration, deep breathing and coughing, facilitate removal of tracheobronchial secretions. These activities should be performed in conjunction with bronchodilator (aerosol) therapy. The frequency and duration of these treatments should be gauged according to the patient's responses and tolerance. Diligent, effective chest physiotherapy and bronchial hygiene may preclude the need for assisted ventilatory therapy.

### Nursing Care of the Patient with Acute Asthma

As an obstructive airway illness, an acute exacerbation of asthma presents with clinical findings similar to those in chronic bronchitis and emphysema (see Chap. 33). As with these disorders, acute asthma has a prolonged expiratory phase (≥3–4 seconds), a productive cough caused by hypersecretions of mucus and usually accompanied by wheezing, and a distinct increase in pulmonary volumes. Overinflation is caused by premature airway closure on expiration and the increased resistance to airflow associated with increased secretions, mucous plugging, and mucosal edema. As is true with the other obstructive airway diseases, the FRC and RV are also increased during an acute asthmatic episode.

Because of these many similarities, therapeutic modalities used in the treatment and management of chronic bronchitis and emphysema can be applied to the care and treatment of patients with acute asthma (see Table 33–2). (For a discussion of the specific modalities used in the care of the patient with respiratory problems, including oxygen therapy, chest physiotherapy–bronchial hygiene, airway management, and mechanical ventilation, see Chap. 32.)

## PLEURA

### Anatomy and Physiology of the Pleura

The pleura is the serous membrane enveloping the lungs and lining the walls of the pleural cavity. It consists of a double layer: the visceral pleura overlies the outer surface of the lungs; the parietal pleura lines the inner surface of the chest wall and reflects over the diaphragmatic and mediastinal borders of the lungs. The visceral pleura also separates the lobes of the lungs from each other, and the two opposing visceral and parietal surfaces define the major fissures (see Fig. 29–7).

The pleura itself consists of mesothelial cells, beneath which is a layer of connective tissue. Malignant mesothelioma is an intrathoracic malignancy that may involve the pleura and is associated with a high mortality (survival rate 10%). Blood vessels and lymphatic vessels course throughout the pleura and play an important role in pleural fluid formation and resorption in the intrapleural space. Sensory innervation to the parietal and diaphragmatic pleura, or adjacent layers, may be responsible for the characteristic "pleuritic" chest pain.

The pleura plays an essential role in the mechanics of respiration. A thin film of pleural fluid within the intrapleural space allows the visceral and parietal pleural surfaces to glide over each other, but resists the separation of these linings from one another. Consequently, as the thoracic cage expands on inspiration, it pulls away from the lung surface, causing intrapleural pressure to become more negative. Because the visceral and parietal pleural surfaces cannot be pulled apart, the lungs are also forced to expand along with the chest cage. The resulting alveolar subatmospheric pressure causes air to flow into the lungs (see Fig. 28–7).

#### *Intrapleural Fluid Formation and Resorption*

The dynamics of pleural fluid formation and its resorption from the intrapleural space are related to the difference in driving pressures at the interface of visceral and parietal pleural surfaces. Whereas the blood supply to the parietal pleura originates from the high-pressure systemic arterial circulation (largely by way of intercostal arteries), the visceral pleura receives its blood supply from the low-pressure pulmonary arterial circulation.

Pleural fluid is formed as the high hydrostatic pressure at the arteriolar end of the parietal pleural capillary bed favors the movement of fluid from the capillaries into the intrapleural space. Pleural fluid is resorbed by the capillaries of the visceral pleura because the low hydrostatic pressure within these vessels is not sufficient to overcome the colloidal osmotic pressure exerted by plasma proteins.

Thus, pleural fluid is filtered from the parietal pleura into the intrapleural space and is reabsorbed by the visceral pleura and lymphatic vessels within the pleura. As a result of these pressure gradients, it has been estimated that 5–10 liters of fluid pass through the intrapleural space each day.[3]

## PLEURAL EFFUSION

### Pathophysiology

Pleural effusion refers to an accumulation of fluid within the intrapleural space that may reflect an increase in pleural fluid formation and/or a decrease in its reabsorption from the intrapleural space. Two mechanisms may underlie pleural effusion: (1) an alteration of the permeability characteristics of the pleural surface, and/or (2) an alteration in the pressure gradients (hydrostatic and/or colloidal osmotic pressure changes) between parietal and visceral pleural surfaces.

#### *Exudative Pleural Fluid*

Exudates are characteristically associated with an increase in permeability of the pleural surfaces with a consequent movement of protein and fluid into the intrapleural space. Inflammatory and neoplastic disease are the two major pathophysiologic processes that may underlie an exudative pleural effusion.

#### *Transudative Pleural Fluid*

Transudates occur as a result of changes in the pressure gradients between parietal and visceral pleura. Such changes may involve an increase in hydrostatic pressure within pleural capillaries (e.g., congestive heart failure) or a decrease in colloidal osmotic pressure (e.g., hypoproteinemia). Because the permeability of the pleural surfaces remains largely intact, a transudate characteristically has a very low protein content.

### Clinical Presentation

Clinical features of pulmonary effusion depend on the size of the pleural effusion and the nature of its pathophysiologic process. A sharp pleuritic chest pain aggravated by breathing is often associated with an inflammatory process involving the pleura. Fever may accompany the pleuritic pain. Dyspnea may be observed if the effusion is large enough to compromise the underlying lung. A dry, irritating cough may also be present.

On physical examination it is important to appreciate that pleural fluid muffles all sounds. Thus, the region overlying the effusion is dull to percussion, and breath sounds may reflect decreased to absent vesicular breath sounds. A bronchial quality breath sound may be heard if fluid compresses the lung. Egophony may sometimes be heard at the upper level of the effusion, reflecting an increase in sound transmission resulting from compression or atelectasis of underlying lung. A scratchy friction rub may be heard over the affected area when an inflammatory process involves the pleural surface.

### Diagnosis

Chest x-ray may be helpful in the diagnosis of pleural effusion, although its presence may not be apparent even with significant accumulation of pleural fluid. Ultrasonography is especially useful in locating a small pleural effusion not apparent on physical examination. It is sometimes used to determine a suitable site for thoracentesis (i.e., withdrawal of fluid from pleural space by needle or catheter).

Sampling of pleural fluid obtained by thoracentesis allows for determination of chemical and cellular characteristics of the fluid. Common chemical criteria used to differentiate an exudative versus transudative effusion include the levels of protein and the enzyme lactic dehydrogenase (LDH), within the pleural fluid. In exudative fluid the levels of these substances are low. Chemical analysis of pleural fluid may also include pH, glucose, and amylase levels.

Analysis of the cellular characteristics of pleural fluid includes the absolute numbers and types of cellular constituents, the presence of microorganisms, and cytologic examination. A pleural biopsy may be performed to obtain a sample of pleural tissue for histologic examination.

### Treatment and Management

The treatment of pleural effusion depends entirely on the nature of the underlying pathophysiologic process. A large accumulation of pleural fluid, which compromises respiratory function or causes respiratory distress, can be promptly relieved by thoracentesis. Use of closed thoracotomy tube drainage may be indicated to treat an empyema (effusion with bacteria) or hemothorax (blood in intrapleural space). A thoracotomy tube may also be used to instill therapeutic agents (e.g., antibiotics, chemotherapy) directly into the pleural space.

### Nursing Care of the Patient with Pleural Effusion

Tentative nursing diagnoses are listed below in the section entitled "Nursing Care of the Patient with Pneumothorax/Pleural Effusion." See Tables 36-2 and 36-3 for nursing care considerations regarding thoracentesis and chest drainage, respectively.

## PNEUMOTHORAX

### Definition

A pneumothorax is created when air is introduced into the intrapleural space by a break in the surface of the pleural lining. Air can also be introduced from outside the lung (e.g., post-trauma; or post-abdominal procedure). The subatmospheric pressure normally present within the pleural space allows air to readily enter into the space whenever communication with the surrounding atmospheric air occurs. Collection of air within the intrapleural space, if sufficiently large, may cause partial or total lung collapse.

### Etiology

A pneumothorax can be caused by the entry of air into the pleural cavity through the chest wall and parietal pleura. Common etiologies include chest trauma (e.g., knife or gunshot wounds; crushing injury) and introduction of air, either intentionally or inadvertently, by a needle or catheter inserted through the chest wall and into the pleural space.

Impairment of the integrity of the visceral pleura, thereby allowing communication of air between the airways and alveoli, and the pleural space, may also create a pneumothorax. Rupture of a subpleural air pocket (e.g., bleb, cyst, or bulla) or necrosis of lung parenchyma adjacent to the visceral pleura (e.g., necrotizing pneumonia, or neoplasm) are examples of etiologies involving the visceral pleura.

Iatrogenic causes of spontaneous pneumothorax may include unintentional puncture (e.g., subclavian insertion site), mechanical ventilation with positive end-expiratory pressure (PEEP) therapy, a tracheostomy, and thoracentesis. It is essential for the critical care nurse to identify patients at risk and to monitor the patient closely for signs and symptoms indicative of pneumothorax.

### Pathophysiology

When the normal subatmospheric intrapleural pressure is lost, there is nothing to counteract the elastic recoil tendency of the lung, and the lung collapses. The degree of collapse and, thus, the pathophysiologic consequences of a pneumothorax depend on its size (i.e., the amount of air within the pleural space). Small amounts of air may cause no symptoms and few, if any, physical signs; while a massive pneumothorax can result in acute cardiovascular collapse.

#### *Tension Pneumothorax*

A tension pneumothorax occurs when air within the pleural space comes under positive pressure or "tension." This tension may be the result of a "check-valve" mechanism by which air freely enters the pleural space during inspiration but is unable to escape on expiration. Such one-way movement of air into the pleural space causes a progressive increase in intrapleural pressure with a concomitant progressive collapse of the underlying lung. When pleural pressures become sufficiently high, a shift of the mediastinum and trachea away from the side of the pneumothorax (i.e., the side with the positive intrapleural pressure) occurs. Of critical importance is that the positive pressure within the pleural space inhibits venous return by way of the superior and inferior venae cavae. This severely compromises cardiac output, and emergency treatment may be required to reverse the cardiopulmonary failure.

At high risk of developing a tension pneumothorax are patients who have sustained chest trauma and patients receiving mechanical ventilation therapy. It is important to appreciate that any pneumothorax, small or large, has the potential to

TABLE 36–2
**Thoracentesis: Nursing Considerations**

| Nursing Considerations | Rationales |
|---|---|
| *Purpose:*<br>1. To remove fluid or air from the pleural space to relieve lung compression and consequent respiratory distress.<br>2. To obtain a fluid specimen for chemical, microbial (bacterial), and cytologic analysis. | When air and/or fluid accumulates in the pleural space, the increase in intrapleural pressure compromises lung expansion; ventilation/perfusion mismatching is increased. |
| *Action:*<br>1. Assess patient/family's understanding of the procedure including: its purpose, indications, expectation of patient's participation.<br>a. Reinforce explanation made by physician.<br>b. Provide opportunity for questions/answers regarding procedure.<br>c. Obtain a signed permission (as per unit protocol). | An informed patient/family promotes cooperation and ease of procedure implementation. |
| 2. Establish baseline assessment database.<br>a. Vital signs: Blood pressure, heart rate, pulses; respiratory rate, pattern and work of breathing.<br>b. Physical examination of the chest.<br>• Palpation: tactile fremitus.<br>• Percussion: Resonance, hyperresonance, dullness.<br>• Auscultation: Breath sounds; adventitious sounds. | Baseline assessment data provide a basis for evaluating the patient's subsequent responses to therapeutic measures. |
| 3. Assemble necessary equipment. | |
| 4. Assist patient to assume an appropriate, but well-supported position:<br>a. Approach to thoracentesis needle/catheter insertion:<br>1) Anterior approach—Used to evacuate *air* from the pleural space.<br>Site: 2nd intercostal space.<br>Positions: Sitting in bed in semi-Fowler's position; supine position with arm positioned under head.<br>2) Posterior approach—Used to remove *fluid* from the pleural space.<br>Site: 8–9th intercostal space at mid- or posterior axillary line.<br>Positions: Dangling on side of bed with arms resting on a bedside table; straddling a chair, if possible, with arms resting on back of chair or overbed table. | Placement of patient in an appropriate position assists in determining landmarks; reduces risk of complications. |
| 5. Monitor use of aseptic technique.<br>a. Use of masks, sterile gowns, and gloves by persons at bedside. | Every effort must be made to minimize risk of infection. |
| 6. Assist physician with procedure as indicated. | |
| 7. Assess patient's condition continuously throughout the procedure. | Spontaneous pneumothorax, hemorrhage with hemothorax, diaphragmatic injury, and abdominal viscera penetration are complications that may require immediate intervention. |
| 8. Encourage shallow, controlled breathing during needle insertion; ask patient to refrain from coughing or making any sudden movements. | Reduces risk of lung trauma. |
| a. Inform physician of patient's complaints of pain, dyspnea, tachypnea, changes in respiratory pattern and rate, and other signs of respiratory distress; nausea, weakness, diaphoresis. | This clinical presentation is highly suggestive of pneumothorax. Within minutes a spontaneous or traumatic pneumothorax can progress to a life-threatening tension pneumothorax. |
| 9. Assist patient to remain immobilized until thoracentesis needle is secured. | Prevents inadvertent or accidental advancement of needle with the potential risk of puncturing the lung. |
| 10. Apply firm pressure to insertion site upon removal of thoracentesis needle.<br>a. Apply povidone-iodine ointment and sterile dressing. | |
| 11. Encourage patient to rest after thoracentesis.<br>a. Monitor patient's vital signs and respiratory function. | |
| 12. Record amount and appearance of pleural fluid removed.<br>a. Label specimens carefully and deliver to appropriate laboratories for prescribed analysis. | |
| 13. Obtain chest x-ray after thoracentesis. | Chest x-ray can detect presence of pneumothorax; when compared with pre-thoracentesis chest x-ray, it assists in evaluating status of pleural effusion. |

TABLE 36–3

## Chest Drainage: Nursing Care Considerations

**Underwater-seal Drainage System**

***Purpose:***

1. To re-expand the involved lung (pneumothorax) and re-establish the physiologic integrity of the intrapleural space.
2. To assess, measure, and record chest drainage.
3. To promote ease of breathing and respiratory excursion.
4. To facilitate more evenly matching of ventilation with perfusion.

***Types of drainage in use:***

1. One-, two-, and three-bottle drainage systems.
2. Pleur-evac (disposable chest drainage unit).
   A. A special feature of the Pleur-evac unit is that it has a positive-pressure release valve, which prevents pressure buildup in the intrapleural space.
   B. This disposable chest drainage unit is used predominantly today because it is less cumbersome, simpler, and safer to use than the bottle chest drainage systems.

***Components of a chest drainage system:***

1. Three chambers:
   A. Collection chamber—Receives fluid draining from intrapleural space.
   B. Water-seal chamber—Allows venting of air displaced from collection chamber, but prevents atmospheric air from entering the intrapleural space.
   C. Suction control chamber—Controls the amount of suction exerted on the chest.
2. Options of straight gravity drainage under low suction (external source) depend on which chambers are used.
   A. Low suction can be applied with the use of 2- and 3-bottle drainage systems, or with the Pleur-evac unit.

***Underlying physical principles of chest drainage systems:***

1. All methods of chest drainage function to allow air and fluid to pass in one direction only (i.e., from an area of greater pressure [intrapleural space] to one of less pressure [collection chamber]).
2. The degree of negative pressure within the water-seal system (i.e., the pressure exerted by the water) is determined by the depth to which the distal end of the chest tube is submerged in the water (Fig. 36–1).
   A. A depth of 2 cm is usually prescribed. If immersed under too much water, pressure accumulating within the intrapleural space cannot escape.
   B. Submersion of distal end of chest tube in water ensures "water-seal," preventing retrograde flow of air and/or fluid into intrapleural space.
   C. Maintenance of negative pressures within the water-seal system facilitates drainage of the air and/or fluid responsible for the disruption of normal pressures within the intrapleural space.

***Setting up chest drainage:***

1. One-bottle system—The bottle acts as both a water-seal and collection chamber (see Fig. 36–1). An air vent in the bottle allows the air drained from the pleural space to escape, preventing pressure buildup within the system.

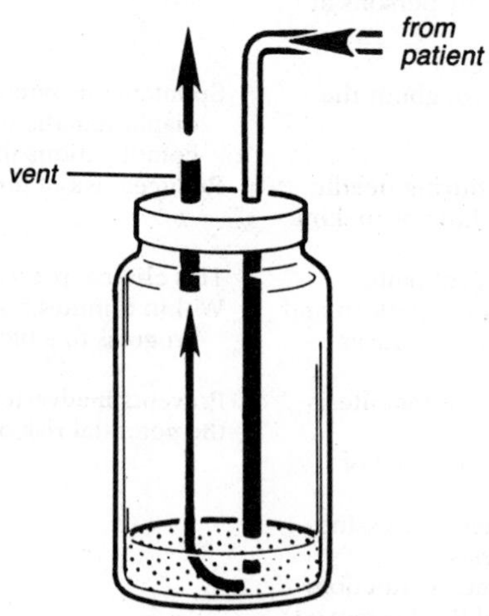


**Figure 36–1.**

   A. This system is used primarily to decompress a pneumothorax; drainage of fluid along with air will cause the fluid level to rise, increasing the pressure within the system and creating a progressive resistance to drainage.
   The end result: A greater effort must be exerted by the patient in order to force air and/or fluid into the drainage system on expiration.

TABLE 36–3
## Chest Drainage: Nursing Care Considerations *(Continued)*

| Nursing Considerations | Rationales |
|---|---|

2. Two-bottle system—In this system the first bottle acts as the drainage chamber and the second bottle as the water-seal chamber (Fig. 36–2). An air vent in the second bottle allows escape of air preventing pressure buildup within the system.

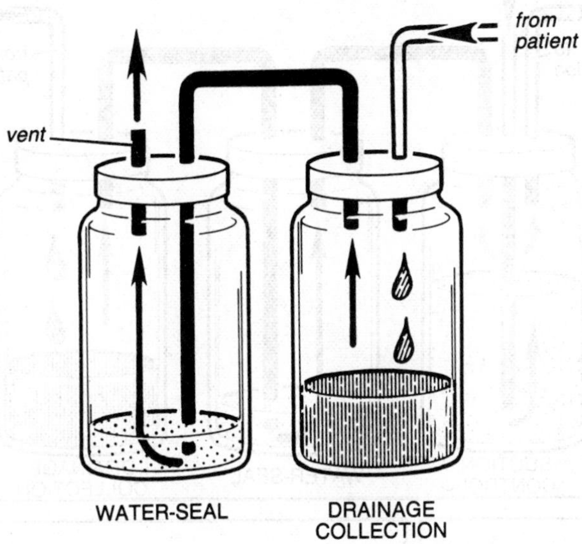


**Figure 36–2.**

   A. An advantage to this system is that the water-seal is kept at a fixed level (bottle 2). This facilitates accurate assessment and recording of the amount and type of drainage.
3. Three-bottle system—In this system there are separate bottles for each chamber: collection, water-seal, and suction control (Fig. 36–3).
   A. Continuous gentle suction may be indicated if there is a considerable amount of air leaking into the intrapleural space.
   B. The amount of suction delivered by way of the chest tube is determined by the depth to which the air vent tube is submerged in the suction control chamber (bottle 3).
4. Pleur-evac (disposable chest drainage unit).
   A. The Pleur-evac is a single molded unit with 3 chambers duplicating the 3-bottle system (see Fig. 36–3).

| Nursing Considerations | Rationales |
|---|---|
| 1. Assisting with chest tube insertion. | See Table 36–2 for nursing considerations in thoracentesis. |
| 2. Additional considerations: | |
| A. Tape all connections securely. | Reduces risk of air leakage or inadvertent disconnection. |
| • A Y connection may be used to connect 2 chest tubes to the drainage system. | Anterior chest tube (2nd intercostal space) = removal of *air.* Posterior axillary chest tube (8th to 9th intercostal space) = removal of *fluid.* |
| B. Maintain drainage system below level of chest tube insertion site. | Facilitates gravity drainage of air and/or fluid from pleural space; prevents retrograde flow of air and/or fluid into pleural space. |
| C. When bottle drainage system is used, all bottles must be secured at bedside either in an appropriate holder or taped to floor. | Prevents accidental separation of tubing connections, or breakage of bottles should they be jarred. |
| • Place calibrated tape on collection bottle to mark level of drainage. | Facilitates monitoring of quantity of drainage. |
| D. Dressing care at chest tubing insertion site: | |
| • Apply occlusive dressing using petroleum jelly gauze and dry sterile gauze pads. | Reduce risk of air leak and infection. |
| • Secure dressing with occlusive cloth tape. | |
| • Secure excess chest drainage tubing loosely to bottom sheet; allow sufficient tubing to enable patient movement in bed. | Prevents kinking of tubing and stress on insertion site. Prevents accumulation of fluid in the lengths of dependent tubing, which may interfere with flow of drainage into collection chamber; or provide a milieu for bacterial growth. |

*(continued)*

TABLE 36-3
**Chest Drainage: Nursing Care Considerations *(Continued)***

| Nursing Considerations | Rationales |
|---|---|

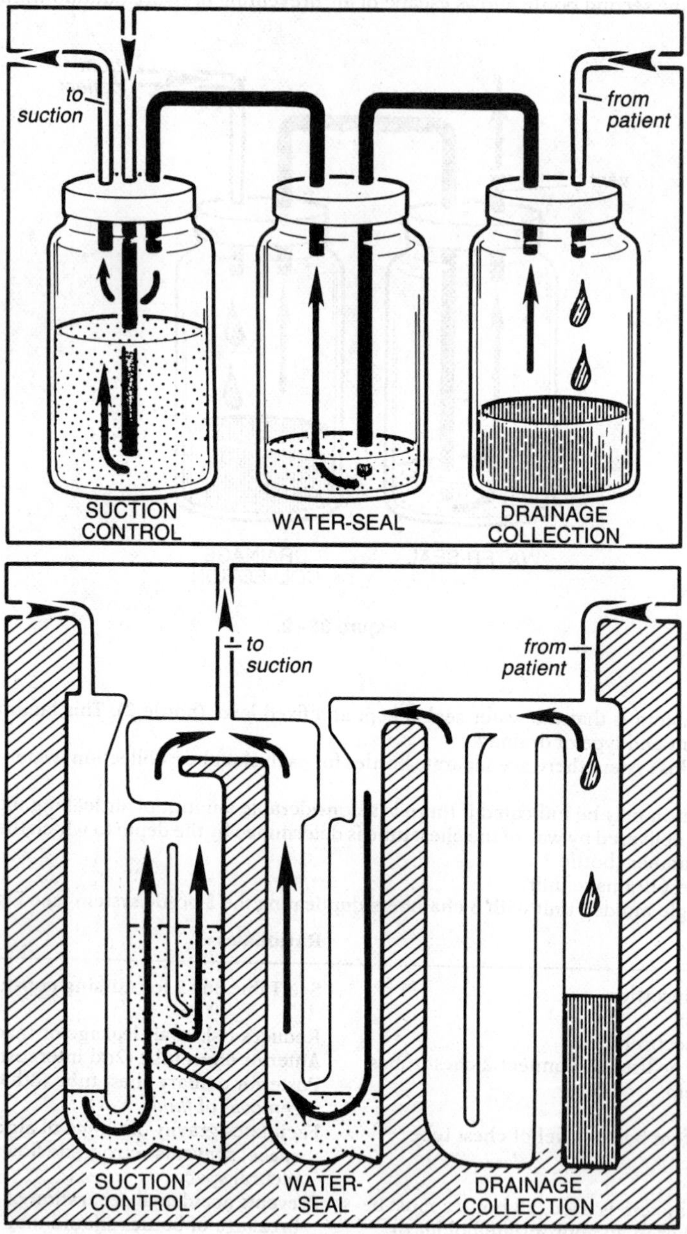


**Figure 36-3.**

| Nursing Considerations | Rationales |
|---|---|
| 3. Maintenance of chest drainage: | Patency of drainage system must be maintained for therapeutic effectiveness. |
| A. Assess collection chamber for amount, rate, and type of drainage.<br>• Mark level of drainage on calibrated tape hourly.<br>• Notify physician if frank bleeding occurs. | A reduction in drainage may reflect an obstruction in the system, pooling of secretions, or lung re-expansion. |
| B. Place patient in semi-Fowler's position (unless contraindicated). | Facilitates both air and fluid removal. |

TABLE 36–3
**Chest Drainage: Nursing Care Considerations *(Continued)***

| Nursing Considerations | Rationales |
|---|---|
| • Turn and reposition at regular intervals. | Helps to mobilize lung secretions and prevent pooling. |
| C. Consider "stripping" or "milking" the tubing if fluid is not draining freely. | The drainage system must remain patent; occlusion can predispose to tension pneumothorax. |
| • Assess patient's status.<br>• Consider unit protocols. | Use of "stripping" technique is controversial; there is some concern that such technique can generate pressures that far exceed those normally applied by gentle suction. |
| 4. Monitoring drainage system: | |
| A. Assess water level in water-seal chamber every 8 hr.<br>• Level usually prescribed is 2 cm. | Too little water increases risk of air entering chest; too much increases the effort necessary to generate intrapleural pressures sufficiently high to force air and/or fluid into the drainage system. |
| B. Observe water-seal chamber for fluctuations:<br>• Percuss and auscultate chest to determine if nonfluctuating water-seal chamber is due to an obstruction in the system or re-expansion of the lung. | Fluctuations result from changes in intrapleural pressure during respirations: with spontaneous breathing an upward movement occurs on inspiration; a downward movement on expiration. (The direction is reversed if the patient is on positive-pressure mechanical ventilation.)<br>Excessive fluctuations may reflect coughing or respiratory distress; decrease in, or cessation of fluctuations suggests a possible obstruction in the system, faulty suction, or lung re-expansion. |
| C. Observe water-seal chamber for intermittent bubbling during expiration. | Persistent continuous bubbling indicates an air leak within the drainage system or the patient; absence of bubbling indicates that evacuation is complete and pressure of the re-expanded lung has sealed the chest tube opening. |
| D. Observe for gentle bubbling in suction control chamber and note level of fluid.<br>• A gentle stream of bubbling is sufficient. | The amount of suction depends on the amount of fluid in the suction control chamber and not on setting of the external suction source. |
| E. In bottle drainage system, check air vent patency; in Pleur-evac system, make sure the small hole in the rubber cap of the suction control chamber is not occluded. | Occlusion increases pressure within the system and can cause tension pneumothorax. The system *must* always be vented to air. |
| F. Keep two clamps at bedside to be used appropriately to:<br>• Clamp the system briefly to locate source of air leak, or to change the collection chamber.<br>• Extra sterile bottle setup, or Pleur-evac, and thoracentesis set should be available at bedside for emergency use. | Clamping of chest tubes for more than a few seconds can lead to life-threatening tension pneumothorax. |
| 5. Implement comfort measures: | |
| A. Turning and positioning at regular intervals. | |
| B. Range-of-motion exercises. | |
| C. Splinting of chest tube insertion site during coughing or turning. | |
| 6. Assisting with chest tube removal: | |
| A. Indications: Signs of lung re-expansion.<br>• Cessation of bubbling in water-seal chamber.<br>• Stable clinical status.<br>• Fully aerated lungs on chest x-ray. | |
| B. Nursing measures: | |
| • Appropriate explanation to patient. | To reduce risk of pneumothorax, the able patient should be instructed to perform a Valsalva's maneuver during chest tube removal (e.g., take a deep breath and bear down). |
| • Pre-medication as prescribed. | Chest tube removal can be painful. |
| • Monitor dressing for bleeding and reinforce if necessary. | Small amount of serosanguineous drainage may occur after chest tube removal; dressing change after initial 48–72 hr. |
| • Assess respiratory function. | |

become a tension pneumothorax when mechanical ventilation is initiated.

## Clinical Presentation

Clinical features of pneumothorax depend largely on its size and on the presence of underlying pulmonary disease (e.g., COPD). If the pneumothorax is small and the patient is without preexisting pulmonary disease, he/she may remain completely asymptomatic.

The most common symptoms of pneumothorax include the acute onset of chest pain and/or dyspnea. Physical findings reflect the presence of free pleural air on the affected side. On palpatory examination of the chest, tactile fremitus and egophony may be decreased to absent as the air-filled pleural space muffles voice and breath sounds. A hyperresonant note may be elicited on percussion; breath sounds may be diminished to absent on auscultation.

The patient with tension pneumothorax presents with severe respiratory distress (apprehension, agitation, dyspnea/tachypnea) accompanied by cardiovascular collapse (tachycardia, profound hypotension, cyanosis). The trachea and mediastinum are shifted away from the affected side; a marked elevation of jugular venous pressure is usually observed. Arterial blood gas values reflect severely compromised gas exchange. In the patient who is mechanically ventilated, ventilation quickly becomes compromised, peak airway pressure rapidly increases, and gas exchange deteriorates.

## Treatment and Management

Treatment of pneumothorax depends on its size and underlying cause. With a small pneumothorax causing few symptoms and no indication of expanding, no treatment other than close observation is usually necessary. Larger symptomatic (dyspnea, tachypnea) pneumothoraces are best treated with chest tube insertion and decompression.[4,5]

Treatment of a hemodynamic compromising tension pneumothorax is immediate. A large-bore needle placed in the second intercostal space (anteriorly) usually helps to relieve the positive intrapleural pressure sufficiently to improve hemodynamics while a chest tube is being inserted. The effectiveness of decompression is reflected by an improvement in cardiac output and a rise in arterial blood pressure.

## Nursing Care of the Patient with Pneumothorax/Pleural Effusion

### *Tentative Nursing Diagnoses*

Tentative nursing diagnoses in the care of the patient with pneumothorax/and pleural effusion may include the following:

1. Anxiety, related to: Sudden, acute respiratory distress; chest/shoulder pain; knowledge deficit regarding illness. (See Table 35-3, Nursing Diagnosis #1.)
2. Breathing pattern, ineffective, related to: Tachypnea, dyspnea; and altered respiratory mechanics. (See Table 34-3, Nursing Diagnosis #2.)
3. Gas exchange, impaired, related to: Ventilation/perfusion mismatch (atelectasis). (See Table 34-3, Nursing Diagnosis #1.)
4. Cardiac output, alteration in, decreased, related to: Altered hemodynamics (reduced preload). (See Table 33-2, Nursing Diagnosis #4, and Table 35-3, Nursing Diagnosis #4.)
5. Comfort, alteration in, related to: Pleuritic pain (chest/shoulder pain). (See Table 35-3, Nursing Diagnosis #7.)
6. Sleep pattern disturbance.
7. Injury, potential for: Infection. (See Table 49-7.)

For nursing care considerations regarding thoracentesis and chest drainage, see Tables 36-2 and 36-3. For specific information related to the above nursing diagnoses, refer to the tables indicated.

# PNEUMONIA

Patients requiring lengthy stays in the intensive care setting are at especially high risk of developing a pneumonia or infection of the lung parenchyma. Pneumonia is a commonly occurring disease, and it is a major cause of death accounting for over 50,000 deaths each year.

## Etiology and Pathogenesis

While pneumonia can occur in essentially normal persons, particularly if the causative organism is virulent, more commonly this disease occurs in persons whose host defense mechanisms of the upper and lower respiratory tract are impaired or overwhelmed by a frank infectious process within the lung parenchyma. Factors contributing to the impairment of host defenses include cigarette smoking, alcohol abuse, viral infection of the upper respiratory tract, a preexisting COPD, and underlying malignancies (e.g., leukemia and lymphoma), particularly when treatment of such disorders involves the use of corticosteroids and cytotoxic drug therapy.

Microorganisms gain entry into the tracheobronchial tree largely by way of small droplet particles that are inhaled; or by aspiration, whereby secretions from the oropharynx pass through the larynx and into the lower respiratory tract. Less commonly, bacteria may reach the lung parenchyma by way of the bloodstream (i.e., bacteremia). The *Staphylococcus* organism is frequently spread by this route.

### *Causative Organisms*

There are many infectious agents associated with the development of pneumonia. The major categories of these causative organisms include bacteria, viruses, and mycoplasma. Of these, bacteria are by far most frequently associated with the development of pneumonia.

**Bacteria[6].** *Streptococcus pneumoniae* (pneumococcus), a normal inhabitant of the oropharynx in a large number of adults, is most frequently associated with pneumonia. Pneumonia caused by *Staphylococcus aureus* usually occurs as a secondary complication of respiratory tract infection of viral origin; in the hospitalized patient whose oropharynx has been colonized by staphylococci; or as a complication of widespread dissemination of the *Staphylococcus* organisms by way of the bloodstream. Hospitalization, underlying disease, compromised host defenses, and recent antibiotic therapy are implicated as predisposing factors to oropharyngeal bacterial colonization.

Anaerobic organisms, normally part of the bacterial flora in the mouth, are implicated as a major cause of pneumonia associated with aspiration of secretions from the oropharynx into the tracheobronchial tree.

Other important organisms implicated in respiratory infections (pneumonia) include *Hemophilus influenzae, Legionella pneumophilia, Enterobacter, Escherichia coli, Klebsiella pneumoniae, Pseudomonas aeruginosa,* and *Proteus,* among others.

**Viruses.** Influenza virus and adenovirus have been diagnosed as the causative agents in some pneumonias. Viruses in general are infrequently identified as a cause of frank pneumonia.[7]

**Mycoplasma.** Mycoplasma are considered to be the smallest known free-living organisms, occurring as a class of organisms intermediate between viruses and bacteria. Unlike viruses, mycoplasma do not require the intracellular biologic processes of the host cell to replicate and, thus, are capable of self-sufficient growth. Unlike bacteria, mycoplasma have no rigid cell wall. These organisms are frequently implicated as a common cause of pneumonia, especially in young, previously normal, nonhospitalized individuals.

## Pathology

The underlying pathologic process involved in pneumonia is infection and inflammation of the lung parenchyma involving distal airways and acini (see Fig. 28–5). Characteristically, there is an influx of inflammatory cells (polymorphonuclear leukocytes), edema fluid, and fibrin, into alveolar spaces as the pulmonary defense system attempts to limit the bacterial invasion and proliferation.

In the past, a distinction was often made with respect to the distribution of the pneumonia as, for example, lobar pneumonia, bronchopneumonia, or interstitial pneumonia. However, it is appreciated that such distinctions are often difficult to make because individual cases of pneumonia frequently do not adhere to any one particular pattern but, rather, can reflect a mixture of all types of pneumonia.

Recovery from pneumonia may occur without any sequelae (i.e., with restoration of relatively normal parenchymal structure; classic example, pneumococcal pneumonia), or a more destructive course may evolve with actual tissue necrosis, abscess formation, and/or scarring of parenchymal tissue.

## Pathophysiology

The pathophysiology underlying pneumonia predominantly involves ventilation/perfusion ($\dot{V}/\dot{Q}$) mismatch. Some right-to-left shunting may occur where alveoli are completely filled with inflammatory exudate. Hypercapnia is usually not a factor (unless COPD is present) because patients with pneumonia commonly *hyper*ventilate.

## Clinical Presentation

Clinical features of pneumonia include fever (possibly with shaking chills, but not always); cough, nonproductive (as in viral or mycoplasmal pneumonias) or very productive (especially in bacterial pneumonias); dyspnea, tachypnea; tachycardia; and pleuritic pain (extension of pulmonary parenchymal inflammation to the pleural surface).

On chest examination, rales (crackles) may be detected over the affected lung; and adventitious breath sounds (bronchial in quality) may be heard over peripheral lung areas. With frank consolidation (sound transmission greatly increased), there may be an increase in fremitus, and egophony may also be present. There is usually a characteristic dullness on percussion of the chest wall overlying the consolidated lung area. Leukocytosis, consisting largely of polymorphonuclear leukocytes (PMNs) with a shift toward immature neutrophils, or bands ("shift to the left"), is a common finding with bacterial pneumonia.

With bacterial pneumonias the onset is usually relatively abrupt with a high fever and shaking chills. Cough may be productive of yellow-green or rust-colored sputum. The clinical history may reveal a recent viral upper respiratory infection.

In contrast to bacterial pneumonias, mycoplasmal pneumonia usually has a slower, more insidious onset. The cough is prominent and commonly nonproductive; fever, if present, is not as high, and shaking chills are uncommon.

Pneumonias caused by anaerobic organisms are usually associated with aspiration and occur in patients with altered level of consciousness or impaired protective reflexes. The onset may be gradual; a cough, productive of sputum with a foul odor, is characteristic.

Diagnosis is based largely on chest x-ray, microscopic examination of sputum, and sputum culture.

## Treatment

### Antibiotic Therapy

Antibiotic therapy is the basis of treatment of bacterial pneumonias. It is important to identify the causative microorganism(s) and determine sensitivity to available antibiotics. Penicillins remain as one of the most effective antibiotics available. For penicillinase-producing organisms (e.g., staphylococcal pneumonia), penicillinase-resistant forms of penicillin are available (e.g., oxacillin or nafcillin). A variety of cephalosporin antibiotics are available including first, second, and third generation-type cephalosporins, which are effective against a variety of microorganisms (see Appendix A). Aminoglycosides (e.g., tobramycin or gentamicin) remain widely used especially against susceptible gram-negative bacteria.

Mycoplasmal pneumonia is usually responsive to treatment with erythromycin. There is currently no specific form of antimicrobial therapy available for the treatment of viral pneumonias.

### Supportive Therapeutic Modalities

Supportive therapeutic modalities include chest physiotherapy and bronchial hygiene to assist in clearance of respiratory secretions. Supplemental oxygen therapy is available to treat hypoxemia (see Chap. 32).

## Complications

Complications of pneumonia include abscess formation, empyema, pleural effusion, bacteremia, and septicemia. Empyema, broadly defined, refers to pus in the pleural space.

## Nursing Care of the Patient with Pneumonia

### Tentative Nursing Diagnoses

Tentative nursing diagnoses in the care of the patient with pneumonia include the following:

1. Airway clearance, ineffective, related to: Copious sputum production (bacterial pneumonia).
2. Gas exchange, impaired, related to: Alveolar hyperventilation, ventilation/perfusion mismatching (predominantly), or right-to-left shunting.
3. Comfort, alteration in, related to: Pleuritic pain; shaking chills, spiking temperature (bacterial pneumonia).
4. Fluid volume deficit, potential, related to: Increased fluid losses via profuse diaphoresis associated with fever; hyperventilation; increase in pulmonary secretions.
5. Nutrition, alteration in, related to: Less than body requirements; reduced oral intake associated with dyspnea, tachypnea, anorexia, nausea, and vomiting; weakened, exhausted state; hypermetabolic state (fever, infection).
6. Sleep pattern disturbance, related to: Anxiety; intensive care setting (sensory overload); excessive coughing, dyspnea, tachypnea.

## REFERENCES

1. Weinberger, SE: Principles of Pulmonary Medicine. WB Saunders, Philadelphia, 1986, p 75.
2. Weinberger, SE: Principles of Pulmonary Medicine. WB Saunders, Philadelphia, 1986, p 77.
3. Weinberger, SE: Principles of Pulmonary Medicine. WB Saunders, Philadelphia, 1986, p 180.
4. Carroll, P: The ins and outs of chest drainage systems. Nursing '86 16(12):26, December 1986.
5. Quinn, A: Thora-Drain III, Closed chest drainage made simpler and safer. Nursing '86 16(9):46, September 1986.
6. Stratton, C: Bacterial pneumonias—An overview with emphasis on pathogenesis, diagnosis, and treatment. Heart Lung 15(3):226, May 1986.
7. Belshe, R: Viral respiratory disease in the intensive care unit. Heart Lung 15(3):222, May 1986.

# UNIT FIVE

# Bibliography


Ahrens, T and Rutherford, K: The new pulmonary math applying the a/A ratio. Am J Nurs 87(3):337, March 1987.

Applefeld, JH: Acute Respiratory Care. Blackwell Scientific, Boston, 1988.

Ayres, S, Schlichtig, R, and Sterling, M: Care of the Critically Ill, ed 3. Year Book Medical Publishers, Chicago, 1988.

Belshe, R: Viral respiratory disease in the intensive care unit. Heart Lung 15(3):222, May 1986.

Bradley, R: Adult respiratory distress syndrome. Focus Crit Care 14(5):48, October 1987.

Brandstetter, R: The acute respiratory distress syndrome—1986. Heart Lung 15(2):156, March 1986.

Broughton, J: Understanding Blood Gases. Ohio Medical Products, A Division of Airco, Inc., Wisconsin, August 1979.

Campbell, M and Greenberg, C: Reading pulmonary artery wedge pressure at end-expiration. Focus Crit Care 15(2):60, April 1988.

Carroll, P: The ins and outs of chest drainage systems. Nursing '86 16(12):26, December 1986.

Chalikian, J and Weaver, T: Mechanical ventilation: For CE credit where it's at, where it's going. Am J Nurs 84(11):1372, November 1984.

Chin, R and Pesce, R: Practical aspects in management of respiratory failure in chronic obstructive pulmonary disease. Crit Care Q 6(2):11, September 1983.

Clinical News. Transtracheal oxygen: The nose knows the difference. Am J Nurs 87(4):421, April 1987.

Code, JF and Pain, MC: Essentials of Respiratory Medicine. Blackwell Scientific, Boston, 1988.

Dennison, R: Managing the patient with upper airway obstruction. Nursing '87 17(10):34, October 1987.

Des Jardins, TR: Cardiopulmonary Anatomy & Physiology, Essentials for Respiratory Care. Delmar Publishers, New York, 1988.

Driedger, A and Sibbald, WJ: Acute Pulmonary Embolism. In Sibbald, WJ (ed): Synopsis of Critical Care, ed 3. Williams & Wilkins, Baltimore, 1988.

Emanuelsen, K and Densmore, MJ: Acute Respiratory Care. Flescher, Bethany, Conn, 1981.

Forshee, T: Systemic origins of chest pain. Nursing '87 17(4):30, April 1987.

Fulmer, J and Snider, G: American College of Chest Physicians, National Heart, Lung and Blood Institute, National Conference on Oxygen Therapy. Heart Lung 13(4):550, September 1984.

Hahn, K: Slow-teaching the COPD patient. Nursing '87 17(4):34, April 1987.

Herrold, R: The drug connection. Am J Nurs 84(11):1389, November 1984.

Hoffman, L, Mazzocco, M, and Roth, J: Fine tuning your chest PT. Am J Nurs 87(12):1566, December 1987.

Jorgenson, S: CE weaning from the ventilator. Am J Nurs 87(9):1173, September 1987.

Kacmerek, R and Stoller, J: Current Respiratory Care. BC Decker, Philadelphia, 1988.

King, G: Respiratory failure in the critically ill. In Sibbald, WJ (ed): Synopsis of Critical Care, ed 3. Williams & Wilkins, Baltimore, 1988.

McHugh, J: Chest physiotherapy perfecting the 3 steps. Nursing '87, 17(11):54, November 1987.

Norton, LC and Neurenter, A: Weaning the long-term ventilator-dependent patient: Common problems and management. Critical Care Nurse 9(1):42, January 1989.

Peil, M and Rubin, L: Therapy of secondary pulmonary hypertension. Heart Lung 15(5):450, September 1986.

Petty, T: Drug strategies for airflow obstruction. Am J Nurs 87(2):180, February 1987.

Quinn, A: Thora-Drain III, closed chest drainage made simpler and safer. Nursing '86 16(9):46, September 1986.

Rarey, K and Youtsey, J: Respiratory Patient Care. Prentice-Hall, Englewood Cliffs, NJ, 1981.

Romanski, S: Interpreting ABGs in four easy steps. Nursing '86 16(9):58, September 1986.

Shapiro, BA: Noncardiogenic Edema, Adult Respiratory Distress Syndrome, and PEEP Therapy, Case Studies in Critical Care Medicine. Year Book Medical Publishers, Chicago, 1985.

Sibbald, WJ: Pulmonary edema. In Sibbald, WJ (ed): Synopsis of Critical Care, ed 3. Williams & Wilkins, Baltimore, 1988.

Slonim, N and Hamilton, L: Respiratory Physiology, ed 5. CV Mosby, St. Louis, 1987.

Stone, KS and Vorst, EC, et al: Effects of lung hyperinflation on mean arterial pressure and postsuctioning hypoxemia. Heart Lung 18(4):377, July 1989.

Stratton, C: Bacterial pneumonias—An overview with emphasis on pathogenesis, diagnosis, and treatment. Heart Lung 15(3):226, May 1986.

Vincent, JE: Medical problems in the patient on a ventilator. Crit Care Q 6(2):40, September 1983.

Weinberger, SE: Principles of Pulmonary Medicine. WB Saunders, Philadelphia, 1986.

Wollschlager, C and Kahn, F: Secondary pulmonary hypertension, clinical features. Heart Lung 15(4):338, July 1986.

# UNIT SIX

# Cardiovascular System

The cardiovascular system, in concert with other major organ systems within the body, functions to maintain the integrity of the internal environment. The cardiovascular system consists of a pump, the heart, and a system of conduits, the blood vessels, which facilitate transport and distribution of oxygen, nutrients, and other substances to the tissues while removing carbon dioxide and other by-products of cellular metabolism.

In the following chapters, the essential aspects of the anatomy and physiology underlying cardiovascular function are closely examined, including the significance of the heart as a pump and the function of the various components of the vascular system in meeting the body's metabolic needs. Emphasis is placed on reviewing the assessment of the various parameters of cardiovascular function, including the clinical history; the physical examination including heart sounds; a review of the diagnostic techniques in current use; and cardiac and hemodynamic monitoring.

The therapeutic modalities used in the treatment of the patient with cardiovascular dysfunction are discussed. These modalities include cardiac pacing, intra-aortic balloon pumping (IABP), percutaneous transluminal coronary angioplasty (PTCA), thrombolytic therapy, and laser angioplasty.

The discussion of cardiovascular pathophysiology includes coronary artery disease, angina, myocardial infarction, pump failure, and shock. Nursing process is examined including the use of pertinent nursing diagnoses. Nursing care plans are based on nursing diagnoses and include specific patient outcomes and nursing interventions.

## UNIT OUTLINE

## UNIT OUTLINE—*CONTINUED*

CHAPTER 37

# Anatomy and Physiology of the Cardiovascular System

*Donna Kemp and Joan T. Dolan*

## CHAPTER OUTLINE



## LEARNING OBJECTIVES

**At the end of this chapter, you should be able to:**

1. Describe the functional anatomy of the heart including its position in the thorax, fibrous skeletal ring, heart chambers, heart valves, conduction system, and tissue layers.
2. Explain how the heart valves function to maintain unidirectional blood flow through the heart.
3. Describe the coronary circulation and its regulation.
4. Describe essential aspects of myocardial electrochemical physiology.
5. Define the following terms: depolarization, repolarization, and absolute and relative refractory periods.
6. Differentiate between the slow-response and fast-response action potentials and their significance in terms of the electrical events of the cardiac cycle.
7. Contrast the action potentials of the cardiac working cell and those of the pacemaker cell in terms of underlying physiology.
8. Describe essential aspects of myocardial mechanical physiology.
9. Describe the structure of the sarcomere and its function as the fundamental contractile unit of the heart.
10. Explain the significance of the functional syncytium in terms of the electrical and mechanical events of the cardiac cycle.
11. Identify the principal determinants of cardiac output and the significance of preload, contractility, and afterload.
12. Identify the major determinants of mean arterial pressure (MAP) and systemic and pulmonary blood flow.
13. Describe the events of the cardiac cycle and electrical and mechanical synchronization.
14. Differentiate the antagonistic effects of sympathetic and parasympathetic innervation to the heart and cardiovascular system.

## FUNCTIONAL ANATOMY OF THE HEART

The heart is a hollow muscular 4-chambered organ located in the thoracic cavity within the mediastinum. It is enclosed within a fibrous sac, the pericardium, which functions to support the heart, to hold it in place, and to protect it from trauma or the spread of infection or neoplasia.

### Position of Heart in the Thorax

The heart is positioned in the thoracic cavity so that its long axis is directed obliquely to the left, downward and forward. Most of its anterior surface is made up of the right ventricle, which is well protected by the overlying sternum (Fig. 37 – 1). The right atrium forms the right heart border to the right of the sternum at about the fourth rib and intercostal space (ICS).

The left ventricle lies largely behind the right ventricle and only the apex of the left ventricle projects anteriorly at about the fifth ICS. The left heart border is formed by the lateral wall of the left ventricle.

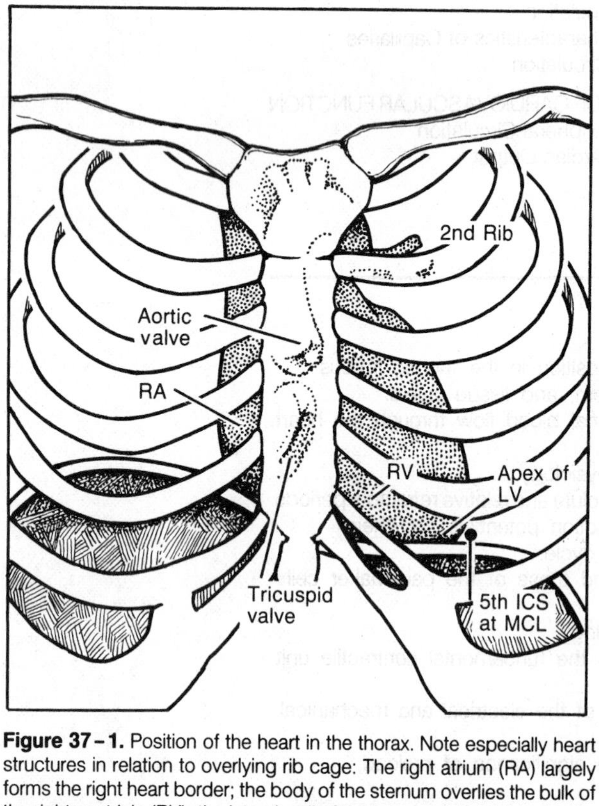


**Figure 37 – 1.** Position of the heart in the thorax. Note especially heart structures in relation to overlying rib cage: The right atrium (RA) largely forms the right heart border; the body of the sternum overlies the bulk of the right ventricle (RV); the lateral wall of the left ventricle (LV) forms the left heart border; and the apex of the heart is seen at the fifth intercostal space (ICS) at the mid-clavicular line (MCL). Note also the approximate location of the heart valves and projection of the aorta, details of considerable importance when auscultating heart sounds (see Chap. 38).

The inferior or diaphragmatic surface of the heart reflects predominantly the left ventricle and a portion of the right ventricle. The heart is suspended within the pericardial sac by the great vessels (aorta and pulmonary artery), which arise from their roots in the fibrous skeletal ring at the base of the heart. The long axis of the heart within the thorax changes with alterations in diaphragmatic excursion and chest cage expansion.

### Structural Components of the Heart

#### *Fibrous Skeleton*

The fibrous skeleton of the heart consists of 4 adjacent rings of dense fibrous connective tissue connected by a central fibrous core (Fig. 37 – 2). It provides the foundation for the 4 cardiac valves and the roots of the great vessels (aorta and pulmonary artery); it also provides the sites of attachment for cardiac muscle fibers, thereby dividing the atria from the ventricles. The conduction system may provide the only continuity between atria and ventricles (see below).

#### *Heart Chambers*

The 4 chambers of the heart are the upper right and left atria and the lower right and left ventricles (Fig. 37 – 3). The two atria are separated by a thin muscular wall called the interatrial septum. The ventricles are separated by the interventricular septum. The upper or membranous portion of this septum is formed by an extension of the fibrous skeleton downward between the right atrium and left ventricle. The remainder of the interventricular septum, which extends from this membranous portion, is comprised of a thick muscle layer (13 – 15 mm) (see Fig. 37 – 3).

The muscle layers of the atria are very thin (2 – 3 mm in thickness), and these chambers serve functionally as reservoirs and conduits for blood that is funneled into the ventricles. In the ventricles, the muscle thickness of the left ventricle is 2 – 3 times that of the right ventricle (13 – 15 mm to 3 – 5 mm, respectively). This reflects the fact that the left ventricle pumps blood into the high-pressure systemic circulation, while the right ventricle pumps blood into the low-pressure pulmonary circulation.

Notable landmarks within the right atrium include the entry points for the great veins (superior and inferior venae cavae), which return deoxygenated blood from the systemic circulation into the right heart. The coronary sinus drains venous blood from the heart muscle itself into the right atrium.

The right ventricle is a thin-walled crescent-shaped cavity that receives venous blood from the right atrium via the tricuspid valve and ejects blood through the pulmonic valve into the low-pressure

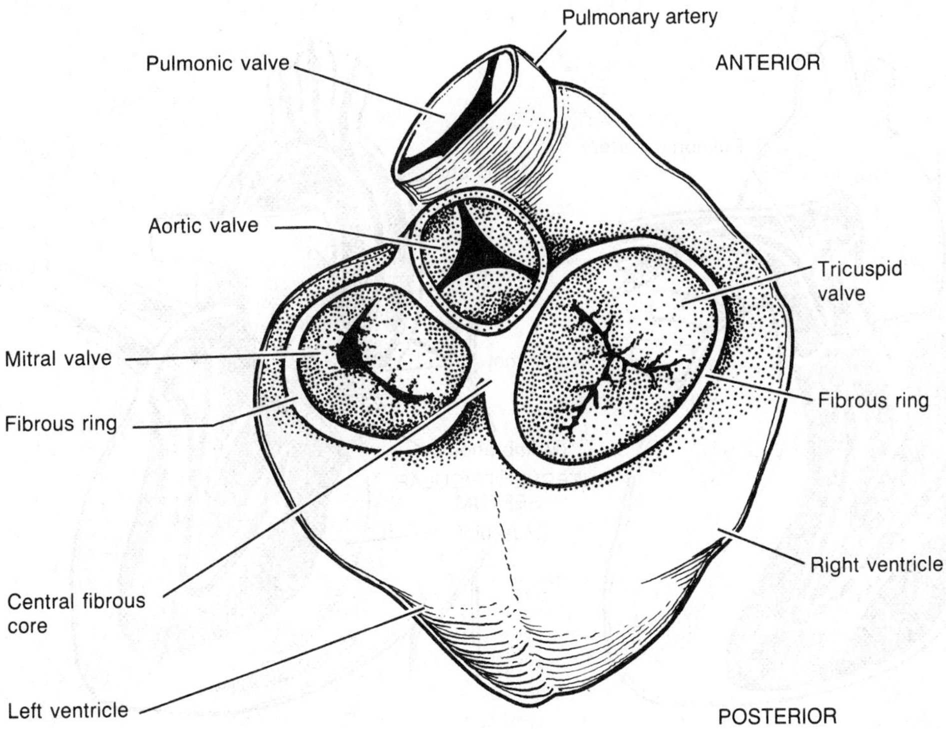


**Figure 37-2.** Fibrous skeleton of the heart (viewed in cross-section from above). Dense fibrous connective tissue forms the base of the heart. It provides the foundation for the heart valves and the roots of the aorta and pulmonary artery, as well as the framework for the attachment of myocardial muscle fibers.

pulmonary circulation. A notable landmark of the right ventricle is the tricuspid (atrioventricular) valve, which forms part of the inferior wall of the right atrium and superior wall of the right ventricle.

The right ventricular chamber can be divided into the posteroinferior *inflow* tract, which contains the tricuspid valve and receives blood funneled into the right ventricle from the right atrium; and the anterosuperior *outflow* tract, through which blood is propelled into the pulmonary artery upon ventricular contraction. The inflow tract is especially well trabeculated with thick muscle bundles attached to the inner wall of the right ventricle (trabeculae carneae cordis). The trabeculae serve as supporting fibers and also help to divide the right ventricle into an inflow tract and an outflow tract.

There are 3 papillary muscles, which function to anchor the leaflets of the tricuspid valve to the wall of the right ventricle by means of fibrous strands called the chordae tendineae. Each papillary muscle receives chordae tendineae from more than one leaflet. For example, the medial papillary muscle receives chordae tendineae from the anterior and septal leaflets of the tricuspid valve; the anterior papillary muscle receives chordae tendineae from the anterior and posterior leaflets of the tricuspid valve.

The pulmonary artery trunk arises superiorly from the right ventricle and passes upward and backward. Upon leaving the pericardial sac, the main pulmonary artery bifurcates into the right and left pulmonary arteries. The pulmonic valve guards the opening between the right ventricle and main pulmonary artery.

The left atrium is a smooth-walled sac that receives the 4 pulmonary veins carrying oxygenated blood from the lungs. Some venous blood from the heart muscle itself drains into the left atrium via the thebesian veins.

The left ventricle is a thick-walled conical-shaped cavity, which can be divided into the left ventricular *inflow* tract formed by the mitral valve and the *outflow* tract formed partly by the anterior surface of the anterior mitral valve leaflet, the interventricular septum, and the left ventricular free wall. Trabeculae carneae appear largely in the apex of the left ventricle, but overall, trabeculae are less prominent in the left ventricle than in the right ventricle. A notable landmark of the left ventricle is the bicuspid or mitral valve through which oxygen-

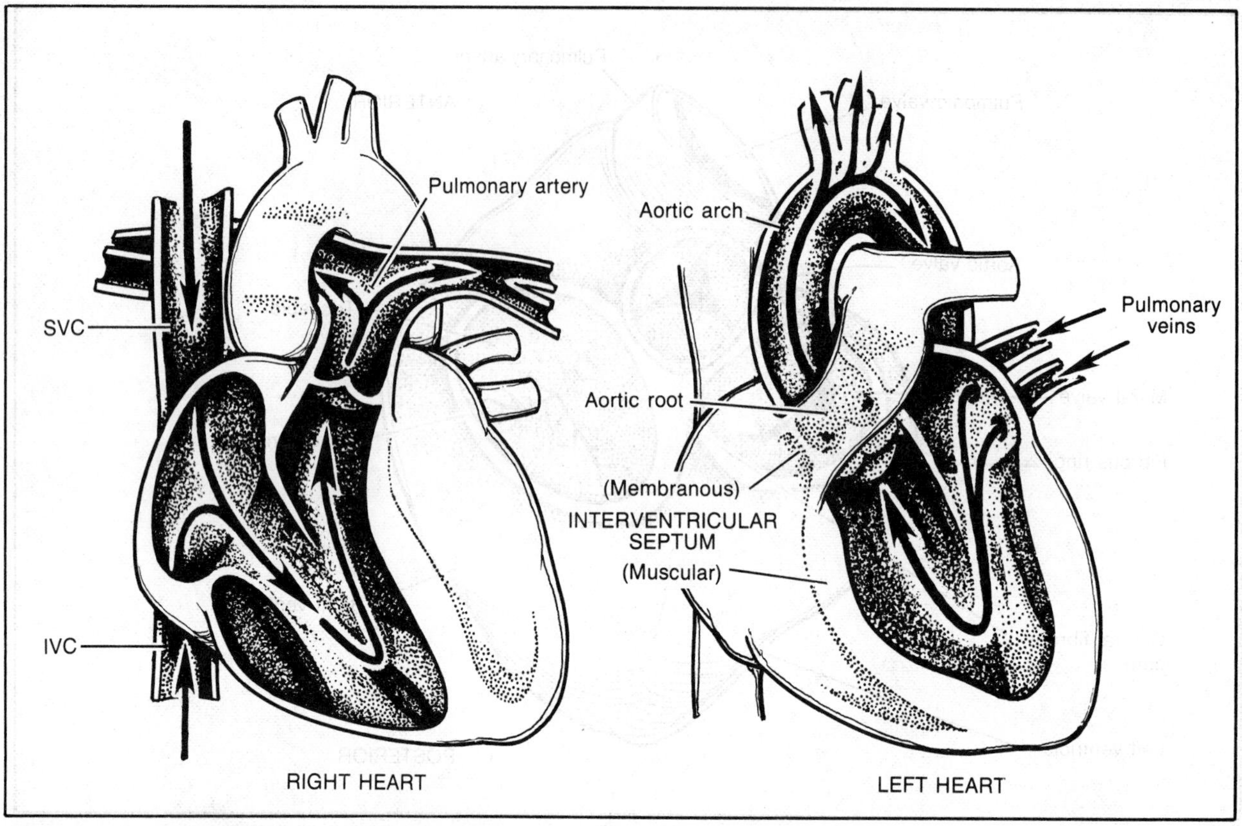


**Figure 37-3.** Functional anatomy of the right and left heart. In the right heart the superior vena cava (SVC) and inferior vena cava (IVC) empty into the right atrium; blood flows from the right atrium into the right ventricle (RV) via the *inflow* tract formed largely by the tricuspid valve. Upon ventricular contraction, blood is propelled out of the RV via the *outflow* tract, through the pulmonic valve and into the pulmonary artery and pulmonary circulation. Blood returns from the lungs via the pulmonary veins to the left heart. It flows from the left atrium through the *inflow* tract formed by the mitral valve and into the left ventricle (LV). During ventricular systole blood is propelled out of the LV via the *outflow* tract, through the aortic valve and into the aorta, from whence it flows throughout the systemic circulation. The *membranous* interventricular septum forms part of the aortic root. It is here that the openings to the right and left coronary arteries are strategically located behind the cusps of the aortic valve. The left ventricular muscle mass is significantly thicker than that of the RV. The *muscular* interventricular septum is largely an integral part of the LV, anatomically and functionally.

ated blood flows from the left atrium into the left ventricle.

There are usually 2 stout papillary muscles within the left ventricle, each receiving chordae tendineae from both major mitral valve leaflets. Anatomically and functionally, the muscular interventricular septum is more an integral part of the left ventricle than of the right ventricle.

The aorta arises superiorly from its root in the left ventricle to form the aortic arch. Upon crossing the bifurcation of the pulmonary artery, the aortic arch gives off its 3 main branches, the brachiocephalic (innominate), left common carotid, and the left subclavian arteries. The aortic valve guards the opening between the left ventricle and the aorta (see Fig. 37-3).

### Heart Valves

There are 4 heart valves, each consisting of flexible, tough, fibrous connective tissue anchored at the base to the dense fibrous skeletal rings (see Fig. 37-2). Each valve consists of leaflets or cusps covered with endothelium. Movements of the leaflets or cusps are largely passive, and their orientation within the heart is responsible for the unidirectional flow of blood through the heart. There are 2 types of valves in the heart: the atrioventricular (AV) valves and the semilunar valves. The atrioventricular-valve apparatus consists of the valve itself, comprised of several cusps or leaflets, the chordae tendineae, and papillary muscles. The semi-lunar valves consist of thick fibrous cuplike cusps without other support structures.

Of the 2 AV valves, the tricuspid valve is situated between the right atrium and right ventricle, and, as its name suggests, it consists of 3 cusps or leaflets; the bicuspid or mitral valve located between the left atrium and left ventricle consists of 2 cusps or leaflets. The total area of the leaflets of each valve is considerably greater than that of the atrioventricular opening, thereby providing for considerable overlap by the leaflets when they are closed.

The chordae tendineae, which arise from the papillary muscles, are attached to the free edges of the valve leaflets and function to prevent eversion of the valves into their respective atria during ventricular contraction (systole). As the myocardium contracts, the papillary muscles likewise contract, thereby preventing any easing of tension on the chordae tendineae. This prevents the valves from everting back into the atria.

The semilunar valves differ considerably in structure from the AV valves, each consisting of 3 cuplike cusps attached to the fibrous connective skeletal rings at the base of the heart. The opening of the right ventricle into the pulmonary artery is guarded by the pulmonic valve; the opening between the left ventricle and the aorta is guarded by the arotic valve (see Fig. 37–3). These valves permit blood flow into the great arteries during ventricular systole (contraction), but prevent any reflux of blood flow in the opposite direction during ventricular diastole (relaxation).

Behind each of the semilunar valves are small outpouches (sinuses of Valsalva) where eddy currents tend to keep the valvular cusps away from the vessel walls. This is especially significant in the aorta where the openings to the right and left coronary arteries are located behind the right and left cusps, respectively. Were it not for blood streaming in and around these small outpouches, the coronary orifices would be blocked by the valve cusps.

The heart valves open and close passively in response to blood flow and pressure changes. During ventricular diastole the AV valves are open and allow blood to be funneled into the ventricles. Late in diastole, the increased intraventricular volume of blood circulating around and behind the valve leaflets helps them to close. An increase in intraventricular pressure greater than the pressure in the atria largely contributes to AV valve closure. Thus, during ventricular systole, the AV valves remain closed, preventing any regurgitation of blood into the atria. Closure of the AV valves signals the onset of ventricular systole and accounts for the first heart sound. ($S_1$). (Heart sounds are discussed in detail in Chap. 38.)

When intraventricular pressure exceeds the pressure in the pulmonary artery and aorta, the cusps of the semilunar valves are thrust open as blood flows to these areas of lower pressure. At the end of ventricular systole when the pressure within the large arteries exceeds that in the ventricles, the cusps snap shut. The closure of the semilunar valves prevents backflow or regurgitation of blood into the ventricles. It signals the onset of ventricular diastole and accounts for the second heart sound ($S_2$).

When pressure within the atria exceeds that in the ventricles during ventricular diastole, the AV valves open and the cycle is repeated. In this way, blood flow through the heart is *uni*directional and always *forward*.

### *Tissue Layers of the Heart*

The major portion of the heart wall is composed of cardiac muscle, the myocardium. The internal surface of this muscular layer is covered by endocardium; its outer surface is covered by epicardium.

**Endocardium.** Endocardium is largely composed of a layer of endothelial cells and is continuous with the endothelial lining of the blood vessels. A small amount of connective tissue and elastic fibers also comprise the inner lining of the heart.

**Epicardium.** Closely applied to the outer surface of the heart is a thin covering, the visceral epicardium. This membrane is continuous with the parietal epicardium, which is reflected over the inner surface of the pericardium. The resulting pericardial sac usually contains about 10–30 ml of thin, clear serous pericardial fluid, which serves as a lubricant to facilitate movement of the heart as occurs with myocardial contraction and relaxation.

**Myocardium.** The myocardium of the atria and ventricles is discontinuous, with muscle fibers of both chambers separated by the fibrous skeleton to which they are attached. Unlike the atria, the ventricles have a thick muscular layer especially in the left ventricle. Current thinking regarding the structure of this muscular layer is that there is a gradual, smooth transition in muscle fiber orientation between the pericardium and endocardium (Fig. 37–4). Based on findings from light microscopy, the mid-wall fibers are more circumferentially oriented, while the subepicardial and subendocardial fibers are more obliquely oriented.[1] Mechanically, this difference in the alignment of cardiac muscle fibers underlies the heart's effectiveness as a pump since the net effect of ventricular contraction reduces the long and short axes of the heart and propels blood into the outflow tracts (see Figs. 37–3 and 37–5).

***Pumping Actions of the Heart.*** Blood flow within the pulmonary and systemic circulations depends upon the pumping actions of the ventricles. Ejection of blood from the thin-walled crescent-shaped right ventricular cavity into the low-pressure pulmonary circuit is accomplished by right ventricular contraction resulting in overall muscle shortening and "bellow-like" compression of the free wall of the chamber toward the interventricular septum (Fig. 37–5). Ejection of blood from the thick-walled conical-shaped left ventricle into the high-pressure systemic circulation involves left ventricular contraction with muscle shortening and an overall decrease in the diameter of this chamber. This allows generation of high intraventricular pressures, which facilitate ejection of blood against the high mean systemic blood pressure.

The almost simultaneous contraction of all muscle fibers, beginning in the septal and apical areas of the heart and moving toward its base, shortens the heart's long and short axes and facilitates ejec-

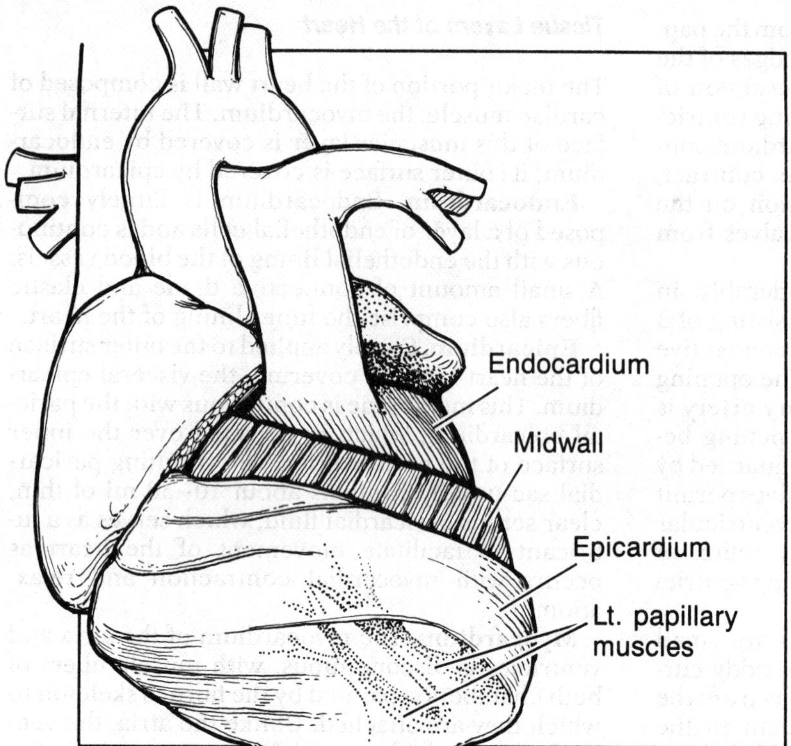


**Figure 37–4.** Myocardium. Muscle fibers of the atria and ventricles are separated by the fibrous skeleton to which they are attached. In contrast to the atria, the ventricular musculature is characterized by its thickness and the gradual transition of muscle fiber orientation from the endocardium, through the midwall, to the epicardium. Fibers of the subendocardial and subepicardial layers are described as being more obliquely oriented in contrast to the more circumferentially oriented fibers of the midwall. This difference in fiber alignment underlies the mechanical effectiveness of the heart as a pump. The net effect of ventricular contraction is to reduce the long and short axes of the heart, thereby facilitating propulsion of blood into the aorta (see Fig. 37–5).

tion for blood superiorly into the great vessels via the outflow tracts. The distinct ventricular muscle mass, the unique arrangement and orientation of the muscle fibers (see Fig. 37–4), and the ability of the muscle fibers to contract almost simultaneously in response to electrical excitation (see below) underlie the efficiency of the heart as a pump.

### *Conduction System*

Cells of the heart have either a mechanical or electrical function. The myocardial working cell, with its ability to generate a contractile force, reflects the former; the pacemaker and nodal cells, which have the inherent ability to generate and conduct electrical impulses, reflect the latter. It is these latter cells that comprise the conduction system within the heart, which includes the sinoatrial (SA) node, the atrioventricular (AV) node/junction, the bundle of His, the bundle branches, and the Purkinje network. The anatomical arrangement of the components of the conduction system influences the timing and sequencing of atrial and ventricular excitation and contraction. Intercalated disks, occurring at the junctions between all cardiac muscle fibers, facilitate impulse transmission throughout the myocardium by permitting rapid conduction of electrical impulses from one cardiac cell to the next.

The SA node lies in the right atrium near the entry point of the superior vena cava (Fig. 37–6). It is referred to as the "pacemaker" of the heart because cells included in the SA node initiate electrical impulses at a more rapid rate than cells elsewhere within the conduction system.

Once generated, the electrical impulse is conducted over interatrial nodal fibers to both atria and to the AV node/junction. The rapid conduction of the impulse over Bachman's bundle is thought to account for the nearly simultaneous contraction of the right and left atria.

The AV node/junction lies in the floor of the right atrium close to the ostium of the coronary sinus. The upper end of the junction is in continuity with the atrial myocardium and fibers of the internodal tracts. At the lower end the conducting fibers converge to form the common bundle, the bundle of His. The His bundle passes along the membranous septum (see Fig. 37–6), which is part of the fibrous skeleton, to the apex of the muscular interventricular septum. The His bundle may provide the only definitive muscular connection between the atria and ventricles. Accessory tracts (e.g., Kent bundles and fibers of Mahaim) that join the atria with the ventricles through connections external to the junction and His bundle have been documented.

At the septum, the common bundle divides into the right and left bundle branches. The right bundle is a well-defined, slender fiber with little branching.

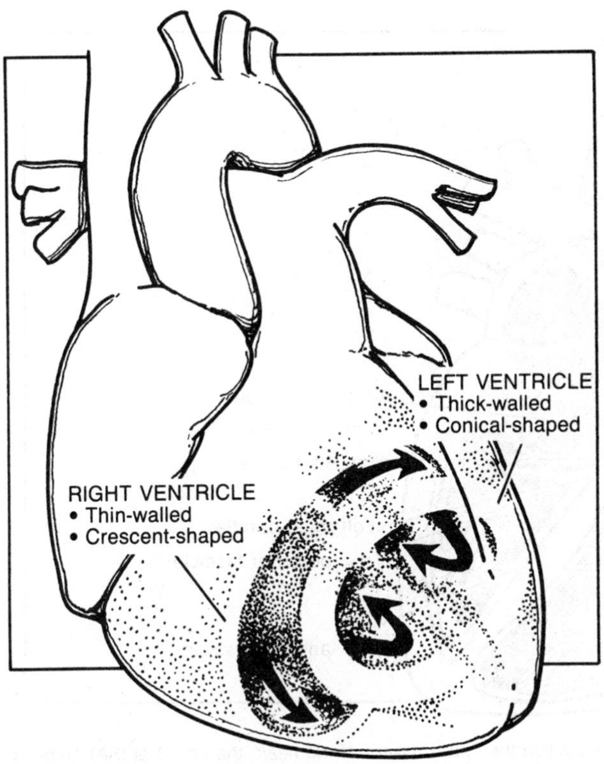


**Figure 37-5.** Ventricular contraction and ejection of blood. Ejection of blood from the less muscular, crescent-shaped right ventricule (RV) into the low-pressure pulmonary circuit occurs largely via "bellows-like" action associated with muscle fiber shortening and compression of this chamber *toward* the interventricular septum. Ejection of blood from the highly muscular, cone-shaped left ventricle (LV) into the high-pressure systemic circulation occurs largely by "circumferential" contraction of muscle fibers, decreasing the diameter of the chamber and its long and short axes. The consequent increase in left ventricular pressure culminates with ejection of blood *cephalad* (upward) into the aorta.

It courses downward along the right side of the interventricular septum, eventually subdividing peripherally to form the subendocardial network of Purkinje fibers.

The left bundle arises from the His bundle and quickly branches into the anterosuperior division (left anterior fascicle) and the posteroinferior division (left posterior fascicle). The left anterior fascicle courses down the left side of the septum in the aortic outflow tract to the anterior papillary muscle and the apex of the left ventricle. Significantly, this fascicle has but a *single* blood supply (via the left anterior descending artery; see below), which contributes to the higher incidence of left anterior hemiblock (especially in the setting of an acute anterior or anteroseptal myocardial infarction; see Chap. 43). Aortic valve dysfunction as well as the fascicle's proximity to the turbulent flow of blood contribute to its vulnerability.

The left posterior fascicle courses inferiorly and posteriorly across the left ventricular inflow tract to the posterior papillary muscle and the posterior inferior free wall of the left ventricle. This fascicle is less vulnerable because of its dual blood supply and its location in a relatively nonturbulent region of the ventricle. As is the case with the right bundle branch, the left anterior and posterior fascicles eventually subdivide peripherally to form the Purkinje network.

Of note, a slight delay in the conduction of the impulse through the junction is attributed possibly to the increased resistance to current flow offered by converging nerve pathways and internodal tracts; the smaller size of these fibers; and to a predominance of slow calcium channel activation (see below). This delay is significant physiologically in that it allows for sequential contraction of atria and ventricles; it allows atrial contraction to occur just prior to ventricular systole, thereby enhancing cardiac output; and it helps to protect the ventricles from abnormally fast heart rates that can be generated in the atria under pathologic conditions.

Once the impulse reaches the bundle branches and the His-Purkinje system, conduction velocities become most rapid. This may be attributed to the large size of Purkinje fibers, providing less resistance to current flow, and to the activation of fast sodium channels. The wave of ventricular excitation involves septal depolarization initially, followed by apical and then, finally, complete ventricular depolarization (Fig. 37-7). The wave of depolarization proceeds from the endocardium outward toward the epicardial surface of the heart.

The fast velocity of impulse conduction throughout the ventricles facilitates the almost simultaneous depolarization of all myocardial working cells, as if but one cell, thereby triggering the almost simultaneous contraction of all myocardial working cells, as if but one "pump."

### *Cardiac Nerves*

Innervation to the heart consists of sensory fibers of cardiac nerves and the sympathetic and parasympathetic branches of the autonomic nervous system. Sensory fibers arise within the ventricular walls, coronary arteries, and the pericardium, and transmit information (e.g., ischemia) from the heart to the central nervous system. Motor responses are transmitted via the sympathetic and parasympathetic fibers from the central nervous system to the heart. Sympathetic adrenergic stimulation accelerates firing of the SA node, enhances conduction through the AV node/junction, and increases contractility; parasympathetic cholinergic stimulation reduces the rate of firing of the SA node and slows conduction through the AV node/junction. Parasympathetic innervation to the ventricles does not seem to affect contractility as does sympathetic innervation. (For further details on the autonomic nervous system, see Chap. 6; see also Chap. 40.)

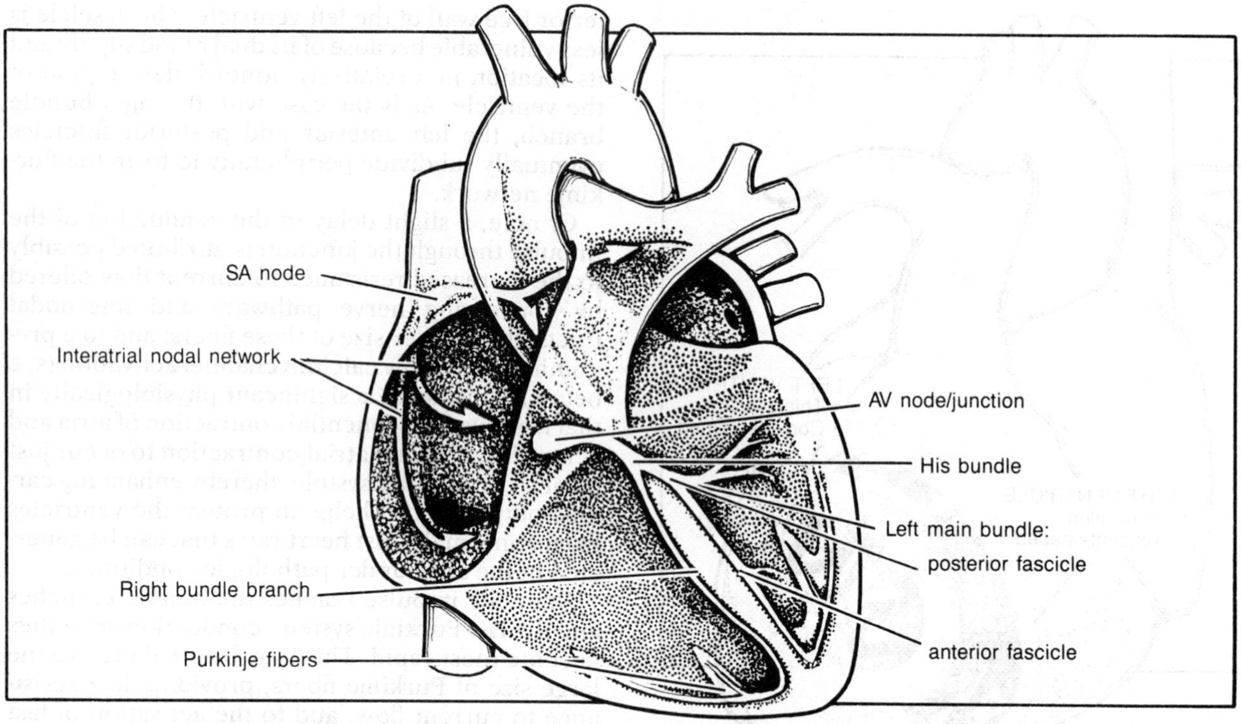


**Figure 37-6.** Conduction system of the heart. An electrical impulse, initiated within the "pacemaker" of the heart, the sinoatrial (SA) node, is conducted over interatrial nodal fibers to both atria, the atrioventricular (AV) node/junction, and the common bundle of His, which, in turn, divides into the right bundle branch and the left main bundle branch. The left main bundle branch quickly divides into the left anterior fascicle (anterosuperior division) and the left posterior fascicle (posteroinferior division). These branches and the right bundle branch subdivide peripherally to form the Purkinje fiber network, which conducts the impulse directly to the myocardial working cells.

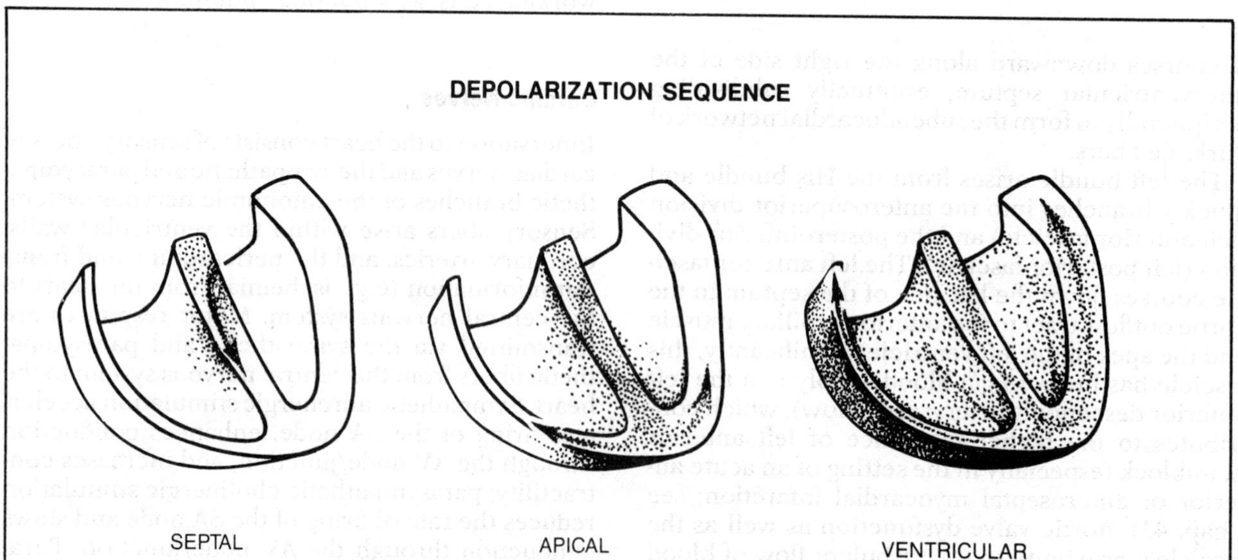


**Figure 37-7.** Normal sequence of ventricular depolarization.

## CORONARY CIRCULATION

### Coronary Arteries

The major regulator of coronary blood flow is the myocardial oxygen demand (see below). Continuously active and largely dependent upon aerobic metabolism, the heart must receive a continuous supply of oxygen and metabolic substrates while having carbon dioxide and other by-products of metabolism continuously removed. The fact that the heart muscle normally extracts about 70% of the oxygen supplied via coronary artery blood flow reflects the degree of aerobic metabolism within the myocardium. Thus, the amount of additional oxygen that the heart can extract from circulating blood is limited. Consequently, myocardial oxygen demands are met primarily by an increase in coronary artery blood flow.

The perfusion of the entire myocardium is supplied by the right and left coronary arteries that arise from the right and left sinuses of Valsalva, respectively, at the aortic root (see Fig. 37–3). These vessels and their branches lie on the epicardial surface and send smaller intramyocardial arteries into the myocardium. The majority of coronary blood flow occurs during ventricular diastole (relaxation). The squeezing effect of the ventricles during systole (contraction) compresses the intramyocardial arteries, permitting only a minimal amount of coronary blood flow to occur during ventricular systole (see below).

#### *Left Main Coronary Artery (LMCA)*

The left main coronary artery (LMCA), having arisen from the aortic root, courses between the left atrial appendage and the pulmonary artery and almost immediately divides into 2 major branches, the left anterior descending artery (LAD) and the left circumflex artery (LCX) (Fig. 37–8). These arteries supply approximately 60% of the total coronary blood flow to the left heart.

#### *Left Anterior Descending Coronary Artery (LAD)*

The left anterior descending coronary artery (LAD) originates from the LMCA and travels along the anterior interventricular sulcus to the cardiac apex and into the posterior interventricular sulcus. The LAD supplies the greatest portion of the left ventricular mass. It gives rise to diagonal and septal perforator branches that supply the anterior free wall of the left ventricle and the bulk of the interventricular septum. The anteroapical portions of the left ventricle, including the anterior papillary muscle, are supplied by the LAD. This artery also supplies a portion of the conduction system including the right bundle branch (RBB), the left anterior fascicle, and, in part, the left posterior fascicle.

#### *Left Circumflex Coronary Artery (LCX)*

The left circumflex coronary artery (LCX) also originates from the LMCA and travels along the left

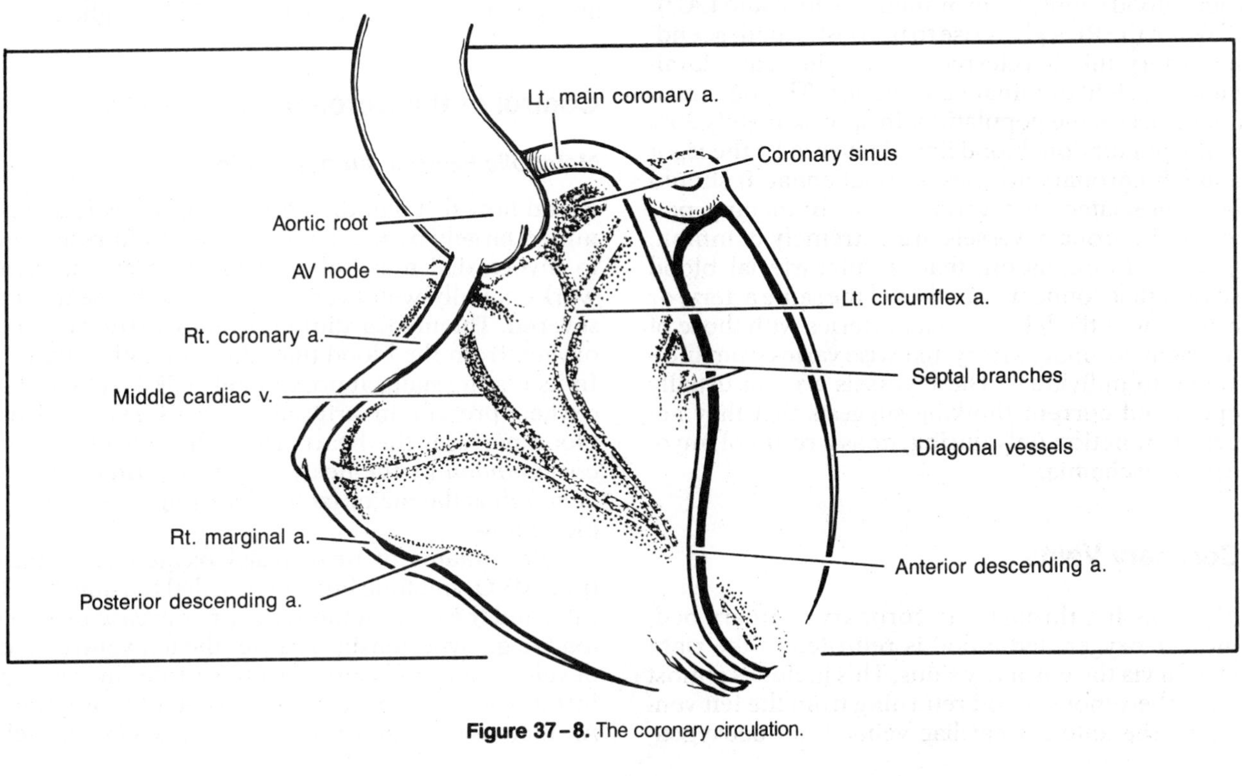


**Figure 37–8.** The coronary circulation.

atrioventricular sulcus to the left heart margin and posteriorly. This artery supplies the left atrium; it gives off marginal branches that supply the apical and lateral walls of the left ventricle and a large portion of the inferior surface of the left ventricle. It supplies, in part, the posterior papillary muscle of the left ventricle.

The LCX also supplies a portion of the conduction system including the SA node in about 45% of the population and the AV node in about 10% of the population. When the LCX gives rise to the posterior descending artery (see Fig. 37–8) this is referred to as left heart dominance or left dominant circulation. This occurs in about 20% of the population.

#### *Right Coronary Artery (RCA)*

The right coronary artery (RCA) arises from the right sinus of Valsalva at the aortic root and courses along the right atrioventricular sulcus (see Fig. 37–8). This artery and its variable branches supply blood to the right atrium and anterior right ventricular wall. The diaphragmatic surface of the heart is largely supplied via the posterior descending artery, as is the posterior one third of the interventricular septum. The posterior papillary muscle of the left ventricle receives a dual blood supply from both the left and right coronary arteries.

The right atrial branches of the RCA are significant in that they supply the SA node in about 55% of the population and the AV node in about 90% of the population. The AV nodal artery also supplies the bundle of His and, in part, the left posterior fascicle (dual blood supply from branches of RCA and LAD).

When the RCA gives rise to the posterior descending artery this is referred to as right heart dominance or right dominant circulation. This occurs in about 50% of the population. In approximately 30% of the population, blood flow delivered by the right and left coronary arteries is about equal. It should be appreciated that variations in branching patterns of coronary vessels are extremely common. *Collateral* circulation, that is, interarterial blood vessels that connect branches of the same artery, or branches of the left coronary arteries with those of the right coronary artery, likewise varies from individual to individual. These vessels are not usually open, and current thinking suggests that they appear to function only during, or as a result of, myocardial ischemia.

## Coronary Veins

After passing through the coronary capillary bed, most deoxygenated blood is returned to the right atrium via the coronary sinus. This includes almost all of the venous blood returning from the left ventricle; the anterior cardiac veins drain deoxygenated blood from the right coronary circulation. Small cardiac veins, thebesian veins, connect capillary beds directly with heart chambers as well as with other cardiac veins. Many collateral vessels are found throughout the heart's venous system, and intercommunication appears to exist among many minute vessels in the form of an extensive subendocardial plexus.

## Coronary Lymphatics

The heart muscle is endowed with an abundant network of lymphatic vessels. Myocardial contraction assists lymphatic drainage into lymph nodes in the mediastinum, which, in turn, empty into the superior vena cava.

## Coronary Blood Flow

Coronary blood flow in the average adult is approximately 250–300 ml/min, or about 4%–5% of the total cardiac output. During ventricular systole, blood flow through the capillaries, especially in the deep subendocardial layers, is greatly reduced as the contracting myocardium compresses these vessels. Upon ventricular diastole, relaxation of the myocardium relieves this compressive force and blood flow during this phase of the cardiac cycle becomes rapid. Because of the greater thickness of the left ventricular musculature and contractile force generated, changes in blood flow through the left heart during systole and diastole are considerably greater than those that occur in the right heart.

## Control of the Coronary Circulation

#### *Metabolic Factors: Autoregulation*

Blood flow through the coronary arteries is determined largely by local autoregulation in response to myocardial metabolic needs. This mechanism works equally well even if nerves to the heart are severed. The myocardium normally extracts more oxygen from the blood than does any other tissue. In its resting state, approximately 65%–70% of the oxygen present in arterial blood is removed as blood perfuses the heart. Thus, the *rate* of *oxygen consumption* by the heart (i.e., *myocardial oxygen demand*) is the major factor determining coronary blood flow.

Determinants of myocardial oxygen consumption ($MVO_2$) include intramyocardial tension, heart rate, and the contractile state. An increase in afterload (e.g., hypertension) causes the left ventricle to develop more pressure during systole, increasing intramyocardial tension and oxygen consumption. An increase in heart rate increases $MVO_2$ as each heart beat reflects the generation of tension by the myocardium. Positive inotropic factors also increase $MVO_2$ (e. g., administration of digoxin or isoproterenol, inotropic agents).

When the force of contraction is increased, regardless of the cause, the rate of coronary blood flow simultaneously increases; conversely, a decrease in myocardial activity is accompanied by a decrease in coronary blood flow. As in the systemic circulation, an increase in metabolic activity within the heart results in a decrease in coronary vascular resistance; a reduction in cardiac metabolism results in an increase in coronary vascular resistance. Thus, the heart *intrinsically* can adjust its blood flow over a wide range of blood pressures (60–180 mmHg) to meet its energy requirements.

The link between cardiac metabolic rate and coronary blood flow remains unsettled but a number of physiologic mediators have been implicated including, among others, adenosine, histamine, prostaglandins, and bradykinin. It is speculated that a decrease in blood oxygen tensions within the heart causes these substances to be released from myocardial cells, and they, in turn, cause coronary arterioles to dilate.

Other factors exerting a vasodilating effect on the coronary vasculature include hypoxemia, hypoxia, and hypercapnia. An increase in hydrogen-ion concentration associated with hypercapnia and/or accumulation of lactic acid and other metabolites may be a contributing factor. Potassium, released by myocardial cells, accounts for some initial decrease in coronary vascular resistance, but its effect is transitory and cannot be responsible for the increased coronary blood flow associated with prolonged and heightened cardiac metabolism.

It is important to note that when coronary artery perfusion pressure drops below 60 mmHg, blood vessels are fully dilated and the capacity for autoregulation is exceeded. At this point, coronary blood flow becomes largely pressure-dependent.

#### Neurogenic Factors

Although coronary vascular resistance and, thus, coronary blood flow are predominantly under nonneural (metabolic) control, direct sympathetic stimulation to the coronary arteries and to the heart muscle itself can also affect coronary blood flow. Direct sympathetic stimulation of the coronary arteries tends to cause slight vasoconstriction. Sympathetic stimulation directly to the heart muscle itself increases both the heart rate and the force of myocardial contraction. These latter activities increase the myocardial oxygen demand, which tends to cause vasodilation of coronary arteries. Thus, direct vasoconstriction effect of sympathetic innervation is generally overridden by its effect on the cardiac muscle, which indirectly can cause considerable vasodilation with a consequent increase in coronary perfusion.

Parasympathetic innervation to the coronary vasculature is negligible. Vagal stimulation directly to the SA and AV nodes may indirectly reduce coronary blood flow primarily by decreasing the heart rate.

## FUNCTIONAL MICROANATOMY OF THE HEART

The heart's primary function is a mechanical one. It is a pump responsible for delivering oxygenated blood to body tissues to meet their metabolic demands and for removing the waste products of metabolism. To accomplish this, the heart generates an electrical impulse, conducts the impulse throughout the heart, and contracts in response to the electrical stimulation.

This pumping action of the heart results from the activities of the individual cells of which it is composed. Cardiac cells are of 2 types: the myocardial working cells and the pacemaker cells. Myocardial working cells comprise the bulk of the atrial and ventricular musculature and function to generate the heart's contractile force (contractility); pacemaker cells are somewhat smaller in size and are concerned primarily with initiating (automaticity) and conducting electrical impulses throughout the heart (conductility).

### Myocardial Mechanical Physiology

Myocardial working cells are characteristically long, narrow, and highly branching (Fig. 37–9). Each cell is surrounded by a plasma membrane, the sarcolemma. Intercalated disks separate adjacent myocardial cells at right angles to their long axis. They provide low-resistance pathways that facilitate the rapid spread of excitation across the myocardium. Because of these junctions, all myocardial working cells contract almost simultaneously, as if but one cell or as a *syncytium* of cells. This activity is critical to the pumping action of the heart.

Each myocardial working cell contains an energy-generating system (the mitochondria), an intracellular transportation and storage system for calcium and other ions (transverse tubular system and sarcoplasmic reticulum), and an electromechanical apparatus (the myofibrils) (Fig. 37–10).[2] The myofibrils extend the full length of each cell and insert into the intercalated disks. Each myofibril is divided into a series of repeating units, the *sarcomeres*, which are the structural and functional unit of contraction. The arrangement of the sarcomeres within each myocardial working cell ac-

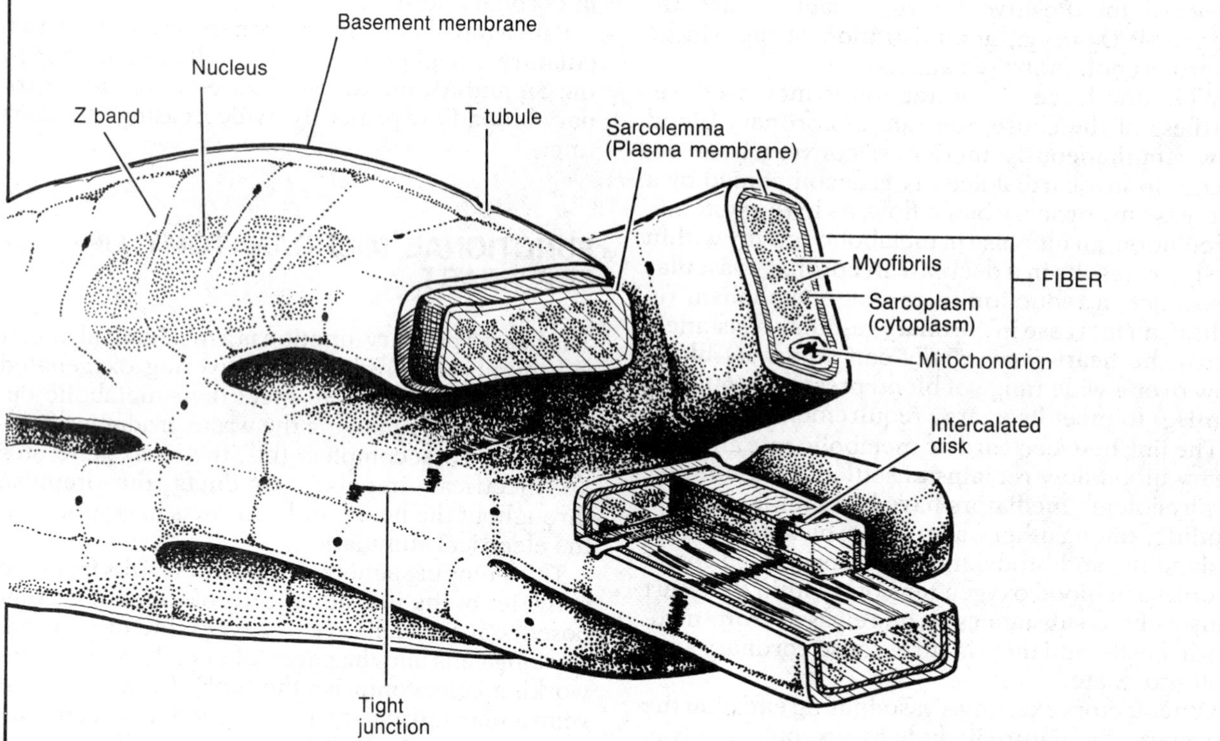


**Figure 37-9.** Myocardial working cells are characteristically long, narrow, and highly branching, with each cell surrounded by a plasma membrane, the sarcolemma, and separated from one another by intercalated disks, which provide low-resistance pathways facilitating the rapid spread of excitation across the myocardium.

counts for the cross-striations observed on microscopy.

### *Sarcomere: Contractile Unit*

The sarcomeres are composed of longitudinally arranged thick and thin filaments. Thin filaments consist primarily of actin, a protein, arranged as 2 intervening globular chains with binding sites at regular intervals. Two other proteins, troponin and tropomyosin, are located on the thin filament at periodic intervals and function to block the actin-binding sites (myocardial relaxation) (Fig. 37-11).

The thick filaments consist of many molecules of the protein myosin. Each myosin is rod-like, with a globular arrangement, or head, at one end. The myosin head is thought to contain the enzyme that breaks down the high-energy molecule adenosine triphosphate (ATP). The chemical energy released is converted to the mechanical energy of contraction.

According to the sliding filament theory of muscle contraction, "cross-bridges" or links are formed between the protuberant myosin head and the actin binding site. The swiveling, stroking motions of the cross-bridges, repeated many times over, "slide" the thin filaments toward the center of the sarcomere, thereby causing the muscle to shorten, or "contract" (Fig. 37-12).

When the muscle is relaxed (diastole) the interaction between myosin and actin is inhibited by tropomyosin and troponin. When stimulated by an electrical impulse, the influx of calcium from extracellular fluid by way of the T-tubules and release from intracellular stores within the sarcoplasmic reticulum triggers contraction (systole). Calcium binds to troponin, which induces a conformational change in tropomyosin, thereby exposing actin binding sites. The sites become accessible to myosin, and cross-bridges are formed (see Fig. 37-11).

Following contraction, troponin releases its bound calcium, enabling tropomyosin to assume the position in which the myosin and actin interaction is blocked. Calcium removal from the sarcoplasm occurs via active transport mechanisms. The sarcoplasmic reticulum pumps calcium back into its core; the sarcolemma actively pumps calcium out of the cell into the extracellular fluid. Thus,

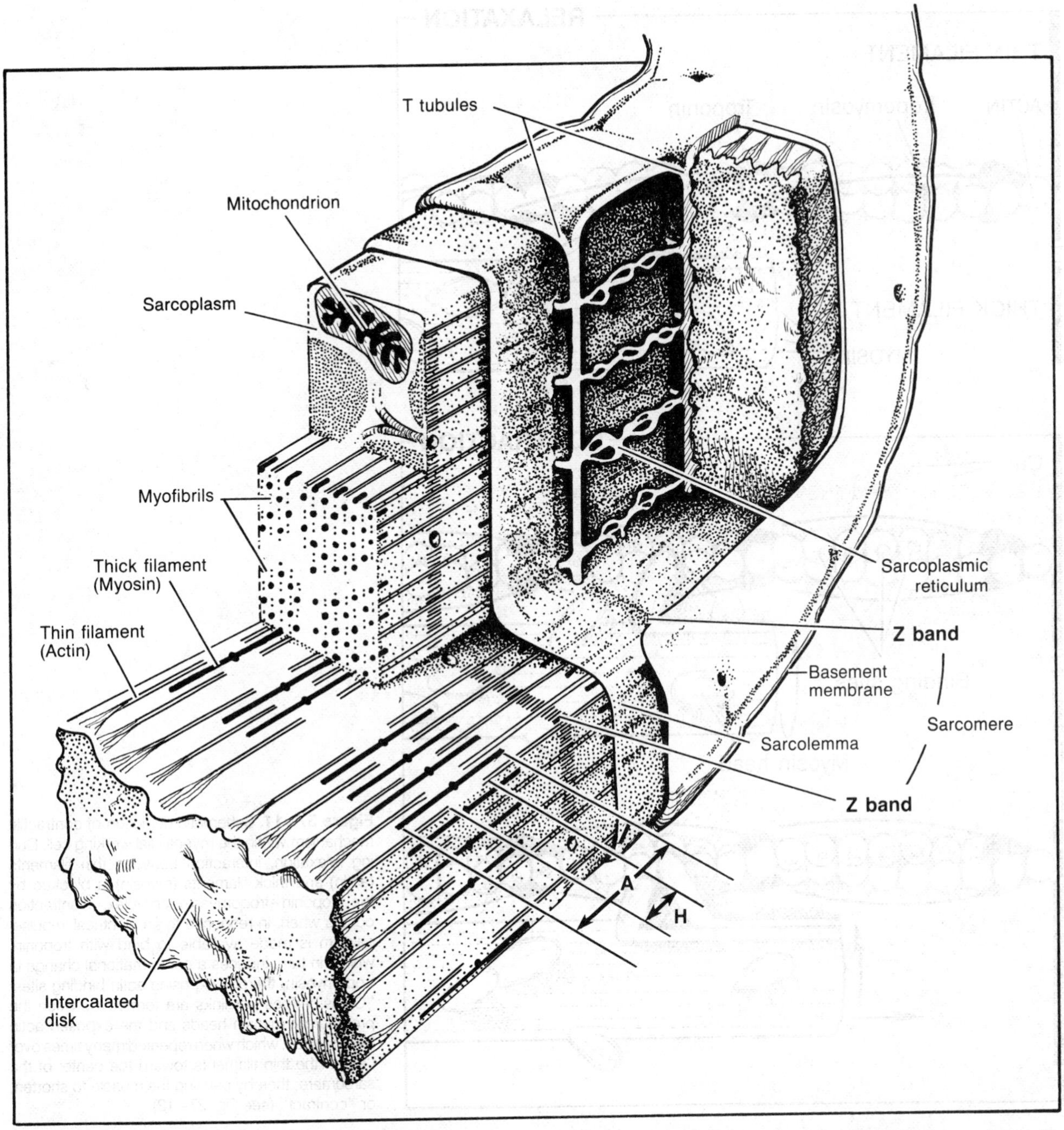


**Figure 37-10.** Ultrastructure of the myocardial working cell depicting the myofibrils (the electromechanical apparatus), their intimate association with the transverse (T) tubules and sarcoplasmic reticulum (intracellular transportation and storage system for calcium), and mitochondria (the energy-generating system). The myofibrils extend the full length of each cell, inserting into the intercalated disks. Each myofibril consists of a series of repeating units, the sarcomeres, the arrangement of which accounts for the cross-striations seen on microscopy. The sarcomere is the structural and functional unit of contraction.

energy (ATP) is essential for the separation of cross-bridges between myosin and actin filament, thereby allowing muscle relaxation to occur.

Structurally, the intimate arrangement of the sarcolemma and its invaginations (transverse or T-tubules) within the myocardial cell facilitates the release of calcium for use in muscle contraction and relaxation. Such an arrangement ensures that all cellular structures are in contact with the sarcolemma and extracellular fluid. An abundance of mitochondria within the cell fuels these high-energy-requiring activities.

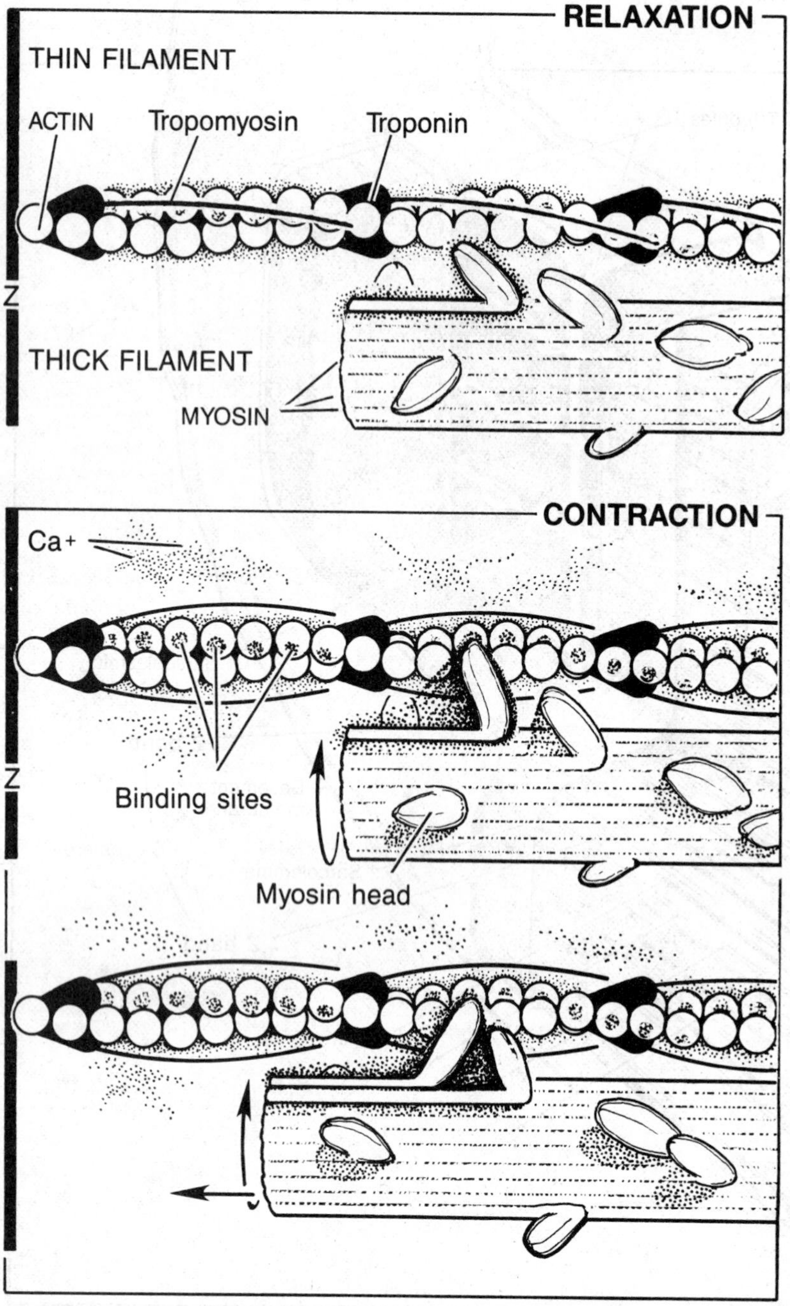


**Figure 37-11.** Schematic depiction of contractile mechanism within the myocardial working cell: During relaxation, interaction between thin filaments (actin) and thick filaments (myosin) is blocked by the troponin-tropomyosin complex. Contraction occurs when, in response to an electrical impulse, calcium is made available to bind with troponin, which, in turn, induces a conformational change in tropomyosin, thereby exposing actin binding sites. "Cross-bridges" or links are formed between the protuberant myosin heads and the exposed actin binding sites, which when repeated many times over "slide" the thin filaments toward the center of the sarcomere, thereby causing the muscle to shorten, or "contract" (see Fig. 37-12).

## Myocardial Electrochemical Physiology

The capacity for the heart to function as a pump depends upon the intimate interaction between an electrical stimulus and a mechanical response. Normally, the SA node initiates an electrical impulse (action potential), which is transmitted through the conduction system of the atria and ventricles. This impulse triggers the sequential contraction of atria and ventricles, resulting in the "pumping" of blood. To ensure that the chambers of the heart contract sequentially, that is, contraction of the atria is followed by contraction of the ventricles, it is necessary that each individual myocardial cell be stimulated to contract in proper sequence. This is achieved by organized depolarization and conduction over the conduction pathway and along the sarcolemma.

### *Transmembrane Potential*

Intracellular and extracellular fluids contain electrolytic solutions having approximately the same concentrations of positively and negatively charged

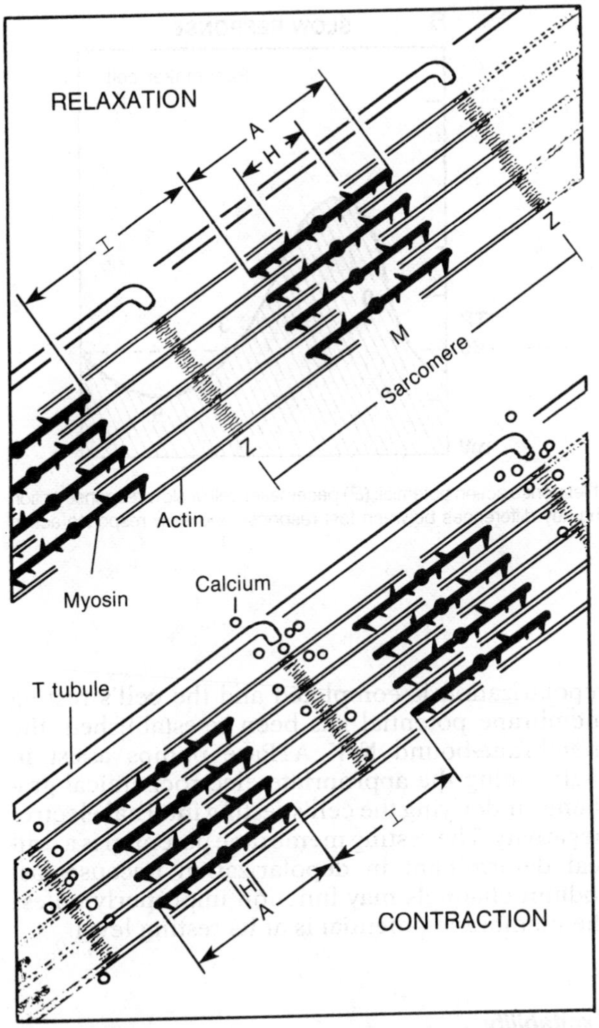


**Figure 37–12.** Sliding filament mechanism of muscle contraction. The lengths of neither the thick nor thin filaments change during muscle shortening, or contraction. Rather, these two sets of filaments "slide" past each other as "cross-bridges," or links, are formed between the myosin heads and actin binding sites (see Fig. 37–11). This is reflected by the constant width of the A band during both muscle relaxation and contraction. The width of the A band corresponds to the length of the thick filament. Similarly, the distance from the edge of the H zone to the nearest Z line, which reflects the length of the thin filament, also remains constant. Only the widths of the H zone and the I band decrease upon muscle shortening (contraction) as the thin filaments from opposing ends of the sarcomere approach each other. As more and more of the thin filament overlaps the thick filament, fiber shortening, or contraction, results.

ions (150–160 mEq/liter). Generally, a slight excess of negative ions (anions) accumulates along the inner surface of the plasma membrane, and an equal number of positive ions (cations) accumulates along the outer surface of the membrane. The result is the establishment of a *transmembrane potential* between the inside and outside of the cell.

Contributing to this transmembrane potential are the electrochemical gradients largely involving potassium and sodium ions, and the presence of a selectively permeable plasma membrane. To a lesser extent, membrane-based Na/K ATPase pumps also contribute to the transmembrane potential by helping to maintain appropriate electrochemical gradients.

The normal intracellular concentration of potassium ions is approximately 140 mEq/liter, and the extracellular concentration normally ranges between 3.5–5.5 mEq/liter. Conversely, the intracellular concentration of sodium ions is approximately 14 mEq/liter and the extracellular concentration is about 142 mEq/liter. Under resting conditions, the plasma membrane is relatively permeable to potassium but largely impermeable to sodium.

Under these circumstances, potassium diffuses out of the cell along its electrochemical gradient, leaving behind negatively charged proteins, organic phosphates, sulfates, and other ions that are too large to diffuse through the membrane. Therefore, the intracellular potential becomes increasingly negative while that of the extracellular fluid becomes increasingly positive, until an electrochemical equilibrium potential is reached. When measured within a resting myocardial working cell, this potential is found to be approximately −90 millivolts (mV) inside the cell with respect to the outside, and the cell is said to be *polarized.*

### Myocardial Working Cell Action Potential (Fast Response)

The myocardial working cell (fast response) action potential is generated by the movement of ions across the sarcolemma of myocardial cells when stimulated. The total net movement of ions across this membrane determines the membrane potential of the cell at any specific point in time. The cardiac fast response action potential has been described as having 5 phases, each phase reflecting particular electrochemical events. These phases include: depolarization (Phase 0), early repolarization (Phase 1); plateau phase (Phase 2); repolarization (Phase 3); and resting membrane potential (Phase 4) (Fig. 37–13, *A*).

**Depolarization (Phase 0).** Under resting conditions, the sarcolemma is practically impermeable to sodium despite a large electrochemical gradient. When an electrical impulse of sufficient magnitude causes an increase in the membrane's permeability to sodium to reach a critical threshold (i.e., threshold potential), sufficient sodium channels within the membrane open and an action potential is generated. The rapid influx of sodium ions into the cell along its electrochemical gradient causes a sudden reversal in polarity such that the potential inside the cell becomes positive with respect to the outside, and the cell is said to be *depolarized* (see Fig. 37–13, *A*). Because these sodium channels allow a rapid entry of sodium ions into the cell, they are called "fast channels" or fast sodium channels.

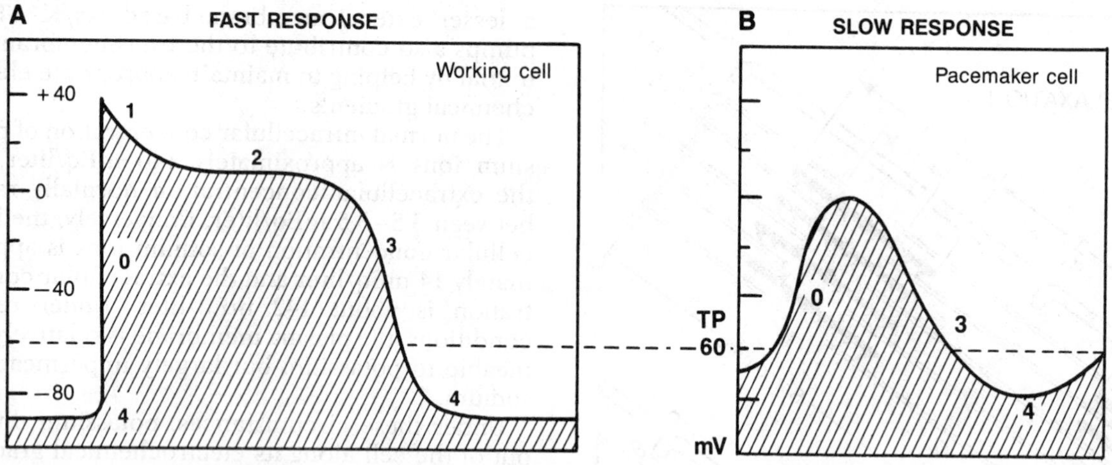


**Figure 37–13.** Myocardial action potentials. (*A*) Myocardial working cell or fast response action potential; (*B*) pacemaker cell or slow response action potential. See text for a description of each phase, and a discussion as to the key differences between fast response and slow response action potentials.
(TP = threshold potential.)

Fast sodium channels, which open to cause depolarization, close almost immediately. However, the inward rush of positive sodium ions is so rapid that sufficient positive ions enter the cell to cause the intracellular membrane potential to rise above 0 to about +30 mV. This is sometimes referred to as "overshoot" and is characteristic of the fast-response action potential.

**Early Repolarization (Phase 1).** The return of the intracellular potential to its resting membrane potential (i.e., −90 mV) is termed repolarization. Early repolarization is identified as Phase 1 and results from rapid closure of fast sodium channels, a rapid but brief influx of chloride ions, and an efflux of potassium ions. During this phase, intracellular membrane potential may be reduced to approximately 0 mV.

**Plateau Phase (Phase 2).** As part of repolarization, another type of channel is opened, characterized by the relatively slow inward movement of calcium ions into the cell. In contrast to the fast sodium channels, these channels are called "slow channels" (slow calcium channels). In the myocardial working cell, this influx of positively charged calcium ions helps to maintain the cell in a depolarized state. A decrease in potassium efflux also contributes to the maintenance of the depolarized state as the membrane permeability to potassium is reduced during this phase (*anomalous rectification*).

**Repolarization (Phase 3).** The return of the membrane to its resting potential (−90 mV) is accomplished largely by the rapid efflux of potassium along its electrochemical gradient as the membrane again becomes relatively permeable to potassium.

**Resting Membrane Potential (Phase 4).** Once repolarization is completed and the cell's resting membrane potential has been re-established, the membrane-bound N/K ATPase pumps assist in maintaining the appropriate electrochemical gradients underlying the cell's resting internal electronegativity. The resting membrane potential is a critical determinant in depolarization because fast sodium channels may function improperly unless the membrane potential is at its resting level.

### *Excitability*

**Threshold Potential.** All cardiac cells are *excitable*, that is, they are capable of responding to a stimulus by depolarizing. Depolarization occurs when the resting potential within the cell is reduced to a critical value. This value is called the threshold potential and is found to be between −65 and −50 mV in the myocardial working cell. If the stimulus is of threshold potential, an action potential is fired, and it does so in an "all or none" fashion.

**Refractory periods.** After a cell is depolarized, it cannot respond to another stimulus for a specific time period regardless of the intensity of the stimulus. This is called the *absolute* (effective) refractory period. In the myocardial working cell, this period encompasses Phase 0, Phase 1, and Phase 2, and it concludes at the midpoint of the repolarization phase (Phase 3) (Fig. 37–14). The period from the midpoint of Phase 3 extending to the beginning point of Phase 4 is called the *relative* refractory period. The cell is capable of generating an action potential provided the stimulus is stronger than that required during Phase 4. There is a brief period following the completion of Phase 3 and ending with Phase 4, called the *supranormal* period, during

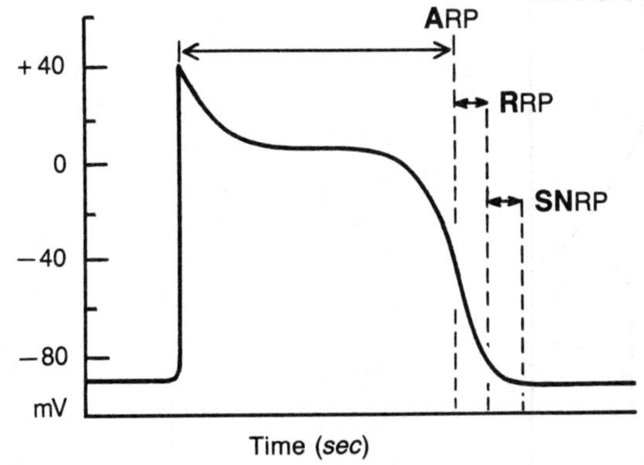


**Figure 37-14.** Myocardial working cell action potential: Degrees of excitability. (ARP—absolute refractory period = zero excitability; RRP—relative refractory period = excitable, providing the stimulus is stronger than that required during Phase 4; SNP—supranormal period = excitable with a stimulus that is slightly less than normal.) See text for discussion.

which a stimulus that is slightly less than normal can initiate an action potential.

The basis for the refractory periods is possibly related to the inactivation of fast sodium channels during repolarization. The closer the membrane is to resting potential when stimulated, the greater the number of fast sodium channels that can be reactivated. In general, the later in Phase 3 that a stimulus occurs, the greater the amplitude and velocity of the action potential fired. During Phase 4, myocardial working cells become maximally excitable. However, action potentials generated during the supranormal period usually have a reduced amplitude.

To this point, the discussion has centered on the action potential of a myocardial working cell, that is, *fast response* action potential. In the following section, an effort is made to closely examine the action potential (*slow response* action potential) of a pacemaker cell, which differs from that of the myocardial working cell in several respects.

### Pacemaker Cell Action Potential (Slow Response)

**Automaticity.** The SA node, AV node/junction, and His-Purkinje system contain specialized cells, called *pacemaker* cells, which demonstrate the property of automaticity. *Automaticity* is the ability of a cell to spontaneously and automatically reach threshold potential and depolarize, in the absence of an external stimulus. A comparison of the action potential of a pacemaker cell with that of the myocardial working cell reveals several key differences (refer to Fig. 37-13, *B*): The resting membrane potential can be seen to be less negative in the pacemaker cell; the upstroke in Phase 0 is more sluggish, and the amplitude of the action potential is significantly less with no overshoot as occurs in the myocardial working cell. There is no plateau phase.

Unique to the pacemaker cell is that it exhibits an unstable resting potential (Phase 4), which causes it to depolarize spontaneously to threshold, eliciting an action potential. This is in contrast to the Phase 4 of the myocardial working cell wherein the resting membrane potential remains constant at about a −90 mV.

The mechanism underlying spontaneous depolarization involves the slow inward movement of sodium ions coupled with a decrease in the outward movement of potassium ions. Unlike the myocardial working cell, the plasma membrane of the pacemaker cell is somewhat permeable to sodium ions. Thus, these ions slowly leak into the cell during Phase 4, causing the cell to depolarize automatically without a preceding stimulus.

### "Pacemaker" of the Heart

When pacemaker cells spontaneously depolarize they stimulate adjacent cells. Once initiated, propagation of the impulse occurs in all directions, leading ultimately to depolarization of the entire myocardium. The rate at which pacemaker cells fire action potentials depends on the movement of positively charged ions during Phase 4. When comparing the action potentials of pacemaker cells in the SA node, AV node, and His-Purkinje system, and that of the myocardial working cell (refer to Fig. 37-15), it can be seen that the pacemaker cells of the SA node exhibit the steepest spontaneous depolarization during Phase 4, and therefore they fire before other pacemaker cells and the myocardial working cell. Furthermore, SA nodal pacemaker cells fire at a faster inherent rate than do other cardiac cells (about 60-80 beats/min). Thus, the SA node is said to be the "pacemaker" of the heart, initiating the wave of excitation that depolarizes all other cardiac cells.

Should the SA node fail to generate an impulse, or should the impulse, if generated, fail to be conducted to adjacent cells and other cells in the conduction system, subsidiary pacemakers capable of automaticity but at slower inherent rates would assume the pacemaker responsibility and take over control of the heart. Following the SA node, the next fastest pacemaker is the AV node/junction with an inherent rate of 40-60 beats/min. Should the AV node fail, pacemaker cells in the His-Purkinje system could kick in at an inherent rate of 20-40 beats/min.

## Excitation-Contraction Coupling

As discussed above, the 2 major physiologic processes underlying cardiac function include electrical excitation initiated by pacemaker cells and

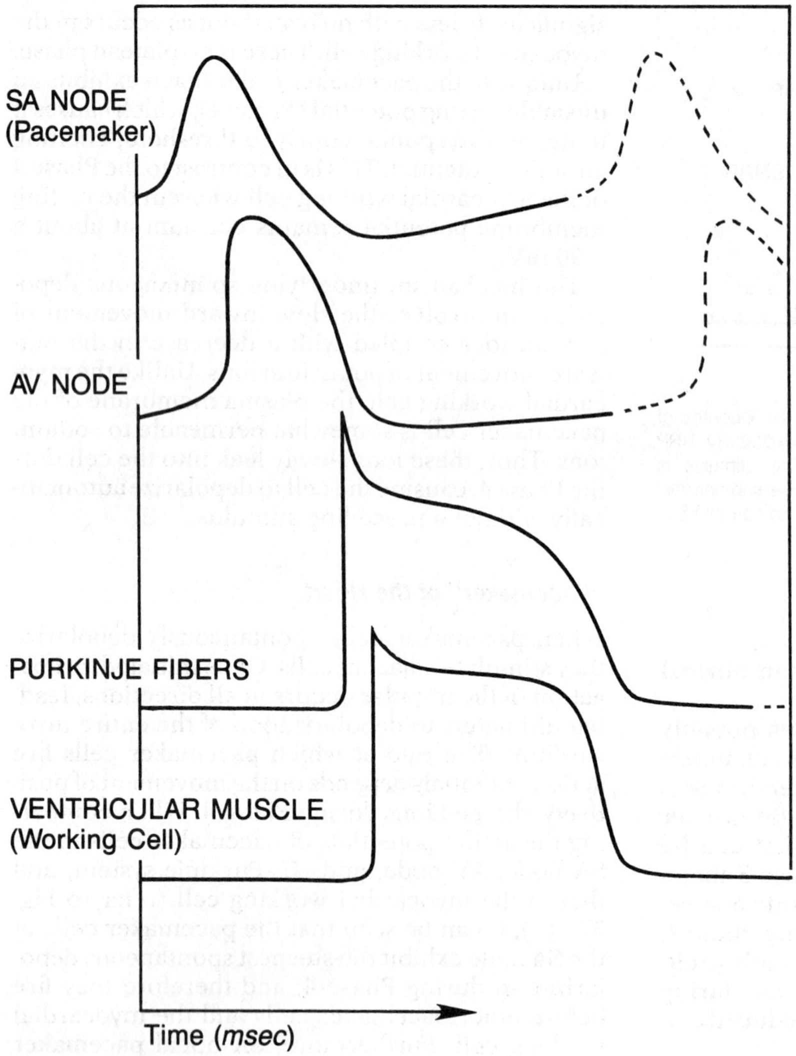


**Figure 37 – 15.** Action potentials of 3 types of pacemaker cells, including the SA node, AV node, and Purkinje fiber; and action potential of the myocardial working cell. The pacemaker cells of the SA node exhibit the steepest spontaneous depolarization during Phase 4, thereby firing before other pacemaker cells and the myocardial working cell. This factor, in conjunction with its faster inherent rate, underlies the role of the SA node as the "pacemaker" of the heart. (Dark line = 1 full cycle.)

conducted via a specialized conduction system throughout the myocardium; and mechanical contraction produced by shortening of the contractile units, the sarcomeres, within the myocardial working cells. These 2 processes occur in sequence with each heart beat.

The sequence of events by which the stimulation of the sarcolemma by an electrical impulse leads to cross-bridge activity and myocardial contraction is referred to as *excitation-contraction coupling*. Significantly, the one functional link between these 2 physiologic processes is the calcium ion.

## CARDIAC CYCLE

The function of the heart is to generate pressures that propel blood through the pulmonary and systemic circulations. To pump blood effectively, a synchronization of electrical and mechanical events within the heart is essential. In the discussion that follows, electrical and mechanical events are defined and the sequence of events as they occur within the left heart during the cardiac cycle is examined. The reader is advised to refer to Figure 37 – 16 during this discussion.

The electrical events of the heart as reflected on the surface of the body are recorded on the electrocardiogram (ECG). As depicted in Figure 37 – 16 the ECG configuration reflects the following: the P wave reflects spread of depolarization throughout atria; the PR interval reflects the conduction of electrical impulse through the AV junction, His bundle, and His-Purkinje system; the QRS complex reflects ventricular depolarization; the ST segment is isoelectric (i.e., there is no net current flow); and the T wave reflects ventricular repolarization (see Chap. 40).

Mechanical events within the heart are reflected by pressure waveforms as recorded via hemody-

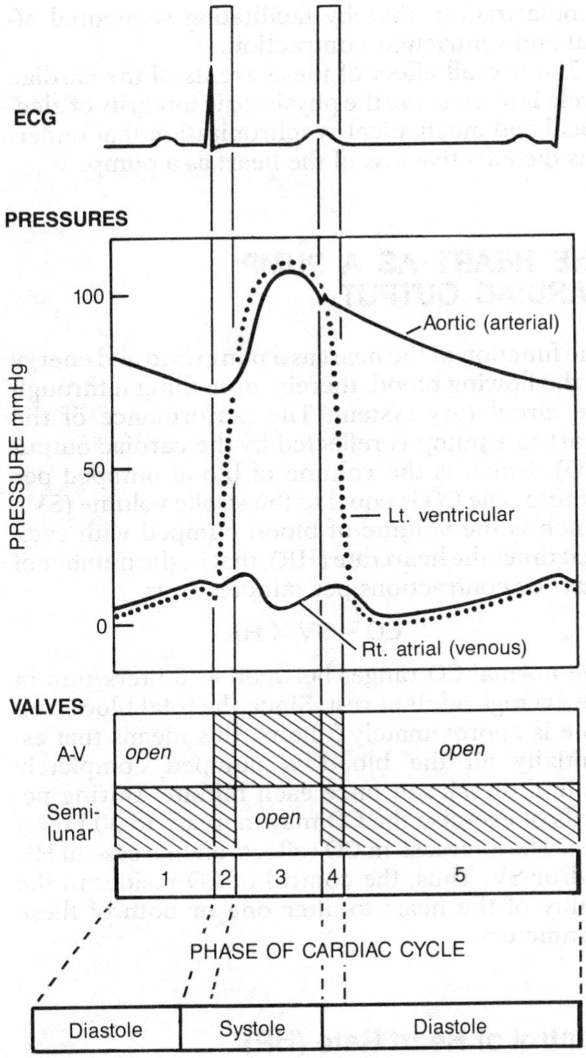


**Figure 37–16.** Phases of the cardiac cycle illustrating the relationship between electrical (ECG) and mechanical (aortic, left ventricular, and right atrial pressures, and valve opening and closure) events in the heart. See text for discussion. (From Vander, A, Sherman, J, and Luciano, D: Human Physiology: The Mechanisms of Body Function, ed 4. 1985, p 325, with permission.)

namic monitoring techniques (see Chap. 41). The aortic (arterial), right atrial (venous), and left ventricular pressures are depicted in Figure 37–16. Also indicated are the mitral ($S_1$) and aortic ($S_2$) valve closures. These create the heart sounds that help to distinguish systolic and diastolic phases of the cardiac cycle (see Chap. 38).

## Ventricular Systole

Ventricular systole is divided into 2 phases: isometric (isovolumic) ventricular contraction and ventricular ejection.

### *Isometric Ventricular Contraction*

This phase marks the onset of ventricular systole (contraction). Electrically, it coincides with the R wave on the ECG and reflects ventricular depolarization. Mechanically, the mitral valve has just closed as ventricular pressure exceeded atrial pressure. Mitral valve closure underlies the first heart sound ($S_1$); the aortic valve has not yet opened. The aortic (mean arterial) pressure is about 80 mmHg. Significantly, there is a rapid, progressive increase in left ventricular pressure reflecting the increasing tension generated by the muscle fibers. There is no fiber shortening; thus, this phase is termed *isometric* contraction. Since all 4 valves are all momentarily closed, the contracting muscle fibers generate increasing ventricular pressures without a change in volume. Thus, this phase has also been termed *isovolumic* contraction.

### *Ejection Phase*

The ejection phase of ventricular systole involves rapid and reduced ventricular ejection. *Rapid* ejection phase reflects rapid expulsion of blood from the ventricle into the aorta as ventricular pressure exceeds that in the aorta. This forces the aortic valve to open. Characteristically, there is a sharp rise in aortic pressure; ventricular pressure continues to rise rapidly during the initial part of this phase and less rapidly during the latter part of this period. An abrupt decrease in intraventricular volume occurs. Approximately two thirds of the stroke volume is ejected during this rapid phase.

*Reduced* ejection phase is defined as the slow expulsion of blood from the left ventricle into the aorta. This period of reduced ventricular ejection comprises the later two thirds of the total ejection period. Blood continues to flow from the left ventricle into the aorta because of the momentum of forward blood flow. Both aortic and ventricular pressures decline, but the ventricular pressure becomes less than that in the aorta and the aortic valve closes (dicrotic notch). This creates the second heart sound ($S_2$), and signals the beginning of ventricular diastole. Atrial pressures during this phase slowly increase, reflecting atrial diastolic filling.

Electrically, the ejection phase coincides with the ST segment on the ECG. Normally, there is no current flow recorded during this time because the ventricle is completely depolarized and in the contractile state. (See Fig. 37–13, myocardial working cell action potential, plateau phase [Phase 2].)

## Ventricular Diastole

Ventricular diastole can be divided into 4 phases: isometric ventricular relaxation, rapid and slow ventricular filling, and atrial systole.

### Isometric Ventricular Relaxation

Isometric ventricular relaxation begins with closure of the aortic valve and reflects the time period when both valves are closed and ventricular diastole (relaxation) has begun. Left ventricular pressure decreases; aortic pressure increases momentarily with closure of the aortic valve, as valve closure prevents backflow of blood into the left ventricle. Atrial pressure continues to rise. Electrically, this phase coincides with the downslope of the T wave on the ECG.

### Rapid Ventricular Filling Phase

This phase is initiated with the opening of the mitral valve as atrial pressure exceeds that in the left ventricle. The ventricle fills rapidly with blood that has accumulated in the atrium. The bulk of ventricular filling occurs during this phase, but intraventricular pressure continues to diminish as ventricular relaxation continues.

### Slow Ventricular Filling Phase

During this phase (also referred to as *diastasis*), the mitral valve remains open and intra-atrial and intraventricular pressures begin to approximate one another. During both rapid and slow ventricular filling phases, aortic pressures diminish slightly but maintain a mean arterial pressure of about 80 mmHg. Significantly, this is the phase of maximum coronary perfusion.

Electrically, there is no measurable activity recorded on the ECG until the very end of this phase when atrial depolarization occurs. This is reflected by the upslope of the P wave on the ECG.

### Atrial Systole

Atrial systole (contraction) follows atrial depolarization. This is reflected by the slight increase in atrial pressure. Atrial systole signals the last phase of ventricular diastole and is responsible for contributing an additional 20% of the total left ventricular filling volume, often referred to as the "atrial kick."

Following atrial contraction there is a decrease in atrial pressure. When pressure in the left ventricle exceeds that in the atrium, the mitral valve closes, signaling the onset of ventricular systole, and the cycle repeats itself.

Electrically, atrial systole begins at the peak of the P wave and continues until the peak of the R wave. During this PR interval, conduction of the electrical impulse is delayed as it moves through the conduction system—AV junction, bundle of His, and His-Purkinje system. Mechanically, this delay in impulse conduction is significant. It allows for atrial contraction to occur prior to ventricular depolarization, thereby facilitating sequential atrial and ventricular contraction.

The overall effect of these events of the cardiac cycle is to preserve the physiologic integrity of electrical and mechanical synchronization that underlies the effectiveness of the heart as a pump.

## THE HEART AS A PUMP: CARDIAC OUTPUT

The function of the heart as a pump is to add energy to the flowing blood, thereby propelling it through the circulatory system. The performance of the heart as a pump is reflected by the cardiac output (CO), which is the volume of blood pumped per minute. The CO is equal to the stroke volume (SV), which is the volume of blood pumped with each beat times the heart rate (HR), that is, the number of beats or contractions per minute. Thus,

$$CO = SV \times HR$$

The normal CO ranges between 4–8 liters/min in the average adult at rest. Since the total blood volume is approximately 5 liters, this means that essentially all the blood is pumped completely around the circuit once each minute. During periods of exercise the CO may increase to 30 liters/min. This increase in CO reflects an increase in HR and/or SV. Thus, the control of CO resides in the ability of the heart to alter one or both of these parameters.

### Control of Heart Rate (HR)

Changes in HR are primarily controlled via the parasympathetic and sympathetic branches of the autonomic nervous system. With sympathetic stimulation, the HR increases; with parasympathetic stimulation, the HR decreases. In the resting state the parasympathetic influence is dominant and the resting HR in the average resting adult is approximately 60–80 beats/min. When the need for an increase in CO arises (e.g., as occurs with exercise), the HR increases abruptly, and may progressively increase to a maximal rate as much as 3 times the normal resting rate, or about 180–200 beats/min.

### Control of Stroke Volume

The second variable that determines cardiac output is stroke volume (SV), the volume of blood ejected by the ventricles with each contraction. Determinants of SV include the degree of ventricular filling during diastole, or preload; the pressure against which the ventricles must pump to eject blood during systole, or afterload; and the myocardial contractile state.

### Preload

**Length-Tension Relationship.** The force of myocardial contraction is a function of its initial muscle fiber length. The more these fibers are stretched, the more forcefully they contract, within physiologic limits. If stretched excessively, these muscle fibers develop less tension, resulting in a decrease in contractility.

The sliding-filament theory explains, in part, the length-tension relationships of myocardial muscle fibers. The lengths of neither the thick filaments nor the lengths of the thin filaments change during shortening (see Fig. 37–12). Rather, these 2 sets of filaments overlap (via cross-bridge formation) and *slide* past one another. Stretching a muscle fiber changes the degree of overlap between thick and thin filaments.

When muscle fiber length is too short, thin filaments overlap one another and this interferes with cross-bridge formation between thin and thick filaments (Fig. 37–17). At the other extreme, if fiber length is too long the extent of cross-bridge formation and overlapping is reduced and less tension is developed. Maximum tension develops when fiber lengths are established at which there is maximum cross-bridge formation and overlapping.

Clinically, this length-tension relationship of cardiac muscle is known as the Frank-Starling law of the heart, which simply states that an increase in left ventricular end-diastolic volume results in the generation of increased pressure with a consequent increase in the volume of blood ejected during the ensuing contraction. Beyond a certain volume, however, this mechanism becomes compromised and an increase in end-diastolic volume results instead in decreased pressures generated and decreased volume of blood ejected.

Preload refers to the distending force stretching the ventricular muscle just prior to contraction. While the increase in pressure generated is related to the volume of blood in the ventricle and thus to the length of the ventricular muscle fibers, the term preload is used clinically as an index of ventricular volume. This term is frequently used interchangeably to reflect left ventricular filling pressures or *venous return* to the heart. The significance of this intrinsic mechanism is that any increase in venous return to the heart (i.e., an increase in ventricular filling pressure) automatically forces an increase in CO by increasing the stroke volume. In the absence of mitral valve dysfunction, preload, or left ventricular end-diastolic volume (LVEDV), can be assessed clinically by monitoring the pulmonary capillary wedge pressure (PCWP). (For a detailed discussion of hemodynamic pressure monitoring, the reader is referred to Chap. 41.)

### Afterload

Afterload is defined as the load against which the heart muscle must exert its contractile force. The heart's ability to contract is influenced by the

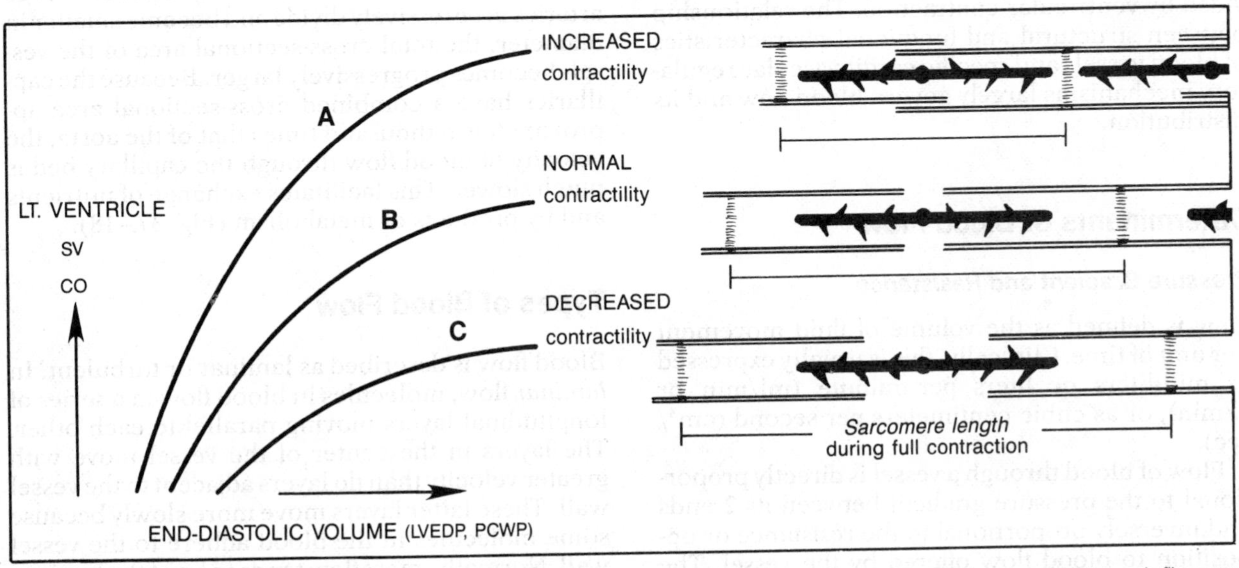


**Figure 37–17.** Length–tension relationship of the heart: The end-diastolic volume determines the end-diastolic length of myocardial muscle fibers and is proportional to the strike volume and cardiac output. Within physiologic limits, stretching of myocardial fibers as occurs with an increase in end-diastolic volume produces an augmentation of ventricular contraction. Beyond a certain volume, this mechanism is no longer operational and any further increase in end-diastolic volume results instead in a decrease in tension developed and volume ejected. Clinically, this phenomenon is known as the Frank-Starling law of the heart.

amount of wall tension above the preload that it must generate to eject blood. Clinically, afterload is largely determined by aortic end-diastolic pressure. It is also influenced by other factors such as aortic distensibility and peripheral vascular resistance. With a smaller afterload (i.e., low aortic pressure), the heart is able to contract more rapidly; against a large afterload (i.e., high aortic pressure), contraction is much slower. This is referred to as the *force-velocity* relationship. This relationship can be altered by changes in the initial muscle fiber length (i.e., preload), or by changes in contractility.

#### Myocardial Contractility

Contractility refers to the intrinsic capacity of myocardial muscle fibers to shorten and/or develop tension. Clinically, there is no single measurement that defines contractility. Rather, it can be inferred through clinical assessment and trends established via hemodynamic monitoring. An increase in contractility is referred to as positive inotropism, a decrease as negative inotropism.

## THE VASCULAR SYSTEM

The vascular system is composed of the systemic and pulmonary circulations serially connected in a closed system. These systems consist of arteries, capillaries, and veins, which function, respectively, to distribute blood to the tissues, facilitate exchange of metabolic substrates and by-products, and return blood to the heart. The driving force for blood flow throughout the vascular system is provided by ventricular contraction. The relationship between structural and functional characteristics of blood vessels and specific cardiovascular regulatory mechanisms largely govern blood flow and its distribution.

### Determinants of Blood Flow

#### Pressure Gradient and Resistance

*Flow* is defined as the volume of fluid movement per unit of time. Clinically, this is usually expressed as milliliters or liters per minute (ml/min or L/min), or as cubic centimeters per second ($cm^3$/sec).

Flow of blood through a vessel is directly proportional to the pressure gradient between its 2 ends and inversely proportional to the resistance or opposition to blood flow offered by the vessel. The relationship between flow (Q), pressure gradient (ΔP), and resistance (R) can be expressed mathematically as follows:

$$Q = \frac{\Delta P}{R} \qquad \text{Equation 1}$$

*Pressure* is defined as force per unit area or, in the case of blood, as the force exerted on the liquid per unit area. Because fluid moves from a region of greater pressure to one of lower pressure, flow is proportional to the inflow *minus* the outflow pressure differences.

*Resistance* is defined as a hindrance or opposition to force. Hemodynamically, it is a measure of the friction resulting from collisions between vessel wall and flowing blood; between cells and particulate matter in blood; and between the fluid molecules themselves. Vascular resistance is proportional to blood viscosity and vessel length, and inversely proportional to vessel radius. Thus, *vessel radius* is the major factor determining resistance in the vascular system; that is, small changes in vessel radius can lead to large changes in resistance.

The effect that these relationships have on blood flow is expressed by the following equation, known as Poiseuille's law:

$$Q = \frac{\Delta P\, r^4}{8\eta l} \qquad \text{Equation 2}$$

It relates blood flow (Q) to the change in pressure (P), the radius (r), the length of the vessel (l), and viscosity of the fluid ($\eta$).

### Velocity of Blood Flow

*Velocity* is the rate of fluid movement per unit time and is expressed as $cm^3$/sec. It varies inversely with the total cross-sectional area. As the aorta and large arteries progressively divide and become smaller in diameter, the total cross-sectional area of the vessels becomes progressively larger. Because the capillaries have a combined cross-sectional area approximately a thousand times that of the aorta, the velocity of blood flow through the capillary bed is much slower. This facilitates exchange of nutrients and by-products of metabolism (Fig. 37–18).

### Types of Blood Flow

Blood flow is described as laminar or turbulent. In *laminar* flow, molecules in blood flow in a series of longitudinal layers moving parallel to each other. The layers in the center of the vessel move with greater velocity than do layers adjacent to the vessel wall. These latter layers move more slowly because some molecules in the blood adhere to the vessel wall. Normally, most flow tends to be of the laminar type, and very quiet.

*Turbulent* flow consists of both laminar and cross-wise flow, forming whirlpools, swirls, and

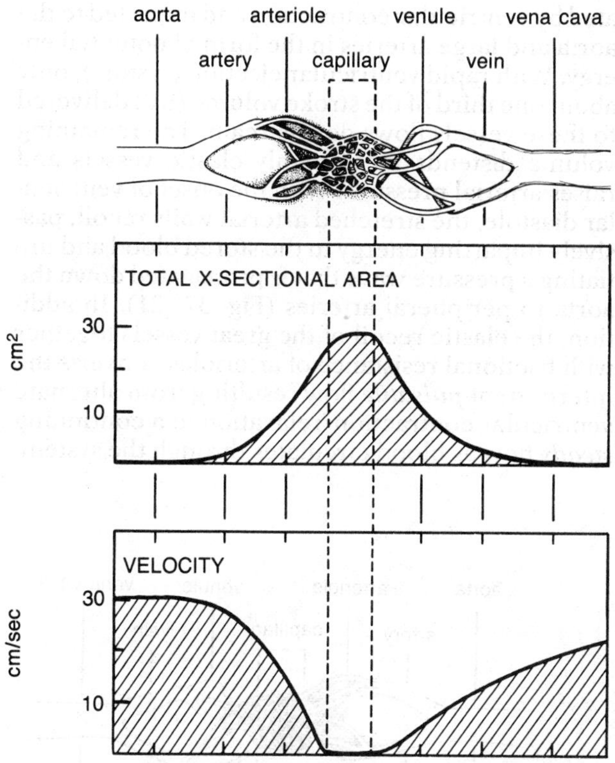


**Figure 37–18.** Relationship between total cross-sectional area and velocity of blood flow in the various vessels comprising the systemic circulation. The length–tension relationship of myocardial muscle fibers can be viewed in terms of sarcomere length, or the degree of overlap or cross-bridging between actin and myosin filaments. On the *A* length–tension curve, thin filaments overlap one another, thereby interfering with cross-bridge formation between actin and myosin filaments; on the *B* curve, maximum cross-bridging occurs between actin and myosin filaments; and on the *C* curve, actin and myosin filaments are stretched beyond maximum cross-bridging with fewer actin receptor sites available for binding with myosin filaments. (CO = cardiac output; SV = stroke volume; PCWP = pulmonary capillary wedge pressure; LVEDP = left ventricular end-diastolic pressure.)

eddy currents. Normally, such flow occurs in the ventricles and in the aorta during rapid ventricular ejection. It may also occur at bifurcations of blood vessels and in areas where the integrity of the blood vessel is disrupted by atheromatous plaques or dilatations.

Clinically, turbulent flow within the ventricles may give rise to a palpable *thrill* over the precordium and/or to third and fourth heart sounds or murmur on auscultation; when auscultated over a blood vessel (e.g., carotid artery or abdominal aorta), such flow is referred to as a *bruit*.

## Systemic Circulation

### *Structural Characteristics*

With each ventricular contraction blood is ejected into the aorta and large vessels and propelled downstream. Structurally, the walls of most blood vessels, including arteries and veins, are composed of 3 tissue layers: the tunica intima (elastic tissue, and the innermost vascular lining, the endothelium); tunica media (largely smooth muscle layer); and tunica adventitia (elastic and loose connective tissue). The size of each of these layers within the blood vessels varies based on their underlying function (Fig. 37–19).

The walls of the aorta and large arteries consist largely of elastic tissue, which befits their major functions as high-pressure reservoirs and conduits between the heart and arterioles. The arterioles and precapillary sphincters largely function to regulate distribution of blood to various capillary beds. Well endowed with smooth muscle layers, these structures are the major sites of change in radius, and thus resistance, within the vascular system. Approximately 80% of the pressure drop that occurs between the aorta and capillaries occurs in the arterioles (Fig. 37–20, *A*). Because these vessels offer the greatest frictional resistance to blood flow, they are referred to as "resistance" vessels.

Precapillary sphincters figure prominently in autoregulation, that is, local control of tissue perfusion (see below).

Capillaries are distinctly different from all other blood vessels as they consist of but a single layer of endothelial cells without any surrounding smooth muscle or elastic tissues. Capillaries differ structurally from organ to organ. In the brain, capillaries have extremely tight junctions, which function as part of the blood–brain barrier (see Fig. 6–11). In the kidney and gastrointestinal tract, the capillaries are distinguished by having fenestrations or pores that are well suited for the filtration and absorptive functions of these organs (see Fig. 21–3). The discontinuous capillaries, or sinusoids, of the liver are the most permeable, allowing movement of particles that are smaller than cells. These include all substances transported to the liver from the gut via the portal vein (see Chap. 47).

Blood flows from the capillaries into venules, which have some smooth muscle, the contraction of which can influence capillary pressure (see below). In the medium-sized and larger veins the walls are thinner than those in the arteries with a more prominent elastic layer. These vessels have the capacity to pool large volumes of blood with minimal changes in blood pressure, and they are frequently referred to as "capacitance" vessels. The muscular layer of the larger veins assists these vessels to act as reservoirs returning blood to the right heart in amounts necessary to meet body needs. The presence of one-way valves within the veins helps to prevent backward flow of blood, thereby assisting return of the blood to the heart. At any given point, about 75% of the total blood volume is within the venous system; about 20% in the low-

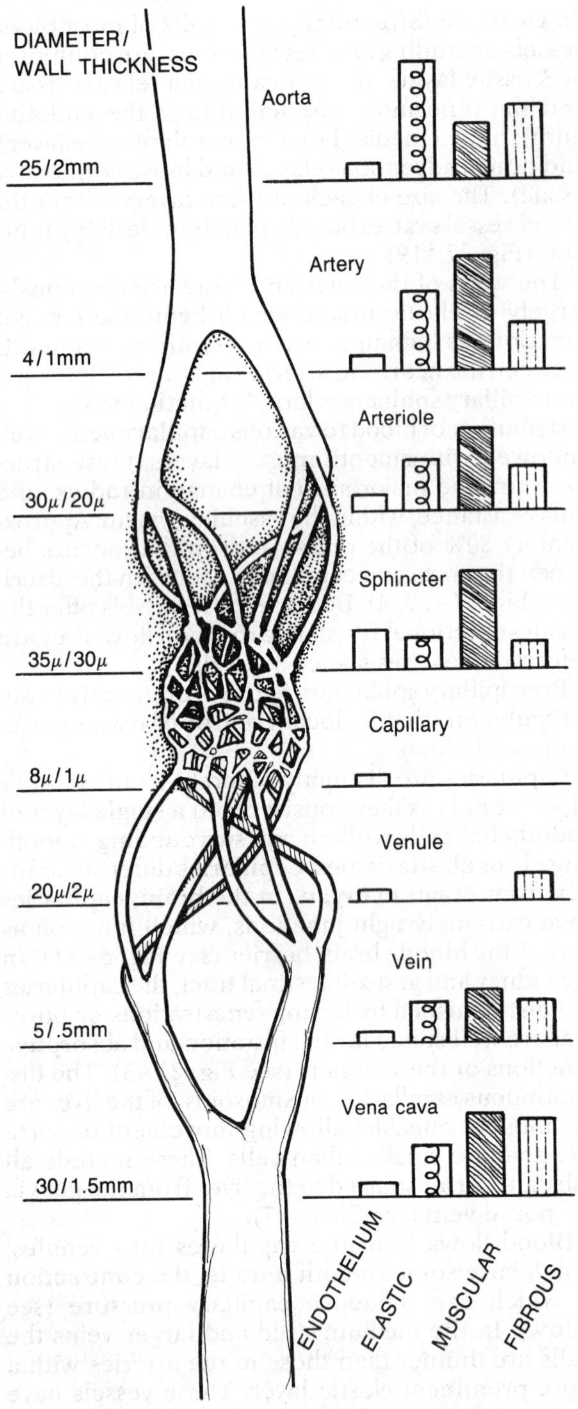


**Figure 37-19.** Structural characteristics of blood vessels in the systemic circulation including a comparison of the endothelial, elastic, muscle, and fibrous layers.

compliant arterial system; and 5% in the capillaries (Fig. 37-20, *B*).

### *Functional Characteristics*

**Arterial Pressure.** The energy necessary for the flow of blood through the vascular circuit is generated by ventricular contraction and imparted to the aorta and large arteries in the form of potential energy. With rapid ventricular ejection (systole), only about one third of the stroke volume (SV) delivered to these vessels flows downstream. The remaining volume distends these highly elastic vessels and raises arterial pressure. With the onset of ventricular diastole, the stretched arterial walls recoil, passively imparting energy to the stored blood and initiating a pressure wave that is propagated down the aorta to peripheral arteries (Fig. 37-21). In addition, the elastic recoil of the great vessels together with frictional resistance of arterioles converts the intermittent *pulsatile* flow resulting from alternate ventricular contraction/relaxation to a continuing *steady* flow as blood circulates through the system.

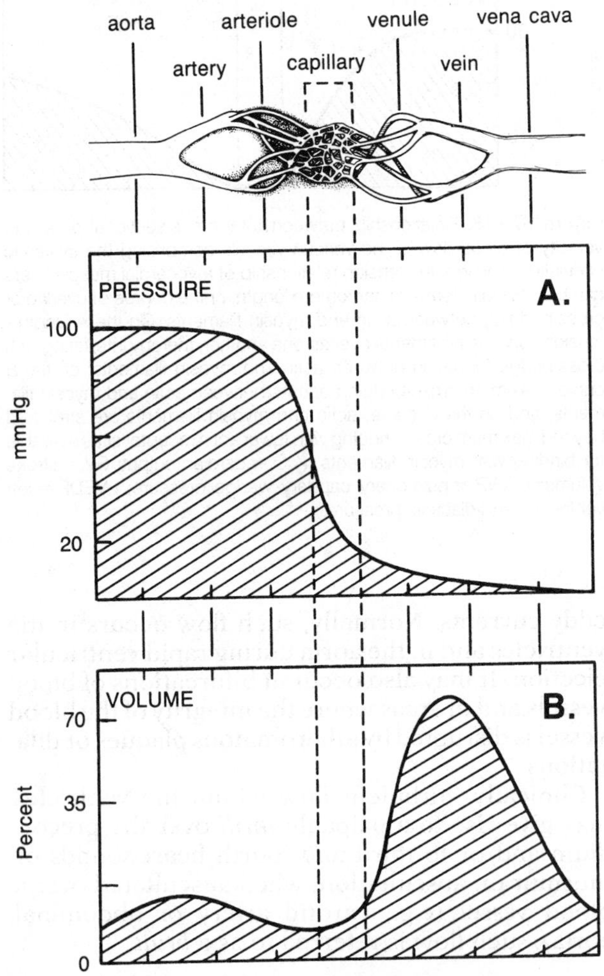


**Figure 37-20.** (*A*) The greatest decrease in systemic blood pressure occurs at the level of the arterioles, also referred to as "resistance" vessels because they offer the greatest frictional resistance to blood flow. Pressure is at its lowest in the venous system. (*B*) At any given moment, the greatest percentage of total blood volume is found within the venous system. These vessels are known as "capacitance" vessels because they can accommodate a large volume of blood with minimal rise in pressure.

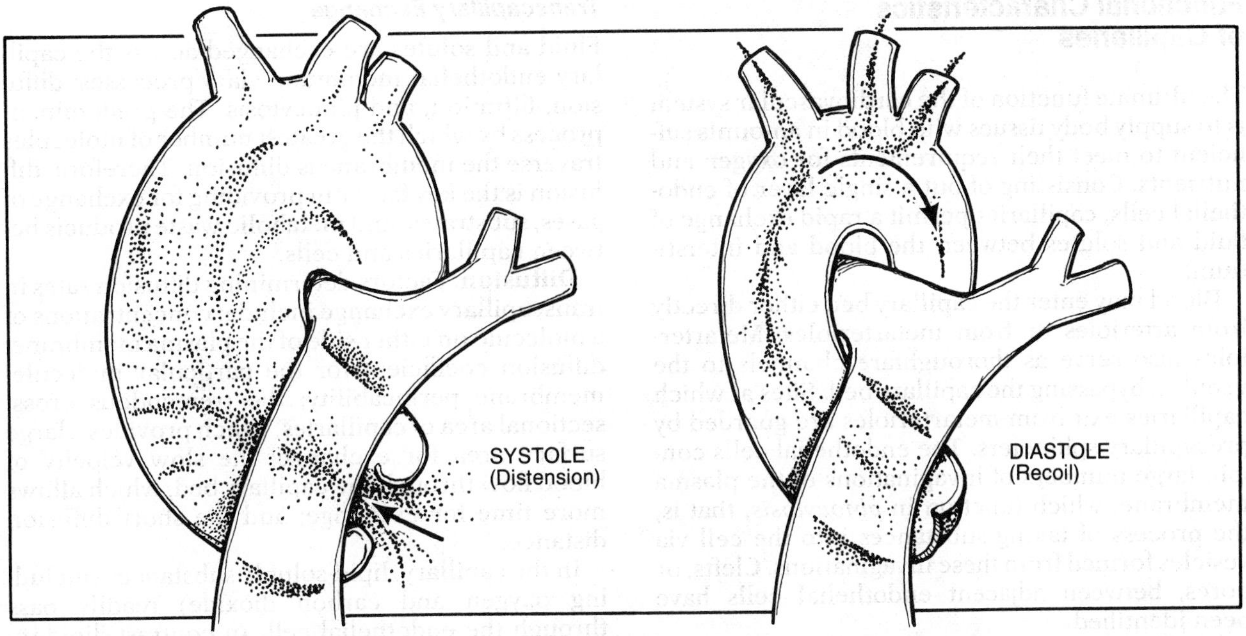


**Figure 37–21.** During peak systolic ejection only about one third of the stroke volume delivered to the aorta and great vessels flows downstream. The remaining volume distends these highly elastic vessels, which, with the onset of ventricular diastole, recoil, passively imparting energy to the stored blood and initiating a pressure wave that drives blood throughout the systemic circulation. The elastic recoil of the great vessels coupled with the frictional resistance offered by the arterioles is instrumental in converting the pulsatile blood associated with the cardiac cycle to a continuing steady blood flow as blood circulates throughout the system.

***Arterial Pressure Waveform.*** The arterial pressure waveform reflects the pressure changes that occur in the large arteries during the cardiac cycle (Fig. 37–22). The maximum pressure reached during peak ventricular ejection is called *systolic* pressure; the minimum pressure occurs just before ventricular ejection begins and is called *diastolic* pressure. The minimal diastolic pressure is determined by the systolic pressure, the arterial recoil, systemic vascular resistance, and the length of diastole.

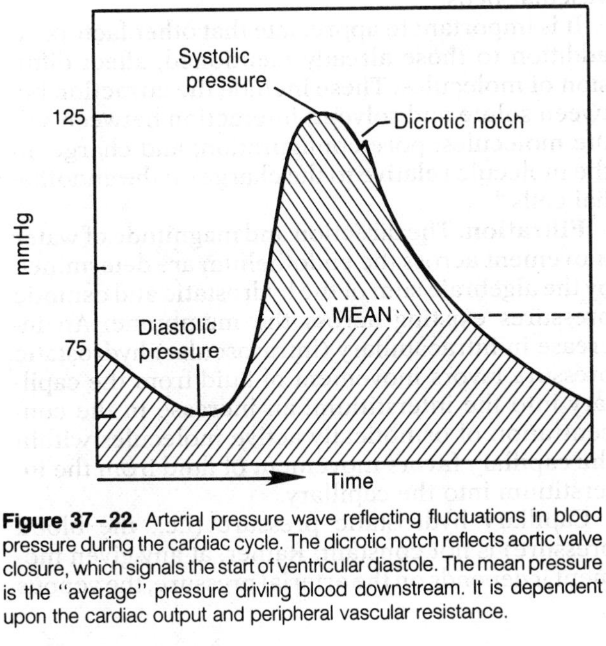


**Figure 37–22.** Arterial pressure wave reflecting fluctuations in blood pressure during the cardiac cycle. The dicrotic notch reflects aortic valve closure, which signals the start of ventricular diastole. The mean pressure is the "average" pressure driving blood downstream. It is dependent upon the cardiac output and peripheral vascular resistance.

***Pulse Pressure.*** The pulse pressure is the difference between the systolic and diastolic pressures. The magnitude of the pulse pressure is determined by the stroke volume, the rapidity of ventricular ejection, and the arterial capacitance. Pressures will be increased if the volume of blood ejected is increased; if the volume is ejected more quickly, or if arteries are resistant to expansion as occurs, for example, in atherosclerosis.[3]

***Mean Arterial Pressure.*** The mean arterial pressure (MAP) is the *average* pressure driving blood downstream throughout the cardiac cycle. It is dependent upon the cardiac output (SV × HR) and peripheral vascular resistance (elasticity of large arteries; contractile state of arterioles), and both of these parameters are closely regulated via basic cardiovascular control mechanisms (see below). The MAP can be approximated by adding the diastolic pressure to one third of the pulse pressure. This takes into consideration that diastole lasts longer than systole.

## Functional Characteristics of Capillaries

The ultimate function of the cardiovascular system is to supply body tissues with blood in amounts sufficient to meet their requirements for oxygen and nutrients. Consisting of but a single layer of endothelial cells, capillaries permit a rapid exchange of fluid and solutes between the blood and interstitium.

Blood may enter the capillary bed either directly from arterioles or from metarterioles. Metarterioles also serve as thoroughfare channels to the venules, bypassing the capillary bed. Sites at which capillaries exit from metarterioles are guarded by precapillary sphincters. The endothelial cells contain large numbers of invaginations of the plasma membrane, which function in *pinocytosis*, that is, the process of taking substances into the cell via vesicles formed from these invaginations. Clefts, or pores, between adjacent endothelial cells have been identified.

Capillary distribution is variable from tissue to tissue. Capillaries are found to be more numerous in metabolically active tissues (e.g., cardiac and skeletal muscle, and glands); less active tissues (e.g., subcutaneous tissue, cartilage) have a lower capillary density. (Structural differences of capillaries from organ to organ were mentioned earlier.)

Blood flow through the capillaries is not uniform but depends upon the contractile state of arterioles and metarterioles. Through rhythmic alternate dilation and constriction (*vasomotion*) of the precapillary sphincter, blood flow is controlled, in part, based on the metabolic needs of the various tissues. Vasomotion of precapillary sphincters may also fluctuate in response to intravascular pressures (myogenic theory of autoregulation; see below). According to the theory, an increase in arterial pressure stretches the smooth muscle layer of metarterioles and precapillary sphincters, thereby inducing vasoconstriction. In this way, high arterial pressures may be prevented from being applied to the capillary bed.

While capillaries are very narrow in structure, the total resistance to flow offered by capillaries is not as significant as that of the arterioles. This is so for at least 2 reasons: first, the total number of capillaries provides a great cross-sectional area for flow; and second, in contrast to arterioles, there is an absence of smooth muscle and innervation in capillary walls.

Velocity of blood flow through the capillary bed is exceedingly slow and attributed to the tremendous cross-sectional area presented by the capillaries (see Fig. 37–18). This reduced velocity of flow facilitates exchange between the blood and the tissues.

### *Transcapillary Exchange*

Fluid and solutes are exchanged across the capillary endothelial membrane via 3 processes: diffusion, filtration, and pinocytosis. The predominant process by which the greatest number of molecules traverse the membrane is diffusion. Therefore, diffusion is the key factor in providing for exchange of gases, substrates, and metabolic waste products between capillaries and cells.

**Diffusion.** Factors determining diffusion rates in transcapillary exchange include: concentrations of a molecule on either side of the plasma membrane; diffusion coefficient for the particular molecule; membrane permeability; the tremendous cross-sectional area of capillaries, which provides a large surface area for exchange; the slow velocity of blood flow through the capillary bed, which allows more time for exchange; and the short diffusion distance.

In the capillary, lipid-soluble substances (including oxygen and carbon dioxide) readily pass through the endothelial cell. In contrast, lipid-insoluble molecules do not pass freely, and their passage through the endothelium is largely restricted to clefts, or pores, located within the membrane or between adjacent cells. Water and water-soluble molecules (e.g., electrolytes, glucose, and urea) traverse the endothelium in this manner. Even so, capillary pores offer little restriction to the movement of small molecules such as water, and diffusion is very rapid.

With lipid-insoluble molecules of increasing size, diffusion through the capillaries becomes progressively more restricted, becoming minimal at molecular weights of about 60,000 and above. In general, the size of the pores limits movement of larger substances; and the size of molecules that easily penetrate capillary endothelium varies in different vascular beds.

It is important to appreciate that other factors, in addition to those already mentioned, affect diffusion of molecules. These include the attraction between solute and solvent; interaction between solute molecules; pore configuration; and charge on the molecule relative to the charge on the endothelial cells.[4]

**Filtration.** The direction and magnitude of water movement across the endothelium are determined by the algebraic sum of the hydrostatic and osmotic pressures existing across the membrane. An increase in intracapillary (intravascular) hydrostatic pressure favors movement of fluid from the capillary into the interstitium; an increase in the concentration of osmotically active molecules within the capillary favors movement of fluid from the interstitium into the capillary.

Capillary hydrostatic pressure (i.e., the blood pressure) is not constant. Rather, at any given moment it depends on the arterial pressure, the venous pressure, and on the precapillary (arterioles and precapillary sphincters) and postcapillary (venules) contractile state. An increase in arterial or venous pressures increases capillary hydrostatic pressure, whereas a reduction in these pressures decreases capillary hydrostatic pressure. An increase in resistance offered by the arterioles or by closure of precapillary sphincters decreases capillary pressure, whereas greater venous resistance increases capillary pressure. Additionally, a given increase in venous pressure produces a greater effect on capillary hydrostatic pressure than a similar increase in arterial pressure. Approximately 80% of the increase in venous pressure is transmitted back to the capillary bed.

Although capillary hydrostatic pressure varies from organ to organ and is subject to gravitational forces, an average pressure at the arteriolar end of a capillary is about 32 mmHg, whereas at the venule end the pressure is approximately 15 mmHg. This net capillary hydrostatic pressure is the principle force underlying filtration across the endothelium. It is opposed by the interstitial fluid pressure, that is, tissue pressure outside the capillary, which more recently has been determined to be from −1 to −7 mmHg. The result is a greater hydrostatic force for capillary filtration.

**Osmotic Forces.** Maintenance of intravascular volume is the very basis of capillary dynamics. The major factor that acts as a counterforce to capillary hydrostatic pressure, thereby restraining fluid loss from the capillaries, is the osmotic pressure exerted by the plasma proteins. The average osmotic pressure is about 25 mmHg. Because plasma proteins are essentially confined to the intravascular space, the small osmotic pressure they exert plays an important role in the fluid exchange across the capillary wall. This is especially so because electrolytes, which are responsible for the major fraction of plasma osmotic pressure, are practically in equal concentrations on either side of the capillary endothelium. The relative permeability of the membrane influences the actual magnitude of the osmotic pressure.

Of the plasma proteins, albumin is the major protein in determining osmotic pressure. The normal concentration of albumin in blood ranges between 3.5–5.0 g/100 ml. At higher plasma concentrations the osmotic force albumin exerts becomes disproportionately greater, whereas at low plasma concentrations (as occurs in interstitial fluid), the osmotic force exerted by albumin becomes weak to absent. One explanation for this behavior of the albumin molecule is its net negative charge at normal blood pH, and thus its attraction and retention of cations (principally sodium) in the intravascular space (the Gibbs-Donnan effect). While the endothelium is largely impermeable to albumin, small amounts do escape into the interstitial fluid where they exert a very small osmotic force (0.1–5.0 mmHg).

**Starling Hypothesis.** The Starling hypothesis describes the relationship between hydrostatic and osmotic pressures and the role these forces play in regulating fluid movement across the capillary endothelium. It can be expressed mathematically as the following:[5]

$$\text{Fluid movement} = k[(P_c - \pi_i) - (P_i + \pi_p)] \qquad \text{Equation 3}$$

where:

$P_c$ = capillary hydrostatic pressure
$P_i$ = interstitial fluid hydrostatic pressure
$\pi_p$ = plasma protein osmotic pressure
$\pi_i$ = interstitial fluid osmotic pressure
k = filtration constant for the capillary membrane

*Filtration*, that is, movement of fluid out of the capillary and into the interstitium, occurs when the algebraic sum is positive; and *absorption* occurs when it is negative (i.e., movement of fluid from the interstitium into the capillary).

Classically, it has been thought that filtration occurs at the arteriolar end of the capillary and absorption at the venule end (Fig. 37–23). However, more recent observations have revealed that in some capillary beds (e.g., renal glomerulus) filtration occurs for the entire length of the capillary bed; in others (e.g., intestinal mucosa), only absorption occurs. In the lungs, capillary hydrostatic pressure is estimated to be about 8 mmHg, while

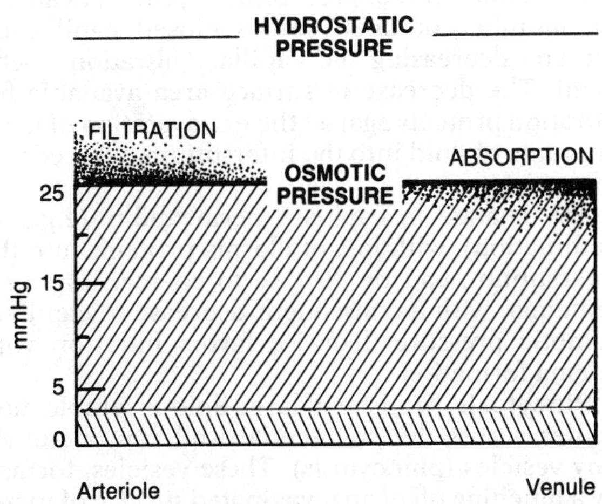


**Figure 37–23.** Capillary fluid dynamics. Forces regulating fluid movement across the capillary endothelium include: (1) capillary hydrostatic pressure; (2) interstitial fluid hydrostatic pressure; (3) plasma protein osmotic pressure; and (4) interstitial fluid osmotic pressure. Net forces exerted at the arteriole end of the capillary favor *filtration*; forces at work at the venule end favor fluid *reabsorption*.

osmotic pressure is 28 mmHg. Thus, these forces across the membrane favor absorption. Normally, fluid and a small amount of protein that leaks out of the pulmonary capillaries are removed via the lymphatics and returned to the blood.

**Capillary Filtration Coefficient.** The rate of movement of fluid across the endothelium depends on other factors in addition to the algebraic sum of hydrostatic and osmotic forces across the endothelium. These factors, collectively referred to as the capillary filtration coefficient, include the surface area available for filtration; distance across the capillary wall; and the viscosity of the filtrate.

**Alterations in Hydrostatic-Osmotic Balance.** Normally, changes in arterial pressure have little effect on filtration because such changes are compensated for by adjustments of precapillary resistance vessels (autoregulation). Therefore, capillary hydrostatic pressure remains essentially unchanged. In the scenario of a severe drop in arterial pressure as occurs, for example, in hemorrhage, a decrease in capillary hydrostatic pressure may occur. In this case, arteriolar vasoconstriction (as by the sympathetic nervous system), coupled with a fall in venous pressure resulting from the blood loss, may underlie the decrease in capillary hydrostatic pressure. Concomitantly, the consequent decrease in perfusion, and hence decreased oxygen supply to the tissues, results in release of vasodilator metabolites, which induce relaxation of the arterioles. The decrease in capillary hydrostatic pressure as a consequence of these several factors causes absorption to predominate over filtration, thereby serving to restore blood volume.

An increase in venous resistance distal to the capillary bed causes an increase in capillary hydrostatic pressure, thereby favoring filtration. However, vasomotion of precapillary sphincters affects the number of open versus closed capillaries, thereby decreasing the capillary filtration coefficient. The decrease in surface area available for filtration protects against the extravasation of large amounts of fluid into the interstitium, with edema formation.

Any change in capillary permeability (e.g., inflammation), with loss of plasma proteins into the interstitium, can predispose to edema. Hypoproteinemia, with a consequent decrease in capillary osmotic pressure, likewise favors filtration with edema formation.

**Pincytosis.** Transfer of large lipid-insoluble molecules across the endothelial wall can occur via tiny vesicles (pinocytosis). These vesicles, formed by a pinching off of an invaginated surface of membrane, can take up substances on one side of the endothelial wall (*endocytosis*) and move across the cell and extrude their contents on the other side (*exocytosis*). The extent of this pinocytotic activity varies from tissue to tissue and increases from the arteriolar to the venule end of the capillary.

### Venous Pressure

The venous system serves as the final conduit through which blood flows in returning to the right heart. The driving force for venous return to the heart is the pressure difference between peripheral venules (approximately 15 mmHg) and the right atrium (approximately 0-6 mmHg), also referred to as *central venous pressure* (CVP). While this pressure difference is small, it is adequate because of the low resistance to blood flow offered by the thin-walled, large-diameter veins.

At any given moment in time, approximately 70% of the blood volume is present in the systemic venous system (see Fig. 37-20), but the venous pressure averages less than 10 mmHg. In contrast, systemic arteries contain less than 15% of the total blood volume but at pressures of approximately 100 mmHg. This ability of the veins to accommodate large volume increases with but small increases in pressure is referred to as *venous capacitance*.

Venous return to the heart is enhanced by several mechanisms. Sympathetic stimulation causes contraction of venous smooth muscle, thereby increasing venous pressure and driving more blood out of the veins and into the right heart. The venous "skeletal pump" functions to increase venous return. During skeletal muscle contraction in the extremities, veins within the muscles are compressed. This decreases venous capacity and forces more blood back to the heart. The presence of valves in the venous system also enhances venous return by helping to maintain forward flow of blood toward the heart. In this respect, valves play an especially important role in counteracting the effects of gravity in the upright posture, which might otherwise cause blood to pool in the lower extremities.

Venous return to the heart is also enhanced by the "respiratory pump." During quiet inspiration, the thoracic cavity expands, causing intrathoracic pressures to become more negative. Concomitantly, with the descent of the diaphragm, intra-abdominal pressures become more positive. The net effect of these pressure gradients is to increase venous return on inspiration, thereby enhancing cardiac output.

### Lymphatics

The lymphatic system consists of a closed-end network of highly permeable lymph capillaries anchored to surrounding connective tissue by fine filaments. The lymph capillaries drain into larger vessels that eventually return the plasma capillary filtrate to the systemic circulation via the right and left subclavian veins. This process is facilitated by intermittent skeletal muscle activity, contraction of lymphatic vessels, and the presence of one-way valves. Significantly, the lymphatics provide the only means whereby protein (albumin) that leaves the intravascular space is returned to the blood. Were it not for the lymphatic system, protein accumulation in the interstitium would increase the interstitial osmotic force, drawing fluid from the blood capillaries and resulting in edema.

The lymphatic system also plays a significant role in the absorption of fats from the gastrointestinal tract (principally chylomicrons) to the circulating blood (see Chap. 47).

### Pulmonary Circulation

The pulmonary circulation occurs in concert with the systemic circulation and receives approximately the same cardiac output. Its primary function is to perfuse the lungs, facilitating the exchange of gases between the alveoli and pulmonary capillaries (see Fig. 28–11).

Structurally, the pulmonary vasculature is a highly capacitant system, its capacitance being largely attributed to its thin-walled blood vessels with minimal smooth muscle and to the tremendous cross-sectional area of the capillary bed. These features underlie its status as a low-resistance, low-pressure system. It also acts as a low-pressure reservoir capable of transiently increasing left ventricular end-diastolic volume and thus cardiac output.

Pulmonary capillary hydrostatic pressures are approximately 8–12 mmHg, while capillary osmotic pressure is the same as that of the systemic circulation, about 28 mmHg. Consequently, these pressures do *not* favor filtration, thereby preventing fluid from accumulating in the pulmonary interstitium and entering the alveoli under normal circumstances. In addition, there is an extensive lymphatic system throughout the pulmonary system that functions to return to the blood any capillary filtrate or plasma proteins that leak out of the pulmonary capillaries.

## REGULATION OF CARDIOVASCULAR FUNCTION

The major variable being regulated via the control and integration of cardiovascular function is the mean systemic arterial blood pressure (MAP). MAP is determined by 2 factors: cardiac output and systemic vascular resistance.

$$\text{MAP} = \text{Cardiac output} \times \text{systemic vascular resistance} \qquad \text{Equation 4}$$

The cardiac output reflects flow (per minute); the systemic vascular resistance reflects total arteriolar resistance (in dynes/sec/cm$^{-5}$). Thus, there is an intimate relationship among pressure, flow, and resistance. It is obvious from the equation that any condition that increases either CO or SVR (assuming the other factor remains constant) will cause an increase in MAP; conversely, any decrease in CO or SVR (if the other factor remains unchanged) will decrease MAP.

The cardiovascular system has intricate mechanisms for regulating these parameters in such a way that changes in MAP are minimized. Some of these mechanisms (neural and hormonal) act swiftly (within seconds) to restore and/or maintain MAP; others (renal-body fluid, renin-angiotensin system) act more slowly (several days and longer). Commonly, peripheral perfusion involves a dual control mechanism mediated centrally by the central nervous system and locally via autoregulation.

In this section the control of the peripheral circulation is discussed, following which the factors involved in the control of cardiac output are addressed.

### Control of Peripheral Circulation

The peripheral circulation is basically under dual control; centrally it is controlled by the nervous system and locally by autoregulation. The blood vessels primarily involved in regulating blood flow throughout the body are the arterioles (resistance vessels). These vessels offer the greatest resistance to flow of blood and therefore play a significant role in the maintenance of MAP.

#### Vascular Smooth Muscle

Structurally, vascular smooth muscle comprises a high percentage of the arteriolar walls, and it is the contractile state of this tissue layer that is largely responsible for the control of vascular tone, total peripheral resistance, and the distribution of blood throughout the body. Vascular tone is maintained through innervation of arteriolar smooth muscle by the sympathetic nervous system. In addition, vascular smooth muscle also responds directly to hormones and other humoral substances (e.g., norepinephrine, epinephrine, histamine, angiotensin, and prostaglandins), without evidence of electrical excitation. Vascular smooth muscle is also sensitive to local environmental changes. Alterations in pH, $PaO_2$, and body temperature, for example, have a direct effect on vascular tone (autoregulation).

#### Intrinsic Control of Peripheral Blood Flow: Autoregulation

Blood flow appears to be adjusted to the existing metabolic demands in various tissues, thereby maintaining a constancy of blood flow. This mechanism is referred to as *autoregulation*. The mechanism underlying this activity is not known, but 3 explanations have been suggested, including the tissue pressure hypothesis, myogenic hypothesis, and metabolic hypothesis.[6]

With respect to the *tissue pressure* theory, an increase in blood flow to the tissues increases hydrostatic blood pressure, thereby increasing capillary filtration. There is a net transfer of fluid from the intravascular to interstitial spaces. The consequent increase in interstitial (tissue) pressure (turgor) is believed to compress tiny, thin-walled blood vessels, thereby reducing blood flow to the tissue. A decrease in blood flow would elicit the opposite response.

The *myogenic* concept suggests that arteriolar smooth muscle responds directly to an increased stretch associated with an abrupt elevation in arterial pressure by increasing its tone. Conversely, decreased stretch associated with a reduction in arterial pressure causes vascular smooth muscle to decrease its tone. This mechanism may be at work when one changes position, as, for example, from lying to standing. With this change in position, a large change in hydrostatic pressure occurs in the lower extremities. Arterioles and precapillary vessels constrict in response to this imposed stretch, resulting in decreased blood flow to the capillary bed. As flow decreases, capillary filtration diminishes until the intravascular osmotic pressure and the increase in interstitial fluid pressure balance the elevated capillary hydrostatic pressure associated with the position change. Without an increase in arteriolar vascular tone upon standing, capillary hydrostatic pressure in the lower extremities would reach such high levels that large fluid volumes would be filtered from the capillaries into the interstitium, with consequent edema formation.

According to the *metabolic* hypothesis, blood flow is governed by the metabolic demands of the tissue. Any activity that reduces the oxygen supply to the tissues results in the formation and secretion of vasodilator metabolites (e.g., adenosine, lactic acid, carbon dioxide, histamine, potassium ions, hydrogen ions, etc.) by the tissues. These metabolites act locally to dilate blood vessels, thereby increasing tissue perfusion. When blood supply to a tissue has been interrupted, the reduced blood flow triggers activities that result in local vasodilatation. When flow is re-established in these tissues a *reactive* hyperemia results.

Similarly, when any tissue becomes highly active (e.g., exercising muscle), the rate of blood flow through the tissue increases. The enhanced metabolism rapidly uses up oxygen and nutrients. In response, the tissue releases large quantities of vasodilator substances, which in turn dilate local blood vessels, thereby increasing local blood flow. This response is referred to as *active* hyperemia.

### *Extrinsic Control of Peripheral Blood Flow*

Within the central nervous system, cardiovascular reflex responses are mediated by centers in the medulla (cardiac and vasomotor centers), hypothalamus, and other brain centers. Such responses are based upon sensory (afferent) input received from baroreceptors, chemoreceptors, and other peripheral receptors located within the heart, blood vessels, and lungs; these, in turn, act on cardiac and vascular smooth muscle to influence heart rate, myocardial contractility, systemic vascular resistance, and venous capacitance.

**Neural Regulation: Sympathetic Vasoconstriction.** Neural regulation of peripheral circulation is accomplished via the autonomic nervous system. Of its 2 branches, the sympathetic and parasympathetic systems, the sympathetic regulation of circulation is more important. Sympathetic innervation is accomplished primarily by alteration of the number of impulses passing from central vasoconstrictor regions of the vasomotor center via the vasoconstrictor fibers of sympathetic nerves to the blood vessels. The vasoconstrictor regions are tonically active and the usual tone of peripheral blood vessels is one of slight vasoconstriction.

Stimulation of vasoconstrictor centers, whether via reflexes or humoral stimuli (e.g., norepinephrine, epinephrine, and antidiuretic hormone, among others), enhances their tonic activity, resulting in an increase in the frequency of impulses reaching the small arteries and arterioles. This enhanced sympathetic activity in turn elicits vasoconstriction of these resistance vessels, and by doing so, changes the flow of blood to the tissues. Inhibition of vasconstrictor areas reduces their tonic activity, thereby diminishing the frequency of impulses to the blood vessels, resulting in vasodilatation.

Vasomotor innervation of large vessels, particularly veins, makes it possible for sympathetic stimulation to change the volume of these vessels, and thereby to alter the distribution of blood volume in the peripheral circulation. One consequence of these activities is the increase in venous return to the heart, which in turn enhances cardiac output, thereby impacting on overall cardiovascular function.

The medullary vasomotor center, in addition to controlling peripheral circulation (i.e., the degree of vasoconstriction), also controls heart activity. It does so via both sympathetic and parasympathetic innervation. Sympathetic stimulation to the heart increases heart rate and contractility; parasympathetic stimulation decreases heart rate and contractility. Thus, the vasomotor center can regulate the degree of heart activity and usually does so in conjunction with its effect on the peripheral circulation.

It is important to note that the role played by the parasympathetic innervation in the direct regulation of peripheral circulation is minor. The parasympathetic system does supply blood vessels of the head, viscera, genitalia, bladder, and large bowel, but it does not innervate skeletal muscle and skin. Thus, because only a small portion of the resistance vasculature receives parasympathetic stimulation, its effect on total systemic resistance is small. Rather, parasympathetic influence is largely exerted via its direct effects on cardiac function.

Activity of the vasomotor center is modulated by higher brain centers, including areas in the cerebral cortex, hypothalamus, and brainstem. These areas have a profound effect on the activities of the vasomotor center and, in turn, on the sympathetic vasoconstrictor system of the body. Stimulation of the vasoconstrictor system by these areas of the brain can further enhance systemic vasoconstriction; inhibition can reduce the degree of vasoconstrictor tone, thereby causing vasodilatation.

**Vascular Reflexes.** The medullary vasomotor center, which mediates sympathetic and parasympathetic influence on both the heart and the circulatory system, is in turn influenced by impulses arising in baroreceptors, cardiopulmonary baroreceptors, and chemoreceptors.

***Baroreceptors.*** Baroreceptors are sensory organs especially sensitive to stretch and located in the carotid sinus and aortic arch. Since the degree of stretch is directly related to pressure within the artery, baroreceptors are actually *pressure* receptors. Impulses generated within these receptors travel via afferent (sensory) neurons to the vasomotor center in the medulla. The input received determines the outflow via the parasympathetic system to the heart and the sympathetic system to the heart, arterioles, veins, and adrenal medulla. The effect generated by this system is exerted transiently, within seconds, and helps to maintain MAP within its narrow physiologic range (90–100 mmHg) on a moment-to-moment basis.

If a decrease in MAP occurs, the baroreceptors, sensing a change in the degree of stretch, send impulses into the medullary centers and elicit the following responses: (1) increase in heart rate as sympathetic stimulation to the heart is enhanced, while parasympathetic stimulation is decreased; (2) increase in myocardial contractility because of direct stimulation to the ventricular myocardium; (3) increase in systemic vascular resistance associated with enhanced vasoconstriction of resistance vessels; and (4) increase in venous vasoconstriction due to increase in sympathetic output to venous smooth muscle, thereby increasing venous return to the heart.

The net result of these activities is to increase cardiac output (via increased heart rate and stroke volume) and to increase total systemic vascular resistance (via arteriolar vasoconstriction).

$$MAP = CO \times SVR \qquad \text{Equation 5}$$

In considering this equation it is easy to appreciate how these events return MAP to within the normal physiologic range. In contrast, when MAP increases for whatever reason, it causes increased firing of the baroreceptors, which decreases output from the medullary vasomotor center. The result is a compensatory decrease in cardiac output and systemic vascular resistance, thereby reducing MAP.

***Cardiopulmonary Baroreceptors.*** In addition to the carotid sinus and aortic body baroreceptors, there are also cardiopulmonary baroreceptors with sympathetic and parasympathetic innervation. Located in the atria, ventricles, and pulmonary vasculature, these receptors are tonically active and can alter peripheral resistance with changes in intracardiac, venous, or pulmonary vascular pressures.

***Chemoreceptors.*** Chemoreceptors are sensory receptors located peripherally in the carotid body and aortic arch; they monitor plasma levels of oxygen, carbon dioxide, and hydrogen ions, and plasma pH. Although more intimately concerned with regulation of respiration (see Chap. 28), they do influence cardiovascular function as well. For example, a reduction in blood oxygen tension ($PaO_2$) is sensed by the chemoreceptors, which send impulses to the medullary vascular centers. The vasomotor response results in an increased tone of resistance and capacitance vessels, thereby increasing arterial pressure and peripheral blood flow.

**Humoral Regulation of Peripheral Blood Flow.** Humoral regulation of peripheral circulation involves regulation by substances found in body fluids, such as hormones and vasodilator agents, as well as the effect of ions and other chemical factors on vascular control. Epinephrine and norepinephrine are hormonal substances secreted by the adrenal medulla in response to sympathetic stimulation. These substances exert a profound effect on peripheral blood vessels. In skeletal muscle, the action of epinephrine is dose related. In low concentrations it dilates resistance vessels; in high concentrations it produces vasoconstriction. In the skin, epinephrine's effect is one of vasoconstriction alone. The primary effect of norepinephrine in all vascular beds is vasoconstriction.

Other humoral agents include angiotensin and vasopressin. In response to a decrease in arterial pressure, the kidneys secrete renin, which initiates a series of reactions resulting in the formation of angiotensin II (see Fig. 21–9). Angiotensin II exerts a potent pressor effect by causing vasoconstriction of blood vessels throughout the body.

In addition to its pressor effect, angiotensin stimulates secretion of the hormone aldosterone by the adrenal cortex. This hormone in turn stimulates sodium reabsorption by the renal tubules along with an obligatory reabsorption of water. In so doing, in conjunction with antidiuretic hormone (ADH), it contributes significantly to the maintenance of body fluid volume.

ADH (vasopressin) exerts an even more powerful vasoconstrictor effect on the peripheral vasculature than does angiotensin II. In addition, ADH plays an all-important role in the maintenance of body fluid volume by its effect on water reabsorption in the cells of the distal renal tubules and collecting ducts (see Chap. 21).

Vasodilator agents usually exert a more localized effect and consequently their role may be more important in autoregulation. Specific agents include, among others, bradykinin, histamine, and prostaglandins.

Bradykinin triggers a very powerful dilatation of resistance vessels as well as an increase in capillary permeability. Histamine is similar to bradykinin in its overall effect, causing intense arteriolar vasodilatation and increased capillary porosity. This enables large quantities of fluid to leak out of the intravascular space into the tissues. Prostaglandins may exert either a vasoconstrictor or vasodilator effect, but most of the important prostaglandins seem to exert the latter effect.

## Control of Cardiac Output

Cardiac output (CO) is the product of the heart rate (HR) times the stroke volume (SV).

$$CO = HR \times SV \qquad \text{Equation 6}$$

Stroke volume in turn is determined by preload, afterload, and contractility. Consequently, factors to be considered in the control of CO include HR, myocardial contractility, preload, and afterload.

Of these factors, HR and myocardial contractility are basically limited to the heart itself. HR is directly controlled by sympathetic and parasympathetic stimulation. Sympathetic stimulation increases HR and contractility; parasympathetic stimulation decreases HR and the heart's contractile force. Contractility is also dependent upon other variables such as the inherent degree of overlap of actin and myosin filaments and the rate of tension development and myocardial muscle fiber shortening.

Preload and afterload depend on *both* the heart and the vascular system. On the one hand, preload and afterload are important determinants of CO; on the other hand, these parameters are themselves determined by CO and the status of the vascular system. Berne and Levy designate preload and afterload as "coupling factors" because they constitute the functional coupling between the heart and blood vessels. The heart provides the pump to circulate blood through the vascular system; the blood vessels, in turn, determine in part the preload (venous return) and afterload (aortic end-diastolic volume) and therefore regulate the quantity of blood that the heart ultimately pumps throughout the cardiovascular system per unit of time.

When considering the control of CO, it is important to recall the Frank-Starling law of the heart (see Fig. 37–17), which states that within its physiologic limit the heart will pump whatever amount of blood that enters the right atrium, *automatically*. The volume of blood that can be pumped without extrinsic sympathetic stimulation can reach as high as 10–13 liters/minute. In other words, the heart is capable of pumping far more than the 4–8 liters/minute that normally returns to it from the peripheral circulation under resting conditions. Thus, it is the *rate of venous return* (i.e., the preload), and not the pumping action of the heart, that determines CO. This phenomenon has been described by Guyton as the "permissive" role of the heart.

Factors that determine the rate of blood return to the right heart include arterial pressure and total peripheral vascular resistance. As long as arterial blood pressure remains within normal physiologic range, the ultimate control of CO actually occurs at the tissue level where each organ adjusts its own blood supply (via vasoconstriction and vasodilatation of its vascular bed) to meet its specific needs. The venous return to the heart actually represents the sum of all the local blood flows throughout the body.

## REFERENCES


1. Cohn, PF: Clinical Cardiovascular Physiology. WB Saunders, Philadelphia, 1985, p 13.
2. Wilson, RF: Critical Care Manual. FA Davis, Philadelphia, in preparation.
3. Guyton, AC: Textbook of Medical Physiology, ed 7. WB Saunders, Philadelphia, 1986, p 262.
4. Berne, R and Levy, M: Cardiovascular Physiology, ed 5. CV Mosby, St Louis, 1986, p 143.
5. Berne, R and Levy, M: Cardiovascular Physiology, ed 5. CV Mosby, St Louis, 1986, p 148
6. Berne, R and Levy, M: Cardiovascular Physiology, ed 5. CV Mosby, St Louis, 1986, p 156.

CHAPTER 38

# Cardiovascular Assessment

## CHAPTER OUTLINE



## LEARNING OBJECTIVES

**At the end of this chapter, you should be able to:**

1. Outline essential aspects of the clinical history as they pertain to cardiovascular function and dysfunction.
2. List the cardinal signs and symptoms reflective of cardiopulmonary dysfunction.
3. Identify assessment data based upon knowledge of functional health patterns.
4. Locate and describe specific anatomical landmarks and imaginary lines of the anterior chest and how they relate to the position of the heart in the chest and to the heart sounds.
5. List the components of the physical examination of cardiovascular function including the general survey, vital signs, examination of arteries and veins, and the heart itself.
6. Identify physiologic and mechanical factors to be considered in the examination of arterial pulses.
7. Describe the appropriate procedure for assessing the carotid pulse.
8. Identify physiologic and mechanical factors to be considered in the examination of jugular venous pressure and pulses.
9. Describe the significance of edema and thrombophlebitis in terms of overall cardiovascular function and mechanisms underlying their occurrence.
10. Describe essential information to be obtained on inspection and palpation of the heart and precordium.
11. State the functions of the bell and diaphragm of the stethoscope in discerning low-pitched and high-pitched heart sounds.
12. Describe the technique of auscultation of heart sounds.
13. Discuss the assessment of the following heart sounds and their clinical significance: splitting; extra heart sounds, $S_3$ and $S_4$; murmurs; and pericardial friction rub.

The ubiquitous nature and overwhelming prevalence of cardiovascular disease in our society make it essential to include an assessment of cardiovascular function as part of the patient's overall assessment. Effective cardiovascular function is necessary for survival. Thus, regardless of whether the patient's underlying problem is cardiovascular in origin or whether cardiovascular function is compromised by disease involving another organ system, appropriate and effective clinical management dictates that a thorough and comprehensive cardiovascular assessment be performed. Furthermore, as the initial step in nursing process, valid assessment is necessary to develop and implement the plan of patient care.

Assessment of respiratory function (see Chap. 29) and cardiovascular function is discussed separately in this text, but the intimate physiologic relationships between these 2 systems warrants an assessment of *cardiopulmonary* function as a whole. The reader is encouraged to refer to Chapter 29 for additional details regarding the assessment of overall cardiopulmonary function.

Major components of a thorough, comprehensive cardiovascular diagnostic workup include the clinical history and physical examination; laboratory tests and radiologic studies; graphic recordings (12-lead ECG, stress test, phonocardiogram); ultrasonography, radionuclide studies (thallium imaging, Te-PYP scan); electrophysiologic studies; cardiac catheterization; cardiac and hemodynamic monitoring; and new techniques including digital subtraction angiography and magnetic resonance imaging.

The focus of this chapter is the patient's clinical history and physical examination; cardiac monitoring and hemodynamic monitoring are discussed in Chapters 40 and 41, respectively; the remaining diagnostic studies are discussed in Chapter 39. A care plan for the clinical management of the patient post-cardiac catheterization is presented in Table 39–3; care plans for the patient with a cardiac monitor and for the patient undergoing hemodynamic monitoring are presented in Tables 40–1 and 41–7, respectively.

The reader is also referred to Appendix E for the monograph on assessment of the critically ill cardiovascular patient. This monograph describes an alternative approach to assessment based upon the nursing framework of the 9 human response patterns including exchanging, communicating, relating, valuing, choosing, moving, perceiving, knowing, and feeling. A human response pattern assessment guide is included in the monograph.

## THE CLINICAL HISTORY

The clinical history includes the patient's chief complaint or presenting health problem, the circumstances surrounding the complaint, pertinent past medical and family history, and an examination of the patient's functional health patterns. (Refer to Appendix C for definitions of specific functional health patterns.)

In performing the cardiopulmonary assessment, it is essential to first determine the patient's current status to ascertain if he or she is experiencing distress. The extent and thoroughness of the initial history and examination should be modified accordingly. When assessing signs and symptoms it is important to establish the *onset, progression* since onset, and the *current status* of the illness or unhealthful state. A careful examination of all symptomatology requires that the severity, frequency, and duration of symptoms be assessed; influencing factors including precipitating, aggravating, alleviating, or associated factors should be identified. (See the SLIDT tool in Table 7–1.)

### Cardinal Cardiopulmonary Signs and Symptoms

Cardinal signs and symptoms of cardiopulmonary dysfunction include chest pain, dyspnea, fatigue, palpitations, dizziness and syncope, pedal edema, cyanosis, clubbing, intermittent claudication, and anemia.

#### *Chest Pain*

Although chest pain is usually associated with the cardiovascular system, it may also be reflective of a variety of other disorders. These may be of pulmonary origin (e.g., pneumonia, pulmonary embolic disease, spontaneous pneumothorax); chest wall or skeletal trauma (e.g., rib fractures, costochondritis, cervical osteoarthritis); gastrointestinal disorders (e.g., esophageal spasm, hiatal hernia); dissecting aortic aneurysm; infection (e.g., herpes zoster); and anxiety. It may be the site of *referred* pain associated, for example, with peptic ulcer disease, cholecystitis, pancreatitis, subdiaphragmatic mass or abscess, or abdominal aortic aneurysm. Disorders in the differential diagnosis of chest pain are listed in Table 43–2.

**Chest Pain of Cardiac Origin.** The numerous cardiac-related causes of chest pain must be distinguished carefully by assessing the characteristics of the pain using the SLIDT tool (see Table 7–1). Cardiac disorders implicated as the cause of chest pain include ischemic heart disease syndromes (e.g., angina pectoris, unstable angina pectoris, coronary insufficiency, and Prinzmetal's angina); myocardial infarction; cardiomyopathy; mitral valve prolapse; and pericarditis. Differential diagnosis as to the underlying cause of chest pain based on its characteristics is presented in Table 38–1. See Table 43–3 for specific characteristics of angina pectoris, including its response to sublingual nitroglycerin.

**Chest Pain of Pulmonary Embolus.** The pain of a large pulmonary embolus that produces infarction of lung tissue is usually easily diagnosed based on the sudden onset of sharp pleuritic chest pain, dyspnea, hemoptysis, and tachycardia. More commonly, pulmonary emboli do not produce infarction and the diagnosis of the underlying cause of the chest pain may be more difficult to establish.

TABLE 38–1
## Differential Diagnoses of Chest Pain

| Characteristics | Angina | Myocardial Infarction | Pericarditis | Pulmonary Embolism |
|---|---|---|---|---|
| Onset/duration | Sudden, but may build in intensity. Usually lasts less than 10–20 minutes; may have an initial period of significant pain followed by a lingering achiness or chest discomfort. | Sudden. Lasts at least 30 minutes and usually 1–2 hours; residual achiness in chest over several days. | Sudden. Continuous (sometimes intermittent), usually lasting over several days. | Sudden. Continuous for several hours or longer. |
| Severity (intensity) | Varies considerably from subtle, vague chest discomfort to an intense pain that immediately grips and immobilizes the patient. Usually not unbearable or intolerable. | Frequently unbearable or intolerable; pain may be gripping and immobilizing. | Usually tolerable or bearable; sometimes more severe. | Usually not severe unless major pulmonary infarction. |
| Location/radiation | Substernal or retrosternal spreading over precordium (anterior chest) and not distinctly localized; may radiate to jaw, shoulders, arms, and/or back. | Usually substernal and over precordium; may radiate to neck, jaw, one or both arms, and/or back. | Substernal or over precordium; may radiate down arm, back, or epigastrium; frequently to left shoulder. | Anterior chest, shoulder, and/or neck; inferior borders of pleura; may radiate to costal margins. |
| Influencing factors | | | | |
| Precipitating | Physical exertion; emotional stress; heavy eating; extreme cold or hot, humid weather. | May be associated with physical, mental, or emotional stress; may occur at rest. | Usually not triggered by activity. Upper respiratory infection; myocardial infarction (transmural). | Heart failure; myocardial infarction; atrial fibrillation. Venostasis; coagulopathy. |
| Aggravating | Stress, exertion, cold; emotions such as anger, fear, tension; Valsalva maneuver (e.g., straining at stool). | Activity; anxiety. | Coughing or swallowing; motion (rotation) of upper trunk. | Anxiety. |
| Ameliorating | Rest; sublingual nitroglycerin (relief usually occurs within 3–5 minutes). | May require morphine to relieve pain; sublingual nitroglycerin may be ineffective. | Shallow breathing; sitting up and leaning forward. | Rest, reassurance; analgesic. |
| Associated | Palpitations, dizziness, nausea. | Nausea/vomiting; diaphoresis, dizziness, syncope; palpitations; dyspnea. Sensation of impending doom. | Pericardial friction rub heard best with diaphragm of stethoscope during inspiration. | Unexplained dyspnea; hemotypsis; cyanosis, tachycardia (in presence of pulmonary infarction); syncope. |
| Type (quality) | Feeling of tightness, squeezing, heaviness, pressure, or constriction in chest; may not be experienced as "pain" but rather described as a burning or cramping sensation; like "gas" or indigestion. | Crushing, vise-like, choking. | Sharp, often accentuated by deep breathing and/or lying in a recumbent position. May also be described as stabbing or burning, or a deep dull ache. Friction rub, if present, may be described as grating, scraping, or scratchy; it is usually heard best in third ICS to left of sternum (Erb's point). | Sharp, pleuritic-type chest pain. |

The diagnosis of pulmonary embolism should be highly suspected when a pleuritic type chest pain accompanied by unexplained dyspnea occurs in the setting of venostasis, venous injury, or altered blood coagulation. Important information to ascertain this diagnosis includes a prior history of pulmonary emboli; presence of leg or calf tenderness; recent surgery, trauma, pregnancy, bedrest, or long car trip or plane ride; or the use of birth control pills. (Refer to Chap. 35 for a detailed discussion of pulmonary embolism.)

### Dyspnea

Dyspnea refers to shortness of breath or the uncomfortable awareness of one's own sensation of breathlessness. Dyspnea associated with cardiac disease may be difficult to distinguish from other causes of dyspnea. Dyspnea caused by left ventricular failure may present with characteristic features. For example, dyspnea that becomes apparent during the performance of activities of daily living or when walking several blocks or climbing stairs is called *exertional* dyspnea. It is important to establish the extent of a given activity that precipitates the dyspnea.

*Orthopnea* is the inability of the person to breathe easily when lying flat. The person may need to use 2 or 3 pillows (e.g., 3-pillow orthopnea) to elevate the head in order to breathe comfortably. It is important to establish how many pillows are used, why they are necessary, and when the patient found it necessary to use multiple pillows. The patient who is suddenly awakened from sleep by a smothering sensation and gasping for breath may be experiencing *paroxysmal nocturnal* dyspnea, a frequent complaint associated with left-sided heart failure. However, this type of dyspnea may occur in response to the slow mobilization of body fluids as, for example, from peripheral or dependent edema. Dyspnea wherein patients are unable to sleep on the left side is termed *trepopnea*. It is a complaint sometimes verbalized by patients with cardiac disease.

Patients with severe left ventricular failure may develop *pulmonary edema*, which is characterized by overwhelming pulmonary congestion with transudation (i.e., movement of fluid through a membrane) of fluid into the alveoli. In its advanced stage it is characterized by the gurgling forth of frothy, pink-tinged sputum, accompanied by an exaggerated respiratory effort. *Wheezing* commonly accompanies pulmonary edema; however, other causes of wheezing need to be ruled out (e.g., asthma, hyperventilation). Unexplained dyspnea is a symptom of a variety of cardiopulmonary disorders. It is essential to determine its significance in terms of the patient's overall clinical presentation. (Refer to the section on dyspnea in Chap. 29 for further discussion.)

### Fatigue

Fatigue is a common complaint associated with the stress and anxiety of everyday life. It takes on added significance as an early symptom of heart disease when the patient who previously enjoyed unlimited exercise tolerance complains of progressive increase in fatigue. It is important to establish prior activity tolerance, and when the patient became aware of increasing fatigue with activity. What was the patient's level of activity 6 months ago? What has changed? Questions such as, "How far did you jog 6 months ago?" and "How far do you jog now?" may help to establish a trend of decreasing activity tolerance. Often, patients with heart disease will decrease their activities so gradually that they are unaware of underlying cardiac disease.

### Palpitations

Complaints of palpitations, skipping of heart beat, flutter in chest, or rapid pulsation in the chest frequently reflect irregularities of heart beat, or dysrhythmias. Sometimes the sensation reflects a heightened awareness of one's normal heart beat, noticed especially while lying quietly in bed. Isolated premature heart beats are common and usually go unnoticed. Irregular, forceful contractions may be perceived, whether extrasystoles or an abrupt onset and termination of a run of beats as occurs with a paroxysmal atrial tachycardia; or as a rapid ventricular response in atrial fibrillation. Frequently occurring ventricular premature beats or a brief run of ventricular tachycardia may likewise be perceived as palpitations or fluttering feeling in the chest.

In assessing palpitations it is important to determine when the episode began and what was the patient doing at the time. Did it begin and end abruptly? How long did it last? Was the rhythm regular or irregular? Did the patient count the rate? Did the patient experience any associated symptoms such as chest pain or discomfort, feeling of lightheadedness, dizziness, fainting, or diaphoresis? Did the patient take any medications? If so, what medication, and why? It is also important to ascertain how much coffee, tea, or soda was consumed in the period of time preceding the episode of palpitations. Was there alcohol or beer consumption at the time? How much? Was the patient smoking cigarettes at the time? More than usual? How many cigarettes over how long a period of time? How many packs per day does the patient usually smoke? For how many years?

If the patient has experienced prior episodes of palpitations it is important to elicit the details surrounding these episodes, how frequently they occur, and whether the patient has been examined or had an ECG rhythm strip done at the time of the attack. Does the patient take any prescribed medications because of episodes of palpitations? Is there a prior history of heart disease, hypertension, anxiety, or recent emotional stress? Does the patient have a thyroid disorder? Does the patient take thyroid medications?

### *Dizziness and Syncope*

Dizziness as a symptom is perceived in a multitude of ways by different persons. It may be described as a feeling of faintness, unsteadiness, lightheadedness, spinning, vertigo, or blacking out. Syncope implies that a blackout or loss of consciousness has occurred. Causes of dizziness or syncope include dysrhythmias, orthostatic hypotension, vasovagal effect, coronary artery occlusion, cerebrovascular disease, and hyperventilation, among others.

Symptomatic cardiac dysrhythmias, such as heart blocks or rapid ventricular rates (supraventricular tachycardia or runs of ventricular tachycardia), are possible underlying causes of syncope because they reduce cardiac output. Heart block reduces cardiac output by decreasing the heart rate; tachydysrhythmias reduce cardiac output by decreasing diastolic filling time, with a consequent reduction in stroke volume. (Dysrhythmias are discussed in Chap. 40).

Orthostatic hypotension (i.e., a reduction in blood pressure occurring upon sudden positional changes, such as rising quickly from a recumbent position) is frequently implicated as a cause of dizziness or syncope. It is associated with reduced venous return, reduced circulating blood volume, or possibly autonomic nervous system dysfunction. It is commonly seen in the elderly, in dehydrated states, and in patients taking antihypertensive medications, vasodilators, propranolol, or calcium channel blockers. When assessing the patient with dizziness or syncope, it is important to take the patient's blood pressure both when lying down and immediately upon sitting up, or from a sitting to a standing position. A careful drug history should also be elicited.

*Vasovagal* syncope is usually associated with an intense emotional experience ("emotional" fainting). It reflects an enhanced excitation of the parasympathetic (vagal) innervation to the heart resulting in a slowing of the heart rate. The consequent reduction in cardiac output may reduce cerebral blood flow and cause the patient to faint. Prior to fainting the patient may experience nausea, weakness, diaphoresis, blurred vision, tinnitus, and dizziness. Upon recovery, weakness, dizziness, and nausea may persist but the patient remains alert and oriented. Eliciting details as to the patient's emotional status at the time of the fainting spell may help in the differential diagnosis.

Other causes of dizziness or syncope include cerebrovascular disease; hyperventilation; and hypersensitive carotid sinus wherein hyperextension of the neck, turning of the head, or pressure over the area of the carotid sinus may precipitate syncope. In this latter circumstance, the syncope is usually associated with a slowing of the heart rate (vasovagal response) and/or a drop in blood pressure. Coronary artery occlusion has also been implicated as a cause of syncopal episodes.

### *Pedal Edema*

Pedal edema is commonly associated with fluid and salt retention resulting from heart disease. It is manifested as soft tissue swelling usually in dependent areas such as the feet and ankles or over the sacral area in the bedridden patient. Gravity promotes fluid extravasation from the intravascular space into the interstitium, and the edema becomes worse as the day progresses. With night-time recumbency, the return of fluid to the vascular system predisposes to nocturia and paroxysmal nocturnal dyspnea (see above). A careful history of increasing tightness of shoes and clothing, frequent night-time urination, or episodes of sudden awakenings feeling short of breath is highly suggestive of underlying cardiopulmonary dysfunction.

### *Intermittent Claudication*

Intermittent claudication refers to pain experienced in the foot, calf, thigh, and buttocks upon walking. It reflects an inadequate blood supply to exercising muscles usually associated with significant atherosclerotic obstruction to the lower extremities. Embolization and arteritis have also been implicated as possible etiologic factors. Clinically, the patient usually describes a muscle cramp, "charley horse," or weakness with exercise. The pain disappears when the patient rests, but recurs when the exercise is resumed. The obstruction may become progressively more severe and eventually the patient may experience a boring, aching, intense, or steady pain even at rest.

It is important to determine what type of and how much exercise predispose to the pain. Questions to be asked may include: "How far can you walk without resting?" "What kind of discomfort do you feel when you have to stop walking?" "Does resting help to relieve the pain?" "Does it recur when the exercise is resumed?" "Has there been a progressive decrease in the amount of exercise that can be performed before precipitating pain?"

Other factors associated with the clinical presentation of cardiopulmonary dysfunction include the presence of a cough with or without hemoptysis, cyanosis, and clubbing. (The reader is referred to Chap. 29 for a discussion of these factors.) Anemia, which reduces the oxygen-carrying capacity of the blood, is commonly associated with cardiopulmonary disorders.

## Past Medical History

Eliciting events in the patient's past medical history may contribute information regarding the current problem. Information regarding childhood diseases, mumps, maternal rubella, group A beta-hemolytic streptococcal infections, and rheumatic fever may have significance in terms of the patient's overall health status. Rheumatic fever in childhood may underlie heart valve dysfunction in an adult; prior type A beta-hemolytic streptococcal infections may explain the occurrence of subacute bacterial endocarditis.

It should be determined if the patient has had previous hospitalizations, when, and for what reason. Has the patient had surgery? If so, for what reason? Have there been any previous accidents or injuries? Is there a history of heart murmur, hypertension, hyperlipidemias, diabetes mellitus, renal disease, anemia, bleeding disorder, thrombophlebitis, or varicosities? Has the patient previously experienced chest pain, heart attack, chronic obstructive pulmonary disease, or other pulmonary disease? Has the patient had an ECG done? When? For what reason? What were the results? Does the patient take medication? What type, in what dose and frequency, and for what reason? Who prescribed the medication? Is it effective in treating the problem? Does the patient have any allergies? Drug, food, other? What kind of allergic reaction is experienced?

## Family History

It is important to determine the past and current health status of each member of the immediate family. Is there a history of congenital heart disease? Is there a recurring familial history of coronary artery disease, angina pectoris, or myocardial infarction? Are hypertension, hypercholesterolemia, hyperlipoproteinemia, stroke, obesity, or diabetes mellitus significant factors in terms of overall family health? Ascertain who in the family have died, their age at death, and the immediate cause of death.

## Functional Health Patterns

### *Health Perception/Health Management*

It is important to determine the overall health status of the patient and family and their attitudes regarding the importance of health in their lives. How do they feel about cigarette smoking, alcohol consumption, diet, exercise, self-medication (use of over-the-counter drugs)? What amounts of caffeine, coffee, tea, or soda are consumed daily? What are their past health practices in these areas? Has the patient followed prescribed treatment for past and/or current illness or unhealthful state? What are the concerns about current illness and how it may impact on the patient and other family members? What have been previous experiences with hospitalization? What are the expectations regarding the current hospitalization?

No one becomes ill in a vacuum. Rather, the occurrence of illness reflects a "family" disease, which impacts on each member of the family. For example, the patient who is recuperating from a myocardial infarction may be making a concerted effort to stop cigarette smoking. Should he return home only to have his wife blowing cigarette smoke across the dinner table, this behavior is hardly conducive to his health or hers. Thus, it is important to assess the family as a whole and to involve all family members in examining their attitudes and behavioral health practices, so as to initiate behaviors conducive to the health of all.

### *Nutritional/Metabolic*

Nutrition is especially significant in cardiovascular disease because many of its major risk factors reflect dietary intake and therefore are *controllable* factors (see Chap. 43). Hyperlipidemia (hypercholesterolemia and triglyceridemia) is well documented as being an essential risk factor in the development of coronary artery disease (CAD). Low-density lipoproteins are highly atherogenic, whereas high-density lipoproteins have been found to have a negative correlation in this regard.

Hyperglycemia may increase the risk of CAD. Atherosclerosis in general and coronary atherosclerosis in particular are more extensive in patients with diabetes mellitus, especially in those with uncontrolled hyperglycemia. In addition, fluid and salt retention is commonly associated with heart disease, and reduction in salt intake is usually indicated. Hydration status can best be monitored by daily weights (at the same time each day and with the same scale) and by carefully documented daily intake and output.

In assessing nutritional status it is important to ascertain patient and family attitudes about nutrition and their dietary patterns. Food intolerances should be identified; if there are food restrictions, determine what they are, and why. A thorough comprehensive diet history, performed in collaboration with the staff nutritionist, is essential in the treatment of hyperlipidemic states, which should include patient and family education.

### Activity/Exercise

Evaluation of activity tolerance is especially significant because fatigue can be an early symptom of the presence and/or progression of heart disease (see above). Some patients with heart disease may decrease their activities so gradually that they may not be aware of the underlying problem. It is helpful to ask patients to compare what they could do in the past, and how that may have changed currently. (Functional and therapeutic classifications of patients with diseases of the heart are listed in Table 38-2).

### Sleep/Rest

In patients with cardiopulmonary disease it is important to determine what their usual sleeping patterns have been and how they may have changed. It is necessary to determine how many pillows the patient requires to elevate the head during sleep (orthopnea) and whether the patient becomes short of breath when lying on left side (trepopnea). (Refer to the section on dyspnea, above). Does the patient suddenly awaken from a sound sleep, gasping for breath. Paroxysmal nocturnal dyspnea is highly suggestive of underlying heart disease.

TABLE 38-2

**Functional and Therapeutic Classifications of Patients with Diseases of the Heart***

| Functional Classification | Therapeutic Classification |
|---|---|
| *Class I:* Patients with cardiac disease but without limitations of physical activity. Ordinary physical activity does not cause undue fatigue, palpitation, dyspnea, or anginal pain. | *Class A:* Patients with cardiac disease whose physical activity need not be restricted in any way. |
| *Class II:* Patients with cardiac disease resulting in slight limitation of physical activity. They are comfortable at rest. Ordinary physical activity results in fatigue, palpitation, dyspnea, or anginal pain. | *Class B:* Patients with cardiac disease whose ordinary physical activity need not be restricted, but who should be advised against severe or competitive efforts. |
| *Class III:* Patients with cardiac disease resulting in marked limitation of physical activity. They are comfortable at rest. Less than ordinary physical activity causes fatigue, palpitation, dyspnea, or anginal pain. | *Class C:* Patients with cardiac disease whose ordinary physical activity should be moderately restricted, and whose more strenuous efforts should be discontinued. |
| *Class IV:* Patients with cardiac disease resulting in inability to carry on any physical activity without discomfort. Symptoms of cardiac insufficiency or of the anginal syndrome may be present even at rest. If any physical activity is undertaken, discomfort is increased. | *Class D:* Patients with cardiac disease whose ordinary physical activity should be markedly restricted. |
| | *Class E:* Patients with cardiac disease who should be at complete rest, confined to bed or chair. |

*New York Heart Association

### Elimination

Usual bowel and bladder habits should be determined. Nocturia frequently occurs in congestive heart failure because fluid in dependent areas of the body is redistributed when the patient assumes a recumbent position for sleep. A tendency toward constipation should be ascertained. Valsalva maneuvers, such as straining at stool, can trigger a vagal response that slows the heart rate, and this may not be well tolerated by the patient with compromised cardiovascular function.

### Cognitive/Perceptual

It is important to establish baseline data regarding the patient's mental status and level of consciousness. Inquire as to the level of knowledge and insight the patient may have regarding: (1) changes in bodily functions and the significance of these changes; (2) the impact of cardiovascular disease on individual and family lifestyles; and (3) the motivation and readiness to learn how to cope with the limitations of the disease so as to maintain an optimal level of health. Establishing these baseline data will help to facilitate patient/family teaching.

### Coping/Stress Tolerance

Personality type (Type A) and behavior patterns have long been implicated as a factor in the development of coronary artery disease. Characteristically, Type A individuals are highly ambitious, competitive, and impatient, and constantly struggling to achieve more and more in less and less time. Underlying pathogenesis of coronary artery disease in such individuals may involve excess sympathetic arousal with increased levels of circulating catecholamines.

In assessing the coping/stress tolerance pattern it is important to identify the patient's usual response to stress and past behaviors that were helpful in coping with stress. Questions to be asked might include, "Who is most helpful in discussing concerns and problems?" "What did you do when previously confronted with a stressor?" "What worked in the past?" "Are there currently any major stressors, personally, job-related?" "Have there been any recent changes in overall lifestyle, what kind of changes, and why?" "How did the patient/family respond?"

### *Self-Perception/Self-Concept*

It is important to ascertain the patient's sense of self. How does the patient describe and feel about himself/herself? What are his/her strengths and weaknesses? Is there anger, denial, depression? In the early stages following myocardial infarction, denial may be a therapeutic mechanism in some patients and needs to be supported accordingly. Often patients are unaware of their anger. Allowing patients to verbalize their anger at the appropriate time may help them gain insight into their feelings so that they may cope better.

### *Value/Belief*

What kinds of things are important to the patient/family? Do they have short-term and long-term goals? Are the goals realistic? Are their values/beliefs compromised by the patient's illness? This is an area of considerable importance for the patient with significant cardiovascular disease, because it often requires considerable adjustments in lifestyle (see Table 38-2).

### *Sexuality/Reproductive*

It is important to ascertain attitudes about sexual activity and the importance of such activity to the patient. The effect of the physical exertion associated with sexual activity on cardiac function may create some concerns for the patient and partner. The patient may be afraid to engage in sexual activity for fear of another heart attack; the partner may feel responsible for having caused the heart attack. Both may need assistance in working through their feelings. Often this is an area that both patient and nurse feel uncomfortable about. Nurses may need to examine their own feelings about sexuality before trying to be of assistance to their patients.

### *Role/Relationships*

Questions related to role and relationships are concerned with family structure and support systems, home environment, roles in family, and occupation, among others. What role does the patient play in the family? Breadwinner? Decision-maker? What impact will heart disease have on this role? Will it be necessary for the patient to seek new employment?

In summary, the clinical history is never considered to be complete. As physical findings are discovered and information from laboratory and diagnostic studies is ascertained, the original database is reevaluated and expanded accordingly.

## PHYSICAL EXAMINATION

The physical examination includes the general survey or overall inspection, assessment of vital signs, examination of arteries and peripheral pulses, examination of veins, and an examination of the heart. Examination techniques used include inspection, palpation, and auscultation. The examination should be organized and systematic. The extent of the initial examination depends upon the patient's condition. Throughout the examination, be cognizant of underlying tissues including the location of lung lobes and the position of the heart in the chest.

When assessing cardiovascular function it is important to recall the factors that influence mean arterial pressure (MAP) including cardiac output (stroke volume × heart rate); elastic recoil of the great arteries; peripheral vascular resistance (total arteriolar resistance); blood volume; and blood viscosity (hematocrit). (Refer to the appropriate sections in Chap. 37 for an indepth discussion of these physiologic factors.)

For a review of thoracic landmarks, imaginary lines, and the overall position of lung lobes within the thoracic cavity, the reader is encouraged to study Figures 29-2 through 29-7; refer to Figure 37-1 to appreciate the position of the heart in the thorax and its relationship to adjacent structures, thoracic landmarks, and imaginary lines.

### General Survey

The general survey or inspection of the patient involves a quick "head-to-toe" overview, taking into consideration the following details: What is the apparent state of health? Does the patient appear acutely or chronically ill? Does the patient appear to be the stated age? Is the patient cachetic? Debilitated? Obese?

Are there signs of distress? Dyspnea, labored noisy breathing, use of accessory muscles? Rib retraction? Pursed-lip breathing? Is the patient wide-eyed and anxious? Is the patient in pain? Is the patient diaphoretic? Skin cool to touch, mottled appearance? Is there cyanosis (circumoral)? Or clubbing of nailbeds? (See Fig. 29-1.) Is there neck vein distention? Dependent edema?

What is the patient's mental status? Alert and oriented? Confused? Are there speech difficulties? Is there good eye contact? Is the patient's behavior appropriate? How is the patient dressed and groomed?

Information obtained on a quick "head-to-toe" inspection assists in determining overall acuity of the patient's condition. The extent of the physical examination should be modified accordingly.

## Vital Signs

Vital signs include body temperature; pulse rate and rhythm; respirations, including rate, rhythm, and depth (see Chap. 29); and blood pressure (both arms; sitting and recumbent, if possible).

Arterial blood pressure varies with the events of the cardiac cycle, reaching a systolic high during peak left ventricular ejection and a diastolic trough as blood is driven downstream through the vascular system. The difference between the systolic and diastolic pressures is the *pulse* pressure (see the section on arterial pressure in Chap. 37). Normally it is 30–40 mmHg. A *widened* pulse pressure may reflect both systolic and diastolic hypertension; it is seen in thyrotoxicosis and aortic regurgitation; or it may be associated with extreme emotional distress. A *narrowed* pulse pressure may be associated with tachycardia, aortic stenosis, or pericardial effusion and cardiac tamponade.

## Examination of Arterial Pulses

The arterial waveform (Fig. 38–1) reflects pressure changes as they occur within the large arteries during the cardiac cycle. The pressure wave is initiated with peak left ventricular ejection and is transmitted throughout the peripheral vascular system, where it can be palpated as pulses.

Assessment of the arterial pulse includes determining rate and rhythm, amplitude and contour of the pressure wave, and bilateral equality. The status of the vessel wall can also be determined. Normally, arterial vessel walls are elastic on palpation; when abnormal, they may be described as hardened, thickened, beaded, inelastic, or calcified.

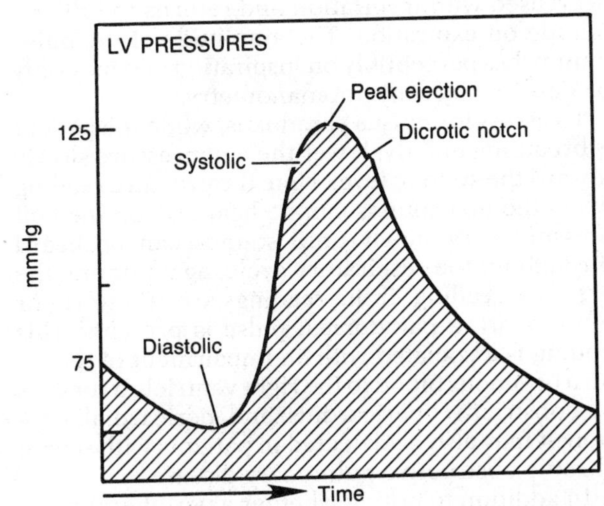


**Figure 38–1.** Arterial pressure waveform reflecting pressure changes as they occur within the large arteries during the cardiac cycle. The pressure wave reaches its peak during ventricular systole (LV peak ejection), and its low point during ventricular diastole. The dicrotic notch reflects closure of the aortic valve.

### *Peripheral Pulses*

The rate reflects the number of heart beats per minute; rhythm reflects the regularity of their occurrence. The radial pulse is used conveniently to assess heart rate and rhythm. The pads of the index and middle fingers are used to gently compress the artery until a maximum pulsation is detected. The rate is counted and any variations in rhythm noted. An irregular pulse reflects an underlying cardiac dysrhythmia. If a beat is dropped or apparently absent, this usually reflects a premature ventricular contraction, particularly when the dropped beat is followed by an especially full or forceful beat. The rhythm of atrial fibrillation is especially irregular, reflecting the irregular conduction of impulses through the AV junction and the consequent irregular ventricular response.

The amplitude and contour of the arterial pulse reflect the pressure wave that reaches its peak during ventricular systole and its low point during ventricular diastole (see Fig. 38–1). The amplitude of the pulse refers to the extent of divergence between the systolic and diastolic pressure waves, and is usually described as strong or weak (Fig. 38–2). A strong pulse is associated with an increase in cardiac output; a weak pulse reflects a decrease in cardiac output, or partial occlusion of an artery. In the presence of an occlusion, the weak pulse will be palpated distal to the occlusion. Pulses are evaluated bilaterally for equality.

The arterial pressure waveform undergoes changes as it is transmitted toward the capillary beds (Fig. 38–3). Systolic pressures in the extremities are higher than in the aorta; systole becomes shorter, and the pressure decrease following systole is faster. This creates a waveform that becomes more sharply elevated and narrower. Diastolic pressures decrease slightly more in the extremities, thereby increasing the pulse pressure. These changes reflect in part the aortic capacitance and increased frictional resistance of arterioles as blood flows downstream.

Abnormal pulses are sometimes described, including pulsus alternans, bigeminal pulse, and pulsus paradoxus (see Fig. 38–2). *Pulsus alternans* is a pulse with a regular rhythm wherein the amplitude fluctuates from beat to beat. This pulse may be evident in left heart failure. A *bigeminal* pulse is usually produced by a normal beat alternating with a premature ventricular contraction. The decreased amplitude of the premature beat reflects

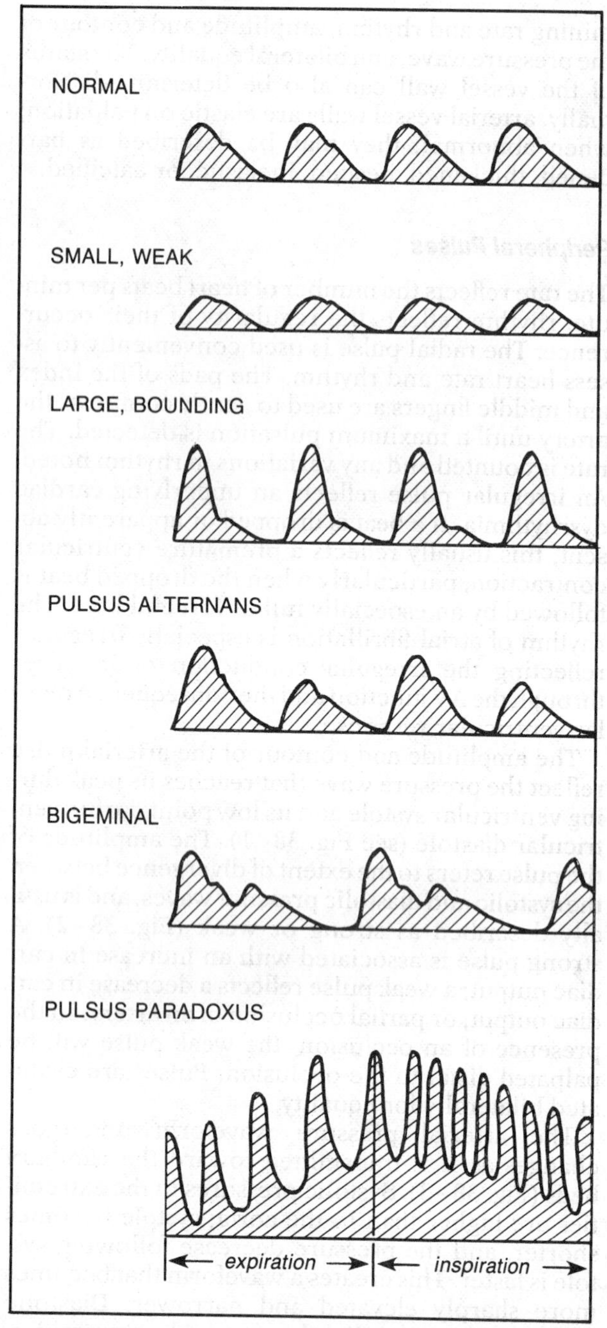


**Figure 38–2.** Normal and abnormal arterial pulses. Differences in amplitude and contour distinguish the variable pulses encountered clinically. Amplitude of a pulse reflects the extent of divergence between the systolic and diastolic pressure waves. This difference reflects the pulse pressure, which is normally about 30–40 mmHg. Normal contour is smooth and rounded, reflecting a strong upstroke and peak ventricular ejection. Pulses are assessed bilaterally for rate, rhythm, amplitude, contour, and equality. See text for discussion. (From Bates, B: A Guide to Physical Examination, ed 4. JB Lippincott, Philadelphia, 1988, p 297, with permission.)

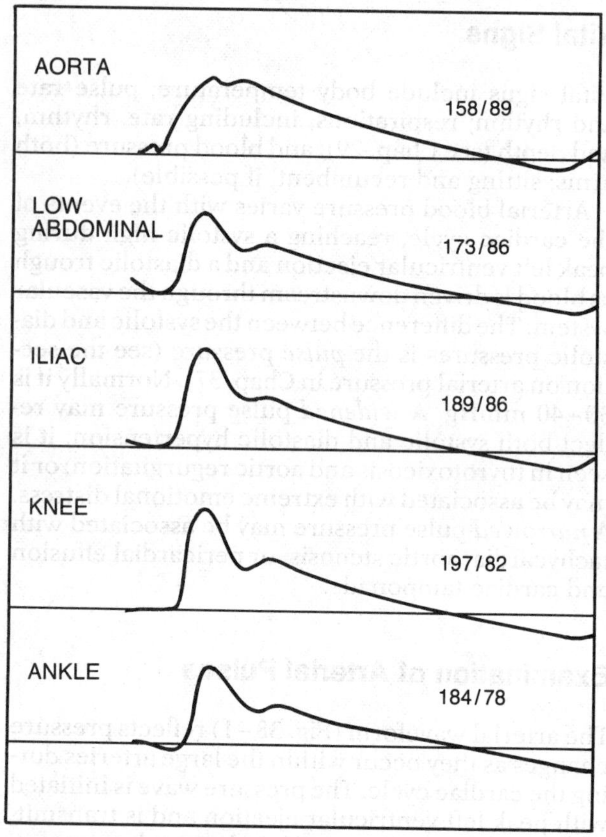


**Figure 38–3.** Changes in the arterial pressure and arterial pressure waveform from the aorta distally to the ankle. (From Remington, JW, O'Brien, LJ: Changes in arterial pressure wave. Am J Physiol 218:437, 1970, with permission.)

the reduced cardiac output, a consequence of a decrease in left ventricular end-diastolic filling pressure. *Pulsus paradoxus* reflects a change in the amplitude with respirations. The amplitude is decreased with inspiration and returns to full amplitude on expiration. The amplitude of the pulse diminishes perceptibly on inspiration and may only be detected by sphygmomanometry.

To assess for pulsus paradoxus, while the patient is breathing quietly, lower the cuff pressure slowly toward the systolic level. Note the pressure reading when the first sounds can be heard. Drop the cuff pressure very slowly until sounds can be heard throughout the respiratory cycle, again noting the pressure reading. If the readings are 10 mmHg or more apart, a paradoxical pulse is present.[1] This finding is associated with an impairment of the return of venous blood to the right ventricle as occurs in constrictive pericarditis and pericardial effusion; it may also be detected in patients with severe chronic obstructive pulmonary disease.

In addition to noting whether a peripheral pulse is strong or weak, these pulses may be given a rating on a scale of 0–3:

0 = No pulse.
1+ = Pulse is thready, weak, difficult to palpate; may be easily obliterated with pressure.

2+ = "Normal" pulse; it is easily palpable and not obliterated with pressure.
3+ = Pulse is strong and bounding.

### Carotid Pulse

When assessing the carotid pulse, first inspect the neck for pulsations. Carotid pulsations may be visible just medial to the sternomastoid muscles. With the patient's head elevated about 15–30 degrees on a pillow, turn the head slightly toward the side being examined. (This will relax the sternomastoid muscle.) Palpate the pulse by placing the pads of the index and middle fingers along the medial border of the sternomastoid muscle in the *lower* half of the neck; press down and feel the carotid pulsations. One side at a time is palpated, taking care to avoid the carotid sinus, which is located at the level of the thyroid cartilage just below the angle of the jaw. Pressure over the carotid sinus may cause a reflex decrease in blood pressure and heart rate. Note any palpable thrills.

Auscultate over the arteries using the bell of the stethoscope. Ask the patient to hold the breath and listen for the presence of a bruit. A bruit suggests narrowing of the artery. It may also reflect a systolic murmur from the aortic area. While palpating the carotid pulse, listen simultaneously over the base of the heart to assess the amplitude of the pulse and variations from beat to beat and with respirations. Normally, the upstroke is smooth and rapid and immediately follows the first heart sound. The downstroke is less abrupt than the upstroke. Any variations from beat to beat could reflect a pulsus alternans; variations with respirations suggest a pulsus paradoxus.

## Examination of Jugular Venous Pressure and Pulses

The venous pressure waveform (Fig. 38–4) reflects the central venous pressure (CVP), that is, the pressure of blood in the right atrium. Although CVP is dependent upon left ventricular pressure, other determinants include blood volume and the capacity of the right heart to receive blood and eject it through the pulmonic valve into the pulmonary vascular circuit. Any changes in these variables will cause a corresponding change in venous pressure. For example, when cardiac output or blood volume is significantly reduced, venous pressure falls; if the right heart fails, CVP is increased. Pericardial effusion or tamponade may impede blood flow into the right heart, thereby increasing venous pressure.

A reliable estimate of CVP, and thus of right heart pressures, can be obtained by the examination of the internal and external jugular veins. (The internal jugular veins are more reliable in this respect.) The patient should be positioned in a relaxed and comfortable position. A pillow placed under the patient's head will relax the sternomastoid muscle. The head of the patient's bed is elevated to maximize venous pulsations. Usually, a low semi-Fowler's position (15–30 degrees) is sufficient to visualize the venous pulsations in the neck; however, if venous pressures are elevated it may be necessary to place the patient in a high-Fowler's (>45 degrees), or seated upright (90 degrees).

Using tangential (oblique) lighting, examine both sides of the neck. Identify the external jugular veins, and look for the pulsations of the internal jugular vein. The internal jugular vein lies deep to the sternomastoid muscle and therefore cannot be observed directly. What can be seen are the venous pulsations transmitted through the surrounding tissues. Observe for the *a*-wave and *v*-wave of the venous pressure waveform; the *c*-wave, if visible, is a reflected wave from the nearby carotid artery.

When observing the pulsation, consider the right heart hemodynamics. The *a*-wave reflects the slight increase in right atrial pressure caused by atrial contraction. This wave will be almost synchronized with $S_1$ (AV valve closure). The *v*-wave occurs during ventricular contraction and largely reflects right atrial filling pressures. The occurrence of this wave is almost synchronized with $S_2$ (semilunar valve closure).

Respirations also affect central venous pressures. The fall in intrathoracic pressure during normal inspiration causes the level of the pulse in the neck veins to descend. The increase in intrathoracic pressure during expiration causes the level of the neck pulsations to rise.

Three pulsations may be seen in the suprasternal notch, above the clavicle, or just posterior to the sternomastoid muscle. Turning the patient's head away from the side being examined may help to make the pulsations more visible. To differentiate venous pulsations from that of the carotid artery, apply light pressure over the neck veins just above the sternal end of the clavicle. Pulsations of the jugular veins are easily eliminated with relatively light pressure, whereas much greater pressure is

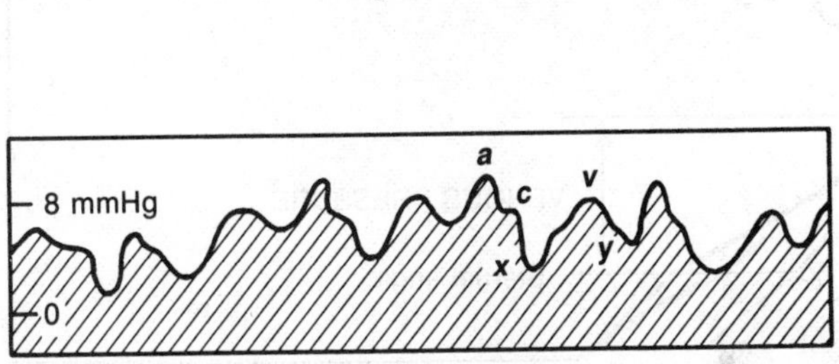


**Figure 38–4.** Venous pressure waveform. The *a*-wave reflects slight increase in right atrial pressure that occurs with atrial contraction; the *v*-wave largely reflects right atrial filling pressures and occurs during ventricular contraction; the *c*-wave, if present, is a reflected wave from the nearby carotid artery. The *x* descent reflects decrease in right atrial pressure associated with atrial relaxation that occurs upon closure of the tricuspid valve; *y* descent reflects drop in right atrial pressure that occurs at the beginning of diastole upon opening of the tricuspid valve.

required to eliminate carotid artery pulsations.

### Hepatojugular Reflux

In the presence of right-sided heart failure the increase in central venous pressure is reflected by the increased level of venous pressure in the neck veins and consequent exaggeration of venous pulsations. A sustained compression with the palm of the hand over the right upper quadrant for 30–60 seconds will cause venous pressure to rise. This rise in venous pressure will cause the venous pulsations in the neck to become more prominent and their level in the neck will also rise. This maneuver is referred to as the *hepatojugular reflux*. It is sometimes performed to determine the presence of right heart failure. A rise greater than 1 cm above the pressure level is abnormal. During this maneuver it is important for the patient not to hold the breath or perform a Valsalva maneuver, which may cause an increase in central venous pressures and invalidate the findings.

### Measurement of Venous Pressure

To measure the venous pressures identify the highest point at which venous pulsation within the neck can be seen. Using a centimeter ruler, measure the vertical distance between that point and the sternal angle (Fig. 38–5). Congestive heart failure is the most frequent cause of abnormally increased venous pressures.

### Examination for Edema and Thrombophlebitis

Edema may be associated with *systemic* causes, including congestive heart failure, hypoalbuminemia, or excessive renal salt and water retention; or with *local* causes, including venous stasis associated with thrombophlebitis, immobility, and/or prolonged dependent positions. The edema of congestive heart failure appears initially in dependent areas where capillary hydrostatic pressure is highest, as, for example, the feet and ankles in the upright position or the sacral area in the bedridden individual. Edema associated with hypoalbuminemia and/or excessive salt and water retention appears initially in the subcutaneous tissue of the eyelids (e.g., periorbital edema), as well as dependent areas.

Local edema associated with thrombophlebitis is usually limited to the extremity in which venous drainage is partially or completely interrupted. Most commonly, this involves one lower extremity. Prolonged immobility, sitting, or standing usually results in edema in dependent areas.

Superficial thrombophlebitis most commonly involves the lower extremities. Redness, edema,

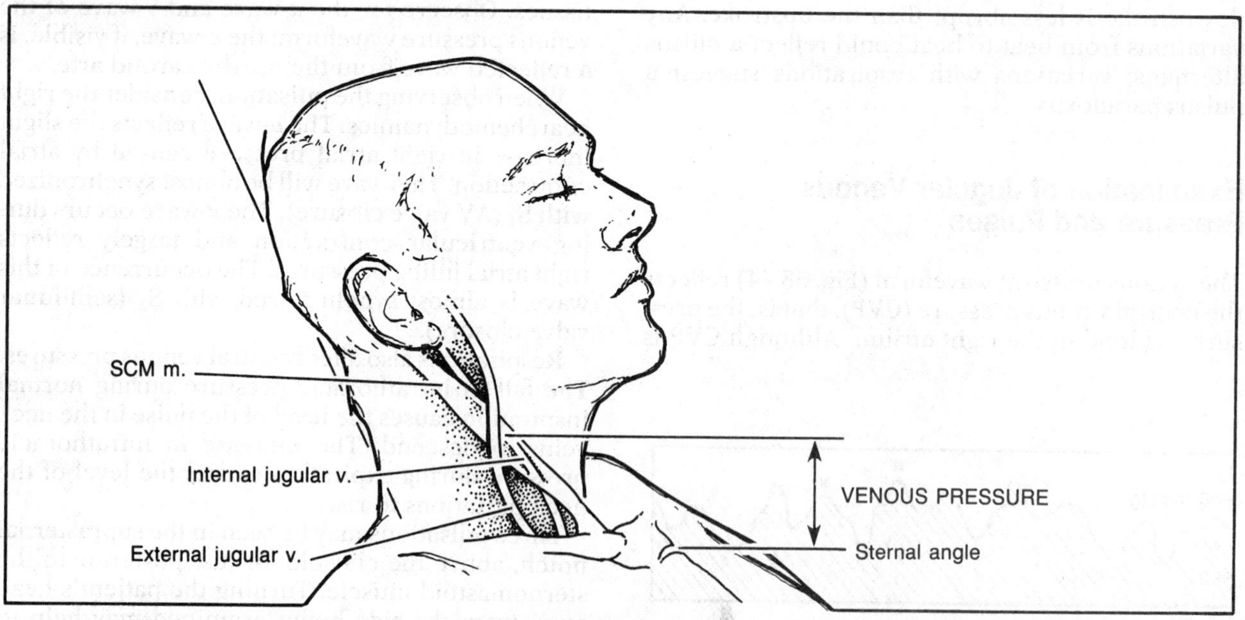


**Figure 38–5.** Measurement of venous pressure. Venous pressure is best estimated from the internal jugular; the external jugular may be used but is less reliable. The level of venous pressure is determined by locating the highest point of pulsation in the internal jugular. Since the internal jugular lies deep to the sternocleidomastoid muscle (SCMm), use of tangential lighting helps in identifying the pulsations reflected from the internal jugular. If the external jugular is used, the point above which the external jugular appears collapsed, is used. The vertical distance between either of these points and the sternal angle (zero point) is recorded as the venous pressure. In order to see the venous pressure level as reflected by the jugular veins, it may be necessary to alter the patient's position. Pressure more than 3 cm to 4 cm above the sternal angle is considered elevated. When discerning pulsations, it is important to be aware that those of the nearby carotid artery must be differentiated.

and tenderness may be observed over the inflamed vein. The calf should be palpated for signs of deep thrombophlebitis. It is important to feel for any increased firmness or tension of calf muscles. In the presence of deep thrombophlebitis of the lower leg the patient may be assessed for the presence of *Homans' sign*. This sign is positive when forceful dorsiflexion of the leg produces pain in the calf muscles. When thrombophlebitis is suspected, daily measurement of bilateral midcalf and midthigh circumferences may be helpful in diagnosing the presence of deep venous thrombosis.

## Examination of the Heart

The examination of the heart includes inspection, palpation, and auscultation. Inspection and palpation of the anterior chest are best performed with the patient lying in the supine or a low-Fowler's position. It is important to visualize the position of the heart within the chest (see Fig. 37-1) including the location of heart chambers and great vessels. The examination of the heart should be conducted from the patient's right side. It should be systematic, proceeding in an orderly fashion from the following areas: aortic, pulmonic, right ventricular (tricuspid) and apical, or left ventricular (mitral) areas (Fig. 38-6). It is in these areas that heart sounds produced at each of the valves are heard most distinctly over the precordium (see below).

### Inspection and Palpation

The entire anterior chest (precordium) should be visible and inspected for the presence of any abnormal pulsations or chest wall movements. Use of tangential or oblique lighting helps to detect pulsations. Finger pads are most helpful in detecting pulses; the palmar surface at the base of the finger is most sensitive to vibrations or thrills. A *thrill* is a palpable vibration usually associated with the turbulent flow of blood through a narrowed opening or stenosis. Pulsation and thrills should be timed in relation to the cardiac cycle, that is, systole and diastole. These time periods can be discerned by feeling the carotid pulse or auscultating the heart as you palpate. The carotid pulse is felt to rise just as $S_1$ ends, or the $S_1$ just precedes the carotid pulse.

Aortic valve function is assessed by inspection and palpation of the *aortic* area, the second intercostal space to the right of the sternum (see Fig. 38-6). Pulsations or thrills detected here may reflect the presence of an aortic aneurysm or aortic stenosis.

Examination of the *pulmonic* area, the second intercostal space to the left of the sternum (see Fig. 38-6), allows assessment of pulmonic valve function. A palpable thrill detected at Erb's point, the third intercostal space at the left sternal border, may reflect increased pressure or flow in the pulmonary artery; accentuated pulsation in this area may be due to sharp closure of the pulmonic valve often associated with pulmonary hypertension.

The *right ventricular* or *tricuspid* area is located in the fourth intercostal space at the left sternal border (see Fig. 38-6). Lifts or heaves associated with forceful cardiac action, as occurs with right ventricular hypertrophy, may be detected here. In the presence of enhanced cardiac output, as occurs for example in anxiety states, hyperthyroidism (thyrotoxicosis), fever, and anemia, an accentuated ventricular impulse may be felt. The presence of a thrill in this area may reflect ventricular septal defect.

The apical pulse may be palpated in the *apical* or *left ventricular* area in the fifth intercostal space just medial to the midclavicular line (see Fig. 38-6). The apical impulse should be assessed in terms of its amplitude, duration, and location. The amplitude of the apical impulse is normally small, light, or absent; its duration is usually less than half of systole; and it is usually palpable in the fifth intercostal space approximately 7-9 cm from the midsternal line. In the presence of left ventricular hy-

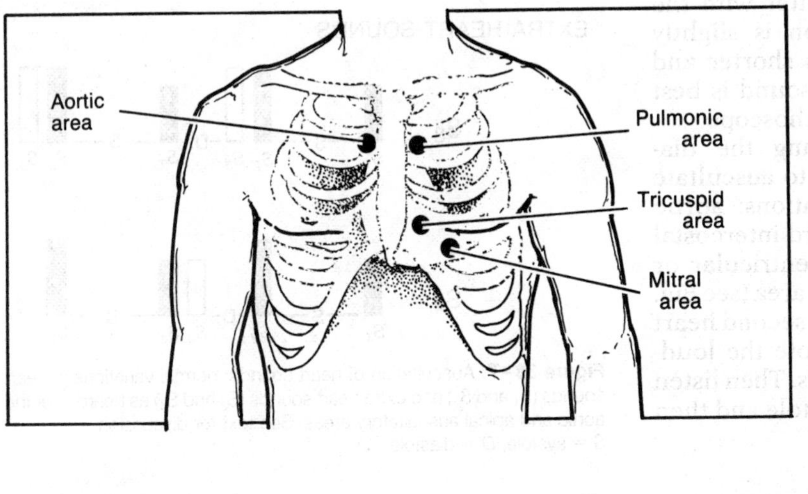


**Figure 38-6.** Auscultatory areas for assessment of heart sounds: Aortic area (second ICS to right of sternum); pulmonic area (second ICS to left of sternum); tricuspid area (fourth or fifth ICS at left sternal border); and mitral area (fifth ICS at MCL). (ICS = intercostal space; MCL = midclavicular line.)

pertrophy the amplitude of the apical pulse is larger and more forceful; its duration extends throughout most of systole; and its location may be displaced lateral to the midclavicular line and downward. Extra pulses detected in the apical area may reflect extra heart sounds, $S_3$ and $S_4$; thrills palpated in this area suggest a mitral stenosis or regurgitation.

Assess the *epigastric* area at the base of the sternum for any pulsations. Pulsations of the abdominal aorta may often be seen here especially in thin persons. Increased aortic pulsations may reflect an abdominal aortic aneurysm.

### Auscultation

To properly auscultate the heart it is essential to use a stethoscope equipped with a diaphragm and a bell. The diaphragm amplifies and transmits higher-pitched sounds; the bell transmits lower-pitched sounds. To appreciate heart sounds, it is important to "tune in" to specific events of the heart during the cardiac cycle, and to concentrate on one feature at a time. Concentrate first on the second heart sound ($S_2$) and listen to it *alone*; then shift to the first heart sound ($S_1$) and listen to it *alone*; next concentrate on the systolic interval between $S_1$ and $S_2$—try to hear nothing else; next concentrate on the diastolic interval between $S_2$ and $S_1$, in the same manner.

It is important to associate heart sounds with the mechanical events of the cardiac cycle: the first sound ($S_1$) is produced by closure of the AV valves (tricuspid and mitral); the second sound ($S_2$) is produced by closure of the semilunar valves (pulmonic and aortic). Normally, heart sounds are not heard during the interval between $S_1$ and $S_2$ (i.e, systole); or between $S_2$ and $S_1$ (i.e., diastole).

The first and second heart sounds are heard throughout the precordium. The second heart sound ($S_2$) is louder in the *aortic* area; the first heart sound ($S_1$) is louder in the *tricuspid* and *mitral* areas. Listening for the particular heart sound in the area where it is distinctly louder enables one sound to be distinguished from the other. Normally on auscultation, $S_1$ ("lup") is heard as a duller, lower-pitched sound often heard better with the bell of the stethoscope; its duration is slightly longer than that of $S_2$. $S_2$ ("dup") is shorter and snappier than $S_1$; its higher-pitched sound is best heard using the diaphragm of the stethoscope.

**Technique of Auscultation.** Using the diaphragm of the stethoscope, proceed to auscultate systematically in the following locations: aortic area; pulmonic area; Erb's point (third intercostal space at left sternal border); right ventricular or tricuspid area; and the apical or mitral area (see Fig. 38–6). When listening to the first and second heart sounds in each auscultatory area, note the loudness, pitch, and quality of these sounds. Then listen for extra heart sounds first during systole and then during diastole.

Beginning in the aortic area, identify $S_2$, which is louder in this area; then concentrate your full attention on $S_1$. Compare these two sounds and establish how they relate and the expected normal characteristics (Fig. 38–7). Next concentrate on the *systolic* interval between $S_1$ and $S_2$, followed by the *diastolic* interval between $S_2$ and $S_1$. Normally, there should be no sounds during these intervals.

Shift the diaphragm of the stethoscope to the pulmonic area and proceed as above. $S_2$ should be shorter, snappier, higher-pitched, and louder than $S_1$ in this area. Splitting of $S_2$ may be heard (see below). Compare the loudness of $S_2$ in the aortic area with that in the pulmonic area. In adults, $S_2$ is usually louder in the aortic area. The finding of $S_2$ pulmonic sound louder than $S_2$ aortic sound in an adult over 40 years of age is abnormal. This may result from factors that increase pulmonary pressures (pulmonary hypertension) such as longstanding COPD.

Having identified the heart sounds at the base of the heart, move or "inch" the stethoscope down along the left sternal border to the tricuspid area. The first sound, $S_1$, may be normally louder than $S_2$, or both may be equal. Shift to the bell to see if the lower-pitched sounds are heard better than with the diaphragm. Once again, examine $S_1$, $S_2$, systole, and diastole, assessing the sounds and then the intervals for any abnormalities.

Move the bell slowly toward the apex of the heart. The sounds are loudest in the mitral, or apical, area.

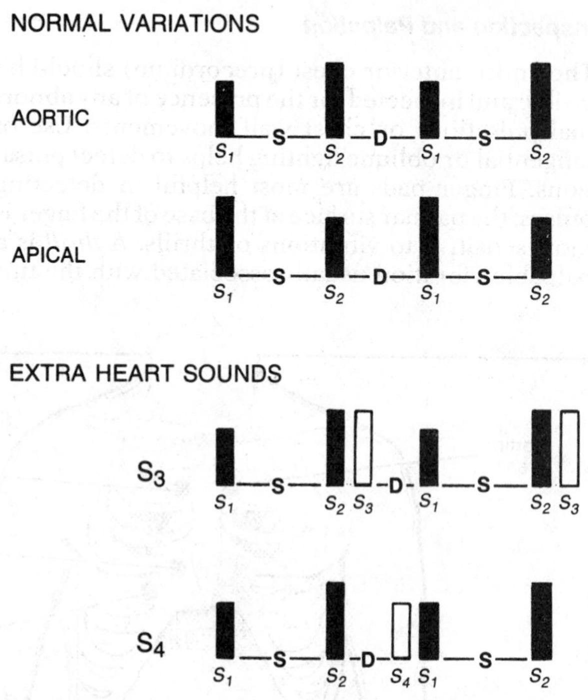


**Figure 38–7.** Auscultation of heart sounds: normal variations in heart sounds ($S_1$ and $S_2$) and extra heart sounds ($S_3$ and $S_4$) as heard over the aortic and apical auscultatory areas. See text for discussion. $S$ = systole, $D$ = diastole

Commonly, $S_1$ is louder than $S_2$ in this area. Proceed to examine the sounds and intervals for any abnormalities.

It should be appreciated that all heart sounds may be diminished in certain clinical circumstances. For example, an increase in chest wall thickness associated with obesity, pleural effusion, or a highly developed thoracic musculature has been associated with diminished heart sounds; an increase in the anterior/posterior diameter of the chest and/or hyperinflated lungs as occurs in chronic obstructive pulmonary disease decreases breath sounds as well as heart sounds; an increase in intrapleural air associated with a pneumothorax may likewise diminish heart sounds.

### Splitting

The valves of the right and left sides of the heart snap shut almost simultaneously so that the sound produced is usually heard as but a single sound. Should a delay occur in the closure of one valve, the resulting sound will be heard with two distinct components, and it is said to *split* (Fig. 38–8). Splitting of the first heart sound is more distinctly heard at the apex; splitting of the second heart sound is most often heard at the base of the heart. The split sound should be assessed for loudness, pitch, and quality. The split sound is distinguished by having the same characteristic features as the unsplit sound except that it consists of 2 distinct components, one occurring immediately after the other.

Physiologically, right-sided events involving closure of tricuspid and pulmonic valves usually occur slightly later than corresponding events in the left heart. Therefore, slight splitting of the normal heart sounds may occur, particularly of $S_2$. The splitting of $S_2$ is especially accentuated on inspiration. Venous return to the right heart is increased, thereby prolonging right ventricular ejection and delaying pulmonic valve closure ever so slightly. On expiration, when blood flow through the right heart is reduced, the splitting disappears. This normal splitting of $S_2$, which is heard to widen on inspiration and to disappear on expiration, is referred to as *physiologic* splitting.

Variations in splitting may reflect underlying pathology. *Wide* splitting heard throughout the respiratory cycle may be caused by delayed pulmonic valve closure associated with pulmonic stenosis. Wide splitting of both $S_1$ (mitral and tricuspid valve closure) and $S_2$ is often caused by right bundle branch block in which the left ventricle depolarizes before the right ventricle. *Fixed* splitting refers to wide splitting that does not vary with respirations. This type of splitting may occur in right ventricular failure or atrial septal defect. *Paradoxical* splitting refers to splitting that appears on expiration and disappears on inspiration. This is contrary to physiologic splitting discussed above. A common cause of paradoxical splitting is left bundle branch block resulting in unusually delayed closure of the aortic valve.

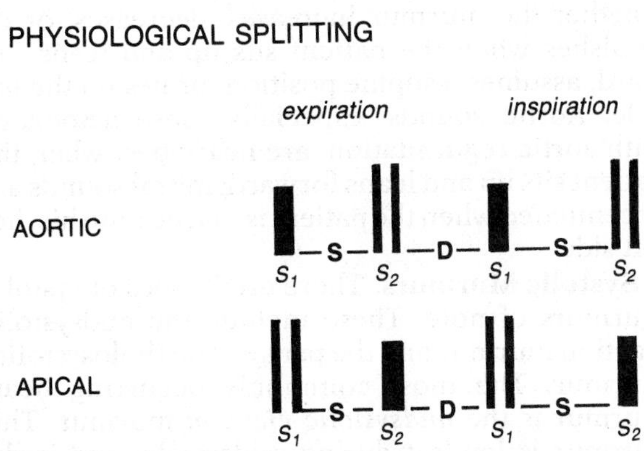


**Figure 38–8.** Auscultation of heart sounds: physiologic splitting as heard over the aortic and apical auscultatory areas during inspiration and expiration. See text for discussion.
$S$ = systole, $D$ = diastole

### Extra Heart Sound: $S_3$

A physiologic third heard sound ($S_3$) may be heard in children and it may persist in young adults under 30–40 years of age. It is largely associated with flow of blood from atria into ventricles. The $S_3$ is a lower-pitched sound heard best over the apex of the heart using the bell of the stethoscope. It usually becomes louder on inspiration and is accentuated in the left lateral decubitus (or side-lying) position. At rapid heart rates (tachycardia), the sound produced becomes that of a ventricular *gallop* rhythm ($S_3$ gallop), reflecting the cadence produced by the 3 heart sounds ($S_1$, $S_2$, and $S_3$). Sometimes, repeating the word "Ken-*tuck*-y" in time with the cadence helps to distinguish the third heart sound as $S_3$, which occurs *early* in diastole immediately following $S_2$ (see Fig. 38–7).

The presence of $S_3$ is considered pathologic in individuals over 40 years of age. It has been associated with conditions that create volume overloading of the ventricles as occurs in aortic, mitral, or tricuspid regurgitation, or during periods of rapid ventricular filling.

### Extra Heart Sound: $S_4$

The occurrence of a fourth heart sound ($S_4$) is usually associated with atrial contraction. Atrial contraction occurs prior to closure of AV valves ($S_1$), which signals the onset of ventricular contraction. Thus, the fourth heart sound will be heard at the end of diastole, just before $S_1$ (see Fig. 38–7). The $S_4$ is a lower-pitched sound heard best at the left sternal border, or apex of the heart, using the bell of the stethoscope. It can usually be distinguished from the $S_3$ sound by its appearance *late* in diastole, just prior to $S_1$. At rapid heart rates, the occurrence of a third heart sound may result in a "gallop" rhythm. To distinguish an $S_4$ gallop from an $S_3$ gallop (described above), try to repeat the word, "Tenne-*see*" in time with the cadence.

The appearance of an $S_4$ is abnormal. It is associated with increased resistance to ventricular filling, as occurs in congestive heart failure. It has been identified in patients with hypertensive heart disease, coronary artery disease, or aortic stenosis. It may also be associated with anemia and hyperthyroidism.

Other abnormal extra heart sounds that may be heard on auscultation include ejection clicks heard in early systole and opening snaps heard in early diastole. *Ejection clicks* may be associated with pathologic conditions involving the aortic valve; *opening snaps* are most often associated with stenotic mitral and, to a lesser extent, stenotic tricuspid valves. For further description and assessment of these sounds, the reader is referred to the appropriate texts on this subject.

### Murmurs

Murmurs are abnormal sounds resulting from turbulent blood flow within the heart. Such sounds may be associated with various mechanisms including the following: (1) valvular dysfunction including a forced forward flow of blood through a narrowed opening (stenosis), or backward flow of blood associated with defective valve closure (regurgitation); (2) septal defects with shunting of blood from a high-pressure chamber through an abnormal opening (atrial or ventricular septal defects); and (3) increased velocity of blood flow through normal structures as occurs, for example, in anemia (aortic systolic murmur).

Murmurs may be described as *functional* (i.e., altered physiologic function with or without heart disease) or *organic* (i.e., associated with a structural abnormality). It should be noted that all murmurs do not indicate pathology, nor do all cardiac structural defects produce murmurs. In general, murmurs occurring during diastole are considered pathologic.

Murmurs may occur at various times during the cardiac cycle (systole and diastole), and should be assessed for the following characteristics: timing, location, radiation, intensity, pitch, quality, and changes with respiration, movement, or position.

The *timing* of murmurs is based upon when they occur during the cardiac cycle and in relation to the first and second heart sounds. By definition, systolic murmurs occur between $S_1$ and $S_2$; diastolic murmurs occur between $S_2$ and $S_1$. Systolic murmurs may be described as occurring in early, mid-, or late systole; or they may be heard throughout systole (pansystolic or holosystolic). Similarly, diastolic murmurs are classified as early, mid-, and late diastolic (presystolic).

The *location* of a murmur is the point at which it is heard the loudest (i.e., location of maximal intensity). Location of murmurs is usually described in terms of their relationship to imaginary lines and intercostal spaces (see Figs. 29–2 through 29–4). *Transmission* or *radiation* of the murmur from the point of maximal intensity may be auscultated. Aortic murmurs commonly radiate to the neck and down the left sternal border; mitral valve murmurs often radiate to the left axilla.

Murmurs may also be graded in terms of their *intensity* and *loudness*, and are usually recorded using the following scale:

Grade I: Very faint, heard only after the examiner has listened carefully.
Grade II: Quiet, but heard immediately with the stethoscope.
Grade III: Moderately loud, not associated with a thrill (i.e., a fine vibration palpated with the ball of the hand).
Grade IV: Loud, may be associated with a thrill.
Grade V: Very loud, may be heard with the stethoscope partly off the chest; associated with a thrill.
Grade VI: May be heard with the stethoscope off the chest; associated with a thrill.

The intensity of a murmur is written as a Roman numerical fraction. For example, if a Grade III murmur is heard, it is documented as Gr III/IV. Loudness or intensity may also be described in terms of *crescendo* (i.e., building to a climax) and *decrescendo* (i.e., starting at a climax or maximum, and dropping off or diminishing).

The *pitch* of a murmur is described as low, medium, or high pitched. In general, high-pitched murmurs are heard best using the diaphragm of the stethoscope; low-pitched murmurs are more clearly auscultated using the bell. The *quality* of a murmur is described as blowing, rumbling, harsh, or musical.

It is important to note if there is any variation in murmurs with respiration. Right heart murmurs tend to change more with respirations than do left heart murmurs. Body position also affects auscultation of murmurs. It may be helpful to determine whether the murmur increases, decreases, or diminishes when the patient sits up and leans forward, assumes a supine position, or lies on the left side. Aortic sounds, especially those associated with aortic regurgitation, are heard best when the patient sits up and leans forward; mitral sounds are accentuated when the patient is placed onto his/her left side.

**Systolic Murmurs.** There are 2 types of systolic murmurs of note. These include the midsystolic ejection murmur and the pansystolic (holosystolic) murmur. The most commonly occurring heart murmur is the *midsystolic ejection* murmur. This murmur is loudest during midsystole, and is described as a diamond-shaped crescendo-decrescendo murmur (Fig. 38–9). It is heard best over

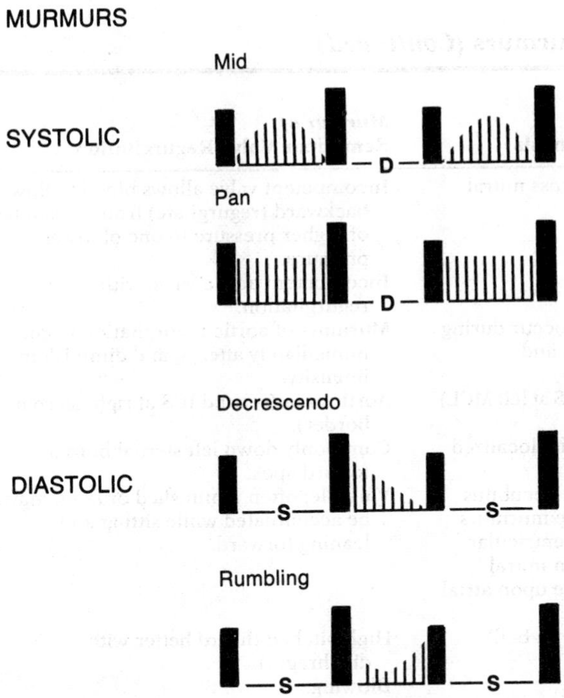


**Figure 38-9.** Auscultation of heart sounds: differentiation of systolic and diastolic murmurs. See text for discussion. *S* = systole, *D* = diastole.

the aortic area; radiation to the neck and down the left sternal border may also be auscultated. The midsystolic ejection murmur is usually associated with altered forward flow of blood through the semilunar valves, as occurs, for example, in aortic stenosis. Less commonly, it may be produced by pulmonic stenosis or by flow of blood into an aorta *dilated* by atherosclerotic and/or syphilitic changes.

The *pansystolic* (*holosystolic*) murmur is heard throughout systole beginning with $S_1$ and continuing up to $S_2$ (see Fig. 38-9). It is most frequently associated with an incompetent mitral valve wherein blood flows from a chamber of higher pressure to one of lower pressure (e.g., mitral regurgitation during ventricular contraction). This murmur is high pitched and is heard best using the diaphragm of the stethoscope placed over the mitral or apical area. Radiation into the left axilla may also be noted. The quality of the sound produced is that of a "blowing" characteristic. (Refer to Table 38-3 for a comparison of the characteristics of these murmurs.)

Systolic murmurs may also be described as crescendo or decrescendo depending upon when in systole they are heard the loudest.

**Diastolic Murmurs.** Diastolic murmurs are almost always indicative of underlying heart disease. The 2 commonly described types of diastolic murmurs are *diastolic rumbling* murmur of mitral stenosis and the *early diastolic* murmur of aortic regurgitation.

In the case of mitral stenosis, blood flow across the affected valve is disrupted. The consequent murmur is low pitched and rumbling in quality, and is heard best with the bell of the stethoscope placed lightly over the tricuspid and apical areas. These murmurs are loudest during periods of rapid ventricular filling, including in early diastole upon

TABLE 38-3
**Characteristics of Common Systolic and Diastolic Murmurs**

| **Systolic Murmurs** / *Characteristics* | *Murmur of* **Semilunar Valve Stenosis** | *Murmur of* **Atrioventricular Valve Regurgitation** |
|---|---|---|
| Pathophysiology | Usually associated with altered blood flow through semilunar valves. | Incompetent valve allows blood to flow (regurgitate) from a chamber of higher pressure to one of lower pressure. |
| Underlying pathology | Aortic stenosis (most common). Pulmonic stenosis. | Incompetent mitral valve with regurgitation (most common); may also occur with tricuspid regurgitation and ventricular septal defect. |
| Timing | Midsystolic ejection murmur (diamond-shaped crescendo-decrescendo murmur) occurs midway between $S_1$ and $S_2$ | Pansystolic (holosytolic) murmur occurs throughout systole, beginning with $S_1$ and continuing through to $S_2$. |
| Location | Aortic area (second ICS at right sternal border). | Tricuspid and mitral areas (fourth and fifth ICs at left sternal border; and apical area). |
| Radiation | Neck and/or down left sternal border. | Left axillary area with mitral valve pathology; left sternal border to left MCL with tricuspid valve defect. |
| Intensity (loudness) (*Scale:* Grades I through VI; see text) | Variable; if loud, a thrill may be palpated over aortic area. | Variable; if loud, it may be associated with thrill over apical area. |
| Pitch | Medium to low. | High. |
| Quality | Harsh. | Blowing. |

*(continued)*

TABLE 38–3
**Characteristics of Common Systolic and Diastolic Murmurs *(Continued)***

**Diastolic Murmurs**

| *Characteristics* | ***Murmur of* Atrioventricular Valve Stenosis** | ***Murmur of* Semilunar Valve Regurgitation** |
|---|---|---|
| Pathophysiology | Disruption of blood flow across mitral valve. | Incompetent valve allows blood to flow backward (regurgitate) from a chamber of higher pressure to one of lower pressure. |
| Underlying pathology | Mitral valve stenosis. | Incompetent aortic valve with regurgitation. |
| Timing | Murmurs of mitral stenosis occur during early diastole following $S_2$ and continuing to $S_1$. | Murmurs of aortic regurgitation begin immediately after $S_2$ and diminish in intensity. |
| Location | Mitral or apical area (fifth ICS at left MCL). | Aortic area (second ICS at right sternal border). |
| Radiation | Minimal radiation; tends to be localized to apical area. | Commonly down left sternal border toward apex. |
| Intensity (loudness) (*Scale:* Grades I through VI) | Variable; accentuated in left decubitus (side-lying) position. These murmurs are loudest during rapid ventricular filling (early diastole) upon mitral valve opening; late diastole upon atrial contraction). | Variable; often diminished or faint. May be accentuated while sitting and leaning forward. |
| Pitch | Low-pitched (heard better with bell). | High-pitched (heard better with diaphragm). |
| Quality | Rumbling. | Blowing. |

mitral valve opening and in late diastole during atrial contraction (see Fig. 38–9).

In the presence of a regurgitant aortic valve, blood flows backward from the aorta as it recoils during ventricular diastole. Sounds of these murmurs are described as high pitched and blowing, in contrast to the low rumbling of mitral valve murmurs. Murmurs of aortic regurgitation commence immediately after the second heart sound ($S_2$), and diminish in intensity (see Fig. 38–9). They are best heard with the diaphragm of the stethoscope firmly placed over the aortic area. Radiation down the left sternal border toward the apex of the heart may be discerned. Refer to Table 38–3 for a comparison of the characteristics of these murmurs.

### *Pericardial Friction Rub*

A friction rub is a distinct grating or scraping sound associated with inflammation of the visceral and parietal epicardial layers of the heart (see Chap. 37). The inflammatory process disrupts the normal gliding of these membranes over each other during the heart's pumping actions. The consequent increase in friction accounts for the "friction rub." The actual sound produced may be similar to that produced by rubbing 2 inflated balloons together.

A friction rub can often be heard over the lower sternum and apical areas; it may be heard during both systole and diastole, or points therein; and the sound may vary with respirations as inflammation of the pleura often occurs in conjunction with the pericarditis. Characteristically, a pericardial friction rub is transient and disappears as the pericarditis subsides.

## REFERENCES

1. Bates, B: A Guide to Physical Examination, ed 4. JB Lippincott, Philadelphia, 1987, p 297.

CHAPTER 39

# Cardiovascular Diagnostic Techniques

*Sheila M. Keller*

## CHAPTER OUTLINE

RADIOLOGIC TESTING: THE CHEST X-RAY

GRAPHIC RECORDING: STRESS TEST OR GRADED EXERCISE TEST (GEX)

PHONOCARDIOGRAM

ULTRASONOGRAPHY: ECHOCARDIOGRAM

RADIONUCLIDE STUDIES
- Thallium Imaging (Cold Spot Myocardial Imaging Thallium Scintigraphy)
- Tc-PYP Heart Scan
- Gated Blood Pool Scans (Blood Pool Imaging)

CARDIAC CATHETERIZATION

ELECTROPHYSIOLOGIC STUDIES (EPS)
- His Bundle Electrography
- Ventricular Mapping or Programmed Electrical Stimulation (PES)

NEW TECHNIQUES
- Digital Substraction Angiography (DSA)
- Magnetic Resonance Imaging (MRI)

## LEARNING OBJECTIVES

**At the end of this chapter, you should be able to:**

1. Explain the purpose of specific cardiovascular diagnostic techniques.
2. Describe cardiovascular diagnostic procedures in terms that the patient/family can comprehend.
3. Identify situations for which the procedures would be contraindicated.
4. Discuss interfering factors that may alter proper interpretation of test results.
5. Describe patient preparation needed pre- and post-procedure, including desired patient outcomes.
6. Prioritize nursing care measures pre- and post-procedure.
7. Analyze tests results, identifying abnormalities and their significance in terms of patient outcomes.

The clinical history and physical examination of the cardiac patient are of primary importance in the diagnosis and/or evaluation of cardiovascular disease. These findings are frequently augmented with additional diagnostic studies. The sophistication in testing techniques has greatly improved over the years, increasing the accuracy of diagnostic tests/studies and thereby decreasing the morbidity and mortality rates. Nurses must keep abreast of rapid technological advances in order to provide safe and effective nursing care. To assist the nurse in this regard, specific and pertinent diagnostic tests/studies in current use are discussed in the text that follows. For simplicity and comparison, the purpose, contraindications, normal findings and results, complications, patient preparation, and nursing care implications pre- and post-procedure, are presented in Table 39–1. The reader is encouraged to refer to this table while studying the text.

## RADIOLOGIC TESTING: THE CHEST X-RAY

The chest x-ray is one of the most frequently used diagnostic tests. Routinely, posteroanterior (PA) and left lateral views are taken. These provide a

TABLE 39-1
## Cardiovascular Diagnostic Tests

| Diagnostic Test | Purpose | Contraindications | Normal Findings | Complications | Patient Preparation | Nursing Care: Pre-test | Nursing Care: Post-test |
|---|---|---|---|---|---|---|---|
| Chest x-ray | To evaluate/detect cardiac disease and abnormalities that change the size, shape, position, and appearance of the heart, lungs, and great vessels.<br>To ensure correct positioning of catheters, i.e., pulmonary artery lines, subclavian lines, pacemaker wires, chest tubes, and endotracheal tubes. | Pregnancy<br>Young children and infants | Normal size (PA view—the heart is less than 50% of the thoracic diameter)<br>No calcifications<br>No masses<br>No pericardial effusions<br>Lungs clear<br>No pleural effusions<br>No infiltrates | None | Explain the procedure and purpose.<br>Emphasize the procedure is painless and that there is little radiation given off.<br>Have the patient remove all clothing from the neck to the waist and put on a hospital gown (with ties, not snaps).<br>Have the patient remove all jewelry and other metal objects. | Patient teaching. | Review findings.<br>Update nursing care plan. |
| Fluoroscopy | To evaluate cardiac wall motion and movement of prosthetic heart valves. | Pregnancy<br>Young children and infants | Normal heart motion<br>Normal prosthetic valve function<br>No evidence of ventricular aneurysms | None | Same as the chest x-ray. | Patient teaching. | Review findings.<br>Update nursing care plan. |
| Stress testing | To assess cardiac response to an increased workload.<br>To help diagnose the cause of chest pain.<br>To determine the functional capacity of the heart after cardiac surgery or a myocardial infarction.<br>To establish readiness for, or set limitations for, an exercise program. | New or changing chest pain, hypertension, uncontrolled heart failure, acute pericarditis, acute myocarditis, severe anemia, serious dysrhythmias, severe valvular disease, ventricular or dissecting aneurysm, known high-grade left main coronary artery disease | Little or no change in the ECG/rhythm strip with exercise<br>The heart rate increases in proportion to the workload.<br>Attainment of the target heart rate<br>Systolic blood pressure increases in proportion to the workload.<br>Absence of dysrhythmias with exercise | Dysrhythmias<br>Hypotension<br>Bradycardia<br>Myocarcardial infarction<br>Cardiac arrest | Explain the procedure and purpose.<br>Ensure that consent form is signed.<br>Reassure that the physician is available at all times.<br>Tell patient to avoid strenuous exercise 24 hours before the test.<br>Patient is not allowed to eat, smoke, or drink alcohol or caffeine 2–3 hr | Patient teaching.<br>Check consent form.<br>Check with the physician concerning cardiac medications.<br>Check for the history and physical examination. One must be done within 1 week of the test.<br>Check for a baseline 12-lead ECG.<br>Have emergency | Assist the patient to a chair.<br>Continue monitoring heart rate, blood pressure, and rhythm strips until parameters return to baseline.<br>Monitor for signs of intolerance.<br>Remove all electrodes, and clean sites.<br>Tell patient to wait 1 hr before taking a *warm* shower (hot water may |

| | | | | | | | |
|---|---|---|---|---|---|---|---|
| | To identify exercise-related dysrhythmias.<br>To evaluate the effectiveness of antidysrhythmics or antianginal drugs.<br>Exercise stress testing may be done within 72 hours post-myocardial infarction in some patients. | Patients severely limited by neurologic, peripheral-vascular, or musculoskeletal disease, hyperthyroidism | | | prior to the test.<br>Patient must continue medications unless physician specifies otherwise.<br>Tell patient to wear loose comfortable clothing (shorts or slacks). Men usually don't wear a shirt. Women should wear a bra and a light, loose short-sleeve blouse that buttons down the front or a patient gown with a front closure.<br>Patient should wear comfortable shoes and socks, not slippers. Sneakers are best but any rubber-soled shoes will do. | equipment on standby. | make him/her feel faint or dizzy).<br>Tell patient to resume usual diet and activity.<br>Review findings.<br>Update nursing care plan. |
| Phonocardiogram | To augment auscultation in differentiating normal and abnormal heart sounds.<br>To aid in the timing of the cardiac cycle.<br>To calculate ventricular function.<br>To identify structural defects. | None | Normal heart sounds | None | Explain the procedure and purpose.<br>Explain that the procedure is safe and painless.<br>There is no need to restrict food and fluids. | Patient teaching. | Review findings.<br>Update nursing care plan. |

*(continued)*

TABLE 39–1
**Cardiovascular Diagnostic Tests *(Continued)***

| Diagnostic Test | Purpose | Contraindications | Normal Findings | Complications | Patient Preparation | Nursing Care: *Pre-test* | Nursing Care: *Post-test* |
|---|---|---|---|---|---|---|---|
| Echocardiogram | To diagnose and evaluate valvular disorders.<br>To aid in the diagnosis of hypertrophic and related cardiomyopathies.<br>To detect atrial tumors.<br>To evaluate cardiac function post-myocardial infarction.<br>To detect pericardial effusions, septal defects, and ventricular aneurysms.[1]<br>To evaluate prosthetic valve function. | None | Normal motion pattern and structure of the valves<br>Ventricles are echo-free.<br>No effusion<br>No septal defects<br>Normal prosthetic valve function | None | Explain the procedure and purpose.<br>Reassure the patient that the procedure is safe and painless.<br>Explain that some discomfort may be felt due to the amount of pressure needed on the transducer to keep it in contact with the skin.<br>There is no need to restrict food or fluids. | Patient teaching. | Remove the conductive jelly from the patient's chest.<br>Review the findings. Update nursing care plan. |
| Radionuclide studies | | | | | | | |
| Thallium imaging ("cold spotting") | To evaluate myocardial blood flow and the status of the myocardial cells.<br>To determine ejection fraction and velocity. | Children and pregnancy | Blood flow equal throughout the myocardium<br>Ejection fraction >70%<br>Normal velocity<br>No area of ischemia; no cold spots<br>No hot spots; only the sternum and ribs should be visible.<br>Improved regional perfusion | None | Explain the procedure and purpose.<br>Ensure that consent form is signed.<br>Reassure the patient that there is no known radiation danger.<br>If the patient has to return for additional scanning, tell him/her to rest and restrict diet to clear liquids until the scanning is completed. (If a stress thallium scan is being done, refer to Stress Testing, | Patient teaching. | Tell patient to resume pre-study orders concerning diet, activity, and medications unless otherwise ordered by the physician.<br>Review findings.<br>Update nursing care plan. |
| Tc-PYP heart scan ("hot spotting") | To assess myocardial scarring and perfusion.<br>To distinguish if myocardial infarction is old or new.<br>To evaluate patency of grafts.<br>To evaluate the effectiveness of balloon angioplasty. | | | | | | |

| | | | | | | | |
|---|---|---|---|---|---|---|---|
| | To determine the ejection fraction.<br>To determine the effectiveness of antianginal therapy. | | | | above, for additional preparations.) | | |
| Blood-pool imaging | To evaluate left ventricular function.<br>To detect aneurysms and other myocardial abnormalities.<br>To detect intracardiac shunting.<br>To determine the ejection fraction. | | No aneurysms or muscle wall dysfunction<br>No intracardiac shunting<br>Ejection fraction >70% | | | | |
| Cardiac catheterization | To evaluate cardiac wall motion.<br>To evaluate valve function.<br>To determine cardiac output.<br>To determine presence of cardiac defects/abnormalities.<br>To determine the presence of coronary artery disease.<br>To determine candidates for balloon angioplasty, fibrinolytic therapy, bypass surgery, heart transplantation, and for the artificial heart.<br>To determine the presence of intracardiac shunting.<br>To evaluate patency of bypass grafts. | Acute myocardial infarction<br>Acute debilitating conditions<br>Gross cardiomegaly<br>Poor renal function<br>Special conditions:<br>Right-sided catheterization: Left bundle branch block (LBBB) unless a temporary pacemaker is inserted<br>Patients with valvular disease: Prophylactic antibiotics to guard against subacute bacterial endocarditis (SBE) | Normal wall motion<br>Normal valve movement<br>Coronary arteries: Smooth, with regular outline<br>Pressures: RA—0–8 mmHg<br>RV—15–25 mmHg systolic; 0–8 mmHg diastolic<br>PA—15–30 mmHg systolic; 8–15 mmHg diastolic<br>LA—4–12 mmHg<br>LV—100–140 mmHg systolic; 0–10 mmHg diastolic<br>Ao—100–140 mmHg systolic; 60–80 mmHg diastolic<br>PCWP—8–12 mmHg<br>Stroke Index: 30–65 ml/beat/$m^2$<br>Cardiac index: 2.5–4.0 ml/min/$m^2$ | General:<br>MI<br>Cardiac tamponade<br>Dysrhythmias.<br>Pneumothorax<br>Infection: local and/or systemic<br>Hypovolemia<br>Pulmonary edema<br>Hemorrhage/hematoma at the site of insertion<br>Arterial spasm<br>Allergic reaction to the contrast medium<br>Cardiac arrest<br>Left-sided:<br>Arterial emboli<br>Thrombus<br>CVA<br>Right-sided:<br>Thrombophlebitis<br>Pulmonary emboli<br>Vasovagal reaction | Explain the procedure and purpose.<br>Ensure that consent form is signed.<br>Restrict foods and fluids 6–12 hr prior to the test (may be allowed to take oral medications with sips of water).<br>Reinforce the need for complete cooperation. Must follow orders immediately, e.g., cough.<br>Reinforce that he/she will be awake throughout the procedure but a sedative or tranquilizer will be given.<br>Reinforce that there will be talking among the professionals and that when they talk to him/her they will call him/her by name. | Check history and physical examination.<br>Check pre-procedure studies: Chest x-ray, ECG, coagulation values, cardiac enzymes, CBC, and electrolytes.<br>*Check for allergies* especially to seafood, iodine, and other contrast media.<br>Patient teaching.<br>Encourage to practice breathing and coughing.<br>Provide emotional support.<br>Administer sedative/tranquilizer unless the patient has respiratory compromise.<br>Mark peripheral pulses for easier location post-procedure.<br>Monitor vital signs for baseline parameters. | Monitor vital signs every 15 minutes ×4 until stable.<br>Check periphreral pulses every 1/2 hr.<br>Observe insertion site for bleeding or hematomas.<br>Have patient wiggle fingers and toes every 1/2 hr.<br>Enforce bedrest for 6–12 hr.<br>Keep extremity straight for 6–8 hr.<br>Support the extremity during transfer from the stretcher to the bed especially if the Judkin's technique was used; apply pressure during transfer.<br>Encourage fluid intake; maintain IVs.<br>Measure I&O.<br>Obtain a post-procedure ECG.<br>Review medica- |

*(continued)*

TABLE 39–1
**Cardiovascular Diagnostic Tests *(Continued)***

| Diagnostic Test | Purpose | Contraindications | Normal Findings | Complications | Patient Preparation | Nursing Care | |
|---|---|---|---|---|---|---|---|
| | | | | | | *Pre-test* | *Post-test* |
| | | | Ejection fraction 70% or greater<br>Oxygen saturation:<br>Right side: 75% ± 14<br>Left side: 95% ± 19<br>Valve Orifices:<br>Mitral: 5–6 $cm^2$<br>Aortic: 2.5–3.5/$cm^2$ | | He/she may wear dentures, glasses, and hearing aid. | Have patient void and put on a hospital gown before leaving for the procedure.<br>**When the procedure is ordered by the physician, check about any anticoagulants that the patient may be receiving and if cardiac drugs are to be given prior to the procedure.** | **tions with the physician for resumption.<br>Review test results.<br>Update nursing care plan.<br>Start discharge teaching.** |
| Electrophysiologic studies (EPS)<br>His bundle electrography<br>Ventricular mapping (PES)<br>Epicardial mapping | To measure discrete conduction intervals.<br>To localize disturbances within the atrioventricular conduction system.<br>To pinpoint ectopic pacemakers.<br>To evaluate for implantation of permanent pacemaker.<br>To evaluate effectiveness of antidysrhythmic therapy. | Severe coagulopathy<br>Recent thrombophlebitis<br>Acute pulmonary embolism<br>Valvular/subvalvular infection | H-V interval: 35–55 msec<br>A-H interval: 45–150 msec | Prolonged, sustained dysrhythmias<br>Phlebitis<br>Pulmonary emboli<br>Thromboemboli<br>Hemorrhage at the insertion site<br>Perforation of the ventricular or septal wall<br>Damage to the tricuspid valve<br>Damage to the catheterized vein (occlusion)<br>Infection: Local/systemic<br>Pneumothorax | Explain the procedure and purpose.<br>Ensure that consent form is signed.<br>Restrict food and fluids for at least 6 hr prior to procedure.<br>Refer to Cardiac Catheterization, above. | **Patient teaching.**<br>Check consent form.<br>Check patient history and ongoing drug therapy.<br>Emergency equipment on standby.<br>Refer to Cardiac Catheterization, above. | **Refer to Cardiac Catheterization, above.** |

| | | | | | | | |
|---|---|---|---|---|---|---|---|
| New techniques | | | | | | | |
| Digital subtraction angiography (DSA) | To analyze ventricular wall motion.<br>To calculate ejection fraction.<br>To evaluate patency and perfusion of bypass grafts.<br>To detect vascular abnormalities, i.e., plaques, tumors, aneurysms, emboli. | None | Normal wall motion<br>Patent bypass grafts with good perfusion<br>Ejection fraction: >70%<br>Negative tumors, plaques, aneurysms, emboli | Dysrthythmias<br>Allergic reaction to the contrast medium<br>Bleeding at insertion site<br>Infection | May be done on an outpatient basis.<br>Explain procedure and purpose.<br>Ensure that consent form is signed. | Patient teaching.<br>Check patient history.<br>Check consent form.<br>Check for allergies. | Monitor vital signs every 15 minutes until stable.<br>Check for bleeding and infection.<br>Force fluids.<br>Discharge teaching must include signs and symptoms for which patient should seek immediate medical attention<br>Review results.<br>Update nursing care plan. |
| Magnetic resonance imaging (MRI) | To visualize blood flow.<br>To visualize cardiac chambers.<br>To visualize the interventricular septum and valcular areas.<br>To detect vascular lesions, i.e., plaque, tumors, clots, and myocardial infarction. | Permanent pacemakers | No impedance of blood flow<br>No abnormalities in the interventricular septum<br>Normal valves—no calcification<br>No evidence of tumors, plaques, clots, or myocardial infarction. | Affects pacemaker function | Explain procedure and purpose.<br>Removal of all metal objects.<br>Ensure that consent form is signed. | Patient teaching.<br>Check consent form.<br>Check for removal of metal objects. | Review results.<br>Update nursing care plan. |

sharper and less distorted image of the heart. If the patient is unable to be transported to the x-ray department, a portable x-ray can be used. The portable equipment provides an anteroposterior (AP) view, which may distort the relative size of the heart and great vessels as reviewed and interpreted. Vascular markings in the AP view may appear increased.

### *Procedure and Nursing Care Implications*

The PA view is obtained by having the patient stand erect with the chin resting on top of the cassette holder and the chest and shoulders resting against the holder. The x-ray machine is approximately 6 feet behind the patient. The patient is told to take a deep breath and to hold it until the picture is taken. The technician advises the patient when to again breathe. The patient holds the breath but for a few seconds. Post-myocardial infarction patients should be warned not to bear down while holding their breath (Valsalva maneuver), as this may precipitate a vagal response resulting in bradycardia or other cardiac dysrhythmias. Full cooperation on the part of the patient is necessary for a clear picture.

The AP view is taken by placing the cassette behind the patient's back with the head of the bed either flat or in a high Fowler's position. The upright position is best since the patient's diaphragm will not interfere with the visualization of the heart and lungs. The x-ray machine is placed in front of the patient approximately 2 feet away from the patient's chest. The patient is told to take a deep breath and to hold it until told to breathe again. If patients are unable to hold their breath, the technician times the exposure to take place at the end of inspiration. The AP view is the view obtained when a portable x-ray is desired.

### *Abnormal Findings*

Cardiac enlargement, pericardial effusions, pericardial tamponade, valve calcification, ventricular and aortic aneurysms, and coarctation of the aorta are some of the abnormalities that can be found on a PA and lateral chest x-ray.

### *Interfering Factors*

Interfering factors include: poor technique or exposure, patients unable to hold their breath, and patient movement.

## GRAPHIC RECORDING: STRESS TEST OR GRADED EXERCISE TEST (GEX)

There are a variety of stress tests. The oldest approach is the Master's double 2-step test, but it is not frequently used. In this test the patient walks up and down a set of 9-inch steps. This activity usually is not adequate to increase the heart rate to the target limit.

The bicycle ergometry test measures the effects of arm and leg exercises applied against a calibrated amount of resistance. The amount of resistance is gradually increased as the patient tries to maintain a constant speed. The patient sits on the bicycle, and the seat and handlebars are adjusted so that the patient is comfortable and able to maintain balance.

The multistage treadmill test measures the effects of graduated exercise at adjusted speeds and inclines. The patient is shown how to step on the treadmill moving at a slow speed, and how to use the support rails to maintain balance only. The patient then steps on to the treadmill and continues walking at a slow rate until familiar with walking on it; then the speed and incline are gradually increased. The patient is always informed prior to any changes.

### *Procedure and Nursing Care Implications*

In general, the procedure for stress testing or exercising includes cleaning (and shaving, if necessary) several areas on the patient's chest and possibly the back. The skin is abraded and the monitor electrodes are applied in selected leads. (Reassure the patient that no current will be felt from the electrodes.) The electrodes are secured and the lead cable placed over the patient's shoulder and secured with tape or pinned to the clothing. A baseline tracing is obtained, as well as a baseline heart rate (HR) and blood pressure (Bp). The patient's heart and lungs are auscultated, noting the presence of extra heart sounds (e.g., $S_3$ or $S_4$ gallop) and/or adventitious breath sounds (e.g., rales, or crackles). (Refer to Chaps. 29 and 38). The test is cancelled if any pre-test abnormalities are noted.

Once the test is begun, the patient's rhythm, heart rate, and blood pressure are monitored throughout the test, usually at predetermined intervals. The test level and elapsed time are noted with each set of parameters. The test takes approximately 30 minutes although the patient may be in the laboratory for 1 – 1½ hours.

The test is usually stopped when the target heart rate is reached. The target heart rate may vary among institutions. It is usually based upon age and sex; a general rule of thumb calculation is 220 minus the patient's age. The test can also be terminated for reasons other than the patient reaching the target heart rate. Table 39 – 2 lists these reasons according to subjective and objective data.

Upon termination of the test, speed of the treadmill or bicycle is slowed for several minutes; then the patient is assisted off the equipment and helped to a chair. An ECG is performed, and rhythm strips are obtained at 2 – 3 minute intervals until parameters return to the patient's baseline levels. The

TABLE 39-2
**Reasons to Terminate Stress Testing**

| |
|---|
| **Subjective Data** |
| Chest pain |
| Extreme fatigue |
| Extreme weakness |
| Severe dyspnea |
| Dizziness or syncope |
| Ataxia |
| Claudication |
| **Objective Data** |
| Gallop heart sounds ($S_3$, $S_4$) |
| Valvular regurgitation murmur |
| Abnormal chest pulsations or heaves |
| ST-segment elevation or depression of 1 mm or more |
| Dysrhythmias |
| Target heart rate is reached |
| Heart rate > 80% – 85% of maximum rate |
| Failure of the blood pressure to rise above resting level |
| Elevation in systolic blood pressure > 250 mmHg |
| Drop in systolic blood pressure > 10 mmHg after elevation |
| Rise in diastolic blood pressure |
| Confusion |
| Cold sweat |
| Glassy stare |
| Change in skin color |

Adapted from Kenner, CV, Guzzetta, CE, and Dossey, B (eds): Critical Care Nursing: Body-Mind-Spirit, Little, Brown & Co, Boston, 1985.

blood pressure and heart rate are monitored at 5–10 minute intervals, and more frequently if they are abnormal.

### *Abnormal Results*

A positive test consists of a flat or downsloping of the ST segment (i.e., J point depression) of 1 mm or more for more than .08 second. If there was initial ST segment depression on the resting ECG, the depression must be 1 mm or more over the baseline depression during exercise to be of significance. There is controversy concerning the extent of ST segment changes that constitutes an abnormal response to exercise.

### *Interfering Factors*

Interfering factors include patient failure to observe pre-test restrictions; fatigue; uncooperativeness; the use of beta-blockers or digitalis; bundle branch block, Wolff-Parkinson-White syndrome (see Chapter 40), or Lown-Ganong-Levine syndrome; vasoregulatory asthesia; anemia; hypoxia; electrolyte imbalance; and hyperventilation.

## PHONOCARDIOGRAM

The phonocardiogram is a safe, painless, noninvasive study that is used to augment auscultation. It is usually recorded simultaneously with the ECG to aid in timing of the cardiac cycle. It also can be recorded with carotid (and sometimes jugular) pulse wave tracings, as well as with apexcardiography, to give precise timing of heart sounds and cardiac events.

### *Procedure and Nursing Care Implications*

The procedure entails placing the patient in a supine position in a bed or on a table with pillows under the head. Small microphones are applied to the chest and secured. Sometimes the chest has to be shaved to ensure direct contact. The patient must remain still and quiet during the procedure. He or she will be told when to change position, perform isometric exercises, perform the Valsalva maneuver, breathe slowly, or hold the breath. These maneuvers are done to accentuate $S_3$, $S_4$, or murmurs, if present. The patient may be asked to inhale amyl nitrate (sweet odor), which may cause an increase in heart rate (tachycardia), flushing, dizziness, and palpitations. These effects last only a short time. The overall test takes 15–30 minutes.

### *Abnormal Results*

The presence of an $S_3$, $S_4$, and/or a murmur suggests underlying cardiac pathology.

### *Interfering Factors*

Interfering factors include: incorrect placement of the microphone; incorrect amount of pressure on the microphone; background noise; patient movement (voluntary or involuntary); and abnormal chest thickness and shape (e.g., obesity and chronic obstructive pulmonary disease).

## ULTRASONOGRAPHY: ECHOCARDIOGRAM

The echocardiogram is a safe, painless, noninvasive procedure that shows the size, shape, and movement of cardiac structures and the dimensions of the heart chambers and cardiac output. Sound waves of high frequency and short duration are directed through the chest wall, which then reflects waves to a transducer and a recording device at various frequencies depending on the density and mobility of the cardiac tissue.[1]

There are various techniques utilized in performing the procedure. The motion mode (M-mode) involves a thin ultrasound beam striking the heart. This produces a vertical or "ice pick" view of the heart and structures. This mode is especially useful in recording the motion of the intracardiac structures. Frequently, it is done in time-sequence–time-motion mode (TM-mode).

The other technique, 2-dimensional mode (2-D mode), involves a rapid sweeping of the ultrasound beam in an arc, thereby producing a cross-sectional or fan-shaped view of the cardiac structures. This mode is useful for recording lateral motion and providing a correct spatial relationship between the cardiac structures.[1]

### Procedure and Nursing Care Implications

The procedure entails placing the patient in a quiet, darkened room. The patient is supine or lying on the left side. Conductive jelly is applied to the chest and a special dime-sized transducer is placed directly over the chest at the acoustic window (i.e., the area where bone and lung tissue are absent), at approximately the third to fourth intercostal space to the left of the sternum. The transducer is systematically angled to view different parts of the heart. Patients may be told to change their position, breathe slowly, hold their breath, or inhale amyl nitrate, while heart function is being recorded. The procedure usually takes 15–60 minutes.

### Abnormal Results

Abnormal findings are indicative of valvular disorders, left ventricular hypertrophy, cardiomyopathies, myxomas, ventricular aneurysms, or pericardial effusions.

### Interfering Factors

Interfering factors include: incorrect placement of the transducer, patient movement, and abnormally shaped or thickened chest walls. Technical problems can also arise in patients with small hearts.

# RADIONUCLIDE STUDIES

## Thallium Imaging (Cold Spot Myocardial Imaging Thallium Scintigraphy)

Thallium imaging can be done at rest in order to detect abnormalities in perfusion, or it can be done in conjunction with stress testing (stress thallium test) in order to evaluate ischemic areas or areas with decreased perfusion related to the exercise. The radionuclide is absorbed by healthy myocardial tissue, which appears dark on the scan. Ischemic or necrotic areas do not absorb the radionuclide and appear white or as "cold spots."

### Procedure and Nursing Care Implications

The resting thallium test involves the injection of the radionuclide, thallium-201, into a vein. The patient lies supine on the x-ray table; after 3–5 minutes, scanning begins. The patient may be repositioned so that anterior, left anterior oblique at 45 and 60 degrees, and left lateral views can be evaluated. The resting thallium test can detect a myocardial infarction within the first few hours of the onset of symptoms. This procedure takes 30–40 minutes to complete.

The thallium stress test involves the same procedure as the stress test. Thallium-201 is injected after the patient reaches a peak stress level (usually within 10–30 minutes). The patient continues to exercise for an additional 45–60 seconds to allow the radionuclide to circulate. Scanning then begins 10–15 minutes after the injection. The patient may have to return to the laboratory 1–24 hours posttest so that resting films can be taken.

### Abnormal Findings

Persistent defects in perfusion indicate a myocardial infarction. Transient defects (i.e., those present during peak exercise but not at rest) usually indicate ischemia secondary to coronary artery disease.

### Interfering Factors

False-positives ("cold spots") may occur secondary to ventricular aneurysms; metastatic carcinoma; skin lesions; sarcoidosis; myocardial fibrosis; cardiac contusions; apical clefts; coronary spasms; or attenuation due to soft tissue and artifact such as the diaphragm, breast implants, or electrodes. False-negatives may be due to insignificant obstruction, inadequate stress, delayed imaging, single vessel disease especially involving the right or left circumflex arteries, and the presence of collateral circulation. Other interfering factors include mechanical malfunction, technician error, and patient movement.

## Tc-PYP Heart Scan

Tc-PYP heart scan involves the injection of technetium-99m stannous pyrophosphate (Tc-99), a radionuclide that is absorbed by damaged or ischemic myocardial cells. The radionuclide appears as dark or "hot spots" on the film. The PYP heart scan is helpful in detecting the location and age (recent or old) of a myocardial infarction. The test must be performed within 72 hours of the onset of symptoms in order to determine onset of the infarct. The scan can also be performed in conjunction with a stress test to aid in the diagnosis of coronary artery disease.

### Procedure and Nursing Care Implications

The procedure is like that of the thallium imaging, the only difference being that scanning must take place 3 hours after injection of the radionuclide (as opposed to 3–5 minutes post-injection in the thallium scan). Once the patient returns 3 hours after injection of the radionuclide, the test usually takes from 30–60 minutes to perform, during which time the patient may lay still for 15–30 minutes.

#### Abnormal Findings

Uptake of the radionuclide occurs in areas of valve calcification, damage/ischemia of the myocardium, viral myocarditis, and ventricular aneurysm.

#### Interfering Factors

Interfering factors include: hypotension; scanning done within 3 hours of injection; previous infarction; subendocardial infarctions and small infarcted areas of necrosis (less than 3 g);[2] renal insufficiency; and patient movement.

### Gated Blood Pool Scans (Blood Pool Imaging)

The gated blood pool scan is a radionuclide test that involves various techniques. These techniques include the first-pass scanning, the 2-frame gated scanning, and the multiple-gated acquisition scanning (MUGA), which can be done in conjunction with the stress test (stress MUGA) or with the administration of nitroglycerin (nitro MUGA).

#### Procedure and Nursing Care Implications

These tests involve an intravenous injection of nonradioactive pyrophosphate, which attaches itself to, or "tags," the red blood cells (RBCs). After 30 minutes, an intravenous injection of radioactive technetium is given, which combines with the pyrophosphate on the RBCs, thus creating a radioactive pool. Scintillation cameras record the initial passage of the radionuclide through the heart (first pass). Then, in synchrony with the electrocardiogram, the camera records the left ventricular end-systolic and left ventricular end-diastolic phases for 500–1000 cardiac cycles (i.e., 2-framed gated imaging). This allows visualization of the left ventricle for the presence of akinesia, dyskinesia, or the presence of intracardiac shunts.

The MUGA scan records 14–64 points of a single cardiac cycle, thereby giving sequential images in order to evaluate wall motion and calculate the ejection fraction. When done in conjunction with the stress test, it detects changes in the ejection fraction, cardiac output, and wall motion related to exercise or stress. The nitro MUGA is done to evaluate the effect of nitroglycerin on ventricular function. The blood-pooling imaging tests take 60–90 minutes to perform.

#### Abnormal Findings/Interfering Factors

Abnormal findings and interfering factors associated with the MUGA scan are similar to those presented for the Tc-PYP heart scan.

## CARDIAC CATHETERIZATION

Cardiac catheterization is a frequently performed invasive technique requiring expert nursing care. Nurses not only have to know what the procedure entails in order to implement patient teaching, but they also need to monitor the patient carefully post-procedure to prevent complications.

#### Procedure and Nursing Care Implications

The patient is wheeled to the cardiac catheterization lab on a stretcher and placed on a padded x-ray table where he or she is strapped in place. An intravenous line is started if one does not already exist, and the chart is carefully checked for appropriate consents and for any abnormal results (e.g., laboratory data including electrolytes, liver/renal function studies, hematology profile, prothrombin and partial thromboplastin times, chest x-ray, and ECG). Patients who have any allergies to iodine, fish, shell fish, or contrast medium may be given an antihistamine or steroid to lessen the reaction to the contrast medium. (In some institutions, the patient may be started on steroids or antihistamines a few days prior to the procedure.) Electrodes are placed on the patient's extremities to allow for continuous monitoring of the patient's rhythm during the procedure.

The site to be used for catheter insertion is shaved and cleansed with an antiseptic solution, and a sterile milieu within which to implement the procedure is established and maintained. An antecubital vein is usually utilized for a right-sided catheterization; the femoral artery is the preferred site for left-sided catheterization. When local anesthesia is given, the patient may experience a transient stinging sensation. The catheter can be inserted either by a percutaneous stick or by means of a cutdown. As the artery is entered, the patient may experience a slight "shock" or pain, similar to that experienced when hitting the "funny" bone. As the catheter is advanced under fluoroscopy, the patient may feel slight pressure, but it should not be painful. Sometimes the catheter has to be reinserted because of blockage or obstruction in the vessel, anatomical abnormalities, or severe vessel spasms. Once the catheter reaches the heart, pressure readings and blood samples for oxygenation determination are taken from the various chambers and vessels.

Throughout the procedure the patient may be moved into various positions to enhance catheter advancement and visualization. Two frequently used positions are the right anterior oblique, which allows visualization of the anterior, basal, apical, and inferior walls and vessels, and the basal wall segments of the left ventricle; and the left anterior oblique position, which allows visualization of the septum and posterior wall of the left ventricle. The patient may also be asked to deep breathe, which aids in placement of the catheter into the pulmonary artery and into a wedge position in a branch of the pulmonary artery. Deep breathing may also aid catheter placement into the coronary arteries. Visualization may be enhanced by depression of the diaphragm during deep breathing. Throughout the procedure the patient's cardiac rhythm, blood pressure, and heart rate are continuously monitored.

A right-sided or left-sided catheterization can be done singularly, or both sides may be catheterized. If both sides are to be catheterized, the right side is usually done first and the catheter is kept in place so that pulmonary artery and pulmonary capillary wedge pressures (as a reflection of left heart pressures) can be monitored and measured simultaneously. The right-sided catheter is subsequently removed.

Cardiac catheterization is usually done in conjunction with angiography, which involves the injection of a radiopaque dye. Various studies can be performed including: ventriculography, which is used to assess ventricular contraction; aortography, used to assess the ascending aorta and aortic valve function; and coronary arteriography, used to determine coronary artery patency. When the contrast medium is injected, the patient may experience a feeling of warmth, flushing, lightheadedness, or nausea, due to the vasodilation effect of the contrast medium. The sensation passes within a few seconds.

In response to the injection of the contrast medium, the patient may become hypotensive, bradycardic, or develop dysrhythmias. Under these circumstances, the patient may be asked to cough deeply to help propel the dye through the heart or coronary arteries. It is important to instruct the patient to cough immediately when asked to do so. If hypotension persists, a pressor agent may be prescribed.

Other drugs may be administered during an angiographic procedure. Nitroglycerin (NTG) may be given sublingually or intravenously, especially if the patient develops chest pain during the procedure. Nitroglycerin is used to eliminate catheter-induced spasms; to assess its effect on coronary artery perfusion, thereby assisting in determining candidacy for coronary artery by-pass surgery; and to augment left ventricular contractility.

Ergonovine maleate is another drug that may be used in conjunction with cardiac catheterization. It is valuable in diagnosing Prinzmetal's angina (see Chap. 43) because its vasoconstrictive action produces coronary artery spasm. Systemic heparin may be administered during left-sided catheterization to decrease the possibility of clot formation at the tip of the catheter. Its effects are reversed with the administration of protamine sulfate. Direct pressure must be applied to the site for at least 15 minutes after removal of the catheter. The procedure takes between 2–4 hours to complete. For specific nursing care considerations refer to Table 39–3, Care Plan for the Patient Post-Cardiac Catheterization.

#### *Abnormal Findings*

Constriction or irregularity of the coronary arteries indicates coronary artery disease. Constriction greater than 60% is significant especially in the proximal portion of the left main coronary artery and high in the left anterior descending coronary artery. The decision can be made concerning the need for revascularization, angioplasty, or fibrinolytic therapy, based on findings determined on cardiac catheterization.

Valvular disorders are diagnosed based on differences in pressures on both sides of the valves. The greater the pressure difference (gradients), the greater the degree of stenosis. Incompetent valves are determined by the retrograde blood flow across the valves during systole, as visualized on ventriculography.

Septal defects are confirmed by measurement of the blood oxygen content on both sides of the heart. Elevated blood oxygen levels on the right are indicative of a left-to-right shunt; a decrease in blood oxygen levels on the left is indicative of a right-to-left shunt. Ejection fraction under 55% is indicative of myocardial incompetency; ejection fractions less than 35% are generally indicative of poor surgical prognosis. (Note: The *ejection fraction* is defined as the ratio of the volume of blood ejected from the left ventricle per beat [stroke volume], to the volume of blood in the left ventricle at the end of diastole.)

#### *Interfering Factors*

Interfering factors include: equipment malfunction, poor technique, patient anxiety causing a vasovagal reaction, dysrhythmias, and an increase in chamber pressures.

## ELECTROPHYSIOLOGIC STUDIES (EPS)

### His Bundle Electrography[1]

His bundle electrography is an invasive procedure that is performed in the cardiac catheterization laboratory.[1] It can be performed in conjunction with a cardiac catheterization, ventricular mapping, and epicardial mapping. The study involves insertion of

## TABLE 39–3. CARE PLAN FOR THE PATIENT POST-CARDIAC CATHETERIZATION

| Nursing Diagnoses | Desired Patient Outcomes | Nursing Interventions | Rationales |
|---|---|---|---|
| ***Nursing Diagnosis #1*** Cardiac output, alteration in: Decreased (actual and potential), related to underlying cardiac disease, hemorrhage, cardiac perforation, myocardial infarction, dysrhythmias. | The patient will:<br>1. Maintain effective cardiovascular function as measured by:<br>A. Stable blood pressure—systolic pressure between 100–145 mmHg (or baseline for patient).<br>B. Regular heart beat with rate between 60–100 beats per minute.<br>C. Absence of angina.<br>D. Absence of pulmonary edema or neck vein distention.<br>E. Minimal bleeding at the catheterized site.<br>F. Optimal cardiac indices including skin, warm and dry, usual skin color; brisk capillary refill; alert and oriented; following commands. | • Perform a comprehensive cardiopulmonary assessment. | |
| | | ○ Monitor blood pressure observing for a drop in systolic pressure, a narrowing pulse pressure, and pulsus paradoxsus. | ○ Changes in blood pressure may reflect a reduced cardiac output possibly related to left ventricular failure, hypovolemia, or cardiac tamponade. |
| | | ○ Monitor heart rate and regularity. | ○ Dysrhythmias can compromise cardiac output and increase the risk of ischemia and life-threatening dysrhythmias. |
| | | ○ Monitor ECGs and rhythm strips for abnormalities. | ○ Provides a basis for comparison in the detection of dysrhythmias, ischemia, or infarction. |
| | | ○ Monitor heart sounds. | ○ Presence of $S_3$ (after age 40) is indicative of heart failure; a murmur may be indicative of valvular dysfunction; and a pericardial friction rub is indicative of pericarditis. |
| | | ○ Monitor for neck vein distention. | ○ An increase in neck vein distention warns of increasing heart failure, fluid overload, or cardiac tamponade. |
| | | ○ Monitor breath sounds. | ○ The presence of rales is indicative of fluid overload or an increase in left ventricular failure. Decreased breath sounds may indicate pulmonary emboli or pneumothorax. |
| | | ○ Monitor the respiratory rate. | ○ An increase in the respiratory rate may indicate extreme anxiety, pain, hypoxia, or an acid–base imbalance. |
| | | ○ Monitor the amount of bleeding from the catheter site. | ○ Uncontrolled bleeding would lead to hypovolemia, which would further decrease the cardiac output, increasing the workload of the heart and decreasing myocardial oxygenation. |
| | | ○ Monitor the skin and nailbeds for color, warmth, and capillary refill. | ○ These are indices of peripheral vascular perfusion and may be one of the first signs of a decrease in cardiac output. |
| | | ○ Monitor the level of consciousness. | ○ A decrease in the level of consciousness may be indicative of hypoxia, a decrease in cardiac output, cerebral emboli. |
| | | ○ Monitor for the presence of angina, evaluating its quality, location, and radiation. | ○ Angina may be indicative of myocardial ischemia or infarction, or of a pulmonary embolus. |

*(continued)*

**TABLE 39–3. CARE PLAN FOR THE PATIENT POST-CARDIAC CATHETERIZATION *(Continued)***

| Nursing Diagnoses | Desired Patient Outcomes | Nursing Interventions | Rationales |
|---|---|---|---|
| ***Nursing Diagnosis #1 (con't.)*** | | | |
| | | ○ Notify the physician immediately of any abnormalities. | ○ Immediate medical treatment can be initiated to prevent further complications and deterioration in the patient's condition. |
| | | • Institute prescribed therapies and monitor responses:<br>○ Administer intravenous fluids. | ○ Adequate fluids are necessary to prevent hypovolemia and subsequent renal failure due to the osmotic effect of the contrast medium. If oliguria/anuria occurs, the rate of infusion may have to be decreased to prevent fluid overload. The IV also provides an access through which emergency drugs can be administered. |
| | | ○ Administer antidysrhythmics, diuretics, pain medications, as prescribed, and monitor responses to therapy. | ○ Prompt administration of precribed medications can help prevent further decrease in cardiac output and prevent cardiopulmonary, neurologic, and renal complications. |
| | | • Be prepared to institute emergency treatment.<br>○ Have crash cart available nearby. | ○ Immediate emergency actions may be necessary to prevent cardiac injury and to treat life-threatening complications (e.g., dysrhythmias). |
| ***Nursing Diagnosis #2***<br>Tissue perfusion, alteration in: Peripheral, related to the insertion of catheter into an artery or vein. | The patient will:<br>1. Maintain adequate perfusion in the catheterized extremity as evidenced by:<br>A. Warmth of the extremity.<br>B. Pink color.<br>C. Baseline pulses bilaterally.<br>D. Intact movement and sensation. | *LEFT-SIDED CATHETERIZATION–ARTERIAL INSERTION*<br>• Monitor pulses in the extremity distal to the insertion site. Report any changes immediately to the physician. | • Distal artery can rapidly become thrombosed and ischemia of the extremity may occur. If the thrombosis or arterial spasm is not treated immediately, ischemia can lead to tissue necrosis eventuating the need for amputation. |
| | | • Monitor color and warmth of the extremity, comparing it with the opposite extremity. | • Color and warmth are indices of peripheral perfusion. Pale/mottled skin indicates a compromised blood supply to the extremity. |
| | | ○ Notify the physician immediately if any signs of decreased perfusion occur. | ○ Immediate action must be taken to preserve the circulatory integrity of the affected extremity. |
| | | ○ Heat may be applied to the opposite extremity. Never apply heat to the affected extremity. | ○ Heat applied to the opposite extremity will produce a reflex vasodilatation, thereby increasing the blood supply to the extremity. |

| | |
|---|---|
| | Heat applied to the affected extremity will only further compromise oxygenation of the limb due to enhanced cellular metabolism. |
| • Administer heparin as prescribed. | • Heparin will prevent further clots from forming. |
| • Keep the catheterized extremity straight for 6–8 hr, as prescribed. | • Movement can disrupt the clot at the insertion site and hemorrhage or embolization may occur. |
| • Maintain bedrest for 6–12 hr, as prescribed. | • Allows the patient to rest and regain his/her strength. Prevents the dislodgment of the clot at the insertion site. |
| • Administer pain medication as ordered. Monitor effectiveness in relieving pain. | • Pain medications will keep patient comfortable and allow him/her to relax. This will break the pain–fear–anxiety cycle, which could cause a sympathetic response. This response can precipitate an increase in BP and HR causing the heart to work harder and increasing risk of bleeding at insertion site. |
| • Monitor the insertion site for increasing edema and bleeding. | • Enlargement of the limb could indicate bleeding into the soft tissue. |
| ○ Apply a sand bag to femoral insertion sites immediately post-procedure. | ○ The weight of the sand bag applies continuous direct pressure to the site, thereby decreasing bleeding. |
| ○ Apply direct pressure to the insertion site for moderate to large amounts of bleeding. | ○ Direct pressure slows the blood flow around the insertion site, thereby allowing the normal clotting mechanism to occur. |
| ○ Notify the physician immediately of any active bleeding, excessive swelling, or hematoma formation. | ○ Immediate intervention is needed to stop the bleeding, maintain the patient's blood volume, and maintain perfusion to the extremity. |
| *RIGHT-SIDED CATHETERIZATION–VENOUS INSERTION* | |
| • Monitor the pulses distal to the insertion site. | • Sometimes during a cutdown, the vein is tied off, causing venous blood to become trapped in the tissues. Consequent edema formation may exert pressure against the adjacent arteries, causing occlusion and compromising circulation to tissues distal to the occlusion. |
| • Elevate the extremity. | • Elevation will facilitate venous return and fluid absorption. |
| • Apply an ice bag to the insertion site. | • Ice will decrease the amount of edema |
| • Maintain bedrest for 4–6 hr as ordered. | • Same as for arterial insertion. |
| • Keep catheterized extremity straight for 3–6 hr. | • Same as for arterial insertion. |
| • Monitor insertion site for bleeding or hematoma. | • Same as for arterial insertion. |

*(continued)*

**TABLE 39–3. CARE PLAN FOR THE PATIENT POST-CARDIAC CATHETERIZATION *(Continued)***

| Nursing Diagnoses | Desired Patient Outcomes | Nursing Interventions | Rationales |
|---|---|---|---|
| ***Nursing Diagnosis #3*** Fluid volume deficit: Potential (refer to Table 23–3). | The patient will:<br>1. Maintain blood pressure at patient's baseline.<br>2. Maintain a urinary output > 30 ml/hr for adults.<br>3. Show no signs of bleeding.<br>4. Show no signs of dehydration.<br>5. Maintain a normal hemoglobin and hematocrit. | • Monitor the blood pressure every 1 hr until stable. Notify the physician of any abnormality. | • Timely detection of abnormalities enables timely intervention, thereby reducing the risk of complications. |
| | | • Monitor urinary output and I&O closely for the first 24 hr.<br>◦ Assess urine specific gravity. | • Urinary outputs of less than 30 ml/hour are highly suggestive of renal failure.<br>◦ Renal excretion of contrast dyes requires ample fluid intake to reduce risk of renal dysfunction. Initial specific gravity determinations will be high, reflecting the presence of contrast dye in the urine. |
| | | • Monitor for signs of dehydration (dry mucous membranes, poor skin turgor, a decrease in urinary output with a high specific gravity). | • Astute observation for signs of dehydration can prevent the occurrence of renal and/or cardiac complications by identifying the need for fluids. These changes may occur before there is a change in blood pressure. |
| | | • Monitor for bleeding at the insertion site. | • Blood loss can cause a decrease in cardiac output because of hypovolemia. |
| | | • Monitor the hemoglobin and hematocrit. | • If the fluid deficit is related to the blood loss, the hemoglobin will be decreased; if related to hypovolemia, the hematocrit will be decreased. |
| ***Nursing Diagnosis #4*** Infection: Potential for (refer to Table 49–7, Potential for Infection). | The patient will:<br>1. Demonstrate no signs of infection as evidenced by: | • Monitor insertion site for the presence of redness, heat, or exudate. | • Redness and heat are responses of the body's defense system against infection and trauma. They are indicative of infection especially in the presence of exudate. |

| | | | |
|---|---|---|---|
| | A. Maintaining a normal body temperature (~98.6°F [~37°C])<br>B. Wound clean and dry without redness, heat, or exudate. | • Monitor body temperature every 4 hr.<br>◦ Obtain wound and blood cultures if the temperature rises above 101°F (38.3°C) and notify the physician.<br>• Monitor for signs of endocarditis (high fever, hematuria, and the presence of a new murmur).<br>• Monitor for signs of pericarditis (decreased heart sounds and the presence of a pericardial friction rub). | • Temperature elevation is a normal response to infection.<br>◦ Temperatures above 101°F (38.3°C) are indicative of bacterial invasion, and immediate treatment with the appropriate antibiotic is necessary to prevent sepsis. Antibiotic therapy should not be initiated until the appropriate cultures have been obtained.<br>• Endocarditis and pericarditis are possible complications of cardiac catheterization. This is related to the introduction of a foreign object (the catheter) into the heart especially in patients with valvular disease. |
| ***Nursing Diagnosis #5***<br>Knowledge deficit. | The patient will:<br>1. Verbalize understanding of prescribed treatment plan including medications, diet, exercise, and follow-up care after discharge. | • Provide patient and family with verbal and written instructions concerning wound care, signs of infection, activity restrictions, medications, and follow-up appointments.<br>• Discuss the implications of the catheterization, the results, and the physician recommendations with the patient and family. Evaluate their perception and correct any misconceptions they may have. | • Information decreases the patient's anxiety and facilitates participation in self-care; it may help to prevent the occurrence of serious complications.<br>• Knowledge decreases anxiety. Correcting misconceptions allows the patient greater ability to make objective decisions. |

an electrode-tipped catheter into the right side of the heart in order to record activity of the conduction system.

Assessment of atrioventricular conduction times can be achieved by determining the A-H interval and H-V interval. The A-H interval reflects the conduction time from the right atrium, through the AV node/junction, to the His bundle. The A-H interval is measured from the initial deflection of the atrial electrogram to the earliest deflection of the His bundle electrogram. Normally, this interval ranges between 45–150 msec (Fig. 39–1).

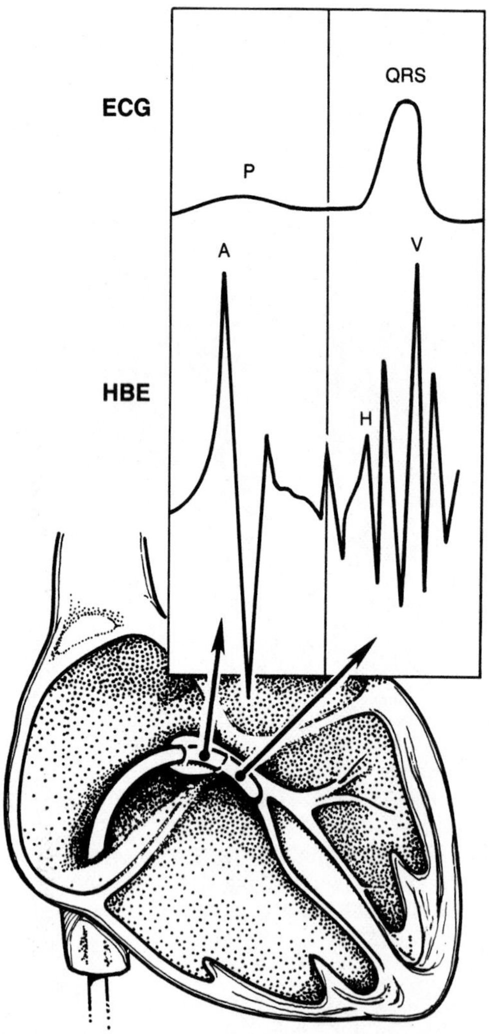


**Figure 39–1.** Intracardiac electrogram revealing atrial (A), His bundle (H), and ventricular (V) activity. The A–H interval reflects conduction time from the right atrium through the AV node/junction, to the His bundle; the H–V interval reflects conduction time from the proximal His bundle to the initial deflection of ventricular activity. The A–H interval normally ranges from 45–150 msec; the H–V interval ranges from 35–55 msec. Complexes of surface ECG appear elongated because of rapid recording speed, greater than 25 mm/sec.

The H-V interval reflects conduction time from the proximal His bundle to the ventricular myocardium. The H-V interval is measured from the initial deflection of the His bundle electrogram to the initial deflection of the ventricular electrogram. The normal H-V interval ranges between 35–55 msec.

### *Procedure and Nursing Care Implications*

The procedure involves shaving and prepping the groin or antecubital fossa for catheter placement, and insertion of an intravenous line to administer medications, especially emergency drugs. The patient is also connected to a cardiac monitor and/or ECG machine (limb leads only). Local anesthesia is given and the electrode is inserted through either the femoral or brachial vein. The catheter is advanced into the right ventricle under visualization by fluoroscopy. The catheter is slowly withdrawn from the tricuspid area and simultaneous and sequential recordings of the conduction intervals are performed. The catheter is removed and a pressure dressing is applied. The procedure takes 1–3 hours to complete.

### *Abnormal Findings*

Abnormal prolongation of the A-H interval (>150 msec) indicates atrioventricular nodal delays as seen in atrial pacing, chronic conduction system disease, carotid sinus pressure, recent myocardial infarction, and pharmacologic therapy. Abnormal prolongation of the H-V interval (>55 msec) is indicative of acute or chronic disease of the conduction system.

### *Interfering Factors*

Interfering factors include: malfunctioning of the recording equipment, improper catheter positioning, and patient intolerance (e.g., cardiac arrest).

## Ventricular Mapping or Programmed Electrical Stimulation (PES)[3,4]

Ventricular mapping or programmed electrical stimulation is an invasive procedure performed on patients with dysrhythmias refractive to pharmacologic therapy, syncope of unknown etiology, cardiac conduction system disease, and sinus node dysfunction.

### *Procedure and Nursing Care Implications*

The procedure is similar to that for His bundle electrography but involves insertion of up to 6 catheters into the heart. The 3 most common catheter placement sites are high in the right atrium, just below the triscuspid area, and the right ventricular apex.[4] If the dysrhythmia is associated with a preexcitation syndrome, for example, Wolff-Parkinson-White (WPW) or Lown-Ganong-Levine (LGL) syndrome, a catheter may be positioned in the coronary sinus. Catheter position is confirmed by fluoroscopy and baseline recordings are taken.

The conduction system is stressed by rapidly pacing it or administering extra stimuli. If a dysrhythmia is induced, its origin, that is, atrial, supraventricular, or ventricular, is determined by computer analysis. Pharmacologic agents may be administered to control the induced dysrhythmias. If the pharmacologic agents cannot control the dysrhythmia, the situation is evaluated for the possible effectiveness of surgical intervention. Such surgery may involve coronary artery bypass graft if due to ischemia; ventricular aneurysmectomy if caused by ventricular aneurysm; or surgical ablation of the ectopic focus or reentrant pathway. In those patients in whom surgical intervention is successful their antidysrhythmia medications may be altered or stopped.

Once the site is identified, the catheter is removed and pressure is applied to the venipuncture site. The test takes 2–6 hours to complete. Other types of mapping include epicardial mapping, which is similar to ventricular mapping; and endocardial mapping, which is similar but performed during open heart surgery.

#### Interfering Factors

Interfering factors include: malfunction of the recording equipment; computer malfunctioning; inability to induce the dysrhythmia; or patient intolerance as seen with cardiopulmonary arrest.

## NEW TECHNIQUES

### Digital Subtraction Angiography (DSA)

Digital subtraction angiography is a new relatively noninvasive technique that involves computer-assisted imaging.[2,4,5] DSA is presently being utilized to localize regions of peripheral arterial disease; assess ventricular function, including ventricular wall motion and calculation of ejection fractions; identify and quantify intracardiac shunts; visualize coronary artery bypass grafts and congenital cardiac malformations; and evaluate vascular tumors.[2] The scope of the DSA as a diagnostic tool is unlimited. It can be utilized alone or in conjunction with standard arteriographic techniques.

#### Procedure and Nursing Care Implications

There are 2 methods of DSA: the serial or static mode, and the continuous or dynamic mode. The serial or static mode involves obtaining an image of the area to be studied prior to injection of the contrast medium. This is stored in memory as the "mask image." The contrast medium is then power-injected and a second series of images is obtained as the dye passes through the area being studied. A computer subtracts all of the background layers such as bone and soft tissue, leaving only the image of the contrast-filled vessels. The images are recorded at a rate of 1–4 images/second.

The continuous or dynamic mode is similar to the static mode but the serial images are obtained at a rapid rate of 30 images per second. Images are stored on a videotape or videodisc, which can be viewed on a screen. Prior to formal interpretation, hard copies are produced for permanent storage.

An advantage of the DSA over conventional arteriographic studies is that lower doses of contrast media are required to present consistent images, thereby decreasing the possibility of an allergic response to the dye.

#### Abnormal Findings

Abnormal findings include any abnormal anatomy or function of the cardiovascular system.

#### Interfering Factors

Patient movement appears to be the only interfering factor for both modes of DSA, thereby reinforcing the need for careful preprocedure patient education. A problem that arises with the continuous mode is the storage of the large quantities of information.

### Magnetic Resonance Imaging (MRI)

Magnetic resonance imaging is the absorption and reemission of radiofrequency electromagnetic energy by certain nuclei when placed in a strong magnetic field.[2,4,5] This principle is utilized to generate spatial and 3-dimensional image data in order to diagnose structural and biochemical abnormalities without the risk of ionizing radiation.

MRI is safe to use in children and pregnant women. Because of the magnetic field it cannot be used in patients with implants of metal clips because of the danger of displacement. Use of MRI is likewise contraindicated in patients with permanent pacemakers because of the danger of pacemaker reprogramming, or switch to the fixed-rate mode.[2]

#### Procedure and Nursing Care Implications

The patient is placed in a large super-cooled electromagnetic scanner that produces a magnetic field. Normally the protons (i.e., nuclei of hydrogen atoms) move at random, but when placed inside the magnetic field they line up. A short radiofrequency is applied and the protons become tilted out of alignment. They realign due to the external magnetic field itself emitting a radio signal that can be detected by an antenna and located by a computer recording the spatial information into the 3-dimensional image.

### Abnormal Findings

Abnormal findings may include the following: myocardial ischemia; infarction size and age; ventricular function, including wall motion and ejection fractions; presence of atherosclerotic plaques in proximal coronary artery disease; ventricular aneurysms; valvular disorders; papillary muscle dysfunction; pericarditis; hypertrophic cardiomyopathy; vascular lesions in dissecting aneurysms; blood clots; and tumors.

### Interfering Factors

Large moving objects, as, for example, elevators, can interfere with the study. This appears to be the only interfering factor known currently. There are disadvantages in using this technique, including its expense; the amount of space needed for the equipment; interference with the operation of other equipment because of the magnetic field; and, most significant, the conversion of small ferromagnetic objects into dangerous projectiles.[2]

## REFERENCES


1. Cahill, M, DiCarlantonio, M, and Leibrandt, T: Diagnostics: Patient Preparation, Interpretation, Sources of Error, Post-Test Care. Intermed Communications, Horsham, PA, 1981.
2. Come, PC: Diagnostic Cardiology: Non-Invasive Imaging Techniques. JB Lippincott, Philadelphia, 1985, p 89.
3. Kenner, CV, Guzzetta, CE, and Dossey, BM: Critical Care Nursing: Body-Mind-Spirit, ed 2. Little, Brown & Co, Boston, 1985, p 382.
4. Hudak, CM, Gallo, BM, and Lohr, TS: Critical Care Nursing: A Holistic Approach, ed 4. JB Lippincott, Philadelphia, 1986, p 96.
5. Hamilton, HK (ed): Nurse's Clinical Library: Cardiovascular Disorders. Springhouse Corporation, Springhouse, PA, 1984.


## SELECTED READINGS


Fishbach, FT: A Manual of Laboratory Diagnostic Tests, ed 2. JB Lippincott, Philadelphia, 1984.

Hamilton, H (ed): Combating Cardiovascular Disease Skillfully. Intermed Communications, Horsham, PA, 1987.

Hamilton, HK (ed): Nurses Clinical Library: Cardiovascular Disorders. Springhouse Corporation, Springhouse, PA, 1984.

Lamb, JI and Carlson, VR (eds): Handbook of Cardiovascular Nursing. JB Lippincott, Philadelphia, 1986.

Lewis, SM and Collier, IC: Medical-Surgical Nursing: Assessment and Management of Clinical Problems. McGraw-Hill, New York, 1983.

Patrick, ML, Woods, SL, Craven, RF, et al: Medical-Surgical Nursing: Pathophysiological Concepts. JB Lippincott, Philadelphia, 1986.

Sadler, D: Nursing for Cardiovascular Health. Appleton-Century-Crofts, Norwalk, CT, 1984.

Thompson, JM, McFarland, GK, et al: Clinical Nursing. CV Mosby, St Louis, 1986.

Tilkian, A and Daily, E: Cardiovascular Procedures Diagnostic Techniques and Therapeutic Procedures. CV Mosby, St Louis, 1986.

West, RS (ed): Nursing Photobook: Giving Cardiac Care. Springhouse Corporation, Springhouse, PA, 1981.


## Journal Articles


Barta, KJ and Vacek, JL: Transesophageal atrial pacing with stress echocardiography. Focus on Crit Care 16(1):12, February 1989.

Cole, FL: The electrophysiology study. Critical Care Nurse 4:2, 1984.

Haughey, CW: Preparing your patient for echocardiography. Nursing '84 14:5, 1984.

Johnston, BL: Exercise testing for patients after myocardial infarction and coronary by-pass surgery: Emphasis of pre-discharge phase. Heart Lung 13:1, 1984.

Loeb, JM: Cardiac electrophysiology: Basic concepts and arrhythmogenesis. Crit Care Q 7:2, 1984.

Tydall, A: A nursing perspective of the invasive electrophysiologic approach to treatment of ventricular arrhythmias. Heart Lung 12:6, 1983.

Ventura, B: What you need to know about cardiac catheterization. RN 47:9, 1984.

Winters, WL and Cashion, WR: Imaging techniques in patients with acute myocardial infarction. Heart Lung 14:3, 1985.

Yacone, L: Cardiac diagnostic studies: Nuclear scanning and cardiac catheterization. RN 47:5, 1984.

CHAPTER 40

# Electrocardiography: An Overview

*Laura Toledo and Joan T. Dolan*

## CHAPTER OUTLINE



## LEARNING OBJECTIVES

**At the end of this chapter, you should be able to:**

1. Define the electrophysiologic basis of transmembrane and action potentials.
2. Describe the conduction system of the heart.
3. Define electrocardiography.
4. List the basic ECG waves, complexes, and deflections.
5. Describe ECG paper and its standardization.
6. Define morphology of the components of the P-QRS-T configuration.
7. Describe the 12 standard ECG leads.
8. Differentiate standard limb leads from the precordial (chest) leads.
9. Describe 2 cardiac monitoring lead systems.
10. Define basic principles of electrocardiography.
11. Describe the normal ECG configuration.
12. Examine the pathogenesis of cardiac dysrhythmias.
13. Define the basic steps in dysrhythmia identification.
14. Describe criteria for differentiating fast-rate dysrhythmias, and their clinical significance and treatment.
15. Describe criteria for differentiating slow-rate dysrhythmias and conduction blocks, and their clinical significance and treatment.
16. Differentiate types of ventricular ectopy and their clinical significance and treatment.
17. Differentiate supraventricular tachycardia with aberrancy from ventricular tachycardia.
18. Describe electrocardiographic evidence of electrolyte disturbances.

In the intensive care setting, cardiac monitoring is the most frequently used noninvasive mode of assessing the patient. Few other pieces of information predict and guide the course of patient care better than the cardiac monitor. To provide safe and effective patient care, critical care nurses must be able to assess and interpret data reflected on the patient's bedside cardiac monitor, and to determine their significance in terms of the patient's overall clinical status. An understanding of the heart's synchronized electrical and mechanical phenomena provides the basis for timely decision-making and the implementation of necessary therapeutics.

In the following discussion, emphasis is placed on examining the electrical events of the heart as reflected by the bedside electrocardiogram, and relating these events to the heart's mechanical and hemodynamic performance. Components of the normal ECG configuration are reviewed; mechanisms in the pathogenesis of abnormal ECG configurations reflective of dysrhythmias are discussed. Major types of dysrhythmias and their defining characteristics, treatment, and implications for nursing care are examined.

## CARDIAC CELL TYPES

There are basically 2 cell types in the heart: myocardial working cells and pacemaker cells. *Myocardial working* cells are the cardiac cells responsible for contractility; that is, they respond to electrical excitation by contracting. *Pacemaker* cells occur within the conduction system of the heart and are responsible for initiating and conducting electrical impulses to all myocardial cells.

## ELECTROPHYSIOLOGY

All myocardial cells share the ability to respond to stimuli (excitability), and to do so with regularity (rhythmicity); and once stimulated, to conduct an action potential throughout the entire heart (conductivity). In addition, cardiac pacemaker cells located throughout the heart's conduction system have the ability to spontaneously discharge inherent electrical impulses (automaticity), that is, action potentials that excite myocardial working cells; these cells in turn respond to action potentials by shortening or contracting (contractility), which provides the basis for the heart's pumping action.

The sinoatrial (SA) node normally initiates an electrical impulse (action potential), which is transmitted throughout the conduction system of the atria and ventricles. The electrical impulse in turn triggers the sequential contraction of myocardial working cells (i.e., contraction of the atria followed by ventricular contraction), resulting in *excitation–contraction coupling.* This phenomenon involves the linking of the electrical and mechanical events in the heart. The synchronization of these electrical and mechanical events is achieved by organized depolarization and conduction of electrical impulses over the conduction pathway and along the sarcolemma (plasma membrane) of myocardial working cells (see Figs. 37–9 and 37–10).

To appreciate the significance of the ECG as a diagnostic tool it is essential to review basic myocardial electrochemical physiology. (For a detailed review of basic electrophysiologic principles, the reader is referred to the section on myocardial electrochemical physiology in Chap. 37.) Underlying the ability of myocardial cells to initiate, respond to, and conduct electrical impulses is the movement of positively and negatively charged ions across the semipermeable sarcolemma. Some ions (potassium) move freely across the membrane, while others (sodium, calcium) require the presence of special conditions before they are able to move into or out of the myocardial cells. The movement of these ions across the membrane creates differences in electrical potential between the inside and outside of the cell. It is these differences in potential that constitute a flow of electrical current; and it is this flow of electrical current that is reflected on the body's surface and recorded on the electrocardiogram (ECG).

### Transmembrane Potential

In their resting state myocardial cells have a difference in electrical potential across the plasma membrane oriented so that the inside of the cell is negatively charged with respect to the outside, and the cell is said to be *polarized* (Fig. 40–1, A). The resting membrane potential within a myocardial working cell is found to be approximately −90 mV. The basis of this transmembrane potential is reflected by dif-

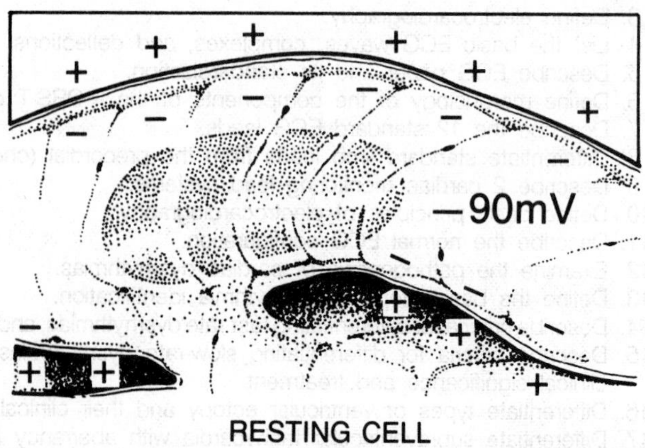


**Figure 40–1.** (*A*) Resting cell—polarized.

ferences in electrochemical gradients largely involving sodium and potassium ions on either side of the membrane, and by the presence of a semipermeable membrane. (For further details regarding the electrochemical basis of the resting membrane potential the reader is referred to the section on transmembrane potential in Chap. 37.)

## Action Potential

When an action potential is initiated in the heart, the permeability of the sarcolemma is altered so that it becomes more permeable to sodium ions. The consequent inward rush of sodium ions along electrochemical gradients and into the cell causes the inside of the cell to become positively charged with respect to the outside, and the cell is said to be *depolarized* (Fig. 40-1, B).

Almost immediately, a reversal in permeability of the membrane occurs wherein the membrane becomes again impermeable to sodium while allowing the continued efflux of potassium ions out of the cell. It is this efflux of potassium ions out of the cell that primarily accounts for *repolarization,* that is, the return of the membrane to its resting potential (Fig. 40-1, C). (For a description of the specific phases of the cardiac action potentials refer to sections on myocardial working cell action potential and pacemaker cell action potential in Chap. 37.)

## Threshold Potential

Threshold potential is the critical voltage level within the cell that must be achieved before the cell can become fully depolarized. In the myocardial working cell this voltage is between −65 and −50

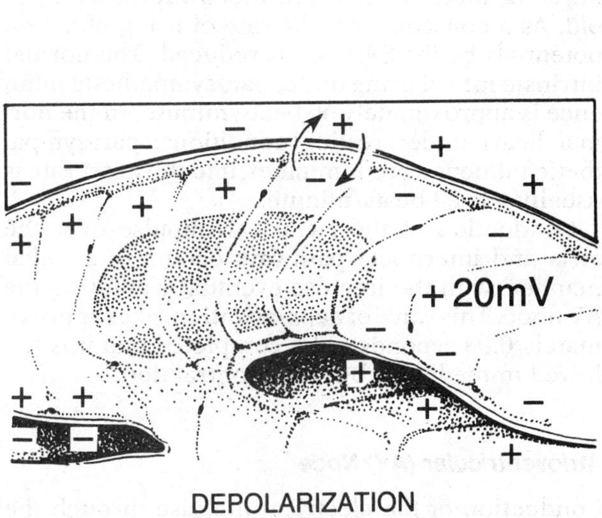


DEPOLARIZATION

**Figure 40-1.** (*B*) Depolarization.

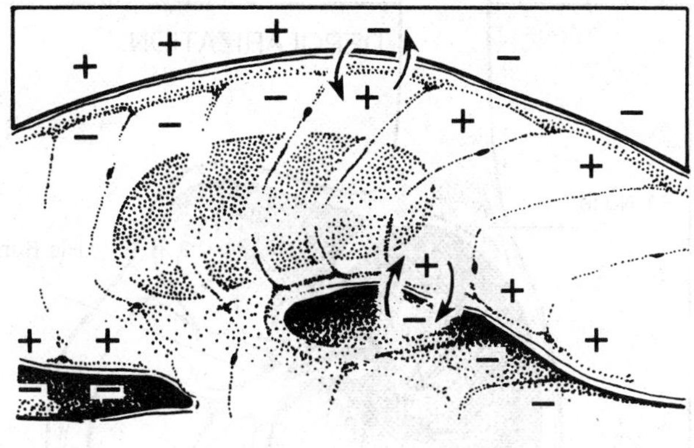

REPOLARIZATION

**Figure 40-1.** (*C*) Repolarization.

mV (see Fig. 37-13). If a stimulus is of threshold potential, an action potential is fired, and it does so in an "all-or-none" fashion.

## Refractory Periods

Once a myocardial cell is depolarized it cannot respond to another stimulus for a specific time period regardless of the magnitude of the stimulus. This is referred to as the *absolute* refractory period. Immediately following this is a period during which the cell is capable of generating an action potential if the stimulus is stronger than the usual stimulus for depolarization. This is called the *relative* refractory period. Finally, there is a period, occurring just prior to complete repolarization, during which a stimulus that is slightly less than normal can generate an action potential. This is referred to as the *supranormal* period (see Fig. 37-14).

## Action Potential Propagation

Once the action potential is initiated within the pacemaker cell it is conducted to adjacent cells, to other pacemaker cells within the conduction system, and to the atrial and ventricular myocardial working cells. The spread of this wave of depolarization occurs in all directions and without any additional stimulation. The inward flow of positively charged sodium ions reverses cellular polarity and an *activation front* is established, which serves as a boundary between the depolarized and polarized regions of the membrane (Fig. 40-2, *A*). As the activation front moves away from depolarized regions, cellular polarity in these areas is again reversed resulting in repolarization (Fig. 40-2, *B*). The consequent differences in potential underlie the flow of electrical current, and it is this current that is reflected on the surface of the body and recorded by the lead system of the electrocardiogram (ECG).

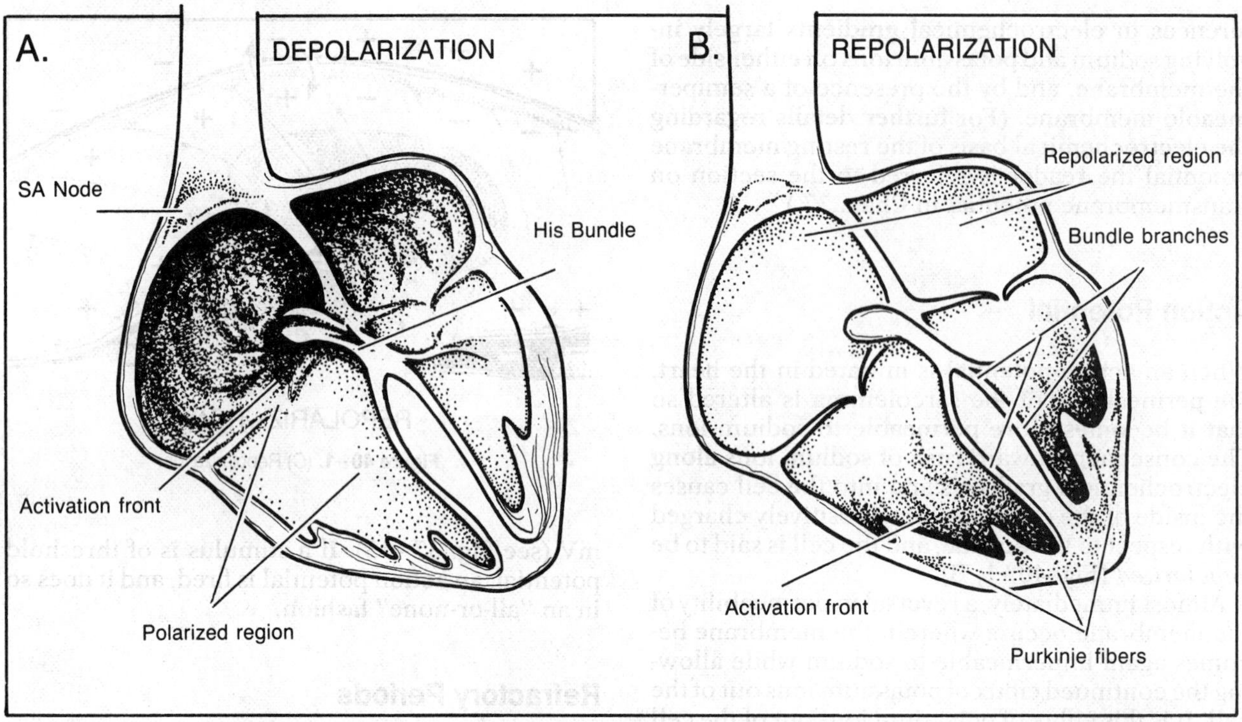


**Figure 40-2.** Propagation of electrical forces within the heart. Upon impulse initiation in the SA node, an *activation front* (a reversal in cellular polarity associated with an inward flow of positively charged sodium ions) is established, and this wave of *depolarization* (*A*) spreads in all directions, initially throughout the atria and AV node/junction, and subsequently through the His bundle, bundle branches, Purkinje fibers, and throughout the myocardial working cells. As the activation front moves away from the depolarized regions, cellular polarity in these areas is again reversed (there is an outward flow of sodium and potassium ions) resulting in *repolarization* (*B*). (See also, Fig. 37-7 which depicts sequential depolarization of the ventricles, and Figures 40-19 and 40-20).

## Action Potential Conduction

### *Sinoatrial (SA) Node*

The speed with which the action potential spreads throughout the heart depends upon the inherent properties of the cells within the different segments of the specialized conduction system and within the myocardium itself. Under normal conditions, the action potential is fired automatically by pacemaker cells in the SA node, which lies within the right atrium at its junction with the superior vena cava (see Fig. 37-6).

The frequency of firing of action potentials by the SA node is influenced by the sympathetic and parasympathetic branches of the autonomic nervous system. Sympathetic stimulation increases heart rate by increasing membrane permeability to sodium. This enables cells within the SA node to reach threshold potential more quickly, thereby increasing the rate of firing. The normal intrinsic rate of firing under sympathetic influence is approximately 100 beats/minute. In addition to increasing the heart rate, sympathetic stimulation also increases conduction velocity (i.e., how rapidly an action potential is conducted) and the excitability and contractility of myocardial cells.

Parasympathetic stimulation produces the opposite effect. It decreases the heart rate and conduction velocity, and its overall effect on the heart is to decrease excitability and contractility. Parasympathetic influence decreases heart rate by increasing membrane permeability to potassium. The efflux of positively charged potassium ions out of the cell causes the potential within the cell to become more negative, thereby moving further away from threshold. As a consequence, the rate of firing of action potentials by the SA node is reduced. The normal intrinsic rate of firing under parasympathetic influence is approximately 60 beats/minute. In the normal heart under resting conditions, parasympathetic influence predominates, and the heart rate is usually 60-80 beats/minute.

Conduction of the electrical impulse over the atria and internodal pathways occurs in a radial manner, with the impulse eventually entering the AV node. This wave of depolarization takes approximately 0.08 seconds to be completed and it is followed immediately by atrial contraction.

### *Atrioventricular (AV) Node*

Conduction of the electrical impulse through the AV node/junction to the His bundle occurs with some delay. This delay may be attributed in part to the increased resistance to current flow offered by converging internodal pathways and by the smaller size of fibers contained therein.

In addition, the AV node/junction exhibits the property of *decremental conduction* whereby transmission of some impulses through the junction is blocked. This property serves as a protective measure preventing the ventricles from having to respond to rates of firing that are overly rapid, as may occur, for example, in some supraventricular tachycardias and atrial fibrillation (see below). Electrically, the length of time for transmission of the impulse through the junction ranges between 0.12–0.2 second. Mechanically, this delay of impulse conduction through the junction allows atrial contraction to occur prior to ventricular systole. The amount of blood delivered to the ventricles via atrial contraction (also referred to as the "atrial kick") helps to ensure adequate ventricular filling.

As is the case with the SA node, the AV node receives sympathetic and parasympathetic innervation. Sympathetic stimulation increases excitability and conduction times; parasympathetic stimulation decreases excitability and conduction times through the junction.

### His-Purkinje System

The His-Purkinje system is responsible for ventricular depolarization, which is facilitated by the exceedingly rapid transmission of the action potential over the Purkinje network. The velocity of impulse conduction is greatest in this segment of the conduction system. Such rapid impulse propagation enables all ventricular myocardial working cells to become depolarized as if but one cell. This in turn facilitates a sequential coordinated response by myocardial working cells as if but one fiber. Synchronization of these 2 events, electrical (depolarization) and mechanical (contraction), underlies the effectiveness of the heart as a pump.

## ELECTROCARDIOGRAPHY

The body acts as a conductor of electricity. As the wave of depolarization is transmitted throughout the heart, electrical currents spread into tissues surrounding the heart and to the surface of the body. The placement of electrodes on the skin on opposing sides of the heart enables the electrical current generated by the heart to be recorded. The recording is known as the *electrocardiogram* (ECG).

### Basic ECG Waves and Complexes

The normal ECG is composed of distinct waves or deflections reflective of the heart's electrical activity as the wave of depolarization, followed by the wave of repolarization spread through the atria and ventricles, with the eventual return of the cardiac transmembrane potential to its resting state. The basic ECG waves are labeled alphabetically and include the P wave, QRS complex, a T wave, and, infrequently, a U wave. The QRS complex is often seen as 3 separate waves, the Q wave, R wave, and S wave (Fig. 40–3).

The P wave reflects the electrical current generated during atrial depolarization. The QRS complex reflects the current generated during ventricular depolarization. The P wave and QRS complex are therefore *depolarization* waves. The T wave represents currents generated as the ventricular potential returns to its resting state (ventricular repolarization). Less commonly, a U wave may be observed following the T wave. Although its significance is not known, it is considered to reflect the final phase of ventricular repolarization. Thus, the T wave and U wave, if present, are *repolarization* waves.

Note that in the normal ECG configuration (i.e., P-QRS-T), there are no waves or complexes representative of *atrial* repolarization. One reason for this is that currents generated during atrial repolarization are of low voltage (amplitude) and therefore are obscured by the greater currents generated during ventricular depolarization (QRS complex). Similarly, the normal ECG is not sufficiently sensitive to record any electrical activity as the impulse is transmitted through the AV node/junction. The time it takes for these events to occur is reflected by the PR interval (see below).

The ECG configuration (i.e., P-QRS-T-U se-

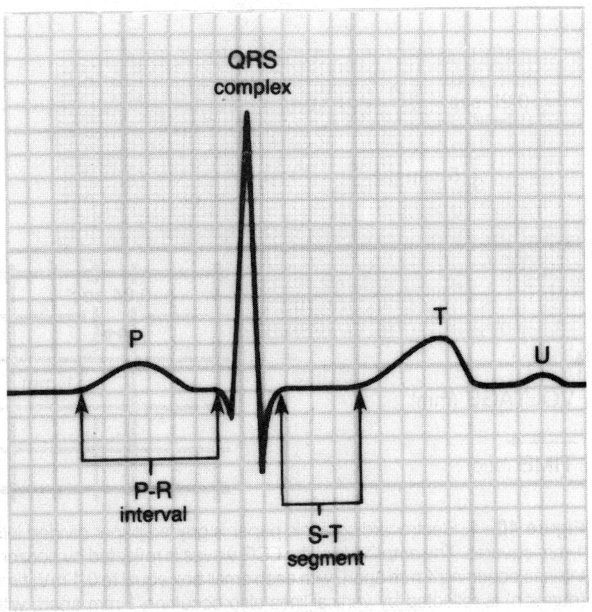


**Figure 40–3.** Normal electrocardiogram configuration. The P wave represents atrial depolarization, the PR interval reflects time from initial stimulation of atria to initial stimulation of ventricles. The QRS complex reflects ventricular depolarization. The ST segment, T wave, and U wave, if present, reflect ventricular repolarization.

quence) represents 1 complete cycle of the heart's electrical activity beginning with the initiation of an action potential within the SA node with conduction through the atria and ventricles (P wave and QRS complex, respectively), and ending with the return to resting membrane potential in the myocardial working cell (ST segment, T wave, and U wave).

## ECG Paper/Standardization/ Deflections

The P-QRS-T sequence is recorded on graded electrocardiographic paper. Each small box is a 1-mm square with every fifth small box marked by a darker line (Fig. 40–4). The darker lines, in turn, form a large square incorporating 25 smaller boxes.

The electrocardiograph is calibrated to inscribe on the ECG paper, thereby providing a means of measuring 2 key features of electrocardiographic waves/deflections: amplitude (or voltage) and duration (or time). The horizontal lines occurring 1 mm apart are used to measure the *amplitude* of the ECG waves in millivolts (mV), with each small box equal to 0.1 mV; the vertical lines, also occurring 1 mm apart, are used to measure *duration*, or time of the ECG events in seconds. At the usual ECG recording speed of 25 mm/second, each small box is equal to 0.04 second, and each large box is equal to 0.20 second.

By convention, the ECG is *standardized* so that the amplitude of an electrical impulse of 1.0 mV causes a deflection of 10 mm, or 2 large boxes. Thus, in this instance, each 1-mm deflection equals 0.1 mV. Should the amplitude of the deflection recorded from the heart be too large for the ECG paper, the standardization must be halved. In this case, an impulse of 1.0 mV results in a deflection of 5 mm, or 1 large box. Whenever the standardization is halved, it must be noted on the ECG paper. Conversely, if the amplitude of the recording from the heart is too small, the standardization can be doubled. The appropriate standardization mark should always be indicated on the ECG. It is usually indicated on the ECG just prior to recording the first lead.

Standardization of the ECG enables any part of the P-QRS-T configuration to be described in terms of amplitude (voltage) in millimeters and width (duration) in seconds. Determining the amplitude and width of each deflection is essential to meaningful ECG analysis and interpretation.

In addition to amplitude and width, it is important to specify whether a wave or deflection is positive or negative. By convention, an *upward* deflection is called *positive;* a *downward* deflection is called *negative.* Deflections partly above the baseline and partly below it are termed *biphasic.* A deflection that rests on the baseline is termed *isoelectric* (Fig. 40–5).

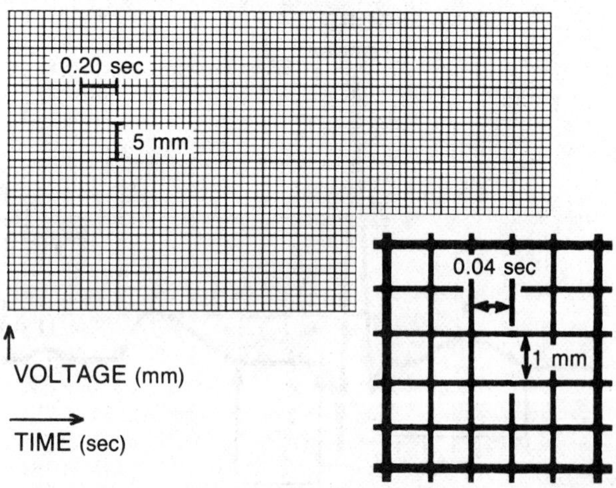


**Figure 40–4.** Electrocardiographic paper is graded paper divided into 1-mm squares. The *amplitude* of the ECG waves is reflected by horizontal lines occurring 1 mm apart, with each small box equal to 0.1 mV; *time* (duration) is reflected by vertical lines also occurring 1 mm apart, with each small box equal to 0.04 second. Each larger box is equal to 0.20 second at the usual ECG recording speed of 25 mm/second. The ECG machine is usually calibrated so that the standardization mark is 10 mm in height.

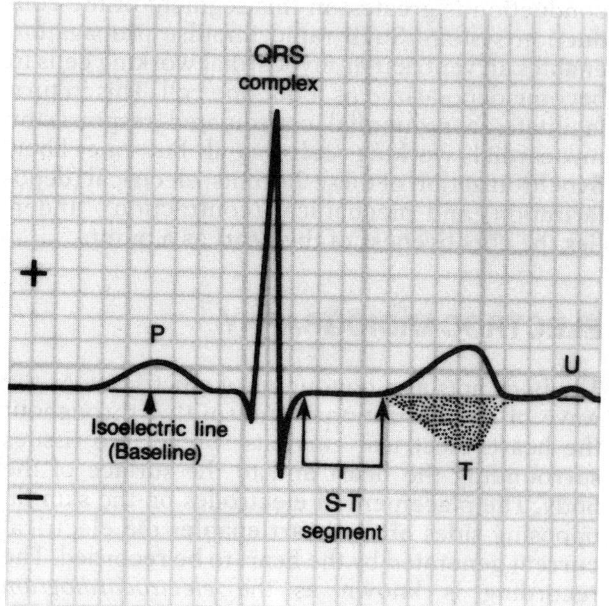


**Figure 40–5.** Positive and negative complexes. An upward deflection from the isoelectric line is *positive*; a downward deflection is *negative*. The **P wave** is deflected upward and therefore is positive; the **T wave** deflected downward is negative; the **QRS complex** is *biphasic*, that is, partly positive and partly negative; the **S–T segment** is *isoelectric* (that is, on the baseline).

## Basic ECG Morphology and Measurements

### P Wave

The P wave reflects atrial depolarization. When it is a positive (upward) deflection, the P wave is measured in millimeters from the upper edge of the baseline, where the P wave begins, to its peak; when it is a negative (downward) deflection, the P wave is measured from the lower edge of the baseline to the lowest point of the P wave (Fig. 40–6). These measurements reflect amplitude (voltage). The width (duration) of the P wave is measured from the point the P wave leaves the baseline to the point at which it returns to the baseline. Normally, the P wave precedes the QRS complex. Its amplitude should not exceed 2–3 mm; its width should be less than 0.12 second (or 3 small boxes).

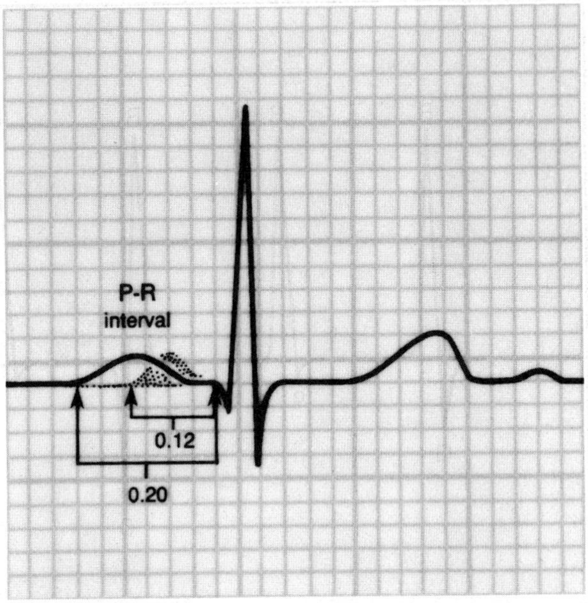


**Figure 40-7.** PR interval measures between 0.12–0.20 second.

### PR Interval

The PR interval reflects conduction time through the atria and AV node/junction, and is measured from the beginning of the P wave to the beginning of the QRS complex. In the adult, the PR interval measures between 0.12–0.2 second (or 3–5 small boxes) (Fig. 40–7). Prolongation of the PR interval above 0.2 second is termed first-degree heart block (see below).

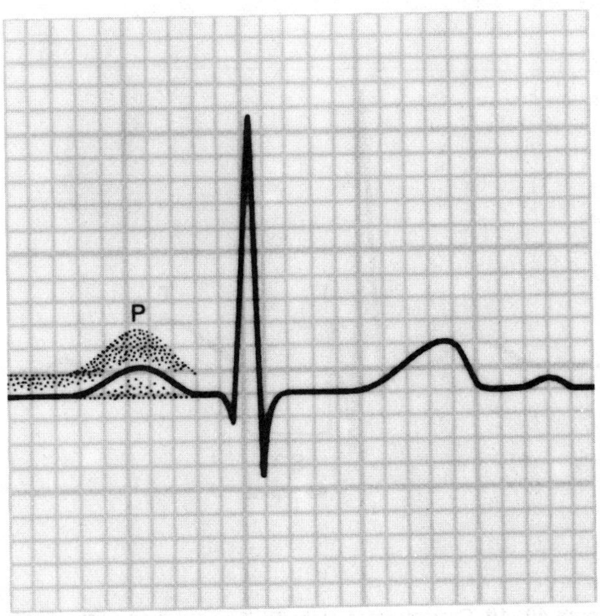


**Figure 40-6.** Normal P wave. It does not exceed 3 mm in height (voltage) and is less than 0.12 second in width (duration).

### QRS Complex

The QRS complex in general reflects ventricular depolarization. However, not every QRS complex contains a Q wave, an R wave, and an S wave. Components of the QRS complex will vary depending upon which ECG lead is used for recording. The following rules prevail (Fig. 40–8):

| | |
|---|---|
| Q wave: | Initial negative deflection preceding an R wave. |
| R wave: | First positive deflection. |
| S wave: | Negative deflection following an R wave. |
| R′ wave: | Second positive deflection. |
| S′ wave: | Negative deflection following an R′ wave. |
| QS wave: | Totally negative deflection. |

By convention, capital letters Q, R, and S are used to designate waves of relatively large amplitude; lower case letters q, r, and s are used to label relatively small waves.

When examining the QRS complex it is important to determine its width (duration). The width of the QRS reflects the time required for ventricular depolarization to be completed, which is normally 0.10 second or less. A width of 0.12 second or more reflects a delay in ventricular depolarization (Fig. 40–9).

### ST Segment

The ST segment represents the time interval during which the ventricles have been completely depolarized and are beginning repolarization. It is mea-

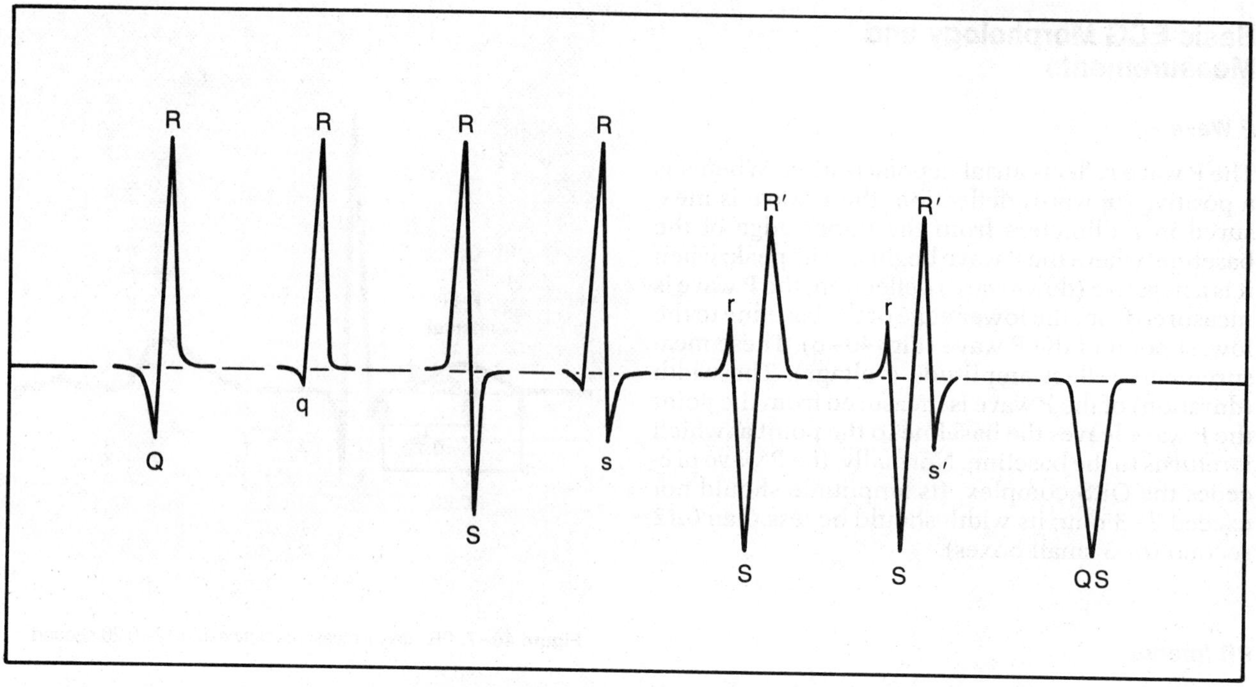


**Figure 40-8.** QRS nomenclature. See text for discussion.

sured from the junction between the end of the QRS complex and the beginning of the ST segment (sometimes called the J point) to the beginning of the T wave (Fig. 40-10). Usually, the ST segment is isoelectric (i.e., at baseline), but it may normally deviate between −0.5 and +1.0 mm, below and above the baseline, respectively. A downward deflection greater than 0.5 mm or an upward deflection greater than 0.1 mm is generally considered to be abnormal. Elevation of the ST segment is determined by measuring from the upper edge of the isoelectric line to the upper edge of the ST segment;

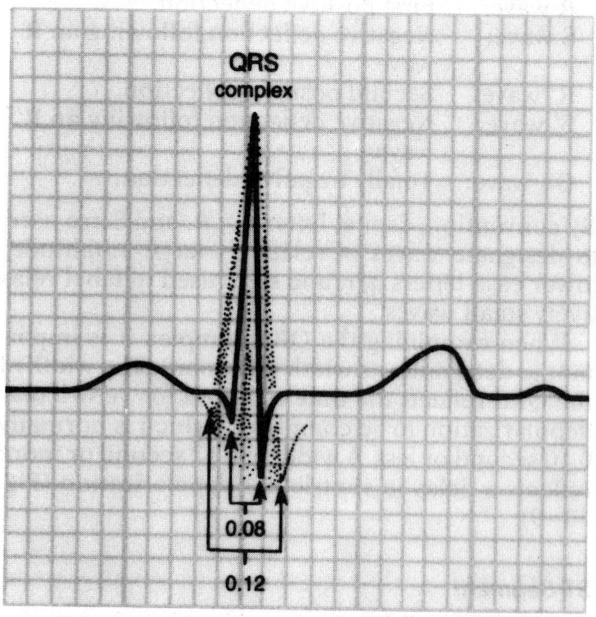


**Figure 40-9.** QRS measurement: Normally it is 0.10 second or less in duration; if 0.12 second or greater in duration, a delay in ventricular depolarization is reflected.

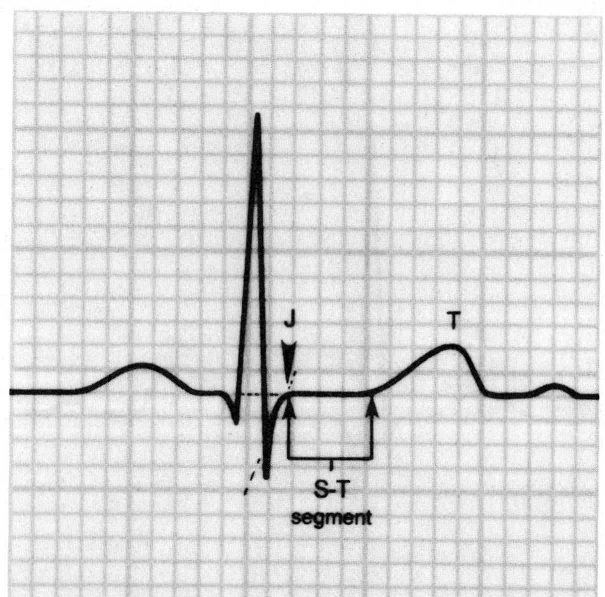


**Figure 40-10.** Characteristics of the **S-T segment** and **T wave**. The **J point** marks the beginning of the S-T segment; the T wave is normally asymmetrical.

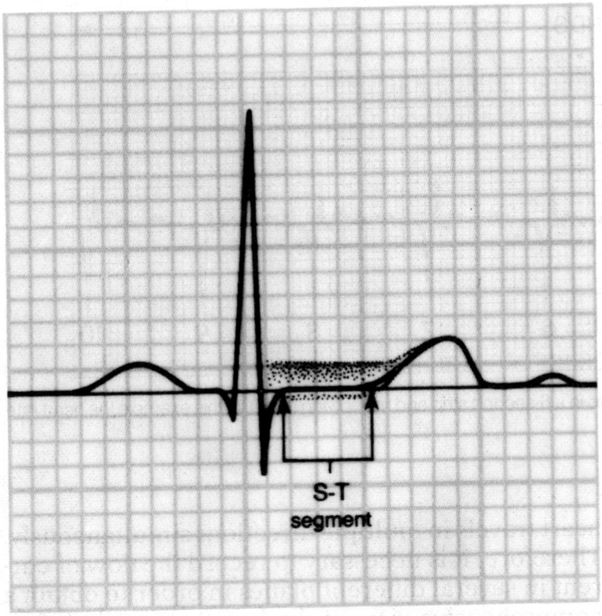


**Figure 40–11.** ST segment measurement. See text for discussion.

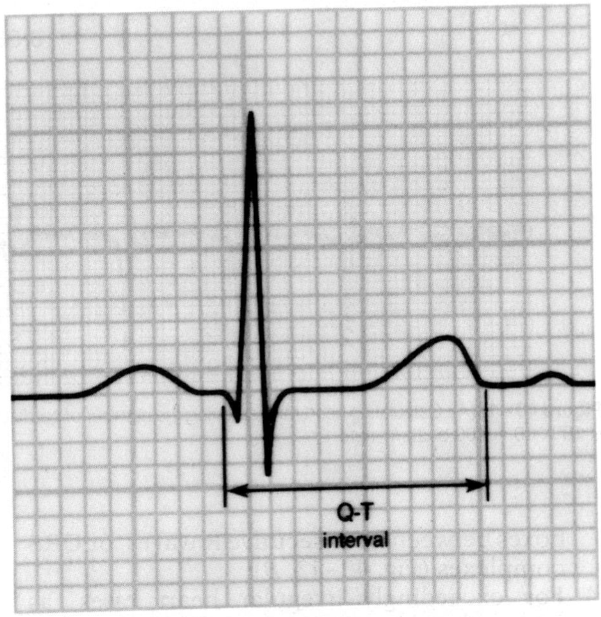


**Figure 40–12.** QT interval measurement. See text for discussion.

ST segment depression is determined by measuring from the lower edge of the isoelectric line to the lower edge of the ST segment (Fig. 40–11).

### *T Wave*

The T wave reflects, in part, ventricular repolarization. It is normally slightly rounded and asymmetrical. Positively deflected (upright) T waves are measured from the upper edge of the isoelectric line to the peak of the T wave; negatively deflected (or inverted) T waves are measured from the lower edge of the isoelectric line to the lowest point of the T wave. T wave duration is measured from the point at which the T wave leaves the baseline to the point at which it returns to the baseline (see Fig. 40–10). Normally, the T wave should not exceed 5 mm in amplitude in the standard ECG leads or 10 mm in the precordial leads. (The ECG lead system is discussed below.)

### *QT Interval*

The QT interval is measured from the beginning of the QRS complex to the end of the T wave (Fig. 40–12). It reflects the time interval of ventricular depolarization and repolarization. The normal values for the QT interval depend upon heart rate and differ between men and women. As the heart rate increases (R to R interval shortens), the QT interval normally shortens; as the heart rate decreases (R to R interval lengthens), the QT interval lengthens. For example, a heart rate of 100 yields a QT interval of 0.31 second in men and 0.34 second in women; a heart rate of 60 yields a QT interval of 0.40 second in men and 0.44 second in women.

### *U Wave*

The U wave is usually of low amplitude. If present, the U wave follows the T wave and is deflected in the same direction as the T wave. Although its exact significance is unknown, a prominent U wave may be associated with hypokalemia, that is, a lower than normal serum potassium (discussed below).

## Calculation of Heart Rate and Rhythm Determination

Heart rate is the number of heart beats per minute. There are several ways to calculate the heart rate on the ECG. These commonly used methods are presented here:

1. If the cardiac rhythm is regular (i.e., the R to R interval is constant), the heart rate can be quickly determined by counting the number of QRS complexes in a 6-second strip, and multiplying this number by 10 (Fig. 40–13, *A*).
2. If the cardiac rhythm is regular, the heart rate can be determined by dividing the total number of large boxes (0.20 sec) per minute (i.e., 300) by the number of large boxes between 2 consecutive R waves, or QRS complexes (Fig. 40–13, *B*).
3. To determine heart rate more accurately, divide the total number of small boxes (0.04 sec) per minute (i.e., 1500) by the number of small

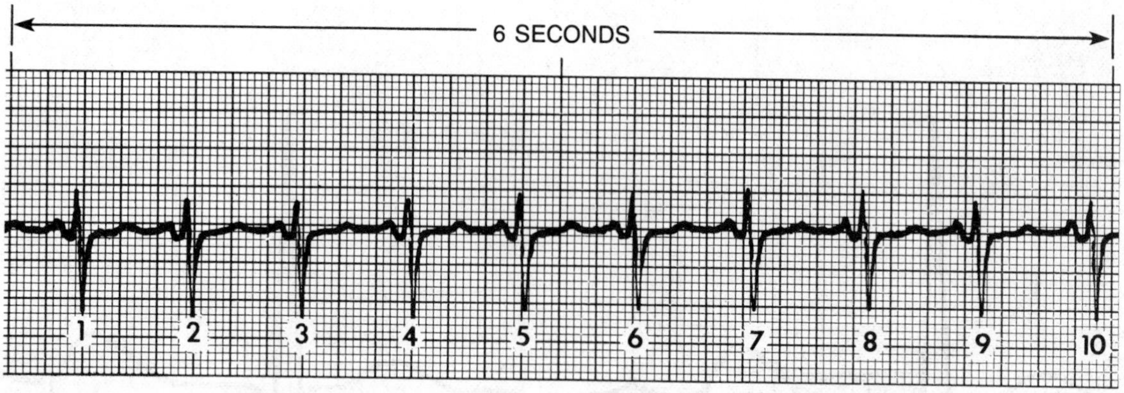


**Figure 40–13**(*A*). Calculating heart rate: counting the number of cardiac cycles in a 6-second strip and multiplying by 10, in this example the heart rate is 10 × 10 = 100 beats/minute.

boxes between 2 consecutive R waves, or QRS complexes (Fig. 40–13, *B*).

4. For exceedingly irregular heart rates, as occurs for example in atrial fibrillation (see below), it may be necessary to run a 1-minute strip and count the number of heart beats, or to take an apical pulse for 1 full minute.

The regularity of cardiac rhythm can be determined by measuring the R-R intervals to determine if they are constant in length. This can be accomplished by using calipers, or by simply marking the R to R length on a piece of paper and using it to compare the length of subsequent R-R intervals. Rhythm is considered regular if the lengths of the shortest and longest R-R intervals vary less than 0.12–0.14 second.

## ECG Leads

The electrocardiogram is a recording of the electrical activity of the heart as reflected on the body's surface. Electrical current generated within the heart travels in multiple directions simultaneously. Therefore, it is necessary to record the flow of current in several different planes in order to obtain a comprehensive view of the heart's overall electrical activity.

The usual method of recording current flow from the heart is with the 12 standard ECG *leads.* By convention, each lead has a positive and negative electrode connected to the body on opposite sides of the heart. The *direction* from the negative to the positive electrode of each lead is called the *axis* of the lead. Each lead's axis is oriented in a specific direction depending on the *location* of the positive and negative electrodes.

Of the 12 standard ECG leads, 6 measure the heart's electrical activity in the *frontal* plane, that is, the electrical forces of the heart directed from the superior to inferior surfaces. These leads include the standard limb leads—I, II, and III; and the augmented leads—$aV_R$, $aV_L$, and $aV_F$. The remaining 6 leads determine the heart's electrical activity in the *horizontal* plane, that is, how far anteriorly or posteriorly from the frontal plane the electrical forces of the heart are directed. These include the chest, or precordial, leads $V_1$ through $V_6$.

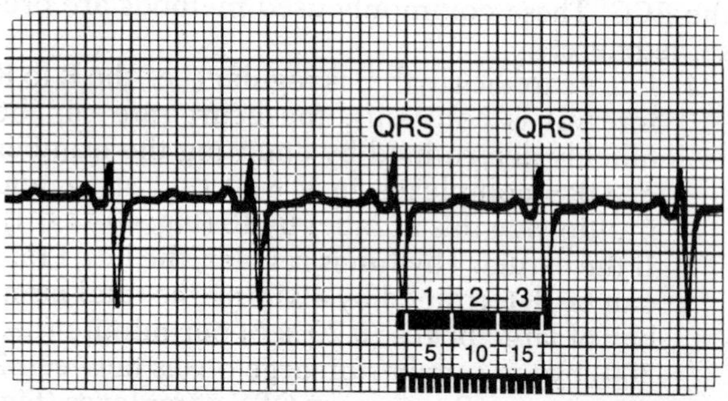


**Figure 40–13**(*B*). Calculating heart rate: counting the number of large boxes between 2 QRS complexes and dividing into 300, in this example the heart rate is 300 divided by 3 = 100 beats/minute. Counting the number of small boxes between 2 QRS complexes and dividing into 1500, in this example the heart rate is 1500 divided by 15 = 100 beats/minute.

### Standard (Bipolar) Leads (Limb Leads)

The standard (bipolar) limb leads are designated as leads I, II, and III. They are referred to as "bipolar" because differences in electrical potential are recorded from 2 specific electrodes placed on the body surface, in this case on the extremities (limbs). Specifically, leads I, II, and III are recorded by placing electrodes on the right arm, left arm, and left leg. The right leg serves as the ground electrode. For lead I, the negative electrode is placed on the right arm and the positive electrode on the left arm; for lead II, the negative electrode is on the right arm and the positive electrode on the left leg; and for lead III, the negative electrode is on the left arm and the positive electrode is on the left leg.

**Standard Bipolar Leads:**

| | | | |
|---|---|---|---|
| I | Right arm negative | —— to —— | Left arm positive |
| II | Right arm negative | —— to —— | Left leg positive |
| III | Left arm negative | —— to —— | Left leg positive |

Leads I, II, and III can be represented schematically in terms of a triangle, *Einthoven's triangle* (after Willem Einthoven, the Dutch physiologist who invented the electrocardiograph), wherein each lead is electrically equidistant from the heart, with the heart in the center of the electrical field that it generates. These leads record the *differences* in electrical potential between the 2 electrodes, with the heart representing *zero potential* (Fig. 40–14, *A*).

Einthoven's triangle can be converted to a *triaxial* figure by shifting the axes of the standard leads to the center of the triangle, as represented by the heart itself. The axes of these leads occur 60 degrees apart (Fig. 40–14, *A*).

### *Augmented (Unipolar) Leads*

The augmented (unipolar) leads are designated as leads $aV_R$, $aV_L$, and $aV_F$. The **a** refers to augmented; the V stands for voltage; and the R, L, and F for the right arm, left arm, and left leg, respectively. These leads are referred to as "augmented" because they have a low electrical potential and are augmented electronically by the ECG machine. They are termed "unipolar" because they record electrical potential at *one* location relative to zero potential rather than relative to the electrical potential at another location (electrode), as is the case of the bipolar lead system.

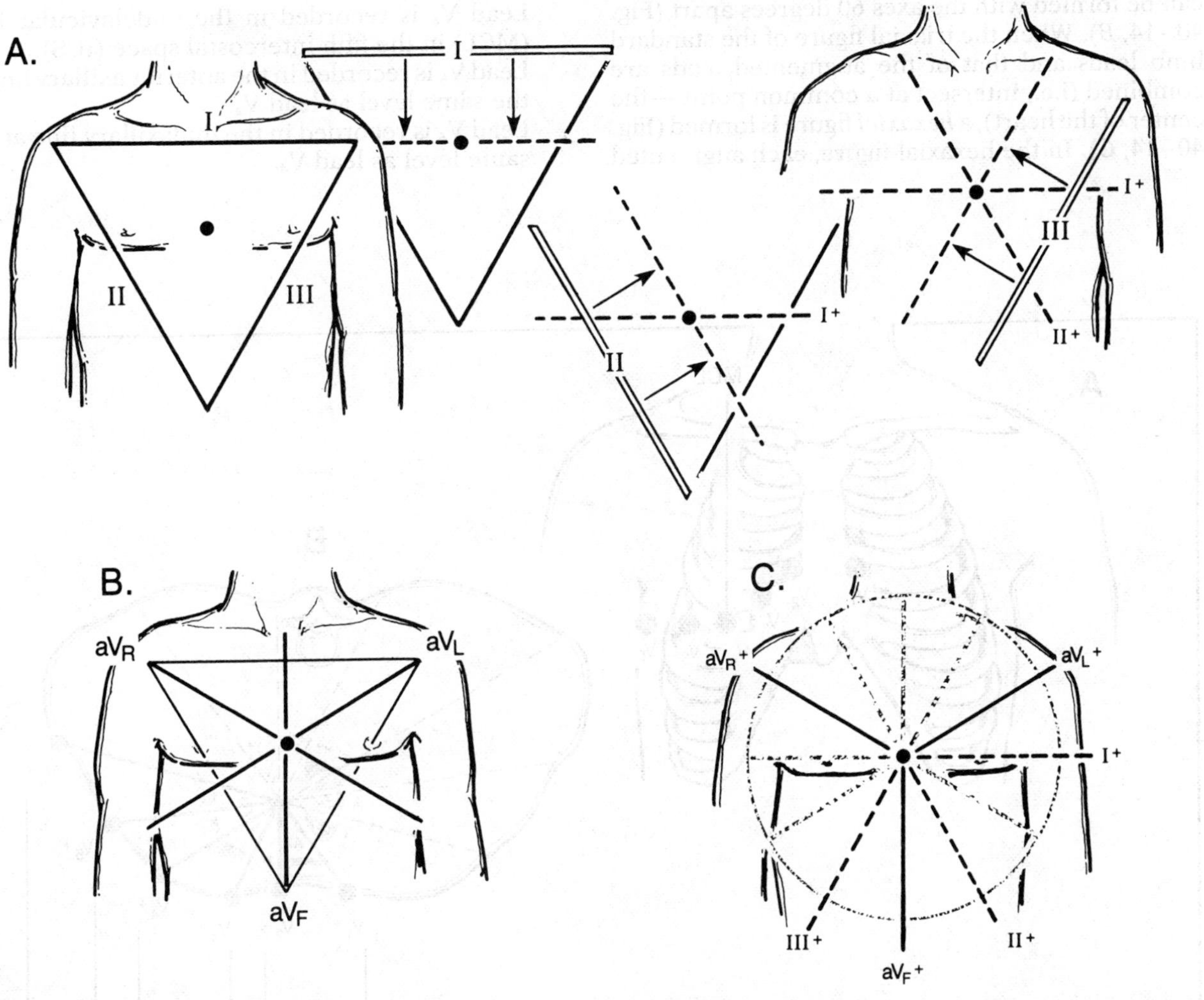


**Figure 40–14.** (*A*) Einthoven's triangle with each bipolar standard limb lead equidistant from the heart at its center. A triaxial figure is produced by shifting the axes of the three standard limb leads (I, II and III) to the center of the triangle (the center of the heart) where they intersect. The axes of these leads occur 60 degrees apart. (*B*) A triaxial figure reflecting the axes of the unipolar augmented leads can be drawn by intersecting the axis of each lead at the center of the triangle. Each augmented lead (aVR, aVL, and aVF) is drawn from the limb (positive lead) to the center of the equilateral triangle. The axis of each of these leads occur 60 degrees apart. (*C*) When the triaxial figure of the standard limb leads and that of the augmented leads intersect at a common point (taken as the center of the heart) a hexaxial figure is formed. In the hexaxial figure each augmented lead is perpendicular to a standard limb lead. Each lead is labeled at its positive electrode. The hexaxial figure is used to plot mean cardiac electrical forces (See Fig. 40–50).

The positive electrode of each augmented lead is placed in the same location as for the standard bipolar leads, that is, the right arm ($aV_R$), the left arm ($aV_L$), or the left leg ($aV_F$); the negative electrode is formed by combining leads I, II, and III, the algebraic sum of which amounts to zero potential. This zero potential, which actually reflects the center of the electrical field as generated by the heart, is obtained within the electrocardiograph by joining the three limb leads to a central terminal.

Thus, the augmented leads measure the difference in potential between the limbs (extremities) and the center of the heart. The positive electrode of lead $aV_R$ projects upward from the heart to the right arm; that of lead $aV_L$ projects upward to the left arm; and the positive pole of lead $aV_F$ points downward toward the left foot.

When the axis for each augmented lead is drawn from the extremity (positive electrode) to the center of the equilateral triangle, a triaxial figure can be formed with the axes 60 degrees apart (Fig. 40–14, *B*). When the triaxial figure of the standard limb leads and that of the augmented leads are combined (i.e., intersect at a common point—the center of the heart), a *hexaxial* figure is formed (Fig. 40–14, *C*). In the hexaxial figure, each augmented lead is perpendicular to a standard limb lead. The hexaxial figure is helpful in plotting mean cardiac electrical forces in the frontal plane.

### *Precordial or Chest (Unipolar) Leads*

In the horizontal plane, precordial or chest leads ($V_1$ through $V_6$) are used to record the electrical potential of the heart as reflected on the chest wall. These leads are unipolar in that they measure current in any one direction (location), relative to zero potential at the heart's center. By convention, placement of these leads is as follows (Fig. 40–15):

$V_1$ is recorded with the electrode in the fourth intercostal space at the right sternal border.
Lead $V_2$ is recorded with the electrode in the fourth intercostal space at the left sternal border.
Lead $V_3$ is recorded on a line midway between $V_2$ and $V_4$.
Lead $V_4$ is recorded in the midclavicular line (MCL) in the fifth intercostal space (ICS).
Lead $V_5$ is recorded in the anterior axillary line at the same level as lead $V_4$.
Lead $V_6$ is recorded in the midaxillary line at the same level as lead $V_4$.

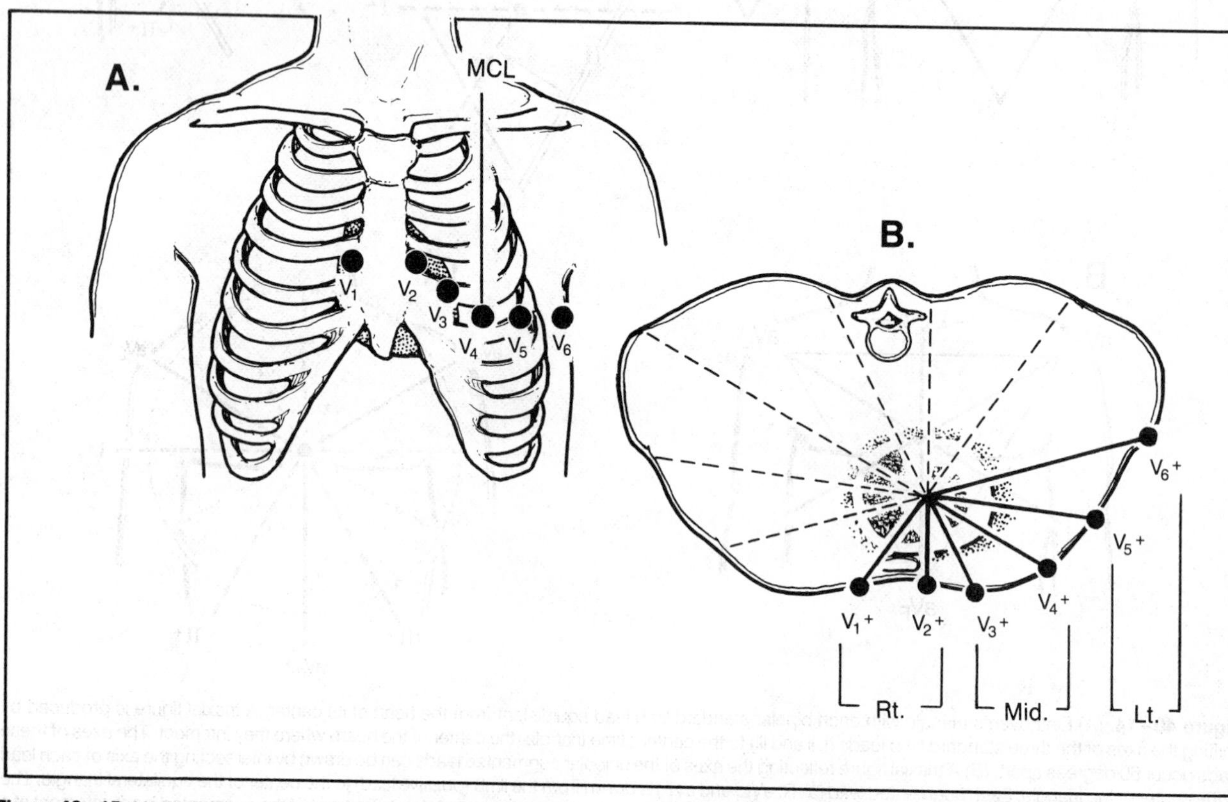


**Figure 40–15.** (*A*) Electrode positions of precordial or chest (unipolar) leads. (See text for discussion.) (*B*) Precordial reference figure: leads $V_1$ and $V_2$ are right-sided precordial leads; leads $V_3$ and $V_4$ are mid-precordial leads; leads $V_5$ and $V_6$ are left-sided precordial leads.

## Cardiac Monitoring Lead Systems

Up to this point, the discussion has centered primarily on the 12-lead ECG. Patients in coronary care and intensive care units require continuous cardiac monitoring. This is accomplished by continuously recording the heart's electrical activity using *1* lead. The monitor lead is obtained via 3 disk electrodes placed on the chest wall.

There are 2 electrode positions that are usually used as monitoring leads: the conventional electrode position similar to standard lead II; and the *modified chest* lead ($MCL_1$), which is equivalent to lead $V_1$. The $MCL_1$ lead is bipolar with the positive electrode in the $V_1$ position and the negative electrode in the left arm position. The electrode positions for each of these monitoring leads are depicted in Figure 40–16.

Advantages of lead $MCL_1$ include the following:

- Depolarization of atrial tissue is seen more clearly.
- Lead placement is not in the way should the patient require defibrillation.
- Muscle artifact is diminished.
- Right and left bundle branch block patterns can be readily defined.
- Supraventricular complexes with aberration are easily differentiated from ventricular complexes.

These monitoring leads are useful for detecting the majority of dysrhythmias; however, by no means can all rhythm disturbances be readily detected. The ECG tracing seen on the monitor depends upon specific lead placement. In addition, cardiac monitors are built with electronic filters, which may distort components of the ECG tracing, as, for example, the ST segment. If ST segment elevation or depression is suspected, it is necessary to document this using the conventional 12-lead ECG.

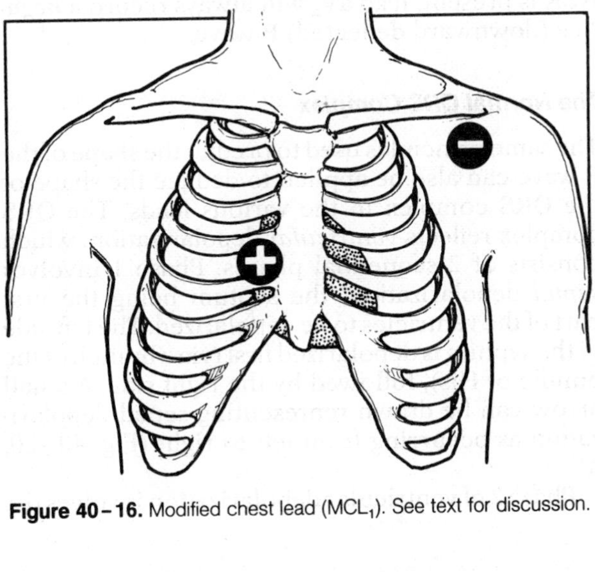

**Figure 40–16.** Modified chest lead ($MCL_1$). See text for discussion.

### *Cardiac Monitoring: Implications for Nursing Care*

Patients placed on a cardiac monitor often experience some special concerns. While they may feel somewhat comfortable knowing they are being carefully observed, they may also conclude that their condition must be very serious to warrant such close monitoring, and this becomes a major source of anxiety. Fear of dying is a feeling frequently experienced by patients in the ICU. With the placement of the electrodes on the chest, patients often become afraid of experiencing an electrical shock. Unexpected sounding of monitor alarms can be especially upsetting.

In caring for these patients it is essential to take the time to explain why their cardiac status is being monitored, and how the equipment works. Patients and families need to be reassured that the patient will not experience any electrical shocks. The alarm system should be explained, and, if appropriate, the sound should be reduced. However, alarms should *never* be turned off.

Assessment of the patient's skin for any irritation at electrode sites should be performed each shift. Sites for lead attachments should be rotated, usually every 24 hours. Additional key points regarding the nursing care of the patient with a cardiac monitor are included in Table 40–1.

## The Normal ECG

The electrical activity generated within the heart during atrial and ventricular depolarization and repolarization is recorded in the form of a P-QRS-T pattern on the ECG. A full 12-lead ECG is shown in Figure 40–17. It can readily be observed that the actual recording of the P-QRS-T pattern differs in each of the 12 leads. Based upon placement of positive and negative electrodes, each lead records current flow from the heart in a different direction.

### *Fundamental Principles of ECG*

To appreciate why the electrocardiographic waves or deflections differ from lead to lead, it is essential to understand the following fundamental principles:

1. When the wave of depolarization (current flow) spreads *toward* a positive electrode of a lead, a positive (upward) deflection is recorded on the ECG.
2. When the wave of depolarization spreads *away* from a positive electrode, a negative (downward) deflection is recorded on the ECG.

TABLE 40-1
**Nursing Care Plan for the Patient with a Cardiac Monitor**

| Nursing Diagnosis | Desired Patient Outcomes | Nursing Interventions | Rationales |
|---|---|---|---|
| 1. Anxiety | Patient will demonstrate via facial expression, heart rate, and blood pressure a decrease in anxiety level. | Reassure regarding ease of placing monitor leads, a part of routine care.<br>Reassure regarding monitors electrical safety.<br>Administer medication for relief of anxiety as prescribed. Monitor response to therapy. | Alleviating stress decreases sympathetic stimulation, which may in itself promote a tachycardia and/or an ectopic rhythm. |
| 2. Knowledge deficit | Patient will verbalize an understanding of the cardiac monitor as an adjunct to ICU care. | Describe the purpose of the monitor and its operational parts. | Alleviate fear and anxiety regarding equipment. |
| | | Demonstrate function of high-low alarms, muscle artifact, lead displacement, and electrical interference. | Anxiety is decreased with an increased understanding of equipment. |
| 3. Potential impairment of skin integrity | Patient will demonstrate healthy, intact skin underneath electrode sites. | Adequately prepare the skin surface by washing, cleansing with an alcohol swab, and shaving hair. | Proper skin preparation enhances skin-electrode contact and ensures a good tracing. |
| | | Replace ECG disks every 24 hours and prn. | Prepping the skin decreases the chances of entrapping contaminants such as dirt or hair under the disk. |
| | | Rotate sites of disks slightly every 24 hours. | Rotation of disk sites gives the skin a chance to "breathe" and lessens the opportunities for skin breakdown. |

3. When the mean path of depolarization is directed at right angles (perpendicular) to any lead, a *biphasic* deflection (i.e., one consisting of positive and negative deflections of equal size) is recorded (Fig. 40-18).

By applying these principles, it is only necessary to know the location of the positive and negative poles of each lead, and the direction in which depolarization spreads throughout the heart at any one time, to predict what the P wave and QRS complex will look like in any one lead.

### The Normal P Wave

With normal sinus rhythm (NSR) the SA node initiates the action potential and the resultant wave of depolarization spreads over the atria in a direction from right to left, and downward toward the AV node. This spread of atrial depolarization can be represented by an arrow that points downward and toward the left (Fig. 40-19). In lead II, the positive pole is oriented downward and toward the left leg. Therefore, the normal path of atrial depolarization is directed *toward* the positive electrode of lead II. When NSR is present, lead II will always record a *positive* (upward deflected) P wave.

Conversely, in lead $aV_R$, the positive pole is oriented upward toward the right shoulder. The normal path of atrial depolarization is directed *away* from the positive electrode of lead $aV_R$. Thus, when NSR is present, lead $aV_R$ will always record a *negative* (downward deflected) P wave.

### The Normal QRS Complex

The same principles used to predict the shape of the P wave can also be applied to deduce the shape of the QRS complex in the various leads. The QRS complex reflects *ventricular* depolarization, which consists of 2 sequential phases. Phase 1 involves *septal* depolarization, the septum being the first part of the ventricles to be depolarized. The left side of the septum is depolarized first (via a branch of the bundle of His), followed by the right side. A small arrow can be drawn representing septal depolarization as occurring from left to right (Fig. 40-20, *A*).

Phase 2 of ventricular depolarization involves the

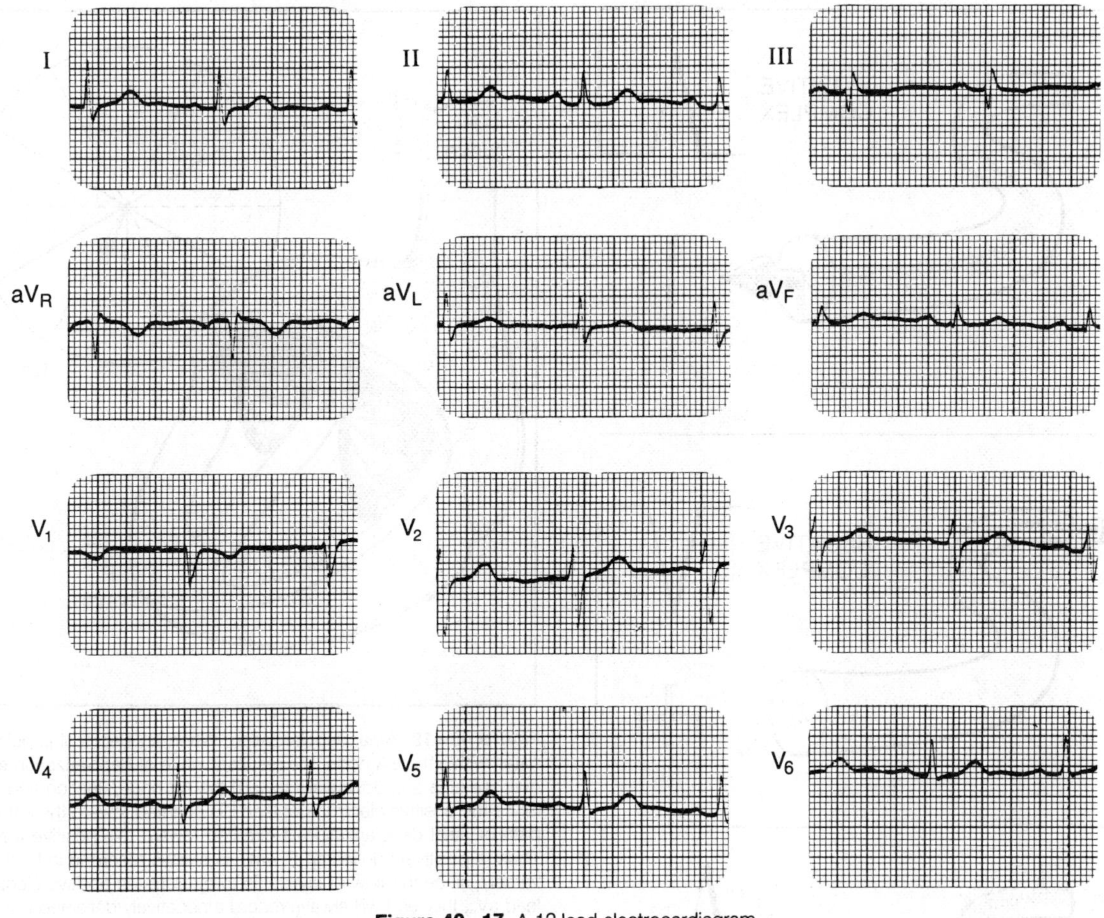


**Figure 40-17.** A 12-lead electrocardiogram.

simultaneous depolarization of the main muscle mass of both the left and right ventricles, occurring from inside the heart (endocardium) to the outside (epicardium). In the normal heart, the muscle mass of the left ventricle is considerably greater than that of the right ventricle. Consequently, the electrical current generated within the left ventricle predominates over that of the right. A large arrow representing phase 2 of ventricular depolarization can be drawn pointing toward the left ventricle and downward in the direction of the left leg. This arrow reflects the heart's *mean electrical axis* (mean cardiac axis), that is, the main *direction* and *magnitude* of current flow within the ventricles (Fig. 40-20, *B*).

Predicting the shape of the QRS complex based upon overall ventricular current flow is not nearly as easily accomplished as that of the P wave. In the standard limb leads there is normally considerable variation in the QRS complex configuration. This is based in part on the position of the heart in the chest and on the mean cardiac axis.

In general, with NSR, lead II usually records a positively deflected QRS complex as the mean ventricular current flow (mean cardiac axis) is directed downward to the left and *toward* the positive electrode of lead II. Lead $aV_R$ will normally record a predominantly negatively deflected QRS complex because the mean cardiac axis is directed *away* from the positive electrode of lead $aV_R$, which is oriented upward toward the right shoulder.

The QRS pattern can more accurately be described by assessing the precordial or chest leads ($V_1$ to $V_6$). The left-to-right depolarization of the septum (phase 1) will produce a small r wave (septal r wave) in lead $V_1$ and a small q wave (septal q wave) in lead $V_6$. Depolarization of the remaining ventricular mass (phase 2) is reflected by a deep (negatively deflected) S wave in lead $V_1$ as the flow of current is directed *away* from the positive electrode; and a tall (positively deflected) R wave in lead $V_6$ as the flow of current is *toward* the positive electrode (Fig. 40-21). As one moves across the chest from $V_1$ through $V_6$ (i.e., in the direction of the electrically predominant left ventricle), there is usually an increase in the size of the R wave, becoming maximal around $V_5$. This increase in the R wave as one moves from right to left is called normal *R wave progression across the precordium* (Fig. 40-22).

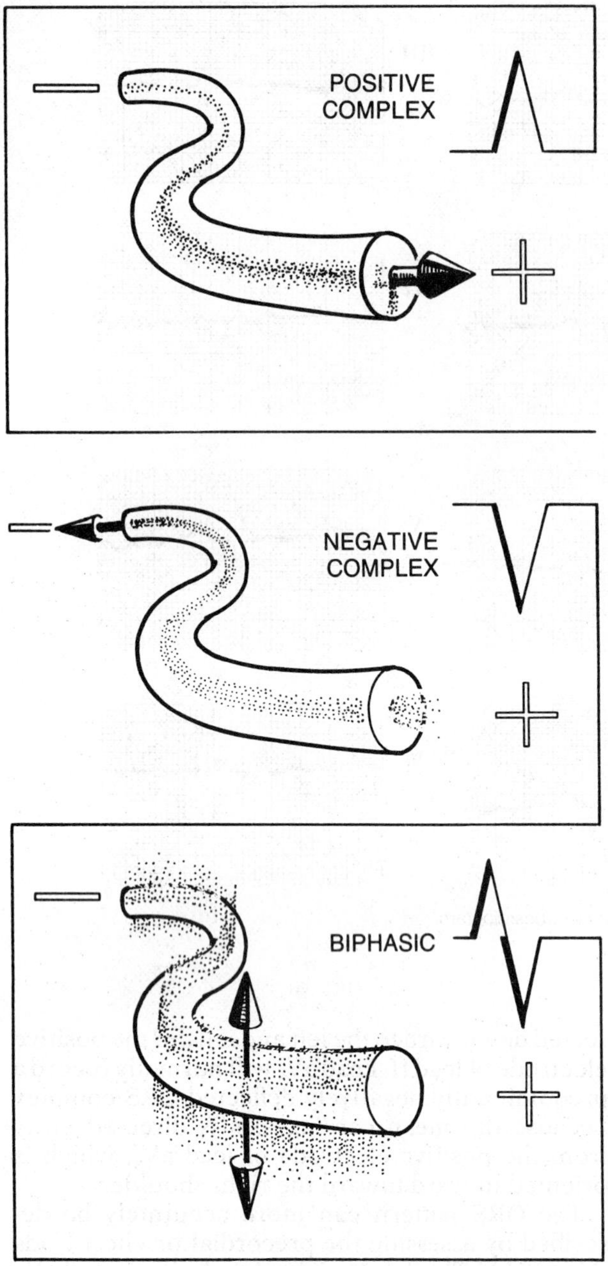


**Figure 40–18.** Fundamental principles of electrocardiography: (*1*) A positive complex (upward deflection) is recorded when the wave of depolarization spreads *toward* the positive electrode of a lead. (*2*) A negative complex (downward deflection) is recorded when the wave of depolarization spreads *away* from the positive electrode of a lead. (*3*) A biphasic complex (one consisting of positive and negative deflections of equal size) is recorded when the mean path of depolarization is directed at right angles (perpendicular) to the lead.

### *The Normal ST Segment and T Wave*

The return of the heart to its resting state, that is, repolarization, is reflected on the ECG by the ST segment and T wave (U wave if present). As discussed earlier, the ST segment reflects early ventricular repolarization and is usually at the isoelec-

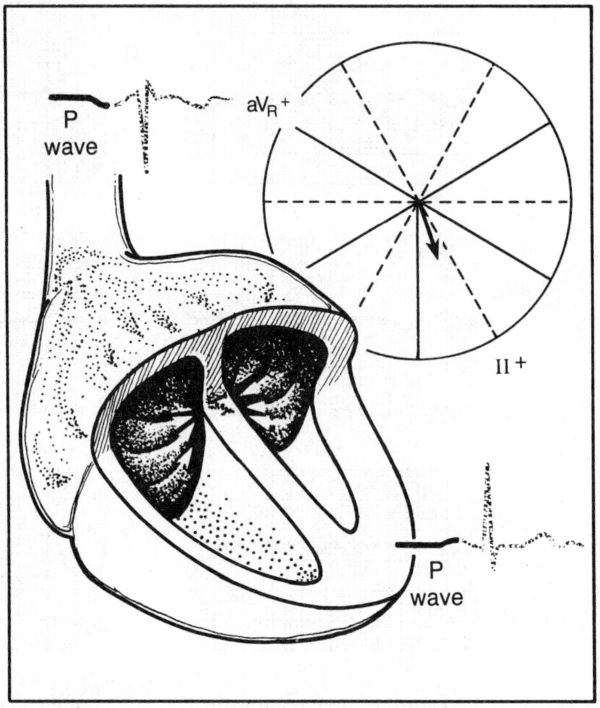


**Figure 40–19.** Atrial depolarization. When an electrical impulse originates within the SA node, the resultant wave of depolarization spreads over the atria and downward toward the AV node/junction and left leg. Since the positive electrode of lead II is oriented toward the left leg, the path of atrial depolarization is directed *toward* this positive electrode. Thus, a positively deflected P wave is always recorded in lead II. Conversely, since the flow of current is *away* from the positive electrode of lead $aV_R$, this lead will always record a negatively deflected P wave.

tric line on the ECG. Slight elevation of less than 1 mm or depression of less than 0.5 mm may be seen normally.

The T wave, as a rule, follows the direction of the QRS complex deflection. When the QRS is positively deflected, the T wave is likewise positively deflected (upright). When the QRS is negatively deflected, the T wave is also negatively deflected (inverted). With NSR, the T wave in lead II is normally positive; in lead $aV_R$ it is always negative. Left-sided chest leads ($V_4$ to $V_6$) normally display a positive T wave; in other leads, the T wave deflection is variable.

## Dysrhythmias: Pathogenesis

Under normal circumstances, the SA node, as the pacemaker of the heart, dominates all other cardiac cells and spontaneously depolarizes at a rate to meet the physiologic needs of body tissues. This is reflected by normal sinus rhythm, which occurs at a rate of 60–80 beats/minute. Any disturbance in the origin, rate, rhythm, or conduction of the cardiac action potential results in a dysrhythmia.

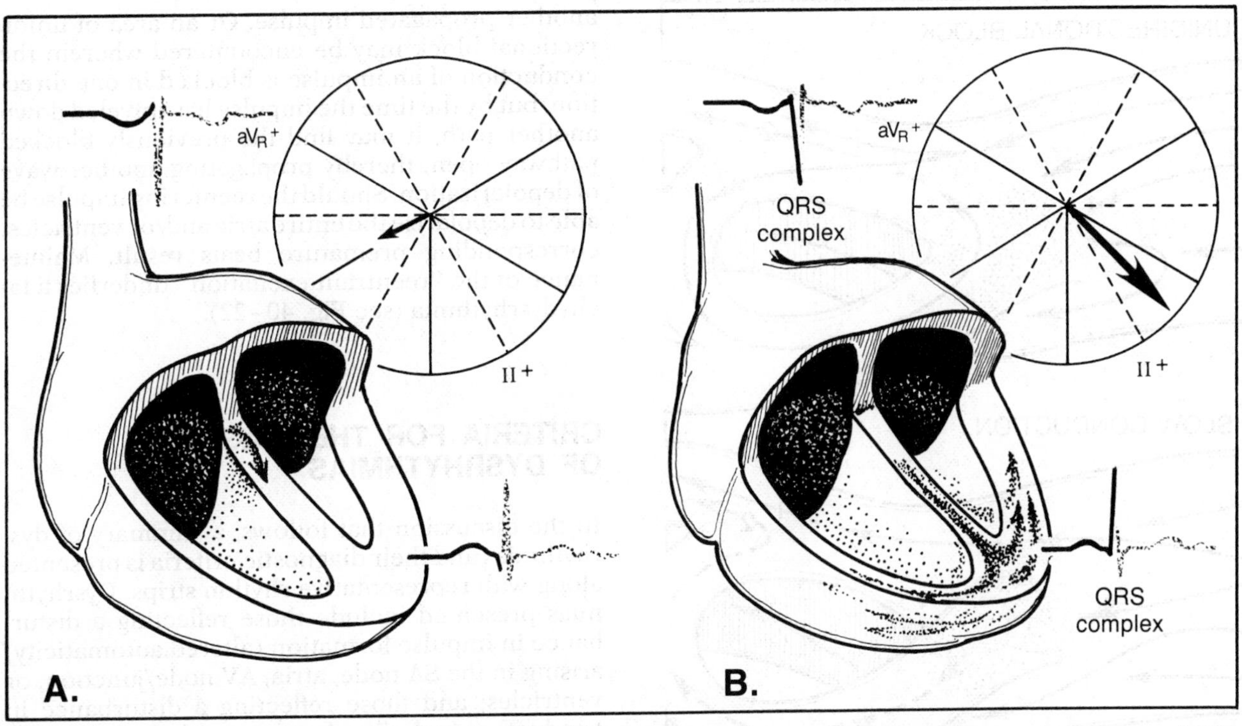


**Figure 40–20.** Ventricular depolarization occurs in 2 sequential phases: (*1*) Phase 1: Septal depolarization proceeds across the septum in a direction from *left* to *right* (indicated by *arrow*). (*2*) Phase 2: Depolarization of main ventricular muscle mass occurs in a direction from right to left and *toward* the left leg (lead II). Note that the magnitude of current flow as reflected by the arrow is directed *toward* the positive electrode of lead II. Thus, this lead usually records a positively deflected QRS complex. Conversely, since current flow is directed *away* from the positive electrode of lead $aV_R$, this lead will record a negatively deflected QRS complex.

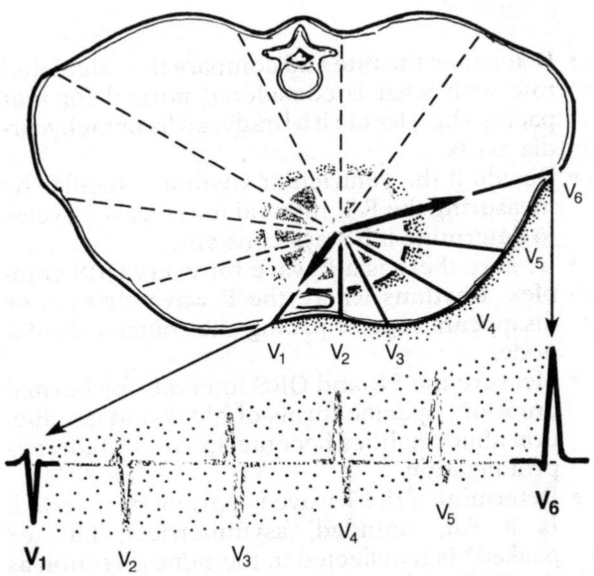


**Figure 40–21.** Ventricular depolarization as recorded by precordial (chest) leads $V_1$ through $V_6$. Note the progressive increase in the amplitude of the R waves as one moves from right to left across the chest. This reflects the recording of current flow as the wave of depolarization moves across the chest in the direction of the electrically predominant left ventricle and toward the positive electrodes of the left chest leads. This is referred to as *R wave progression across the precordium*.

Dysrhythmias can be categorized largely into 2 main groups based on their underlying mechanisms: disorders of impulse formation (altered automaticity) and disorders of impulse conduction (reentry phenomenon).

### *Altered Automaticity*

As discussed earlier, pacemaker cells exhibit the property of automaticity; that is, they have the inherent ability to depolarize spontaneously to threshold potential without any external stimulation, thereby firing an action potential. Pacemaker cells in the SA node normally depolarize to threshold potential sooner than other lower subsidiary pacemaker cells, thereby enabling the SA nodal cells to assume the role as the pacemaker of the heart (see Fig. 37–15).

Should automaticity be enhanced in subsidiary pacemaker cells (i.e., those below the SA node) these cells may fire before the SA nodal pacemaker cells, thereby resulting in premature beats or tachycardia. This is referred to as *enhanced automaticity*. The origin of these extra beats may be atrial, ventricular, or junctional. Conversely, should automaticity be decreased or depressed, bradycardia and

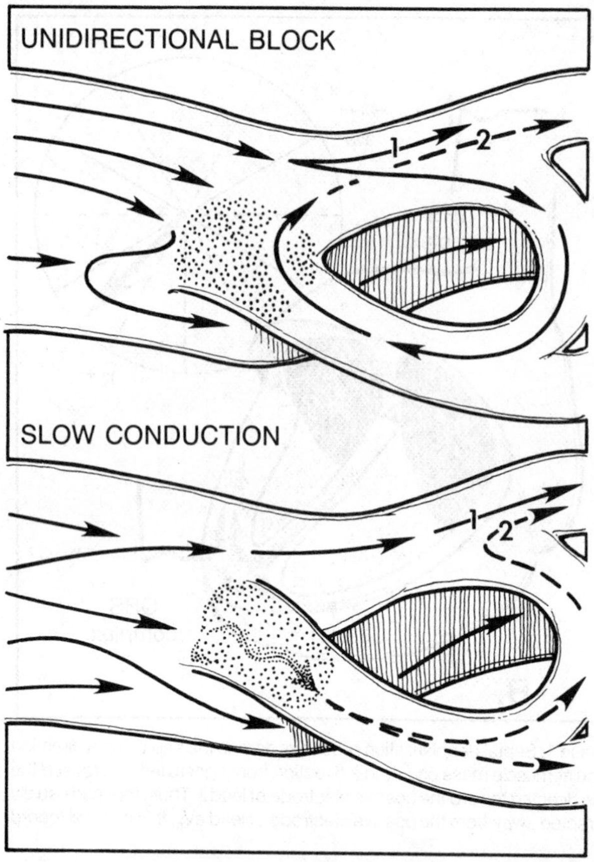


**Figure 40-22.** Disturbances in impulse conduction, reentry phenomena. *Unidirectional block*: The conduction of an impulse (*solid arrows*) is blocked in one direction, but by the time the impulse travels down the open pathway and depolarizes the surrounding myocardium, it may find the previously blocked or refractory pathway excitable, thereby generating another wave of depolarization (*broken arrow*). *Pathway of slow conduction*: an impulse (*solid arrows*) traveling through an area of slow conduction may emerge to find the surrounding myocardium repolarized, and therefore capable of generating another wave of depolarization (*broken arrows*).

escape rhythms may result. (Note: *Escape* rhythms occur when the formation and conduction of sinus impulses are delayed or blocked, enabling a subsidiary pacemaker action potential to "escape." The escape impulse is then conducted and depolarizes the myocardium.)

#### *Reentry Phenomena*

Reentry phenomena are associated with disturbances in conduction wherein an action potential is delayed sufficiently long within a pathway of slow conduction so that it is still active when the surrounding myocardium repolarizes. The impulse can then *reenter* the repolarized tissue and initiate another propagated impulse. Or an area of unidirectional block may be encountered wherein the conduction of an impulse is blocked in one direction, but by the time the impulse has traveled down another path, it may find the previously blocked pathway open, thereby propagating another wave of depolarization. Should the reentering impulse be able to depolarize the entire atria and/or ventricles, corresponding premature beats result. Maintenance of the "reentrant excitation" underlies a tachydysrhythmia (see Fig. 40-22).

## CRITERIA FOR THE DIAGNOSIS OF DYSRHYTHMIAS

In the discussion that follows, a summary of dysrhythmias and their diagnostic criteria is presented along with representative rhythm strips. Dysrhythmias presented include those reflecting a disturbance in impulse formation (altered automaticity) arising in the SA node, atria, AV node/junction, or ventricles; and those reflecting a disturbance in conduction including first-, second-, and third-degree heart block. A discussion of the clinical significance and treatment of these dysrhythmias is also presented.

### Key Steps in Dysrhythmia Identifications

- Determine the rate and compare the calculated rate with what is considered normal for that pacing site. Decide if a bradycardia or tachycardia exists.
- Decide if the ventricular rhythm is regular by measuring the R-R interval for at least 3 cycles to determine if it stays constant.
- Be sure there is a P wave for every QRS complex. Rhythms where the P wave changes or disappears suggest pacing sites outside the SA node.
- Measure the PR and QRS intervals for normal duration. Specific forms of block and conduction abnormalities become apparent if there is prolongation.
- Determine if the T wave is upright or inverted. Is it flat, rounded, asymmetrical, tall, or peaked? Is it deflected in the same direction as the QRS complex?
- Identify whether the ST segment is isoelectric, elevated, or depressed.
- Look for beats or runs of beats that interrupt the dominant rhythm and create an abnormality.

## Dysrhythmias: Specific Criteria and Representative Strips*†

**Sinus Rhythm** (Fig. 40–23)

| Rate | | Rhythm | | Duration | |
|---|---|---|---|---|---|
| Ventricular | 60–100 | R-R | regular | PR Interval | .12–.20 sec |
| Atrial | 60–100 | P-P | regular | QRS Complex | .06–.10 sec |

INTERVENTIONS: None

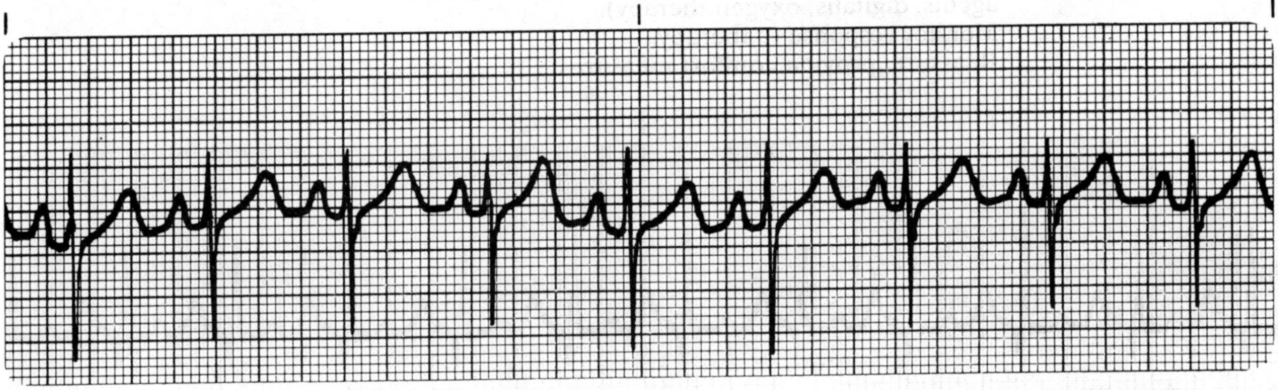

Lead II

**Sinus Bradycardia** (Fig. 40–24)

| Rate | | Rhythm | | Duration | |
|---|---|---|---|---|---|
| Ventricular | less than 60 | R-R | regular | PR Interval | .12–.20 sec |
| Atrial | same as ventricular | P-P | regular | QRS Complex | .06–.10 sec |

INTERVENTIONS:
- ◦ Assess vital signs, clinical status; document ECG strip.
- ◦ Administer atropine as prescribed for symptomatic bradycardia.
- ◦ Monitor response to therapy.

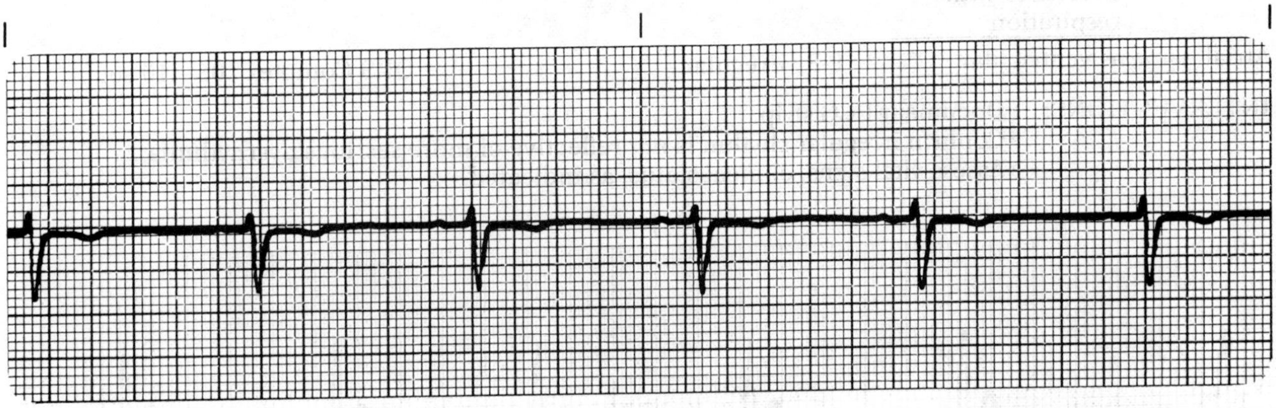

Lead II

*Adapted from American Heart Association: Textbook of Advanced Cardiac Life Support, American Heart Association, National Center, Dallas, Texas, 1987, p. 97–126.

†Representative ECG strips from the nursing staff of Massapequa General Hospital, Intensive Care Unit, Seaford, N.Y.

**Sinus Tachycardia** (Fig. 40–25)

| Rate | Rhythm | Duration |
|---|---|---|
| Ventricular greater than 100 | R-R regular | PR Interval .12–.20 sec |
| Atrial same as ventricular | P-P regular | QRS Complex .06–.10 sec |

INTERVENTIONS:
- Assess vital signs, clinical status; document ECG strip
- Assess to determine underlying cause (e.g., fever, anxiety, pain, congestive heart failure).
- Record 12-lead ECG in the presence of chest pain.
- Administer prescribed medications (e.g., antipyretics, analgesics, antianxiety agents, digitalis, oxygen therapy).
- Monitor response to therapy.
- Reassure; provide comfort measures.

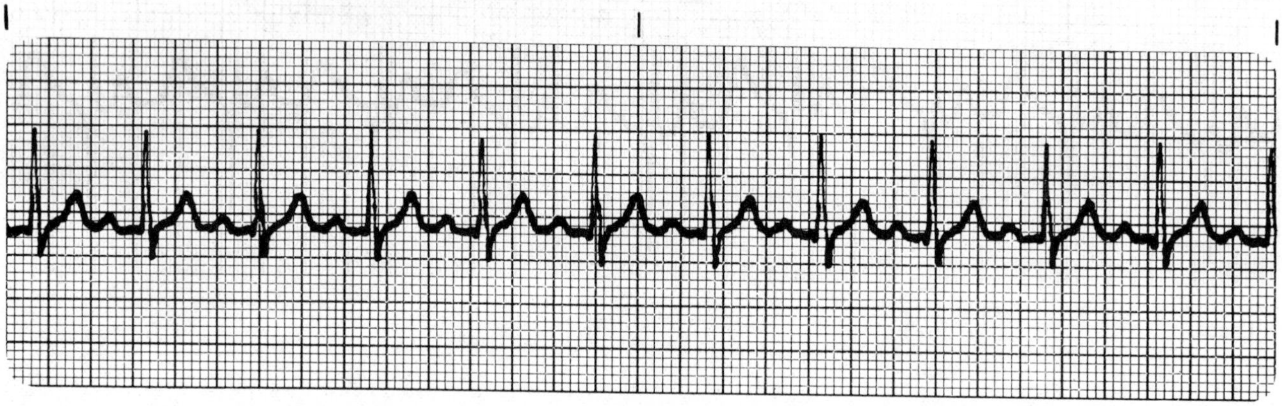

Lead II

**Sinus Arrhythmia** (Fig. 40–26)

| Rate | Rhythm | Duration |
|---|---|---|
| Ventricular increases and decreases with respiration | R-R irregular | PR Interval .12–.20 sec |
| Atrial same as ventricular | P-P irregular | QRS Complex .06–.10 sec |

INTERVENTIONS:
- Document ECG strip.
- Confirm irregular rhythm is *not* reflective of more sesrious dysrhythmia.
- Assess vital signs, clinical status, as indicated.

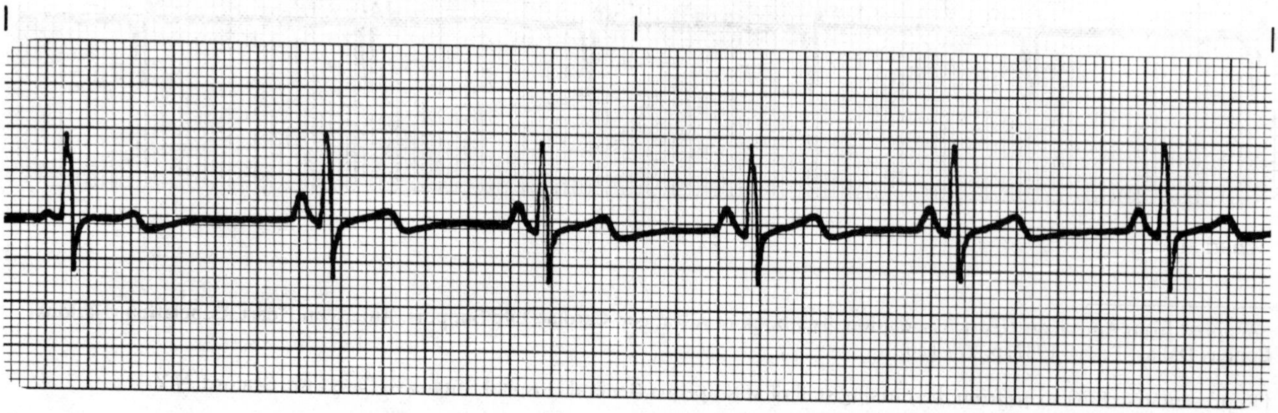

Lead II

**Atrial Fibrillation** (Fig. 40–27)

| Rate | | Rhythm | | Duration | |
|---|---|---|---|---|---|
| Ventricular | 100 controlled<br>100 uncontrolled | R-R | irregular | PR Interval | absent due to fibrillation waves |
| Atrial | greater than 350 | P-P | absent | QRS Complex | .06–.10 sec |

INTERVENTIONS:
- Assess vital signs, clinical status; document ECG strip.
- Notify physician if dysrhythmia develops abruptly and/or patient becomes symptomatic (e.g., faint, lightheaded, shortness of breath, chest pain).
- Prepare for intravenous digitalization; elective cardioversion.
- Prepare for intravenous calcium blocking agent (e.g., verapamil).
- Monitor serum digitalis levels for overdosage.

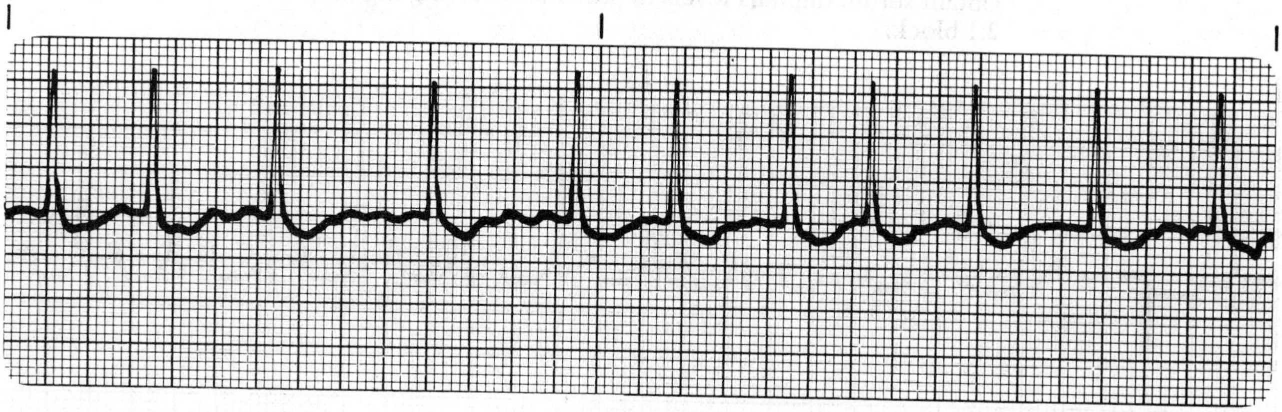

Lead II

**Atrial Flutter** (Fig. 40–28)

| Rate | | Rhythm | | Duration | |
|---|---|---|---|---|---|
| Ventricular | variable depending on degree of block | R-R | regular/irregular | PR Interval | absent due to flutter waves |
| Atrial | less than or equal to 350 | P-P | absent | QRS Complex | .06–.10 sec |

Note: A variable flutter rate will cause the R-R interval to become *irregular*. Ventricular response can be less than or greater than 100.

INTERVENTIONS:
- Assess vital signs, clinical status; document ECG strip.
- Prepare for elective cardioversion.
- Administer prescribed medications (e.g., digitalis).
- Monitor response to therapy.

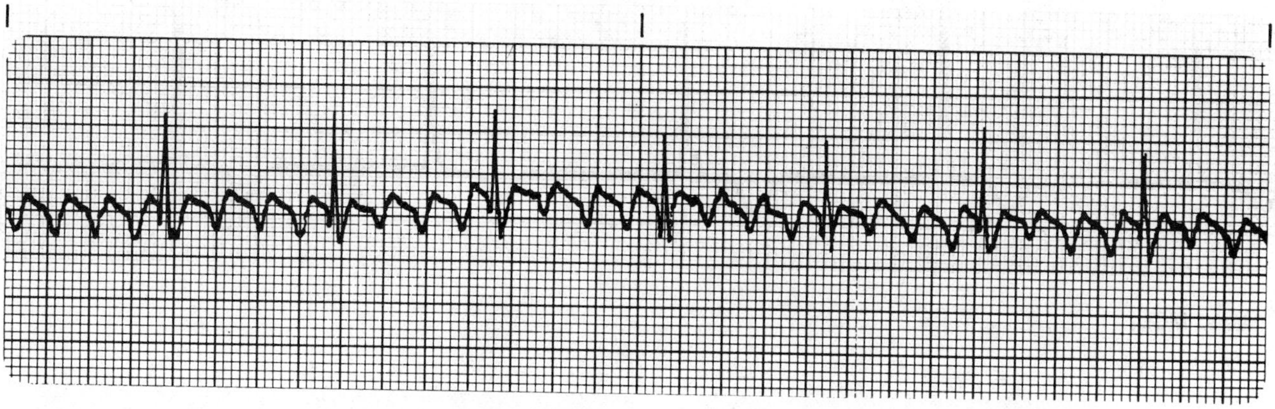

Lead II

**Paroxysmal Atrial Tachycardia** (Fig. 40–29)

| Rate | Rhythm | Duration |
|---|---|---|
| Ventricular 150–250 | R-R regular | PR Interval .12–.20 sec |
| Atrial same as ventricular | P-P regular | QRS Complex .06–.10 sec |

Note: This rhythm is always of sudden onset.

INTERVENTIONS:
- Assess vital signs, clinical status; document ECG strip.
- Notify physician.
- Administer prescribed medications (e.g., oxygen, calcium blocker, beta blocker, digitalis).
- Monitor response to therapy.
- Prepare for elective cardioversion.
- Obtain serum digitalis levels in patients receiving digitalis who develop PAT with 2:1 block.

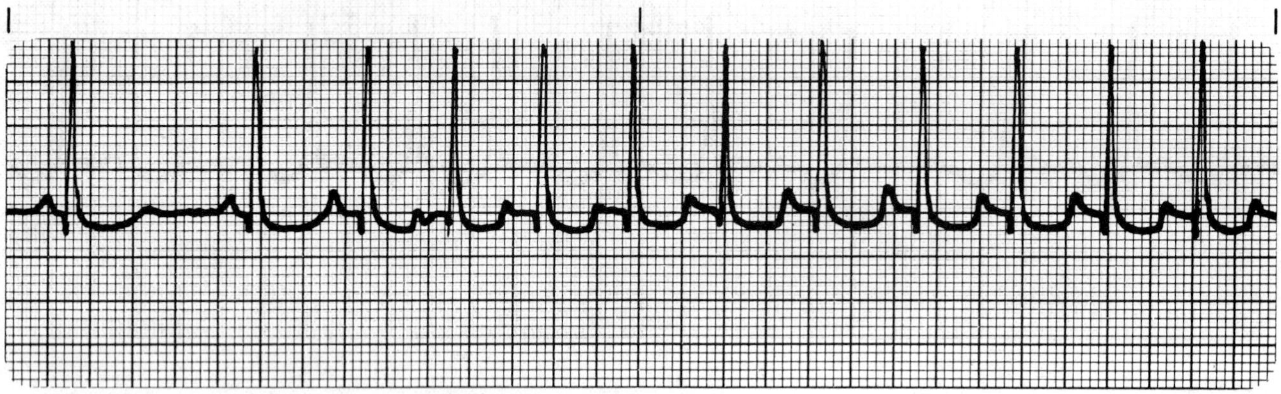

Lead II

**Junctional Rhythm** (Fig. 40–30)

| Rate | Rhythm | Duration |
|---|---|---|
| Ventricular 40–60 | R-R regular | PR Interval absent |
| Atrial usually less than or equal to ventricular rate | P-P absent; inverted in leads II, III, $aV_F$; or "buried" in QRS complex | QRS Complex .06–.10 sec |

INTERVENTIONS:
- Assess vital signs, clinical status; document ECG strip.
- Distinguish dysrhythmia from heart block or ventricular dysrhythmias.
- Monitor patient's tolerance of slow ventricular response.

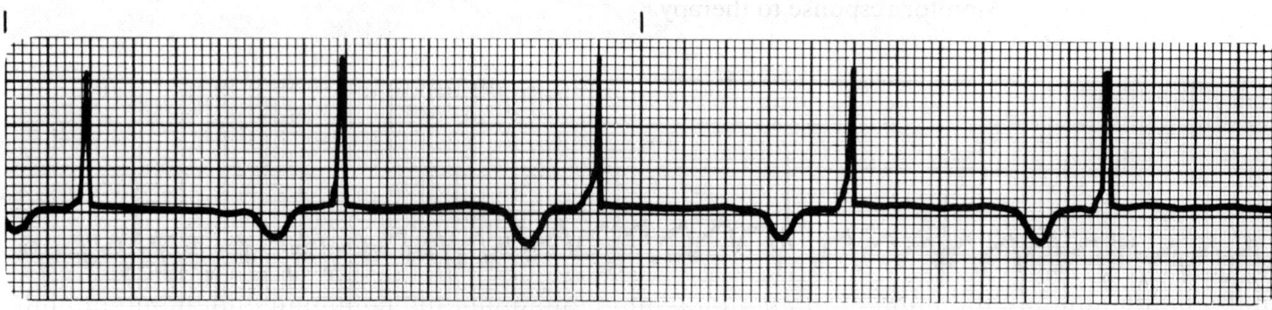

Lead $MCL_1$

**Junctional Tachycardia** (Fig. 40–31)

**Rate**

Ventricular 60–130

Atrial same as ventricular (if visible)

**Rhythm**

R-R regular

P-P same as in junctional rhythm

**Duration**

PR Interval absent

QRS Complex .06–.10 sec may show widening

INTERVENTIONS:
- Assess vital signs, clinical status; document ECG strip.
- Monitor serum digitalis level for digitalis toxicity.
- Prepare for transvenous pacemaker insertion if patient becomes symptomatic.

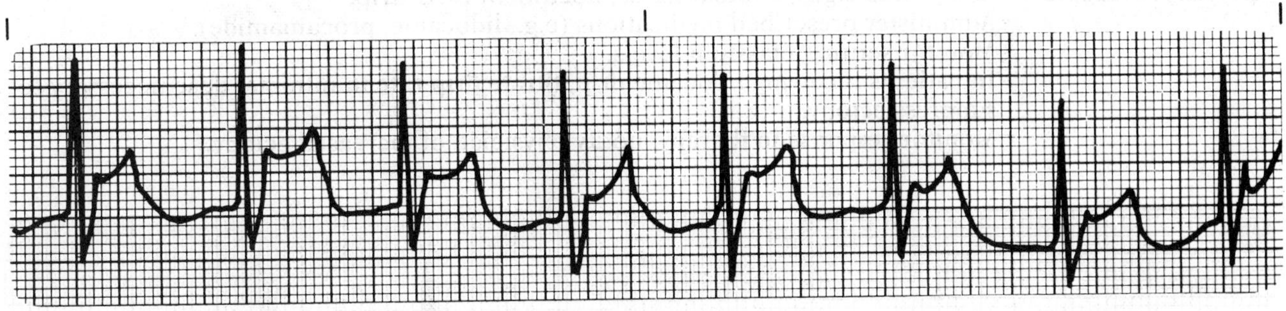

Lead II

**Paroxysmal Junctional Tachycardia** (Fig. 40–32)

**Rate**

Ventricular greater than 130

Atrial same as ventricular (if visible

**Rhythm**

R-R regular

P-P same as in junctional rhythm

**Duration**

PR Interval absent

QRS Complex .06–.10 sec

Note: This rhythm is always of sudden onset.

INTERVENTIONS:
- Assess vital signs, clinical status; document ECG strip.
- Notify physician.
- Record 12-lead ECG if chest pain.
- Administer prescribed medications (e.g., digitalis, beta blocker, calcium blocker).
- Prepare for elective cardioversion.
- Monitor response to therapy.

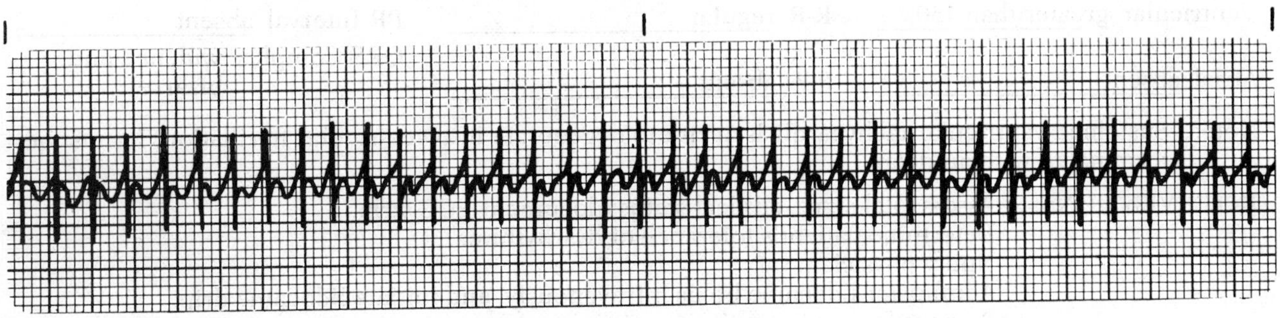

Lead II

**Premature Ventricular Contraction** (Fig. 40–33; refer also to Figs. 40–42, 40–43, 40–44, and 40–45)

| | **Rhythm** | **Duration** |
|---|---|---|
| Ventricular 60–100 | R-R irregular due to PVCs | PR Interval absent in ectopic beats; remaining beats conducted normally |
| Atrial 60–100 | P-P irregular due to PVCs | QRS Complex PVCs widened greater than .12 sec |

INTERVENTIONS:
- Assess vital signs, clinical status; document ECG strip.
- Administer prescribed medications (e.g., lidocaine, procainamide).
- Monitor serum potassium levels.
- In patients receiving lidocaine drip, titrate drip rate to minimal dose necessary to suppress ectopy.
- Monitor response to therapy; notify physician of increased ectopy.

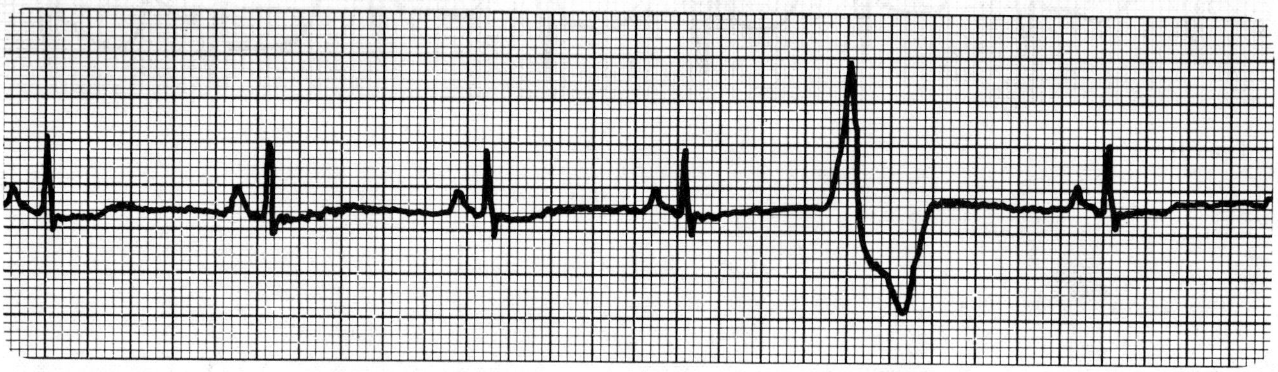

Lead II

**Ventricular Tachycardia** (Fig. 40–34)

| **Rate** | **Rhythm** | **Duration** |
|---|---|---|
| Ventricular greater than 150 | R-R regular | PR Interval absent |
| Atrial absent | P-P absent | QRS Complex widened and bizarre |

Note: Sustained ventricular tachycardia is at risk to degenerate into ventricular fibrillation. It must be terminated without delay.

INTERVENTIONS:
- Assess vital signs, clinical status; document ECG strip.
- Determine patient's tolerance of dysrhythmia.
- Notify physician.
- Administer lidocaine bolus intravenously, and initiate lidocaine drip.
- Prepare for cardioversion.
- Monitor response to therapy.
- If unresponsive, call Code Blue and initiate CPR.

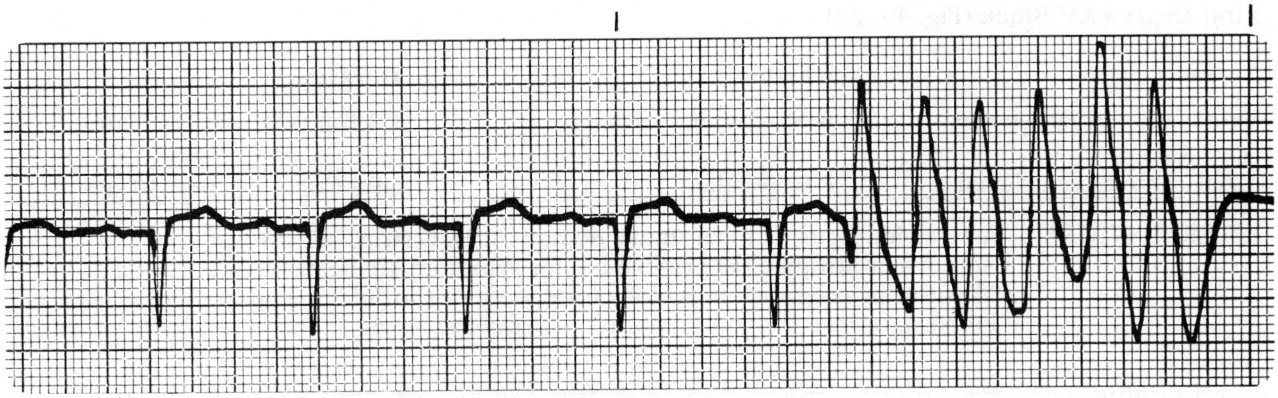

Lead $MCL_1$

**Ventricular Fibrillation** (Fig. 40–35)

**Rate**

Ventricular indeterminable

Atrial absent

**Rhythm**

R-R chaotic rhythm

P-P absent

**Duration**

PR Interval absent

QRS Complex bizarre in configuration; no uniformity

INTERVENTIONS:

- Establish consciousness, breathing, pulse. (Note: If patient is conscious, ventricular fibrillation is *not* the problem.)
- If unconscious, apneic, and pulseless, initiate Code Blue and CPR. (Allow ECG to run to record events.)
- Prepare for defibrillation; endotracheal intubation.
- Establish IV access if not present.
- Administer prescribed medication. (Medications may include: atropine, bretylium tosylate, calcium chloride, dopamine, epinephrine, isoproterenol, lidocaine, procainamide, and sodium bicarbonate.)
- Carefully document sequence of events including events preceding, during, and following code. All drugs, dosages, times, and patient's response to therapy should be documented.

(For additional details regarding the clinical significance and treatment of *fast-rate dysrhythmias*, see section below.)

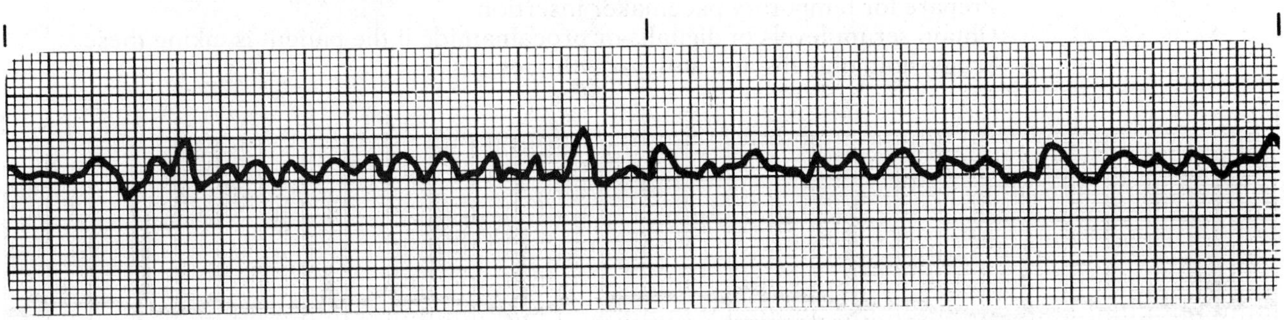

Lead $MCL_1$

**First-Degree AV Block** (Fig. 40–36)

| Rate | Rhythm | Duration |
|---|---|---|
| Ventricular usually normal | R-R regular | PR Interval greater than .20 sec |
| Atrial same as ventricular | P-P regular | QRS Complex .06–.10 sec |

INTERVENTIONS:
- Assess vital signs, clinical status; document ECG strip.
- Administer atropine (as prescribed) for symptomatic heart block.
- Monitor for progression of block to second- or third-degree heart block.
- Prepare for insertion of temporary pacemaker.

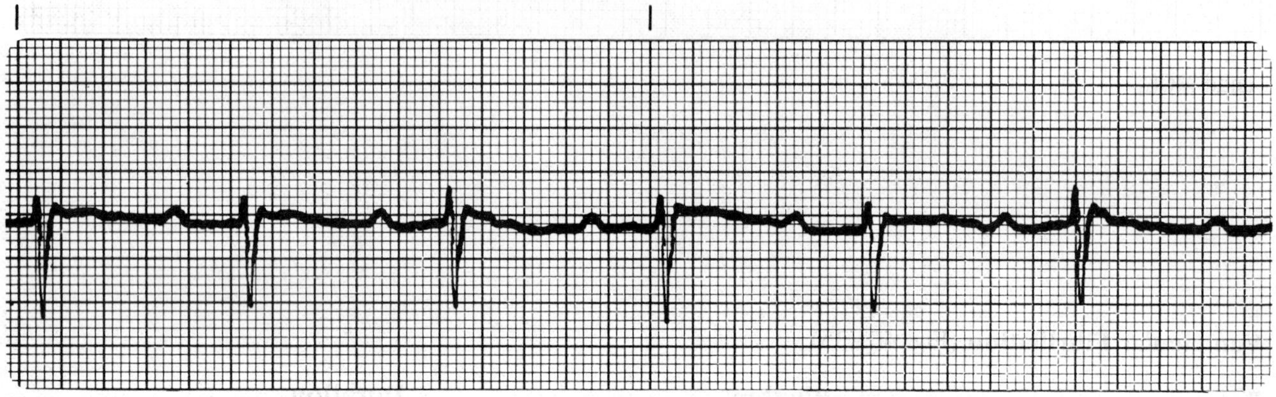

Lead $MCL_1$

**Second-Degree AV Block (Wenckebach, Mobitz Type I)** (Fig. 40–37)

| Rate | Rhythm | Duration |
|---|---|---|
| Ventricular normal or slow | R-R irregular | PR Interval progressive lengthening until one P wave is blocked, and the cycle repeats |
| Atrial greater than ventricular | P-P regular | QRS Complex .06–.10 sec |

INTERVENTIONS:
- Assess vital signs, clinical status; document ECG strip.
- Determine degree of heart block and frequency of nonconducted beats.
- Notify physician.
- Administer prescribed medications (e.g., atropine, isoproterenol).
- Monitor response to pharmacotherapeutics.
- Prepare for temporary pacemaker insertion.
- Obtain serum levels of digitalis or procainamide if the patient is taking these drugs; hold digitalis and antidysrhythmics.

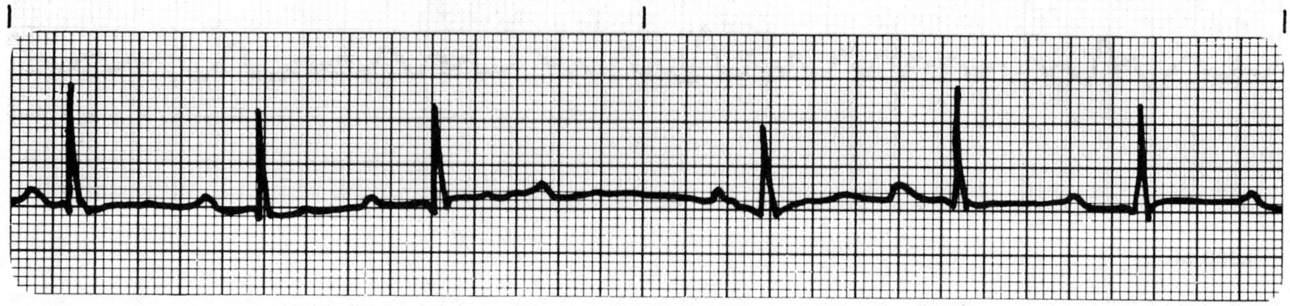

Lead II

**Second-Degree AV Block (Mobitz Type II)** (Fig. 40–38)

| Rate | Rhythm | Duration |
|---|---|---|
| Ventricular usually slow | R-R irregular | PR Interval normal or prolonged |
| Atrial greater than ventricular | P-P regular | QRS Complex normal |

INTERVENTIONS:
- ◦ Assess vital signs, clinical status; document ECG strip.
- ◦ Notify physician.
- ◦ Prepare for insertion of temporary pacemaker.
- ◦ Administer prescribed medication (e.g., atropine, isoproterenol, epinephrine).
- ◦ Monitor response to therapy.
- ◦ Withhold digitalis and antidysrhythmics.

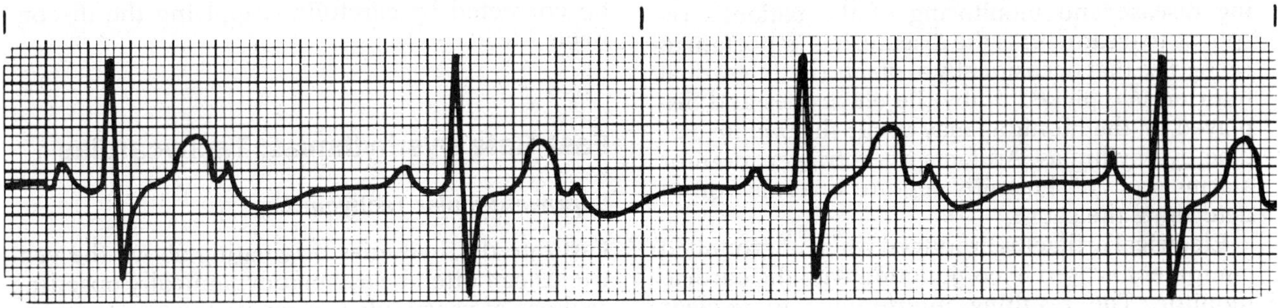

Lead II

**Third-Degree AV Block (Complete Heart Block)** (Fig. 40–39)

| Rate | Rhythm | Duration |
|---|---|---|
| Ventricular usually 20–40 | R-R regular | PR Interval constantly changing |
| Atrial usually 60–100 | P-P regular | QRS Complex normal or widened |

INTERVENTIONS:
- ◦ Assess clinical status.
- ◦ Notify physician.
- ◦ Prepare for insertion of temporary pacemaker (this is the only dependable treatment for complete heart block).
- ◦ Administer medications as prescribed (e.g., epinephrine, intravenous infusion of isoproterenol).
- ◦ Monitor for ventricular ectopy (PVCs). (The occurrence of PVCs may forewarn of ventricular tachycardia or ventricular fibrillation).

(For additional details regarding the clinical significance and treatment of *slow-rate* dysrhythmias, see section below.)

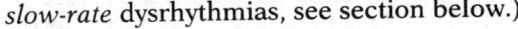

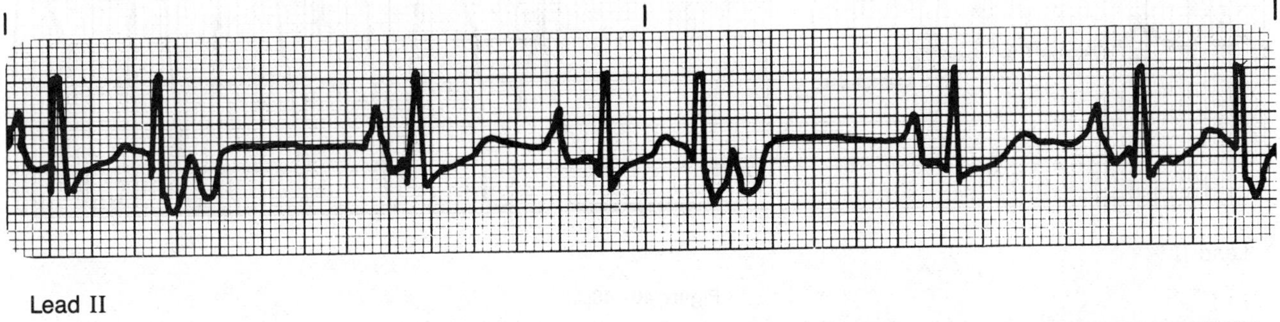

Lead II

## DYSRHYTHMIAS: CLINICAL SIGNIFICANCE AND TREATMENT

In discussing the clinical significance and treatment of dysrhythmias it is helpful to group them into categories of tachycardia/bradycardia, and supraventricular versus ventricular dysrhythmias. Additionally, it is important to stress that there are certain clinical *non-events* that may *mimic* a dysrhythmia on the bedside monitor.

### Artifact and False Alarms

While electronic monitoring provides vast dividends in terms of diagnosis of the patient's underlying disease and monitoring of the patient's response to treatment of the disease, it is important to recognize that occasionally artifacts (i.e., electrical interference picked up by the electrodes and displayed on the monitor) may occur that *mimic* cardiac dysrhythmias. Artifacts often trigger monitor alarms and consequently require investigation to determine the cause.

Electrical artifact is produced when ungrounded equipment is used in conjunction with the cardiac monitor. The resulting interference to a clear transmission on the ECG most often takes the form of a blurred baseline and complexes. When such interference is present, it may be necessary to remove extraneous wiring from the patient and bed, piece by piece until the offending appliance is isolated.

Artifact can also be caused by the patient's own muscle movement, respiratory rate and excursion, and other physical activity. In the tracing shown in Figure 40–40(*A*), the computerized monitor detected a run of ventricular tachycardia. However, patient assessment revealed an alert subject in bed, scratching his chest. In this instance, ventricular tachycardia was simulated by physical activity and interference with lead transmission. In Figure 40–40(*B*) what appears to be an atrial flutter was also caused by patient movement in bed. The appearance of such tracings, whether reflective of artifact or an actual dysrhythmia, necessitates *immediate* patient assessment. Subsequent therapy is always based on the patient's response to any supposed or real dysrhythmia.

Another frequently encountered false alarm situation is caused by *lead displacement.* Without a functioning bipolar system sending signals, the monitor will not pick up a heart beat at all. In this case the screen records a straight line or false asystole. These situations require immediate investigation. Once the problem has been discovered it can be corrected by carefully reapplying the disconnected lead.

### Fast-Rate Dysrhythmias: Tachycardias

#### *Supraventricular Tachycardia*

Fast-rate dysrhythmias originating above the ventricles can often be as hemodynamically upsetting as those of ventricular origin. As the heart rate accelerates certain significant physiologic responses occur:

1. Myocardial oxygen consumption ($\dot{M}VO_2$) increases.
2. Diastole decreases, decreasing the time available for coronary artery perfusion.
3. Fast rates reduce ventricular filling time with loss of the "atrial kick," that is, the extra volume of blood delivered to the ventricles upon atrial contraction. The consequence is a decrease in cardiac output.

It is therefore of great importance to slow or stop fast-rate supraventricular rhythms. The patient

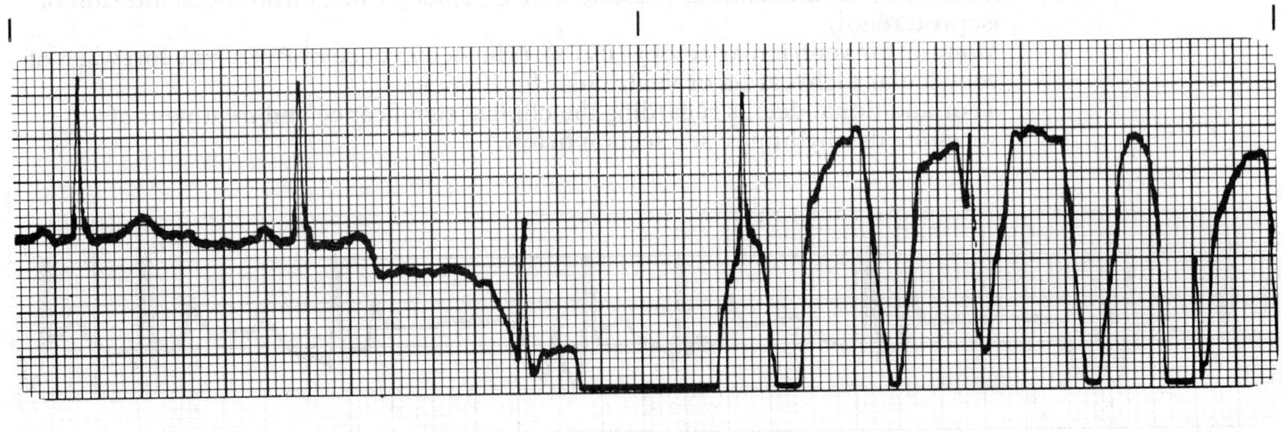


Figure 40–40(*A*).

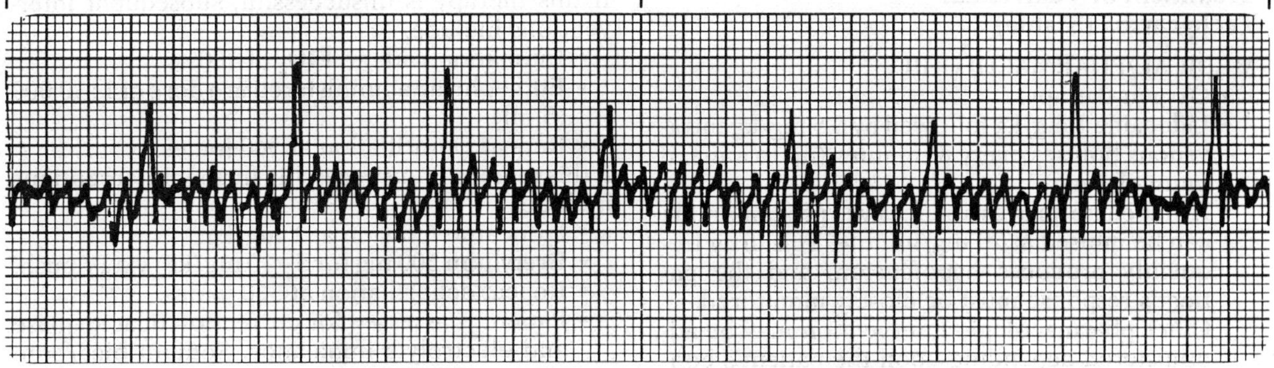

Lead MCL$_1$

Figure 40-40(*B*).

should be assessed for signs of any physical cause of the tachycardia (e.g., fear, anxiety, pain, or temperature elevation), and these conditions should be treated accordingly. Fast-rate supraventricular rhythms may also be due to conduction abnormalities. Treatment of these latter dysrhythmias may require medical and/or pharmacologic interventions. Figure 40-41 reflects a supraventricular tachycardia with a rapid ventricular response.

### Treatment of Supraventricular Tachycardia

MEDICAL:

- Valsalva maneuver or carotid massage (conducted by the physician if the patient's condition is stable).
- Synchronous cardioversion in increasing doses as indicated—initially 75-100 joules, increased to 200-360 joules as needed.
- Overdrive pacing (i.e., electrical pacing at a rate that supercedes the rate of the ectopic focus, thereby nullifying its role as pacemaker).

PHARMACOLOGIC:

(As per physician's order and/or unit protocol)

- Verapamil 5 mg. (Dose may be increased to 10 mg intravenously within 15-20 minutes if dysrhythmia does not resolve.)
- Beta blockers (e.g., propranolol, metoprolol) may be tried.
- Digoxin may be indicated.

### *Ventricular Dysrhythmias*

The classification of "life-threatening" dysrhythmias is usually reserved for 2 specific rhythms both involving the ventricles: *ventricular tachycardia* and *ventricular fibrillation.*

**Ventricular Tachycardia** (See Fig. 40-34). Ventricular tachycardia (VT) is classified as *stable* or *unstable*. While some patients can tolerate sustained runs of VT (i.e., stable), many others, particularly the patient with an acute myocardial infarction, will quickly decompensate into ventricular fibrillation (unstable), without appropriate and timely intervention.

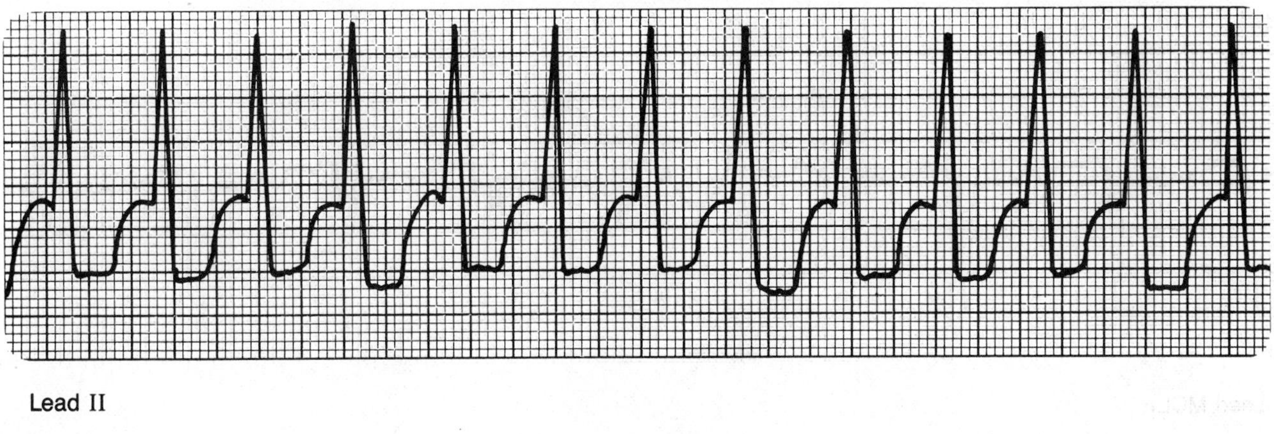

Lead II

Figure 40-41.

### Treatment of Ventricular Tachycardia (Stable)

MEDICAL/PHARMACOLOGIC:

- Oxygen therapy.
- Lidocaine 1 mg/kg followed by 0.5 mg/kg intravenous boluses every 8 minutes (up to a maximum of 3 mg).
- If lidocaine proves ineffective, procainamide can be infused at 20 mg/minute. This drug frequently produces hypotension, and the patient's response must be closely monitored.
- Other pharmacologic intervention may be administered depending upon the patient's condition, physician's preference, and/or unit protocol.
- If the above therapy is ineffective, cardioversion may be indicated and administered in the manner described for the treatment of unstable VT (see below).

### Treatment of Ventricular Tachycardia (Unstable)

MEDICAL/PHARMACOLOGIC:

- Oxygen therapy.
- Cardioversion initially at a dose of 50 joules, increasing to doses up to 360 joules, as indicated for the patient.
- Sedation therapy. (It should be noted that in both stable and unstable ventricular tachycardia, sedating the patient should be considered prior to cardioversion.)

**Ventricular Fibrillation** (See Fig. 40–35). Ventricular fibrillation is most clearly synonymous with biologic death as there is no cardiac output with this dysrhythmia. Immediate action is always necessary to restore cardiovascular function. A representative approach to therapy in the monitored patient includes the following:

- Defibrillation at 200 joules.
- Defibrillation at 300 joules.
- Defibrillation at 360 joules.

If this therapy is unsuccessful, subsequent interventions include:

- Intubation with an $FIO_2$ of 100%.
- Epinephrine administered in a dose of 1 : 10,000 (5 ml).
- Repeat defibrillation at 360 joules.

If this therapy is unsuccessful, further interventions include:

- Lidocaine infusion at 1 mg/kg.
- Bretylium 500 mg (or 5–10 mg/kg) via IV push.
- Repeat defibrillation at 360 joules.
- Patient is assessed for correction of acid–base and electrolyte imbalance. Sodium bicarbonate is administered as indicated.
- CPR should be in progress throughout the entire resuscitation period.

**Ventricular Ectopy (Premature Ventricular Contractions — PVCs).** Both ventricular tachycardia and ventricular fibrillation may be preceded by an increase in premature ventricular contractions (PVCs). PVCs that are *multifocal* (Fig. 40–42) (i.e., originate in more than one ectopic focus) or that occur in a *bigeminal* pattern (Figs. 40–43, 40–44) (i.e., in pairs or couplets) place the patient at greater risk of developing ventricular tachycardia or fibrillation. The more PVCs per minute, the greater the possibility that these electrical events will degenerate into a life-threatening dysrhythmia.

***Treatment of PVCs.*** Patients exhibiting multiple ventricular ectopics should be assessed to rule out the following: serum potassium imbalances, overdigitalization, drug toxicity, or a concomitant bradycardia-promoting ectopy.

When none of these factors need to be corrected, primary treatment of PVCs consists of lidocaine 1 mg/kg bolus. This initial dose may be repeated at half dose every 2–5 minutes (up to a maximum total dose of 3 mg). If the ectopy resolves, a lidocaine drip should be established to protect against further "break through" dysrhythmias.

PVCs intractable (i.e., unresponsive) to lidocaine are treated with procainamide (20 mg/minute) or

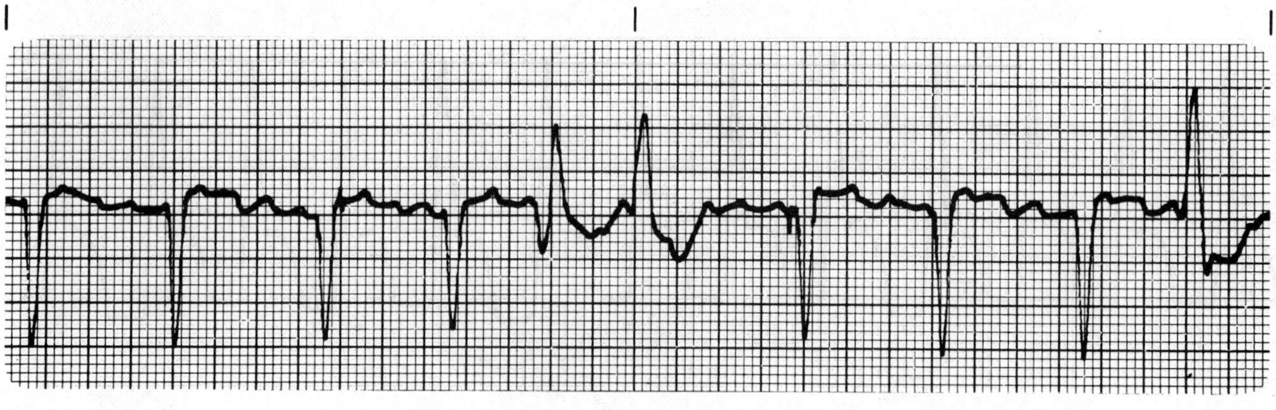

Lead $MCL_1$

**Figure 40–42.**

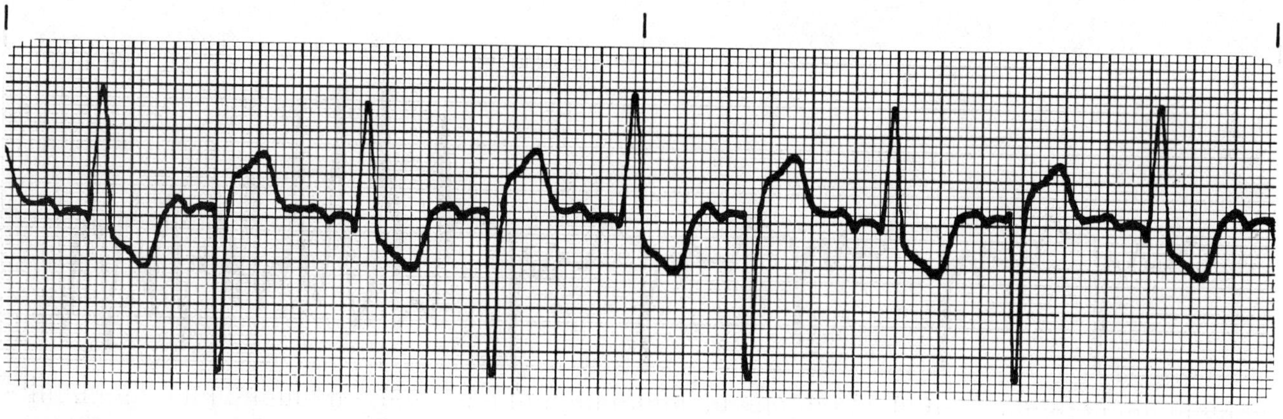


Figure 40-43.

bretylium (5–10 mg/kg over 8–10 minutes). Both of these drugs have been associated with hypotension. Such therapy should only be administered to patients who are being continuously monitored. (The pharmacotherapeutics administered depend upon the patient's condition and response to therapy, physician's preference, and/or unit protocol.)

**R-on-T Phenomenon.** The R-on-T phenomenon (Fig. 40–45) refers to the occurrence of a PVC on the downslope of the T wave of the preceding beat. Electrically, the myocardium is especially vulnerable at this time as the muscle fibers have not completely repolarized but are at varying stages of depolarization and repolarization. An action potential of sufficient magnitude fired during this vulnerable period can cause rhythm degeneration without any further warning and precipitate electrical chaos and ventricular fibrillation. Preventative treatment requires close cardiac monitoring of patients at risk. The treatment for ventricular fibrillation is described above.

## Slow-Rate Dysrhythmias: Bradycardias and Heart Blocks

Any rhythm that is too slow to supply the patient's basic metabolic requirements (i.e., symptomatic bradydysrhythmias) necessitates therapy. Most commonly encountered are sinus bradycardia and second- and third-degree AV heart block (see Figs. 40–24, 40–36, 40–37, 40–38, and 40–39). Sinus bradycardia is usually defined as a heart rate of less than 50–60 beats/minute. Heart block refers to an interruption in the conduction of an impulse from the SA node through the AV node/junction and over the His-Purkinje system to the myocardial muscle fibers. Heart block can occur at any level of the conduction system (see Fig. 37–6).

Clinically, these disorders are significant because they lead to a reduction in cardiac output, thereby compromising cardiovascular function. Hemodynamic instability and an altered level of consciousness are early signs frequently encountered in

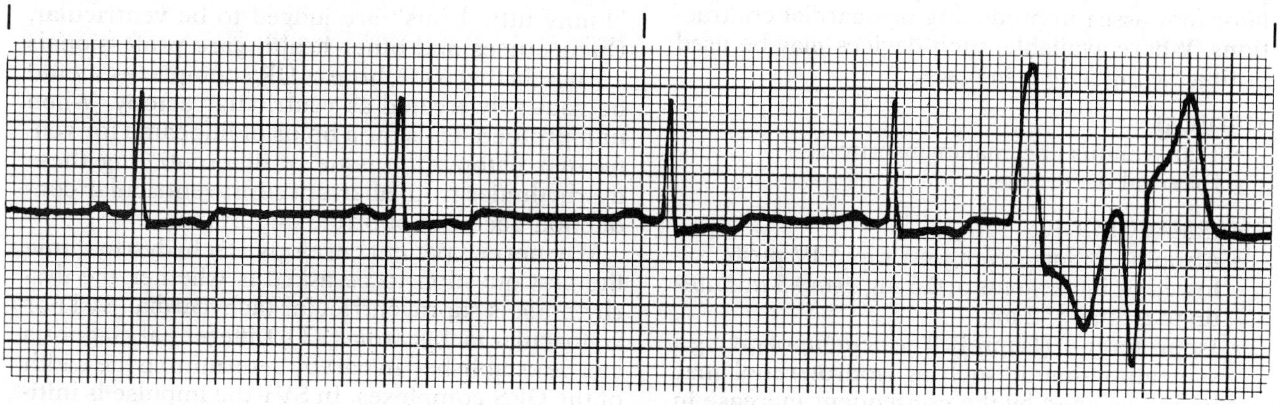


Figure 40-44.

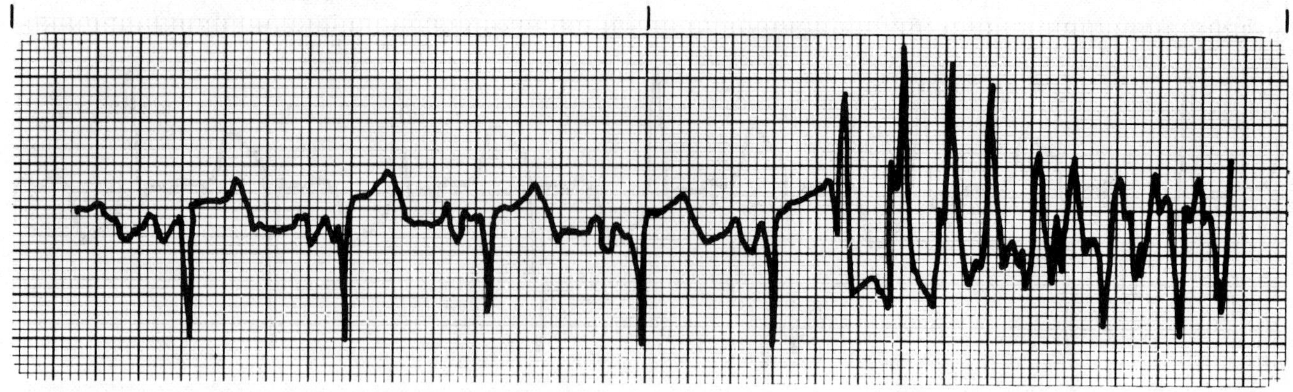


**Figure 40-45.** Premature ventricular contraction: R on T phenomenon.

patients experiencing these dysrhythmias. Furthermore, the presence of a bradycardia may enable a more excitable extopic focus to usurp pacemaker function within the heart. Early detection and timely treatment are imperative to prevent a seemingly innocous bradycardia from progressing to complete heart block and cardiac standstill.

#### *Treatment of Bradydysrhythmias*

Initial intervention usually involves the administration of atropine sulfate. As an anticholinergic agent (see Chap. 6), atropine blocks parasympathetic stimulation to the SA and AV nodes, thereby allowing sympathetic influence to become dominant. The expected response to atropine is an increase in heart rate.

While atropine therapy may work transiently to increase heart rate, the treatment of choice in patients with heart block (especially in the scenario of an anteroseptal myocardial infarction) is *cardioacceleration.* Long-term cardioacceleration is best achieved by insertion of a temporary pacemaker. In some institutions an external pacemaker or stimulator may assist in producing myocardial contractions. Where available, such devices may be used until a pacing wire is in place.

MEDICAL:

- Transvenous pacemaker insertion.
- External pacemaker.

PHARMACOLOGIC:

- Atropine sulfate 0.5 mg via rapid IV push, followed by increments of 0.5 mg every 5 minutes up to a total of 2 mg.
- Isoproterenol (Isuprel). The benefits of giving a sympathomimetic such as isoproterenol may be outweighed by the consequent increase in myocardial oxygen demand ($MVO_2$). This consideration is especially important in patients with anteroseptal and anteroseptal lateral myocardial infarctions.
- Rule out digitalis toxicity. In patients with bradycardia, the possibility of digitalis toxicity must always be ruled out. (Refer to Appendix A for detailed information on specific drugs.)

## Miscellaneous Dysrhythmias

#### *Aberrant Supraventricular/ Ventricular Conduction*

The term *aberrancy,* simply defined, means that some abnormality in ventricular activation is present causing widened, bizarre QRS complexes. This abnormality in intraventricular conduction is usually temporary. It results when a supraventricular impulse arrives in the ventricles before the conduction pathway has completely recovered from a previous impulse.

Clinically, it is essential to determine the origin of a widened QRS complex, that is, whether it is supraventricular (above the ventricles) or ventricular in origin. It has been estimated that up to 50% of these "funny little beats" are judged to be ventricular. Often nurses and other health care professionals are taught that wide, bizarre QRS complexes should be routinely treated as ventricular ectopy. When unit protocol calls for a bolus of lidocaine for ventricular ectopy, the issue of differentiating these dysrhythmias from aberrant supraventricular conduction becomes of prime importance.

Whenever a patient develops a tachydysrhythmia the first question to be asked is whether the dysrhythmia is supraventricular tachycardia (SVT) or ventricular tachycardia (VT). Differential diagnosis can be established in part by determining the width of the QRS complexes. In SVT the impulse is initiated above the ventricles, and is conducted to the ventricles over the normal conduction pathways.

This normal intraventricular conduction is reflected on the ECG by a *narrow* QRS complex (0.06–0.10 sec). SVTs classified in this category include sinus tachycardia, paroxysmal atrial tachycardia (PAT), atrial fibrillation, atrial flutter, and multifocal atrial tachycardia (MAT).

Tachydysrhythmias with *widened* QRS complexes (0.12 sec and above), include 2 possible causes. The first and more significant is VT, a life-threatening dysrhythmia. VT can be defined as a run of 3 or more consecutive PVCs, at a rate between 150 and 200 beats/minute, with a rhythm that is usually regular. The second cause is SVT with aberration.

There are 2 major mechanisms underlying aberrancy with an SVT that assist in differentiating this rhythm from that of VT. These include a bundle branch block (BBB) pattern and the Wolff-Parkinson-White (WPW) preexcitation syndrome. To appreciate the significance of bundle branch block in this regard, a brief review of RBBB and LBBB follows.

**Right Bundle Branch Block (RBBB).** The normal sequence of ventricular depolarization is discussed earlier in this chapter and consists of 2 sequential phases: septal depolarization and ventricular depolarization. (See Figs. 37–7 and 40–20.) *Septal* depolarization normally occurs in a left-to-right direction, reflecting the fact that the left bundle branch (LBB) depolarizes slightly before the right bundle branch (RBB). Thus, in lead $V_1$, as current flows *toward* its positive electrode, an initial r wave is recorded normally; whereas in lead $V_6$ as current initially flows *away* from its positive electrode, an initial s wave is recorded (see Fig. 40–21).

With *ventricular* depolarization, although both ventricles depolarize nearly simultaneously, the left ventricle is electrically predominant because of its greater mass. Therefore, a deep S wave occurs in lead $V_1$ as the bulk of current flows away from its positive electrode; whereas in lead $V_6$, the flow of current toward the positive electrode is recorded as a tall R wave (see Fig. 40–20, *B*).

In right bundle branch block (RBBB), septal depolarization remains undisturbed as it normally occurs via the LBB. A small r wave is written in lead $V_1$, and a small s wave in lead $V_6$. During the early part of ventricular depolarization, the bulk of current flows toward the left ventricle resulting in a deep S wave in lead $V_1$ and a tall R wave in lead $V_6$. An RBBB affects mainly the terminal phase of ventricular depolarization. This delayed depolarization of the remaining right ventricle is reflected by an R′ wave in lead $V_1$ as current again flows toward its positive electrode, and an S wave recorded in lead $V_6$ as current flows away from its positive electrode (Fig. 40–46).

The resultant triphasic pattern of RBBB is characterized by an rSR′ pattern in lead $V_1$ with a broad R′ wave; in lead $V_6$ a qRS type complex is written, with a broad S wave. The additional time taken to complete depolarization of the right ventricle is reflected by a QRS duration of greater than 0.12 sec. Thus, a diagnosis of RBBB can be made by examining the chest leads, $V_1$ and $V_6$, in particular.

**Left Bundle Branch Block (LBBB).** Left bundle branch block (LBBB) (Fig. 40–47) also produces a pattern with widened QRS complex. Understandably, the shape of the QRS complex with LBBB is very different from that of RBBB. In this case, the normal pattern of septal depolarization is disrupted and the septum is depolarized from right to left and not left to right as it is normally. Thus, there is loss of the septal r wave in lead $V_1$ and of the q wave in lead $V_6$. The total time for depolarization of the left ventricle is prolonged resulting in a widened R wave in lead $V_6$, and a QS complex in lead $V_1$. As is the case with RBBB, the diagnosis of LBBB can be made by examining leads $V_1$ and $V_6$. Lead $V_1$ shows a widened entirely negative QS complex with no septal r wave; while lead $V_6$ records a widened tall R wave without a septal q wave.

**SVT with Bundle Branch Block.** Patients with an underlying tachydysrhythmia, in association with a BBB, will record a wide-complex tachycardia that may be mistaken for VT. For example, in patients with sinus tachycardia, paroxysmal atrial tachycardia (PAT), atrial fibrillation, or atrial flutter, who also have a RBBB or LBBB, a wide QRS complex will be observed on the ECG. This is demonstrated in Figure 40–48. An atrial fibrillation

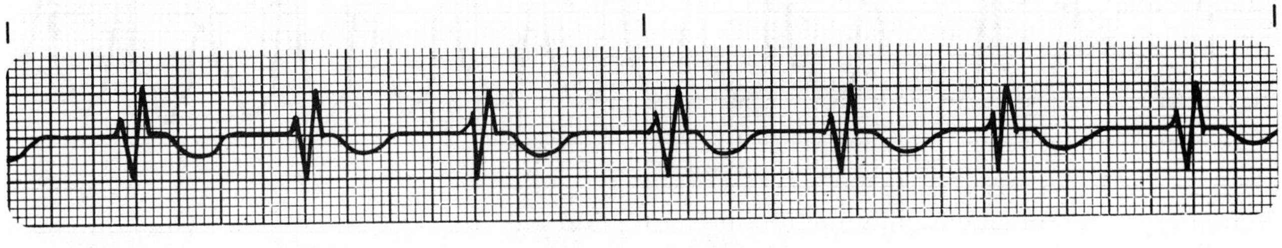

Lead $MCL_1$

**Figure 40–46.** Right bundle branch block.

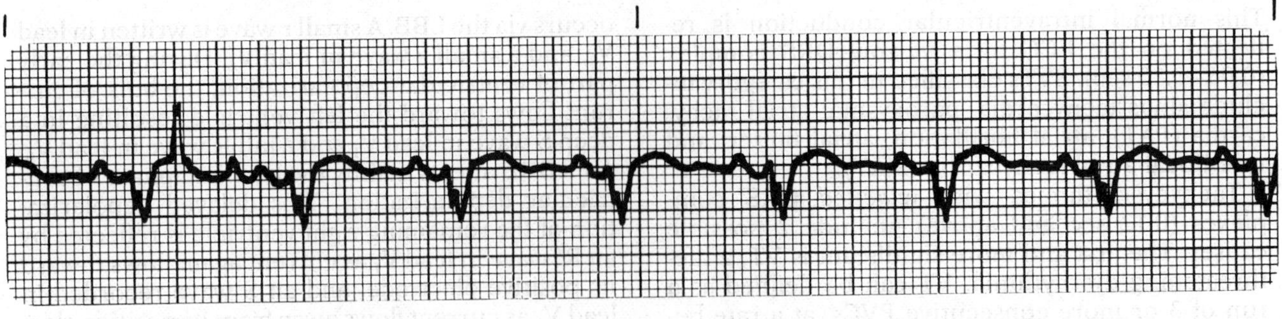


**Figure 40–47.** Left bundle branch block.

with a rapid ventricular response and an associated BBB offers a startling similarity to the actual VT pattern reflected in Figure 40–49. In this case, a distinguishing feature is the *irregularity* of the atrial fibrillation, as opposed to the regular rhythm observed with the VT. However, in this example, the absence of P waves complicates the differentiation (see below).

**SVT with Wolff-Parkinson-White (WPW) Syndrome.** SVT with Wolff-Parkinson-White (WPW) syndrome is a second mechanism underlying a wide-complex tachycardia. An accessory pathway connecting the atria with either ventricle, thereby bypassing the AV node/junction, is thought to be responsible for WPW preexcitation. Conduction over the accessory pathway at very high rates may result in a wide QRS complex tachycardia that may mimic VT. The possible diagnosis of WPW with atrial fibrillation should be strongly suspected if a wide-complex tachycardia is encountered that is irregular and has a very high rate.

### *ECG Criteria for Differentiating Aberrant Supraventricular Beats from Ventricular Ectopy*

Aberrant supraventricular beats (ASBs) are defined as impulses of supraventricular origin whose conduction to the ventricles is *partially,* and usually temporarily, blocked. This "aberrant" conduction causes the QRS complex of these beats to be abnormal and different from the QRS complexes of sinus-conducted beats. This phenomenon is also referred to as *ventricular aberration.* The following discussion identifies ECG criteria that assist in differentiating aberrant supraventricular beats from those of ventricular origin.

**The P-QRS Relationship.** In the absence of P waves and a full compensatory pause (i.e., a long pause after a bizarre beat, usually a PVC), it is necessary to closely examine the P-QRS relationship for additional distinguishing clues. Ideally, when the patient goes into a run of wide, bizarre beats, it would be helpful to identify a P wave. The presence of a P wave *in front of* the first beat of the paroxysm of beats suggests the run is *supra*ventricular in origin, with aberrant conduction. However, the absence of a P wave does not always mean the rhythm is ventricular. During a fast rate, the P wave can be buried in the preceding T wave or QRS complex.

On the other hand, a P wave *following* the initial beat of the run is due to *retrograde* (backward) depolarization of the atria from a site below the SA node. Such a presentation is strongly suggestive of *ventricular* tachycardia.

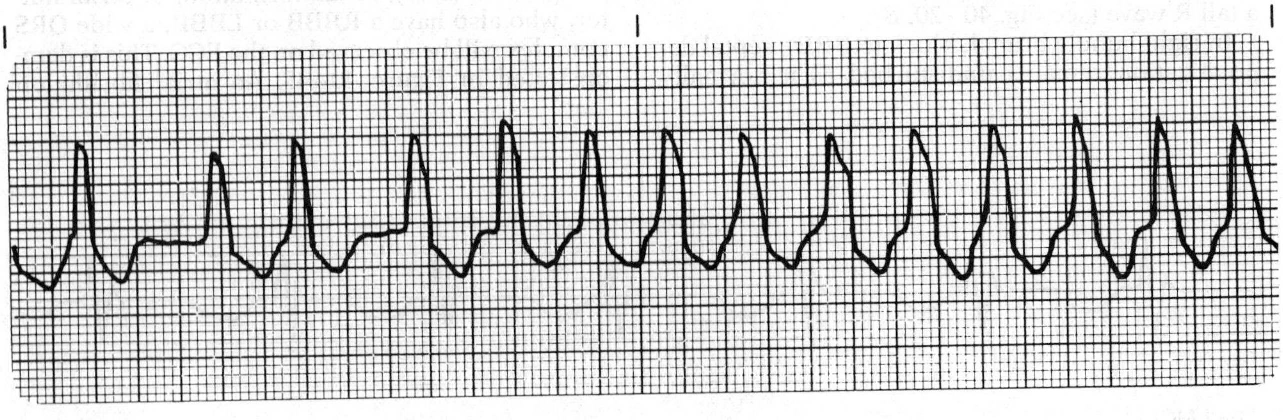


**Figure 40–48.** Atrial fibrillation in association with bundle branch block.

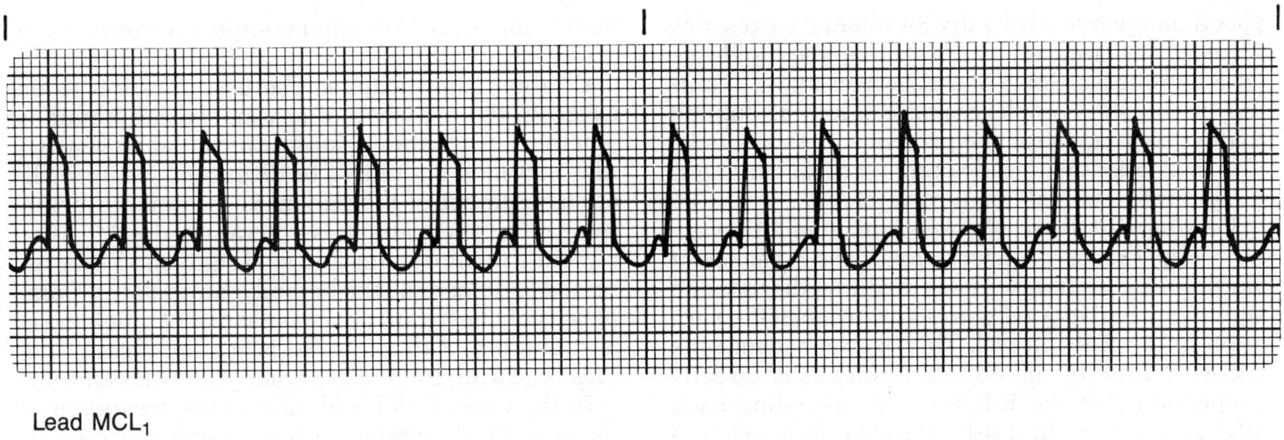


**Figure 40–49.** Ventricular Tachycardia.

This information is helpful in weeding out aberrant supraventricular beats (ASBs) from ventricular beats and rhythms. It is important to appreciate that fast rates are notorious for obscuring P waves and the P-QRS relationship. In addition, it should be noted that rhythms susceptible to ASBs may have no clear P wave, as, for example, in atrial fibrillation and atrial flutter.

Therefore, the majority of criteria for differentiating supraventricular premature beats with aberrant conduction from those of ventricular origin have to do with the presentation of the QRS.

**The Configuration of the QRS.** In assessing a patient with ASBs versus ventricular tachycardia, it is imperative to have access to a 12-lead ECG. In the clinical setting a patient who is known to have ASBs *and* ventricular ectopic beats should be constantly monitored using the $MCL_1$ lead. The $MCL_1$ lead mimics the $V_1$ lead and will provide more information regarding the configuration of ASBs than the standard monitoring leads.

***Axis Determination.*** As discussed earlier, the mean flow of current within the heart (i.e., the mean electrical axis) is directed from right to left across the chest and downward toward the left leg (see Fig. 40–20). If the direction of normal current flow (i.e., mean cardiac vector) is plotted on the hexaxial figure, the mean cardiac axis would occur in the quadrant between 0 degrees and +90 degrees (Fig. 40–50). By convention, each of the 6 standard limb leads has an angular designation, with lead I at 0 degrees; all leads above lead I have negative angular values while those below it have positive values. (Note: A detailed discussion of axis and its determination is beyond the scope of this text, and the reader is referred to the Suggested Readings list at the end of this chapter or to a text on electrocardiography.)

Suffice it to say that in general the following rules apply: (1) Despite abnormal intraventricular conduction, an impulse of supraventricular origin will generate an axis within the normal quadrant of the hexaxial figure, that is, between 0 and +90 degrees; (2) ventricular ectopy is more often associated with abnormal vectors (i.e., those projected in a direction outside of the normal quadrant of 0 to +90 degrees).

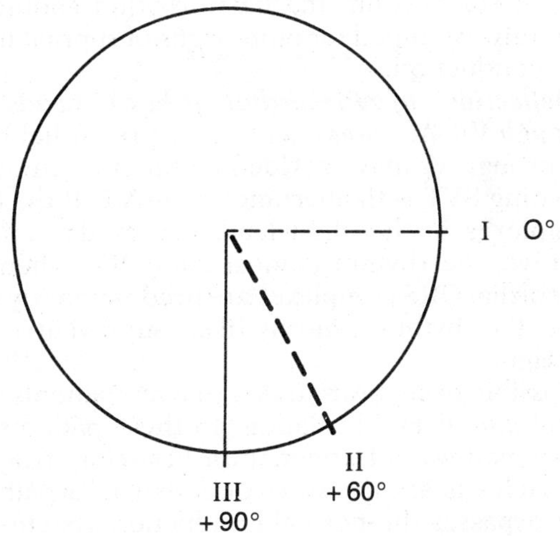


**Figure 40–50.** Mean cardiac axis plotted (*heavy dotted line*) on hexaxial figure.

***Interpretation of QRS Complex in Lead $V_1$.*** An important clue in the differential diagnosis of SVT with aberrancy from ventricular tachycardia is the shape of the QRS complex in lead $V_1$. In general, the presence of an RS wave, an R wave, or an RSr′ pattern in lead $V_1$ suggests VT; whereas an rSR′ pattern in lead $V_1$ favors SVT with aberrancy.

***AV Dissociation.*** The presence of AV dissociation (i.e., when atrial activity as reflected by the presence of P waves is independent of ventricular activity) strongly favors VT. In this circumstance, the ventricles are paced at a rapid rate by an ectopic site within the ventricles, while the atria continue to be paced independently by the SA node. P waves may be seen to occur at a slower rate than the rapid-rate QRS complexes. Some of the P waves may be "buried" in the QRS complexes and thus may be difficult to discern. In general, the presence of AV dissociation in a patient with wide complexes, occurring at a rapid rate, is highly suggestive of VT.

***Varying R-R Intervals.*** Another conduction abnormality that favors aberration is the presence of varying R-R intervals. Those rhythms disposed to supraventricular conduction are all subject to variation in the R-R interval. This occurs because the recovery time of the bundle branches is directly proportional to the R-R interval preceding each QRS complex. A short R-R interval is followed by a short refractory period; a long R-R interval is consistent with a longer refractory period. A premature, wide bizarre beat that follows a lengthening R-R interval within the basic rhythm should be carefully examined for other signs of supraventricular conduction.

***Deflection of Precordial (Chest) Leads ($V_1$ through $V_6$).*** An assessment of the precordial leads $V_1$ through $V_6$ may provide helpful clues in differentiating SVT with aberrancy from VT. If the QRS complexes in the chest leads are predominantly positive, the rhythm is most likely VT; when the precordial QRS complexes are predominantly negative, the rhythm is mostly likely supraventricular in origin.

Possible exceptions to this rule are patients with WPW *and* atrial fibrillation. In these patients the major pathway of conduction between atria and ventricles is an *accessory* one, that is, a pathway that bypasses the normal conduction system (see Fig. 40–48).

**Summary: Key Factors Differentiating SVT with Aberrancy from VT.** There are several features visible on the ECG that assist in differentiating SVT with aberrancy from VT. If a dysrhythmia begins with an ectopic premature P wave, it is either atrial or junctional in origin. If the dysrhythmia is initiated with a QRS complex that is followed by a retrograde P wave, it may be supraventricular (junctional) or ventricular in origin. If the time from the QRS to the retrograde P wave is 0.10 second or less, this favors aberration because the time period is too brief to be of ventricular origin.

Other differentiating factors include the rate of occurrence of the abnormal QRS complexes. If the rate of the wide QRS complex dysrhythmia is the same as the rate of the known supraventricular rhythm, this favors aberration. In the presence of AV dissociation, wherein the atrial rate is independent of the ventricular rhythm, VT is very likely the underlying rhythm. Occasionally, the SA nodal beat may transiently "capture" a ventricular beat, resulting in a QRS complex of normal duration; or a "fusion" beat may occur, in which case the resulting QRS complex is a hybrid of both the sinus and ventricular beat. This latter complex is often seen in VT.

**Clinical Significance.** The first question to be asked in the presence of any tachydysrhythmia is whether the rhythm is supraventricular or ventricular in origin. Should VT be diagnosed, an immediate assessment of the patient is essential to determine how the patient is tolerating the VT. The patient's mental status and vital signs should be assessed to determine the hemodynamic status. Complaints of chest pain or the presence of crackles on auscultation of the lung fields are significant findings requiring immediate emergent intervention.

In the case of SVT with aberrancy, treatment of the tachydysrhythmia will depend upon the clinical circumstance. SVTs associated with PAT, rapid-response atrial fibrillation, or atrial flutter may be treated with cardioversion and/or drug therapy. As is true of patients with VT, it is essential to assess the patient with tachydysrhythmia to determine how well the patient is tolerating it. Should the patient become hemodynamically unstable, or should angina or pulmonary edema be diagnosed, emergent treatment may be necessary.

An important question to be raised in a patient with a tachydysrhythmia is whether the patient is taking digitalis. PAT with block is a major dysrhythmia associated with digitalis toxicity, for which cardioversion is contraindicated. In patients with atrial fibrillation, it is helpful to ascertain whether the rhythm is chronic or acute. In general, chronic atrial fibrillation is not responsive to cardioversion. Conversion to normal sinus rhythm is usually short lived, with the rhythm usually reverting back to the underlying atrial fibrillation.

### *Electrolyte Disturbances and the ECG**

The 2 most important electrolytes concerned with proper function of the heart are potassium and calcium. They help to produce normal contraction of the cardiac muscle. They are also important in the propagation of the electrical impulse in the heart, and an excess or insufficient concentration of either electrolyte may cause changes in the ECG. Recognition of these ECG changes by the nurse may enable electrolyte abnormalities to be suspected before clinical symptoms appear or hazardous dysrhythmias occur.

**Hyperkalemia.** Normal serum potassium levels usually range between 3.5–5.5 mEq/liter. Hyperkalemia reflects a serum potassium level in excess of 5.5 mEq/liter. Hyperkalemia is most likely to occur because of oliguria, tissue injury, or an excessive intake. Under normal conditions, about 90%–95% of the potassium lost from the body is

*For an in-depth discussion of electrolyte balance, see Chapter 23.

excreted in the urine. Thus, renal failure with oliguria eventually will cause progressively rising serum potassium levels.

The main physiologic effects of hyperkalemia appear in muscle, particularly the myocardium. As potassium levels rise above 6.5–7.0 mEq/liter, an intracardiac block is produced, first in the atria, then in the AV node, and ultimately in the ventricles, where the heart finally stops in diastole. Muscle contractility is also weakened at higher potassium levels. The sensitivity of the heart to digitalis is *inversely* proportional to the amount of potassium present; thus, the effect of digitalis is reduced in patients with hyperkalemia. Hyperkalemia is diagnosed primarily by examining the serum electrolytes and ECG. The presence of a tall, tented, and symmetrical T wave is characteristically associated with hyperkalemia (Fig. 40–51; see also Fig. 23–2).

***Emergency Treatment of Hyperkalemia.*** Emergency treatment of hyperkalemia may involve the following treatment modalities:

1. Calcium chloride 10%—5–20 ml in 10–20 minutes. Calcium directly antagonizes the effect of hyperkalemia.
2. Sodium bicarbonate—1–2 ampules intravenously in 10–20 minutes. Sodium bicarbonate causes alkalosis that reduces serum potassium levels as potassium is driven into cells in exchange for hydrogen ions.
3. Glucose and insulin administration (50 ml 50% Glucose/water, or 250 ml 10% G/W with 5–10 units of insulin). As glucose enters the cells under the influence of insulin, the glucose "pulls" potassium into the cells, thereby reducing serum potassium levels.

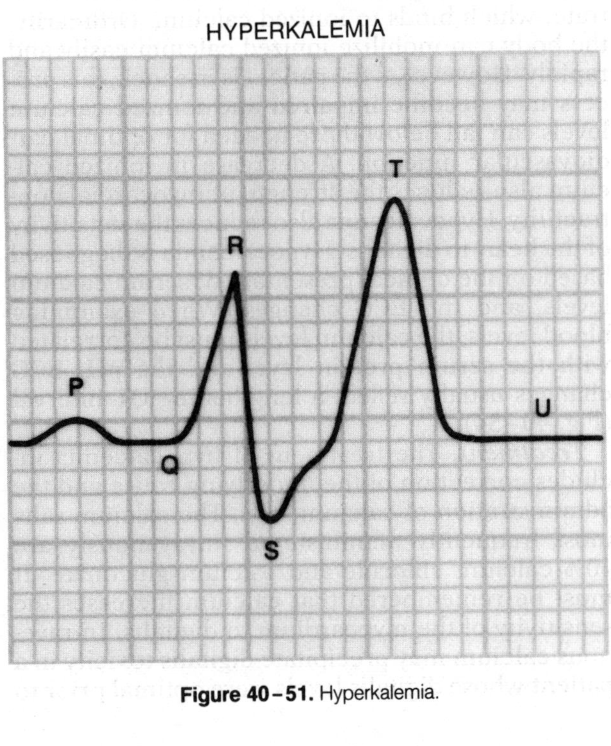


**Figure 40–51.** Hyperkalemia.

4. Cation exchange resins (sodium polystyrene sulfonate). When administered by mouth or retention enema, the resin helps to "pull" potassium out of the body by an ion-exchange mechanism.
5. Peritoneal dialysis or hemodialysis.

***Nonemergency Treatment of Hyperkalemia.*** With potassium levels less than 6.5 mEq/liter and no ECG changes evident, treatment may proceed somewhat more slowly. Whenever possible, all potassium-containing solutions should be discontinued or a sodium salt substituted. Diuresis may also be helpful.

**Hypokalemia.** Hypokalemia reflects a serum potassium level of less than 3.5 mEq/liter. Hypokalemia may be caused by alkalosis and/or by increased potassium losses from the body. A rise of 0.1 in pH generally causes a 0.5 mEq/liter fall in serum potassium levels.

Increased losses of potassium from the body can occur with excessive diuresis, severe diarrhea, severe trauma, or excessive steroid administration. Adrenocorticoid steroids tend to cause kidneys to excrete potassium and to retain sodium via the action of aldosterone on the cells of the distal tubules. During treatment of diabetic acidosis, hypokalemia can develop rapidly and can be severe. As the diabetic acidosis is corrected and the pH rises toward normal, the potassium level tends to fall. In addition, as insulin becomes effective, glucose enters the cells and takes potassium with it.

Hypokalemia may cause muscle weakness, metabolic alkalemia, and increased excretion of hydrogen ions in the urine. Hypokalemia increases the sensitivity of the heart to digitalis.

Hypokalemia is diagnosed primarily from the analysis of the serum electrolyte concentration and the ECG. It may be suspected in patients who are unusually weak, who have a severe ileus, or who have digitalis toxicity. The ECG tracing in hypokalemia is characterized by low-voltage QRS complexes, flattened T waves, depressed ST segment, prominent U waves, and prolonged QT intervals (Fig. 40–52; see also Fig. 23–2).

***Treatment.*** Acute, severe hypokalemia is usually treated by administering 10–20 mEq/liter of potassium chloride per hour by constant infusion. It generally takes 40–60 mEq/liter to raise the serum potassium level by 1.0 mEq/liter. In general, there should be no more than 40–80 mEq/liter of potassium in each liter of intravenous fluids, and no more than 40 mEq/liter should be given each hour.

**Hypercalcemia.** Calcium occurs in plasma in 3 forms:

1. Protein-bound, which accounts for 40%–50% of total calcium.
2. Ionized calcium, which accounts for 50%.
3. Complexed (i.e., non-protein-bound, nonionized calcium), which accounts for 5%–10%.

The ionized calcium fraction is the most important

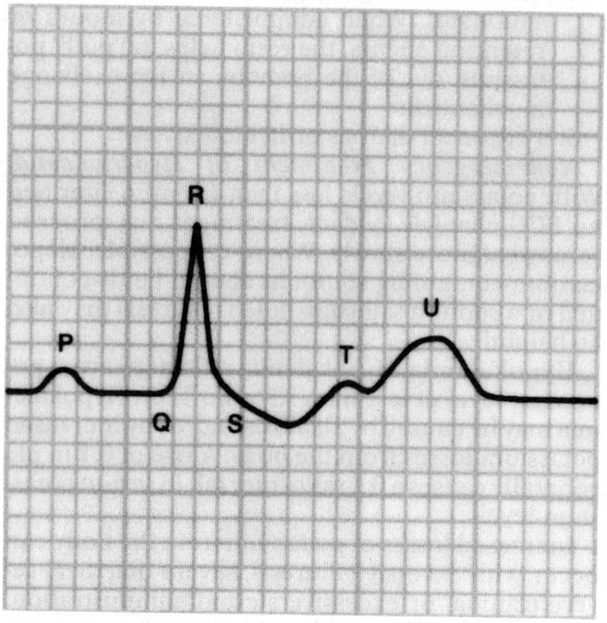


**Figure 40–52.** Hypokalemia.

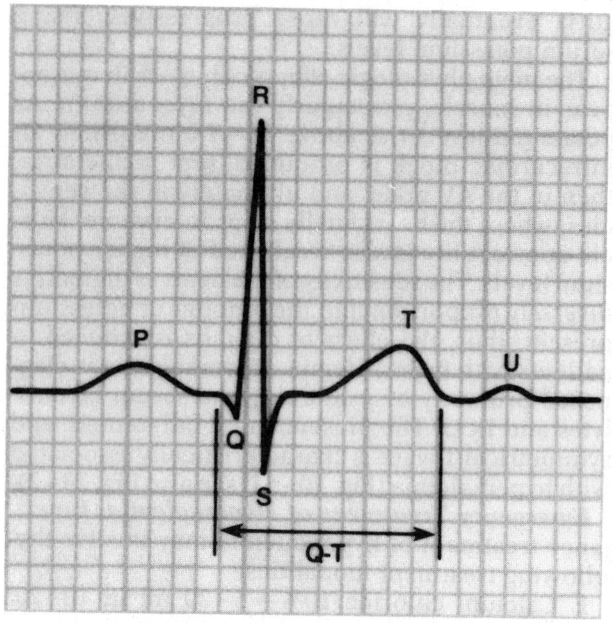


**Figure 40–53.** Hypercalcemia.

of these forms, because it is the cause of virtually all the physiologic effects of calcium. Total calcium in the blood is about 8.5–10.5 mg/100 ml.

The most frequent causes of hypercalcemia are metastatic bone disease, particularly in the presence of carcinoma of the breast, lung, or kidney; multiple myeloma and lymphomas; and immobilization. Additional etiologic factors underlying hypercalcemia are listed in Table 24–4.

Hypercalcemia is associated with weakness, lethargy, fatigue, confusion, and depression. Gastrointestinal symptoms include anorexia, nausea, and vomiting. Polyuria, tachycardia, and increased thirst may also be present. Hypercalcemia increases the sensitivity of the myocardium to digitalis and can precipitate digitalis toxicity. If calcium levels become very high (in excess of 11.0 mg/100 ml), the heart may stop in systole. Hypercalcemia is suspected on the basis of the patient's clinical presentation, and confirmed with serum calcium levels and ECG changes. ECG changes usually reflect a shortened QT interval (Fig. 40–53).

***Treatment.*** Treatment of severe symptomatic hypercalcemia includes the following:

1. Rapidly infusing intravenous fluids that lower serum levels by hemodilution and forced diuresis.
2. Reducing the ionized fraction by making the patient alkalotic.
3. Giving diuretics to increase renal excretion of calcium.
4. Dialysis.

**Hypocalcemia.** Hypocalcemia reflects a plasma level of less than 8.5 mg/100 ml. Hypocalcemia may be seen in hypoparathyroidism, osteomalacia, acute pancreatitis, renal insufficiency, vitamin D deficiency, and magnesium deficiency. Pancreatic lipase converts mesenteric and omental neutral fat into free fatty acids. The fatty acids and calcium combine to form calcium salts and soaps. Additional etiologic factors underlying hypocalcemia are listed in Table 24–4.

Decreased ionized calcium levels are seen most frequently in patients with alkalosis and in those who have had rapid, massive transfusion, particularly if shock is present. Banked blood contains citrate, which binds to ionized calcium. Ordinarily, the body can mobilize ionized calcium easily and rapidly. However, if the patient is in shock, this process may become impaired and ionized calcium levels can fall below those needed for optimal cardiovascular function. A decrease in ionized calcium also reduces the strength of myocardial contractility. Hypocalcemia also reduces the sensitivity of the heart to digitalis. Hypocalcemia is diagnosed based on the clinical presentation, serum calcium levels, and the ECG changes. When examining blood levels, the calcium levels must be correlated with the serum protein level and the pH. ECG changes usually reflect a lengthening QT interval (Fig. 40–54).

***Treatment.*** The treatment of hypocalcemia includes correction of the underlying cause and the administration of calcium salts. The calcium salts most frequently administered intravenously are 10% calcium chloride and calcium gluconate. It must be remembered that calcium increases the sensitivity of the myocardium to digitalis. Intravenous calcium may precipitate digitalis toxicity in a patient whose digitalis levels were optimal prior to

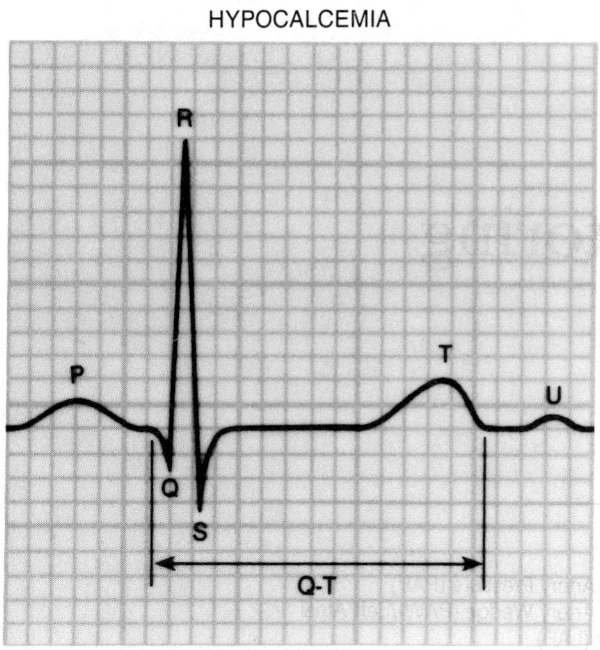


**Figure 40–54.** Hypocalcemia.

calcium therapy. Consequently, the rate of calcium infusion in these patients should not exceed 2 ml/minute.

## SUMMARY

Dysrhythmias are by far the most common complication encountered in the critical care setting. The presence of dysrhythmias largely becomes known through ongoing cardiac monitoring and by 12-lead electrocardiographic interpretation. To provide safe and effective care, it is essential for critical care nurses to be able to assess and interpret information reflective of the electrical events within the heart, and to relate this information to the heart's mechanical and hemodynamic performance.

In the discussion above, an attempt is made to examine the electrical events of the heart as reflected by the patient's bedside monitor. Components of the normal ECG configuration are reviewed, and pathogenic mechanisms underlying dysrhythmias are discussed. Major types of dysrhythmias and their defining characteristics, treatment, and implications for nursing care are presented.

It is important for the reader to appreciate that it is not possible in a work of this type to comprehensively cover electrocardiography. Rather, the intent here is to present a minimal but sufficient amount of basic information regarding cardiac monitoring that assists in the overall assessment of the patient's cardiovascular status. For an in-depth treatment of electrocardiography, the reader is referred to the following Suggested Readings list.

## SUGGESTED READINGS


Andreoli, K, Zipes, D, et al: Comprehensive Cardiac Care, ed 6. CV Mosby, St Louis, 1987.

Brown, K and Jacobsen, S: Mastering Dysrhythmias: A Problem-Solving Guide. FA Davis, Philadelphia, 1988.

Conover, M and Zalis, E: Understanding Electrocardiography, ed 5. CV Mosby, St Louis, 1988.

Goldman, M: Principles of Clinical Electrocardiography. Appleton & Lange, Los Altos, CA, 1986.

Goldberger, AL and Goldberger, E: Clinical Electrocardiography, A Simplified Approach, ed 3. CV Mosby, St Louis, 1986.

Marriott, H: Practical Electrocardiography, ed 8. Williams & Wilkins, Baltimore, 1988.

Marriott, H and Conover, M: Advanced Concepts in Arrhythmias, ed 2. CV Mosby, St Louis, 1989.

Sabetti, K: Distinguishing between ectopic ventricular activity and aberrant ventricular conduction of supraventricular impulses. Heart Lung 8(5):949–952, 1979.

Schamroth, L: An Introduction to Electrocardiography, ed 6. Blackwell Scientific Publications, St Louis, 1982.

CHAPTER 41

# Hemodynamic Monitoring

*Elaine Kiess Daily*

## CHAPTER OUTLINE



## LEARNING OBJECTIVES

**At the end of this chapter, you should be able to:**

1. State the purpose of hemodynamic monitoring.
2. Identify components of a hemodynamic monitoring system and their functions.
3. Review major nursing care considerations in the preparation, insertion, and implementation of hemodynamic monitoring.
4. Explain the physiologic significance of monitoring hemodynamic parameters.
5. Examine waveforms, normal values, clinical applications, and abnormalities with respect to the following hemodynamic pressures:
   a. Central venous pressure (CVP).
   b. Right atrial pressure (RAP).
   c. Right ventricular pressure (RVP).
   d. Pulmonary artery pressure (PAP).
   e. Pulmonary artery wedge pressure (PAWP).
   f. Systemic arterial pressure.
6. Consider major complications associated with hemodynamic monitoring techniques.
7. Investigate the physiologic significance of cardiac output in terms of cardiac performance and overall tissue perfusion, and methods of determining cardiac output.
8. Explain how continuous monitoring of the oxygen saturation of mixed venous blood ($SvO_2$) reflects the adequacy of tissue oxygenation.
9. List important hemodynamic parameters that can be derived or calculated using directly measured hemodynamic data.
10. Delineate the nursing process in the care of the patient undergoing hemodynamic monitoring, including:
    Assessment
    Diagnosis
    Planning: Desired patient outcomes
    Nursing interventions.

Invasive hemodynamic monitoring dates back to 1733 when Stephen Hales cannulated the carotid artery of a horse and measured how high the resulting column of blood rose in a brass pipe.[1]

Monitoring blood volume levels in war-injured patients by means of central venous pressure (CVP) was first described by Wilson and associates[2] in 1962. This method gained widespread popularity in the care and management of critically ill patients. In fact, for many years, hemodynamic monitoring of the critically ill consisted of continuous ECG monitoring, along with intermittent measurements of blood pressure via Korotkoff sounds and CVP.

Hemodynamic monitoring was revolutionized when Doctors Swan and Ganz developed the balloon-tip flotation pulmonary artery (PA) catheter in the late 1960s. This catheter permitted continuous direct measurement of right heart pressures in addition to indirect measurement of the filling pressures of the left side of the heart. Further development of the PA catheter provided the ability to measure cardiac output, perform atrial or ventricular pacing, and continuously measure the oxygen saturation of mixed venous blood ($SvO_2$).

The usefulness of hemodynamic monitoring in defining pathophysiologic conditions and managing the care of critically ill patients was described by Swan and co-workers in 1970.[3] Since then, bedside hemodynamic monitoring has become an integral part of the care and management of acutely ill patients. Hemodynamic parameters are used to assess the response of the cardiovascular system to injury and disease as well as to therapeutic interventions.

## PURPOSE

The function of the heart is to pump blood returning from the body to the lungs and into the aorta. This process delivers oxygenated blood and nutrients to the tissues and removes metabolic waste products. How well the heart performs its function is determined primarily by the heart rate, the ventricular end-diastolic volume (preload), the ventricular afterload, and ventricular contractility. The purpose of bedside hemodynamic monitoring is to survey and optimize these determinants by directing appropriate therapeutic interventions for the purpose of providing adequate oxygen delivery to tissues. This is achieved with the aid of data obtained from the balloon-flotation pulmonary artery (PA) catheter and the arterial catheter, which permits direct monitoring of arterial blood pressure. From these measured pressures various other hemodynamic parameters can be obtained and used to assess the response of the cardiovascular system to injury and disease as well as to therapeutic interventions.

Critical care nurses are responsible for obtaining accurate, valid hemodynamic data and, frequently, are responsible for decision-making regarding initiation or titration of certain pharmacologic agents or therapies used to manipulate hemodynamic parameters. This requires not only knowledge of cardiovascular physiology and pharmacology, but a clear understanding of the principles, equipment, and techniques of hemodynamic monitoring. These principles, as well as ways to optimize hemodynamic data collection, interpret hemodynamic waveforms, perform cardiac output measurements, and monitor mixed venous oxygen saturation ($SvO_2$), are discussed in this chapter.

## HEMODYNAMIC PRESSURE MONITORING PRINCIPLES AND TECHNIQUES

### Equipment

The measurement of any physiologic signal requires: (1) a catheter to relay the signal; (2) a transducer to transform the biophysical event into an electrical signal; (3) an amplifier to energize the transducer and amplify the electrical signal from the transducer; and (4) a monitor screen and/or paper recorder to display the resultant waveform.

#### *Catheters*

Transmission of a pressure signal from the patient to a transducer occurs through a fluid-filled catheter. If the catheter is insufficiently long to provide practical attachment to the external transducer, its length can be extended by the placement of additional fluid-filled tubing. It must be remembered, however, that the closer the transducer is to the physiologic signal, the more accurate the data obtained. Thus, all efforts should be directed toward minimizing all connections (tubing and stopcocks) between the catheter and the transducer.

Catheters used to measure pressures within the right side of the heart are usually multi-lumened, balloon-tipped, flow-directed catheters made of polyvinylchloride. Inflation of the balloon of the catheter with air allows the catheter to be carried through the heart by the forward flow of blood. Right heart catheters for bedside monitoring are available in sizes 5, 7, or 7.5 French with 2, 3, 4, or 5 separate lumens. One lumen provides access to the balloon for inflation or deflation. The balloon capacity varies with the size of the catheter, from 0.5–1.5 ml.

The 2-lumen catheter has a distal port for monitoring PA or PAW* pressures, as well as a lumen for balloon inflation. The 3-lumen catheter has an additional lumen whose port is located more proxi-

*PAW (pulmonary artery wedge) is synonymous with PCWP (pulmonary capillary wedge pressures) as used in this text.

mally, allowing monitoring of right atrial (RA) pressure. The 4-lumen catheter has all of these features plus a thermistor and computer connecting port for measurement of thermodilution cardiac output measurements. The 5-lumen PA catheter has a second proximal port, also terminating in the RA, for infusion of fluids or drugs without interruption during cardiac output measurements.

A recent technological addition to the conventional PA catheters involves fiberoptics for continuous monitoring of the oxygen saturation of mixed venous blood ($SvO_2$) when the catheter is attached to a bedside microprocessor.

While increases in the number of lumens within the PA catheter expand the functional capabilities of the catheter, they also decrease the accuracy of the transmitted pressure waveform and increase the risk of lumen occlusion.

Catheters used for percutaneous arterial cannulation are usually short Teflon catheter-over-needle type.

### *Transducers*

Intravascular or intracardiac pressure signals are transmitted via the fluid-filled catheter and tubing to a transducer that converts the mechanical signal to an electrical signal. Most external transducers are strain gauge transducers wired to form a Wheatstone bridge beneath the diaphragm. When pressure is applied to the diaphragm of the transducer, the wires of the bridge physically change in length and diameter, resulting in changes in the resistance to the flow of current through the wires.

Disposable pressure transducers consist of an etched silicone diaphragm with a single transverse voltage piezo resistor diffused into it. While these transducers work on the same general principle as the nondisposable transducers, their high-frequency response, ease of use, and reduced risk of infection have popularized their use.

Both disposable and nondisposable transducers are electrically energized and are therefore a potential source of current leakage. In addition, defibrillation may damage the diaphragm of these transducers, and therefore they should be changed following defibrillation.

### *Monitor*

Bedside monitoring systems consist of an amplifier (or preamplifier), an oscilloscope, and a digital display or paper recorder.

The purpose of the amplifier is to energize the transducer as well as to amplify, filter, and process the transduced electrical signal. Most transducers produce only about 6 mV when reproducing the systolic arterial pressure, whereas most monitors require a signal of several *volts* to operate. Therefore, an amplifier is necessary to boost the size of the electrical signal by approximately 1000.

The modified electrical output from the amplifier is intelligible only when it is converted into a readable form and displayed on an oscilloscope or paper recorder. Calibration of the light beam on the oscilloscope, or the ink pen on the paper recorder, allows accurate assessment of hemodynamic pressure values in relationship to the respiratory cycle.

Digital displays on monitors provide numerical values of pressure changes during specific times of the cardiac cycle. Selection of systolic, diastolic, or mean pressure values is available on most digital display devices. However, the numerical value displayed on the monitor represents an average of either a certain number of beats or a certain period of time, and therefore does not reflect the pressure value at a certain period of the respiratory cycle. For example, accurate measurement of hemodynamic pressures at end-expiration can only be obtained with the use of a calibrated oscilloscope (preferably with a freeze mechanism) or, more ideally, with a calibrated paper write-out.[4]

## Preparation

Table 41–1 lists the necessary equipment to be assembled for PA or arterial hemodynamic pressure monitoring.

Initiation of hemodynamic monitoring requires careful preparation and set-up of the previously discussed monitoring equipment. Failure to properly prepare the necessary equipment can result in erroneous data and improper patient care and management. Preassembled kits are now available, which contain all the necessary equipment for hemodynamic monitoring and therefore minimize the time required for gathering and assembling the equipment.

TABLE 41–1
**Equipment for Hemodynamic Monitoring**

| |
|---|
| Catheter of choice (balloon flotation PA cathter and/or 22-gauge arterial catheter) |
| Catheter/sheath introducer (for PA catheter) |
| Catheter sterility sleeve (for PA catheter) |
| Percutaneous or cutdown tray with necessary instruments |
| Sterile transducer (disposable or reusable) |
| Sterile transducer dome (if reusable transducer is used) |
| Heparinized IV solution in a collapsible bag |
| IV tubing with pediatric drip chamber |
| Continuous flush device |
| Three-way stopcocks |
| Pressure tubing |
| Pressurized cuff or pump |
| Electronic monitor with oscilloscope and paper recorder |
| Cardiopulmonary resuscitation equipment |

### Disposable Transducer and Flush Solution Assembly

1. Heparinize the IV solution in a collapsible bag by adding 1–2 units of heparin/ml IV fluid. Label the infusion bag with the date, time, and amount of heparin added. Premixed solutions are also available.
2. Remove all the air from the infusion bag.
3. Insert IV tubing into the bag, and squeeze the drip chamber to fill approximately ½ inch. Allow the distal tubing to fill with fluid.
4. Attach the preassembled flush device and disposable transducer to the IV tubing and completely fill with IV fluid by activating the fast-flush device. (This should not be done while the fluid is under pressure in order to prevent the development of air bubbles.)
5. If necessary, connect the pressure tubing to the stopcock attached to the transducer and fill with IV fluid.
6. Carefully check to make sure all air bubbles are removed from the tubing and transducer.
7. Replace all vented stopcock caps with nonvented dead-ender caps.
8. Place the IV bag into a pressure cuff and pressurize to 300 mmHg.
9. Attach the distal IV tubing to the hub of the catheter.
10. Connect the electrical cable of the disposable transducer to the amplifier of the monitor.

### Nondisposable Transducer Preparation

Reusable transducers are generally used with disposable domes, which have a thin flexible membrane separating the diaphragm of the transducer from the flush solution. Because infectious outbreaks have occurred with the use of disposable domes, sterilization of reusable transducers with gas (ethylene oxide) or chemicals (glutaraldehyde preparations) is recommended prior to each patient use.[5] The fluid used to interface between the dome and the diaphragm of the transducer should also be sterile and, preferably, without glucose.

### Monitor Preparation

Turn on the power on the monitor system, and allow the system to warmup for 15–20 minutes prior to use. Check the oscilloscope and/or paper recorder to ensure proper function.

### Transducer/Monitor Zero and Calibration

To eliminate the effects of atmospheric pressure as well as hydrostatic pressure differences, the monitoring system is "zeroed" to atmospheric air. This is done by positioning the air-reference stopcock at the patient's mid-chest level (Fig. 41–1) or phlebostatic axis (the presumed level of the catheter tip), opening the side arm of the stopcock to air and checking that the digital display on the monitor

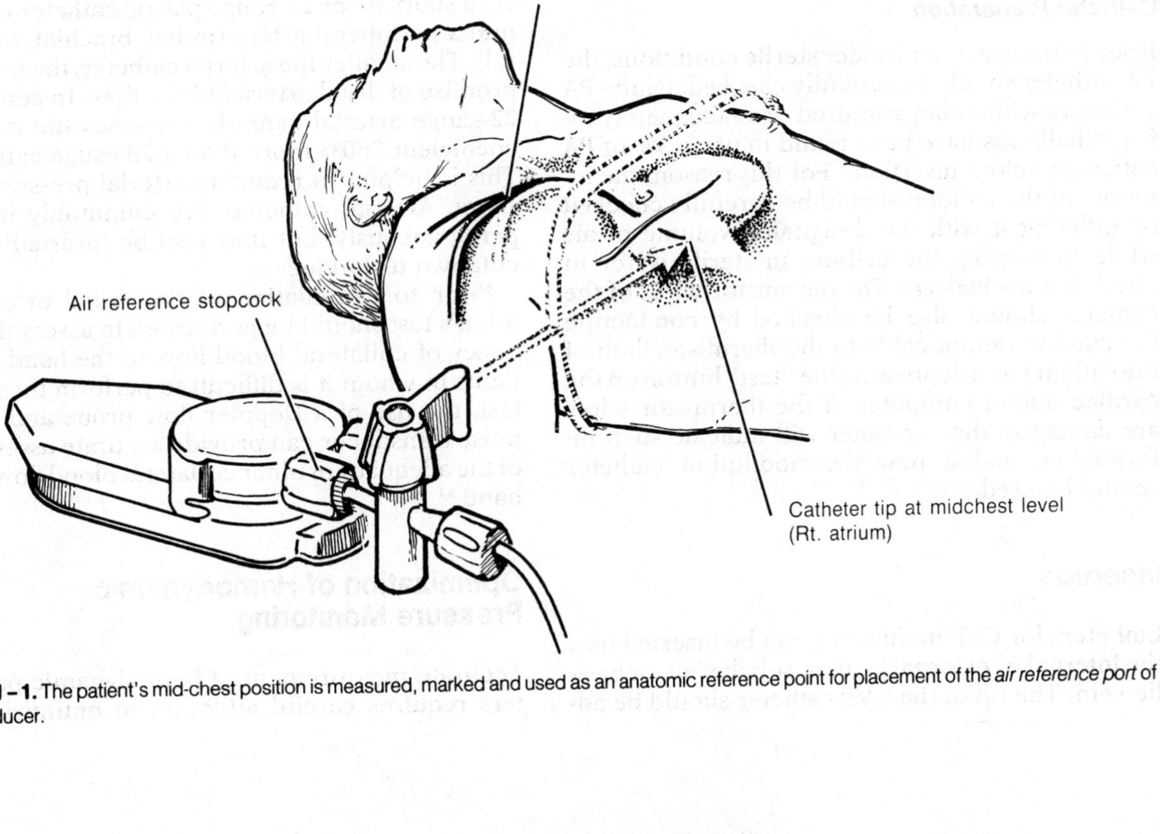


**Figure 41–1.** The patient's mid-chest position is measured, marked and used as an anatomic reference point for placement of the *air reference port* of the transducer.

reads "zero." If necessary, adjust the zero control knob on the monitor to obtain a zero reading. At the same time, adjust the tracing on the oscilloscope or paper recorder to the correct zero position.

The calibration of the monitor should also be checked by simply pressing and holding the calibration knob on the monitor to read the precalibrated value (e.g., 40, 100, or 200 mmHg). Adjust the calibration knob, if necessary, to obtain the correct reading. At the same time, adjust the light beam on the oscilloscope or paper recorder, if necessary.

When using a nondisposable transducer, it is necessary to also check its calibration and sensitivity by applying a known pressure (with either mercury or water) to the transducer and correlating it with the pressure read-out. Transducer calibration should be performed before patient use and whenever suspicion exists regarding the accuracy of the transducer. Special caution must be taken if the calibration check is performed after patient monitoring is instituted to avoid contamination and possible entry of air into the system. Disposable transducers are calibrated by the manufacturer, and since they are not reused, their calibration is usually not checked.

All transducers are sensitive to changes in environmental temperature, resulting in some drift of the zero baseline. For this reason, rezeroing should be performed before critical measurement readings are recorded, whenever there is a sudden change in a pressure reading, whenever there is a change in transducer reference placement, or at least every 4 hours. This is true for both disposable and reusable transducers.[6]

### *Catheter Preparation*

Prior to insertion, and under sterile conditions, the PA catheter should be carefully checked. Faulty PA catheters with either ruptured or inadequately inflated balloons have been found in up to 3% of PA catheters before insertion.[7] For this reason, the integrity of the balloon should be carefully checked by inflating it with the designated volume of air while immersing the balloon in sterile water to check for any leakage. The thermistor wires of the catheter should also be checked by connecting the cardiac output cable to the thermistor hub of the catheter and depressing the "test" button on the cardiac output computer. If the thermistor wires are damaged, the computer will indicate such information, and a new thermodilution catheter should be used.

## Insertion

Catheters for CVP monitoring can be inserted into the internal or external jugular, subclavian, or basilic vein. The tip of the CVP catheter should be advanced to the superior vena cava, just above the right atrium.

The PA catheter can be inserted into the same veins as the CVP. The femoral vein can also be used for PA catheterization, although traversal of the catheter out to the PA is more difficult via this route. The passage of the catheter through a sterile sleeve that covers the skin exit portion of the catheter is very useful should later manipulation of the catheter be required. If inserted under meticulous, aseptic technique, catheter sleeves can provide short-term sterility of the PA catheter for 1 – 2 days.[8] Although either catheter can be inserted via a surgical cutdown or percutaneously, the latter method is more common and is associated with fewer infectious complications.

During insertion and manipulation of the PA catheter, the nurse must carefully monitor the patient to determine the chamber location of the catheter according to the waveform and to note the possible occurrence of any dysrhythmias. The development of PVCs during manipulation of the catheter in the right ventricle (RV) is a common occurrence and usually resolves when the catheter is advanced out to the PA. Occasionally, sustained VT may develop, necessitating drug therapy or prompt cardioversion. Rarely, VF may occur, requiring immediate defibrillation. The development of ventricular dysrhythmias is more frequently associated with shock states, acute MI, hypokalemia, hypocalcemia, hypoxemia, acidosis, and prolonged catheter insertion times.[9] The nurse should be aware of this increased risk and prepared to act accordingly.

The arterial pressure can be measured directly via a short 20- or 22-gauge plastic catheter inserted into a peripheral artery (radial, brachial, or femoral). The smaller the arterial catheter, the less compromise of distal arterial blood flow. In addition, a 22-gauge arterial cannula increases the damping coefficient 260% more than a 20-gauge catheter.[10] This is helpful in reducing arterial pressure overshoot. Arterial catheters are commonly inserted percutaneously, but may also be inserted via the cutdown technique.

Prior to cannulation of the radial artery, the Allen's test should be performed to assess the adequacy of collateral blood flow to the hand. In patients in whom it is difficult to perform the Allen's test, the use of a Doppler flow probe and finger-pulse transducer can provide accurate assessment of the adequacy of ulnar collateral blood flow to the hand.[11]

## Optimization of Hemodynamic Pressure Monitoring

Accurate measurement of hemodynamic parameters requires careful attention to optimizing the fluid-filled monitoring system. Bedside monitoring systems are generally second-order, underdamped systems with numerous artifacts.[12] To faithfully reproduce the pressure signal, the system should be optimally damped and the natural resonant frequency of the plumbing system should be at least 10 times the fundamental frequency of the signal being measured.[13] This can be accomplished by:

1. Minimizing the distance between the transducer and the catheter.
2. Minimizing the number of stopcocks used.
3. Using very stiff, high-pressure tubing in the system.
4. Carefully removing all air bubbles from the system at the time of set-up and periodically during the monitoring period.
5. Continuously flushing the catheter to discourage formation of blood clots.

A low natural frequency of the plumbing system can result in either accentuation or attenuation (damping) of the pressure signal. The damping coefficient or dynamic response of the system can and should be checked at the bedside with the "snap-test," which provides a sudden increase and decrease in pressure. This is performed by quickly activating the fast-flush of the continuous flush device for approximately 1 second and then sharply releasing it.[14] With an optimally damped system, the produced square wave should show a sharp rise in pressure followed by a rapid decrease in pressure with a quick return to baseline (Fig. 41–2).

If optimal damping cannot be obtained by following steps 1 through 5 listed above, commercially available damping devices can be added to the system. However, they should be used with some caution and awareness of the fact that the pressure may become overly damped and thus underestimate the true pressure.

In addition to the plumbing and monitoring equipment, certain physiologic factors can affect the accuracy of hemodynamic data and require special consideration. One major factor affecting the recorded hemodynamic pressure is the intrapleural pressure surrounding the heart and great vessels. Measurement of all hemodynamic pressures at end-expiration, when there is no air flow and the intrapleural pressure is unchanging, minimizes the effect of changes in intrapleural pressure on recorded hemodynamic pressures.[15–17] However, determination of the point of end-expiration may, at times, be difficult. Use of a paper print-out with a marker indicating end-expiration is the most valid way to obtain these data.[4] The digital display value is inaccurate because most monitors simply average a certain number of beats, regardless of the respiratory phase, and thus should not be relied on. However, newer monitoring systems have addressed this issue and now include an algorithm to identify the end-expiratory pressure.[18] The onus of obtaining accurate hemodynamic data falls on the critical care nurse, who must make every effort to ensure that all hemodynamic parameters obtained are as accurate as possible.

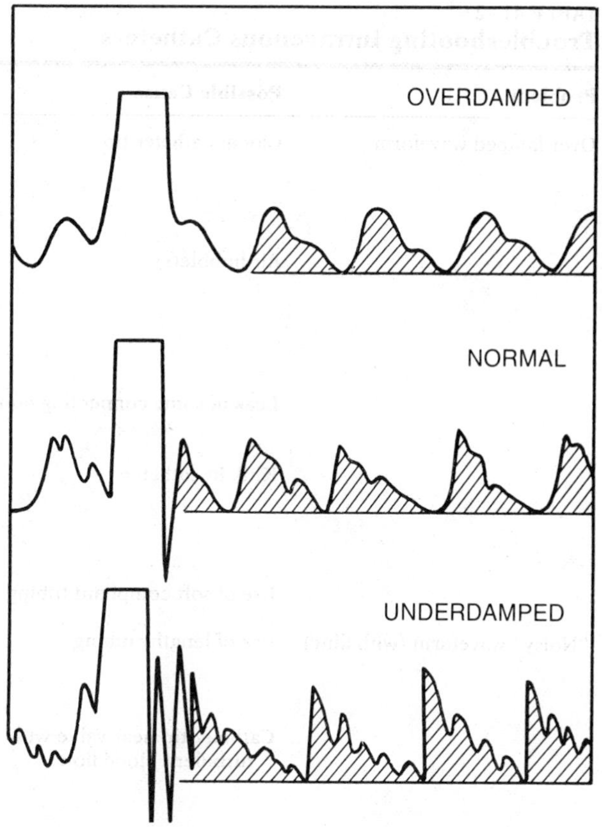


**Figure 41–2.** Square waves produced in response to a rapid change in pressure initiated by activating the fast flush device. (From Tilkian, A and Daily, EF: Cardiovascular Procedures. CV Mosby, St. Louis, 1986, p. 90, with permission.)

Table 41–2 lists problems commonly encountered in hemodynamic monitoring as well as preventive and remedial steps.

## HEMODYNAMIC PRESSURES

### Central Venous Pressure (CVP)

The CVP measures pressure within the superior vena cava (SVC), which represents pressure in the right atrium. Along with the mean arterial pressure, CVP is an important determinant of both venous return and cardiac output. Monitoring of the CVP is used to determine changes in right ventricular function and the adequacy of vascular volume. The CVP may be measured with a water manometer (in $cmH_2O$) or with an electronic transducer (in mmHg). To convert $cmH_2O$ to mmHg, simply divide the CVP value (in $cmH_2O$) by 1.36.

Since CVP represents pressure in the right

TABLE 41-2
**Troubleshooting Intravenous Catheters**

| Problem | Possible Cause | Prevention | Remedy |
| --- | --- | --- | --- |
| Overdamped waveform | Clot at catheter tip | Use continuous flush device.<br>Use heparinized IV solution.<br>Use heparinized catheters.<br>Hand flush occasionally. | Aspirate, then flush catheter with heparin solution (*not* when in PA wedge position).<br>Remove catheter if unable to clear. |
| | Air bubble(s) | Give care and attention to remove all air bubbles during equipment setup, particularly in the pressure transducer.<br>Use macrodrip vs. pedidrip. | Flush system carefully (*not* to patient). |
| | Leak at some connecting point | Use Luer-Lok connectors and stopcocks.<br>Tighten securely. | Check all connections and tighten if necessary. |
| | Kink in catheter | Loosely coil excess catheter.<br>Immobilize arm, if arm insertion.<br>Exercise caution during patient movement. | Try to straighten kink.<br>Replace catheter if necessary. |
| | Use of soft compliant tubing | Use stiff connecting tubing. | Replace soft tubing with stiff connecting tubing. |
| "Noisy" waveform (with fling) | Use of lengthy tubing | Use no more than 2 or 3 feet of connecting tubing (preferably 18 inches or less).<br>Use stiff connecting tubing. | Decrease tubing length.<br>Use stiff connecting tubing. |
| | Catheter tip near valve with turbulent blood flow | Position catheter distal to valve. | Check catheter position by radiograph, and reposition if necessary.<br>Use commercial damping device. |
| | Very rapid heart rate | | Slow heart rate, if possible. |
| Abnormally low or high pressures | Improper air-reference level | Place air-reference at mid-chest level (see Fig. 41-1) | Remeasure phlebostatic axis or mid-chest and reset air-reference level accordingly. |
| | Incorrect zero or calibration | Zero and calibrate monitor correctly. | Recheck zero and calibration of monitor. |
| | Faulty transducer | Calibrate transducer with known pressure; replace if necessary. | Recheck transducer calibration with mercury or water manometer. |
| "Overwedged" or damped, elevated PAWP | Overinflation of the balloon | Slowly inflate balloon while closely observing waveform; inflate *only* enough to obtain PAWP; use a 3-ml plastic syringe with holes punctured at 1.5 ml to avoid injecting >1.5 cc air. | Deflate balloon; reinflate slowly with only enough air to obtain PA wedge waveform. |
| | Eccentric inflation of the balloon | Check balloon inflation before insertion.<br>Do not inflate 7 French catheter with more than 1.0-1.5 cc air. | Deflate balloon; reposition catheter and slowly reinflate. |
| | Location of catheter tip in zone 1 or 2 of the lung (see Fig. 41-7) | Position catheter in zone 3 below the left atrium.<br>Maintain adequate LA pressure through volume administration.<br>Reduce airway pressure. | Obtain lateral chest film to confirm catheter tip location; if in zone 1 or 2, reposition in zone 3, administer volume, or reduce airway pressure. |
| PAWP with balloon deflated | Forward migration of catheter tip due to excessive looping in RV or RA; inadequate suturing of catheter at insertion site; or excessive arm movement of catheter in antecubital vein | Advance, catheter carefully, avoiding excessive catheter insertion.<br>Check catheter position on radiograph.<br>Suture catheter securely at insertion site.<br>Insert catheter in vein proximal to shoulder. | Slowly withdraw catheter until PA waveform appears.<br>Obtain chest radiograph to determine excessive looping of catheter in RV or RA. |

(continued)

TABLE 41-2
**Troubleshooting Intravenous Catheters *(Continued)***

| Problem | Possible Cause | Prevention | Remedy |
|---|---|---|---|
| PA balloon rupture | Overinflation of the balloon<br>Frequent balloon inflation<br>Active balloon deflation by withdrawing air into syringe | Inflate slowly with only enough air to obtain PAWP.<br>Monitor PAedp as reflection of PAWP and LVedp.<br>Allow balloon to deflate passively through stopcock.<br>Remove syringe after inflation. | Remove syringe and apply tape over stopcock to prevent further air injection.<br>Monitor PAedp. |
| Drastic change in pressure | Actual change in hemodynamic state | | Carefully assess patient. |
| | Air-reference or transducer level changed | Maintain air-reference at mid-chest level; re-zero before each reading. | Reposition air-reference mid-chest level; re-zero. |
| | Air or blood in transducer dome | Carefully remove all air bubbles during initial set-up; maintain adequate pressure (300 mmHg) in infusion bag. | Carefully flush system to remove all air or blood (*not* into patient). |
| | Change in temperature of environment or IV solution | Use room temperature flush solution. | Re-zero and calibrate. |
| | Broken transducer cable | Carefully handle transducer and cable | Check transducer with known pressure of mercury or water; replace if faulty. |
| No pressure | Power off | Check power. | Turn power on. |
| | Stopcock open to air | Always turn stopcock off to air after zeroing. | Turn stopcock off to air; open to catheter/transducer. |
| | Transducer dome loose | Carefully tighten dome during set-up and check periodically. | Tighten transducer dome. |
| | Tubing connections loose | Carefully tighten all connections during set-up and check periodically. | Tighten all connections. |
| | Loose cable connections between transducer/monitor/oscilloscope | Carefully and firmly insert all connecting jacks during initial set-up. | Check all connecting jacks. |
| | Transducer attached to wrong module or monitor | Provide careful and accurate transducer and monitor set-up. | Attach transducer to appropriate module. |
| | Gain setting too low | Correctly adjust gain setting of oscilloscope during initial monitor calibration. | Reset gain on the oscilloscope. |
| | Incorrect scale selection | Select appropriate scale to correspond to the monitored pressure. | Select appropriate scale. |
| | Faculty transducer | Check transducer with known pressure of mercury or water before patient use. | Check transducer with known pressure of mercury or water; if faulty, replace. |

(From Tilkian, AG and Daily, EK: Cardiovascular Procedures. CV Mosby, St Louis, 1986; with permission.)

atrium, the following discussion of the right atrial pressure (RAP) applies to the CVP.

## Right Atrial Pressure (RAP)

### *Waveform*

The typical RAP consists of 3 positive waves, an *a* wave, a *c* wave, and a *v* wave, followed by the *x*, $x^1$, and *y* descents, respectively (Fig. 41-3, *A*). The *a* wave is due to atrial contraction and therefore occurs just after the P wave of the ECG. (This wave is not present in patients with atrial fibrillation and absent P waves on the ECG.) The *c* wave occurs as a result of tricuspid valve closure. The *v* wave results from an increase in pressure due to an increase in volume as the atrium fills with blood from the SVC and inferior vena cava (IVC). The *v* wave occurs after the T wave of the ECG (see Fig. 41-5).

The *a* wave of the RAP waveform is often slightly higher (1-3 mmHg) than the *v* wave. However, because the *a* and *v* waves are similar in value, a mean or average pressure is usually recorded.

### *Normal Value*

The normal RA mean pressure is 0-6 mmHg.

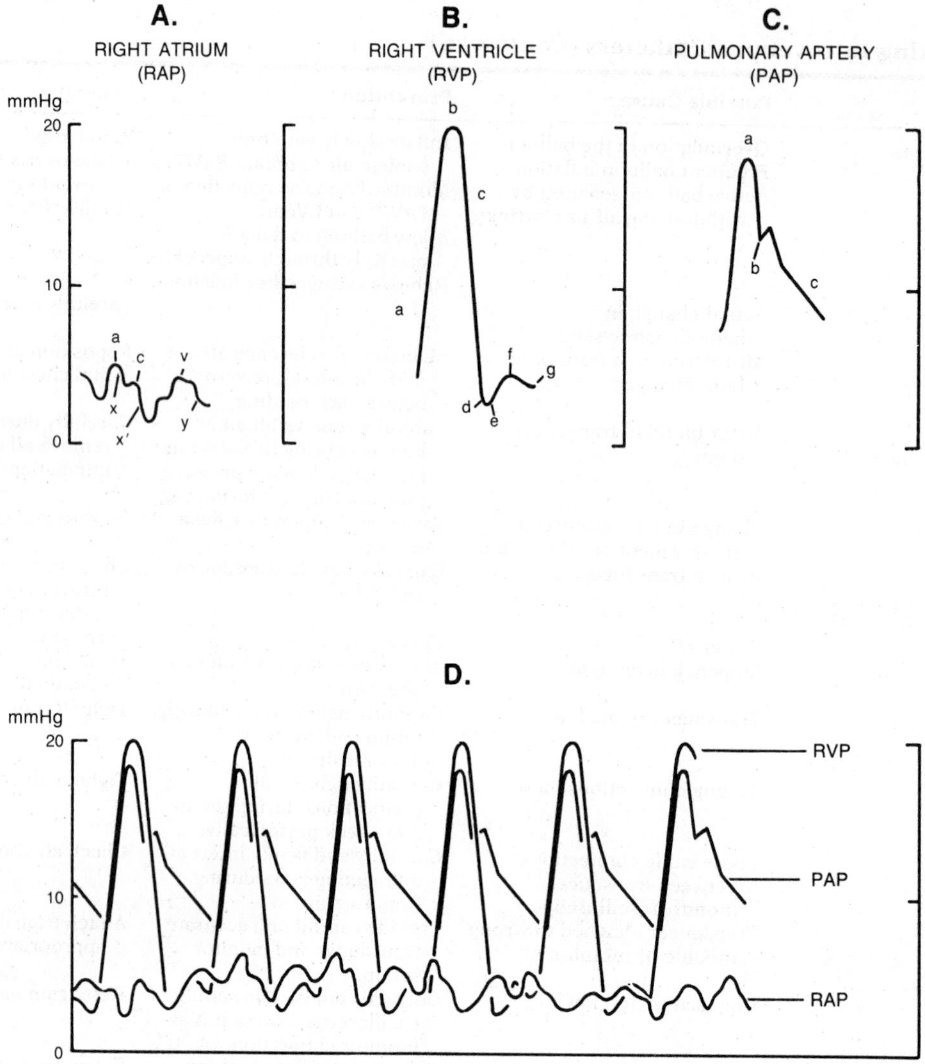


**Figure 41-3.** (*A*) Normal right atrial pressure (RAP) waveform showing an a wave, c wave and v wave, followed by the x, x' and y descents. For the relationship of the atrial waveform to ECG see Figure 41-5. (*B*) Normal right ventricular pressure (RVP) waveform showing: *a.* isovolumetric contraction, *b.* rapid ejection, *c.* reduced ejection, *d.* isovolumetric relaxation, *e.* early diastole, *f.* atrial systole (atrial kick), and *g.* end-diastole. (*C*) Normal pulmonary artery pressure (PAP) waveform showing *a.* systole, *b.* dicrotic notch, and *c.* end-diastole. (*D*) Shows all three pressures (RAP, RVP and PAP) superimposed on one another. All three pressures reflect low-pressure systems of right-heart and pulmonary circulation.

### Clinical Application

The CVP or RAP represents filling of the right side of the heart (preload). As an indicator of the patient's intravascular volume, the CVP or RAP is used as a guide to volume replacement. In addition, the response of the RAP to fluid challenges provides important information regarding the patient's volemic and cardiovascular status.

### Abnormalities

The *a* wave of the RAP may be exaggerated and elevated in any situations that increase resistance to forward blood flow. This includes RV failure, pulmonic stenosis, and pulmonary hypertension.

The *v* wave of the RA waveform becomes dominant and elevated in tricuspid regurgitation due to a reflux of blood backward into the atrium during RV systole. Functional tricuspid regurgitation commonly occurs in patients with RV failure and dilatation. Resolution of the failure is associated with reduction of the size of the *v* wave to more normal levels.

Elevation of both the *a* and *v* waves of the RA waveform occurs with hypervolemia, tamponade, and constrictive pericarditis.

## Right Ventricular Pressure (RVP)

When the catheter is carried across the tricuspid valve into the right ventricle (RV), the pressure suddenly becomes much higher with a sharp, pointed appearance as displayed on the monitor screen or recorder printout. Ventricular ectopy usually occurs transiently.

### *Waveform*

The RVP reflects the pulsatile, pumping nature of the ventricle with a rapid rise to systolic pressure and a drop to or near zero during diastole. The systolic and diastolic phases can be further delineated according to specific cardiac events (Fig. 41–3, *B*). The systolic events include isovolumetric contraction, rapid ejection, and reduced ejection. The diastolic events include isovolumetric relaxation, early diastole, atrial systole (atrial kick), and end-diastole.

### *Normal Values*

| | |
|---|---|
| RV systolic pressure | 20–30 mmHg |
| RV diastolic pressure | 0–5 mmHg |
| RV end-diastolic pressure | 2–6 mmHg |

### *Clinical Application*

Because of the risk of dysrhythmias the RVP is not directly monitored at the bedside. However, the RV systolic pressure is indirectly monitored via the PA systolic pressure, which should be the same as the peak RV systolic pressure in the absence of pulmonic stenosis. The RV diastolic, or filling, pressure is also indirectly monitored via the RAP or CVP, which should be the same as the RV diastolic pressure in the absence of tricuspid stenosis. Thus, both the systolic and diastolic functions of the RV are indirectly monitored at the bedside.

If an RV waveform becomes apparent on the monitor, the balloon of the flotation catheter should be inflated, allowing the catheter to float on out to the PA. It may not always float sufficiently far to obtain an acceptable PAW pressure, and thereafter the PA end-diastolic pressure must be used as a reflection of the LV filling pressure. If the catheter will not float out to the PA, despite balloon inflation, it may be coiled in the RV. In this instance, deflate the balloon and pull the catheter back into the RA. The catheter tip is never allowed to remain in the RV because of the risk of ventricular dysrhythmias.

### *Abnormalities*

The RV systolic pressure is elevated in pulmonary hypertension (either primary or secondary), as well as in ventricular septal defects (VSD) and in pulmonic stenosis. The RV diastolic pressure is elevated with RV failure, cardiac tamponade, or constrictive pericarditis.

## Pulmonary Artery Pressure (PAP)

Inflation of the balloon of the catheter allows it to float along with the flow of blood from the RV to the PA. This is evidenced on the oscilloscope as a sudden increase in the diastolic pressure, with little or no change in the systolic pressure level.

### *Waveform*

The pressure in the PA represents pulsatile blood flow through the pulmonary artery. Systole begins with the opening of the pulmonic valve and rapid ejection of blood into the PA. This is seen as a rapid rise in pressure followed by a gradual decline as the volume of ejected blood is reduced (Fig. 41–3, *C*). Diastole begins with the dicrotic notch, which occurs when the leaflets of the pulmonic valve snap shut. The further decline in diastolic pressure represents the runoff of blood into the pulmonary vasculature. The peak systolic pressure, the end-diastolic pressure, and the mean or average PA pressure are usually recorded.

### *Normal Values*

| | |
|---|---|
| PA systolic pressure | 20–30 mmHg |
| PA end-diastolic pressure | 8–12 mmHg |
| PA mean pressure | 10–20 mmHg |

### *Clinical Application*

As mentioned earlier, the PA systolic pressure reflects the RV peak systolic pressure (in the absence of pulmonic valve disease). Therefore, the PA systolic pressure reflects the *afterload* of the right side of the heart. At the very end of diastole, when the pulmonic valve is closed and the mitral valve is still open, the pressures in the LV, left atrium (LA), pulmonary veins, and PA essentially equilibrate. Therefore, in the absence of increased pulmonary vascular resistance (PVR) or mitral valve disease, the PA end-diastolic pressure (PAedp) reflects LV end-diastolic pressure (LVedp) (within 1–4 mmHg).[19] Because of this, many clinicians routinely monitor the PAedp rather than the pulmonary artery wedge pressure (PAWP) as a reflection of LV filling pressure, or preload.[20] In this way, the risks associated with inflation of the balloon of the catheter and cessation of blood flow to a segment of the PA are avoided. However, in patients with lung disease or increased pulmonary vascular resistance (PVR), the PAP will be elevated due to the increase in resistance to blood flow through the pulmonary system. The PAedp may also be higher than the

PAWP in patients with fast heart rates (>120 bpm) due to the decreased diastolic filling time.[20] Therefore, in these patients, it is necessary to obtain a PAWP as a reflection of LVedp.

The mean PAP is used to calculate PVR (the afterload of the right heart) according to the formula:

$$PVR = \frac{PAm - PAWm \times 80}{CO}$$

where
PVR = pulmonary vascular resistance
PAm = pulmonary artery mean pressure
PAWm = pulmonary artery wedge mean pressure
CO = cardiac output
80 = conversion factor from mmHg/minute/liter to dynes/sec/cm$^{-5}$

Many clinicians prefer to index both pulmonary and systemic vascular resistance to compare patients of varying body size (particularly pediatric patients).[21] This is done by simply dividing the PVR or SVR by the patient's body surface area (BSA).

### *Abnormalities*

The PA systolic pressure becomes elevated (pulmonary hypertension) with any increase in PVR, such as with pulmonary disease, pulmonary embolus, hypoxemia, or primary pulmonary hypertension. Mitral valve disease, as well as LV failure, increases pulmonary venous pressure, which, in turn, increases the PAedp.

## Pulmonary Artery Wedge (PAW)/Left Atrial Pressure (LAP)

### *Waveform*

The PAWP is obtained by inflating the balloon of the PA catheter sufficiently to occlude the branch of the PA in which the catheter tip lies. This blocks off any pressure effects from the right heart and allows the catheter tip, which extends beyond the inflated balloon, to sense only the retrograde pressure generated by the left atrium (LA) (Fig. 41–4). (The left atrial pressure [LAP] can also be measured directly in patients undergoing a thoracotomy with placement of a catheter in the LA appendage.) Therefore, the PAWP is an indirect LAP and is morphologically identical to the RAP consisting of an *a* wave, a *v* wave, and, occasionally, a *c* wave (Fig. 41–5). The *a* wave is produced by LA contraction and is followed by the *x* descent, representing atrial relaxation. The *c* wave that occurs as result of mitral valve closure may not always be evident on the PAW or LA waveform. The *v* wave is produced by filling of the LA from the pulmonary veins, and is followed by the *y* descent, which represents opening of the mitral valve and passive emptying of the LA.

As with the RA waveform, the *a* wave of the LAP or PAWP occurs after the P wave of the ECG, while the *v* wave follows repolarization, or the T wave of the ECG. However, because the PAW measures LAP in a retrograde manner, there may be a greater time delay between the electrical and associated mechanical event.

Alterations in the contour of the PAW or LA waveform may be related to changes in cardiac rhythm, as with the RAP waveform. The *a* wave is absent in

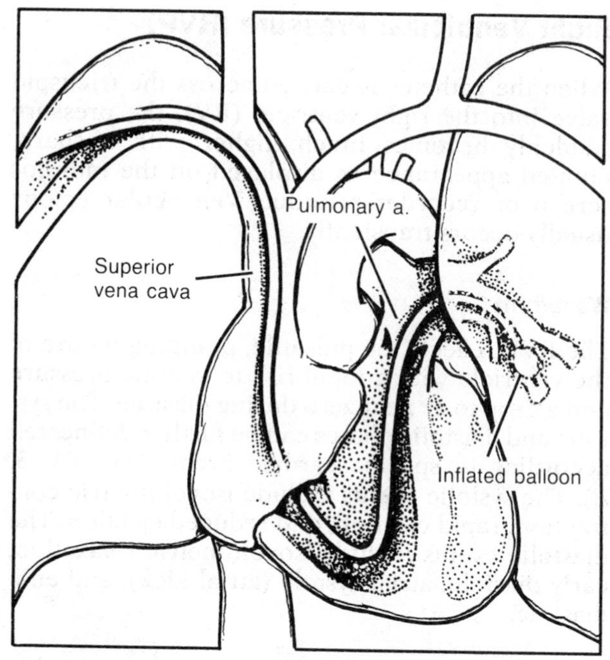


**Figure 41–4.** With the catheter tip in the pulmonary artery, and the balloon inflated to prevent forward flow, the tip of the catheter senses that pressure generated by the left atrium. In the absence of mitral valve disease, this pressure reflects the filling pressure of the left ventricle.

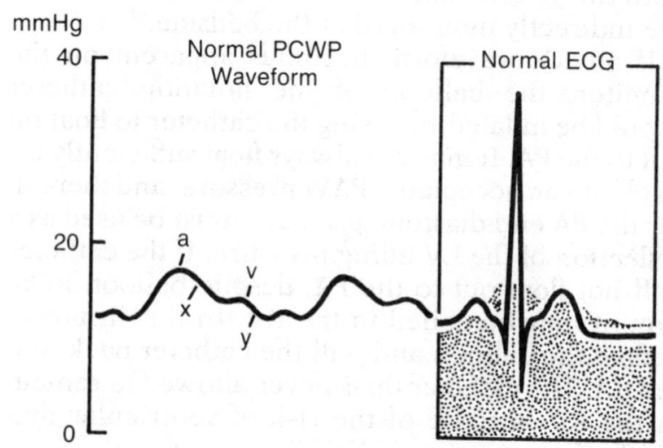


**Figure 41–5.** Normal pulmonary artery wedge pressure waveform showing an a wave and v wave, and the x and y descents. It is morphologically identical to the RAP (see Fig. 41–3(*A*)). The a wave is due to atrial contraction and therefore occurs just after the P wave on ECG. The v wave results from an increase in left atrial pressure due to an increase in volume as the atrium fills with blood from the pulmonary veins. The v wave occurs after the T wave on ECG.

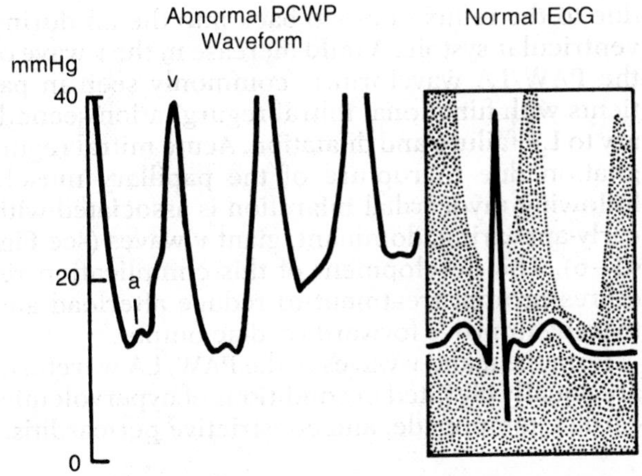


**Figure 41-6.** Pulmonary artery wedge pressure showing elevated and dominant v wave due to mitral regurgitation. The consequent increase in left atrial pressure is seen to occur after ventricular systole and following the QRS complex on ECG.

patients with atrial fibrillation and may be exaggerated (cannon *a* waves) with regularity or intermittently in patients with junctional rhythm or paroxysmal atrial tachycardia with block.

Normally, the *a* and *v* waves of the PAW/LA waveform are of approximately the same value (within a few mmHg), and therefore a mean or average of the 2 pressure rises is taken. If, however, the *v* wave is dominant and elevated, the *a* wave should be measured as a more accurate reflection of LVedp, because the mean will be falsely elevated due to the high *v* wave (Fig. 41-6).

### Normal Values

PAW/LA mean pressure 8-12 mmHg

### Clinical Application

LVedp has traditionally been held as the standard to define the pump function of the left ventricle.[22] In the absence of mitral valve disease, the mean LAP equals LVedp. Because the PAW is a retrograde measurement of the LAP, it indirectly reflects LV filling or LVedp (preload of the left heart). In most patients, the PAWP correlates closely with the LVedp over a fairly wide range of filling pressures (5-25 mmHg).[23] However, with LVedp >25 mmHg, the PAWP may underestimate the true LV filling pressure. In contrast, elevations in the LAP or PAWP overestimate the true LVedp in patients with mitral stenosis or LA myxoma. Decreases in the compliance of the LV alter the relationship between pressure and volume, which also produces an elevated PAWP that does not reflect the volume filling the LV during diastole.[24]

The PAWP also indicates the pressure within the pulmonary capillaries, which is responsible for movement or transfer of fluid between the vessels and the interstitial or intra-alveolar spaces. PAW mean pressures of 20-30 mmHg are usually associated with clinical manifestations of pulmonary congestion due to fluid in the interstitial or intra-alveolar spaces.

Accurate indirect measurement of LAP via the wedged catheter (PAW) relies on an open continuum between the catheter tip and the LA. This may not be the case when airway pressure is increased (PEEP, CPAP), the tip of the catheter lies in zone 2 or 3 of the lung field, and the LAP is low (Fig. 41-7).[25-28] In this situation, the airway pressure can be greater than the pulmonary venous pressure, resulting in collapse of the microvasculature. The recorded PAWP will be inaccurately elevated (perhaps even higher than the PAP) and will lack the normal contour and characteristics of a PAWP. Placement of the catheter tip below the level of the LA permits the hydrostatic pressure to maintain the vasculature open and a true PAWP can be obtained. Confirmation of the position of the catheter relative to the LA is made via a lateral chest film. However, suspicion regarding the possibility of location of the catheter tip in zone 1 or 2 should occur when:

- The PAWP value exceeds the PAedp.
- The PAWP lacks all characteristics of a PAW waveform.
- The value of the PAWP is similar to the level of the PEEP.

Some ways to alter the situation and thereby obtain an accurate PAWP include:

- Turn the patient onto the side in which the catheter tip lies.
- Decrease airway pressure by reducing the level of PEEP.
- Increase the LAP via volume administration.
- Reposition the catheter.
- Use the PAedp as a reflection of LVedp.

Fortunately, because PA catheters are flow-directed, they are most frequently carried out to a zone 3 position, where lung perfusion is the greatest.[29]

In patients with cardiac dysfunction, the PAWP is usually optimized between 14 and 18 mmHg to obtain the best cardiac output, according to Starling's law. However, the limits to which the PAWP can be raised are dictated by the oncotic pressure. Elevations of the PAWP to levels that cause pulmonary edema, and therefore hypoxemia, can decrease oxygen delivery to the tissues, despite apparent increases in cardiac output.

### Abnormalities

The *a* wave of the PAW/LA waveform becomes dominant and elevated in conditions that increase resistance to ventricular filling, such as mitral stenosis or LV failure.

The *v* wave of the PAW/LA waveform becomes exaggerated and elevated with mitral regurgitation

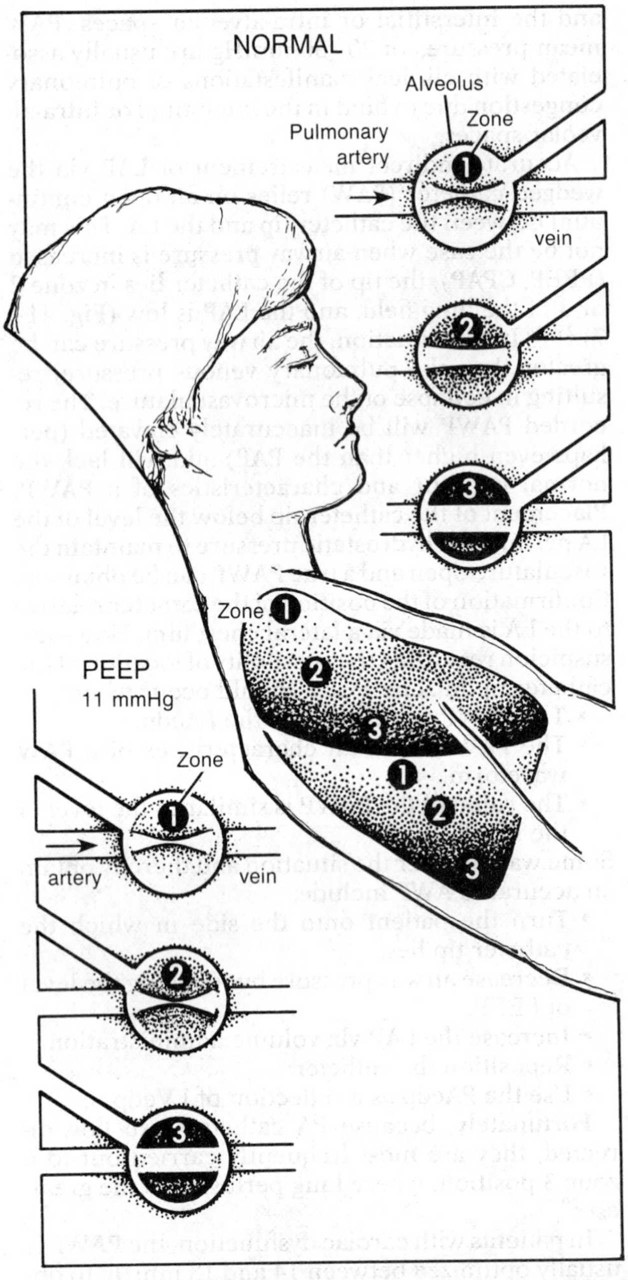


**Figure 41-7.** Schematic illustration of pressure/flow relationships in zones 1, 2, and 3 of the pulmonary circulation under conditions of normal spontaneous breathing and with positive end-expiratory pressure (PEEP). Zone 1 reflects the physiologic areas of the lung (upper one-third) in which alveolar pressure is greater than perfusion pressure and flow is minimal under both normal and PEEP conditions. Balloon inflation in this zone would reflect only alveolar pressures. In zone 2, under normal conditions pulmonary artery pressure is slightly greater than alveolar pressures and flow is increased. However, balloon inflation in this zone interrupting flow is likely to collapse the capillary and the PAWP recorded here would also reflect alveolar pressures. Under conditions of PEEP the capillary is collapsed by the higher alveolar pressures and only the alveolar pressures would be reflected on balloon inflation. In zone 3, perfusion pressure exceeds alveolar pressure under both normal and PEEP conditions. Balloon inflation in zone 3 most accurately reflects the pulmonary artery pressure and thus, left atrial pressures. Note the effect of positioning on pressure/flow relationships in the various areas of the lungs. (Adapted from Daily, EK and Schroeder, JS: Techniques in Bedside Hemodynamic Monitoring. CV Mosby, St. Louis, 1985.)

due to the reflux of blood back into the LA during ventricular systole. A mild increase in the *v* wave of the PAW/LA waveform is commonly seen in patients with functional mitral regurgitation secondary to LV failure and dilatation. Acute mitral regurgitation due to rupture of the papillary muscle following myocardial infarction is associated with early-appearing, dominant, giant *v* waves (see Fig. 41-6). The development of this complication requires prompt treatment to reduce afterload and thereby improve forward cardiac output.

Both the *a* and *v* waves of the PAW/LA waveform are equally elevated in conditions of hypervolemia, cardiac tamponade, and constrictive pericarditis.

## Systemic Arterial Pressure

Continuous direct monitoring of arterial pressure is frequently performed in critically ill patients for prompt detection of changes in cardiovascular function and for assessment of arterial blood gases.

### *Waveform*

Direct measurement of the arterial blood pressure is commonly obtained from a cannula placed in a peripheral artery. The systemic arterial waveform resembles the PA waveform in contour, with a pressure value approximately 6 times greater than that of the PA. Systole begins with the opening of the aortic valve and rapid ejection of blood into the aorta, producing a sharp upstroke on the waveform (Fig. 41-8; see also Fig. 38-1). Diastole begins with the closure of the aortic valve, which is evidenced on the downslope of the peripheral arterial waveform by the dicrotic notch. (In the aortic root pressure, systole and diastole are separated by the incisura, which becomes the dicrotic notch in the

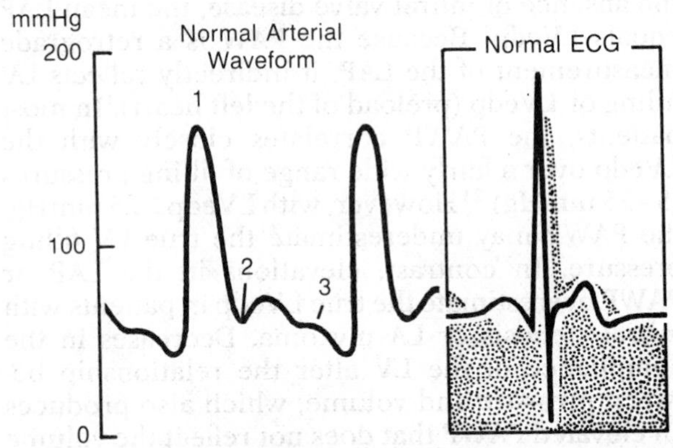


**Figure 41-8.** Normal arterial pressure waveform showing (*1*) systole; (*2*) dicrotic notch; and (*3*) end-diastole. The arterial waveform occurs immediately following the QRS on ECG as the mechanical event of contraction follows the electrical depolarization of the ventricles.

peripheral arteries.[30]) The decline in pressure following the dicrotic notch represents runoff of blood into the arterial circulation. The peak systolic, diastolic, and mean values of the arterial waveform are recorded (see Fig. 37–22).

Because of wave reflection and the tapering diameter of peripheral arteries, the more distal from the aorta the arterial cannula is located, the higher the systolic pressure (by as much as 15–30 mmHg) and the lower the diastolic pressure. The mean pressure, however, remains the same[31] (see Fig. 38–3). Additionally, the more distal the location of the arterial catheter, the sharper the upstroke, the narrower the waveform, and the less defined the dicrotic notch, which virtually disappears into the diastolic pressure in the femoral artery waveform.[32] These changes in systolic pressure may account for some of the disparity encountered between cuff blood pressure measured at the brachial artery and direct arterial pressure measured at the radial or femoral artery.[32]

### Normal Values

| | |
|---|---|
| Arterial systolic pressure | 100–140 mmHg |
| Arterial diastolic pressure | 60–80 mmHg |
| Arterial mean pressure | 70–90 mmHg |

### Clinical Application

In the absence of aortic stenosis, the arterial systolic pressure reflects the peak pressure generated by the LV. It also reflects the compliance of the large arteries, the total peripheral resistance. In general, the systolic pressure is a clinical indication of the amount of work the LV generates during systole. The upstroke of the aortic root arterial waveform is often used as an indication of the inotropic state of the ventricle.

The arterial diastolic pressure represents the runoff of blood into the arterial system, and is determined by the velocity of runoff as well as by the elasticity of the arterial system, particularly the arterioles (see Figs. 37–19 and 37–21). The level to which the arterial diastolic pressure falls is also affected by the patient's heart rate, which determines the duration of diastole. The slower the heart rate, the longer the diastolic period, and the greater the fall in the diastolic pressure.

The *mean* arterial pressure refers to the average pressure in the arterial system during systole and diastole. This pressure can be mathematically calculated (Table 41–3) or, more commonly, is electronically integrated via the bedside monitor, which displays a numerical mean. The mean arterial pressure reflects the driving or perfusion pressure and is determined by the volume of blood flow in the arterial system (cardiac output) and the elasticity or resistance of the vessels (SVR). This can be mathematically expressed as:

$$MAP = SVR \times CO$$

TABLE 41–3
**Calculated Hemodynamic Parameters**

| Parameter | Formula | Normal Values |
|---|---|---|
| Arteriovenous oxygen difference ($a\text{-}vDO_2$) | Arterial $O_2$ content − venous $O_2$ content | 3.5–5.5 vol% |
| Cardiac output (CO) | Heart rate × stroke volume | 4–8 liters/minute |
| Cardiac index (CI) | $\frac{\text{Cardiac output}}{\text{BSA}}$ | 2.5–4 liters/minute |
| Coronary artery perfusion pressure (CAPP) | MAP − LVedp (or PAWm) | 60–80 mmHg |
| Left ventricular stroke work index (LVSWI) | SI × (MAP − PAWm) × 0.0136 | 30–50 g/beat/$m^2$ |
| Mean arterial pressure (MAP) | $\frac{\text{Systolic Blood Pressure} + (\text{diastolic pressure} \times 2)}{3}$ | 70–90 mmHg |
| Oxygen content of blood | % Saturation × hemoglobin × 1.34 | 17.5–20.5 vol% (arterial)<br>12.5–16.5 vol% (venous) |
| Oxygen consumption ($VO_2$) | CO × hemoglobin × 1.34 × (arterial $O_2$ saturation − venous $O_2$ saturation) × 10 | 200–250 ml/minute |
| Oxygen delivery ($DO_2$) | CO × arterial $O_2$ content | 900–1100 ml/minute |
| Right ventricular stroke work index (RVSWI) | SI × (PAm − RAm) × 0.0136 | 5–10 g/beat/$m^2$ |
| Stroke index (SI) | $\frac{\text{Stroke volume}}{\text{BSA}}$ | 40–50 ml/beat/$m^2$ |
| Stroke volume (SV) | $\frac{\text{CO}}{\text{Heart rate}}$ | 70–130 ml/beat |

where
MAP = mean arterial pressure
SVR = systemic vascular resistance
CO = cardiac output

SVR is primarily determined by the change in radius of the major resistance vessels (the arterioles), although other factors such as blood viscosity and vessel length also affect it. SVR cannot be directly measured, but can be calculated by rearranging the previous formula:

$$SVR = \frac{MAP}{CO} \times 80$$

More accurate calculation of systemic vascular resistance includes dividing the pressure difference between the proximal and distal ends of the circulatory system (i.e., arterial and venous) by the CO. This is expressed by the following formula:

$$SVR = \frac{MAP - RA\ mean}{CO} \times 80$$

However, since the RA mean pressure is usually quite low compared to the MAP, it can be eliminated from the calculation of SVR. If, however, the RA mean is significantly elevated, it should be subtracted from the MAP when calculating SVR. SVR is a clinical reflection of the *afterload* of the left side of the heart, that is, the resistance to left ventricular ejection. Afterload levels are manipulated with the use of vasoconstricting or vasodilating agents and therapies.

The mean arterial blood pressure determines tissue perfusion. While some organs can partially autoregulate the amount of blood flow, the myocardium of the LV, which receives most of its blood flow during diastole, requires an arterial driving pressure of 60–80 mmHg to maintain perfusion of the coronary arteries. When the MAP falls, coronary blood flow decreases. When the MAP falls to 40 mmHg or less, coronary blood flow virtually ceases, and the coronary arteries collapse.[33] Therefore, in patients with coronary artery disease, every effort is made to maintain coronary perfusion pressure at 60–80 mmHg.

The *pulse* pressure refers to the difference between peak systolic and end-diastolic pressures of the arterial pressure. The pulse pressure is primarily determined by the volume of blood ejected with each heart beat (stroke volume) and the elasticity or compliance of the arterial system. Increases in the arterial pulse pressure occur with increases in the stroke volume, while narrow pulse pressures are usually associated with a decreased stroke volume.

### *Abnormalities*

The arterial blood pressure is elevated in the following pathologic conditions:

1. Systemic hypertension.
2. Arteriosclerosis.
3. Renal failure.
4. Aortic regurgitation.

The presence of aortic regurgitation is classically associated with a wide pulse pressure (due to a large stroke volume) and an absent dicrotic notch in the arterial waveform (Fig. 41–9).

The arterial blood pressure is reduced in the following conditions:

1. Low cardiac output (from any cause).
2. Aortic stenosis.
3. Dysrhythmias.
4. Vasodilator therapy.

It is important to remember that initially the blood pressure is maintained at normal, or near normal, levels in the presence of hypoperfusion due to the sympathetic nervous system response. Eventually, however, the blood pressure will fall in low cardiac output states.

In aortic stenosis, the arterial pressure waveform exhibits a low pressure with a slow upstroke, poorly defined dicrotic notch, and narrow pulse pressure. Its appearance closely resembles a very damped arterial pressure waveform (Fig. 41–10).

Vasodilator therapy reduces the resistance to ejection of blood, producing a rapid upstroke of the arterial systolic pressure, a rapid decline in pressure during the shortened ejection phase, and a smaller change in the pressure during diastole (Fig. 41–11).

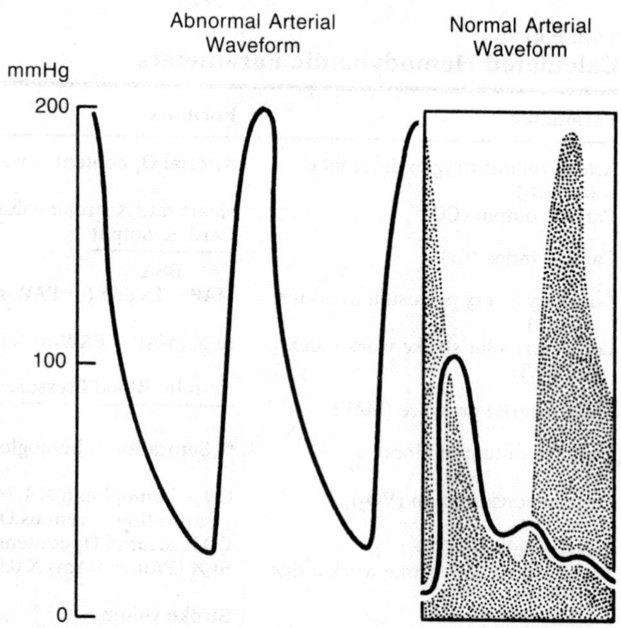


**Figure 41–9.** Arterial pressure tracing in a patient with aortic regurgitation. Note the wide pulse pressure with elevated systolic pressure of 200 mmHg and low diastolic pressure of 50 mmHg. Note the comparison of this pressure waveform with the normal arterial waveform and pressure range.

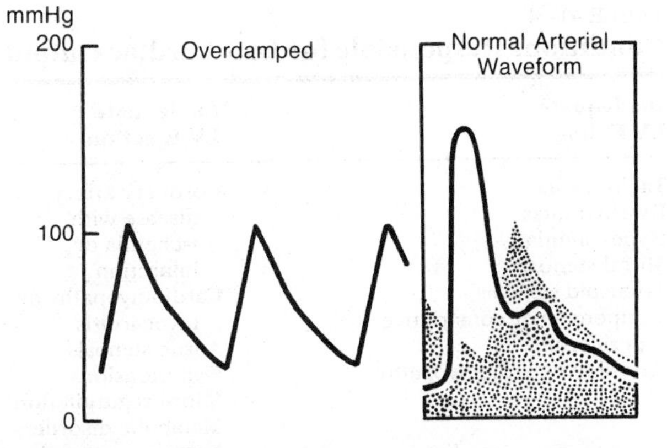


**Figure 41-10.** Overdamped arterial pressure waveform with poor upstroke and loss of dicrotic notch. Compare this pressure waveform with the normal arterial pressure waveform. (Adapted from Daily, EK and Schroeder, JS: Techniques in Bedside Hemodynamic Monitoring. CV Mosby, St. Louis, 1985.)

Regular, alternating changes in the value of the arterial systolic pressure may be seen in patients with severe LV failure. This condition, termed *pulsus alternans*, likely represents a regular alternating change in the inotropic state of the ventricle. Pulsus alternans can be felt at the radial artery as a regular pattern of strong, weak, strong, weak pulsations (see Fig. 38-2).

## DERIVED HEMODYNAMIC PARAMETERS

From directly measured hemodynamic data, other important hemodynamic parameters can be derived or calculated. Table 41-3 lists the formulas

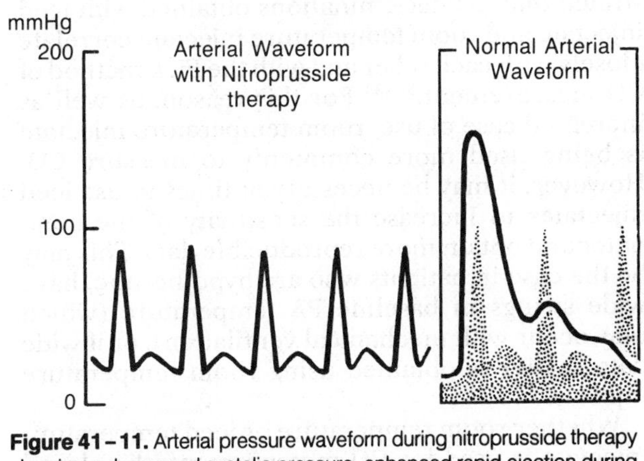


**Figure 41-11.** Arterial pressure waveform during nitroprusside therapy showing a decreased systolic pressure, enhanced rapid ejection during systole, and rapid runoff during diastole. Note comparison of this pressure waveform to normal arterial pressure waveform. (Adapted from Daily, EK and Schroeder, JS: Hemodynamic Waveforms: Exercises in Identification and Analysis. CV Mosby, St. Louis, 1983.)

for obtaining certain hemodynamic parameters, as well as the normal values for those parameters.

## CARDIAC OUTPUT DETERMINATION

### Principle

Cardiac output (CO) refers to the rate at which blood is ejected by the heart and is expressed in liters/minute. Since blood is ejected with each heart beat, the CO is a product of the stroke volume (SV) times the heart rate (CO = SV × HR). Although minor discrepancies may occur, the RV and the LV pump the same volume of blood, unless an intracardiac shunt exists. Thus, measurements of blood flow from one ventricle can be assumed to be the same for the other ventricle.

Cardiac output measurements can be made by (1) the Fick method; (2) the indicator-dilution (dye) method; and (3) the thermodilution method. The thermodilution method correlates closely with both the Fick and the dye-dilution methods of determining CO, except in the presence of intracardiac shunts or tricuspid regurgitation. Because of this, and because of the technical ease with which it can be performed, the thermodilution method is the technique most commonly used at the bedside to measure CO. Discussion here will be limited to this method.

#### *Normal Values*

Normal resting CO is 4-8 liters/minute. This wide range reflects the variations that can occur from person to person as a result of body size. A more specific measurement is the cardiac index (CI), which individualizes the flow rate by taking into account the patient's body size. The patient's body size or surface area (BSA) can be obtained from Dubois' height-weight formula (available as a nomogram), and dividing this into the CO value to obtain the CI (CI = CO ÷ BSA). A normal resting CI is 2.6-4 liters/minute/$m^2$. This is true for both adults and children over 10 years of age. Because of their increased metabolic and heart rates, children under 10 years of age normally have about a 25% greater CI, that is, 3.4-5 liters/minute/$m^2$.[34]

#### *Clinical Application*

Tissue function and viability depend on an adequate supply of oxygen and nutrients from the circulating blood. This supply is dependent on the flow rate (CO) and local tissue perfusion. Measurement of CO provides essential information regarding overall cardiac performance in providing adequate perfusion of the tissues.

CO measurement is a reflection of the systolic performance of the ventricle. According to the

Starling principle, the systolic performance is determined by the diastolic function (preload). The Frank-Starling law states that the greater the fiber length or stretch during diastole (preload), the greater the fiber shortening and ejection during systole, within physiologic limits. This relationship between the diastolic and systolic function of the ventricle can be graphically plotted to form a ventricular function curve (see Fig. 37–17). The LV diastolic measurement of performance (on the horizontal axis) could include LVedp, LAm, PAWm, or PAedp. The systolic measurement of performance (on the vertical axis) could include the CO, CI, SV, stroke volume index (SVI), left ventricular stroke work (LVSW), or left ventricular stroke work index (LVSWI). Although flow rates (CO, CI, SV, or SVI) are more commonly used to plot ventricular function curves at the bedside, LVSW or LVSWI provide a more accurate assessment of changes in cardiac performance irrespective of changes in afterload.[21]

Normally, the ventricular function curve shows a linear increase in systolic performance as preload increases, up to a certain level (see Fig. 37–17). After this level is reached, further increases in preload no longer improve systolic performance. The entire ventricular function curve may be shifted upward and to the left due to increased ventricular contractility, or downward and to the right due to depressed ventricular function and contractility.

Individual ventricular function curves should be plotted for each patient by the critical care nurse in order to determine the *optimum* preload (i.e., that filling pressure which produces the maximum cardiac output) for that particular patient. Adjustment of preload levels can be obtained with administration of volume, diuretics,or nitrate preparations.

Alterations in afterload or the resistance to ejection of blood from the aorta also affect the cardiac output (CO). Conditions that produce vasoconstriction increase the resistance and thus decrease CO. On the other hand, vasodilatation reduces resistance and increases SV or CO. This is the underlying principle of afterload-reducing therapy with arterial vasodilators or counterpulsation.

Since $CO = SV \times HR$, changes in heart rate also affect CO. CO values are greater with faster heart rates, although SV may remain unchanged. However, at very fast heart rates, the decreased duration of diastole prevents adequate filling, and thus stroke volume falls. Slower heart rates will usually improve the stroke volume as well as reduce myocardial oxygen demands.

Low CO values can be due to inadequate ventricular filling or inadequate ventricular ejection, or both. Table 41–4 lists some of the pathologic conditions responsible for low CO.

High CO values at rest can be seen in hyperdynamic states (postoperatively or with increased thyroid function) or with severe vasodilatory states associated with sepsis or anaphylaxis.

TABLE 41–4
**Conditions Responsible for Low Cardiac Output**

| Inadequate LV Filling | Inadequate LV Ejection |
|---|---|
| Tachycardia | Coronary artery disease with ischemia or infarction |
| Dysrhythmias | Cardiomyopathy or myocarditis |
| Hypovolemia | Aortic stenosis |
| Mitral stenosis | Hypertension |
| Tricuspid stenosis | Mitral regurgitation |
| Tamponade or constrictive pericarditis | Metabolic disorders |
| Restrictive cardiomyopathy | Negative inotropic agents |

## Techniques of Thermodilution Cardiac Output Measurement

The thermodilution CO method was first described by Fegler in 1954.[35] This method applies the indicator-dilution method using a solution of exact known temperature as the indicator. The change in blood temperature produced downstream (from the RA to the PA) is recorded by a thermistor near the catheter tip. The change in temperature over time is inversely proportional to blood flow. A special CO computer analyzes the resultant temperature/time curve and applies appropriate constants to calculate the rate of blood flow through the heart.

Since the indicator used in the thermodilution method consists of a known temperature, it is important that the injectate be quite different from the temperature in the PA (at least 12° or more). Initially, chilled injectates with temperatures close to zero were used in order to maximize the difference and thus increase the physiologic noise/signal ratio. However, numerous studies have demonstrated that CO determinations obtained with iced injectate and room temperature injectate correlate closely with each other and with the Fick method of CO measurement.[36–38] For this reason, as well as increased ease of use, room temperature injectate is being used more commonly to measure CO. However, it may be necessary at times to use iced injectates to increase the sensitivity of the computer and obtain more reproducible data. This may be the case in patients who are hypothermic, have wide swings in baseline PA temperature (which may occur with mechanical ventilation), or if wide data scatter is obtained using room temperature injectate.

Whether room temperature or iced temperature injectate is used for CO measurement, the closed system of delivery is recommended to reduce thermal loss and to reduce the risk of contamination or infection.

All CO curves should be recorded on a paper write-out and inspected for accuracy. The upstroke of the CO curve reflects the injection technique and should be smooth and even (Fig. 41–12). Bumps or steps on the upstroke indicate an uneven injection, and the value of such a CO curve should be discarded. The downslope determines the area under the curve, which is inversely proportional to the CO. If the downstroke is rapid (see Fig. 41–12), the area under the curve is small, indicating a high CO. With a low CO, the downslope is very slow and gradual, resulting in an increased area under the curve. If the numerical value displayed by the cardiac output computer does not agree with the displayed CO curve, troubleshooting of the cardiac output computer and equipment should be performed. Table 41–5 lists troubleshooting techniques for various problems encountered with thermodilution CO measurements.

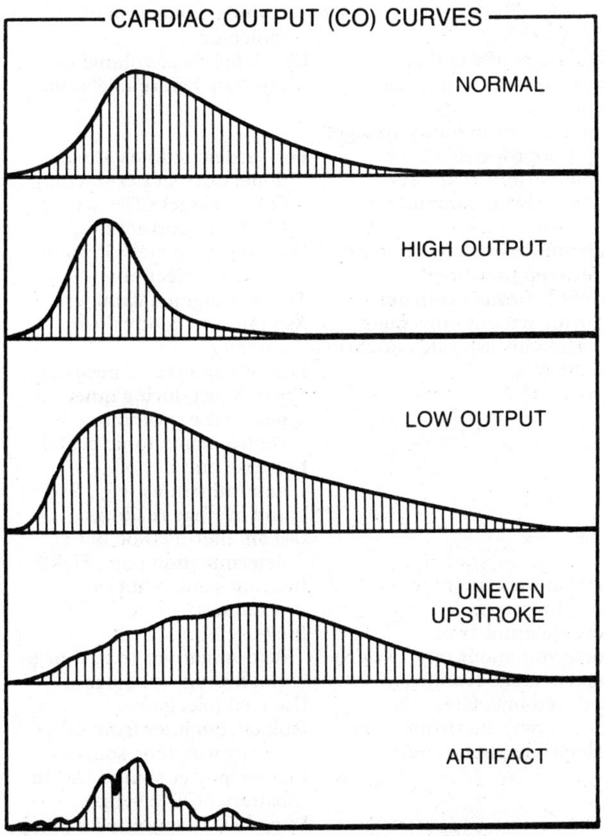


**Figure 41–12.** Schematic representation of various thermodilution cardiac output curves. (*A*) normal cardiac output curve showing a smooth upstroke, (*B*) small area beneath the curve as seen in patients with high cardiac outputs, (*C*) large area beneath the curve as seen in patients with low cardiac outputs, (*D*) uneven injection indicated by uneven upstroke on curve, and (*E*) artifact in both upstroke and decline of curve resulting in erroneous cardiac output measurement. (From Tilkian, A and Daily, EK: Cardiovascular Procedures. CV Mosby, St. Louis, 1986, with permission.)

### Equipment

Equipment needed for thermodilution CO determinations using room temperature injectate consists of:

- Thermodilution PA catheter.
- Sterile IV solution (saline or $D_5W$) in a collapsible bag.
- IV tubing.
- 10-ml syringes.
- Cardiac output computer with connecting cable and temperature probe.

### Preparation

1. Assemble the injectate solution using a closed system. (Follow manufacturer's directions.)
2. Connect the injectate solution tubing to the proximal lumen port of the thermodilution PA catheter via a 3-way stopcock.
3. Attach the in-line temperature probe and a 10-ml syringe to the side port of the stopcock at the proximal lumen port.
4. Connect the thermistor connector hub of the PA catheter to the cardiac output computer via the appropriate connecting cable.
5. Prepare the cardiac output computer (including entry of the correct constant) according to the manufacturer's directions.

### Technique

1. Close the stopcock to the proximal lumen of the catheter and carefully fill the syringe with *exactly* 10 ml from the IV solution bag. (Slow filling of the syringe minimizes the occurrence of any air bubbles, which must be purged before injection.)
2. Activate the CO computer, and wait for a READY signal.
3. Start the paper recorder.
4. Check the PA waveform from the distal lumen of the catheter to verify the PA position.
5. Turn the stopcock closed to the IV solution, press the START button on the CO computer, and immediately inject the contents of the syringe into the proximal lumen. The injection must be done rapidly (within less than 4 seconds) and smoothly. The CO reading should be displayed in approximately 10–30 seconds.
6. Check the paper write-out of the curve to verify a fast, even injection evidenced by a smooth and rapid upstroke (see Fig. 41–12).

Usually at least 3 successive cardiac output measurements are taken and averaged to obtain a mean value. However, if considerable variation among the readings is present, it may be necessary to average 5 or 6 cardiac output measurements. With the use of 10 ml of iced injectate, the first in a series of 3 sequential thermodilution CO measurements was found to be significantly higher than the following 2

TABLE 41–5
## Cardic Output Troubleshooting

| Problem | Cause(s) | Prevention | Remedy |
|---|---|---|---|
| Cardiac output (CO) reading higher than expected | Inaccurate injectate volume caused by air bubbles or loss of injectate | Carefully check for bubbles and expel, if any. | Check for *exact* volume of injectate before injection. |
| | Wrong computation constant (CC) | Check appropriate CC on catheter insert and set correctly on computer. | For cardiac outputs already done: Correct CO = wrong CO × correct CC ÷ wrong CC. Enter correct CC. |
| | Warming of iced injectate in syringe before injection | If syringe method is used, handle syringe only briefly and hold only plunger and syringe flanges during injection. | Perform outputs rapidly with minimal handling of syringe. Use CO-SET with in-line temperature probe. |
| | Migration of catheter tip toward PA wedge | Ascertain catheter tip position with radiograph. Closely monitor PA pressure. | Withdraw catheter a few centimeters. |
| | Thermistor against wall of artery | | Withdraw catheter a few centimeters. |
| | Uneven injection | Use 2 hands to deliver fast, even bolus. Use automatic injector. | Use automatic injector. Analyze curve on strip-chart recorder. |
| | Right-to-left shunt | None. | Use another method of cardiac output determination (such as Fick). |
| | Low stroke volume with long lag time before onset of curve | None. | Press START button *after* complete injection of indicator. |
| Cardiac output reading lower than expected | Inaccurate injectate volume (more than indicated) | Use syringe of size that corresponds to injectate volume. Exercise care in filling syringe. | Check for *exact* volume of injectate before injection. |
| | Wrong computation constant (CC) | Check appropriate CC on catheter insert and set correctly on computer. | For cardiac outputs already done: Correct CO = wrong CO × correct CC ÷ wrong CC. Enter correct CC. |
| | Iced injections spaced <1 minute apart | Wait approximately 1 minute between injections. | Wait approximately 1 minute between injections. |
| | Catheter kinked or partially obstructed by clot | Carefully protect catheter during patient movement. Occasionally aspirate and flush manually. | Try to straighten catheter. Aspirate and gently flush catheter. Remove catheter if necessary. |
| Scattered CO readings (poor reproducibility) | Cardiac dysrhythmias (ventricular ectopic beats, atrial fibrillation, etc.) | None. | Try to inject during quiet period (i.e., without ventricular ectopic beats). Increase number of determinations (e.g., 5 or 6) and average readings. |
| | Tricuspid regurgitation | None. | Use another method of CO determination (e.g., Fick). |
| | Wide swings in intrapleural pressure (spontaneous respiration or mechanical ventilation) | Inject at same point in respiratory cycle. Increase number of determinations (e.g., 5 or 6) and average readings. Used iced injectate. | Inject at same point in respiratory cycle. Increase number of determinations (e.g., 5 or 6) and average readings. Use iced injectate. |
| | Electromagnetic interference | Isolate computer from other electromagnetic sources. | Isolate computer from other electromagnetic sources. Change power source (AC to battery or vice versa). Wipe CO computer with damp cloth. |
| | Migration of catheter tip toward PAW or thermistor against artery wall | Ascertain catheter tip location with radiograph. Closely monitor PAP. | Withdraw catheter several centimeters to position in main PA. |
| | Catheter looped in RV | Advance catheter carefully, avoiding excessive catheter insertion. Confirm catheter position with radiograph. | Withdraw and reposition catheter. |

(From Tilkian, AG and Daily, EK: Cardiovascular Procedures. CV Mosby, St Louis, 1985, with permission.)

values.[39] This situation, which is frequently observed in the clinical setting, is often handled by eliminating the results of the first CO determination and averaging the values of 3 more successive CO determinations. However, this may not be appropriate when fluid restriction is a concern.

Consistently injecting the solution at a specific point in the patient's respiratory cycle may improve reproducibility of data.[36] However, such data may be erroneously skewed and not reflect the patient's true cardiovascular status.

## CONTINUOUS $SvO_2$ MONITORING

The recent addition of fiberoptic technology to the balloon-flotation PA catheter permits continuous monitoring of the oxygen saturation of mixed venous (PA) blood. While hemodynamic parameters provide essential information regarding cardiac performance and, in part, oxygen delivery, monitoring the $SvO_2$ provides information regarding the adequacy of tissue oxygenation.

### Principle

Oxygen is taken up in the lungs and delivered to the tissues by the hemoglobin molecules in blood. Each hemoglobin molecule can carry approximately 1.34 ml of oxygen. The rate of oxygen delivery depends on the flow rate, or CO. Thus, the formula for calculation of oxygen delivery is:

$$\text{Oxygen delivery} = \text{CO} \times \text{hemoglobin} \times 1.34 \times \text{arterial oxygen saturation} \times 10$$

Normally, the hemoglobin becomes fully saturated with oxygen, resulting in an arterial saturation of 95%–99%. Therefore, in a patient with a normal CO of 5 liters/minute, a hemoglobin of 15 g/dl, and an arterial saturation of 97%, the oxygen delivery would be:

$$975 \text{ ml } O_2 \text{ delivery} = 5 \text{ liters/minute} \times 15 \text{ g/100 ml} \times 1.34 \times .97 \times 10$$

This represents a normal delivery of oxygen to the tissues and is a commonly used index of the performance of the cardiopulmonary system. However, it does not indicate the adequacy of oxygen delivery in relation to tissue oxygen needs. While low oxygen delivery values are usually associated with tissue hypoxia, normal or even high oxygen delivery values can also be present with tissue hypoxia.[40]

Previously, intermittent mixed venous oxygen saturation samples were obtained to assess the adequacy of tissue oxygenation. When oxygen consumption is constant and arterial oxygen saturation is maintained, $SvO_2$ varies directly with CO.

### Normal Values

Mixed venous blood in the PA is normally from 65%–77% saturated with oxygen. Venous blood obtained from other sites (RA, RV, peripheral vein) has not adequately mixed and cannot be used as a reflection of overall tissue oxygenation.

### Clinical Applications

As mentioned previously, $SvO_2$ reflects the balance between oxygen supply and demand. Alterations in oxygen supply can be caused by changes in CO, hemoglobin, or arterial oxygen saturation. Anemia or hypoxemia will reduce $SvO_2$ unless the CO can increase sufficiently to maintain the balance between supply and demand. A reduction in hemoglobin, unless as a result of massive hemorrhage, usually occurs slowly and is less commonly responsible for sudden decreases in $SvO_2$. Hypoxemia can be evaluated by arterial blood gas determination. However, in most clinical situations in which the patient is receiving oxygen therapy or mechanical ventilation, the arterial saturation rarely changes more than 10%.[31]

Low CO, therefore, is the most common cause of inadequate tissue oxygenation, as reflected by an $SvO_2$ of less than 60%.[41] Sustained reductions in $SvO_2$ of 10% or greater over 3–5 minutes should prompt an immediate assessment of the patient's cardiovascular status, including cardiac output measurement.[42,43] In this way, CO determinations are performed when hemodynamically indicated, rather than at some pre-set, routine, or arbitrary time.

Increases in the tissues' demand for oxygen may also result in low $SvO_2$ readings, despite normal oxygen delivery values. Increases in oxygen consumption may occur with increases in the patient's metabolic rate, temperature, pain, and so forth. However, this is usually quite evident clinically, and if no apparent increase in oxygen consumption is observed, the components of oxygen supply (CO, hemoglobin, arterial saturation) should be assessed.

Rises in $SvO_2$ readings to levels above normal (80%–95%) may be due to distal wedging of the PA catheter in which postcapillary arterialized blood is monitored. This is evidenced by a change in the light intensity on the strip recorder, as well as by the appearance of a PAW waveform from the distal lumen of the catheter. Slight withdrawal of the catheter tip back into the PA corrects such a situation. High $SvO_2$ values (>77%) may also occur in those situations in which tissue oxygen demands are reduced, such as marked hypothermia, induced muscular paralysis, or anesthesia. However, an elevated $SvO_2$ reading is usually seen in the presence of sepsis; in fact, a rising $SvO_2$ may be the first indication of a septic condition.[41] Table 41–6 lists pathologic conditions associated with alterations in $SvO_2$.

TABLE 41-6
## Various Causes of Alterations in $SvO_2$

| | $SvO_2$ Reading | Physiologic Alteration | Clinical Causes |
|---|---|---|---|
| High | 80%–95% | ↓$O_2$ consumption | Hypothermia<br>Anesthesia<br>Induced muscular paralysis<br>Sepsis |
| | | ↑$O_2$ delivery | Hyperoxia |
| | | Mechanical interference | Wedged catheter<br>Left-to-right shunt |
| Normal | 60%–80% | $O_2$ supply = $O_2$ demand | Adequate perfusion |
| Low | <60% | ↑$O_2$ consumption | Shivering<br>Pain<br>Seizures<br>Activity/exercise<br>Hyperthermia<br>Anxiety |
| | | ↓$O_2$ delivery | Hypoperfusion (↓cardiac output)<br>Anemia<br>Hypoxemia |

(From Tilkian, AG and Daily, EK: Cardiovascular Procedures. CV Mosby, St Louis, 1986, with permission.)

In summary, a normal $SvO_2$ of 65%–77% represents adequate tissue perfusion and oxygenation, while $SvO_2$ readings less than 60% or decreases in $SvO_2$ of 10% or more usually indicate a compromise in at least one of the determinants of oxygen delivery (CO, hemoglobin, or arterial saturation). Since hypoperfusion is the most common cause of decreases in $SvO_2$ in the critical care setting, a CO measurement should be immediately performed to determine and appropriately treat the cause of the reduced oxygen delivery. If the CO is within normal limits, an arterial blood sample should be drawn for blood gases and hemoglobin level. Brief, minor changes in $SvO_2$ readings may be caused by some type of interference. These nonsustained changes are clinically insignificant and likely do not represent changes in CO. Figure 41-13 shows an example of a print-out obtained with continuous $SvO_2$ monitoring.

### *Technique*

The $SvO_2$ catheter is a modified 7.5 or 8 French PA thermodilution catheter that additionally contains optic fibers that transmit and receive light reflected from the bloodstream. The light signal is converted to an electrical signal and transmitted to a remote data processor that displays the signal on a slow-speed paper recorder or a liquid crystal display (LCD) screen. A digital value is also continuously displayed and updated every 1–2 seconds.

Calibration of the light signal should be performed prior to catheter insertion according to each manufacturer's directions. After catheter insertion, calibration of the oximeter with a blood sample of a known saturation (determined by the blood gas laboratory) should be performed daily and whenever there are any doubts regarding the displayed $SvO_2$ reading. Calibration with a known saturation should be performed at a time when the patient's saturation values are relatively stable, according to the manufacturer's directions.

Because of the fiberoptics within $SvO_2$ catheters, they should be handled with care, avoiding any sharp angles or bends in the catheter. Breakage of the fiberoptics of the catheters eliminates the ability to continuously monitor $SvO_2$; however, the catheter may be continued to be used to obtain routine hemodynamic data.

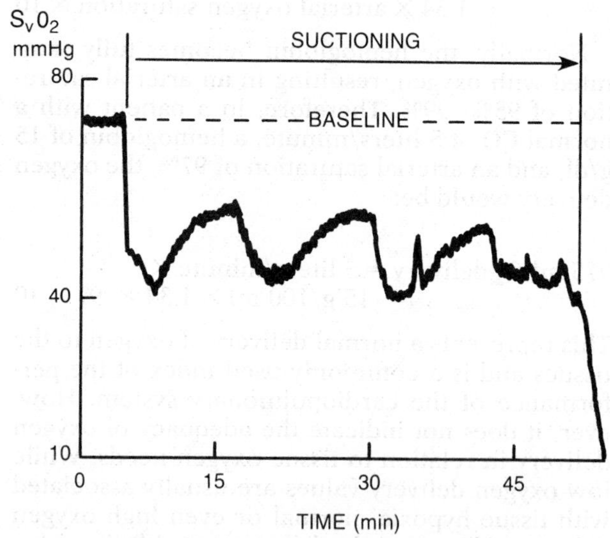


**Figure 41-13.** Example of continuous $SvO_2$ recording showing reductions in $SvO_2$ associated with repeated suctioning. Note that the $SvO_2$ did not return to baseline between suctioning procedures. Ventricular fibrillation occurs as the $SvO_2$ falls to 40 percent and lower. (From Tilkian, A and Daily, EK: Cardiovascular Procedures. CV Mosby, St. Louis, 1986, with permission.)

**TABLE 41-7. CARE PLAN FOR THE PATIENT UNDERGOING HEMODYNAMIC MONITORING**

| Nursing Diagnoses | Desired Patient Outcomes | Nursing Interventions | Rationales |
|---|---|---|---|
| ***Nursing Diagnosis #1*** Alteration in cardiac output: Decreased. | Patient will demonstrate optimal hemodynamic function by:<br>CI 2.5–4 liters/minute/$m^2$<br>PAedp/PAWm* or LAm 15–20 mmHg<br>RAm 4–8 mmHg<br>MAP 70–80 mmHg<br>HR 50–100 bpm without ectopy<br>SVR <1400 dynes/sec/$cm^{-5}$<br>PVR <250 dynes/sec/$cm^{-5}$<br>Normal arterial blood gases<br>Normal hemoglobin level<br>Urinary output ≥40 ml/hr<br>Oxygen delivery to tissues of ≥900 ml/minute | • Monitor preload (RA and PAedp, PAW or LAm) and administer appropriate medications and fluids as prescribed, and monitor response to therapy. | • Optimize preload to systolic ejection according to Starling's law. |
| | | • Measure CO and CI and calculate SVR and/or PVR. Administer appropriate medications as prescribed, and monitor response to therapy.<br>○ Plot ventricular function curves.<br>○ Calculate LVSWI and/or RVSWI. Administer appropriate medications as prescribed, and monitor response. | ○ High LVSWI or RVSWI indicates increased heart work and $O_2$ need ($MVO_2$). |
| | | • Monitor ECG for rate, rhythm, and ectopy, and determine patient's hemodynamic response to changes in rate or rhythm. Treat according to protocol. Implement emergency measures as necessary. | • Very fast heart rates may lower SV by decreasing LV filling. Very low heart rates (<50) may produce inadequate CO (CO = HR × SV). Dysrhythmias reduce CO. |
| | | • Physically assess patient (vital signs, heart and lung sounds, skin color and temperature, fluid balance, mentation, jugular vein distention), and report any significant changes. | • Baseline heart and lung sounds are necessary to determine onset of new sounds associated with cardiac pathology. Decreased mentation or increased restlessness may be early indications of decreased CO. |
| | | • Measure arterial blood gases and hemoglobin levels; report significant changes. Administer therapy as prescribed and monitor response. | • Optimize $O_2$ delivery by maintaining CO, arterial saturation, and Hgb at normal levels. |
| | | • Measure hourly urine output and report if <30 ml/hour. | • To determine renal perfusion and function and prevent dysfunction due to ischemia. |
| | | • Monitor $SvO_2$ and report reductions >10% for 2–3 minutes, or if <60%.[2] | • Decreases in $SvO_2$ indicate inadequate tissue perfusion. $SvO_2$ < 60% is associated with poor prognosis. |
| | | • Reduce patient's activity and stress. | • Reduced activity and stress will decrease $O_2$ demands. |

*(continued)*

**TABLE 41–7. CARE PLAN FOR THE PATIENT UNDERGOING HEMODYNAMIC MONITORING *(Continued)***

| Nursing Diagnoses | Desired Patient Outcomes | Nursing Interventions | Rationales |
|---|---|---|---|
| ***Nursing Diagnosis #2*** Tissue perfusion (peripheral), alteration in, related to compromised circulation associated with invasive monitoring. | Patient will demonstrate:<br>1. Optimal skin integrity.<br>2. Normal skin color and temperature.<br>3. Equal arterial pulses in all extremities. | • Assess catheter insertion site qd; cleanse site and apply iodophor ointment and new sterile dressing (as per unit protocol).<br>• Assess skin color, temperature, and sensitivity in area around catheter insertion site. Report any significant changes. | • Inflammation at catheter insertion site is associated with infection and/or thrombophlebitis.<br>• Alteration in tissue perfusion may result in elevated skin temperature below catheter site. An elevation in skin temperature with pain or tenderness is associated with thrombosis or thrombophlebitis. |
| | | • Palpate and compare pulses in each extremity. Report any changes. | • A decrease or loss in arterial pulsation distal to the catheter insertion site is associated with arterial insufficiency secondary to thrombus formation. |
| | | • Assess catheterized extremity for evidence of edema by measuring the contralateral extremity at the same anatomic location and comparing results from both extremities. | • Edema is characteristic manifestation when tissue perfusion is due to venous interference. |
| ***Nursing Diagnosis #3*** Infection, potential for, related to invasive monitoring. (Refer to Table 49–7, Potential for Infection, Nursing Care Considerations.) | Patient will be free of infection as demonstrated by:<br>1. Baseline temperature (normal).<br>2. Baseline WBC.<br>3. Negative cultures of blood or catheter tip. | • Check patient's temperature q 4 hr and prn and report any significant changes.<br>• Change catheter and catheter site q 4 days or as per unit protocol.<br>• Change IV fluid, tubing, stopcocks, and disposable transducer q 48–72 hr or as per unit protocol. | • Increase in patient's temperature may be associated with an infectious process.<br>• Risk of infection increases with duration of catheter placement >5 days.<br>• Static fluid is a potential source for bacterial growth. |
| | | • Inspect and cleanse catheter insertion site every day, and apply iodophor ointment and clean sterile dressing.<br>• Do not use IV solution containing glucose. | • Skin, old blood, and other such substances are potential sources for infection. Iodophor ointment reduces bacterial growth.<br>• Glucose solutions promote growth of bacteria. |
| | | • Place sterile dead-ender caps on all stopcocks. | • Open stopcock port allows bacteria to enter. |
| | | • Use aseptic technique when withdrawing from or flushing the catheter. | • Prevents contamination of system. |
| | | • If reusable transducers are used, sterilize transducer before patient use. | • Minute flaws in disposable transducer domes allow contact between infusing fluid and transducer, contaminating IV fluid. |
| | | • Carefully remove all traces of blood from stopcock ports after obtaining blood sample from catheter. | • Old blood promotes growth of bacteria. |
| | | • Use sterile plastic catheter sleeve over PA catheter. | • Maintain external portion of catheter sterile to permit catheter advancement, if necessary. |

| | | | |
|---|---|---|---|
| ***Nursing Diagnosis #4***<br>Injury, physiologic, related to:<br>A. Hemorrhage.<br>B. Thromboemboli.<br>C. Venous air embolism.<br>D. Pulmonary infarction or hemorrhage.<br>E. Cardiac dysrhythmias or conduction disturbances. | A. Patient will remain without hemorrhage:<br>1. Stable vital signs.<br>2. Stable hematology profile. | • Keep all catheter connecting sites visible and observe frequently for possible hemorrhage. | • Major blood loss can occur without notice from stopcocks or loose connections that are hidden beneath dressings or bed linens. |
| | | • Tighten all catheter connecting sites and stopcocks q 4 hr and prn. | • Plastic connections become loose over time and leakage can occur. |
| | | • Restrain patient, if necessary. | • A restless or confused patient may pull catheter out or connecting tubing apart. |
| | | • After removal of artrial catheter, apply firm pressure to insertion site for 10 minutes before checking and applying pressure dressing. | • This allows clot to form at insertion site to seal vessel opening. |
| | B. Patient will remain without thromboemboli as evidenced by:<br>1. Patient catheter.<br>2. Unimpeded infusion or flush.<br>3. Undamped waveform. | • Use heparinized IV solution with continuous flush device to continuously infuse all catheter ports *and* side port of sheath, if used. | • Continuous forward flow and use of heparin are associated with decreased thrombus formation at catheter tip or around catheter in sheath. |
| | | • Always aspirate and discard the aspirant before gently flushing any catheter. If unable to aspirate, do not flush catheter. Periodically aspirate and manually flush catheter or activate flush device (q 4–6 hr). | • This removes any fibrin or clot from within or at tip of catheter to prevent injection of clot material. Forward movement or heparinized fluid prevents a clot formation. |
| | | • Do not fast flush arterial catheter for longer than 2 seconds; manually flush arterial catheter by gently tapping plunger of flush syringe with no more than 2–4 ml. | • Vigorous flushing of arterial catheter with large amounts of fluid can result in cerebral embolization.[45] |
| | | • Maintain 300 mmHg pressure on IV cuff. | • 300 mmHg or greater is required to maintain foward flow of heparinized solution via flush device. |
| | | • Remove all traces of blood from catheter, tubing, and stopcocks after withdrawing blood, and flush completely. | • Residual blood in catheter, tubing, or stopcock can form small clots, which can occlude catheter or be injected into patient. |
| | C. Patient will remain without venous air embolism (PA monitoring):<br>1. Absence of pain.<br>2. Arterial blood gases within normal range. | • Tighten all catheter connecting sites and stopcocks q 4 hr and prn and check frequently. | • Plastic connections become loose over time permitting intake of air into system. |
| | | • Place dead-ender caps on all stopcock ports. | • Open or vented ports permit intake of air. |
| | | • Keep all connections or possible openings into system below level of heart. | • Air intake is more likely to occur through a loose connection or open port when the patient is in an upright position and takes a deep breath. |
| | | • Remove all air from IV solution bag. | • Air in bag and solution enters tubing and catheter. |
| | | • Have patient hum or suspend respirations when system is open or near or above heart. | • Air intake through open port occurs during inspiration. |
| | | • After removal of venous catheter that was in place for a long period of time, apply Vaseline and occlusive dressing to site. | • Air intake can occur through the open track formed by long-dwelling catheter, especially in thin person with little subcutaneous tissue. |

*(continued)*

**TABLE 41-7. CARE PLAN FOR THE PATIENT UNDERGOING HEMODYNAMIC MONITORING *(Continued)***

| Nursing Diagnoses | Desired Patient Outcomes | Nursing Interventions | Rationales |
|---|---|---|---|
| | D. Patient will be free of pulmonary infarction or hemorrhage as evidenced by:<br>1. Normal respirations.<br>2. No hemoptysis.<br>3. Normal ABGs. | • Continuously monitor PA waveform at distal tip of PA catheter. | • Forward migration of catheter into a wedged position will be evidenced by PAW waveform. |
| | | • Inflate balloon to wedge catheter briefly (−20 seconds). | • This minimizes cessation in blood flow to reduce risk of pulmonary ischemia and/or infarction. |
| | | • Leave balloon of PA catheter deflated with stopcock open and syringe removed. | • Open stopcock with syringe off permits passive deflation should any air remain in balloon. |
| | | • Monitor PAedp instead of PAW (if closely correlated). | • This reduces risks due to inflation of balloon and cessation of blood flow in branch of PA. |
| | | • Check location of catheter tip after insertion and prn via posteroanterior chest film. | • Catheter tip may migrate forward along with blood flow into a wedge position (particularly during first 24 hours). |
| | | • Continuously observe waveform during slow balloon inflation; stop inflation at *first* appearance of PAW waveform. Do not inflate 7 French catheter with more than 1.5 cc air. | • Overinflation of balloon can cause rupture of vessel. |
| | | • Do not inflate balloon with air if resistance is met. | • Catheter may be in a small branch of the PA and already mechanically wedged; or balloon may already be inflated. |
| | E. Patient will remain free of life-threatening dysrhythmias or conduction disturbances. | • Continuously monitor waveform from distal port of catheter. | • Appearance of RV waveform indicates catheter tip has fallen into RV and could cause ventricular dysrhythmias. |
| | | • Monitor chest film daily. | • Check for coiling of catheter in RV or RA, which could cause dysrhythmias. |
| | | • If RV waveform appears, quickly inflate balloon of catheter. | • Catheter tip in RV can produce ventriclar dysrhythmias. With balloon inflation, catheter should float to PA. |
| | | • To remove catheter, deflate balloon actively and completely with syringe and quickly remove catheter. | • Rapid removal of catheter with fully deflated balloon should result in few, if any, dysrhythmias. |
| | | • Follow emergency protocols for occurrence of life-threatening dysrhythmias. | |

| | | | |
|---|---|---|---|
| ***Nursing Diagnosis #5*** Anxiety, related to fear of technologic equipment and procedures associated with hemodynamic monitoring. | Patient will:<br>1. Verbalize feelings.<br>2. Demonstrate a relaxed manner.<br>3. Verbalize familiarity with hemodynamic monitoring procedures and equipment. | • Initiate interventions to reduce anxiety. | • Anxiety interferes with learning.<br>• Readiness to learn facilitates meaningful learning and retention of knowledge. |
| | | ◦ Assess ability and readiness to learn the following, when appropriate:<br>– Reasons for hemodynamic monitoring.<br>– Function and purpose of hemodynamic monitoring equipment.<br>– Explanation of procedures related to hemodynamic monitoring. | ◦ Knowing rationale and purpose of hemodynamic monitoring reduces anxiety. |
| | | ◦ Instruct patient in relaxation techniques. | ◦ Use of energy release techniques helps reduce anxiety. |
| | | ◦ Listen attentively, encourage verbalization, and provide a caring touch. | ◦ This provides reassurance to patient that he/she is not alone. |
| ***Nursing Diagnosis #6*** Sleep pattern disturbance, related to invasive monitoring procedures. | Patient will verbalize having restful sleep. | • Do not awaken or reposition patient to obtain hemodynamic parameters. | • Hemodynamic measurements may be obtained with patient in supine right or left lateral positions or 45-degree semi-Fowler's position as long as air-reference stopcock is adjusted to mid-RA level and transducer is re-zeroed. |
| | | • Instruct in relaxation techniques. | • Energy release techniques help relax patient and aid in sleep. |
| | | • Provide quiet, dimly lit environment. | • Quiet, dark environment is more conducive to sleep. |

* PAW (pulmonary artery wedge) pressure is synonymous with PCWP (pulmonary capillary wedge pressure) as used in this text.

## NURSING CARE OF THE PATIENT UNDERGOING HEMODYNAMIC MONITORING

Nursing diagnoses, desired patient outcomes, and nursing interventions in the care of the patient undergoing hemodynamic monitoring are presented in the Care Plan in Table 41–7.

## REFERENCES


1. Hales, S: Statistical Essays: Hemostaticks, ed 3, Vol 2. W Innys and R Manby, London, 1978.
2. Wilson, JN et al: Central venous pressure in optimum blood volume maintenance. Arch Surg 85;563, 1962.
3. Swan, HJC, Ganz, W, and Forrester, JS: Catheterization of the heart in man with the use of a flow-directed balloon-tipped catheter. N Engl J Med 283:447, 1970.
4. Gardner, RM and Hollingsworth, KW: Optimizing the electrocardiogram and pressure monitoring. Crit Care Med 14(7):651, 1986.
5. Centers for Disease Control: Nosocomial bacteremia from intravascular pressure monitoring systems. In National Nosocomial Infections Study Report, 1977. US Department of Health, Education, and Welfare, Atlanta, 1979.
6. Disposable pressure transducers. Health Devices 13:267, 1984.
7. Sise, MJ, Hollingsworth, P, and Brimm, JE: Complications of the flow-directed pulmonary artery catheter: A prospective analysis in 219 patients. Crit Care Med 9:315, 1981.
8. Johnston, WE, Prough, DS, and Royster, RL, et al: Short-term sterility of the pulmonary artery catheter inserted through an external plastic shield. Anesthesiology 61:461, 1984.
9. Iberti, TJ, Benjamin, E, Gruppi, L, and Raskin, JM: Ventricular arrhythmias during pulmonary artery catheterization in the intensive care unit. Am J Med 78:451, 1985.
10. Scott, WAC: Haemodynamic monitoring measurement of systemic blood pressure. Can Anaesth Soc J 32(3):294, 1985.
11. Kelly, J, Braverman, B, Land, PC, and Ivankovich, AD: Comparison of Allen test, Doppler and finger-pulse transducer to assess patency of ulnar artery. Anesthesiology 59 (Suppl):A178, 1983.
12. Boutros, A and Albert, S: Effect of the dynamic response of transducer-tubing system on accuracy of direct blood pressure measurement in patients. Crit Care Med 11:124, 1983.
13. Whalley, DG: Haemodynamic monitoring: Pulmonary artery catheterization. Can Anaesth Soc J 32:1299, 1985.
14. Gardner, RM: Direct blood pressure measurement: Dynamic response requirements. Anesthesiology 54:227, 1981.
15. Bromberger-Barnea, B: Mechanical effects of inspiration on heart functions. A review. Fed Proc 40:2172, 1982.
16. King, EG: Influence of mechanical ventilation and pulmonary disease on pulmonary artery pressure monitoring. Can Med Assoc J 121:901, 1979.
17. Labrousse, J, Tenaillon, A, and Lissac, J: Influence of artificial ventilation on the pulmonary capillary wedge pressure. Chest 74:693, 1978.
18. Ellis, DM: Interpretation of beat-to-beat blood pressure values in the presence of ventilatory changes. J Clin Monitoring 1:65, 1985.
19. Bouchard, RJ, Goult, JH, and Ross, J Jr: Evaluation of pulmonary arterial end-diastolic pressure as an estimate of left ventricular end-diastolic pressure in patients with normal and abnormal left ventricular performance. Circulation 44:1072, 1971.
20. Daily, EK and Schroeder, JS: Techniques in Bedside Hemodynamic Monitoring, ed 4. CV Mosby, St Louis, 1989.
21. Keefer, JR and Barash, PG: Pulmonary artery catheterization. In Blitt, C (ed): Monitoring in Anesthesia and Critical Care Medicine. Churchill-Livingstone, New York, 1986.
22. Braunwald, E: On the difference between the heart's output and its contractile state. Circulation 43:171, 1971.
23. Walston, A and Kendall, ME: Comparison of pulmonary wedge and left atrial pressure in man. Am Heart J 86:159, 1973.
24. Calvin, JE, Driedger, AA, and Sibbald, WJ: Does the pulmonary capillary wedge pressure predict left ventricular preload in critically ill patients? Crit Care Med 9:437, 1981.
25. Tooker, J, Huseby, J, and Butler, J: The effect of Swan-Ganz catheter height on the wedge pressure relationship in edema during positive-pressure ventilation. Am Rev Respir Dis 117:721, 1978.
26. Shasby, DM et al: Swan-Ganz catheter location and left atrial pressure when positive end-expiratory pressure is used. Chest 80:666, 1981.
27. Scharf, SM, Brown, R, and Saunders, N, et al: Effects of normal and loaded spontaneous inspiration on cardiovascular function. J Appl Physiol 47(3):582, 1979.
28. Berryhill, RE and Benumof, JL: PEEP-induced discrepancy between pulmonary arterial wedge pressure and left atrial pressure: The effects of controlled vs. spontaneous ventilation and compliant vs. noncompliant lungs in the dog. Anesthesiology 51:303, 1979.
29. Benumof, JL, Saidman, LJ, Arkin, DB et al: Where pulmonary arterial catheters go: Intrathoracic distributions. Anesthesiology 46:336, 1977.
30. Hurst, JS: The Heart: Arteries and Veins. McGraw-Hill, New York, 1982.
31. Gore, JM et al: Handbook of Hemodynamic Monitoring. Little, Brown & Co, Boston, 1985.
32. Bedford, RF: Invasive blood pressure monitoring. In Blitt, C (ed): Monitoring in Anesthesia and Critical Care Medicine. Churchill-Livingstone, New York, 1986.
33. Mueller, H et al: Trans NY Acad Sci, Series II, 34(4):309, 1972.
34. Webster, H: Hemodynamic monitoring in children. In Daily, EK and Schroeder, JS: Techniques in Bedside Hemodynamic Monitoring. CV Mosby, St Louis, 1985.
35. Fegler, G: Measurement of cardiac output in an anesthetized animal by the thermodilution method. Q J Exp Physiol 39:153, 1954.
36. Shellock, FG and Reidinger, MS: Reproducibility and accuracy of using room temperature vs. ice temperature for thermodilution cardiac output determination. Heart Lung 12:175, 1983.
37. Daily, EK and Mersch, J: Comparison of Fick method with thermodilution method using two indicators. Heart Lung 16(3):294, May 1987.
38. Stetz, CS, Miller, RG, Kelly, GE, and Raffin, TA: Reliability of the thermodilution method in determination of cardiac output in clinical practice. Am Rev Respir Dis 126:1001, 1982.
39. Kadota, LT: Reproducibility of thermodilution cardiac output measurements. Heart Lung 15:618, 1986.
40. Miller, MJ: Tissue oxygenation in clinical medicine: An historical review. Anesth Analg 61:527, 1982.
41. McMihan, JC: Continuous monitoring of mixed venous oxygen saturation. In Schweiss, JF (ed): Continuous Measurement of Blood Oxygen Saturation in the High Risk Patient, Vol 1. Beach International Inc, San Diego, 1983.
42. White, KM: Completing the hemodynamic picture: $SvO_2$. Heart Lung 14:272, 1985.
43. Jaquith, SM: Continuous measurement of $SvO_2$: Clinical applications and advantages for critical nursing. Crit Care Nurse 5:40, 1985.
44. Tilkian, AG and Daily, EK: Cardiovascular Procedures: Diagnostic Techniques and Therapeutic Procedures. CV Mosby, St Louis, 1986.
45. Lowenstein, E, Little, JW, and Lo, HH: Prevention of cerebral emobilization from flushing radial-artery cannulas. N Engl J Med 285:1414, 1971.

CHAPTER 42

# Therapeutic Modalities in the Treatment of the Patient with Cardiovascular Dysfunction

*Ellen Strauss McErlean and Gayle R. Whitman*

## CHAPTER OUTLINE



## LEARNING OBJECTIVES

**At the end of this chapter, you should be able to:**

1. Identify 2 indications for artificial pacing.
2. Discuss methods and modes of artificial pacing.
3. Describe nursing interventions in the care of the patient receiving a temporary or permanent pacemaker.
4. Discuss 2 primary goals of intra-aortic balloon pumping.
5. Review 5 underlying principles of intra-aortic balloon pumping.
6. Identify 3 potential complications of intra-aortic balloon therapy.

## LEARNING OBJECTIVES—*CONTINUED*

7. Outline nursing interventions in the care of the patient receiving intra-aortic balloon therapy.
8. Identify the major goal of percutaneous transluminal angioplasty.
9. Explain the mechanics of the PTCA procedure.
10. Identify 3 potential complications of the PTCA procedure.
11. Specify nursing interventions in caring for the patient following angioplasty.
12. Identify 2 major goals of thrombolytic therapy.
13. Explain 3 criteria for clinical eligibility for thrombolytic therapy.
14. Describe 3 relative contraindications for treatment with streptokinase.
15. Discuss 3 common complications encountered with administration of thrombolytic agents for coronary artery disease (CAD).
16. Explain the goal of laser angioplasty.
17. Describe the current indications for the use of laser angioplasty in the treatment of CAD.
18. Identify 2 major complications of laser angioplasty.
19. Specify 2 nursing considerations for the patient receiving laser angioplasty.

## GOAL OF THERAPEUTIC MODALITIES

The heart is a complex organ that provides the pumping activity necessary to maintain circulation of blood to all the tissues of the body, distributing oxygen and nutrients and removing cellular waste products. Cardiac activity is achieved through integration of electrical and mechanical mechanisms that ensure the forward flow of blood throughout the vasculature. Many conditions occur clinically that impair the heart's intrinsic ability to pump blood and that require a variety of therapeutic interventions. These treatment modalities are aimed at supporting the mechanical pumping activity required for adequate tissue perfusion. This chapter highlights the most current interventions that affect both the electrical and mechanical cardiac activity, and examines the goals of treatment, clinical indications, physiologic principles guiding the therapy, relative contraindications, technical aspects of each intervention, potential complications, and nursing considerations.

## CARDIAC PACEMAKERS

### Purpose of the Conduction System: Impulse Transmission

As previously discussed, the conduction system within the heart is a collection of specialized tissue that transmits impulses throughout the myocardium in a rapid and organized fashion (Fig. 42–1). This causes simultaneous depolarization of the atrium and then of the ventricles, which allows for synchronization of contraction and optimal ejection of blood with every beat. Failure of the conduction system to transmit impulses to the ventricle diminishes the heart's ability to maintain adequate tissue perfusion.

The conduction system also possesses the unique property of *automaticity*, which allows the cells to spontaneously depolarize without being stimulated by an outside source. This important property provides a series of backup mechanisms for pacing the heart should the primary pacemaker, usually the sinus node, fail to discharge impulses at its set rate.

At times, other cells within the myocardium exhibit automaticity and attempt to control the pacing function of the heart (i.e., ectopic pacemakers). If the ectopic pacemaker fires impulses at a rate that exceeds the sinus node discharge rate, the ectopic site then depolarizes the ventricles and assumes the primary pacing function of the heart. Often, depolarization of the ventricles from an ectopic site decreases the ability of the heart to allow for adequate ventricular filling and limits synchronous contractile efforts that normally provide for optimal ejection of blood.

### Indications for Artificial Pacing

Artificial pacing is indicated whenever there is a failure of the conduction system to transmit impulses from the sinus node to the ventricles, to generate an impulse spontaneously, or to maintain primary control of the pacing function of the heart. Table 42–1 summarizes the primary indications for artificial pacing.

Many pathophysiologic and iatrogenic conditions are encountered clinically that affect the conduction system's ability to function normally, creating circumstances for which pacing is indicated. These conditions, summarized in Table 42–2, may temporarily or permanently impair cellular activity, prohibiting normal generation and transmission of impulses.

#### *Goals of Artificial Pacing*

Artificial pacing is intended to provide a physiologic "backup" for the heart during failure of the conduction system to depolarize the myocardium

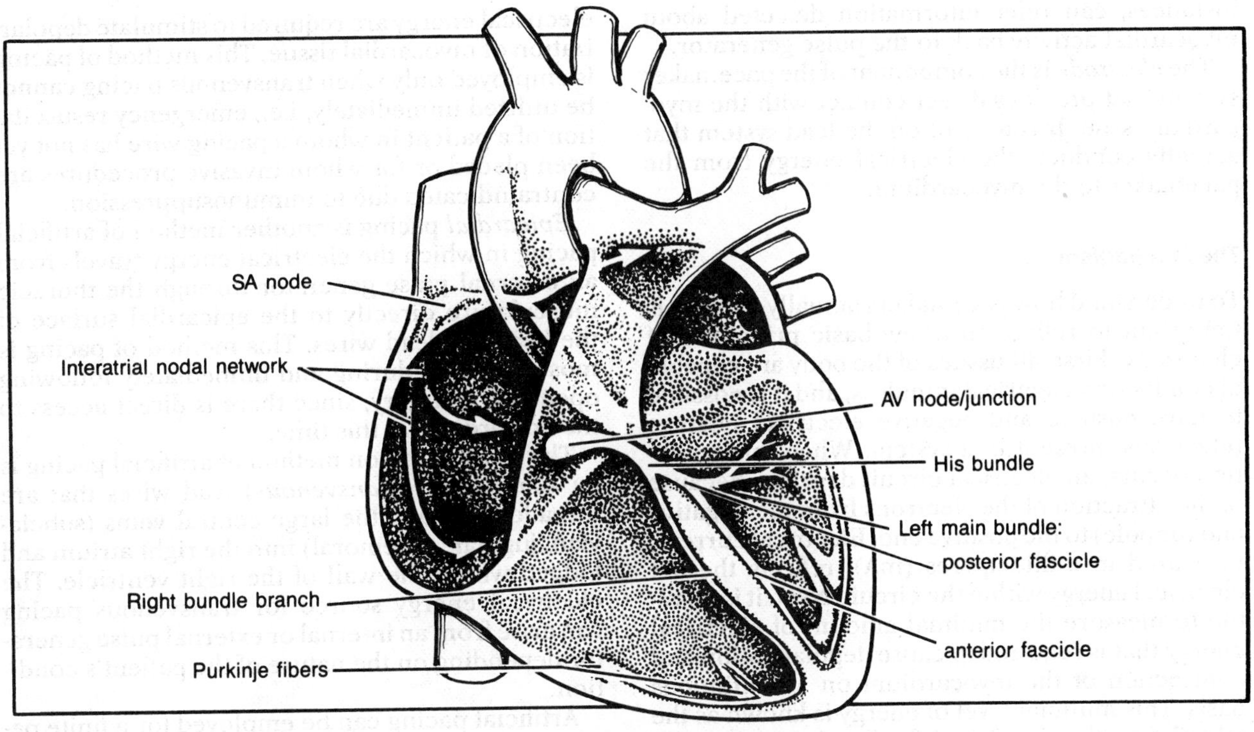


**Figure 42-1.** The conduction system of the heart. (See Fig. 37-6 for discussion.)

and maintain an adequate cardiac output. When cardiac output is diminished because of lack of depolarization of the ventricles, artificial pacing will provide the necessary stimulus directly to the ventricles for contraction to occur. If cardiac output is compromised because an ectopic pacemaker is causing the ventricles to depolarize and contract at a rate that does not promote adequate ventricular filling, artificial pacing will compete with the ectopic pacemaker to assume the primary pacing function of the heart.

## Principles of Artificial Pacing

### *The System*

An artificial pacemaker provides an external source of energy for impulse formation and delivery, and stimulation of myocardial tissue. In any pacemaker, there are several key components that are integrated within the system: the pulse generator with circuitry, the lead, and the electrode system.

The *pulse generator* is the component that houses the energy source and the electronics that control the pacemaker function. Depending on the type of pacemaker employed, the pulse generator may be capable of controlling the discharge of impulses to the myocardium, the timing of the impulse discharge, and recognition of intrinsic electrical activity within the myocardium.

The *lead* is the component that provides communication between the pulse generator and the myocardium. It can carry the impulse created by the pulse generator to the myocardium and, in some

TABLE 42-1
**Primary Indications for Artificial Pacing**

| |
|---|
| *Disruption of the Ability to Generate and Transmit Impulses* |
| Bradyarrhythmias |
| Heart block |
| Sick sinus syndrome |
| Sinus arrest |
| Asystole |
| *Control of Dysrhythmias Related to Ectopic Pacemakers* |
| Atrial tachyarrhythmias |
| Ventricular tachyarrhythmias |

TABLE 42-2
**Common Conditions that Impair Cardiac Conduction**

| |
|---|
| *Pathophysiologic* |
| Acute myocardial infarction |
| Myocardial ischemia |
| Autonomic nervous system failure |
| Electrolyte imbalance |
| *Iatrogenic* |
| Drug toxicity (antiarrhythmics) |
| Cardiac surgery |
| Ablation |

instances, can refer information detected about myocardial activity back to the pulse generator.

The *electrode* is the component of the pacemaker system that provides direct contact with the myocardial tissue. It is a point on the lead system that actually conducts the electrical energy from the pacemaker to the myocardium.

### The Mechanism

To understand how pacemakers actually work, it is important to reflect on a few basic principles of electricity. First, all tissues of the body are capable of conducting electrical impulses, and it is possible to have positive and negative electrical charges (electrons) present in a system. When this condition occurs, an electrical circuit develops because of the attraction of the electrons from the negative end (or pole) to the positive end. Electrical current, measured in milliamperes (mA), reflects the net electrical energy within the circuit. Next, it is possible to measure the minimal amount of electrical energy that is required to cause depolarization and contraction of the myocardium on a continuous basis. This minimal level of energy is known as the *stimulation threshold*. And finally, the stimulation threshold can be affected by a number of factors, including quality of communication with the myocardial tissue, ability of the tissue to propagate impulses, and the characteristics of the lead itself.

Pacemakers rely on the above principles in their delivery of energy to the myocardium. Because the goal of impulse delivery is to have electrical energy travel from the lead to the myocardium, there is always a negative pole on the lead itself. The location of the positive pole within the system defines the type of lead configuration employed. In a *unipolar* lead system, the positive pole is located outside the myocardium, either on the pulse generator itself or on a positive electrode or on the skin. In this type of system, the energy travels from the lead (negative pole) through the myocardium and thoracic musculature back to the positive electrode. In a *bipolar* system both the positive and negative poles are located within the myocardium itself, creating an electrical circuit that does not leave the heart. This is by far the most common lead system used.

## Methods of Artificial Pacing

There are 3 major methods of delivering energy to the myocardial tissue for the purpose of artificial pacing: external (transthoracic), epicardial (transthoracic), or endocardial (transvenous). *External transchest* pacing delivers energy to the heart through the thoracic musculature via 2 surface electrode patches. Because these electrodes have no direct contact with the heart, large amounts of electrical energy are required to stimulate depolarization of myocardial tissue. This method of pacing is employed only when transvenous pacing cannot be utilized immediately, i.e., emergency resuscitation of a patient in whom a pacing wire has not yet been placed or for whom invasive procedures are contraindicated due to immunosuppression.

*Epicardial* pacing is another method of artificial pacing in which the electrical energy travels from an external pulse generator through the thoracic musculature directly to the epicardial surface of the heart via lead wires. This method of pacing is most common during and immediately following open-heart surgery, since there is direct access to the epicardium at this time.

The most common method of artificial pacing is by *endocardial* (*transvenous*) lead wires that are threaded through the large central veins (subclavian, jugular, or femoral) into the right atrium and lodged within the wall of the right ventricle. The electrical energy source for transvenous pacing can arise from an internal or external pulse generator depending on the nature of the patient's condition.

Artificial pacing can be employed for a finite period of time, such as when the disruption of the conduction system is thought to be *temporary*, or the artificial pacer can be implanted as a *permanent* backup for cardiac function when the disruption of the conduction system is thought to be irreversible.

## Modes of Artificial Pacing

There are a variety of ways in which an artificial pacemaker can function to complement the intrinsic electrical activity of the heart. The most basic type of pacemaker fires at a set rate, regardless of the heart's ability to generate spontaneous impulses. This type of pacemaker is known as an *asynchronous*, *fixed-rate*, or *non-demand* pacemaker. This mode of pacing is appropriate in the absence of any electrical activity (asystole), but is dangerous in the presence of an intrinsic rhythm because of the potential of the pacemaker to fire during the vulnerable period of repolarization and initiate lethal ventricular arrhythmias.

The more common type of pacemaker senses the natural electrical activity of the heart and fires only when intrinsic activity is not sensed for a predetermined interval of time. This mode of pacing is known as *demand* pacing, because it initiates pacing only when needed.

A pacemaker is also able to pace different chambers of the heart, depending on placement of the lead/electrode system. If the integrity of the conduction system is not impaired through the AV node to the ventricles, it is possible to pace the atria and send impulses normally to the ventricles. This type of pacing would be indicated in the presence of sinus node disease. The electrocardiographic indicator of atrial pacing is a pacer spike followed by a P wave and a normal QRS complex. Atrial pacemakers are beneficial because they preserve the normal synchrony of depolarization and contraction, allowing the atria to contribute to ventricular filling, which can account for 20%–30% of the total cardiac output.

The ventricles can be stimulated by a pacemaker when a lead wire is placed directly into the right ventricle. This is a common type of pacing seen in critical care, particularly when the pacing is for a temporary situation. Ventricular pacing is indicated when transmission of impulses from the atria is being blocked before depolarization of the ventricles. Electrocardiographic indicators of ventricular pacing include a pacer spike followed immediately by a wide QRS complex. Ventricular pacemakers do not permit synchrony of the atrial activity with ventricular contraction and thus result in a loss of the atrial contribution to cardiac output.

Because this synchrony of atria and ventricles is vital in certain patients, pacemakers are available that mimic the physiologic depolarization of the heart by synchronizing an atrial impulse with a ventricular impulse at predetermined intervals. These pacemakers are known as *AV sequential pacemakers.* Examples of artificial pacing on the electrocardiogram are depicted in Figure 42–2.

In addition to these capabilities, permanent pacemakers now have special programmable and antitachyarrhythmic functions that are quite complex. In order to communicate all the functions of the individual pacemakers, an international code was developed by the Inter-Society Commission for Heart Disease (ICHD). This code is summarized in Table 42–3. The term "chamber paced" (first letter in the code) indicates which chamber(s) of the heart will be stimulated. The term "chamber sensed" (second letter in the code) indicates the chamber(s) of the heart in which the lead is capable of recognizing intrinsic electrical activity. "Mode of response" (third letter in the code) indicates how the pacemaker will act based on the information it senses. "Programmability" (fourth letter in the code) indicates ability to change function once the pacemaker has been implanted. "Tachyarrhythmic" functions (fifth letter in the code) list specific methods of interrupting tachyarrhythmias. Although the last 2 letters contain pertinent information, commonly a pacemaker will be referred to only by its first 3 letters (i.e., VVI, DDD). For example, a VVI pacemaker is one in which only the ventricle will be paced when the unit discharges an impulse and is inhibited from firing when intrinsic ventricular activity is sensed (V—chamber paced; V—chamber sensed, I—mode of response is inhibition). Another common pacemaker mode is the DDD pacemaker. Because D represents both atrial and ventricular (dual) chambers, this unit is able to deliver pacing stimuli to both the atrium and ventricle, detect intrinsic atrial and ventricular activity, and then respond to the sensed activity with inhibition of output or atrial triggering (ventricular pacing when atrial activity is sensed).

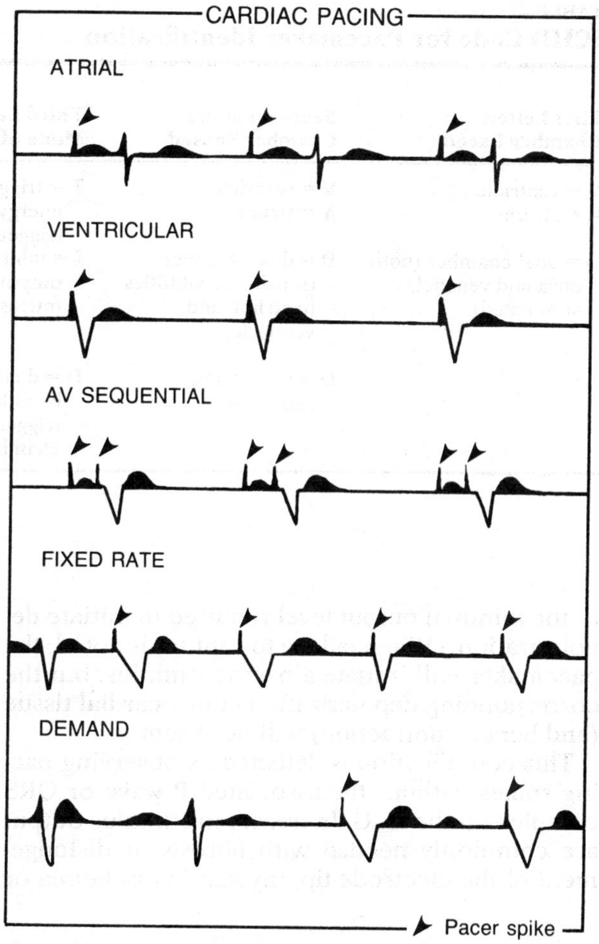


**Figure 42–2.** Electrocardiographic examples of artificial cardiac pacing. (See text for discussion. ➤ indicates pacer spike.)

## Complications of Artificial Pacing

The many complications that can result from artificially pacing the heart relate to the method and technique utilized in insertion, mechanical failure of the pacemaker, and the patient's underlying myocardial disease. These complications are summarized in Table 42–4.

Two complications, common to all forms of pacing, require further discussion. "Failure to capture" and "failure to sense" are problems that indicate that the pacemaker is not able to perform according to specification, requiring adjustment of the settings.

"Capture" refers to the ability of the heart muscle to respond to stimulus output. ("Threshold" refers

TABLE 42-3
## ICHD Code for Pacemaker Identification

| First Letter: Chamber Paced | Second Letter: Chamber Sensed | Third Letter: Mode of Response | Fourth Letter: Programmable Functions | Fifth Letter: Tachyarrhythmic Functions |
|---|---|---|---|---|
| V = ventricle<br>A = atrium | V = ventricle<br>A = atrium | T = triggered (may have energy output triggered) | P = programmable for 1 or 2 functions | B = bursts of pacing |
| D = dual chamber (both atria and ventricles stimulated) | D = dual chamber (sensing capabilities in atrium and ventricle) | I = inhibited (pacing output inhibited by intrinsic activity) | M = multiprogram-mable ability to change functions other than the rate or output | N = normal rate competition |
| | O = no sensing capability | D = dual chamber (may be either inhibition or triggering of both chambers) | | S = scanning |

to the minimal output level required to initiate depolarization.) When failure to capture is noted, the pacemaker will initiate a pacing stimulus, but the corresponding depolarization of myocardial tissue (and hence contraction) will be absent.

This complication is detected by observing pacing spikes without the associated P wave or QRS complex on the ECG. Increases in stimulus output are commonly needed with fibrosis or dislodgement of the electrode tip, myocardial ischemia or infarction, antiarrhythmic therapy, or electrolyte imbalance. Adjustment of the voltage, current (mA), or pulse duration will correct this problem.

"Sensing" refers to the ability of the pacemaker to detect intrinsic electrical activity and respond according to the programmed mode. Failure to sense describes a circumstance in which the detection system does not recognize intrinsic electrical activity, responding in ways that might actually compete with the patient's own rhythm. This is recognized on the ECG by pacemaker spikes falling at intervals that are different from the programmed escape interval (that period of time between the last sensed beat and the paced beat). This condition predisposes the heart to discharge of an impulse during a vulnerable phase of the electrical cycle (i.e., the latter half of the T wave), which might precipitate life-threatening ventricular arrhythmias. Adjustment of the sensitivity setting (decreasing the amplitude at which electrical activity is recognized) or repositioning the catheter may alleviate this complication.

TABLE 42-4
## Complications of Artificial Pacing

| Method | Complication |
|---|---|
| External transthoracic pacing | Pain with impulse delivery<br>Skin burns<br>Muscular twitching<br>Psychological reactions<br>*Failure to capture<br>†Failure to sense |
| Epicardial pacing | Dislodgement of lead<br>Microshock<br>Cardiac tamponade<br>Infection<br>Psychological reactions<br>*Failure to capture<br>†Failure to sense |
| Endocardial (transvenous) pacing | Myocardial irritability<br>Perforation of chamber or septum<br>Electromagnetic interference<br>Infection<br>Embolism<br>Abdominal twitching<br>Hiccups<br>Pacer-induced dysrhythmias<br>*Failure to capture<br>†Failure to sense |

*Failure to capture: Inability of impulse to initiate a contraction.

†Failure to sense: Inability of pacemaker to sense intrinsic electrical activity.

## Nursing Considerations for Artificial Pacing

Although the principles for pacing are the same whether temporary or permanent pacing is employed, each has distinct nursing implications that should be considered. Areas of focus for the patient receiving a temporary pacemaker include the following:

1. Explanation of the procedure for the patient and family.
2. Monitoring the patient's response to the procedure.
3. Maintaining electrical safety.
4. Monitoring pacing parameters (sensing, capture, threshold).

5. Protecting the patient from injury and infection.

Tables 42–5 and 42–6 summarize procedures for insertion of a temporary pacemaker and checking the threshold.

The patient receiving a permanent pacemaker also has unique needs upon which the nurse must focus. These include:

1. Psychological adaptation.
2. Patient education.
3. Follow-up care.
4. Infection.

(See the care plans for patients with temporary and permanent pacemakers in Tables 42–7 and 42–8.)

## INTRA-AORTIC BALLOON PUMPING (IABP)

### Goal of Intra-aortic Balloon Pumping

Intra-aortic balloon pumping, or counterpulsation, is a method of providing assistance to the left ventricle during periods of acute cardiac failure.

TABLE 42–5
**Sample Procedure for Insertion of a Temporary Pacemaker**

| Action | Rationale |
|---|---|
| 1. Explain procedure to patient and family. | 1. Usually semi-emergent situation. Communication allays fears, anxieties. |
| 2. Obtain informed consent. | 2. Patient must give permission for procedure after hearing all options, risks, and benefits. |
| 3. Assemble necessary equipment. Include:<br>Pacing wire<br>Sterile drapes<br>IV $D_5W$ or normal saline<br>Razor<br>Cordis introducer<br>10-ml syringes<br>Betadine swabs<br>Needles (5/8", 1½")<br>2% Xylocaine<br>Pacemaker generator<br>100 mg Lidocaine IV | 3. Pacemaker may be inserted with* or without fluoroscopy, at the bedside or in the cardiac catheterization laboratory. |
| 4. Prepare the site for insertion (may shave if necessary) by swabbing with Betadine and draping with sterile towels. | 4. Most common sites include subclavian and internal jugular veins. |
| 5. Assist physician with insertion. | 5. The physician will infiltrate the area with 2% Xylocaine, isolate the vein, insert the intravenous cordis introducer, and insert the pacing wire under aseptic conditions. |
| 6. Establish the external pulse generator settings (mA sensitivity, mode, heart rate) and attach to lead wires. | 6. Pacemaker settings are determined by the physician. |
| 7. Monitor patient's response to insertion. Note the patient's vital signs, heart rhythm, and comfort level during the advancement of the pacing wire. Have Lidocaine 100 mg IV bolus available for pacemaker-induced ventricular dysrhythmias. | 7. Introduction of a wire through the right atria and ventricle may stimulate dysrhythmias. The patient's hemodynamic status must be evaluated at frequent intervals to ensure adequate perfusion. Patient should not feel more than pressure at insertion site. |
| 8. Reassure patient during procedure. | 8. Patient will be draped with sterile towels and unable to see the activities. Conversation with patient communicates that your primary interest is with his or her response. |
| 9. Initiate pacing after right ventricular position has been established. | 9. Correct position of pacing wire is determined by fluoroscopy. |
| 10. Monitor pacemaker function. Monitor the ECG to note pacing at set rate. Determine presence of patient pulse with each paced beat. Ensure that there is capture with each paced stimulus and that the pacemaker appropriately senses intrinsic electrical activity. | 10. Testing of pacer is important to assess proper functioning. It is possible to have electrical cardiac activity without the associated contraction. Catheter position and stimulus output can be adjusted to ensure adequate delivery of pacing impulse. Sensitivity can be manipulated to prevent competition with the patient's intrinsic rhythm. |
| 11. Document threshold, pacing mode, and ability to sense and capture. | 11. This is important information to have as baseline reference. |
| 12. Apply sterile dressing to site. | 12. Asepsis prevents infection; the dressing stabilizes pacing wire. |
| 13. Obtain ECG strip. | 13. This serves as baseline reference. |
| 14. Obtain portable chest x-ray. | 14. Chest x-ray can confirm placement of wire and rule out pneumothorax. |
| 15. Check patient's vital signs, breath sounds, hemodynamic response to pacing. | 15. Vital signs should remain the same or improve from baseline. Breath sounds should be present and equal bilaterally, unchanged from baseline assessment. Hemodynamic response to pacing should be favorable. |

*This procedure outlines the most common form of insertion with fluoroscopy.

TABLE 42–6
**Sample Procedure for Checking Threshold**

| Action | Rationale |
|---|---|
| 1. Make sure pacer is on the demand mode. | 1. This prevents competition with the patient's intrinsic rhythm. |
| 2. Turn pacemaker rate up slowly until capture is seen for every beat. (This will be evidenced by a pacemaker spike firing at the set rate, followed by a QRS complex for each spike.) | 2. The patient has to be pacing continuously to be able to assess the level of energy at which the myocardium is "captured" by the pacing stimulus. |
| 3. Slowly decrease mA or the current output level until loss of capture is noted. This will be demonstrated by pacemaker spikes without associated QRS complexes on the ECG. | |
| 4. Increase mA until capture is noted for every beat. | 4. The minimal level of energy necessary to stimulate and depolarize the myocardium with each beat is known as the "threshold." |
| 5. Document this energy level and compare with previous threshold. | 5. Monitor for increased tolerance to energy levels. The amount of energy required to depolarize the myocardium is influenced by a number of factors, including electrolyte balance, concurrent drug therapy, and quality of lead contact with the myocardium. |
| 6. Set the mA 1.5–2 points above the threshold. | 6. The setting of output should be adjusted to ensure continuous pacing despite changes in the dynamic system of the body. |
| 7. Check threshold daily. | 7. Threshold can change due to fibrosis at lead tip, ischemia, electrolyte balance, hypoxia. |

The intra-aortic balloon pump (IABP) provides support by improving perfusion of the myocardium and reducing the workload of the left ventricle. Major goals of IABP include:

1. Improving cardiac output by decreasing myocardial work.
2. Decreasing myocardial ischemia.
3. Reducing the amount of myocardial damage.
4. Providing hemodynamic stability until definitive treatment can be initiated.

## Indications for Intra-aortic Balloon Pumping

Intra-aortic balloon pumping can be used in both medical and surgical settings to support the injured myocardium. Table 42–9 summarizes the most common indications for IABP.

## Technique of Counterpulsation

The intra-aortic balloon is an oblong, polyurethane receptacle that is attached to a catheter. The catheter may contain a central lumen that communicates directly with the arterial blood in the aorta, providing exact measurements of central aortic root pressures from which balloon inflation and deflation can be timed. The balloon itself is attached to tubing from the pneumatic system, which regulates the shuttling of gas to inflate and deflate the balloon. Two gases are commonly used for balloon pumping: helium and carbon dioxide. Helium is used in most of the newer-model balloon pump systems because it is a lighter gas and more efficient at faster heart rates. The pneumatic drive system is housed in a console, from which all interaction with the balloon occurs.

## Principles of Counterpulsation

Intra-aortic balloon pumping must coordinate with the cardiac cycle so as not to impede the ejection of blood. Counterpulsation can be thought of as a completely *diastolic event,* where inflation of the balloon occurs at the beginning of diastole and deflation occurs just prior to the next systolic ejection.

Because inflation and deflation must coincide with systole and diastole, a method of *triggering* balloon activity must be selected by the nurse. Most commonly the patient's ECG, or, more specifically, the R wave, is used to signal the beginning of systole. Another triggering mode that can be used is the arterial waveform (see Fig. 37–22), in which the balloon responds to the upstroke of the wave. This mode is particularly helpful when 60-cycle interference is encountered or when ECG leads are being changed. A third mode of triggering, called internal trigger, is used in the absence of any intrinsic electrical or mechanical activity such as when the patient is on cardiopulmonary bypass. With internal triggering inflation and deflation occur at a preset rate. This helps to prevent clot formation on a stagnant noninflating balloon.

Although the triggering signal provides the balloon with general information about inflation and deflation, its action must be *timed* precisely with the mechanical cardiac events to optimize the ef-

**TABLE 42-7. CARE PLAN FOR THE PATIENT RECEIVING TEMPORARY PACEMAKER THERAPY**

| Nursing Diagnoses | Desired Patient Outcomes | Nursing Interventions | Rationales |
|---|---|---|---|
| ***Nursing Diagnosis #1*** Alteration in cardiac output, related to pacer malfunction, dysrhythmias. | 1. Patient will demonstrate clinical behaviors consistent with an adequate cardiac output:<br>• Alert and oriented to person, place and time.<br>• Systolic blood pressure greater than 90 mmHg.<br>• Lungs clear to auscultation.<br>• Capillary refill less than 2 sec.<br>• Urine output greater than 30 ml/hour.<br>• Lack of subjective complaints verbalized prior to the pacer insertion (i.e., dizziness, fatigue).<br>• Strong peripheral pulses.<br>• Absence of jugular venous distention. | • Monitor the pacemaker parameters every shift and document:<br>○ Sensing ability.<br>○ Capture frequency.<br>○ Threshold (check level every day).<br>○ Current setting.<br>○ Mode. | • Failure of the pacemaker in any one of these functions can jeopardize patient safety.<br>–Documentation provides baseline data from which trends in condition can be detected. |
| | 2. Patient will not demonstrate pacer malfunction as evidenced by ECG analysis. | • Perform comprehensive cardiovascular assessment at least once per shift. Include:<br>○ Heart rate, rhythm.<br>○ Quality of peripheral pulses.<br>○ Heart sounds.<br>○ Color, temprature of skin. | • Baseline assessment will provide data from which comparisons can be made.<br>○ Development of additional heart sounds may reflect decreased myocardial compliance or incompetence of valves. |
| | | ○ Presence of pulsus paradoxus (a drop of the systolic blood pressure more than the normal 10 mmHg during inspiration). | ○ Decreased or muffled heart sounds, jugular venous distention, and the presence of pulsus paradoxus may reflect tamponade. |

*(continued)*

**TABLE 42–7. CARE PLAN FOR THE PATIENT RECEIVING TEMPORARY PACEMAKER THERAPY** *(Continued)*

| Nursing Diagnoses | Desired Patient Outcomes | Nursing Interventions | Rationales |
|---|---|---|---|
| ***Nursing Diagnosis #1 (cont.)*** | | ○ Blood pressure.<br>○ Quantity of urine output.<br>○ Presence of JVD.<br>○ Subjective comments. | ○ Quality of pulses, urine output, temperature, color of skin reflect tissue perfusion.<br>○ Jugular venous distention reflects elevation of right-sided heart pressures, which can be associated with tamponade. |
| | | ○ Level of consciousness.<br>○ ECG strip interpretation. | ○ First symptom of decreased cardiac output may be a change in mentation. |
| | 3. Patient will be free of hemodynamically significant dysrhythmias. | • Check pacemaker system every shift including:<br>○ Integrity of lead connections.<br>○ Battery.<br>○ Pacer generator.<br>○ Pacer settings. | • Pacemaker function may be closely assessed through strip analysis.<br>○ Ensure all components of system are functioning appropriately. |
| | | • Monitor patient for presence of dysrhythmias and document type, patient's response, any associated activity, pacer activity (i.e., inability to sense). | • Dysrhythmias may or may not be hemodynamically significant or related to pacer activity. The pacemaker may need to be adjusted. |
| | | • Notify physician at onset of any dysrhythmias. Keep Lidocaine at bedside. Ensure patent IV line is present. | • Physician may want to reposition pacing wire or initiate antiarrhythmic therapy. |
| ***Nursing Diagnosis #2***<br>Potential for injury from microshock. | 1. Patient's environment will be free of microshock hazards.<br>2. Patient will not receive microshock. | • Cover any exposed lead wires with rubber gloves, finger cots, or scotch tape.<br>• Wear rubber gloves if handling exposed wires. | • Insulating the lead wires will decrease the risk of conduction. |
| | | • Use only properly grounded equipment, including the electric bed.<br>• Inspect all electric equipment in room for signs of cord fraying. | • Improperly grounded equipment poses serious threat to patient safety. |
| | | • Do not touch patient while handling electrical equipment. | • It is possible for energy to travel through you from the equipment to the patient. |
| ***Nursing Diagnosis #3***<br>Anxiety, related to invasive procedure, "heart failure." | 1. Patient will demonstrate decreased anxiety as evidenced by:<br>• Subjective comments. | • Assess patient's understanding of situation, reasons for anxiety.<br>• Provide information in supportive manner. | • Pattern interventions to patient's level of comprehension.<br>• Establishing calm rapport will reassure patient. |
| | | • Assess patient's understanding of information provided. | • Patient's level of anxiety may prevent integration of information. |

| | | | |
|---|---|---|---|
| | • Decreased restlessness.<br>• Facial expressions.<br>• Nonverbal behavior.<br>• Ability to concentrate. | ○ Observe patient's response.<br>• Assess past coping.<br>○ Establish calm, quiet environment.<br>• Provide sedation if needed. | • Assessing past coping skills will help you develop a more effective plan of care.<br>• Sedation may be appropriate if nonpharmacologic interventions are ineffective. |
| ***Nursing Diagnosis #4***<br>Knowledge deficit, related to need for pacemaker, procedure for insertion. | 1. Patient/family will verbalize understanding of:<br>• Need for pacemaker.<br>• How pacemaker is helping the heart.<br>• Procedure for insertion. | • Assess patient/family's level of knowledge with pacemakers.<br>• Establish teaching plan, including:<br>○ Need for pacemaker.<br>○ How the pacemaker will help.<br>○ How long the procedure will take.<br>○ Sensations of events expected during insertion.<br>○ Post insertion events.<br>• Provide only necessary information.<br>• Encourage questions. | • Assessing prior level of knowledge will help in developing a more effective teaching plan.<br>○ Including family will help their understanding of events.<br>• Clarification of questions improves understanding. |
| ***Nursing Diagnosis #5***<br>Potential for infection: Invasive line placement. (See Table 49–7.) | 1. Patient will be infection-free, as evidenced by:<br>• Normal temperature.<br>• Lack of redness, heat, swelling, discharge at insertion site. | • Monitor insertion site every day and document findings.<br>• Monitor patient's temperature every 8 hr; every 4 hr if an elevation is noted.<br>• Change dressing using sterile procedure every 24 hr or per unit protocol.<br>• Change IV solution every 24 hr if a central line is present.<br>○ Culture any drainage from site, and notify the physician.<br>• Culture all catheter tips if spike in temperature is noted (i.e., central line, pacing catheter).<br>• Do not administer antipyretics for pain. | • Signs/symptoms of infection often begin at local level.<br>• Temperature elevation is a clinical sign of the immune system's activity in combating pyrogens.<br>• Frequent sterile dressing changes can prevent infections by providing an aseptic barrier once the skin integrity has become impaired.<br>• Changes in IV solution will decrease medium for bacterial growth.<br>• Identification of organism involved in the infectious process is vital for determining course of treatment.<br>• Antipyretics may mask temperature elevation and signs of infection. |
| ***Nursing Diagnosis #6***<br>Alteration in comfort, related to invasive line insertion. | 1. Patient will verbalize statements of comfort. | • Assess patient's level of comfort (verbal and nonverbal cues).<br>• Reposition patient frequently using pillows for support.<br>• Rub areas of discomfort with lotion.<br>• Provide medication for pain as needed. | • Patient may not openly admit discomfort.<br>• Repositioning will prevent development of pressure areas and fatigue of dependent sites.<br>• Rubbing areas of discomfort promotes relaxation of sore muscle groups and enhances circulation to the area.<br>• Medication can provide analgesia necessary to improve the patient's level of comfort. |

## TABLE 42–8. CARE PLAN FOR THE PATIENT WITH A PERMANENT PACEMAKER

| Nursing Diagnoses | Desired Patient Outcomes | Nursing Interventions | Rationales |
|---|---|---|---|
| ***Nursing Diagnosis #1*** Alteration in cardiac output, related to:<br>1. Pacemaker malfunction.<br>2. Pacemaker-induced dysrhythmias.<br>3. Electromagnetic interference. | 1. Patient will demonstrate clinical behaviors consistent with an adequate cardiac output:<br>• Alert and oriented to person, place, and time.<br>• Systolic blood pressure greater than 90 mmHg.<br>• Lungs clear on auscultation.<br>• Capillary refill less than 2 sec.<br>• Urine output greater than 30 ml/hr.<br>• Lack of the subjective complaints that might have been verbalized before the pacemaker insertion, indicative of low cardiac ouput (i.e., dizziness, fatigue, nausea).<br>2. Patient will not demonstrate pacemaker malfunction as evidenced by ECG analysis. | • Monitor ECG continuously for 24–48 hr after pacemaker insertion for:<br>○ Sensing ability.<br>○ Ability to capture.<br>○ Firing rate that is consistent with settings.<br>○ Frequency of pace-assist.<br>○ Presence of dysrhythmias. | • The pacemaker may "oversense" (i.e., become inhibited by other electrical potential in the body) or it may "undersense" and not recognize intrinsic cardiac activity.<br>• Conditions may develop that can increase the threshold and decrease the pacemaker's ability to capture (i.e., fibrosis at the pacing catheter tip, hypoxia, dislodgement of pacing catheter, concurrent drug therapy, electrolyte imbalance). |
| | | • Confirm that the pacemaker is firing at the preset rate. | • Determining how frequently the patient's rhythm requires pacemaker assistance will provide you with pertinent clinical information. |
| | | • CV assessment same as temporary pacer (see Table 42–7). | ○ Foreign object in ventricle can irritate the myocardium and cause dysrhythmias. |
| | 3. Patient will be free of hemodynamically significant dysrhythmias. | • Assess patient's response to dysrhythmias and communicate with physician for appropriate treatment regimen. | • The pacemaker-induced dysrhythmias may be self-limiting and hemodynamically insignificant, or they might be life-threatening. The physician should be made aware of their occurrence to determine if therapeutic intervention is warranted. |
| | | • Rule out any other potential cause of dysrhythmias (i.e., electrolyte imbalance, ischemia, hypoxia). | • Other variables in the patient's clinical picture may be causing the dysrhythmias and should be excluded before the pacing catheter is implicated. |

| | | | |
|---|---|---|---|
| | | • If cardioversion/defibrillation is required, do not place sternal paddle directly over pulse generator. Keep current approximately 10 cm away from pulse generator at all times. Anteroposterior paddle placement is strongly recommended if possible.<br>• Do not expose patient to any conditions known to cause interference:<br>◦ Nuclear magnetic resonance.<br>◦ Cautery.<br>◦ Electroconvulsive therapy.<br>◦ Electric razors. | • Discharge of high amounts of energy over the electrical circuitry can damage the pacemaker and cause malfunction.<br>• Electrical and magnetic fields can alter pacer function. |
| ***Nursing Diagnosis #2***<br>Potential for infection, related to the surgical procedure. | 1. Patient will be infection-free as evidenced by:<br>• Approximation of surgical incision.<br>• Lack of elevation of temperature.<br>• Lack of redness, swelling, discharge, heat at site of incision. | • Monitor incision site and document findings.<br>• Cleanse incision with Betadine daily; keep open to air after 24 hr.<br>• Monitor patient's temperature every 8 hr, every 4 hr if elevation noted.<br>• Do not administer antipyretics for pain. | • Signs/symptoms of infection often begin at local level.<br>• Washing the wound with antibacterial solution will prevent infection. Keeping the incision open to air will promote granulation of tissue.<br>• Temperature elevation is an accurate clinical sign of the immune system's activity in combating pyrogens.<br>• Antipyretics may mask temperature elevation and signs of infection. |
| ***Nursing Diagnosis #3***<br>Alteration in mobility, related to the surgical procedure. | 1. Patient will be able to demonstrate full range of motion in affected extremity. | • Encourage patient to perform ROM exercises 24–48 hr after the insertion to prevent stiffness of shoulder; provide passive ROM if unable. | • Stiffness in affected shoulder occurs because of surgical manipulation of large supportive muscle groups. |
| ***Nursing Diagnosis #4***<br>Anxiety, related to surgical procedure. | 1. Patient will demonstrate decreased levels of anxiety as evidenced by:<br>• Subjective comments.<br>• Decreased restlessness.<br>• Facial expressions.<br>• Nonverbal behavior.<br>• Ability to concentrate. | • Assess patient's understanding of situation, reasons for anxiety.<br>• Provide information in calm, supportive manner.<br>◦ Assess patient's understanding of information provided.<br>– Observe patient's response.<br>• Assess past coping behaviors.<br>• Establish calm, quiet environment.<br>• Provide sedation if needed. | • Pattern interventions to patient's level of comprehension.<br>• Establishing calming rapport will reassure patient.<br>◦ Patient's level of anxiety may prevent integration of information.<br>• Assessing patient's coping skills will help you develop a more effective plan of care.<br>• Sedation may be appropriate if nonpharmacologic interventions are ineffective. |

(continued)

**TABLE 42–8. CARE PLAN FOR THE PATIENT WITH A PERMANENT PACEMAKER *(Continued)***

| Nursing Diagnoses | Desired Patient Outcomes | Nursing Interventions | Rationales |
|---|---|---|---|
| ***Nursing Diagnosis #5***<br>Potential disturbance in self-concept after dependence on the pacemaker, disfigurement. | 1. Patient will verbalize acceptance of the pacemaker as integral part of body. | • Assess patient's level of comfort with the pacemaker. Note comments related to:<br>∘ Dependence on "a machine."<br>∘ Fear of malfunction.<br>∘ Insecurity, embarrassment about cosmetic appearance.<br>∘ Loss of self-control and independence.<br>• Encourage patient to ventilate concerns; reassure and counsel to dispel misconceptions.<br>• Assess past coping mechanisms and apply if pertinent.<br>∘ Consult psychiatry if necessary.<br>• Have patient speak with another recipient of permanent pacemaker.<br>• Refer to support group (if applicable). | • Patients often have difficulty accepting the pacemaker because it is a continual reminder that they have a cardiac condition and because of its limited lifespan.<br>• Many patients have misunderstandings that promote disturbances.<br>• Past coping mechanisms will indicate adaptive/maladaptive behavior.<br>• Recognition that problems are not unique provides comfort and strength for recovery. |
| ***Nursing Diagnosis #6***<br>Knowledge deficit, related to:<br>1. Indication for permanent pacer.<br>2. How it will function.<br>3. Monitoring pacer function.<br>4. Signs and symptoms of malfunction.<br>5. Return to prior lifestyle.<br>6. Changes in lifestyle. | 1. Patient/family will verbalize understanding of:<br>• Indication for permanent pacer.<br>• How it will function.<br>• Signs and symptoms of malfunction.<br>• Monitoring pacer function.<br>• Return to prior lifestyle. | • Assess patient/family level of knowledge regarding pertinent information.<br>• Develop teaching plan specific to their learning needs.<br>• Provide written information for reference of the material covered.<br>• Explain in layman's terms:<br>∘ Purpose of conduction system.<br>∘ Why patient needs pacer.<br>∘ How it will work to *supplement* the patient's cardiac activity. | • Written materials are helpful references when at home.<br>• Understanding will improve patient's ability to care for self.<br>∘ A common misperception is that the pacer is *replacing* patient's own heart function.<br>∘ Must be able to identify specifics about pacemaker should it malfunction. |

| | | | |
|---|---|---|---|
| 7. Medical alert information.<br>8. Electrical precautions.<br>9. Follow-up care. | • Changes in lifestyle.<br>• Medical alert information.<br>• Electrical precautions.<br>• Follow-up care.<br>2. Patient and/or family member will demonstrate how to measure pulse rate with 100% accuracy. | – Signs and symptoms of malfunction (relate to signs/symptoms patient presented with if applicable).<br>– Changes in lifestyle required.<br>– Need to carry Medic-Alert card with pacer information at all times—use of bracelet or necklace.<br>– Follow-up care.<br>○ Electrical precautions:<br>– Magnetic fields (i.e., store theft devices, some microwaves, radar).<br>– Electrical fields (i.e., electric razors, cautery).<br>• Demonstrate to patient/family how to check pulse.<br>○ Have patient/family do return demonstration with 100% accuracy. | ○ Magnetic/electrical fields may cause interference with electrical circuitry; ability of pacemaker to function.<br>• Patient needs to monitor appropriate functioning of the pacemaker. |

TABLE 42-9
**Indications for Intra-aortic Balloon Pumping**

| Clinical Condition | Rationale |
|---|---|
| 1. Preinfarction angina<br>2. Acute myocardial infarction<br>3. Cardiogenic shock | To improve coronary perfusion, decrease left ventricular work, and reduce the amount of myocardium that is damaged. |
| 4. Refractory ventricular arrhythmias related to ischemias | To improve perfusion to the ischemic area causing firing of an ectopic focus. To reduce myocardial oxygen demand. |
| 5. Severe mitral regurgitation<br>6. Severe ventricular septal defect | To improve left ventricular emptying, encouraging forward flow of blood, and reduce the severity of regurgitation or shunting. |
| 7. Pre-open-heart surgery or cardiac transplantation. | To support the heart until surgical intervention can ameliorate the underlying problem. |
| 8. Intra-operative open heart surgery/weaning from cardiopulmonary bypass<br>9. Post-open-heart surgery | To support the ventricle until it recovers from surgery. |
| 10. Low cardiac output syndromes<br>11. Septic shock | To promote adequate tissue perfusion by assisting left ventricular emptying. |
| 12. Prophylaxis | To prevent cardiac decompensation, myocardial damage in high-risk situations (i.e., noncardiac surgeries in the presence of severe left ventricular dysfunction, high-risk PTCA). |

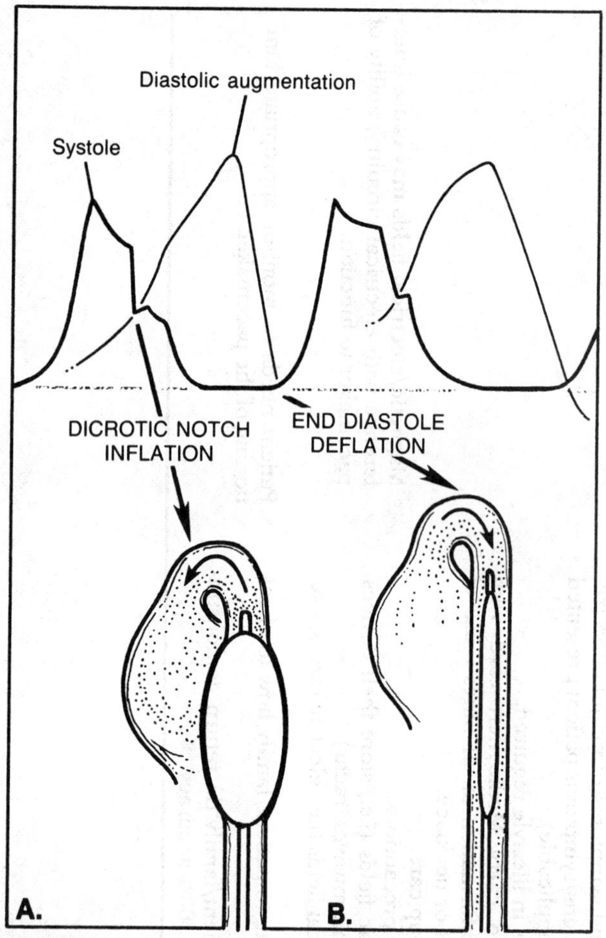


**Figure 42-3.** Intra-aortic balloon pumping and the cardiac cycle reflecting systole and diastole. Balloon inflation and deflation is depicted with inflation occurring at the dicrotic notch, and deflation occurring just prior to the next upstroke of the systolic wave. Diastolic augmentation reflects the increase in aortic pressures afforded by an inflated balloon during left ventricular diastole thereby increasing coronary artery perfusion pressures.

fects of counterpulsation. It is important to remember that the electrical events reflected on the surface ECG occur before mechanical events are recorded on the arterial tracing. It is therefore essential to monitor a continuous arterial waveform to allow for minute adjustments in balloon inflation and deflation (Fig. 42-3A). Ideally, when monitoring an arterial pressure waveform, inflation should occur at the dicrotic notch. The dicrotic notch reflects closure of the aortic valve. Deflation should occur just prior to the next upstroke of the systolic wave, as illustrated in Figure 42-3B.

When the balloon inflates at the beginning of diastole, the blood located in that segment of the aorta is forced back into the aortic arch, increasing the amount of pressure with which the coronary arteries are perfused. This increase in aortic pressure during diastole is known as *diastolic augmentation.* Augmentation of coronary perfusion during ischemic events is critical in offsetting the imbalance between oxygen supply and demand. The myocardium is extremely efficient in its extraction of oxygen, such that the *only* way to meet greater metabolic needs is to increase the amount of blood circulating through the tissue. In the presence of occlusive coronary artery disease, it becomes increasingly difficult to meet these demands.

Upon deflation of the balloon before systole, there is a redistribution of blood away from the aortic root, thereby decreasing the pressure against which the left ventricle must work in order to open the aortic valve. This reduction in afterload is known as *diastolic unloading.* Diastolic unloading also decreases myocardial oxygen demands significantly, thereby assisting a jeopardized ischemic myocardium from becoming more ischemic.

## Insertion of the Balloon

There are two techniques used for initiating balloon pumping: surgical and percutaneous. The surgical technique requires the performance of a femoral arteriotomy and is usually done in the operating room. This method is relatively time consuming and exposes the patient to greater risks due to the surgical nature of the incision. The advent of the percutaneous technique made balloon pumping a much more attractive treatment modality because of the relative ease with which insertion could occur.

The percutaneous insertion procedure can be performed at the bedside, with or without fluoroscopy, and takes approximately 15–20 minutes. The pre-wrapped balloon is placed via a large-lumen introducer sheath into the left common femoral artery and threaded into the thoracic descending aorta to lie just below the left subclavian artery. Once the balloon has been placed, it is filled with gas and pumping is initiated. Placement of the balloon is then confirmed by fluoroscopy and/or x-ray.

Balloon pumping can occur at a number of frequencies relative to the cardiac cycle depending on the amount of support required by the left ventricle. The balloon can inflate and deflate with each ejection (1:1 frequency), with every other ejection (1:2), or with every third ejection (1:3). The usual frequency of balloon pumping initially is 1:1 since the left ventricle is generally in need of significant support during the early hours or days of balloon pumping. As the myocardium recovers, the frequency of assist is decreased to 1:2, and then to 1:3. On average, the intra-aortic balloon pump is utilized for a period of 2–4 days, during which time hemodynamic support with pharmacologic agents is maximized. Once the patient's condition has remained stable for a 24-hour period and stable hemodynamic parameters have been achieved, balloon support is withdrawn.

Because the work of the left ventricle has been assisted for a period of time, it is important to *wean* the patient from the IABP gradually. This is usually accomplished by decreasing the frequency with which balloon pumping occurs (i.e., 1:2, then 1:3). Reduction of the total filling volume of the balloon may also be used as a method to wean the patient off balloon assist.

Clinical parameters utilized in determining when a patient is capable of being weaned from the IABP include:

1. Evidence of adequate cardiac function.
   a. Cardiac index greater than 2.0 liters/min-ute/$m^2$.
   b. Pulmonary capillary wedge pressure less than 18–20 mmHg.
   c. Urine output greater than 30 ml/hour.
   d. Return of peripheral pulse quality to patient baseline.
   e. Absence of subjective complaints of shortness of breath.
   f. Breath sounds clear.
   g. Skin warm and dry.
   h. Mentation returned to baseline.
2. Evidence of resolution of myocardial ischemia.
   a. Absence of chest pain.
   b. ECG reflects absence of acute ischemia.
   c. Dysrhythmias related to ischemia have resolved.

During the weaning period, the patient's clinical response must be closely monitored for signs of left ventricular failure or recurrence of myocardial ischemia, since it is possible to develop dependence on the balloon for hemodynamic support and augmentation of coronary perfusion. Once weaning has occurred successfully, the deflated balloon is withdrawn from the aorta along with the introducer sheath and direct pressure is maintained at the femoral site for approximately 30 minutes.

## Contraindications for Intra-aortic Balloon Pumping

Intra-aortic balloon pumping is initiated as a temporary adjunct to conventional methods of therapy to improve coronary perfusion and support the left ventricle during acute cardiac events. As with any method of treatment, there are certain conditions that preclude use of counterpulsation. Patient benefit, end goal of treatment regimen, and risks posed by insertion of the balloon catheter must be considered before the IABP is placed. Table 42–10 summarizes these absolute and relative contraindications to IABP therapy.

TABLE 42–10
**Contraindications for Intra-aortic Balloon Pumping**

| Clinical Condition | Rationale |
|---|---|
| ***Absolute Contraindications*** | |
| Aortic aneurysm | High risk of aortic dissection. |
| Bypass grafting from the aorta to peripheral vessels | |
| Aortic insufficiency | Inflation of the intra-aortic balloon during diastole will exacerbate the regurgitant flow into the left ventricle. |
| ***Relative Contraindications*** | |
| Peripheral or central atherosclerosis | High risk of vascular compromise distal to the balloon.<br>High risk of plaque dislodgement.<br>Inability to pass catheter. |
| Age<br>Severe left ventricular dysfunction<br>Multisystem failure<br>Chronic, debilitating disease | Ethical considerations are necessary to determine whether there is a treatment regimen available that will improve the current quality of life before intervention with IABP is instituted. |
| Bleeding disorders | High risk for hemorrhage. |
| History of embolic phenomena | High risk for thromboembolic events with IABP catheter. |

### Complications of Intra-aortic Balloon Pumping

There are a number of complications that can occur from insertion and maintenance of the IABP in the aorta. Upon insertion, it is possible that the balloon catheter may dissect any part of the arterial system through which it travels (femoral, iliac, aorta), or it may dislodge a plaque, causing embolization. The placement of the balloon itself may cause problems once inserted. If the catheter is too advanced, it can occlude the left subclavian artery, causing diminished flow to the left arm, or it can hinder flow cephalad. If the catheter is not advanced far enough, it can occlude the renal arteries, compromising perfusion of the kidneys. It is also possible, because of a severe state of atherosclerosis, that the catheter cannot be threaded at all in some patients.

Once the balloon has been placed, possible complications include balloon rupture, embolization, arterial occlusion, mechanical destruction of RBCs because of pumping, or inability to wean from the pump.

During removal of the catheter, it is again possible to fragment or puncture the intima of the vessel, cause embolization, or cause a hematoma at the insertion site.

### Nursing Considerations

The care of the patient requiring intra-aortic balloon support is complex and requires specific training to coordinate all aspects of hemodynamic support. Much attention is centered around monitoring the patient's response to treatment, identifying and treating actual problems, and preventing potential problems. Because of all the equipment and treatments required for the critically ill people who need IABP therapy, it is often possible to lose sight of the human factor in care. These patients are usually alert and frightened by the technical support that is required to sustain them. It is imperative for the nurse to provide support and comfort to the patient and family in addition to coordinating other aspects of care. (See Table 42–11, Care Plan for the Patient Requiring Intra-aortic Balloon Pumping.)

## PERCUTANEOUS TRANSLUMINAL CORONARY ANGIOPLASTY (PTCA)

### Goal of PTCA

Percutaneous transluminal coronary angioplasty (PTCA) is a nonsurgical method of revascularizing myocardial tissue. Goals of treatment include:

1. Prevention of myocardial necrosis.
2. Reduction of myocardial ischemia.
3. Limitation of myocardial infarct size.
4. Improvement of left ventricular function.
5. Reduction in morbidity and mortality associated with CAD.

### Indications for PTCA

Percutaneous transluminal coronary angioplasty has become a major treatment modality for occlusive coronary artery disease and can be used as an alternative to coronary bypass surgery or medical therapy. It is indicated for prophylactic treatment of severe CAD before infarction has occurred, in the presence of symptomatic coronary artery disease, or during an acute infarction. PTCA is a viable treatment option for stenosis of grafted vessels. It is possible to revascularize multiple vessels at once, but the occlusive lesions must be amenable to dilatation.

Selection of the patients for angioplasty is somewhat dependent upon the institution and the preference of the interventional therapist. Several clinical situations are common indications for resolution of coronary stenosis by PTCA. Single-vessel or multiple-vessel disease associated with recent onset of angina and clinical signs of ischemia with distinct, subtotal lesions not located at the orifice or bifurcation of a coronary artery can benefit from dilatation. Patients with acute evolving myocardial infarctions may be treated with PTCA alone or in conjunction with thrombolytic therapy. Stenotic lesions in bypass grafts may be amenable to dilatation if the lesion is not diffuse and not located in an anatomically difficult location. Many patients who receive angioplasty reocclude and require 2 or 3 redilatations. However, benefit to the patient or safety in performing a PTCA cannot be ensured in certain clinical conditions.

### Relative Contraindications

Percutaneous transluminal coronary angioplasty is contraindicated in the setting of severe diffuse coronary atherosclerosis because of the tissue's inability to revascularize. Persons who are considered for treatment with PTCA must be suitable candidates for coronary artery bypass grafting should PTCA fail or complications ensue necessitating emergent open heart surgery. The presence of severe central (i.e., aortic, iliac) and peripheral atherosclerotic diseases presents difficulties because of the need to cannulate the femoral artery and pass a catheter into the aorta.

**TABLE 42-11. CARE PLAN FOR THE PATIENT REQUIRING INTRA-AORTIC BALLOON PUMPING**

| Nursing Diagnoses | Desired Patient Outcomes | Nursing Interventions | Rationales |
|---|---|---|---|
| ***Nursing Diagnosis #1*** Potential alteration in tissue perfusion, related to myocardial ischemia, peripheral vascular disease, embolic phenomena. | 1. The patient will demonstrate adequate tissue perfusion as evidenced by:<br>• Absence of angina.<br>• Capillary refill of less than 2 sec.<br>• Warm extremities.<br>• No change in baseline peripheral pulse quality.<br>• Normal respiratory effort.<br>• Sensorium alert and oriented. | • Check peripheral pulse quality, compare with baseline every hour, and document findings. | • Peripheral ischemia or occlusion may occur due to embolization or diminished flow distal to the catheter. |
| | | • Place patient in vascular position (reverse Trendelenburg). | • Vascular position promotes blood flow to the peripheral bed. |
| | | • Monitor patient for complaints of chest pain, shortness of breath, peripheral pain. | • Complaints of pain can be indicative of ischemia or embolization.<br>◦ Sudden onset of shortness of breath can indicate development of pulmonary edema or pulmonary embolism. |
| | | • Assess color and temperature of extremities with peripheral pulse checks, and compare bilaterally. | • The circulation distal to the IABP catheter is most at risk for compromised flow. |
| | | • Avoid flexion of patient at hips. | • This may cause migration of balloon catheter upward in the aorta.<br>◦ If the balloon catheter migrates forward it will occlude the left subclavian or carotid artery, causing diminished flow to the areas they service. |
| | | • Monitor left radial pulse quality (or arterial waveform if present), mentation, complaints of dizziness. | |
| | | • Place a sheet over the leg in which the balloon is inserted for restraint of movement. | • This will minimize the possibility of catheter migration cephalad. |
| ***Nursing Diagnosis #2*** Impaired physical mobility, related to cannulation of femoral artery. | 1. Patient will maintain range of motion in all extremities except cannulated leg. | • Position patient with head of bed at 30-degree angle. | • This will permit swallowing and performance of some self-care activities. Elevation of head of bed greater than 30 degrees will cause hip flexion and may encourage migration of the IABP catheter. |
| | | • Encourage patient to perform ROM exercises in all extremities except the cannulated leg. | • Maintenance of muscular tone. |
| | | • Reposition patient frequently, log-rolling from side to side. | • Repositioning of patient will maintain use of muscle groups. The patient must be log-rolled to maintain alignment of the cannulated extremity. |
| | | • Have patient continue ankle and foot exercises in affected leg. | • Ankle and foot exercises will help maintain full ROM of these areas without jeopardizing the catheter placement. |

*(continued)*

**TABLE 42-11. CARE PLAN FOR THE PATIENT REQUIRING INTRA-AORTIC BALLOON PUMPING *(Continued)***

| Nursing Diagnoses | Desired Patient Outcomes | Nursing Interventions | Rationales |
|---|---|---|---|
| ***Nursing Diagnosis #3***<br>Potential alteration in cardiac output, related to left ventricular dysfunction, dysrhythmias | 1. Adequate cardiac output will be maintained as evidenced by:<br>• MAP 70–90 mmHg.<br>• Urine output >30 ml/hour.<br>• Cardiac index >2.0 liters/minute/$m^2$.<br>• PCWP <20 mmHg.<br>• SVR 800–1200 dyne-seconds/$cm^{-5}$. | • Monitor the following hemodynamic parameters every 15–30 minutes:<br>○ Systolic and diastolic blood pressure, mean arterial pressure, diastolic augmentation.<br>○ Heart rate.<br>○ Pulmonary artery systolic, diastolic, and mean pressures.<br>○ Urine output every hour.<br>○ CVP, PCWP.<br>○ CO/CI, SVR. | • Ongoing assessment of clinical data is necessary to detect changes in left ventricular function. |
| | | • Check balloon timing every hour or more frequently with changes in heart rate +10%.<br>• Monitor for dysrhythmias. Note patient's hemodynamic response.<br>• If patient is tachycardic (HR greater than 150 bpm) it may be necessary to change IABP frequency to 1:2.<br>• If CPR is required, turn balloon to 1:3 frequency and decrease the volume to minimal level. | • Timing must be precise to optimize effects of IABP.<br>• Dysrhythmias may or may not affect cardiac output.<br>• At high heart rate, shuttling of gas and ability of IABP to inflate and deflate may be compromised.<br>• It is impossible to coordinate IABP with resuscitative efforts, but the balloon should never remain still in the aorta because of the risk of thrombus formation. |
| ***Nursing Diagnosis #4***<br>Anxiety (patient/family). | 1. Patient/family will verbalize feelings of anxiety.<br>2. Patient/family will demonstrate relaxed demeanor as evidenced by verbal and nonverbal clues. | • Explain all aspects of treatment or care to patient/family.<br>• Explain/describe all expected equipment, sounds before they occur.<br>• Maintain interpersonal contact throughout performance of technical care.<br>• Approach patient and family with confident, calm, professional behavior. | • Understanding of patient care activities minimizes misconceptions and fears.<br>• Anticipation of sights and sounds helps prepare the patient.<br>• Recognition of human factor amidst technology is vital.<br>• Patient/family must have confidence in caregivers. |
| ***Nursing Diagnosis #5***<br>Potential alteration in sensory perception, related to sensory overload | 1. Patient will demonstrate lucid mentation as evidenced by:<br>• Appropriate conversation.<br>• Orientation to person, place, and time. | • Maintain quiet, soothing environment.<br>• Attempt to preserve day/night sleep cycle.<br>• Ensure patient has adequate sleep periods.<br>• Restrict traffic around patient's bed; coordinate care to minimize disruptions.<br>• Assess patient's mentation.<br>• Reorient as necessary. | • Interventions are designed to minimize overstimulation, which can contribute to disorientation. |

| | | | |
|---|---|---|---|
| ***Nursing Diagnosis #6*** Potential for infection, related to indwelling catheters. (See Table 49–7.) | 1. Patient will be free of infection as evidenced by:<br>• Lack of temperature elevation.<br>• Lack of redness, heat, swelling, or discharge at catheter insertion site. | • Maintain meticulous handwashing.<br>• Change femoral dressing with aseptic technique.<br>○ Observe insertion site for signs and symptoms of infection.<br>• Monitor temperature every 4–8 hr.<br>○ Do not administer antipyretics for pain.<br>• Meticulous perineal and Foley care. | • Handwashing decreases incidence of nosocomial infections.<br>• Sterile dressings protect site from organisms.<br>• Temperature elevation is an accurate clinical sign of the immune system's activity in combating pyrogens.<br>○ Antipyretics may mask temperature elevation and signs of infection.<br>○ Signs and symptoms of infection often begin at a local site.<br>• Maintain area free of contamination. |
| ***Nursing Diagnosis #7*** Potential for physiologic injury: Bleeding, related to:<br>1. Indwelling arterial catheter.<br>2. Concomitant anticoagulation. | 1. Patient will not have active bleeding as evidenced by:<br>• Stable hematocrit, hemoglobin levels.<br>• Guaiac-free stools.<br>• Absence of hematoma, bruising, or ecchymosis.<br>• Stable blood pressure and heart rate. | • Monitor laboratory values indicative of bleeding status (PTT, hematocrit, hemoglobin).<br>• Monitor all stools for presence of occult blood.<br>• Inspect the patient for oozing and hematoma formation at the catheter insertion site.<br>○ Inspect the flank area for retroperitoneal ecchymosis. Generally inspect the skin for evidence of bleeding.<br>• Apply pressure dressing, direct pressure manually or with a C-clamp if bleeding is noted at the insertion site.<br>• Monitor the patient's blood pressure and heart rate for evidence of diminished intravascular volume. | • PTT will identify the ability of patient's blood to form clots. The hematocrit and hemoglobin will identify the level of circulating red blood cells.<br>• Anticoagulation can promote internal bleeding.<br>• Most common site of bleeding is the catheter insertion site.<br>○ Retroperitoneal ecchymosis may indicate dissection of the iliac artery upon insertion.<br>• Stasis of blood can be achieved by application of pressure to the site of bleeding.<br>• Unexplained drop in systolic pressure with concurrent rise in heart rate may indicate active bleeding. |

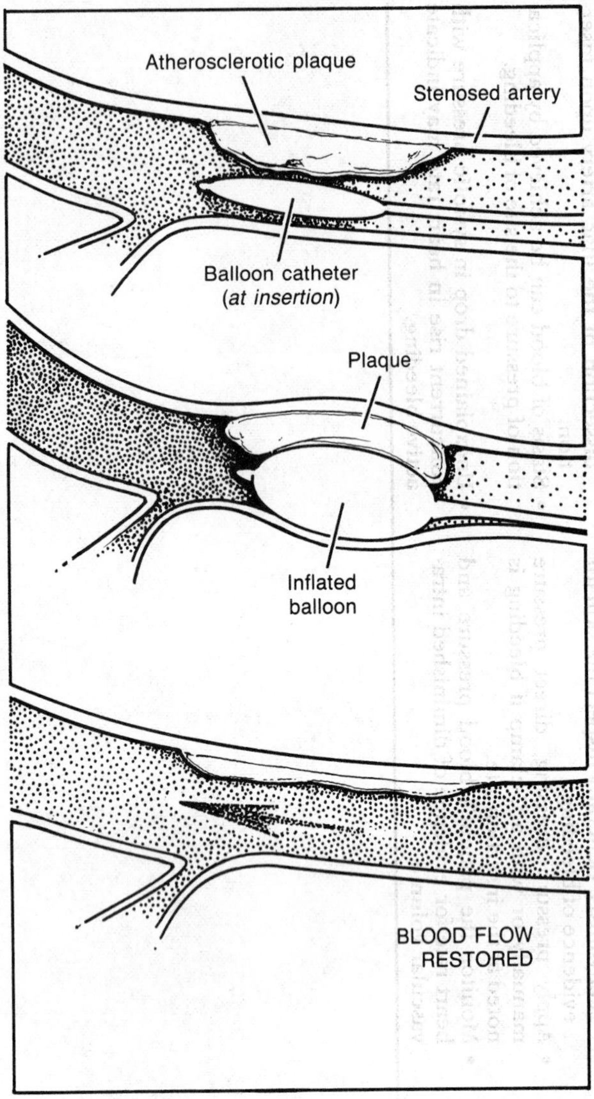


**Figure 42-2.** Electrocardiographic examples of artificial cardiac pacing. (See text for discussion. ■ indicates pacer spike.)

## Technique

PTCA is a relatively simple procedure that is performed under fluoroscopy in the cardiac catheterization laboratory. Using aseptic technique, the femoral artery and vein are cannulated with introducer sheaths via a percutaneous approach.

A steerable catheter very similar to the one utilized for cardiac catheterization with a balloon at the tip is threaded into the coronary artery through the femoral arterial sheath. Once the catheter has passed into the coronary artery, it must be positioned so that the balloon is resting at the site of coronary stenosis (Fig. 42-4). The balloon is expanded over the plaque for 10-15 seconds to actually compress or flatten the plaque. During this inflation period, blood flow distal to the balloon is compromised. This sequence of inflation and deflation is repeated until improved coronary artery perfusion is noted.

## Complications of PTCA

Complications of PTCA have been the subject of intense study and can often be correlated with the complexity of the specific case. The occurrence of complications with this procedure can be attributed to many factors. Inflation of a balloon at the site of a stenotic, fixed lesion within a coronary artery can lead to rupture or dissection of the vessel. Catheter manipulation of vascular obstructions can lead to embolic events. Concurrent anticoagulation helps to minimize the risk of thromboembolism, but predisposes the patient to bleeding events, ranging from oozing of blood or hematoma formation at the insertion site to significant blood loss. Insertion of a catheter within the vascular system can cause dissection at any location. Dysrhythmias can occur from catheter irritation of the myocardium or temporary occlusion of a coronary artery during inflation, or may be related to reperfusion of ischemic tissue. Table 42-12 lists the potential complications that may result from a PTCA.

The patient is monitored in the hospital for 1 or 2 days following PTCA to ensure that acute reocclusion does not occur. Pharmacologic therapy is typically initiated to prevent coronary vasospasms, assist coronary artery flow, and reduce the risk of platelet aggregation at the site of the dilated lesion. Commonly prescribed medications include calcium channel blockers, nitrates, and aspirin or dipyridamole (Persantine).

## Nursing Considerations

The patient requiring a PTCA has a disease that is often difficult to accept because of the inability to "see" something wrong. Unless acute symptoms of severe coronary artery disease allow the patient to

TABLE 42-12
**Potential Complications of Percutaneous Transluminal Coronary Angioplasty**

| |
|---|
| Acute coronary occlusion-myocardial infarction |
| Internal tear of the coronary vessel wall |
| Dissection of coronary artery |
| Inability to dilate the stenosis |
| Embolization of plaque fragments |
| Restenosis of the coronary artery: Acute, chronic |
| Bleeding/hematoma |
| Dissection of the aorta, iliac, or femoral arteries |
| Compromise of peripheral circulation |
| Dysrhythmias |

perceive a health threat, it may be hard for the patient to integrate the notion that lifestyle changes are required because of a risk of a severe heart attack. It is a challenge for the nurse to address these educational issues as well as monitor the patient for actual and potential complications of the procedure. (See Table 42–13, Care Plan for the Patient with Percutaneous Transluminal Coronary Angioplasty.)

## THROMBOLYTIC THERAPY

### Goals of Thrombolytic Therapy

Thrombolytic therapy is a therapeutic modality used for occlusive coronary artery disease in which a pharmacologic agent is administered for the purpose of dissolving thrombi formed at the site of an atherosclerotic lesion. The major goals of thrombolytic therapy are very similar to any other method of revascularization, and include:

1. Improving coronary artery perfusion.
2. Limiting the extent of myocardial ischemia/infarction.
3. Improving left ventricular function.
4. Limiting dysrhythmias related to ischemia.
5. Improving morbidity and mortality related to CAD.

### Indications

Because myocardial necrosis can begin within 20 minutes after onset of ischemia, and progresses through the myocardial layers within 3–6 hours, thrombolytic therapy is indicated for that patient population in which complete myocardial necrosis has not occurred (i.e., patients in the early stages of an acute myocardial infarction). Specific clinical criteria have been established based on clinical research studies to identify those patients who are most likely to benefit from thrombolytic therapy. These criteria are:

1. Acute chest pain with clinical presentation of acute myocardial infarction.
2. ECG changes that reflect acute myocardial ischemia.
3. Lack of relief of chest pain with nitroglycerin administration.
4. Initiation of treatment within the first 6 hours after symptom onset.

The use of a thrombolytic agent is merely a temporizing measure for reperfusion of the myocardium since it has been noted that fresh coronary thrombi are present at the site of atherosclerotic lesions in a majority of patients experiencing an acute myocardial infarction. Oftentimes, more conventional methods of treating the underlying coronary artery disease are then required (i.e., coronary bypass grafting or PTCA).

### Types of Thrombolytic Agents

Ideally, a thrombolytic agent must be able to specifically dissolve the clot within the coronary artery without disrupting the integrity of the patient's blood clotting system. The 2 pharmacologic agents currently used for thrombolytic therapy of coronary artery occlusions are streptokinase and tissue-plasminogen activator (tPA).

Streptokinase, an enzyme produced by beta-hemolytic streptococci, has been the primary coronary thrombolytic agent used. It acts by stimulating the conversion of plasminogen to plasmin within the circulation, thereby promoting the destruction of fibrin clots.

Tissue plasminogen activator (tPA or Activase), recently approved for use in the setting of coronary artery thrombosis, is a naturally occurring human enzyme that acts with greater fibrin specificity by converting plasminogen to plasmin *after* it binds to fibrin clots. It is believed to achieve clot lysis more rapidly and with greater efficacy than streptokinase, and its positive effect in salvaging left ventricular function has been conclusively demonstrated in clinical trials.

### Relative Contraindications

Thrombolytic agents not only interfere with the blood's ability to form clots, they are also unable to differentiate the offensive coronary artery thrombus from other protective clots that develop in response to vascular injury. Additionally, because streptokinase is produced by the beta-hemolytic streptococci, it is antigenic to many individuals. Table 42–14 summarizes the conditions that may preclude the use of thrombolytic agents in the treatment of acute myocardial ischemia.

### Technique of Thrombolytic Therapy with Streptokinase

Streptokinase may be given by intracoronary or intravenous routes of administration. Each of these approaches has its relative merits. Intracoronary administration of the drug is ideal because the drug is delivered right to the site of the thrombus, and this may improve the drug's thrombolytic effect. This requires a cardiac catheterization, which is time consuming, requires greater medical resources, and poses increased risk to the patient.

Because time is of the essence in this treatment modality, the use of intravenous streptokinase has

## TABLE 42-13. CARE PLAN FOR THE PATIENT WITH PERCUTANEOUS TRANSLUMINAL CORONARY ANGIOPLASTY

| Nursing Diagnoses | Desired Patient Outcomes | Nursing Interventions | Rationales |
|---|---|---|---|
| ***Nursing Diagnosis #1***<br>Anxiety, related to upcoming procedure. | 1. Patient will demonstrate decreased anxiety as evidenced by:<br>• Subjective comments.<br>• Decreased restlessness.<br>• Facial expressions.<br>• Nonverbal behavior.<br>• Ability to concentrate. | • Assess patient's understanding of the procedure, any past experiences or misconceptions, and reasons for anxiety.<br>• Provide information based on assessment in a calm, concise manner.<br>• Assess the patient's understanding of the information provided, noting nonverbal cues.<br>• Assess patient's past coping behaviors.<br>• Establish calm, quiet environment.<br>• Provide sedation if needed. | • Identifying patient's level of comprehension and contributing factors to anxiety will allow for clarification through provisions of meaningful information.<br>• Information will be integrated if it is perceived as meaningful.<br>• Patient's anxiety level may prevent integration of information.<br>• Assessing patient's coping skills will help you develop a more effective plan of care<br>• Environmental stimuli can add to anxiety level.<br>• Sedation may be appropriate to decrease catecholamine release and minimize myocardial oxygen demand if nonpharmacologic interventions are ineffective. |
| ***Nursing Diagnosis #2***<br>Potential alteration in comfort, related to: Myocardial ischemia, immobility. | 1. Patient will remain pain-free as evidenced by lack of verbalization of symptoms of angina.<br>2. Patient will promptly report any symptoms of angina and will verbalize rapid relief after intervention.<br>3. Patient will verbalize comfort during period of immobility. | • Instruct patient to report immediately any discomfort. Emphasize the importance of this responsibility.<br>• Assess the patient for signs and symptoms of angina.<br>• Assess type of discomfort along with associated symptoms and compare with presenting symptoms.<br>• Perform stat ECG; note ST segment changes.<br>• Notify physician immediately of any complaints of chest pain or changes in condition.<br>• Administer sublingual nitroglycerin, procardia, or IV nitroglycerin as per protocol.<br>• Instruct patient that although he/she must lie flat during the time interval that the introducer sheaths remain in and for 6 hours after sheaths are removed, there are measures that can be taken to improve his/her comfort level.<br>○ Place eggcrate or air mattress on bed.<br>○ Elevate head of bed 30 degrees. | • Many patients are afraid or do not understand the implications of chest pain after the procedure.<br>• Manifestations of angina may mimic gastric distress.<br>• It is important to differentiate pain of cardiac angina.<br>• ECG will reflect changes consistent with ischemia.<br>○ May need to repeat procedure.<br>• Vasodilation with nitrates and antispasmodic medication is needed to improve coronary perfusion.<br>• Reassurance that this immobility is limited promotes compliance, tolerance.<br>○ Interventions are patterned to minimize time lying flat on back. |

| | | | |
|---|---|---|---|
| | | ◦ Reposition patient on side with pillows. Place rolled towel under small of back.<br>◦ Medicate as necessary.<br>◦ Provide diversional activities. | |
| ***Nursing Diagnosis #3***<br>Potential alteration in tissue perfusion, related to cannulation of femoral artery. | 1. Patient will demonstrate adequate tissue perfusion of extremities as evidenced by:<br>• No change in peripheral pulse quality from baseline.<br>• No change in color, sensitivity, or movement from baseline.<br>• Brisk capillary refill (less than 2 seconds). | • Check bilateral pedal pulse quality every 15–30 minutes until sheaths are pulled.<br>◦ After sheaths are pulled, check pulse quality every 30 minutes times 4 then every hour for 6 hours. Mark location of pulse with pen.<br>◦ Compare findings with baseline.<br>• Place patient in mild vascular position (reverse Trendelenburg)<br>• Remind patient not to bend at waist.<br>• Instruct patient to report any pain, tingling, or numbness immediately. | • The circulation of the extremity distal to the sheath insertion is at high risk for compromise of flow during the period of time that the sheaths remain in and immediately after their removal.<br>• Vascular position promotes flow to lower extremities.<br>• Bending at waist could cause puncture of cannulated artery.<br>• Pain, tingling, or numbness of the cannulated extremity can indicate vascular compromise and decreased tissue perfusion. |
| ***Nursing Diagnosis #4***<br>Potential for physiologic injury: Bleeding, related to:<br>1. Cannulation of an artery.<br>2. Concomitant anticoagulation. | 1. Patient will evidence no bleeding at site of sheath insertion or retroperitoneal area. | • Check femoral insertion site every 15–30 minutes with pulse checks.<br>• Assess the integrity of the sheaths. Ensure that the dilator remains within the arterial cannula.<br>• Assess for oozing, hematoma formation.<br>• Place 5-lb sandbag over site of insertion.<br>• Instruct patient to report any warmth in groin or leg area or sharp flank pain.<br>• Monitor PTT levels.<br>• Assess patient for retroperitoneal ecchymosis. Notify physician immediately if present.<br>• Place direct pressure over site for 20 minutes, or until bleeding stops. | • Bleeding frequently occurs at the sheath insertion site.<br>• The dilator prevents blood from flowing out of the arterial cannula. If the dilator is not in completely, blood loss can occur.<br>• Frank oozing can occur around the cannulae, or hematomas can occur within the subcutaneous tissue.<br>• Sandbag promotes hemostasis at insertion site by providing direct pressure.<br>• Warmth may indicate unintentional blood flow from the cannulae. Flank pain may indicate iliac dissection, peritoneal bleeding.<br>• PTT is indicative of clotting ability and will help direct therapy with heparin. The goal of treatment is to prevent reocclusion of the artery that was dilated.<br>• May indicate femoral or iliac dissection, internal bleeding.<br>• Direct pressure prevents blood loss and promotes hemostasis. |

(continued)

**TABLE 42–13. CARE PLAN FOR THE PATIENT WITH PERCUTANEOUS TRANSLUMINAL CORONARY ANGIOPLASTY *(Continued)***

| Nursing Diagnoses | Desired Patient Outcomes | Nursing Interventions | Rationales |
|---|---|---|---|
| ***Nursing Diagnosis #5***<br>Potential alteration in cardiac output, related to:<br>1. Left ventricular dysfunction.<br>2. Sheath removal.<br>3. Dysrhythmias.<br>4. Orthostatic hypotension. | 1. Patient will exhibit cardiac output adequate for tissue perfusion as evidenced by:<br>• Systolic blood pressure greater than 90 mmHg.<br>• No change in mentation.<br>• Brisk capillary refill time less than 2 seconds.<br>• Urinary output greater than 30 ml/hour. | • Assess vital signs, rhythm, mentation, capillary refill every 15–30 minutes until sheath removal, then every 30 minutes for 6 hours. Notify physician with status changes.<br>• Assess urinary output every hour.<br>• Assess peripheral circulation with vital signs.<br>• Assess patient's mentation along with vital signs.<br>• Encourage fluid intake after procedure.<br>• Monitor patient's response to sheath removal, direct groin pressure. Observe for bradycardia, hypotension, complaints of dizziness. Administer normal saline or other rapid volume replacement; place patient in Trendelenburg position and administer atropine, 1 mg IVP, as per protocol.<br>• Check blood pressures in lying and sitting positions once patient is able to get out of bed, and note decrease in systolic blood pressure greater than 20 mmHg or complaints of dizziness. Return patient to lying position if this occurs. | • Frequent assessment of patient status promotes detection of subtle changes in condition.<br>• Urinary output is a consistent noninvasive measure of cardiac output, renal perfusion.<br>• Vasoconstriction is a compensatory mechanism for decreased CO.<br>• Mentation is one of the most sensitive indicators of altered tissue perfusion.<br>• Fluids are important in maintaining intravascular volume.<br>• It is common to observe a vasovagal reaction to the removal of femoral arterial sheaths.<br>• Orthostatic changes are common after PTCA due to prolonged bedrest, venodilation with nitrates. |

| | | | |
|---|---|---|---|
| ***Nursing Diagnosis #6*** Knowledge deficit, related to coronary artery disease post PTCA expectations. | 1. Patient/family will be able to verbalize an understanding of:<br>• What CAD is.<br>• Why this is a problem for the patient.<br>• Purpose of PTCA.<br>• Immediate post PTCA care.<br>• Risk factors of CAD that the patient can modify.<br>• Name, dosage, and purpose of homegoing medications.<br>• Follow-up care (appointments).<br>• What to do in an emergency. | • Determine patient/family understanding of coronary artery disease, and how it affects them.<br>• Develop comprehensive teaching plan in conjunction with patient and family, based on learning needs.<br>◦ Utilize diagrams and audiovisuals to enhance understanding of CAD.<br>◦ Supply patient with written instructions for information pertaining to medications, risk factors, expected behavioral changes, and emergent care.<br>• Reinforce teaching during care and evaluate level of understanding.<br>• Encourage questions and verbalization of feelings. | • Identification of baseline level of knowledge is necessary in providing individualized teaching.<br>• Mutual agreement on what information is needed is helpful in meeting perceived needs and providing meaningful information.<br>◦ Levels of anxiety during hospitalization as well as quantity of information communicated necessitate written instructions for clarity.<br>• It is important to assess patient's understanding after any teaching to identify any misconceptions. |

TABLE 42-14
**Relative Contraindications for Use of Thrombolytic Therapy**

| |
|---|
| Traumatic cardiopulmonary resuscitation |
| Acute trauma |
| Current anticoagulation |
| Bleeding disorders |
| *Recent exposure to beta-hemolytic streptococci |
| Recent intra-arterial or biopsy procedures |
| Recent aneurysm or cerebrovascular accident |
| Recent surgery (within 10 days of treatment) |
| Uncontrolled hypertension (systolic >180 mmHg and/or diastolic >110 mmHg) |

* Specific to streptokinase only.

become more popular, although the drug's efficacy by this route has not been consistently demonstrated. Commonly, a loading dose of 1.5 million units is administered, followed by a maintenance infusion of heparin to prevent reocclusion.

## Technique of Thrombolytic Therapy with tPA

Tissue plasminogen activator is administered intravenously in 2 phases: the *lytic* phase and the *maintenance* phase. The drug is reconstituted with nonbacteriostatic sterile water to a concentration of 1 mg/ml. The lytic dose is delivered by giving an initial bolus of 6–10 mg by IV push over 1–2 minutes followed by an infusion that would deliver a total of 60 mg in the first hour (i.e., 10-mg bolus followed by 50-mg infusion). The maintenance dose is delivered by infusing 20 mg over the second and third hours, to equal a total dose of 100 mg. Concurrent administration of heparin therapy is usually initiated to prevent rethrombosis.

## Complications of Thrombolytic Therapy

The nurse caring for the patient receiving a thrombolytic agent must consider a number of major complications, including bleeding, allergic response, reocclusion or reinfarction, and reperfusion dysrhythmias.

Bleeding is the most common complication encountered during thrombolytic therapy because of the intentional alteration in the patient's blood-clotting ability. The bleeding incidents have ranged from superficial to severe internal hemorrhage.

The most frequent bleeding complication observed has been oozing or hematoma formation at the catheterization site. Other commonly observed locations for superficial bleeding have included venous or arterial puncture sites; gingival bleeding; cuts or abrasions; and ecchymosis from patient manipulation. The more severe, less frequently occurring bleeding incidents have included intracranial, gastrointestinal, retroperitoneal, and genitourinary bleeding. Many of these bleeding complications can be minimized or avoided by careful pretreatment assessment of the patient for risk of bleeding.

Because many adults have had prior exposure to the beta-hemolytic streptococcal bacteria, it is extremely common for a person receiving streptokinase to exhibit some manifestation of an allergic response. (Tissue plasminogen activator is naturally occurring and is nonantigenic.) The severity of this response can range from a mild elevation of body temperature and itching to severe hives and anaphylaxis, depending on the extent of prior sensitization.

There is always a risk of reocclusion of the treated coronary artery following thrombolytic therapy because of the relatively short duration of effect of the therapy. Once the clot has been successfully dissolved, a high-degree atherosclerotic lesion may remain, predisposing the patient to recurrence of the occlusion and possible infarction. The risk of reocclusion is greatest within the first 24 hours after recanalization. It has therefore become standard practice to initiate concurrent anticoagulant therapy with heparin to decrease the risk of reocclusion.

Another phenomenon that has been observed following thrombolytic therapy is the occurrence of dysrhythmias upon reperfusion of the ischemic myocardium, termed "reperfusion dysrhythmias." The mechanism for these dysrhythmias is not clear, but a variety of rhythm disturbances have been manifested, including accelerated idioventricular rhythm, ventricular tachycardia, premature ventricular contractions, sinus bradycardia, and high-grade AV blocks.

## Nursing Considerations

The patient receiving thrombolytic therapy is at risk for a multitude of actual and potential health problems that the nurse must address in developing a plan of care. Of primary concern is the stabilization of the patient's condition and preservation of myocardial function. Specific nursing diagnoses, desired patient outcomes, and nursing interventions in the care of the patient receiving thrombolytic therapy are presented in the Care Plan in Table 42–15.

# LASER ANGIOPLASTY

## Goals of Laser Angioplasty

Laser angioplasty is the most recent therapeutic modality used for occlusive coronary artery dis-

## TABLE 42–15. CARE PLAN FOR THE PATIENT RECEIVING THROMBOLYTIC THERAPY: STREPTOKINASE AND TISSUE PLASMINOGEN ACTIVATOR

| Nursing Diagnoses | Desired Patient Outcomes | Nursing Interventions | Rationales |
|---|---|---|---|
| ***Nursing Diagnosis #1***<br>Potential for physiologic injury: Bleeding, related to manipulation of clotting cascade. | 1. Patient will not have active bleeding as evidenced by:<br>• Stable hematocrit, hemoglobin levels.<br>• Guaiac-free stools, secretions.<br>• Absence of hematoma, bruising, ecchymosis.<br>• Stable blood pressure.<br>• Stable mentation. | • Perform complete assessment of patient at least every 4 hr including:<br>◦ Neurologic assessment.<br>◦ Inspection of skin for areas of discoloration.<br>◦ Quality of peripheral pulses.<br>◦ Guaiac results of secretions, excretions.<br>◦ Evaluation of current laboratory values (hemoglobin, hematocrit, PTT, fibrinogen levels). | • Complete assessment will allow for rapid detection of any possible bleeding complications.<br>◦ Hemoglobin and hematocrit will determine the volume and oxygen-carrying capacity of red blood cells in the circulation. PTT will estimate the blood's ability to clot. Fibrinogen will estimate the amount of coagulation proteins available to make clots. |
| | | • Monitor vital signs and clinical status every 15–30 minutes until stable, then every 24 hr.<br>• Inspect insertion sites for bleeding when taking vital signs | • Frequent clinical assessment will allow for rapid detection of bleeding.<br>• Previous sites of clotting frequently are dissolved during administration of thrombolytic agent. |
| | | • Observe for retroperitoneal ecchymosis and severe lower back pain when taking vital signs. | • Catheterization via the femoral artery predisposes patient to iliac or femoral dissection. |
| | | • Avoid patient care activities that would predispose patient to bleeding or bruising:<br>◦ Shaving.<br>◦ Venipuncture.<br>◦ Vigorous toothbrushing.<br>◦ Aggressive patient manipulation.<br>◦ Use of noninvasive blood pressure cuffs. | • Hemostatic mechanisms are impaired after thrombolytic therapy, preventing rapid resolution of bleeding. |
| | | • Maintain alignment of extremity involved in the procedure and place 5–10-lb sandbag over site. | • Movement of extremity may dislodge newly formed clots. Direct pressure promotes hemostasis. |
| | | • Coordinate blood work if venipuncture is required, or maintain large-bore IV with saline lock for blood sampling. | • Maintenance of vascular integrity is critical in preventing uncontrolled bleeding. |
| | | • Monitor patient's laboratory work:<br>◦ Thrombin time.<br>◦ Prothrombin time.<br>◦ Partial thromboplastin time.<br>◦ Fibrinogen split products.<br>◦ Fibrinogen levels.<br>◦ Hematocrit. | • All indicators of clotting will be prolonged for 6–12 hr after administration of streptokinase.<br>◦ Indicators of bleeding should not decrease during post-procedure period. |

*(continued)*

**TABLE 42–15. CARE PLAN FOR THE PATIENT RECEIVING THROMBOLYTIC THERAPY: STREPTOKINASE AND TISSUE PLASMINOGEN ACTIVATOR** *(Continued)*

| Nursing Diagnoses | Desired Patient Outcomes | Nursing Interventions | Rationales |
|---|---|---|---|
| ***Nursing Diagnosis #1 (cont.)*** | | ○ Hemoglobin.<br>• Alert all personnel that patient is anticoagulated by placing a sign at bedside.<br>• If invasive procedures are required, avoid noncompressible vessels.<br>○ Subclavian vein.<br>○ Internal jugular vein. | • Increased communication among health care team minimizes risk of complications.<br>• Predisposes patient to uncontrolled bleeding. |
| ***Nursing Diagnosis #2***<br>Potential for physiologic injury: Bleeding, related to thrombolytic therapy (diminished clotting ability). | 1. Patient will remain hemodynamically stable and bleeding will be controlled with minimal blood loss as evidenced by:<br>• No change in blood pressure.<br>• No change in hemoglobin, hematocrit levels. | • Hold pressure to site for at least 1/2–3/4 hr.<br>• Notify physician immediately of any bleeding.<br>• Monitor vital signs and document.<br>• Be prepared to administer blood products containing clotting factors (FFP, Packed RBC, cryoprecipitate).<br>• Administer aminocaproic acid as prescribed, and monitor response to therapy.<br>• Administer fluid and plasma expanders. | • Hemostasis is prolonged due to manipulation of clotting cycle.<br>• Blood pressure will drop and heart rate increase if significant volume loss has occurred.<br>• Supplementing clotting cycle is effective in maintaining hemostasis.<br>• Aminocaproic acid is a hemostatic agent used to prevent excessive formation of plasmin. This helps to control bleeding caused by thrombolytic agents.<br>• May require volume to maintain adequate cardiac output. |
| ***Nursing Diagnosis #3***<br>Potential alteration in comfort, related to allergic response (specific to streptokinase only). | 1. Patient will not demonstrate discomfort related to manifestations of an allergic response (i.e., itching, musculoskeletal pain, respiratory distress, fever, anaphylaxis). | • Monitor temperature every 4 hr.<br>○ Inspect skin every 30 minutes–1 h for 6 h, then every 4 h.<br>○ If febrile, administer medication that does not affect hemostasis (i.e., acetaminophen).<br>• Monitor patient closely if signs/symptoms of reaction occur and document.<br>• Be prepared to administer corticosteroids, Benadryl, or life-support measures if reaction is severe. | • Manifestations of allergic response will occur soon after administration of streptokinase as antigen is encountered.<br>○ Aspirin may contribute to patient's inability to clot.<br>• Patient who has recently had exposure to beta-hemolytic streptococcal proteins will develop a severe response to the therapy. |

| | | | |
|---|---|---|---|
| ***Nursing Diagnosis #4***<br>Potential alteration in cardiac output, related to dysrhythmias. | 1. Patient will remain hemodynamically stable as evidenced by:<br>• Maintenance of MAP greater than 70 mmHg.<br>• Lack of signs and symptoms of decreased cardiac output: dizziness, nausea, shortness of breath. | • Monitor patient's rhythm continuously, noting and documenting any change from baselines.<br>• Treat all dysrhythmias with standard protocols, noting patient's response.<br>• Reassure patient that this is not unexpected and signals success of the procedure. | • Reperfusion dysrhythmias occur frequently after successful thrombolysis.<br>• Patients often fear that dysrhythmias mean the procedure has been unsuccessful. |
| ***Nursing Diagnosis #5***<br>Potential alteration in tissue perfusion, related to reocclusion of coronary arteries. | 1. Patient will remain pain-free or chest pain will be alleviated, with resolution of ECG changes indicative of ischemia, infarction. | • Instruct patient to notify nurse immediately at onset of chest pain; reinforce significance of time.<br>• Observe patient for nonverbal signs of discomfort.<br>• Obtain a 12-lead ECG with any patient discomfort and observe for ischemic changes.<br>  ○ Notify physician immediately.<br>  ○ Administer standard medications for myocardial ischemia.<br>• Prepare patient for possibility of repeat procedure, emergent IABP, or open-heart surgery. | • Patients may not understand the importance of communicating chest pain or are afraid to admit that the problem has not resolved.<br>• Electrocardiographic indicators of ischemia differentiate true angina from other kinds of discomfort.<br>• It may be necessary to revascularize the myocardium by more conventional methods if reocclusion occurs.<br>  ○ Counterpulsation will help with coronary artery perfusion and minimize myocardial demands. |

ease. Currently this therapy remains investigational. It shares the goals of percutaneous transluminal coronary angioplasty and thrombolytic therapy and revascularizes the myocardium by vaporizing the atherosclerotic lesion with direct laser penetration.

## Indications

Clinical indications for laser angioplasty are the same as those for patients eligible for PTCA. Laser angioplasty may provide a viable option for the revascularization of stenosed vessels.

## Technique

The actual technique of laser angioplasty is very similar to that of percutaneous transluminal angioplasty. Once access to the arterial system has been obtained, a flexible catheter is threaded to the site of the coronary occlusion. Instead of inflation of a balloon, however, a laser beam is directed at the plaque on various energy levels until circulation is restored distal to the occlusion. Currently, the quantity and type of laser energy for effective angioplasty are under investigation.

## Complications of Laser Angioplasty

Because laser angioplasty involves the direction of high-intensity energy at the vessel wall, there is always a possibility of perforating the artery during the procedure. It has also been observed that a majority of arteries reocclude or experience spasms shortly after the procedure, limiting its overall efficacy at this time in the treatment of coronary artery disease.

## Nursing Considerations

The nurse caring for the patient receiving laser angioplasty must focus on many of the same problems as encountered in caring for the patient post-PTCA, since the procedures are very similar in approach. (See Table 42-13, Care Plan for the Patient with Percutaneous Transluminal Coronary Angioplasty.) Areas of concern include alteration in comfort related to reocclusion and potential alteration in myocardial tissue perfusion related to perforation, spasm, or reocclusion. Review the data presented in the case study in Table 42-16; then, using the information in Table 42-13, identify nursing diagnoses, desired patient outcomes, and nursing interventions pertinent to this clinical circumstance.

TABLE 42-16
**Case Study: Acute MI/PTCA**

Mr. Adams is a 42-year-old factory worker who experienced acute-onset chest pressure while loading pallets this afternoon. At first he thought it was indigestion, but when he became diaphoretic, dizzy, and short of breath, he notified his foreman, who sent for an ambulance immediately. On arrival to the Coronary Intensive Care Unit, Mr. Adams experienced continued substernal crushing pain, which radiated to his jaw and left shoulder. He was alert and oriented, his color ashen, his skin cool and clammy. The monitor showed sinus tachycardia with occasional premature ventricular contractions. His ECG demonstrated changes reflective of acute anterior ischemia. He was rushed to the cardiac catheterization lab for an emergent catheterization and possible PTCA.

Mr. Adams had a 90% stenosis of the left anterior descending artery, which responded to PTCA. Upon return to CIC, Mr. Adams remarked "how wonderful it is to be cured." He had right femoral venous and arterial sheaths in place and was receiving intravenous nitroglycerin, heparin, and normal saline. His vital signs were stable and his monitor showed normal sinus rhythm without ectopy. He denied any further chest pain but complained of chronic low back pain from lying flat.

**Nursing Diagnoses**

*Actual:* Alteration in comfort, related to immobility.
Knowledge deficit, related to coronary artery disease.

*Potential:* Alteration in cardiac output, related to left ventricular dysfunction, sheath removal, dysrhythmias, and orthosatic hypotension.
Alteration in tissue perfusion, related to cannulation of tissue femoral artery.
Potential for injury, physiologic: Bleeding, related to cannulation of femoral artery and anticoagulation.
Alteration in comfort, related to myocardial ischemia. (See Table 42-13.)

To assist in planning Mr. Adams' care, see the Care Plan in Table 42-13.

## SUGGESTED READINGS


Abela, GS, Seeger, JM, Barbieri, E, et al: Laser angioplasty with angioscopic guidance in humans. J Am Coll Cardiol 8(1):184-192, 1986.

Alspach, J and Williams, S (eds): Core Curriculum for Critical Care Nursing, ed 3. WB Saunders, Philadelphia, 1985.

Bell, WR, Roberts, R, Ludbrook, PA, and Markis, JE: Efficacy of thrombolytic therapy for acute myocardial infarction: A round table discussion. Pract Cardiol 12(10):51-67, 1986.

Blaisdell, MW, Good, L, and Gentzler, MD: Percutaneous Transluminal Valvuloplasty. Crit Care Nurse 9(3):62, March 1989.

Bolooki, H: Current status of circulatory support with an intra-aortic balloon pump. Medical Instrumentation 20(5):226-276, 1986.

Bullas, JB: Care of the patient on the percutaneous intra-aortic counterpulsation balloon. Crit Care Nurse 2(4):40-48, July/August, 1982.

Crea, F, Davies, G, McKenna, W, et al: Percutaneous recanalization of coronary arteries. Lancet, 214-215, July 26, 1986.

Cumberland, DC, Oakley, GDG, Smith, GH, et al: Percutaneous laser-assisted coronary angioplasty. Lancet, 214, July 26, 1986.

Goldsmith, MF: Laser angioplasty: Progressing, but opinions, forecasts vary. JAMA 250(23):1522-1538, 1985.

Gunby, P: "Poof" goes the plaque with experimental laser angioplasty. JAMA 250(23):3135-3141, 1983.

Haak, SW: Intra-aortic balloon pump techniques. Dimensions of Critical Care Nursing 2(4):196-204, 1983.

Haywood, DL: Temporary AV sequential pacing using epicardial lead system. Crit Care Nurse 5(3):21-29, 1985.

Lee, G, Chan, MC, Ikeda, RM, et al: Applicability of laser to assist coronary balloon angioplasty. Am Heart J 110(6):1233–1236, 1985.

Mathewson, M and Dusek, JL: DC countershock does not harm today's internal pacemakers. Crit Care Nurse 4(2):48, March/April 1984.

Phibbs, B and Marriott, HJL: Complications of permanent transvenous pacing. N Engl J Med 342(22):1428–1432, 1985.

Purcell, JA and Burrows, SG: Pacemakers. Am J Nurs 85(5):554–568, May 1985.

Purcell, JA, Pippin, L, and Mitchell, M: IABP therapy. Am J Nurs 83(5):776–790, May 1983.

Reeder, GS and Vliestra, RE: Coronary angioplasty: 1986. Modern Concepts of Cardiovascular Disease 50(10):49–53, 1986.

Shillinger, FL: Percutaneous transluminal angioplasty. Heart Lung 12(1):45–51, 1983.

Slusarczyk, SM and Hicks, FD: Helping your patient live with a permanent pacemaker. Nursing '83 13(4):58–63, 1983.

Spielman, SR: New advances in cardiac pacemaking. In Hakki, AH (ed): Ideal Cardiac Pacing, pp 219–261. WB Saunders, Philadelphia, 1984.

Stevens, L, Redd, R, and Buckingham, T: An alternative to electric countershock for terminating ventricular arrhythmias. Crit Care Nurse 9(3):38, March 1989.

Strauss, E and Rudy, EB: Tissue-plasminogen activator: A new drug in reperfusion therapy. Crit Care Nurse 6(3):30–41, 1986.

The ISAM Study Group: A prospective trial of intravenous streptokinase in acute myocardial infarction (I.S.A.M.). N Engl J Med 314(23):1465–1471, 1986.

Whitman, G: Intra-aortic balloon pumping and cardiac mechanics: A programmed lesson. Heart Lung 7(6):1034–1050, 1978.

CHAPTER 43

# Nursing Management of the Patient with Coronary Artery Disease, Angina Pectoris, or Myocardial Infarction

*Patricia Markmann Naji*

## CHAPTER OUTLINE



## LEARNING OBJECTIVES

**At the end of this chapter, you should be able to:**

1. Identify the major risk factors associated with coronary artery disease.
2. Identify risk factors that may be modified and the factors involved in accomplishing this.
3. Define angina pectoris.
4. Discuss pertinent clinical factors that differentiate stable angina from unstable angina.
5. Discuss pertinent clinical findings used in the differential diagnosis of chest pain.
6. Describe pathophysiologic mechanisms involved in angina pectoris.
7. Describe pathophysiologic mechanisms involved in a myocardial infarction.
8. Discuss hemodynamic alterations that occur with a myocardial infarction.
9. List pertinent clinical factors involved in making the diagnosis of myocardial infarction.
10. Discuss ECG changes that occur with a myocardial infarction.
11. Identify principles of treatment of myocardial infarction.
12. Identify specific interventions involved in the management of the patient having a myocardial infarction.
13. Describe the 4 types of complications associated with myocardial infarction.
14. Relate pertinent nursing diagnoses, desired patient outcomes, and nursing interventions to the therapeutic goals in the care of the patient having a myocardial infarction.

## CORONARY ARTERY DISEASE

Despite major scientific and technologic advances in the field of cardiovascular health care, coronary heart disease remains a national epidemic. The National Center for Health Statistics estimates that 5 million persons in the nation are afflicted with coronary heart disease, and of these nearly one half are limited in activity because of it. It remains the nation's leading cause of death, accounting for 550,000 deaths per year, and often strikes down persons in their most productive years. The National Heart, Lung and Blood Institute estimates that in 1981 national health expenditures and lost productivity attributed to coronary heart disease amounted to 44 billion dollars.

Critical care nurses are confronted daily with caring for individuals who are victims of some form of this devastating disease. In fact, coronary artery disease, either as a primary or a secondary diagnosis, is probably the most common problem encountered by nurses in our nation's intensive care units (ICU). Thus, to function effectively, ICU nurses must have an understanding of coronary artery disease (CAD), including its risk factors, pathogenesis, symptomatology, and possible complications.

## RISK FACTORS

A risk factor is defined as a factor associated with the development of a condition and suspected to be causative.[1] Since the first description of a myocardial infarction in the medical literature in the early 20th century, numerous causative factors for coronary artery disease have been intensively studied and several clear relationships have been established. These factors may be divided into those over which an individual has no control and those which can potentially be modified.

### Noncontrollable Factors

Data from the Framingham Study[2] revealed that the incidence of morbidity and mortality from CAD increases with age in each sex and race group. Male mortality rates from CAD are much higher than those for females, and by age 55–64, 35% of all deaths among men are related to CAD. Unfortunately, the probable normal hormonal protection women enjoy in their younger years decreases with the onset of menopause. Women in their 40s and 50s who are postmenopausal have 3 times the incidence of CAD as those who are still menstruating.[3]

There may also be a familial or genetic predisposition to CAD that is independent of other risk factors.[4] Although genetic predisposition is not a controllable factor, individuals who inherit this tendency need to be made all the more cognizant of modifiable risk factors. Finally, various other factors have been reviewed and some interesting relationships found. The incidence of CAD is higher in industrialized countries, in areas with colder climates and more snowfall,[5] and also in areas with lower altitudes.[6] The importance of all of these findings is still under investigation.

### Controllable Factors

Decades of follow-up of the 5,209 men and women who participated in the Framingham Study starting in 1948 have defined 4 risk factors in the development of CAD: Hypertension, cigarette smoking, elevated serum cholesterol levels, and hyperglycemia. These factors may be considered as major, causative, and potentially modifiable, with such modification capable of substantially reducing the risk of development of the disease. Other factors that may be related to CAD development, such as exercise, obesity, diet, personality type, alcohol, and caffeine, have also been extensively studied and will be discussed briefly.

#### *Hypertension*

Hypertension, either systolic or diastolic, has been demonstrated to be the most significant predictor of an increased risk of developing CAD.[7] Several factors contribute to the link between hypertension and CAD. Chronic hypertension injures the endothelial layer of the arterial wall, which promotes platelet adhesion and aggregation in the injured area. When serum lipid levels are elevated, these exposed subendothelial surfaces become available for fatty deposits as well. Thus, reduction of serum lipid levels (see later) along with blood pressure management must also be addressed. It is important to note that adults with systolic pressure of 120–140 mmHg have twice the risk of developing heart disease as do adults with systolic pressures below 120 mmHg.[8] Therefore, aggressive management of even mild to moderate levels of hypertension seems warranted in preventing future cardiac disease.

#### *Cigarette Smoking*

Unequivocal evidence shows that cigarette smoking has a significant relationship to myocardial infarction and sudden death, particularly in men. Male smokers have an incidence of CAD and mortality rate that is 1.6 times higher than male nonsmokers.[9] Data also support that the risk of developing CAD is directly related to the number of cigarettes smoked per day and that discontinuing smoking diminishes this risk.[10] Various mechanisms have been postulated to explain the adverse effects of cigarette smoking on the heart and blood vessels, including a nicotine-induced increased myocardial oxygen demand, interference of oxygen supply by carboxyhemoglobin, increased adhesiveness of platelets, and a lowering of the threshold for ventricular fibrillation. Whatever the mechanisms, the proven reversibility of the effects of nicotine on the heart and circulatory system has significant implications for health care providers in promoting risk factor modification.

### *Serum Cholesterol Levels*

The essential role of hyperlipidemia in the development of coronary artery disease is well documented. Treatment of this risk factor alone significantly reduces both the number of deaths from coronary heart disease as well as the rate of myocardial infarction. Thus, modification of this risk factor is particularly important.

Cholesterol and trigylcerides are plasma lipids that are transported in the blood by complexes known as lipoproteins. Lipoproteins are classified according to their composition, density, and electrophoretic mobility. Five classes have been identified: Chylomicrons, very low density lipoprotein (VLDL), intermediate-density lipoprotein (IDL), low-density lipoprotein (LDL), and high-density lipoprotein (HDL). The 3 lipoproteins that are most significant in coronary heart disease are LDL, VLDL, and HDL.

LDL is the most atherogenic of the lipoproteins. It is the major cholesterol-carrying molecule in the plasma, accounting for 70% of the total plasma cholesterol. LDL functions in the transport of cholesterol from liver to peripheral tissues where it is taken up by specific receptors. LDL is formed as a breakdown product from the metabolism of VLDL. Thus, an increased level of LDL, which is directly associated with CAD, may be due to an overproduction of VLDL or to defective clearance of LDL. Normal LDL cholesterol level is less than 150 mg/100 ml.

VLDL is composed primarily of triglycerides and is produced by the liver. Ingestion of a high carbohydrate diet will cause an elevation in the triglyceride level. However, the significance of this to the development of CAD is still unknown.

HDL is often referred to as the "good" cholesterol because of its negative correlation with CAD. The mechanisms involved in this relationship remain unclear. Possibly it helps to transport cholesterol from peripheral tissues, including from arterial walls, to the liver for excretion. What is evident is that higher levels of HDL may have a protective effect in the development of vascular disease. Thus, patients need to be encouraged to take steps to raise their HDL levels to greater than 50 mg/100 ml. Aerobic exercise is particularly helpful in this regard.[11] Weight reduction is also probably beneficial in the obese individual, and cessation of cigarette smoking is beneficial in all individuals.

In assessing risk for CAD development based on the lipid profile, serum levels of cholesterol, triglycerides, LDL, VLDL, and HDL are measured. Lipid disorders have been categorized into 5 types based on cholesterol, triglyceride, and lipoprotein patterns. Table 43-1 lists types, patterns, and dietary and pharmacologic therapy indicated for each type. The 3 most common lipid risk patterns associated with CAD are types IIA, IIB, and IV.

Treatment of hyperlipidemia depends on the lipid profile and involves diet alone or diet plus medication. All dietary programs focus on reduc-

TABLE 43-1
**Classification and Treatment of Hyperlipidemias Based on Lipid and Lipoprotein Abnormalities**

| Type | Lipid and Lipoprotein Abnormality | Treatment |
|---|---|---|
| I | Chol ↑, Tg ↑↑<br>VLDL N or ↑, LDL ↓ | Diet |
| IIA | Chol ↑, Tg N<br>LDL ↑, VLDL N or ↓ | Cholestyramine, colestipol, nicotinic acid |
| IIB | Chol ↑, Tg ↑<br>LDL ↑, VLDL ↑ | Cholestyramine, colestipol, clofibrate, nicotinic acid |
| III | Chol ↑, Tg ↑<br>VLDL ↑, LDL ↑ | Clofibrate |
| IV | Chol N or ↑, Tg ↑<br>VLDL ↑, LDL N or ↓ | Clofibrate, gemfibrozil, nicotinic acid |
| V | Chol ↑, Trig ↑↑<br>VLDL ↑, LDL ↓ | Clofibrate, gemifibrozil, nicotinic acid |

Chol = cholesterol; Tg = triglycerides; N = normal.

ing the intake of cholesterol and saturated fats and increasing polyunsaturated fat intake.[12] This usually involves a major change in dietary habits, which requires a great deal of motivation by the patient, support by the family, and detailed explanations by the nurse if it is to be successful. The inclusion of omega-3 polyunsaturated fatty acids, which are found in fish and are also now available in capsule form, should be encouraged. These have a cardio-protective effect. Fish oil intakes of 20–30 g/day effectively lower triglyceride concentrations in individuals with abnormal plasma lipids.[13]

Drug therapy for hyperlipidemia involves the use of 2 types of drugs. Medications are initiated when diet alone has been unsuccessful after a 3–6 month trial. Nicotinic acid, a vitamin in the body, inhibits lipoprotein synthesis. It lowers cholesterol, triglyceride, and LDL, and it also raises HDL levels. Its major side effects are severe flushing of the skin and gastrointestinal upset. One aspirin taken one-half hour prior to the dose may prevent the flushing episodes.

Bile acid sequestrants are the next type of drug used to treat hyperlipidemia. These drugs act by binding bile acids in the intestine to form an insoluble complex that is then excreted in the feces. This serves to increase metabolism of LDL. Cholestyramine and colestipol are 2 examples of this type of drug. Gastrointestinal side effects are also common with these drugs, and patient compliance is often affected because of this. These drugs also interfere with the absorption of many other drugs, and the manufacturer's guidelines for administration with other drugs should be adhered to. This often further complicates an already complex medical regimen in the patient with CAD, and patient compliance may be affected further.

### Hyperglycemia

Although the mechanism linking hyperglycemia with an increased risk of CAD is unclear, numerous studies have shown that atherosclerosis in general and coronary atherosclerosis in particular are more extensive and severe in diabetics than in nondiabetics.[14–16] The interrelationships of obesity, hypertension, and hyperlipidemia, especially hypertriglyceridemia, with each other and with hyperglycemia as an etiologic mechanism for the increased incidence of CAD in diabetics have been studied. No definitive causative mechanism has yet been found. Also uncertain is the significance of the level of blood sugar in predisposing a diabetic to vascular complications and whether tight control of blood sugar level has any major impact on preventing or reducing these. Despite the current lack of conclusive research in this area, most clinicians believe that poorly controlled blood glucose levels may be detrimental, particularly when other risk factors are present, and should be appropriately managed.

### Other Factors

**Exercise.** Numerous studies have supported an association between physical inactivity and an increased incidence of CAD in men. While exercise appears to clearly play a role in the prevention of CAD in men, the mechanism by which it does this remains unclear. Maintenance of optimum body weight, lowering of heart rate and resting blood pressure, and directly improving myocardial function and coronary circulation have all been postulated. Despite the positive effects of exercise, the Framingham Study demonstrated that the modification of other risk factors (i.e., hypertension, cigarette smoking, and hyperglycemia) has more significant effects,[17] suggesting that a program of multiple risk factor modification, including exercise, is warranted.

**Obesity.** The role of obesity in the development of cardiovascular disease remains controversial. Evidence exists that obesity promotes glucose intolerance, hypertriglyceridemia, hypertension, raised LDL-C level, and reduced HDL cholesterol level.[18,19] What is not clear is whether obesity is itself an independent risk factor or whether its role in promoting CAD lies in its contribution to these other risk factors. Whichever is true, appropriate weight reduction should be advocated in the obese individual since studies have shown weight reduction has favorable effects on reducing the aforementioned atherogenic traits.

**Diet.** In discussing the relationship of diet to CAD, the intake of cholesterol and saturated fat, salt, carbohydrate, alcohol, and caffeine is usually considered.

***Cholesterol and Saturated Fat.*** The incidence of coronary heart disease is higher in Western countries where diets tend to be rich in cholesterol and saturated fats than in areas of the world where a low-cholesterol, low-fat diet is consumed.[20] It has also been established that there is a direct relationship between serum cholesterol and triglyceride levels and the intake of saturated fat and cholesterol in the diet. Likewise, there is little dispute over the fact that dietary fat and cholesterol are significant factors in the genesis of atherosclerosis. Since it is also known that reduction in fat intake produces a predictable decrease in serum lipids, modification of this risk factor is probably one of the easiest to achieve and should be strongly advocated.

***Salt.*** The role of sodium restriction in the prevention and/or treatment of hypertension is still ambiguous. Despite this, many clinicians advise prudent salt ingestion on the basis of the studies that suggest that this may be helpful.

***Carbohydrate.*** American diets, which are high in sugars, have generally been cited as another causal agent in the development of CAD. A transitory rise in serum triglyceride levels has been noted after the ingestion of large amounts of carbohydrates, the significance of which is still uncertain. It has been suggested that the significant factor here may be the type of carbohydrate ingested. Sucrose and glucose consumption probably needs to be decreased in the American diet, and fiber-containing complex carbohydrates like grains, cereal products, and legumes need to be increased. The accomplishment of this goal would obviously involve a major change in most American diets.

***Alcohol.*** When taken in large amounts, alcohol appears to have a direct cardiotoxic effect, particularly in the development of cardiomyopathies. Its relationship to CAD is less clear. The current literature suggests that ingestion of alcohol in moderate amounts may beneficially raise HDL cholesterol levels and thus serve some protective purpose in preventing CAD;[21] however, this relationship is still being studied.

***Caffeine.*** While large doses of caffeine have been implicated in the pathogenesis of cardiac dysrhythmias, the data from prospective studies, including the Framingham Study, have failed to show any consistent relationship between it as an independent risk factor and the development of CAD. It has been suggested, however, that caffeine may play a role in association with other risk factors, such as hypertension and cigarette smoking, and thus its intake should probably be eliminated or at least moderated in high risk individuals.

***Personality Type.*** The Type A behavior pattern was conceived by Friedman and Rosenman who felt that a person's personality type was related to the occurrence of CAD.[22] Persons with a Type A behavior pattern are characterized by ambitiousness, impatience, competitiveness, rapid and emphatic speech, and a chronic struggle to achieve more and more in less and less time. Two major studies, the Western Collaborative Group Study and the Framingham Study, have confirmed that the Type A personality trait serves as an independent risk factor in the development of CAD.[23,24]

The pathogenic mechanisms mediating this relationship are being explored. It has been proposed that a stress response to environmental demands unique to Type A individuals may be a factor. Also, excess sympathetic arousal including greater elevations of catecholamine levels, more rapid blood clotting times, increased platelet aggregation, and greater elevations in blood pressure and heart rate have all been noted when Type A persons are exposed to stressors. Definitive evidence of reduced risk for CAD because of modification of this behavior pattern is currently lacking and numerous intervention strategies, particularly stress management and exercise programs, continue to be studied.

## ANGINA PECTORIS

Angina pectoris, which usually accompanies coronary artery disease, was first described in the medical literature in 1772 by Dr. William Heberden.[25] Unlike the word "dolor," which means pain, "angina" was intended to indicate a sense of "strangling." Dr. Heberden noted that a fear of death often accompanied this sensation of discomfort in the breast, and he also described its association with walking and eating, as well as its relief with cessation of the precipitating activity. Recognition of the pathophysiologic mechanism involved in angina also dates back to the 18th century. In 1799, C. H. Parry correctly hypothesized that an imbalance existed between the heart's demand for oxygen and its ability to meet this demand during periods of increased activity.[26] Despite this early recognition and understanding of the syndrome of angina pectoris, much remains to be accomplished in these areas as well as in the prevention and treatment of angina pectoris.

### Definition

Angina may be defined as an imbalance between myocardial oxygen supply and demand. It may be divided into the categories of stable angina, unstable angina, variant or Prinzmetal's angina, and myocardial infarction. Similarities and differences exist in each of these groups.

***Stable Angina.*** Stable angina (also called chronic angina) may be viewed as a syndrome of at least several weeks' duration that is provoked by predictable activities that increase myocardial oxygen demands. The episodes of angina should not be increasing in number or severity and they are routinely relieved by ceasing the precipitating activity or by nitroglycerin.

Management of patients with chronic stable angina begins with patient education. Risk factors need to be discussed including suggestions for their modification. Discontinuation of smoking needs to be particularly emphasized since nicotine increases heart rate and blood pressure and may constrict coronary vessels. Nicotine is also known to shift the oxyhemoglobin dissociation curve, thus making oxygen less available to body tissues (see Fig. 28–15).

Patient education also needs to include helping the patient and his/her family to understand the etiology of angina and that it can often be managed medically indefinitely. They do need, however, to be aware of signs and symptoms of possible progression of the disease, which may indicate a change to an unstable pattern (see below). Proper management of medication regimen needs to be included in discussion with these patients since medications used may be many in number and thus confusing to some patients. (See Appendix A for information on cardiac drugs.)

Particular attention should be paid to discussing with angina patients how and when to take nitroglycerin tablets for relief of angina attacks. When an episode of angina occurs the patient should be instructed to lie down and to take a nitroglycerin tablet under his/her tongue. If the pain persists, 2 or 3 nitroglycerin tablets may be taken 5 minutes apart. If the pain is not relieved following this, the patient should contact his/her health care provider for further instructions. Patients also need to know that nitroglycerin may be taken prophylactically prior to engaging in activities known to produce angina (e.g., sexual intercourse, eating, physical exertion).

### Unstable Angina

Unstable angina pectoris, also known as crescendo angina, pre-infarction angina, acute coronary insufficiency, and by various other terms, is viewed as a relative medical emergency warranting hospitalization. Patients whose angina should be classified as unstable are those with new-onset effort angina; those with an acceleration or a change in pattern of previously stable angina; and those with angina at rest. Patients with this syndrome will often relate that the chest discomfort that they are experiencing is similar to their usual effort-induced discomfort except that it is more intense and has lasted longer (usually longer than 30 minutes.)

Unstable angina has long been related to an increased demand for oxygen by the myocardium that cannot be met by the available supply, which has been compromised by significant fixed obstructive lesions in the coronary vessels. More recent evidence suggests that the mechanism is more complex and implicates coronary *vasospasm* as a causative factor, particularly in the development of rest angina. This concept has several implications in the management of patients with unstable angina. Traditional treatment has consisted of rest and the administration of nitrates and beta-blocking drugs, the latter of which might have potentially adverse effects if spasm is present, allowing unopposed alpha-adrenergic vasoconstrictor activity that could enhance spasm. Thus, current management of unstable angina that may have a vasospastic component should include vasodilating drugs and/or calcium-channel blockers. It must be noted, however, that the majority of patients with unstable angina do have significantly obstructive coronary lesions that limit oxygen supply in the face of an increased demand. A vasospastic component may exist as a part of this syndrome.

Angiographic studies of patients with unstable, particularly new-onset, angina, have demonstrated another interesting finding; that is, that these patients have fewer collateral vessels in their coronary systems.[27] Collateral vessels may be present and unused under normal circumstances, or they may develop de novo in the face of ischemia.[28] While they would seem in theory to afford some protection to ischemia or potentially ischemic myocardium if present, their functional significance in humans is still controversial and under investigation currently.

As noted previously, unstable angina is a potentially life-threatening condition. Patients should be hospitalized and put to rest, both physical and psychological. Pain relief is usually achieved using nitrates and/or narcotics. Sedatives and anti-anxiety drugs are helpful in achieving emotional rest. Patients are placed on continuous electrocardiographic monitoring to observe for dysrhythmias. Tests are done to rule out a myocardial infarction. These include serial cardiac enzyme determinations as well as serial ECGs. Beta-adrenergic blockers and/or calcium channel blockers are used in conjunction with nitrates to promote pain relief and prevent further ischemia. Patients who are refractory to medical management may require intra-aortic balloon pump counterpulsation to achieve pain relief (see Chap. 42).

Early angiographic study is recommended for patients with unstable angina, particularly those refractory to medical management. Those who are persistently unstable despite maximum medical therapy and who have suitable coronary anatomy are referred for coronary artery bypass surgery or for percutaneous transluminal angioplasty, whichever is most appropriate based on the number and type of coronary lesions found. Long-term survival appears to be improved with bypass surgery in those patients who have triple vessel or left main coronary artery disease.

### Variant or Prinzmetal's Angina Pectoris

In 1959 Prinzmetal and his co-workers[29] described a type of cardiac pain that occurs primarily at rest and was noted to be associated with ST segment elevations on the electrocardiogram. The pain is not routinely preceded by blood pressure and heart rate increases, as with effort-induced angina, and in fact is seldom related to emotional stress or physical activity of any kind. These episodes often occur during sleep or in the early morning; the pain is usually severe and syncope may occur. The pathophysiologic mechanism believed to be responsible for this syndrome is a primary decrease in coronary blood flow secondary to coronary artery spasm. Patients with this syndrome may have normal coronary arteries or fixed obstructive lesions in one or more vessels. Those with vasospasm superimposed on fixed lesions may have a mixed anginal syndrome that includes effort-induced as well as rest angina.

When coronary artery spasm is suspected, ergonovine maleate is administered in the cardiac catheterization laboratory to confirm the diagnosis. This drug, which stimulates both alpha-adrenergic and serotonergic receptors, has a constrictive effect on vascular smooth muscle and thus is effective in inducing coronary artery spasm in patients with Prinzmetal's angina when administered in the laboratory. Whether induced pharmacologically or occurring spontaneously, prolonged episodes of spasm can cause myocardial infarctions, ventricular dysrhythmias, heart block, or sudden death. Thus, prompt intervention is essential. Nitroglycerin, by promoting coronary vasodilation, is frequently effective in abolishing attacks. Calcium-channel blockers have recently been found to be quite effective in preventing coronary artery spasm and are now often used in conjunction with nitroglycerin for an added vasodilator effect. The use of beta-blockers is controversial. They may be indirectly helpful in patients with fixed lesions and superimposed spasm because they decrease myocardial oxygen demands. However, they also may promote coronary artery vasoconstriction as beta blockade allows alpha receptors to operate unopposed and thus may generate vasoconstriction and spasm. Coronary artery bypass surgery is useful only in those patients with significant fixed obstructive lesions. Medical management of the vasospastic component is often more effective after the fixed lesions are bypassed.

## Differential Diagnosis of Chest Pain

While chest discomfort is common to each of the above groups, it is also a feature of many other medical problems (Table 43–2). Thus, the initial evaluation of a patient presenting with chest discomfort involves ascertaining whether or not its origin is cardiac. Factors to be included in this are a thorough history and physical examination and an electrocardiogram.

### Clinical History

A thorough clinical history can provide valuable information to guide one's index of suspicion as to whether or not cardiac chest discomfort is present. The patient should be prompted to discuss the characteristics of his/her pain including its quality, location, duration, precipitating factors, sites of radiation, and relief with nitroglycerin (Table 43–3). A pertinent history should also include the presence of risk factors and whether or not the patient has a previous history of myocardial infarction. Based on this profile, the nurse can decide whether or not the patient's symptoms are typical of angina pectoris. (Refer to Chap. 38 for a discussion of the assessment of cardiovascular function.)

TABLE 43–2
**Differential Diagnosis of Chest Pain**

1. Ischemic heart disease syndromes, including angina pectoris, unstable angina pectoris, acute coronary insufficiency, Prinzmetal's angina (variant angina), or acute myocardial infarction
2. Dissecting aortic aneurysm
3. Mitral valve prolapse
4. Pneumonia
5. Atelectasis
6. Spontaneous pneumothorax
7. Pulmonary embolic disease
8. Pulmonary hypertension
9. Cardiomyopathy
10. Valvular aortic stenosis, idiopathic hypertrophic subaortic stenosis, supravalvular aortic stenosis
11. Aortic aneurysm
12. Costochondritis
13. Chest wall or skeletal trauma, including rib fractures
14. Malignancies resulting in marked marrow packing with neoplastic cells, including multiple myeloma and leukemia
15. Anxiety
16. Carcinoma of the lung
17. Esophageal spasm or hiatal hernia
18. Cervical osteoarthritis
19. Thoracic outlet syndrome
20. Herpes zoster (either before or after the development of skin lesions)
21. Pericarditis

**Referred Pain into the Chest**

1. Peptic ulcer disease
2. Cholecystitis
3. Pancreatitis
4. Subdiaphragmatic mass or abscess
5. Abdominal aortic aneurysm

(From Willerson, JT, Hillis, LD, and Buja, LM: Ischemic Heart Disease, Clinical and Pathophysiologic Aspects. Raven Press, New York, 1982, p 115, with permission.)

### Physical Examination

Even after a careful history is obtained, more information is often needed to make a conclusive diagnosis. The patient's vital signs should be taken, with particular attention paid to noting the presence of hypertension and ectopic beats, especially during episodes of chest pain. While examining the patient, the nurse needs to inspect carefully for signs of hyperlipidemia, particularly in patients under 50 years of age. These include xanthomas and arcus cornea. Xanthomas are waxy, yellowish-brown skin lesions. They are usually seen on the dorsum or palmar aspects of the hands and on elbows, knees, Achilles tendons, or the inner canthus of the eye. Arcus cornea, which is a normal finding in the elderly, results from fatty deposits in the cells of the cornea. It is seen as an opaque, gray ring around the outer edges of the cornea. The presence of a diagonal earlobe crease should also be noted while in-

TABLE 43–3
**Characteristics of Angina Pectoris**

**Quality**
- Sensation of pressure or heavy weight on the chest
- Burning sensation
- Feeling of tightness
- Shortness of breath with feeling of constriction about the larynx or upper trachea
- Visceral quality (deep, heavy, squeezing, aching)
- Gradual increase in intensity followed by gradual fading away

**Location**
- Over the sternum or very near to it
- Anywhere between epigastrium and pharynx
- Occasionally limited to left shoulder and left arm
- Rarely limited to right arm
- Limited to lower jaw
- Lower cervical or upper thoracic spine
- Left interscapular or supracapsular area

**Duration**
- 0.5–30 minutes

**Precipitating Factors**
- Relationship to exercise
- Effort that involves use of arms above the head
- Cold environment
- Walking against the wind
- Walking after a large meal
- Emotional factors involved with physical exercise
- Fright, anger
- Coitus

**Nitroglycerin Relief**
- Relief of pain occurring within 45 seconds to 5 minutes of taking nitroglycerin

**Radiation**
- Medial aspect of left arm
- Left shoulder
- Jaw
- Occasionally right arm

(From Helfant, RH and Banka, VS: A Clinical and Angiographic Approach to Coronary Heart Disease. FA Davis, Philadelphia, 1978, p 48, with permission.)

specting the patient. This is a somewhat controversial sign[30] but has been associated with an increased incidence of coronary artery disease in some studies.[31] In patients with coronary artery disease, an examination of eye grounds may reveal retinal arteriolar changes. These include an abnormal light reflex, increased vessel tortuosity, and decreased vessel caliber.[32]

Finally, on auscultation, various sounds may be heard that may or may not be indicative of the presence of CAD and angina pectoris. A fourth heart sound may be heard in many apparently normal individuals over 45 years old, especially those with hypertension or aortic stenosis; however, if it develops or gets louder with chest pain, it is compatible with ischemic heart disease. A third heart sound, a paradoxically split second sound, and/or a murmur of mitral or tricuspid insufficiency heard during chest pain are also consistent with ischemia. The presence of a third or fourth heart sound is related to the functional state of the left ventricle, especially its compliance, which is reduced during diastole, while paradoxical splitting of the second sound is related to asynergy and prolongation of left ventricular contraction. Finally, it should be noted that the absence of any of the above sounds does not exclude angina as the cause of the patient's chest pain. (For discussion of heart sounds and their assessment, refer to the appropriate section in Chap. 38.)

### *Electrocardiogram*

The 12-lead electrocardiogram (ECG) is often a helpful tool in evaluating the patient with chest pain. The resting ECG may be entirely normal in individuals with ischemic heart disease even during episodes of chest pain. However, the development of 1 mm or more of horizontal or downsloping ST depression and/or T wave inversion during chest pain is highly suggestive of ischemia.[33] Thus, obtaining an ECG during an anginal episode can help to definitively diagnose CAD. Location of changes on the ECG is also often helpful in diagnosing which coronary arteries are diseased, since the location of ECG changes often correlates with the specific coronary arteries involved. Other abnormalities may be seen on the electrocardiogram, including left bundle branch block, left anterior hemiblock, ventricular premature beats, and other ST and T wave changes. All of these are nonspecific findings and are common in CAD as well as in other conditions.

## Pathophysiology of Angina Pectoris

As noted previously, angina occurs when the demand for oxygen by the myocardium exceeds the available supply. Since the amount of oxygen extracted from the blood by the heart is nearly maximal at rest, only by increasing oxygen delivery can increased myocardial demands be met. Thus, augmenting coronary blood flow is the major mechanism by which the need for an increased blood supply is met. When atherosclerotic lesions are present in the coronary vessels, this mechanism is effectively diminished or abolished. Other factors that affect oxygen supply via the coronary arteries to the myocardium include coronary thrombosis or embolization, the tone of the coronary vessels (general and focal), circulating blood volume, hemoglobin, and the extent of coronary collateral circulation.

### *Regulation of Coronary Blood Flow*

Coronary blood flow, the major determinant of myocardial oxygen supply, is related to the perfusion pressure (essentially the aortic diastolic pressure) and the duration of diastole and is inversely related to the resistance of the coronary vascular bed.[34] Resistance can be affected by metabolic, neural, pharmacologic, or autoregulatory factors that alter the vascular tone of the vessel smooth muscle. It can also be affected by mechanical factors, particularly myocardial compression of intramyocardial vessels during systole. For this reason, most coronary blood flow occurs in diastole. Finally, atheromatous lesions also offer resistance to blood flow. Such lesions must cause greater than 60% obstruction of vessel diameter before they interfere with blood flow at rest. With lesions that are 60%–85% obstructive, compensatory vasodilation of distal vascular beds maintains near normal flow to rest; however, when lesions obstruct greater than 85% of the vessel diameter, this adaptive mechanism fails to compensate, although some vasodilatory reserve is still present.[35]

### *Myocardial Oxygen Demand*

While coronary blood flow is the major determinant of myocardial oxygen supply, myocardial oxygen consumption ($MVO_2$) determinants are more complex. There are 3 major factors involved: (1) systolic left ventricular wall stress or tension; (2) heart rate; and (3) myocardial contractility. An alteration in any of the above (for example, giving an inotropic drug to increase myocardial contractility) causes an increase in $MVO_2$. Since direct measurement of these variables in the clinical setting is not yet feasible, an indirect system of calculating $MVO_2$ is often used. This index of $MVO_2$ is determined by multiplying the systolic blood pressure by the heart rate. This so-called double product has been proven to reliably correlate with the development of angina, particularly effort-induced angina.[36,37] This means that during exertion, most patients with angina have a predictable, constant, and reproducible angina threshold for this product.

## Treatment

Since angina has been assumed to be associated with alteration of either side of the supply/demand equation, treatment has historically been directed at affecting one of these. Various medications, including nitrates, beta blockers, calcium-channel blockers, antihypertensives, and diuretics, are all employed alone or in various combinations to try to decrease the $M\dot{V}O_2$. More invasive interventions used to augment coronary blood supply include coronary revascularization, percutaneous transluminal coronary angioplasty, and lysis of coronary lesions with various thrombolytic agents (see Chap. 42).

In the 1970s it became apparent that factors affecting the supply side of the equation were more complex that simple obstruction of a vessel by atheromatous plaques (static obstruction) causing a decrease in flow. Angiographic and myocardial perfusion studies have demonstrated that there is a dynamic component to vessel obstruction. That is, that even with fixed atherosclerotic lesions increased vasomotor tone or spasm can occur (Fig. 43–1). This mechanism has been increasingly invoked to explain non-Prinzmetal's rest angina. Calcium-channel blockers are added to therapy when this phenomenon is felt to exist.

# ACUTE MYOCARDIAL INFARCTION

Each year approximately 1.5 million persons in the United States have a myocardial infarction. More than 40% of these people die. Primary ventricular dysrhythmias are the cause of most of these deaths, the majority of which occur before the patient reaches the hospital.

Advanced dysrhythmia detection systems in today's modern coronary care unit have greatly decreased in-hospital mortality. Improvement in the pre-hospital phase of emergency cardiac care, including training more individuals to perform bystander CPR, continues to be a priority in efforts to further decrease myocardial infarction-related mortality.

Myocardial infarction (MI) results when cardiac cells are irreversibly damaged secondary to an episode of prolonged ischemia. It occurs primarily in patients with significant coronary artery disease, although it may also occur in individuals without atheromatous luminal narrowing who may have coronary artery spasm, coronary artery dissection, coronary emboli, or vasculitis. MIs are more common in individuals whose risk factors include hyperlipidemia, hypertension, smoking, a family history of CAD, and sedentary lifestyles.

## Type and Location

There are 2 major types of myocardial infarction: *subendocardial* or non-transmural infarcts, which involve the subendocardial and/or the intramural myocardium; and *transmural* infarcts, which involve the full thickness of the ventricular wall including the epicardial layer.

Numerous factors determine the size and location of a myocardial infarction. These include the location and extent of atheromatous lesions within the coronary vessels, the extent and quality of collateral blood vessels, the amount of jeopardized myocardium produced by the diseased vessels, the presence of coronary vasospasm, the rate of development of the obstruction, the degree of stenosis in the coronary vessels, and the level of myocardial metabolism.[38] Collateral coronary blood vessels are particularly important in determining the site

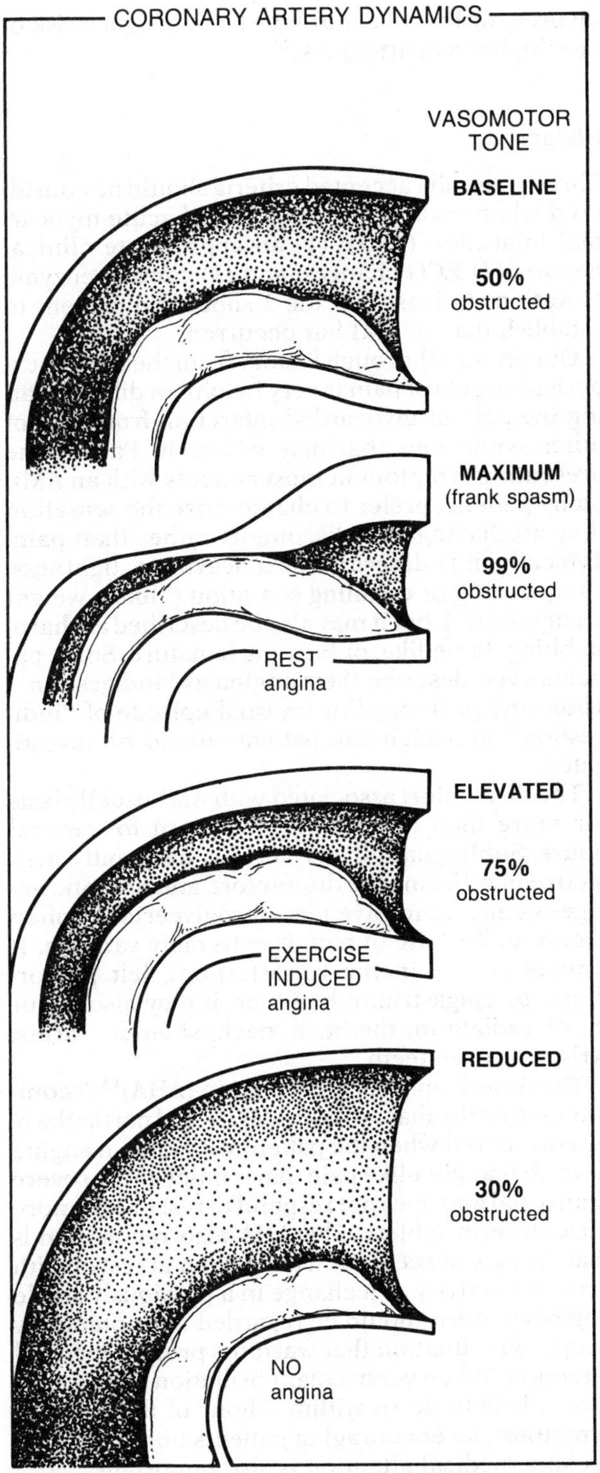


**Figure 43–1.** Demonstrates how the underlying tone of a coronary vessel can influence type of angina in the presence of a 50 percent obstructive lesion. Rest angina, exercise-induced angina, or no angina may occur as muscle tone varies. (Adapted from Epstein, SE and Talbot, TL: Dynamic coronary tone in precipitation, exacerbation, and relief of angina pectoris. Am J Cardiol 48:797, 1981.)

and size of an infarction and even play a role in determining whether or not an infarction will occur after a vessel occludes. That is, if the collateral network is extensive, no necrosis may occur despite an occlusive thrombotic event, or non-transmural damage may occur. Physiologic mechanisms that prompt the development and function of collaterals remain speculative.

## Pathophysiology

Acute myocardial infarction is generally caused by severe ischemia after complete or almost complete occlusion of a coronary artery in patients with significant coronary artery disease. There are 2 major situations in which such an ischemic episode is provoked. First, anything that increases myocardial oxygen needs beyond the ability of the coronary supply to meet the increased need because of fixed obstructive lesions enhances one's vulnerability for myocardial cell injury and necrosis to occur. Prolonged episodes of tachycardia, increased contractility, and increased myocardial wall tension are the most common precipitating factors here. Second, an MI can occur when there is a primary interruption or significant decrease of blood, and thus oxygen supply, to the myocardium. Causative factors in this instance include coronary arterial thrombosis, coronary vessel spasm, hemorrhage into an atherosclerotic plaque, or a significant episode of systemic arterial hypotension.

Acute thrombosis of a coronary vessel has been found to be the most prevalent precipitator of acute ischemic heart disease, particularly in the genesis of transmural myocardial infarction.[39] In these patients the coronary thrombi are usually superimposed on, or adjacent to, atherosclerotic plaques. The mechanism by which this occurs is still unclear. Possibly tissue damage associated with atherosclerotic lesions results in plaque rupture, which may precipitate an intramural hemorrhage. The increased size of the plaque that is caused by this process may by itself produce occlusion of the lumen. Alternatively, thrombus formation can occur because the hemorrhage may cause the plaque's internal layer, which contains collagen, to be exposed to flowing blood, which is known to precipitate thrombus formation.[40] Likewise, ulceration or erosion of an atherosclerotic plaque, which exposes collagen and other thrombogenic agents to the blood stream, is also a precursor of thrombus formation. Hemodynamic trauma, coronary vasospasm, inflammatory or chemical damage to coronary artery endothelium, and blood infiltration, which increases intraplaque pressure, are the chief causes of ulceration or erosion of plaques.[41]

Subendocardial or non-transmural MIs are not usually caused by sudden, complete thrombotic occlusion of a coronary vessel. More commonly they are associated with vessels that are severely narrowed but still patent to some flow. Conditions that are known to precipitate increased myocardial oxygen demands or decreased supply, such as anemia, hypertension, hypotension, and others, can promote non-transmural necrosis when vessels are already compromised by significant lesions.

### *Hemodynamic Alterations in Myocardial Infarctions*

Obstruction of a coronary vessel prompts a series of hemodynamic consequences of variable magnitude. Figure 43-2 depicts a diagrammatic representation of this series of events. When coronary occlusion occurs, it causes a regional area of ischemia and ultimately, infarction if the ischemia is prolonged. If this area is large enough, left ventricular (LV) function is compromised, causing its stroke volume (SV) to fall. If LV function is significantly depressed, aortic pressure and subsequently coronary perfusion pressure will diminish. This further intensifies myocardial ischemia. As less efficient LV emptying occurs secondary to this, filling pressures start to rise.

As the uninvolved segments of the LV wall dilate in response to the increased filling pressures (preload), stroke volume is temporarily restored. However, excess elevation of preload stimulates an increase in afterload, which tends to diminish SV as the ventricle attempts to empty in the face of this increased resistance to LV ejection. This increase in wall tension serves to increase myocardial oxygen requirements, which further intensifies myocardial ischemia. If the damage is not excessive, the remaining uninfarcted myocardial muscle compensates and adequate cardiac function will ensue. With extensive necrosis (>40% of the LV wall), compensatory mechanisms will usually fail and cardiogenic shock is the outcome.

## Diagnosis of Acute Myocardial Infarction

### *Precipitating Events*

A broad spectrum of events may precipitate a myocardial infarction. Many patients are at rest or asleep when the event occurs, while others are engaged in some form of physical activity, usually mild to moderate exertion. The importance of strenuous activity as a precipitator of MI remains controversial. The combination of strenuous activity with excessive fatigue or emotional upset has been noted to be more likely to precede a myocardial infarction than strenuous activity alone. There is also some evidence to suggest that individuals who have recently sustained an upsetting event in their lives (e.g., death of a significant other person, divorce, or loss of a job) may be at a higher risk of developing a heart attack.[42]

### *History*

Three generally accepted criteria should be considered when making the diagnosis of acute myocardial infarction (AMI): (1) an appropriate clinical history; (2) ECG changes; and (3) cardiac enzyme elevation. At least 2 of the 3 should be present to establish that an AMI has occurred.

Obtaining a thorough history from the patient experiencing chest pain is very helpful in differentiating the pain of myocardial infarction from that of other syndromes that may mimic it. Pain is the presenting symptom in most patients with an AMI. Many patients prefer to characterize the sensation they are having as a discomfort rather than pain. Typically, it is described as a heaviness, tightness, or squeezing or crushing sensation ("like a weight on my chest"), but it may also be described as sharp, stabbing, knife-like, or burning in nature. Some patients even describe their angina as "indigestion." Thus, any prolonged or unusual episode of "indigestion" in a high-risk patient should be investigated.

The discomfort associated with AMI usually lasts for more than 30 minutes and often for several hours. Sublingual nitroglycerin is frequently ineffective in relieving the discomfort, and narcotic analgesics and/or intravenous nitroglycerin are often required. The site of pain is extremely variable. It usually occurs in the retrosternum, left precordium, or epigastrium; however, it may also occur in, or radiate to, the back, neck, shoulder, arms, wrists, or even teeth.

The American Heart Association (AHA)[43] recommends that the diagnosis of AMI should particularly be considered when the patient with known angina describes angina-like pain that is much more severe than usual and does not respond to rest or 3 or more nitroglycerin tablets. The AHA also recommends that the new onset of chest pain either at rest or with ordinary activity or a change in a previously stable anginal pattern should be regarded as a potentially dangerous situation that warrants prompt medical attention. When ventricular fibrillation occurs, it is most likely to do so within 1 hour of the onset of symptoms, so encouraging patients not to delay in seeking medical attention is also important.

While pain is the presenting symptom with most AMIs, it should also be noted that infarctions can occur painlessly. These so-called silent MIs are known to occur in individuals with insulin-independent diabetes mellitus and are felt to be related to their systemic neuropathies. They have also recently been noted in individuals who have undergone cardiac transplantation and are presumably

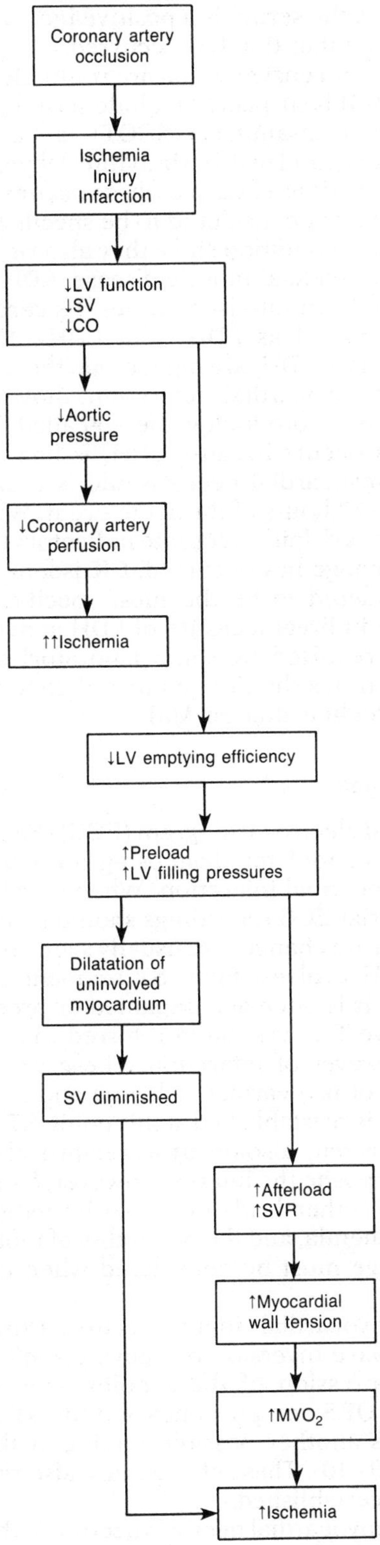


**Figure 43-2.** Hemodynamic consequences prompted by myocardial ischemia associated with coronary artery occlusion.

related to the nerve transections that have been done during the procedure. Although true painless MIs do occur, approximately one-half of patients in whom silent MIs are detected on routine electrocardiographic examinations do relate symptoms in retrospect that are compatible with those of an AMI.

### *Physical Examination*

The behavior of patients who are sustaining an AMI is quite variable. Some patients will lie or sit quietly while the pain persists whereas others may be extremely anxious and restless. Most appear to be in some distress and many will hold a clenched fist over their chest (Levine's sign) to describe their discomfort.

The process of palpation and auscultation in the individual having an AMI also reveals variable findings that are primarily related to the extent of myocardial damage sustained. When myocardial necrosis is severe, more significant physical findings are present, whereas with minimal damage there may be no abnormal findings on physical examination.

When the patient suspected of having an AMI is admitted, he/she should be connected to a cardiac monitor, and vital signs should be obtained immediately. Hypertension is seen in some patients and is usually related to pain and anxiety. Hypotension, or at least a decrease in blood pressure, is probably more common and is related to depressed myocardial function. It often increases again to normal levels as the infarct heals. Extensive myocardial necrosis produces profound hypotension (<80–90 mmHg) along with other shock symptoms including cold clammy skin, oliguria, and mental status changes (see Chaps. 44 and 46 for further discussion of cardiogenic shock). Previously hypertensive patients who sustain significant damage are often normotensive after their MI.

Sinus tachycardia may be seen after an AMI and may be related to pain and agitation. However, it also occurs as a compensatory mechanism to increase cardiac output when extensive damage has occurred. Sinus bradycardia is common after inferior or posterior infarcts and is due to sinus node ischemia. It usually resolves within the first few days.

Cardiac and pulmonary auscultation may also reveal abnormal findings in the individual having an MI, but this part of the physical examination may also be completely normal. Heart sounds are often quiet and even difficult to hear in the individual having a myocardial infarction. Normal intensity gradually returns as healing progresses. (See Chap. 38 for a discussion of heart sounds.)

Fourth heart sounds are common in patients with an AMI and are the result of reduced left ventricular compliance. However, fourth heart sounds are also common in healthy older individuals and thus are not a specific finding in AMI. Third heart sounds, which are more common after anterior infarcts than after inferior or non-transmural infarcts,[44] reflect greater reductions in left ventricular compliance and are indicative of significant myocardial damage. The presence of a third heart sound during the acute phase of myocardial infarction is associated with high mortality rates.

Transmural inferior or lateral infarctions may cause damage to the mitral valve, particularly the papillary muscle structure. In this instance, a systolic murmur of mitral regurgitation will be heard. The patient who sustains an anterior infarction is more likely to develop a defect or hole in the ventricular septal wall (VSD). While this is fortunately not a common occurrence after an AMI, it is a serious one and should be suspected when one detects a new holosystolic murmur heard best along the left sternal border and possibly radiating to the cardiac apex.

Another auscultatory finding in the peri-infarct or post-infarct period is a pericardial friction rub. These occur primarily in transmural myocardial infarctions. They are usually best heard along the left sternal border, although loud rubs may be heard across the entire precordium and even the back. The discomfort associated with friction rubs tends to be constant and can often be intensified by having the patient take a deep breath and diminished by having the patient lean forward. They are usually responsive to anti-inflammatory agents. These factors help to differentiate a rub from post-infarction angina.

Finally, auscultation should include an examination of the lung fields. The presence of rales is indicative of some degree of left ventricular failure. Patients with extensive infarcts may present in frank pulmonary edema with rales and possibly wheezes throughout their lung fields. (See Chap. 29 for a discussion on the assessment of breath sounds).

### *Cardiac Enzymes*

Enzymes are catalytic proteins that damaged tissues release into the blood stream. They are helpful in determining which organ is damaged and to some extent the amount of damage. When a myocardial infarction is suspected, serial serum enzyme levels are checked. Creatinine phosphokinase (CK) is the enzyme that is the most specific indicator of myocardial cell damage, although it can also rise after intramuscular injections, strenuous exercise, or in conditions such as polymyositis or muscular dystrophy. To identify heart muscle damage more specifically, CK is broken down in the laboratory into its isoenzymes: MM, BB, and MB. MB-CK is found almost exclusively in heart muscle, and its elevation in the serum is a positive indicator that a myocardial infarction has occurred.

Other serum enzymes that are routinely checked when an AMI is suspected include serum glutamic-oxaloacetic transaminase (SGOT), lactic dehydrogenase (LDH), and hydroxybutyrate dehydrogenase (HBD). Elevations of each of these occur with AMI, but they are not considered to be specifically diagnostic of this condition since they also rise in liver, kidney, and skeletal muscle disease. LDH can also be broken down into isoenzymes. Its cardiac fraction is reported as $LDH_1$ and $LDH_2$. Normally, serum levels of $LDH_2$ are higher than those of $LDH_1$. Following myocardial infarction, however, the ratio reverses, producing the so-called LDH flip pattern. It occurs because $LDH_1$ is liberated as a result of myocardial necrosis and is usually seen within 12–72 hours of the acute event. While LDH isoenzymes are fairly accurate indicators that myocardial damage has occurred, CK isoenzymes are still considered to be the most specific. Finally, HBD is an indirect measure of LDH activity and is routinely reported by some laboratories. Figure 43–3 illustrates the time course of enzyme elevation and decline after an AMI.

### *ECG Changes*

The 12-lead electrocardiogram (ECG) (Fig. 43–4) is an excellent tool for diagnosing an acute transmural myocardial infarction. When an AMI is suspected, serial ECG recordings should be obtained. Characteristic changes are usually seen on the ECG as the AMI evolves. First, ST segment elevation occurs. This is often accompanied or preceded by tall positive T waves, often referred to as "hyperacute" T waves of infarction. These changes are indicative of myocardial ischemia and are reversible if flow is reestablished at this point. ST segment depressions may also occur as reciprocal changes in leads opposite the infarct. However, ST segment changes in other leads may also be indicative of further ischemia, and the possibility of more extensive damage must be considered when these are seen.

Next, myocardial injury occurs. During this phase, T wave inversion or "cove-plane" T waves occur. Depression of the J point—the point at which the QRS complex ends and the ST segment begins—is another possible finding at this stage (see Fig. 40–10). These changes are also reversible if flow is reestablished.

Finally, myocardial necrosis occurs. At this stage, the ECG will show significant changes in the initial forces of the QRS complex. This is due to a loss of electrical forces from the infarcted area causing the initial QRS forces to move away from the infarct. An initial negative deflection (Q wave $>.04$ second) is created over the area of infarct. A decrease in R

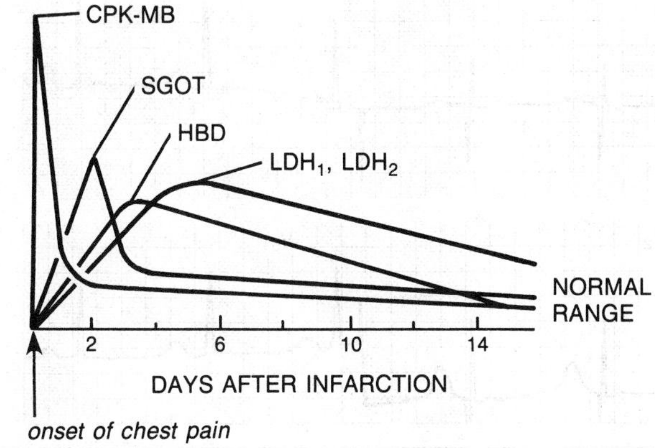


**Figure 43-3.** Evolution of enzyme changes after myocardial infarction.

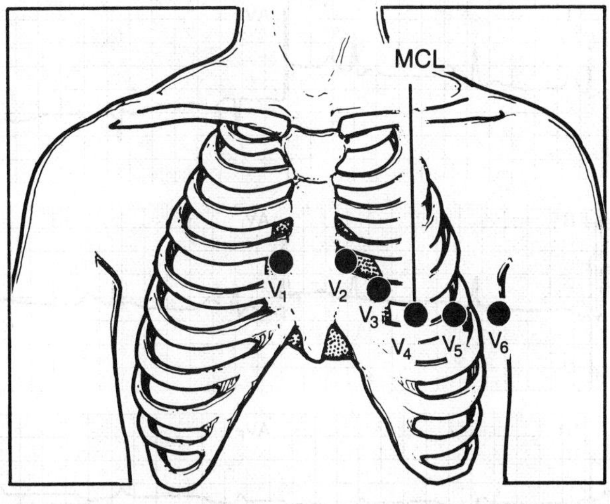


**Figure 43-4.** Twelve-lead electrocardiogram (ECG). To obtain a 12-lead ECG attach limb electrodes to the patient's extremities as labeled. Chest electrodes are positioned as follows: $V_1$ fourth intercostal space (ICS), to the right of the sternum; $V_2$ fourth intercostal space (ICS), to the left of the sternum; $V_3$ halfway between $V_2$ and $V_4$; $V_4$ fifth intercostal space (ICS), at the midclavicular line (MCL); $V_5$ anterior axillary line, (halfway between $V_4$ and $V_6$); $V_6$ fifth intercostal space at the mid-axillary line.

wave amplitude (>30% loss) may also be seen in leads facing the infarcted area because of this negative shift in electrical forces.

The time course over which ECG changes occur is variable. ST segment elevations and peaked T waves develop early and usually return to baseline in a few days to 1-2 weeks. ST segment elevations that persist may be indicative of the development of a ventricular aneurysm. T wave inversions are usually seen within the first few hours and may last for weeks to months. Q waves and R wave amplitude changes usually last indefinitely.

Infarct site is determined by looking for the above ECG changes in leads that face the area of damage. Table 43-4 describes ECG leads associated with the types of various infarcts. It should be noted that since none of the routine 12 leads faces the true posterior surface of the heart, this diagnosis is inferred from reciprocal changes occurring in anterior leads, which are opposite the posterior surface. Leads $V_1$ and $V_2$ are particularly helpful in making this diagnosis. Figure 43-5 demonstrates typical changes associated with posterior myocardial damage and Figures 43-6 and 43-7 illustrate serial changes seen with anterior and inferior infarcts, respectively.

Besides localization by ECG leads, infarcts have also often been categorized as being transmural or non-transmural (subendocardial) based on whether or not Q waves develop on the electrocardiogram. It is now known that Q waves may be seen with non-transmural infarctions and that transmural infarctions do not always develop Q waves. Q wave and non-Q wave infarcts are the preferable terms and the patient's clinical course and evolutionary changes in serial records are used to estimate depth of necrosis.

TABLE 43-4
## Location of Infarct by ECG Leads

| Infarct Area | ECG Leads | ECG Changes |
|---|---|---|
| Anterior wall | $V_1$-$V_6$ | QS pattern<br>Poor R wave progression |
| Anteroseptal | $V_1$-$V_3$ or $V_4$ | QS pattern<br>Poor R wave progression |
| Anterolateral | I, $aV_L$, $V_1$-$V_6$ | Abnormal Q waves |
| Inferior wall (diaphragmatic) | II, III, $aV_F$ | Abnormal Q waves |
| Inferolateral | II, III, $aV_F$, $V_5$, $V_6$ | Abnormal Q waves |
| Posterior wall | $V_1$, $V_2$ | Tall wide R wave |
| Posterolateral | $V_1$, $V_2$<br>I, $aV_L$, $V_5$, $V_6$ | Tall wide R wave<br>Abnormal Q wave |
| Lateral wall | I, $aV_L$, $V_5$, $V_6$ | Abnormal Q waves |

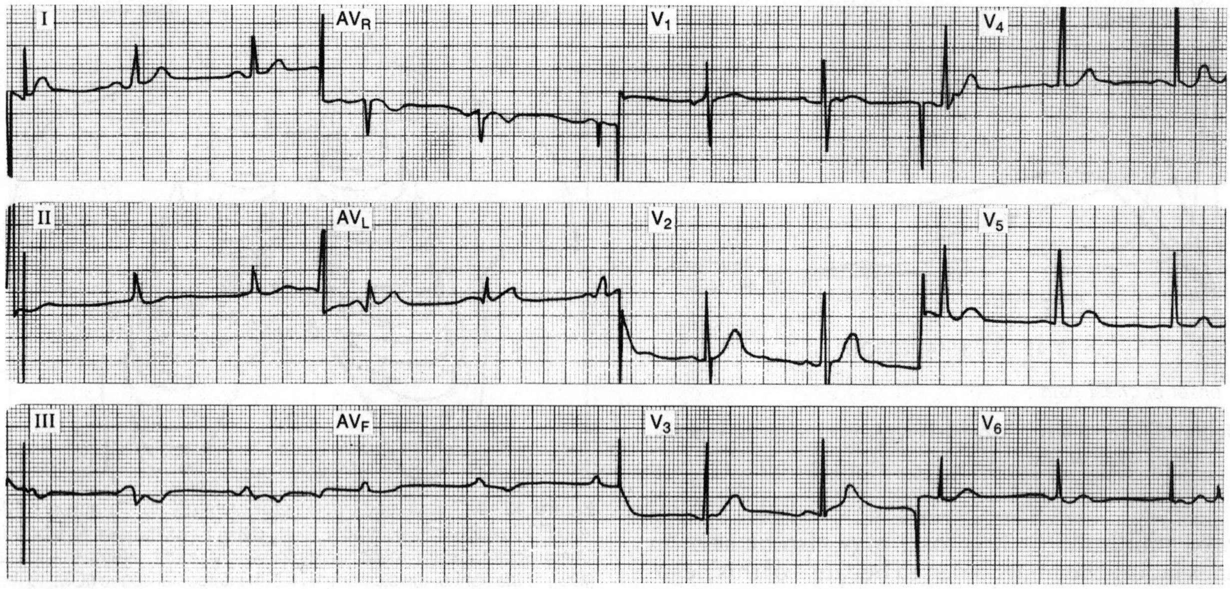


**Figure 43-5.** ECG in posterior myocardial infarction. Note the tall R waves in leads $V_1$ and $V_2$, the upright T wave in lead $V_1$, and flipped T waves in inferior leads III and aVF. (From Cohn, PF: Diagnosis and Therapy of Coronary Artery Disease. Martinus Nijhoff Publishing, Hingham, MA, 1985, p 270, with permission.)

## Treatment of Myocardial Infarction

Treatment of AMI is guided by the following principles: (1) prevention of lethal dysrhythmias or, if this is unsuccessful, their rapid detection and treatment; (2) prevention of other complications; (3) limitation of infarct size; and (4) returning patient to pre-infarct physical and psychologic health status. To accomplish these goals, the following measures are usually employed in the care of the patient who has had an AMI.

### *Monitoring*

Dysrhythmic deaths associated with AMI usually occur within the first hour of the onset of symptoms. Therefore, ECG monitoring should be initiated as rapidly as possible when AMI is suspected. This allows life-threatening dysrhythmias such as ventricular tachycardia and ventricular fibrillation to be rapidly detected and treated. The prophylactic administration of the antiarrhythmic drug lidocaine, which can suppress reentrant activity responsible for ventricular dysrhythmias in ischemic settings, is common in most ICUs. It is usually initiated by administering a bolus injection of 50–100 mg (or 1 mg/kg) intravenously, followed immediately by an infusion of 1–4 mg/minute (20–50 μg/kg/minute).

Vital signs (blood pressure, heart rate, and pulse) should be assessed every 15 minutes until the patient is stable. The patient can be progressed to 1-hour intervals for a few hours and then to 2-hour intervals if stability continues. At nighttime 4-hour intervals are acceptable to promote rest if the patient's condition is satisfactory.

### *Oxygen*

The routine administration of oxygen to patients having a myocardial infarction has recently been questioned. Prior studies have shown that oxygen may increase systemic vascular resistance and arterial blood pressure and thus lower cardiac output, possibly compromising peripheral delivery of oxygen to the tissues.[45,46] On the other hand, there is literature to suggest that elevating arterial oxygen tension ($P_aO_2$) by oxygen inhalation may protect ischemic myocardium and thus reduce infarct size.[47,48]

Hypoxemia secondary to ventilation-perfusion abnormalities, which occur as a consequence of left ventricular failure, is common in AMI patients, particularly in those having a moderate to large infarct. Routine administration of oxygen to these patients is clearly beneficial. In those individuals whose MI is uncomplicated by failure and hypoxemia, the need for oxygen remains less clear. Because of this, some physicians advocate delivering oxygen therapy to these patients based on arterial blood gas results. Other physicians, however, recommend that oxygen still be administered to all patients experiencing chest pain, shortness of breath, or an MI until research on its effects is more definitive.

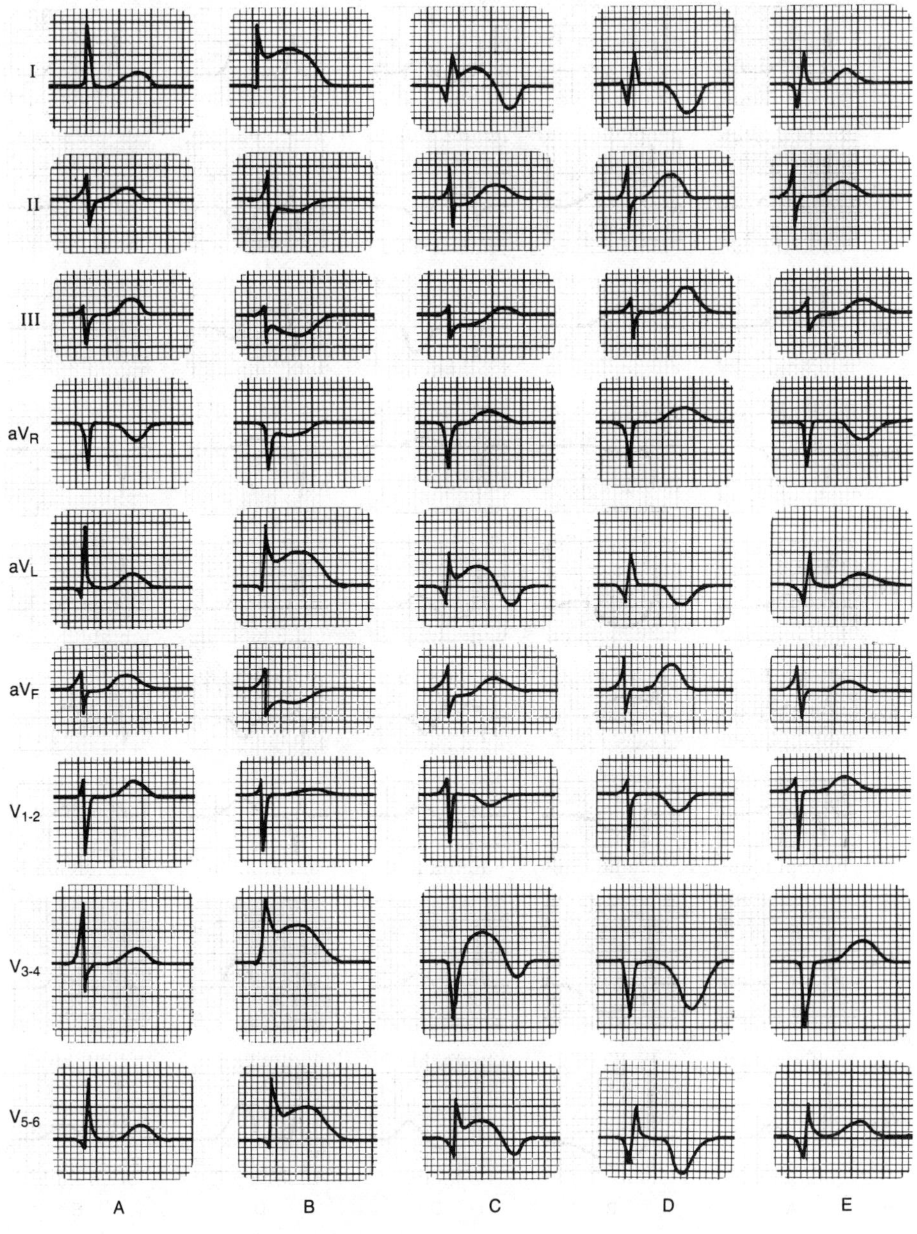


**Figure 43–6.** Diagrammatic illustration of serial electrocardiographic patterns in anterior wall myocardial infarction. (*A*) Normal tracing. (*B*) Early pattern. There is ST segment elevation in leads I, aVL, and $V_3$ to $V_6$ and ST depression in leads II, III, and aVF (the ST depression might reflect inferior wall ischemia or reciprocal depression). (*C*) Later pattern (hours to days). Q waves are present in leads I, aVL, and $V_5$ to $V_6$. QS complexes are present in leads $V_3$ and $V_4$, indicating that the major area of infarction underlies the area recorded by leads $V_3$ and $V_4$. ST segment changes persist but to a lesser degree, and the T waves are beginning to invert in those leads in which ST segment elevation is present. (*D*) Late (established) pattern (days to weeks). The Q waves and QS complexes persist. The ST segments are isoelectric. The T waves are deeply and symmetrically inverted in the leads that showed ST elevation and tall in the leads that showed ST depression. This pattern may persist for the remainder of the patient's life. (*E*) Very late pattern (months to years). The abnormal Q waves and QS complexes persist, but the T waves have returned to normal. Without the benefit of serial ECGs, it is not possible to determine when myocardial infarction occurred. Therefore, no conclusions should be drawn as to the age of the process on the basis of a single ECG. (Adapted from Goldschlager, W and Goldman, MJ: Electrocardiography: Essentials of Interpretation. Appleton & Lange, Los Altos, CA, 1984, p 89.)

### *Analgesia*

Pain relief should be a high priority in managing the patient having an AMI. Sublingual nitroglycerin is usually given initially. It has several beneficial effects in the ischemic setting, including coronary vasodilation, a decrease in myocardial oxygen demand, and possibly an increase in collateral blood flow to the myocardium. It may also cause a drop in blood pressure with a resultant decrease in coronary perfusion pressure and precipitate a compensatory reflex tachycardia, which may increase myocardial oxygen demands. Thus, frequent assessment of blood pressure (BP) and heart rate is mandatory when nitroglycerin is given. It should never be used unless the patient's systolic BP is greater than 100 mmHg. Sublingual isosorbide dinitrate, which has actions similar to those of nitroglycerin, is increasingly being prescribed to manage patients having an AMI.

For severe pain that is unrelieved by sublingual nitroglycerin, morphine sulfate is the drug of choice. Besides providing pain relief, it is also helpful in alleviating patient anxiety and restlessness as well as having beneficial hemodynamic effects. It decreases afterload (systemic vascular resistance), thus enhancing ventricular emptying. It also increases venous capacitance, which reduces venous return to the heart. This action is helpful in enabling the ischemic and/or infarcted myocardial

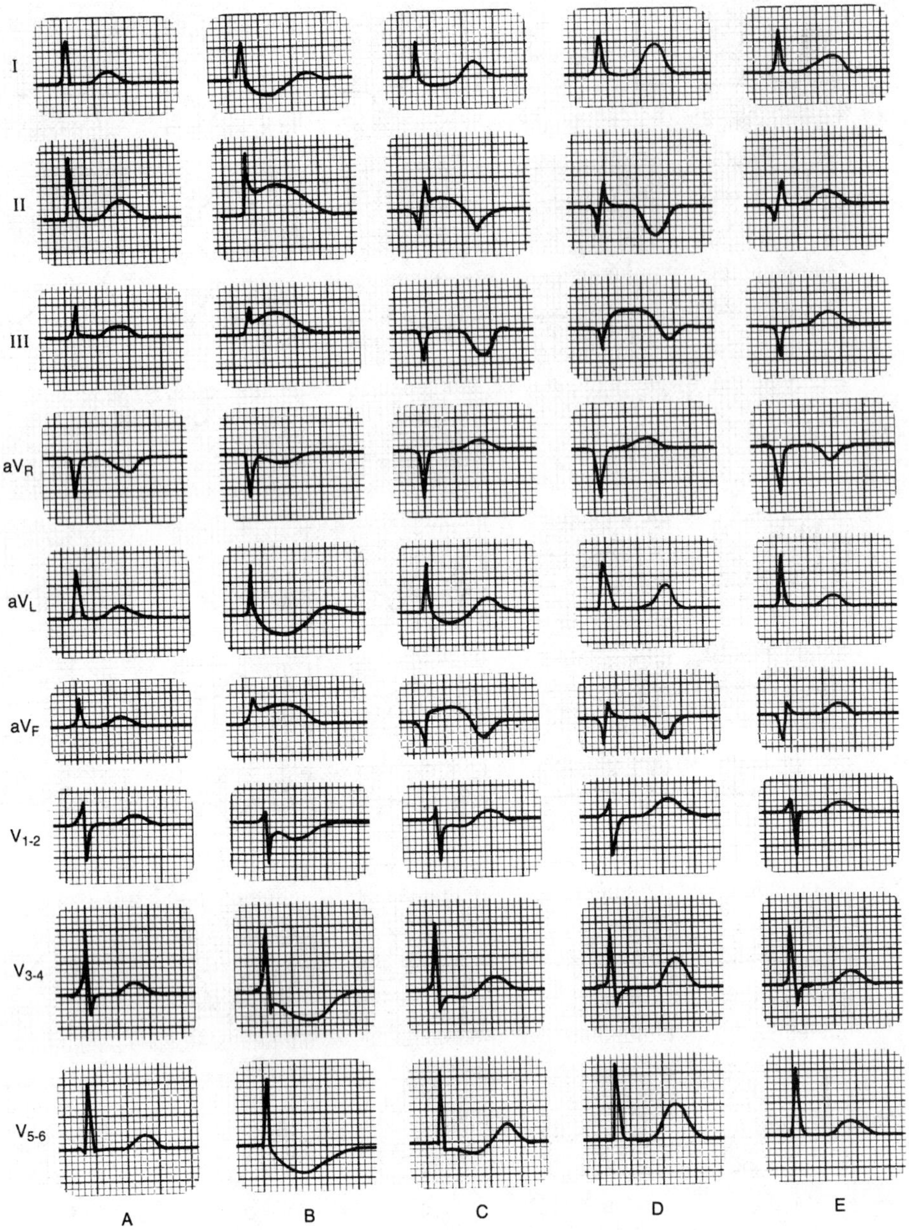


**Figure 43-7.** Diagrammatic illustration of serial electrocardiographic patterns in inferior myocardial infarction. (*A*) Normal tracing. (*B*) Very early pattern (hours after infarction). There is ST segment elevation in leads II, III, and aVF and ST segment depression in leads I, aVL, and aVR, as well as in the precordial leads. (*C*) Later pattern (hours to days). Abnormal Q waves have appeared in the inferior leads. There is less ST elevation in these leads and less ST depression in the anterior leads. The T waves are becoming inverted in leads II, III, and aVF. (*D*) Late (established) pattern (days to weeks). The ST segments are isoelectric. Deep, symmetrically inverted T waves are seen in leads II, III, and aVF. The T waves are abnormally tall and symmetric in leads I and aVL and in the precordial leads. This pattern may persist for the remainder of the patient's life. (*E*) Very late (months to years) pattern. The abnormal Q waves persist, but the T waves have become normal. (Adapted from Goldschlager, W and Goldman, MJ: Electrocardiography: Essentials of Interpretation. Appleton & Lange, Los Altos, CA, 1984, p 92.)

muscle to pump more effectively, particularly in those patients in congestive heart failure.

Finally, intravenous nitroglycerin is employed in the management of patients whose angina is refractory to the above-mentioned measures. Like other forms of nitroglycerin (sublingual, topical, or oral), intravenous nitroglycerin decreases pulmonary capillary wedge pressure and right atrial pressure. Arterial blood pressure may also be lowered, which may have detrimental effects on myocardial perfusion, thus promoting further ischemia. Therefore, hemodynamic monitoring to detect significant changes in cardiac indices is essential during vasodilator therapy. (See Appendix A for further discussion of nitroglycerin.) (The effect of vasodilator therapy on arterial pressure dynamics is depicted in Fig. 41-11.)

### *Activity and Diet*

Bedrest is generally prescribed for the first 24 hours after an MI. Those individuals whose MI is uncomplicated may be allowed out of bed to a chair on the first post-MI day, and their activity level is gradually increased after this. Activity progression must be slower when post-MI complications such as congestive heart failure, dysrhythmias, shock, or postinfarction angina occur. It is important to consider the need for emotional as well as physical rest for all MI patients. The ICU environment should be quiet, families should be urged to avoid controversial issues, and sedation should be provided to promote rest.

The uncomplicated MI patient may be discharged from the ICU in 2–3 days and from the hospital within as few as 5 days (commonly 7–10 days). Discharge of the patient with complications is primarily dependent on their severity.

Rehabilitation, which should be started during the patient's hospitalization, proceeds gradually at home. Patients are usually advised that they may return to work in 4–6 weeks provided that no heavy lifting is required.

In regard to diet, it is advisable to keep patients NPO for the first 4–6 hours and then on clear liquids only for 24 hours. This helps to diminish the possibility of aspiration during this high-risk period if a cardiac arrest should occur. A low-cholesterol diet should then be provided with appropriate explanations about its benefits. Salt restriction should also be provided for patients with heart failure. Caffeine intake should be limited because of its potential arrhythmogenic effects. Finally, a stool softener is routinely administered to prevent constipation and straining.

### *Anticoagulation*

The role of systemic anticoagulation in the AMI patient remains controversial. However, minidose heparin (5000 units subcutaneously) every 8–12 hours has been shown to substantially diminish the incidence of deep vein thrombosis and pulmonary embolism in these patients.[49] It is routinely prescribed and continued until the patient is fully ambulatory.

## Complications

The complications associated with myocardial infarction can be divided into 4 types of disorders: (1) hemodynamic, (2) inflammatory, (3) embolic, and (4) rhythm.

### *Hemodynamic Disorders*

The hemodynamic states seen after myocardial infarctions have been divided into 5 clinical classifications: (1) normal hemodynamics, (2) hyperdynamic circulatory state, (3) hypovolemic hypotension, (4) left ventricular failure, and (5) cardiogenic shock[50,51] (Table 43–5).

The patient who has a small myocardial infarction usually has stable vital signs and no evidence of congestive heart failure. These individuals normally will do well with continuous ECG monitoring, pain relief, frequent assessments for evidence of complications, and reassurance.

When a hyperdynamic circulatory state exists, the patient will present with a sinus tachycardia, hypertension (in a previously normotensive individual), and bounding pulses. Since myocardial oxygen consumption can be significantly increased in this state, treatment with beta-adrenergic blocking agents is usually initiated. Beta-blockers decrease cardiac index, stroke index, heart rate, and blood pressure with a net effect of decreased myocardial oxygen consumption in the setting of increased circulating catecholamines associated with AMI.[52]

Hypotension in the post-MI patient requires careful evaluation in order to ensure appropriate treatment. Hypovolemia, which may be due to vomiting, severe diaphoresis, or aggressive treatment with diuretics or nitrates, is one potential cause of hypotension. When it is suspected or documented (i.e., pulmonary capillary wedge pressure less than 14 mmHg) treatment consists of fluid replacement with 50-ml intravenous bolus infusions with a crystalloid solution until the wedge pressure is between 14 and 18 mmHg. Because of the reduced left ventricular compliance associated with acute ischemia, these higher than normal filling pressures may be required to achieve normotension. Red blood cells, rather than crystalloid solution, should be infused in the patient with a low hematocrit.

A relative state of hypovolemia may exist when systemic vascular resistance (SVR) is reduced after an AMI. Activation of left ventricular wall baroreceptors mediated by systolic bulging of the infarcted segment is felt to account for this abnormal reduction in SVR.[53] Careful administration of nor-

TABLE 43–5
**Classification of Hemodynamic States following Myocardial Infarction**

| Classification | LVFP | CI | HR | CVP | BP |
|---|---|---|---|---|---|
| Normal | Normal | Normal | Normal | Normal | Normal |
| Hyperdynamic | Decreased | Normal | Normal or increased | Normal or decreased | Increased |
| Hypovolemia | Decreased | Decreased | Increased | Decreased | Normal or increased |
| Pump failure, shock | Increased | Decreased | Increased | Normal or decreased | Decreased |

LVFP = left ventricle filling pressure; CI = Cardiac index; HR = heart rate; CVP = central venous pressure; BP = blood pressure.

epinephrine is the treatment of choice here despite epinephrine's known effects on increasing $MVO_2$ through dual alpha- and beta-adrenergic stimulating actions. Hopefully, its elevation of coronary perfusion pressure will offset its negative effects on $MVO_2$.

Hypotension on the basis of a relative hypovolemia is also seen in patients who have had a right ventricular (RV) infarct. RV infarcts are most common in inferior or inferoposterior AMIs. They are diagnosed when the patient has an elevated jugular venous pressure, a right ventricular gallop, ST segment elevations in ECG leads $V_1$, $V_{3R}$, and $V_{4R}$, and central venous pressure elevation that is disproportionate to the pulmonary capillary wedge pressure. Volume administration in these patients augments RV preload, which ultimately serves to augment LV preload and finally cardiac output. Vasodilators, which decrease impedance to RV and LV outflow, may also be administered, particularly when LV infarct accompanies RV infarct, which often occurs. Positive inotropic agents such as dobutamine are also often needed.

The last 2 clinical classifications of hemodynamic states seen after AMI are left ventricular failure and cardiogenic shock. The reader should refer to Chapter 44 for further discussion of these topics. Mitral regurgitation that is caused by papillary muscle dysfunction or rupture in the post-MI patient is also discussed in Chapter 44.

Ventricular septal defects (VSD) develop in approximately 1% of patients who have had an MI. They can cause right and left ventricular failure, particularly if not detected and treated promptly. Rupture of a portion of the ventricular septum usually produces a holosystolic murmur and systolic thrill along the left sternal border. Left-to-right shunting occurs through the defect. The degree of shunting is primarily influenced by the ratio of the pulmonary to systemic vascular resistance. A greater reduction in systemic vascular resistance than in pulmonary vascular resistance will produce a reduction in left-to-right shunting and an improvement in systemic cardiac output. The intra-aortic balloon pump is the treatment of choice because of its ability to selectively lower systemic vascular resistance. Early surgical intervention is then recommended to repair the defect.

### Inflammatory Disorders

Pericarditis, an inflammation of the pericardial lining of the heart, occurs in up to 15% of patients who have transmural infarctions. It is recognized by auscultation of a pericardial friction rub, which is usually best heard along the left sternal border or just inside the PMI. The discomfort associated with pericarditis is generally continuous, which helps to differentiate this syndrome from post-infarction angina.

Dressler's syndrome, which is characterized by pericarditis, pericardial and pleural effusion, and fever, usually occurs several weeks to many months after infarction. Its etiology is unclear. It is usually responsive to aspirin or indomethacin, although occasionally steroids are required for symptom relief. Anticoagulation should be avoided in all patients with pericarditis to reduce the risk of hemorrhagic pericardial effusion.

### Embolic Disorders

A variety of embolic disorders may occur as a complication of myocardial infarction. Large infarctions, particularly those that develop a ventricular aneurysm, predispose the patient to the development of a mural thrombus, which can embolize systemically. Pulmonary embolization is another possibility. Immediate anticoagulation followed by long-term administration is indicated if either of these develops.

### Rhythm Disorders

Tachydysrhythmias, bradydysrhythmias, and conduction defects may occur after a myocardial infarction. Treatment of any rhythm disorder in this setting is indicated when myocardial oxygen requirements are increased, hemodynamic compromise occurs, or the patient is at risk of developing a more lethal dysrhythmia.

Tachydysrhythmias limit the diastolic filling time, and thus reduce coronary vessel perfusion during diastole. They are also detrimental because of their deleterious effect on myocardial oxygen consumption. Bradydysrhythmias and conduction defects can produce a significant decrease in cardiac output. When the normal atrioventricular (AV) conduction sequence is disturbed by these rhythm disorders, further compromise of cardiac output occurs as the atrial contribution to ventricular filling is lost. Finally, hypotension may result from any of these dysrhythmias. It is particularly damaging to the ischemic myocardium and should be treated promptly. For further discussion of the etiology and treatment of dysrhythmias and conduction defects after AMI, see Table 43-6 (see also Chapter 40).

## Nursing Care

### Therapeutic Goals

The following therapeutic goals provide the framework upon which the critical care nurse bases care:

1. Perform a thorough and ongoing assessment.
2. Limit energy expenditure to minimize myocardial oxygen consumption.

TABLE 43-6
**Dysrhythmia and Conduction Defect Etiology and Treatment after Myocardial Infarction**

| | Etiology | Treatment |
|---|---|---|
| **Atrial Dysrhythmias** | | |
| Sinus tachycardia | Hypovolemia, hypotension | Volume replacement |
| | Pain, anxiety | Analgesia, sedation |
| | Hypertension | Beta-adrenergic blockade |
| | Extensive myocardial damage | Assess hemodynamic parameters to determine need for inotropes, vasodilators, volume, diuretics |
| | Pericarditis | Indomethecin, aspirin |
| | Anemia | Administer RBCs to keep hemoglobin >10 g/100 ml |
| | Hypoxemia | Oxygen |
| | Electrolye, acid-base disturbance | Correct disturbances |
| Atrial flutter or fibrillation | Left atrial dilatation (especially with extensive anterior infarction) | Prompt treatment with D/C synchronized cardioversion or rapid atrial stimulation (atrial flutter only) if hemodynamic compromise occurs |
| | Heart failure | Digitalis, beta blocker, or verapamil; treat faillure |
| Supraventricular tachycardia | Catecholamine stimulation of ischemic myocardium | D/C synchronized cardioversion or rapid atrial stimulation if hemodynamic compromise occurs |
| | AV nodal reentry | Manual carotid sinus pressure<br>Edrophonium (Tensilon)<br>Digitalis |
| Premature atrial contractions | Atrial dilatation | Treatment of failure |
| | Heart failure | Analgesia, sedation |
| | Excessive autonomic stimulation | |
| **Ventricular Dysrhythmias** | | |
| Ventricular premature contractions (>6/minute, multifocal pairs, R on T) | Ischemia, infarct (reentry mechanism in first hour; enhanced automaticity thereafter) | Lidocaine<br>Procainamide if lidocaine is ineffective |
| Accelerated idioventricular rhythm | Sinus node slowing or ectopic site acceleration | Atropine or atrial pacing to increase sinus rate and suppress ventricular pacemaker<br>Lidocaine |
| Ventricular tachycardia | Ischemia, infarct (mechanism may be enhanced automaticity or reentry) | If hemodynamically stable:<br>Bolus lidocaine therapy<br>If hemodynamically unstable:<br>Precordial thump<br>D/C synchronized cardioversion<br>D/C defibrillation if rate too rapid for synchronized shock |
| Ventricular fibrillation | Ischemia, infarct | Prophylactic lidocaine<br>D/C defibrillation |
| **Bradyarrhythmias and Conduction Defects** | | |
| Sinus bradycardia | Vagal hyperactivity in first 6 hours | No treatment if patient is asymptomatic |
| | Sinus node dysfunction or atrial ischemia after first 6 hours | Atropine if symptomatic |
| **Atrioventricular (AV) Block** | | |
| First-degree AV block | Digitalis toxicity | Discontinue digitalis |
| | Vagal hyperactivity | Atropine if symptomatic |
| | AV node ischemia (inferior MI or RV infarct) | |
| Second-degree AV block Mobitz Type I or Wenckebach | Same as above | Same as above, plus temporary transvenous pacemaker insertion if ventricular rate falls below 60/minute, or patient develops ventricular irritability, heart failure, or bundle branch block |
| Second-degree AV Block Mobitz Type II | Same as above<br>Seen rarely in AMI | Temporary transvenous pacemaker insertion |
| Complete AV Block | Anterior infarction (poor prognosis)<br>Inferior infarction | Temporary ventricular or atrioventricular sequential transvenous pacing |
| **Intraventricular Block** | | |
| Left bundle branch block (LBBB) | Usually anterior MI | Temporary pacemaker prophylactically because of 40%–60% risk of complete heart block |

*(continued)*

TABLE 43-6
**Dysrhythmia and Conduction Defect Etiology and Treatment after Myocardial Infarction *(Continued)***

| | Etiology | Treatment |
|---|---|---|
| Right bundle branch block (RBBB) | Usually anterior MI | Observation |
| Bilateral bundle branch block<br>Left axis deviation + RBBB<br>Right axis deviation + RBBB<br>First-degree AV block + LBBB | Usually anterior MI (poor prognosis) | Temporary pacemaker—high risk of complete heart block |

3. Maintain hemodynamic stability to facilitate cardiac output and tissue perfusion.
4. Identify and promptly treat complications of myocardial infarction.
5. Provide emotional support to patient and family.
6. Provide appropriate education to patient and family.

Implementation of the nursing process with nursing diagnoses, desired patient outcomes, and nursing interventions and their rationales are presented in Table 43-7.

## CASE STUDY WITH SAMPLE CARE PLAN: PATIENT WITH MYOCARDIAL INFARCTION*

Mr. M.T. is a 45-year-old white male who developed right-sided chest pain that radiated down both arms and to his jaw, at 8:40 a.m. while shopping. The pain was associated with shortness of breath. He denied nausea, vomiting, dizziness, or palpitations.

*6/6, 9:40 a.m.* M.T. was admitted to the Emergency Room of University Hospital while continuing to complain of right-sided chest pain. Vital signs on admission: BP 180/110; heart rate 50 beats/minute; sinus bradycardia, respiratory rate 20/minute, non-labored; 12-Lead ECG showed 2-mm ST segment elevation in leads $V_1$ through $V_4$ and 1-mm ST segment elevation in leads $V_5$ and $V_6$, and in leads I and $aV_L$. He was given a total of 1 nitroglycerin sublingually and 1 inch of nitropaste, with no relief of pain.

*6/6, 10 a.m.* M.T. was transferred to the Coronary Care Unit to rule out an anterolateral wall MI, where he arrived continuing to complain of chest pain. Vital signs on admission to the CCU: BP 140/96; heart rate 60 beats/minute in normal sinus rhythm, without ectopy; respiratory rate 16/minute, nonlabored; temperature 97.6°F (36.4°C) orally; 12-lead ECG continued to show ischemic changes. Patient is mildly anxious, asking if he has had any heart damage.

*By Kathleen Daley White and Margaret Connelly

## Assessment

Cardiovascular: Normal $S_1$ and $S_2$; no murmurs or rubs on auscultation. No peripheral edema or jugular venous distention observed. All peripheral pulses present and strong in quality.

Respiratory: M.T. is placed on oxygen at 2 liters via nasal cannula. ABGs are within normal limits. Lungs are clear to auscultation; he denies shortness of breath.

Gastrointestinal: Abdomen is soft with no palpable masses. Bowel sounds are normal. He denies nausea or indigestion. He is placed on a clear-liquid diet.

Renal/Urinary: The patient is voiding clear, amber urine. A urinalysis is within normal limits. An intravenous 5% dextrose and water at 20 ml/hour is initiated.

Past Medical History: M.T. has a past history of subendocardial MI 5 years prior to this admission. Six months after the initial MI, he developed angina at rest and was started on 10 mg propranolol 3 times/day. He has been free of chest pain since that time. He also has a 6-year history of hypertension controlled on Minipress, 1 mg twice a day.

Family History: His family history is significant for heart disease. His father is alive at age 74 with hypertension. Mother died at age 71 from congestive heart failure.

M.T. is given 3 doses of IV push metoprolol (Lopressor) at 5-minute intervals with complete relief of chest pain. A 12-lead ECG shows persistent changes but now with T wave inversion in lead I and then in lead $aV_L$. He is started on low-dose nitroglycerin infusion, titrated to maintain systolic

## TABLE 43-7. CARE PLAN FOR THE PATIENT WITH AN ACUTE MYOCARDIAL INFARCTION

| Nursing Diagnoses | Desired Patient Outcomes | Nursing Interventions | Rationales |
|---|---|---|---|
| ***Nursing Diagnosis #1*** Tissue perfusion, alteration in, related to:<br>1. Coronary artery occlusion resulting in decreased myocardial tissue perfusion.<br>2. Ventricular dysfunction resulting in decreased perfusion to brain, kidneys, lungs, liver.<br>3. Thromboembolism resulting from deep venous thrombosis or mural thrombi. | Patient will:<br>1. Maintain hemodynamic stability:<br>• BP within 10 mmHg of baseline.<br>• HR 60–80/minute.<br>• Absence of dysrhythmias.<br>• Cardiac output 4–8 liters/minute.<br>• Brisk capillary refill (within 2 sec).<br>• Urine output >30 ml/hr.<br>• Mental status: alert, oriented.<br>2. Remain without thromboembolic events or, if they occur, thromboembolism will resolve without significant sequelae.<br>• Extremities warm to touch; pulses palpable and equal bilaterally.<br>• Absence of positive Homan's sign.<br>• Circumference of extremities equal bilaterally. | • Initiate rest-promoting activities: Bedrest until hemodynamically stable, quiet environment; limit visitors if needed to ensure patient rest. | • Rest decreases myocardial oxygen consumption. |
| | | • Allow bedside commode privileges if hemodynamically stable.<br>• If MI is uncomplicated, patient should be allowed out of bed to the chair for periods of 1–2 hours and should be allowed to use the commode instead of a bedpan from the time of admission. | • Use of bedside commode is associated with less stress than use of a bedpan.<br>• Prolonged bedrest is associated with many complications (fluid shifting, orthostatic intolerance, increased heart rate, progressive decalcification resulting in osteoporosis and urolithiasis, and thromboembolism). Early ambulation is the most effective means to combat these.[54] |
| | | • For patient with complicated MI, initiate activities to counteract effects of bedrest.<br>○ Elevate head of bed when possible.<br>○ Have patient turn frequently in bed.<br>○ Teach footboard exercises (limit contraction durations to less than 10 seconds when performing these).<br>○ Apply anti-embolism stockings.<br>○ Consult with physician regarding initiation of mini-dose heparin (5,000 units subcutaneously q 8–12 hr). | • Footboard exercises may decrease venous stasis. Contractions less than 10 seconds in duration cause no significant detrimental cardiovascular response.[55] |
| | | • Allow to feed self if able and if patient desires.<br>• Assist with bathing the first day and as needed on subsequent days. | • Self-feeding is less stressful for most patients.<br>• Bed bathing is associated with insignificant cardiovascular responses in terms of blood pressure, ECG, heart sounds, oxygen uptake.[56] |
| | | • Monitor for factors that may cause an increase in myocardial oxygen consumption and institute measures to correct these. | • Hypotension, hypertension, increased heart rate, increased contractility, pain, fever, anemia, volume depletion, and psychologic stress cause an increase in myocardial oxygen consumption and may increase infarct size.[57] |
| | | • Administer pharmacologic therapy as ordered (nitrates, nitroprusside, beta-blockers, calcium channel blockers) to increase myocardial oxygen supply or decrease $MVO_2$. | • Pharmacologic measures to increase myocardial oxygen supply or to decrease demand may help to limit infarct size. |

*(continued)*

**TABLE 43-7. CARE PLAN FOR THE PATIENT WITH AN ACUTE MYOCARDIAL INFARCTION *(Continued)***

| Nursing Diagnoses | Desired Patient Outcomes | Nursing Interventions | Rationales |
|---|---|---|---|
| ***Nursing Diagnosis #1 (cont.)*** | | | |
| | | • Administer oxygen as prescribed.<br>○ Monitor for possible negative effects of $O_2$ therapy including increased HR and systemic vascular resistance. | • Oxygen may have negative cardiovascular effects. |
| | | • Monitor for signs and symptoms of pulmonary embolus including tachypnea, tachycardia, shortness of breath, anxiety, hypotension, deteriorating oxygenation, pulmonary artery pressure elevation, jugular venous distention. | • Early detection and treatment of thromboembolic events may aid in more successful recovery. |
| | | • Monitor for signs of deep vein thrombosis:<br>○ Positive Homan's sign.<br>○ Change in color, temperature, or girth of extremity.<br>○ Presence of tenderness and/or cords. | • Early detection and treatment of thromboembolic events may aid in more successful recovery. |
| ***Nursing Diagnosis #2***<br>Alteration in cardiac output, related to:<br>1. Dysrhythmias, conduction disturbances.<br>2. Left ventricular dysfunction.<br>3. Hypovolemia. | Patient will:<br>1. Maintain electrophysiologic stability.<br>• Absence of dysrhythmias.<br>• 12-lead ECG return to baseline.<br>2. Maintain hemodynamic stability.<br>• HR 60–80/min.<br>• BP within 10 mm Hg of baseline.<br>3. Be normovolemic.<br>• Cardiac output 4–8 liters/min.<br>• Brisk capillary refill (2 seconds). | • Attach to cardiac monitor as soon as possible. | • Early detection of dysrhythmia allows for early treatment. |
| | | • Select best lead to monitor based on type of MI patient is having, type of conduction disturbance, and needs of monitor, especially if a computerized dysrhythmia detection system is used. Multiple lead monitoring is preferable. | • Appropriate lead monitoring allows ECG changes (i.e., ST segment, T wave, PR or QRS interval prolongation) to be seen and treated properly. |
| | | • Treat lethal dysrhythmias immediately (V-tach, V-fib, asystole) per unit protocols. Notify physician. | • Prompt treatment of lethal dysrhythmias is more successful than delayed treatment. |
| | | • Be aware of potential significance of warning dysrhythmias—VPBs >6/minute, R-on-T VPBs, coupling. | • "Warning dysrhythmias" may precipitate episodes of V-tach, V-fib. These dysrhythmias may also occur without warning. |
| | | • Notify physician and institute treatment of tachyarrhythmias and bradyarrhythmias as soon as possible. | • Bradyarrhythmias and tachyarrhythmias may compromise CO, and increase myocardial oxygen consumption. |
| | | • Check vital signs (BP, HR, PAP, CVP, CO) with any change in rhythm or conduction. | • Rhythm or conduction changes may be associated with hemodynamic compromise, particularly in a patient with marginal left ventricular function. |
| | | • Allow hot or cold beverages in small quantities if patient desires. Elevate head of bed during ingestion. | • Hot or cold beverages in small quantities (1 glass) consumed in a sitting position (at least semi-Fowler's) are not associated with dysrhythmias, ECG changes.[58] |

| | | | |
|---|---|---|---|
| | | • Take oral temperature routinely; rectal temperature may be taken if necessary. | • Taking oral temperature is less stressful to the patient.<br>• Rectal route is not associated with vagal stimulation and thus may be used if necessary.[59] |
| | | • Assess for signs and symptoms of left ventricular dysfunction. These include sinus tachycardia; dyspnea, orthopnea; pulmonary rales; $S_3$ gallop, pulsus alternans; jugular venous pressure elevation, positive hepatojugular reflex, peripheral or sacral edema; hypotension, elevated pulmonary capillary wedge pressure, elevated central venous pressure, decreased cardiac output and cardiac index. | • Myocardial ischemia and/or infarct predisposes patient to left ventricular dysfunction.<br>• Degree of LV dysfunction is a major determinant of post-MI mortality. |
| | | • See Chapter 44 for further discussion of ventricular dysfunction related to cardiogenic shock, mitral valve dysfunction. | |
| | | • Assess for signs of ventricular septal defect (VSD) including a holosystolic murmur heard best at the lower left sternal border; left-to-right shunting; signs of heart failure as above with the degree dependent on the size of the VSD. | • Myocardial damage may result in a defect in the ventricular septal wall. |
| | | • Assess patient for signs of hypovolemia. These include hypotension (BP may be increased initially); decreased central venous pressure; decreased pulmonary capillary wedge pressure; tachycardia; oliguria; decreased cardiac output and cardiac index. | • Vomiting, severe diaphoresis, aggressive treatment with diuretics or nitrates may deplete intravascular volume. |
| ***Nursing Diagnosis #3***<br>Alteration in comfort: Pain, related to:<br>1. Myocardial ischemia, necrosis.<br>2. Extension of infarct.<br>3. Pericarditis.<br>4. Dressler's syndrome (late pericarditis). | Patient will:<br>1. Be pain free.<br>2. Notify staff immediately of chest pain episodes.<br>3. Maintain hemodynamic stability:<br>• BP within 10 mmHg of baseline.<br>• HR at rest: 60–80/minute without dysrhythmias.<br>• Mental status: Alert and oriented to person, place, and time. | • Have patient describe pain, including location, radiation, associated symptoms (nausea, vomiting, diaphoresis, shortness of breath, palpitations), precipitating factors, quality, duration, relief mechanisms, association with movement, respiration, or palpation. | • Description helps to determine etiology of chest pain.<br>◦ See Table 7–1 for SLIDT tool. |
| | | • Administer nitrates and/or narcotic analgesia as needed and monitor response to therapy. | • Nitrates help to relieve pain by means of coronary vasodilatation and both preload and afterload reduction. Narcotics act centrally to relieve pain and also have some afterload reducing effects. |
| | | • Monitor vital signs before and per unit protocol after medication administration. Assess for hypotension, tachycardia, and respiratory depression. Assess for relief of pain. | • Significant change in vital signs (BP decrease > 10 mmHg and/or HR increase > 20 beats/minute and/or respiratory rate < 10/minute) may necessitate discontinuation of medication. |

*(continued)*

**TABLE 43-7. CARE PLAN FOR THE PATIENT WITH AN ACUTE MYOCARDIAL INFARCTION *(Continued)***

| Nursing Diagnoses | Desired Patient Outcomes | Nursing Interventions | Rationales |
|---|---|---|---|
| ***Nursing Diagnosis #3 (cont.)*** | • Urinary output greater than 30 ml/hr. | • Obtain 12-lead ECG prior to medication administration, particularly if this is undiagnosed or new-onset chest pain, or recurrence of chest pain in a patient who has been pain free for 24 hours.<br>• Stay with patient until ischemic chest pain is relieved. | • Documentation of changes on a 12-lead ECG helps to make the diagnosis of cardiac chest pain (vs. other types of chest discomfort), and also helps to diagnose infarct extension, Printzmetal's angina, or pericarditis.<br>• Presence of caring, supportive, knowledgeable nurse may reduce patient anxiety, which reduces stress response. This causes reduced circulating catecholamines (epinephrine), which help to increase the pain threshold, thereby reducing myocardial oxygen consumption. |
| | | • Assess patient for pericarditis or Dressler's syndrome (depending on time interval after MI) if recurrent MI and infarct extension have been ruled out. Symptoms of pericarditis or Dressler's syndrome may include:<br>○ Chest pain increased by deep inspiration.<br>○ Chest pain alleviated by leaning forward.<br>○ Presence of a pericardial friction rub.<br>○ ECG changes associated with pericarditis (diffuse or localized ST segment elevation, with upward concavity).<br>○ Atrial arrhythmias.<br>○ Persistent fever >101°F. (38.3°C.).<br>○ Symptoms of pleuritis, pericardial effusion, or tamponade.<br>○ Response to aspirin or indomethacin. | • Either condition may occur following myocardial infarction, particularly following transmural MIs. Symptoms are similar. Time courses are somewhat similar and overlap does occur, sometimes making it difficult to distinguish between these two syndromes. |
| | | ○ If patient is on anticoagulant medication, check with physician about continuation. | ○ Anticoagulants may precipitate cardiac tamponade. |
| ***Nursing Diagnosis #4***<br>Anxiety, related to:<br>1. Knowledge deficit regarding illness and its prognosis.<br>2. Pain. | Patient will:<br>1. Verbalize basic understanding of his/her illness. | • Assess level of understanding of disease process and readiness to learn.<br>○ Provide patient with appropriate information on coronary artery disease and myocardial infarction when patient is ready. | • Fear and anxiety initiate the stress response. This causes increased catecholamine release, which causes increased myocardial oxygen consumption ($MVO_2$), as well as decreasing the pain threshold, which further increases $MVO_2$.[60] |

| | | | |
|---|---|---|---|
| 3. Intensive care setting.<br>4. Disruption of daily life activities, role and self-image changes, family concerns. | 2. Verbalize feeling less anxious.<br>3. Describe pain and verbalize when it is relieved.<br>4. Verbalize familiarity with ICU routines and practices. | ○ Reassure patient appropriately regarding prognosis.<br>○ Initiate other anxiety-relieving measures; remain with patient during stressful periods or when patient needs to talk; encourage to verbalize fears and anxieties; listen attentively; explain all procedures and equipment involved in the patient's care; involve in decision-making whenever possible; instruct in relaxation techniques; limit nursing personnel caring for patient to increase continuity; orient patient and family to all ICU routines. | ○ Presence of a caring supportive individual may help to increase patient's ability to cope.<br>○ Knowing what to expect helps to reduce anxiety.<br>○ Maintaining some sense of control helps to reduce anxiety.<br>○ Use of relaxation techniques helps to promote a sense of control over situation. |
| | | • Assess for signs and symptoms of anxiety: restlessness, agitation, tachycardia, tachypnea, diaphoresis, crying, uncooperative or noncompliant behavior, verbalization of fears, concerns, inability to concentrate. | • Underlying cause of anxiety must be determined in order to provide appropriate intervention.<br>○ Some behaviors may be helpful during the acute phase of an MI, as for example, denial. (Refer to Chapter 3 for discussion of psychosocial implications of MI.) |
| | | • Administer nitrates and/or narcotic medications until pain is relieved or until significant decrease in BP occurs (<90–100 mmHg). | • Pain precipitates and/or aggravates anxiety.<br>• Narcotics alleviate chest discomfort and also decrease anxiety and increase the patient's sense of well-being. |
| | | ○ Administer sedatives as needed. | • Mild sedation helps to decrease anxiety and increase sense of well-being. |
| | | • Manipulate ICU environment to promote as much rest for patient as possible. | • Physical rest reduces myocardial oxygen consumption, promotes a sense of well-being, and reduces anxiety. |
| | | • Assess family members' coping abilities.<br>• Support family members in dealing with their own as well as patient's needs.<br>• Encourage family members to avoid stressful and controversial issues at this time. | • Family coping behaviors influence patient's coping abilities and may positively or negatively affect patient's level of anxiety.[61] |
| | | • Assess family members' level of knowledge and educate appropriately when they are ready.<br>• Allow family members to verbalize fear, concerns. | • Family members' lack of knowledge may influence their level of anxiety and ultimately patient's anxiety level.[62] |
| | | • Facilitate family visiting by individualizing visiting hours to patient and family needs. | • Short, artificially terminated visiting hours are arousing to patient's cardiovascular system[63–64] and may increase anxiety and myocardial oxygen consumption. |
| | | • Assess need for spiritual counselor. | • Spiritual support is helpful to some patients to decrease anxiety. |

*(continued)*

## TABLE 43-7. CARE PLAN FOR THE PATIENT WITH AN ACUTE MYOCARDIAL INFARCTION *(Continued)*

| Nursing Diagnoses | Desired Patient Outcomes | Nursing Interventions | Rationales |
|---|---|---|---|
| ***Nursing Diagnosis #5***<br>Coping, potential ineffective individual, related to:<br>1. Diagnosis and fear of death. | Patient will:<br>1. Verbalize feelings of fear and depression.<br>2. Use denial (if he/she chooses) as a defense mechanism to control fear and anxiety but not to interfere with ultimate acceptance of prognosis and rehabilitation program. | • Assess for symptoms of depression, including anorexia, insomnia, listlessness, crying, expression of feelings of hopelessness, lack of self-esteem.<br>• Encourage to verbalize feelings.<br>• Assess use of denial as a defense mechanism; signs of this include explicit verbal denial, inappropriate cheerfulness, unrealistic noncompliance with medical regimen.<br>• Support appropriate use of denial by the patient.<br>• Monitor physiologic parameters (HR + BP) closely during conversations that deal with potentially stressful topics. | • Depression may interfere with patient's ability to deal realistically with situation and may compromise patient's recovery.<br>• Denial is commonly used by patients after an MI to deal with the overwhelming anxiety associated with having an MI. Survival rate during the first few days of CCU care is higher in patients who effectively deny their illness.[65,66]<br>• HR and rhythm changes may occur when patient engages in conversations about stressful topics[67] (pain, symptoms before admission, concerns about death, the consequences of death for their dependents, the consequences of continued survival, the life problems that await them after discharge, the difficulties they had with compliance, and guilt about noncompliance and its contribution to their present illness). |
| ***Nursing Diagnosis #6***<br>Sexual patterns, potentially altered, related to:<br>1. Fear and lack of knowledge about sexual activity after a myocardial infarction. | Patient and/or significant other will:<br>1. Feel comfortable expressing concerns about sexuality.<br>2. Verbalize that sexual activity is a form of exercise.<br>3. Be able to verbalize criteria for "safe sex" after an MI.<br>4. Be able to verbalize practices to be avoided. | • Answer patient's (or significant other's) questions regarding sex directly and honestly.<br>• Describe the following guidelines to patient:<br>∘ Sex may be resumed when patient can climb 20 steps in 10 seconds without symptoms or when HR rises to 110–120 bpm without causing chest pain or shortness of breath.[68]<br>∘ Encourage foreplay before intercourse.<br>∘ Inform patient that intercourse in a familiar place, with a familiar partner, and in a familiar position has very little risk.<br>• Describe the things to avoid:<br>∘ Anal intercourse.<br>∘ Sex when fatigued or after a large meal or heavy alcohol intake.<br>∘ Sex in very hot or cold environment. | • Patient who brings this up during ICU stay is obviously anxious about it. Answering questions directly and honestly should decrease anxiety.<br>∘ These activities are the metabolic equivalent of sexual intercourse and can be used as guidelines for when the patient is physically ready to resume sexual activities.<br>∘ Foreplay allows HR and BP to increase gradually.<br>∘ Familiarity with place, partner, and position is associated with less anxiety.<br>∘ Anal intercourse may precipitate vagal stimulation and bradycardia.[68]<br>∘ These increase metabolic demands and workload on the heart.<br>∘ Same as above. |

## SAMPLE CARE PLAN FOR THE PATIENT WITH MYOCARDIAL INFARCTION

| Nursing Diagnoses | Desired Patient Outcomes | Nursing Interventions | Rationales |
|---|---|---|---|
| ***Nursing Diagnosis #1*** Alteration in comfort, related to:<br>1. Myocardial ischemia. | Patient will verbalize feeling free of pain. | • Assess for presence of chest discomfort. | • Continuous assessment of patient to determine verbal and nonverbal cues of pain episodes is essential as patient may be experiencing denial of his condition. |
| | | ◦ Have patient rate discomfort on a scale of 1–10, with 10 being most severe. | ◦ Patient may not appear to be in distress, but because he may mask signs of pain as a result of such factors as stoicism and cultural differences, pain may be severe. A scaling system is a more objective tool. |
| | | ◦ Notify physician of any episodes of chest pain and take appropriate actions: Obtain vital signs, get a 12-lead ECG. | ◦ Enhanced sympathoadrenal response associated with pain and anxiety may increase heart rate and oxygen demand, and may provoke myocardial ischemia. |
| | | • Minimize discrepancy between $O_2$ supply and demand.<br>◦ Provide periods of rest.<br>◦ Regulate activities.<br>◦ Maintain a quiet environment. | • Goal in treatment is to maximize $O_2$ supply and minimize $O_2$ demand. |
| ***Nursing Diagnosis #2*** Potential for anxiety, related to:<br>1. CCU environment.<br>2. Newly diagnosed disease. | Patient will:<br>1. Verbalize anxiety and/or fears.<br>2. Demonstrate behavior suggesting decreased anxiety: Relaxed facies and demeanor.<br>3. Heart rate 60–80 beats/minute.<br>4. Blood pressure within 10 mmHg of baseline. | • Assess for verbal and nonverbal cues of anxiety. | • Patient may verbalize he is not feeling anxious but may be demonstrating anxious behavior. |
| | | ◦ Provide patient/family with information regarding diagnosis, diagnostic procedures. | ◦ Family members can be helpful in relaxing patient but must be included when giving information regarding care. |
| | | • Orient patient and family to CCU environment: Staff, equipment, visiting hours, when and whom to call for information about the patient's condition. | • Knowing what to expect assists in coping; family may feel reassured knowing when they can visit or whom to call to get progress reports on the patient's condition. |
| | | • Sedate as necessary, and monitor response. | • Quiet rest and relaxation are essential especially during acute phase when oxygen demands need to be reduced. |
| ***Nursing Diagnosis #3*** Alteration in cardiac output: Decreased, related to:<br>1. Dysrhythmias.<br>2. Left ventricular dysfunction. | Patient will:<br>1. Maintain electrophysiologic stability:<br>• Heart rate 60–80 beats/minute.<br>• Rhythm: Regular. | • Initiate continuous cardiac monitoring.<br>◦ Monitor rate, rhythm. | • Early detection of serious dysrhythmias allows early treatment and prevention of complications. |
| | | • Treat serious or "warning" dysrhythmias as per unit protocol. | • "Warning dysrhythmias" may precipitate episodes of ventricular tachycardia and/or fibrillation. |

*(continued)*

## SAMPLE CARE PLAN FOR THE PATIENT WITH MYOCARDIAL INFARCTION *(Continued)*

| Nursing Diagnoses | Desired Patient Outcomes | Nursing Interventions | Rationales |
|---|---|---|---|
| ***Nursing Diagnosis #3 (cont.)*** | | | |
| | 2. Maintain hemodynamic stability:<br>• Blood pressure within 10 mmHg of baseline.<br>• Mental status: Alert, oriented to person, time, and place.<br>3. Skin warm, usual color.<br>4. Urine output greater than 30 ml/hr. | • Initiate hemodynamic pressure monitoring as prescribed/indicated: Arterial pressure, central venous pressure; PAP, PCWP, CO should the patient's condition become complicated. | • Rhythm and conduction disturbances may be associated with hemodynamic compromise, particularly in the patient with marginal left ventricular function. |
| | | • Monitor for signs and symptoms of left ventricular dysfunction: Sinus tachycardia, dyspnea, orthopnea, crackles, $S_3$ gallop, jugular venous distention; hypotension, elevated pulmonary pressures, and decreased cardiac output. | • Myocardial ischemia and/or infarction predisposes patient to left ventricular dysfunction. |
| | | • Initiate treatment protocol should left ventricular dysfunction occur:<br>○ Administer vasopressors as prescribed and monitor response to therapy.<br>○ Administer antidysrhythmics as prescribed and monitor response to therapy.<br>○ Administer vasodilator therapy and monitor response to therapy. | • Prompt treatment to reduce ischemia and decrease oxygen demand may prevent myocardial injury and necrosis and preserve left ventricular function.<br>○ Dysrhythmias may reduce cardiac output and compromise coronary artery perfusion.<br>○ Should left ventricular function become compromised, therapy to reduce preload and afterload may be initiated to reduce the work of the left ventricle and, thus, oxygen demand. |
| ***Nursing Diagnosis #4***<br>Coping, potentially ineffective (individual), related to:<br>1. Diagnosis, and fear of dying. | Patient will:<br>1. Verbalize feelings of depression, fears about heart disease.<br>2. Use denial as a | • Assess for signs and symptoms of depression: Withdrawal, insomnia, listlessness, crying, lack of self-esteem, feelings of hopelessness, anorexia.<br>• Encourage verbalization of feelings. | • Depression may interfere with patient's ability to deal realistically with situation, and may compromise recovery. |

| | | | |
|---|---|---|---|
| 2. Necessary changes in lifestyle, occupation. | mechanism to help control fear and anxiety, but not to interfere with ultimate acceptance of diagnosis and rehabilitation. | • Assess use of denial as a defense mechanism.<br>◦ Support appropriate use of denial by the patient.<br>• Monitor physiologic parameters (heart rate, blood pressure, pulse) closely during conversations that involve potentially stressful topics. | • Denial is commonly used by patients who have myocardial infarctions; this mechanism can reduce overwhelming anxiety and enable the patient to progress through the acute phase without further physiologic compromise.<br>• Potentially distressful topics include pain, fear of dying, and consequences of death for family members, as well as changes in lifestyle and occupation as may be necessitated by the myocardial infarction.<br>◦ Such topics can cause changes in physiologic parameters, and may reflect the patient's coping ability. |
| ***Nursing Diagnosis #5***<br>Knowledge deficit regarding:<br>1. Coronary artery disease. | Patient will have knowledge of disease:<br>• Risk factors.<br>• Medications.<br>• Rest/exercise.<br>• Changes in lifestyle.<br>• Follow-up care. | • Assess knowledge base and learning needs of patient and family.<br>◦ Utilize resources in patient teaching (pamphlets, video tapes, as appropriate).<br>• Document knowledge base, teaching, and patient's response to teaching in progress notes. | • Patient has a cardiac history and may have received teaching previously. Assessment of learning needs is essential at this time.<br>◦ Patient may not be ready for teaching while in the CCU, but the foundation for learning can begin.<br>• This facilitates continuity of care. |

blood pressure > 100 mmHg. The patient is bolused with 2 doses of lidocaine and started on a 2 mg/minute lidocaine infusion prophylactically.

*6/6, 6 p.m.* The cardiac enzyme screen of CPK, LDH, and SGPT blood levels reveals CPK 1,000 with CP-MB 12%. There is a total LDH elevation, but LDH1 is less than LDH2.

## Initial Nursing Diagnoses

1. Alteration in comfort, related to myocardial ischemia.
2. Potential for anxiety, related to CCU environment and newly diagnosed disease.
3. Alteration in cardiac output: Decreased, related to dysrhythmias and left ventricular failure (potential).
4. Coping, potentially ineffective (individual), related to diagnosis of heart disease and fear of dying; and necessary changes in lifestyle, occupation.

## Additional Nursing Diagnoses

6. Sexual patterns, potentially altered, related to fear and lack of knowledge regarding sexual activity post myocardial infarction.
7. Activity intolerance, related to myocardial ischemia.
8. Potential for dysrhythmias, related to myocardial ischemia.

# CASE STUDY WITH SAMPLE CARE PLAN: PATIENT WITH ACUTE MYOCARDIAL INFARCTION*

H.R. is a 52-year-old male who came to the hospital Emergency Department (ED) after 2 hours of chest discomfort. The episode began as "indigestion" while he was driving to work, and progressed to severe, substernal chest pain described as "an elephant sitting on my chest." Pain was unrelieved by sublingual 1/150 nitroglycerin, but controlled with intravenous (IV) morphine sulfate administered in 2-mg doses. An electrocardiogram (ECG) showed 3-mm ST segment elevation in leads $V_1$ through $V_4$, diagnostic of an acute anteroseptal myocardial infarction (MI).

Laboratory analysis of room air arterial blood gases (ABGs), serum creatine kinase (CK), MB-CK and LDH isoenzymes, PTT, and plasma fibrinogen was done. ABGs revealed $PaO_2$ 76, $PaCO_2$ 28, pH 7.52, and oxygen saturation 90%; 2 liters oxygen per nasal prongs were ordered. CK was 132 IU/liter; LDH was normal. The PTT was normal at 32 seconds, and plasma fibrinogen was 260 mg/100 ml.

No contraindications to thrombolytic therapy were noted, so 3 IV lines were carefully started in preparation for tPA infusion. Prophylactic lidocaine 1 mg/kg bolus was administered followed by a 2 mg/minute drip and a 0.75 mg/kg bolus 15 minutes later to prevent reperfusion dysrhythmias. A 1 : 1 infusion of 100 mg of tPA in sterile water, based on body size, was begun after 10 mg (10% of the dose) was given by slow IV bolus over 12 minutes.[69] An IV bolus of 5,000 units of heparin was administered followed by an infusion at 800 IU/hour to keep the PTT between 50 and 80 seconds. The patient was then transferred to the coronary care unit (CCU).

Initial assessment in the CCU revealed an anxious patient with nonradiating chest pain. Transfer from the guerney to the bed increased his already present shortness of breath and diaphoresis. Vital signs were: BP 110/70 mmHg; pulse 112/minute; respirations 22/minute and labored; temperature 98.9°F (37.1°C). Cardiac monitoring revealed sinus tachycardia with 3-mm ST segment elevation and 2–3 premature ventricular contractions (PVCs)/minute. His skin was cool to the touch. Auscultation revealed bibasilar rales in the lower third of the lung fields, weak heart tones with a summation gallop, no murmurs or rubs. Peripheral pulses were 1+; no evidence of peripheral edema was noted. Abdomen was soft with hypoactive bowel sounds. The patient denied nausea.

H.R. was monitored closely during the 3½ hours of thrombolytic therapy for bleeding, dysrhythmias, chest pain, and changes in coagulation parameters. An hour and 15 minutes after the tPA was started, an 8-beat run of ventricular tachycardia (VT) suggested that reperfusion had occurred. The patient's chest pain resolved. CK levels peaked early at 2400 IU/liter 10 hours following initiation of tPA therapy. PTT following the infusion was prolonged to 80 seconds, and fibrinogen decreased to 100 mg/100 ml. The heparin infusion was continued for 36 hours. No bleeding occurred. An ECG taken after the VT and pain resolution showed ST segment normalization and T wave inversion in the anteroseptal leads.

## Initial Nursing Diagnoses

1. Alteration in comfort (pain), related to myocardial ischemia.
2. Potential for injury, related to lytic state.
3. Alteration in cardiac output, related to stunned and damaged myocardium.
4. Activity intolerance, related to myocardial ischemia.
5. Anxiety, related to sudden onset of illness, knowledge deficit, pain.

---

*By Barbara Riegel

## SAMPLE CARE PLAN FOR THE PATIENT WITH ACUTE MYOCARDIAL INFARCTION

| Nursing Diagnoses | Desired Patient Outcomes | Nursing Interventions | Rationales |
|---|---|---|---|
| ***Nursing Diagnosis #1*** Alteration in comfort, related to: 1. Myocardial ischemia manifested by verbal reports of pain. | Patient will notify nurse immediately when pain recurs and will experience relief within 10 minutes after treatment. | • Ask patient about the presence of pain at least q 2 hr. Teach about the importance of reporting pain immediately. | • Pain may increase myocardial oxygen consumption and extend infarct size.[70] Patient may not want to "bother" the nurse, or may not think the pain is severe enough to warrant treatment. |
| | | • Document ECG changes with pain. | • Pain with ischemic changes warrants aggressive therapy. |
| | | • Administer nitroglycerin 1/150 SL. If no relief within 5 minutes, give 2 mg IV morphine sulfate q 5 minutes until pain is relieved (as prescribed). | • Rapid relief of pain is required to avoid sympathetic nervous system stimulation and infarct extension. |
| | | • Notify physician immediately of recurrence of chest pain. | • Recurring chest pain following thrombolytic therapy suggests reocclusion and the need for cardiac catheterization. |
| | | • Use alternate methods of pain relief to potentiate pharmacologic interventions. | • Reassurance, relaxation, repositioning, distraction, and enhancement of the placebo effect may facilitate pain management.[71] |
| ***Nursing Diagnosis #2*** Potential for injury, related to: 1. The lytic state caused by thrombolytic therapy manifested by lengthened PTT and lowered fibrinogen levels. | Patient will be free of major bleeding complications defined as more than 250 ml volume or intracranial bleeding[69] throughout the duration of thrombolytic and anticoagulant therapy. | • Monitor BP, pulse, and neurologic signs q 15 minutes during thrombolytic therapy and q 1 hr during anticoagulant therapy. | • BP and heart rate changes may provide the earliest signs of concealed bleeding.[69] Neurologic changes may indicate intracranial hemorrhage requiring immediate intervention. |
| | | • Avoid trauma such as excess needle punctures or falls. | • Even minor trauma may cause bleeding that is difficult to control. |
| | | • Monitor coagulation studies carefully. | • The PTT must be kept approximately 2 times normal to avoid reocclusion; values greater than this place the patient at increased risk of bleeding. |

(continued)

## SAMPLE CARE PLAN FOR THE PATIENT WITH ACUTE MYOCARDIAL INFARCTION *(Continued)*

| Nursing Diagnoses | Desired Patient Outcomes | Nursing Interventions | Rationales |
|---|---|---|---|
| ***Nursing Diagnosis #3*** Alteration in cardiac output (decreased), related to: 1. Stunned myocardium and dysrhythmias. (Manifestations include rales, increased respiratory rate, tachycardia, ABG evidence of uncompensated respiratory alkalosis, low normal BP, and summation gallop.) | Patient will maintain a balance of cardiac output and physiologic requirements as evidenced by: 1. Decreased pulmonary rales. 2. Normalized ABGs. 3. Stabilized vital signs. 4. Resolved summation gallop. | • Assess vital signs, lung and heart sounds q 2 hr.<br>• Administer medications ordered to increase contractility, decrease afterload, optimize preload.<br>• Administer $O_2$ as prescribed and monitor response. | • Note changes in physiologic parameters that may require intervention.<br>• Medications that optimize the balance of contributors to myocardial oxygen consumption minimize the risk to jeopardized myocardium.[72]<br>• Supplemental oxygen at low doses increases the circulating oxygen supply in a fixed system unable to augment oxygen supply in other ways.[70,73] |
| ***Nursing Diagnosis #4*** Activity intolerance, related to: 1. Myocardial ischemia manifested by shortness of breath and diaphoresis with movement. | Patient will be able to tolerate minor activity such as getting out of bed for toileting within 24 hours as evidenced by absence of pain, shortness of breath, diaphoresis, or dysrhythmias with activity. | • Assess the patient's response to movement in bed.<br>• Teach the need to rest, especially during and immediately after activities such as eating or treatments. | • Accentuated changes in symptoms and vital signs with even minor movement in bed suggest that getting out of bed may not be well tolerated.[74]<br>• Some limitation of activity is required immediately following an MI. The combination of activities such as eating and getting out of bed, especially if the patient removes $O_2$ therapy for such activities, may cause an imbalance of oxygen supply and demand.[74] |
| ***Nursing Diagnosis #5*** Anxiety, related to: 1. Sudden onset of illness, knowledge deficit, pain manifested by attention deficit, agitation, shortness of breath. | Patient will be able to control his anxiety as evidenced by verbal report of low anxiety, normal vital signs. | • Establish a primary relationship with the patient, checking on him frequently and communicating your availability and concern.<br>• Orient the patient to the unit with short sentences and brief messages.<br>• Allow liberal visiting privileges if the family seems to calm the patient. | • Communicating concern and availability makes patients feel safe in the foreign and frightening environment of the CCU.<br>• Attention span is shortened with anxiety.[75]<br>• Some patients may feel safer and calmer, and demonstrate a more stable hemodynamic profile when in the presence of their loved ones.[76] |

## REFERENCES


1. Stokes, J III, Noren, J, and Shindell, S: Definition of terms and concepts applicable to clinical preventive medicine. Journal of Community Health 8:33, 1982.
2. Kannel, WB, McGee, D, Gordon T, et al: A general cardiovascular risk profile: The Framingham Study. Am J Cardiol 38:46, 1976.
3. Kannel, WB, Hjortland, MC, McNamara, PM, et al: Menopause and risk of cardiovascular disease: The Framingham Study. Ann Intern Med 85:447, 1976.
4. Neufeld, HN and Goldbourt, U: Coronary heart disease: Genetic aspects. Circulation 67:943, 1983.
5. Rogot, E and Padgett, SJ: Association of coronary and stroke mortality with temperature and snowfall in selected areas of the United States, 1962–1966. Am J Epidemiol 103:565, 1976.
6. Fabsitz, R and Feinleib, M: Geographic patterns in county mortality rates from cardiovascular diseases. Am J Epidemiol 111:325, 1980.
7. Kannel, WB: Role of blood pressure in cardiovascular disease: The Framingham Study. Angiology 26:1, 1975.
8. Kannel, WB: Role of blood pressure in cardiovascular morbidity and mortality. Prog Cardiovasc Dis 17:5, 1974.
9. Feinleib, M and Williams, RR: Relative risks of myocardial infarction, cardiovascular disease and peripheral vascular disease by type of smoking. Proc Third World Conf Smoking and Health I:243, 1976.
10. Gordon, T, Kannel, WB, McGee, D, et al: Death and coronary attacks in men after giving up cigarette smoking. A report from the Framingham Study. Lancet 2:1345, 1974.
11. Quaal, S: A study of fitness and cardiovascular risk factors in male office workers. West J Nurs Res Summer:9, 1981.
12. Smith, A: Physiology, diagnosis, and life-style modifications for hyperlipidemia. J Cardiovasc Nurs 1(4):15, 1987.
13. Herold, P and Kinsella, J: Fish oil consumption and decreased risk of cardiovascular disease: A comparison of findings from animal and human feeding trials. Am J Clin Nutr 43:566, 1986.
14. Walter, BF, Palumbo, PJ, Lee, JT, et al: Status of the coronary arteries at necroscopy in diabetes mellitus with onset after 30 years: Analysis of 229 diabetic patients with and without clinical evidence of coronary heart disease and comparison to 183 control subjects. Am J Med 69:498, 1980.
15. Dortimer, AC, Sheony, PN, Shiroff, RA, et al: Diffuse coronary artery disease in diabetic patients: Fact or fiction? Circulation 57:133, 1978.
16. Partamian, JO and Bradley, RF: Acute myocardial infarction in 258 cases of diabetes: Immediate mortality and five year survival. N Engl J Med 273:455, 1975.
17. Kannel, WB and Sorlee, PD: Some health benefits of physical activity: The Framingham Study. Arch Intern Med 139:857, 1979.
18. Little, JA, Birchwood, BL, Simmons, DA, et al: Interrelationship between the kinds of dietary carbohydrate and fat in hyperlipoproteinemic patients. Atherosclerosis 11:173, 1970.
19. Levy, RI and Gluech, CJ: Hypertriglyceridemia, diabetes mellitus and coronary vessel disease. Arch Intern Med 123:220, 1969.
20. Connor, WE and Connor, SL: The key role of nutritional factors in the prevention of coronary heart disease. Prev Med 1:49, 1972.
21. Gordon, T, Ernst, N, Fisher, M, et al: Alcohol and high-density lipoprotein cholesterol. Circulation 64(Suppl III):III-63, 1981.
22. Friedman, H and Rosenman, RH: Type A Behavior and Your Heart. Alfred A Knopf, New York, 1974.
23. Rosenman, RH, Brand, RJ, Sholtz, RI, et al: Multivariate prediction of coronary heart disease during 8.5 year follow-up in the Western Collaborative Group Study. Am J Cardiol 37:903, 1976.
24. Haynes, SG, Feinleib, M, and Kannel, WB: The relationship of psychosocial factors to coronary heart disease in the Framingham Study: III. Eight-year incidence of coronary heart disease. Am J Epidemiol 111:37, 1980.
25. Heberden, W: Some account of a disorder of the breast. Med Trans R Coll Physicians (London) 2:59, 1772.
26. Parry, CH: An inquiry into the symptoms and causes of the syncope anginosa, commonly called angina pectoris, Vols 3 and 4. R Cuttwell, Bath, England, 1799.
27. Oliva, PB: Unstable rest angina with ST-segment depression: Pathophysiologic considerations and therapeutic implications. Ann Intern Med 100:424, 1984.
28. Cohen, MV: The functional value of coronary collaterals in myocardial ischemia and therapeutic approach to enhance collateral flow. Am Heart J 95:396, 1978.
29. Prinzmetal, M, Kennamer, R, Merliss, R, et al: A variant form of angina pectoris. Am J Med 27:375, 1959.
30. Fisher, JR and Sieves, ML: Ear-lobe crease in American Indians. Ann Intern Med 93:512, 1980.
31. Lichstein, E, Chapman, I, Gupta, PK, et al: Diagonal ear lobe crease and coronary artery sclerosis. Ann Intern Med 85:337, 1976.
32. Michaelson, EL, Morganroth, J, Nichols, CW, et al: Retinal arteriolar changes as an indicator of coronary artery disease. Arch Intern Med 139:1139, 1979.
33. Blomqvist, CG and Mitchell, JH: Heart disease and dynamic exercise testing. In Willerson, JT and Sanders, CA (eds): Clinical Cardiology. Grune & Stratton, New York, 1977, p 94.
34. Cohn, PF and Vokonas, PS: Pathophysiology of coronary artery disease in humans. In Cohn, PF (ed): Diagnosis and Therapy of Coronary Artery Disease, ed 2. Martinus Nijhoff, Boston, 1985.
35. Gould, LK, Lipscomb, K, and Calvert, C: Compensatory changes of the distal coronary vascular bed during progressive coronary artery occlusion. Circulation 51:1085, 1975.
36. Gobel, FL, Nordstrom, LA, Nelson, RR, et al: The rate-pressure product as an index of myocardial oxygen consumption during exercise in patients with angina pectoris. Circulation 57:549, 1978.
37. Robinson, BF: Relation of heart rate and systolic blood pressure to the onset of pain in angina pectoris. Circulation 35:1073, 1967.
38. Betriu, A, Costoner, A, Santz, GA, et al: Angiographic findings 1 month after myocardial infarction: A prospective study of 259 survivors. Circulation 65:1099, 1982.
39. Buja, LM and Willerson, JT: Clinicopathologic findings in 100 episodes of acute ischemic heart disease (acute myocardial infarction or coronary insufficiency) in 83 patients. Am J Cardiol 47:343, 1981.
40. Ridolfi, RL and Hutchins, GM: The relationship between coronary artery lesions and myocardial infarcts: Ulceration of atherosclerotic plaques precipitating coronary thrombosis. Am Heart J 93:468, 1977.
41. Alpert, JS and Braunwald, E: Acute myocardial infarction: Pathologic, pathophysiologic, and clinical manifestations. In Braunwald, E: Heart Disease. WB Saunders, Philadelphia, 1984.
42. Rake, RH, Romo, M, Bennett, L, et al: Recent life changes, myocardial infarction, and abrupt coronary death. Arch Intern Med 133:221, 1974.
43. McIntyre, KM, Lewis, AJ, Parker, MR, et al: Myocardial infarction. In Textbook of Advanced Cardiac Life Support. American Heart Association, Dallas, 1983.
44. Riley, CP, Russell, RO, Jr, and Rachey, CE: Left ventricular gallop sound and acute myocardial infarction. Am Heart J 86:598, 1973.
45. Sukumalchantra, Y, Levy, S, Danzig, R, et al: Correcting arterial hypoxemia by oxygen therapy in patients with acute myocardial infarction. Effect on ventilation and hemodynamics. Am J Cardiol 24:838, 1969.
46. Ganz, W, Donoso, R, Marcus, H, et al: Coronary hemodynamics and myocardial oxygen metabolism during oxygen

breathing in patients with and without coronary artery disease. Circulation 45:763, 1972.
47. Maroko, PR, Radvany, P, Braunwald, E, et al: Reduction of infarct size by oxygen inhalation following acute coronary occlusion. Circulation 52:360, 1975.
48. Madias, JE and Hood, WB, Jr: Reduction of precordial ST-segment elevation in patients with anterior myocardial infarction by oxygen breathing. Circulation 53(Suppl 1):1-198, 1976.
49. Wray, R, Maurer, B, and Shillingford, J: Prophylactic anticoagulation therapy in the prevention of calf vein thrombosis after myocardial infarction. N Engl J Med 288:815, 1973.
50. Forrester, JS, Diamond, G, Chatteyee, K, and Swan, HJC: Medical therapy of acute myocardial infarction by application of hemodynamic subsets (first of two parts). N Engl J Med 295:1356, 1976.
51. Forrester, JHS, Diamond, G, Chatteyee, K, and Swan, HJC: Medical therapy of acute myocardial infarction by application of hemodynamic subsets (second of two parts). N Engl J Med 295:1404, 1976.
52. Braunwald, E, Muller, JE, Kloner, RA, and Maroko, PR: Role of beta adrenergic blockade in the therapy of patients with myocardial infarction. Am J Med 74:113, 1983.
53. Ross, J, Jr, Frahn, CJ, and Braunwald, E: The influence of intracardiac baroreceptors on venous return, systemic vascular volume, and peripheral resistance. J Clin Invest 40:563-572, 1962.
54. Winslow, EH: Cardiovascular consequences of bed rest. Heart Lung 14:236, 1985.
55. Ahrens, WD, Kenney, MR, and Carter, R: The effect of antistatis footboard exercise on selected measures of exertion. Heart Lung 12:366, 1983.
56. Johnston, BL, Watt, EW, and Fletcher, CF: Oxygen consumption and hemodynamic and electrocardiographic responses to bathing in recent post-myocardial infarction patients. Heart Lung 10:666, 1981.
57. Riegel, BJ: The role of the nurse in limiting myocardial infarct size. Heart Lung 14:247, 1985.
58. Kirchoff, KT: An examination of the physiologic basis for "coronary precautions." Heart Lung 10:874, 1981.
59. Yu, PN, Bielski, MT, Edwards, A, et al: Report of inter-society commissions for heart disease resources: Resources for the optimal care of patients with acute myocardial infarction. Circulation 43:A-171, 1971.
60. Bramwell, L and Whall, A: Effect of role clarity and empathy on support role performance and anxiety. Nurs Res 35(5):282, 1986.
61. Royle, J: Coronary patients and their families receive incomplete care. Canadian Nurse 69(2):21, 1973.
62. Brown, AJ: Effect of family visits on the blood pressure and heart rate of patients in the coronary care unit. Heart Lung 5:291, 1976.
63. Kirchoff, KT: Visiting policies for patients with myocardial infarction: A national survey. Heart Lung 11:571, 1982.
64. Johanson, BC, Dungca, CU, Hoffmeister, D, et al: Standards for Critical Care, ed 3. CV Mosby, St. Louis, 1988.
65. Hachett, TP, Cassem, NH, and Wishnie, H: Psychological hazards of coronary care units. N Engl J Med 297:1365, 1968.
66. Thomas, SA, Sappington, E, Gross, HS, et al: Denial in coronary care patients—an objective assessment. Heart Lung 12:74, 1983.
67. Puksta, NS: All about sex . . . after a coronary. Am J Nurs 77:602, 1977.
68. Baggs, J: Nursing diagnosis: Potential sexual dysfunction after myocardial infarction. Dimensions Crit Care Nurs 5:178, 1986.
69. Emde, K and Searle, L: Current nursing practices with thrombolytic therapy. J Cadiovasc Nurs 4(1), in press.
70. Riegel, B: The role of nursing in limiting myocardial infarct size. Heart Lung 14(3):247, 1985.
71. Altice, NF and Jamison, GB: Interventions to facilitate pain management in myocardial infarction. J Cardiovasc Nurs 3(4):49, August 1989.
72. Dix-Sheldon, DK: Pharmacologic management of myocardial ischemia. J Cardiovasc Nurs 3(4):17, August 1989.
73. Enger, EL and Schwertz, DW: Mechanisms of myocardial ischemia. J Cardiovasc Nurs 3(4):1, 1989.
74. Riegel, B: Acute myocardial infarction: Nursing interventions to optimize oxygen supply and demand. In Kern, L: Cardiac Critical Care Nursing. Aspen, Rockville, MD, 1988.
75. Leavitt, M and Minarik, P: The agitated, hypervigilant response. In Riegel, B and Ehrenreich, D: Psychological Aspects of Critical Care Nursing. Aspen, Rockville, MD, 1989.
76. Riegel, B: Families of the critically ill. In Riegel, B and Ehrenreich, D: Psychological Aspects of Critical Care Nursing, Aspen, Rockville, MD, 1989.

## SUGGESTED READINGS

Brest, AN: Antihypertensive therapy in perspective, Part 1. Modern Concepts of Cardiovascular Disease 57(12), December, 1988.
Caplin, MS: Stresses experienced by spouses of patients in a coronary care unit with myocardial infarction. Focus on Critical Care 15:5, October, 1988.
Helgason, C: Blood glucose and stroke. Current Concepts of Cerebrovascular Disease and Stroke 23(1), January-February, 1988.
Owens-Jones, S and Hopp, L: Viral myocarditis. Focus on Critical Care 15:1, February, 1988.
Pattilio, M and Knox, TL: Postmyocardial infarction syndrome: A case study. Focus on Critical Care 14:5, October, 1987.
Perchalski, DL and Pepine, CJ: Patient with coronary artery spasm and role of the critical care nurse. Heart Lung 16(4), July, 1987.
Schmeck, HM Jr: The revolution in heart treatment, Part 2. The Good Health Magazine, The New York Times Magazine, October 9, 1988.
Thadani, U: Current status of nitrates in angina pectoris. Modern Concepts of Cardiovascular Disease 56(9), September, 1987.
Watson, JE: The National Cholesterol Education Program: The role of nursing. Cardiovascular Nursing 24(3), May/June, 1988.
Winslow, EH (ed): Nursing research in cardiovascular risk reduction. Cardiovascular Nursing 24(6), November/December, 1988.

CHAPTER 44

# Nursing Management of the Patient with Heart Failure

*Patricia L. Wallace*

## CHAPTER OUTLINE



## LEARNING OBJECTIVES

**At the end of this chapter, you should be able to:**

1. Identify the primary hemodynamic alteration associated with heart failure.
2. Differentiate between the signs and symptoms of right heart failure and left heart failure.
3. Describe the normal compensatory mechanisms associated with a fall in cardiac output.
4. Describe the pathologic conditions associated with the development of heart failure.
5. Outline the pertinent clinical assessment and hemodynamic findings of the specific disorders associated with the development of heart failure.
6. Identify the predisposing factors associated with the development of cardiogenic shock.
7. Relate the role of pharmacologic intervention to the treatment and management of heart failure.
8. Discuss the role of supportive care measures in the management of heart failure.
9. Relate pertinent nursing diagnoses, desired patient outcomes, and nursing interventions to the therapeutic goals in the care of the patient with heart failure.

Heart failure is a pathophysiologic state in which the heart is unable to eject an amount of blood sufficient to meet the metabolic demands of the body. The onset of heart failure can be precipitous in certain clinical conditions and gradual in others. The rapidity with which this syndrome develops and whether sufficient time has elapsed for compensatory mechanisms to have developed distinguish acute from chronic heart failure.

Heart failure is the result of a variety of underlying pathologic processes whose primary manifestation is a reduced cardiac output. This can result from a loss of myocardial contractile function, an abnormal volume load, an abnormal pressure load, or conditions that restrict ventricular filling (Table 44-1). Conditions associated with an increased metabolic demand do not cause heart failure but can be precipitants of a decompensation when an underlying cardiac condition exists. These conditions are noted in Table 44-2.[1] Regardless of the pathologic condition that results in heart failure, the common threat that runs throughout these disorders is that they cause a decrease in cardiac out-

TABLE 44–1
**Conditions Responsible for the Development of Heart Failure**

| Loss of Myocardial Contractility | Abnormal Volume Load | Abnormal Pressure Load | Filling Disorders |
|---|---|---|---|
| Cardiomyopathies | Valvular incompetence | Systemic hypertension | Mitral stenosis |
| Myocardial infarction | Left-to-right shunts | Pulmonary hypertension | Tricuspid stenosis |
| Myocarditis | | Aortic stenosis | Atrial myxomas |
| Cardiogenic shock | | Pulmonic stenosis | |
| | | Pulmonary embolism | |

put and an increase in myocardial oxygen consumption, disrupting the delicate balance of myocardial oxygen supply and demand.

A variety of descriptive terms associated with heart failure require clarification. These include right- and left-sided failure, forward versus backward failure, and acute versus chronic failure, as previously discussed. Left and right ventricular failure are terms used to identify the ventricle of primary involvement. Right ventricular failure occurs when the volume of blood returning to the right side of the heart exceeds right ventricular cardiac output. This can cause an elevation in the systemic venous pressure, which then gives rise to the clinical manifestations of right-sided heart failure, as noted in Table 44–3. Left ventricular failure occurs when left ventricular cardiac output is less than the volume of blood received from the pulmonary circulation. As a result, pulmonary filling pressures rise while systemic filling pressures fall. This is clinically manifested as dyspnea, fatigue, confusion, pulmonary congestion, and hypotension (see Table 44–3). Although the terms right ventricular failure and left ventricular failure are used in the clinical setting, unilateral heart failure can exist in pure form for only a short period of time. Because the cardiopulmonary system is a closed circuit, the effects of any abnormal volume load will eventually be transmitted from the affected to the unaffected side of the heart.

The *forward* theory of heart failure states that the failure is caused by an inadequate delivery of blood to the arterial system. This stimulates compensatory mechanisms to increase perfusion by augmenting the extracellular fluid volume. Over time, this increases the workload of the heart and causes congestion of vital organs. The *backward* theory of failure states that as the ventricle cannot empty its contents adequately, pressure rises in the ventricle and atria, and in the venous circulation that empties into them. The rise in venous pressure causes transudation of fluid across the capillary membranes into the extracellular spaces and is responsible for the clinical picture of edema.[2]

The syndromes and manifestations associated with heart failure encompass some of the most frequently encountered situations in critical care settings today. For appropriate patient management, the critical care nurse must understand the etiology, pathophysiology, and hemodynamic consequences of heart failure in order to implement a therapeutic plan of care. Without appropriate recognition and intervention, heart failure heralds the onset of a vicious downward spiral that can rapidly lead to the death of the individual.

TABLE 44–2
**Precipitating Factors in the Development of Heart Failure**

| | |
|---|---|
| Anemia | Pregnancy |
| Dysrhythmias | Hypervolemia |
| Infection | Endocrine disorders |
| Fever | Thyrotoxicosis |
| Thiamine deficiency | Myxedema |
| Overexertion | Cushing's syndrome |

TABLE 44–3
**Clinical Presentation of the Patient with Heart Failure**

| Left Heart Failure | Right Heart Failure |
|---|---|
| Tachycardia | Tachycardia |
| ↑Pulmonary artery diastolic pressure | ↑Right atrial pressure |
| ↑Pulmonary capillary wedge pressure | ↑Central venous pressure |
| Pulsus alternans | Jugular venous distention |
| Gallop rhythm | Dependent pitting edema |
| Basilar rales | Ascites |
| Cyanosis or pallor | Weight gain |
| Dyspnea | Hepatojugular reflux |
| Orthopnea | Hepatosplenomegaly |
| Cough | Jaundice |
| Nocturnal dyspnea | Complaints of vague abdominal discomfort |
| Anxiety | Nocturia |
| Diaphoresis | |
| Oliguria | |
| Weakness, fatigue | |

## COMPENSATORY MECHANISMS

Regardless of the specific pathologic condition that caused the initial reduction in cardiac output, there are 3 mechanisms by which the heart and vascular system attempt to compensate: the Frank-Starling phenomenon, sympathoadrenergic stimulation, and myocardial hypertrophy. Once the limits of the compensatory mechanisms have been exceeded, the clinical manifestations of heart failure develop.

## Frank-Starling Phenomenon

The initial consequence of acute ventricular dysfunction is incomplete left ventricular emptying resulting in an increase in the residual volume in the left ventricle (LV).[3] Because the diastolic filling of the heart remains essentially the same, there is an increase in left ventricular end-diastolic volume (LVEDV) and left ventricular end-diastolic pressure (LVEDP). The greater diastolic distention improves stroke volume and ejection and maintains a normal cardiac output by the Frank-Starling phenomenon. This is clinically represented by a left ventricular function curve, plotting cardiac output as a measure of contractility on the vertical axis and pulmonary capillary wedge pressure (PCWP) as a measure of preload and LVEDP on the horizontal axis (Fig. 44–1; see also Fig. 37–17). The Frank-Starling mechanism demonstrates that as preload (LVEDV) is increased, the stroke volume and cardiac output are increased, achieving optimal contractility between 12 and 18 mmHg.

In the patient with heart failure, the initial ventricular function curve shifts to the left as the effects of sympathoadrenergic stimulation on heart rate and contractility increase cardiac output with little or no change in filling pressures. As the myocardial dysfunction progresses, however, the effects of the compensatory mechanisms result in an increase in vascular tone, increased blood volume, and decreased ventricular compliance. This causes a shift of the curve to the right and a greater increase in filling pressures that is not associated with an additional improvement in cardiac output.

With the persistently elevated filling pressures and the increase in the degree of myocardial dysfunction, the compensatory mechanism is no longer effective and the physiologic limits of the Frank-Starling mechanism are exceeded. Filling pressures continue to rise, ventricular compliance diminishes, and cardiac output falls, resulting in systemic and pulmonary venous congestion and impaired perfusion to peripheral tissues.[4]

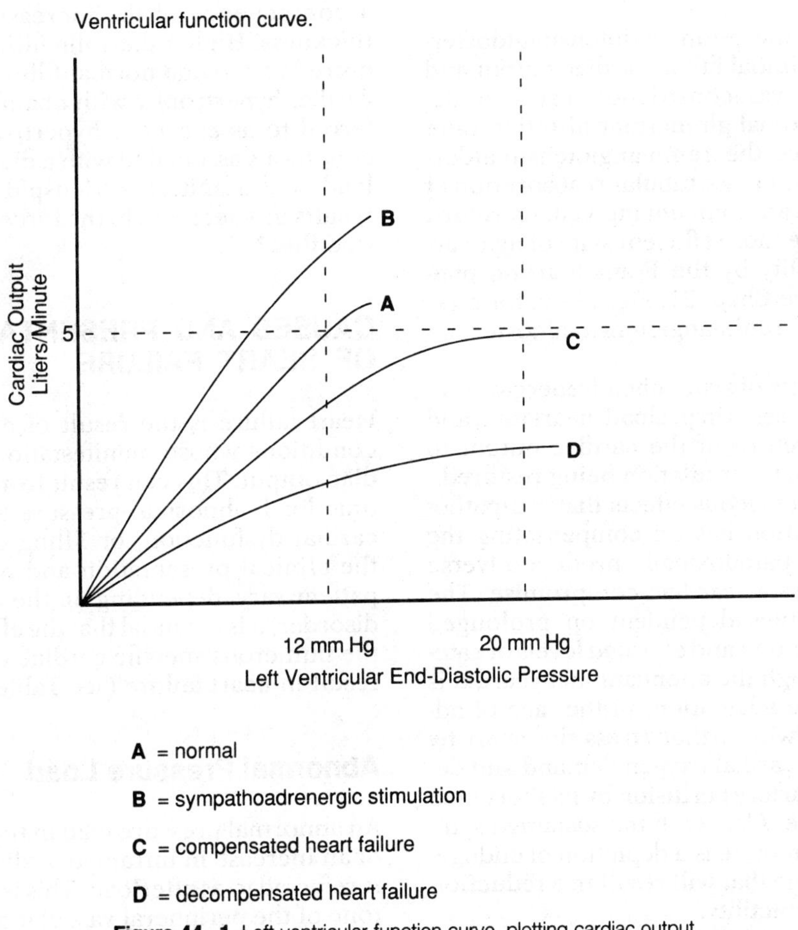


**Figure 44–1.** Left ventricular function curve, plotting cardiac output.

## Sympathoadrenergic Stimulation

The 2 major effects of sympathetic nervous system stimulation that operate in the compensation of heart failure are the cardiac and peripheral vascular mechanisms. Responding to a momentary decrease in cardiac output, the pressure-sensitive baroreceptors transmit impulses to the cardioregulatory centers in the brain. This results in generalized sympathetic efferent nerve stimulation that has the following effects:

1. Vasoconstrictor response in the cutaneous, muscular, renal, and splanchnic circulation. Because coronary muscle and cerebrovascular smooth muscle are not part of this vasoconstrictor response, blood is redistributed from peripheral tissues to these organs. The hemodynamic effects of this vasoconstriction are increased systemic vascular resistance, increased mean aortic pressure, and increased venous return to the heart.
2. The release of epinephrine and norepinephrine from the adrenal medulla. In combination with circulating catecholamines, this stimulates the cardiac beta receptors to increase heart rate and contractility, resulting in an increased stroke volume and increased cardiac output.
3. Activation of the renin-angiotensin-aldosterone axis. The initial fall in cardiac output and the resultant vasoconstriction cause a decrease in the renal glomerular filtration rate. This stimulates the renin-angiotensin-aldosterone axis to increase tubular reabsorption of sodium and water, enhancing venous return and fostering a more efficient state of myocardial contractility by the Frank-Starling phenomenon. (See Chap. 21, Fig. 21–9, for a review of the renin-angiotensin-aldosterone axis.)

The beneficial effects of sympathoadrenergic stimulation include increases in preload, heart rate, and contractility and return of the cardiac output to normal with adequate circulation being restored.

Despite the advantageous effects that sympathoadrenergic stimulation has on compensating the failing heart, it can, paradoxically, produce adverse effects and progressive cardiac compromise. The myocardium becomes dependent on prolonged sympathetic stimulation and elevated levels of catecholamines. Although the attendant tachycardia is initially a favorable adaptation, in the face of advancing disease it will further stress the heart by increasing the myocardial oxygen demand and decreasing coronary artery perfusion by its shortened diastolic filling time. Also, with the sustained sympathetic stimulation there is a depletion of endogenous norepinephrine that will result in a reduction in myocardial contractility.

The vasoconstrictive effects also extract a large toll on the failing heart. With an increase in circulating blood volume, there is an increase in cardiac output. However, with the failing heart, the cardiac output falls. Additionally, the persistent elevation in systemic vascular resistance increases myocardial wall tension and myocardial oxygen demand, and further impedes the ejection of blood from an already compromised ventricle.

## Myocardial Hypertrophy

The process of myocardial hypertrophy, with or without cardiac chamber dilatation, is not an acute compensatory adjustment to stress. It develops as the result of a sustained, elevated myocardial workload. This workload is then distributed across a greater amount of muscle mass. Initially, this decreases the myocardial energy requirements and improves contractility. Over time, the muscle of the chamber pumping against the resistance can hypertrophy to such a degree that it outgrows its blood supply and becomes ischemic.

Myocardial hypertrophy without chamber dilatation is known as *concentric* hypertrophy and occurs most frequently in the setting of an increased afterload. This results in a poorly compliant ventricle as a consequence of the increased ventricular wall thickness. Higher diastolic filling pressures are required to provide normal filling of the heart. Myocardial hypertrophy with chamber dilatation is referred to as *eccentric* hypertrophy and occurs in conditions associated with a diastolic volume overload, such as mitral or tricuspid incompetence, and results in a decrease in the force of myocardial contractility.[5]

# CAUSES AND PRESENTATION OF HEART FAILURE

Heart failure is the result of a variety of cardiac conditions whose manifestation is a reduced cardiac output. This can result from an abnormal volume load, abnormal pressure load, primary myocardial dysfunction, or filling disorders. Because the clinical presentation and management of the patient vary, depending on the underlying cardiac disorder, it is essential that the clinician understand the numerous specific cardiac conditions that can result in heart failure (see Table 44–1).

## Abnormal Pressure Load

An abnormal pressure load in the heart is the result of an increase in intramyocardial wall tension and is referred to as afterload. This is determined by the tone of the peripheral vascular system, viscosity of the blood, and condition of the aortic and pulmonic valves. With an abnormal pressure load, the ventricles must generate higher contractile pressures to overcome the impedance to forward blood flow. Clinically, afterload is measured by arterial blood pressure and calculation of the systemic vascular resistance.

### Aortic Stenosis

**Description and Underlying Pathophysiology.** Aortic stenosis represents an obstruction to the ejection of blood from the ventricle during systole. It may be the result of a congenital malformation above or below the valve, congenital bicuspid valve, rheumatic inflammation, or degenerative calcification, and can occur in 1 of 3 places; valvular, which is the most common; supravalvular; and subvalvular.

Normally the size of the aortic valve is 2.5–3.5 $cm^2$. Clinically significant stenosis occurs when the aortic valve opening has decreased to one third its normal size and is considered severe when the valve orifice is less than .75 $cm^2$.[6] Aortic stenosis can exist for many years before the patient becomes symptomatic because of the left ventricle's ability to compensate to the increased pressure load and maintain cardiac output by concentric hypertrophy. A strong atrial systole is also an important factor in maintaining cardiac output since it increases the LVEDV and LVEDP. This causes the ventricular muscle fibers to stretch and, by the Frank-Starling phenomenon, increases the force of ventricular contraction. Because a forceful atrial systole contributes 20% of the cardiac output, the loss of this contribution, as happens in atrial fibrillation, can cause a precipitous deterioration in the patient's condition.

As a result of the hypertrophic response, the left ventricle becomes stiff and noncompliant and higher end-diastolic pressures are necessary to maintain cardiac output. The sustained pressure load eventually leads to left ventricular dilatation, resulting in a diminished stroke volume, ejection fraction, and cardiac output. With the failing hypertrophic response there is an elevation in mean left atrial pressure that is ultimately reflected backward to the pulmonary vascular bed and right side of the heart.

**Clinical Presentation.** Angina is one of the most common clinical findings in patients with aortic stenosis. The hypertrophied LV and elevated afterload increase myocardial oxygen requirements. The pressure compressing the coronary arteries may exceed coronary perfusion pressure, with a resultant interference in coronary blood flow. Dyspnea is the result of the elevated LVEDP that leads to an increased left atrial pressure (LAP) and increased PCWP. Syncope is usually reported during or immediately following physical activity and is the consequence of a decline in arterial blood pressure caused by vasodilatation of skeletal muscles and a fixed cardiac output. As the disease progresses, advanced signs of right and left ventricular failure occur.[7]

***Physical Examination.*** Physical examination reveals a normal arterial blood pressure except in cases of advanced disease at which time the systolic blood pressure and pulse pressure falls. A forceful, sustained apical impulse, displaced laterally and downward, is the result of the hypertrophy. A systolic *thrill* is palpable at the base of the heart, noted best with the patient leaning forward. Auscultation reveals a soft first heart sound and a noticeable fourth heart sound indicative of the vigorous atrial contraction and left ventricular hypertrophy (LVH). The third heart sound may occur when left ventricular dilatation and failure develop. Aortic stenosis is characterized by a harsh mid-systolic aortic ejection murmur that is heard best at the base of the heart and is transmitted along the carotid arteries. It has a characteristic diamond-shaped, crescendo-decrescendo quality (see Fig. 38–9).

**Diagnostic Considerations.** Diagnostic considerations include obtaining an electrocardiogram (ECG) that indicates LVH; a chest x-ray (CXR) that reveals left ventricular enlargement and pulmonary congestion in the later stages of the disease; and an echocardiogram and cardiac catheterization to determine the severity of the stenosis, evaluate LV function, and evaluate for the presence of other valvular or coronary artery disease.

**Treatment.** Treatment is aimed at alleviating symptoms with digitalis glycosides, diuretics, sodium restriction, and activity restriction. Nitrates are generally contraindicated since patients can develop syncope and severe orthostatic hypotension. Prompt surgical replacement of the valve is indicated in patients with heart failure, angina, or exertional syncope and significant valvular stenosis.[8] Endocarditis prophylaxis is employed in all patients with valvular disease.

### Pulmonic Stenosis

**Description and Underlying Pathophysiology.** Pulmonic stenosis is predominantly congenital in origin but can also be caused by rheumatic fever. The obstruction of right ventricular outflow causes a reduction in pulmonary blood flow. As a compensatory mechanism, right ventricular hypertrophy (RVH) develops and pulmonary perfusion temporarily remains sufficient to meet metabolic demands. The right ventricular systolic pressure elevates as the result of the pressure overload and there is subsequent development of right ventricular failure, at which point the cardiac output is compromised. The resultant elevated right ventricular end-diastolic pressure (RVEDP) is reflected back through the right atrium with the development of signs of systemic congestion.

**Clinical Presentation.** Pulmonic stenosis may not cause symptoms in mild cases. With a moderate degree of stenosis the resting cardiac output is near normal, although it does not rise appropriately with exercise and asymptomatic patients can rapidly deteriorate and manifest symptoms of right ventricular failure (RVF).

Auscultatory findings reveal a normal first heart sound, a split second heart sound, and a fourth heart sound indicative of the vigorous atrial contraction. A harsh systolic, diamond-shaped ejection murmur is noted at the upper left sternal border. The classic finding in pulmonic stenosis is a systolic thrill, best noted in the second intercostal space along the left sternal border.

**Diagnostic Considerations.** In cases of severe pulmonic stenosis, the ECG reveals a right axis deviation and RVH. High-amplitude P waves in leads $V_1$ and II indicate right atrial enlargement. The CXR is usually normal in mild to moderate stenosis. In severe stenosis, dilatation of the main and left pulmonary arteries may be evident. Right atrial and ventricular enlargement can also be seen. Cardiac catheterization is necessary to determine the site and severity of the obstruction.

**Treatment.** Prophylaxis for infective endocarditis is prescribed for these patients. Symptoms of RVF are usually treated with digitalis glycosides, diuretics, and sodium restriction. Pulmonary valve commissurotomy or valvuloplasty may be done to relieve the stenosis.[9] (Refer to Chap. 45 for discussion of the cardiac surgical patient.)

### *Pulmonary Hypertension*

**Description and Underlying Pathophysiology.** Pulmonary hypertension is a disorder of the pulmonary vasculature that is diagnosed when the pulmonary artery systolic pressure exceeds 30 mmHg. It is characterized as either primary hypertension, which is predominantly idiopathic and typically seen in females between the ages of 20 and 40 years, or as secondary hypertension, which is the result of cardiac or pulmonary disease. The causes of pulmonary hypertension are outlined in Table 44–4.

A reduction in the size of the vascular bed or intense pulmonary vasoconstriction secondary to alveolar hypoxia causes the small pulmonary arteries to develop medial muscle layer hypertrophy and thickening of the intimal lining of the vessels, sometimes with fibrosis, which results in the noncompliance of the pulmonary vascular bed. This in turn creates a pressure buildup in the right heart secondary to the impedance to right ventricular outflow.[10]

**Clinical Presentation.** Generally, the patients are asymptomatic until late in the disease process, at which time they exhibit symptoms of right heart failure, fatigue, chest pain, exertional dyspnea, and effort syncope as a result of the accompanying hypoxemia and diminished cardiac output. Hoarseness is occasionally noted secondary to compression of the left recurrent laryngeal nerve by the enlarged pulmonary artery. The pulmonary artery pressure is markedly elevated, sometimes nearing the systemic arterial pressure. The PCWP is normal with primary pulmonary hypertension. The mean right atrial (RA) pressure is elevated. Auscultation reveals the presence of an atrial gallop at the left lower sternal border, a narrowly split second heart sound, and an ejection click at the second left intercostal space at the sternal border. Precordial palpation reveals a right ventricular *heave* as well as an impulse over the main pulmonary artery. The ECG shows evidence of RVH and a right axis deviation, and the CXR shows cardiac enlargement with right atrial and ventricular prominence and a dilated pulmonary artery.

TABLE 44–4
**Causes of Pulmonary Hypertension**

| |
|---|
| Diffuse alveolar hypoxia |
| Obesity |
| High-altitude hypoxia |
| Alveolar hypoventilation |
| Smoke inhalation |
| Reduction of the pulmonary vascular bed |
| Recurrent emboli |
| Widespread interstitial diseases |
| Cardiac disorders |
| Mitral stenosis |
| Atrial myxoma |
| Congenital heart disease |
| Left-to-right shunts |

**Treatment.** Medical management includes supportive treatment for systemic venous congestion with diuretics, digitalis glycosides, and sodium and water restriction. Anticoagulant therapy is used in the presence of pulmonary emboli. Oxygen therapy helps to reverse the hypoxic vasoconstriction. Vasodilator therapy is used to reduce the tone in the pulmonary vascular bed, with varying degrees of success, and largely remains a trial-and-error effort. Surgical correction of mitral, aortic, or intracardiac defects is used and heart-lung transplantation is an option for the patient with severe disease.

### *Systemic Hypertension*

**Description and Underlying Pathophysiology.** Systemic hypertension continues to be a common cause of cardiovascular mortality and morbidity as well as a strong etiologic factor in the development of heart failure. Initially, the peripheral vascular resistance (PVR)* may be normal and the cardiac output is normal or elevated. With the progression

*Peripheral vascular resistance (PVR) is synonymous with systemic vascular resistance (SVR) as used in this text.

of the disease, the peripheral vasculature becomes less compliant, PVR rises, and the left ventricle increases the force of its contraction in order to open the aortic valve against the elevated aortic diastolic pressure. This results in LVH. Although the elevated systolic pressure and LVH initially compensate for the increased PVR, this also results in an increase in myocardial oxygen consumption. When the compensatory mechanisms can no longer meet the oxygen demands, signs of heart failure develop.

Clinical evidence of systemic hypertension requires serial (3 or more) blood pressure readings, obtained in an unstressed environment, with systolic blood pressures above 140 mmHg and diastolic pressures above 90 mmHg. Clinically, hypertension is asymptomatic. Therefore, patient complaints of headache, restlessness, feelings of apprehension, dizziness, tinnitus, fatigue, and vague chest discomfort are usually due to another problem and not the hypertension. The ECG may reveal left ventricular hypertrophy (LVH) and the chest x-ray may show cardiomegaly. Medical management is directed at modifying risk factors, and includes sodium restriction, diuretics, and antihypertensive therapy. Current literature suggests sodium restriction is not effective in all hypertensives. Use of diuretics is recommended only in certain subtypes.

## Filling Disorders

A second group of diseases that contribute to the development of heart failure consists of conditions characterized by an inadequate filling of the ventricles from the atria due to a reduction in the size of the valvular orifice. Initially, cardiac output is maintained through the development of eccentric hypertrophy, but it does so at the expense of markedly elevating myocardial oxygen demand. With the progression of the disease, the hypertrophic response fails and the patient develops signs of heart failure.

### *Mitral Stenosis*

**Description and Underlying Pathophysiology.** The most common cause of mitral stenosis is rheumatic fever, with symptoms developing over the 2 decades that follow the initial attack. Other causes of mitral stenosis include thrombus formation, bacterial vegetation, degenerative calcification, and atrial myxomas.[11]

When the mitral valve becomes stenotic, the valvular leaflets fuse, the valve becomes scarred or thickened, and there is a fusion and shortening of the chordae tendineae, all of which make it difficult for the left atrium (LA) to eject blood into the left ventricle during diastolic filling. Because of a compensatory rise in LA pressure, cardiac output is maintained and the diastolic pressure of the left ventricle remains normal.

The elevated LA pressure causes left atrial dilatation and hypertrophy. This increased pressure is then reflected backward, elevating the pressure in the pulmonary circulation. As the PCWP increases, it eventually exceeds oncotic pressure, and fluid is forced out of the capillary bed, into the lung tissue. This results in pulmonary edema, which is described in detail in Chapter 34 (see Fig. 34-1). The pulmonary capillaries undergo hypertrophy and hyperplasia; this decreases arteriolar lumen size and thus creates an obstruction to right ventricular outflow. Over time, mitral stenosis leads to right ventricular and atrial enlargement, RVF, and signs of systemic congestion. Left ventricular function begins to deteriorate in response to the diminished left ventricular diastolic filling.[12]

**Clinical Presentation.** The most common symptom of mitral stenosis is dyspnea resulting from pulmonary venous hypertension. Orthopnea and paroxysmal nocturnal dyspnea (PND) occur at night when blood is shifted from the trunk and legs. This can be accompanied by a cough, which is a result of the enlarged left atrium irritating the left main bronchus. Dysphagia can occur from the posterior displacement of the esophagus by the enlarged left atrium, and hoarseness develops from pressure on the left recurrent laryngeal nerve from an enlarged pulmonary artery.

In severe mitral stenosis there is often a resting tachycardia, an increased respiratory rate, and a narrow pulse pressure as a consequence of the reduced cardiac output and peripheral vasoconstriction. The neck veins will be distended if right ventricular function is impaired.

Auscultation in mitral stenosis is enhanced by the patient assuming a left lateral decubitus position and will reveal a loud first heart sound, an opening snap caused by the forced opening of the mitral valve in the face of an elevated LA pressure, and a soft, low-pitched diastolic murmur with a rumbling quality.

The ECG will reveal a right axis deviation and tall R waves in the right precordial leads when pulmonary hypertension and RVH are found. Evidence of left atrial enlargement is noted in lead II by the presence of a broad, notched P wave. Atrial fibrillation and atrial dysrhythmias are common findings in mitral stenosis.

**Treatment.** Medical management is supportive and includes antibiotic prophylaxis, digitalis glycosides for atrial dysrhythmias with a rapid ventricular response, and reducing the manifestations of right heart failure with activity restriction, diuretics, and sodium restriction to minimize the symptoms of pulmonary venous congestion. Surgical repair with a commissurotomy or valvular replacement is the only definitive method to alter the obstruction of flow through the stenotic valve.[13]

### Tricuspid Stenosis

**Description and Underlying Pathophysiology.** Tricuspid stenosis is most frequently caused by rheumatic fever although it can be the result of right atrial myxomas and the carcinoid syndrome. Tricuspid stenosis is an uncommon valvular disorder and generally is seen in patients with multivalvular disorders, particularly with mitral stenosis and combined mitral and aortic stenosis.

An obstruction of right atrial emptying develops as a result of the narrowed tricuspid valve orifice. Cardiac output is compromised from the restriction to right ventricular filling. Mean right atrial pressure increases due to the stenotic tricuspid valve, and this pressure is reflected backward into the systemic venous circulation.

**Clinical Presentation.** Signs and symptoms noted with tricuspid stenosis include fatigue and effort intolerance as the result of the reduced cardiac output, hepatomegaly, peripheral edema, and ascites. Lung fields are clear despite the presence of jugular venous distention. Auscultation reveals a diastolic, rumbling murmur at the left lower sternal border. The ECG will frequently show a prolonged PR interval and tall peaked P waves.

**Treatment.** Medical management includes antibiotic prophylaxis to prevent endocarditis. Digitalis glycosides, diuretics, and sodium restriction are used to manage the symptoms of systemic venous congestion. Tricuspid commissurotomy can be done in cases of severe stenosis.

### Atrial Myxomas

Atrial myxomas are benign cardiac tumors that intermittently block the atrioventricular orifice, producing a functional mitral or tricuspid stenosis. The signs, symptoms, and manifestations of the myxomas are the same as those found in mitral or tricuspid stenosis. The myxoma is surgically removed if the patient is symptomatic as a result of the obstruction.

## Abnormal Muscle Conditions

The myocardium is a muscle that functions as a pump. The actin-myosin mechanism is responsible for muscle contractility (see Figs. 37–9 through 37–12). Factors that interfere with the actin-myosin mechanism produce a less forceful contraction and result in a diminished cardiac output. Additionally, the efficiency of the contractility can be manipulated by alterations in preload and/or afterload such as the Frank-Starling mechanism (see Fig. 37–17).

### Cardiomyopathies

Cardiomyopathies are subacute disorders of the heart muscle. All cardiomyopathic diseases affect cardiac function, involve one or both ventricles, and can result in heart failure. Cardiomyopathies are divided into 3 major groups based on pathophysiologic abnormalities: dilated, hypertrophic, and restrictive. The causes of cardiomyopathies are numerous and are listed in Table 44–5.

#### Dilated Cardiomyopathy

***Description and Underlying Pathophysiology.*** The term congestive cardiomyopathy was first used in the 1960s when the patient would initially present with symptoms of congestive heart failure. However, the predominant feature of the disease is 4-chamber dilatation, not congestion, so the term *congestive* cardiomyopathy has been replaced with *dilated* cardiomyopathy. It occurs more frequently in men between the ages of 40 and 60, with an increased incidence in blacks. After the symptoms of heart failure develop, death usually occurs within 6 months to 5 years.[14]

The underlying pathologic mechanism is an interference with the calcium uptake by the mitochondria of the myocardial cell, which reduces cellular contractility and impairs the pumping ability of the heart. This causes a substantial reduction in the left ventricular ejection fraction with a resultant decrease in stroke volume and an increase in LVEDV. The elevated LVEDV results in increased pressure in the left atrium, pulmonary veins, and pulmonary capillaries.

In an attempt to increase contractility, there is a compensatory dilatation of all 4 cardiac chambers, with the ventricles being more dilated than the atria. This results in an increased ventricular radius and, according to the law of LaPlace, increases ventricular wall tension and myocardial oxygen consumption, thereby limiting the efficacy of the compensatory response. The dilated ventricles cause a

TABLE 44–5
**Causes of Cardiomyopathies**

| |
|---|
| **Hypertrophic Cardiomyopathy** |
| Genetic |
| **Dilated Cardiomyopathy** |
| Alcohol |
| Peripartum |
| Viral |
| Bacterial |
| Chemotherapy |
| Hypersensitivity to penicillin, tetracycline, and sulfonamides |
| **Restrictive Cardiomyopathy** |
| Amyloidosis |
| Sarcoidosis |
| Hemochromatosis (accumulation of iron in body tissues) |
| Infiltrative neoplastic disease |

further reduction in ventricular ejection and an increase in LVEDP, resulting in signs of left-sided heart failure. Symptoms of right ventricular failure can develop as the result of chronically elevated pulmonary vascular pressures.[15]

***Diagnostic Findings.*** Auscultation will reveal evidence of cardiac enlargement. The apical impulse will be displaced laterally, third and fourth heart sounds are commonly heard, and an apical systolic murmur of a functional mitral regurgitation may be heard. The ECG may reveal a sinus tachycardia, intraventricular conduction disturbance, and signs of left or biventricular and left or biatrial enlargement. Echocardiography and radionuclide angiography are used for diagnostic confirmation. Cardiac catheterization may be indicated to assess therapeutic interventions and to evaluate co-existent valvular or coronary artery disease.

***Treatment.*** Because the etiology of most causes of dilated cardiomyopathy is unknown, the principles of management are largely supportive. Digitalis glycosides and sympathomimetic amines provide inotropic support; sodium restriction, diuretics, and nitrates will reduce preload; and afterload is reduced through vasodilator therapy. Anticoagulants are frequently employed for the prevention and/or treatment of mural thrombi that may develop from the stasis that develops because of the incomplete ventricular emptying. Cardiac transplantation may be explored in severe cases of dilated cardiomyopathy.

### Hypertrophic Cardiomyopathy

***Description and Underlying Pathophysiology.*** Hypertrophic cardiomyopathy is usually genetically transmitted. There are a variety of descriptive terms used to describe this disorder, the most common of which include hypertrophic cardiomyopathy, asymmetrical septal hypertrophy, idiopathic hypertrophic subaortic stenosis, and hypertrophic obstructive cardiomyopathy. Hypertrophic cardiomyopathy is the preferred term.

Left ventricular hypertrophy, thickening of the anterior and posterior leaflets of the mitral valve, hypertrophy of the papillary muscles and left ventricular free wall, and thickening of the endocardial lining located in the ventricular outflow tract are the classic features of this disorder. Because of the disproportionate hypertrophy, the left ventricular cavity has a bizarre shape and may appear slit-like. This causes malalignment of the papillary muscles. As the papillary muscles contract, they cause the anterior mitral valve leaflet to be pulled abnormally forward toward the hypertrophied ventricular septum, causing an obstruction to left ventricular outflow. Events that increase contractility or decrease left ventricular volume intensify this type of obstruction.[16] Blood not ejected during the initial phase of systole is trapped in the left ventricle, resulting in an elevated LVEDP. The increased LVEDP and non-compliant nature of the left ventricle impede left atrial emptying and contribute to a diminished cardiac output and atrial dilatation.

***Clinical Presentation.*** Dyspnea, syncope, dizziness, angina, and palpitations are the most frequently reported symptoms. The primary auscultatory finding is a harsh, crescendo-decrescendo systolic murmur caused by the turbulent blood flow through the narrowed left ventricular outflow tract. The ECG discloses evidence of LVH in 86% of the patients with hypertrophic cardiomyopathy.[17] Atrial and ventricular dysrhythmias are common. The high incidence of sudden death in these patients has been attributed to an arrhythmogenic origin.

***Treatment.*** Surgical management of this disorder includes myectomy with muscle resection or transaortic ventriculomyotomy to relieve the outflow obstruction. Medical management includes antiarrhythmic agents, antibiotic prophylaxis for bacterial endocarditis, and anticoagulation in the setting of atrial fibrillation. Recent evidence indicates that verapamil may be effective in reducing symptoms of hypertrophic cardiomyopathy by regressing the hypertrophic response.[18] Beta-adrenergic blocking agents, particularly propranolol, are used extensively although their exact mechanism of action has not been fully described. Drugs that increase contractility or decrease left ventricular volume are generally contraindicated, since they intensify the degree of the obstruction. Therefore, digitalis is generally reserved for the management of rapid atrial fibrillation that is unresponsive to beta-adrenergic blockade. Diuretics should be used with caution so as not to lead to hypovolemia. Nitrate therapy is usually ineffective in relieving the angina and is contraindicated.[19]

### Restrictive Cardiomyopathy

***Description and Underlying Pathophysiology.*** Restrictive cardiomyopathy is the least common type of myopathy. It is a syndrome with features simulating, and therefore it is often misdiagnosed as, constrictive pericarditis. Restrictive cardiomyopathies are caused by a variety of specific processes associated with fibrotic or infiltrative pathologic processes. The most frequent causes are myocardial fibrosis, amyloidosis, sarcoidosis, and endomyocardial fibrosis.

The infiltration of the myocardium makes it rigid and less distensible in diastole. The ventricular noncompliance causes an impairment in ventricular filling. Because the ventricle is noncompliant, small increase in diastolic volume results in a marked increase in diastolic pressure. A persistent tachycardia is a limited compensatory mechanism; however, there is an eventual decline in cardiac output, atrial dilatation develops, and symptoms of systemic and pulmonary venous congestion ensue.

***Clinical Presentation/Treatment.*** The signs and

symptoms are those of pulmonary and systemic venous congestion, with the notable exception of the absence of cardiomegaly. Treatment of the restrictive cardiomyopathy is similar to that of a dilated cardiomyopathy except that vasodilator therapy has not proven to be effective; the tachycardia is beneficial in maintaining cardiac output and, unless it is severe, is generally not treated; any attempt to reduce venous pressure must be done with caution so as not to precipitate a sharp reduction in blood pressure and cardiac output.[20]

### *Myocarditis*

Myocarditis is an inflammation of the myocardium that can be an acute or chronic process and can occur at any age. It is most frequently idiopathic in origin, but can also be caused by rheumatic fever, radiation therapy, drugs, chemicals, metabolic disorders, or viruses.

The pathologic mechanisms responsible for myocarditis include direct myocardial invasion by the causative agent, production of a myocardial toxin, and/or the stimulation of antibody production. The involvement of the myocardium can be focal or diffuse, and the clinical course is determined by the extent and location of the myocardial involvement. Diffuse myocardial involvement may result in heart failure, and focal lesions in the conduction pathways may lead to dysrhythmias and bundle branch blocks. Medical management includes antibiotic therapy and supportive management of heart failure and dysrhythmias.

### *Coronary Artery Disease/Myocardial Infarction*

Ventricular myocardial ischemia/infarction causes a reduction in the number of functional muscle fibers. This results in diminished stroke volume and cardiac output. The development of altered hemodynamic functioning and the propensity for the development of heart failure attributed to CAD and myocardial infarction are described in detail in Chapter 43.

### *Cardiogenic Shock*

**Description.** Cardiogenic shock, or severe heart failure, is a complex syndrome characterized by systemic hypotension, arterial vasoconstriction, and impaired tissue and organ perfusion. It develops when there is an insufficient amount of myocardium to adequately support systemic perfusion. Pathologic studies demonstrate that cardiogenic shock occurs when at least 40% of the left ventricular myocardium has been destroyed.[21] Cardiogenic shock develops in 10% of the patients hospitalized with an acute myocardial infarction and has a mortality approaching 85%. The onset of cardiogenic shock can occur within hours to days after a myocardial infarction, although 50% of its victims develop symptoms within the first 24 hours post-infarction.

**Etiology.** Etiologic factors associated with the development of cardiogenic shock can be divided into 3 categories, as shown in Table 44–6. The most frequent cause of cardiogenic shock continues to be impaired muscular function associated with a massive myocardial infarction. Such massive myocardial necrosis and ischemia occurs when there is an occlusion of the proximal portion of the left anterior descending artery with the consequence of a large dyskinetic segment of the anterior, septal, and apical regions of the left ventricle. With the exception of left main coronary artery lesions or proximal lesions of the left anterior descending artery, isolated single-vessel disease is infrequently associated with cardiogenic shock.[21]

**Underlying Pathophysiology.** The basic physiologic condition that results in cardiogenic shock is a severe depression of myocardial contractility in which the cardiac output is markedly diminished. The physiologic limits of the normal compensatory mechanisms are exceeded, and evidence of circulatory failure develops.

The hemodynamic profile of the patient in cardiogenic shock is presented in Table 44–7, and the signs and symptoms are listed in Table 44–8. In addition to the impaired myocardial contractility, the compliance of the ventricle is impaired. This increases the resistance to ventricular filling and causes an elevated LVEDP and further impairs the cardiac output. The increase in systemic vascular resistance from sustained sympathetic stimulation further compromises LV ejection and cardiac output. Additionally, the intense vasoconstriction reduces perfusion to the skin and kidneys, lactic acid production is accelerated, and the resultant aci-

TABLE 44–6
**Causes of Cardiogenic Shock**

| |
|---|
| **Electrical Factors** |
| Bradyarrhythmias |
| Tachyarrhythmias |
| **Mechanical Factors** |
| Cardiac tamponade |
| Left ventricular aneurysm |
| Myocarditis |
| Dilated cardiomyopathy |
| Hypertension |
| Post-cardiac surgery pump failure |
| Myocardial infarction |
| **Structural Factors** |
| Atrial myxomas |
| Aortic stenosis |
| Mitral stenosis |
| Mitral regurgitation |
| Aortic regurgitation |
| Ruptured intraventricular septum |

TABLE 44–7
**Hemodynamic Profile of Cardiogenic Shock**

| Hemodynamic Parameter | Value in Cardiogenic Shock | Normal Value |
|---|---|---|
| Heart rate | ↑ | 60–90 beats/minute |
| Pulmonary artery pressure | ↑ | 20–25 mmHg / 8–12 mmHg |
| Pulmonary wedge pressure | ↑ | 8–12 mmHg |
| Systemic vascular resistance | ↑ | 800–1200 dynes/sec/cm$^{-5}$ |
| Blood pressure | ↓ | 110–120 mmHg / 70–80 mmHg |
| Cardiac output | ↓ | 4–8 liters/minute |
| Cardiac index | ↓ | 2.5–3.5 liters/minute/m$^2$ |
| Stroke volume | ↓ | 50–100 ml/beat |
| Stroke work index | ↓ | 45–75 g/m$^2$/beat |

dosis further depresses myocardial contractility.[22] With prolonged sympathetic stimulation, systemic and myocardial norepinephrine stores are depleted, which interferes with contractility and peripheral vascular tone. This results in the pooling of blood in the peripheral vasculature, further intensifying the diminished cardiac output state.

As the shock progresses, the severe vasoconstriction impairs cellular functioning in all organs. Renal perfusion is markedly impaired, and acute tubular necrosis develops. Mental status changes are the result of the depressed cardiac output. There is visceral ischemia and necrosis, which can lead to ulceration of intestinal mucosa and spillage of bacteria and toxins into the circulation, intensifying the shock state. As the pancreatic cells become ischemic and necrotic they release an enzyme that assists in the formation of a polypeptide, *myocardial depressant factor* (MDF), which depresses myocardial contractility even further. The pulmonary system is also affected by the vasoconstriction. Necrotic pulmonary parenchymal cells release serotonin and histamine, which increase pulmonary capillary permeability and vasoconstriction. This intensifies the ventilation-perfusion mismatch and aggravates the acidosis and hypoxia. Fluid migrates from the pulmonary vasculature into the interstitium, resulting in interstitial edema. Atelectasis develops as the result of the alveoli's inability to produce enough surfactant to maintain adequate surface tension.[23]

TABLE 44–8
**Clinical Presentation of the Patient with Cardiogenic Shock**

| Body System | Signs/Symptoms |
|---|---|
| Cardiovascular | Systolic blood pressure <90 mmHg<br>Tachycardia<br>Weak, thready pulses<br>$S_3$, $S_4$<br>Decreased pulse pressure<br>Palpitations<br>Chest pain |
| Renal | Urine output ≤30 ml/hr<br>Decreased urine osmolality |
| Integumentary | Cool, clammy skin<br>Decreased capillary refill<br>Peripheral edema<br>Pallor or cyanosis |
| Neurologic | Restlessness, agitation<br>Confusion<br>Altered level of consciousness<br>Dilated pupils |
| Pulmonary | Tachypnea<br>Dyspnea<br>Rales |
| Gastrointestinal | Decreased bowel sounds<br>Nausea/vomiting<br>Melena<br>Hematemesis |

Early recognition and prompt aggressive management are crucial to enhancing the patient's survival and interrupting the vicious, downward spiralling course of patients with cardiogenic shock.

**Treatment.** Medical management includes volume management, sympathomimetic drugs to increase myocardial contractility, vasodilator agents to maximize preload and afterload, mechanical circulatory assist (see Chap. 42), and mechanical ventilation (see Chap. 32).

## Abnormal Volume Load

An abnormal diastolic volume load in the heart (preload) refers to the length of myocardial fibers prior to ventricular contraction. Preload is determined by ventricular compliance, blood volume, venous tone, the condition of the mitral valve, and the timing and force of atrial contraction. Diastolic overload is initially reflected by an elevated LVEDV. Over a period of time, the filling pressures exceed those of the normally compliant heart, causing a decrease in the strength and efficacy of ventricular function.

### *Aortic Regurgitation*

Aortic regurgitation can be acute or chronic and occurs most frequently in men. It can be congenital or caused by infective endocarditis, rheumatic fever, dissecting aortic aneurysm, connective tissue diseases, and anatomic aortic valvular abnormalities.

**Underlying Pathophysiology.** Aortic regurgitation is the result of an incompetent aortic valve during ventricular diastole. Blood ejected into the aorta regurgitates back into the LV through an incompetent valve, imposing a large volume overload on the LV. As much as 60% of the forward stroke volume can be regurgitated.[24]

In acute aortic regurgitation, the increase in LVEDV causes a rise in LVEDP. As the LVEDP exceeds left atrial pressure, the mitral valve closes early in diastole, protecting the pulmonary circulation from the elevated pressure.

In chronic aortic regurgitation, there is a gradual increase in LVEDV, and LVEDP does not initially become elevated. As a compensatory mechanism, left ventricular stroke volume increases to maintain a normal cardiac output. Over time, however, there is a gradual decline in contractility, the LVEDV and LVEDP increase, and the pressure is transmitted back through the pulmonary vasculature, eventually to the right side of the heart. Peripheral vasodilatation occurs in chronic aortic regurgitation as a compensatory mechanism to decrease afterload and minimize the regurgitant volume. This is manifested by a low diastolic blood pressure and warm, flushed appearance.

**Clinical Presentation.** Physical findings include a blowing diastolic murmur. As the disease progresses, the patient might have sweating, flushing, a widened pulse pressure with an elevated systolic and diminished diastolic blood pressure, and a diastolic thrill palpable at the left lower sternal border. The apical impulse is displaced laterally and the heart is hyperdynamic with a prolonged systolic thrust. An $S_3$ gallop is commonly heard. A blowing, high-pitched decrescendo diastolic murmur is heard at the second right intercostal space and radiates to the left sternal border. A rapidly rising and collapsing ("water-hammer" or Corrigan's)* pulse is noted peripherally in the patient with significant aortic regurgitation. With significant regurgitation, the ECG reveals evidence of LVH and left atrial enlargement. Physical findings and an echocardiogram are sufficient to establish the diagnosis of aortic regurgitation although a cardiac catheterization is necessary to quantify the extent of the regurgitation.

**Treatment.** Treatment includes antibiotic prophylaxis against bacterial endocarditis. Digitalis glycosides, sodium restriction, diuretics, and vasodilators provide symptomatic relief of the pulmonary congestion. Valve replacement is the only effective long-term corrective therapy.

### *Mitral Regurgitation*

Mitral regurgitation (MR) can be caused by rheumatic fever, dysfunction of the papillary muscles, calcification of the mitral annulus, conditions causing left ventricular dilatation, congenital anomalies, and connective tissue disorders. Acute MR may involve rupture of the chordae and/or papillary muscles and perforation of a mitral valve leaflet.

**Underlying Pathophysiology.** MR results in systolic volume overload. As the left ventricle attempts to eject its contents into the aorta, there is also a backflow of blood into the left atrium through the incompetent mitral valve. The left atrium dilates and hypertrophies in order to compensate for the enhanced systolic blood volume. The left ventricle also hypertrophies and dilates in an attempt to compensate for the volume lost to the left atrium during systole. This is a limited compensatory mechanism to maintain cardiac output, and left ventricular failure develops with progressive dilatation. Signs of pulmonary and systemic congestion develop secondary to the prolonged elevation in left atrial pressure.

In acute MR the left atrium is of normal size. The regurgitant volume causes a rapid, marked increase in left atrial pressure. This is rapidly transmitted back to the pulmonary veins, capillaries, and arteries with the rapid development of pulmonary edema.

**Clinical Presentation.** Patients with mild MR are usually asymptomatic. With advancing disease, symptoms of fatigue and exhaustion are the result of the diminished cardiac output. When pulmonary hypertension and RVH develop, evidence of RV failure is apparent, including hepatomegaly and peripheral edema. With the development of left atrial dilatation, atrial fibrillation frequently develops. Evidence of systemic embolization can occur as a consequence of blood stagnating in the dilated left atrium.

The apical impulse is displaced laterally and caudally and is abnormally large. The murmur of MR is pansystolic, best heard at the apex, and radiates to the left axilla. Splitting of the second heart sound is a common finding, and an $S_3$ gallop is noted in severe MR. The ECG may be normal even in patients with hemodynamically significant MR. Evidence of LVH is not always present. Left atrial and ventricular enlargement can be noted on the CXR. Ventriculography via cardiac catheterization is re-

*Water-hammer pulse is characterized by a rapid rise in arterial pressure during systole followed by a rapid fall in pressure during diastole.

quired for calculating the mitral valve area and the percentage of the insufficiency.

**Treatment.** Medical treatment of MR includes digitalis glycosides, vasodilators, diuretics, and sodium restriction for symptoms of pulmonary congestion; activities that produce fatigue and dyspnea are restricted; anticoagulation is utilized in chronic MR; and antiarrhythmics are employed if the patient develops atrial fibrillation. Various surgical methods have been employed to repair specific portions of the valve apparatus, including leaflet plication and placement of artificial chordae, although the results of these procedures have varied. Replacement of the mitral valve continues to be the treatment of choice for symptomatic, severe MR[25] (see Chap. 45).

### *Pulmonic Regurgitation*

The primary cause of pulmonic valve regurgitation is congenital malformation of the valve or the absence of one of the leaflets. Acquired causes of the disease arise from conditions associated with pulmonary hypertension that results in valvular ring dilation. Pulmonic regurgitation imposes a volume overload on the right ventricle, increasing RVEDV and RVEDP. Decreased ventricular compliance is the result of the compensatory RV hypertrophy and dilatation. Ultimately the right ventricular diastolic pressure equals the pulmonary artery diastolic pressure, and right ventricular failure develops with symptoms of systemic venous congestion and impaired cardiac output.

Auscultation reveals an early diastolic decrescendo murmur heard best in the fourth or fifth intercostal space at the left sternal border. Treatment includes antibiotic prophylaxis for bacterial endocarditis. If heart failure exists, diuretics, digitalis glycosides, and sodium restriction are prescribed.

### *Tricuspid Regurgitation*

Tricuspid regurgitation is characterized by incomplete valve closure during systole. As the right ventricle attempts to eject its contents into the pulmonary artery, there is a regurgitant flow of blood back into the right atrium through the incompetent tricuspid valve. This elevation in right atrial pressure causes an increased pressure in the systemic circulation. During diastole, the normal contents of the atrium and also the regurgitant volume flow into the right ventricle, increasing RVEDV. Right ventricular hypertrophy and dilatation develop as an adaptive mechanism but are limited, and tricuspid regurgitation results in a diminished cardiac output.

Generally tricuspid regurgitation develops secondary to right ventricular dilatation, which causes distortion of the chordae tendineae and papillary muscles as well as of the valvular ring. It can also develop from infective endocarditis, trauma, or carcinoid syndrome.

Tricuspid regurgitation is well tolerated, but the symptoms that develop in advanced cases are the result of a reduced cardiac output and systemic venous congestion. Common symptoms include marked hepatomegaly, ascites, pleural effusions, edema, hepatojugular reflux, and jugular venous distention with observable systolic pulsations. A pansystolic murmur may be heard at the left sternal border in the fourth intercostal space. The ECG may show atrial fibrillation or right bundle branch block. Treatment includes a sodium-restricted diet, diuretics, and digitalis glycosides. Tricuspid valve replacement is done when tricuspid stenosis and tricuspid regurgitation co-exist.

## THERAPEUTIC INTERVENTIONS

The goals of therapeutic intervention in the patient with heart failure are to support cardiac output and enhance ventricular emptying. This can be accomplished by drug therapy, dietary restriction of sodium, activity restriction, mechanical circulatory assist devices, and surgical intervention. All these interventions attempt to manipulate 1 or more of the components of myocardial function: preload, afterload, and/or contractility. In the critical care setting, the use of bedside hemodynamic monitoring provides necessary diagnostic information and is essential in guiding therapeutic interventions.

### Drug Therapy

#### *Diuretics*

The goals of diuretic therapy include enhancing the excretion of sodium and water, reducing preload and filling pressures, and reducing the signs of systemic and pulmonary venous congestion. There are 5 groups of diuretics that accomplish these goals by their actions on specific sites of the nephron. Thiazide diuretics are the diuretics of choice in patients with right ventricular failure with peripheral, dependent edema and in patients with mild to moderate left ventricular failure. Potassium-sparing diuretics have a long onset of action, thereby limiting their usefulness in the management of acute heart failure, but they are used successfully in the treatment of chronic heart failure especially when combined with other diuretics. Carbonic anhydrase inhibitors have limited value in the treatment of heart failure since they have a very small degree of sodium excretion and are frequently used with other diuretics. Osmotic compounds are used with extreme caution in the heart failure patient. The increased solute load of the osmotic diuretics could potentiate a cardiovascular volume overload and therefore osmotic diuretics are contraindicated in the patient with pulmonary edema. The most frequently used diuretics in the acute care setting continue to be the loop diuretics. They are potent, rapid-acting agents that can be given intravenously or orally. Furosemide possesses vasodilating and diuretic properties that are particularly advantageous in reducing preload and filling pressures in patients with acute left ventricular failure and pulmonary edema.[26]

Two of the main concerns when using diuretic therapy are electrolyte depletion and overdiuresis, which may result in hypovolemia and hypotension. Electrolyte depletion, particularly hypokalemia, is a particular concern in the patient receiving digitalis therapy as this increases the patient's susceptibility to developing dysrhythmias.

### *Inotropic Agents*

The decreased contractility seen in heart failure provides the basis for the use of inotropic agents. Digitalis glycosides continue to be the most widely used oral inotropic agents but their ability to increase the contractile force of the myocardium and improve depressed ventricular function is limited by their modest potency, narrow therapeutic range, and associated toxicities. The hemodynamic effects associated with digitalis administration include a decrease in central venous and pulmonary capillary wedge pressures, an increased stroke volume, and decreased ventricular end-diastolic volume and filling pressures. The increased contractility is associated with an increase in myocardial oxygen consumption. However, this may be offset by the beneficial hemodynamic effects described above. Because digitalis glycosides have a narrow range of therapeutic efficacy and a wide variety of side effects, sympathomimetic agents are more frequently used in the management of the patient with acute heart failure. Digitalis is commonly reserved for the patient in acute congestive failure precipitated by rapid atrial fibrillation.

Sympathomimetic amines are positive inotropic agents that stimulate sympathetic nervous system (SNS) activity and are used to treat severe low-output failure. The SNS attempts to compensate for a fall in cardiac output by the release of endogenous catecholamines, which causes vasoconstriction and tachycardia. Over time, however, the myocardium develops a resistance to the effects of sympathetic stimulation and requires higher levels of catecholamines to maintain heart rate and contractility. This is further complicated by a reduction of endogenous stores of myocardial catecholamines. The combination of these factors contributes to a decrease in the efficiency of the myocardial pumping action. The administration of sympathomimetic amines provides an exogenous method of supporting myocardial function. Although sympathomimetic amines improve myocardial functioning by increasing the heart rate and contractility, there is also an associated increase in myocardial oxygen consumption. An understanding of the response of specific adrenergic receptors to these drugs assists in manipulating combinations and dosages of these drugs so as to minimize their adverse effects and maximize their therapeutic effects (Table 44–9).

TABLE 44–9
**Sympathomimetic Therapy: A Hemodynamic Comparison**

| Drug | Receptor Site Stimulated | Hemodynamic Effects | | | | | |
|---|---|---|---|---|---|---|---|
| | | *HR* | *MAP* | *CO* | *Contractility* | *SVR* | *RBF* |
| Dobutamine | Beta$_1$<br>Beta$_2$ (slight) | 0/↑ | 0/↑ | ↑ | ↑ | 0/↑ | |
| Dopamine | | | | | | | |
| <2–5 μg/kg/minute | Beta$_1$ dopaminergic | 0 | 0 | ↑ | ↑ | 0 | ↑↑ |
| 5–10 μg/kg/minute | Beta$_1$<br>Alpha<br>Beta$_2$ | ↑↑ | ↑ | ↑ | ↑↑ | ↑ | ↑ |
| >10 μg/kg/minute | Alpha<br>Beta$_1$ | ↑↑ | ↑↑ | ↑ | ↑↑ | ↑↑ | 0/↓ |
| Epinephrine | Beta$_1$<br>Alpha (large doses)<br>Beta$_2$ (small doses) | ↑↑ | ↑ | ↑↑ | ↑ | ↑ | ↓↓ |
| Isoproterenol | Beta$_1$<br>Beta$_2$ | ↑↑↑ | 0/↑/↓ | ↑↑ | ↑ | ↓↓ | 0/↑/↓ |
| Norepinephrine | Alpha<br>Beta$_1$ (small amount) | ↑ | ↑↑ | 0 | ↑ | ↑↑ | |
| Phenylephrine | Alpha | ↓ | ↑↑ | ↓ | 0 | ↑↑ | |

*Key: HR*, heart rate; *MAP*, mean arterial pressure; *CO*, cardiac output; *SVR*, systemic vascular resistance; *RBF*, renal blood flow; *O*, unchanged; ↑, increased; ↓, decreased; ↑↑↑, greatest effect; ↓↓↓, least effect.

Alpha-adrenergic receptors are located in the smooth muscle of all vascular tissue. Stimulation of alpha receptors causes cutaneous, renal, and splanchnic vasoconstriction, resulting in an increased systemic vascular resistance (SVR) and elevated blood pressure. $Beta_1$ receptors are found in the heart and their stimulation causes an increase in myocardial contractility, automaticity, and heart rate. $Beta_2$ receptors are principally found in the smooth muscle in the bronchi and skeletal muscle arterioles. $Beta_2$ stimulation results in bronchodilatation and increased blood flow to skeletal muscle beds.

The primary contraindication to the use of sympathomimetic amines is in the management of subvalvular and valvular stenosis. The anticipated increase in heart rate and contractility will adversely increase myocardial oxygen consumption.[26]

### *Vasodilator Agents*

The goal of vasodilator therapy is to limit venous return, maximize filling pressures and contractility by the Frank-Starling mechanism, and decrease impedance to left ventricular outflow. This is accomplished by altering the tone of the peripheral vascular system.

An elevated preload, manifested by an increased LVEDP, can be reduced through the administration of agents with venodilating properties. This causes a redistribution of the circulating blood volume (see Fig. 37–20) from the central to the peripheral circulation and results in decreased filling pressures and elimination or diminution of pulmonary venous congestion. However, venodilating agents can have deleterious effects in the patient with a normal preload state and can cause hypotension and a further decrease in cardiac output. Venodilator therapy is most commonly used in patients with LV failure with pulmonary edema or chronic severe heart failure refractory to diuretics and digitalis.[26]

Afterload is reduced by the administration of arteriolar dilators, which directly decrease the impedance to LV ejection and ultimately decrease intramyocardial wall tension, resulting in an improved stroke volume, cardiac output, and peripheral perfusion. If there is sufficient improvement in stroke volume, the blood pressure will remain unchanged or fall only slightly, indicating an overall improvement in myocardial pump function.[26]

In addition to the drugs that act either on the venous or arteriolar vascular beds, there is a group of drugs that possess both venous and arteriolar dilating properties. The hemodynamic effects of the combined agents are an improved cardiac output and a reduction in cardiac filling pressures. Table 44–10 presents the vasodilator agents and their specific vascular responsiveness.

Morphine sulfate is frequently administered intravenously in small, intermittent doses in the patient with acute heart failure. This causes peripheral pooling of blood with redistribution of the blood away from the congested pulmonary circulation, resulting in a decreased preload. Additionally,

TABLE 44–10
**Vasodilator Therapy: A Hemodynamic Comparison**

| | | Hemodynamic Effects | | | | | | | |
|---|---|---|---|---|---|---|---|---|---|
| **Drug** | **Vasospecificity** | ***HR*** | ***SVR*** | ***MAP*** | ***CO*** | ***PCWP*** | ***RAP*** | ***SV*** | **Indications** |
| Nitroprusside | Arterial and venous vasodilator | 0/↑ | ↓↓ | ↓ | ↑ | ↓ | ↓ | ↑↑ | Acute left ventricular failure with ↑ pulmonary pressures, ↓ CO |
| Nitroglycerin | Venous vasodilator | 0 | 0/↓ | ↓ | 0/↑ | ↓↓↓ | ↓↓↓ | ↑ | Acute left ventricular failure with severe pulmonary congestion and/or ischemia |
| Phentolamine | Arterial and venous vasodilator | ↑↑ | ↓↓↓ | ↓ | ↑↑ | ↓↓ | ↓↓ | ↑↑ | LV failure with low CO; requires high doses for sustained vasodilatation and causes ↑ HR |
| Hydralazine | Arterial vasodilator | 0/↑ | ↓↓↓ | ↓ | ↑↑↑ | 0/↓ | 0/↓ | ↑↑↑ | Chronic severe heart failure |
| Captopril | Arterial and venous vasodilator | 0 | ↓↓ | ↓↓ | ↑↑ | ↓↓↓ | ↓↓↓ | ↑↑ | Chronic refractory heart failure |
| Nifedipine | Arterial and venous vasodilator | 0/↑ | ↓↓↓ | ↓↓ | ↑↑ | ↓↓ | 0/↓ | ↑↑ | Heart failure with coronary vasospasm or acute infarction |
| Prazosin | Arterial and venous vasodilator | 0/↓ | ↓↓ | ↓↓ | ↑↑ | ↓↓↓ | ↓↓↓ | ↑↑ | Chronic severe heart failure |
| Minoxidil | Arterial vasodilator | ↑ | ↓↓↓ | ↓↓ | ↑↑↑ | 0/↓ | 0 | ↑↑ | Chronic heart failure; hypertension |

*Key: HR*, heart rate; *SVR*, systemic vascular resistance; *MAP*, mean arterial pressure; *CO*, cardiac output; *PCWP*, pulmonary capillary wedge pressure; *RAP*, right atrial pressure; *SV*, stroke volume; *O*, unchanged; ↑, increased; ↓, decreased; ↑↑↑, greatest effect; ↓↓↓, least effect.

Adapted from Chatterjee, K.[29]

morphine helps to decrease the anxiety and tachypnea noted in the acute heart failure patient and also helps relax airway smooth muscle to facilitate gas exchange.

Vasodilators are generally not used in the management of valvular stenosis. The hemodynamic consequences of mitral stenosis include an elevation in the left atrial pressure and pulmonary venous pressures. There is a mechanical obstruction to LV filling and little evidence of LV failure; therefore, afterload reduction would have little effect on LV function. In aortic stenosis associated with LV failure, extreme caution must be used with vasodilator therapy. Although cardiac output could be improved by afterload reduction, there is a risk of the vasodilator precipitating hypotension, which would impair coronary perfusion.

Vasodilator therapy has a limited value in the treatment of right ventricular failure and in the management of pulmonary hypertension because vasodilators have a greater effect on systemic vascular beds than on pulmonary vascular beds. This necessitates the use of high doses of vasodilator agents to achieve a reduction in the impedance to right ventricular outflow, and systemic hypotension generally precludes the administration of such high doses.[26]

## Supportive Therapy

### Oxygen Therapy

Impaired gas exchange develops as a consequence of LV failure with the transudation of fluid from the pulmonary vascular system into the interstitial and alveolar spaces of the lung. Also, a diminished cardiac output leads to impaired perfusion and gas exchange at the cellular level, resulting in tissue hypoxia. Contractility is impaired by hypoxia as the result of an ineffective myocardial cellular metabolism that develops with the shift from an aerobic to an anaerobic state. Supplemental oxygen is provided to reduce the workload of the heart and to support cellular energy requirements.

### Dietary Sodium Restriction

Dietary restriction of sodium is also an important part of the management of the patient with heart failure. As a result of sympathoadrenergic stimulation, the renin-angiotensin-aldosterone mechanism results in an increased tubular reabsorption of sodium and water (see Fig. 21–9). In severe cases, the body can retain as much as 10 liters of extra fluid and 80 g of sodium. This causes an increase in cardiac workload and can increase filling pressures and precipitate the development of pulmonary edema. The amount of sodium and water retained by the body can be altered by decreasing the amount of sodium ingested in the diet.

Normally, the average American diet contains 2.5–6 g of sodium. Omitting the use of table salt reduces the sodium intake to 1.6–2.8 g. However, in cases of severe heart failure, it may be necessary to restrict the sodium intake to 0.2–1 g sodium per day. This would require patients to eliminate the use of table salt and salt in cooking, as well as purchasing and preparing foods with a low sodium content.[27]

### Activity

The modification of activity is also an important part of the prescriptive plan for patients with heart failure in order not to place excessive workload demands on the heart. The activity plan is highly individualized and the degree of restriction is based on the severity of the heart failure. It is generally recommended that the highest level of activity be maintained that does not produce symptoms. Isometric exercises are discouraged since they do not promote cardiovascular conditioning and cause an increase in blood pressure and cardiac workload. Aerobic activities are good for cardiovascular conditioning but must not be too strenuous.

The teaching plan should include an assessment of the severity of the patient's heart failure and prior activity pattern; teaching the importance of environmental factors on cardiac function; explaining the importance of rest periods and the timing of activity to avoid exercise after a meal or alcohol; and teaching the patient to identify the end points of activity intolerance. These usually include the sensation of fatigue, chest discomfort, shortness of breath, palpitations, or a heart rate that exceeds the resting heart rate by more than 25 beats/minute.

### Mechanical Support

Mechanical support of the failing heart may be fundamental to improving the pumping action of the myocardium and reducing the heart's workload. Mechanical support devices are usually reserved for the treatment of intractable heart failure. The intra-aortic balloon pump (IABP) is the most frequently used device to temporarily support the failing heart and systemic circulation. The beneficial hemodynamic effects anticipated with the use of the IABP include an elevation of the aortic pressure and improved coronary artery perfusion by augmentation of arterial diastolic pressure. As the balloon is deflated during isovolumetric contraction, there is a decrease in intra-aortic volume, a diminished resistance to LV ejection, and a decrease in ventricular workload and myocardial oxygen consumption. This is evidenced by an improved cardiac output, increased stroke volume, and a reduction in LVEDP.

The left ventricular assist device (LVAD) is a mechanical device that is used predominantly in post-

## TABLE 44–11. CARE PLAN FOR THE PATIENT WITH HEART FAILURE

| Nursing Diagnoses | Desired Patient Outcomes | Nursing Interventions | Rationales |
|---|---|---|---|
| ***Nursing Diagnosis #1***<br>Cardiac output, alteration in, decreased, related to:<br>1. Impaired myocardial contractile functioning.<br>2. Filling disorders.<br>3. Abnormal volume load.<br>4. Abnormal pressure load. | Patient will:<br>1. Demonstrate signs of hemodynamic stability:<br>• Cardiac output 4–8 liters/minute.<br>• Heart rate $<100$ beats/minute.<br>• Systolic blood pressure $>110$ mmHg or within 10 mmHg of baseline.<br>• Pulmonary capillary wedge pressure 8–12 mmHg (mean).<br>• Absence of $S_3$ and $S_4$.<br>2. Maintain electrophysiologic stability.<br>• Absence of dysrhythmias.<br>3. Maintain state of normovolemia.<br>• Good skin turgor.<br>• Absence of peripheral edema.<br>• Absence of jugular venous distention.<br>• Absence of rales on auscultation.<br>• Stable baseline body weight. | • Ongoing assessment of signs and symptoms of *left* ventricular failure: | • Provides a systematic approach to data collection to gauge the severity of the disease and the efficacy of therapeutic intervention. |
| | | ○ Rales (crackles). | ○ Fluid in alveoli, the result of pressure increases in the pulmonary capillary bed. |
| | | ○ Bronchial wheezing. | ○ Bronchiolar constriction from excess fluid. |
| | | ○ Dyspnea. | ○ Result of elevation in pulmonary interstitial edema. |
| | | ○ Paroxysmal nocturnal dyspnea. | ○ Serum proteins are at lowest level in early morning; redistribution of volume secondary to recumbent position; nocturnal respiratory depression. |
| | | ○ Nocturia. | ○ Increased renal perfusion secondary to postural redistribution of blood flow. |
| | | ○ Orthopnea. | ○ Result of increased venous return from postural redistribution of pulmonary blood flow. |
| | | ○ Anxiety, restlessness, disorientation. | ○ Decreased cerebral perfusion and cerebral hypoxia. |
| | | ○ Pulsus alternans (see Fig. 38–2). | ○ Secondary to variation in strength of ventricular contraction. |
| | | ○ Gallop rhythms. | ○ $S_3$ associated with increased LVEDP, left atrial pressure, and PCWP.<br>○ $S_4$ related to decreased ventricular compliance. |
| | | ○ Peripheral cyanosis. | ○ Secondary to decreased cardiac output and decreased peripheral circulation; blood stays in peripheral tissues longer to extract more oxygen, and when blood reaches distal vascular bed, it has a markedly diminished $O_2$ content. |
| | | ○ Central cyanosis. | ○ Results when alveolar edema impairs $O_2$ diffusion. |
| | | ○ Blood-tinged sputum. | ○ Rupture of bronchiolar capillaries due to increased hydrostatic pressure in capillaries. |
| | | ○ Cheyne-Stokes respirations. | ○ Decreased cardiac output causes prolonged circulation time, which in turn causes the respiratory center in the brainstem to be underperfused and underoxygenated. |

*(continued)*

### TABLE 44-11. CARE PLAN FOR THE PATIENT WITH HEART FAILURE *(Continued)*

| Nursing Diagnoses | Desired Patient Outcomes | Nursing Interventions | Rationales |
|---|---|---|---|
| ***Nursing Diagnosis #1** (cont.)* | | | |
| | | • Ongoing assessment of the signs and symptoms of *right* ventricular failure: | |
| | | ○ Jugular venous distention. | ○ Result of elevated venous pressures. |
| | | ○ Peripheral edema.<br>○ Weight gain. | ○ May gain as much as 10–15 lb of extracellular fluid before edema is readily apparent. |
| | | ○ Ascites.<br>○ Hepatojugular reflux. | ○ Pressure on right upper quadrant compresses liver and acts as a temporary fluid challenge; dysfunctional right heart will show a visible increase in pressure in jugular veins; competent right heart will not show a visible increase in pressure. |
| | | ○ Anorexia, nausea, vomiting. | ○ Increased pressure in capillaries of abdominal organs results in edema; nausea is secondary to stretching of liver capsule secondary to edema. |
| | | • Identify and correct (if possible) precipitating factors of heart failure. | • Any factor that increases metabolic demand of body stresses the cardiovascular system, which can precipitate the development of heart failure in the patient with cardiac dysfunction. Identification fosters early, more effective intervention. |
| | | • Monitor fluid balance:<br>○ Measure weight daily.<br>○ Document intake and output, urine specific gravity.<br>○ Maintain fluid restriction as indicated.<br>○ Use microdrip or infusion pump for fluid administration. | |
| | | • Monitor hemodynamic parameters. | • Provide best indication of patient's response to therapy. |
| | | ○ Arterial blood pressure. | ○ Decreased systolic pressure or narrowed arterial *pulse* pressure indicative of decreased cardiac output; increased diastolic blood pressure indicates increased peripheral vascular resistance. |

| | |
|---|---|
| ◦ Pulmonary capillary wedge pressure. | ◦ Pulmonary edema develops when PCWP exceeds plasma osmotic pressure (>28 mmHg).<br>◦ Measure of LVEDP-preload; optimal PCWP maximizes contractility via Frank-Starling mechanism (see Fig. 37–17). Elevated in aortic stenosis and regurgitation, mitral stenosis and regurgitation, cardiogenic shock, dilated cardiomyopathy, hypertropic cardiomyopathy, and restrictive cardiomyopathy. |
| ◦ Cardiac output and cardiac intake.<br>◦ Systemic vascular resistance. | ◦ Determinant of afterload; increased impedance to left ventricular ejection increases intramyocardial wall tension; result of sympathoadrenergic stimulation; increased SVR increases myocardial oxygen requirements and decreases myocardial contractility. |
| ◦ Right atrial pressure. | ◦ Elevated in pulmonary hypertension, tricuspid and pulmonic stenosis, tricuspid regurgitation, right heart failure, and hypervolemia. |
| • Monitor laboratory/diagnostic data.<br>◦ Arterial blood gases. | ◦ Increased work of breathing secondary to pulmonary congestion leads to hypoxia and hypercapnia, which further depress myocardial contractility. |
| ◦ Electrolytes. | ◦ BUN, Na—reflect hydration status; hypokalemia—diuresis-induced; hyperglycemia—secondary to stress-related catecholamines. |
| ◦ ECG. | ◦ May reveal evidence of ischemia, LVH, RVH, dysrhythmias. |
| ◦ Chest x-ray. | ◦ Presence of pleural effusion, usually right-sided or bilateral (rarely on the left); interstitial pulmonary edema; enlarged cardiac silhouette. |
| ◦ Circulation time. | ◦ Prolonged secondary to decreased contractility of ventricles leading to decreased cardiac output. |
| ◦ Elevated bilirubin, SGOT, and LDH. | ◦ Result of hepatic congestion in right heart failure. |
| ◦ Proteinuria, increased specific gravity, increased BUN and creatinine. | ◦ Indicate renal dysfunction as a result of decreased cardiac output and decreased glomerular filtration rate. |
| • Implement measures to reduce cardiac workload:<br>◦ Place patient in semi-Fowler's position if blood pressure tolerates. | ◦ Diminishes venous return and promotes adequate lung expansion. |

*(continued)*

**TABLE 44–11. CARE PLAN FOR THE PATIENT WITH HEART FAILURE *(Continued)***

| Nursing Diagnoses | Desired Patient Outcomes | Nursing Interventions | Rationales |
|---|---|---|---|
| ***Nursing Diagnosis #1 (cont.)*** | | | |
| | | ○ Allow for frequent rest periods. | ○ Reduces fatigue, decreases myocardial oxygen consumption. |
| | | ○ Administer oxygen as prescribed. | ○ Reduces workload of heart and supports cellular energy requirements.<br>○ Correction of hypoxia related to pulmonary congestion.<br>○ Myocardial tissue hypoxia predisposes to dysrhythmias and further decreases myocardial contractility. |
| | | ○ Institute measures to allay anxiety (see Nursing Diagnosis #4). | |
| | | • Administer prescribed medication regimen to maximize effects of preload, afterload, and myocardial contractility.<br>○ Cardiac glycosides. | ○ Positive inotropic and negative chronotropic agent = improved cardiac output. |
| | | ○ Diuretics:<br>– Monitor I&O; daily weights.<br>– Monitor for side effects of diuretic therapy (hypokalemia, hyponatremia, fatigue, muscle cramps, hypotension, tachycardia). | ○ Decrease intravascular volume by their direct action on the kidney and by reducing sodium reabsorption; increase venous capacitance, reduce preload to maximize Frank-Starling mechanism.<br>○ Increased venous capacitance provides beneficial effect in patients with left heart failure and pulmonary edema; in patients with right heart failure with vigorous diuresis, this may be detrimental as it contributes to systemic venous pooling, thereby limiting venous return and right ventricular filling and further contributing to a decreased cardiac output. |
| | | ○ Vasodilators:<br>– Monitor for side effects and efficacy of therapy (headache, dizziness, hypotension, postural hypotension, muscle weakness, syncope; ↓SVR, ↓PCWP, ↓RA pressure, diuresis, increased exercise tolerance, resolution of heart failure symptoms). | ○ Vasodilators increase cardiac output by decreasing SVR and/or reducing LVEDP by decreasing vascular tone. Vasodilators reduce myocardial oxygen demand, which may help minimize ischemia and infarction size. |

| | |
|---|---|
| ◦ Sympathomimetics. | ◦ Positive inotropic agents that increase cardiac output by increasing stroke volume and contractility; myocardium becomes dependent on circulating catecholamines in heart failure, and sympathomimetic administration provides an exogenous source of catecholamines to support myocardial contractility. |
| • Assess the effects of systemic congestion and decreased cardiac output on drug therapy. | • Hepatic congestion and renal dysfunction may alter drug metabolism and excretion, predisposing the patient to toxic side effects. |
| • Assess medication regimen for drugs with negative inotropic effects; discuss with physician before discontinuing. | • Such drugs may cause further compromise of cardiac function but may be controlling dysrhythmias, which may also precipitate a deterioration in patient's condition and in cardiac output. |
| • Monitor for dysrhythmias.<br>◦ Maintain continuous ECG monitoring.<br>◦ Monitor conditions that precipitate dysrhythmias (hypoxia, acidosis, alkalosis, digoxin toxicity, electrolyte imbalance) and implement corrective action. | ◦ Increased irritability of myocardium predisposes to dysrhythmias. |
| ◦ Document rhythm changes and assess for hemodynamic compromise; notify physician of patient response. | ◦ Bradyarrhythmias may decrease cardiac output secondary to decreased stroke volume.<br>◦ Tachyarrhythmias reduce diastolic filling time and increase myocardial oxygen consumption. Loss of atrial kick contributes to a decreased cardiac output. |
| ◦ Administer treatment to correct dysrhythmias (may include pacing, antiarrhythmics, and/or cardioversion). | |
| • Identify factors that exacerbate structural abnormalities of cardiac function and institute appropriate therapy.<br>◦ Hypertrophic cardiomyopathy: Avoid conditions that increase the degree of obstruction and/or decrease ventricular volume (digitalis, diuretics, nitrates, exercise, sudden postural changes, Valsalva maneuvers, beta-antagonists). | ◦ Digitalis, exercise, beta-agonists, and Valsalva maneuvers increase contractility and the degree of obstruction and should be avoided. Diuretics, nitrates, sudden postural changes decrease ventricular volume. |
| ◦ Encourage factors that increase cardiac output (alpha-stimulants, supine or squatting position). | |
| • Prepare for insertion of mechanical circulatory assist devices (see Chap. 42). | |
| • Maintain properly functioning emergency equipment and ensure its availability on each shift. | |

(*continued*)

**TABLE 44-11. CARE PLAN FOR THE PATIENT WITH HEART FAILURE *(Continued)***

| Nursing Diagnoses | Desired Patient Outcomes | Nursing Interventions | Rationales |
|---|---|---|---|
| ***Nursing Diagnosis #2***<br>Tissue perfusion, alteration in, related to:<br>1. Severely impaired myocardial contractility. | Patient will:<br>1. Demonstrate signs of hemodynamic stability:<br>• Systolic BP >90 mmHg.<br>• Diastolic BP 60–90 mmHg.<br>• PCWP 8–12 mmHg (mean).<br>• Cardiac output 4–8 liters/minute.<br>• Heart rate <100 beats/minute.<br>• SVR 800–1200 dynes/sec/cm$^{-5}$.<br>2. Maintain adequate tissue perfusion.<br>• Patient awake, alert, oriented.<br>• Urine output >30 ml/hr.<br>• Skin warm and dry.<br>• Absence of peripheral edema.<br>• Absence of rales (crackles) on auscultation.<br>3. Maintain electrophysiologic stability.<br>• Absence of dysrhythmias.<br>4. Maintain arterial blood gases within normal limits.<br>5. Verbalize anxieties and concerns. | • Identify patients at risk of developing cardiogenic shock (see Table 44-6). | • Early recognition and intervention are crucial determinants to patient survival. |
| | | • Assess signs of inadequate tissue perfusion.<br>○ Coronary:<br>○ Blood pressure. | ○ Decreased pulse pressure, increased diastolic blood pressure, systolic pressure less than 90 mmHg: Indicative of increased SVR and decreased cardiac output. |
| | | ○ Heart rate. | ○ Compensatory tachycardia. |
| | | ○ Cardiac output/cardiac index. | ○ Decreased in heart failure; indicator of tissue perfusion. |
| | | ○ SVR. | ○ Measurement of afterload; increased secondary to sympathetic nervous system stimulation. |
| | | ○ $\overline{MAP}$. | ○ Decreased $\overline{MAP}$ and increased LVEDP (PCWP) result in decreased coronary artery perfusion potentially resulting in myocardial ischemia and necrosis. |
| | | ○ Right atrial pressure. | ○ Measurement of adequacy of central venous return. |
| | | ○ PAP, PCWP. | ○ Increased secondary to impaired myocardial contractility; maintained slightly higher than normal to maximize Frank-Starling mechanism; serial measurements to evaluate left ventricular function and response to therapy. |
| | | ○ Monitor for signs of left or right ventricular failure and dysrhythmias. | ○ See Nursing Diagnosis #1. |
| | | ○ Evaluate medication regimen for any treatments that may cause myocardial depression. | ○ See Nursing Diagnosis #1. |
| | | ○ Assess for signs and symptoms indicative of myocardial ischemia and necrosis. | ○ Refer to Chapter 43 for discussion of myocardial infarction. |
| | | ○ Renal:<br>○ Measure urine output hourly; notify physician <30 ml/hr.<br>○ Measure intake and output.<br>○ Monitor BUN and creatinine.<br>○ Assess for increased tolerance to diuretic therapy. | ○ Decreased cardiac output results in decreased renal perfusion and function; the afferent arterioles vasoconstrict and glomerular filtration decreases, which results in a decreased ability of the kidneys to filter, excrete, and reabsorb. |

| | |
|---|---|
| ○ Cerebral:<br>○ Assess neurologic status: LOC; restlessness, agitation, confusion, and somnolence; response to verbal and tactile stimuli; EOMs and pupillary responses. | ○ Decreased cardiac output causes diminished carotid and vertebral artery blood flow. Blood flow to medulla remains normal until late in the stages of shock; midbrain, cerebellum, and cerebral cortex are underperfused. |
| ○ Respiratory. | ○ For respiratory assessment, interventions, and rationales see Nursing Diagnosis #3, below). |
| ○ Cutaneous:<br>○ Assess capillary refill.<br>○ Assess warmth, color, and moistness of skin. | ○ Cool, moist skin indicates decreased perfusion secondary to redistribution of blood flow to central circulation. |
| ○ Assess quality of peripheral pulses. | ○ Weak, thready peripheral pulses are indicative of vasoconstriction. |
| ○ Visceral:<br>○ Monitor bowel sounds.<br>○ Assess for abdominal discomfort. | ○ Indicative of decreased perfusion and ischemia to splanchnic area secondary to a profound decrease in cardiac output. |
| ○ Laboratory data (see Nursing Diagnosis #1):<br>○ Arterial blood gases. | ○ Acidosis depresses myocardial contractility; acidosis indicates inadequate tissue perfusion and accumulation of lactic acid. |
| ○ Venous blood saturations. | ○ Increased arterial-venous $O_2$ difference indicates increased $O_2$ extraction by tissues in response to a decreased cardiac output. |
| ○ Electrolytes. | ○ Hyponatremia and hyperkalemia are myocardial depressants. |
| ○ Serum lactate level. | ○ Elevated secondary to anaerobic metabolism. |
| ○ Assess for hypovolemia (hydration status).<br>○ Intake and output including extrarenal (insensible) losses; urine output; PCWP; and weight changes.<br>○ Keep physician informed of patient's status.<br>○ Monitor effects of fluid challenge if ordered. | ○ Contraindicated for PCWP $>20$ mmHg; CVP $>12$ $cmH_2O$. |
| ○ Administer fluid challenge (0.9% normal saline) rapidly: 100 ml every 5–10 minutes. | ○ Ensures intravascular expansion. |
| ○ Determine CVP or PCWP after each bolus. | ○ End points of challenge are hypotension; PCWP at 20 mmHg; CVP increase by 2 $cmH_2O$. |

(continued)

**TABLE 44–11. CARE PLAN FOR THE PATIENT WITH HEART FAILURE *(Continued)***

| Nursing Diagnoses | Desired Patient Outcomes | Nursing Interventions | Rationales |
|---|---|---|---|
| ***Nursing Diagnosis #2 (cont.)*** | | | ○ PCWP >20 mmHg increases likelihood of precipitating pulmonary edema. |
| | | • Administer medications as prescribed.<br>○ Monitor medications for efficacy and toxicity. | ○ Hypotension, redistribution of blood volume, impaired renal and hepatic perfusion may impair absorption and metabolism. |
| | | ○ Monitor hemodynamic parameters to assess efficacy of pharmacologic therapy. | ○ Best indices to LV function and systemic perfusion. |
| | | ○ Monitor arterial pH. | ○ Most vasoactive therapy has decreased efficacy in an acidotic or alkalotic environment. |
| | | • Prepare for use of mechanical circulatory assistance if above measures are ineffective in restoring tissue perfusion. | • Decreases afterload during systole and increases perfusion by increasing aortic pressure during diastole (see Chap. 42). |
| | | • Institute measures to allay anxiety. | • See Nursing Diagnosis #4, below). |
| ***Nursing Diagnosis #3***<br>Gas exchange, impaired, related to:<br>1. Pulmonary congestion with increased ventilation/perfusion mismatching, and shunting. | Patient will:<br>1. Demonstrate signs of adequate cerebral oxygenation: Alert mental status; oriented to person, time, and place.<br>2. Demonstrate normal respiratory effort:<br>• Rate <25/minute; pattern—eupneic.<br>3. Maintain optimal arterial blood gases:<br>• pH 7.35–7.45.<br>• $PaO_2$ >60 mmHg.<br>• $PaCO_2$ 35–45 mmHg.<br>4. Maintain breath sounds clear to auscultation.<br>5. Demonstrate clear lung fields on chest x-ray.<br>6. Maintain effective cardiovascular function:<br>• HR 60–80/minute. | • Perform ongoing mental status assessment: Confusion, restlessness, anxiety, stupor, loss of consciousness. | • Hypoxemia may predispose to cerebral tissue hypoxia. |
| | | • Monitor respiratory function on ongoing basis.<br>○ Respiratory rate and rhythm. | ○ Reflects work of breathing: Increased work of breathing increases oxygen consumption and myocardial oxygen demand. |
| | | ○ Dyspnea. | ○ Secondary to increased pulmonary interstitial edema. |
| | | ○ Orthopnea. | ○ Increased venous return secondary to postural redistribution of pulmonary blood flow. |
| | | ○ Cough. | ○ Usually nonproductive, periodic, and nocturnal. |
| | | ○ Status of weakness and fatigue. | ○ Secondary to decreased perfusion to skeletal muscles; increased work of breathing further fatigues the patient and predisposes to alveolar hypoventilation with hypercapnia and respiratory acidemia. |
| | | ○ Secretions: Quality, quantity, presence of blood (frequently pink and frothy secretions). | ○ Result of capillary hydrostatic pressure exceeding pulmonary capillary oncotic pressure, which allows fluid to leak into pulmonary interstitium; when this cannot be reabsorbed via the pulmonary lymphatic system, fluid fills the alveoli. |

| | | |
|---|---|---|
| • Cardiac output 4–8 liters/minute. | ◦ Cyanosis, pallor. | |
| | ◦ Auscultation of lungs for presence of adventitious sounds: Rales, bronchial wheezing. | ◦ Frequent assessments allow for early intervention, minimizing deleterious effects of respiratory compromise. |
| | • Monitor diagnostic tests and studies: | |
| | ◦ Arterial blood gases. | ◦ Reflect effectiveness of gas exchange; decreased $PaO_2$ result of alveolar flooding; $PaCO_2$ initially decreases secondary to hyperventilation; then it elevates secondary to patient fatigue (see Fig. 32–4). |
| | ◦ Chest x-ray. | ◦ Butterfly distribution of pulmonary infiltrates; may take 24 hr after symptoms develop to become apparent on chest x-ray. |
| | ◦ ECG. | ◦ May reflect signs of myocardial ischemia. |
| | • Assess cardiovascular function frequently: | |
| | ◦ Heart rate. | ◦ Initial tachycardia is the result of sympathetic nervous system stimulation; return of heart rate to baseline may be indicative of resolving pulmonary edema. |
| | ◦ Hemodynamic parameters: | |
| | ◦ Systemic blood pressure. | ◦ May become hypertensive from sympathetic stimulation. |
| | ◦ Cardiac output. | ◦ Reflects tissue perfusion. |
| | ◦ PCWP. | ◦ Increased LVEDP reflected back to pulmonary capillary bed, increasing pulmonary intravascular hydrostatic pressure; PCWP >20 mmHg. |
| | ◦ Jugular venous distention; peripheral edema, sacral edema; presence of $S_3$, $S_4$; gallop rhythm; pulsus alternans; palpitation, chest pain. | ◦ Affords noninvasive evaluation of changes in venous pressure (see Nursing Diagnosis #1). |
| | • Implement measures to allay patient anxiety. | • Anxiety causes patient to become tachypneic, which causes him/her to consume more oxygen. |
| | ◦ Assess patient's anxiety. | |
| | ◦ Explain treatment plan and procedures. | |
| | ◦ Maintain calm, reassuring approach to care. | |
| | • Implement measures to increase gas exchange. | |
| | ◦ Administer oxygen as prescribed and monitor response to therapy. | ◦ $O_2$ is given to raise $PaO_2$ above 60 mmHg when there is hypoxemia without hypercapnia. |
| | | ◦ Hypoxia enhances likelihood of dysrhythmia development, depresses myocardial contractility, and causes pulmonary vasoconstriction, which increases the workload of the right side of the heart; elevating the $PaO_2$ will minimize and/or reverse these processes. |

*(continued)*

**TABLE 44–11. CARE PLAN FOR THE PATIENT WITH HEART FAILURE *(Continued)***

| Nursing Diagnoses | Desired Patient Outcomes | Nursing Interventions | Rationales |
|---|---|---|---|
| ***Nursing Diagnosis #3 (cont.)*** | | ○ Reassure patient of the need for oxygen and its temporary nature.<br>○ Administer positive pressure as needed. | ○ Most patients tolerate administration of oxygen by mask poorly and frequently fear suffocation.<br>○ Increases mean lung volume (functional lung capacity), allowing more alveoli to participate in gas exchange. |
| | | ○ Assess hemodynamic parameters meticulously during positive pressure therapy (PEEP). | ○ Positive pressure can impede venous return, thereby decreasing cardiac output. |
| | | ○ Initiate intubation and mechanical ventilation as necessary. | ○ See Tables 32–7 and 32–9. |
| | | • Implement measures to decrease preload and afterload.<br>○ Place patient in high Fowler's position with dependent lower extremities if blood pressure allows. | ○ Dilates peripheral arteries and veins and causes venous pooling, thereby decreasing venous congestion. |
| | | ○ Administer morphine sulfate IV.<br>○ Monitor for respiratory depressant effects; have morphine antagonist at bedside. | ○ Reduces patient's anxiety, decreases tachypnea, causes peripheral pooling of blood, decreases preload and afterload.<br>○ Respiratory depression occurs in approximately 7 minutes. |
| | | ○ Monitor blood pressure for hypotension. | ○ Hypotension, the result of baroreceptors' vasoconstrictive reflexes, is inhibited by morphine. |
| | | ○ Administer intravenous vasodilators such as nitroprusside and nitroglycerin. Carefully monitor arterial blood pressure while administering these drugs. | ○ Reduce vascular hydrostatic pressure and reduce PCWP; these drugs have systemic venous and arterial vasodilatory properties. |
| | | ○ Administer intravenous diuretics as ordered (usually potent loop diuretics such as furosemide and ethacrynic acid). Carefully monitor for hypotension and tachycardia, and check for signs of hypokalemia. | ○ Reduce total blood volume and increase venous capacitance.<br>○ Cause reduction in sodium reabsorption in loop of Henle; direct effect on arterial and venous dilatation.<br>○ Evidence of circulatory intolerance and potassium wasting is associated with use of these diuretics. |
| | | ○ Apply rotating tourniquets as ordered (automatic tourniquet machine) following appropriate procedure:<br>○ Connect to upper portion of arms and legs; only 3 cuffs should be inflated simultaneously. | |

| | | | |
|---|---|---|---|
| | | **∘ Inflate blood pressure cuffs to 10 mmHg below the diastolic pressure.** | **∘ Higher pressures will cause fluid loss into the patient's peripheral extravascular spaces.**<br>**∘ Should not occlude arterial blood flow.**<br>**∘ Pulse should be palpable with cuff inflated.** |
| | | **∘ Check for presence of peripheral pulses, warmth, and color of extremities.**<br>**∘ Make certain tourniquets rotate every 15 minutes.** | |
| | | **∘ When discontinuing tourniquets, remove one by one in a counterclockwise direction every 15 minutes.**<br>**∘ Assess patient's tolerance to discontinuance of treatment.** | **∘ Avoids excessive increase in venous return.** |
| | | • Implement measures to improve left ventricular contractility. | • Increased myocardial contractility leads to increased cardiac output with a reduction in LVEDP and PCWP. |
| | | ∘ Administer cardiac glycosides as prescribed.<br>∘ Administer dopamine, dobutamine in low doses as prescribed. | ∘ Stimulate myocardial beta-receptors to enhance contractility. |
| | | ∘ Administer aminophylline as prescribed (observe for hypotension, dysrhythmias). | ∘ Bronchodilator; also increases myocardial contractility and enhances diuresis. |
| ***Nursing Diagnosis #4***<br>Anxiety, related to:<br>1. Potential for lifestyle modification.<br>2. Powerlessness (see Chaps. 3 and 5).<br>3. Intensive care setting.<br>4. Uncertainty related to illness and diagnosis. | Patient will:<br>1. Verbalize anxieties and fears.<br>2. Verbalize feeling less anxious.<br>3. Demonstrate a relaxed demeanor. | • Obtain baseline assessment of anxiety level and coping patterns from patient, family members, or significant others.<br>• Assess level of anxiety; include heart rate, blood pressure, increased muscle tension, increased startle response, a change in sleeping patterns, nightmares, irritability, diaphoresis, nausea, diarrhea, repetitive behaviors. | • Baseline data are essential in evaluating the effectiveness of therapeutic interventions and the patient's ability to cope.<br>∘ Assists in determining the underlying cause of anxiety and provides a basis for intervention. |
| | | • Ascertain what the patient or family member is experiencing; eliminate a physiologic basis of symptoms.<br>• Determine what the individual's needs are and what resources can be mobilized to decrease feelings of anxiety; provide positive reinforcement when appropriate.<br>• Implement therapeutic measures to decrease anxiety. | • Hypoxemia, hypercarbia, decreased cardiac output, and pain precipitate and intensify feelings of apprehension and anxiety.<br>• Positive feedback helps nurture confidence. |
| | | ∘ Encourage the patient and/or family to verbalize anxieties and concerns; encourage them to ask questions; listen attentively; provide a caring environment. | ∘ Helps to create a trusting relationship; reassures patient he/she is not alone. |
| | | ∘ Explain procedures and limitations to patient/family. Relate to nature of heart disease. | ∘ See Nursing Diagnosis #7, below. |

*(continued)*

**TABLE 44–11. CARE PLAN FOR THE PATIENT WITH HEART FAILURE *(Continued)***

| Nursing Diagnoses | Desired Patient Outcomes | Nursing Interventions | Rationales |
|---|---|---|---|
| ***Nursing Diagnosis #4 (cont.)*** | | | |
| | | ◦ Familiarize patient with ICU staff, routines, equipment. | ◦ Knowing what to expect will help to reduce anxiety. |
| | | ◦ Mobilize appropriate resources:<br>◦ Consult with social services, chaplaincy program, financial advisor, or other such services, as appropriate.<br>◦ Modify the environment to decrease anxiety; modify the policy regarding visitors; increase or decrease environmental stimuli as indicated; increase frequency of nurse/patient contacts. | ◦ Removal or modification of precipitating factors may reduce anxiety; social interaction helps modify feelings of depersonalization that accompany hospitalization (see Chaps. 3 and 5). |
| | | ◦ Involve patients in their own care within physical limitations. | ◦ Will decrease anxiety by re-establishing sense of control and purpose. |
| ***Nursing Diagnosis #5***<br>Infection, potential for, related to:<br>1. Decreased mobility.<br>2. Invasive lines.<br>3. Pulmonary congestion.<br>4. Valvular heart disease.<br>(See Table 49–7, Potential for Infection.) | Patient will:<br>1. Demonstrate absence or resolution of infection as indicated by:<br>• White blood cell count within normal limits.<br>• Normal body temperature (37°C, 98.6°F).<br>2. Demonstrate understanding of importance of antibiotic prophylaxis (as patient's condition warrants).<br>3. Remain without complications of infectious process (e.g., embolization associated with infective endocarditis). | • Identify patients at high risk of developing an infection: Elderly; rheumatic heart disease; prosthetic heart valves; valvular lesions; intravenous drug abuse; hypertrophic cardiomyopathy; multiple invasive lines; immunocompromised; chronic debilitating diseases. | • Patients with heart disease are at high risk due to alterations in endothelial integrity on cardiac valves secondary to surgical, congenital, or rheumatic causes. Early detection and treatment may improve prognosis. |
| | | • Maintain strict aseptic technique during insertion and changing of hemodynamic monitoring lines; strict adherence to handwashing protocols. | • Minimizes likelihood of airborne and contact organisms entering sterile field. |
| | | ◦ Maintain closed system; use sterile stopcocks with caps. | ◦ Stopcocks that are not maintained as a closed system contribute to 5%–10% of the infections associated with intravascular catheters. |
| | | ◦ Change pressure tubing and flush solutions every 48 hr or as per unit protocol.<br>◦ Change dressings and observe for signs of infection, as per unit protocol. | ◦ Has proven sufficient for minimizing incidence of line-related septicemia. |

| | |
|---|---|
| ◦ Record date of insertion of each line; arterial, CVP, and PA lines should be changed every 3–4 days, or as per unit protocol.<br>◦ Culture tips of catheters when removed, if indicated. | ◦ Irritation of vessel or endocardium predisposes to thrombophlebitis and infective endocarditis. |
| • Monitor for signs of infection.<br>◦ Monitor temperature every 4 hr; report elevation to physician.<br>◦ Monitor WBC count.<br>◦ Observe for tachycardia, chills, or diaphoresis. Keep patient warm and dry. | ◦ Fever increases basal metabolic rate and causes tachycardia and increase in cardiac output to meet tissue metabolic demands. This hyperdynamic response is likely to precipitate severe heart failure by markedly elevating myocardial oxygen demand and reducing the time for diastolic filling.<br>◦ Early detection of an inflammatory or infectious process encourages prompt intervention to minimize deleterious effects of the causative organism on the heart and other body processes. |
| • Administer antibiotics and antipyretics as prescribed and monitor response to therapy. | |
| • Turn every 2 hr while on bedrest. | • To maintain skin integrity and mobilize pulmonary secretions. |
| • Initiate measures to prevent atelectasis.<br>◦ Encourage hourly deep breathing while awake and during periods of immobility.<br>◦ Teach use of incentive spirometer if appropriate. | ◦ Maximizes alveolar inflation and minimizes atelectasis and hypoventilation. |
| ◦ Progress activity as tolerated.<br>◦ Note color, quantity, character of secretions (pulmonary). | ◦ Pulmonary edema results in frothy, blood-tinged sputum; pneumonia results in thick, purulent sputum. |
| ◦ Auscultate breath sounds every 4 hr and prn. | ◦ Assessment for atelectasis, increasing left heart failure, or pneumonia. |
| • Assess for potential source of infection:<br>◦ Urine: Hematuria, cloudy, flank pain.<br>◦ Sputum: Character, color, quantity.<br>◦ Monitor cultures and sensitivities. | ◦ Assists in assessing response to therapy. |
| • Assess for signs and symptoms of infective endocarditis:<br>◦ Change in murmur. | • Infective endocarditis can precipitate the development of heart failure.<br>◦ Murmurs are usually absent in patients with right-sided endocarditis, particularly with tricuspid valve involvement.<br>◦ Murmurs that develop with endocarditis are usually regurgitant; vegetative lesion (if large enough) can cause stenotic murmur.<br>◦ New or changing murmur may indicate erosive complications of valve. |

*(continued)*

**TABLE 44–11. CARE PLAN FOR THE PATIENT WITH HEART FAILURE *(Continued)***

| Nursing Diagnoses | Desired Patient Outcomes | Nursing Interventions | Rationales |
|---|---|---|---|
| *Nursing Diagnosis #5 (cont.)* | | | |
| | | ○ Fever. | ○ *Staphylococcus* is usually associated with acute infectious process and causes temperature elevations with high fever spikes and rigors; *Streptococcus* usually produces a subacute process with moderate temperature elevations. |
| | | ○ Hematuria. | ○ Result of renal emboli and infarction. |
| | | ○ Petechiae. | ○ One of the most frequent signs noted in neck, conjunctivae, clavicles, wrists, ankles, and mucous membranes. |
| | | ○ Osler's nodes. | ○ Painful, red subcutaneous nodules noted in the pads of the fingers or toes. |
| | | ○ Roth's spots. | ○ Retinal hemorrhages with white or pale center, located near optic disc. |
| | | ○ Janeway nodes. | ○ Non-tender hemorrhagic lesions 1–5 mm in diameter; occur on arms, legs, palms, and soles; intensify when extremity is elevated. |
| | | ○ Nailbed splinter hemorrhages. | ○ In distal one third of nail; thought to be result of an allergic vasculitis of the arterioles. |
| | | • Assess for complications of embolization: | |
| | | ○ Change in level of consciousness, visual disturbances, headache. | ○ CNS embolization from *left* heart endocarditis. |
| | | ○ SOB, chest pain, hemoptysis. | ○ Result of *right*-sided endocarditis causing pulmonary infarction. |
| | | ○ Hematuria, decreased urine output, increased BUN and creatinine. | ○ Embolization to renal vasculature. |
| | | ○ Dysrhythmias, pericardial friction rub, sudden hemodynamic compromise. | ○ Left heart endocarditis; result of erosive vegetations. Can cause VSD, fistulas, pericarditis, cardiac tamponade, or myocardial infarction. |
| | | ○ Left upper quadrant pain radiating to left shoulder. | ○ Spleen is most common site of embolic infarction in bacterial endocarditis. |
| | | • Instruct patient with valvular heart disease regarding importance of antibiotic prophylaxis. | • See Nursing Diagnosis #7, below. |

| | | | |
|---|---|---|---|
| ***Nursing Diagnosis #6*** Potential for activity intolerance, related to compromised cardiac reserve. | Patient will:<br>1. Maintain normal muscle tone.<br>2. Maintain highest level of activity that does not produce symptoms of myocardial dysfunction.<br>3. Identify end-points of activity tolerance. | • Perform assessment of activity and exercise tolerance. | • Initial assessment provides pertinent data that will guide individualized activity prescription from acute to rehabilitative phase. |
| | | ○ Age. | ○ Physical endurance decreases with age; older patients will tolerate less activity. |
| | | ○ Weight. | ○ Obesity increases myocardial burden. |
| | | ○ Gender. | ○ Females have more endurance; men can tolerate workload of higher intensity secondary to the increased ratio of muscle mass : total body weight. |
| | | ○ Cardiovascular disorder. | ○ Cardiovascular history may influence the attitude of the patient to activity (i.e., if angina or palpitations developed on exertion, this may influence the patient's attitude toward exercise). |
| | | ○ Previous activity and motivation. | ○ Identifies patients who may need encouragement to exercise. |
| | | • Initiate gradual activity progression in the critical care setting. | • Minimizes the deleterious effects of deconditioning, which include a decreased work capacity, tachycardia, orthostatic hypotension, venous thrombosis, and feelings of hopelessness and dependency. |
| | | ○ Encourage to participate in ADL (feed self, wash hands, shave, active ROM). | ○ Such activities improve circulation and help to prevent phlebitis or thromboembolism. |
| | | ○ Maintain bedrest with commode privileges during acute phase of heart failure. | ○ Physical activity redistributes blood from viscera and kidneys to the skeletal muscle and skin. Bedrest allows for a limited cardiac output and decreases myocardial oxygen demand. However, myocardial oxygen consumption is greater when a patient uses bedpan than during commode use. |
| | | ○ Prevent complications of immobility.<br>○ Assist with frequent position change.<br>○ Provide frequent back care and skin care. | ○ Maintenance of skin integrity and muscle tone. |
| | | ○ Encourage hourly deep breathing while awake. | ○ Minimizes development of atelectasis. |
| | | ○ Maintain in semi-Fowler's position. | ○ Reduces venous return to the heart; increases ability to expand lungs during deep breathing exercises. |

*(continued)*

**TABLE 44-11. CARE PLAN FOR THE PATIENT WITH HEART FAILURE (*Continued*)**

| Nursing Diagnoses | Desired Patient Outcomes | Nursing Interventions | Rationales |
|---|---|---|---|
| ***Nursing Diagnosis #6 (cont.)*** | | | |
| | | • Assess tolerance to activity progression by checking blood pressure, heart rate, and respiratory rate 1 minute and 4 minutes after the activity. Indicators of poor tolerance include dyspnea, syncope, angina, diaphoresis, cyanosis, fatigue, weakness, dysrhythmias; heart rate should return to baseline within 4 minutes. Heart rate should not exceed 20 beats/minute above resting heart rate and it should not exceed 110 beats/minute. | • Physical activity increases venous return to the heart, increases myocardial workload, and increases metabolic heat production, i.e., one fifth of cardiac output is shunted to skin in thermoregulation and the patient with impaired myocardial function cannot compensate for this with a tachycardia or increased contractile force; symptoms of pulmonary venous congestion and decreased cardiac output intensify. |
| | | ○ Monitor systolic blood pressure. | ○ Fall of 20 mmHg below resting level and failure of systolic blood pressure to increase above the resting level suggest poor exercise tolerance. |
| | | • Assess readiness to learn and instruct regarding indicators of activity intolerance, as noted above. | • Readiness to learn facilitates meaningful learning. |
| | | ○ Teach patient how to take own pulse. | |
| | | ○ Isometric exercises should be discouraged. | ○ Result in increased blood pressure and cardiac workload; do not improve cardiovascular conditioning. |
| | | ○ Encourage gradual resumption of aerobic activity when free of heart failure. | ○ Increases functional capacity and cardiovascular conditioning. |
| | | ○ Reemphasize to patient that activity will be progressed gradually and will be supervised during the initial stages; provide positive reinforcement when appropriate; gradually transfer supervision of tolerance from health care personnel to patient and family. | ○ Builds and reinforces self-confidence; helps minimize deleterious effects of psychophysiologic responses to stress (increased myocardial oxygen consumption). |
| ***Nursing Diagnosis #7***<br>Knowledge deficit, related to:<br>1. Underlying heart disease, treatment, and follow-up. | Patient will:<br>1. Describe underlying disease process and relationship to heart failure. | • Assess knowledge of heart failure, underlying disease process, and expectations of disease progression. | • Readiness to learn varies because of differences in general educational background, intellectual ability, and motivation. Assessment establishes baseline data from which to build or determines need to alter misconceptions. |

| | | |
|---|---|---|
| 2. Identify own risk factors or precipitating conditions that require modification.<br>3. Identify importance of follow-up care and symptoms requiring medical intervention.<br>4. Describe the importance of medications, diet, and activity to the overall treatment plan.<br>5. Identify signs and symptoms of activity intolerance.<br>6. Identify indications for endocarditis prophylaxis (if patient is in high-risk profile.) | • Encourage verbalization of patient/family concerns and their learning needs. | • Fosters establishment of open, trusting relationship. Learning is enhanced when patient participates in goal setting. Heart failure affects patient and his/her lifestyle and impacts on the entire family to varying degrees. |
| | • Assess readiness to learn. | • Readiness facilitates more effective learning. |
| | • Implement teaching plan, which should include:<br>○ Explanation of normal heart function, heart failure, and underlying disease process.<br>○ Explanation of signs and symptoms and appropriate action regarding their development.<br>○ Explanation of risk factors and factors that will aggravate the symptoms of heart failure and methods to modify these factors.<br>○ Explanation of medication regimen (including name, dosage, frequency, action, and side effects).<br>○ Explanation of diet modification if indicated.<br>○ Activity prescription and signs and symptoms of activity intolerance. | • Patient and family have a right to receive information about the disease, treatment, and prognosis; understanding enhances compliance; knowledge allays anxieties and the adverse effects associated with psychophysiologic stress. |
| | • Assist patient/family in identifying family strengths and resources. | • Engenders self-confidence. |
| | • Initiate referral to appropriate resources if indicated (social services; community resources). | • It is reassuring to have support services available. |

operative cardiac surgery patients with severe heart failure. The LVAD functions as a reservoir. A pneumatically driven pump diverts blood from the left ventricle and pumps it into the ascending thoracic aorta, almost totally relieving the left ventricle of its workload. The beneficial physiologic effects associated with LVAD include a reduction in myocardial wall tension and myocardial oxygen consumption as a result of a reduction in preload; a reduced afterload is accomplished by the mechanical pumping of blood into the aorta, allowing a period of rest for the failing heart.[28] A detailed discussion of mechanical support devices can be found in Chapter 42.

## NURSING CARE

### Therapeutic Goals

The therapeutic goals listed below provide the framework on which the critical care nurse bases patient care. Implementation of the nursing process with nursing diagnoses, desired patient outcomes, interventions, and their rationales is presented in the Care Plan in Table 44–11.

1. Perform a thorough and ongoing assessment.
2. Reduce cardiac workload.
3. Provide hemodynamic support to maintain cardiac output and tissue perfusion.
4. Provide ventilatory support and oxygenation to relieve hypoxia associated with pulmonary venous congestion.
5. Maintain fluid and electrolyte balance.
6. Identify and treat conditions that aggravate the development of heart failure.
7. Prevent infection.
8. Provide emotional and psychologic support to patient and family.
9. Initiate patient/family health education pertinent to heart failure, clinical manifestations, and treatment regimens.

## REFERENCES


1. Michaelson, CR: Pathophysiology of heart failure: A conceptual framework for understanding clinical indicators and therapeutic modalities. In Michaelson, CR (ed): Congestive Heart Failure. CV Mosby, St Louis, 1983, p 45.
2. Dossey, BM: The person with heart failure. In Guzzetta, CE and Dossey, BM: Cardiovascular Nursing, Body Mind Tapestry. CV Mosby, St Louis, 1984, p 517.
3. Donat, WE and Weiner, BH: Syndromes of left ventricular failure. In Rippe, JM, Irwin, RS, Alpert, JS, and Dalen, JE (eds): Intensive Care Medicine. Little, Brown & Co, Boston, 1985, p 326.
4. Michaelson, CR: Pathophysiology of heart failure: A conceptual framework for understanding clinical indicators and therapeutic modalities. In Michaelson, CR (ed): Congestive Heart Failure. CV Mosby, St Louis, 1983.
5. Michaelson, CR: Pathophysiology of heart failure: A conceptual framework for understanding clinical indicators and therapeutic modalities. In Michaelson, CR (ed): Congestive Heart Failure. CV Mosby, St Louis, 1983, p 64.
6. Cohn, PF: Clinical Cardiovascular Physiology. WB Saunders, Philadelphia, 1985, p 204.
7. Cohn, PF: Clinical Cardiovascular Physiology. WB Saunders, Philadelphia, 1986, p 251.
8. Cavallo, GAO: The person with valvular heart disease. In Guzzetta, CE and Dossey, BM: Cardiovascular Nursing, Body Mind Tapestry. CV Mosby, St Louis, 1984, p 631.
9. Walls, JJ, Lababidi, Z, Curtis, JJ, and Silver, D: Assessment of percutaneous balloon pulmonary and aortic valvuloplasty. J Thorac Cardiovasc Surg 88:352–356, 1984.
10. Pura, LS and Sam, CS: Underlying causes and precipitating factors in heart failure. In Michaelson, CR (ed): Congestive Heart Failure. CV Mosby, St Louis, 1983, p 93.
11. Cavallo, GAO: The person with valvular heart disease. In Guzzetta, CE and Dossey, BM: Cardiovascular Nursing, Body Mind Tapestry. CV Mosby, St Louis, 1984, p 623.
12. Cavallo, GAO: The person with valvular heart disease. In Guzzetta, CE and Dossey, BM: Cardiovascular Nursing, Body Mind Tapestry. CV Mosby, St Louis, 1984, p 624.
13. Cavallo, GAO: The person with valvular heart disease. In Guzzetta, CE and Dossey, BM: Cardiovascular Nursing, Body Mind Tapestry. CV Mosby, St Louis, 1984, p 626.
14. Torp, A: Incidence of congestive cardiomyopathies. Postgrad Med J 54:435, 1978.
15. Wingate, S: Dilated Cardiomyopathy, Part I. Focus 11(4):49–56, 1984.
16. Dossey, BM: The person with cardiomyopathy or myocarditis. In Guzzetta, CE and Dossey, BM: Cardiovascular Nursing, Body Mind Tapestry. CV Mosby, St Louis, 1984, p 739.
17. Shah, PM: Cardiomyopathies. In Shine, KI: Cardiology. John Wiley & Sons, New York, 1983, p 85.
18. Shah, PM: Cardiomyopathies. In Shine KI: Cardiology. John Wiley & Sons, New York, 1983, p 88.
19. Shah, PM: Cardiomyopathies. In Shine, KI: Cardiology. John Wiley & Sons, New York, 1983, p 88.
20. Dossey, BM: The person with cardiomyopathy or myocarditis. In Guzzetta, CE and Dossey, BM: Cardiovascular Nursing, Body Mind Tapestry. CV Mosby, St Louis, 1984, p 739.
21. Resnekov, L: Cardiogenic Shock. Chest 83:893, 1983.
22. Niles, NA and Wills, RE: Heart failure. In Underhill, SL, Woods, SL, Sivarajan, ES, and Halpenny, CJ: Cardiovascular Nursing, ed 2. JB Lippincott, Philadelphia, 1988, p 387.
23. Dossey, BM: The person in cardiogenic shock. In Guzzetta, CE and Dossey, BM: Cardiovascular Nursing, Body Mind Tapestry. CV Mosby, St Louis, 1984, p 553.
24. Goldberger, E: Textbook of Clinical Cardiology. CV Mosby, St Louis, 1981.
25. Rippe, JM and Howe, JP: Acute mitral regurgitation. In Rippe, JM, Irwin, RS, Alpert, JS, and Dalen, JG (eds): Intensive Care Medicine. Little, Brown & Co, Boston, 1985, p 261.
26. Taormina Paplanus, LM, Strebel, CA, and Michaelson, CR: Drug therapy for congestive heart failure. CV Mosby, St Louis, 1983, pp 272, 274, 285, 290.
27. Gawlinski, A: Diet therapy in heart failure. In Michaelson, CR (ed): Congestive Heart Failure. CV Mosby, St Louis, 1983, pp 354–355.
28. Brannon, PHB and Towner, SB: Ventricular failure: New therapy, using the mechanical assist device. Crit Care Nurse 6(2):76, 1986.
29. Chatterjee, K: Vasodilator therapy for heart failure. In Cohn, JN (ed): Drug Treatment of Heart Failure. Yorke Medical Books, New York, 1983, p 157.

CHAPTER 45

# Nursing Management of the Cardiac Surgical Patient

*Sheila M. Keller*

## CHAPTER OUTLINE



## LEARNING OBJECTIVES

**At the end of this chapter, you should be able to:**

1. Identify common causes of valvular defects in the adult, approaches to surgical intervention, and potential complications.
2. Describe how nursing care in valve replacement surgery differs from that in coronary artery bypass (CABG) surgery.
3. Describe nursing care considerations unique to the patient with an artificial heart, and those unique to the patient with a heart transplant.
4. List indications and contraindications for coronary artery bypass surgery.
5. Examine the significance of anxiety in terms of postoperative complications.
6. Identify major aspects of preoperative teaching for the cardiac surgical patient.
7. Identify major aspects of the postoperative assessment in the immediate postoperative period and implications for nursing care.
8. Prioritize postoperative nursing care for the cardiac surgical patient.
9. Delineate the nursing process in the care of the cardiac surgical patient, including:
   Assessment
   Nursing Diagnoses
   Planning: Desired patient outcomes.
   Nursing interventions.

Cardiac surgery has long been associated with the repair of congenital defects, largely in infants and children. More recently, surgical procedures have been developed to repair *acquired* defects, including repair of ventricular-septal defects, ventricular aneurysmectomy, pericardiectomy, valvular repair or replacement, coronary artery bypass, implementation of the artificial heart, and heart transplantation.

Along with advances in cardiac surgical techniques have come the development and expansion of cardiovascular nursing. Nursing's role has become an integral component in the care of the cardiac surgical patient. Preoperative and postoperative teaching, so vital to the successful outcome of cardiac surgery, is largely the responsibility of the patient's nurse.

In this chapter, specific cardiac surgical procedures are briefly examined, with emphasis placed on coronary artery bypass surgery. The discussion of nursing care of the patient having coronary artery bypass surgery in particular may serve as a template for the care of the cardiac surgical patient in general. Nursing care plans concerned with the preoperative and postoperative care of the cardiac surgical patient are included.

Protocols and procedures regarding care of the cardiac surgical patient differ among hospitals nationwide. Therefore, with this in mind, only generalizations regarding specific nursing care are presented. Since the discussion that follows is limited to the adult patient, readers interested in the care of the pediatric cardiac surgical patient are referred to an appropriate pediatric text.

## VALVULAR DEFECTS

Over the past 2 decades significant advances have been made in the treatment of valvular defects. Common causes of valvular dysfunction include rheumatic fever and endocarditis. Additional causes include cardiomyopathies, Marfan's syndrome, myomatous degeneration of the mitral valve, myocardial infarction, congenital defects, and trauma. Pathophysiology and medical management of valvular defects are presented in Chapter 44. Valvular disorders frequently treated with surgical intervention include aortic stenosis, aortic regurgitation, mitral stenosis, and mitral regurgitation.

Patients with valvular dysfunction are treated initially with a medical regimen of inotropic agents (e.g., digitalis) and diuretics (e.g., furosemide). Antidysrhythmics and anticoagulants may be prescribed for patients with atrial dysrhythmias, particularly atrial fibrillation. Valvular surgery is performed when medical management is no longer effective in controlling heart failure or in preventing the formation of thromboemboli.

### Approaches to Valvular Surgery

Valvular surgery may involve closed or open heart surgery. Specific procedures involving closed heart surgery include annuloplasty and commissurotomy. Annuloplasty involves the trimming of the valve ring with insertion of a Carpentier ring into the annulus; commissurotomy involves the trimming of the valve leaflets to increase the size of the valve opening. Although these techniques are safer than open heart procedures, usually their results do not remain functional and the patient eventually requires valve replacement.

Valve replacement, which involves the surgical removal of a diseased valve and insertion of a prosthetic valve, requires open heart surgery. The choice of the prosthesis is determined by the design of the valve, its durability, potential for thromboemboli, and hemodynamic properties. In addition, the patient's age, size, medical history, activity level, and tolerance to anticoagulant therapy are of prime importance in the decision-making process.

### Types of Prosthetic Heart Valves

There are 2 types of prosthetic heart valves: mechanical and biologic.[1] Mechanical valves, or lateral flow valves, are highly durable and highly responsive to changes in chamber pressure. Biologic valves are less durable than mechanical valves but have a lower incidence of thromboemboli. Table 45–1 compares the various types of valves in current use.

### Complications of Valve Replacement

General complications of valve replacement include thromboembolism, prosthetic malfunction, paravalvular leaks, hemolysis, hemolytic anemia, and prosthetic valve endocarditis. The mortality rate of prosthetic valve replacement is 5% to 10% depending on the patient's overall condition.

### Nursing Care in Valve Replacement Surgery

The preoperative and postoperative care of the patient with a valve replacement is similar to that for the patient with coronary artery bypass graft (CABG) surgery (see below), with 2 major differences.[2] First, the patient having valve replacement surgery is placed on anticoagulant therapy prophylactically. Postoperatively, the patient's prothrombin time and partial thromboplastin time are closely monitored. Vigilant nursing care is essential in assessing for signs of bleeding or increased clotting time as reflected by the appearance of petechiae, ecchymosis, oozing at puncture sites, bleeding gums, increased chest tube drainage, or frank bleeding.

Second, as is the case with coronary artery bypass surgery, the patient with a valve replacement is placed on intravenous antibiotics, but the course of antibiotic therapy is usually for a longer period of time. It is essential that the patient receive the appropriate dosages at the appropriate intervals, and for the prescribed duration, to ensure that optimal therapeutic serum levels of antibiotics are maintained.

Discharge planning specific for the patient with a valve replacement begins early on in the recupera-

TABLE 45–1
## Artificial Valves: A Comparison

| Type | Name | Special Information | Advantages | Disadvantages |
|---|---|---|---|---|
| ***Mechanical Valves*** | | | | |
| Caged-Ball Valve 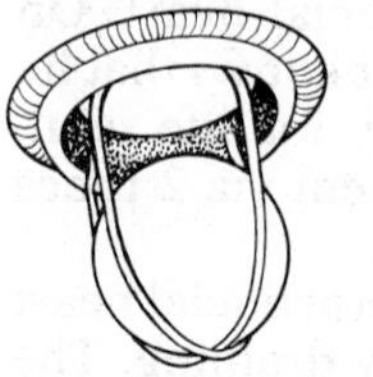 | Starr-Edwards | Blood flows through the cage and around the ball/poppet | Durable<br>Valve malfunction infrequent | High incidence of thromboemboli<br>Requires long-term anticoagulant therapy<br>Noisy |
| Tilting Disk Valve 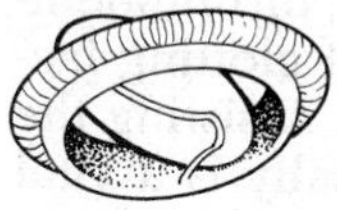 | Bjork-Shiley<br><br>Lillehei-Kaster | Disk tilts open 60 degrees to allow blood to flow through<br>Disk tilts open 80 degrees to allow blood to flow through | Durable<br>Offers less obstruction to blood flow | High incidence of thromboemboli<br>Requires long-term anticoagulation<br>Valve malfunction more frequent than with Starr-Edwards valve |
| Bileaflet 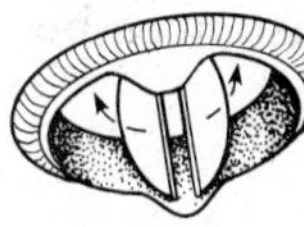 | St. Jude | Disk or leaflets open perpendicularly | Durable<br>Offers minimum obstruction to blood flow<br>Used in patients with small orifices, especially children | Thromboembolism<br>Requires long-term anticoagulation |
| ***Biologic Valves*** | | | | |
| Porcine Xenograft 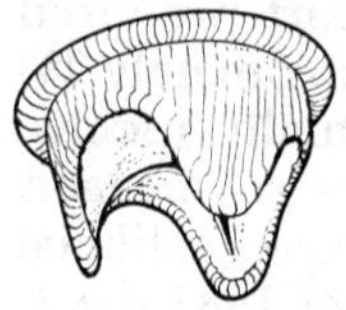 | Hancock Carpentier-Edwards | Aortic valve of a pig, harvested intact<br>Preserved with glutaraldehyde* and mounted on a sew ring | Blood flows almost unobstructed through a central opening<br>Biocompatible | Prone to tissue degeneration and calcification, which causes the orifice to decrease in size and therefore leads to an increased gradient and obstruction to flow<br>Requires short-term anticoagulation therapy† |
| Pericardial Xenograft 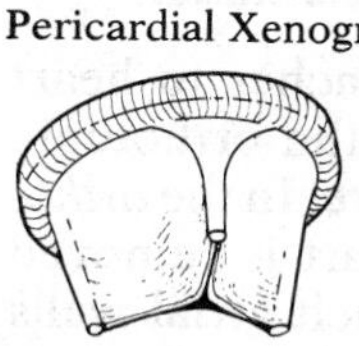 | Ionescu-Shiley | Calf pericardium preserved in glutaraldehyde and mounted on a Dacron frame | Blood flow is unobstructed<br>Biocompatible<br>Non-thrombogenic | Same as above<br>Space restricted |
| Homograft 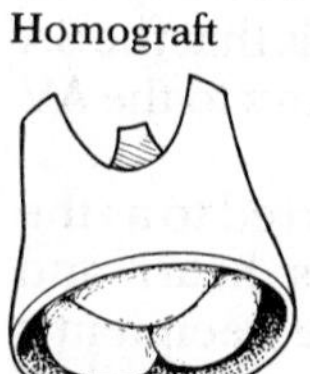 | | Aortic valve of a human cadaver | Excellent hemodynamics<br>Non-thrombogenic<br>No need for anticoagulation therapy | Not used for mitral valve or tricuspid valve replacement<br>Not always readily available |

Adapted from Kretten, CK and Baas, L: Valvular heart disease: Surgery and post-op care. RN, December 1987.
*Glutaraldehyde is a preservative used to increase the strength of the collagen tissue, thereby decreasing the degeneration process.
†Biologic valves generally require a short course of anticoagulation therapy, approximately 3 months after which it is discontinued unless the patient has atrial fibrillation or atrial enlargement.

tive period. It entails patient and family education regarding the signs and symptoms of valve dysfunction, which include sudden chest pain, fatigue, and dyspnea, among others. The patient and family must understand the immediate need to seek health care when such symptoms appear. The patient must also know the importance of informing health care providers (especially dentists) of the valve replacement because of the higher risk of infective endocarditis. Prior to any invasive procedure a course of prophylactic antibiotic therapy is essential.

Depending on the type of valvular prosthesis and the presence of atrial fibrillation (or the risk of its occurrence), the patient may be placed on long-term anticoagulant therapy. It is essential for the patient and family to be taught the signs and symptoms of overcoagulation. Because bleeding is the most significant side effect of anticoagulant therapy, the patient and family should be alerted as to signs of bleeding, which include ecchymoses, hematuria, uterine bleeding melena, hematoma, gingival bleeding, hemoptysis, and hematemesis. The importance of medical follow-up must be emphasized.

It is important for the patient and family to understand that initially on discharge there may be some physical restrictions (e.g., no lifting of heavy objects or driving a car). Such restrictions are usually temporary to allow for the sternal bone and musculature to heal properly. Within a few weeks following discharge the patient can usually resume most daily activities. The patient should be encouraged to participate in a controlled exercise program.

## ARTIFICIAL HEART AND HEART TRANSPLANT

The insertion of an artificial heart and heart transplantation are usually last resorts for the failing irreparable heart. These approaches to therapy have provoked many ethical questions and entail high risks, many complications, and a course of complex long-term care. The cost of hospitalization, surgery, and postsurgical rehabilitation can be prohibitive.

### Artificial Heart

A number of artificial hearts have been developed over the last decade, probably the most famous of which is the Jarvik 7 artificial heart. In general, the artificial heart is made up of mechanical ventricles that are sewn to the patient's pulmonary artery, aorta, and atria, and placed within the mediastinum. The mechanical heart is powered by compressed air, which activates the internal valves and diaphragms thereby simulating the pumping action of the heart.

In addition to the high economic costs entailed with insertion of an artificial heart are the immense emotional costs to the patient and family. The patient must decide not only to have surgery to live but must also accept the drastic change in lifestyle intrinsic to this type of therapy. Preoperatively, it is explained that the patient's ventricles will be removed and replaced with the artificial heart. On awakening from surgery, the patient knows that he or she is dependent on machinery for life, connected to 2 large pieces of equipment via 2 tubes emerging from the abdomen.

Nursing care of the patient with an artificial heart is highly technical and emotionally draining. The nurse must constantly monitor the patient for complications such as mechanical failure, thromboemboli, infection, seizures, depletion of clotting factors, and pneumonia, among others. Assisting the patient and family to cope emotionally is a vital component of nursing care. Because of the constant life-threatening atmosphere, the patient, family, and nurses involved in the patient's care tend to develop very close bonds, in some instances becoming like family.

### Heart Transplantation

Heart transplantation involves the replacement of the patient's heart with a donor heart procured from a brain-dead patient. Only approximately 2% of those awaiting donor hearts actually receive them, largely because the supply is so meager. Some patients awaiting donors have artificial hearts implanted in the interim. As of 1983 the 1-year survival rate for the heart transplant patient was 70%–80%. Of these patients, approximately 90% returned to normal activity levels. The 5-year survival rate was 50%.

#### *Surgical Approaches to Heart Transplantation*

There are mainly 2 surgical approaches to heart transplantation and these include the orthotopic procedure and the parallel procedure. In the *orthotopic* procedure the recipient's heart is removed except for the posterior right and left atrial walls and their venous connections. The donor heart is trimmed to match the recipient's heart and sewn in place. The advantage of this procedure is that the SA node and most of the internodal pathways to the AV node are preserved.

In the *parallel* procedure (often referred to as the "piggy-back" procedure) the donor's heart and major blood vessels are sewn to the recipient's heart and major vessels so that there are literally 2 hearts within the chest. The major advantage of this approach is that there is a lower incidence of pulmonary hypertension and rejection. It has been reported in some cases that the recipient's own heart has recovered after being allowed to rest.[3]

### Criteria for Heart Transplantation Candidacy

The potential heart transplant candidate must meet certain criteria to be considered for heart transplant surgery. Although variations in these criteria may exist from center to center, these criteria usually include those listed in Table 45-2. Fulfillment of these criteria helps to ensure a more successful outcome following transplantation. Medical evaluation prior to acceptance for heart transplantation includes a thorough health history, physical examination, and routine laboratory and roentgenographic studies. A complete workup is initiated to determine the status of pulmonary, renal, and hepatic function. Evaluation of pulmonary hemodynamics is especially critical. If pulmonary vascular resistance exceeds 600 dynes/cm$^{-5}$, a healthy donor heart may be unable to significantly increase its workload to overcome such high pulmonary vascular resistance, thereby predisposing to right ventricular failure early after surgery.

Assessment of cardiovascular function entails cardiac catheterization to evaluate right and left heart hemodynamics. A thorough evaluation of the patient's immunologic status, including compatibility between the donor heart and recipient, is vital. The presence of donor-specific cytotoxic antibodies is a distinct contraindication for transplant surgery. (The reader is referred to Chaps. 27 and 57 for further details related to transplant immunology.)

The presence of infection is also a contraindication to heart transplantation. The necessary immunosuppressant therapy post-surgery greatly increases the likelihood of life-threatening infection during the postoperative phase.

Nursing evaluation of the transplant candidate involves an assessment of the patient's functional health patterns. It is important to establish how the patient perceives health and to identify those activities performed by the patient and family that reflect the level of health care desired. An assessment of roles and relationships may assist in determining psychological stability and available family support systems. Identifying how the patient and family cope with stress may be of assistance during the preoperative and postoperative periods. Reinforcement of formerly effective coping mechanisms may be vital to the patient's recuperation during the postoperative and rehabilitative phases of care.

TABLE 45-2
**Criteria for Heart Transplantation Candidacy***

1. End-stage cardiac disease irreparable or irremedial to medical or other cardiac surgery.
2. Less than 55 years of age.
3. No evidence of current pulmonary infarction.
4. Pulmonary hypertension less than 600 dyne/cm$^{-5}$.
5. No active infection.
6. No insulin-dependent diabetes mellitus.
7. No multisystem disease (including severe kidney or hepatic dysfunction, and pulmonary failure).
8. No neoplastic disease.
9. Absence of donor-specific cytotoxic antibodies.
10. No major psychosocial dysfunction (history of alcohol or drug abuse, depression or psychosis).
11. Commitment and compliance on the part of the patient and family.

*Criteria may vary somewhat from institution to institution.

### Donor Procurement

Heart donors are individuals who have sustained an irreversible brain injury usually as a result of a traumatic event. Ideally, the heart donor is less than 30 years of age with a heart that is healthy and largely free of advanced atherosclerotic disease.

Upon procurement of brain death (see Table 57-2 for brain death criteria) and the family's desire for organ donation, a complete assessment of cardiac function is initiated. Cardiac catheterization and angiography studies are performed as indicated, and usually in all donors over 35 years of age. If a compatible recipient is found for the donor's heart, transplantation surgery is scheduled as soon as possible. The hemostatic instability of the brain-dead individual makes timely matching of the donor heart to a compatible heart transplant recipient imperative.

Nursing care of the heart transplant patient is similar in many respects to that of the coronary artery bypass surgical patient (see below). Unique to the postoperative care of heart transplant patients is that they require immunosuppressant therapy and are at extreme risk of infectious complications. In some institutions the heart transplant patient is provided a room with strict isolation. Vigilant nursing care is essential to prevent infection or to recognize its presence early on so that timely and aggressive therapy can be instituted.

Once the heart transplant patients are stabilized hemodynamically they are transferred to a stepdown unit. Barring complications, a heart transplant patient can be discharged as early as 3 weeks after surgery. The patient is monitored closely for the first several weeks, and then monthly for at least 3-6 months. Post-transplantation, right ventricular endomyocardial biopsies are performed at intervals determined by the recipient's overall condition, as a means of monitoring for and diagnosing organ rejection. A complete cardiac assessment, including a right and left cardiac catheterization, is done on a yearly basis.[4]

Discharge teaching includes the conventional discharge teaching of the coronary artery bypass patient (see below), as well as patient and family education about preventing infection and signs and symptoms to look for which may indicate the presence of infection or rejection. Patient education regarding immunosuppressant therapy and other medications, including dosage, desired actions, side effects, and precautions, is essential. (For additional factors of significance to the nursing care of the transplant surgical patient, the reader is referred to Chap. 27.)

## CORONARY ARTERY BYPASS SURGERY

The most common type of cardiac surgery over the past 2 decades has been the coronary artery bypass graft (CABG). In this procedure a blood vessel (usually the saphenous vein or internal mammary artery) is anastomosed to a coronary artery distal to the point of occlusion and to the ascending aorta (if the saphenous vein is used), thereby bypassing the area of vessel obstruction and reestablishing effective coronary artery perfusion.

The purpose of the CABG is to relieve angina and preserve myocardial function. Bypass surgery can also be used to prevent myocardial infarction in patients in whom angioplasty or fibrinolytic therapy is contraindicated or has failed.

What type of patient should have a CABG and what lesions should be grafted remain controversial. The consensus seems to be that life expectancy is increased when CABG is performed on patients with left main coronary artery disease or severe triple-vessel disease. The obstruction should be greater than 70% of the diameter of the artery with good distal runoff. Surgery should not be performed on only 1 vessel unless it is the left main coronary artery or possibly a high-grade proximal left anterior descending coronary artery obstruction[5] (see Fig. 37–8).

The mortality rate for the CABG is 1%–2% with 90% of the post-CABG patients demonstrating an improvement in cardiac function and 60% of the patients demonstrating elimination of anginal episodes.

A CABG is contraindicated in patients with bleeding disorders or acute cerebrovascular accident (CVA). Patients with cardiomegaly, severe congestive heart failure, recent myocardial infarction, high left ventricular end-diastolic pressure, or inadequate ejection fractions are at higher risk. More specifically, patients with an ejection fraction of 30%–35% are at poor risk; those with ejection fractions of 20%–25% are inoperable.

### Preoperative Anxiety: Clinical Significance

A patient generally waits 1–6 weeks for surgery to be scheduled and/or performed. Normally there is some degree of preoperative anxiety associated with the psychologic adjustment to, and/or acceptance of, the necessity for the procedure. Depression, a low self-esteem, and withdrawal are not uncommon in patients about to have heart surgery. As the waiting increases, so does the intensity of the adjustment difficulties. Frequently, the patient must draw on inner strengths and coping mechanisms that have proved reliable in the past. A thorough assessment of the patient's functional health patterns may assist the patient and family to identify their strengths and to cope more effectively.

Prior to surgery, some patients appear to cope best by seeking information. Members of the health team become highly supportive and helpful in this regard. Individuals who have had similar surgery can be helpful, especially if surgery has been effective for them.

Other patients become more anxious if they perceive that they are being bombarded with information regarding the details of the upcoming surgery. These patients may prefer not to know what to expect or what is expected of them. They may experience more adjustment difficulties, which in turn may complicate the postoperative phase of care.

Excessive preoperative anxiety can have a negative influence on the patient's postoperative recovery. Anxiety stimulates the sympathetic nervous system, causing an increase in circulating catecholamines (norepinephrine and epinephrine), which in turn increase heart rate and therefore the workload of the heart just at a time when it needs to rest.

There is also a direct relationship between the amount of anxiety and the occurrence of post-cardiotomy delirium (PCD). The greater the patient's preoperative anxiety, the greater the chance of the patient becoming disoriented to time and place and developing sensory distortions or hallucinations postoperatively. These symptoms are usually manifested during the immediate postoperative period, lasting 2–3 days.

### Preoperative Teaching

The preoperative teaching of the cardiac surgical patient should be individualized to the patient's specific needs. Sadler[6] identifies 4 areas of preoperative teaching: (1) teaching the patient about the normal function of the heart; (2) providing a description of the disease process and risk factors that have necessitated surgery; (3) providing a description of the surgery and the preoperative physical preparation; and (4) preparing the patient and family for the postoperative course.

Teaching the patient about the normal function of the heart should include the specific areas of the heart that are to be repaired. In the case of a CAGB, this includes how the heart is nourished by the coronary arteries; in patients having valve replacement surgery, it includes the function of the heart valves.

A description of the disease process that has necessitated the surgery should include the risk factors associated with heart disease. Included among these are hypertension, smoking, high serum cholesterol and triglyceride levels, obesity, stress, and diabetes mellitus. (The reader is referred to Chap. 43 for an indepth discussion of risk factors in coronary artery disease.)

An overall description of the surgery to be performed should be made simple and easy for patient and family members to understand. Individualization is determined by the patient's outlook on surgery and readiness to learn. Since cardiac surgery (i.e., CABG) is *not* a *cure*, it is imperative that patient and family learn as much as possible so that they may adjust lifestyles to minimize the underlying pathophysiologic process. Discharge teaching and planning begin on admission.

Preparation of the patient and family for surgery includes attention to several factors. The role of each member of the cardiac surgical team should be described, and the patient should understand that consultants from the cardiology and anesthesia departments will be visiting preoperatively. These physicians are responsible for evaluating the patient's status to ensure a stable preoperative condition. The patient is instructed that informed consents must be obtained for the operative procedure, transfusions, and injections.

Physical preparation of the patient for surgery involves skin preparation. The patient should understand that shaving the skin helps to remove the bacteria that tend to cling to the hair and thereby helps decrease the risk of infection. Showering with povidone-iodine (Betadine) or other special soap further decreases the number of organisms on the skin, thereby decreasing the risk of infection.

The patient is instructed regarding NPO status preoperatively. No eating or drinking is permitted after midnight on the day of surgery to ensure that the stomach will be empty prior to surgery. The night before surgery the patient may receive a laxative and/or enema to empty the lower bowel to avoid a bowel movement early in the postoperative phase. The patient must also understand that on the day of surgery, dentures (unless the anesthesiologist requests that they be left in place), prostheses, and nailpolish should be removed, and all the patient's effects should be given to the family to take home.

The patient should understand that pre-anesthesia medications will be prescribed. These usually include a sleeping medication to be given the evening before surgery to assist the patient in attaining a good night's sleep. Medications are also given immediately prior to the move to the operating room to help relax the patient and to minimize oropharyngeal secretions. Nasal oxygen may also be prescribed to enhance the effects of preoperative medications.

As part of the preoperative teaching the ICU routine should be described, including average length of stay, monitoring equipment, and intensive nursing care. Family members should be made aware as to visiting hours and number of visitors, and told the telephone extension to call regarding the patient's condition.

Specific instructions should be provided regarding IV therapy, including the need for an arterial line to be used to monitor blood pressure and to provide an easy access for blood sampling.

The patient's respiratory status should be discussed in detail so that the patient may know what to expect in terms of respiratory care and, in turn, what is expected of him/her in maintaining optimal respiratory function. The patient and family should know that an endotracheal tube will be inserted in the operating room after the patient is asleep; this provides a patent airway through which the patient will be assisted with breathing while under anesthesia and serves as a conduit through which accumulated secretions can be removed via suctioning. The patient should understand that speaking is not possible while the endotracheal tube is in place. A system of communication to be used while the patient is intubated should be established prior to surgery.

Extubation occurs when the patient is able to breathe without assistance. A sore throat may be experienced post-extubation. Coughing and deep breathing exercises and use of incentive spirometry are essential postoperative activities requiring patient participation. Essentials of respiratory physiotherapy including pre- and postoperative examination and treatment are included in Table 45–3.

Other important aspects included in preoperative teaching of the cardiac surgical patient include details regarding incisional lines. A mid-sternal incision is made for heart surgery. Patients having CABG surgery wherein the superficial saphenous veins are used as the grafts will also have an incisional line along the inner aspect of one or both legs. Ace bandages are usually applied for bypass patients, whereas full leg length antiembolic stockings are applied in patients having valve replacement surgery.

Patients should be instructed regarding chest tubes and their function in draining blood and fluid that has accumulated during and after surgery. Chest tubes are attached to underwater-seal drainage (see Table 36–3), with 20–40 $cmH_2O$ suction. An indwelling urinary catheter is placed in the operating room and is left in place during the early postoperative period to assist in monitoring renal function and hydration status. Hourly urine outputs are closely monitored. Infrequently, a perioperative hypotensive episode may precipitate prerenal failure.

A temporary cardiac pacemaker is utilized in patients having valve replacement surgery and in certain bypass surgical patients. Pacing wires are inserted at the conclusion of the operation and removed 1 or 2 days prior to discharge. Edema of

TABLE 45–3
**Respiratory Physiotherapy: Preoperative and Postoperative Phases***

The overall goal of instruction in techniques of respiratory physiotherapy is to assist the patient to utilize these techniques post-surgery to facilitate alveolar ventilation and secretion removal, prevent complications, and enhance postoperative recovery. Such instruction involves the preoperative phase and the postoperative phase.

**Preoperative Phase**

***Preoperative Examination***

1. Evaluate the patient's breathing pattern. Are the respirations short or long? Is there shortness of breath or hyperventilation?
2. Perform auscultation. Listen for abnormal breath sounds and signs of pulmonary congestion.
3. Observe the shape of the patient's chest. Look for abnormalities such as scoliosis, kyphosis, funnel chest, and barrel chest. They can frequently be the cause or the result of abnormal breathing patterns and pulmonary dysfunction.

***Preoperative Treatment***

Primary goal is to get the patient in optimum pulmonary condition before surgery. This can be achieved by patient education in the following methods:

1. Instruct the patient in deep breathing exercises to promote lung aeration.
2. Instruct the patient in cough techniques to help remove unwanted secretions.
3. Remove secretions through postural drainage, cupping, and percussion, if indicated.
4. Instruct the patient in ROM exercises to maintain joint mobility and promote circulation.
5. Instruct the patient in postoperative treatment.

Deep breathing exercises are most important. Patients should inhale through the nose, if feasible, and expand the diaphragm and lower parts of the chest. They should exhale through the mouth. The expiratory phase should take twice as long as the inspiratory phase. In this way adequate alveolar ventilation can be achieved. Instruct patient to perform this frequently. Set up a disciplined time frame, such as 15 breaths at a time, every 30 minutes. Have the patient place his or her hands over the diaphragm and lower chest area. This will provide tactile stimuli. The patient will push against the hands on inspiration and inflate the chest cavity, and then relax on expiration. In conjunction with deep breathing exercises, teach use of incentive spirometry and encourage its use on an hourly basis (see Table 32–2).

Coughing ability is essential. The vibrations of a cough will expel secretions. Encourage the patient to cough strongly with a double cough. It should emanate from the chest, not the throat. Have the patient cough in a forward flexed position, preferably sitting at the edge of the bed. Have the patient use a towel or pillow to give counterforce and to support the chest, particularly over the incisional area.

Postural drainage, cupping, and percussion are only performed if indicated. The patient's overall pulmonary status will indicate if these methods are necessary.

Encourage the patient to move and, if ambulatory, to walk. Instruct in basic ROM exercises for the arms and legs.

Discuss postoperative details with the patient. Prepare the patient for what to expect after surgery. Post-cardiac surgery patients are returned to the recovery room and/or intensive care units. They will awaken from surgery with a multitude of apparatuses attached to them, which may be frightening. Inform patients that postoperative pulmonary care will begin immediately upon awakening from anesthesia.

**Postoperative Phase**

The objectives of postoperative treatment are essentially the same as for the preoperative state, namely, to maintain effective alveolar ventilation and facilitate secretion clearance.

Treatment should begin as soon as possible post-surgery. Upon recovery from anesthesia and even with the endotracheal tube in place, patients should be encouraged to begin deep breathing exercises learned during the preoperative phase.

***Postoperative Examination***

1. Upon transfer to the ICU setting it is necessary to receive a report regarding the patient's condition, paying particular attention to the results of the surgery. Were there any complications or unexpected findings?
2. Evaluate the patient's breathing pattern, and compare it to the preoperative performance. What effects has the surgery had on it? Once again, are the respirations long or short? Is there shortness of breath or hyperventilation?
3. Perform auscultation. Listen for abnormal breath sounds and signs of pulmonary congestion. Determine the results of the most recently drawn arterial blood gases.
4. Observe the patient's condition. Take note of mental status and endurance. Fatigue may be a major factor. Note all bodily attachments such as catheters, IVs, and so forth.

***Postoperative Treatment***

1. Have the patient perform deep breathing exercises. Follow the same procedure as in preoperative deep breathing, including the use of the incentive spirometer.
2. Have the patient cough. If possible, get the patient to sit up and compress the incisional area with a pillow or blanket to diminish pain. Once again, encourage a double cough from the chest, not the throat. Encourage the patient to cough up any secretions, which can then be accessible to suctioning while the artificial airway is in place.
3. Perform cupping, percussion, and postural drainage, if indicated or per physician's guidelines.
4. Review ROM exercises. Have the patient perform active extremity exercises. When ambulatory, have the patient get out of bed and walk.

*This information has been contributed by Robert DiBartolo, P.T.

the skeletal ring associated with valve placement may impinge on the AV node/junction located therein, predisposing to dysrhythmias (bradycardias and heart blocks). If the heart rate becomes too slow the pacemaker can be activated to ensure an optimal heart rate.

The patient and family should be advised that blood transfusions may be provided to offset a lowered blood count, which sometimes occurs post-surgery.

Finally, the patient should be assured that pain medication is available. Pain experienced post-cardiac surgery is usually incisional and the patient should be encouraged to request pain medication when needed. The patient's nurse should closely monitor the degree of discomfort and the effectiveness of the analgesic therapy in relieving the patient's pain.

In general, the preoperative teaching protocol should be modified to meet the individual needs of the patient and family. The patient's nurse needs to be sensitive to the feelings of the patient and family, and to closely monitor their tolerance of stress. Refer to the care plan in Table 45–4 for specific details related to preoperative preparation of the cardiac surgical patient.

## Postoperative Teaching

Postoperative teaching serves to reinforce information presented to the patient preoperatively and to expand on those factors essential to postoperative recuperation, rehabilitation, and home health care. It is necessary to assess patients and their support systems to gain a clear understanding of the patient and family members as individuals and collectively, the environment in which they live and work, and their health management and rehabilitation concerns. Assessment of functional health patterns enables specific needs and problems to be identified, explored, and mutually acted upon. Areas of particular emphasis include the patient's emotional status, activities of daily living, exercise, diet, sexual activity, prevention of infection, medication regimen, follow-up care, and instruction regarding the underlying disease process that necessitated surgery.

Postoperatively, it is not unusual for patients to feel anxious, irritable, and depressed. Often these feelings are related to concerns regarding changes in body image and to fears of the "chest opening." Sleep disturbances post-surgery are not unusual and may last for as long as 4–6 weeks. Appropriate explanations and reassurance can defuse some of these feelings and assist the patient to better understand the healing process.

Activity is an essential factor in the patient's recuperation and needs to be addressed in postoperative instruction. Immediately post-surgery, the patient can be expected to change positioning while in bed and to progress to getting into and out of bed, sitting in a chair, and then walking. The patient should demonstrate leg exercises that assist in returning blood to the heart (i.e., "skeletal muscle pump"). He or she should be taught to elevate the legs while out of bed to minimize fluid accumulation, and to avoid crossing legs to ensure adequate circulation. Support stockings should be worn during the first few weeks post-surgery since they help to improve circulation and prevent fluid accumulation and venostasis.

Over the long term, the patient should be able to understand progression of activity level as well as necessary restrictions. Cardiac surgical patients should avoid driving for 4–6 weeks post-surgery and to avoid lengthy care rides. For car trips longer than an hour, frequent rest stops should be planned to allow ambulation. This helps to promote good circulation to the legs. Heavy lifting (no objects over 10 lbs) or straining is to be avoided to prevent injury to the chest. Resumption of sexual activity should be discussed with the physician.

After the initial 2 weeks at home the patient can gradually return to household chores and activities. Frequent rest periods and an afternoon nap should be planned. Excessive visitors should be avoided since extensive socialization causes fatigue.

Regularly planned exercise is necessary to promote cardiovascular fitness. Slow, progressive ambulation is recommended. Thus, the patient may walk 1 block the second postoperative week, increasing the distance gradually to 1 mile as tolerated. The patient should avoid extremes of outside temperatures, and should not exercise for 30 minutes to 2 hours after meals to prevent competition for oxygen needs between gastrointestinal organs and muscle. Ideally, participation in a cardiac rehabilitation program would optimize physical, psychologic, and mental recuperation.

In conjunction with a planned progressive exercise program, the patient and family should receive appropriate diet instruction. Such instruction should take into consideration who in the family shops for food and prepares meals. Alcohol consumption should be minimal (less than 1–2 oz daily). The patient should monitor body weight at least once weekly. Changes in body weight most closely reflect hydration status, including fluid retention, weight loss, and response to diuretic therapy.

Following cardiac surgery, the patient's medication regimen frequently changes. Patients who are post-CABG surgery are often placed on aspirin or dipyridamole (Persantine); patients with valve replacement may be placed on long-term coumadin therapy. The patient and family should be instructed regarding the specific medications, their names, purpose, dosage, schedule, and side effects. Special instruction may be necessary. For example,

## TABLE 45–4. CARE PLAN FOR PREOPERATIVE CARE OF THE CARDIAC SURGICAL PATIENT

| Nursing Diagnoses | Desired Patient Outcomes | Nursing Interventions | Rationales |
|---|---|---|---|
| ***Nursing Diagnosis #1*** Anxiety, related to: 1. Upcoming cardiac surgery. | The patient will demonstrate decreased anxiety by indicating willingness to discuss the following: 1. Normal function of the heart. 2. Disease process, including: a. Risk factors. b. Surgical procedure. c. Expected outcomes of the surgery. | • Teach the patient about the normal function of the heart; underlying disease process including risk factors; the surgical procedure; and the expected outcomes of the surgery. | • Teaching provides a basic understanding of the problem, the solution, and what to expect, thereby decreasing the patient's anxiety. However, not all patients experience a decreased level of anxiety when bombarded with new information. |
| | | • Use simple terms or explain medical terms used. | • Using simple terms or explaining medical terms enhances learning because the patient can understand the explanations. Using medical terms sometimes confuses and overwhelms the patient. |
| | | • Utilize posters, models, and handouts/pamphlets. | • Visualization aids learning. |
| | | • Teach in short blocks if time allows. | • Allows assimilation of information before more is added, and thus enhances learning. |
| | | • Observe patient's nonverbal cues. | • Enables the nurse to evaluate patient's understanding and anxiety level. The nurse can determine whether to proceed, reiterate, or stop. |
| | | • Allow time for questions. | • Relieves anxiety, clarifies information, and prevents misconceptions. |
| | | • Answer questions honestly. | • Establishes a trusting relationship and attains patient cooperation. |
| | | • Maintain a calm, relaxed, nonrushed atmosphere with little or no interruptions. | • Enhances the learning experience. |
| | | • Have the patient discuss the information in his/her own words. | • Assists in evaluating what has been learned. |
| | | • Correct any misconceptions. | • Patient knows what to expect, thereby reducing some of his/her anxiety. |
| ***Nursing Diagnosis #2*** Knowledge deficit regarding preoperative and postoperative expectations. | Patient will verbalize an understanding of the preoperative routine: 1. Tests, procedures. 2. Medications. 3. The night before the surgery. 4. The day of the surgery. | • Provide information regarding the following: | |
| | | ◦ Tests and procedures that will be performed before surgery. | ◦ This is a time when the patient needs and wants to be with family but is frequently interrupted, causing frustration and sometimes anger. Knowing about these studies ahead of time will help in coping with the interruptions. |

| | | |
|---|---|---|
| 5. The immediate postoperative care. | ○ Blood studies: CBC, serum electrolytes, BUN, creatinine, cardiac enzymes, clotting time, prothrombin time, fibrinogen levels, platelets, type and cross-match of blood, arterial blood gases. | ○ To evaluate baseline values. If any abnormal values are present, treatment can be initiated so as to prevent complications intraoperatively and postoperatively. Patient is typed/cross-matched to ensure blood is available if needed. |
| | ○ ECG. | ○ Provides a baseline for comparison. |
| | ○ Chest x-ray. | ○ To examine for abnormalities; provides a baseline for comparison. |
| | ○ Urine analysis. | ○ To evaluate for signs of infection. |
| | ○ Pulmonary function tests (PFTs). | ○ To evaluate patient's pulmonary status. |
| | ○ Changes in medication regimen and necessary preoperative medication: | ○ Changes in medication regimen can cause anxiety. Understanding of what the changes will be helps decrease anxiety and enhance patient cooperation. |
| | ○ Sedation the evening before/prior to surgery. | ○ Decreases anxiety, allows a good night's sleep. |
| | ○ All aspirin, anticoagulants, and anti-inflammatory drugs should be discontinued at least 2 days prior to surgery. | ○ Prevents bleeding due to altered coagulation studies. |
| | ○ Digitalis is usually held 1–2 days prior to the surgery unless the patient is in uncontrolled atrial fibrillation. | ○ Digitalis toxicity is a common complication postoperatively, related to low potassium levels. If given to control atrial fibrillation, the patient must be monitored closely for signs of toxicity postoperatively, especially in the immediate postoperative phase. |
| | ○ Propranolol is tapered 24 hr–2 weeks prior to surgery. | ○ Negative chronotropic and inotropic action postoperatively further decreases the cardiac output. If needed early in the postoperative period, dopamine, epinephrine, isoproterenol, and/or glucagon can be given. |
| | ○ Diuretics are discontinued 24–48 hours prior to the surgery if congestive heart failure is controlled. | ○ Diuretics increase the loss of fluids and potassium, which could cause adverse reactions postoperatively (i.e., hypovolemia, acidemia, hyponatremia, digoxin toxicity). |
| | ○ Nitroglycerin is kept at the bedside and can be taken for chest pain (as per protocol). | ○ Relieves chest pain associated with anxiety. |
| | ○ Long-acting insulin is changed to regular insulin and patient is placed on a sliding-scale coverage 24 hr prior to the surgery. | ○ Insulin requirements change due to the stress of the surgery and NPO status. Administration of insulin on a sliding scale provides a more precise dosage to meet the patient's needs, thereby preventing hyperglycemia/hypoglycemia. |

*(continued)*

**TABLE 45–4. CARE PLAN FOR PREOPERATIVE CARE OF THE CARDIAC SURGICAL PATIENT *(Continued)***

| Nursing Diagnoses | Desired Patient Outcomes | Nursing Interventions | Rationales |
|---|---|---|---|
| ***Nursing Diagnosis #2 (cont.)*** | | | |
| | | ○ Potassium supplements are given to maintain the patient's potassium level at 4.0 mEq/liter. | ○ To prevent intraoperative and postoperative complications (i.e., acidemia, digoxin toxicity, dysrhythmias). |
| | | ○ Norpace may be discontinued 24 hr prior to the surgery. | ○ Norpace may cause heart failure in the postoperative phase. |
| | | ○ Antidysrhythmics are maintained to control the dysrhythmias. | ○ Prevent further decrease in the cardiac output related to the dysrhythmias; help to prevent serious or life-threatening dysrhythmias. |
| | | ○ Antihypertensive medications are maintained. | ○ Maintain the patient's blood pressure. Nitroprusside (Nipride) can be given intraoperatively. |
| | | ○ Prophylactic antibiotics are given prior to the surgery and continued for 2 days postoperatively. | ○ Prevent infection. |
| | | ○ Check the patient for allergies to any medications, especially antibiotics, iodine preparations, or fish. | ○ Prevents anaphylaxis. |
| | | • The night before the surgery, the patient will: | |
| | | ○ Receive a light dinner, then nothing to eat or drink after midnight. | ○ Prevents aspiration of the stomach contents. |
| | | ○ Be shaved from the chin to the toes (CABG) or chin to shins (valve replacement). | ○ Decreases the possibility of infection since skin and hair harbor bacteria. |
| | | ○ Shower with an antibacterial agent (i.e., Betadine). | ○ Decreases the possibility of infection by decreasing the bacteria on the skin. |
| | | • The morning of the surgery, the patient will: | |
| | | ○ Shower again with the antibacterial agent. | |
| | | ○ Put on a hospital gown. | |
| | | ○ Receive a preoperative sedative. | ○ Decreases anxiety and helps the patient to relax. |
| | | ○ Receive family for a brief visit (according to hospital policy). | ○ Allays anxiety of patient and family. |
| | | ○ Give valuables to the family to take home. | ○ There is little room in the ICU for the patient's personal effects. Family will be told what to bring in when it is needed. |
| | | ○ Be transferred to a stretcher and transported to the OR. | |
| | | • Explain the immediate postoperative care: Inform the patient of the ICU routine: | • Knowing what to expect decreases the patient's anxiety and enhances cooperation. |
| | | ○ Patients remain in the ICU for 2–3 days if no complications occur. | |

| | |
|---|---|
| ◦ The unit may be noisy and the lights left on.<br>◦ Patients are checked frequently for vital signs and assessments.<br>◦ Visiting hours are restricted to brief periods.<br>◦ A tour of the unit is offered to those who want it. Patient may be able to meet the nurse who will be taking care of her/him in the ICU. | ◦ The patient should understand that frequent assessments are part of usual ICU protocols. It does not mean that anything is wrong.<br>◦ Awareness of the unit's environment will decrease the anxiety level for some patients. The patient will not become alarmed in response to the noise, frequency of vital signs, and absence of family except during brief visits. |
| • Explain expectations of postoperative period (e.g., equipment/routines). Patient will: | • Knowledge regarding expectations of care enables the patient to be cooperative and participate in care (e.g., not trying to pull the tubes out, fighting procedures, afraid of moving). The patient needs to know that needs will be anticipated and a method of communication worked out. This serves to reduce anxiety. |
| ◦ Have an endotracheal tube connected to a ventilator that will help with breathing. | ◦ The endotracheal tube is usually left in place for 8–24 hr. |
| ◦ Be unable to talk. | ◦ An alternate means of communication should be set up (i.e., mouthing words, finger writing, sign language). |
| ◦ Experience breathlessness when suctioned. | ◦ The patient should know that the feeling of breathlessness, should it occur, will last only a few seconds.<br>◦ The patient should be encouraged to breathe with the ventilator and not to "fight" the ventilator. |
| • The patient will:<br>◦ Have a Foley catheter postoperatively. | ◦ Allows for accurate measurement of urine output. |
| ◦ Have peripheral, jugular, and subclavian IVs. | ◦ Access for emergency medications, fluids, blood and blood products, and plasma expanders as needed. Once stabilized postoperatively, all but one will be discontinued while in the ICU. |
| ◦ Have an arterial line for approximately 1 day. | ◦ Access for arterial blood gases and other blood specimens. Allows for continuous monitoring of arterial blood pressure. |
| ◦ Be connected to a cardiac monitor. | ◦ To monitor heart rhythm and rate. |
| ◦ Have a rectal temperature probe in place postoperatively until temperature stabilizes (usually 8 hr). | ◦ Allows frequent monitoring of the patient's temperature. In the absence of a temperature probe, rectal temperatures can be taken hourly until stabilized. |
| ◦ Have chest tubes in place for approximately 2 days. | |

*(continued)*

**TABLE 45-4. CARE PLAN FOR PREOPERATIVE CARE OF THE CARDIAC SURGICAL PATIENT *(Continued)***

| Nursing Diagnoses | Desired Patient Outcomes | Nursing Interventions | Rationales |
|---|---|---|---|
| ***Nursing Diagnosis #2 (cont.)*** | | | |
| | | | ○ Allows evaluation of bleeding in the chest, which may indicate improper closure of a graft, cardiac tamponade, or coagulation abnormality.<br>○ The drainage will be bloody initially and then gradually become serous. |
| | | • Explain the various suture lines. | • Patient will have a midline chest incision (medial sternotomy) that will be dressed initially. The dressing is usually removed 24 hr postoperatively. Patient may have some chest discomfort related to the sternum being opened; this pain differs from the chest pain experienced previously. Pain medication will be available.<br>• Patient will have an incision in one or both legs. It may extend from the thigh to the knee, the thigh to the ankle, or the knee to the ankle, depending on the amount of graft needed, the surgeon's preference, and the condition of the vein.<br>*Note:* When a mammary artery is used as bypass graft, incisions in lower extremities are unnecessary. |
| | | ○ Advise that postoperatively Ace bandages or elastic stockings are applied. | ○ Ace bandages/elastic stockings aid in the venous return from the legs; they are also used to prevent thrombi. |

| | | |
|---|---|---|
| Patient will demonstrate activities expected to be performed in the postoperative period:<br>1. Coughing and deep breathing (see Table 45–3).<br>2. Splinting the chest incision.<br>3. Use of the incentive spirometer (see Table 32–2).<br>4. Arm and leg exercises.<br>5. Turning side to side.<br>6. Getting out of bed the day after the surgery. | • Demonstrate, and have the patient return the demonstration, activities to be performed postoperatively:<br>◦ Coughing and deep breathing: Take 4–5 deep breaths, then cough.<br>◦ Pain medication will be given prior to the exercises (as indicated).<br>◦ Splinting the chest incision.<br>◦ Arm exercises—range of motion and walking up the wall.<br>◦ Leg exercises—ankle range of motion, "ankle pump," and dorsiflexion.<br>◦ Turning side to side every 2 hr.<br>◦ Getting out of bed—splint chest.<br>◦ Inch legs over the side of the bed. Sit up straight on the edge of the bed, then ease the feet down to the floor. Nurses will be present for support and guidance of tubings. | • Enhances cooperation in the postoperative activities needed to prevent complications. Ensures that the patient knows what must be done, why, and how it is to be done.<br>◦ Prevent atelectasis and pneumonia.<br>◦ Deep breaths loosen the secretions so they can be mobilized.<br>◦ Decreases the amount of pain so the exercises can be done effectively.<br>◦ Decreases the amount of pain.<br>◦ Prevent frozen shoulder.<br>◦ Increase circulation in the lower extremities and prevent stasis and thrombosis. Range of motion also prevents foot drop.<br>◦ Early ambulation helps prevent many complications, especially pneumonia and thrombosis. It is not as simple a task postoperatively as patients may believe. |

patients placed on coumadin therapy must understand the importance of ongoing follow-up care. They should know to contact the physician immediately should any of the following signs and symptoms be noted: black or tarry stool, pink or red urine, excessive bruising or unexplained swelling, severe headache, abdominal pain, coffee-ground vomitus, or epistaxis. The patient should be instructed to take only the prescribed medications and to avoid use of over-the-counter drugs. The patient should carry a card listing all his/her medications with dosage and time of administration, at all times.

Patients with valve replacements are at especially high risk of infection (e.g., bacterial endocarditis). These patients should contact their physician regarding the need for prophylactic antibiotics when dental work, surgery, invasive procedures, or self-injection of drugs is anticipated.

The patient's return to work should be discussed with the physician. Depending on the type of work (e.g., laborer versus clerical worker), the patient may be able to resume work within 4–6 weeks. Encourage the patient to verbalize concerns regarding livelihood. Assist the patient and family to identify effective coping mechanisms and the family support systems. Instruction in relaxation techniques may be initiated early on in the postoperative phase.

Finally, it is essential to teach patient and family regarding the underlying disease process and risk factors associated with heart disease. Discuss the function of the heart as a pump; the significance of coronary artery perfusion; and the nature of the atherosclerotic process. Patients with valve replacement should be able to describe the heart chambers and the role played by the valves in the unidirectional flow of blood through the heart. Patients should be able to identify risk factors for cardiovascular disease in general (see Preoperative Teaching, above) and their own risk factors in particular. Physical conditions and living habits that contribute to the process of coronary artery disease should be discussed and modifications in the patient's and family's lifestyle should be determined so as to control some of the identified risk factors (e.g., stress management, diet, weight reduction).

## General Review of CABG Procedure

The actual and sequential events occurring within the operating room may vary from center to center, but overall, the approach to cardiac surgery is quite similar. The patient is placed on the operating room table, cardiac monitor electrodes and ground panel are applied, and intravenous and arterial lines are inserted. A narcotic anesthesia (e.g., morphine sulfate or fentanyl) is usually administered and the patient is immediately intubated. A flow-directed pulmonary catheter may be inserted at this time and baseline data are established. The skin is prepped and a midline sternotomy is performed, splitting the sternum and separating the ribs to allow full visualization of the heart. The pericardium is then opened fully to expose the heart.

While the chest is being entered, another surgical team works on the legs, excising the superficial saphenous vein. The saphenous vein is used because there are collateral veins available in the leg to do the work of returning blood to the heart; also, this vein is accessible to surgical removal. The length of vein excised is determined by the number of grafts to be performed. Once removed, the veins are checked for patency and for the presence of disease. Side channels to other vessels are tied off and the vessel is tested for leakage. Sometimes it is necessary to remove the saphenous veins from both legs. If the internal mammary artery is to be used rather than the saphenous vein, it is localized and prepared at this time.

### *Cardiopulmonary Bypass*

While the veins are being harvested, preparations are made to place the patient on the cardiopulmonary bypass machine. The function of the bypass machine is to provide oxygenation, circulation, and hypothermia during induced cardiac arrest. By diverting blood flow away from the heart, it also helps to provide a bloodless field for surgeons to do their work. The machine is initially primed with Ringer's lactate or an electrolyte solution, thereby reducing the need for transfusions. This helps to reduce the risk of transfusion reactions, hepatitis, and transmission of acquired immune deficiency virus (AIDS virus).

The bypass machine is connected to the patient via venous and arterial cannulae. The venous cannula is inserted into the vena cava or right atrium. The arterial cannula is inserted into the ascending aorta or femoral artery. As the blood enters the machine, heparin is administered to prevent clot formation. The blood travels through the tubing to the oxygenator where it receives oxygen while carbon dioxide is removed. Oxygenators come into various styles, the most commonly used ones being the rotating disk, the bubble, and the membrane.

As blood is pumped through the bypass machine, formed elements (including RBCs, WBCs, and platelets) and unformed elements (e.g., plasma proteins) of the blood are traumatized by direct contact with the surface of the pump, its mechanical and consequent turbulent flow, and by the intracardiac suction system. The free hemoglobin released in conjunction with trauma to RBCs is eventually cleared via the kidneys. Administration of mannitol and furosemide (Lasix) facilitates the clearance process. Patients usually tolerate this disturbance postoperatively as long as the bypass time is under 3 hours.

Complications related to the use of cardiopulmonary bypass usually include blood dyscrasias leading to loss of clotting factors or thromboembolism formation; reduction in pulmonary surfactant leading to pulmonary edema and atelectasis; and showers of microemboli to the brain causing cerebral hypoxia and strokes.

The arteriolized (oxygenated) blood travels to the heat exchanger where it is cooled to 25°-30°C. Prior to returning to the patient, the blood travels through a filter or bubble trap where it is filtered of clots, fat debri, air, and other particulate matter. The blood then returns to the patient through an arterial cannula placed in the femoral or iliac artery, or commonly in the ascending aorta. The mean arterial pressure is maintained by adjusting the rate of perfusion and blood volume flow through the machine or by administering vasopressors.

The aorta is cross-clamped and the heart is cooled by an infusion of cold, hyperkalemic cardioplegic solution into the aortic root or coronary artery ostia, causing the heart to stop in diastole. To further lower the temperature of the myocardium, the pericardium may be filled with Ringer's lactate at 4°C. This induced hypothermia reduces the oxygen requirements of the body as well as of the myocardium. In some cases an additional catheter is inserted into the left ventricle to prevent ventricular distention.

Once the heart is arrested, grafting begins. The saphenous vein is inverted, with the proximal end anastomosed to the aorta and the distal end to the coronary artery distal to the point of occlusion. The grafts are measured for flow rates. The basal flow rates should be greater than 40 ml/minute, and peak flow rates greater than 80-100 ml/minute.

Upon completion of grafting, the heart is slowly rewarmed and the cardioplegic solution is flushed from the heart and mediastinum. As blood circulates through the heart, the heart muscle regains its rate, rhythmicity, and strength of contraction; or the heart may be defibrillated to resume function. The blood is rewarmed and the rate of return from the cardiopulmonary bypass machine is decreased. As the patient is weaned from the cardiopulmonary bypass machine, the grafts are assessed for leakage at the suture sites and for patency, before the patient is removed from bypass. Protamine sulfate is given to counteract the effect of the heparin as weaning occurs.

Once satisfactory arterial pressure and cardiac function are achieved, the patient is taken totally off the bypass machine, and the cannulae are removed. Anesthesia is discontinued and the patient is ventilated for a time with 100% oxygen. The patient is suctioned as necessary.

The pericardium may be left open to prevent tamponade should postoperative bleeding occur. Mediastinal chest tubes are placed and connected to water seal drainage. Atrial and ventricular pacemaker wires may be sewn to the epicardium if electrical malfunctioning of the heart is anticipated in the immediate postoperative period. This is a special consideration for patients who have valvular repair or replacement surgery because of the anatomic proximity of the AV node to the tricuspid and mitral valves.

The sternum is closed with stainless steel wire and the chest is sutured closed. A sterile dressing is applied. The patient is then transferred to a postoperative bed and accompanied to the recovery room or ICU by the anesthesiologist, surgeon, and operating room nurses.

Close monitoring of the patient's vital signs, heart rhythm, arterial blood gases, serum electrolytes, coagulation studies, and urinary output is performed throughout the operative procedure. Bypass time is also closely monitored and kept to a minimum (less than 3 hours) since the longer the patient is on bypass, the greater the risk of complications. Uncommonly, some patients are difficult to wean from the bypass machine and require the assistance of the intra-aortic balloon pump (see Chap. 42) to augment left ventricular function.

## Postoperative Nursing Management

Immediately upon return from the operating room the patient is connected to various bedside monitoring devices, such as thoracic suction, intravenous infusion pumps, and a mechanical ventilator. A portable chest x-ray is obtained to check placement of the endotracheal tube; pulmonary, cardiovascular, neurologic, and abdominal assessments are performed. Baseline laboratory studies are drawn including arterial blood gases, serum electrolytes, complete blood count and hematology profile, cardiac enzymes, and coagulation studies. Baseline hemodynamic values are obtained. These include arterial blood pressure, central venous pressure, pulmonary artery pressure, pulmonary capillary wedge pressure, and left atrial pressure, if monitoring accesses and equipment are available. Cardiac rhythm, body temperature, and hourly urine outputs are closely monitored.

### Therapeutic Goals

The goals of care for the cardiac surgical patient include the following: (1) maintain adequate cardiac output and tissue perfusion; (2) prevent complications; and (3) assist the patient and family to initiate rehabilitative activities.

To maintain adequate cardiac output and tissue perfusion the nurse must constantly analyze assessment data, identifying trends and initiating timely and appropriate interventions. It is often necessary to manipulate the determinants of cardiac output —preload, afterload, contractility, and heart rate —to maintain an optimal cardiac output without undue strain on the heart.

A low cardiac output syndrome is reflected by systemic hypotension, peripheral vasoconstriction (cool, clammy, pale, or mottled skin), oliguria, and neurologic changes (mental status and orientation). In the majority of post-cardiac surgical patients the low cardiac output is associated with hypovolemia (i.e., reduced preload) and responds well to fluid volume expansion. If the hematocrit or hemoglobin is low, part of the fluid volume expansion can be accomplished by the transfusion of blood or blood products.

A low cardiac output state may also be caused by an increase in afterload and is characterized by increased systemic vascular resistance and arterial hypertension. Reduction in afterload is accomplished with vasodilator therapy (e.g., nitroprusside) providing the preload is adequate. Patients who have received beta-adrenergic antagonists (e.g., propranolol) prior to surgery may experience depressed cardiac contractility postoperatively. These patients are usually responsive to dopamine. If pharmacotherapeutics are unsuccessful in improving cardiac output, the intra-aortic balloon pump (IABP) may be used (see Chap. 42). The IABP decreases afterload and increases coronary artery and tissue perfusion.

Cardiac dysrhythmias may also cause a low cardiac output. Bradydysrhythmias and AV blocks are frequently associated with valve replacement surgery. These abnormalities may be responsive to chronotropic therapy; more commonly, atrioventricular (AV) sequential pacing is the therapy of choice as the "atrial kick" (i.e., the volume of blood delivered to the ventricles with atrial contraction just prior to ventricular systole) is preserved. Tachydysrhythmias are usually controlled with antidysrhythmic agents. It is essential to monitor serum electrolytes and the acid–base status because premature ventricular contractions may evolve into lethal dysrhythmias in the presence of hypokalemia. Replacement potassium chloride is added to intravenous therapy to maintain serum potassium within its normal, physiologic range. Abnormalities in serum potassium may stem from hemodilution, nasogastric suction, diuretic therapy, and the overall response of the body to the stress of surgery.

A major postoperative complication of cardiac surgery is hemorrhage. Excessive bleeding may occur at the site of surgery (e.g., anastomoses of graft vessels); be associated with insufficient reversal of heparinization with protamine sulfate; or be caused by a decrease in clotting factors. Chest tubes must be kept patent and the amount and characteristics of the drainage closely monitored. Should the tubes become occluded by clots, accumulation of blood and fluid in the pericardial sac may precipitate cardiac tamponade. Cardiac tamponade is reflected by the classical signs, including rising central venous pressures with neck vein distention, falling arterial pressure with hypotension, and distant, muffled heart sounds. This triad of symptomatology is described as *Beck's triad*. Additional signs may include presence of pulsus paradoxus and a narrowing pulse pressure as filling volumes and stroke volume become reduced. Timely and aggressive intervention is imperative.

In the postoperative phase the patient is also at risk of developing other complications including pulmonary emboli, pneumonia, and fluid overload. Frequent position changes, range-of-motion exercises, and early ambulation help in preventing thromboembolic episodes. Ace bandages or antiembolic stockings applied to the lower extremities help to promote venous return and prevent venostasis. In patients in whom the saphenous vein is harvested for grafting, elastic bandages applied to the lower extremities prevent oozing from the incisional site and hematoma formation.

The patient's cardiopulmonary status must be evaluated at frequent intervals. Serial arterial blood gases and chest x-rays help to monitor pulmonary function. Coughing, turning, and deep breathing are essential to raising secretions and preventing atelectasis (see Table 45–3). Splinting of the chest incision may assist the patient in coughing. Incentive spirometry is used to support deep breathing. Special attention to these details helps to prevent pulmonary complications (e.g., pneumonia). Refer to Table 45–5 for additional potential postoperative complications in the cardiac surgical patient.

Following the stabilization of the patient in the immediate postoperative period, the focus of nursing care becomes the patient's rehabilitation and discharge. The rapport and support systems established preoperatively assist the patient and family during the recuperative period. The adjustment of moving from the ICU setting to the step-down unit or general acute floor can be a highly anxious experience for both patient and family. If the patient doesn't experience a dramatic improvement in overall body function, he/she may become depressed. It should be emphasized that each case is different, and it sometimes takes 3–6 months for an individual to experience any significant improvement in overall physical and psychologic status. The achievement of strength, stamina, and optimal well-being may take longer than the patient's preoperative expectations.

Patients are generally discharged 7–10 days after surgery. Discharge teaching is very important to help ease the transition. Some hospitals offer a callback system where patients and their families can call for advice if they are experiencing difficulties or have questions. This system not only helps ease the psychologic transition to home, but it also helps prevent severe complications by advising the patient to seek medical assistance in a timely fashion.[7]

As discussed earlier in the sections on preoperative and postoperative teaching, it is essential to discuss the underlying cause of coronary artery disease. Cigarette smoking, weight gain, and lack of

TABLE 45-5
**Postoperative Complications in the Cardiac Surgical Patient**

**I. Cardiovascular Dysfunction**
1. Low cardiac output syndrome
   A. Reduced preload
      Hypovolemia
      Hemorrhage
         Surgical site
         Overheparinization
         Depleted clotting factors
   B. Increased afterload
      Increased systemic vascular resistance
      Arterial hypertension
   C. Cardiac dysrhythmias
      Bradydysrhythmias
      Conduction defects
      Tachydysrhythmias
2. Congestive heart failure
3. Cardiogenic shock
4. Cardiac tamponade
5. Acute myocardial infarction
6. Electrolyte disturbances
   A. Hypokalemia
      Extracorporeal circulation
      Hemodilution
      Diuretic therapy
      Nasogastric decompression

**II. Pulmonary Dysfunction**
1. Pneumothorax
2. Hemothorax
3. Atelectasis
4. Pneumonia
5. Pulmonary edema (cardiogenic versus noncardiogenic pulmonary edema; see Table 34-2)
6. Pulmonary embolism

**III. Renal Dysfunction**
1. Prerenal failure

**IV. Gastrointestinal Dysfunction**
1. Stress ulcer
2. Paralytic ileus

**V. Neurologic Dysfunction**
1. Post-pericardiotomy syndrome (postcardiotomy delirium associated with cardiopulmonary bypass and manifested by behavioral changes ranging from confusion to frank psychosis)
2. Cerebral vascular accident (CVA)

**VI. Infection**
1. Endocarditis
2. Mediastinitis
3. Sepsis

**VII. Miscellaneous**
1. Thromboembolic disorder
2. Disseminated intravascular coagulation (DIC)

exercise should all be explored with the patient and family, as they have all been identified as risk factors (Chap. 43). The atherosclerotic process does not stop after bypass surgery. The CABG itself is only palliative therapy and this should be understood by patient and family. The family involvement is especially important because no one becomes ill in a vacuum. Rather, illness evolves out of the total interaction between the individual, the family, and environment. Nurses need to consider how they may influence the patient/family/environment so that when the patient is discharged, he or she does not return to the same lifestyle that predisposed to the illness in the first place. Enrollment in a cardiac rehabilitation program is of utmost importance.

### Nursing Diagnoses, Desired Patient Outcomes, and Nursing Interventions

For pertinent nursing diagnoses, desired patient outcomes, and nursing interventions/rationales in the postoperative care of the cardiac surgical patient, refer to Table 45-6.

## TABLE 45-6. CARE PLAN FOR EARLY POSTOPERATIVE CARE OF THE CARDIAC SURGICAL PATIENT

| Nursing Diagnoses | Desired Patient Outcomes | Nursing Interventions | Rationales |
|---|---|---|---|
| ***Nursing Diagnosis #1***<br>Cardiac output, alteration in: Decreased, related to:<br>1. Cardiopulmonary bypass.<br>2. Low cardiac output syndrome. | Patient will demonstrate stabilization of body function as supported by monitoring and life-support systems:<br>1. Arterial blood pressure within 10 mmHg of patient's baseline.<br>2. Stable pulmonary artery pressures:<br>• PAP <25 mmHg.<br>• PCWP 8–12 mmHg.<br>• CVP 0–8 mmHg.<br>3. Cardiac output ~5 liters/minute.<br>• Heart rate >60 <100 beats/minute.<br>4. Urine output >30 ml/hour.<br>5. Alert mental status; oriented to person, place, time.<br>6. Electrolyte balance.<br>7. Acid–base balance:<br>• pH 7.35–7.45.<br>• $PaO_2$ >80 mmHg.<br>• $PaCO_2$ 35–45 mmHg.<br>8. Stable hematology profile:*<br>• Hct: male, 45–52%; female, 37–48%.<br>• Hgb: male, 13–18 g/100 ml; female, 12–16 g/100 ml.<br>• Platelet count: 150,000–350,000/mm³. | • Monitor vital signs (BP, heart rate, respiratory rate, and temperature) q 5 minutes while rewarming, then q 15 minutes until stable, then q 1 hr × 12. | • Frequent monitoring of the vital signs allows early detection of abnormalities, and treatment can be initiated to prevent complications. |
| | | • Assess the patient q 1 hr until stable, including heart sounds; ECG changes; cardiac rhythm; neck veins; lung sounds; peripheral pulses; capillary refill; skin turgor, color, and temperature; movement and sensation. | • Changes may indicate hemodynamic decompensation or complications. Signs of low cardiac output syndrome include a decrease in arterial pressure, urine output below 30 ml/hr, signs of vasoconstriction (cool, pale, or cyanotic skin and mucous membranes), tachycardia, dysrhythmias, tachypnea, narrow pulse pressure, weak peripheral pulses, decrease in level of consciousness, restlessness. |
| | | • Monitor hemodynamic parameters: Mean arterial pressure (MAP), pulmonary artery pressure (PAP), pulmonary capillary wedge pressure (PCWP), central venous pressure (CVP), or right atrial pressure (RAP), and left atrial pressure (LAP). | • Parameters will reflect left ventricular function, fluid status, and arterial perfusion. |
| | | • Assess the pacemaker concerning type (fixed or demand), the rate it is set at, the milliamperes (mA), and whether it is functioning properly. (Pacing wires are commonly used in valve replacement surgery.) | • Need to be familiar with equipment in order to use it properly, identify if it is functioning properly, and how to trouble-shoot problems. Pacemaker is usually kept on standby to keep the patient's heart rate above 60 beats/minute and to treat other dysrhythmias. (Cardiac pacing is discussed in detail in Chapter 42.) |
| | | ○ Keep exposed wires wrapped in gauze and place in a plastic covering. | ○ Prevents the possibility of electrical shock or short circuit. |
| | | • Report any abnormalities in vital parameters to physician immediately: | • Immediate intervention can be ordered to prevent further deterioration/complications. |
| | | ○ BP: Systolic <80, >180.<br>Diastolic >100.<br>○ MAP: <60, >100. | ○ Pressures below 80 mmHg could cause graft closure or indicate shock; pressures above 180 mmHg could cause the graft to "blow," or could cause a CVA. |
| | | ○ CVP: <5, >15. | ○ CVP readings below 5 $cmH_2O$ indicate inadequate intravascular fluid; readings above 15 $cmH_2O$ indicate fluid overload. |

* Some hemodilution is expected with bypass and fluid retention; thus, lower hematocrits may be acceptable.

| | | | |
|---|---|---|---|
| | | ○ Heart rate: <60, >100. | ○ Heart rates below 60 could cause graft closure; rates above 100 will decrease the oxygenation to the myocardium and increase the workload of the heart. |
| | | ○ Temperature: Remains hypothermic or rises above 101°F. | ○ Hypothermia prolongs vasoconstriction, adding to low cardiac output syndrome. Temperatures above 101°F may indicate infection. |
| | | ○ Excessive or bloody chest tube drainage >100 ml/hr. | ○ Excessive and/or bloody drainage suggests bleeding at surgical site. |
| | | ○ Urine output <30 ml/hr. | ○ Reduced urine output warns of prerenal failure. |
| | | ○ Extremities: Cool, moist, mottled, with sluggish capillary refill and poor or absent peripheral pulses. | ○ Signs of decreased peripheral perfusion related to emboli or decreased cardiac output. If accompanied by pain, arterial occlusion of the extremity may have occurred. |
| | | ○ A decrease in movement or sensation. | ○ May indicate possible neurologic involvement or may be due to the effect of the anesthesia. |
| | | ○ Presence of anginal pain or ECG changes: ST segment elevation or depression; T wave peaked/inverted. | ○ Indicative of myocardial ischemia. |
| ***Nursing Diagnosis #2***<br>Breathing pattern, ineffective, related to:<br>1. General anesthesia.<br>2. Incisional pain with splinting.<br>(See Table 44–11, Nursing Diagnosis #3.) | The patient will maintain:<br>1. A patent airway.<br>2. Respiratory rate <25–30/minute; eupneic rhythm.<br>3. ABGs within normal range:<br>• pH 7.35–7.45.<br>• $PaO_2$ >80 mmHg.<br>• $PaCO_2$ 35–45 mmHg.<br>• $HCO_3$ 22–26 mEq/liter. | • Assess respiratory function: Rate, rhythm, pattern, chest excursion, use of accessory muscles; breath sounds; presence of adventitious sounds. | • It is essential to establish baseline function with which to compare subsequent findings; assists in following trends. |
| | | • Maintain patient on ventilator at prescribed settings. | • Maintains patient's respirations when the respiratory center is depressed due to the anesthesia and narcotics. Provides adequate oxygenation. Decreases the workload of the heart. |
| | | ○ Check the endotracheal cuff for adequate inflation. | ○ Improper cuff inflation reduces tidal volume and may compromise ventilation. |
| | | • Administer pain medications to decrease pain and prevent "fighting" the ventilator. | • Pain and "fighting" the ventilator can lead to hyperventilation, which may predispose to respiratory alkalosis. Acid–base imbalances can cause dysrhythmias.<br>○ Tachycardia related to pain can increase workload of the heart. |
| | | • Suction prn. Sigh the patient before and after suctioning. (Sigh is a deeper than normal breath with 100% oxygen.)<br>○ Use hand resuscitator to ventilate and preoxygenate prior to and following each suction pass (some mechanical ventilators have "sigh" capability.) | • Remove secretions for adequate oxygenation and gas exchange. Sighing the patient before and after expands the alveoli, mobilizes the secretions, and prevents drastic drops in the patient's oxygen levels. |

**TABLE 45-6. CARE PLAN FOR EARLY POSTOPERATIVE CARE OF THE CARDIAC SURGICAL PATIENT *(Continued)***

| Nursing Diagnoses | Desired Patient Outcomes | Nursing Interventions | Rationales |
| --- | --- | --- | --- |
| ***Nursing Diagnosis #2 (cont.)*** | | | |
| | | • Monitor ABGs q 1–4 hr as the patient's condition warrants; or continuously monitor mixed venous gases ($S\bar{v}O_2$) as prescribed. (*Note:* $S\bar{v}O_2$ is discussed in Chap. 41.) | • Respiratory and metabolic alterations are reflected in the ABGs. Adjustment in the ventilator settings or pharmacologic interventions can be initiated to prevent severe imbalances. |
| | | • Wean patient off the ventilator as prescribed, when alert, breathing spontaneously, and demonstrating adequate ABGs and appropriate ventilatory parameters (i.e., inspiratory pressure, expiratory pressure, tidal volume, minute volume, and vital capacity). | • The patient must be able to breathe spontaneously with adequate respiratory excursion, tidal volume, minute ventilation, and peak inspiratory pressure. (See Chap. 32, section on mechanical ventilation.) |
| | | • Administer oxygen through a heated humidified face mask or tent after weaning. | • Provides oxygenation with humidification to assist in thinning the secretions and thereby facilitating deep breathing and coughing. |
| | | • Encourage patient to cough and deep breathe hourly; administer chest percussion; encourage the use of the incentive spirometer q 1–2 hr while awake.<br>◦ Have respiratory therapist administer IPPB and nebulizer treatments as ordered. | • Loosens and mobilizes the secretions, thereby preventing atelectasis and pneumonia. Incentive spirometer provides patients with a visual feedback as to how well they are breathing. |
| | | • Assess breath sounds q 2 hr and/or when indicated. | • Decreased breath sounds may indicate atelectasis, pneumonia, or poor breathing technique due to splinting. Absence of breath sounds on one side suggests atelectasis or malpositioning of the endotracheal tube. Endotracheal tube may have slipped down into right bronchus. Pneumothorax, if present, is usually accompanied by unequal chest excursion and shifting of trachea to opposite side. |
| | | • Notify the physician of any significant abnormalities in respiratory parameters. | • Interventions may be taken expeditiously to prevent complications. |

| | | | |
|---|---|---|---|
| ***Nursing Diagnosis #3*** Fluid volume deficit, actual and potential, related to:<br>1. Surgery-related blood loss or hemorrhage.<br>2. NPO status.<br>3. Peripheral vasodilation associated with rewarming (disproportion between size of vascular bed and intravascular blood volume).<br>(See Tables 23–1, 23–2, and 23–3). | Patient will:<br>1. Maintain stable hemodynamic parameters:<br>• BP, pulses, CVP, PAP, PCWP (see Nursing Diagnosis #1, above).<br>2. Demonstrate adequate peripheral perfusion; peripheral pulses 2+ bilaterally; brisk capillary refill; skin warm, no cyanosis of nailbeds or mucous membranes.<br>3. Be alert and oriented.<br>4. Maintain urinary output above 30 ml/hour with no hematuria.<br>5. Show no sign of hemorrhage (stable vital signs).<br>6. Maintain a hematocrit above 30%. | • Monitor vital signs q 15 minutes while the patient is rewarming. | • The vascular bed increases during rewarming, causing a disproportion in the vascular volume and the vascular bed size. If the disproportion is great enough the patient will become hypotensive, predisposing to shock. Under these circumstances, there is a risk that the grafts may close off. In response to the hypotension the patient may develop myocardial ischemia with dysrhythmias, prerenal failure, or DIC. |
| | | • Administer fluids as ordered. (Usually less than 100 ml/hr total volume unless the patient is hypovolemic). | • Adequate fluids are necessary to prevent hypovolemia; overhydration can cause the patient to develop pulmonary edema. |
| | | • Monitor the patient's intake and output carefully. Weigh daily. | • Patient may be retaining fluid if fluid intake is greater than output plus the insensible losses. Daily weighing is a reliable indicator of hydration status (2.2 lb is equal to 1 liter of fluid). |
| | | • Monitor urine output q 1 hr; specific gravity q 2 hr. | • Urine output less than 30 ml/hr may indicate decreased cardiac output, hypovolemia, or renal failure. A decrease in specific gravity indicates hypovolemia. |
| | | • Monitor BUN and creatinine. | • The BUN is an indicator of renal function and fluid status, the creatinine is an indicator of renal function. The physician should be notified of an increase in either, or of any change in BUN/creatinine ratio. |
| | | • Assess skin turgor and mucous membranes for hydration status. | • Tenting of the skin when pinched indicates dehydration. Edema indicates fluid excess or decreased cardiac output. Dry mucous membranes indicate dehydration; moist mucous membranes indicate adequate hydration. |
| | | • Monitor hemodynamic parameters especially when rehydrating the patient. | • PAP, LAP, and CVP will be decreased in volume depletion. As fluids are administered the pressures also will increase. Pressures will be elevated in fluid overload.<br>• Low Hgb and Hct are indicative of blood loss or hemodilution; an elevated Hct is indicative of hemoconcentration. |
| | | • Monitor serum electrolytes and hemoglobin and hematocrit (Hgb and Hct). Administer potassium to maintain level within 3.5–5.5 mEq/liter. | • Elevation of potassium may be related to renal failure, cardiopulmonary bypass, or acid–base imbalance. Abnormal potassium levels can cause dysrhythmias. |

*(continued)*

**TABLE 45–6. CARE PLAN FOR EARLY POSTOPERATIVE CARE OF THE CARDIAC SURGICAL PATIENT *(Continued)***

| Nursing Diagnoses | Desired Patient Outcomes | Nursing Interventions | Rationales |
|---|---|---|---|
| ***Nursing Diagnosis #3 (cont.)*** | | • Monitor amount and color of chest tube drainage. | • Chest tube drainage greater than 100 ml/hr for the first 4 hr is indicative of abnormal bleeding, which could be related to platelet destruction, inadequate reversal of the heparin, inadequate suturing of arteries during the surgery, or diffuse intrathoracic ooze. |
| | | ○ Observe the dressings and bedding for signs of hemorrhage. | ○ Bleeding may occur at the suture line. Excessive bleeding may ooze down the patient's side and pool under him. |
| | | • Monitor coagulation studies. | • Abnormal coagulation caused by anticoagulants or DIC can cause hemorrhage related to oozing at injection sites, suture lines, insertion sites of IVs. |
| | | • Administer blood, plasma expanders, and clotting factors as prescribed. | • Blood and plasma expanders are given to maintain the intravascular volume. Fresh-frozen plasma and cryoprecipitate may be administered to bolster concentration of clotting factors to ensure appropriate blood coagulation and prevent hemorrhaging. |
| ***Nursing Diagnosis #4***<br>Tissue perfusion, alteration in peripheral, related to:<br>1. Low cardiac output syndrome. | Patient will:<br>1. Demonstrate normotension (MAP within 10 mmHg of patient's baseline).<br>2. Demonstrate normothermia (98.6°F, 37.0°C).<br>3. Maintain palpable peripheral pulses and brisk capillary refill.<br>4. Exhibit warm, dry skin, pink in color with good turgor.<br>5. Maintain heart rate >60, <100.<br>6. Maintain urine output >30 ml/hr. | • Assess peripheral pulses. Compare right with left. Note characteristics: Rate, rhythm, quality (bounding, weak, and thready), and equality.<br>○ Mark sites of pulses if difficult to palpate. | • Peripheral pulses are indicators of the arterial flow through the extremity. An absence or decrease in the pulse may indicate occlusion of the vessel due to emboli.<br>○ Marking the sites makes it easier to find the pulse, especially if the pulse is weak. |
| | | • Assess the skin for temperature, color, capillary refill, breakdown, and sensation. | • Indicators of peripheral perfusion. A decrease may be indicative of poor perfusion. |
| | | • Have patient perform leg and arm exercises as taught in the preoperative phase. | • Exercises increase circulation. |
| | | • Apply elastic stockings or Ace bandages to lower extremities as prescribed.<br>○ Check size of elastic stockings and apply properly; check pulses q 4 hr, administer skin care. Remove stockings once each shift. | • Properly applied elastic stockings and Ace bandages assist in venous return, reducing risk of venous stasis. |
| | | • Assess the patient for calf tenderness, swelling, and a positive Homan's sign. | • Signs of thrombophlebitis. |

| | | | |
|---|---|---|---|
| | | • Measure girth of calves and thighs bilaterally. | • Often the means of detecting that a deep venous thrombosis is present is by monitoring the circumference. |
| | | • Do not gatch the bed or use pillows under the knee. Discourage the patient from crossing knees and/or ankles. | • Applies pressure under the knee, thereby decreasing circulation to the lower leg. |
| ***Nursing Diagnosis #5***<br>Tissue perfusion, alteration in cerebral, related to:<br>1. Anesthesia.<br>2. Cardiopulmonary bypass.<br>3. Narcotics.<br>4. Postcardiotomy delirium (PCD). | Patient will:<br>1. Demonstrate an intact, direct, and consensual pupillary light reflex bilaterally.<br>2. Demonstrate an intact gag reflex.<br>3. Be alert and oriented to person, place, and time.<br>4. Follow commands/behavior appropriately.<br>5. Speak clearly and understandably.<br>6. Demonstrate movement in all extremities equal to preoperative state. | • Assess neurologic status at least every 2–4 hr, or when indicated: Pupils—size and equality, reaction to light; level of consciousness; orientation; speech, obeys commands; movement of all extremities. | • Abnormal neurologic findings may be indicative of permanent or temporary alterations related to the anesthesia, intraoperative stroke, cardiopulmonary bypass machine, hypothermia, decreased cardiac output. Abnormal findings may occur in the immediate postoperative phase but they should gradually return to baseline within the initial 4–8 hr postoperatively. |
| | | • Assess the patient's behavior every shift. Orient to person, place, and time. Provide frequent explanations. Allow family to visit. Reinforce normality of the disorientation (if no other signs of neurologic deficit are present). | • Confusion and disorientation may be indicative of postcardiotomy delirium (PCD). Frequent explanations, reorientation, and visits from family help the patient cope with PCD. Postcardiotomy delirium is associated with cardiopulmonary bypass and is manifested in some patients post-bypass by changes in behavior, confusion, and frank psychosis. |
| ***Nursing Diagnosis #6***<br>Infection, potential for, related to:<br>1. Interruption in integrity of skin barrier (surgical incision).<br>2. Invasive monitoring.<br>3. Chest tubes, Foley catheter. | The patient will remain infection free:<br>1. Temperature at baseline (98.6°F, 37.0°C).<br>2. WBC at baseline.<br>3. Incisional area clean, dry, and healing. | • Assess incision, IV sites, intravascular lines for signs of infection (warmth, redness, swelling). | • The skin is the first line of defense against infection. Any break in the skin's integrity is prone to infection. |
| | | • Change IV lines and hemodynamic lines per hospital protocol. Maintain sterility of the lines. | • These are access sites through which bacteria enter. |
| | | • Change dressings daily or according to hospital protocol. | • Dressing changes permit visualization of the surgical site. Redness, warmth, and swelling suggest infection. |
| | | • Administer antibiotics as prescribed. | • Timely and accurate administration of antibiotics helps to maintain therapeutic blood levels. |
| | | • Culture any draining wound. | • Detection of the causative organism is necessary so that appropriate antibiotic therapy can be prescribed. |
| | | • Assess breath sounds and appearance of sputum. | • Presence of adventitious sounds and sputum production can signal possible onset of pneumonia. |
| | | • Maintain the Foley catheter as a closed system. Discontinue as soon as possible. | • Foley catheters are a common source of infection and can lead to gram-negative sepsis. |

*(continued)*

**TABLE 45–6. CARE PLAN FOR EARLY POSTOPERATIVE CARE OF THE CARDIAC SURGICAL PATIENT *(Continued)***

| Nursing Diagnoses | Desired Patient Outcomes | Nursing Interventions | Rationales |
|---|---|---|---|
| ***Nursing Diagnosis #6 (cont.)*** | | | |
| | | • Assess the patient for signs of systemic infection (sepsis): Change in behavior, hyperthermia/hypothermia, chills, diaphoresis. | • The first sign of sepsis is a change in behavior. Timely and aggressive intervention is necessary to prevent septic shock and multisystem organ dysfunction. (Septic shock is discussed in Chap. 66.) |
| | | • Practice good handwashing technique. | • Good handwashing technique is the main way to prevent inspection or its spread. |
| ***Nursing Diagnosis #7*** Anxiety, related to: 1. Outcome of surgery. 2. Recuperative period. 3. Lack of sleep/rest. 4. Noisy ICU environment. | Patient will verbalize: 1. Feeling less anxious. 2. Ability to rest and to sleep. 3. Progress made in recuperation. 4. Willingness to cooperate in care. 5. Desire to make decisions concerning care. | • Familiarize with ICU environment: Equipment, procedures, and protocols. | • Appropriate explanation decreases anxiety. |
| | | • Explain condition and treatments. Stress the patient's progress. | • Reassures the patient. Gives positive reinforcement. |
| | | • Administer pain medication as needed. Withhold if the patient is hypotensive, is being weaned off the ventilator, or has neurologic changes. | • Decreasing the pain will decrease the patient's anxiety by breaking the pain-fear-anxiety triangle. Narcotics are not given if they will interfere with assessment or stabilization of the patient. |
| | | • Provide rest periods. Administer sedatives/pain medication to enhance sleep at night. | • Sleep and rest deprivation causes irritability, which increases anxiety. |
| | | • Allow the patient to take an active part in care; allow patient to make decisions concerning care. | • Decision-making and active participation in care give positive feedback to the patient that he/she is making progress, as well as giving the patient a sense of self-worth. |
| | | • Allow the family to visit as much as possible according to unit/hospital policy. | • The family is a support system that the patient depends on. Family interaction helps prevent social isolation and gives the patient a sense of being needed. |

## REFERENCES


1. Weiland, AP: A review of cardiac valve prostheses and their selection. Heart Lung 12(5):498, September 1983.
2. Kretten, CK and Bass, L: Valvular heart disease: Surgery and post-op care. RN 50(12):38, December 1987.
3. Painvin, GA, Frazier, OH, Chandler, LB, et al: Cardiac transplantation: Indications, procurement, operation and management. Heart Lung 14(5):485, September 1985.
4. Zochoche, DA (ed): Mosby's Comprehensive Review of Critical Care, ed 3. CV Mosby, St Louis, 1986, pp 498–504.
5. Lewis, S and Collier, I: Medical-Surgical Nursing: Assessment and Management of Clinical Problems. McGraw-Hill, New York, 1983, pp 784–791.
6. Sadler, D: Nursing for Cardiovascular Health. Appleton-Century-Crofts, Norwalk, Connecticut, 1984, pp 138; 297–298; 311.
7. Nicklin, WM: Postdischarge concerns of cardiac patients as presented via a telephone callback system. Heart Lung 15(3):268, 1986.


## SELECTED READINGS


Artinian, NT: Family member perceptions of a cardiac surgery event. Focus on Critical Care 16(4):301, August 1989.

Blaisdell, MW, Good, L, and Gentzler, RD: Percutaneous transluminal valvuloplasty. Crit Care Nurse 9(3):62, March 1989.

Carabello, BA: Mitral regurgitation, Part 1: Basic pathophysiological principles. Mod Conc Cardiovasc Dis 57(10), October, 1988.

Carabello, BA: Mitral regurgitation, Part 2: Proper timing of mitral valve replacement. Mod Conc Cardiovasc Dis 57(11), November, 1988.

Carden, S and Clark, S: A Nursing diagnoses approach to the patient awaiting cardiac transplant. Heart Lung 14:5, 1985.

Cisar, NS and Morphew, SF: Preoperative teaching: Aortocoronary by-pass patients. Focus on Critical Care 10:1, 1983.

Cromwell, V, Huey, R, Korn, R, et al: Understanding the needs of your coronary bypass patient. Nursing '80, 10:3, 1980.

Flynn, MK and Frantz, R: Coronary artery bypass surgery: Quality of life during early convalescence. Heart Lung 16(2) March, 1987.

Fuller, E: Stress testing: From whom? Patient Care 20:8, 1986.

Fütterman, LG: Cardiac transplantation: A comprehensive nursing perspective, Part 1. Heart Lung 17(5), September, 1988.

Gillis, CL: Reducing family stress during and after coronary artery bypass surgery. Nurs Clin North Am 19:1, 1984.

Grady, KC: Development of a cardiac transplantation program: Role of the clinical nurse specialist. Heart Lung 14:5, 1985.

Grady, KL: Evolution of a cardiac transplantation program: Role of the clinical nurse specialist. Focus on Critical Care 16(2):130, April, 1989.

Gurevich, I: Infectious complications after open heart surgery. Heart Lung 10:5, 1984.

Kretten, CK and Baas, L; Valvular heart disease: Its causes, symptoms, and consequences. RN 50:11, 1987.

Kronick-Mest, C: Postpericardiotomy syndrome: Etiology, manifestations, and interventions. Heart Lung 18(2):192, March, 1989.

Lamb, IS and DiGiacomo, BM: What to expect when your patient's scheduled for mitral valve replacement. Nursing '85 15:1, 1985.

Marshall, J, Penckofer, S, and Llewellen, J: Structured postoperative teaching and knowledge and compliance of patients who had coronary artery bypass surgery. Heart Lung 15:1, 1986.

Murdock, DK, Collins, EG, et al: Rejection of the transplanted heart. Heart Lung 16(3), May, 1987.

Ohler, L, Fleagle, DJ, and Lee, BI: Aortic valvuloplasty: Medical and critical care nursing perspectives. Focus on Crit Care 16(4):275, August 1989.

Pieper, B, Lepczyk, M, and Caldwell, M: Perceptions of the waiting period before coronary artery bypass grafting. Heart Lung 14:3, 1985.

Rodgers, CD: Needs of relatives of cardiac surgery patients during the critical care phase. Focus on Critical Care 10:15, 1983.

Stradtman, JC and Ballenger, MJ: Nursing implications in sternal and mediastinal infections after open heart surgery. Focus on Crit Care 16(3):178, June 1989.

# CHAPTER 46

# Nursing Management of the Patient in Shock

## CHAPTER OUTLINE



## LEARNING OBJECTIVES

**At the end of this chapter, you should be able to:**

1. Define shock and its classifications.
2. Describe the pathophysiology underlying the effect of shock on body organ systems.
3. Identify the major compensatory mechanisms triggered in response to shock, including neural, hormonal, and chemical influences.
4. Identify key factors to be assessed in the early recognition and treatment of shock.
5. Describe hypovolemic shock, its etiology, pathophysiology, diagnosis, treatment, and management.
6. Delineate the nursing process in the care of the patient with hypovolemic shock, including:
   Assessment
   Diagnosis
   Planning: Desired patient outcomes
   Nursing interventions.

## SHOCK: A DEFINITION

Shock is a state of impaired cellular metabolism, or an "acute nutritional insufficiency at the cellular level," which occurs as a consequence of inadequate tissue perfusion and/or the inability of cells to metabolize nutrients appropriately.[1] It is a pathophysiologic state involving a circulatory disturbance characterized by a systemic imbalance between oxygen supply and demand. Shock is a critical illness that begins as a compensatory response to some insult or trauma and rapidly progresses to multisystem organ failure. Without timely, skilled, and aggressive intervention based on the trends and responses obtained clinically via astute observation and serial objective measurements, shock can be life-threatening.

## PATHOPHYSIOLOGY

The shock state impacts on virtually every organ system of the body. In the early stages of shock, compensatory mechanisms are triggered that function to maintain vital bodily processes while the shock state is diagnosed and its cause eliminated. With timely and aggressive intervention, the underlying pathophysiologic insult is resolved and cellular injury is averted. Should the shock state remain unresolved and the compensatory capabilities of the body exceeded, a progressive deterioration of circulatory and cellular function occurs, leading ultimately to a final, irreversible stage, and the patient eventually succumbs to the effects of shock.

## Impact on the Body's Organ Systems

### *Cardiovascular*

Initial compensatory mechanisms activated in response to shock include those of the cardiovascular system. A fall in the arterial blood pressure is sensed by baroreceptors located within the aortic arch and carotid sinus. These sensory nerve endings are sensitive to the degree of stretch of the vessel wall caused by pressure exerted by the volume of circulating blood (see Chap. 37). When a drop in mean arterial pressure occurs, the consequent reduction in the degree of stretching causes the baroreceptors to send impulses to the vasomotor center in the medulla.

An immediate sympathetic response occurs with the release of norepinephrine at adrenergic synapses. Stimulation of the vasomotor center also reflexly stimulates the adrenal medulla to secrete epinephrine and, to a lesser extent, norepinephrine.

Physiologically, the body's overall response to increased sympathetic activity involves an increase in heart rate (chronotropic effect); an increase in the force of myocardial contraction (inotropic effect); an increase in systemic vascular resistance associated with heightened vasoconstriction of resistance vessels (arterioles and metarterioles); and an increase in vasoconstriction of capacitance vessels (venules and veins), thereby increasing venous return to the heart. The net result of these activities is to increase cardiac output (via increased heart rate and stroke volume), and to increase total systemic vascular resistance (via arteriolar vasoconstriction). The increase in cardiac output and systemic vascular resistance results in a return of the mean arterial pressure to within the physiologic norm.

Stimulation of beta-adrenergic receptors underlies the chronotropic and inotropic effect on the heart, as well as the slight vasodilation of the coronary circulation and that of skeletal muscle. Alpha-adrenergic stimulation to the skin, splanchnic circulation, and kidneys causes these vessels to vasoconstrict, thereby shunting blood to the priority organs, the heart and brain. Sympathetic stimulation does not cause significant vasoconstriction of the cerebral vasculature, as blood flow through the cerebral circulation is largely intrinsically regulated via the phenomenon of autoregulation (see Chap. 37).

The body's ability to compensate for a significant reduction in arterial blood pressure has its limitations. As shock progresses, these compensatory mechanisms begin to fail and circulatory and cellular deterioration begins. As stores of energy utilized to maintain the vasoconstrictive state become depleted, the heart itself becomes weakened and unable to maintain the necessary cardiac output. The reduction in cardiac output decreases coronary artery perfusion, thereby leading to ischemia, serious dysrhythmias, and heart failure; the consequent reduction in peripheral blood flow predisposes to tissue hypoxia.

Reduced tissue perfusion necessitates that cells produce energy (ATP) via anaerobic glycolysis. A major end-product of this series of reactions is lactic acid, which is responsible for the metabolic acidemia associated with the shock state. Lactic acidosis depresses the myocardium and decreases the peripheral vascular responsiveness to catecholamines (e.g., epinephrine, norepinephrine, and dopamine).

Tissue hypoxia also triggers the release of chemical mediators, which potentiate the severity of the shock state. Two of these mediators, bradykinin and histamine, are especially potent vasodilators that contribute to the pooling of blood in the vascular bed. Disruption of the integrity of the vascular bed leads to transudation of fluid from the capillaries into the interstitium. This not only contributes to the pooling of blood, but, very importantly, it reduces blood volume and diminishes venous return to the heart.

Relaxation of precapillary sphincters causes blood to sequester in the microcirculation. As oxygen and energy stores become depleted, metabolic waste products accumulate and contribute to the development of metabolic acidosis. There is an accumulation of the cellular elements of blood, platelet microaggregates, and other particulate matter, all of which lead to the sludging of blood within the microcirculation. Such sludging eventually predisposes to thrombosis and intravascular coagulation (see Chap. 63).

### *Respiratory*

Hyperventilation is generally observed in the early stages of shock. Although the tidal volume ($V_T$) may be reduced, the respiratory rate increases by 2- or 3-fold, resulting in a minute ventilation that is often 1½–2 times normal.

Underlying respiratory dysfunction is a disruption in pulmonary capillary dynamics predisposing to pulmonary edema (see Fig. 34–1). In patients with cardiogenic shock, a cardiogenic (hydrostatic) pulmonary edema evolves. As the volume of blood in the left ventricle at the end of diastole increases, there is a consequent increase in left ventricular end-diastolic pressure, which is reflected back to the pulmonary capillary bed. The increase in pulmonary hydrostatic pressure favors the transudation of fluid out of the pulmonary capillaries and into the lung interstitium, predisposing to pulmonary congestion. Early on, the lymphatic system can effectively drain off excess fluid. However, when the drainage capacity of the pulmonary lymphatic system is exceeded, fluid begins to accumulate in the alveoli, causing acute pulmonary edema. In this clinical circumstance, the permeability of the microvascular membrane remains intact, limiting movement of protein out of the capillaries.

In contrast to cardiogenic (hydrostatic) pulmonary edema, *noncardiogenic* pulmonary edema is associated with an increase in the permeability of the alveolar-capillary membrane, frequently in the presence of *normal* pulmonary capillary hydrostatic pressure. The disruption in the integrity of this membrane causes leakage of fluid, plasma proteins, and cellular elements into the interstitium, thereby altering interstitial osmotic pressure. Involvement of alveolar epithelial cells results in alveolar edema, atelectasis, and decreased lung compliance, with adult respiratory distress syndrome (ARDS) as the end result (see Chap. 34).

**Chemically Activated Compensatory Mechanisms.** Closely associated with pulmonary function are chemically activated compensatory mechanisms, which respond largely to chemical stimuli including those directly related to the serum concentrations of oxygen, carbon dioxide, and hydrogen ions. When cardiac output is reduced, blood flow to the lungs is also reduced. This contributes to an increase in ventilation-perfusion imbalance, the consequence of which is a decreased oxygen tension ($PaO_2$) in the blood leaving the lungs.

Chemoreceptors located in the aortic arch and carotid bodies sense this reduced oxygen tension and send impulses to the vital centers in the medulla. The physiologic response is an increase in the rate and depth of respirations. The consequent increase in alveolar ventilation reduces the carbon dioxide tension while increasing the oxygen tension of blood leaving the lungs to within an acceptable physiologic range.

Chemoreceptors also respond to increases in carbon dioxide and the hydrogen ion concentrations of circulating blood, and elicit a response similar to that described for oxygen. The increase in the rate and depth of respirations eliminates carbon dioxide, and the hydrogen ion concentration is reduced accordingly. This response is reflected in the following equation:

$$H^+ + HCO_3^- \rightleftharpoons H_2CO_3 \rightleftharpoons CO_2 + H_2O$$

As $CO_2$ is eliminated by the lungs, the reaction shifts to the *right,* thereby reducing the hydrogen ion concentration. The result is a rise in the pH (see Chap. 30).

### Renal/Endocrine

In response to shock, the kidneys function to restore tissue perfusion by conserving sodium and water. Cells of the juxtaglomerular apparatus secrete renin, a proteolytic enzyme, which triggers the crucial series of events of the renin-angiotensin-aldosterone system (see Fig. 21–9). Angiotensin II, the end-product of this series of reactions, exerts a potent vasoconstrictor effect on both arteries and veins. The consequent increase in systemic vascular resistance raises blood pressure and increases the venous return to the heart.

Angiotensin II also stimulates secretion of aldosterone by the adrenal cortex. Aldosterone, in turn, acts on the distal renal tubules to increase reabsorption of sodium. The reabsorption of sodium is accompanied by the reabsorption of water. In this way, the body's compensatory mechanisms attempt to overcome the effects of the shock state.

Under normal conditions, the kidneys respond to a reduced cardiac output and mean arterial pressure by shunting blood flow from cortical nephrons to the juxtaglomerular nephrons. These latter nephrons largely function to establish and maintain the osmolality of the renal medullary interstitium creating osmotic gradients essential for the reabsorption of water and the concentration of urine (see Chap. 21).

Reabsorption of water is facilitated by the action of antidiuretic hormone (ADH), which is released from the posterior pituitary gland (neurohypophysis) in response to an increase in the osmolality of the circulating blood. This hormone acts on the cells of the distal kidney tubules and collecting ducts to increase the permeability of these cells to water, facilitating its passive reabsorption in conjunction with enhanced sodium reabsorption. ADH, or vasopressin, also exerts the body's most potent vasoconstrictor effect on the systemic vasculature.

The increase in sympathetic activity in response to shock also stimulates the anterior pituitary gland (adenohypophysis) to release adrenocorticotropic hormone (ACTH). This hormone acts directly on the adrenal cortex to increase release of glucocorticoids. The glucocorticoids act to elevate the serum glucose concentration, which provides a ready source of energy for cellular metabolism and contributes to the osmolality of circulating blood.

### Gastrointestinal

The gastrointestinal mucosa is particularly vulnerable to the shock state. Erosions and ulcerations of the mucosal lining can potentially precipitate significant gastrointestinal bleeding. In the stomach, these alterations may be associated with a back-diffusion of hydrogen ions across the friable mucosa. Maldistribution of blood flow to the mucosal lining may also contribute to this pathogenic mechanism because the absorptive processes occurring therein consume large amounts of oxygen and are particularly vulnerable to ischemia.

Hepatic complications may also develop in response to the shock state. Fatty infiltrates and centrolobular necrosis have been identified. Prolonged impairment of hepatic blood flow in shock can increase the tendency to severe acute failure of other organ systems. Furthermore, as liver metabolism becomes progressively impaired there is also concurrent impairment of the hepatic reticuloendothelial system (RES). Disruption of Kupffer cells compromises a large segment of the body's RES phagocytic components. The liver plays a key role in the removal of a large number of potentially toxic substances absorbed from the gastrointestinal tract and splanchnic tissues during shock. Many of these substances cause further impairment of cardiovascular function, and a vicious downward cycle of progressive hepatic and cardiovascular failure is perpetuated.

#### *Neurologic*

Because blood flow to the brain is largely autoregulated, neurologic function is usually well preserved until late in the shock process. As long as the arterial pressure remains above approximately 70 mmHg, cerebral blood flow is usually maintained essentially at normal levels.

### Thrombosis of the Microcirculation

Under normal conditions, the processes of clot formation (thrombosis) and clot dissolution (fibrinolysis) occur sequentially at a localized site of injury. As a result of these processes, bleeding is prevented, healing is promoted, and patency of the vessel is eventually reestablished. In the shock state, sluggish blood flow and altered cellular metabolism predispose to the formation of thrombi in the microcirculation. Damage to the endothelial lining and platelet aggregation give rise to intravascular coagulation with subsequent deposition of fibrin and accumulation of microthrombi. Agglutination of erythrocytes and leukocytes may also occur. As the shock state progresses these processes occur throughout the microcirculation and result in a significant bleeding diathesis. (For a detailed discussion of disseminated intravascular coagulation [DIC], see Chap. 63.)

### Disruption of Cellular Function

As the shock state persists, cellular metabolism becomes progressively disturbed. The sluggish microcirculation diminishes the availability of oxygen to the tissues, and cells must shift from aerobic to anaerobic metabolism. This is a significant factor because anaerobic metabolism is almost 20 times *less* effective in generating ATP than is aerobic metabolism. In addition, anaerobic glycolysis involves the conversion of pyruvate to lactate, thereby predisposing to metabolic lactic acidosis and other metabolic derangements.

Mitochondrial oxidative phosphorylation, the mechanism by which the transfer of electrons along the respiratory chain is used to generate ATP, requires a continuous supply of oxygen. When the demand for oxygen cannot be met, mitochondrial activity becomes significantly depressed. The consequent reduction in ATP stores is reflected by failure of the Na/K-ATPase pump. Active transport of sodium and potassium through the cell membrane is greatly diminished. As a result, sodium and water accumulate within the cell, while potassium effluxes out of the cell. Cells may begin to swell.

As stores of ATP diminish and cellular membranes become increasingly disrupted, cAMP production declines. This occurs because the formation of cAMP requires the presence of ATP and membrane-bound adenyl cyclase. The reduction in cAMP is significant because this molecule plays a pivotal role in numerous cellular reactions, including, for example, cellular responsiveness to catecholamines and calcium regulation.

Alteration in calcium regulation is especially critical because the consequent elevation in cytoplasmic levels of calcium inhibits mitochondrial release of ATP and interferes with the activity of adenyl cyclase, thereby decreasing production of cAMP.

As the shock state evolves, further deterioration in cellular function occurs. Lysosomal disruption causes the release of hydrolytic enzymes within the cell, thereby initiating cell autolysis (i.e., self-dissolution or self-digestion of a cell by enzymes from within the cell itself). The end result is cellular death.

## CLASSIFICATION/ETIOLOGY

Shock can be classified based on its underlying pathophysiologic mechanism(s), which involves one or more of the major components of the cardiovascular system. These include (1) the heart, which functions as a pump; (2) the blood vessels, which function as conduit that distribute blood to various tissues, facilitate transcapillary exchange, and return blood to the right heart; and (3) the relationship between blood volume and the size of the vascular space.

Shock occurs when there is an inadequate cardiac output due to the inability of the heart to pump effectively; or when there is a decrease in the venous return to the heart, whether due to a depleted circulating blood volume or to peripheral vasodilation. There are several classifications of shock. The classification presented here includes (1) cardiogenic; (2) vasogenic, including anaphylactic, neurogenic, and septic; and (3) hypovolemic (hemorrhagic) shock.

## Cardiogenic Shock

Cardiogenic shock is caused by the inability of the heart to function as a pump to maintain adequate tissue perfusion. It occurs most commonly in the scenario of acute myocardial infarction in patients with severe coronary artery disease, wherein the primary problem is diseased or atherosclerotic coronary arteries leading to inadequate oxygen delivery to the myocardium itself. Damage to 40% or more of the left ventricular mass predisposes to cardiogenic shock.

Less commonly, cardiogenic shock may develop in patients with acute MI who develop associated mechanical dysfunction as, for example, papillary muscle rupture resulting in a regurgitant mitral valve, or a perforated interventricular septum. End-stage cardiomyopathies associated, for example, with vitamin deficiencies, excessive thyroid hormones, or myocarditis secondary to a viral or bacterial infection may underlie pump failure with consequent cardiogenic shock. Cardiogenic shock may also occur following cardiac surgery in a heart muscle depressed by hypothermia and cardioplegia, or in the scenario of serious, potentially life-threatening dysrhythmias.

Clinically, patients with cardiogenic shock experience a fall in mean systemic blood pressure associated with an inadequate cardiac output and an increase in systemic vascular resistance (SVR). Stroke volume (SV) is reduced and the heart rate increased. With the increase in heart rate, there is a consequent decrease in ventricular diastolic filling time and coronary artery perfusion. Reflex sympathetic activity is further detrimental because an increase in heart rate and myocardial contractility increases myocardial oxygen consumption, potentiating myocardial ischemia. The increase in afterload associated with systemic vasoconstriction similarly increases the work of the heart.

With progressive heart failure, left ventricular end-diastolic pressure (LVEDP) increases, and this increase is passively transmitted to the pulmonary capillary bed, predisposing to pulmonary edema. As the pulmonary capillary wedge pressure rises ($>$18–20 mmHg) and the cardiac index falls ($<$2.2 liters/minute), cardiogenic shock becomes definitive. (For a detailed discussion and care plan for the patient with heart failure, see Chap. 44.)

## Distributive (Vasogenic) Shock

Distributive, or vasogenic, shock is a broad category that includes several types of shock, all of which are characterized by peripheral vasodilation with a disproportion between the usual circulating blood volume and the size of the vascular bed. This alteration in blood vessel radius leads to a decrease in systemic vascular resistance and an increase in vascular capacity. Subclassifications of distributive, or vasogenic, shock include (1) anaphylactic, (2) neurogenic, and (3) septic shock.

### *Anaphylactic Shock*

Anaphylactic shock is an uncommon yet dramatic clinical event associated with a severe allergic reaction in which an antigen-antibody reaction is the precipitating event. It involves an immediate systemic normovolemic, vasogenic reaction that occurs when an individual who has been sensitized to an antigen from a previous exposure (i.e., an individual who has preformed antibody) is again exposed to the antigen in question. The consequent interaction between the antigen and preformed antibody causes mast cells to release their chemical mediators (e.g., histamine, serotonin, and slow-reacting substance of anaphylaxis [SRS-A]). On release, these chemical mediators, among other actions, cause vasodilation and an increase in vascular permeability. The consequent fluid shifts and vasodilatation result in a "relative hypovolemia" predisposing to a significant, symptomatic hypotensive state. (For a detailed discussion and care plan for the patient with anaphylactic shock, see Chap. 67.)

### *Neurogenic Shock*

Neurogenic shock is characterized by an abnormal distribution of blood volume caused by massive vasodilation of the systemic vasculature as a result of an interruption or loss of sympathetic innervation. Loss of sympathetic vasoconstrictor tone in arterioles, metarterioles, and venules results in a significant decrease in peripheral vascular resistance. Consequently, there is a reduction in venous return to the heart, a decrease in stroke volume, and symptomatic hypotension.

Neurogenic shock is associated with injury or disease of the upper spinal cord or involvement of the brainstem. It may occur following general anesthesia or spinal anesthesia that extends upward in the spinal cord. (See Chap. 12 for further discussion of neurogenic shock.)

### *Septic Shock*

Septic shock is a consequence of an abnormal distribution of intravascular blood volume caused by massive vasodilation associated with an overwhelming infection or septicemia. Specifically, endotoxin(s) released by the causative microorganism(s) acts to trigger a variety of biochemical reactions that adversely affect the body and predispose to the shock state. Included among these reactions is the activation of the complement, clotting, and kinin systems. In addition, endotoxin(s) triggers the release of vasoactive mediators from the damaged tissues.

Clinically, septic shock is seen to progress through the stages of preshock, hyperdynamic or "warm" shock, hypodynamic or "cold" shock, and multisystem organ failure. Early in the course of the illness, activation of the sympathetic nervous system is reflected clinically by an increase in heart rate and cardiac output and by a heightened systemic vascular resistance. With progression to the preshock stage, a decrease in systemic vascular resistance occurs, but the cardiac output and mean arterial pressure remain within normal limits.

The hyperdynamic stage, or "warm" shock, is characterized by profound peripheral vasodilation with a reduced systemic vascular resistance. The consequent reduction in afterload promotes an increase in cardiac output. However, the patient becomes hypotensive despite the increase in cardiac output because of the disproportion between blood volume and the size of the vascular bed. Clinically, the patient presents with warm, flushed skin and hyperthermia ("warm" shock).

Hypodynamic shock, or the "cold" shock stage, is characterized by an increase in systemic vascular resistance, a reduction in cardiac output, and hypotension. Tissue perfusion is compromised and the patient presents clinically with cool, clammy skin and hypothermia ("cold" shock). Without timely and aggressive intervention, the patient rapidly decompensates and progresses to multisystem organ failure involving a disruption of cardiopulmonary, renal, and hepatic function. (For a detailed discussion and care plan for the patient with septic shock, see Chap. 66.)

## Hypovolemic Shock

Hypovolemic shock is characterized by a significant reduction in effective circulating intravascular volume relative to the vascular capacity. In the scenario of hemorrhagic shock (usually a blood loss of 15%–25%) a decrease in the oxygen-carrying capacity of the blood will also be experienced. (The remainder of this chapter will include an in-depth discussion of hypovolemic shock, its etiology, diagnosis, treatment, and nursing care.)

### *Etiology*

Hypovolemic shock reflects a depletion of extravascular fluid volume caused either directly or indirectly by a variety of conditions, including one or more of the following: (1) an actual decrease in blood volume (i.e., hemorrhagic shock) associated with bleeding related to trauma or with gastrointestinal bleeding; (2) a decrease in intravascular fluid volume associated with fever or profuse diaphoresis; gastrointestinal dysfunction, including a reduction in fluid intake, severe vomiting or continuous nasogastric suctioning, diarrhea, or fistula or wound drainage; (3) renal dysfunction (e.g., tubular damage with sodium and protein depletion, or overzealous use of diuretics); (4) endocrine dysfunction (e.g., diabetes insipidus); (5) hypoproteinemia, or reduction in plasma volume as occurs in severe burns; and (6) third-spacing (i.e., a shifting of fluid into transcellular spaces as occurs with ascites, pleural effusion, or intestinal obstruction with mobilization of fluid within the proximal intestinal lumen), thus depleting the intravascular volume (see Table 23–3).

### *Pathophysiology*

Hypovolemic shock occurs in stages, with progressive deterioration of essential body functions unless timely and aggressive interventions are instituted. In the *initial* stage of hypovolemic shock there is a decrease in venous return to the heart and cardiac output as a direct consequence of a reduction in circulating blood volume (usually less than 500 ml). While subtle changes may be occurring at the cellular level, there are no clearly evident clinical manifestations to suggest the presence of an underlying pathophysiologic process.

With the onset of the *compensatory* stage, the body responds to the fluid volume deficit via the activation of neural, hormonal, and chemical mechanisms in an attempt to restore cardiac output, mean arterial pressure, and tissue perfusion. The response of the nervous system occurs within seconds and is influenced by negative feedback control mechanisms. Signals from baroreceptors located in the aortic arch and carotid sinus trigger sympathetic outflow to the heart and vasculature. An increase occurs in heart rate and in myocardial contractility as well as in vascular tone.

Hormonal responses, also triggered at this time, function to restore intravascular fluid volume in several ways. Activation of the renin-angiotensin-aldosterone system stimulates the reabsorption of sodium in the distal renal tubules, and water reabsorption in the distal renal tubules and collecting ducts is facilitated by the secretion of antidiuretic hormone (see Figs. 21–9 and 21–10). Together, these 2 processes play a significant role in reestablishing and maintaining adequate intravascular fluid volume. Angiotensin II also functions to raise mean arterial blood pressure via its potent vasoconstrictor activity.

Chemoreceptors located in the aortic arch and

carotid bodies monitor concentrations of oxygen and carbon dioxide in circulating blood, as well as the pH of the blood, and send signals to the vital centers in the medulla. In the presence of reduced blood oxygen tensions, the central nervous system output results in an increase in the rate and depth of respirations, thereby increasing alveolar ventilation and raising the $PaO_2$ to within acceptable physiologic range.

If the underlying cause is not corrected, shock evolves into the *progressive* stage. In this stage, compensatory mechanisms progress to beyond being helpful and begin to fail in maintaining cardiac output. Vasoconstriction, which was so very important initially, when prolonged and severe, predisposes to adverse affects on cellular function, capillary dynamics, and overall systemic circulation.

**Disruption of Cellular Function.** With a significant reduction in circulating blood volume and oxygen delivery to the tissues, cells must utilize anaerobic metabolism, which predisposes to a state of metabolic acidosis. Mitochondrial activity becomes depressed, reducing stores of ATP and disrupting active transport mechanisms (e.g., Na/K-ATPase pump). Metabolism of carbohydrates, fats, and proteins likewise becomes depressed. Under these circumstances of altered metabolism, cellular lysosomal membranes become impaired, allowing release of various intracellular substances, such as enzymes, ions, and vasoactive agents, into the extracellular space. These substances, in turn, cause local damage to adjacent tissues and capillaries.

**Deterioration of the Microcirculation.** Localized pathophysiologic changes cause precapillary sphincters to relax, allowing the capillary bed to fill with blood. Postcapillary venules are less responsive to local metabolic changes and consequently offer resistance to the flow of blood out of the capillary bed. This results in stasis of blood within the capillary bed. As capillary hydrostatic pressure rises, fluid is forced out of the capillaries and into the interstitium. Concomitantly, the integrity of the capillary endothelium becomes impaired, allowing serum proteins and other molecules in blood to leak into the interstitial space. The shifting of fluid from the intravascular to the interstitial space (often referred to as third-spacing) results in a further reduction in circulating blood volume, and in the formation of peripheral edema.

As shock progresses to its *final* stage, the body's response to shock is characterized by severe acidemia/acidosis associated with impaired cellular function. Failure of the major organ systems (cardiovascular, pulmonary, renal, and hepatic) develops in conjunction with inadequate tissue perfusion, with consequent cellular ischemia and tissue necrosis. Disseminated intravascular coagulation (DIC) frequently occurs as a bleeding diathesis associated with depletion of clotting factors and thrombosis of the microcirculation. Death eventually ensues as a result of vasomotor failure and severely compromised cerebral perfusion.

### Diagnosis

The diagnosis of hypovolemic shock must be made swiftly and precisely so that appropriate and aggressive treatment may be initiated. The diagnosis is based on the clinical history, physical findings, laboratory data, and diagnostic studies, and efforts in this regard are undertaken after the patient's condition is sufficiently stabilized so that there is no imminent danger of ventilatory and/or circulatory compromise. Essential information to elicit during the early phase of treatment includes the time when the triggering event occurred, the circumstances surrounding the episode, the patient's status during the interval since the onset, and the patient's current physiologic, psychologic, and emotional state.

In the scenario of acute blood loss, regardless of the underlying cause, it is necessary to estimate the magnitude of the loss based on the patient's initial clinical presentation. Findings in this regard are listed in Table 49–1.

It is important to keep in mind that the normal blood volume in the average adult amounts to about 4–5 liters, of which RBCs constitute 45% of the volume and plasma constitutes 55%. Under normal conditions, about 75% of the total blood volume is contained within the low-pressure venous capacitant vessels, while only about 20% is contained within the arteries. Despite a large cross-sectional area, the maximal volume of blood in the capillaries at any given moment is about 5% of the total blood volume (see Chap. 37, Fig. 37–20).

The parameters most commonly assessed in the diagnosis of shock include blood pressure, urine output, acid–base status, and the degree of tissue perfusion.[2]

**Blood Pressure.** The components of the arterial blood pressure include the pulse pressure, the diastolic pressure, and the systolic pressure. The *pulse* pressure is the difference between the systolic and diastolic pressures and primarily reflects stroke volume and the capacitance of the aorta and larger arteries. The pulse pressure correlates quite well with changes in stroke volume. For example, if blood pressure changes from 120/80 mmHg to 120/100 mmHg, it is likely that the stroke volume has decreased by about 50%. The *diastolic* pressure largely reflects the degree of arteriolar vasoconstriction. The *systolic* pressure is determined by a combination of these factors (see Figs. 37–22 and 38–1).

In all cases of shock there is a decrease in mean arterial blood pressure. The pattern reflected by changes in these 3 components (i.e., pulse pressure, systolic pressure, and diastolic pressure) varies based on the underlying cause of the shock state. In hypovolemic shock, major decreases in stroke volume and pulse pressure may occur long before there is a significant fall in systolic pressure. The diastolic pressure may increase slightly in the early stage due to enhanced sympathoadrenal activity, and the pulse pressure is seen to narrow. These pressure findings, although subtle, may be an early indication of underlying hemodynamic changes. As the shock state progresses and the compensatory mechanisms become exceeded, both the systolic and diastolic pressures fall and the pulse pressure remains constant.

**Hemodynamic Parameters.** Early recognition and treatment of shock require a clinical assessment of the determinants of cardiac output, including heart rate, preload, afterload, and contractility. Assessment of these parameters assists in delineating the etiology of the shock state and provides baseline data that help both in determining initial therapy and evaluating the patient's response to therapy.

Heart rate is determined by simple auscultation of the heart. In patients with hypovolemic shock, a sinus tachycardia (greater than 120 beats/minute) is commonly experienced and largely reflects the body's attempt to compensate for the decrease in cardiac output. It is important to appreciate that as heart rate increases, the time available for left ventricular filling and coronary artery perfusion decreases.

In addition to changes in heart rate, patients with hypovolemic shock may experience dysrhythmias (especially premature ventricular contractions). This is especially so in patients with coronary artery disease who experience myocardial ischemia in response to tachycardia. Dysrhythmias may also be precipitated by severe metabolic derangements associated with acid–base imbalance and tissue hypoxia.

Preload reflects the venous return to the right heart and can usually be accurately determined by monitoring direct hemodynamic parameters, including central venous pressure (CVP), pulmonary artery pressure (PAP), and pulmonary capillary wedge pressure (PCWP). The PCWP most closely reflects left ventricular end-diastolic pressure in the presence of a functioning mitral valve. Since left ventricular end-diastolic volume reflects the preload of the left heart, monitoring the PCWP helps to assess how well the left heart is managing the volume presented to it. In the patient with hypovolemic shock, all of these parameters are decreased largely as a result of the decreased intravascular blood volume.

Afterload is reflected by the mean arterial blood pressure, and it may be normal to slightly elevated in the patient with hypovolemic shock due to extensive vasoconstriction. The systemic vascular resistance is a derived parameter reflective of the degree of vasoconstriction and is calculated as follows:

$$\text{SVR} = \frac{\text{MAP} - \text{CVP}}{\text{CO}} \times 80$$

where SVR is the systemic vascular resistance calculated in dynes/sec/cm$^{-5}$, MAP is the mean arterial blood pressure, CVP is the central venous pressure, and CO is the cardiac output.

Two additional derived parameters include:

*Cardiac output:*

$$\text{CO} = \text{stroke volume (SV)} \times \text{heart rate (HR)}$$

$$\left(\text{SV} = \frac{\text{CO}}{\text{HR}}\right)$$

*Cardiac index:*

$$\text{CI} = \frac{\text{CO}}{\text{body surface area}}$$

Contractility is more difficult to assess, but palpation of the heart at its point of maximal impulse (PMI) may provide some appreciation as to the heart's thrust.

**Urine Output and Composition.** In the scenario of shock, the renal system is not viewed as a vital organ. Consequently, regardless of its underlying cause, the presence of a shock state will cause blood to be shunted *away* from the kidneys to the heart and brain, resulting in *renal hypoperfusion.* This decrease in renal blood flow is reflected clinically by a prompt reduction in urine output. Since renal perfusion depends on the cardiac output, any alteration in this parameter will greatly influence urine output. Thus, if cardiac output falls precipitously, the consequent decrease in renal perfusion will be reflected by a corresponding precipitous fall in urine output.

With a gradual fall in cardiac output and renal perfusion, the *composition* of the urine may change prior to changes in urine output. Urine sodium concentration will often fall and urine osmolality may rise before there is any significant change in the urine output. The renal arterioles tend to constrict with any decrease in renal blood flow, thereby reducing glomerular filtration. In addition, blood flow tends to shift from the cortical nephrons to the juxtaglomerular nephrons, thereby further reducing glomerular filtration. The juxtaglomerular nephrons, because of their larger loops of Henle (see Fig. 21–2), are better able to conserve more water and sodium than the cortical nephrons, and the urine becomes more concentrated.

The decrease in renal perfusion also stimulates cells in the juxtaglomerular apparatus (see Fig. 21–8) to secrete renin, thereby initiating a series of reactions that culminates in the retention of even more sodium and water. In this way, the body tries to compensate for the decrease in cardiac output.

**Acid–Base Changes.** In the early stages of hypovolemic shock, the patient may present with a respiratory alkalemia associated with tachypnea (air hunger) and an increase in minute ventilation. Such findings are usually related to the degree of blood loss and/or the status of the intravascular volume relative to the vascular capacity. As shock progresses, local changes in cellular metabolism eventually result in the development of metabolic acidosis. Compromised oxygen delivery to the tissues causes cells to shift from aerobic to anaerobic metabolism, with the consequent production and accumulation of lactic acid.

In the early stage of hypovolemic shock, the acid–base abnormality can usually be corrected by improving tissue perfusion and oxygenation. Later in the course, treatment of the acidemia may require the administration of sodium bicarbonate.

**Tissue Perfusion.** Tissue perfusion can be evaluated by assessing the following parameters: skin changes, mentation, mixed venous oxygen saturation ($S\bar{v}O_2$), urine output, pulse pressure, and cardiac output. (Urine output and hemodynamic parameters are discussed above.)

***Skin Changes.*** Widespread peripheral vasoconstriction in response to intense sympathoadrenal stimulation causes the skin to appear pale and mottled, and cool to the touch. Increased sweat gland activity causes the skin to feel clammy and moist. These findings become apparent once the shock state is well established.

However, it should be appreciated that in shock complicated by sepsis the patient may present with skin that is relatively warm and dry, without apparent vasoconstriction. In the septic patient, the release of vasoactive substances in response to the endotoxin(s) underlies the vasodilatation (see Chap. 66).

***Mentation.*** The effectiveness of cerebral perfusion is reflected by the patient's demeanor and general cerebral functioning (e.g., mental status; orientation to person, time, and place). Reduced cerebral perfusion is exhibited by an altered level of consciousness, apathy, lethargy, confusion, or an increasingly cloudy sensorium. As the shock state deepens and coma ensues, the patient's response to pain may progress from flexion, to extension, to no response. Severe cerebral ischemia leads to depression of the vasomotor center and sympathetic activity. The loss of sympathetic tone causes the systemic vasculature to dilate, resulting in the pooling of blood in the periphery. This further reduces venous return to the heart and cardiac output.

***Mixed Venous Oxygen Saturation ($S\bar{v}O_2$).*** Trends in cardiac output and tissue perfusion can be evaluated by monitoring mixed venous oxygen saturation as obtained via the pulmonary artery catheter. Normally, the $S\bar{v}O_2$ is about 75%. A decrease of 5% or more may provide early warning of deteriorating cardiopulmonary function; less than 60% suggests compromised tissue perfusion or increased oxygen extraction/consumption by the tissues.

***Urine Output.*** If urine output and urine sodium concentrations are decreasing, and the urine osmolality is rising, this is usually indicative of renal hypoperfusion commonly associated with the hypovolemic state. A urine output less than 30 ml/hour is indicative of decreased renal perfusion, and thus decreased cardiac output.

**Diagnostic Tests/Studies.** In the scenario of shock or trauma, the principal diagnostic tests include radiographic and laboratory studies. A simple chest x-ray provides immediate information about intrathoracic injury. Pneumothorax, hemothorax, mediastinal or diaphragmatic injury, and rib fractures can usually be determined on chest x-ray. The chest x-ray is also helpful in determining underlying pulmonary congestion as exhibited by pulmonary infiltrates and lymphatic enlargement. Depending on the underlying condition and a high index of suspicion, other radiographic studies may be requested, including computed tomography (CT scan) and magnetic resonance imaging (MRI). Contrast imaging studies such as intravenous pyelography and angiography may also be requested.

Implementation of hemodynamic monitoring is invaluable both in determining the patient's hemodynamic status and in managing the shock state. As discussed previously, use of a pulmonary artery catheter facilitates assessment of left heart function and mixed venous oxygen saturation; central venous pressure measurements reflect venous return and right heart function. Arterial pressure monitoring enables ongoing assessment of mean arterial pressure; evaluation of the arterial pressure waveform; and, very importantly, blood sampling for arterial blood gases, hematology profile (CBC, hematocrit, hemoglobin), serum electrolytes, glucose, BUN and creatinine, and prothrombin and thromboplastin times.

### *Treatment and Management*

Basic resuscitative measures that may have to be implemented prior to determining the underlying problem include establishing and/or maintaining an airway to ensure adequate ventilation and oxygenation; correction of electrolyte abnormalities (e.g., hyperkalemia) and acidosis; treatment of obvious fluid volume deficit with rapid infusions of crystalloids, colloids, and blood/blood products; and initiation of pharmacologic therapy, titrated to maintain blood pressure at the desired level.

Once the underlying diagnosis is established, goals of therapy are directed toward the following: (1) reduction in anaerobic cellular metabolism with correction of consequent acidosis; (2) a reduction in intrapulmonary shunting and improved gas exchange as reflected by an increase in arterial oxygenation ($PaO_2$ >80 mmHg); (3) improvement in tissue perfusion with increased cerebral blood flow as determined by improvement in mental status and state of consciousness, increased renal perfusion as reflected by an increase in hourly urine outputs, and increased peripheral perfusion as reflected by pink, warm, dry skin; and (4) treatment of the underlying cause (e.g., gastrointestinal bleeding associated with peptic ulcer disease; thoracic, abdominal, or long bone trauma).

**Ventilation/Oxygenation.** Oxygen deprivation to the tissues is considered to be a major mechanism underlying the pathophysiology of the shock state. The inability to maintain tissue perfusion and oxygenation leads to metabolic acidosis and tissue hypoxia. Therefore, establishing and maintaining a patent airway with the necessary ventilation and oxygenation are of prime importance.

Patients in early shock can be observed to be hyperventilating and tachypneic, with a minute volume ($\dot{V}$) twice the normal and a $PaCO_2$ that usually ranges between 25–35 mmHg. These are anticipated compensatory responses to enhanced chemoreceptor stimulation in the presence of a lowered $PaO_2$, a raised $PaCO_2$, and a decreasing pH. If the patient in shock is not seen to be hyperventilating early in its course, the presence of a significant ventilatory problem should be considered and the need for ventilatory support determined. Indications for endotracheal intubation and implementation of ventilatory assistance in patients with shock are listed in Table 46–1.

In all patients in shock, including those in whom spontaneous ventilation is adequate, oxygen therapy should be administered during the initial 4–6 hours of the resuscitative period, to maintain a $PaO_2$ greater than 80 mmHg.

**Fluid Volume Replacement.** Timely and aggressive administration of fluids is by far the simplest and most effective treatment for the patient with hypovolemic shock. Fluid volume replacement helps to reestablish hemodynamic stability essential for adequate tissue perfusion, and administration of blood/blood products is necessary to assist in maintaining the oxygen-carrying capacity of the intravascular volume.

TABLE 46–1
**Criteria for Mechanical Ventilatory Assistance for Patients in Shock**

1. Minute ventilation less than 6–8 liters/minute (or greater than 15 liters/minute)
2. Tidal volume less than 4–5 ml/kg
3. Vital capacity less than 10–12 ml/kg
4. $PaCO_2$ greater than 45 mmHg if a metabolic acidosis is present or $PaCO_2$ greater than 50–55 mmHg with normal bicarbonate
5. $PaO_2$ less than 60 mmHg on 40% $O_2$ *or* $PaO_2$ less than 200 mmHg on 100% $O_2$
6. Respiratory rate greater than 35 per minute
7. Excessive ventilatory effort

(Adapted from Wilson, RF: Critical Care Manual, ed 2. FA Davis, Philadelphia, in preparation.)

***Crystalloids.*** Crystalloids include those solutions consisting of dextrose dissolved in water or electrolytes dissolved in water. If the goal is fluid volume expansion of both the intravascular and interstitial compartments, crystalloid solutions may be indicated. However, it is important to appreciate that approximately one fourth of the volume infused remains in the intravascular space, the remainder moving into the interstitial space. Therefore, if the goal is predominantly to expand the intravascular fluid volume, then these agents are not the solutions of choice. In addition, in the presence of altered capillary permeability, movement of the fluid into the interstitial compartment is enhanced and may predispose to peripheral edema.

Administration of 0.9% normal saline, an isotonic solution, may be indicated when extracellular fluid volume expansion is desired because it increases intravascular volume. It is necessary to cautiously monitor serum electrolytes during therapy because normal saline can disrupt serum electrolyte balance and predispose to hypernatremia, hypokalemia, and metabolic acidosis.

Administration of lactated Ringer's solution is especially indicated in the treatment of hypovolemic shock. In addition to volume replacement, this agent helps to buffer the acidosis since the lactate contained therein is converted to bicarbonate in the liver. In the presence of cardiac disease, half normal saline (0.45%) may be indicated because of its lower sodium content.

Dextrose in water ($D_5W$) is the solution of choice in hypovolemic shock and in states of severe dehydration because this solution is evenly distributed throughout the body. As is the case with all replacement fluid, serum electrolytes need to be closely monitored because such solutions tend to dilute serum concentrations of these molecules.

***Colloids.*** In contrast to crystalloids, the capillary endothelium is largely impermeable to colloids. Thus, these agents play a pivotal role in maintaining the osmotic pressure within the vascular space and are therefore ideal for intravascular fluid volume expansion in patients with hypovolemic shock. Colloid solutions of importance include albumin (available in 5% and 25%), hetastarch, and dextran. Hetastarch is similar to albumin in its plasma volume expansion capability, and its effect can last up to 36 hours. Dextran preparations are frequently used for rapid volume expansion. Use of these agents has been associated with coagulation and bleeding complications because they reduce platelet adhesiveness. Prothrombin time, partial thromboplastin time, and platelet count should be monitored.

***Blood/Blood Products.*** Replacement of blood

and blood products may be indicated in cases of hypovolemic shock associated with hemorrhage. For details related to assessment of the extent of blood loss and accompanying clinical manifestations, the reader is referred to Table 49-1. Available blood and blood products include fresh whole blood, stored whole blood, packed red cells, fresh-frozen red cells, platelet concentrate, fresh-frozen plasma, plasmanate, and cryoprecipitate. For details related to the constituents of each of these blood products, indications for administration, method of administration, advantages/disadvantages, complications, and nursing care considerations, the reader is referred to Table 49-2. Additionally, precautions to be taken in the actual administration of blood/blood products are identified in Table 49-3. The ultimate goal of blood replacement therapy is to keep the hematocrit at 30%-35%, and hemoglobin levels between 12.5 and 14.5 g/100 ml, depending on the needs of each patient.

***Artificial Blood.*** Two types of artificial blood currently being investigated include stroma-free hemoglobin (SFH) and fluorocarbons. The difficulty experienced with SFH is caused by its very high affinity for oxygen, thereby reducing the amount of oxygen released for use by the tissues. Fluosol-DA 20% (Flusol) has been used to treat life-threatening blood loss in patients who refused blood therapy for religious reasons. Complications of fever, leukocytosis, diffuse pulmonary infiltrates, and hypoxemia have been encountered in its use. While current use of artificial blood products is largely still investigational, there is the promise of conventional use of these products in the future.

**Pharmacologic Support.** The mainstay of treatment of the patient with hypovolemic shock is fluid volume replacement, with the type of fluid used (crystalloids, colloids, and/or blood and blood products) depending on the nature of the fluid loss. Use of vasopressors is usually contraindicated because of the intense vasoconstriction of the microcirculation associated with shock-induced enhanced sympathoadrenal activity. If fluid volume replacement therapy and the inherent sympathetic response are inadequate in maintaining blood pressure, a vasopressor such as dopamine may be prescribed. At low doses (1-2 $\mu$g/kg/minute), dopamine acts selectively on the peripheral vascular beds particularly in the renal and splanchnic areas, improving blood flow (*dopaminergic* effect). Its inotropic effect increases cardiac contractility and improves cardiac output.

Furosemide may be indicated if urine output does not increase with fluid volume replacement therapy. In severe acid-base disturbances (pH <7.20), sodium bicarbonate may be prescribed. It is important to administer sodium bicarbonate carefully so as not to overcorrect the acidosis and to avoid precipitating an alkalotic state. Patients who receive transfusions of stored whole blood may require calcium therapy because a reduction in serum ionized calcium may occur. Antiarrhythmic agents may be prescribed for patients experiencing dysrhythmias.

**Military Antishock Trousers (MAST).** The MAST is an external counterpressure device consisting of an inflatable unit with 3 chambers—an abdominal chamber and 2 leg chambers—each chamber inflating separately from the others. The MAST—also called the pneumatic antishock garment (PASG)—is a form of circulatory assistance and is particularly indicated in the scenario of severe hemorrhage and hypovolemic shock. The device assists in increasing arterial pressure in 2 ways: compression of vascular beds by the inflatable layers increases SVR; compression also redistributes blood flow from the peripheral circulation, making it available for the perfusion of vital organs.

In addition to stabilizing arterial blood pressure and redistributing blood flow to vital organs, the equipment has also been used as a tamponade to stop bleeding and as a splint for fractures of the pelvis or long bones of the lower extremities.

***Nursing Care Considerations.*** Key nursing considerations for the patient receiving treatment with the MAST device include careful monitoring of the patient's arterial blood pressure and respiratory function, and vigilant maintenance of the equipment to ensure optimal effect while minimizing complications. A baseline cardiopulmonary assessment should be performed prior to inflation of the device. Prior to inflation, it is useful to pad all bony prominences and pressure points. This helps to prevent an impairment in skin integrity. When applying the garment, it is important to avoid positioning it over the lower costal margins so as not to interfere with respiratory excursion. Sudden deflation must be avoided to prevent a precipitous fall in blood pressure. If the garment is to be used for a prolonged period it is useful to insert a nasogastric tube. Pressure on the abdominal viscera may cause vomiting, as well as defecation and urination. A Foley catheter is indicated.

While in use, the patient should be assessed for compartment syndrome reflected by pain, redness, swelling, and tenderness. Loss of peripheral pulses is an ominous sign. During the course of therapy the patient should also be monitored for signs of the need to discontinue counterpressure. This may be indicated by an adequate volume replacement or control of bleeding. When the therapy is to be discontinued, it must be done gradually, with sequential release of pressure in each compartment, beginning with the abdomen. Blood pressure should be monitored closely and volume replacement instituted immediately if the blood pressure drops by 5 mmHg. Subsequent deflation should proceed only if the patient remains hemodynamically stable.

## TABLE 46-2. CARE PLAN FOR THE PATIENT WITH HYPOVOLEMIC SHOCK

| Nursing Diagnoses | Desired Patient Outcomes | Nursing Interventions | Rationales |
|---|---|---|---|
| ***Nursing Diagnosis #1***<br>Tissue perfusion, alteration in: Cerebral, renal, and peripheral, related to:<br>1. Reduced circulating blood volume.<br>2. Fluid volume deficit. | Patient will maintain adequate tissue perfusion:<br>1. Arterial blood pressure within 10 mmHg of baseline.<br>2. Heart rate less than 100 beats/minute.<br>3. Mental status: Alert; oriented to person, time, and place.<br>4. Skin warm, dry to touch; usual color, good turgor, good capillary refill (<2 seconds).<br>5. Urinary output greater than 30 ml/hr.<br>6. Arterial blood gases within normal range:<br>• $PaO_2$ >80 mmHg<br>• $PaCO_2$ 35–45 mmHg<br>• $HCO_3$ 22–26 mEq/liter<br>• pH 7.35–7.45<br>7. $S\bar{v}O_2$ about 75%. | • Assess for signs/symptoms of hypovolemic shock: | • A baseline assessment is necessary to establish stage of shock and to determine emergent measures indicated; serves as a measure of the patient's response to therapy. |
| | | ◦ Assess cardiovascular function:<br>◦ Blood pressure (orthostatic). | ◦ A drop in blood pressure of 10–15 mmHg from supine to sitting/standing position suggests blood loss of about 1 liter (see Table 49–1). |
| | | ◦ Heart rate, rhythm. | ◦ Reflects effect of altered intravascular volume on cardiac function. |
| | | ◦ Resting peripheral pulses. | ◦ Peripheral pulses, if palpable, may be weak and thready due to decrease in stroke volume and peripheral vasoconstriction. |
| | | ◦ Skin color, moisture, temperature, and turgor. | ◦ When tissue perfusion is decreased, skin becomes cool and clammy to the touch and pale in color; cyanosis may occur if reduced hemoglobin concentration exceeds 5 g/100 ml. |
| | | ◦ Assess neurologic function:<br>– Mental status.<br>– Orientation. | ◦ Appropriateness of patient's behavior and responses reflects adequacy of cerebral tissue perfusion. |
| | | ◦ Assess renal function:<br>– Urine output.<br>– Intake and output. | ◦ Reduced circulating blood volume and hypotensive state compromise renal perfusion. Urine output is a reliable indicator of renal perfusion. |
| | | ◦ Assess gastrointestinal function:<br>– Bowel sounds, abdominal distention, pain. | ◦ Decrease in blood flow to splanchnic area depresses bowel motility and peristalsis. |
| ***Nursing Diagnosis #2***<br>Cardiac output, alteration in: Decreased, related to:<br>1. Decreased venous return (preload). | Patient will maintain stable hemodynamics:<br>1. Central venous pressure 0–8 mmHg.<br>2. Pulmonary artery pressure <25 mmHg (systolic).<br>3. Pulmonary capillary wedge pressure 8–12 mmHg.<br>4. Cardiac output 4–8 liters/minute.<br>5. Systemic vascular resistance (SVR) 800–1200 dynes/sec/$cm^{-5}$. | • Establish/maintain 1 or more large-gauge intravenous access sites. | • Rapid administration of fluids and fluid volume expanders and blood and blood products may be necessary to restore circulating blood volume. |
| | | • Initiate timely and aggressive fluid replacement therapy and monitor response to therapy:<br>◦ Administer crystalloids, colloids. | |
| | | ◦ Transfuse blood/blood products. | ◦ See Tables 49–2, 49–3, and 49–4 for nursing care considerations in blood/blood product administration. |

*(continued)*

**TABLE 46–2. CARE PLAN FOR THE PATIENT WITH HYPOVOLEMIC SHOCK *(Continued)***

| Nursing Diagnoses | Desired Patient Outcomes | Nursing Interventions | Rationales |
|---|---|---|---|
| ***Nursing Diagnosis #2 (cont.)*** | | • Initiate hemodynamic monitoring: Arterial, pulmonary artery, and pulmonary capillary wedge pressures. | • Insertion of systemic arterial and pulmonary artery catheters in the setting of massive hemorrhage and/or fluid loss with massive fluid volume replacement is essential to accurately follow trends and evaluate patient's response to therapy. |
| | | ○ Initiate monitoring of mixed venous blood ($S\bar{v}O_2$). | ○ Status of mixed venous blood reflects adequacy of peripheral tissue perfusion. |
| | | • Monitor hydration status during fluid replacement therapy:<br>○ Assess respiratory function:<br>– Respiratory rate, rhythm, chest excursion, breath sounds, use of accessory muscles; status of neck veins. | ○ Detection of adventitious breath sounds (crackles, rhonchi) in previously clear lungs suggests overhydration. |
| | | ○ Obtain daily weight.<br>○ Monitor intake and output. | ○ Most accurate measure of hydration status. |
| | | • Insert Foley catheter to measure hourly urine output. | • Hourly urine outputs reflect status of renal perfusion and underlying hemodynamic status. |
| | | • Insert nasogastric tube. | • Decompresses stomach to facilitate respiratory excursion and prevent aspiration of stomach contents, and affords means to monitor for gastrointestinal bleeding. (See Table 49–6.) |
| | | • Monitor hematology profile:<br>○ Hematocrit, hemoglobin, RBCs, platelets | • Reflects hemoglobin oxygen-carrying capacity; decrease in hemoglobin levels compromises oxygen delivery to tissues. |

| | | | |
|---|---|---|---|
| ***Nursing Diagnosis #3***<br>Anxiety, related to:<br>1. Hemorrhage.<br>2. Transfusion therapy.<br>3. Inherent sympatho-adrenal activity (enhanced).<br>4. ICU setting. | Patient will:<br>1. Verbalize feeling less anxious.<br>2. Demonstrate relaxed demeanor.<br>3. Perform relaxation techniques with assistance.<br>4. Verbalize familiarity with ICU setting. | • Assess signs/symptoms of anxiety:<br>◦ Restlessness, agitation, diaphoresis; tachypnea, tachycardia, palpitations; uncooperative or noncompliant behavior; verbalization of fears and concerns. | • Thorough assessment assists in discerning underlying cause of anxiety and provides a basis for therapy. Patients with hypovolemic shock may experience anxiety associated with massive sympathoadrenal output. |
| | | • Examine circumstances underlying anxiety. | • Removal of precipitating cause may reduce anxiety. |
| | | ◦ Manipulate ICU environment to provide calm, restful periods. | ◦ Reduction in stimuli is essential to assist patient to relax. This is especially important in the patient at risk of bleeding or rebleeding. |
| | | • Assess patient coping behaviors and their effectiveness in dealing with current stressors. | • Experiencing a bleeding episode can be very distressing. |
| | | ◦ Provide positive reinforcement when desired outcome is achieved. | ◦ Positive feedback and reassurance nurture self-confidence and confidence in health team. |
| | | • Initiate interventions to reduce anxiety:<br>◦ Relieve pain or other discomfort.<br>– Medication for pain; monitor response.<br>– Comfort measures. | ◦ Pain precipitates and/or aggravates anxiety. |
| | | ◦ Monitor effectiveness of ventilation and oxygenation.<br>◦ Serial arterial blood gases. | ◦ Inadequate gas exchange, "air hunger," hypoxemia, and/or hypercapnia may cause the patient to experience a "sense of doom." |
| | | ◦ Listen attentively, encourage verbalization, provide a caring touch. | ◦ These nursing activities reassure the patient that he/she is not alone. |
| | | ◦ Let the patient know it's okay to feel anxious and afraid.<br>◦ Remain with patient during periods of acute stress. | ◦ Reassurance helps patient to focus on feelings and to work them through. |
| | | • Assess readiness to learn and implement the following when appropriate: | • Readiness to learn facilitates meaningful learning and a sense of accomplishment. |
| | | ◦ Orient patient to environment, ICU equipment and routines, and staff.<br>– Explain all procedures and activities involving patient. | ◦ Knowing what to expect helps to reduce anxiety. |
| | | ◦ Involve patient in decision-making regarding care when possible and appropriate. | ◦ Helps patient to maintain some degree of control of health management. |
| | | ◦ Assist in establishing short-term goals and desired patient outcomes. | ◦ Builds and reinforces self-confidence. |
| | | ◦ Instruct patient in relaxation techniques when it is prudent to do so. | ◦ Use of energy-release techniques allows an outlet for pent-up feelings; enables patient to have some control over anxiety. |

*(continued)*

**TABLE 46–2. CARE PLAN FOR THE PATIENT WITH HYPOVOLEMIC SHOCK *(Continued)***

| Nursing Diagnoses | Desired Patient Outcomes | Nursing Interventions | Rationales |
|---|---|---|---|
| ***Nursing Diagnosis #4***<br>Fluid volume, alteration in, related to:<br>1. Hemorrhage.<br>2. Fluid shifts associated with loss of plasma proteins (hypoproteinemia, hypoalbuminemia). | Patient will:<br>1. Maintain body weight within 5% of baseline.<br>2. Balance fluid intake and output.<br>3. Exhibit good skin turgor, absence of peripheral edema, absence of jugular venous distention, absence of adventitious breath sounds.<br>4. Maintain serum electrolytes within normal limits. | • Maintain fluid and electrolyte balance.<br>◦ Administer prescribed fluid volume.<br>◦ Document intake and output, urine specific gravity.<br>◦ Record daily weight.<br>◦ Monitor serum electrolytes. | • Fluid therapy is the mainstay of treatment of hypovolemic shock to restore/maintain tissue perfusion.<br>◦ Close monitoring of urine output helps to evaluate renal perfusion and assess overall hemodynamics.<br>◦ Rapid and massive fluid volume replacement therapy can dilute electrolytes and precipitate electrolyte imbalance. |
| | | • Monitor hemodynamic parameters:<br>◦ Arterial blood pressure.<br>◦ Pulmonary artery pressure parameters.<br>◦ Central venous pressure.<br>◦ Cardiac output. | • These measures best reflect the patient's status and response to therapy. Rapid administration of crystalloids and colloids may precipitate fluid shift between extracellular and intracellular compartments. |
| | | • Implement nursing measures to improve and/or maintain cardiac output:<br>◦ Assist patient into positions of comfort that facilitate breathing.<br>– Head of bed elevated to 20–30 degrees. | ◦ Placing patient with hypovolemic shock into Trendelenburg's position (i.e., the legs higher than the head) may be of little value to hemodynamics or to improvement of cardiac output. Optimal ventilation/perfusion matching occurs in dependent areas of lungs. |
| | | ◦ Maximize patient activities in accordance with the acuity and limitations of the illness. | ◦ Nursing interventions are implemented to maximize circulation, prevent pooling or stasis of blood, ensure adequate venous return, and promote comfort. |
| | | ◦ Provide special care to back and to skin over joints and pressure points.<br>◦ Assist with passive range-of-motion exercises. | ◦ Compromised circulation in a patient with reduced tissue perfusion increases the risk of tissue ischemia and stasis of blood predisposing to venous thrombosis, and reduces venous return and cardiac output. |

## NURSING CARE OF THE PATIENT WITH HYPOVOLEMIC SHOCK

The immediate goal in the treatment of the patient with hypovolemic shock is to control bleeding (if present) and stabilize hemodynamic function. It is critical to restore an adequate intravascular volume so that tissue perfusion can be maintained and the metabolic needs of the cells fulfilled. In the patient with hypovolemic shock this is achieved by timely and aggressive fluid and/or blood replacement therapy.

It is essential to establish baseline assessment data when caring for the patient with hypovolemic shock. Such data are used to assess the patient's subsequent responses to treatment and to determine the effectiveness of that therapy in meeting the patient's desired outcomes. Identifying trends, or series of patient responses over time, is of greater clinical significance than any isolated responses.

### Therapeutic Goals

Implementation of the nursing process in the care of the patient with hypovolemic shock involves consideration of the following therapeutic goals:

1. Restore/maintain hemodynamic stability via fluid and blood replacement therapy to improve tissue perfusion.
2. Maintain adequate ventilation and oxygenation.
3. Restore/maintain fluid and electrolyte balance.
4. Reduce anxiety and apprehension.
5. Maintain therapeutic milieu with optimal rest and comfort to minimize bleeding or rebleeding.
6. Provide hydration and nutritional support to maintain ideal weight.
7. Prevent and/or monitor for complications of shock, including ARDS, acute renal failure, and DIC.
8. Prevent infection.
9. Provide emotional and psychologic support to patient and family.
10. Initiate activities to assist the patient in health management.

### Nursing Diagnoses, Desired Patient Outcomes, and Nursing Interventions

Pertinent nursing diagnoses, desired patient outcomes, nursing interventions, and their rationales are presented in Table 46–2, Care Plan for the Patient with Hypovolemic Shock. In addition, see Table 49–6, Care Plan for the Patient with Acute Upper Gastrointestinal Hemorrhage.

## REFERENCES

1. Sibbald, WJ: Synopsis of Critical Care, ed 2. Williams & Wilkins, Baltimore, 1984, p 34.
2. Wilson, RF: Critical Care Manual, ed 2. FA Davis, Philadelphia, in preparation.

## SELECTED READINGS

Ayres, S, Schlichtig, R, and Sterling, M: Care of the Critically Ill, ed 3. Year Book Medical Publishers, Chicago, 1988.

Chernow, B, and Roth, B: Pharmacologic manipulation of the peripheral vasculature in shock: Clinical and experimental approaches. Circulatory Shock 18:141, 1986.

Ledingham, IM and Ramsey, G: Hypovolemic shock. Br J Anaesth 58:169, 1986.

Maclean, LD: Shock: A century of progress. Ann Surg 201:407–414, 1985.

Perry, AC and Potter, PA: Shock: Comprehensive Nursing Management. CV Mosby, St Louis, 1983.

Rice, V: Shock management, Part I. Fluid volume replacement. Crit Care Nurse, 4:69–82, 1985.

Rice, V: Shock management, Part II. Pharmacologic intervention. Crit Care Nurse 5:42–47, 1985.

Sibbald, WJ: Synopsis of Critical Care, ed 3. Williams & Wilkins, Baltimore, 1989.

Whitman, GR: Tissue Perfusion, AACN's Clinical Reference for Critical-Care Nursing, ed 2. McGraw-Hill, New York, 1988.

# UNIT SIX

# Bibliography


Abela, GS, Seeger, JM, Barbieri, E, et al: Laser angioplasty with angioscopic guidance in humans. J Am Coll Cardiol 8(1):184–192, 1986.

Ahrens, WD, Kenney, MR, and Carter, R: The effect of antistasis footboard exercise on selected measures of exertion. Heart Lung 12:366, 1983.

Alpert, JS and Braunwald, E: Acute myocardial infarction: Pathologic, pathophysiologic, and clinical manifestations. In Braunwald, E: Heart Disease. WB Saunders, Philadelphia, 1984.

Andreoli, K, Zipes, D, Wallace, A, et al: Comprehensive Cardiac Care, ed 6. CV Mosby, St Louis, 1987.

Baggs, J: Nursing diagnosis: Potential sexual dysfunction after myocardial infarction. Dim Crit Care Nurs 5:178, 1986.

Bates, BA: A Guide to Physical Examination: The Clinical History, ed 4. JB Lippincott, Philadelphia, 1987.

Bedford, RF: Invasive blood pressure monitoring. In Blitt, C (ed): Monitoring in Anesthesia and Critical Care Medicine. Churchill-Livingstone, New York, 1986.

Bell, WR, Roberts, R, Ludbrook, PA, and Markis, JE: Efficacy of thrombolytic therapy for acute myocardial infarction: A round table discussion. Practical Cardiology 12(10):51–67, 1986.

Benumof, JL, Saidman, LJ, Arkin, DB, et al: Where pulmonary arterial catheters go: Intrathoracic distributions. Anesthesiology 46:336, 1977.

Berne, R and Levy, M: Cardiovascular Physiology, ed 5. CV Mosby, St Louis, 1986.

Berryhill, RE and Benumof, JL: PEEP-induced discrepancy between pulmonary arterial wedge pressure and left atrial pressure: The effects of controlled vs. spontaneous ventilation and compliant vs. noncompliant lungs in the dog. Anesthesiology 51:303, 1979.

Betriu, A, Costoner, A, Santz, GA, et al: Angiographic findings 1 month after myocardial infarction: A prospective study of 259 survivors. Circulation 65:1099, 1982.

Blomqvist, CG and Mitchell, JH: Heart disease and dynamic exercise testing. In Willerson, JT and Sanders, CA (eds): Clinical Cardiology. Grune & Stratton, New York, 1977.

Bolooki, H: Current status of circulatory support with an intraaortic balloon pump. Medical Instrumentation 20(5):226–276, 1986.

Borg, N, Nikas, D, Stark, J, and Williams, S (eds): Core Curriculum for Critical Care Nursing, ed 3. Philadelphia, WB Saunders, 1985.

Bouchard, RJ, Goult, JH, and Ross, J Jr: Evaluation of pulmonary arterial end-diastolic pressure as an estimate of left ventricular end-diastolic pressure in patients with normal and abnormal left ventricular performance. Circulation 44:1072, 1971.

Boutros, A and Albert, S: Effect of the dynamic response of transducer-tubing system on accuracy of direct blood pressure measurement in patients. Crit Care Med 11:1214, 1983.

Bramwell, L and Whall, A: Effect of role clarity and empathy on support role performance and anxiety. Nurs Res 35(5):282, 1986.

Brannon, PHB and Towner, SB: Ventricular failure: New therapy, using the mechanical assist device. Crit Care Nurse 6(2):76, 1986.

Braunwald, E: On the difference between the heart's output and its contractile state. Circulation 43:171, 1971.

Braunwald, E, Muller, JE, Kloner, RA, and Maroko, PR: Role of beta adrenergic blockade in the therapy of patients with myocardial infarction. Am J Med 74:113, 1983.

Bromberger-Barnea, B: Mechanical effects of inspiration on heart functions. A review. Fed Proc 40:2172, 1982.

Brown, AJ: Effect of family visits on the blood pressure and heart rate of patients in the coronary care unit. Heart Lung 5:291, 1976.

Brown, K and Jacobson, S: Mastering Dysrhythmias: A Problem-Solving Guide. FA Davis, Philadelphia, 1988.

Buja, LM and Willerson, JT: Clinicopathologic findings in 100 episodes of acute ischemic heart disease (acute myocardial infarction or coronary insufficiency) in 83 patients. Am J Cardiol 47:343, 1981.

Bullas, JB: Care of the patient on the percutaneous intra-aortic counterpulsation balloon. Crit Care Nurse, 2(4):40–48, July–August, 1982.

Cahill, M, DiCarlantonio, M, and Leibrandt, T: Diagnostics: Patient Preparation, Interpretation, Sources of Error, Post-Test Care. Intermed Communications. Horsham, PA, 1981.

Calvin, JE, Driedger, AA, and Sibbald, WJ: Does the pulmonary capillary wedge pressure predict left ventricular preload in critically ill patients? Crit Care Med 9:437, 1981.

Cavallo, GAO: The person with valvular heart disease. In Guzzetta, CE and Dossey, BM: Cardiovascular Nursing, Body Mind Tapestry. CV Mosby, St Louis, 1984.

Centers for Disease Control: Nosocomial bacteremia from intravascular pressure monitoring systems. In National Nosocomial Infections Study Report, 1977. US Dept of Health, Education and Welfare, Atlanta, 1979.

Chatterjee, K: Vasodilator therapy for heart failure. In Cohn, JN (ed): Drug Treatment of Heart Failure. Yorke Medical Books, New York, 1983.

Cohen, MV: The functional value of coronary collaterals in myocardial ischemia and therapeutic approach to enhance collateral flow. Am Heart J 95:396, 1978.

Cohn, PF: Clinical Cardiovascular Physiology. WB Saunders, Philadelphia, 1985.

Cohn, PF and Vokonas, PS: Pathophysiology of coronary artery

disease in humans. In Cohn, PF (ed): Diagnosis and Therapy of Coronary Artery Disease, ed 2. Martinus Nijhoff, Boston, 1985.
Cole, FL: The electrophysiology study. Crit Care Nurse 4:2, 1984.
Come, PC: Diagnostic Cardiology: Noninvasive Imaging Techniques. JB Lippincott, Philadelphia, 1985.
Connor, WE and Connor, SL: The key role of nutritional factors in the prevention of coronary heart disease. Prev Med 1:49, 1972.
Conover, M: Understanding Electrocardiography: Arrhythmias and the 12-Lead ECG, ed 5. CV Mosby, St Louis, 1988.
Crea, F, Davies, G, McKenna, W, et al: Percutaneous recanalization of coronary arteries. Lancet, pp 214–215, July 26, 1986.
Cumberland, DC, Oakley, GDG, Smith, GH, et al: Percutaneous laser-assisted coronary angioplasty. Lancet, p 214, July 26, 1986.
Daily, EK and Mersch, J: Comparison of Fick method with thermodilution method using two indicators. Heart Lung 16(3):294, May 1987.
Daily, EK and Schroeder, JS: Techniques in Bedside Hemodynamic Monitoring, ed 4. CV Mosby, St Louis, 1989.
Disposable pressure transducers. Health Devices 13:267, 1984.
Donat, WE and Weiner, BH: Syndromes of left ventricular failure. In Rippe, JM, Irwin, RS, Alpert, JS, and Dalen, E (eds): Intensive Care Medicine. Little, Brown & Co, Boston, 1985.
Dortimer, AC, Sheony, PN, Shiroff, RA, et al: Diffuse coronary artery disease in diabetic patients: Fact or fiction? Circulation 57:133, 1978.
Dossey, BM: The person with heart failure. In Guzzetta, CE and Dossey, BM: Cardiovascular Nursing, Body Mind Tapestry. CV Mosby, St Louis, 1984.
Dossey, BM: The person with cardiomyopathy or myocarditis. In Guzzetta, CE and Dossey, BM: Cardiovascular Nursing, Body Mind Tapestry. CV Mosby, St Louis, 1984.
Ellis, DM: Interpretation of beat-to-beat blood pressure values in the presence of ventilatory changes. J Clin Monitoring 1:65, 1985.
Fabsitz, R and Feinleib, M: Geographic patterns in county mortality rates from cardiovascular diseases. Am J Epidemiol 111:325, 1980.
Fegler, G: Measurement of cardiac output in an anesthetized animal by the thermodilution method. Q J Exp Physiol 39:153, 1954.
Feinleib, M and Williams, RR: Relative risks of myocardial infarction, cardiovascular disease and peripheral vascular disease by type of smoking. Proc Third World Conf Smoking and Health I:243, 1976.
Fisher, JR and Sieves, ML: Ear-lobe crease in American Indians. Ann Intern Med 93:51;2, 1980.
Forrester, JS, Diamond, G, Chattejee, K, and Swan, HJC: Medical therapy of acute myocardial infarction by application of hemodynamic subsets (first of two parts). N Engl J Med 295:1356, 1976.
Forrester, JS, Diamond, G, Chattejee, K, and Swan, HJC: Medical therapy of acute myocardial infarction by application of hemodynamic subsets (second of two parts). N Engl J Med 295:1404, 1976.
Friedman, H and Rosenman, RH: Type A Behavior and Your Heart. Alfred A Knopf, New York, 1974.
Ganz, W, Donoso, R, Marcus, H, et al: Coronary hemodynamics and myocardial oxygen metabolism during oxygen breathing in patients with and without coronary artery disease. Circulation 45:763, 1972.
Gardner, RM: Direct blood pressure measurement: Dynamic response requirements. Anesthesiology 54:227, 1981.
Gardner, RM and Hollingsworth, KW: Optimizing the electrocardiogram and pressure monitoring. Crit Care Med 14(7):651, 1986.
Gawlinski, A: Diet therapy in heart failure. In Michaelson, CR (ed): Congestive Heart Failure. CV Mosby, St Louis, 1983.
Gobel, FL, Nordstrom, LA, Nelson, RR, et al: The rate-pressure product as an index of myocardial oxygen consumption during exercise in patients with angina pectoris. Circulation 57:549, 1978.
Goldberger, AL and Goldberger, E: Clinical Electrocardiography: A Simplified Approach, ed 3. CV Mosby, St Louis, 1986.
Goldberger, E: Textbook of Clinical Cardiology. CV Mosby, St. Louis, 1981.
Goldsmith, MF: Laser angioplasty: Progressing, but opinions, forecasts vary. JAMA 250(23):1522–1538, 1985.
Golman, M: Principles of Clinical Electrocardiography. Lange Medical Publishers, Los Altos, CA, 1986.
Gordon, T, Ernst, N, Fisher, M, et al: Alcohol and high-density lipoprotein cholesterol. Circulation 64(Suppl III):III-63, 1981.
Gordon, T, Kannel, WB, McGree, D, et al: Death and coronary attacks in men after giving up cigarette smoking. A report from the Framingham Study. Lancet 2:1435, 1974.
Gould, LK, Lipscomb, K, and Calvert, C: Compensatory changes of the distal coronary vascular bed during progressive coronary artery occlusion. Circulation 51:1085, 1975.
Grady, KL: Evolution of a cardiac transplantation program: Role of the clinical nurse specialist. Focus on Critical Care 16(2):130, April, 1989.
Gunby, P: "Poof" goes the plaque with experimental laser angioplasty. JAMA 250(23):3135–3141, 1983.
Guyton, AC: Textbook of Medical Physiology, ed 7. WB Saunders, 1986.
Haak, SW: Intra-aortic balloon pump techniques. Dim Crit Care Nurs 2(4):196–204, 1983.
Hachett, TP, Cassem, NH, and Wishnie, H: Psychological hazards of coronary care units. N Engl J Med 297:1365, 1968.
Hales, S: Statistical Essays: Hemostaticks, vol 2, ed 3. London, W. Innys and R. Manby, 1978.
Hamilton, HK (ed): Nurses' Clinical Library: Cardiovascular Disorders. Springhouse, Springhouse, PA, 1984.
Haughey, CW: Preparing your patient for echocardiography. Nursing '84 14:5, 1984.
Haynes, SG, Feinleib, M, and Kannell, WB: The relationship of psychosocial factors to coronary heart disease in the Framingham Study: III. Eight-year incidence of coronary heart disease. Am J Epidemiol 111:37, 1980.
Haywood, DL: Temporary AV sequential pacing using epicardial lead system. Crit Care Nurse 5(3):21–29, 1985.
Heberden, W: Some account of a disorder of the breast. Med Trans R Coll Physicians (London) 2:59, 1772.
Herold, P and Kinsella, J: Fish oil consumption and decreased risk of cardiovascular disease: A comparison of findings from animal and human feeding trials. Am J Clin Nutr 43:566, 1986.
Hudak, CM, Gallo, BM, and Lohr, TS: Critical Care Nursing: A Holistic Approach, ed 4. JB Lippincott, Philadelphia, 1986.
Hurst, JS: The Heart: Arteries and Veins. McGraw-Hill, New York, 1982.
Iberti, TJ, Benjamin, E, Gruppi, L, and Raskin JM: Ventricular arrhythmias during pulmonary artery catheterization in the intensive care unit. Am J Med 78:451, 1985.
Jaquith, SM: Continuous measurement of $SVO_2$: Clinical applications and advantages for critical nursing. Crit Care Nurse 5:40, 1985.
Johanson, BC, Dungca, CU, Hoffmeister, D, et al: Standards for critical care, ed 3. CV Mosby, St Louis, 1988.
Johnston, BL: Exercise testing for patients after myocardial infarction and coronary by-pass surgery: Emphasis of pre-discharge phase. Heart Lung 13:1, 1984.
Johnston, BL, Watt, EW, and Fletcher, CF: Oxygen consumption and hemodynamic and electrocardiographic responses to bathing in recent post-myocardial infarction patients. Heart Lung 10:666, 1981.
Johnston, WE, Prough, DS, Royster, RL, et al: Short-term sterility of the pulmonary artery catheter inserted through an external plastic shield. Anesthesiology 61(4):461, October 1984.
Kadota, LT: Reproducibility of thermodilution cardiac output measurements. Heart Lung 15:168, 1986.
Kannel, WB: Role of blood pressure in cardiovascular disease: The Framingham Study. Angiology 26:1, 1975.
Kannel, WB: Role of blood pressure in cardiovascular morbidity and mortality. Prog Cardiovasc Dis 17:5, 1974.

Kannel, WB, Hjortland, MC, McNamara, PM, et al: Menopause and risk of cardiovascular disease: The Framingham Study. Ann Intern Med 85:447, 1976.

Kannel, WB, McGree, D, Gordon, T, et al: A general cardiovascular risk profile: The Framingham Study. Am J Cardiol 38:46, 1976.

Kannel, WB and Sorlee, PD: Some health benefits of physical activity: The Framingham Study. Arch Intern Med 139:857, 1979.

Keefer, JR and Barash, PG: Pulmonary artery catheterization. In Blitt, C (ed): Monitoring in Anesthesia and Critical Care Medicine. Churchill-Livingstone, New York, 1986.

Kelly, J, Braverman, B, Land, PC, and Ivankovich, AD: Comparison of Allen test, Doppler and finger-pulse transducer to assess patency of ulnar artery. Anesthesiology 59(Suppl):A178, 1983.

Kenner, CV, Guzzetta, CE, and Dossey, BM: Critical Care Nursing: Body-Mind-Spirit, ed 2. Little, Brown, & Co, Boston, 1985.

King, EG: Influence of mechanical ventilation and pulmonary disease on pulmonary artery pressure monitoring. Can Med Assoc J 121:901, 1979.

King, KB: Measurement of coping strategies, concerns and emotional response in patients undergoing coronary artery bypass grafting. Heart Lung 14:6, 1985.

Kirchoff, KT: An examination of the physiologic basis for "coronary precautions." Heart Lung 10:874, 1981.

Kirchoff, KT: Visiting policies for patients with myocardial infarction: A national survey. Heart Lung 11:571, 1982.

Kreeten, CK and Baas, L: Valvular heart disease: Surgery and post-op care. RN 50:12, 1987.

Kronick-Mest, C: Postpericardiotony syndrome: Etiology, manifestations, and interventions. Heart Lung 18(2):192, March, 1989.

Labrousse, J, Tenaillon, A, and Lissac, J: Influence of artificial ventilation on the pulmonary capillary wedge pressure. Chest 74:693, 1978.

Lee, G, Chan, MC, Ikeda, RM, et al: Applicability of laser to assist coronary balloon angioplasty. Am Heart 110(6):1233–1236, 1985.

Levy, RI and Gluech, CJ: Hypertriglyceridemia, diabetes mellitus and coronary vessel disease. Arch Intern Med 123:220, 1969.

Lewis, SM and Collier, IC: Medical-Surgical Nursing: Assessment and Management of a Clinical Problem. McGraw-Hill, New York, 1983.

Lichstein, E, Chapman, I, Gupta, PK, et al: Diagonal ear lobe crease and coronary artery sclerosis. Ann Intern Med 85:337, 1976.

Little, JA, Birchwood, BL, Simmons, DA, et al: Interrelationship between the kinds of dietary carbohydrate and fat in hyperlipoproteinemic patients. Atherosclerosis 11:173, 1970.

Loeb, JM: Cardiac electrophysiology: Basic concepts and arrhythmogenesis. Crit Care Q 7:1, 1984.

Lowenstein, E, Little, JW, and Lo, HH: Prevention of cerebral embolization from flushing radial-artery cannulas. N Engl J Med 285:1414, 1971.

Madias, JE and Hood, WB, Jr: Reduction of precordial ST-segment elevation in patients with anterior myocardial infarction by oxygen breathing. Circulation 53(Suppl 1):1–198, 1976.

Maroko, PR, Radvany, P, Braunwald, E, et al: Reduction in infarct size by oxygen inhalation following acute coronary occlusion. Circulation 52:360, 1975.

Marriott, H: Practical Electrocardiography, ed 8. Williams & Wilkins, Baltimore, 1988.

Marriott, H and Conover, M: Advanced Concepts in Arrhythmias, ed 2. CV Mosby, St Louis, 1989.

Mathewson, M and Dusek, JL: DC countershock does not harm today's internal pacemakers. Crit Care Nurse, 4(2):48, March/April, 1984.

McIntyre, KM, Lewis, AJ, Parker, MR, et al: Myocardial infarction. In Textbook of Advanced Cardiac Life Support. American Heart Association, Dallas, 1983.

McMihan, JC: Continuous monitoring of mixed venous oxygen saturation. In Schweiss, JF (ed): Continuous Measurement of Blood Oxygen Saturation in the High Risk Patient, vol 1. Beach International, San Diego, 1983.

Michaelson, CR: Pathophysiology of heart failure: A conceptual framework for understanding clinical indicators and therapeutic modalities. In Michaelson, CR (ed): Congestive Heart Failure. CV Mosby, St Louis, 1983.

Michaelson, EL, Morganroth, J, Nichols, CW, et al: Retinal arteriolar changes as an indicator of coronary artery disease. Arch Intern Med 139:1139, 1979.

Miller, MJ: Tissue oxygenation in clinical medicine: An historical review. Anesth Analg 61:527, 1982.

Mueller, H, et al: Trans NY Acad Sci (Series II) 34(4):309, 1972.

Neufeld, HN and Goldourt, U: Coronary heart disease: Genetic aspects. Circulation 67:943, 1983.

Nicklin, WM: Postdischarge concerns of cardiac patients as presented via a telephone callback system. Heart Lung 15:3, 1986.

Niles, NA and Wills, RE: Heart Failure. In Underhill, SL, Woods, SL, Sivarajan, ES, and Halpenny, CJ: Cardiovascular Nursing, ed 2. JB Lippincott, Philadelphia, 1988.

Oliva, PB: Unstable rest angina with ST-segment depression: Pathophysiologic considerations and therapeutic implications. Ann Intern Med 100:424, 1984.

Painvin, GA, Frazier, OH, Chandler, LB, et al: Cardiac transplantation: Indications, procurement, operation and management. Heart Lung 14:5, 1985.

Parry, CH: An Inquiry into the Symptoms and Causes of the Syncope Anginosa, Commonly Called Angina Pectoris, Vols 3 and 4. R. Cuttwell, Bath, England, 1799.

Partamian, JO and Bradley, RF: Acute myocardial infarction in 258 cases of diabetes: Immediate mortality and five year survival. N Engl J Med 273:455, 1975.

Phibbs, B and Marriott, HJL: Complications of permanent transvenous pacing. N Engl J Med 342(22):1428–1432, 1985.

Prinzmetal, M, Kennamer, R, Merliss, R, et al: A variant form of angina pectoris. Am J Med 27:375, 1959.

Puksta, NS: All about sex . . . after a coronary. Am J Nurs 77:602, 1977.

Pura, LS and Sam, CS: Underlying causes and precipitating factors in heart failure. In Michaelson, CR (ed): Congestive Heart Failure. CV Mosby, St Louis, 1983.

Purcell, JA and Burrows, SG: Pacemakers. Am J Nurs 85(5):554, May 1985.

Purcell, JS, Pippin, L, and Mitchell, M: IABP therapy. Am J Nurs 83(5):776, May 1983.

Quaal, S: A study of fitness and cardiovascular risk factors in male office workers. West J Nurs Res Summer:9, 1981.

Rake, RH, Romo, M, Bennett, L, et al: Recent life changes, myocardial infarction, and abrupt coronary death. Arch Intern Med 133:221, 1974.

Reeder, GS, and Vliestra, RE: Coronary angioplasty: 1986. Mod Conc Cardiovasc Dis 50(10):49–53, 1986.

Resnekov, L: Cardiogenic shock. Chest 83:893, 1983.

Ridolfi, RL and Hutchins, GM: The relationship between coronary artery lesions and myocardial infarcts: Ulceration of atherosclerotic plaques precipitating coronary thrombosis. Am Heart J 93:468, 1977.

Riegel, BJ: The role of the nurse in limiting myocardial infarct size. Heart Lung 14:247, 1985.

Riley, CP, Russell, RO, Jr, and Rachey, CE: Left ventricular gallop sound and acute myocardial infarction. Am Heart J 86:598, 1973.

Rippe, JM and Howe, JP: Acute mitral regurgitation. In Rippe, JM, Irwin, RS, Alpert, JS, and Dalen, JG (eds): Intensive Care Medicine. Little, Brown & Co, Boston, 1985.

Robinson, BF: Relation of heart rate and systolic blood pressure to the onset of pain in angina pectoris. Circulation 35:1073, 1967.

Rogot, E and Padgett, SJ: Association of coronary and stroke mortality with temperature and snowfall in selected areas of the United States, 1962–1966. Am J Epidemiol 103:565, 1976.

Rosenman, RH, Brand, RJ, Sholtz, RI, et al: Multivariate prediction of coronary heart disease during 8.5 year follow-up in the

Western Collaborative Group Study. Am J Cardiol 37:903, 1976.

Ross, J, Jr, Frahn, CJ, and Braunwald, E: The influence of intracardiac baroreceptors on venous return, systemic vascular volume, and peripheral resistance. J Clin Invest 40:563–572, 1962.

Royle, J: Coronary patients and their families receive incomplete care. Canadian Nurse 69:2:21, 1973.

Sabetti, K: Distinguishing between ectopic ventricular activity and aberrant ventricular conduction of supraventricular impulses. Heart Lung 8(5):945, 1979.

Sadler, D: Nursing for Cardiovascular Health. Appleton-Century-Crofts, Norwalk, CT, 1984.

Schamroth, L: An Introduction to Electrocardiography. Blackwell Scientific Publications, St Louis, 1976.

Scharf, SM, Brown, R, Saunders, N, et al: Effects of normal and loaded spontaneous inspiration on cardiovascular function. J Appl Physiol 47(3):582, 1979.

Scott, WAC: Haemodynamic monitoring measurement of systemic blood pressure. Can Anaesth Soc J 32(3):294, 1985.

Shah, PM: Cardiomyopathies. In Shine, KI: Cardiology. John Wiley & Sons, New York, 1983, p 85.

Shasby, DM, et al: Swan-Ganz catheter location and left atrial pressure when positive end-expiratory pressure is used. Chest 80:666, 1981.

Shellock, FG and Reidinger, MS: Reproducibility and accuracy of using room temperature vs. ice temperature for thermodilution cardiac output determination. Heart Lung 12:175, 1983.

Shillinger, FL: Percutaneous transluminal angioplasty. Heart Lung 12(1):45–51, 1983.

Sise, MJ, Hollingsworth, P, and Brimm, JE: Complications of the flow-directed pulmonary artery catheter: A prospective analysis in 219 patients. Crit Care Med 9:315, 1981.

Slusarczyk, SM and Hicks, FD: Helping your patient live with a permanent pacemaker. Nursing '83 13:58–63, April, 1983.

Smith, A: Physiology, diagnosis, and life-style modifications for hyperlipidemia. J Cardiovasc Nurs 1(4):15, 1985.

Spielman, SR: New advances in cardiac pacemaking. In Hakki, AH (ed): Ideal Cardiac Pacing. WB Saunders, Philadelphia, 1984, pp 219–261.

Stetz, CS, Miller, RG, Kelly, GE, and Raffin, TA: Reliability of the thermodilution method in determination of cardiac output in clinical practice. Am Rev Respir Dis 126:1001, 1982.

Stokes, J III, Noren, J, and Shindell, S: Definition of terms and concepts applicable to clinical preventive medicine. J Commun Health 8:33, 1982.

Strauss, E and Rudy, EB: Tissue-plasminogen activator: A new drug in reperfusion therapy. Crit Care Nurse 6(3):30–41, 1986.

Sukamalchantra, Y, Levy, S, Danzig, R, et al: Correcting arterial hypoxemia by oxygen therapy in patients with acute myocardial infarction. Effect on ventilation and hemodynamics. Am J Cardiol 24:838, 1969.

Swan, HJC, Ganz, W, and Forrester, JS: Catheterization of the heart in man with the use of a flow-directed balloon-tipped catheter. N Engl J Med 283:447, 1970.

Taormina Paplanus, LM, Strebel, CA, and Michaelson, CR: Drug therapy for congestive heart failure. CV Mosby, St Louis, 1983.

The ISAM Study Group: A prospective trial of intravenous streptokinase in acute myocardial infarction (I.S.A.M.). N Engl J Med 314(23):1465–1471, 1986.

Thomas, SA, Sappington, E, Gross, HS, et al: Denial in coronary care patients—an objective assessment. Heart Lung 12:74, 1983.

Tilkian, AG and Daily, EK: Cardiovascular Procedures: Diagnostic Techniques and Therapeutic Procedures. CV Mosby, St Louis, 1986.

Tooker, J, Huseby, J, and Butler, J: The effect of Swan-Ganz catheter height on the wedge pressure relationship in edema during positive-pressure ventilation. Am Rev Respir Dis 117:721, 1978.

Torp, A: Incidence of congestive cardiomyopathies. Postgrad Med J 54:435, 1978.

Tyndall, A: A nursing perspective of the invasive electrophysiologic approach to treatment of ventricular arrhythmias. Heart Lung 12:6, 1983.

Ventura, B: What you need to know about cardiac catheterization. RN 47:9, 1984.

Walls, JJ, Lababidi, Z, Curtis, JJ, and Silver, D: Assessment of percutaneous balloon pulmonary and aortic valvuloplasty. J Thorac Cardiovasc Surg 88:352–356, 1984.

Walston, A and Kendall, ME: Comparison of pulmonary wedge and left atrial pressure in man. Am Heart J 86:159, 1973.

Walter, BF, Palumbo, PJ, Lee, JT, et al: Status of the coronary arteries at necroscopy in diabetes mellitus with onset after 30 years: Analysis of 229 diabetic patients with and without clinical evidence of coronary heart disease and comparison to 183 control subjects. Am J Med 69:498, 1980.

Webster, H: Hemodynamic monitoring in children. In Daily, EK and Schroeder, JS: Techniques in Bedside Hemodynamic Monitoring. CV Mosby, St Louis, 1985.

Weiland, AP: A review of cardiac valve prostheses and their selection. Heart Lung 12:5, 1983.

Whalley, DG: Haemodynamic monitoring: Pulmonary artery catheterization. Can Anaesth Soc J 32:1299, 1985.

White, KM: Completing the hemodynamic picture: $SVO_2$. Heart Lung 14:272, 1985.

Whitman, G: Intra-aortic balloon pumping and cardiac mechanics: A programmed lesson. Heart Lung 7(6):1034–1050, 1978.

Wilson, JN: Central venous pressure in optimum blood volume maintenance. Arch Surg 85:563, 1962.

Wilson, RF: Critical Care Manual. FA Davis, Philadelphia, in preparation.

Wingate, S: Dilated Cardiomyopathy, Part I. Focus II(4):49–56, 1984.

Winslow, EH: Cardiovascular consequences of bed rest. Heart Lung 14:236, 1985.

Winters, WL and Cashion, WR: Imaging techniques in patients with acute myocardial infarction. Heart Lung 14:3, 1985.

Wray, R, Maurer, B, and Shillingford, J: Prophylactic anticoagulation therapy in the prevention of calf vein thrombosis after myocardial infarction. N Engl J Med 288:815, 1973.

Yacone, L: Cardiac diagnostic studies: Nuclear scanning and cardiac catheterization. RN 47:5, 1984.

Young, L: Coronary artery bypass surgery: Commonplace yet complicated. Crit Care Nurse pp 15–22, November/December, 1981.

Yu, PN, Bielski, MT, Edwards, A, et al: Report of inter-society commissions for heart disease resources: Resources for the optimal care of patients with acute myocardial infarction. Circulation 43:A-171, 1971.

Zochoche, DA (ed): Mosby's Comprehensive Review of Critical Care, ed 3. CV Mosby, St Louis, 1986.

UNIT SEVEN

# Gastrointestinal System

Maintenance of the life processes of the human body in an equilibrated state requires energy. The source of this energy is the food we eat. Such food taken into the body must be broken down into a suitable form for digestion and absorption. It is the role of the gastrointestinal system to perform these functions and to facilitate movement of energy-containing nutrients into the circulation for transport to the cells.

The significance of the gastrointestinal system is reflected by the fact that a large population of patients present clinically with symptoms of gastrointestinal dysfunction. Common symptoms such as anorexia, nausea, vomiting, heartburn, indigestion, abdominal discomfort, constipation, and diarrhea may be indicative of underlying gastrointestinal disease or may be associated with a disease process involving another organ system. Often, symptoms of gastrointestinal dysfunction occur in conjunction with the treatment regimen for an unrelated disorder, as, for example, use of chemotherapeutic agents to treat cancer.

The following chapters examine the functional structure of the gastrointestinal system, identify key aspects of the gastrointestinal assessment, and investigate specific pathophysiologic states. These include upper gastrointestinal bleeding (acute hemorrhagic, hypovolemic shock), hepatic failure, pancreatitis, and inflammatory bowel disease. Nutritional support of the critically ill patient is addressed.

Nursing process in the diagnosis and management of the patient with gastrointestinal dysfunction is explored, including the use of pertinent nursing diagnosis. Nursing care plans are based on nursing diagnosis and include specific patient outcomes and nursing interventions.

## UNIT OUTLINE

## UNIT OUTLINE—*CONTINUED*

CHAPTER 47

# Anatomy and Physiology of the Gastrointestinal System

## CHAPTER OUTLINE



## LEARNING OBJECTIVES

**At the end of this chapter, you should be able to:**

1. Describe the microstructure of the gastrointestinal tract.
2. Identify the mechanisms underlying gastrointestinal motility and its functional significance.
3. Describe the mechanisms underlying digestion, absorption, and assimilation of ingested foodstuffs.
4. Define the neural and hormonal control and regulation of gastrointestinal functions.
5. Describe the functional anatomy of the upper and lower gastrointestinal tract.
6. Contrast secretory functions of stomach, small and large intestines.
7. Differentiate digestive and absorptive pathways for the major nutrients.
8. Describe the microstructure of the liver and exocrine pancreas.
9. Define the significance of the dual blood supply to the liver.
10. List the major functions of the liver and exocrine pancreas.

The major processes by which the gastrointestinal system functions to prepare nutrients for energy use by the cells include digestion and absorption. Digestion is the preparation of ingested foods for use by the body and involves a number of physiologic activities including mastication (chewing), deglutition (swallowing), gastrointestinal motility, and secretion of various enzymes and hormones. Absorption involves the actual movement of digestive nutrients, vitamins, and minerals from the gastrointestinal tract into the bloodstream, which transports these substances throughout the body, making them available to cells for their metabolic activities.

## GASTROINTESTINAL TRACT—BASIC CONSIDERATIONS

The gastrointestinal tract consists of a tube that extends from the mouth to the anus and includes the oropharynx, esophagus, stomach, small and large intestines (Fig. 47–1). Each part of this tube is adapted for specific functions. In the mouth, chewing effectively breaks up large food particles and mixes these chewed particles with salivary secretions. The esophagus acts as a conduit of food from the oral cavity to the stomach; the stomach and colon act as storage chambers for food and end-products of digestion, respectively. The stomach and the entire small intestine are involved in the actual processes of digestion and absorption. The colon also functions in a limited but highly significant absorptive capacity.

The salivary glands, pancreas, liver, and gallbladder are accessory organs of the gastrointestinal system. They empty their secretions directly into the lumen of the gastrointestinal tract at specific points.

## Microstructure of the Gastrointestinal Tract

The overall microstructure of the gastrointestinal tract consists of 4 distinct layers of tissues. Proceeding from the lumen outward, they include the mucosa, submucosa, muscularis externa (circular and longitudinal smooth muscle layers), and the serosa. Structural modifications of these layers occur in different parts of the gastrointestinal tract depending on the underlying function (e.g., transfer, digestion, absorption, storage).

### *Mucosa*

The mucosa consists of the innermost lining of epithelial cells and a mucosal layer, the lamina propria, which consists of loose connective tissue and a fine network of elastic fibers, which afford distensibility and provide structural support. Blood vessels contained within the lamina propria nourish the epithelial layer and serve as conduits for water-soluble substances absorbed by the epithelial cells.

### *Submucosa*

The submucosa consists of areolar connective tissue, elastic fibers, blood vessels, which receive the absorbed nutrients from the intestinal lumen, and a network of nerve fibers, Meissner's plexuses.

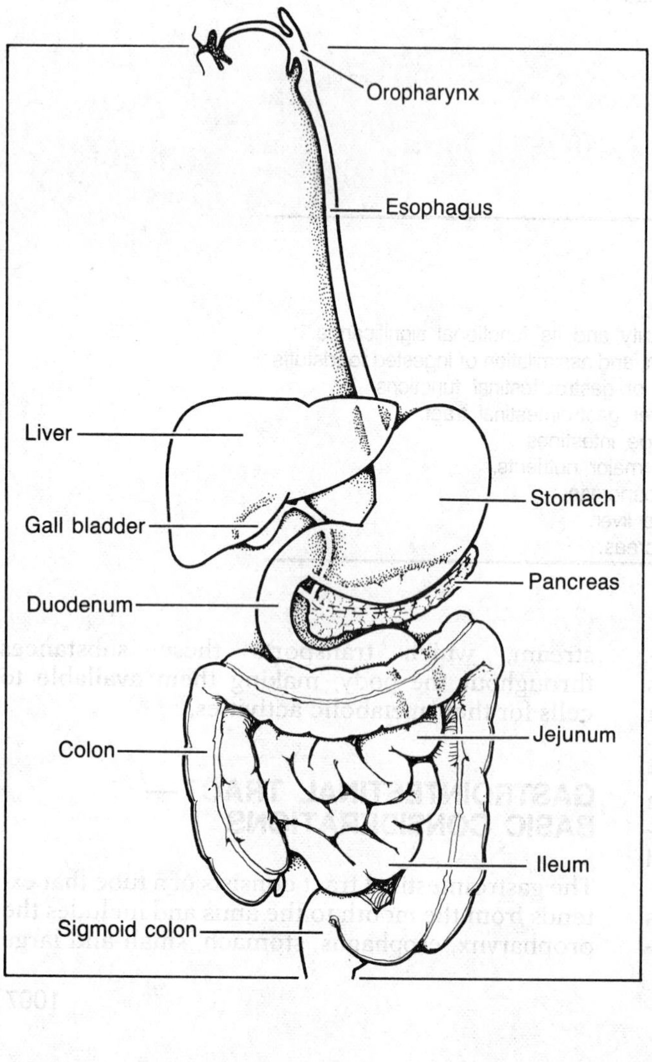


**Figure 47–1.** The digestive system, including the gastrointestinal tract and accessory organs, pancreas, liver, and gallbladder.

### Muscularis Externa

The muscularis externa consists of 2 smooth muscle layers, described as circular and longitudinal. These muscle layers occur throughout the gastrointestinal tract and facilitate gastrointestinal motility, a critical component of the digestive process.

The muscularis externa of the stomach differs from that elsewhere in the gastrointestinal tract in that it has 3 muscle layers, an outer longitudinal, middle circular, and an inner oblique layer. This unique muscular arrangement facilitates the mixing, churning functions of the stomach as it reduces the semisolid food, resulting from mastication in the oral cavity, to a fluid mass.

### Serosa

The serosa (tunica adventitia) is the outermost surface of the gastrointestinal tract, which anchors it to surrounding tissues/organs by loose connective tissue.

## Gastrointestinal Functions

### Motility

Optimal digestion, absorption, and assimilation of nutrients by the gastrointestinal tract require coordinated motor activity that facilitates an orderly intraluminal propulsion of ingested food, at a rate that ensures maximal mixing of food with digestive secretions. The muscle layers of the gastrointestinal tract consist of striated muscle (under voluntary control) found within the pharynx, upper one third of the esophagus, the upper esophageal sphincter, and the anal sphincter. The remainder of the gastrointestinal tract is richly endowed with smooth muscle layers. This smooth muscle coat provides the basis for well coordinated gastrointestinal motility.

Characteristically, the smooth muscle coat is arranged in 2 layers: an inner, thicker circular layer, and a thinner, outer longitudinal layer. Fundamental to smooth muscle cells is the presence of gap junctions or nexi between these cells, which provide a low-resistance pathway for the movement of ions, thereby facilitating conduction of electrical impulses from cell to cell. These nexi are especially demonstrable in circular smooth muscle cells. This arrangement of electrical and contractile properties of gastrointestinal smooth muscle results in 3 patterns of motility: rhythmic segmentation, peristalsis, and tonic contractions.[1]

**Rhythmic Segmentation.** Rhythmic segmentation is attributed largely to the activity of the circular muscle layer. Distention of the intestinal wall caused by the food within it causes localized contractions to occur, spaced at intervals along the gastrointestinal tract and lasting for several seconds. As these contractions wane, similar rings of contraction appear in the previously inactive intervening segments (Fig. 47-2). Occurring at a frequency of 7 to 12 times per minute, these actions promote progressive mixing of solid and semisolid food particles with digestive secretions.

**Peristalsis.** Peristalsis consists of a wave of circular smooth muscle contractions, which are responsible for the bulk of forward movement (analward) of intraluminal contents within the gastrointestinal tract. Peristaltic waves also function to spread out the semifluid mass of partly digested food along the intestinal tract to increase the surface area of the gut to which it is exposed. This activity may also help to avoid areas of unusual hypertonicity and hypotonicity, which might result in unexpected fluid shifts.

**Tonic Contractions.** Tonic contractions of sphincters, alternating with their intermittent relaxation, serve to regulate movement of intraluminal contents. The term *sphincter* is applied to specialized areas of muscle occurring at strategic points along the gastrointestinal tract. With the ex-

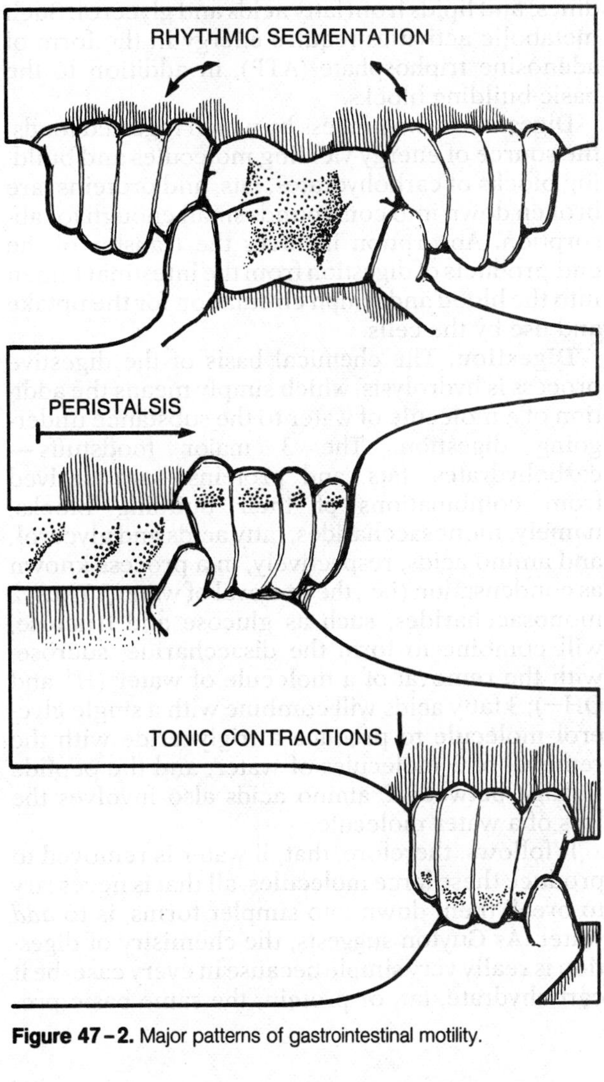


**Figure 47-2.** Major patterns of gastrointestinal motility.

ception of the upper esophageal and external anal sphincters, both of which are comprised of striated, skeletal muscle cells, all other sphincters consist of smooth muscle cells. These sphincters function to regulate movement of digestive contents between adjacent luminal compartments.

In general, gastrointestinal motor activity is enhanced by parasympathetic influence, while sympathetic discharge tends to reduce it. The hormones gastrin, cholecystokinin, and insulin stimulate smooth muscle contraction; secretin and glucagon depress contractile activity.

### *Digestive and Absorptive Processes*

Intestinal digestion and absorption are the physiologic processes by which essential foods, water, vitamins, minerals, and other substances are taken into the body and made available to cells for their metabolic activities.

An integral part of cellular metabolism is the biosynthesis of large molecules from more simple molecules, as, for example, proteins from amino acids; polysaccharides from simple sugars, glucose, and fructose; DNA-RNA from purines and pyrimidines; and lipids from fatty acids and glycerol. Such metabolic activities require energy in the form of adenosine triphosphate (ATP), in addition to the basic building blocks.

Digestion is the process by which ingested foods, the source of energy-yielding molecules and building blocks of carbohydrates, fats, and proteins, are broken down into compounds small enough for absorption. Absorption involves the transfer of the end-products of digestion from the intestinal lumen into the blood and lymph circulation for the uptake and use by the cells.

**Digestion.** The chemical basis of the digestive process is hydrolysis, which simply means the addition of a molecule of water to the substance undergoing digestion. The 3 major foodstuffs—carbohydrates, fats, and proteins—are derived from combinations of their building blocks, namely, monosaccharides, fatty acids and glycerol, and amino acids, respectively, in a process known as condensation (i.e., the removal of water). Thus, 2 monosaccharides, such as glucose and fructose, will combine to form the disaccharide, sucrose, with the removal of a molecule of water ($H^+$ and $OH-$); 3 fatty acids will combine with a single glycerol molecule to produce a triglyceride with the removal of 3 molecules of water; and the peptide linkage between 2 amino acids also involves the loss of a water molecule.

It follows, therefore, that, if water is removed to produce these large molecules, all that is necessary to break them down into simpler forms, is to *add* water. As Guyton suggests, the chemistry of digestion is really very simple because in every case, be it carbohydrate, fat, or protein, the same basic process of hydrolysis is involved (i.e., the addition of water).[2] The only difference involves the specificity of enzymes essential to the digestion of each food type.

**Absorption.** Once food is broken down by the various digestive enzymes, the end-products must be transported from the intestinal lumen into the blood, eventually to be metabolized by the cells. The route of absorption is determined by the characteristics of the substances and includes molecular size, charge, if present, and the relative aqueous and lipid solubilities.

***Mechanisms of Absorption.*** The basic processes involved in the absorption of nutrients from the gastrointestinal tract are diffusion and active transport. Diffusion is a passive process involving the movement of molecules through a membrane. There are 2 subprocesses of diffusion: simple diffusion and facilitated diffusion.

*Simple Diffusion.* Simple diffusion involves movement of molecules or ions through a membrane either directly through the lipid bilayer, and/or by way of protein channels or pores within the membrane. Water molecules, for example, because of their small size, diffuse through membranes with astonishing ease, passing through the lipid bilayer, as well as protein channels. Lipid-soluble molecules cross the lipid portion of the membrane with relative ease by passive diffusion in accordance with their concentration gradients.

Hydrogen ions and electrolytes (e.g., sodium, potassium, and chloride), while very small molecules, penetrate the membrane less rapidly because of their charge. Interaction between these charged ions and the negative and positive charges within the membrane actually causes the ions to be repulsed. Consequently, transport of these ions occurs predominantly through protein channels or pores.

The rate of simple diffusion depends on molecular size, net charge on the molecule, concentration gradient across the membrane, lipid solubility, the total cross-sectional surface area for diffusion to occur, and the diffusion distance.

*Facilitated Diffusion.* Facilitated diffusion, also referred to as carrier-mediated diffusion, requires a specific carrier protein to assist or facilitate movement of the molecule across the membrane. Larger water-soluble molecules, for example, are unable to cross the membrane by simple diffusion and are obliged to use an alternative pathway involving carrier proteins within the membrane. Such carriers "facilitate" the diffusion of these substances through the lipid portion of the membrane, in which they would otherwise be insoluble.

As with simple diffusion, facilitated diffusion of molecules occurs in accordance with their concentration gradients. These processes differ in that facilitated diffusion depends on a fixed number of carrier sites, thus limiting the rate of diffusion.

Once these sites become maximally occupied with the specific molecules, further diffusion is limited. Glucose and amino acids are 2 very important molecules that cross cell membranes by facilitated diffusion.

*Active Transport.* No substances can diffuse passively against an electrochemical gradient, either a concentration gradient or an electrical gradient. In other words, molecules cannot diffuse "uphill." To move molecules uphill, energy is required. This process is termed *active transport.* Thus, active transport differs from simple and facilitated diffusion in that it can move substances against an electrochemical gradient with the expenditure of energy. The exchange of sodium and potassium across the cell membrane is an example of a primary active transport process in which the energy that fuels the process is derived from ATP.

***Intestinal Absorption of Water.*** Water absorption from the gastrointestinal tract deserves special mention because up to 10 liters of water daily are normally transported from the lumen into the blood. Much of this water is absorbed in conjunction with osmotic pressure gradients created by electrolyte secretion, as, for example, the active transport of sodium (sodium pump).

## Circulatory and Lymphatic Distribution of Digestive Organs

Perfusion of digestive organs plays an important role inasmuch as the processes of digestion and absorption involve the transport of large volumes of solute and fluids between the gastrointestinal lumen and the blood. Three major arteries perfuse the digestive organs—celiac, superior and inferior mesenteric arteries. The venous drainage from these organs empties directly into the portal vein, which, in turn, perfuses the liver.

Key features of the microcirculation of digestive organs that facilitate movement of large amounts of fluid, nutrients, and electrolytes between the blood and mucosal epithelial cells include (1) the extensive surface area available for absorption and secretion; (2) presence of fenestrated-type capillaries (i.e., characterized by having an enormous pore area for exchange of water and solutes); and (3) an increased permeability to smaller-sized molecules, while remaining relatively impermeable to macromolecules. For example, glucose readily gains access to the blood while movement of larger-sized plasma protein molecules is largely restricted by the capillary endothelium.

Approximately 1–2 liters of lymph reaching the thoracic duct every 24 hours are derived from the gastrointestinal tract. Lymph is the major pathway for fat transport into the systemic circulation.

## Control of Gastrointestinal Functions

### Innervation

The gastrointestinal tract is extensively innervated by the sympathetic and parasympathetic divisions of the autonomic nervous system (*extrinsic* innervation), and by a network of ganglia and nerve fibers located within its walls (*intrinsic* innervation). In addition, motor fibers from the somatic (voluntary) division of the peripheral nervous system innervate the skeletal muscles of the oropharynx, upper one third of the esophagus including the upper esophageal sphincter, and the external anal sphincter. This somatic innervation accounts for the voluntary control of such activities as chewing, initiation of swallowing, and defecation.

**Intrinsic Innervation.** Intrinsic innervation consists of 2 networks of nerve fibers. The myenteric plexus (Auerbach's) is located between the circular and longitudinal muscle and submucosal layers. These plexuses receive sensory input from a variety of receptors (e.g., stretch, pain) located within the intestinal wall. The myenteric plexus influences gastrointestinal muscle tone and motility as its fibers terminate on circular and longitudinal smooth muscle cells.

Efferent fibers from the submucosal plexus terminate directly on the muscularis mucosa and mucosal epithelial cells. This latter plexus primarily influences the secretory functions of epithelial cells. There are many neuronal connections between these plexuses, and afferent fibers from these plexuses relay sensory information (e.g., stretch, distention, pain) to the central nervous system.

**Extrinsic Innervation.** Extrinsic innervation occurs by way of the parasympathetic and sympathetic divisions of the autonomic nervous system, which function to regulate secretory activity, gastrointestinal motility, and sphincter tone. In general, fibers from these 2 divisions exert contrasting effects. Parasympathetic stimulation increases secretory activity and gastrointestinal motility, and relaxes sphincters; sympathetic stimulation reduces secretory activity, decreases motility, and increases sphincter tone.

The central nervous system is able to exert an influence on gastrointestinal function by efferent fibers in the vagus (parasympathetic) and spinal (sympathetic) nerves. Afferent fibers in these nerves, in turn, transmit information from gastrointestinal organs to the central nervous system. In this way, psychologic and emotional factors can influence overall gastrointestinal function.

### Gastrointestinal Hormones

Scattered throughout the gastrointestinal mucosa are cells that synthesize and secrete hormones. These hormones regulate important physiologic functions of the gastrointestinal tract. Cholecystokinin (CCK), for example, is synthesized and secreted from mucosal cells in the small intestine in response to ingestion of dietary fat. CCK reaches the gallbladder by way of the blood and stimulates it to contract and empty its bile contents into the duodenum. The presence of bile within the gut facilitates fat digestion.

Other major gastrointestinal hormones include gastrin, which is structurally similar to CCK but exerts its major influence on parietal cells of the stomach; and secretin, which stimulates pancreatic bicarbonate secretion. It is now recognized that the principal physiologic stimuli for release of gastrointestinal hormones are the intraluminal hydrolyzed products of foods—carbohydrates, fats, and proteins. Blood levels of these hormones fluctuate in accordance with the passage of food through the gastrointestinal tract. These hormones and other related biologically active substances within the gastrointestinal tract will be discussed in greater detail later in this chapter.

# FUNCTIONAL ANATOMY OF THE UPPER GASTROINTESTINAL TRACT

## Structural Components and Their Functions

### *Oral Cavity*

Initiation of the digestive process begins with the oral ingestion of food. The activities of the structures within the oral cavity (cheeks, gums, teeth, palate, and tongue) are coordinated primarily to prepare food for swallowing and transport to the stomach by the esophagus. The tongue, by virtue of its ability to change shape rapidly and extensively, plays a key role in various digestive activities including mastication, salivation, and swallowing.

### *Salivary Glands*

The salivary glands include the parotid, sublingual, and submandibular glands, and numerous small salivary glands widely scattered throughout the submucosal lining of the oral cavity (e.g., buccal glands).

The salivary secretions produced and secreted by these glands are important to hygiene, comfort, and normal digestion. Mucins, secreted largely by the sublingual and submandibular salivary glands, reduce frictional interaction between ingested food and the oral and esophageal mucosa, and facilitate chewing and swallowing. The enzyme, $\alpha$-amylase (ptyalin), secreted largely by the parotid gland, initiates carbohydrate digestion by converting much of the starch digested to the disaccharide form. The remaining starch is digested by pancreatic $\alpha$-amylase when it reaches the duodenum.

Saliva has the highest potassium level of any digestive juice. Clinically, it may be necessary to provide supplemental parenteral potassium therapy to patients with draining neck or facial fistulas, who may be unable to eat.

The salivary glands are innervated by the autonomic nervous system. Parasympathetic stimulation promotes a copious secretion of watery saliva; sympathetic innervation causes a decreased secretion of a thick saliva. Anticholinergic agents (e.g., atropine) greatly reduce salivation.

### *Pharynx*

The pharynx consists of 3 sections—the oropharynx, nasopharynx, and laryngeal pharynx—all of which participate in swallowing.

### *Esophagus*

**Motility.** The primary function of the esophagus is to transfer ingested solids and liquids from the pharynx to the stomach. Each end of the esophagus is guarded by sphincters. The cricopharyngeal muscle forms the upper esophageal sphincter and consists of skeletal striated muscle fibers. Its contraction relaxes the esophageal opening, allowing the bolus to enter the esophagus, while its relaxation facilitates peristaltic movement. Peristalsis is largely regulated by impulses from the vagus nerve.

The lower esophageal sphincter, while not anatomically distinct, nevertheless functions to prevent reflux of gastric contents into the esophagus. The normally alkaline milieu within the esophagus is unable to tolerate highly acidic gastric secretions.

**Secretion.** The esophagus does not have any digestive or absorptive functions. Glands within the lamina propria and submucosa secrete mucus, which serves to lubricate the bolus of food as it passes into the stomach.

### *Stomach*

The stomach is an expanded portion of the gastrointestinal tract that functions to store food and to process it in a preliminary manner to facilitate its transfer into the duodenum. The stomach initiates some definitive digestive processes that alter the foodstuffs chemically in preparation for further digestion and absorption in the small intestine. Although the absorptive function of the stomach is limited, some water and lipid-soluble substances (e.g., ethanol) are absorbed at this level of the gastrointestinal tract. The major role of the stomach is to regulate the rate at which the chyme is delivered to the duodenum.

The anatomical divisions of the stomach include the fundus, cardia, corpus (body), and the pylorus area, which is further divided into the pyloric antrum and pyloric canal (Fig. 47–3). The innermost

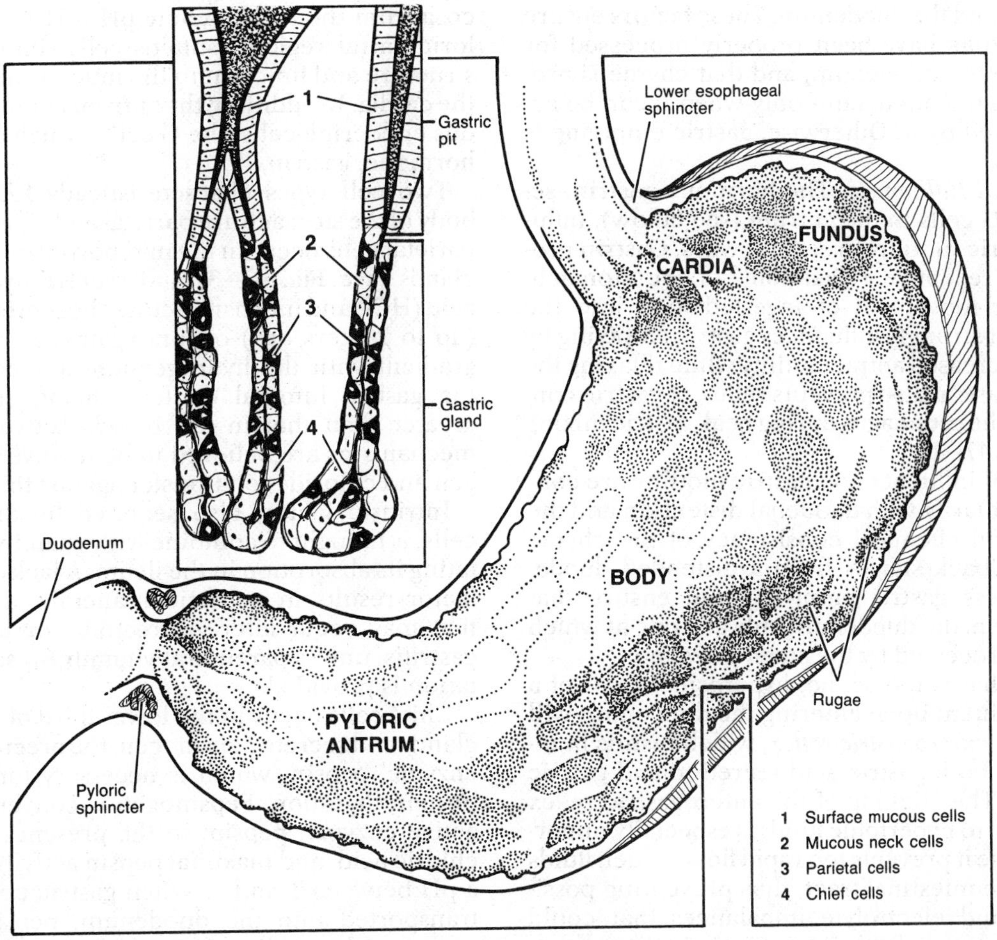


**Figure 47–3.** Macroscopic and microscopic anatomy of stomach. Grossly depicted are the major areas of the stomach, including the fundus, cardia, body, and pylorus; rugae occur throughout the inner lining of the stomach; the entrance to and exit from the stomach are guarded by the lower esophageal and pyloric sphincters, respectively. Microscopically, the gastric gland is depicted, and the major cell types included therein are identified.

surface throughout the entire stomach is found to be thrown into longitudinal folds or *rugae*. These function to increase surface area for digestion and absorption, enhance expansion/distention, and provide friction to the movement of food, which facilitates mechanical activities of the stomach (e.g., mixing, churning, and breaking down of foodstuffs).

The stomach is guarded at its two ends by sphincters, the lower esophageal sphincter at the upper end and the pyloric sphincter at its lower end (see Fig. 47–3). These 2 sphincters function to prevent retrograde reflux of digestive contents into the esophagus and stomach, respectively. Clinically, the pyloric sphincter is frequently involved in the pathophysiology of peptic ulcer disease.

**Gastric Motility.** Gastric motility facilitates the mechanical functions of the stomach. These include the expansion and distention of the stomach to accommodate large volumes of ingested foods; contraction of the gastric musculature to break down foodstuffs, and to mix them with gastric juice so that the digestive process can be initiated; and organized propulsion of the partially digested gastric contents into the duodenum.

The unique motility characteristics of the stomach are a result of the arrangement of its 3 muscle layers in the muscularis externa: outer longitudinal, middle circular, and inner oblique layers. The circular layer is the most prominent and strongest of the 3 layers. It is continuous throughout the wall of the stomach and is intimately involved in forming the muscular ring that makes up the pyloric sphincter.

The mixing and churning activities of the stomach reduce the semisolid food resulting from mastication in the oral cavity to a fluid mass. The upper part of the stomach temporarily stores this semifluid mass for a time following a meal, while, in the more distal regions of the stomach, the semisolid contents are reduced mechanically and chemically into chyme, which is of the soft, fluid consistency necessary for transport to the duodenum.

***Regulation of Gastric Motility.*** Regulation of gastric motility involves neural and hormonal influences, including intrinsic signals from the stomach, itself, and the duodenum. These factors ensure that foodstuffs have been properly processed for delivery to the duodenum, and that chyme is propelled into the duodenum only when it can be accommodated by it. Otherwise, gastric emptying is prohibited.

*Hormonal Influences.* The hormone gastrin, secreted by G cells in the antrum (see below), influences gastric motility in several ways. Gastrin promotes a "receptive relaxation" of the stomach, facilitating movement of ingested food into the stomach. It strongly influences gastric emptying by causing increased antral motility while relaxing the pylorus. Gastrin also prevents reflux of gastric contents into the esophagus during peak gastric mixing (see Table 47-1).

Duodenal influences on gastric motility are concerned primarily with duodenal distention and the physical and chemical consistency of the chyme itself. Feedback signals from a distended duodenum depress gastric emptying and ensure that chyme enters the duodenum only at a rate at which it can be processed by the small intestine.

Chyme that is too acidic, hyperosmolar, or of a high fat content upon entering the duodenum will initiate the *enterogastric reflex*, which results in inhibition of both gastric acid secretion and gastric emptying. The eliciting of the enterogastric reflex in response to hypertonic fluids is especially important because it prevents too rapid flow of such fluids through the intestinal tract, thus preventing possible fluid and electrolyte imbalances that could occur during the absorption of intestinal contents.

Hormonal inhibition of gastric emptying includes the effect of cholecystokinin (CCK), which is released from the mucosa in the jejunum in response to fatty substances entering the duodenum. This hormone blocks the effect of gastrin, which is to increase gastric motility. Secretin, secreted by cells in the duodenum in response to the presence of acidic chyme, also has the effect of decreasing gastric motility.

**Gastric Secretion.** The epithelium of the gastric mucosa is concerned chiefly with the secretory and digestive processes of the stomach, and its distinctive structure is well correlated with these functions. The mucosal surface is lined with mucus-secreting, simple columnar epithelium; there occurs within it numerous involutions and convolutions known as gastric pits. The gastric pits function to increase surface areas and give rise to the gastric glands that house the various secretory cells of the stomach (see Fig. 47-3).

***Distinct Cell Types.*** Histologically, each major anatomical region of the stomach (i.e., the cardia, corpus [body], and antrum) contains distinctive cell types that elaborate the gastric secretions. In the cardia, mucous neck cells secrete mucus, which serves to moisten further the foodstuffs entering the stomach and to protect the gastric mucosa from the highly acidic pH (pH 1-3). The pyloric antral region contains cells similar in both structure and function to the mucous neck cells of the cardia. In addition, the antrum contains numerous endocrine cells, the G cells, which secrete the hormone, gastrin.

Two cell types characteristically found in the body of the stomach are parietal and chief cells. The parietal cells occur in the mid-portion of the gastric glands (see Fig. 47-3) and secrete hydrochloric acid (HCl) and intrinsic factor. The secretion of HCl (up to 2 liters/day) occurs against a tremendous gradient with the hydrogen-ion concentration of the gastric luminal contents being enormously greater than that in the blood. Active transport mechanisms are believed to be involved in hydrogen and chloride-ion transfer against this gradient.

Intrinsic factor, also secreted by the parietal cells, is thought to combine with vitamin $B_{12}$, facilitating its absorption in the ileum. A lack of intrinsic factor results in pernicious anemia, a condition that may occur after gastrectomy or in atrophic gastritis, unless parenteral vitamin $B_{12}$ supplementation is provided.

Chief cells occur in the lower third of the gastric glands and secrete pepsinogen, the precursor to the enzyme, pepsin, which is necessary for initiating protein digestion. Pepsinogen is converted to the active enzyme, pepsin, in the presence of hydrochloric acid, and maximal pepsin activity occurs at a pH between 1 and 3. When gastric contents are transported into the duodenum, pepsin activity ceases as the acidity of gastric contents is neutralized by alkaline pancreatic and duodenal secretions.

***Control Mechanisms.*** Regulation of digestive events in the stomach involves both nervous and hormonal mediation and can be subdivided into the cephalic, gastric, and intestinal phases. The cephalic phase, which is largely neurogenic, includes secretory responses to sensory stimuli at the level of the cerebral cortex (e.g., sight, smell, sound, thoughts of food) and/or the appetite center. Sympathetic innervation to the stomach provides the mechanism whereby psychologic and emotional factors can influence gastric secretions.

The gastric phase is so named because stimuli occur in the stomach itself and are of 2 types, mechanical and chemical. Distention, caused by the entrance of the food bolus into the stomach, provides the most significant mechanical stimulus. (The presence of a nasogastric tube does not stimulate gastric secretion because it does not cause distention.) Chemical stimuli include the contents of ingested foods (e.g., polypeptides), alcohol ingestion, or the presence of an alkaline pH, for example.

Both mechanical and chemical stimuli evoke gastric secretion by contact with pyloric antral cells, resulting in the secretion of gastrin. Although some vagal stimulation occurs, the gastric phase is

TABLE 47-1
**Gastrin: Summary of Hormonal Actions**

| Stomach | Duodenum | Pancreas | Liver |
|---|---|---|---|
| ↑HCl secretion<br>↑pepsinogen/pepsin<br>↑"receptive relaxation"<br>↑lower esophageal tone<br>↑pylorus sphincter tone<br>↑gastric motility<br>↑intrinsic factor secretion | ↑intestinal motility<br>↑bicarbonate secretion (Brunner's glands)<br>↓secretin secretion<br>↓cholecystokinin secretion | ↑bicarbonate secretion<br>↑pancreatic enzyme secretion<br>↑insulin secretion | ↑hepatic bile flow |

considered to be primarily hormonal in nature as gastrin release becomes the primary stimulus for gastric secretion. Table 47-1 summarizes the major actions of gastrin in promoting digestion.

The intestinal phase of gastric secretion regulation is mainly inhibitory, causing a reduction in gastric secretion as chyme enters the duodenum. This phase is mostly hormonal.

Neural mediation does occur by the myenteric plexus and autonomic nerve fibers in response to distention of the small intestine. Stretch or increased tension in the intestinal wall initiates the enterogastric reflex, resulting in inhibition of gastric secretion and gastric emptying.

## FUNCTIONAL ANATOMY OF THE LOWER GASTROINTESTINAL TRACT

### Structural Components and Their Functions

#### *Small Intestine*

The bulk of digestion and absorption of essentially all major foodstuffs takes place in the small intestine. Its major divisions, based on structural and functional differences, include the duodenum, the jejunum, and the ileum. The pyloric sphincter separates the stomach from the duodenum; it allows entry of chyme into the duodenum and prevents retrograde reflux of duodenal contents into the stomach. The *ileocecal* valve occurs at the junction of the ileum with the cecum and allows exit of digested foodstuffs into the colon, while preventing reflex of colonic contents back into the small intestine.

The free surfaces of organs in the abdominal cavity are covered by peritoneum (lesser and greater omentum), which protects the abdominal contents and provides support for abdominal viscera. The mesentery is a fold of peritoneum that functions to suspend and support the small intestine and provides a rich blood and lymphatic supply to the jejunum and ileum. The manner in which it suspends the intestine allows for considerable motility of the bowel, facilitating mixing actions and peristalsis.

**Intestinal Motility.** Intestinal motility of the small intestine is essential to the digestive and absorptive processes. Not only is it necessary for chyme to be moved through the gastrointestinal tract, but it must be thoroughly mixed so that all portions of it may be exposed to digestive enzymes and absorptive surfaces. Mixing and propulsive contractions characterize motility of the small intestine. Specific patterns of motility include rhythmic segmentation, peristalsis, and tonic contractions. These patterns were examined previously (see Fig. 47-2).

Characteristically, intestinal peristalsis is greatly increased after a meal. This increase in intestinal motor activity is mediated by the *gastroenteric reflex* in response to gastric distention. Peristaltic waves within the ileum intensify, and this, accompanied by relaxation of the ileocecal valve, enables chyme to be emptied into the colon.

***Control of Intestinal Motility.*** Control of intestinal motility involves a combination of neural and hormonal factors. Intrinsic innervation (Auerbach's myenteric plexus) occurs throughout the intestinal tract so that activity in the upper gastrointestinal tract can impact on that in the more distal areas. Parasympathetic innervation (extrinsic) increases muscle tone and stimulates intestinal motility; sympathetic effect decreases muscle tone. Strong sympathetic innervation may even block movement of chyme through the gastrointestinal tract.

*Hormonal Influence.* Hormonal influence on intestinal motility involves the action of gastrin. Secreted by gastric antral cells in response to the mechanical and chemical stimuli of ingested food entering the stomach, gastrin stimulates intestinal motility and promotes digestion. Cholecystokinin (CCK), secreted by jejunal endocrine cells in response to the presence of fat in the duodenum, blocks the action of gastrin by inhibiting gastric motility. Concomitantly, CCK stimulates contraction of gallbladder smooth muscle. By limiting gastric emptying and, therefore, the volume of chyme in the small intestine, and by enhancing bile secretion, CCK facilitates fat digestion and absorption. The hormone, secretin, exerts a mild inhibitory effect on motility throughout most of the gastrointestinal tract.

**Secretion.** Digestive and absorptive functions of the intestinal tract are related to its unique structure. The duodenum is a critical segment because it is anatomically situated to receive the connecting ducts of the liver, gallbladder, and pancreas (see Fig. 47–8). Endocrine cells within the duodenum and jejunum secrete hormones that facilitate digestion and absorption. The ileum has enhanced absorptive capabilities, including the absorption of nutrients, vitamin $B_{12}$, and bile salts.

***Microstructure.*** The mucosal layer comprising the luminal surface of the small intestine is structured to provide a large surface area for digestive and absorptive activities. It consists of three anatomical modifications, including the plicae circularis (valvular conniventes), fingerlike projections called villi, depressions called crypts (of Lieberkühn), and microvilli. The plicae circularis are permanent structures involving both the mucosal and submucosal layers and are found predominantly in the distal duodenum and proximal jejunum (Fig. 47–4).

The intestinal villi are minute fingerlike projections of mucosa present in enormous numbers and covering the entire surface of the mucosa. They are most numerous in the duodenum and proximal jejunum. In addition to the villous surface projections, the mucosal surface area is further increased by invaginations of the mucosa, which form tubular intestinal glands, the crypts of Lieberkühn (see Fig. 47–4). The microvilli are projections on the luminal surface of absorptive cells. The combination of the plicae circularis, villi, crypts, and microvilli enhances total intestinal surface area by as much as 600-fold.

*Functional Unit of the Small Intestine.* The villus is considered to be the main structural and functional unit of the small intestine. There may be as many as 25 million villi throughout the small intestine, and

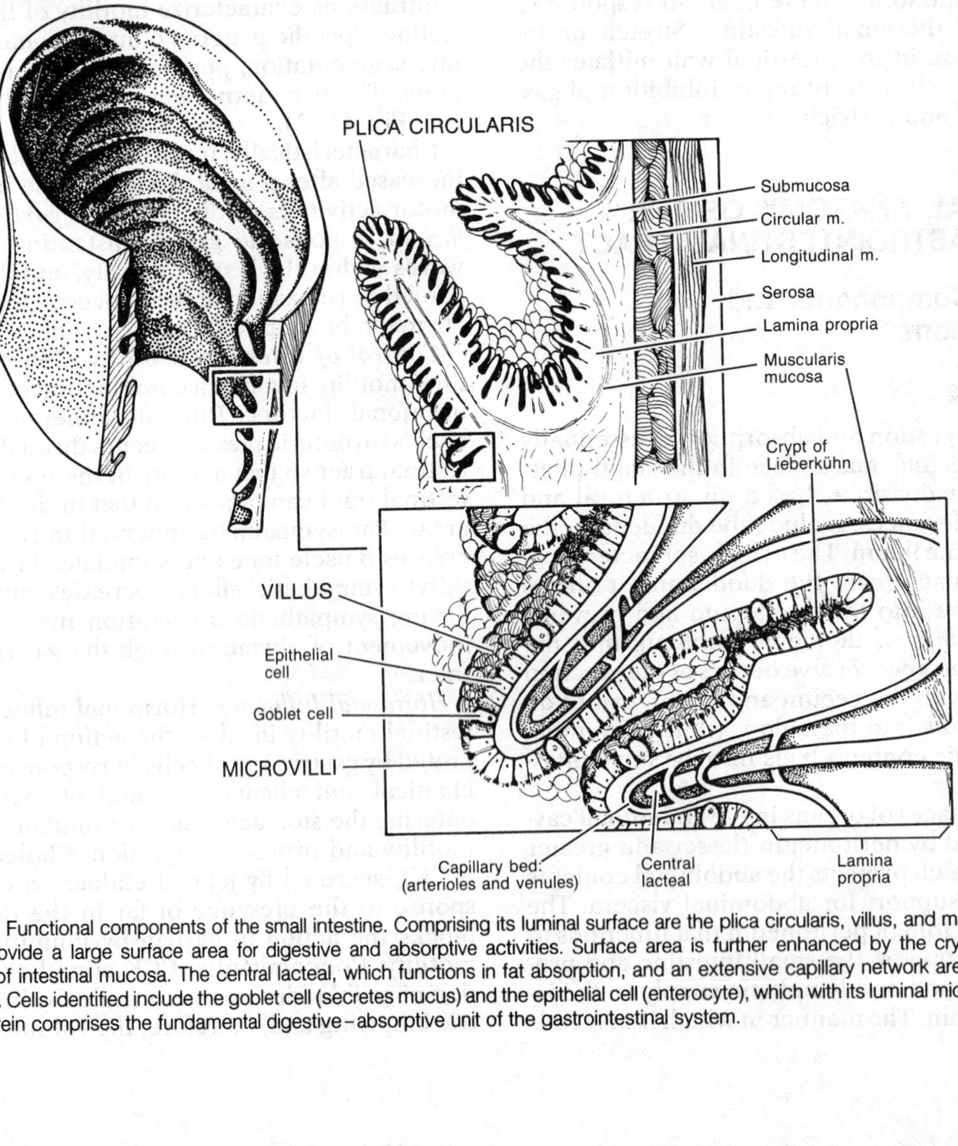


**Figure 47–4.** Functional components of the small intestine. Comprising its luminal surface are the plica circularis, villus, and microvilli, all of which function to provide a large surface area for digestive and absorptive activities. Surface area is further enhanced by the crypts of Lieberkühn, invaginations of intestinal mucosa. The central lacteal, which functions in fat absorption, and an extensive capillary network are found within each intestinal villus. Cells identified include the goblet cell (secretes mucus) and the epithelial cell (enterocyte), which with its luminal microvilli and enzymes contained therein comprises the fundamental digestive–absorptive unit of the gastrointestinal system.

they vary in shape from the duodenum to the ileum. Each villus consists of a central lymph channel, the lacteal, surrounded by a network of capillaries and lymphoid tissue (see Fig. 47–4).

The outermost (luminal) epithelial lining of the villus is comprised of simple columnar absorptive cells, or enterocytes. The most striking feature of the enterocyte is the presence of many microvilli on its luminal surface (see Fig. 47–4). The plasma membrane of the microvilli is covered with a brush border (glycoprotein-containing substance), and this combination is viewed as the fundamental digestive–absorptive unit of the enterocyte. In addition to increasing total intestinal surface area, microvilli also contain digestive enzymes (e.g., maltase, sucrase, and lactase), which complete the process of digestion as absorption is taking place (see below).

In addition to the absorptive cell, the enterocyte, the intestinal mucosal epithelium also contains goblet cells and endocrine cells (see Fig. 47–4). Goblet cells are found to be scattered among the enterocytes. These cells secrete a viscous mucus, which may function to protect the intestinal mucosa and facilitate movement of digested material along the gastrointestinal tract. Endocrine cells, which elaborate and secrete hormones (e.g., cholecystokinin and secretin), are found dispersed among the enterocytes lining the villi. Goblet cells and endocrine cells are also found in the crypts.

A noteworthy consideration regarding the intestinal submucosal layer is the presence of Brunner's glands within the duodenum. These glands secrete a clear, viscous, and distinctly alkaline fluid (pH 8.2–9.3), which functions to neutralize the acidity of gastric chyme. These glands serve to protect the duodenal mucosa from the irritating effects of acidic gastric juice.

**Digestion–Absorption.** Upon arrival in the duodenum, chyme is immediately mixed with a combination of intestinal secretions including: a viscous mucus (goblet cells), alkaline secretions (Brunner's glands and pancreas), digestive enzymes (intestinal mucosal cells and pancreas), and bile (liver and gallbladder).

***Carbohydrate.*** Carbohydrate digestion is completed within the duodenum and jejunum by the pancreatic enzyme, α-amylase. The alkaline intestinal milieu is conducive to α-amylase activity. The hormone secretin, secreted by endocrine cells in the duodenum in response to the entrance of chyme into the duodenum, functions to enhance pancreatic secretion of digestive juices with a high bicarbonate content. This hormone also stimulates Brunner's glands in the duodenum to secrete another bicarbonate-rich fluid.

The neutralization of acidic chyme performs two essential functions: one, it protects the duodenal mucosa from the digestive action of gastric juices; and, two, it provides an appropriate pH for action of pancreatic enzymes, which function optimally in an alkaline milieu. This protective mechanism afforded by secretin is considered to be essential in preventing duodenal (peptic) ulcers.

Final hydrolysis of carbohydrates takes place within the brush border of the epithelial absorptive cells (enterocytes), which contain a number of enzymes (e.g., lactase, sucrase, and maltase). The action of these enzymes splits the appropriate disaccharide sugars into their monosaccharides (e.g., the enzyme sucrase splits the disaccharide sucrose into a molecule of glucose and a molecule of fructose). It is in their monosaccharide form (glucose, galactose, and fructose) that carbohydrates are absorbed into the blood. Once within the blood, these end-products of carbohydrate digestion are carried to the liver by the portal venous system.

***Protein.*** Protein digestion is initiated in the stomach. The enzyme involved in the hydrolysis of protein is pepsin, which is secreted as pepsinogen by the chief cells within the gastric mucosa. The activity of pepsin is optimal at a pH of 1–3. Its activity is terminated when the stomach contents reach the alkaline milieu of the duodenum.

The presence of food within the duodenum enhances the secretion of pancreatic enzymes, an effect mediated by the hormone, cholecystokinin (CCK), which is secreted by endocrine cells in the jejunum. Upon gastric emptying, the hormone, gastrin, also stimulates CCK secretion.

CCK stimulates pancreatic secretion of proteolytic enzyme precursors into the small intestine where they are activated by enzymes located within the microvilli (brush border). For example, trypsinogen is converted to its active enzymatic form, trypsin, by enterokinase, an enzyme thought to reside within the brush border. Once activated, trypsin functions to convert other precursors to their active enzymatic form and, in doing so facilitates protein digestion.

The end-products of protein metabolism include free amino acids, dipeptides, and tripeptides. Absorption of peptides may constitute the predominant mechanism for intestinal assimilation of dietary protein.

***Fat.*** Fat digestion and absorption occur in the small intestine and differ from that of carbohydrates and proteins by virtue of the size and lipid-solubility of fat molecules. Triglycerides, cholesterol esters, phospholipids, and lipid-soluble vitamins (A, D, E, and K) are the primary forms of dietary fat.

Hydrolysis of fats requires an initial process of emulsification (i.e., the physical dispersion of large fat globules into minute droplets; Fig. 47–5). Emulsification facilitates fat digestion by increasing the total surface area available for the action of the pancreatic enzymes, which act only at the surface of the minute fat droplet. Cholecystokinin (CCK), secreted in response to the presence of fat in the duodenum, stimulates pancreatic secretion of lipase and other essential fat-digesting enzymes.

Absorption of the end-products of fat metabolism requires the solubilization or dissolution of these products in the aqueous phase of the luminal contents. This is achieved by micelle formation in the presence of bile salts. Bile salts are amphipathic molecules, that is, they contain both hydrophilic (attracted to water) and lipophilic (attracted to lipids) properties. As such, they facilitate micelle formation by aggregating lipid molecules so that their lipophilic portion faces the interior of the resultant micelle, while the hydrophilic portion faces the aqueous phase of the luminal contents within which it dissolves (see Fig. 47–5).

At the luminal surface of the absorptive cells, fatty acids and monoglycerides leave the micelle and diffuse passively across the plasma membrane into the cell. The bile salts remain within the intestinal lumen and continue to participate in the solubilization of fat. Eventually, the bile salts pass to the distal ileum where they are readily absorbed (up to 95%).

Although some short-chain fatty acids are absorbed directly into the blood, the bulk of fatty acids and monoglycerides is resynthesized into triglycerides within the absorptive cell and packaged into complexes called chylomicrons. This new complex is extruded from the absorptive cell and passes into the central lacteal of the intestinal villus. The chylomicrons ultimately gain access to the circulatory blood by way of the thoracic duct, which empties into the subclavian vein.

The absorptive cell also forms small lipoproteins called very low density proteins (VLDL), which contain more cholesterol and protein than do the chylomicrons. The processes of VLDL synthesis and release are similar to those of the chylomicrons. The very low density lipoproteins may be a major route of transport of dietary cholesterol into the blood.

***Vitamins.*** Absorption of vitamins can be considered on the basis of their solubility properties. The fat-soluble vitamins (A, D, E, and K) are assimilated in much the same way as are fats. They are incorporated into chylomicrons for transport into the lacteal, eventually to reach the systemic circulation. Any disorder causing a malabsorption of fat will likewise alter absorption of fat-soluble vitamins.

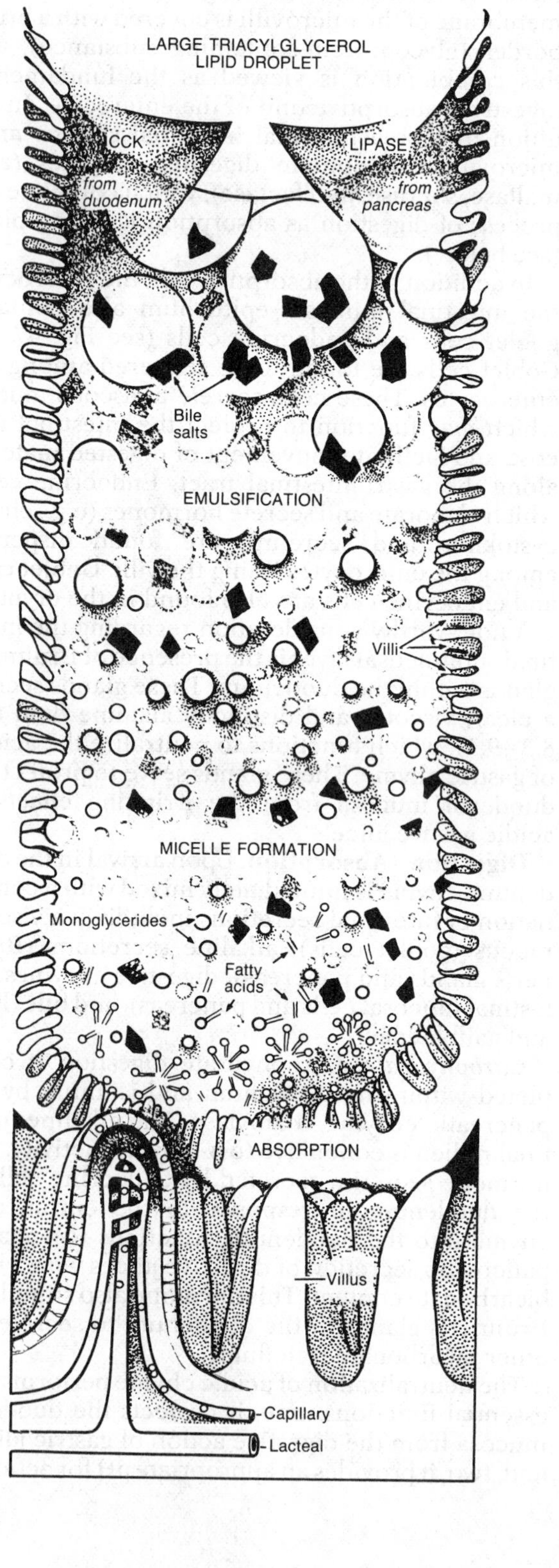


**Figure 47–5.** Digestion and absorption of fats. Bile salts emulsify large lipid droplets into smaller lipid droplets, and they combine with fatty acids and monoglycerides, products of enzymatic action of water-soluble lipase, to form water-soluble complexes called micelles. Micelles consist of bile salts, fatty acids, phospholipids, and monoglycerides, all clustered together with the polar ends of each molecule oriented toward the micelle surface, and the nonpolar portion forming the core of the micelle. At the luminal surface, fatty acids and monoglycerides leave the micelle and are absorbed into the intestinal epithelial cell. Bile salts remain within the intestinal lumen to continue to participate in the solubilization of fats. Eventually, they are reabsorbed in the distal ileum. Fatty acids and monoglycerides in the micelles are in equilibrium with those in free solution. As the concentration of free fatty acids falls (because of their diffusion into epithelial cells), there is a shift of more lipids out of the micelle into the free phase. In this way, micelles provide a means of "storing" products of fat metabolism within the intestinal lumen until absorption is completed.

TABLE 47–2
**Net Fluid Volume Entering Gastrointestinal Tract Daily**

| Source | Fluid Volume (liters, approximate) |
|---|---|
| Oral ingestion: foods and fluid intake | 1.5 to 2.5 |
| Salivary glands | 1.0 to 1.5 |
| Gastric secretions | 2.0 to 2.5 |
| Small intestinal secretions | 1.0 to 2.0 |
| Pancreatic secretions | 1.0 to 1.5 |
| Bile | 0.7 to 1.0 |

Absorption of water-soluble vitamins is less well defined but largely occurs within the duodenum and jejunum. Absorption of vitamin $B_{12}$ requires intrinsic factor, which is secreted by the gastric parietal cells. Absorption of vitamin $B_{12}$ occurs largely in the distal ileum.

***Water and Electrolyte Absorption.*** As much as 10 liters of fluid enter the gastrointestinal tract daily (Table 47–2) with all but 200–300 ml reabsorbed, the remainder being excreted in the feces. Movement of water through the intestinal mucosa occurs by passive diffusion that follows osmotic or hydrostatic pressure gradients. If the chyme is *hyper*tonic, transport of water occurs from the blood into the lumen; if the chyme is *hypo*tonic, movement of water occurs in the opposite direction, from intestinal lumen into the blood. An osmotic equilibrium is established within the proximal intestine, and the chyme remains isosmotic with the blood during its transit through the gastrointestinal tract.

Factors that contribute to the driving force for water absorption include: permeability of intestinal mucosal cells to the movement of water; and osmotic gradients associated with active transport of electrolytes (sodium, potassium, chloride) and solutes (glucose, amino acids, other nutrients). Because water diffuses rapidly in both directions across the intestinal wall in response to changes in osmotic pressure gradients, the gastrointestinal tract has a tremendous capacity to move large volumes of water into and out of the intestinal lumen.

This capacity to move large volumes of water within the gastrointestinal tract can impact on other organ systems. For example, movement of fluid out of the blood and into the lumen of the gut in response to a hypertonic load may compromise cardiovascular dynamics by significantly reducing blood volume. Hypotension may rapidly ensue. Alterations in electrolyte transport into and out of the intestinal lumen occur in the presence of an intestinal obstruction. The consequent disruption in osmotic pressure gradients may predispose to retention and pooling of fluid within the gut, causing marked distention of the intestinal wall, disruption of blood flow, and ischemia of visceral organs.[3]

***Electrolytes and Trace Metals.*** Absorption of electrolytes and trace metals occurs by passive diffusion and active transport mechanisms. Active transport of an electrolyte creates an electrochemical gradient, which facilitates the passive diffusion of another electrolyte. Active transport of sodium, for example, facilitates chloride absorption by simple, passive diffusion. Other mechanisms may be involved. The active and selective absorption of calcium requires the presence of vitamin D and the influence of parathormone (see Chap. 24). In general, the amount of absorption of any one electrolyte or trace metal (e.g., magnesium) is related ultimately to the body's needs. Table 47–3 lists the absorption sites of the nutrients.

**Control Mechanisms.** Regulation of intestinal digestive secretions follows a similar pattern to that described for gastric secretion. The cephalic phase

TABLE 47–3
**Gastrointestinal Absorption Sites of Major Nutrients**

| Duodenum–Jejunum | Ileum | Colon |
|---|---|---|
| Water | Water | Water |
| Electrolytes: Sodium, potassium; Chloride, bicarbonate | Chloride | Potassium |
| Calcium (requires vitamin D) | Bile salts (95% reabsorbed) | |
| Folic acid | Vitamin $B_{12}$ (requires intrinsic factor) | |
| Water-soluble vitamins: Thiamine, niacin, ascorbic acid | | |
| Fat-soluble vitamins: (A, D, E, K) | | |
| Simple sugars: Glucose, fructose; Galactose | | |
| Amino acids, small peptides | | |
| Triglycerides, fatty acids | | |

of intestinal digestion is mediated largely by neuronal pathways. Responses to sensory stimuli (sight, smell, sounds, taste, thoughts of food) are generated within the cerebral cortical and subcortical levels and carried by the vagus nerve to stimulate directly the pancreas to secrete digestive juices. Much overlap exists between gastric and intestinal phases, but the predominant control is hormonal, as reflected by the actions of gastrin, secretin, and cholecystokinin (CCK).

An appreciation of such factors controlling digestive secretions becomes critical when planning patient care. For example, in the patient with acute pancreatitis, the major goal is to prevent stimulation of the pancreas. Therefore, ways of minimizing mental, emotional, physical, and chemical stimuli must be carefully considered.

### *Large Intestine–Colon*

The divisions of the colon include the cecum, ascending colon, hepatic flexure, transverse colon, splenic flexure, descending colon, sigmoid, rectum, and anus. The ileocecal valve separates the small intestine (ileum) from the proximal colon (Fig. 47–6). Internal and external anal sphincters guard the distal end of the colon and play an important role in defecation (see Fig. 12–1 and Table 12–10).

The most important function of the colon is water and electrolyte absorption. Of the total amount of water received daily (½–1 liter), the colon absorbs 80%–90%. This is a significant factor in reducing intestinal contents from a semifluid to a semisolid mass.

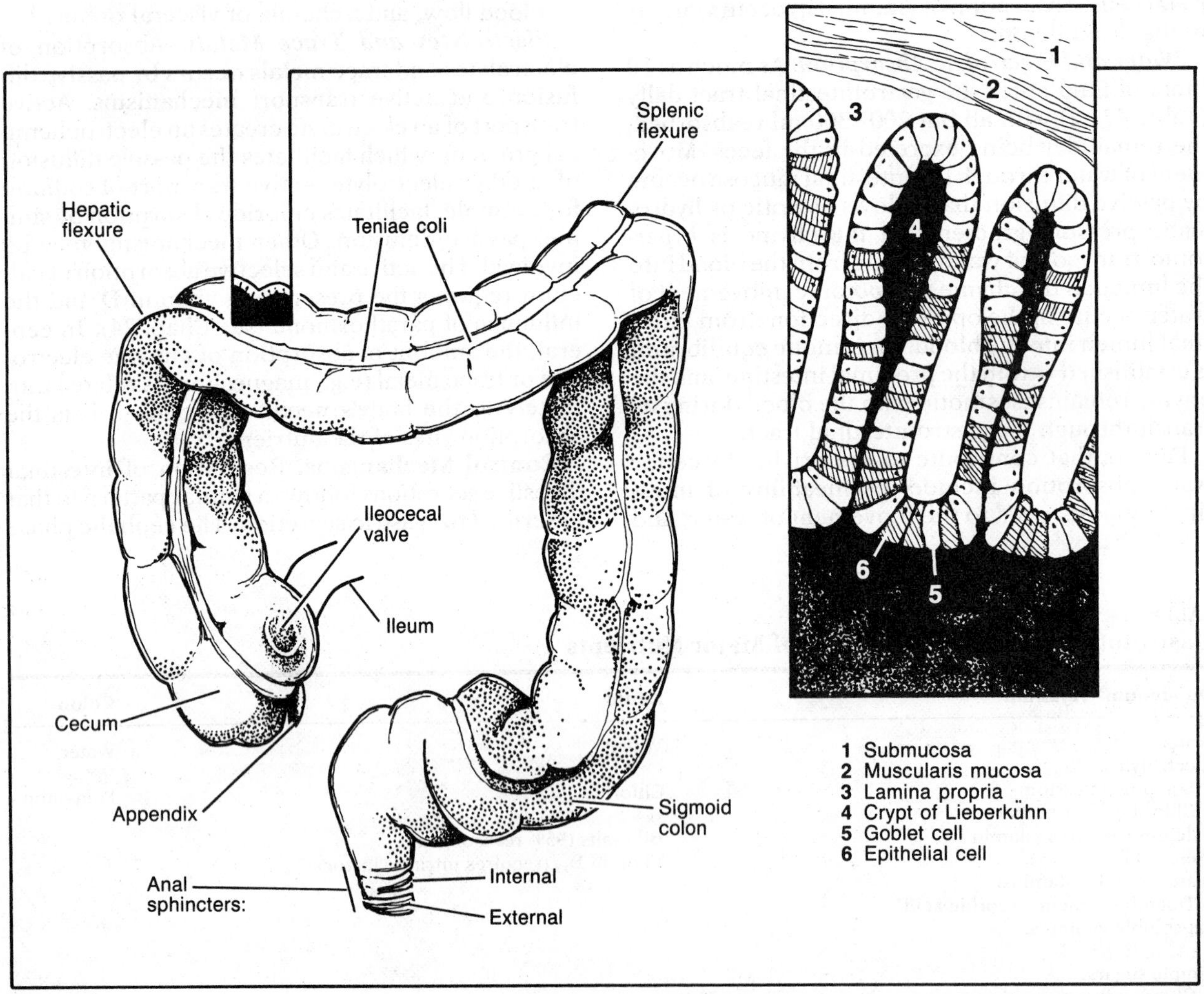


**Figure 47–6.** Macroscopic and microscopic anatomy of the large intestine. Its major divisions are depicted on the left, as are the ileocecal valve and anal sphincters. Microscopic structures are depicted on the right including the crypts of Lieberkühn and specific cells contained therein. In contrast to the small intestine (see Fig. 47–4), the predominant cells lining the colon are goblet cells, which secrete mucus. The epithelial cells are fewer in number, and they contain no enzymes.

The colon has the capacity to absorb as much as 2 liters daily. If the amount of fluid within the colon exceeds this amount, or if inflammation and infection of the bowel exists, diarrhea may be precipitated, with loss of both water and electrolytes. Bacterial infection (enteritis), intense inflammation, or irritation causes mucosal cells to secrete large volumes of water and mucus to dilute the irritating effect. Water and electrolyte losses (potassium and bicarbonate) can be significant and predispose to dehydration, electrolyte imbalance, and acid–base disturbances.

**Intestinal Motility.** As with the more proximal gastrointestinal tract, the large intestinal motility is characterized by mixing and propulsive movements. Mixing movements are very similar to the segmentation movements that occur in the small intestine. Combined contractions of longitudinal smooth muscle strips (teniae coli) and the circular muscle layer cause different portions of the colon to bulge outward into sacs or segments, in a process referred to as haustrations. Such movements have a kneading and churning effect on the intestinal contents, which serves to mix fully and mold the stool as it travels analward. The uncoordinated manner in which these movements occur in various parts of the colon serves to slow down intestinal movements, providing more time for absorption to occur.

Peristaltic waves of the type seen in the small intestine probably rarely occur in the large intestine. Most of the propulsive force is generated by the haustrations, which, like the segmentation of the small intestine, have some net forward movement of chyme. The movement is very slow, taking as many as 10–12 hours for chyme arriving at the ileocecal valve to move into the transverse colon.

Propulsion of chyme over the distal half of the colon occurs by mass movement. These strong peristaltic movements may occur only a few times each day, most often during the hour after eating. They can move the colonic contents en masse over long distances. When feces is forced into the rectum from its storage depot in the sigmoid colon, the urge for defecation is experienced.

**Secretions.** Secretions of the large intestine are scant with no digestive function. The epithelial cells lining the crypts of Lieberkühn are fewer in number than in the small intestine and contain no enzymes. The predominant cells lining the colon are goblet cells, which secrete mucus (see Fig. 47–6). In the large intestine, mucus has several functions. It acts as a lubricant and protects the intestinal mucosa from injury or excoriation as the forming stool moves toward the rectum. It provides a viscous medium that helps to hold fecal matter together in a semisolid mass. In combination with a rich bicarbonate supply, mucus protects the mucosal wall from any acids that may be formed from bacterial activity within the feces. In the presence of inflammation, secretion of mucus may be increased greatly, predisposing to loss of protein in the stool.

The large intestine contains a significant, flourishing bacterial flora, which makes a distinct contribution to body physiology. Vitamin K, essential for blood coagulation, is synthesized by bacteria within the intestinal flora. Any alteration in, or destruction of, the intestinal bacterial flora, as occurs, for example, with the administration of large doses of antibiotics, may cause a vitamin K deficiency. While a small amount of vitamin K does occur in ingested foods, it is not nearly enough to meet the body's daily need for this nutrient.

Malabsorption disorders can also predispose to vitamin K deficiency and deficiency of the other fat-soluble vitamins (A, D, E) as well. Folic acid and some of the B vitamins are also derived from bacterial metabolism and are subject to deficiency states when there is an alteration in bowel function.

Colonic bacteria are also involved in continuous putrefaction activity, which serves to break down undigested and/or unabsorbed substances. This process of putrefaction accounts for much of the gas present within the gut on a daily basis. Production of ammonia from the putrefaction of blood in the gut is a significant consideration in cirrhosis of the liver (see Chap. 50).

Other functions of the colon include excretion of heavy metals (silver, zinc, mercury) and unabsorbed substances such as calcium and phosphate. The sigmoid portion of the colon acts as a storage chamber for feces until such time as defecation occurs.

## ACCESSORY ORGANS OF DIGESTION

### Liver

The liver, the largest gland in the body, is involved intricately in numerous and complex biochemical functions essential in maintaining the life processes of the body in an equilibrated state.

#### *Microstructure*

The functional unit of the liver is the liver lobule. Classically, the liver lobule is described as roughly hexagonal in shape and composed of rows or plates of hepatic cells (hepatocytes) arranged radially around a central vein which drains it (Fig. 47–7). The central vein empties blood into the hepatic veins and, thence, into the vena cava.

Located at the periphery of each lobule are the portal triads, which mark the intersection of several lobules. Each portal triad consists of at least one branch of the hepatic artery and portal vein, a bile duct, and supportive connective tissue. The spaces between the plates of hepatocytes are lined with

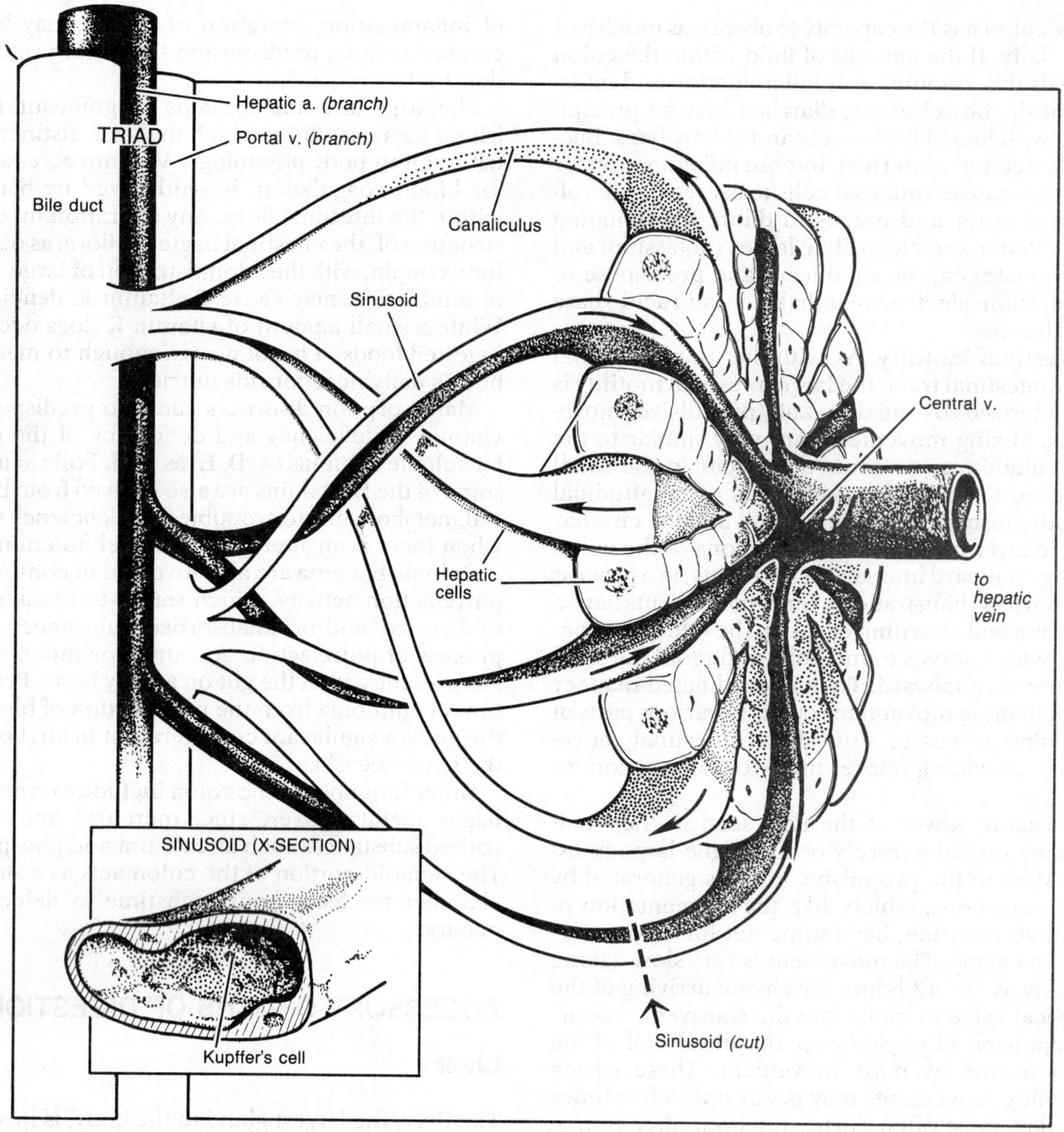


**Figure 47-7.** Ultrastructure of liver lobule. Diagrammatic representation of the radial disposition of liver cell plates and sinusoids around the central vein. There is centripetal flow of blood from branches of the hepatic artery and portal vein and centrifugal flow of bile to small bile ducts in the portal triad. A sinusoid is depicted in cross-section, and a Kupffer's cell, contained therein, is identified.

specialized capillaries called sinusoids, which are branches of the portal vein and hepatic artery.

The structure of the sinusoids is unique in 2 respects: one, extremely large pores, or fenestrations, exist between the endothelial cells of the sinusoids, enabling a variety of substances (including plasma proteins) to be filtered freely into and out of the sinusoids; and, two, the sinusoids are lined with Kupffer cells, which are cells of the reticuloendothelial system capable of phagocytizing bacteria and other foreign matter in the blood. This is an important feature because the portal system drains blood directly from the gastrointestinal tract where bacteria and other substances may have been absorbed. Kupffer cells provide a major mechanism of defense against bacterial invasion and/or other substances toxic to the body.

**Hepatocyte.** The functional unit of the liver is the hepatocyte, which comprises 70%–80% of the total mass of the liver. The hepatocyte is the only cell in the liver responsible for many of the metabolic processes, both anabolic and catabolic, essential for life. Its close anatomical approximation to both biliary and sinusoidal vascular systems enables the hepatocytes to carry out many of its sophisticated metabolic functions. Major functions of the hepatocyte are listed in Table 47-4.

**Hepatic Biliary System.** The bile duct located in

TABLE 47-4
## Major Functions of the Liver—Hepatocyte

| Function | Underlying Process/Mechanism |
|---|---|
| ***Carbohydrate Metabolism*** | ***Glycogenesis*** |
| Maintenance of serum glucose levels: 70–110 mg/100 ml | Conversion of glucose that is not used immediately by the cells for energy, to its storage form, glycogen. |
| | ***Glycogenolysis*** |
| | Breakdown of glycogen into glucose molecules with subsequent release into bloodstream for use as an energy source by the cells. |
| | When serum glucose levels rise above the normal level (e.g., at mealtimes—digestive periods), the excess glucose is quickly taken up by hepatocytes, converted to glycogen and stored in the liver. |
| | When serum glucose levels drop below the normal level (e.g., in between meals—interdigestive periods), the hepatocytes rapidly split stored glycogen into glucose molecules, which are released into the circulating blood and made available as an energy source for cells throughout the body. |
| | The ability to convert glycogen into glucose molecules that can easily pass into extracellular fluid and circulating blood is a function unique to the hepatocyte. |
| | ***Gluconeogenesis*** |
| | Synthesis of glucose molecules from protein and fats. |
| ***Protein Metabolism*** | ***Transamination/Deamination Reactions*** |
| Synthesis of nonessential amino acids | Synthesis of eleven nonessential amino acids from the ten essential amino acids obtained from exogenous sources (diet). |
| Synthesis of serum proteins | Synthesis of serum proteins including:<br>• Albumin—function to maintain colloidal osmotic pressure<br>• Globulins—alpha, beta and gamma globulins (gamma globulins are synthesized by plasma cells in lymphoid tissue predominantly in the gastrointestinal tract).<br>• Fibrinogen—source of fibrin, which forms basis of clot formation. |
| Synthesis of clotting factors | Clotting factors II, VII, IX, and X require vitamin K for synthesis. |
| Removal of waste products of protein metabolism. | ***Conversion of Ammonia to Urea*** |
| | Two molecules of ammonia plus one molecule of carbon dioxide are combined to produce urea and water. |
| | Urea diffuses out of hepatocytes into the blood and is eliminated via the kidneys. |
| | Moderate amounts of ammonia are continuously being formed in the gut secondary to metabolic activities of the intestinal bacterial flora. Without a normally functioning liver, concentrations of ammonia in the blood would rise, predisposing the patient to hepatic encephalopathy. |
| Regenerative capability of the liver | The synthesis of serum proteins by hepatocytes is so significant that should their concentrations become depleted for whatever reason, hepatocytes undergo mitosis with rapid regeneration and proliferation in order to increase the protein-synthesizing capacity of the liver to meet the demand. |
| ***Fat Metabolism*** | |
| Maintenance of serum lipid levels | The liver is the principal site for synthesis and degradation of lipids. |
| Energy source | ***Beta Oxidation Reactions*** |
| | Formation of acetoacetic acid, a potent energy source made available by hepatocytes to cells throughout the body. |
| Synthesis of structural components of plasma membranes | Cholesterol and phospholipid (lecithin) synthesis.<br>Most membranous structures throughout the body contain predominant amounts of cholesterol and phospholipids. |
| Major component of bile synthesis | Eighty percent of cholesterol synthesized by the liver is converted to bile salts.<br>Phospholipids may facilitate absorption of fatty acids by the intestinal mucosa and contribute to the structural framework of intracellular organelles. |
| Synthesis of lipoproteins. | *Lipoprotein Synthesis* |
| | Aggregates of lipid molecules partially coated by protein, lipoproteins play a strategic role in the transport of lipids in the blood.<br>Types of liproproteins include:<br>• Very low density lipoproteins (VLDL)<br>• Low density lipoproteins (LDL)<br>• High density lipoproteins (HDL) |
| Synthesis and use of triglycerides as energy source | *Triglyceride Synthesis* |
| | Formation of acetoacetic acid.<br>Conversion of carbohydrates into fat.<br>Conversion of protein into fat. |
| ***Drug Metabolism*** | Hepatocytes are responsible for the metabolism of a large variety of lipid-soluble drugs (e.g., barbiturates). |
| | Administration of such drugs induces an increase in drug-metabolizing enzymes, which enhance the efficiency with which the hepatocytes can eliminate such drugs. |

*(continued)*

TABLE 47-4
**Major Functions of the Liver—Hepatocyte *(Continued)***

| Function | Underlying Process/Mechanism |
| --- | --- |
| ***Detoxification*** Detoxification of endogenous and exogenous substances | Oxidation, reduction, acetylation and conjugation are some of the chemical reactions occurring within hepatocytes that render potentially harmful substances inactive and amenable to excretion via the bile and kidneys. These chemical reactions similarly metabolize a variety of hormones secreted within the body. |
| ***Hormonal Metabolism*** All major steroids Thyroxine Other | |
| ***Vitamin and Mineral Utilization and Storage*** | Hepatocytes play a key role in absorption, utilization and storage of fat-soluble vitamins A, D, E and K. Stores of vitamin A may last as long as two years. Stores of vitamins D and $B_{12}$ are sufficient to last up to four months. |
| ***Storage of Iron, Copper, Calcium*** | Hepatocytes contain large amounts of the protein apoferritin, which combines with iron to form ferritin, the form in which it is stored in the liver. The liver also stores copper. The major route for the excretion of calcium is via bile, and then the feces. |
| ***Bile Synthesis*** | Bile, which is essential for digestion and absorption of fats and fat-soluble vitamins, is continuously produced by hepatocytes, stored in the gallbladder, and released into the duodenum in response to appropriate stimuli (fatty chyme in duodenum, secretion of cholecystokinin). |
| ***Bilirubin Metabolism*** Bilirubin metabolism and elimination in the bile | Hepatocytes play a key role in the uptake, conjugation and excretion of bilirubin in bile. |
| ***Synthesis of Coagulation Factors*** | Hepatocytes play a strategic role in blood coagulation through synthesis of proteins essential for blood clotting, and for fibrinolysis (clot lysis). |
| ***Blood Filtration and Storage*** | The liver, by virtue of its size and strategic position in the circulatory system, has the important functions of blood filtration and storage. The unique structure of the sinusoids and the presence of Kupffer cells throughout enable blood received from the gastrointestinal tract to be filtered of intestinal or exogenous bacteria, endotoxins, and other absorbed substances. Thus, blood returning to the systemic circulation from the liver is cleared of potentially harmful material. |
| ***The Liver as a Reservoir ("Hepatic Reserve")*** | The liver receives about 25 percent of the cardiac output each minute via its dual circulation—hepatic artery and portal vein. Of this amount approximately 500 ml is held within the sinusoids and hepatic vessels. This large volume present in the liver at any given time enables this organ to act as a reservoir for blood, storing it if it occurs in excess (right sided congestive heart failure), or relinquishing it to the systemic circulation if its volume becomes depleted (dehydration, hypovolemia). |

the portal triad drains the bile produced by the hepatocytes. The flow of bile occurs through a system of bile canaliculi (tiny bile capillaries) found between the plates of hepatocytes, in a direction that is from the more central areas of the liver lobule to its periphery. All bile eventually empties into the main hepatic duct, which merges with the cystic bile duct from the gallbladder to form the common bile duct. The common bile duct enters the duodenum at the ampulla of Vater (Fig. 47-8).

A muscular sphincter (sphincter of Oddi) guards the duodenal opening of the common bile duct as it enters the intestinal lumen. The sphincter relaxes, largely in response to the presence of chyme (fat) in the duodenum and to the effects of the hormone, cholecystokinin (CCK). A relaxed sphincter of Oddi, coupled with contractions of the gallbladder (also stimulated by CCK), enables the appropriate amount of bile to be emptied into the duodenum where it is available for the digestion of fats. When the sphincter is closed, bile, which is continuously secreted by the liver, is directed to the gallbladder where it is concentrated and stored.

Bile salts facilitate digestion and absorption of fats by their role in emulsification and micelle-formation processes. Without the presence of bile salts in the gastrointestinal tract, up to 40%–50% of ingested fat would be lost in the stool.

### Blood and Lymphatic Circulation

The liver enjoys a dual blood supply accounting for up to 25% of the cardiac output each minute. Of this amount, approximately 1 liter is supplied by the portal vein, while the remainder is supplied by the hepatic artery.

An important feature of the portal system is the low resistance to hepatic blood flow. Hydrostatic pressure of blood in the portal system as it enters the liver is approximately 9 mmHg, while the pressure within the hepatic vein leaving the liver is approximately zero.

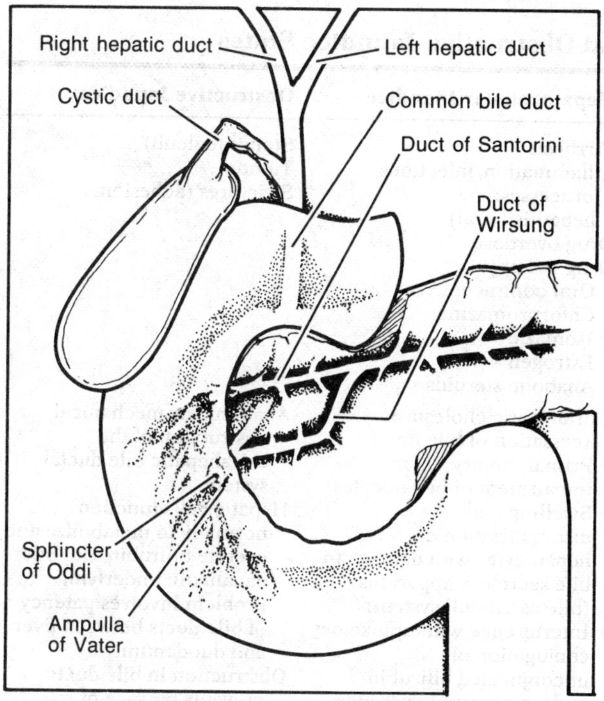


**Figure 47-8.** Depiction of structural relationships of biliary system, pancreas, and duodenum. The right and left hepatic ducts join to form the common bile duct, which eventually drains bile into the intestinal lumen (duodenum). Bile not used for digestion drains by way of the cystic duct into the gallbladder where it is stored. Pancreatic secretions drain by way of the ducts of Wirsung and Santorini into the duodenum. The sphincter of Oddi guards the opening of the common bile duct as it enters the intestinal lumen.

The portal vein, formed by the union of the splenic and superior mesenteric veins, carries venous blood, rich in absorbed nutrients and metabolic products, from the capillaries of the gastrointestinal tract into the liver. The uniqueness of the "portal" system is that the portal vein is interposed between 2 capillary beds, that of the gastrointestinal tract, which it drains, and that of the sinusoids.

### *Bilirubin Metabolism*

In addition to secretory functions, the hepatocytes are also involved in the excretion of substances formed elsewhere in the body. One of the more important of these is bilirubin, a major metabolic end-product of the degradation of hemoglobin. As senescent red blood cells are sequestered within cells of the reticuloendothelial system, hemoglobin is catabolized with the heme portion converted first to biliverdin, and, subsequently, to unconjugated bilirubin. In this reaction, the iron is liberated and enters the circulation by a carrier molecule, transferrin. It may be used in the production of new red blood cells or stored in a variety of tissues until needed.

Unconjugated bilirubin circulates in the blood tightly bound to albumin. The concentration of unconjugated bilirubin occurring in the blood is reflected by the indirect serum bilirubin level. Excessive hemolysis of red blood cells is often associated with elevated indirect serum bilirubin levels.

Eventually, unconjugated bilirubin is transported to the liver where it is metabolized in a series of reactions to its conjugated form. The significance of the conjugation reactions is that the previously water-*in*soluble bilirubin (unconjugated form) is rendered water-soluble and capable of being excreted by the liver into the bile. Once delivered to the small intestine in the bile, bilirubin conjugates are acted on by the normal intestinal bacterial flora to form urobilinogen.

Urobilinogen is highly soluble, and some of it is reabsorbed into the bloodstream and, subsequently, excreted as urobilin in the urine. A small fraction of conjugated bilirubin does remain in the blood, and this is reflected by the direct serum bilirubin levels. The remaining urobilinogen found in the intestine is oxidized to stercobilin and excreted in the feces. The presence of urobilin and stercobilin gives the urine and stool their characteristic colors. Elevated direct serum bilirubin levels reflect parenchymal liver disease or biliary obstruction.

**Hyperbilirubinemia — Jaundice States.** Jaundice (icterus) refers to the yellowish tint or staining of the skin, sclerae, deeper tissues, and body secretions (urine and feces). It is usually due to the presence of large quantities of bilirubin in the extracellular fluid. The normal serum bilirubin concentration, including the direct (conjugated) and indirect (unconjugated) forms, averages 0.5 mg/100 ml. Jaundice may begin to appear at serum bilirubin levels greater than 1.5–2.0 mg/100 ml.

Four pathophysiologic mechanisms may predispose to hyperbilirubinemia and jaundice. They include: bilirubin overproduction, decreased uptake by hepatic cells, impairment of hepatic conjugation reactions, and decreased excretion of bilirubin into bile. The resulting disease (jaundice) states include hemolytic jaundice, hepatocellular jaundice, and obstructive or cholestatic jaundice. The contrasting features of these jaundice states are presented in Table 47-5.

## Pancreas

Next to the liver, the pancreas is considered to be the largest gland connected with the gastrointestinal tract. It is located in the retroperitoneal space deep within the epigastrium at the level of the first and second lumbar vertebrae. Of importance, the pancreas has no defined external capsule as does the liver, and, therefore, infections and other pancreatic disorders may not be well contained. Disease of surrounding tissue (e.g., perforated duodenal ulcer) may directly involve the pancreas,

TABLE 47–5

## Contrasting Features: Hemolytic, Hepatocellular and Obstructive Jaundice States

| Features | Hemolytic Jaundice | Hepatocellular Jaundice | Obstructive Jaundice |
|---|---|---|---|
| ***Etiology*** | Hemolytic disease (anemia)<br>Ineffective erythropoiesis<br>Massive tissue infarction:<br>• Pulmonary embolism<br>• Ruptured aneurysm<br>• Profuse hemorrhage | Cirrhosis<br>Inflammation/infectious processes:<br>• hepatitis (viral)<br>Drug overdose<br>Drug therapy:<br>• Oral contraceptives<br>• Chlorpromazine<br>• Isoniazid<br>• Estrogen<br>• Anabolic steroids | Stones (calculi)<br>Tumors<br>Strictures (adhesions) |
| ***Pathophysiology*** | Increased production of bilirubin beyond the capacity of liver to metabolize and excrete it in the bile.<br>Increased red blood cell hemolysis, and hemoglobin degradation.<br>Metabolic and excretory hepatic functions remain unimpaired and intact. | Intrahepatic cholestasis (cessation of bile flow)<br>• Primary injury to, or impairment of hepatocytes.<br>• Swelling and disorganization of hepatocytes with damage to bile secretory apparatus (bile canaliculi system).<br>• Interference with uptake or conjugation of unconjugated bilirubin and/or impaired excretion of conjugated bilirubin. | Anatomic or mechanical obstruction of the extrahepatic bile ductal system.<br>Hepatic cells function normally to metabolize and excrete bilirubin into bile canaliculi; underlying problem involves patency of bile ducts between liver and duodenum.<br>Obstruction in bile duct prevents passage of bilirubin-containing bile into duodenum.<br>***Complete Bile Duct Obstruction***<br>Back up of pressure in biliary system.<br>Interference with secretion of conjugated bilirubin by hepatocytes into bile canaliculi system.<br>Accumulation of bile within hepatocytes and Kupffer cells.<br>Entrance of bile into bloodstream via sinusoids and lymphatic circulations.<br>Interference with uptake and conjugation of unconjugated bilirubin. |
| ***Clinical Presentation*** | | | |
| Skin color | Mild pale yellow jaundice | Deep yellow to orange | Deep yellow-green hue (biliverdin) |
| Pruritus | None | Variable | Present-persistent pruritus is associated with deposition of bile salts in the skin. |
| Urine color | Normal to dark | Dark (conjugated bilirubin) | Dark (conjugated bilirubin) |
| Stool color | Normal to dark<br>• Darker colored urine and stool are due to increased levels of urobilinogen formed in the gut and absorbed into the blood. | Light-colored | Clay-colored |
| Other | Anemia | | Digestive disturbances due to inability to digest fats. |
| ***Laboratory*** | | | |
| *Serum Bilirubin* | | | |
| Total | Rarely >5 mg/100 ml | >50 mg/100 ml | 30–40 mg/100 ml |
| Indirect (unconjugated) | Increased | Increased | Increased<br>Pronounced cholestasis interferes with uptake and conjugation, and serum levels of unconjugated bilirubin also rise. |

TABLE 47-5
**Contrasting Features: Hemolytic, Hepatocellular and Obstructive Jaundice States *(Continued)***

| Features | Hemolytic Jaundice | Hepatocellular Jaundice | Obstructive Jaundice |
|---|---|---|---|
| Direct (conjugated) | Normal | Increased (predominantly) Impaired excretion of bilirubin into the bile canalicular circulation accounts for conjugated hyperbilirubinemia. | Increased |
| Serum alkaline phosphatase | Normal | Increased ↑ | Increased ↑↑ |
| Serum SGOT | Normal | Increased | Increased ↑ |
| Other | Reticulocytes with abnormal erythrocytes | Elevated serum cholesterol | |
| Urine bilirubin | Absent Unconjugated bilirubin is water-insoluble. | Increased Evidence of conjugated hyperbilirubinemia as conjugated bilirubin is water-soluble. | Increased |

causing inadvertent release of digestive enzymes into adjacent tissues with consequent abscess formation.

### Microstructure

The pancreas functions as both an endocrine and exocrine gland with these functions carried out by different groups of cells. The endocrine pancreas consists of isolated clumps of cells, the islets of Langerhans, which are scattered throughout the organ. Functionally, these islet cells are unrelated to the exocrine pancreas; rather, as true endocrine glands, they secrete the hormones insulin and glucagon directly into the bloodstream. These hormones, which are essential for the metabolism of fats, proteins, and especially carbohydrates, are discussed in detail in Chapter 19.

**Exocrine.** The exocrine pancreas consists of groups or clusters of cells called acini, which are responsible for the production of pancreatic digestive juices. Small ducts from these acini empty their contents directly into the main pancreatic duct (duct of Wirsung), which extends throughout the length of the pancreas, joining the common bile duct within the ampulla of Vater before its entrance into the duodenum (see Fig. 47-8). The exocrine pancreatic glands elaborate approximately 1200-1500 ml of digestive juices each day.

### Secretion

Pancreatic digestive juice contains enzymes of their precursors, for digesting all 3 major food types: carbohydrates (α-amylase), proteins (trypsin, chymotrypsin, elastase, carboxypeptidases, and aminopeptidases), and fats (lipase, phospholipase $A_2$, and cholesterol esterase). Trypsin is a pivotal enzyme because, once it is activated, it is responsible for activating other enzymatic precursors. The pancreas also contains specific enzymes (nucleases, for example, ribonuclease) for metabolism of nucleic acids.

Most proteolytic enzymes synthesized within the pancreatic acinar cells are secreted by the acini in an inactive form. They become activated only after they reach the alkaline milieu of the duodenum. Perhaps this is nature's way of protecting the pancreas from self-digestion.

Two other important components of pancreatic juice are bicarbonate and water. This highly alkaline juice serves to neutralize the acid chyme emptied into the duodenum from the stomach and, thus, protects the sensitive mucosal cells of the small intestine from the intense digestive action of gastric juice. Secretion of bicarbonate ions is essential to provide an appropriate alkaline pH for the catalytic activity of pancreatic enzymes.

### Regulation of Pancreatic Secretion

Regulation of pancreatic secretion involves both nervous and hormonal mechanisms. During the cephalic and gastric phases of stomach digestion, the pancreas receives parasympathetic stimulation by the vagus nerve, which increases enzyme secretion. There is little concomitant secretion of water and electrolytes to facilitate movement of enzymes through the pancreatic ductal system. Therefore, pancreatic enzymes are stored in the acini during these phases of digestion.

After chyme enters the duodenum (intestinal phase), pancreatic secretion becomes copious, mainly in response to 2 hormones: secretin and cholecystokinin (CCK). Secretion of secretin by intestinal mucosal cells in response to presence of acid chyme in the duodenum precipitates copious secretions of bicarbonate by the pancreas, which functions to neutralize the acid chyme. Secretin also stimulates Brunner's glands within the duodenum to secrete a bicarbonate-rich fluid, further neutralizing the acidity.

Cholecystokinin (CCK), secreted by intestinal mucosal cells in response to presence of partially digested proteins and fats in the duodenum, directly stimulates the pancreas to secrete digestive enzymes. This hormone also stimulates the musculature of the gallbladder to contract, propelling bile into the duodenum for the digestion of fats.

Gastrin, secreted by antral cells in the stomach, also stimulates pancreatic secretion, but its effect is quantitatively less important than that of CCK.

## REFERENCES

1. Granger, DN, Barrowman, J, and Kvietys, P: Clinical Gastrointestinal Physiology. WB Saunders, Philadelphia, 1985, p 17.
2. Guyton, AC: Textbook of Medical Physiology, ed 7. WB Saunders, Philadelphia, 1986, p 787.
3. McConnell, E: Meeting the challenge of intestinal obstruction. Nursing '87 17(7):34, 1987.

CHAPTER 48

# Gastrointestinal Assessment

## CHAPTER OUTLINE

CLINICAL HISTORY
- Components of the Clinical History

PHYSICAL EXAMINATION
- Components of the Physical Examination

DIAGNOSTIC STUDIES
- Laboratory Tests
- Diagnostic Studies and Procedures
- Nursing Considerations

## LEARNING OBJECTIVES

**At the end of this chapter, you should be able to:**

1. Identify essential aspects of the clinical history as they pertain to gastrointestinal function and dysfunction.
2. List the cardinal symptoms of gastrointestinal dysfunction.
3. Elicit assessment data based on knowledge of functional health patterns.
4. Describe the four abdominal quadrants and the anatomical relationships of organs within each quadrant.
5. List the four techniques used in the physical examination of the abdomen, and the order in which they are performed.
6. Define essential information to be obtained on inspection of the mouth and pharynx, neck and abdomen.
7. Describe the techniques of auscultation of the abdomen and expected findings.
8. State the significance of percussion in determining size and location of abdominal organs, distribution of air within the gastrointestinal tract, and presence of solid, or fluid-filled masses, and ascites.
9. Describe key aspects of the palpatory examination of the gastrointestinal system.
10. Outline key diagnostic tests and studies for gastrointestinal disorders.
11. Identify key nursing considerations in the diagnostic workup for gastrointestinal disorders.

The critical care nurse assesses the patient with altered gastrointestinal function by collecting data from history-taking and astute observation, physical assessment, laboratory tests, and pertinent diagnostic studies. The assessment and diagnosis of gastrointestinal disorders can be perplexing and formidable tasks. It may be difficult to differentiate systemic manifestations of underlying gastrointestinal disease from systemic disease involving other organ systems that is complicated by gastrointestinal dysfunction. Such cardinal gastrointestinal signs and symptoms as anorexia, nausea, vomiting, diarrhea, or abdominal pain may be indicative of a number of markedly different etiologies (e.g., severe metabolic derangement, fluid and electrolyte imbalance, renal disease, cancer, adverse drug reactions).

Often, what may appear to be an innocuous gastrointestinal symptom (e.g., heartburn or indigestion) may, in fact, signal the occurrence of serious underlying pathology in another organ system (e.g., myocardial infarction). It is important to determine whether assessment data are related to the established diagnosis or reflect a change in the patient's condition. Establishing baseline assessment data is invaluable in differential diagnosis. It is essential to always consider the patient as a whole and to evaluate clinical manifestations and responses in terms of total body function.

## CLINICAL HISTORY

In initiating the patient's gastrointestinal assessment, it is essential to consider the patient's immediate status and whether the patient is experiencing distress. The extent and comprehensiveness of the initial history and examination should be modified accordingly.

### Components of the Clinical History

#### *Chief Complaint*

In eliciting the patient's history, it is necessary to establish the chief complaint (i.e., the single, most important reason as to why the patient has sought health care at this point in time).

#### *History of Present Illness*

The history of present illness serves to elaborate the details surrounding the chief complaint and should include its *onset*, the *course since onset*, and *current status*. Use of the "SLIDT" tool assists in eliciting specific information about the nature of the gastrointestinal complaint, which may otherwise seem vague. It is important to determine the *S*everity of the symptom; its *L*ocation (radiation); *I*nfluencing factors, which include precipitating event, factors that aggravate or ameliorate the complaint, and associated factors and events including the setting within which it occurs; *D*uration of the complaint and its timing in terms of events or patterns surrounding the patient; and *T*ype or quality of the complaint, or its descriptive characteristics (e.g., bright red hematemesis). (See Table 7-1.)

**Cardinal Symptoms of Gastrointestinal Dysfunction.** The cardinal symptoms of gastrointestinal dysfunction include anorexia, nausea, vomiting, dysphagia, diarrhea, constipation, and abdominal and referred pain.

***Anorexia.*** Anorexia is a nonspecific symptom associated with many acute and chronic illnesses. It is defined as an aversion to eating despite an existing hunger (i.e., craving for food). It is significant clinically in that it predisposes to malnutrition. Regulation of food intake occurs primarily within the hypothalamus and involves the interaction of the neural networks within the "feeding" (hunger) center and the "satiety" center. (*Satiety* is defined as the lack of desire to eat that occurs after food is ingested.)

Factors that stimulate the "feeding" center (increase appetite) include hypoglycemia and the hormone, insulin; factors that stimulate the "satiety" center (decrease appetite) include hyperglycemia, gastric distention, and the hormone, cholecystokinin. Emotional factors also impact on appetite and eating patterns probably by neuronal connections between the cerebral cortex, subcortical areas, and the hypothalamus.

***Nausea.*** Nausea is the conscious awareness of the need to vomit. It occurs largely as a premonition of vomiting and is associated with distention and/or irritation of the gastrointestinal tract, motion sickness (brainstem neuronal activity), and/or altered autonomic system activity. It is usually accompanied by hypersalivation and a reduction in gastric tone with a concomitant increase in intestinal muscle tone. Diaphoresis, skin pallor, and hypotension may also occur.

***Vomiting.*** Vomiting is the forceful expulsion of gastric and duodenal contents. It involves strong contractions of abdominal muscles, which increase intra-abdominal pressure, forcing the diaphragm and cardia portion of the stomach up into the thorax. This increases intrathoracic pressure. When intrathoracic pressure overcomes the resistance of the upper esophageal sphincter, gastrointestinal contents are expelled. Vomiting is thought to be controlled by a "vomiting" or "emetic" center within the brainstem (medulla), which is closely approximated, both anatomically and functionally, with respiratory and vasomotor medullary centers. The major stimulus for vomiting is gastric and duodenal overdistention and/or excessive irritation.

Clinically, major sequelae of severe vomiting include dehydration and malnutrition associated with reduced fluid and food intake; metabolic alkalemia with hypokalemia associated with loss of gastric secretions; and an increased risk of aspiration in patients who have compromised protective reflexes (e.g., gag and swallowing reflexes).

Documentation of the vomiting episode should include precipitating or associated factors, whether it was projectile, the amount, and characteristics of the vomitus (e.g., bright red blood, coffee-grind, bilious, or feculent).

***Dysphagia.*** Dysphagia is difficulty in swallowing. In assessing this symptom, it is important to appreciate that its clinical presentation will vary according to the anatomical location of the difficulty. Disturbances at the level of the oropharynx may result in nasal regurgitation, choking, aspiration, and the inability to move the bolus into the esophagus. Disruptions at the level of the esophagus may involve ineffective, diminished, or absent peristalsis, preventing movement of the bolus through the esophagus. The patient may complain of retrosternal fullness on swallowing. Dysfunction of the lower esophageal sphincter (*achalasia*) may disrupt esophageal motility, prevent movement of the bolus into the stomach, and result in the accumulation of food within the esophagus.

It is important to pinpoint where the discomfort occurs during swallowing and whether it occurs with liquids, solid foods, or both. The "swallowing" center in the medulla coordinates the highly complex and intricate nature of the events involved in swallowing. Most muscles involved in swallowing are innervated by the vagus nerves. Dysphagia is often a consequence of neurologic or neuromuscular disease.

***Diarrhea.*** Diarrhea refers to an increase in frequency and fluidity of the stool. The stool should be assessed for the presence of abnormal constituents such as blood (inflammation), mucus (irritable colon), or greasy, bulky, or foul-smelling stools (fat malabsorption). Influencing factors, such as pattern of bowel movements (e.g., constipation alternating with diarrhea), ingestion of foods that seem to precipitate the diarrhea, and associated symptoms such as abdominal cramping, pain, weakness, diaphoresis, and vomiting, should all be evaluated.

The significance of diarrhea is the impact it can have on fluid and electrolyte balance. Of the nearly 10 liters of fluid that enters the gastrointestinal tract daily, 2–3 liters reflect exogenous sources (ingested foods and fluids), while the remainder reflects endogenous sources (salivary, gastric, pancreatic, biliary, and intestinal secretions). All but a few hundred milliliters of this amount is reabsorbed. Active absorption of electrolytes (especially sodium) plays a significant role in establishing electrochemical, osmotic, and hydrostatic gradients, which facilitates absorption of nutrients, vitamins, minerals, and water.

Any abnormal increase in gastrointestinal secretions and/or alteration in the absorptive efficiency of the gastrointestinal tract can predispose to diarrhea. *Secretory* diarrhea is characterized by a net loss of sodium and bicarbonate ions, and the 24-hour stool volume may exceed 1 liter. *Osmotic* diarrhea occurs when the absorptive capabilities of the gastrointestinal tract are exceeded. It is characterized primarily by potassium and water depletion. The 24-hour stool volume is usually less than 1 liter. Frequently, a combination of both types of diarrhea occurs. Hypermotility and excessive peristalsis throughout the gastrointestinal tract are often implicated as underlying causes.

***Constipation.*** Constipation refers to a decrease in the usual frequency of bowel evacuation. It may imply excessive straining during a bowel movement and is usually characterized by a small volume of stone-hard stools. It is important to determine the patient's pre-illness bowel routine, and how it may have changed. The acuity or chronicity of the constipation should be established. Chronic constipation is associated with a low residue diet. It is a frequent occurrence in patients with a longstanding pattern of voluntary inhibition of the defecation reflex.

Documentation should include the size, volume, character, and frequency of bowel movements; the presence or absence of flatulence; the presence of associated symptoms such as abdominal cramps or pain, and abdominal distention; and whether or not there has been any recent change in the patient's lifestyle.

***Abdominal and Referred Pain.*** Pain is a factor in the clinical presentation of a variety of disorders. A thorough, comprehensive history is often helpful in differential diagnosis. Use of the SLIDT tool (see Table 7–1) is especially helpful when assessing pain.

*Referred Pain.* Referred pain is pain in a part of the body that is distant to the tissues in which the pain originates. Commonly, such pain is initiated in a visceral organ and referred to an area of the body surface. Branches of visceral pain fibers synapse in the spinal cord with afferent neurons transmitting pain impulses from the skin surface along dermatomal distribution. The resulting pain sensation may be perceived as originating in the skin rather than within a viscus. Referred pain may be the only symptom of underlying visceral pathophysiology. It is usually described as sharp and is well-localized.

*Visceral Pain.* Visceral pain originates in abdominal or thoracic viscera. It differs from body surface pain in that it is poorly localized. It is frequently described as a dull, gnawing, or cramping sensation. Widespread stimulation of visceral pain nerve endings, as occurs with ischemia, stretching, or overdistention of the gut, or smooth muscle spasm of a hollow viscus (e.g., intestines, gallbladder, bile ducts, ureter), can precipitate severe pain. Injury caused by chemical stimuli (e.g., leakage of proteolytic enzymes into surrounding tissues, as occurs in acute pancreatitis or perforated peptic ulcer) can cause extremely severe abdominal pain. Cramping pain may assume a rhythmic pattern, waxing and waning in severity in conjunction with peristaltic smooth muscle contraction and relaxation.

*Parietal Pain.* Parietal pain is associated with inflammation of underlying viscera with extension to parietal membranes lining body cavities (e.g., pleura, pericardium, peritoneum). These linings and/or adjacent tissues are richly endowed with pain nerve endings, which, when irritated, can cause very sharp pain (e.g., pleuritis, peritonitis).

Additional significant gastrointestinal symptomatology may include gastrointestinal bleeding as demonstrated by bright red to coffee-grind vomitus (*hematemesis*), bloody stool (*hematochezia*), or tarry stool (*melena*); jaundice (see Table 47–5) accompanied by pruritis (hyperbilirubinemia); *ascites* (i.e., an accumulation of serous fluid in the peritoneal cavity); and bleeding or bruising tendency (onset, duration, extent).

### Functional Health Patterns

Assessment of the patient's functional health patterns (see Appendix C) is essential to elicit information of significance to nursing diagnosis and treatment, including patient/family education and discharge planning.

**Nutritional–Metabolic.** The nutritional–metabolic assessment may reveal changes in the patient's general state of health. It involves such questions as: Has there been a weight gain or loss? How much, over how long a period of time? Is there loss of stamina? Does the patient tire easily? Is there an increased susceptibility to infection? Is wound healing sluggish?

Has the patient experienced any intolerance to foods? Are there complaints of heartburn, indigestion, or belching associated with eating? An intolerance to foods high in fat content, for example, may suggest a gallbladder problem. Is there evidence of a "pain–food–relief" pattern commonly associated with peptic ulcer disease? Does the patient take antacid medications? Why, how much, how frequently, for how long? Are the symptoms relieved?

The nutritional assessment should help to determine patient/family attitudes regarding diet and eating, and how they view themselves nutritionally and weightwise. What is a typical daily diet? Who prepares the food? Do socioeconomic constraints impact on daily food intake? Are there emotional or psychologic considerations that may impact on the patient's nutritional status (e.g., depression)?

**Elimination Pattern.** Assessment of the patient's bowel function, diet, and bowel habits is essential. Such information may provide the initial often subtle clues as to the presence of underlying gastrointestinal pathophysiology. Important questions to be asked are: Have there been recent changes in the patient's bowel elimination pattern? Is excessive straining required to move the bowels? Are the bowel movements painful? Are there changes in the frequency and consistency of bowel movements—diarrhea? constipation? What is the appearance of the stool—bloody, tarry, fatty (steatorrhea), mucoid, clay-colored, foul-smelling? Is there use of enemas, laxatives, other medications? What medications, over-the-counter or prescribed? Reason for taking medication, dose? Does the patient have hemorrhoids, for how long?

Assessment of urine elimination should include frequency, amount, color. A dark or orange urine suggests hyperbilirubinemia.

**Health Perceptions—Health Management.** It is important to determine what the patient's overall health status has been and whether there have been any significant changes in health or lifestyle. Patient/family attitudes about health, and the optimal level of health desired can be helpful in planning care. The patient's use of medications, prescriptions, and over-the-counter, should be ascertained. Data about use of such drugs as aspirin, steroids, and anticoagulants are critical in the patient who presents with gastrointestinal bleeding. Use of antibiotics can alter the intestinal bacterial flora disrupting bowel motility, and digestive and absorptive functions of the gastrointestinal tract. Alcohol or other drug use and abuse may provide a clue to underlying hepatic insufficiency.

#### *Past Medical History*

It is important to ascertain if the patient has had any previous gastrointestinal surgery—dental surgery, cholecystectomy, gastric or intestinal resection, appendectomy, hemorrhoidectomy, other? Has there been previous hospitalizations—why, when? Is there a past history of any of the following: Peptic ulcer disease (gastric, duodenal, stress)[1]; gastrointestinal hemorrhage; hepatic disease (cirrhosis, hepatitis, blood transfusions); abdominal trauma; pancreatitis; renal disease (renal colic, lithiasis–calculi formation); or diabetes mellitus?

#### *Family History*

It is important to determine if a predisposition exists for any disease that may be transmitted genetically or along ethnic lines. Examples of such diseases include peptic ulcer disease, ulcerative colitis, reginal enteritis (Crohn's disease), diverticulitis, gastric or colonic cancer, pernicious anemia, malabsorption syndromes, lactose intolerance, and alcoholism.

## PHYSICAL EXAMINATION

### Components of the Physical Examination

Components of the physical examination of the gastrointestinal assessment include an examination of the mouth and pharynx, the neck, and abdomen.

#### *Examination of the Mouth and Pharynx*

Techniques used to examine the mouth and pharynx include inspection and palpation. The face, lips, and jaw are inspected for signs of swelling or asymmetry. While the patient opens and closes his/her mouth, the temporomandibular joint is examined for tenderness, crepitus, and limitation of movement (see Table 7–3).

The lips are inspected for any abnormal color, dryness, cracking, lumps, ulceration, or other lesions. Using a rubber glove, the nurse should inspect the inner lip, buccal membranes and gums for color, pigmentation, inflammation (swelling and/or tenderness), excessive salivation, white patches, plaques, and ulceration; these tissues are palpated for lumps or nodules. Gums should also be examined for evidence of hypertrophy or retraction. Teeth are observed for malocclusion, dental caries, and general state of repair.

The tongue is inspected for color, moisture, unusual smoothness, abnormal movement, deviation, or paralysis (12th cranial nerve, hypoglossal). Grasping the tongue with a gauze pad enables inspection and palpation of the superior and lateral surfaces of the tongue for ulcerations or other lesions, lumps, or nodules. The floor of the mouth is inspected by asking the patient to touch the roof of the mouth with the tongue.

The pharynx can be examined by holding the tongue down with a tongue depressor and tilting the head backwards. When the patient is asked to say "ah," the uvula and soft palate should rise and remain in the midline (9th cranial nerve, or glossopharyngeal; 10th cranial nerve, or vagus). The anterior or posterior pharyngeal pillars, tonsils, if present, and posterior pharynx are examined for color, symmetry, inflammation, plaques, exudation, petechiae, and ulceration. Mouth odors, if unusual, should be described (e.g., sweet or fruity smell). (For cranial nerve examination, see Table 7-3.)

### Examination of the Neck

Examination of the neck is performed using inspection and palpation, and good lighting. The neck is inspected for symmetry, swelling, masses, and scars. Lymph nodes are systematically examined, noting size, shape, mobility, consistency, and tenderness. It is important to appreciate the regions drained by the lymph nodes (Fig. 48-1). The trachea should be inspected for any deviation from its midline position. The thyroid gland is palpated by an anterior or posterior approach, noting its size, shape, symmetry, tenderness, and the presence of any lumps or nodules (see Fig. 17-1).

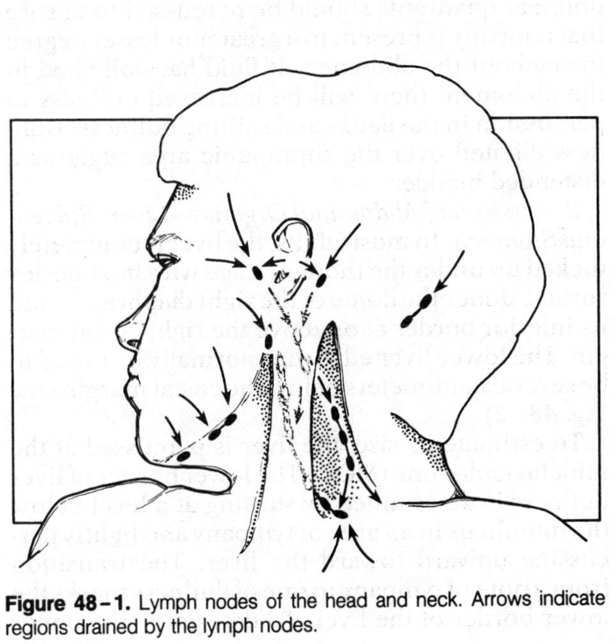

**Figure 48-1.** Lymph nodes of the head and neck. Arrows indicate regions drained by the lymph nodes.

The carotid arteries and jugular veins may be examined. The presence of jugular venous distention should be assessed with the patient in a sitting position. Auscultation may detect a thyroid or carotid bruit, or a jugular venous hum (see Chap. 38).

### Examination of the Abdomen

**Abdominal Quadrants.** For descriptive purposes, the abdomen is usually divided into 4 quadrants by imaginary lines, which cross at the umbilicus (Fig. 48-2). It is important to visualize underlying organs and their structural relationships within each quadrant.

**Techniques of Examination.** The techniques of examination include inspection, auscultation, percussion, and palpation, *in that order.* A systematic approach ensures thoroughness of examination. The examination should be conducted with the examiner at the patient's bedside.

To facilitate the examination, it is important to make appropriate explanations regarding the examination, and to help the patient to relax. The patient should not have a full bladder. The supine position is assumed, with a pillow for the patient's head and another under the knees. The arms should be at the patient's side. This position helps to relax abdominal musculature. The patient should be appropriately draped to ensure privacy, with full exposure of the abdomen. Good lighting is essential.

It is important to ask the patient to point to areas of pain or tenderness; these areas should be examined last. Throughout the abdominal examination,

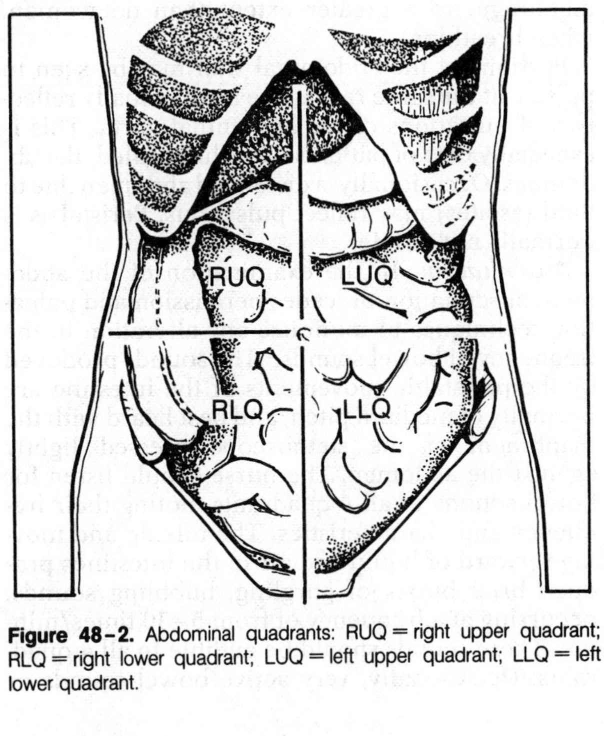


**Figure 48-2.** Abdominal quadrants: RUQ = right upper quadrant; RLQ = right lower quadrant; LUQ = left upper quadrant; LLQ = left lower quadrant.

it is important to watch the patient's face and expression for clues as to the presence of any discomfort.

***Inspection.*** When inspecting the abdomen for pulsations or peristaltic movements, it is important to bend down so that the abdominal surface can be viewed at eye level, and tangentially. The nurse should visualize the underlying organs. The position of the umbilicus should be noted, and the contour of the abdomen should be observed. Normally, the abdomen should be flat; there should be no bulging of the flanks. The skin is inspected for scars, texture, color, wounds, masses, or lesions. Bluish discolorations, bruises, or petechiae should be viewed with suspicion.

*Spider angiomas* (i.e., small red blood vessels radiating from a central point) suggest liver disease. Veins are normally not visible or prominent. When veins are prominent, the direction of blood flow should be noted. Normally, blood flows away from the umbilicus.

The abdomen should be inspected for hernias (i.e., a protrusion of tissue or an organ through an abnormal opening). Locations where hernias are prone to occur include the umbilicus, surgical scars, and above or below the inguinal ligament. Small protrusions may be checked by having the patient strain or perform a Valsalva's maneuver, which increases intra-abdominal pressure. Palpation helps to confirm the presence of a hernia.

The motion of the abdominal wall should be observed during respiration. Often the initial finding indicative of peritonitis is "splinting" (i.e., holding the diaphragm still) to reduce abdominal pain. This may be especially significant in men because they tend to be "abdominal breathers" (i.e., they use the diaphragm to a greater extent than do women, when breathing).

Portions of the abdominal wall may be seen to pulsate at the same rate as the heart, usually reflective of pulsations of the abdominal aorta. This is especially true of patients with thin-walled, flat abdomens. Occasionally, a distended abdomen due to fluid (ascites) may reflect pulsations. Peristalsis is normally not visible.

***Auscultation.*** In the examination of the abdomen, auscultation precedes percussion and palpation techniques to minimize any alteration in the frequency of bowel sounds.[2] The sounds produced by the peristaltic movements of the intestine are normally of medium pitch, and best heard with the diaphragm of the stethoscope pressed lightly against the abdomen. The nurse should listen for bowel sounds in all 4 quadrants, noting their frequency and characteristics. The mixing and moving forward of liquid and air in the intestines produce brief bursts of gurgling, bubbling sounds, occurring at a frequency of from 5–30 times/minute. These sounds should be audible in all 4 quadrants. Occasionally, very active bowel sounds or *borborygmi* (i.e., loud, prolonged gurgles of hyperperistalsis; "growling stomach") may be heard.

Bowel sounds may be described as hypoactive or hyperactive. In the presence of a paralytic ileus, the frequency of bowel sounds may only be 1/minute or less. This reflects abnormally slow bowel activity and is described as *hypo*active.

With increased bowel activity as occurs in bouts of gastroenteritis, diarrhea, or partial intestinal obstruction, bowel sounds may be heard occurring every 2–3 seconds. These sounds are described as *hyper*active. In the case of obstruction, the character of bowel sounds also changes in that they become more high-pitched than normal, taking on a "tinkling" quality.

It is important to listen for bruits in all 4 quadrants and over the midline in the epigastrium. A bruit in this area most often arises from lesions of the abdominal aorta, celiac artery, or the renal arteries. If a bruit is detected, the area should be palpated very gently so as not to injure atherosclerotic vessels. Occasionally, a cardiac murmur may be transmitted along the aorta. In this instance, it may be difficult to differentiate the murmur from the abdominal bruit.

A venous hum is a continuous sound that, when heard, may reflect an increase in collateral circulation between the portal system and the systemic venous system.

***Percussion.*** Percussion is a useful technique for determining the size and location of organs, detecting air in the stomach and bowel, and identifying solid or fluid-filled masses, or ascites. The presence of a large amount of air (swallowed) in the stomach and intestines produces a hollow percussion note called *tympany; dullness* is the percussion note elicited over solid or fluid-filled masses, or ascitic fluid. Tympany usually predominates. Each of the abdominal quadrants should be percussed to ensure that tympany is present to a greater or lesser degree throughout the abdomen. If fluid has collected in the abdomen, there will be increased dullness to percussion in the flanks and shifting dullness. Dullness elicited over the suprapubic area suggests a distended bladder.

*Percussion of Abdominal Organs—Liver, Spleen, and Stomach.* In most adults, the liver is completely tucked up under the thoracic cage with its superior surface under the dome of the right diaphragm, and its inferior border at or above the right costal margin. The lower liver edge may normally be found to be several centimeters below the costal margin (see Fig. 48–2).

To estimate its size, the liver is percussed at the midclavicular line (MCL). The lower border of liver dullness is determined by starting at a level below the umbilicus in an area of tympany and lightly percussing upward toward the liver. The transition from a note of tympany to one of dullness marks the lower border of the liver. To determine the upper border of the liver at the MCL, lightly percuss downward from an area of lung resonance toward liver dullness. The transition from a note of resonance to dullness marks the upper border of the liver. Between its upper and lower borders at the MCL, the liver measures approximately 6–12 cm. If the liver appears enlarged, it may be necessary to outline the boundaries of liver dullness using the midsternal and right anterior axillary lines.

The presence of a right pleural effusion or consolidated lung adjacent to the liver may falsely increase the estimated size of the liver; gas in the overlying colon may produce a note of tympany in the right upper quadrant (RUQ) and may falsely decrease the estimated size of the liver.

Percussion over the left upper quadrant (LUQ) is usually performed to rule out enlargement of the spleen. The small area of splenic dullness near the left 10th rib posterior to the midaxillary line is often obscured by gastric or colonic air. A full stomach or feces-filled colon may exaggerate the area of splenic dullness.

Any increase in the size of the gastric air bubble (i.e., an increased area of tympany in the LUQ), accompanied by upper abdominal distention, suggests gastric dilatation.

***Palpation.*** When eliciting the patient's clinical history, it is important to have the patient identify any areas of pain. These areas are left for last in palpation to avoid producing spasm and rigidity of the abdominal wall, which would interfere with the abdominal assessment. It is important to observe the patient's expression throughout the examination.

*Light Palpation.* Light palpation assists in identifying muscle resistance, detecting areas of tenderness, and locating superficial organs and masses. It is performed by pressing the abdominal wall with the pads of the fingers, lightly, but firmly enough to indent the wall. No attempt should be made to press deeply. All areas of the abdomen should be palpated, comparing the resistance on one side with that on the other. Areas of tenderness should be palpated last and as gently as possible to avoid muscle guarding. If resistance is detected, it is important to determine whether it is voluntary or involuntary. An effort should be made to help the patient relax. The abdominal rectus muscle should be checked for relaxation, which occurs with expiration. If the abdominal wall remains rigid in spite of these maneuvers, it is probably involuntary. Involuntary spasm of the abdominal musculature is indicative of peritonitis.

*Deep Palpation.* Deep palpation is helpful in delineating abdominal organs and masses, and in identifying areas of deep pain or tenderness. The palmar surfaces of the fingers are used to explore all 4 quadrants. It is essential for the patient to be relaxed. Appropriate explanations regarding the examination should be made. The patient should know that deep palpation may cause some discomfort. Deep abdominal breathing may help the patient relax.

All areas of the abdomen should be examined thoroughly and systematically. If any masses are identified, it is important to note the location, size, shape, consistency, tenderness, pulsations, and mobility. If tenderness is detected, the abdomen should be checked for rebound tenderness. *Rebound tenderness* is elicited by firmly and slowly pressing into the abdominal wall, then quickly letting go. If pain is elicited during the quick release, rebound tenderness is present, indicating peritoneal inflammation.

*Bimanual* palpation (using 2 hands) can be used for deep palpation, particularly when there is obesity or muscular resistance. One hand is placed on top of the other. Pressure is applied with the outer hand, while the nurse concentrates on what the fingers of the inner hand are feeling.

Several approaches can be used in palpating the liver, spleen, kidneys, and abdominal aorta. The reader is referred to an appropriate text for a detailed discussion regarding the techniques used. Normally, the spleen is not palpable unless it is 3 times its normal size. The kidneys are usually not palpable except in children or very thin adults. A blunt blow to the *costovertebral angle* is performed to elicit tenderness caused by inflammation of the kidneys (see Fig. 22–1).

### Summary of the Abdominal Assessment

To assess the abdomen thoroughly, the nurse must:

1. Have a solid understanding of underlying anatomy and physiology.
2. Elicit a thorough clinical history.
3. Appreciate structural relationships of abdominal organs and their location in each quadrant.
4. Be skilled in the techniques of inspection, auscultation, percussion, and palpation.
5. Document the findings accurately and precisely.

### Rectal Examination

The rectal examination is an essential component of the assessment of the gastrointestinal system in the adult. Omitting this part of the examination increases the risk of missing an asymptomatic carcinoma. The anus is inspected for inflammation, excoriation, hemorrhoids, fissures, and lesions. With a well-lubricated glove, the nurse should palpate the rectum for tenderness, nodules, masses, and fecal impaction. Appropriate explanations should be made to the patient prior to the examination. The examination should be conducted with gentleness and a calm demeanor.

## DIAGNOSTIC STUDIES

In patients with gastrointestinal disorders, the diagnosis can be elusive. Many types of studies may be employed to determine the underlying cause. These studies may include laboratory tests, radiologic studies, cytologic studies, and endoscopy procedures. In many instances, it is the nurse's responsibility to prepare patients for specific diagnostic studies. Appropriate explanations need to be made, dietary restrictions may be necessary, and bowel preparation and evacuation may be indicated. Tests may need to be scheduled so as not to conflict with one another and, thus, invalidate results.

### Laboratory Tests

Blood and urine tests can be of considerable diagnostic value, especially in the presence of liver and pancreatic dysfunction, biliary disorders, and intestinal malabsorption. Serum enzyme studies assist in differential diagnosis. Each organ of the body contains its own characteristic enzymes, which function to catalyze numerous metabolic activities. In the presence of tissue injury or necrosis, these enzymes are released from the damaged tissues into the blood. Their concentrations in the blood provide inferential or confirmatory evidence of the underlying disease process.

The ability to differentiate *isoenzymes* (i.e., enzymes occurring in more than one organ, having a similar function but uniquely different structural and physical characteristics) further assists in the differential diagnosis. A list of these and other specific laboratory tests for gastrointestinal disorders is presented in Table 48-1.

### Diagnostic Studies and Procedures

Other helpful diagnostic studies frequently used in gastrointestinal liver, biliary, and pancreatic dis-

TABLE 48-1
**Laboratory Tests for Gastrointestinal Dysfunction**

| Test | Purpose | Clinical Significance |
|---|---|---|
| ***Liver Function Tests*** | | |
| *Biliary System* | | |
| Serum bilirubin | Measures the liver's ability to conjugate and excrete bilirubin, a product of hemoglobin degradation within the reticuloendothelial system. | Hyperbilirubinemia is associated with heptocellular disease; hemolytic jaundice, hepatic jaundice, and obstructive jaundice. |
| • Total | Normal level: 1.0 mg/100 ml. | |
| -Direct | Normal level: 0.4 mg/100 ml. Reflects level of conjugated bilirubin in the blood. | Increased in obstructive disease of the biliary system. |
| -Indirect | Normal level: Total minus direct bilirubin. Measures concentration of unconjugated bilirubin in the blood. | Increased in hemolytic disorders (increased erythrocyte destruction). Increased in hepatocellular disease. |
| Serum alkaline phosphatase | Normal levels: (vary depending upon laboratory and procedure used). Enzyme most often measured to indicate bile duct obstruction. Measures enzyme activity in bone, intestine, and in liver and biliary systems. Overall clinical picture usually provides sufficient discriminative evidence as to underlying pathology; it is possible to partition this enzyme into its isoenzymes if more definitive data are required for diagnosis. | Increased in cholestasis (i.e., an arrest in bile flow); biliary obstruction; liver metastasis; viral, drug-induced, or chronic hepatitis. Increased in bone disease. Results must be evaluated in terms of complete clinical picture. |
| Serum cholesterol | Normal levels: 120-220 mg/100. ml. Measures liver metabolism and synthesis of this bile acid precursor. Cholesterol is a basic constituent of structural elements (e.g., plasma membrane), and hormones and other metabolites. | Increased levels are associated with cholestasis resulting from biliary disease; bile duct obstruction; hepatitis; lipid disorders; and pancreatitis. Decreased levels may occur with hepatocellular damage, cirrhosis. |
| Urine bilirubin | Measures conjugated (water-soluble) form of bilirubin. | Increased with liver disease and/or biliary obstruction; increased when levels of conjugated bilirubin are increased. |
| Urine bilinogen | Measurement reflects patency of biliary ducts, and the hepatocellular capacity to process and excrete bilirubin. | Characteristically increased in hemolytic disorders and states of large hemoglobin turnover; increased in hepatocellular disease; absent in complete obstructive biliary disease. |
| Fecal urobilinogen | Measurement reflects patency of biliary ducts; quantity of bilirubin processed. | Increased levels with hemolysis; or with soft-tissue bleeding requiring resorption and degradation of hemoglobin. |

*(continued)*

TABLE 48-1
## Laboratory Tests for Gastrointestinal Dysfunction *(Continued)*

| Test | Purpose | Clinical Significance |
|---|---|---|
| ***Liver Function Tests (cont.)*** | | |
| *Hepatocellular Function: Serum Enzyme Studies* | | |
| Amino transferases | These enzymes are stored in the liver and released when liver cells are damaged. | The two enzymes SGOT and SGPT are most often associated with hepatocellular damage. |
| Serum glutamic oxaloacetic transaminase (SGOT) | Normal levels: 10-40 U/ml.<br>This enzyme is also called aspartate aminotransferase (AST). | SGOT levels serve as an indication of the extent and severity of tissue damage. They need to be evaluated in terms of the complete clinical picture because this enzyme is also released from heart, kidneys, lungs, pancreas, and skeletal muscle. |
| Serum glutamic pyruvic transaminase (SGPT) | Normal levels: 6.0-36.0 U/ml.<br>This enzyme is also called alanine aminotransferase (ALT). | SGPT is more specifically associated with the liver than is SGOT. It occurs in high concentrations in the liver; lesser concentrations occur in kidney, heart, and skeletal muscle.<br>Increased SGOT and SGPT occurs in biliary obstruction; cirrhosis, acute or drug-induced hepatitis; liver metastasis; and pancreatitis. |
| Gamma glutamyl transpeptidase (GGT) | This enzyme is active in amino acid transport. Measurements reflect enzyme activity in liver, biliary tract epithelium, pancreas and kidney tubules. | Increased in acute liver disease, particularly that associated with chronic alcohol abuse; obstructive biliary disease, liver metastasis; acute pancreatitis. This test requires 24-hour alcohol abstention. |
| Lactic dehydrogenase (LDH) | Normal levels and distribution of isoenzymes:<br>• $LDH_1$—heart, brain, RBC 18-33%<br>• $LDH_2$—heart, brain, RBC 28-40%<br>• $LDH_3$—lung, spleen, pancreas, thyroid, adrenals, kidneys, RBC 16-30%<br>• $LDH_4$—liver, skeletal muscle, brain, kidneys 6-16%<br>• $LDH_5$—liver, skeletal muscle, kidneys 2-13%<br>Total LDH: 60 to 120 U/ml | This enzyme is found in nearly all cells with especially high concentration in liver, heart, brain, kidney, blood and skeletal muscle.<br>Isoenzymes provide more specific information regarding the source of LDH. |
| *Hepatocellular Function: Protein Metabolism* | | |
| Serum total protein | Normal level: 6.0-8.4 gm/100 ml. Reflects a quantitative measure of albumin and globulins in the blood. | Longstanding hepatocellular dysfunction decreases levels of circulating serum proteins. |
| Albumin | Normal level: 3.5-5.0 gm/100 ml. Reflects capacity to synthesize protein. | Hypoalbuminemia is associated with gradual progressive diseases including cirrhosis, tumors; malnutrition; protein-wasting renal or gastrointestinal diseases; severe catabolic states such as burns or acute and chronic infections.<br>Hyperalbuminemia is associated with dehydration (prolonged vomiting or diarrhea) with hemoconcentration. |
| Globulins | Include alpha, beta, and gamma fractions. Beta fraction also includes lipoproteins. | Serum globulins frequently rise above normal values in chronic liver disease.<br>Beta globulin fraction is elevated in viral hepatitis, biliary cirrhosis, and extrahepatic biliary tract obstruction. |
| Serum ammonia | Normal levels: 80-110 $\mu$g/100 ml.<br>Measures ability of liver to detoxify ammonia, an end-product of protein metabolism.<br>Ammonia is normally metabolized to urea by hepatic cells; urea is then eliminated via the kidneys. | Increased in hepatic necrosis; hepatic failure accompanied by portal hypertension with its frequently occurring sequelae of esophageal varices and upper gastrointestinal bleeding, and hepatic encephalopathy; and cirrhosis. |
| Serum urea | | Serum urea levels are reduced in severe liver disease.<br>Impaired sodium and water metabolism, characteristics of hepatocellular and circulatory disorders of the liver, produce dilutional changes reflected by reduced serum urea levels.<br>Severe liver disease reduces the capacity of the liver to degrade proteins, further reducing serum urea levels. |

*(continued)*

TABLE 48-1
**Laboratory Tests for Gastrointestinal Dysfunction *(Continued)***

| Test | Purpose | Clinical Significance |
|---|---|---|
| ***Liver Function Tests (cont.)*** | | |
| | | Degradation of protein by intestinal bacteria generates ammonia, which readily enters the portal circulation to be normally converted to urea. In liver failure and/or portal hypertension, portal blood is diverted to collateral vessels, causing systemic ammonia levels to rise and urea levels to fall.[3] Elevated ammonia levels predispose patient to hepatic encephalopathy. |
| Prothrombin time | Normal values: <2-sec deviation from control. Measures clotting time to determine activity of prothrombin and fibrinogen. | Normal liver synthesizes clotting factors II (prothrombin), VII, IX and X in the presence of adequate vitamin K (fat-soluble vitamin). Synthesis of these four factors declines with hepatocellular dysfunction or inadequate supply of vitamin K. Vitamin K is produced by the intestinal bacterial flora. It requires bile salts for absorption from the gut. Bile duct obstruction preventing bile salts from entering the duodenum may indirectly cause a reduction in vitamin K absorption. Prothrombin time is increased with Vitamin K deficiency; a value >2½ times normal very likely reflects abnormal bleeding. |
| *Other Liver Function Tests:* | | |
| Serum alpha-fetoprotein (AFP) | Normal levels in nonpregnant patients: <30 ng/ml. AFP is the major serum protein in early fetal life with synthesis of large quantities through the 32nd week of gestation. Thereafter synthesis declines to reach its lowest concentrations during the first year of life. | Synthesis of AFP is repressed in normal, resting hepatocytes after the first year of life, but may resume in rapidly multiplying and proliferating hepatocytes. Hepatocellular carcinoma may cause the AFP level to rise a thousand-fold or more. Lesser elevations (~500 ng/ml) may occur in active cirrhosis or in viral or toxic hepatitis. Demonstration of elevated levels of AFP may assist in the differential diagnosis of hepatomegaly, hepatocellular dysfunction, and the jaundice state. |
| Serum hepatitis B surface antigen | Used to screen for latent or active hepatitis B virus. Normal results: negative. | Highly sensitive for hepatitis B antigen (HBsAg); widely available and permit specific diagnosis of hepatitis B in mild, subclinical, or persistent cases. |
| ***Pancreatic Function Tests:*** | | |
| Serum amylase | Normal levels: 4–25 U/ml. Measurement of pancreatic enzyme active in the digestion of starch; it splits starch into smaller carbohydrate units. Amylase activity occurs in many cells but pathologic elevations of serum amylase levels nearly always involve the pancreas. Significant concentrations of amylase also occur in salivary gland secretions. | Increased levels occur in acute pancreatitis and common bile duct obstruction. Elevations in serum amylase levels may be attributed to disruption of pancreatic secretory cells, and to the absorption of extracellular enzyme from intestinal contents and ascites fluid through dilated, permeable peritoneal lymphatic capillaries. Morphine and cholinergic drugs may alter serum amylase levels. |
| Serum lipase | Normal levels: 2 U/ml or less. Measurement of pancreatic enzyme active in digestion of fats. | Significant elevations occur with acute pancreatitis; carcinoma of the pancreas may produce a sustained moderate elevation. Levels may also be increased in pancreatic duct obstruction, biliary duct obstruction, and intestinal obstruction. Morphine and cholinergic drugs may alter serum lipase levls. |
| Secretin test | Measurement of pancreatic secretion. | |

*(continued)*

TABLE 48-1
**Laboratory Tests for Gastrointestinal Dysfunction *(Continued)***

| Test | Purpose | Clinical Significance |
|---|---|---|
| ***Miscellaneous Tests for Gastrointestinal Disorders*** | | |
| Serum glucose | Normal level: (fasting) 70–110 mg/100 ml.<br>Hyperglycemia:<br>• Mild—120–150 mg/100 ml<br>• Moderate—200–500 mg/100 ml<br>• Marked: >500 mg/100 ml<br>• Hypoglycemia: <70 mg/100 ml | Hyperglycemia reflects reduced insulin secretion by islet cells of pancreas; or a crude indication of the liver's capacity to store glycogen and mobilize glucose.<br>Hypoglycemia may reflect excessive secretion of insulin; or it may occur in response to stress in which inadequate sugar is being consumed in proportion to the amount being metabolized. Other causes of hypoglycemia include extensive liver disease, insulin overdose; malnutrition. |
| Oral glucose tolerance test | Reflects metabolic response to glucose load.<br>Normal serum glucose:<br>• 160–180 mg/100 ml in 30–60 minutes.<br>• Return to fasting levels within 2 to 3 hours.<br>Normal urine glucose: negative. | This test is affected by many physiologic variables with many different diagnostic interpretations. |
| Galactose | Reflects ability of liver to convert galactose to glycogen.<br>Normal result: negative. | Absence of tolerance occurs with extrahepatic biliary obstruction or obstructive jaundice. |
| D-xylose test | Evaluates intestinal absorption of xylose, a pentose sugar normally passed through liver and excreted intact. | Reduced levels occur in cirrhosis; regional ileitis; sprue; diverticula. |
| Schilling test | Helps to establish if vitamin $B_{12}$ absorption is defective; or whether intrinsic factor necessary for vitamin $B_{12}$ absorption is deficient. | Decreased absorption may occur in pernicious anemia (lack of intrinsic factor); pancreatic insufficiency; intestinal disorder. |
| ***Fecal Analysis*** | | |
| Occult blood | | Positive tests occur in upper gastrointestinal bleeding; gastritis, gastric carcinoma; bleeding varices; peptic ulcer disease; lower gastointestinal causes: diverticulitis, colitis, carcinoma of colon. |
| Fat (lipids) | Stool analysis to quantitate fat excretion. This test requires a known dietary intake and timed stool collection. | Lipase deficiency commonly associated with pancreatic disease increases the proportion of neutral fat in stool.<br>Steatorrhea can occur in liver and biliary tract disease but jaundice and abnormal blood chemistries occur before steatorrhea becomes a significant diagnostic problem. |

orders are listed in Table 48-2. Results of all of these diagnostic tests, studies, and procedures must be evaluated in terms of the overall clinical presentation.

## Nursing Considerations

A major nursing responsibility is to assist in preparing the patient for the diagnostic workup. Many of these tests are time-consuming, expensive, and not without risks and complications. Often, a series of tests are ordered, and they must be performed in a specific sequence to prevent one test from altering the results of another.

An understanding of the purpose of these tests and the actual procedures involved assists the nurse to better prepare the patient. Preparation begins with an assessment of the patient to determine if there are any contraindications to performing a test (e.g., an allergy to iodine in patients scheduled for tests requiring the use of a contrast medium). Many tests require dietary restriction, bowel preparations, and the administration of appropriate medications. All diagnostic procedures require that the patient have an adequate explanation of what to expect. The patient will probably be more cooperative so that necessary procedures can be carried out.

Upon completion of the diagnostic workup, the nurse assists the patient and family to understand results and their implications in terms of treatment, prognosis, and recovery. The nurse helps to reinforce and to clarify explanations made to the patient and family by the physician. The nurse supports the patient and family in the decision-making process regarding the ultimate level of health desired.

TABLE 48–2
## Diagnostic Studies and Procedures for Gastrointestinal Dysfunction

| Test | Description | Clinical Significance/ Nursing Implications |
|---|---|---|
| ***Radiography*** | | |
| Abdominal series | A three-way view of abdomen: flat plate, erect position, decubitus position. | Useful in differentiating free air in the abdomen from that related to perforated bowel; can detect presence of bowel obstruction and ascites. |
| ***Contrast Radiography*** | | |
| Oral cholecystography | A study of the gallbladder to detect gallstones, tumors, or inflammatory disease. A radiopaque dye is ingested, absorbed by the small intestine, removed from blood by the liver, excreted into the bile, and stored in the gallbladder. | This test should be performed prior to barium swallow; since contrast dye contains iodine, tests such as iodine uptake should be done prior to this study. • Whenever an iodine-based contrast medium is used it is important to establish if the patient is allergic to iodine. • This test permits visualization of gallbladder and biliary system (extrahepatic); it reflects the capacity of the liver to conjugate and excrete the dye (intrahepatic). • Inability to visualize gallbladder suggests biliary duct obstruction, or an inability of the gallbladder to concentrate the dye. |
| Barium enema | Permits visualization of lower intestinal tract including ileocecal junction, colon and rectum. | This test should be performed prior to barium swallow because the slow passage of barium through the gastrointestinal tract may alter the findings. Preparation requires use of laxative and enemas; and appropriate explanation so that patient can cooperate in retaining the barium enema during the procedure. Post-procedure enemas may be required to prevent constipation associated with barium. • This study is of diagnostic value in structural changes of large intestine—diverticula, polyps, colorectal cancer; and in inflammatory disorders of the colon (ulcerative colitis). |
| Barium swallow (upper GI series) | The patient swallows a thick barium sulfate mixture and cineradiography and fluoroscopy are used to record esophageal and gastric action. | This test allows visualization of the upper gastrointestinal tract as the patient swallows. • It is of diagnostic value in detecting esophageal irregularities such as polyps, tumors, diverticula and hiatal hernia; gastric pathology including ulcers and tumors; and intestinal abnormalities such as altered motility, obstruction, masses, polyps, and diverticula. |
| Intravenous cholangiography | Allows direct visualization of cystic, hepatic, and common bile ducts. | This procedure can be performed prior to, during and after surgery. The tests may be performed in patients unable to tolerate oral intake. |
| Percutaneous transhepatic cholangiography | This procedure is performed in the presence of mechanical obstruction of the biliary system causing bile ducts to be dilated. A long needle is used to inject dye directly into a dilated bile duct under fluoroscopy. | This study is used to assess biliary duct obstruction; it helps to differentiate extrahepatic from intrahepatic obstructive jaundice. • Hemorrhage or leakage of bile are potential complications requiring monitoring for 24 hours post-procedure. |
| Angiography studies | Radiographic contrast study of the vascular system. A catheter is placed in either the superior or inferior mesenteric arteries and dye is injected. | These studies are used to locate sites of gastrointestinal and mesenteric bleeding; they are especially helpful in defining aneurysms of the aorta. Areas of ischemia may also be determined. |

*(continued)*

TABLE 48-2
**Diagnostic Studies and Procedures for Gastrointestinal Dysfunction *(Continued)***

| Test | Description | Clinical Significance/ Nursing Implications |
|---|---|---|
| ***Ultrasonography (Echography)*** | This is a noninvasive procedure wherein high-frequency sound waves are emitted from a transducer and spread throughout underlying tissues. Depending upon the density of the tissues, these sound waves bounce back (echoes) and are converted by a receiver into a dot pattern. The dots reflect the location of an "echo" in the body. | This procedure helps to differentiate between obstructive and nonobstructive jaundice. It assists in the diagnosis of cholelithiasis and cholecystitis. • Ultrasonography of the liver can detect hematomas and metastasis. Pancreatic ultrasonography is helpful in detecting pancreatitis, pancreatic carcinoma, pseudocysts. • Ultrasonography can be used in conjunction with liver-spleen scanning to pick up "cold spots", i.e., areas that do not pick up the radionuclide, e.g., tumors or abscesses. |
| ***Nuclear Imaging*** | | |
| Liver/spleen scanning | An injection of a radionuclide is given to the patient, who is then positioned under a scanner that records the distribution of radioactivity in the liver and spleen. | Nuclear imaging is an efficient way to diagnose hepatocellular disease, liver metastasis, hepatomegaly, and splenomegaly; and abdominal hematoma post-trauma. • Local bleeding sites can also be detected using this technique. |
| Computerized tomography (CT scan) | A computer-assisted cross-sectional x-ray that can be used with or without a contrast medium. | CT scan can detect biliary, liver and pancreatic disorders. This study is helpful in differentiating between obstructive and nonobstructive jaundice; it can identify tumors, cysts, hematomas, and abscesses. Barium studies, when ordered, should be performed 4 days prior to or post CT scan. |
| ***Endoscopy*** | | |
| Esophagogastroduodenoscopy | Procedure involves the passing of a fiberoptic endoscope through the patient's mouth, the esophagus, stomach, and into the duodenum. Endoscopy enables taking photographs, obtaining biopsies and cytologic specimens, and removal of polyps. | Enables visualization of luminal lining of upper gastrointestinal tract. The procedure can detect areas of inflammation, ulcerations, varices, hiatal hernia, mucosal lesions and carcinoma. It helps to differentiate between gastric and duodenal ulcers; and between benign and malignant ulcers in conjunction with a barium swallow. |
| Endoscopic retrograde cholangiopancreatography (ERCP) | This procedure involves the passing of catheter with the aid of a fiberscope into the common bile duct and pancreatic duct so that a contrast dye can be introduced and x-rays taken. | ERCP enables radiological visualization of common bile and pancreatic ducts. The patient should be observed for possible complications post-procedure including pancreatitis or cholangitis. This procedure is not without risks. |
| Colonoscopy | This procedure involves insertion of a flexible fiberscope. | This procedure allows for direct visualization of the bowel; biopsy of lesions and/or excision of polyps can be performed. |
| Proctosigmoidoscopy | This procedure permits direct visualization of distal sigmoid colon, rectum, and anal canal. | This procedure is useful in detecting hemorrhoids, polyps, fissures, fistulas, and inflammatory, infectious, and ulcerative bowel disease. |
| ***Paracentesis (Peritoneal Tap with Lavage)*** | | This procedure is useful to determine intra-abdominal hemorrhaging post-trauma; to detect presence of pancreatitis by measurement of amylase and lipase levels in the peritoneal fluid aspirated; and to determine the presence of tumors via cytologic studies. |

## REFERENCES

1. Konopad, E, and Noseworthy, T: Stress ulceration: A serious complication in critically ill patients. Heart Lung 17(4):339, July 1988.
2. Smith, CE: Assessing bowel sounds, more than just listening. Nursing '88 18(2):42, February 1988.
3. Cohn, HO: Complications of portal hypertension. Current Hepatology 1:119-180, 1980.

CHAPTER 49

# Nursing Management of the Patient with Acute Upper Gastrointestinal Hemorrhage

## CHAPTER OUTLINE



## LEARNING OBJECTIVES

**At the end of this chapter, you should be able to:**

1. Differentiate peptic ulcer disease, erosive bleeding, and esophageal/gastric varices, in terms of etiology and pathophysiology.
2. Define classes of blood loss and consequent clinical manifestations, based on the percentage of total blood volume lost.
3. Describe the essential aspects of the diagnostic evaluation of acute upper gastrointestinal hemorrhage.
4. Identify goals of emergency treatment and overall management of acute upper gastrointestinal hemorrhage.
5. Describe implications for nursing care based on nursing process:
   Assessment
   Specific nursing diagnoses
   Planning: Desired patient outcomes
   Nursing interventions.

## ACUTE UPPER GASTROINTESTINAL TRACT HEMORRHAGE

Acute upper gastrointestinal (GI) tract hemorrhage may be the primary reason for admission of a patient into the intensive care setting. Frequently, it occurs as a complication of a critical illness involving another organ system(s). Common causes of the majority of cases of upper gastrointestinal bleeding include peptic ulcer disease, erosive gastritis, and variceal bleeding associated with portal hypertension.

### Etiology and Pathophysiology

#### *Peptic Ulcer Disease*

Two major factors need to be considered in the pathophysiology of peptic ulcer disease. First, all areas of the GI tract exposed to gastric juice (acid pepsin) are well supplied with mucous glands. In the duodenum, added protection against the acidity of gastric juice is afforded by the alkalinity of small intestinal and pancreatic secretions. Second, the GI tract is endowed with a rich, submucosal blood supply with major arteries or branches so situated anatomically that they can be easily eroded in the presence of underlying pathology.

Disruption of the delicate balance between acidic gastric juices and the defensive mucosal barrier may result in duodenal and gastric ulceration, or peptic ulcer disease. Erosion of the peptic ulceration into a major artery or its branches is probably the most common cause of massive upper GI tract bleeding. Predominantly, the majority of these ulcers are situated in the proximal duodenum in an area called the duodenal bulb. The proximity of the gastroduodenal and pancreaticoduodenal arteries in this area frequently results in hemorrhage if the ulcer erodes through the posterior wall. When a patient with a prior history of peptic ulcer presents with an acute upper GI hemorrhage, the ulcer is the most probable site of bleeding.

Breakdown of the gastroduodenal mucosal barrier may be caused by a variety of factors including stress (physiologic stress of trauma, burns, extensive surgery, sepsis, or psychologic stress),[1] ischemia, excess secretion of gastric acid, reflux of bile acids, and drugs (aspirin, alcohol, caffeine, nicotine, corticosteroids, phenybutazone, and indomethacin). A back diffusion or reflux of hydrochloric acid (HCl) through the impaired mucosal barrier destroys mucosal cells and liberates histamine. Histamine stimulates further acid secretion and causes vasodilation of underlying blood vessels. The mucosa becomes edematous, and there is leakage of interstitial fluid into the lumen of the GI tract. Eventually, blood vessels (arterioles) are ruptured and bleeding occurs.

#### *Erosive Gastritis*

Erosive gastritis usually involves a combination of an increase in acid pepsin secretion coupled with another factor such as drug ingestion or stress. Recent heavy alcohol consumption or a history of ingestion of salicylates, corticosteroids, indomethacin, and phenylbutazone has a direct effect on increasing acid secretions. Ingestion of such drugs may also alter the structural integrity of the mucosal layer. Trauma, burns, sepsis, and hypovolemic shock are examples of stressful situations that can predispose to GI bleeding. The consequent bleeding probably reflects ischemic cellular injury and disruption of the defensive mucosal barrier, which prevents neutralization of hydrochloric acid.

#### *Variceal Bleeding Associated with Portal Hypertension*

Esophageal variceal bleeding may result from dilatation of lower esophageal venous plexi in the scenario of portal hypertension, whether associated with cirrhosis or portal venous thrombosis in the absence of cirrhosis. Variceal bleeding may also occur as a result of forceful vomiting, particularly on a full stomach, and when there is an excess of alcohol in the system. Forceful vomiting under these circumstances can cause a traumatic tear of the lower esophageal mucosa into the submucosal layer, rupturing blood vessels in the process.

Commonly, variceal hemorrhage occurs in conjunction with alcoholic cirrhosis and, to a lesser extent, postnecrotic cirrhosis (see Chap. 50). Obstruction at the liver interface causes an increase in portal blood pressure, which opens up existing collateral channels. Included among these are the lower esophageal venous plexi, which soon dilate and become thin-walled veins easily eroded by reflux of the acidic gastric juices.

Bleeding from esophageal varices tends to be abrupt and frequently massive. Minor bleeding may occur for days prior to the acute episode.

## Clinical Presentation

The clinical presentation of acute upper GI hemorrhage depends in large measure on the amount and acuity of the blood loss and the character of blood lost (i.e., whether it presents as bright red blood or coffee-ground material in vomitus [hematemesis], as bloody stool [hematochezia], or as tarry stools [melena]). Table 49 – 1 classifies blood loss according to the approximate amount of blood lost and the consequent clinical manifestations.

## Diagnosis

In the diagnosis of acute upper GI hemorrhage, it is necessary to establish the site of the GI bleeding. This will largely determine the type and sequence of various diagnostic procedures and the management. If blood loss has been extensive (>1200 ml), it may be necessary to stabilize the patient's cardiopulmonary function before initiating diagnostic steps. The orderly sequence of history-taking, diagnostic evaluation, and treatment frequently is adjusted to meet the emergent demands. A meticulous clinical history and physical examination, in conjunction with radiologic and endoscopic investigations, may be necessary to differentiate the underlying cause of the gastrointestinal bleeding.

Complete assessment of the patient's clinical status is necessary because of a variety of systemic disease that may be associated with hemorrhage (e.g., aortic aneurysm, gastric carcinoma, mesen-

TABLE 49-1
**Assessment of the Extent of Blood Loss and Clinical Manifestations[2]**

| Blood Loss Classification | Approximate Amount of Blood Loss* | Percent (%) of Total Blood Volume Lost | Clinical Manifestations |
|---|---|---|---|
| Class I | 500–750 ml | 10–15 | None |
| Class II | 700–1200 ml | 15–25 | 1. Anxiety, tachycardia, tachypnea<br>2. Orthostatic hypotension<br>3. Urine output normal |
| Class III | 1200–1500 ml | 25–35 | 1. Anxiety, tachycardia, tachypnea<br>2. Restlessness, agitation<br>3. Systolic blood pressure 90–100 mmHg in recumbent position (orthostatic hypotension)<br>4. Reduced urine output |
| Class IV | 1500–2000 ml | 35–50 | 1. Anxiety, tachycardia, tachypnea<br>2. Systolic blood pressure ~ 60 mmHg<br>3. Reduced tissue perfusion:<br>• cerebral—confusion, restlessness<br>• renal—oliguria (<30 ml/hour)<br>• skin—diaphoresis, cool, clammy, pallor<br>4. Hypovolemic, hemorrhagic shock state |

*All blood loss estimates are acute losses in 60–70 Kg individual.

teric venous thrombosis, arterial embolic occlusion, blood dyscrasias such as leukemia, thrombocytopenic disorders, and a bleeding diathesis such as disseminated intravascular coagulation). If the patient has known heart, liver, renal, or other serious diseases, such information may be valuable in guiding medical and, if necessary, surgical decisions during the management of GI bleeding.

### Clinical History

A history of known peptic ulcer or the existence of a *pain–food–relief* pattern suggests the possibility of erosive bleeding. Epigastric pain is a cardinal symptom of peptic ulcer disease, and its assessment may be of assistance in differential diagnosis. The patient with a *duodenal* ulcer experiences epigastric pain about 2 hours after a meal and in the middle of the night. These episodes of pain are characteristically relieved by food and/or antacids, and the pain–food–relief pattern of peptic ulcer disease is established.

In the presence of a *gastric* ulcer, the patient may describe the onset of gnawing epigastric pain ½–1 hour after meals. Pain may or may not occur in the middle of the night, and often the pattern of *food–pain* is present, rather than pain–food–relief. Gastric cancer is often characterized by the onset of epigastric fullness or distress shortly after a meal.

A history of cirrhosis, hepatitis, jaundice, and chronic alcoholism suggests possible bleeding esophageal varices, and confirmatory signs of portal hypertension must be sought during the physical examination. Erosive gastritis is suggested by a history of recent consumption of large quantities of alcohol or drugs such as aspirin, indomethacin, steroids, among others.

Additional clinical history that may be of assistance includes the following: Recent medication history including the use of antacids and/or laxatives, in addition to those drugs previously mentioned; dietary habits including complaints of anorexia, food intolerance, indigestion, dysphagia, belching, nausea, and vomiting; occurrence of changes in bowel habits including the character of stools, flatulence, diarrhea, constipation; significant weight change; and the presence of a precipitating cause related to stress.

Additional clinical history that may be of assistance includes the following: Recent medication history including the use of antacids and/or laxatives, in addition to those drugs previously mentioned; dietary habits including complaints of anorexia, food intolerance, indigestion, dysphagia, belching, nausea, and vomiting; occurrence of changes in bowel habits including the character of stools, flatulence, diarrhea, constipation; significant weight change; and the presence of a precipitating cause related to stress.

While a thorough clinical history should be obtained if possible, it is important to be cognizant of the fact that this information may be misleading in determining the bleeding site. For example, nearly two thirds of patients with known esophageal varices who present with acute upper GI hemorrhage will have another lesion in the upper GI tract.

### Physical Examination

The findings on physical examination may reflect the acuity of blood loss. If bleeding is gradual, the patient may present with weakness, fatigue, pallor, and a slightly increased heart rate. Changes in blood pressure and heart rate occur in response to acute blood loss. As intravascular volume is reduced, there is a decrease in venous return with a consequent decrease in cardiac output and systemic blood pressure. As a rule, if, when the patient sits from a supine position, the heart rate increases more than 20 beats/minute and the systolic blood pressure falls more than 10 mmHg, it is likely that the blood loss has exceeded 1 liter. If bleeding is severe, signs of hypovolemic hemorrhagic shock may quickly ensue, characterized by extreme apprehension; pallor; cold, clammy skin; rapid, thready pulse; rapid, shallow respirations; hypotension (systolic ~60 mmHg); and reduced urine output (~30 ml/hour).

The physical examination of a patient with GI bleeding requires a search for signs of liver failure —jaundice, ascites, spider nevi, gynecomastia in men, asterixis ("liver flap"), and hepatic encephalopathy; and portal hypertension — splenomegaly and hemorrhoids. The abdomen should be carefully percussed and palpated to determine liver size and consistency, splenomegaly, and the presence of epigastric tenderness or guarding. Abdominal rigidity and rebound tenderness suggest perforation, especially when preceded by an episode of markedly exacerbated abdominal pain, followed by sudden but temporary relief. The complete physical examination includes a rectal examination. Aside from information that can be obtained regarding the anus, perianal area, and possible rectal masses, polyps, and nodules, the character of the stool can be confirmed.

### Laboratory Tests

Laboratory investigation (see Tables 48-1 and 48-2) should include a determination of the hematocrit, hemoglobin, white blood cell count with differential, platelet count, prothrombin time, and coagulation studies. Establishing baseline parameters assists in monitoring the evolving clinical course of the GI bleeding. However, some patients bleed so rapidly that there is insufficient time for the blood volume to equilibrate, and the hematocrit and hemoglobin may be normal or only slightly reduced. In patients with acute bleeding, changes in vital signs coupled with direct evidence of profuse bleeding are better indicators than the hematocrit and hemoglobin for replacement of blood and electrolyte solutions.[3]

Extensive transfusion will dilute platelets and clotting factors, particularly factors V and VII. This can be treated by infusion of fresh frozen plasma and platelets, as necessary.

Monitoring of the blood urea nitrogen (BUN) may assist in evaluating upper GI bleeding. Because blood in the upper GI tract may be digested and absorbed, an elevated BUN level in a patient who has recently had a normal BUN, or in whom the creatinine level is normal, may provide supportive evidence as to upper gastrointestinal bleeding. Increases in both BUN and serum creatinine levels may reflect impaired renal perfusion associated with the hypovolemia of acute blood loss.

### Nasogastric Tube Insertion

This simple maneuver can quickly confirm the presence of blood in the stomach. The presence of bright red blood confirms ongoing hemorrhage, while the presence of dark and clotted blood (coffee-grounds) is more indicative of an earlier hemorrhage that may have ceased. Once inserted, the nasogastric tube allows for continuing monitoring of the bleeding. It is also used to remove blood clots and to decompress the stomach. An empty stomach will allow the walls to collapse and may contribute to hemostasis.

### Endoscopy

Endoscopy is the primary diagnostic step in the investigation of upper GI bleeding. It enables direct evaluation of the esophagus, stomach, and duodenum. It is especially helpful in diagnosing erosive gastritis, which is a superficial lesion not evident on radiology studies.

### Radiology Studies

Peptic ulceration can usually be demonstrated by contrast radiology (barium swallow). Because blood clots in the gastric lumen or ulcer bed can negate any positive findings, these studies are best performed 12 hours after the bleeding has been controlled.

If bleeding persists and endoscopic and barium studies are inconclusive, emergency selective angiography may be indicated. Angiography may demonstrate the site of active bleeding. In the case of suspected esophageal varices, it may demonstrate the presence of varices as well as portal hypertension.

## Treatment and Management

Overall goals in the treatment and management of the patient with acute upper GI hemorrhage involve the treatment of hypovolemia, hemorrhagic shock, assessment of the severity of blood loss, diagnosis and control of the source of bleeding, and planning for definitive treatment of the underlying disease.

### Initial Management

The initial management in any patient with GI hemorrhage must be *hemodynamic stabilization* by replacement of blood, fluid, and electrolyte losses.

Initial measures require establishing at least 1, and if bleeding is profuse, 2 multiple large-bore intravenous access lines. Blood samples for appropriate laboratory studies, and type and crossmatching are drawn at this time. Normal saline or Ringer's lactate solution is infused rapidly in volumes sufficient to maintain blood pressure and correct tachycardia, until blood for transfusion is available. Albumin or plasma may also be used. With ongoing and/or massive hemorrhage, stabilization requires use of whole blood or packed cells. See Tables 49-2, 49-3, and 49-4 for nursing care considerations, precautions, and summary of adverse reactions in the administration of blood and blood products.

Patients with acute GI hemorrhage must be monitored continuously until bleeding has ceased or a decision has been made to intervene surgically. Frequently, a pulmonary artery catheter (Swan-Ganz) is inserted to evaluate closely the effects of fluid replacement.

Following acute resuscitation and hemodynamic stabilization, a nasogastric tube is placed. If there is evidence of continued bleeding, continuous iced saline lavage may be instituted until the return is clear.

Because gastric acidity plays a pathogenic role in most causes of upper GI bleeding, an approach to treatment is either to neutralize acid with antacids and/or to inhibit acid secretion with histamine$_2$ antagonists. Antacids and histimaine$_2$ antagonists act to reduce the direct harmful effects of acid and pepsin on the bleeding lesion; and they create a milieu in which platelets are more likely to aggregate, thus promoting clotting.[6]

The most efficacious approach to therapy is a combination of *antacid* and *histamine$_2$ antagonists* (e.g., cimetidine or ranitidine—see Appendix A). A sample regimen might include 300 mg cimetidine every 6 hours (q6h), administered by continuous infusion with 600 mg in 1000 ml 5% dextrose in water ($D_5W$).[3]

Antacids, in amounts of 60-90 ml, can be administered every 2 hours (q2h), leaving the nasogastric tube clamped for 30 minutes. Monitoring the pH of the nasogastric aspirate prior to the next dose of antacid or histamine$_2$ antagonist helps to evaluate the effectiveness of therapy. An attempt should be made to keep gastric pH above 4.5.

### *Definitive Treatment of Underlying Disease*

**Peptic Ulcer Disease and Erosive Gastritis.** The majority of patients with peptic ulcer disease and erosive gastritis can usually be controlled with conservative antacid/histamine$_2$ antagonist therapy and require no other treatment than prevention of their recurrence. In patients who have a history of previous GI bleeding or whose conditions fail to respond to conservative medical treatment, other modes of therapy may be considered including:[7]

| | |
|---|---|
| Peptic ulcer disease | Arterial embolization; freezing of the gastric mucosa; laser surgery; intragastric, intra-arterial, or intraperitoneal vasoconstrictors; and surgical procedures such as vagotomy, pyloroplasty, and gastrectomy. |
| Erosive gastritis | Angiography and vasopressin administration; and total gastrectomy. Because erosion is seldom limited to a particular region within the stomach, partial surgical resection even with vagotomy may not be effective. |

**Esophageal Variceal Bleeding.** Treatment of bleeding esophageal varices secondary to alcohol cirrhosis remains controversial. Current available therapies are less than ideal, primarily because of the underlying alcoholic cirrhosis. Mortality remains about 50%.

### Special Therapeutic Considerations[8]

***Esophageal Tamponade.*** Active bleeding should be controlled, if possible, by compression of gastroesophageal varices using balloon tamponade. The *Sengstaken-Blakemore* tube is the prototype of several tubes (including 3-lumen Linton tube, and 4-lumen Minnesota esophagogastric tamponade tube) capable of applying direct pressure to the bleeding area, thereby controlling the bleeding. It is a 3-lumen tube, wherein 1 lumen is comprised of a relatively large-bore gastric tube used to evacuate the stomach, and the second and third lumens lead to the gastric (distal) and esophageal (proximal) balloons, respectively (Fig. 49-1).

The gastric or distal balloon is round and should be situated in the stomach; the esophageal or proximal balloon is sausage-shaped and should lie in the esophagus. The gastric balloon is inflated with 100-150 ml of air, and traction is applied to pull it back into the gastroesophageal junction. The esophageal balloon is then inflated to 25-40 mmHg pressure to tamponade the bleeding vessel. Tamponade should be maintained for 48 hours. See Table 49-5, Sengstaken-Blakemore Tube: Nursing Care Considerations.

***Selective Angiography with Continuous Vasopressin (Pitressin) Infusion.*** When balloon tamponade fails to control bleeding, selective angiogra-

TABLE 49-2
## Blood and Blood Products Administration: Nursing Care Considerations

| Blood Product | Constituents | Clinical Significance/ Nursing Care Considerations |
|---|---|---|
| ***Whole Blood*** | | |
| Fresh whole blood | Contains all components including coagulation (clotting) factors and platelets.<br>Adequate red blood cell (RBC) content of 2,3-diphosphoglycerate (if less than 5 days old).<br>Volume: ~ 500 ml/unit. | Indications: Used in situations requiring viable platelets; used to treat hypovolemic, hemorrhagic shock; severe anemia.<br>Actions: Increases blood volume and oxygen-carrying capacity; provides platelets and clotting factors.<br>Administration: Use of a component/platelet infusion set.<br>Disadvantage: Limited availability in most blood banks. |
| Stored whole blood | RBCs<br>Contains all coagulation factors except factors VIII and V. (The amounts of these factors are considerably reduced in stored whole blood.)<br>Does not contain viable platelets.<br>Anticoagulant used is most commonly citrate-phosphate-dextrose compound (CPD).<br>Volume: ~ 500 ml/unit. | Indications: Hypovolemic, hemorrhagic shock.<br>Actions: Increases blood volume and oxygen-carrying capacity.<br>Administration: Always use blood filter (170 microns). Administer 1 unit fresh frozen plasma after every 4 units of stored whole blood to assure availability of all clotting factors. Before administration, gently but thoroughly mix whole blood to assure uniform suspension.<br>Advantage: Less viscous and therefore infused at faster rate than RBC concentrates.<br>Disadvantages: does not contain all clotting factors and a dilutional coagulopathy can occur. Can contribute to increase in serum ammonia levels.<br>Complications of whole blood administration: Volume overload; infusion of excess electrolytes ($Na^+$ and $K^+$) and anticoagulants (citrate); increased risk of hepatitis and acquired immune deficiency syndrome (AIDS). |
| ***Red Blood Cells (RBCs)*** | | |
| Packed red blood cells (RBC concentrate) | Contains equal number of RBCs as whole blood.<br>Volume: 200–250 ml/unit. | Indications: Anemia; slow blood loss.<br>Actions: Increases oxygen-carrying capacity of blood.<br>Administration: Use macrospore filtration device, which should be changed after every 2 units of packed RBCs or sooner if the rate of blood flow slows. Solutions containing calcium must never be added to a blood product since calcium will initiate clotting.<br>Advantages: Less risk of complications; replaces twice the amount of hemoglobin as the same amount of whole blood; this reduces the risk of circulatory overload, while still providing same oxygen-carrying capacity.<br>A greater supply of RBCs is usually available because blood banks fractionate whole blood into its various components so as to enable maximal utilization of a limited resource.<br>Disadvantages: Slow infusion rate, but this is overcome by adding 150–250 ml of 0.9% saline to cells, infusing them under pressure. |
| Fresh-frozen red blood cells | Same as above.<br>Essentially free of WBCs, plasma proteins and irregular antibodies as fresh-frozen RBCs are washed (deglycerolized) prior to administration. | Same as for packed red blood cells.<br>Indications: Used for patients who are at high risk of transfusion reactions; immunodeficient patients; and for storage of rare blood types. |
| ***Platelet Concentrate*** | Concentration: 4–6 × $10^{10}$ platelets/unit.<br>Volume: 35–50 ml/unit. | Indications: thrombocytopenia due to reduced platelet production or platelet misuse.<br>Actions: Increases platelet count; aids in clot formation.<br>Administration: Can be stored at room temperature for 24–72 hours of preparation. A component filter should be used with rapid infusion over 15–30 minutes. |

*(continued)*

TABLE 49-2
**Blood and Blood Products Administration: Nursing Care Considerations *(Continued)***

| Blood Product | Constituents | Clinical Significance/ Nursing Care Considerations |
|---|---|---|
| ***Platelet Concentrate (cont.)*** | Four to 8 units are usually prescribed. Expected increase in platelets per unit is ~ 10,000/unit/ squared meter. | Precaution: With infusion of multiple units of platelets, there is increased risk of adverse effects such as chills, fever, allergic reactions. Hepatitis risk is the same as for whole blood. Failure of expected increase in platelet numbers may be associated with fever, sepsis, splenomegaly, or DIC. |
| ***Fresh Frozen Plasma*** | Contains all clotting factors but no platelets. Volume: 200–250 ml/unit. Also contains albumin, globulins, water, and electrolytes. | Indications: Coagulopathies. Action: Raises levels of clotting factors. Administration: Stored up to 12 months; takes 20–30 minutes to thaw before using; must be given within 6 hours of thawing. Administer rapidly via blood or component filter. |
| ***Cryoprecipitate*** | Contains factors VIII, fibrinogen, and XIII. Volume: 10–20 ml/unit. | Indications: DIC; hemophilia A; von Willebrand's disease. Actions: Raises blood levels of factors VIII and XIII; prevents and/or controls bleeding in hemophilia A, and in hypofibrinogenemia. Administration: Administer rapidly using a component filter; as many as 4 units can be administered within 15 minutes. Should be administered as soon as possible after thawing. |
| ***Volume Expanders:*** 25% normal serum albumin | Contains 25% protein with ~ 96% albumin; 135 mEq. sodium, and small amounts of chloride. | Indications: Plasma expander in shock; hypoproteinemia; cerebral edema; burns. Contraindications: Avoid use in dehydrated patients. Actions: Solution is hyperosmolar and acts by moving water from extravascular to intravascular space, thus increasing intravascular volume. Administration: Use special administration set with vial: Infuse cautiously, adjusting rate according to clinical response; monitor for any signs of fluid overload or congestive heart failure. Monitor trauma or postoperative wounds because bleeding may occur as intravascular volume is expanded, and systemic blood pressure rises. |
| Plasma protein fraction (plasmanate) | Chemically processed pooled plasma treated with heat to kill hepatic virus. Volume: ~ 250–500 ml increments in shock. | Indications: Same as for 25% normal serum albumin. Actions: Increases intravascular volume and protein level. Administration: Use component filter; compatible with most parenteral intravenous solutions. Infuse carefully, adjusting infusion rate according to clinical response. |

raphy of the left gastric and superior mesenteric arteries can be performed with initiation of a continuous arterial infusion of vasopressin, 0.2–0.4 units/minute (in dextrose 5% water). An infusion pump is used, and vasopressin therapy is continued for 2–3 days, with slow decreases in rate over this time.

Nursing care requires extreme precautions to prevent dislodging of the arterial catheter because arterial bleeding can occur. The leg used for the arterial line insertion should be kept straight and loosely restrained, if necessary. This leg should be assessed hourly for changes in pulse, temperature, mottling. These signs suggest compromised perfusion to the extremity. The cutdown site should be examined for infection, clot, or hematoma formation, and possible infiltration. If infiltration occurs, immediate removal of the line is necessary to prevent tissue sloughing.

Ongoing monitoring of systemic blood pressure is necessary to recognize trends indicative of hypertension. Vasopressin is a potent vasopressor. In addition, it increases water reabsorption in the distal kidney tubules, contributing to an increase in

TABLE 49-3
## Precautions to Be Taken When Administering Blood and Blood Products[4]

| Nursing Action | Rationale |
|---|---|
| 1. Label specimen containers carefully when collecting blood samples for type and crossmatch. | Improper labeling can result in the patient receiving the wrong blood. |
| 2. Verify identification data prior to administration of blood or blood products. | Administering the wrong blood or blood products can precipitate a hemolytic transfusion reaction. |
| 3. Transfuse blood or blood products slowly over the initial 15 minutes. | Transfusion reaction can occur early in the transfusion. |
| A. Monitor patient's response to blood therapy: | |
| 1. Vital signs—prior to, during and post-transfusion therapy. | Baseline vital signs enable evaluation of the patient's response to blood therapy. |
| 2. Blood chemistries: Electrolytes, serum calcium levels. | Hyperkalemia can occur with infusion of blood nearing the end of its expiration period.<br>RBC hemolysis causes release of intracellular potassium.<br>Stored blood contains citrate, which binds to calcium upon infusion; multiple transfusions can predispose to hypocalcemia. |
| B. Monitor for signs of transfusion reaction: | The severity of a transfusion reaction can be proportional to the amount of blood infused. |
| 1. Early signs: Apprehension, headache, muscle cramps, fever, chills, dyspnea, cyanosis, hypotension, nausea/vomiting, urticaria.<br>2. Late signs: Oliguria, jaundice, shock. | It is important to clarify (with a physician) acceptable signs and symptoms of transfusion reaction, and the use of prophylactic medications (antipyretics, antihistamines) prior to and during transfusion. |
| C. Discontinue transfusion if any signs of a transfusion reaction occurs. | |
| 1. Perform the following in the event of transfusion reaction (as per unit protocol):<br>a. Discontinue blood transfusion.<br>b. Maintain patent intravenous line.<br>c. Notify physician.<br>d. Notify blood bank.<br>e. Re-verify identification data on all labels.<br>f. Return to blood bank:<br>• Partially used blood container and transfusion administration set. | |
| • Post-transfusion blood sample. | Direct Coombs' test is performed to detect the presence of antibody or complement molecules on the surface of red blood cells. Because it is never normal for red blood cells to be coated with globulin (antibody), a positive Coombs' test suggests hemolysis associated with transfusion reaction. |
| • Post-transfusion urine sample. | The presence of heme pigments, granular casts, and RBCs in urine provides additional evidence as to the occurrence of a transfusion reaction. |
| • Copies of appropriate records, documentation of transfusion therapy, and transfusion reaction. | |
| 4. Adjust infusion rate so that infusion is complete within 2–4 hours. | Blood or blood products left at room temperature for >4 hours are at risk of increased RBC hemolysis and bacterial proliferation. Blood and blood products should be administered immediately upon arrival from blood bank; they should never be placed into refrigerator on the unit. |
| A. Monitor for circulatory overload. | Use of whole blood increases volume infused (~500 ml) with each unit; in patients with a history of compromised cardiovascular function or anemia, additional fluid may further compromise cardiac function. |
| 5. Monitor flow rate especially with multiple transfusions. | Blood filter becomes clogged with aggregates and debris within the blood; blood filter should be changed at the end of every fourth transfusion or sooner, if flow rate diminishes appreciably. |
| 6. Document patient's response to blood therapy and nursing interventions performed. | |
| A. Complete documentation of transfusion forms as per unit protocol. | Transfusion record is a legal document. |

TABLE 49-4
**Summary of Potential Adverse Effects and Complications of Massive Blood Transfusions**[5]

1. Transmission of disease (e.g., acquired immune deficiency disease; hepatitis).
2. Pyrogenic reactions (fever-producing) associated with contaminated blood containers.
3. Transfusion reactions (fever-producing) associated with infusion of mismatched blood.
4. Allergic reactions (e.g., rash, urticaria, bronchospasm, edema, etc.).
5. *Dilutional coagulopathies* (i.e., blood clotting disorders) associated with a drop in the intravascular concentrations of clotting factors caused by administration of large volumes of crystalloids and red blood cell concentrates.
6. Citrate (anticoagulant used in stored whole blood) toxicity predisposing to hypocalcemia and acidemia.
7. Hyperkalemia (potassium intoxication). Potassium concentration in stored blood may rise as high as 30 mEq/liter, associated with RBC hemolysis.
8. Adult respiratory distress syndrome (ARDS) associated with seeding of the lungs with microaggregates of cellular debris, small fibrin clots, white blood cells, and platelets, which occur in blood and blood products.
9. Compromised oxygen delivery to the tissues caused by low concentrations of 2,3-diphosphoglycerate in stored blood.
10. Acidemia associated with a reduction in pH of stored blood caused by increasing concentrations of lactic acid over time, in stored blood (pH of stored blood ranges from 7.1 to 6.6).
11. Ammonia intoxication, especially in patients with liver disease. Stored blood has high concentrations of ammonia.
12. Hypothermia associated with rapid infusion of large amounts of cold blood. All blood and fluids should be warmed, especially when administered in large volumes.

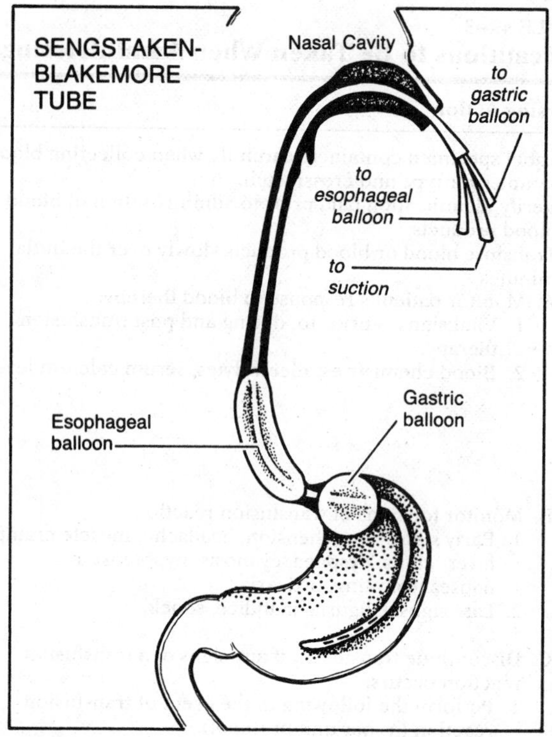


**Figure 49-1.** Sengstaken-Blakemore tube used for esophagogastric tamponade.

intravascular volume, which, in turn, also contributes to an increase in blood pressure. Continuous cardiac monitoring is required to detect the development of dysrhythmias and myocardial ischemic changes.

***Sclerotherapy.*** In patients with uncontrollable bleeding who are poor surgical risks, sclerotherapy may be indicated. Sclerosing solutions may be administered directly to the bleeding site by catheters passed into the portal circulation; or such solutions may be applied by endoscopy. Sclerosing solutions function to create variceal thrombosis and, in this way, curtail bleeding.

***Oral Propranolol Therapy.*** Propranolol has been found to lower portal venous hypertension and may be efficacious in the treatment of cirrhosis complicated by recurrent esophageal and gastric variceal bleeding.

***Surgical Intervention for Bleeding Varices.*** The most common surgical interventions performed for the treatment of bleeding varices include portocaval or splenorenal shunts. The treatment goal is to decompress the portal venous system by shunting blood into nearby, low-pressure venous channels. In general, such surgical procedures have not been found to prolong life. Major complications of surgery include hemorrhage, shunt thrombosis, hepatic encephalopathy, ascites, with edema of lower extremities, among others.

## NURSING CARE OF THE PATIENT WITH ACUTE UPPER GASTROINTESTINAL TRACT HEMORRHAGE AND HYPOVOLEMIC, HEMORRHAGIC SHOCK

Whether the underlying cause is a primary disease of the gastrointestinal system or occurs as a complication of a critical illness involving another organ system(s), the critical care nurse plays a crucial role in the assessment, diagnosis, and management of the patient with acute upper gastrointestinal (GI) tract hemorrhage, complicated by hypovolemic, hemorrhagic shock.

The immediate goals are to treat the shock and control the bleeding. Hemodynamic function can be stabilized and maintained through timely and aggressive fluid and blood replacement therapy. It is essential to reestablish adequate circulatory fluid volume so that tissue perfusion can be maintained and the oxygen delivered to the tissues is sufficient to meet the metabolic demands of the cells. (See Chap. 46 for an indepth discussion of shock.)

Monitoring of a patient with, or at risk of developing, acute upper GI bleeding should be ongoing and continuous. It is necessary to establish a baseline of

TABLE 49–5
## Sengstaken-Blakemore Tube: Nursing Care Considerations

**Purpose**
The Sengstaken-Blakemore tube is used for the emergency control of hemorrhage from esophageal and gastric varices. This tube affords the application of direct pressure to these bleeding blood vessels, thereby compressing them and controlling bleeding.

**Description**
The Sengstaken-Blakemore tube consists of a triple-lumen, double-balloon catheter. One lumen is used for gastric decompression; another for inflation of the gastric balloon, and the third for inflation of the esophageal balloon (see Figure 49–1).

| Nursing Actions | Rationales |
|---|---|
| 1. Patient preparation. | |
| A. Appropriate explanations to patient and family. | Knowing what to expect may help patient to relax and cooperate. |
| B. Pre-insertion sedation. 1. Morphine 2. Diazepam | Administration of sedatives must be done cautiously in patients with hepatic failure because such drugs can precipitate coma in these patients. |
| C. Position patient in left lateral and/or semi-Fowler's position. | Facilitates passage of gastric balloon into stomach. Semi-Fowler's position facilitates breathing and prevents aspiration. |
| D. Physician may attempt gastric lavage prior to insertion. | Minimizes risks of aspiration of stomach contents. |
| 2. Equipment preparation. | |
| A. Inflate both balloons and hold under water to assess for air leaks. | Ensures proper function upon insertion. |
| B. Lubricate entire tube including balloons, thoroughly with a water-soluble lubricant. | Reduces trauma to mucous membranes. |
| C. Have suction readily available. | Patient may vomit during insertion and aspiration is a danger. |
| ***Insertion and Tube Placement*** | |
| 1. Upon insertion, inflate gastric balloon with 50 ml air and clamp. | Prevents air leak. |
| 2. Withdraw tube until gastric balloon sits snugly against cardia of stomach (see Figure 47–3). | |
| 3. Verify tube placement: A. Aspirate gastric contents. B. Auscultate over stomach while injecting air. C. Obtain abdominal x-ray to confirm position of gastric balloon. | Verification of placement of gastric balloon is important to avoid inadvertent inflation of gastric balloon in the esophagus. This could precipitate respiratory distress, cardiac dysrhythmias, tissue necrosis, and perforation. |
| 4. Inflate gastric balloon with 100–150 ml air when tube placement is verified. | |
| 5. Apply gentle traction by taping catheter to a piece of sponge rubber as it emerges from the nostril; or place football helmet on patient and tape tube to face guard. | Prevents movement of tube with peristalsis; maintains continuous pressure to varices. Use of sponge helps to minimize pressure on nostrils caused by traction. |
| 6. Inflate esophageal balloon if bleeding persists. | |
| A. Maintain pressure of 25–40 mmHg with the use of a sphygmomanometer. | |
| B. Maintain pressure for up to 48 hr. | Longer use could cause esophageal tissue injury, necrosis and perforation. |
| C. Suction oropharynx and esophagus frequently: • Assist patient to suction her/his own secretions if the patient is alert and cooperative. | Patient is unable to swallow with esophageal tube inflated. Physician may elect to pass an accessory nasogastric tube into esophagus and apply continuous low suction to prevent fluid accumulation with its increased risk of aspiration. |
| ***Maintenance and Ongoing Care*** | |
| 1. Irrigate gastric tube as frequently as prescribed (q 30–60 min). | |
| A. Perform initial irrigation (with iced saline or water) until returns are clear. | This prevents clotted blood from plugging up gastric lumen. |
| B. Connect gastric lumen to continuous intermittent suction and monitor returns. | With initial evacuation of stomach subsequent assessments can be made as to the effectiveness of the tamponade. |
| C. Observe for persistent bleeding. | This may suggest erosive gastritis or bleeding peptic ulcer. |
| 2. Maintain tamponade for prescribed period of time. | |
| A. Monitor vital signs frequently. | |
| B. Assess neurological status: • Lethargy, drowsiness, confusion, unconsciousness. | |
| C. Assess for chest pain, back pain, respiratory distress. | |
| D. Record intake and output. | |
| E. Monitor serial electrolyte, BUN, Hct, Hgb, clotting factors. | |
| F. Monitor balloon pressures hourly. | |
| G. Double-clamp balloon parts. | This prevents air leaks; prevents gastric balloon from riding up into esophagus as air leaks out. |

*(continued)*

TABLE 49–5
**Sengstaken-Blakemore Tube: Nursing Care Considerations *(Continued)***

**Purpose**
The Sengstaken-Blakemore tube is used for the emergency control of hemorrhage from esophageal and gastric varices. This tube affords the application of direct pressure to these bleeding blood vessels, thereby compressing them and controlling bleeding.

**Description**
The Sengstaken-Blakemore tube consists of a triple-lumen, double-balloon catheter. One lumen is used for gastric decompression; another for inflation of the gastric balloon, and the third for inflation of the esophageal balloon (see Figure 49–1).

| Nursing Actions | Rationales |
|---|---|
| ***Maintenance and Ongoing Care (cont.)*** | |
| H. Keep scissors at bedside at all times. • In a true emergency, e.g., airway obstruction, cut through the entire tube with scissors and remove it. | Airway obstruction and esophageal perforation are major complications. Rupture of gastric balloon will cause entire tube to move up in the esophagus with the danger of airway obstruction. |
| • Notify physician immediately. | Sudden upper abdominal and/or back pains, and altered hemodynamics or shock, suggests esophageal perforation. |
| I. Deflate/inflate esophageal balloon as prescribed. | |
| 3. Provide comfort measures: | |
| A. Frequent and conscientious oral hygiene. B. Examine nostrils frequently and keep cleansed and lubricated. | Prevents mucous membrane encrustation; dryness and cracking; mouth breathing often becomes necessary because of large bore nasal tube. |
| C. Maintain on complete bed rest, avoiding any exertion, e.g., coughing, straining. | These activities increase intra-abdominal pressure and may predispose to further bleeding. |
| D. Maintain in semi-Fowler's position. | |
| E. Stay with patient as this may be a frightening experience. • Provide reassurance. | |
| 4. Continuous monitoring for the following complications: | |
| A. Aspiration of oral secretions or refluxed blood. | |
| B. Airway obstruction. | |
| C. Esophageal rupture. | |
| D. Cardiac dysrhythmias from distended esophagus. | |
| 5. Deflate balloons for a period of ~ 12 hr prior to removal. | |
| A. Monitor for signs of rebleeding. | Evidence of any rebleeding can be assessed. |

assessment data with which the patient's responses to therapy can be assessed and the effectiveness of such therapy in meeting patient outcomes can be evaluated. Clinical findings are not considered separately, but rather, they are examined in terms of the patient's entire clinical status. Furthermore, it is the *trend* or series of responses rather than any single, isolated response that is of clinical significance.

Nurses caring for the patient must be alert for any changes in the patient's condition, however subtle they may be. It is important to appreciate the distinct classes or degrees of blood loss and the associated clinical manifestations (see Table 49–1). In the patient at risk, complaints of weakness, fatigue, apprehension, and shortness of breath, coupled with tachycardia and orthostatic hypotension, take on added clinical significance in terms of possible underlying gastrointestinal bleeding. The extent of blood loss can sometimes be estimated based on the patient's overall clinical presentation.

In patients receiving massive blood transfusions, the nurse has the added responsibility of preventing complications associated with such therapy. An appreciation of the pathophysiology underlying blood incompatibility and transfusion reactions, dilutional coagulopathies, citrate toxicity with hypocalcemia and acidemia, hyperkalemia, and hypothermia is necessary for the prevention and/or early detection and treatment of such complications, should they occur (see Tables 49–2, 49–3, and 49–4).

For the patient with frank upper GI tract hemorrhage and his or her family, fear and apprehension are appropriate responses. The sight of blood can be upsetting regardless of how massive or minuscule the quantity. The critical care nurse provides a calming and stabilizing effect by encouraging patient and family to ask questions and verbalize their fears; offering appropriate explanations and reassurance; being accessible to them; and displaying a competent, efficient demeanor in providing overall patient care. The critical care nurse establishes a working rapport and trusting relationship with the patient and family, which assists them to cope with the immediate crisis situation, and lays the foundation for assisting patient and family to work through their problems, examine their lifestyles, and meaningfully consider the level of health desired.

**TABLE 49–6. CARE PLAN FOR THE PATIENT WITH ACUTE UPPER GASTROINTESTINAL HEMORRHAGE AND HYPOVOLEMIC, HEMORRHAGIC SHOCK**

| Nursing Diagnoses | Desired Patient Outcomes | Nursing Interventions | Rationales |
|---|---|---|---|
| ***Nursing Diagnosis #1*** Fluid volume deficit, actual, related to:<br>1. Acute blood loss—hematemesis, hematochezia.<br>2. Gastric drainage (continuous).<br>(Refer also to Tables 23–2 and 23–3.) | Patient will:<br>1. Maintain an effective circulating blood volume and stable hemodynamic functions:<br>• Heart rate (resting) <100 beats/min.<br>• Central venous pressure 0–8 mmHg.<br>• Pulmonary artery pressure <25 mmHg.<br>• Pulmonary capillary wedge pressure 8–12 mmHg.<br>• Cardiac output ~5 liters/min.<br>• Systemic arterial blood pressure within 10 mmHg of baseline, without orthostatic hypotension.<br>2. Remain alert, and oriented to person, place and time; without weakness and dizziness.<br>3. Maintain urine output >30 ml/hour.<br>4. Remain without signs of rebleeding:<br>• No hematemesis; hematochezia.<br>• Gastric aspirate blood-free.<br>5. Maintain body weight within 5% of baseline.<br>6. Balance intake with output. | • Assess for signs and symptoms of hypovolemic, hemorrhagic shock:<br>○ Observe for signs of acute or subacute hemorrhage: hematemesis, hematochezia; melena; abdominal distention, epigastric pain. | • A baseline assessment is necessary to establish the stage of shock—initial compensatory, progressive or final, and emergent measures indicated; it serves as a measure of the patient's response to therapy. (See Chapter 46 for a discussion of hypovolemic hemorrhagic shock, including the stages of shock.) |
| | | ○ Assess cardiovascular function:<br>○ Hypotension (orthostatic). | ○ A drop in blood pressure of 10–15 mmHg from supine to sitting position suggests blood loss of ~1 liter. |
| | | ○ Resting pulse >100 beats/min. Characteristics—faint, rapid, thready. | ○ Blood loss and enhanced peripheral vasoconstriction underlie diminished to absent pulses, coolness of the extremities, and pallor of conjunctiva, mucous membranes, and nailbeds. |
| | | – Skin color—pallor, cyanosis; skin temperature; delayed capillary refill time (>3 sec.) | |
| | | ○ Signs of dehydration—poor skin turgor; weakness, fatigue. | ○ Skin turgor is best assessed over forehead or sternum. |
| | | ○ Cardiac monitoring: rate and rhythm. | ○ Reflect effect of blood loss on cardiac function. |
| | | • Assess renal function:<br>○ Urine output >30 ml/hour. | • Reduced circulating blood volume and hypotensive state compromises renal perfusion. The consequent reduction in glomerular filtration underlies the reduced urine output associated with hypovolemic shock. |
| | | • Establish baseline abdominal assessment data:<br>○ Presence or absence of bowel sounds (timing and characteristics). | |
| | | ○ Pain and tenderness (location, radiation, quality, severity, duration). (See Table 7–1). | ○ Abdominal pain with muscle guarding and rebound tenderness is highly suggestive of peptic ulcer perforation, especially if preceded by an episode of severe abdominal pain, followed by sudden, but temporary relief, in patients at risk. |

*(continued)*

**TABLE 49–6. CARE PLAN FOR THE PATIENT WITH ACUTE UPPER GASTROINTESTINAL HEMORRHAGE AND HYPOVOLEMIC, HEMORRHAGIC SHOCK *(Continued)***

| Nursing Diagnoses | Desired Patient Outcomes | Nursing Interventions | Rationales |
|---|---|---|---|
| ***Nursing Diagnosis #1 (cont.)*** | | | |
| | 7. Exhibit good skin turgor; moist mucous membranes; minimal thirst. | ∘ Hepatomegaly, ascites, spider nevi, splenomegaly.<br>∘ Abdominal mass or bruit. | ∘ Suggestive of cirrhosis with portal hypertension.<br>∘ Questionable abdominal aneurysm. |
| | 8. Maintain laboratory parameters within acceptable physiological range:<br>• Hematocrit 37–52%.<br>• Hemoglobin 12–18 g/100 ml.<br>• RBC and WBC counts.<br>• BUN, electrolytes, calcium. | • Insert at least one, or more (if bleeding is massive) large gauge angiocatheters for rapid administration of blood and blood products, volume expanders, and fluids (Ringer's lactate, and normal saline).<br>∘ Obtain blood samples for baseline laboratory data. | • A single peripheral intravenous catheter may not be sufficient to provide adequate blood replacement in a profusely bleeding patient.<br>∘ A central venous line or pulmonary artery catheter is indicated to closely monitor the patient's response to volume replacement. |
| | | • Monitor Hct, Hgb; RBC, WBC counts; electrolytes, serum calcium; blood glucose levels. | • In patients bleeding profusely, there may be insufficient time for the blood volume to equilibrate. Thus, Hct and Hgb may not be reliable indicators of the patient's status. In such patients, changes in blood pressure and pulse are better indicators for replacement of blood and blood products.<br>∘ Rapid fluid shifts during GI bleeding, and subsequent infusion of blood, blood products and other fluids, require frequent assessment of serum electrolytes—sodium, potassium, chloride, bicarbonate, and serum calcium. The serum calcium level may become depressed after several units of anticoagulate (citrate)-containing blood have been administered. |
| | | ∘ Monitor BUN and creatinine levels. | ∘ Metabolism of blood by intestinal bacteria, coupled with compromised liver perfusion, causes the BUN level to rise.<br>– A rising BUN in the presence of a normal creatinine is highly indicative of a massive upper GI bleed. |
| | | ∘ Obtain blood samples for type and cross-match. | ∘ Even in acute emergencies, there is usually sufficient time to type and cross-match blood for infusion properly. This reduces the incidence of blood incompatibility and transfusion reactions. |

| | |
|---|---|
| ○ Monitor prothrombin time, clotting factors, fibrin degradation products. | ○ Patients receiving massive fluid and blood replacement therapy are at risk of developing a dilutional coagulopathy; patients with profuse hemorrhaging are at high risk of developing consumptive coagulopathies (e.g., disseminated intravascular coagulation, DIC). |
| • Initiate aggressive infusion of electrolytes, and volume expanders until blood is ready for administration. | |
| • Insert nasogastric tube: | • To decompress the stomach and assist (in conjunction with endoscopy) in determining site, amount, and rate of bleeding); to test gastric aspirate for blood, and pH; and to administer antacids, iced saline lavage (as prescribed). |
| • Check for tube placement: | • Inadvertent placement of the nasogastric tube into the respiratory passage is always a potential complication of this procedure. |
| ○ Auscultate over the gastric area while injecting 50 ml air into the nasogastric tube. | ○ A rush of air should be heard if the tube is properly placed. |
| • Assess gastric aspirate:<br>○ Presence of fresh blood, or a large amount of old blood (coffee-ground material) are indications for gastric lavage. | • Removal of as much clot and intragastric material, as possible, is important; it assists in evaluating continuous bleeding; an empty stomach will allow the walls to collapse and may contribute to hemostasis. |
| • Implement gastric lavage as prescribed. | • Irrigation with iced saline causes vasoconstriction of bleeding vessels; the efficacy of this treatment has yet to be substantiated. |
| ○ Maintain patency of tube by irrigation and repositioning if necessary. | ○ Use saline rather than water for lavage to minimize saline depletion via gastric mucosa. |
| • Maintain the patient NPO, and implement continuous gastric suction, as prescribed.<br>○ Monitor amount and characteristics of gastric drainage.<br>• Maintain a strict intake and output.<br>○ Include amount of fluid lavaged, and that removed via gastric suction.<br>○ Document amount and characteristics of any emesis. | • Continuous gastric suctioning enables close monitoring of bleeding; it minimizes the amount of blood passing into the intestine, where the action of the intestinal bacteria metabolizes blood to ammonia. |
| • Provide comfort measures:<br>○ Provide quiet, calm environment with frequent rest periods; minimize stimuli. | ○ To promote physical and mental rest; stimulation may provoke vomiting, bleeding. |
| ○ Provide mouth care with oral suctioning as necessary. | ○ Aspiration is a potential complication. |

**TABLE 49–6. CARE PLAN FOR THE PATIENT WITH ACUTE UPPER GASTROINTESTINAL HEMORRHAGE AND HYPOVOLEMIC, HEMORRHAGIC SHOCK *(Continued)***

| Nursing Diagnoses | Desired Patient Outcomes | Nursing Interventions | Rationales |
|---|---|---|---|
| *Nursing Diagnosis #1 (cont.)* | | | |
| | | ∘ Secure tube to patient's gown with adequate slack. | ∘ This prevents tugging on tube when patient moves, which can injure nose. |
| | | ∘ Lubricate nares; assess nares for pressure areas caused by nasogastric tube. | |
| | | ∘ Monitor body temperature.<br>– Provide extra blankets if appropriate. | ∘ Continuous iced saline lavage can lower body temperature. |
| | | • Transfuse blood and blood products as prescribed.<br>∘ Consider unit procedure and protocols for:<br>– Administering blood therapy.<br>– Monitoring patient's response to blood therapy.<br>– Recognizing early signs of adverse effects and transfusion reactions.<br>– Procedure to follow in the event of transfusion reaction. | • See Tables 49–2, 49–3, and 49–4 for nursing care considerations, precautions, and summary of adverse reactions (respectively) in the administration of blood and blood products. |
| | | • Insert Foley catheter to measure hourly urine output. | • Hourly urine outputs assist in monitoring renal perfusion and function. |
| | | • Assist with insertion of hemodynamic pressure monitoring lines. | • Insertion of systemic arterial and pulmonary artery flotation (Swan-Ganz) catheters are indicated in the setting of massive upper GI hemorrhage, and massive blood and fluid replacement therapy. |
| | | ∘ Monitor hemodynamics: arterial, and pulmonary artery pressures-CVP, pulmonary artery and pulmonary capillary wedge pressures (PCWP); and cardiac output. | ∘ PCWP is a useful parameter for monitoring for fluid overload, a potential complication of massive, aggressive fluid replacement therapy. |
| | | • Monitor hydration status during fluid replacement therapy. | |
| | | ∘ Assess respiratory function: respiratory rate and rhythm; presence of adventitious sounds. | ∘ The detection of rales in previously clear lungs suggest possible overhydration. |
| | | ∘ Assess signs/symptoms of fluid overload. (See Chapter 23.) | |
| | | ∘ Monitor daily weight. | • Should be maintained within 5% of baseline. |
| | | • Assist with insertion of Sengstaken-Blakemore tube in setting of persistent variceal bleeding. | • See Table 49–5 for nursing care considerations for patients with a Sengstaken-Blakemore tube. |

| | | | |
|---|---|---|---|
| ***Nursing Diagnosis #2***<br>Gas exchange impaired: Ventilation/perfusion imbalance, related to:<br>1. Reduced circulating volume and compromised hemodynamics. | Patient will:<br>1. Be alert and oriented to person, place, time.<br>2. Exhibit appropriate behavior.<br>3. Maintain effective cardiovascular function:<br>• Blood pressure within 10 mmHg of baseline.<br>• Cardiac output: ~5 liters/min.<br>4. Maintain arterial blood gas parameters within acceptable physiological range:<br>• pH 7.35–7.45<br>• $PaO_2$ >60 mmHg<br>• $PaCO_2$ 35–45 mmHg<br>5. Maintain hematologic values within acceptable range.<br>• Hematocrit 37–52%.<br>• Hemoglobin 12–18 g/100 ml.<br>• Red blood cell count. | • Perform neurological assessment.<br>○ Mental status; orientation to person, place, time; level of consciousness; appropriateness of responses/behavior.<br>• Monitor cardiovascular function:<br>○ Cardiac dysrhythmias.<br>○ Tachycardia; rapid, thready peripheral pulses.<br>○ Cyanosis.<br>• Monitor respiratory function:<br>○ Respiratory rate and pattern, breath sounds: normal and adventitious breath sounds.<br>○ Arterial blood gases: pH, $PaO_2$, $PaCO_2$; alveolar-arterial gradient ($AaDO_2$).<br>○ Monitor hematologic profile: hematocrit, hemoglobin, red blood cell count.<br>• Administer prescribed humidified oxygen therapy.<br>○ Monitor arterial blood gas and hematologic parameter as indicated.<br>○ Provide frequent rest periods.<br>○ Evaluate effectiveness of oxygen therapy: assess neurological function and vital signs. | • Hypoxemia coupled with hypovolemic shock can predispose to cerebral tissue hypoxia.<br>○ Hypoxemia is commonly associated with myocardial irritability.<br>○ Commonly associated with blood loss, and consequent reduced circulating blood volume and peripheral vasoconstriction.<br>○ Late sign reflecting desaturation of at least 5 gm/100 ml of hemoglobin; commonly associated with ventilation/perfusion mismatch, and right to left shunting.<br>○ Presence of rales (crackles) may be indicative of fluid overload.<br>○ Most closely reflect effectiveness of gas exchange.<br>○ Reflects hemoglobin oxygen-carrying capacity within blood; reduced hemoglobin levels can compromise oxygen delivery to tissues.<br>• Tissue hypoxia is a common consequence of hypovolemic, hemorrhagic shock due to depleted blood volume, and reduced number of RBCs.<br>○ To reduce oxygen demand by tissues. |
| ***Nursing Diagnosis #3***<br>Anxiety, related to:<br>1. Acute upper gastrointestinal hemorrhage (hematemesis).<br>2. Abdominal pain.<br>3. Transfusion therapy.<br>4. Intensive care setting. | Patient will:<br>1. Verbalize feeling less anxious.<br>2. Demonstrate relaxed demeanor.<br>3. Perform relaxation techniques with assistance.<br>4. Verbalize familiarity with ICU routines and protocols. | For specific Nursing Interventions and their rationales, see Table 35–3, Nursing Diagnosis #1, Anxiety. | |

*(continued)*

**TABLE 49-6. CARE PLAN FOR THE PATIENT WITH ACUTE UPPER GASTROINTESTINAL HEMORRHAGE AND HYPOVOLEMIC, HEMORRHAGIC SHOCK *(Continued)***

| Nursing Diagnoses | Desired Patient Outcomes | Nursing Interventions | Rationales |
|---|---|---|---|
| ***Nursing Diagnosis #4*** | | | |
| Comfort, alteration in: epigastric pain, related to:<br>1. Enhanced gastric acidity.<br>2. Reflex muscle spasm. | Patient will:<br>1. Verbalize pain relief.<br>2. Exhibit relaxed demeanor:<br>• Relaxed facial expression and body posturing.<br>Gastric aspirate: pH >4.5 | • Assess complaints of pain including: severity; location/radiation; influencing factors (e.g., what precipitates, aggravates or ameliorates the pain?; what signs and symptoms are associated with the pain?). | • Use of the "SLIDT" tool (see Table 7-1) assists in eliciting specific information about the nature of the complaints. |
| | | • Assess for nonverbal clues as to the presence of pain (e.g., restlessness, irritability, agitation, diaphoresis, tense facial features; rapid, shallow breathing). | |
| | | • Implement measures to reduce pain:<br>○ Administer the following medications as prescribed: | |
| | | ○ Antacids. | ○ Antacids neutralize gastric acidity. |
| | | ○ Histamine$_2$ antagonist—cimetidine (Tagamet) or ranitidine (Zantac). | ○ Inhibit gastric acid secretion. The combination of antacids/histamine antagonist therapy is more efficacious than either therapy alone in reducing the harmful effects of acid and pepsin on the bleeding lesion. |
| | | ○ Analgesics.<br>– Encourage patient to request medication when pain is first perceived, rather than waiting until it becomes severe.<br>– Evaluate the effectiveness of medication in relieving patient's pain. | |
| | | ○ Mild sedation. | ○ It is absolutely essential to assist the patient to rest and relax, mentally and physically, to reduce danger of continued bleeding, or rebleeding. |
| | | • Determine how patient usually copes with pain or stress:<br>○ Pain tolerance.<br>○ Willingness to discuss pain; or stoically "keeping it within."<br>○ Willingness to use medication for pain.<br>○ Behavior used to reduce level of stress. | • Details elicited at this time regarding patient/family attitudes about pain and stress may help lay the foundation for patient/family education in this regard. |

| | | | |
|---|---|---|---|
| ***Nursing Diagnosis #5***<br>Nutrition, alteration in: less than body requirements, related to:<br>1. Maintenance on NPO with continuous gastric suctioning.<br>(See Chapter 53, Nutritional Support of the Critically Ill Patient.) | Patient will maintain:<br>1. Body weight within 5% of baseline.<br>2. Total serum proteins 6.0–8.4 g/100 ml.<br>3. Laboratory data within acceptable physiological range:<br>• BUN, serum creatinine.<br>• Electrolytes, serum calcium.<br>• Blood glucose levels.<br>• Serum albumin 3.5–5.5 g/100 ml.<br>• Hematology profile.<br>4. Triceps skinfold measurements within normal range. | • Consult with nutritionist in assessing overall nutritional status; and signs and symptoms of malnutrition.<br>∘ Major considerations: General state of health—weakness; body weight; physiological factors—age, height, triceps skin fold; mid-upper arm circumference; food intolerance; allergies.<br>∘ Laboratory data: BUN, serum creatinine; fasting blood glucose; serum electrolytes, total protein (serum albumin); cholesterol; transfusion levels, hematology profile. | • Catabolic state associated with critical illness rapidly depletes body stores of nutrients. |
| | | • Maintain adequate nutrition with prescribed enteral and/or parenteral nutrition.<br>∘ Order prescribed feeding from Pharmacy. | • The purpose of total parenteral nutrition (TPN) is to provide sufficient nutrients intravenously, to achieve anabolism, and to promote weight gain.<br>∘ Solution should be prepared in Pharmacy under a laminar air-flow unit to minimize danger of contamination. |
| | | ∘ Assist with placement of TPN central intravenous catheter.<br>∘ Explain purpose of parenteral therapy.<br>∘ Explain procedure for insertion:<br>∘ Use of Trendelenburg position and Valsalva maneuver.<br>∘ Apply dressing.<br>∘ Prepare patient for chest x-ray. | ∘ Helps to avoid air embolism upon insertion.<br>∘ To confirm correct placement of catheter and rule out potential pneumothorax. |
| | | ∘ Assess patient for signs and symptoms of respiratory distress: Dyspnea, decreased breath sounds; chest pain; hematoma formation. | ∘ Pneumothorax, hemothorax, air embolism, and sepsis are major complications. |
| | | ∘ Initiate prescribed parenteral feedings.<br>∘ Begin infusion at slow rate (60–80 ml/hour); increase infusion by 25 ml/day. | ∘ Allows for physiological adjustments in pancreatic insulin secretion; helps to avoid glucose intolerance. |
| | | ∘ Use flow control device or pump to administer feeding.<br>– Weigh patient daily; record intake and output.<br>– Monitor serum glucose; monitor for signs of hyperglycemia (polyuria, glycosuria, elevated serum glucose). | ∘ This helps to prevent fluid or glucose overload. |
| | | ∘ Wean from TPN therapy slowly. | ∘ This avoids danger of hypoglycemic reaction as pancreatic secretion of insulin is allowed to decline accordingly. |

*(continued)*

**TABLE 49–6. CARE PLAN FOR THE PATIENT WITH ACUTE UPPER GASTROINTESTINAL HEMORRHAGE AND HYPOVOLEMIC, HEMORRHAGIC SHOCK** *(Continued)*

| Nursing Diagnoses | Desired Patient Outcomes | Nursing Interventions | Rationales |
|---|---|---|---|
| ***Nursing Diagnosis #5 (cont.)*** | | • Ongoing monitoring/maintenance:<br>∘ Maintain catheter asepsis. Monitor body temperature at regular intervals and report any temperature elevation to physician. Follow unit protocol in obtaining specimens for culture and sensitivity. | ∘ Consistent monitoring is necessary because there is no single febrile pattern associated with TPN sepsis. Temperature elevation may be low-grade, constant, or intermittent, or characterized by daily spiking. |
| | | ∘ Never use TPN catheter for anything other than parenteral feedings. | ∘ If catheter is used as a central access line in an emergency, it should not be reused for TPN. |
| | | ∘ Provide catheter site care as per unit protocol. | ∘ Cleansing of catheter site minimizes potential complications of sepsis, or mechanical disruption of catheter placement; it helps to preserve skin integrity at insertion site. |
| ***Nursing Diagnosis #6***<br>Infection, potential for, related to:<br>1. Invasive procedures.<br>2. Malnutrition. | Patient will:<br>1. Maintain body temperature within acceptable physiological range.<br>• ~98.6°F (37°C).<br>2. Maintain white blood count:<br>• 5000–10,000/$mm^3$.<br>3. Remain without signs and symptoms of infection; urine free of infection. | For specific Nursing Interventions and their rationales, see Table 49–7, Potential for Infection: Nursing Care Considerations. | |
| ***Nursing Diagnosis #7***<br>Sleep pattern disturbance, related to:<br>1. Frequent interruption for assessment and treatments.<br>2. Intensive care environment and protocols.<br>3. Psychologic stress. | Patient will:<br>1. Verbalize underlying concerns regarding inability to sleep.<br>2. Verbalize familiarity with ICU protocols and environmental stimuli.<br>3. Assist in planning for undisturbed rest periods within the | • Assess sleep pattern and difficulty sleeping:<br>∘ Encourage patient to verbalize concerns regarding sleeplessness.<br>∘ Monitor the amount of time the patient is sleeping or napping.<br>∘ Identify times and circumstances during which sleep seems most restful.<br>∘ Identify factors particularly disturbing to the patient.<br>∘ Observe for signs and symptoms of fatigue, restlessness, apprehension. | • To minimize bleeding and prevent rebleeding, it is essential to provide a clinical milieu that is as calm and quiet as possible, and conducive to patient rest and relaxation. |

| | | | |
|---|---|---|---|
| | constraints of ongoing monitoring, and essential patient care.<br>4. Report a sense of well-being and restfulness. | • Administer prescribed medications for pain and sedation.<br>○ Monitor effectiveness of medications in relieving pain, and relaxing the patient. | • Pain and anxiety undermine efforts to rest and relax. |
| | | • Provide comfort measures:<br>○ Include personal hygiene; back massage, position changes.<br>○ Minimize room noise; dim lighting during rest periods (if possible); maintain comfortable room temperature. | • Comfort measures aid muscle relaxation. |
| | | • Assist patient to establish a pattern conducive to sleep.<br>○ Explain ICU protocols and procedures. | ○ Understanding what to expect, and what is expected of the patient, may help to relieve concerns and apprehension. |
| | | ○ Encourage patient to verbalize feelings; provide an attentive, listening ear.<br>○ Stay with patient at times that are especially stressful.<br>○ Provide reassurance. | ○ Demonstration of caring, concern, and acceptance may be reassuring to patient. |
| | | ○ Allow patient to make some decisions regarding his/her care (e.g., when to rest; or when to have visitors). | ○ Enables patient to assume responsibility for some aspects of overall care. |
| ***Nursing Diagnosis #8***<br>Fear, related to:<br>1. Possibility of bleeding to death. | Patient will:<br>1. Verbalize fear of dying.<br>2. Verbalize knowledge of clinical status and proposed course of therapy.<br>3. Demonstrate behaviors indicative of lessened fear (e.g., relaxed facies and posture). | • Assess degree of fear and patient's perceptions as to the reality of the possibility of dying.<br>○ Encourage patient/family to discuss their perceptions and feelings regarding the patient's health status; to share subjective experiences.<br>○ Observe nonverbal and verbal responses. | • An episode of massive upper GI hemorrhage can be perceived by patient/family as an imminent threat that the patient is going to bleed to death. |
| | | ○ Assess for accompanying changes in patient's physiological status.<br>– Vital signs | ○ Recognize that sympathetic response to fear may actually aggravate bleeding, and needs to be minimized. |
| | | ○ Assess for accompanying changes in patient's psychological status.<br>○ Evidence of denial, anger, depression. | ○ These responses may assist patient/family to cope at least temporarily until patient/family have learned ways to reduce the threat. |
| | | • Assist patient/family to deal with fear:<br>○ Stay with patient/family.<br>○ Allow time for, and encourage expression of feelings and concerns.<br>○ Assist patient/family to identify feelings.<br>○ Clarify questions or misconceptions regarding illness or treatment. | |

*(continued)*

**TABLE 49-6. CARE PLAN FOR THE PATIENT WITH PULMONARY ACUTE UPPER GASTROINTESTINAL HEMORRHAGE AND HYPOVOLEMIC, HEMORRHAGIC SHOCK** *(Continued)*

| Nursing Diagnoses | Desired Patient Outcomes | Nursing Interventions | Rationales |
|---|---|---|---|
| ***Nursing Diagnosis #8 (cont.)*** | | | |
| | | • Assist patient/family to learn from this experience and to problem-solve:<br>○ Identify strengths of family members, individually and collectively.<br>○ Acknowledge usefulness of fear, denial, anger, in coping.<br>○ Promote honest and open communication between family members. | • Recognize that fear can be a motivating factor for learning only if the arousal of fear is accompanied by steps/actions to reduce the threat. |
| | | ○ Involve patient/family in problem-solving and decision-making. | ○ Assists patient/family in coping; this may help to increase self-confidence in their own capabilities. |
| | | • Referral to psychiatric liaison nurse and/or social worker as indicated, and/or requested by patient and/or family. | • Patient/family may feel reassured that other resources are available to lend assistance and support. |

TABLE 49–7
## Potential for Infection: Nursing Care Considerations[9]

| Nursing Actions | Rationales |
|---|---|
| • Define major risk factors for nosocomial infections in ICUs:<br>○ Invasive devices: Pressure monitoring devices, intravascular catheters, urinary catheters, respiratory therapy equipment, continuous ambulatory peritoneal dialysis (CAPD), hemodialysis.<br>○ Resistant microorganisms.<br>○ Altered immune response.<br>○ Antimicrobial therapy.<br>○ Underlying chronic or debilitating disease. | • *Nosocomial* infection is defined as a hospital-borne infection. Most frequently involved organisms (some with highly resistant strains) include: Serratia, pseudomonas, Enterobacter, proteus, Klebsiella, enterococci; Staphylococcus aureus and streptococcus (these latter two strains are frequently implicated in bacterial pneumonias.) Candida infections proliferate in hyperalimentation solutions. |
| • Monitor for urinary tract infection (UTI):<br>○ Avoid inserting catheter when alternative techniques for urinary drainage can be used.<br>○ Remove catheter as soon as possible. | ○ The incidence of UTI is directly related to the length of time a urinary catheter is in the bladder. |
| ○ Assess for signs/symptoms of UTI: urgency, frequency, dysuria, fever, chills, sweats; septic shock may be associated with a secondary bacteremia. | ○ Major complications of UTI include gram-negative sepsis and acute/chronic pyelonephritis. |
| ○ Insert catheter using aseptic technique:<br>○ Use smallest bore possible.<br>○ Secure catheter leaving enough slack to prevent pull on bladder neck and urinary meatus.<br>○ Maintain closed sterile drainage system. | ○ To minimize trauma to urinary tract. |
| • Monitor for intravascular infection.<br>○ Identify risk factors for IV-catheter related infections: Patient's health status and susceptibility (e.g., immunosuppressed)<br>○ Method of insertion: Percutaneous approach; cutdowns; centrally placed catheters (subclavian, CVP). | ○ Percutaneous approach has lower infection rate than cutdown or centrally placed catheters. |
| ○ Duration of cannulation. | ○ Infection rate markedly increases after 48–72 hours of insertion. |
| ○ Degree of manipulation of infusion system: Replacement of infusion solution container upon infusion completion; "piggyback" infusions.<br>○ Stopcocks—hemodynamic monitoring equipment.<br>○ Contaminated infusion solutions. | ○ Bacteremias are most commonly associated with hemodynamic pressure monitoring. |
| • Assess for signs and symptoms of intravascular cannula-related infection:<br>○ Swelling, pain, tenderness, warmth and erythema at insertion site, or over an indurated vessel, suggests phlebitis. | ○ Phlebitis is highly implicated in intravascular infections and bacteremia. |
| ○ Elevation in body temperature. | ○ When cause of elevated body temperature cannot be determined, suspect the IV site. |
| • Note precautions for the insertion and maintenance of intravenous line: Wash hands carefully prior to insertion; use antiseptic to prepare insertion site.<br>○ Anchor line securely.<br>–Apply topical antibiotic and sterile dressing over insertion site.<br>–Avoid use of infusates beyond 24-hr period.<br>○ Follow unit protocols for IV tubing and dressing changes (technique/time interval). | ○ Securing line reduces risk of injury to cannulated vessel. |
| • Note precautions for the insertion and maintenance of pressure-monitoring system.<br>○ Avoid inappropriate use of hemodynamic pressure-monitoring lines.<br>○ Utilize strict aseptic technique (masks, gloves, gowns)<br>○ Utilize closed flush system to maintain patency of line.<br>○ Saline solutions are used. | ○ Glucose solutions support bacterial colonization. |
| • Monitor for respiratory tract infection (RTI):<br>○ Risk factors for RTI include:<br>○ Compromised pulmonary defense mechanisms (e.g., intubation, tracheostomy, suctioning); aspiration of oropharyngeal and/or gastric secretions. | |

*(continued)*

TABLE 49–7

## Potential for Infection: Nursing Care Considerations[9] *(Continued)*

| Nursing Actions | Rationales |
|---|---|
| ○ Antibiotic therapy | ○ Occasionally predisposes to gram-negative infection of mouth and oropharynx. |
| –Hematogenic spread of infection to the lungs from distant foci (e.g. UTI). | |
| –Debilitating disease, multiorgan system failure. | |
| ○ Assess for signs and symptoms of RTI: fever (spiking); dyspnea, tachypnea. | |
| ○ Dullness to percussion. | ○ Suggests lung consolidation in this clinical setting. |
| ○ Abnormal breath sounds (bronchial in place of vesicular); and adventitious sounds (rales, rhonchi) on auscultation. | |
| • Review laboratory data and other studies: | |
| ○ Increase in WBC. | ○ In immunosuppressed patients, WBC may be decreased. |
| ○ Chest x-ray may indicate pulmonary consolidation. | |
| ○ Sputum production. | ○ Purulent sputum production, in conjunction with other clinical findings, is highly suggestive of pneumonia. |
| • Implement care considerations: | |
| ○ Rigorous handwashing. | ○ Common source of cross-contamination. |
| ○ Institution of timely and aggressive chest physiotherapy, and bronchial hygiene; coughing; deep breathing; incentive spirometry. | ○ Facilitates secretion mobilization and removal. |
| ○ Minimize risk of aspiration:<br>–Confirm placement of nasogastric tube prior to tube feeding. | |
| ○ Maintain in semi-Fowler's position. | ○ Reduces risk of aspiration; allows for maximum respiratory excursion. |
| ○ Monitor use and handling of respiratory therapy equipment. | ○ Highly implicated in nosocomial infections. |
| ○ Follow unit protocols in maintenance of artificial airways (endotracheal and tracheostomy tubes). | ○ See Tables 32–3 and 32–4 for Complications of Endotracheal Intubation, and Procedure for Endotracheal Suctioning, respectively. |
| • Appreciate significance of widespread antimicrobial use as a contributing factor in the selection of resistant strains of microorganisms. | • Selection of resistant strains occurs when sensitive microflora is suppressed by an antibiotic, enabling colonization and/or superinfection by resistant bacteria. |
| ○ Mechanisms underlying microbial resistance include: Enzymatic inactivation of antibiotic; alterations in biochemical pathways; alterations in drug-receptor sites; changes in cell-wall binding sites; alterations in genetic coding. | ○ *Candida* is an example of an infectious process, or superinfection, which becomes clinically evident after the antibiotic has eliminated the normal flora. |
| • Nursing care considerations: | • It is essential for nurses to appreciate potential adverse drug interactions. |
| ○ Administer prescribed antibiotics as directed: Avoid too rapid IV infusion; avoid infusion of two different antibiotics via the same line as the drug interaction may alter the desired effects of each drug (e.g., penicillins and aminoglycosides.) | ○ Excessively high levels of some drugs may predispose to drug toxicity. |
| • Appreciate infection control actions by health care providers: | • Health care providers have a responsibility to implement steps necessary to control the spread of infection in the patient population, environment, and in themselves and fellow health care professionals. |
| ○ Elements of the infectious process include: Causative agent, reservoir, portal of exit, transmission, portal of entry, susceptible host. | |
| • Viral hepatitis Type B—the infectious process: | • Viral hepatitis Type B is a commonly occurring infectious disease. |
| ○ Causative agent—hepatitis B virus (HBV). | |
| ○ Reservoir—patients who are hepatitis-B surface-antigen positive. | |
| ○ Portal of exit—primarily blood. | |
| ○ Transmission—by blood (needle stick, blood-soiled particles). | |
| ○ Portal of entry—direct contact by contaminated needle stick or by contact of infected materials with body surfaces, abrasions or other lesions. | |
| • Viral hepatitis Type B—precautions: | • Disease-specific precautions have been established for most known infectious diseases (refer to Hospital's Infection Control Manual). |
| ○ Avoid percutaneous inoculation by contaminated needle stick, or contact of infective blood or secretions (saliva) with scratches, abrasions or other skin lesions. | |
| ○ Avoid contamination of mucosal surfaces (eyes, mouth) by infective material. | |
| • Infection control measures: Disease-specific precautions should be initiated for patients admitted to ICU with a diagnosis or possible diagnosis of an infectious disease. Follow unit specific protocols in this regard. | |

## Therapeutic Goals

Implementation of nursing process in the care of the patient with acute upper gastrointestinal tract hemorrhage, and hypovolemic, hemorrhagic shock revolves around the following therapeutic goals:

1. Reestablish/maintain hemodynamic stability by restoring circulating blood volume, increasing cardiac output, and improving tissue perfusion.
2. Maintain a patent airway.
3. Prevent tissue hypoxia by providing oxygen therapy to maximize oxygen-carrying capacity of the blood and oxygen delivery to the tissues.
4. Establish a thorough, comprehensive assessment database, including clinical history and physical examination.
5. Maintain fluid and electrolyte balance.
6. Reduce anxiety and apprehension.
7. Maintain therapeutic milieu with optimum rest, comfort, and relaxation, to minimize bleeding or rebleeding.
8. Provide nutritional support to maintain ideal body weight.
9. Prevent and/or monitor for complications of shock, including adult respiratory distress syndrome (ARDS), acute renal failure, and disseminated intravascular coagulation (DIC).
10. Prevent infection.
11. Provide emotional and psychologic support to patient and family.
12. Initiate patient/family health education regarding underlying disease process, impact on performance of activities of daily living and overall lifestyle, and decision-making process as to the optimum level of health desired.

## Nursing Diagnoses, Desired Patient Outcomes, and Nursing Interventions

Pertinent nursing diagnoses, desired patient outcomes, nursing interventions and their rationales are presented in Table 49–6. Table 49–7 is concerned with potential for infection: nursing care considerations. See Chapter 46 for an indepth discussion of hypovolemic shock.

## REFERENCES


1. Konopad, E and Noseworthy, T: Stress ulceration: A serious complication in the critically ill patient. Heart Lung 17(4):339, July 1988.
2. Kelton, JG: Management of the bleeding patient. In Sibbald, WJ (ed): Synopsis of Critical Care, ed 3. Williams & Wilkins, Baltimore, 1988, p 245.
3. Zaharopoulos P, Angie, PJ, and Lanigan, K: Managing G.I. bleeding. It takes a two-tract mind. Nursing '88 18(4):68, April 1988.
4. Millar, S, Sampson, L, and Soukup, SM: AACN Manual for Critical Care, ed 2. WB Saunders, Philadelphia, 1985, p 415.
5. Sinclair, DM: Upper gastrointestinal tract bleeding and liver failure. In Cane, RD and Shapiro, BA (eds): Case Studies in Critical Care. YearBook Medical Publishers, Chicago, 1985, p 228.
6. Eastwood, GL: Core Textbook of Gastroenterology. JB Lippincott, Philadelphia, 1984, p 226.
7. Sinclair, DM: Upper gastrointestinal tract bleeding and liver failure. In Cane, RD and Shapiro, BA (eds): Case Studies in Critical Care. YearBook Medical Publishers, Chicago, 1985, p 215.
8. Quinless, FW: Severe liver dysfunction. Client problems and nursing actions. Focus Crit Care 12(1):27–32, February 1985.
9. Goldrick, B: Infection control in the ICU. In Emanuelsen, KL and Rosenlicht, JM (eds): Handbook of Critical Care Nursing. John Wiley & Sons, New York, 1986, p 401.

CHAPTER 50

# Nursing Management of the Patient with Hepatic Failure–Hepatic Encephalopathy

## CHAPTER OUTLINE



## LEARNING OBJECTIVES

**At the end of this chapter, you should be able to:**

1. Differentiate common causes of hepatic failure.
2. Identify types of liver disease and underlying pathophysiology.
3. List the clinical features of hepatic failure.
4. State the major complications of hepatic failure.
5. Define hepatic encephalopathy and the stages of its clinical course.
6. Describe the pathophysiology of hepatic encephalopathy and its consequent clinical presentation.
7. Define treatment priorities in the management of hepatic failure and hepatic encephalopathy.
8. Describe the nursing process in the care of the patient with hepatic failure and hepatic encephalopathy including:
   Assessment
   Nursing diagnoses
   Planning: Desired patient outcomes
   Nursing interventions/rationales.

## HEPATIC FAILURE

Hepatic failure may result from chronic or acute liver disease and is commonly associated with viral, chemical, metabolic, or ischemic injury to hepatic cells (hepatocytes; see Fig. 47–7). Disorders of neurologic, renal, and hematologic function commonly develop. In patients with acute hepatic failure and hepatic encephalopathy, whether superimposed on chronic liver disease (e.g., Laennec's cirrhosis) or occurring in a young patient with a previously healthy liver (fulminant hepatic failure), the mortality rate is at least 80%.

Although there is no specific curative therapy for hepatic failure and treatment is mainly supportive, survivors generally attain full functional recovery of all systems, owing in large measure to the regenerative capability of the liver. The challenge presented to critical care nurses caring for patients with hepatic failure is to provide timely, meticulous, and attentive care to maintain the patient during the critical phase of illness and to prevent complications.

## Etiology

### Viral

Viral hepatitis is the most common cause of fulminant hepatic failure (FHF) and includes both hepatitis A and hepatitis B infections. Acute non-A non-B hepatitis has also been implicated in FHF. Herpes virus, likewise, has been implicated as a cause of acute liver disease.

### Chemical

Drug-related liver disease and hepatic failure have been associated with such drugs as acetaminophen, salicylates, and phenylbutazone (analgesics, antipyretics, and anti-inflammatory agents); halothane (anesthetic agent); tetracycline, sulfonamides, isoniazid, and rifampin (antibiotics); phenytoin (anticonvulsant); and methyldopa and furosemide (anti-hypertensive and diuretic, respectively.) Hepatotoxic reactions in the liver may be enhanced by the concurrent administration of isoniazid and rifampin. Alcohol produces a direct toxic effect on hepatic cells, and chronic alcohol abuse has long been identified as a cause of chronic liver disease (Laennec's cirrhosis). Intoxication with industrial chemicals (e.g., carbon tetrachloride) is another potential cause of liver disease and hepatic failure.

### Metabolic

Malnutrition (often seen in the chronic alcoholic) is associated with fatty degeneration of the liver parenchyma. Normally, the liver synthesizes lipoproteins from ingested protein and triglycerides. Lipoproteins play a strategic role in lipid transport by the blood. When dietary intake of protein is insufficient, there is decreased utilization of triglycerides for the synthesis of lipoproteins. This, coupled with disturbances in fat transport and metabolism, contribute to the development of *fatty* liver early in the course of the disease.

A reduced serum glucose (secondary to malnutrition) may also contribute to fatty infiltration of the liver by stimulating the release of triglycerides from adipose tissue. Less commonly, acute fatty liver of pregnancy and Reye's syndrome are implicated in FHF.

### Ischemic

Ischemic hepatic necrosis is a less common cause of FHF.

## Pathophysiology

### Chronic Liver Disease

Chronic liver disease, or cirrhosis, is characterized by a gradual, insidious, and progressive degeneration of the liver parenchyma, with diffuse hepatocellular necrosis, widespread hepatic fibrosis, and nodular regeneration. Several clinically distinct forms have been identified.

**Laennec's Cirrhosis.** Laennec's cirrhosis is the most commonly occurring chronic liver disease, and it is most closely associated with chronic alcohol abuse. The direct toxic effect of alcohol on hepatocytes, coupled with malnutrition, predisposes to fatty infiltration of the hepatic parenchyma.

**Postnecrotic Cirrhosis.** Postnecrotic cirrhosis is characterized by a significant loss of hepatic cells (hepatic necrosis), collapse of the fibroconnective tissue framework of the liver parenchyma, and the presence of large, irregular nodules of regenerating and degenerating hepatic tissue. Approximately 25% of patients with postnecrotic cirrhosis have a history of acute viral hepatitis. Intoxication with industrial chemicals, drugs, poisons, and certain infections (endotoxins) has been implicated in the etiology of this form of cirrhosis. Postnecrotic cirrhosis has been associated with primary hepatic neoplasm formation (*hepatoma*).

**Biliary Cirrhosis.** Biliary cirrhosis may develop secondary to decreased bile flow and cholestasis, as occurs in intrahepatic and/or extrahepatic biliary obstruction. Stasis of bile within the liver parenchyma and its accumulation result in destruction of hepatic cells (see Fig. 47-7).

**Cardiac Cirrhosis.** Cardiac cirrhosis is relatively rare and associated with severe right-sided congestive heart failure. Severe venous congestion predisposes to ischemia and anoxia with consequent cellular injury and necrosis. Persistence of this process leads to generalized fibrosis.

### Acute Liver Disease

**Fulminant Hepatic Failure.** Fulminant hepatic failure (FHF) involves a rapid, progressive deterioration and degeneration of liver parenchyma, frequently with massive hepatocellular necrosis, resulting in severe hepatic dysfunction. The underlying disease process may precipitate hepatic failure and hepatic encephalopathy within but 4–8 weeks of the onset of symptoms in a person with previously normal liver function.

## Clinical Presentation

Familiarity with the major functions of the liver assists in anticipating and identifying specific dysfunction and consequent clinical manifestations that are likely to occur in acute hepatic failure. When more than 60% of hepatocytes sustain injury and/or necrosis, acute hepatic failure ensues, resulting in the inability of the liver to perform its metabolic functions adequately (see Table 47–4).

### *Metabolic Alterations in Hepatic Failure*[1]

A major role of the liver is to provide for a "metabolic pool" of essential nutrients, which are made available to all other cells in the body.

**Carbohydrate Metabolism.** Hepatic failure may manifest as abnormal carbohydrate metabolism with impairment of glycogenesis, glycogenolysis, and gluconeogenesis. The end result is hypoglycemia marked by weakness, fatigue, lethargy, and weight loss. The serum glucose reflects the hypoglycemic state.

**Fat Metabolism.** Because the liver is the principal site for lipid synthesis and degradation, any alteration in its ability to metabolize fats impacts on all cells of the body. Abnormal lipid metabolism reduces the availability of triglycerides and lipoproteins, the former as an energy source, and the latter for transport of lipids by the blood. Altered cholesterol and phospholipid synthesis predisposes to impairments in the structural integrity of cellular membranes and intracellular organelles. Abnormalities in cholesterol synthesis also disrupt synthesis of bile salts, which contain about 80% of the total cholesterol synthesized by the liver. Altered bile salt synthesis, in turn, disrupts the digestion and absorption of fats and fat-soluble vitamins (A, D, E, K) from the gastrointestinal tract.

Clinically, the patient may experience dyspepsia, a feeling of "bloatedness," and gas pain related to gas accumulation associated with impaired fat digestion and absorption. Complaints of anorexia, nausea and vomiting, and intestinal disturbances (diarrhea or constipation) are common. Impaired vitamin K absorption interferes with the hepatic synthesis of prothrombin and clotting factors VII, IX, and X, and predisposes to bleeding. Serum levels reflect a significant decrease in total cholesterol levels; prothrombin time may be prolonged.

**Protein Metabolism.** The clinical implications of altered protein metabolism are significant.

***Hypoalbuminemia.*** Decreased protein synthesis predisposes to *hypoalbuminemia* with a consequent lowering of the serum colloidal osmotic pressure. Alterations in the colloidal osmotic pressure lead to generalized systemic edema (*anasarca*) and ascites.

*Ascites.* Ascites (i.e., accumulation of fluid in the peritoneal cavity) is a major clinical finding in advanced liver disease. Obstruction to portal blood flow, whether due to extrahepatic or intrahepatic pathology, eventually results in portal hypertension, with a consequent formation of ascites.

Accumulation of ascites occurs when forces favoring movement of fluid into the interstitium (increased *hydrostatic* blood pressure) exceed forces favoring movement of fluid from the interstitium into the intravascular space (*colloidal osmotic* pressure). As increased hydrostatic pressure (portal hypertension) and decreased colloidal osmotic pressure (hypoalbuminemia) occur, there is marked transudation of fluid from the intravascular space into the interstitium. Excess fluid is normally returned to the systemic circulation by the lymphatic system. When this process fails to keep pace with the volume of fluid extravasated into the peritoneal cavity, ascites forms and accumulates.

The consequent depletion of intravascular volume reduces renal perfusion and stimulates the juxtaglomerular apparatus and the renin–angiotensin–aldosterone system. The activity of aldosterone, which is to stimulate sodium reabsorption in the distal tubules, becomes especially heightened in hepatic failure. The resultant increase in sodium and water reabsorption, coupled with hypoalbuminemia, serve to further promote ascites.

Other contributing factors include the inability of damaged liver cells to metabolize aldosterone properly, enabling the serum concentration of this hormone to increase; and the inability of these cells to synthesize sufficient albumin to maintain intravascular colloidal osmotic pressure.

Ascites is an example of *"third-spacing"* of fluid (see Chap. 23). Assessment for the presence of ascites involves inspection of the abdomen for distention, bulging of the flanks, or a protruding misplaced umbilicus; percussion for shifting dullness; and/or palpation for the presence of a fluid wave. Measurements of the abdominal girth should be made using ink marks on the abdomen as guidelines as to where the measurements are made.

***Clotting Factors—Decreased Synthesis.*** A decrease in overall protein synthesis results in a decreased production of clotting factors. The consequent derangement of the blood clotting mechanisms can lead to bleeding tendencies. These may be manifested by epistaxis, gingival bleeding, menorrhagia, purpura, and areas of ecchymosis. The prothrombin time may be prolonged. Coagulopathies may develop because of the liver's inability to metabolize activated coagulation and fibrinolysis factors.

***Ammonia Metabolism—Urea Synthesis.*** Urea

synthesis is commonly depressed in hepatic failure, and this is reflected by a rising serum ammonia and a low blood urea nitrogen (BUN) level. Ammonia ($NH_3$) is formed from metabolism of amino acids and from the action of intestinal bacteria on proteins. It is converted to urea exclusively by the liver and subsequently eliminated by the kidneys. When hepatocytes fail to metabolize ammonia to urea, concentrations of this substance circulating in the blood become greatly increased.

In the patient with portal hypertension, elevation of serum ammonia levels will be augmented because ammonia absorbed from the gastrointestinal tract may bypass the liver by collateral circulation. Hypokalemic metabolic alkalemia, which commonly occurs in hepatic failure, also contributes to rising serum ammonia levels by shifting the balance between ammonia ($NH_3$) and ammonium ($NH_4^+$) in the direction of ammonia (see Chap. 30):

$$\underset{\text{(un-ionized)}}{\text{(ammonia) } NH_3} + H^+ \underset{\uparrow \text{pH (alkalemia)}}{\overset{\downarrow \text{pH (acidemia)}}{\rightleftharpoons}} \underset{\text{(ionized)}}{NH_4^+ \text{ (ammonium)}}$$

It is ammonia (un-ionized form) that readily crosses the blood–brain barrier; it is also more easily reabsorbed from the urine than ammonium (ionized form). Elevated serum ammonia levels contribute to the development of hepatic encephalopathy (see section entitled "Complications").

### Alterations in Hormonal Metabolism

Endocrine disturbances commonly occur in cirrhosis and hepatic failure because this organ is largely responsible for the metabolism and inactivation of hormones of the adrenal cortex, testes, and ovaries. *Hyperaldosteronism* predisposes to fluid and electrolyte imbalance by stimulating sodium reabsorption at the expense of potassium and hydrogen ion secretion. This accounts, in part, for the hypokalemic, metabolic alkalemia commonly associated with hepatic failure. The enhanced reabsorption of sodium is accompanied by the reabsorption of water, predisposing to fluid retention. Clinically, this is reflected by systemic edema and ascites.

Increased levels of estrogen are reflected clinically in several ways. Spider nevi (angiomas) appear on the skin, especially around the chest and neck. These lesions consist of a central arteriole from which numerous small vessels radiate. When pin-point pressure is applied to the central arteriole, the lesion blanches; when pressure is released, blood flow readily returns. Testicular atrophy and gynecomastia (in men), amenorrhea or menstrual irregularity (in women), pectoral and axillary alopecia, and palmar erythema are other clinical manifestations of excess circulating estrogen.

Cirrhosis is derived from the Greek *kirrhos,* which means tan or tawny. In patients with long-standing liver disease, an increased pigmentation of the skin may be observed. This results from excessive activity of melanin-stimulating hormone that is not metabolized by the damaged liver cells.

### Alterations in Bilirubin Metabolism

Jaundice is a common occurrence in liver disease. Hyperbilirubinemia occurs as the hepatocytes fail to metabolize bilirubin, and its increased concentration in the blood stains elastic tissues, especially in skin, sclera, and mucous membrane. Jaundice may be accompanied by pruritus caused by deposition of bile salts in the skin. In biliary cirrhosis, the patient may also experience malabsorption and steatorrhea.

### Alterations in Hematologic Function

Chronic hepatic congestion and portal hypertension predispose to splenomegaly with consequent hematologic disorders including thrombocytopenia, leukopenia, and anemia. The enlarged spleen is very active in the removal of blood cells from the circulation. Leukopenia is clinically significant because it places the patient at added risk of infection.

Anemia may result from deficiencies of folate and vitamin $B_{12}$ because of failure of hepatocytes to process and store these vitamins properly. Iron deficiency due to increased hemolysis of red blood cells, bleeding, and the inability of the liver to store iron (ferritin-storage form) also contributes to anemia.

### Portal Hypertension—Clinical Signs

Whenever portal circulation is obstructed, causing overload of the portal circuit, significant collateral circulation forms to circumvent the obstruction and reduce portal system pressure. Blood may be shunted to the umbilical area where superficial veins of the abdominal wall become dilated and distended (*caput medusa*); hemorrhoids may occur when backflow of blood from the portal system drains into the venous plexus formed by the superior hemorrhoidal veins. The most important collateral circulation that develops in response to portal hypertension occurs in the lower esophagus where the esophageal plexuses merge with the left gastric vein. Dilation of these blood vessels predisposes to esophageal varices, the rupture of which can precipitate massive upper gastrointestinal hemorrhaging. Splenomegaly is considered to be one of the most important diagnostic signs of increased portal vein pressure.

Nonspecific clinical signs in liver disease may include clubbing of the fingers, whitening of nailbeds, and Dupuytren's contracture. In more advanced liver disease, a characteristic odor, *fetor he-*

*paticus,* may be detected. It is thought to arise from mercaptans that are absorbed from the gut and are inadequately metabolized. Fetor must be distinguished from halitosis or other breath odors. For a summary of clinical findings (signs, symptoms, and laboratory data), see Table 50-1.

TABLE 50-1
**Liver Disease: Summary of Clinical Findings**

**Signs and Symptoms**
***Early Findings***
Asymptomatic with hepatomegaly (smooth to palpation).
Malaise, weakness, fatigue, lethargy, weight loss.
Anorexia, nausea, vomiting, indigestion (fat intolerance), flatulence, diarrhea or constipation.

***Later Findings—Hepatocellular Decompensation***
*Dermatologic*
Jaundice, pruritus; dryness, poor skin turgor; low-grade fever.
Spider nevi (angiomas); palmar erythema.
Increased skin pigmentation (tawny appearance).
Pectoral alopecia—loss of axillary and pubic hair (men).
Clubbing of fingers, whitened nailbeds.
Caput medusae; peripheral edema (lower extremities; or sacrum if recumbent).
Muscle wasting.

*Gastrointestinal*
Malnutrition, weight loss.
Dyspepsia, abdominal distention, gastritis, right upper quadrant tenderness.
Splenomegaly; hepatomegaly (irregular and nodular to palpation).
Ascites—shifting dullness on percussion; fluid wave present.
Bleeding esophageal/gastric varices; hemorrhoids.
Fetor hepaticus.
Vitamin K deficiency.

*Cardiovascular*
Generalized edema (anasarca).
Hypovolemia with hypotension; tachycardia.

*Hematologic*
Anemia, thrombocytopenia, leukopenia.
Bleeding diathesis—petechiae; ecchymosis; epistaxis; gingival bleeding.
Coagulopathies.
Deficient clotting factors; capillary fragility.
Poor wound healing.

*Renal*
Urobilinogenuria (dark amber urine)
Oliguria—hepatorenal syndrome (see complications)

*Neurologic*
Peripheral neuritis; asterixis (flapping tremor), hyperactive reflexes, Babinski sign.
Hepatic encephalopathy (see complications).
Hepatic coma.

*Endocrine*
Gynecomastia; testicular atrophy; impotence (men).
Menstrual irregularities (women).

***Laboratory Findings (see Table 48-1)***
*Evidence of Hepatocellular Injury*
Elevated serum enzymes: SGOT, SGPT, gamma-glutamyl transferase (GGT); alkaline phosphatase (elevated in biliary obstruction), lactic dehydrogenase (isoenzyme $LDH_5$ indicative of jaundice, hepatitis, and hepatic metastasis).

TABLE 50-1
**Liver Disease: Summary of Clinical Findings *(Continued)***

*Evidence of Hepatocellular Insufficiency*
Hypoalbuminemia, hypoglycemia, hyperbilirubinemia.
Elevated serum ammonia levels, low BUN.
Low serum cholesterol.
Altered complete blood count:
- Decreased RBC, hematocrit, and hemoglobin (reflect inability of hepatocytes to store hematopoietic factors [folate, vitamin $B_{12}$, and iron]).
- Decreased WBC count and thrombocytopenia (reflect splenomegaly).
- Prolonged prothrombin time; reduced clotting factors.

***Other Findings***
Serum electrolytes: Hypokalemia (secondary to diuretic therapy and hyperaldosteronism).
Serum creatinine.
Arterial blood gases:
- Reduced arterial oxygen saturation.
- Metabolic alkalemia.

Viral serology for hepatitis A and B.
Urine:
- Urobilinogenuria (reflects decreased reabsorption of urobilinogen in liver disease).
- Decreased urine sodium (reflects hyperaldosteronism).

Stool:
- Decreased fecal urobilinogen.
- Positive guaiac (suggests gastrointestinal bleeding).

## Diagnosis

### Clinical History

To assist in the diagnosis and management of the patient with liver disease and hepatic failure, it is essential to elicit pertinent information regarding patient/family health patterns.

### Functional Health Patterns

***Health Perception—Health Management.*** Establish overall health status and recent changes that may have occurred in health or lifestyle: Weight gain or loss; appetite, diet (fatty food intolerance); malnutrition; activity intolerance.

Elicit a thorough history regarding prescribed or self-medication, especially with respect to the following drugs, which have been associated with hepatotoxicity: Acetaminophen, salicylates, phenylbutazone, tetracycline, sulfonamides, rifampin, nitrofurantoin, phenytoin, methyldopa, furosemide, phenothiazines, and oral contraceptives.

Elicit a detailed history regarding alcohol use and abuse. Alcohol is the most common agent implicated as a cause of hepatic injury and cirrhosis. It is associated with a long latent period in the development of cirrhosis; therefore, it is necessary to elicit the past history of alcohol use dating back at least several years. The amount, type, and duration of alcohol consumption should be established. A family history of alcohol use may assist in ascertaining attitudes regarding drinking and its significance in their lifestyle.

It is essential to determine recent illnesses, especially of viral origin (e.g., viral hepatitis, herpes). Viral hepatitis is the most common cause of fulminant hepatic failure occurring in a previously healthy person with apparent normal liver function. Reye's syndrome has been associated with acute liver disease and hepatic failure. A past history of tuberculosis may be significant, especially if the patient was treated with a combination of isoniazid and rifampin therapy. This combination of drugs has been associated with hepatotoxic reactions. A past history of allergies or allergic reactions, especially in conjunction with drug use, may be important and should be documented.

The patient's occupation may furnish clues as to exposure to, or use of, industrial chemicals or other agents that cause hepatotoxicity. Hypertension, treated with furosemide or methyldopa, may be implicated in the etiology of liver disease.

Family history related to alcoholism, liver, and gallbladder disease; gastrointestinal ulceration and bleeding; pancreatic disease; cancer of colon, pancreas, or liver; and malabsorption syndromes should be ascertained and documented.

For additional patient/family history guidelines and tips on physical examination, see Chapter 48. Pertinent physical findings and laboratory data for the patient with liver disease and hepatic failure are listed in Table 50-1.

## Complications

Major complications associated with hepatic failure include encephalopathy, cerebral edema, hepatorenal syndrome, bleeding diathesis, and sepsis. (Hepatic encephalopathy is discussed in the section to follow.)

### *Cerebral Edema*

Cerebral edema has been reported in cases of fulminant hepatic failure. In extreme cases, transtentorial herniation and brainstem compression have occurred. The pathogenesis of this cerebral edema is unknown.

### *Hepatorenal Syndrome*

Hepatorenal syndrome describes the development of a progressive functional renal failure in the setting of fulminant hepatic failure, or advanced end-stage liver disease. The exact pathogenesis of the syndrome is unknown. A possible mechanism involves altered renal perfusion attributed to renal arteriolar vasoconstriction with a consequent increased renal vascular resistance. Clinically, the syndrome may be recognized by the presence of oliguria, azotemia, and a urine of high osmolality and low sodium content in the setting of progressive liver failure.

### *Bleeding Diathesis*

Clinically, significant bleeding usually occurs with erosion of esophageal and gastric varices. Bleeding disorders and coagulopathies (e.g., disseminated intravascular coagulation—DIC) may also result from failure of hepatocytes to synthesize clotting factors or to clear fibrinolysins; dysfibrinogenemia (abnormal fibrinogen), thrombocytopenia, platelet dysfunction, and capillary fragility also predispose to bleeding.

### *Sepsis*

Sepsis is a frequently occurring complication of hepatic failure. The WBC may be elevated, but neutrophil function may be impaired. Corticosteroids may aggravate the problem by depressing the immune response, and their use is contraindicated.

# HEPATIC ENCEPHALOPATHY

## Definition

Hepatic encephalopathy is a major complication of hepatic failure characterized by reversible alterations in mentation, consciousness, and motor function. The neuropsychiatric manifestations of hepatic encephalopathy can dominate the clinical presentation of the underlying hepatic failure.

## Pathophysiology

Hepatic encephalopathy may occur in the setting of chronic, end-stage liver disease, or in acute fulminant hepatic failure (FHF).

### *Portal-Systemic Encephalopathy*

In longstanding liver disease (cirrhosis), the major contributing factor is portal hypertension, and the encephalopathy is often referred to as *portal-systemic encephalopathy (PSE)*. The liver plays a vital role in the metabolism, transformation, and detoxification of both exogenous and endogenous substances. In severe liver disease, almost all the portal circulation can be diverted away from the liver by collaterals. In this event, exogenous and endogenous toxins deprived of hepatic filtration may accumulate in the systemic circulation. The nature of these toxins remains undefined, but most theories suggest that their toxic effect involves one or more of the following: Alteration in brain energy metabolism, alteration in neuronal membrane physiology, or derangement in neurosynaptic transmission (neurotransmitter imbalance, or false neurotransmitters.)[2]

**Mechanisms of Toxicity.** The mechanisms of toxicity likewise remain undefined.

***Altered Ammonia Metabolism.*** Altered ammonia metabolism is most closely identified with hepatic encephalopathy. The bulk of serum ammonia originates in the gastrointestinal tract where it is derived from the metabolism of ingested proteins, breakdown of blood, or degradation of urea secreted into the colon. Most ammonia produced in this manner undergoes detoxification in the liver by the synthesis of urea. When the liver is bypassed, as it is in portal-systemic shunting, the major site of ammonia detoxification is eliminated, and it accumulates in the blood. Because ammonia easily traverses the blood-brain barrier, fragile brain tissues become exposed to exceedingly high concentrations of ammonia.

Patients with longstanding liver disease who develop bleeding of esophageal and gastric varices, secondary to portal hypertension, are especially at high risk of developing encephalopathy. The action of intestinal bacteria on the additional load of blood presented to the gut by bleeding varices further augments the serum concentration of ammonia.

### *Fulminant Hepatic Failure*

Unlike portal-systemic encephalopathy, where portal hypertension is considered to be the major contributing factor, encephalopathy associated with fulminant hepatic failure (FHF) is more directly attributed to hepatocellular necrosis rather than portal-systemic shunting. Such necrosis, itself, causes extensive intrahepatic shunting, but extensive portal-systemic collaterals are lacking. Portal pressure may be elevated in acute, rapidly progressing hepatic failure, but it is elevated to a lesser extent than in longstanding, slowly progressing, chronic liver disease (cirrhosis).

## Clinical Presentation

While there are some subtle differences in the clinical presentations of portal-systemic encephalopathy and the encephalopathy of fulminant hepatic failure, they both reflect disorders of mentation, consciousness, and motor function, and, therefore, are considered together. The progression of hepatic encephalopathy occurs in stages.

### *Stages of Encephalopathy*

For a listing of clinical neuropsychiatric manifestations of hepatic encephalopathy, see Table 50-2.

TABLE 50-2
**Stages of Hepatic Encephalopathy: Neuropsychiatric Manifestations**

| |
|---|
| **Stage I** |
| Mild confusion, decreased intellectual function; slowed mental processes. |
| Sleep disorder; tremor. |
| Personality changes (obtaining a thorough history is paramount to developing baseline data with which the patient's progress can be closely monitored and evaluated) |
| **Stage II** |
| Agitation and euphoria; more commonly, drowsiness. |
| Inappropriate behavior. |
| Slurred speech, incoordination. |
| Asterixis (flapping tremor), bilaterally. (To assess for *asterixis*, ask the patient to hold both arms and hands outstretched with fingers apart. If asterixis is present, a series of rapid, asynchronous forward movements of the hands will occur. Asterixis is not specific for hepatic failure, but may occur in the setting of altered metabolism due to a variety of insults.) |
| **Stage III** |
| Deep coma, unarousable, unresponsive to pain stimuli. |
| Decorticate or decerebrate posturing. |
| Hyperactive deep tendon reflexes. |
| Babinski's sign (bilaterally). |

Depending on the underlying disease process and its course, the neuropsychiatric manifestations of hepatic encephalopathy may dominate the patient's clinical picture.

## Treatment and Management of Hepatic Failure and Hepatic Encephalopathy

### *Goal of Treatment*

The liver has a remarkable capacity for regeneration. The patient who survives is likely to regain normal liver function. Because there is no specific therapy for patients with hepatic failure and hepatic encephalopathy, the major goal of treatment and management is to sustain life until sufficient liver regeneration occurs to restore some minimal level of function.

**Therapeutic Priorities.** Following ventilatory and hemodynamic stabilization, initial treatment is focused on identifying and treating the precipitating cause(s) of hepatic failure. This usually involves intervention to control gastrointestinal bleeding, discontinuing drug therapy especially sedatives and hypnotics (hepatotoxic), treating intercurrent infection to which these patients are especially prone (altered nutritional state, compromised immune system), reducing azotemia and serum ammonia levels, normalizing fluid/blood volume and electrolytes, and correcting acid-base imbalance. Efforts are directed toward preventing secondary complications involving other organ systems.

Specific therapeutic priorities include anti-ammonia regimen; fluid, electrolyte, and acid–base balance; prevention of hepatotoxicity; monitoring of neurologic function; prevention of hypoglycemia; prevention of bleeding diathesis; prevention of infection; and monitoring of renal function.[2] See Table 50–3 for details related to these therapeutic priorities.

Surgical interventions, short of liver transplantation, are, at best, palliative. There are no surgical measures available that can directly treat hepatocellular dysfunction. Peritoneovenous shunting procedures (LeVeen, Denver shunts) may be performed to decompress the portal system and reduce ascites, but they are not without risks or complications (gastrointestinal bleeding, hemodilution, congestive heart failure, wound infection, disseminated intravascular coagulation [DIC], and shunt failure).

Liver transplantation is an approach to treatment available in only a few select medical centers. In spite of recent breakthroughs in tissue matching and immunosuppressive drug therapy, major complications continue to be rejection reactions, infection, and cholestasis. One of every 5 recipients has a survival of 1 year.

## NURSING CARE OF THE PATIENT WITH HEPATIC FAILURE AND HEPATIC ENCEPHALOPATHY

Nursing care of the patient with hepatic failure and hepatic encephalopathy is especially challenging because the liver is involved in so many life-sustaining processes. Hepatic dysfunction affects every organ system in the body. It enacts changes in the patient's psychologic, physiologic, and emotional well-being.

Longstanding, slowly evolving liver disease, as occurs in cirrhosis, may reflect many years of established habits and behaviors (e.g., alcoholism, malnutrition, drug abuse), instrumental in the eventual demise of the patient's health status, and potential obstacles to the patient's full recovery. Acute fulminant hepatic failure (e.g., secondary to acute viral hepatitis) often reflects a sudden, rapidly progressing, frequently fatal illness, which afflicts unsuspecting, commonly young, healthy persons with previously normal liver function.

These clinical circumstances require that the critical care nurse have a keen understanding of basic physiologic and psychologic processes, and the pathophysiologic responses underlying liver disease. Knowing what to expect in hepatic dysfunction assists the nurse to assess the patient thoroughly, to identify actual and/or potential alterations in body processes, and to plan and implement timely and appropriate interventions.

TABLE 50–3
### Hepatic Failure and Hepatic Encephalopathy: Therapeutic Priorities

**Anti-Ammonia Regimen**

Specific therapy to reduce the production of ammonia may include:

1. Gastric decompression to remove blood and assess bleeding.
2. Administration of cathartics and enemas to evacuate blood from the gastrointestinal tract. Intestinal bacteria metabolize the protein in blood to ammonia, which is absorbed into the blood.
3. Administration of lactulose (cephulac) therapy. Lactulose is a synthetic disaccharide (galactose and glucose) that is not absorbed, but is metabolized (acidified) by intestinal bacteria to lactic and acetic acids. It reduces the pH of the intestinal milieu and facilitates the conversion of ammonia ($NH_3$) to ammonium ($NH_4^+$). As a charged ion, $NH_4^+$ is trapped within the bowel and eliminated during catharsis. This reduction in ammonia concentration within the gut allows more ammonia to diffuse from the blood into the gastrointestinal tract.

   Lactulose has a cathartic effect that speeds bowel evacuation; it also stimulates intestinal bacteria to take up ammonia and incorporate it into bacterial protein synthesis. Ideally, 2–3 bowel movements daily is the desired effect; overdosing with lactulose may precipitate diarrhea. When administering lactulose, it is important to monitor serum glucose levels and assess for signs of hyperglycemia. It should be used with caution in patients with diabetes mellitus.

   Major side effects of lactulose include abdominal distention, flatulence, cramping, and diarrhea. Lactulose is available for oral, nasogastric tube, or enema administration.
4. Administration of antibiotic therapy. Antibiotics reduce the intestinal bacterial flora, thereby reducing the number of colonic bacteria that normally convert urea and amino acids into ammonia and other toxic metabolites. The aminoglycoside neomycin is the most commonly used antibiotic, and it is capable of reaching high antibacterial concentrations in the colon without causing systemic toxicity. When treating hepatic encephalopathy, neomycin is given orally, or via nasogastric tube, with only 1–3% of the dose absorbed.

   In patients with renal insufficiency (hepatorenal syndrome), this small amount of neomycin will not be excreted, and will accumulate in the body leading to nephrotoxicity and ototoxicity. Neomycin should not be given with other aminoglycosides as the nephrotoxic and ototoxic effects may be potentiated. It should be used cautiously with furosemide. Lactulose and neomycin should not be used simultaneously. Lactulose requires bacteria for its action, while neomycin destroys the intestinal flora.
5. Restriction or elimination of protein intake; dietary protein may be the source of various harmful substances including ammonia, mercaptans, and amino acids. A reduction in protein intake diminishes a source of hepatotoxins.
6. Elimination of all nitrogen-containing drugs.
7. Administration of levodopa therapy to restore catecholamine neurotransmitters necessary for synaptic transmission.

**Fluid, Electrolyte, and Acid-Base Balance**

Fluid, electrolyte, and acid-base status must be closely monitored. In the setting of profuse upper gastrointestinal tract hemorrhage, with massive blood and fluid replacement therapy, hemodynamic pressure monitoring is indicated. Specific therapy may include:

1. Restriction of sodium and fluids when necessary to limit ascites. Hyperaldosteronism, which commonly occurs in hepatic failure, stimulates sodium reabsorption and contributes to fluid retention and hypokalemia.
2. Cautious administration of diuretics; close monitoring of serum potassium levels is essential. Administration of large volumes of stored blood, which is high in potassium, may predispose to potassium intoxication.

*(continued)*

TABLE 50–3
**Hepatic Failure and Hepatic Encephalopathy: Therapeutic Priorities *(Continued)***

**Fluid, Electrolyte, and Acid-Base Balance (cont.)**
3. Abdominal paracentesis, especially if respiratory effort is compromised. It is important to avoid tapping too much fluid too quickly as this could precipitate hemodynamic instability.

**Prevention of Hepatotoxicity**
To reduce the risk of hepatotoxicity, it is important to consider the following:
1. Avoid administration of sedatives and hypnotics because such drugs may enhance the progression of encephalopathy.
2. Review all drugs that the patient is taking to avoid inadvertent accumulation of drug due to altered liver metabolism, and to reduce the potential for adverse drug interactions.
3. Avoid administration of drugs via the intramuscular route because of increased risk of bleeding. Preferred parenteral routes include intravenous and subcutaneous routes.
4. Adjust drug dosage to assure desired effect and prevent toxicity.

**Monitoring of Neurological Function**
Ongoing assessment of neurological function is necessary to determine the stage of encephalopathy, and the patient's response to therapy.
1. In patients with cerebral edema who are at risk of brain herniation, intracranial pressure monitoring may be initiated; administration of osmotic diuretic (e.g., mannitol) may be indicated.
2. Ventilatory support may also be necessary as hypoxia will predispose to lactic acidosis and carbon dioxide retention. The consequent vasodilation of the cerebral vasculature and increased blood flow will further aggravate the status of intracranial pressure.
3. Parenteral thiamine may be prescribed in the presence of neurological dysfunction, especially that associated with Laennec's cirrhosis (alcoholism).

**Prevention of Hypoglycemia**
Hypoglycemia must be avoided as glucose is the primary fuel for brain cell metabolism.
1. Intravenous infusions of glucose 10% are commonly administered, with serum glucose levels monitored frequently.
2. A minimum of 1400 calories per day as carbohydrate should be administered. Glucose is both an energy source and a protein sparer.

**Prevention of Bleeding Diathesis**
Bleeding, when it occurs in the setting of hepatic failure, is commonly associated with bleeding esophageal and gastric varices, and erosive gastritis. It may occur in response to a deficiency in vitamin K, necessary for the synthesis of factors II, VII, IX, and X. It may also occur as a result of dilutional coagulopathy associated with massive administration of stored whole blood.
1. Monitor prothrombin and partial thromboplastin times frequently as they are good indicators of liver function.
2. Administer vitamin K therapy.
3. During massive stored whole blood replacement therapy, administer sufficient fresh frozen plasma to replace necessary clotting factors.
4. Administer intravenous cimetidine or ranitidine, and antacid (nasogastric tube) therapy prophylactically to maintain gastric pH > 4.5.

**Prevention of Infection**
Patients with hepatic failure are especially susceptible to infection.
1. Strict aseptic technique for pulmonary, invasive lines and catheter care.

TABLE 50–3
**Hepatic Failure and Hepatic Encephalopathy: Therapeutic Priorities *(Continued)***

2. Prompt vigorous search for infection, and initiation of aggressive therapy in the presence of fever or leukocytosis. (The patient in hepatic failure may experience leukocytosis in the absence of infection.)
3. Culture sputum, blood, urine, or wound drainage, as indicated.

**Monitoring of Renal Function**
Hepatorenal syndrome with decreased sodium and water excretion is a frequent complication of chronic hepatic failure.
1. Monitor for oliguria, urine sodium < 10 mEq/L, and azotemia in a volume-repleted patient.
2. Monitor fluid status (right atrial and pulmonary capillary wedge pressures).
3. Adjust sodium and fluid intake to match output.
4. Monitor BUN, creatinine, serum osmolality, and serum electrolytes at frequent intervals.

## Therapeutic Goals

The major therapeutic goal in the setting of liver disease is to assist, support, and sustain the patient and family through the acute phase of illness, and to prevent complications until sufficient liver regeneration has occurred to enable the patient to become self-sustaining. To accomplish this goal, a concerted effort is required to establish a trusting, working rapport with patient and family, and to initiate education activities directed toward promoting and facilitating their eventual rehabilitation.

Often the outcome of liver disease is not so positive. In the terminal stages of illness, the challenge to nursing is to provide support to family members, to assist them to express feelings and frustrations, to promote the grieving process, and to help identify resources to whom the family can turn in their hour of need.

Implementation of nursing process in the care of the patient with hepatic failure and hepatic encephalopathy revolves around the following therapeutic goals:

1. Establish a thorough comprehensive database including:
   A. Clinical history.
   B. Physical examination.
   C. Laboratory data.
2. Maintain fluid, electrolyte, and acid–base balance.
3. Assist in maintenance of effective alveolar ventilation.
4. Monitor cerebral and neurologic functions.
5. Initiate therapeutic activities to maintain serum ammonia levels within acceptable physiologic range.

(*text continues on page 1092*)

## TABLE 50–4. CARE PLAN FOR THE PATIENT WITH HEPATIC FAILURE AND HEPATIC ENCEPHALOPATHY

| Nursing Diagnoses | Desired Patient Outcomes | Nursing Interventions | Rationales |
|---|---|---|---|
| ***Nursing Diagnosis #1***<br>Fluid volume deficit (intravascular, actual), related to:<br>1. Ascites and anasarca ("third spacing").<br>A. Hypoalbuminemia.<br>B. Portal hypertension.<br>C. Hyperaldosteronism (secondary).<br>D. Capillary fragility/increased permeability.<br>2. Bleeding.<br>A. Bleeding varices (hematemesis).<br>B. Erosive gastritis.<br>C. Coagulopathy.<br>(For fluid volume deficit related to hypovolemic, hemorrhagic shock, see Table 49–6, Nursing Diagnosis #1.)<br>***Nursing Diagnosis #2***<br>Electrolyte balance, alteration in: hypokalemia, related to:<br>1. Diuretic therapy.<br>2. Hyperaldosteronism (sodium retention). | Patient will:<br>1. Maintain stable hemodynamics:<br>• Heart rate (resting) <100 beats/min.<br>• Central venous pressure 0–8 mmHg.<br>• Pulmonary artery pressure <25 mmHg.<br>• Pulmonary capillary wedge pressure 8–12 mmHg.<br>• Cardiac output ~5 liters/min.<br>• Systemic arterial blood pressure within 10 mmHg of baseline.<br>2. Maintain baseline mental and neurological status; deep tendon reflexes brisk.<br>3. Achieve resolution of ascites and anasarca.<br>• Body weight within 5% of baseline.<br>• Abdominal girth at baseline measurement.<br>• Functioning peritoneovenous shunt (if inserted).<br>4. Balance intake and output.<br>5. Maintain urine output >30 ml/hour.<br>6. Maintain laboratory parameter as follows:<br>• Serum osmolality 285–295 mOsm/Kg. | • Assess for signs and symptoms of hypovolemia:<br>◦ Assess cardiovascular function:<br>◦ Heart rate (resting). | • Establish baseline assessment data with which to evaluate the patient's response to therapy.<br>◦ An increase in heart rate reflects a compensatory response to maintain cardiac output. |
| | | ◦ Hypotension (orthostatic). | ◦ A decrease in blood pressure of >10–15 mmHg from a supine to sitting position reflects a reduced circulatory (intravascular) volume. |
| | | ◦ Skin color—pallor, mottled appearance; cyanosis; cool to touch; peripheral edema (anasarca). | ◦ Compensatory peripheral vasoconstriction shunts blood from skin and nonvital organs to the heart and brain. |
| | | ◦ Assess for ascites—abdominal assessment:<br>– Inspect for bulging of flanks or a protruding, misplaced umbilicus; skin tautness; new striae.<br>– Percuss for shifting dullness.<br>– Palpate for fluid wave. | ◦ Ascites results from a combination of low intravascular colloidal osmotic pressure (hypoalbuminemia), portal hypertension, overproduction of hepatic lymph, and secondary retention of sodium and water.<br>– When forces favoring movement of fluid from the intravascular space into the interstitium (portal hypetension) exceed forces favoring movement of fluid in the opposite direction (e.g., decreased intravascular colloidal osmotic pressure), fluid accumulates. When the capacity of the lymphatic system to return fluid to the circulating blood is exceeded, ascites results. Of central importance to the formation of ascites is renal sodium and water retention. |
| | | ◦ Measure abdominal girth daily using markings indicated on abdomen. | ◦ Measurement of abdominal girth assists in evaluating the status of the ascites. Markings made on the abdomen help to assure that repeated measurements are made at the same circumference; measure with patient in same position. Clinical findings of ascites are usually demonstrable after >1500 ml of ascites fluid has accumulated. |
| | | ◦ Determine body weight. | ◦ Daily measurement of body weight most closely reflects total body fluid volume. |

*(continued)*

**TABLE 50-4. CARE PLAN FOR THE PATIENT WITH HEPATIC FAILURE AND HEPATIC ENCEPHALOPATHY *(Continued)***

| Nursing Diagnoses | Desired Patient Outcomes | Nursing Interventions | Rationales |
|---|---|---|---|
| ***Nursing Diagnosis #2 (cont.)*** | • Serum sodium >135 and <148 mEq/liter.<br>• Serum potassium 3.5–5.5 mEq/liter.<br>• Serum albumin 3.5–5.5 g/100 ml.<br>• Hematocrit 37–52%.<br>• Hemoglobin 12–18 g/100 ml.<br>• RBC count >4.7–5.9 million/mm³.<br>• Platelet count >150,000 mm³. | ◦ Assess serum albumin levels. | ◦ Serum albumin is largely responsible for maintaining serum colloidal osmotic pressure. |
| | | ◦ Cardiac monitoring. | ◦ Cardiac dysrhythmias may occur in response to ischemia or electrolyte imbalance. |
| | | ◦ Hemodynamic pressure monitoring parameters: Central venous pressure; pulmonary artery pressure; pulmonary capillary wedge pressure; cardiac output; arterial pressure monitoring. | ◦ Monitoring of these parameters is indicated in the setting of hypovolemic shock, hemodynamic instability, and during massive fluid, albumin, and blood replacement, to monitor patient's response to therapy and prevent fluid overload. |
| | | ◦ Assess neurological function: Mental status, orientation; thought processes; motor responses; deep tendon reflexes. | ◦ See Nursing Diagnosis #7, Thought processes, alteration in (below). |
| | | ◦ Assess renal function: Intake and output; hourly urine output; monitor creatinine and BUN. | ◦ Hypovolemia can cause a decrease in renal perfusion; patients with hepatic failure are at risk of developing hepatorenal failure. Renal function is best monitored by serum creatinine; BUN may be altered by G.I. bleeding and impaired liver function. |
| | | ◦ Assess for signs and symptoms of electrolyte imbalance: Hypokalemia—general malaise, fatigue, anorexia, nausea, vomiting, diarrhea; abdominal cramps; muscle weakness; hyporeflexia; cardiac dysrhythmias.<br>◦ Monitor serum electrolytes. | ◦ Excessive sodium reabsorption and retention associated with increased aldosterone secretion, and diuretic therapy, can predispose to hypokalemia and metabolic alkalemia. |
| | | • Implement prescribed measures to reestablish normovolemia: | • Therapeutic goal is to gradually mobilize fluid back into the intravascular compartment and prevent further third-spacing. |
| | | ◦ Maintain fluid restriction (~1000–1500 ml/day). | ◦ To decrease ascites and generalized edema. |
| | | ◦ Maintain sodium restriction (200–500 mg/day).<br>– Avoid use of saline for intravenous therapy, gastric lavage, or other irrigation. | ◦ To reduce fluid retention as ascites and anasarca, and enhance mobilization of excessive fluids from the tissues. |
| | | ◦ Administer diuretic therapy with necessary potassium replacement therapy. | ◦ Controlled diuresis decreases water load with consequent reduction in ascites and edema; it minimizes the risk of renal failure. |

| | |
|---|---|
| ◦ Furosemide, thiazide diuretics. | ◦ Require monitoring of serum potassium with concomitant potassium replacement therapy. |
| ◦ Spironolactone therapy. | ◦ A potassium-sparing diuretic, it inhibits the action of aldosterone on the distal tubular cells, thereby increasing excretion of sodium, chloride and water, while retaining potassium. |
| ◦ Administer inotropic agents and vasopressors (e.g., low-dose dopamine). | ◦ To increase cardiac ouput and maintain effective renal perfusion. |
| ◦ Administer protein supplementation. | ◦ To restore intravascular colloidal osmotic pressure to within acceptable physiological range; and enhance movement of ascitic and edema fluid into the intravascular space, promoting diuresis. |
| ◦ Administer salt-poor albumin intravenously. | ◦ Replaces albumin levels, restores intravascular volume and maintains renal perfusion. Monitor for fluid overload. |
| • Assist with abdominal paracentesis:<br>◦ Key nursing considerations: | • In patients with severe ascites, paracentesis may be necessary to relieve dyspnea and compromised respiratory excursion, and/or urinary frequency. |
| ◦ Have patient urinate prior to procedure. | ◦ Reduces risk of nicking bladder with needle. |
| ◦ Provide necessary explanations.<br>– Position appropriately and as comfortably as possible. | ◦ May help patient to relax. |
| ◦ Note that fluid removal should not exceed 1 – 1.5 liters.<br>– Removal of fluid should be done slowly. | ◦ Sufficient quantity of fluid is removed to decrease intra-abdominal pressure; altered hemodynamics including hypotension and shock can be precipitated by the removal of too large a volume of fluid. |
| ◦ Monitor vital signs pre-, peri- and post-paracentesis. | ◦ Assists in assessing possible intra-abdominal bleeding. |
| ◦ Measure abdominal girth pre- and post-paracentesis, and daily thereafter.<br>– Assess insertion site; monitor for complications of hypotension, bleeding, protein depletion, and infection. | ◦ Assists in assessing for further fluid accumulation. |
| • Implement ongoing monitoring: | • Assists in evaluating the patient's response to therapy; reduces risk of complications. |
| ◦ Cardiovascular status:<br>– Monitor heart rate, pulses, blood pressure, hemodynamic parameters. | ◦ Patients with cirrhosis, ascites and bleeding potential are at high risk of complications. |

## TABLE 50–4. CARE PLAN FOR THE PATIENT WITH HEPATIC FAILURE AND HEPATIC ENCEPHALOPATHY *(Continued)*

| Nursing Diagnoses | Desired Patient Outcomes | Nursing Interventions | Rationales |
|---|---|---|---|
| ***Nursing Diagnosis #2 (cont.)*** | | | |
| | | ○ Respiratory status:<br>○ Monitor respiratory rate and pattern; respiratory excursion, breath sounds (normal and adventitious). | ○ Respiratory embarrassment caused by ascites can lead to pulmonary complications; e.g., compromised alveolar ventilation with $CO_2$ retention ($CO_2$ narcosis may complicate the clinical presentation of hepatic encephalopathy); and pneumonia. |
| | | ○ Monitor arterial blood gases. | ○ Assists in evaluating effectiveness of ventilation; and acid-base balance. |
| | | ○ Renal status: Assess urine output (hourly); BUN, creatinine.<br>○ Assess fluid and electrolyte status: Accurate intake and output; daily weight; daily measurement of abdominal girth.<br>○ Serum studies: Electrolytes; protein (albumin/globulin ratio); osmolality, glucose.<br>○ Urine studies: Electrolytes, specific gravity. | ○ Assists in evaluating the patient's response to therapy. |
| | | • Assist in preparation of patient for peritoneovenous shunt (e.g., LeVeen and Denver shunts):<br>○ Monitor for effectiveness of shunt post-surgery.<br>○ Maintain bed rest as indicated.<br>○ Enhance flow through shunt using abdominal binder and teaching patient to perform breathing exercises.<br>○ Monitor for complications: hemodilution; congestive heart failure; gastrointestinal bleeding; leakage of ascitic fluid from incision site; infection, sepsis, coagulopathy (DIC); shunt occlusion/malfunction. | • This procedure may be indicated for the treatment of intractable ascites. It allows ascitic fluid to flow from the peritoneal cavity through a catheter tunneled under subcutaneous tissues, into the jugular vein or superior vena cava. The patient's own breathing triggers the shunt: On inspiration, the diaphragm descends, increasing intra-abdominal pressure while reducing intrathoracic pressures. This difference in pressures allows the fluid to flow from the peritoneal cavity into the thoracic veins. |

| | | | |
|---|---|---|---|
| ***Nursing Diagnosis #3***<br>Breathing pattern, ineffective, related to:<br>1. Ascites (abdominal distention).<br>2. Weakened, debilitated state. | Patient will:<br>1. Maintain baseline mental status.<br>2. Maintain effective respiratory function:<br>• Respiratory rate <25–30/min.<br>• Tidal volume ($V_T$) >5–7 ml/Kg.<br>• Vital capacity ($V_C$) >12–15 ml/Kg. | • Assess respiratory function: Assess specific parameters—rate, pattern, depth of breathing; symmetry of chest wall and diaphragmatic excursion.<br>○ Assess use of accessory muscles; breath sounds, evidence of adventitious sounds (rales, wheezes); dyspnea, tachypnea, orthopnea.<br>○ Assess effectiveness of cough; sputum production. | • Ascites causes pressure on diaphragm, limiting respiratory excursion and contributing to decreased alveolar ventilation, and atelectasis. The end result is hypoxemia.<br>○ Weakened, debilitated status may compromise patient's respiratory effort, reducing alveolar ventilation and predisposing to hypoxemia.<br>○ Accumulation of fluids and secretions reduces ventilation and predisposes to infection. |
| | | ○ Assess pulmonary volume/capacity: tidal volume ($V_T$); vital capacity ($V_C$).<br>○ Monitor arterial blood gases: $PaO_2$, $PaCO_2$ pH | ○ Reflect effectiveness of ventilation and gas exchange. |
| | | • Assess tissue perfusion and oxygenation.<br>○ Assess cerebral function: mental status—restlessness, apprehension, confusion; drowsiness.<br>○ Assess cardiovascular function: evidence of cyanosis—lips, mucous membranes, nailbeds; vital signs: heart rate, blood pressure, peripheral pulses, cardiac dysrhythmias.<br>○ Assess fluid status: intake and output; body weight.<br>○ Laboratory data: hematocrit, hemoglobin, serum electrolytes; BUN; serum osmolality. | • These signs and symptoms may be reflective of hypoxemia and tissue hypoxia. |
| | | • Assist patient to semi-Fowler's position. | • This position allows for maximal respiratory excursion and lung expansion. Adequate lung expansion facilitates more even distribution of ventilation; it enhances ventilation/perfusion matching. |
| ***Nursing Diagnosis #4***<br>Airway clearance, ineffective, related to:<br>1. Compromised cough reflex.<br>2. Immobility, with decreased mobilization of secretions. | Patient will:<br>1. Verbalize ease of breathing.<br>• Breath sounds audible throughout anterior and posterior chest.<br>• Reduced to absent adventitious sounds.<br>2. Maintain arterial gases:<br>• pH 7.35–7.45. | • Monitor quality, quantity, color, odor, consistency of sputum.<br>○ Obtain sputum for culture as indicated.<br>○ Assess secretions for state of hydration. | ○ Maintaining hydration keeps secretions thin and easily mobilized. |
| | | ○ Monitor body temperature, sputum production, and white blood count profile.<br>○ Obtain baseline cultures: sputum, urine, blood, wounds, IV sites when changed. | ○ Early detection of an infectious or inflammatory process affords prompt intervention to minimize the effect of the insult on pulmonary and other organ functions. |

*(continued)*

**TABLE 50–4. CARE PLAN FOR THE PATIENT WITH HEPATIC FAILURE AND HEPATIC ENCEPHALOPATHY *(Continued)***

| Nursing Diagnoses | Desired Patient Outcomes | Nursing Interventions | Rationales |
|---|---|---|---|
| ***Nursing Diagnosis #4 (cont.)*** | • $PaO_2 > 60$ mmHg.<br>• $PaCO_2$ 35–45 mmHg. | • Initiate chest physiotherapy—bronchial hygiene (as appropriate).<br>○ Encourage coughing and deep breathing; use incentive spirometry if appropriate.<br>○ Turn and position every 2 hr.<br>– Position so as to minimize risk of aspiration, especially in lethargic or semi-comatose patient.<br>○ Provide necessary pharyngeal and tracheal suctioning if patient is unable to handle pulmonary secretions.<br>• Consider endotracheal intubation and mechanical ventilation in the following settings:<br>○ Hypoxemia: $PaO_2 < 60$ mmHg on $FIO_2 > 40\%$.<br>○ Cerebral edema, as a complication of fulminant hepatic failure.<br>○ High risk of aspiration (e.g., patient unable to handle secretions; absent or compromised gag reflex).<br>• Administer prescribed oxygen therapy.<br>○ Humidify inspired oxygen.<br>• Maintain hydrated state.<br>○ Monitor intake and output; weigh daily. | • These activities help to loosen and dislodge secretions and facilitate movement toward trachea, from where they are accessible to removal via cough and/or suctioning.<br>○ Turning and deep breathing assist to mobilize secretions, enhance ventilation and prevent areas of atelectasis.<br>○ See Unit V, Respiratory System, for procedures related to incentive spirometry and suctioning (Tables 32–2, 32–3, and 32–4).<br>○ Tissue hypoxia predisposes to lactic acidosis.<br>○ Carbon dioxide retention ($PaCO_2 > 45$ mmHg) may precipitate cerebral vasodilation and aggravate existing cerebral edema.<br>• Assists in relieving hypoxemia.<br>○ Humidification liquefies secretions.<br>• Adequate hydration moistens, loosens, and liquefies secretions. |
| ***Nursing Diagnosis #5***<br>Potential for infection: pneumonia, related to:<br>1. Prolonged immobility.<br>2. Compromised cough reflex.<br>3. Compromised immune response.<br>(See Table 49–7, Potential for Infection.) | Patient will:<br>1. Remain without signs/symptoms of pulmonary infection:<br>• Body temperature 98.6°F.<br>• WBC at baseline.<br>• Lungs resonant to percussion.<br>• Vesicular breath sounds over peripheral lung fields.<br>2. Demonstrate effective cough | • Monitor patient's environment for potential sources of infection:<br>○ Visitors, staff, other patients.<br>• Administer prescribed antibiotic therapy:<br>○ Obtain necessary cultures prior to initiation of antibiotic therapy. | • Depression of immune response associated with liver disease places patient at increased risk of infection. |

| | | | |
|---|---|---|---|
| ***Nursing Diagnosis #6***<br>Acid-base balance, alteration in: metabolic alkalemia, related to:<br>1. Hypokalemia.<br>2. Diuretic therapy.<br>3. Nausea/vomiting or continuous nasogastric decompression (suctioning).<br>4. Secondary hyperaldosteronism.<br>5. Poor nutrition. | Patient will:<br>1. Maintain serum electrolyte levels:<br>• Sodium $>135 <148$ mEq/liter.<br>• Potassium 3.5–5.5 mEq/liter.<br>• Chloride 100–106 mEq/liter.<br>2. Maintain serum pH 7.35–7.45 (arterial blood gas).<br>3. Maintain serum ammonia within acceptable physiological range: 80–110 $\mu$g/100 ml. | • Monitor laboratory data:<br>∘ Serum electrolytes.<br>– Sodium, potassium, chloride.<br>∘ Arterial blood gas—pH.<br>∘ Serum ammonia levels.<br>∘ Blood urea nitrogen.<br>• Administer prescribed potassium replacement therapy.<br>• Administer spironolactone therapy.<br>• Titrate dietary protein intake. | • Patients with cirrhosis have depleted stores of potassium related to nausea, vomiting, poor nutrition, diuretic usage, and secondary hyperaldosteronism. Hypokalemia contributes to metabolic alkalemia.<br>∘ Alkalemia shifts the ammonia-ammonium ion dissociation equilibrium in favor of ammonia:<br>$NH_3 + H^+ \leftarrow NH_4^+$ ($\uparrow$pH)<br>∘ Ammonia easily crosses blood-brain barrier; high ammonia levels in the setting of liver disease are associated with hepatic encephalopathy (see Nursing Diagnosis #7 below).<br>∘ It is necessary to titrate patient's protein intake so as to keep serum ammonia and BUN at acceptable levels.<br>∘ In hepatic failure the liver is unable to convert ammonia, a by-product of protein metabolism, to urea for elimination.<br>• Use of furosemide and thiazide diuretics should be accompanied by potassium therapy.<br>• This drug is a potassium-sparing diuretic.<br>• Excess dietary protein is an excellent substrate for the generation of $NH_3$. |
| ***Nursing Diagnosis #7***<br>Thought process, alteration in, related to:<br>1. Hepatic encephalopathy associated with high serum ammonia levels caused by the inability of the liver to convert ammonia to urea. | Patient will:<br>1. Maintain baseline mental status:<br>• Level of consciousness: Arousable; oriented to person, place, time.<br>• Mentation: Memory intact; able to concentrate; performs simple calculations; demonstrates abstract reasoning.<br>• Usual personality.<br>• Appropriate behavior. | • Assess for signs and symptoms of hepatic encephalopathy (See Table 50–2):<br>∘ Mental status: level of consciousness; arousable; comatose.<br>∘ Mentation: Memory lapses, shortened attention span; confusion; ability to perform simple calculations; abstract reasoning.<br>∘ Behavior: Appropriate or inappropriate.<br>– Agitation, combativeness; incoherent; drowsiness, lethargy.<br>∘ Personality changes. | • Signs and symptoms of hepatic encephalopathy are categorized into stages; familiarity with the stages of hepatic coma assists in bedside assessment, and in evaluation of response to therapy.<br>• Establishing a baseline and ongoing monitoring is essential to determine the clinical course and the patient's response to therapy.<br>∘ Family and friends may assist in establishing baseline data. |

(continued)

**TABLE 50–4. CARE PLAN FOR THE PATIENT WITH HEPATIC FAILURE AND HEPATIC ENCEPHALOPATHY *(Continued)***

| Nursing Diagnoses | Desired Patient Outcomes | Nursing Interventions | Rationales |
|---|---|---|---|
| ***Nursing Diagnosis #7 (cont.)*** | | | |
| | 2. Maintain baseline neurological function:<br>• Able to write name and draw simple figures/numbers.<br>• Speech intact, without slurring.<br>• Absence of asterixis; deep tendon reflexes brisk.<br>• Without seizure activity. | ○ Neurological status: Status of speech—evidence of slurring; asterixis; tremors; deep coma—unarousable, unresponsive to painful stimuli; pupillary responses, oculocephalic reflexes, decorticate/decerebrate posturing; hyperactive deep tendon reflexes, bilateral Babinski sign. | ○ (See Chapter 7 for essentials of the neurological assessment.) |
| | | ○ Electroencephalogram (EEG). | ○ There is a characteristic but not pathogenic slowing of EEG. These changes may precede clinical deterioration, but are not usually present early in the course. |
| | 3. Maintain serum ammonia levels within acceptable range. | • Monitor serum ammonia levels. | • Increase in circulating serum ammonia levels predisposes to hepatic encephalopathy as ammonia is toxic to cerebral tissues. However, hepatic encephalopathy can occur in the absence of elevated ammonia levels, and mechanisms of toxicity remain undefined.<br>○ Possible toxic effects of ammonia on cerebral tissues include: Alteration in cerebral energy metabolism; disruption of resting membrane potentials; and altered neurotransmission. |
| | | • Implement anti-ammonia regimen:<br>○ Initiate and/or assist with measures to prevent or control bleeding. | • (Refer to Table 50–3, Therapeutic Priorities.)<br>○ Blood in the gastrointestinal tract is metabolized by intestinal bacteria with the production of ammonia. In liver disease, with intrahepatic and portal hypertension, ammonia absorbed from gut bypasses liver and enters the systemic circulation. Ammonia easily traverses the blood-brain barrier. |
| | | ○ Initiate gastric decompression with iced gastric lavage (as prescribed). | ○ Evacuates blood and allows assessment of the extent of bleeding. |
| | | ○ Assist with insertion of Sengstaken-Blakemore tube. | ○ Inserted to control esophageal and variceal bleeding. (See Table 49–5 for nursing care considerations.) |
| | | ○ Assist with selective angiography with continuous vasopressin (pitressin) infusion (as prescribed). | |

| | |
|---|---|
| ◦ Assist with sclerotherapy. | ◦ This therapy may be prescribed for patients with uncontrollable bleeding who are poor surgical risks. |
| ◦ Initiate prescribed therapy to reduce gastric acidity:<br>– Combination of parenteral ranitidine or cimetidine (histamine$_2$ antagonists) and antacid therapy via nasogastric tube. | ◦ Gastric acidity plays a key role in the pathogenesis of upper gastrointestinal bleeding. |
| ◦ Serial monitoring of gastric pH. | ◦ Ideally gastric pH should be maintained at >4.5. |
| ◦ Cautiously administer blood replacement therapy: Packed RBCs should be administered in conjunction with massive blood replacement with stored whole blood.<br>– Monitor hematology profile, prothrombin time, clotting factors. | ◦ Stored whole blood is deficient in some clotting factors and can predispose to dilutional coagulopathy (See Tables 49–2, 49–3, and 49–4). |
| ◦ Implement nursing measures to prevent/control bleeding. | ◦ See Nursing Diagnosis #10, Injury, potential for: bleeding diathesis (below). |
| • Initiate lactulose (cephulic) therapy.<br>◦ Initial dosage: 30–45 ml/hourly (orally or via nasogastric tube) until first bowel movement.<br>◦ Maintenance dose: 30–45 ml 3–4 times daily. Overdose can cause diarrhea. | • Lactulose, in conjunction with the action of intestinal bacteria, creates an acidic milieu within the colon that favors conversion of ammonia to ammonium, which is speedily evacuated by the cathartic action of lactulose.<br>$NH_3 + H^+ \xrightarrow{\downarrow pH} NH_4^+$ |
| ◦ Monitor serial serum glucose. | ◦ Lactulose contains galactose and glucose; it may elevate glucose levels; use with caution with diabetes; contraindicated in patients requiring a low-galactose diet. |
| • Initiate antibiotic therapy:<br>◦ Aminoglycosides used: Neomycin (most commonly) and Kanamycin. | • Antibiotics reduce intestinal bacterial flora, thereby reducing bacterial ammonia production. Note: Lactulose and neomycin should not be administered concurrently. Lactulose requires bacteria for its action; neomycin destroys intestinal bacteria flora. |
| ◦ Avoid use with other aminoglycosides, or other nephrotoxic or ototoxic drugs. | ◦ The nephrotoxic and ototoxic effects may be potentiated. |
| ◦ Contraindicated in the setting or renal insufficiency and hepatorenal failure. | ◦ Approximately 1–3% of drug is absorbed; in the presence of renal failure, the drug can accumulate, predisposing to nephrotoxicity and ototoxicity. |
| ◦ Monitor renal function: BUN, creatinine, urine output (hourly); intake and output. | |
| • Avoid constipation.<br>◦ Lactulose is a good cathartic. | • Intestinal bacteria have a longer exposure and greater bulk to convert to ammonia. |

*(continued)*

**TABLE 50-4. CARE PLAN FOR THE PATIENT WITH HEPATIC FAILURE AND HEPATIC ENCEPHALOPATHY *(Continued)***

| Nursing Diagnoses | Desired Patient Outcomes | Nursing Interventions | Rationales |
|---|---|---|---|
| ***Nursing Diagnosis #7 (cont.)*** | | | |
| | | ○ Administer stool softeners as prescribed. | |
| | | • Restrict or eliminate protein dietary intake. | • To reduce ammonia production and consequent increase in serum ammonia levels. |
| | | ○ Administer high carbohydrate diet (~1400 calories); or intravenous infusion of 10% glucose. | ○ Glucose provides the primary source of energy for cerebral tissues; prevents gluconeogenesis (protein catabolism). |
| | | ○ Provide potassium supplements.<br>– Cautious use of diuretic therapy. | ○ Hypokalemia predisposes to metabolic alkalemia which favors the conversion of ammonium to ammonia.<br>$NH_3 + H^+ \leftarrow NH_4^+$<br>$\downarrow K^+$ |
| | | ○ Maintain fluid and electrolyte balance. | ○ Refer to Nursing Diagnosis #1 above. |
| | | • Prevent hepatotoxicity:<br>○ Avoid use of sedatives, hypnotics and other drugs normally metabolized by the liver, or containing ammonia. | • Compromised hepatocellular function may cause accumulation of drug; some drugs may be toxic to the liver. Such drugs, or combination of drugs, may precipitate or aggravate encephalopathy or mask signs of developing coma. |
| | | ○ Review patient's entire drug regimen:<br>– Dosage may need to be revised in presence of hepatocellular failure.<br>– Potential for adverse drug reactions and toxicity should be monitored.<br>– Assess effect of newly prescribed drugs on neurological function. | |
| | | • Implement nursing interventions in caring for the patient with hepatic encephalopathy:<br>○ Monitor neurologic function hourly (if in coma).<br>○ Monitor serial laboratory studies: Serum ammonia; BUN, creatinine, electrolytes. | ○ Specific parameters are listed under Nursing Interventions at the beginning of Nursing Diagnosis #7, in the section on assessing for signs and symptoms of hepatic encephalopathy, neurological status. |
| | | • Implement specific measures:<br>○ Maintain safe environment: Remove hazardous objects from bedside; use padded rails; keep rails in up position; provide close supervision; initiate seizure precautions.<br>○ Reorient patient to person, place, time.<br>○ Explain procedures clearly. | ○ A confused, agitated, or unreliable patient is at greater risk of injury (e.g., falling out of bed). |

| | | | |
|---|---|---|---|
| | | ∘ Obtain feedback from family and friends regarding mental status, personality and behavior. | |
| | | ∘ Plan for same staff members to care for the patient (if possible). | ∘ This affords continuity of care, and facilitates very close monitoring of the patient's response to therapy. |
| | | ∘ Provide comfort measures: Oral hygiene, back care, gentle passive range of motion exercises. | ∘ Relaxes tired muscles; a caring touch may help to relieve anxiety and apprehension. |
| | | ∘ Plan for undisturbed rest periods.<br>∘ Use calm, reassuring approach: Anticipate patient/family needs for support; be accessible; offer directions and explanations; allow patient/family to verbalize fears and concerns. | ∘ All efforts should be directed toward keeping the patient relaxed and quiet to prevent bleeding or rebleeding. |
| | | ∘ Involve patient/family in decision-making process regarding care when possible. | ∘ Enables patient/family to assume some control and responsibility for their well-being. |
| ***Nursing Diagnosis #8***<br>Nutrition, alteration in, less than body requirements, related to:<br>1. Malnutrition associated with insufficient dietary protein intake.<br>2. Avitaminosis associated with impaired absorption of fat-soluble vitamins.<br>3. Vitamin $B_{12}$ deficiency associated with liver disease.<br>4. Anorexia, nausea/vomiting, weakness and fatigue associated with elevated serum ammonia levels.<br>(See Chapter 53, Nutritional Support of the Critically Ill Patient) | Patient will:<br>1. Maintain stable body weight within 5% of baseline.<br>2. Maintain the following laboratory parameters within acceptable physiologic range:<br>• Total serum protein; serum albumin.<br>• Serum ammonia levels.<br>• Serum cholesterol; fasting serum glucose.<br>• Hematology profile.<br>• Vitamin $B_{12}$, folate.<br>• Transferrin levels.<br>3. Verbalize an increase in strength and improved appetite. | • Collaborate with nutritionist to perform comprehensive nutritional assessment.<br>∘ Assess the following parameters: Total serum protein; serum albumin; fasting serum glucose; serum cholesterol; hematology profile, vitamin $B_{12}$, folate; transferrin levels; body weight (dry), height; skinfold measurements.<br>∘ Assess for anorexia, nausea, vomiting, diarrhea, dyspepsia. | • Assists in determining basic caloric requirements sufficient to meet the energy needs of the body, while limiting protein to that amount which the liver can effectively metabolize. (See Chapter 53, Tables 53–1 through 53–8.) |
| | | • Implement nutritional plan:<br>∘ Acute phase (hepatic encephalopathy) dietary requirements include:<br>– Restriction of protein, sodium and fluid.<br>∘ Protein 20 to 60 gm/day. | • Goal of diet therapy is to reduce dietary protein so that a minimum of protein will remain in the gastrointestinal tract for conversion to ammonia.<br>∘ The degree of protein restriction will depend upon patient's level of consciousness and clinical status.<br>– Except in advanced coma, it is seldom necessary to reduce daily protein intake to less than 20 gm. Further reduction of protein offers little benefit because of consequent catabolism of endogenous proteins. |
| | | ∘ Sodium 250 to 500 gm/day. | ∘ Sodium restriction is necessary because of sodium and water retention associated with secondary hyperaldosteronism. |
| | | ∘ Fluids ~1000 ml/day. | ∘ Degree of fluid restriction depends on degree of third-spacing (ascites and anasarca). |

(continued)

TABLE 50-4. CARE PLAN FOR THE PATIENT WITH HEPATIC FAILURE AND HEPATIC ENCEPHALOPATHY *(Continued)*

| Nursing Diagnoses | Desired Patient Outcomes | Nursing Interventions | Rationales |
|---|---|---|---|
| ***Nursing Diagnosis #8 (cont.)*** | | | |
| | | ◦ High carbohydrate intake. (See Tables 53-9 and 53-10). | ◦ Glucose prevents hypoglycemia and breakdown of energy reserves. |
| | | ◦ Vitamin supplementation:<br>◦ Fat-soluble vitamins: A, D, E, and K. | ◦ Hepatocellular dysfunction alters bilirubin metabolism and bile synthesis; inadequate bile secretion impairs absorption of fat, and fat-soluble vitamins. |
| | | ◦ Folate $B_9$ (parenterally). | ◦ Hepatic stores depleted in liver disease. |
| | | ◦ Vitamin $B_{12}$ (parenterally).<br>– Thiamine (vitamin $B_1$) (parenterally). | ◦ Used to correct anorexia, and neuritis associated with alcoholism (Wernicke-Korsakoff's syndrome). |
| | | ◦ Minerals and trace elements supplementation (refer to Table 53-13). | |
| | | ◦ Methods of dietary intake:<br>◦ Oral: Provide mouth care; pleasant environment; assist to comfortable position.<br>– Minimize nausea/vomiting; eliminate noxious stimuli. | |
| | | ◦ Offer frequent smaller meals; avoid fatigue; plan rest period prior to mealtime.<br>– Consider patient's preference for food choices.<br>– Encourage visit by family at mealtimes if patient desires. | ◦ Large meals may precipitate nausea. |
| | | ◦ Enteral feedings. (Refer to appropriate sections in Chapter 53 for specific details regarding enteral feedings.) | ◦ Enteral approach to feeding may be necessary for patients unable to ingest food normally; bleeding varices necessitate enteral feedings. |
| | | ◦ Assess gag reflex prior to feeding.<br>– Confirm tube placement in stomach prior to feeding.<br>– Assess for signs of gastrointestinal intolerance of feeding (e.g., nausea, vomiting, abdominal distention, hyperactive bowel sounds). | ◦ To avoid pulmonary aspiration. (See Table 53-18 for complications of enteral feedings.) |
| | | ◦ Total parenteral nutrition.<br>– Provides for nutritional needs including: Hypertonic glucose. | ◦ If adequate intake of nutrients is impossible via oral or enteral feedings, total parenteral nutrition may be indicated. |

| | | | |
|---|---|---|---|
| | | ◦ Amino acids; high concentration branched-chain amino acids; low concentration aromatic amino acids.<br>– Electrolytes; minerals, vitamins, trace elements; lipid therapy (when indicated).<br>◦ Document: Type of feeding, amount; how tolerated by patient; adverse effects, if any.<br>◦ Monitor: Weight, intake and output; laboratory data (see "Assess the following parameters" under Nursing Interventions at the beginning of Nursing Diagnosis #8). | ◦ Amino acid imbalance may predispose to synthesis of false neurotransmitters that may be responsible for neurologic changes seen in hepatic encephalopathy. Aromatic amino acids are precursors to false neurotransmitters (e.g., octopamine).<br>◦ (See Table 53–25 for complications of parenteral therapy.) |
| ***Nursing Diagnosis #9***<br>Tissue perfusion, alteration in, hepatorenal syndrome, related to:<br>1. Hypovolemia associated with ascites (third-spacing).<br>2. Renal arteriolar vasoconstriction. | Patient will:<br>1. Maintain adequate hemodynamics:<br>• Systemic arterial blood pressure within 10 mmHg of baseline.<br>2. Maintain adequate renal function:<br>• Urine output $>30$ ml/hour.<br>• Urine specific gravity: 1.010–1.025<br>• BUN, serum creatinine, urinary sodium within acceptable range.<br>3. Maintain body weight within 5% of baseline. | • Assess for signs and symptoms of hepatorenal syndrome:<br>◦ Specific features: Oliguria (urine output $<30$ ml/hr); azotemia; specific gravity $>1.015$; low urinary sodium; increasing ascites; peripheral edema; weight gain; rising BUN, serum creatinine; hyperphosphatemia; hyperkalemia.<br>• Implement prescribed measures to reestablish normovolemia:<br>◦ Specific measures: Restrict fluids and sodium; administer prescribed diuretic therapy and potassium replacement therapy; administer inotropic agent/vasopressor (e.g., low-dose dopamine); administer protein supplementation.<br>◦ Assist with abdominal paracentesis (if indicated).<br>• Monitor patient's response to therapy.<br>• Prepare for dialysis if indicated. | • Hepatorenal syndrome describes development of progressive functional renal failure in the setting of advanced liver disease.<br>• (See "Therapeutic goal . . ." under Rationales column—second major rationale under Nursing Diagnoses #1 and #2.)<br>◦ (See "In patients with severe ascites . . ." under Rationales column—third major rationale under Nursing Diagnoses #1 and #2.) |
| ***Nursing Diagnosis #10***<br>Injury, potential for, bleeding diathesis, related to:<br>1. Massive blood transfusion for treatment of bleeding varices (dilutional coagulopathy). | Patient will:<br>1. Maintain stable vital signs:<br>• Systemic arterial pressure within 10 mmHg of baseline. | • Assess for signs/symptoms of bleeding:<br>◦ Vital signs: Blood pressure (orthostatic), heart rate, peripheral pulses; respiratory rate. | • Increased risk of bleeding in hepatic failure is associated with reduced hepatocellular synthesis of clotting factors (including vitamin K-dependent factors II, VII, IX, X) and reduced inactivation of activated clotting factors. |

*(continued)*

**TABLE 50–4. CARE PLAN FOR THE PATIENT WITH HEPATIC FAILURE AND HEPATIC ENCEPHALOPATHY *(Continued)***

| Nursing Diagnoses | Desired Patient Outcomes | Nursing Interventions | Rationales |
|---|---|---|---|
| ***Nursing Diagnosis #10 (cont.)*** | | | |
| 2. Decreased synthesis of clotting factors related to impaired hepatocellular function, and impaired vitamin K absorption.<br>3. Thrombocytopenia associated with splenomegaly (portal hypertension). | • Heart rate (resting) <100 beats/min.<br>• Respiratory rate <25–30/min.<br>2. Maintain baseline mental status:<br>• Level of consciousness; mentation intact.<br>3. Maintain stable hematologic profile:<br>• Hematocrit; hemoglobin, platelets.<br>4. Maintain stable coagulation profile.<br>5. Remain without signs of bleeding:<br>• No petechiae, ecchymosis.<br>• No hematuria; no occult blood in stool, vomitus, gastric drainage.<br>• No unusual joint pain/swelling.<br>6. Maintain stable abdominal girth. | ◦ Physical signs: Petechiae, ecchymosis; gingival bleeding; epistaxis; hematemesis, melena, hematochezia; expanding abdominal girth; unusual joint swelling; hematuria; oozing from wounds, venipuncture and invasive sites.<br>◦ Neurological signs: Headache, dizziness, confusion, lethargy; deep tendon reflexes.<br>◦ Hematologic profile: Hematocrit, hemoglobin, platelet count.<br>◦ Coagulation profile: Prothrombin time; activated partial thromboplastin time; platelet count; bleeding time. | ◦ In the setting of profuse bleeding with massive blood transfusions, bleeding may be associated with dilutional coagulation. |
| | | • Implement measures to prevent or minimize bleeding: | |
| | | ◦ Specific measures: Use smallest gauge needle possible for venipuncture and subcutaneous injection. | ◦ Minimizes tissue trauma. |
| | | ◦ Avoid intramuscular injections; apply firm, prolonged pressure to venipuncture and injection sites. | ◦ There is a greater tendency to bleed with intramuscular injections. |
| | | ◦ Avoid activities with the potential to cause bleeding: Avoid use of straight razor, use electric razor; avoid gingival bleeding associated with too vigorous tooth brushing; pad bedrails for confused, restless or agitated patients; provide close supervision. | |
| | | • Administer prescribed therapy to improve hemostasis. | |
| | | ◦ Vitamin K (parenterally). | ◦ Necessary for synthesis of clotting factors A, D, E, K. |
| | | ◦ Bile salts. | ◦ Necessary for absorption of vitamin K. |
| | | ◦ Administration of fresh, frozen plasma or packed red blood cells. | ◦ Stored whole blood lacks some of the clotting factors; citrate, used as a blood preservative (anticoagulant) may not be metabolized by hepatocytes. |
| | | • Consider the following if bleeding occurs:<br>◦ Apply firm, prolonged pressure to bleeding site if possible. | |

| | | | |
|---|---|---|---|
| | | ○ Administer fluids and blood products as prescribed.<br>○ Administer prescribed oxygen therapy.<br>○ Maintain gastric decompression.<br>○ Initiate iced gastric lavage (as prescribed).<br>○ Prepare to assist with insertion of Sengstaken-Blakemore tube; if tube is in place, assess its position, balloon inflation, and catheter patency.<br>○ Provide reassurance and support to patient and family.<br>○ Monitor vital signs, neurological status, hourly urine output. | ○ To maintain hemodynamic parameters and hematologic profile within acceptable limits.<br>○ Maximizes arterial blood oxygenation.<br>○ To determine presence of upper gastrointestinal bleeding, and the extent of bleeding.<br>○ For specific nursing care considerations of patients with a Sengstaken-Blakemore tube, see Table 49–5.<br>○ Profuse hemorrhage can be a frightening experience for patient and family. |
| ***Nursing Diagnosis #11***<br>Skin integrity, impairment of, potential, related to:<br>1. Increased skin fragility associated with generalized edema (anasarca) and ascites).<br>2. Malnutrition.<br>3. Immobility associated with stupor and edema.<br>4. Pruritus associated with hyperbilirubinemia. | Patient will:<br>1. Maintain skin intact, no breaks, lesions, irritation or infection; good skin turgor. | • Assess skin, especially reddened areas over bony prominences where skin is thin.<br>○ Assess generalized edema, especially dependent areas (e.g., sacrum, extremities)<br>• Initiate measures to prevent skin breakdown.<br>○ Mobilize extracellular fluid accumulation, especially in dependent areas.<br>○ Turn patient at least every 2 hr; administer backrubs.<br>○ Provide supportive measures and pressure-relief device:<br>– Utilize alternating pressure or egg carton mattress; provide sheepskin; change linen frequently.<br>○ Keep skin well lubricated. If pruritus is present, apply calamine lotion with 1% phenol, or use cholestyramine or cool baking soda bath (as prescribed).<br>○ Assist with range of motion exercises. Handle limbs gently. Apply support stockings.<br>○ Assist with personal hygiene.<br>– Provide oral hygiene frequently, especially when a nasogastric tube or Sengstaken-Blakemore tube is in place.<br>– Provide perineal care, keeping buttocks clean and dry. (Restrict use of soap.) Keep nails trimmed and clean. | ○ Promotes circulation and relieves muscle tension; helps to prevent decubiti.<br>– If reddened areas at pressure points do not blanch within less than 30 minutes, avoid using the position except for shorter periods at less frequent intervals.<br>○ Exercise promotes circulation and prevents venostasis, a contributing factor to the development of a coagulopathy (e.g., disseminated intravascular coagulation, DIC). |

*(continued)*

**TABLE 50–4. CARE PLAN FOR THE PATIENT WITH HEPATIC FAILURE AND HEPATIC ENCEPHALOPATHY** *(Continued)*

| Nursing Diagnoses | Desired Patient Outcomes | Nursing Interventions | Rationales |
|---|---|---|---|
| ***Nursing Diagnosis #11 (cont.)*** | | ○ Instruct patient to apply firm pressure over pruritic areas rather than scratching. | ○ To minimize trauma from scratching. Patient may need gloves or mittens at night while asleep. |
| ***Nursing Diagnosis #12***<br>Self concept, disturbance in, related to:<br>1. Altered physical appearance associated with jaundice, ascites, alopecia, gynecomastia, and other changes associated with chronic liver disease. | Patient will:<br>1. Express feelings about self.<br>2. Participate in decision-making process regarding care.<br>3. Initiate self-care activities. | • Establish a trusting rapport and working relationship:<br>○ Spend time to get to know patient<br>○ Explain all procedures simply and clearly.<br>○ Allow patient participation in procedures whenever possible.<br>○ Encourage patient to participate in decision-making process whenever appropriate.<br>– Assess readiness for decision-making.<br>○ Encourage patient to talk about the illness and how it impacts on self, family and others.<br>– Explain that jaundice, edema, and ascites are usually temporary.<br>○ Help patient to identify strengths, weaknesses, and coping capabilities.<br>– Utilize time during direct patient care to involve patient in discussion of needs, priorities, and how to cope.<br>– Encourage patient to ventilate feelings; provide listening ear and "sounding board."<br>○ Call attention to areas of improvement in the patient's condition.<br>○ Offer immediate praise and feedback for patient's accomplishments no matter how small. | • It is important to encourage/assist the patient to verbalize concerns, to acknowledge and cope with the illness, and to achieve independence in self-care.<br>○ Emphasis is focused on assisting the patient/family to get in touch with their feelings, to identify them, and to begin to deal with them.<br>○ It is important to assist the patient to acknowledge his/her perceptions, and how they differ from those of others, or from the actual situation.<br>○ Praise helps to build self-confidence. |

| | | | |
|---|---|---|---|
| ***Nursing Diagnosis #13***<br>Grieving, dysfunctional, related to:<br>1. End-stage liver disease.<br>2. Altered appearance and lifestyle associated with chronic liver disease. | Patient will:<br>1. Verbalize feelings about liver disease and how it impacts on patient/family.<br>2. Demonstrate progress in dealing with stages of grieving at own pace.<br>3. Participate in self-care activities and in decision-making process regarding care. | • Assess patient's perception of liver disease and how it impacts on patient/family lifestyle.<br>• Identify the stage of grief being experienced by patient/family.<br>○ Assist patient/family to acknowledge that grieving is a process and experiencing the stages of grief is most appropriate and necessary.<br>– Assist patient to acknowledge bodily changes and consequent changes in lifestyle so that the process of grieving can begin.<br>• Assist patient/family to develop a plan for discharge and followup care.<br>○ Be honest and forthright in discussing disease and its ramifications both with patient and family.<br>○ Help patient and family to identify resources.<br>– Assist with referrals to counseling services and support groups. | • Stages of grief include denial, anger, bargaining, depression, and acceptance.<br>○ The nurse must be aware that not every stage is experienced or expressed by each individual; and some individuals will remain in one stage longer than others. In chronic disease, the grief may recur. |

6. Provide nutritional support with adequate calories and limited protein intake.
7. Monitor renal function.
8. Prevent bleeding associated with bleeding varices, erosive gastritis, and altered and/or insufficient clotting factors.
9. Minimize discomfort and promote rest and relaxation.
10. Prevent impairment of skin integrity.
11. Prevent infection.
12. Provide emotional and psychologic support to patient and family.
13. Initiate patient/family education to assist in achieving optimal level of health desired.
14. Promote the grieving process.

## Nursing Diagnoses, Desired Patient Outcomes, and Nursing Interventions

Pertinent nursing diagnoses, desired patient outcomes, and nursing interventions/rationales are presented in Table 50–4 which begins on p. 1075.

## REFERENCES

1. Quinless, F: Severe liver dysfunction, client problems and nursing actions. Focus Crit Care 12(1):24–32, February 1985.
2. Atterbury, CE: Hepatic encephalopathy. In Eastwood G (ed): Core Textbook of Gastroenterology. JB Lippincott, New York, 1984, p 402.

CHAPTER 51

# Nursing Management of the Patient with Acute Pancreatitis

## CHAPTER OUTLINE



## LEARNING OBJECTIVES

**At the end of this chapter, you should be able to:**

1. Define acute pancreatitis and its classifications.
2. Describe the etiology and pathogenesis of acute pancreatitis.
3. Examine underlying pathophysiology associated with acute pancreatitis.
4. Describe the clinical presentation of acute pancreatitis based on underlying pathophysiologic processes.
5. Specify essential components of the assessment of the patient/family health status.
6. List potential complications of acute pancreatitis and the implications for nursing care.
7. Define goals of treatment and treatment priorities.
8. Describe the nursing process in the care of the patient with acute pancreatitis including:
   Assessment
   Nursing diagnosis
   Planning: Desired patient outcomes
   Nursing interventions/rationales.

## ACUTE PANCREATITIS

### Definition/Classification

Acute pancreatitis is an inflammatory disease of the pancreas in which autodigestion of the organ occurs in the presence of activated pancreatic proteolytic enzymes. The 2 main classifications of acute pancreatitis based on pathologic sequelae include *edematous* pancreatitis and *hemorrhagic* or *necrotic* pancreatitis.

#### *Edematous Pancreatitis*

Edematous pancreatitis is more common and is grossly described as a swollen, somewhat indurated pancreas, without evidence of hemorrhage or necrosis.

#### *Hemorrhagic Necrotic Pancreatitis*

Hemorrhagic necrotic pancreatitis is grossly described as a swollen, indurated necrotic pancreas associated with hemorrhage, thrombosis, peripancreatic fat necrosis and accompanied by pseudocyst and abscess formation.

Clinical manifestations of acute pancreatitis depend on the extent of inflammation and destruction of pancreatic tissue. They may vary from mild disorders with rapid and complete recovery, to severe hemorrhagic necrotizing pancreatitis associated with a high mortality rate.

## Etiology and Pathogenesis

The most common etiologic factors associated with pancreatitis include biliary tract disease, with cholelithiasis involving the common bile duct and the ampulla of Vater (see Fig. 47–8); chronic alcoholism (considered to be the most common cause of chronic pancreatitis); and idiopathic pancreatitis.

### *Biliary Tract Disease with Cholelithiasis*

The presence of stones in the common bile duct or ampulla of Vater is thought to predispose to reflux of pancreatic digestive enzymes and bile into the pancreatic duct, which has no sphincter at its duodenal or proximal end. When the amount of digestive juices regurgitating into the pancreas exceeds the capacity of its protective barriers, pancreatic injury and inflammation ensue.

**Pancreatic Protective Barriers.** There are 3 protective barriers that function to prevent injury to pancreatic tissue caused by activated enzymes and bile. These include the sphincter of Oddi, secretion of pancreatic trypsin inhibitor, and an intraductal pressure gradient between the pancreatic and common bile ducts.

The *sphincter of Oddi*, which guards the duodenal opening of the common bile duct as it enters the intestinal lumen at the ampulla of Vater, provides an anatomical barrier to reflux of digestive juices into the pancreas. Normally, this sphincter remains closed except during intraduodenal food digestion, at which time it relaxes to enable passage of bile into the duodenum for the digestion of fats.

Should regurgitation of trypsin bypass the sphincter of Oddi, allowing this activated enzyme to enter the pancreatic duct, it becomes inactivated by *pancreatic trypsin inhibitor*, a second barrier. A third barrier to the reflux of bile into the pancreatic duct involves a pressure gradient between the pancreatic duct and common bile duct. Bile is normally prevented from refluxing into the pancreatic duct because its intraductal pressure is greater than that of the common bile duct.

If the sphincter of Oddi is incompetent or the level of pancreatic trypsin inhibitor is insufficient, or if there is a buildup of pressure in the common bile duct associated, for example, with an impacted stone at the sphincter of Oddi, the regurgitated, activated trypsin can initiate autodigestion of the pancreatic parenchyma. Biliary juices refluxed back into the pancreatic duct along with other digestive juices cause further damage to the pancreas.

### *Chronic Alcoholism*

*Acute* alcohol intake increases the tone of the sphincter of Oddi and inhibits pancreatic secretion of water, bicarbonate, and proteins. In contrast, *chronic* alcoholism is associated with hypersecretion of pancreatic juice, including water, bicarbonate, and enzymes, in response to the stimulation of the hormones, secretin and cholecystokinin (CCK). The pancreatic juice in chronic alcohol consumption is also rich in calcium and unusual proteins such as lactoferrin. While the underlying mechanism remains unknown, the presence of a calcium-containing, protein-rich pancreatic fluid may predispose to pancreatic calculi often seen in the acute alcohol abuser.

Chronic alcoholism is also associated with a decrease in sphincter of Oddi tone, increasing the risk of reflux of digestive juices and bile into the pancreatic duct. A genetic predisposition that allows the development of pancreatic fibrosis and necrosis in chronic alcohol abuse may also be a contributing factor.

### *Idiopathic Pancreatitis/Other Causes*

As the name implies, no known cause of acute pancreatitis has been identified in this instance. Such cases of acute pancreatitis may account for up to 20% of all cases of reported acute pancreatitis.

Other etiologies implicated in acute pancreatitis include postoperative pancreatitis, hyperlipidemia, hypercalcemia, abdominal trauma, pancreatic carcinoma, endoscopic cannulation of the pancreatic duct (ERCP), and drug-induced pancreatitis. While drugs are an uncommon cause of acute pancreatitis, the most frequently cited drugs include azathioprine (Imuran), thiazide diuretics, corticosteroids, furosemide, tetracycline, and oral contraceptives. Oral contraceptives are thought to induce pancreatitis by first provoking hypertriglyceridemia.

Hypercalcemic disorders are associated with acute pancreatitis. Ionic calcium is necessary to convert trypsinogen to trypsin. It is possible that hypercalcemia activates trypsin within the pancreatic parenchyma, triggering acute pancreatitis.

## Pathophysiology

The primary lesion in acute pancreatitis is *chemical inflammation* caused by activated pancreatic enzymes, which leads to necrosis of the pancreatic parenchyma. *Trypsin* is the major culprit. Once activated, this enzyme is known to activate other enzymes including phospholipase A and elastase. *Phospholipase A* digests the phospholipid constituents of cell membranes, damaging pancreatic acinar cells and producing edema, coagulation, and fat necrosis. *Elastase* digests the elastic fibers in the wall of blood vessels leading to hemorrhage, ischemia, and necrosis.

Trypsin also activates the *kallikrein–kallidin–bradykinin* system (a system of serum proteins that amplify the humoral immunologic response), predisposing to edema, vasodilation with increased capillary permeability, infiltration of inflammatory cells, and pain. This inflammatory process results in loss of serum albumin in the exudates. The consequent hypoalbuminemia causes loss of fluid from the intravascular space into the interstitium (pancreatic ascites). This eventually predisposes to hypovolemia, hypotension, and hypovolemic shock.

Biliary juices refluxed back into the pancreatic duct, together with elevated levels of the enzyme lipase, play a key role in fat necrosis within the pancreas. The consequent liberation of large amounts of fatty acids is thought to predispose to hypocalcemia as calcium is taken up in the form of calcium salts by these fatty acids.

Should proteolytic enzymes digest their way through the surface of the pancreas (which, unlike the liver, has no definitive enveloping capsule), causing pancreatic juice to seep into the peritoneal cavity, a *chemical peritonitis* results. Zones of fat necrosis may develop throughout the omenta, and possibly the mesentary, with deposition of calcium. Large abscesses may form.

Diabetes mellitus may become evident during the acute phase and may be irreversible if patients with severe necrosis of the pancreas survive. Occlusion of the common bile duct by edema, adhesions, or calculi may cause jaundice.

## Clinical Presentation

Clinically, signs and symptoms of acute pancreatitis will vary according to the extent of the underlying pathologic process. *Abdominal pain* is the most characteristic feature of acute pancreatitis. The pain is usually epigastric, of a gnawing or boring quality, and unrelenting. It frequently radiates to the back, which corresponds to the location of the pancreas in the retroperitoneal space. Patients with pancreatic pain often find some relief by sitting with knees drawn up against the chest, or by assuming a fetal position in bed.

The pain may begin gradually, usually becoming more severe than the clinical picture might otherwise suggest. The pain is accompanied by restlessness, nausea, vomiting (dry heaves), abdominal distention, and possibly constipation. If hemorrhage or chemical peritonitis occurs, the patient becomes acutely ill with excruciating pain radiating to the back. The pain may be accompanied by spasm or boardlike rigidity of the abdomen, and paralytic ileus. Shocklike symptoms may be associated with hemorrhage or loss of serum proteins into pancreatic parenchyma and surrounding tissues.

Fever, elevation of WBC count, tachycardia, diaphoresis, and jaundice are frequent findings. Uncommonly, signs of respiratory insufficiency (dyspnea, tachypnea, cyanosis) and tetany (marked hypocalcemia) may be present.

## Diagnosis

### Clinical History

**Functional Health Patterns.** Assessment of the patient with possible pancreatitis requires a careful history. It is important to elicit information regarding the following functional health patterns.

***Health Perception–Health Management.*** Establish overall health status and recent changes in the patient's health or lifestyle. Has there been a recent illness, significant weight change, anorexia, nausea, vomiting, or abdominal distention? Has there been recent abdominal surgery or endoscopic examination of the common bile duct? Has the patient sustained recent abdominal trauma? Has there been a recent infection? Is there a history of biliary tract disease, pancreatitis, hepatitis, peptic ulcer disease, hepatic or pancreatic cancer, hyperlipidemia, endocrine disorders, or a hereditary predisposition to any disease?

It is important to elicit a thorough history regarding patient/family use and/or abuse of alcohol and drugs. Data obtained should reflect the amount, type, and duration of alcohol or drug consumption. The patient/family attitudes regarding use/abuse of alcohol and drugs, and their significance in the patient/family lifestyle, should be ascertained.

***Coping–Stress Intolerance.*** Has there been any recent emotional upheaval or stress? It is important to identify how the patient/family cope with stress. What resources are available to assist them in handling stress?

***Cognitive–Perceptual.*** Assessment of patient's perception of pain should be performed. The location, radiation, and duration of the pain, its severity and quality, need to be established. How does the patient describe the pain? Is it gnawing or boring? Is the pain accompanied by nausea and vomiting? Does vomiting relieve the pain? What position does the patient assume in an attempt to reduce the pain? What is the patient's response to analgesic therapy? (See Table 7–1.)

***Nutritional–Metabolic.*** Is there a history of anorexia or weight gain or loss? Inability to tolerate dietary intake? Is the abdominal pain aggravated by thoughts of food or by attempts to ingest foods? Is there a history of hyperlipidemia? Fat intolerance?

***Elimination.*** Has the patient recently experienced changes in bowel habits? Is constipation a problem? Is there steatorrhea? Are there complaints of abdominal bloating?

### *Physical Examination*

The most common clinical findings include epigastric tenderness associated with paralytic ileus. In the setting of acute hemorrhagic pancreatitis, the patient may experience severe pain accompanied by restlessness, anxiety, and distress. The abdomen may become rigid and boardlike with complete cessation of bowel sounds. Abdominal distention may be evident with bulging of the flanks (pancreatic ascites). The presence of periumbilical ecchymosis (*Cullen's* sign) indicates retroperitoneal hemorrhage with dissection along fascial planes to the skin.

Signs of hypovolemic (hemorrhagic) shock may be evident, including hypotension, tachycardia, thready pulse, and cold, clammy and mottled skin of the extremities. A positive *Chvostek's* or *Trousseau's* sign reflects hypocalcemia. Acute pancreatitis can also produce altered respiratory function with atelectasis accompanied by pleural effusion. Adventitious breath sounds (rales/crackles) may be detected on auscultation.

### *Laboratory Tests/Studies*

There is no single accurate diagnostic test for the presence of acute pancreatitis. *Serum amylase* levels, although a sensitive indicator of pancreatic cellular damage, is nonspecific and can be elevated in a number of other conditions. In the presence of acute pancreatitis, the serum amylase levels may only be elevated early in the course of the disease (first 24–48 hours). The determination of serum *isoamylases* may prove to be a more specific diagnostic test.

Another diagnostic test that has been employed is the *amylase/creatinine clearance ratio.* A ratio greater than 5% is highly suggestive of acute pancreatitis. However, this ratio is also elevated in diabetic ketoacidosis, severe burns, and in the postoperative period.

Other laboratory findings may include leukocytosis and elevated serum lipase and urine amylase levels. Liver function studies may be mildly elevated with pancreatitis. Serum bilirubin, alkaline phosphatase, and serum triglyceride levels may all be increased. A decrease in total serum protein with hypoalbuminemia, coupled with serum calcium level of less than 7.5 mg/100 ml, suggests an ominous prognosis. Electrolyte alterations may reflect an altered hydration status. Hyperglycemia and glycosuria may become evident with severe pancreatic cellular damage.

### *Radiologic Studies*

Calcifications in the right upper quadrant (RUQ) depicted on x-ray suggest cholelithiasis, while opacities in the epigastric area suggest pancreatitis. Evidence of paralytic ileus is frequently present. If air is present under the diaphragm, a perforated hollow viscus may be present. Gastrointestinal barium studies may indicate changes in the duodenum consistent with pathology of the head of the pancreas. Chest x-ray may indicate diaphragmatic elevation due to fluid accumulation; atelectasis accompanied by pleural effusion may be evident. Abdominal ultrasonography and computerized tomography of the pancreas are now commonly used to diagnose disorders of the pancreas more specifically.

## Complications

Potential complications of acute pancreatitis are numerous and may be difficult to distinguish from clinical manifestations of the disease. The most serious complications include the development of hypovolemic (hemorrhagic) shock, acute renal failure, adult respiratory distress syndrome, pancreatic abscess or pseudocyst formation, disseminated intravascular coagulation, and malnutrition.

## Prognosis

Early prognostic signs associated with an increased risk of death or major complications have been described by Ronson (Table 51–1). If patients have at

TABLE 51–1
**Prognostic Factors in Acute Pancreatitis[1]**

| Time Frame | Factor | Value |
|---|---|---|
| On admission: | Age | >55 years |
| | Blood glucose | >200 mg/100 ml |
| | White blood cell count | >16,000 mm³ |
| | Serum LDH | >350 μ/ml |
| | SGOT | >250 μ/ml |
| Within 48 hours of admission: | Hematocrit | > 10% decrease |
| | BUN | > 5 mg/100 ml increase |
| | Serum calcium | <8 mg/100 ml |
| | $PaO_2$ | <60 mmHg |
| | Base deficit | >4 mEq/liter |
| | Estimated fluid sequestration | >6000 ml |
| Classification of acuity of pancreatitis based on the number of prognostic factors present: | | |
| | Mild pancreatitis: | <3 factors |
| | Severe pancreatitis: | ≥3 factors |

## TABLE 51-2. CARE PLAN FOR THE PATIENT WITH SEVERE ACUTE PANCREATITIS

| Nursing Diagnoses | Desired Patient Outcomes | Nursing Interventions | Rationales |
|---|---|---|---|
| ***Nursing Diagnosis #1*** Tissue perfusion, alteration in, related to hypovolemic shock. | Patient will:<br>1. Maintain stable hemodynamics:<br>• Blood pressure within 10 mmHg of baseline.<br>• Heart rate < 100 beats/min.<br>• Central venous pressure 0–8 mmHg.<br>• Pulmonary capillary wedge pressure 8–12 mmHg.<br>• Cardiac output ~5 liters/min.<br>• Skin warm with usual color. | • Perform ongoing cardiovascular assessment:<br>∘ Continuous cardiac monitoring.<br>– Establish baseline rate, rhythm, ectopy.<br>∘ Continuous hemodynamic pressure monitoring:<br>– Establish baseline values: Central venous pressure, pulmonary capillary wedge pressure.<br>∘ Assess peripheral pulses: Rate, rhythm, quality.<br>∘ Assess skin temperature, moisture, color, turgor. | • Establishing baseline data assists in evaluating subsequent responses to therapy.<br>∘ Cardiac tissue hypoxia may predispose to dysrhythmias.<br>∘ Offers significant data regarding cardiopulmonary status; affords *trending*, i.e., frequent serial measurements; trending more accurately reflects changes occurring in patient's condition and the patient's response to therapeutic measures.<br>∘ Presence of cool, moist skin with pallor or cyanosis reflects compensatory peripheral vasoconstriction response to permit blood to be shunted to vital organs. |
| | 2. Demonstrate alert mental status, appropriate behavior and neurological function:<br>• Oriented to person, place, time.<br>• Cranial nerves intact.<br>• Deep tendon reflexes brisk. | • Assess ongoing neurological function: Mental status; level of consciousness; behavior—appropriate?; cranial nerves; deep tendon reflexes. | • Compromised hemodynamics (hypotension) and hypoxemia predispose to cerebral hypoxia, reflected by alterations in cerebral function, level of consciousness, responsiveness of cranial nerves, and deep tendon reflexes. |
| | 3. Maintain renal function:<br>• Urine output > 30 ml/hr.<br>• Balanced intake and output.<br>• BUN, serum creatinine within acceptable physiological range. | • Monitor renal function: Hourly urine output; intake and output.<br>∘ Daily weight. | • Reduction in urine output suggests decreased renal perfusion commonly associated with hypovolemic shock. Acute renal failure is a major complication of acute pancreatitis.<br>∘ Most closely reflects hydration status. |

(continued)

## TABLE 51–2. CARE PLAN FOR THE PATIENT WITH SEVERE ACUTE PANCREATITIS *(Continued)*

| Nursing Diagnoses | Desired Patient Outcomes | Nursing Interventions | Rationales |
|---|---|---|---|
| ***Nursing Diagnosis #2***<br>Fluid volume deficit (intravascular), actual, related to:<br>1. Hemorrhage.<br>2. Third-spacing (pancreatic ascites).<br>A. Hypoalbuminemia.<br>3. Dehydration.<br>A. NPO.<br>B. Nasogastric suctioning.<br>C. Vomiting. | Patient will:<br>1. Achieve resolution of edema/ascites:<br>• Body weight within 5% of baseline.<br>• Abdominal girth at baseline measurement. | • Assess gastrointestinal function:<br>○ Abdominal assessment: Abdomen—soft, rigid; rebound tenderness; presence of Cullen or Grey-Turner signs; abdominal girth.<br>○ Nausea/vomiting/constipation, hematemesis, melena. | • Compensatory vasoconstriction of splanchnic circulation (sympathetic response) may result in decreased peristalsis, and ischemia of the gastric and intestinal mucosa.<br>– *Cullen* sign: Bluish umbilicus or faintly blue discoloration of skin associated with hemoperitoneum from any cause.<br>– *Grey-Turner* sign: Ecchymoses on abdomen and flanks possibly associated with infiltration of extraperitoneal tissues with blood. |
| ***Nursing Diagnosis #3***<br>Electrolyte balance, alteration in, related to:<br>1. Diuretic therapy.<br>2. Acid-base imbalance.<br>(See also Table 49–6, Nursing Diagnosis #1, Table 50–4, Nursing Diagnoses #1 and #2.) | Patient will:<br>1. Restore/maintain laboratory parameters within acceptable physiological range:<br>• Serum osmolality 285–295 mOsm/Kg.<br>• Serum sodium >135 <148 mEq/liter.<br>• Serum potassium 3.5–5.5 mEq/liter.<br>• Serum albumin 3.5–5.5 g/100 ml.<br>• Hematocrit 37–52%.<br>• Hemoglobin 12–18 g/100 ml.<br>• CBC.<br>• Urine electrolytes and specific gravity. | • Assess for signs and symptoms of electrolyte imbalance:<br>○ Hypokalemia—cardiac dysrhythmias; hypotension; weakness; fatigue; nausea, vomiting; lethargy, muscle weakness; paresthesias, hyporeflexia.<br>○ Hyponatremia—nausea, vomiting, headache, lethargy, confusion, seizures, coma.<br>○ Hypocalcemia—tremors, paresthesias, tetany, laryngospasm, convulsions, positive Chvostek's and Trousseau's signs.<br>○ Hypochloremia: Alkalemia. | • Acute pancreatitis usually predisposes to electrolyte imbalance. Nasogastric suctioning, vomiting, diarrhea, and extravasation of fluid account for much of the loss of sodium, potassium, and chloride.<br>– It is important to establish baseline blood chemistry values so that replacement therapy may be guided by serial studies, which should include total protein and serum osmolality, in addition to electrolytes. |

| | |
|---|---|
| • Implement prescribed measures to re-establish and maintain normovolemia and electrolyte balance. | |
| ◦ Administer blood products and intravenous fluids. | ◦ To reverse hypovolemia/hypotension. Reestablishing intravascular volume improves circulation, tissue perfusion and oxygenation. Replace fluid losses associated with NPO, vomiting, and nasogastric suctioning.<br>– Irritating and inflammatory effects of acute pancreatitis on the pancreatic parenchyma and surrounding tissues cause extravasation of fluids, electrolytes, and protein into the interstitium and peritoneal cavity (third-spacing). |
| ◦ Replace serum albumin. | ◦ Loss of plasma proteins from the intravascular space disrupts colloidal osmotic pressure, predisposing to even greater fluid loss with interstitial edema and ascites. |
| ◦ Monitor for signs of circulatory overload: Generalized (dependent) edema, weight gain, increased blood pressure, bounding pulses; signs of pulmonary congestion—dyspnea, rales (crackles), elevation of central venous and pulmonary artery pressures; neck vein distention.<br>◦ Monitor for signs of hypovolemia: Hypotension, tachycardia, decreased central venous and pulmonary artery pressures; decreased urine output, increase in urine specific gravity; signs of dehydration—elevated body temperature, poor skin turgor, sunken eyeballs, and dryness of mucous membranes. | ◦ Fluid overload is a complication of aggressive fluid volume replacement. |
| ◦ Administer prescribed inotropic and vasopressor therapy.<br>– Dopamine hydrochloride. | ◦ Increases cardiac output by increasing preload (venous return) and cardiac contractility; enhances tissue perfusion. |
| ◦ Replace serum electrolytes:<br>◦ Sodium.<br>– Hyponatremia/hypernatremia: monitor hydration status, monitor serum/urine sodium levels. | ◦ Hyponatremia is a frequent occurrence in acute pancreatitis.<br>– A decrease in total body sodium predisposes to hypovolemia.<br>– Intravenous replacement of sodium needs to be carefully monitored to prevent sodium excess (hypernatremia) with consequent fluid overload. |

*(continued)*

**TABLE 51-2. CARE PLAN FOR THE PATIENT WITH SEVERE ACUTE PANCREATITIS** *(Continued)*

| Nursing Diagnoses | Desired Patient Outcomes | Nursing Interventions | Rationales |
|---|---|---|---|
| ***Nursing Diagnosis #3 (cont.)*** | | | |
| | | ∘ Potassium.<br>– Hypokalemia/hyperkalemia: Monitor ECG for dysrhythmias, monitor arterial blood gases (acid-base status), monitor serum potassium levels. | ∘ Potassium, an intracellular ion, is closely associated with acid-base balance:<br>– Acidemia—hydrogen ions are driven into cells in exchange for potassium; this increases serum potassium levels.<br>– Alkalemia—hydrogen ions move out of cells in exchange for potassium; this decreases serum potassium levels.<br>– This reciprocal relationship between potassium and hydrogen ions also occurs in the distal tubules, necessitating that kidney function be closely monitored. |
| | | ∘ Calcium.<br>– Hypocalcemia. | ∘ Deposition of calcium into areas of fatty necrosis occurs frequently in acute pancreatitis and requires close monitoring of serum calcium levels. Calcium replacement therapy requires careful administration to prevent complications:<br>– Patent intravenous line needs to be maintained because tissue sloughing and necrosis can occur with extravasation of calcium preparations. |
| | | ∘ Monitor ECG for dysrhythmias. | ∘ Potentiation of digitalis effect by calcium can occur in patients receiving digitalis; this can predispose to digitalis toxicity. Continuous ECG monitoring is essential. |
| | | ∘ Monitor total serum protein and serum albumin levels. | ∘ Calcium is highly bound to serum proteins; alkalemia increases percent calcium bound to protein, thus reducing fraction of ionized calcium. |
| | | ∘ Chloride. | ∘ Chloride is necessary for gastric production of HCl; it plays a major role in acid-base balance. |
| | | – Hypochloremia: monitor acid-base status, monitor serum chloride. | ∘ Hypochloremia is associated with vomiting, and nasogastric suctioning; it predisposes to metabolic alkalosis. |

| | | | |
|---|---|---|---|
| ***Nursing Diagnosis #4***<br>Breathing pattern, ineffective, related to:<br>1. Hypoventilation associated with severe abdominal pain.<br>2. Atelectasis.<br>3. Pleural effusion.<br>***Nursing Diagnosis #5***<br>Airway clearance, ineffective, related to:<br>1. Cough suppression and failure to deep breathe because of severe abdominal pain.<br>2. Immobility. | Patient will:<br>1. Demonstrate effective minute ventilation:<br>• Tidal volume ($V_T$) >5–7 ml/Kg.<br>• Respiratory rate <25–30 per min.<br>2. Achieve vital capacity ($V_C$) >12–15 ml/Kg.<br>3. Verbalize ease of breathing.<br>4. Demonstrate deep-breathing techniques and effective secretion-clearing cough.<br>5. Maintain arterial blood gases within acceptable physiological range:<br>• $PaO_2$ >60 mmHg.<br>• $PaCO_2$ 35–45 mmHg.<br>• pH >7.35 <7.45.<br>• Base excess +2/−2.<br>6. Maintain appropriate responses on respiratory examination:<br>• Tactile fremitus present on palpation.<br>• Resonance throughout lung fields on percussion.<br>• Vesicular breath sounds throughout peripheral lung fields on auscultation.<br>7. Demonstrate an absence of atelectasis and pleural effusion on chest x-ray. | • Assess respiratory function:<br>○ Rate, rhythm, depth and pattern of breathing.<br>○ Symmetry of chest wall and diaphragmatic excursion.<br>○ Use of accessory muscles.<br>○ Auscultation of breath sounds.<br>○ Pulmonary lung volumes: Total minute ventilation; tidal volume, respiratory rate; vital capacity.<br>○ Assess quantity, quality, color, odor and consistency of sputum.<br>○ Assess arterial blood gases. | ○ Abdominal pain causes splinting and hypoventilation; hypoventilation predisposes to hypercapnia and atelectasis; atelectasis predisposes to ventilation/perfusion inequality.<br>– Abdominal pain predisposes to cough suppression and immobility; pooling of secretions predisposes to pneumonia. |
| | | • Implement measures to improve respiratory function:<br>○ Administer prescribed medication for abdominal pain and monitor response.<br>○ Meperidine is drug of choice. | ○ Relief of pain encourages patient to breathe more deeply and to cough more vigorously.<br>○ Meperidine causes less spasm of Oddi's sphincter than does morphine. |

*(continued)*

**TABLE 51–2. CARE PLAN FOR THE PATIENT WITH SEVERE ACUTE PANCREATITIS *(Continued)***

| Nursing Diagnoses | Desired Patient Outcomes | Nursing Interventions | Rationales |
|---|---|---|---|
| ***Nursing Diagnosis #5 (cont.)*** | | | |
| | | ○ Perform measures to reduce anxiety:<br>– Encourage verbalization of fears and concerns.<br>– Provide a caring touch and listening ear.<br>– Provide explanations and feedback regarding care and health status.<br>– Identify patient/family coping strengths and resources. | ○ A reduction in the level of anxiety or stress may help to reduce the level of pain, and facilitate breathing. |
| | | ○ Perform measures to facilitate chest wall expansion and diaphragmatic excursion:<br>– Minimize abdominal distention associated with gastrointestinal gas and fluid accumulation. | ○ Help to improve ventilation and oxygenation, and prevent atelectasis and pooling of secretions. |
| | | ○ Maintain proper placement and patency of nasogastric tube. | ○ Nasogastric suction helps to reduce gastric distention. |
| | | ○ Encourage frequent position changes.<br>– Maintain patient in semi- to high-Fowler's position unless contraindicated. | ○ Patient is inclined to assume a position of greatest pain relief and to remain in that position. Coughing, deep breathing, and position changes may best be performed following administration of analgesics. |
| | | ○ Encourage patient to expel flatus whenever the urge arises. | ○ Deep breathing and position changes may stimulate peristalsis and flatulence. |
| | | ○ Monitor for signs and symptoms of pleural effusion: Shortness of breath; pleuritic pain; splinting to reduce chest excursion; dullness on percussion; and diminished to absent breath sounds over the affected area on auscultation. | |
| | | ○ Perform measures to minimize pancreatic secretory activity. | ○ The pancreas is stimulated by gastric juice in the duodenum; a patent nasogastric tube with suction reduces delivery of HCl to duodenum. |
| | | ○ Administer anticholinergic drugs cautiously, if prescribed. | ○ Blocking parasympathetic stimulation (via vagus) decreases amount of gastric HCl secretion; use of anticholinergics in a patient with paralytic ileus may actually worsen the patient's condition by suppressing pancreatic secretion and allowing enzymes to accumulate within the pancreas. |
| | | ○ Prepare patient and assist with thoracentesis (see Table 36–2). | ○ Decompression of pleural effusion facilitates greater lung expansion. |

| | | | |
|---|---|---|---|
| | | ○ Prepare patient and assist with paracentesis (see Table 50–4, Nursing Diagnosis #1). | ○ Decompression of peritoneal fluid increases diaphragmatic excursion. |
| | | ○ Implement prescribed respiratory support therapy:<br>○ Oxygen therapy.<br>○ Intermittent positive pressure breathing (IPPB). | |
| ***Nursing Diagnosis #6***<br>Comfort, alteration in: Acute pain.<br>(See Table 35–3, Nursing Diagnoses #1 and #7.) | Patient will:<br>1. Verbalize relief of pain.<br>2. Exhibit relaxed demeanor:<br>• Relaxed facial expression and body posturing.<br>• Ease of breathing.<br>3. Identify effective pain relief and coping mechanisms. | Refer to Table 35–3, Nursing Diagnoses #1 and #7, for specific nursing interventions. The following interventions should be considered for the patient with acute pancreatitis: | |
| | | • Implement measures to reduce pancreatic stimulation. | • Stimulation of inflamed pancreatic acinar cells aggravate pain.<br>– Pain and anxiety increase pancreatic secretory activity via enhanced parasympathetic stimulation. |
| | | ○ Maintain the patient NPO. | ○ It is necessary to minimize gastric secretions as they stimulate secretion of the hormones secretin and cholecystokinin, both of which stimulate pancreatic secretion. |
| | | ○ Maintain patency of nasogastric tube with continuous nasogastric suction.<br>– Confirm tube placement every two hours. | ○ Nasogastric suction also relieves nausea, vomiting, and intestinal distention. |
| | | ○ Administer prescribed medications:<br>○ Meperidine is usual analgesic of choice. Evaluate the effectiveness of the prescribed analgesic. | ○ Morphine is avoided because it causes a greater degree of spasm of the sphincter of Oddi than does meperidine. |
| | | ○ Anticholinergics, papaverine: | ○ These drugs function to relax smooth muscle which may help to reduce pain. |
| | | ○ Provide frequent oral care. | ○ Anticholinergic drugs suppress salivary secretion; oral mucous membranes become dry. |
| | | ○ Monitor urine output. | ○ Urinary retention and paralytic ileus are also associated with anticholinergic therapy. |
| | | ○ Provide frequent comfort measures:<br>○ Mouth care; position changes; time periods of quiet and sleep; spending more time with patient:<br>– Provide a listening ear. | |
| | | ○ Involve patient/family in quiet recreational activities. | ○ This may help to distract the patient from thoughts of food and to avoid parasympathetic stimulation associated with the cephalic phase of digestive activity. |
| | | ○ Minimize visitors. | ○ Increased activity may aggravate pain. |
| | | ○ Instruct family members and friends not to take food into the patient's room. | ○ Sight of food can stimulate pancreatic secretory activity (cephalic phase of digestion). |

*(continued)*

## TABLE 51–2. CARE PLAN FOR THE PATIENT WITH SEVERE PANCREATITIS *(Continued)*

| Nursing Diagnoses | Desired Patient Outcomes | Nursing Interventions | Rationales |
|---|---|---|---|
| ***Nursing Diagnosis #7***<br>Nutrition, alteration in, less than body requirements (malnutrition), related to:<br>1. Nausea and vomiting.<br>2. NPO status.<br>3. Malabsorption (altered fat metabolism).<br>4. Altered carbohydrate and protein metabolism.<br>A. Hypoglycemia.<br>B. Hypoalbuminemia. | Patient will:<br>1. Maintain body weight within 5% of baseline.<br>2. Maintain serum albumin within physiological range:<br>• 3.5–5.0 g/100 ml.<br>3. Demonstrate unimpaired integrity of skin and mucous membranes.<br>4. Verbalize feeling of increased strength.<br>5. Triceps skinfold within acceptable range.<br>6. Laboratory parameters within acceptable range:<br>• Hematology profile.<br>• Cholesterol.<br>• BUN, creatinine. | Refer to Chap. 53, Nutritional Support of the Critically Ill Patient, for details related to treatment and prevention of malnutrition. | |
| ***Nursing Diagnosis #8***<br>Oral mucous membranes, alteration in, related to:<br>1. Altered fluid and electrolyte imbalance (dehydration).<br>2. Mouth breathing with nasogastric tube.<br>3. Reduced salivation associated with dehydration and medication regimen (e.g., narcotics, anticholinergics). | Patient will:<br>1. Maintain integrity of mucous membranes:<br>• Mucous membranes moist.<br>• Lips without cracking or fissures. | • Assess and monitor status of mucous membranes: Monitor daily weight, intake and output; monitor dietary intake. | |
| | | • Implement measures to prevent drying and cracking of mucous membranes: | • When nutritional intake is less than body requirements, the patient becomes at risk of infections, and healing capabilities become compromised. |
| | | ◦ Maintain hydration. | ◦ Adequate hydration is necessary to keep mucous membranes moist. |
| | | ◦ Provide frequent oral hygiene, rinsing mouth frequently. | |
| | | ◦ Keep lips well lubricated. | ◦ Prevent cracking and fissure formation. |
| | | ◦ Assess lips, mouth and pharynx for lesions, fissures, or bleeding. | ◦ Ongoing assessment assists in determining changes in the mucosa, and the effectiveness of therapy. |
| | | • Implement measures to treat drying and cracking or oral membranes: Apply topical ointment to keep mucous membranes moist. | |

| | | | |
|---|---|---|---|
| ***Nursing Diagnosis #9***<br>Infection, potential for, related to:<br>1. Malnutrition.<br>2. Invasive procedures.<br>3. Peritonitis associated with autodigestion of adjacent tissues by pancreatic juices. | Patient will:<br>1. Maintain body temperature within acceptable physiological range ~98.6°F.<br>2. Maintain white blood count: ~5000–10,000/mm³.<br>3. Remain without signs and symptoms of infection: Pain, erythema, edema, increased temperature (peripheral sites). | For specific nursing interventions and rationales, see Table 49–7, Potential for Infection: Nursing Care Considerations. | |
| ***Nursing Diagnosis #10***<br>Knowledge deficit regarding:<br>1. Convalescence and followup care.<br>2. Impact on lifestyle.<br>∘ Alcoholism<br>∘ Stress | Patient will:<br>1. Verbalize importance of strict adherence to prescribed dietary regimen:<br>• Total abstinence from alcohol.<br>• High carbohydrate and protein diet; low fat intake.<br>2. Verbalize alternatives in pain relief:<br>• Medication therapy.<br>• Relaxation exercises.<br>3. Identify effective coping mechanisms in stress management. | • Establish a trusting rapport with patient and family members.<br>∘ Verbalize fears and concerns for patient and family. | • An environment of mutual respect and trust can enhance the learning process. Often a long convalescence follows recovery from acute pancreatitis. Discharge planning should begin as early as possible.<br>∘ While the patient may be too ill initially to participate in learning, involvement of family members in the patient's overall care may impact on the progress made by patient and family members alike toward level of health and well-being desired. |
| | | • Assess patient/family baseline knowledge and readiness to learn.<br>∘ Encourage patient/family to assist in identifying needs and learning objectives.<br>• Assist patient/family in problem-solving techniques.<br>∘ Help to identify family strengths and weaknesses.<br>• Determine appropriate teaching strategies to facilitate learning:<br>∘ Encourage open discussions regarding illness and impact on family lifestyle.<br>∘ Consider role of alcohol in lifestyle if appropriate. | • An informed patient/family can participate in care and make necessary adjustments in lifestyle.<br>∘ Assisting patient/family to cope increases self-confidence in their own capabilities.<br>• Learning should occur at a rate that is meaningful to participants. |

*(continued)*

**TABLE 51–2. CARE PLAN FOR THE PATIENT WITH SEVERE PANCREATITIS *(Continued)***

| Nursing Diagnoses | Desired Patient Outcomes | Nursing Interventions | Rationales |
|---|---|---|---|
| ***Nursing Diagnosis #10 (cont.)*** | | | |
| | | • Initiate health teaching concerned with the following:<br>○ Diet management: Emphasize importance of strict adherence to prescribed diet; abstinence from alcohol and high fat intake.<br>○ Consider who in the family is responsible for meal preparation. | ○ It is essential for the family member who cooks to appreciate the patient's diet and its preparation. |
| | | ○ Pain management: Advise patient as to alternatives in pain relief: Medication therapy; surgery; relaxation exercises, recreational therapy.<br>– Support patient/family in their decision.<br>– Include the following in teaching: purpose, action(s), dosage, frequency and route of administration and drug interactions for prescribed medications. | |
| | | ○ Management of stress: Assist patient/family to: Identify sources of stress; identify effective and ineffective coping mechanisms and their usefulness; assist patient/family to become in touch with their feelings, and to communicate these feelings to each other. | ○ Effective stress management may be helpful in reducing pain. |
| | | • Initiate referrals to appropriate resources:<br>○ Nutritionist.<br>○ Social worker.<br>○ Psychiatric liaison nurse.<br>○ Other. | • Successful recovery of all members of the family from the stress of acute illness, and continued health maintenance, requires timely and ongoing support. No one lives in a vacuum. |

least 3 of these 11 risk factors, they are at high risk of having a long, complicated, often fatal course.

## Treatment

There is presently no specific, clinically substantiated, efficacious treatment of acute pancreatitis. The current approach to therapy is supportive and is directed at preventing and/or treating complications of acute pancreatitis. Shock, hemorrhage, fluid and electrolyte imbalances are the most urgent clinical findings that require immediate intervention. Blood, colloids, fluids, and electrolytes are replaced, and the patient's central venous and/or pulmonary artery pressures are closely monitored.

Serial arterial blood gas studies are performed to monitor closely for the development of acute respiratory distress syndrome (ARDS). Assisted mechanical ventilation with positive end-expiratory pressure (PEEP) is initiated with the earliest indications of respiratory failure. Serum calcium levels are monitored, and hypocalcemia is treated with intravenous infusions of calcium. Renal failure may necessitate hemodialysis.

Suspected pancreatic abscess is treated with broad-spectrum antibiotics and is surgically drained. Prophylactic use of antibiotics in the treatment of acute pancreatitis has failed to demonstrate any clinical benefit. Such use of antibiotics may mask the causative organism should sepsis develop.

Pain control is usually maintained by the use of meperidine, with frequent assessments made as to its effectiveness. Morphine use is avoided because it causes a greater spasm of the sphincter of Oddi than does meperidine.

To avoid malnutrition, parenteral nutritional support is prescribed. The daily nutritive requirements can be met in this way with the least stimulation of pancreatic activity.

A variety of treatments of acute pancreatitis have been prescribed, but the efficacy of such therapies has not been substantiated by controlled clinical studies. Of the following medications, none is of proven value: prophylactic antibiotics, cimetidine or ranitidine, anticholinergics, pancreatic enzyme inhibitors (e.g., Trasylol, no longer used), and hormones, including insulin, glucagon, somatostatin, calcitonin, and prostaglandin $E_2$. Nasogastric intubation, suction, and peritoneal lavage are likewise of unproven benefit. Surgery may be indicated in 2 recognized instances; 1) when the diagnosis of acute pancreatitis is in doubt, and an abdominal emergency such as a perforated viscus or infarcted bowel must be ruled out; and 2) in the drainage of a suspected pancreatic abscess.

The definitive treatment of severe acute pancreatitis awaits the development of clinically substantiated efficacious drugs and procedures.

## Nursing Care of the Patient with Severe Acute Pancreatitis

### *Therapeutic Goals*

The overall approach to the nursing care and management of the patient with severe acute pancreatitis is to provide supportive care to maintain optimal function of all body processes, and to prevent complications.[2] To care effectively for such patients, the nurse must have a keen understanding of the underlying anatomy and physiology of the pancreas, liver, biliary system, and upper gastrointestinal tract; and must appreciate the clinical ramifications of the pathophysiology associated with pancreatic disease.

The astute critical care nurse recognizes that the clinical presentation of the patient with acute pancreatitis (e.g., duration/severity of abdominal pain, vomiting, the presence of guarding or rebound tenderness, and increase in the serum amylase levels) does not necessarily correlate with outcome. Patients with severe pain, vomiting, marked guarding, and high serum amylase levels may do quite well; whereas, the patient with seemingly mild pain, no guarding or ileus, and with a slight elevation in serum amylase level may have a fatal course. Detection of even the slightest change and recognition of its clinical significance require that the critical care nurse have sharply honed assessment skills, a sophisticated bedside instinct, the ability to integrate knowledge and skills with the particular clinical circumstances, and the capacity to implement nursing process.

Implementation of nursing process in the care of the patient with acute pancreatitis revolves around the following therapeutic goals:

1. Establish a thorough comprehensive assessment database including:
   a. Clinical history.
   b. Physical examination.
   c. Laboratory/x-ray data.
2. Promote/maintain optimal alveolar ventilation.
3. Promote/maintain optimal oxygenation and tissue perfusion.
4. Promote/maintain fluid, electrolyte, and acid–base balance.
5. Alleviate/control pain.
6. Provide emotional support and reassurance to patient and family.
7. Implement measures to minimize pancreatic secretory activity.
8. Implement nutritional therapy to prevent malnutrition.
9. Prevent complications including:
   a. Cardiovascular: Shock, hemorrhage, cardiac dysrhythmias, disseminated intravascular coagulation (DIC).
   b. Pulmonary: Atelectasis, hypoxia, pleural

effusion, adult respiratory distress syndrome (ARDS).

c. Renal: Acute renal failure.

d. Metabolic: Acid–base disturbance; hyperglycemia or hypoglycemia; hypocalcemia.

e. Infection.

10. Assist patient/family with management of stress.

#### *Nursing Diagnoses, Desired Patient Outcomes, and Nursing Interventions*

Pertinent nursing diagnoses, desired patient outcomes, and nursing interventions/rationales are presented in Table 51–2.

## REFERENCES

1. Ranson, JH, Ritkind, KM, and Turner, JW: Prognostic signs and nonoperative peritoneal lavage in acute pancreatitis. Surg Gynecol Obstet 143(2):212, August 1976.
2. Emanuelsen, K and Rosenlicht, J: Handbook of Critical Care Nursing. John Wiley & Sons, New York, 1986, p 251.

CHAPTER 52

# Nursing Management of the Patient with Gastrointestinal Dysfunction: Intestinal Ischemia, Acute Inflammatory Bowel Disease, and Intestinal Obstruction

## CHAPTER OUTLINE



## LEARNING OBJECTIVES

**At the end of this chapter, you should be able to:**

1. Describe the splanchnic circulation and its regulation.
2. Define intestinal ischemic disease and its classifications.
3. Differentiate classes of intestinal ischemic disease in terms of:
   A. Etiology and pathogenesis.
   B. Pathophysiology.
   C. Clinical presentation.
   D. Diagnosis.
   E. Treatment.
4. List tentative nursing diagnoses pertinent to the care of the patient with intestinal ischemic disease.
5. Define inflammatory bowel disease and the disorders it encompasses.
6. Differentiate regional enteritis (Crohn's disease) and ulcerative colitis in terms of:
   A. Etiology and pathogenesis.
   B. Pathology.

## LEARNING OBJECTIVES—*CONTINUED*

   C. Clinical presentation.
   D. Diagnosis
   E. Complications.
   F. Treatment.
7. List tentative nursing diagnoses pertinent to the care of the patient with inflammatory bowel disease.
8. Describe intestinal obstruction including types, underlying causative mechanisms, pathophysiology, clinical presentation, diagnosis, and treatment.
9. List tentative nursing diagnoses pertinent to the care of the patient with intestinal obstruction.

# INTESTINAL ISCHEMIA—MESENTERIC VASCULAR INSUFFICIENCY

## Splanchnic Circulation

Blood supply to the stomach and intestines is provided by three unpaired arteries—the *celiac* axis, *superior mesenteric* artery, and *inferior mesenteric* artery. These three vessels arise from the abdominal aorta. Nearly 30% of the resting cardiac output is delivered to the intestines by these major splanchnic arteries each minute. Extensive anastomotic connections within the splanchnic vasculature permit the development of collateral circulation, a major consideration in the origin and consequence of intestinal ischemia.

### *Regulation of the Splanchnic Circulation*

The regulation of the splanchnic circulation remains poorly understood. The splanchnic microcirculation, which is responsible for perfusion and the actual delivery of oxygen to the tissues, is under the immediate control of arteriolar wall smooth muscle and precapillary sphincters. These structures, in turn, are influenced by other factors. Cardiac output, mean systemic arterial blood pressure, blood volume, and blood viscosity are factors involved in the regulation of intestinal perfusion. A reduction in blood volume and arterial blood pressure, as occurs for example in acute hemorrhage, can dramatically reduce splanchnic blood flow.

**Autoregulation.** Autonomic nervous system regulation of splanchnic blood flow involves the phenomenon of autoregulation. While sympathetic stimulation initially results in vasoconstriction of the arteriolar smooth muscle, producing an increase in resistance to splanchnic blood flow and a consequent reduction in oxygen tension, a prolonged sympathetic response produces vasodilation of these arterioles as a result of tissue hypoxia. Vasodilation, coupled with a relaxation of intestinal wall muscle tension, promotes blood flow and increases tissue perfusion.

Autoregulation functions to maintain blood flow to the intestines, despite alterations in systemic arterial pressure. Sympathetic stimulation also directs blood flow away from the intestinal mucosa to the muscle layers of the intestinal wall. As a consequence, mucosal ischemia and injury may occur, despite the fact that total blood flow remains unchanged.

Local metabolic factors also help to control splanchnic circulation. By-products of enhanced metabolic activity of intestinal cells (enterocytes) trigger vasodilation, with a resultant increase in blood flow.

## Intestinal Ischemic Disorders

*Intestinal ischemia* or *mesenteric vascular insufficiency* can create a wide spectrum of tissue injury, ranging from completely reversible mucosal damage to transmural infarction and gangrene. The severity of the injury depends on the degree of oxygen deprivation to the tissues and the duration of the insult. Other factors to be considered include the size (diameter) of the involved blood vessel(s) and the length of the intestine that depends on it for its blood supply. The underlying cardiopulmonary and hematologic status of the patient need to be considered. Intestinal vascular injury is ultimately a result of impaired oxygen delivery to the tissues, which, in turn, depends on the oxygen-carrying capacity of the blood, and the perfusion pressure at the level of the intestines.

Specific intestinal ischemic disorders include acute superior mesenteric artery occlusion, chronic mesenteric occlusion ("intestinal angina"), non-occlusive mesenteric ischemia/infarction, and mesenteric venous ischemia. See Table 52–1 for a comparison of these ischemic disorders including their etiology, pathophysiology, clinical presentation, diagnosis, and treatment. Tentative nursing diagnoses pertinent to the care of the patient with intestinal ischemia are also listed.

## Nursing Care Considerations

Nursing care of the patient with ischemic disease is frequently complicated by the age of the patient. These patients are usually elderly with advanced

TABLE 52–1
## Intestinal Ischemic Disorders—Mesenteric Vascular Insufficiency

| | Acute Superior Mesenteric Artery Occlusion | Chronic Mesenteric Occlusion | Nonocclusive Mesenteric Ischemia/ Infarction | Mesenteric Venous Ischemia |
|---|---|---|---|---|
| **Definition** | Sudden, complete occlusion of a major splanchnic artery (most commonly the superior mesenteric artery) caused by embolus or thrombus formation. | Chronic occlusive mesenteric ischemia occurs secondary to atherosclerotic changes within the splanchnic vasculature; patency of blood vessels becomes compromised, more gradually enabling *collateral circulation* to develop. This helps to maintain blood flow and prevent ischemic episodes from occurring. Eventually, blood vessels become progressively occluded, predisposing to ischemia. | Nonocclusive mesenteric ischemia occurs due to reduced blood flow to the splanchnic circulation, but without occlusion. | A result of acute thrombosis. |
| **Incidence** | Occurs most frequently in the elderly, and is complicated by total body disease secondary to atherosclerotic changes. | Same as in acute occlusion. | This syndrome is recognized with increasing frequency and may be the most common cause of small bowel ischemia. It frequently occurs in the elderly. | |
| **Etiological Factors and Pathogenesis** | Embolus secondary to:<br>• Mural thrombus after myocardial infarction.<br>• Atrial fibrillation.<br>• Endocarditis.<br>• Cholesterol plaques dislodged during arteriography.<br>Thrombosis secondary to:<br>• Mesenteric atherosclerosis.<br>• Reduced mesenteric blood flow associated with congestive heart failure and reduced cardiac output.<br>• Intense splanchnic vasoconstriction associated with "shock" state.<br>Other contributing factors:<br>• History of rheumatic heart disease. | Chronic occlusive ischemia develops as a result of gradual changes in the wall of blood vessels leading eventually to total occlusion.<br>• This form is often referred to as *intestinal angina*.<br>• The angina results from:<br>–Progressive narrowing of the major splanchnic vessels (celiac, superior, and inferior mesenteric arteries).<br>–Compression of blood vessels by adjacent structures.<br>–Involvement by an expanding abdominal aortic aneurysm.<br>• In contrast to the | Characteristics of nonocclusive ischemia/infarction include:<br>• Atherosclerotic changes within the splanchnic vasculature.<br>• Vasoconstriction and vasospasm of splanchnic blood vessels predisposing to reduced blood flow and ischemia.<br>• Vasopressors (e.g., dopamine at dose of 15 $\mu$g/Kg/min), although capable of improving cardiac output, may cause further splanchnic vasoconstriction, thereby aggravating the ischemic state.<br>• Beta-agonists such as isoproterenol may be useful in vasodilating | Acute thrombosis may be:<br>• Idiopathic.<br>• Secondary to intra-abdominal suppuration (e.g., appendicitis, pelvic abscess).<br>• Hypercoagulable status (e.g., polycythemia, carcinomatosis).<br>• Local venous congestion or stasis of blood flow.<br>• Secondary to tumor mass or fibrosis (cirrhosis).<br>Other contributing factors:<br>• Low hemoglobin content (<10 g/100 ml); anemic states.<br>• Alveolar hypoventilation with consequent reduced $PaO_2$. |

*(continued)*

TABLE 52-1
**Intestinal Ischemic Disorders—Mesenteric Vascular Insufficiency *(Continued)***

| | Acute Superior Mesenteric Artery Occlusion | Chronic Mesenteric Occlusion | Nonocclusive Mesenteric Ischemia/ Infarction | Mesenteric Venous Ischemia |
|---|---|---|---|---|
| **Etiological Factors and Pathogenesis** *(cont.)* | • Perivascular disorders (e.g., thromboangiitis obliterans).<br>• Systemic vasculitis.<br>• Dissecting abdominal aortic aneurysm.<br>• Low hemoglobin content (<10 g/100 ml); anemic state)<br>• Alveolar hypoventilation with consequent reduced $PaO_2$.<br>• Enhanced metabolic needs of intestinal mucosal epithelial cells after meals increase oxygen demand. | acute occlusive disorder, gradual occlusion of blood vessels allows for collateral circulation to become established, decreasing acuity of oxygen deprivation to tissues distal to the obstruction.<br>Other contributing factors:<br>- Atherosclerotic processes as in acute occlusive disease.<br>- Low hemoglobin content; anemic states.<br>- Alveolar hypoventilation.<br>- Enhanced metabolic needs of intestinal mucosal epithelial cells after meals increase oxygen demands. | splanchnic vasculature along with other vascular beds in the system circulation.<br>Other contributing factors:<br>• Low hemoglobin content (<10 g/100 ml); anemic state.<br>• Alveolar hypoventilation with consequent reduced $PaO_2$.<br>• Enhanced metabolic needs of intestinal mucosal epithelial cells after meals increase oxygen demand. | • Enhanced metabolic needs of intestinal mucosal epithelial cells after meals increase oxygen demand. |
| **Pathophysiology** | Intestinal ischemic changes include:<br>• Initial intense spasm of muscularis externa followed by bowel immobility and paralytic ileus.<br>• Consequent bowel distention with fluid and gas, which eventually culminates in hemodynamic shock, electrolyte imbalance (hyponatremia, hypochloremia) and metabolic acidosis.<br>• Patient is at high risk of developing septic shock secondary to absorption of bacteria and/or toxins through disrupted intestinal membranes.<br>• Gastrointestinal bleeding may also occur. | • Some pathophysiological changes occur during ischemic episodes, but they are not of the severity of those described for acute occlusive ischemia.<br>• The intermittent, discontinuous episodes of ischemia are characteristic of chronic occlusive disease. They are usually associated with eating, during which time the splanchnic demand for oxygen is greatly increased.<br>When oxygen supply temporarily does not meet the oxygen demand, ischemia results.<br>• Chronic intestinal ischemia may cause mucosal damage predisposing to malabsorption, leading to weight | • The ischemic bowel loses protein-rich fluid into the intestinal wall and lumen. Major fluid losses occur because of the great length and surface areas of the intestines.<br>• The increase in catecholamine secretion accompanying the hypotensive state, as well as treatment with vasopressors, further impairs intestinal blood flow. | • Thrombosis of major mesenteric vein predisposes to paralytic ileus with intraluminal accumulation of fluid.<br>- Frequently characterized by local inflammation.<br>- May progress to venous gangrene. |

TABLE 52–1
**Intestinal Ischemic Disorders—Mesenteric Vascular Insufficiency *(Continued)***

| | Acute Superior Mesenteric Artery Occlusion | Chronic Mesenteric Occlusion | Nonocclusive Mesenteric Ischemia/ Infarction | Mesenteric Venous Ischemia |
|---|---|---|---|---|
| **Pathophysiology** *(cont.)* | • Intestinal mucosal epithelial cells are especially sensitive to the availability of oxygen; alterations within these cells occur within minutes of oxygen deprivation.<br>• Sudden arterial occlusion results in an ischemic infarct with intense vasospasm leading to mucosal ulceration; full intestinal wall thickness necrosis may occur with hemorrhagic infarction.<br>• Gangrenous changes occur, and as intraluminal pressure increases, perforation may occur resulting in generalized peritonitis, or localized abscess formation. | loss. Weight loss is further enhanced by the patient who does not eat in order to avoid crampy, abdominal pain that becomes associated with eating. | | |
| **Clinical Presentation**<br>Clinical features depend on:<br>• Length of intestine involved.<br>• Extent of vascular insufficiency.<br>• Rapidity of onset. | Episode is characterized by:<br>• Sudden, severe, colicky abdominal pain in the periumbilical area in response to the initial tense spasm of the small intestine.<br>• As ischemia persists, pain may become continuous and generalized throughout the abdomen.<br>• Urgent bowel movement, which may be diarrheal and bloody.<br>• Hematemesis may occur.<br>• Signs of shock: Hypotension, tachycardia, weakness, prostration, diaphoresis.<br>• Temperature elevation.<br>• Leukocytosis.<br>• Metabolic acidosis.<br>• Elevated phosphate level. | • Abdominal pain is usually the presenting symptom; it is described as crampy, located in the periumbilical area, and accompanied by hyperactive bowel sounds.<br>• If the ischemic episodes progress to infarction, there is the development of paralytic ileus with loss of bowel sounds, intestinal distention; and potentially hypovolemic shock.<br>• Diarrhea, constipation, and occult blood in the stool can occasionally be present.<br>• Abdominal pain accompanied by nonspecific nausea, vomiting, and diarrhea can make differential diagnosis more difficult. | • Clinically, the patient presents with diffuse abdominal pain or cramping; diarrhea, melena.<br>• Fever, dehydration with hemoconcentration; leukocytosis.<br>• Severe fluid and electrolyte imbalance may occur; metabolic acidosis.<br>• These patients may exhibit severe left ventricular failure, shock, or hypoxia. The consequent reduction in cardiac output causes blood to be diverted from the splanchnic circulation to the brain and other vital organs.<br>• Progressive dehydration leads to hypovolemia, tachycardia; reduced urine output. | • May present as abdominal emergency with diffuse pain.<br>• Signs of peritonitis may be evident, along with blood in stool (see "diagnosis" below). |

*(continued)*

TABLE 52-1
**Intestinal Ischemic Disorders—Mesenteric Vascular Insufficiency *(Continued)***

| | Acute Superior Mesenteric Artery Occlusion | Chronic Mesenteric Occlusion | Nonocclusive Mesenteric Ischemia/ Infarction | Mesenteric Venous Ischemia |
|---|---|---|---|---|
| **Clinical Presentation *(cont.)*** | | • Weight loss is frequently present and associated with fear of eating rather than anorexia. | | |
| **Diagnosis Clinical History** | Diagnostic triad:<br>• Sudden, severe abdominal pain.<br>• History of cardiac disease (e.g., myocardial infarction, atrial fibrillation; rheumatic heart disease, valvular disease). Such lesions are likely to produce embolization.<br>• Urgent bowel emptying with bloody diarrhea; hematemesis.<br>• History of previous embolic episodes. | Significant data:<br>• History of episodes of crampy, intermittent abdominal pain associated with eating (*post-prandial pain*).<br>• Weight loss associated with post-prandial pain. These patients become afraid to eat large meals.<br>• Malabsorption may occur with steatorrhea, weight loss, anemia. | Significant data:<br>• May mimic that of chronic occlusive disease. | Significant data:<br>• May present as abdominal catastrophe with an acute onset as seen in arterial infarction.<br>• Other cases may present more insidiously with a gradual and progressive course characterized by abdominal discomfort, anorexia, changes in bowel routine. |
| **Physical Examination** | Significant findings:<br>• "Surgical" abdomen with marked peritoneal signs (rebound tenderness, guarding, rigidity); absence of bowel sounds. | Significant findings:<br>• Abdominal tenderness (diffuse).<br>• Hyperactive bowel sounds.<br>If infarction occurs, there will be absent to hypoactive bowel sounds associated with ileus. | Significant findings:<br>• Abdominal pain/ tenderness.<br>• Bowel sounds may be hyperactive, reflecting initial spasm of the intestine. With progressive ischemia, the spasm relaxes and the bowel becomes atonic. | • Abdominal findings may be nonspecific; serosanguinous ascites may be detected; or<br>• An acute "surgical" abdomen may be seen.<br>• Blood in stool. |
| **Laboratory** | • Severe leukocytosis<br>• Severe metabolic acidosis.<br>• Elevated serum phosphate levels; urine and peritoneal fluid may likewise indicate elevated phosphate levels. | • Laboratory data similar to that of acute occlusion if ischemia progresses to infarction.<br>• Occasionally, occult blood in the stool. | • Elevated hematocrit reflects fluid loss (hemoconcentration)<br>• Marked leukocytes.<br>• Hyperkalemia associated with gut necrosis. | Sigmoidoscopy: May reveal a dusky, ischemic bowel with early signs of mucosal injury including edema and bleeding. |
| **Special Procedures** | Doppler ultrasonic flow detection and fluorescein fluorescence.<br>After injection with sodium fluorescein (IV), the bowel is examined under ultraviolet light to detect fluorescence. If the bowel fluoresces, perfusion is adequate. | | | |

TABLE 52-1
**Intestinal Ischemic Disorders—Mesenteric Vascular Insufficiency *(Continued)***

| | Acute Superior Mesenteric Artery Occlusion | Chronic Mesenteric Occlusion | Nonocclusive Mesenteric Ischemia/ Infarction | Mesenteric Venous Ischemia |
|---|---|---|---|---|
| **Arteriography** | Diagnosis must be confirmed by emergent, selective abdominal arteriography studies. | Because of the possibility of developing a full-blown intestinal infarction, arteriography studies are usually considered. Collateral circulation needs to be determined. | Arteriography can distinguish occlusive and nonocclusive intestinal ischemia. | • High degree of suspicion is imperative.<br>• Emergent, selective arteriography may be essential. |
| **Treatment** | Immediate goals:<br>• Reestablish hemodynamic stability and hemostasis.<br>• Prevent further progress of the underlying cause of the ischemia.<br>• Prevent complications.<br>Supportive measures:<br>• Blood product and fluid replacement therapy.<br>• Close monitoring of: Vital parameters (CVP, PCWP, cardiac output, systemic blood pressure, urine output, neurological status).<br>• Implement antibiotic therapy to treat sepsis.<br>Surgical interventions (based on arteriography studies):<br>• Endarterectomy.<br>• Embolectomy.<br>• Revascularization procedures.<br>Ultimate goals:<br>• Reestablish bowel continuity and gastrointestinal function. | Major concerns:<br>• If undiagnosed, and untreated, ischemia may progress to infarction.<br>• Decision to operate is difficult to make because such patients are poor surgical risks, and mortality is high.<br>• Risk of the operative procedure must be weighed against the high morality of the disease itself.<br>• Patients in whom arteriography studies confirm the diagnosis of intestinal infarction should have definitive treatment with surgical removal of the vascular obstruction, or bypass surgery.<br>• Selective surgical intervention. | Medical/conservative treatment directed toward:<br>• Reestablishing homeostasis.<br>• Improvement of pulmonary and cardiovascular function.<br>• Prevention of sepsis.<br>• Careful use of vasoconstrictor drug therapy to prevent further depression of splanchnic blood flow.<br>• Intra-arterial infusion of vasodilators such as papaverine and thrombolytic agents may be efficacious.<br>Supportive therapy:<br>• Broad spectrum antibiotics.<br>• Nasogastric suction and decompression to relieve vomiting and reduce abdominal distention. This may help to improve intramural blood flow.<br>• Fluid therapy to maximize cardiac output.<br>Surgical therapy:<br>• Resection of necrotic bowel.<br>• Embolectomy, endarterectomy, bypass grafting. | Acute mesenteric thrombosis is usually treated with bowel resection. |

*(continued)*

TABLE 52-1
**Intestinal Ischemic Disorders—Mesenteric Vascular Insufficiency *(Continued)***

| | Acute Superior Mesenteric Artery Occlusion | Chronic Mesenteric Occlusion | Nonocclusive Mesenteric Ischemia/ Infarction | Mesenteric Venous Ischemia |
|---|---|---|---|---|
| **Potential Complications** | Sepsis. Perforation. Peritonitis. Malnutrition. | Same as in acute occlusion. | Same in presence of infarction. | Same as in acute occlusive disease. |
| **Mortality** | • 60–70%. • Age and other organ system disease present greatest risk. | Same as in acute occlusion. | Poor prognosis is usually related to circumstances involving delays in diagnosis, and concomitant multiorgan complications (sepsis, renal failure). | Same as in cute occlusive disease. |

**Tentative Nursing Diagnoses**

1. Airway clearance, ineffective, related to:
   A. Ineffective cough.
2. Breathing pattern, alteration in, related to:
   A. Hypoventilation.
   B. Reduced mobility.
3. Anxiety related to:
   A. Lack of understanding regarding disease.
   B. Unfamiliar surroundings.
4. Fluid volume deficit, potential, related to:
   A. Vomiting, diarrhea.
   B. Inadequate oral fluid intake.
5. Electrolytes, alteration in, potential, related to:
   A. Vomiting, diarrhea.
   B. Inadequate dietary intake.
   C. Metabolic acidosis.
6. Tissue integrity impaired: integumentary; mucous membranes, related to:
   A. Nutritional deficit.
   B. Fluid deficit (dehydration).
   C. Immobility, activity intolerance.
7. Nutrition, alteration in: less than body requirements, related to:
   A. Anorexia.
   B. Malabsorption.
   C. Fear of precipitating abdominal pain by eating.
8. Comfort, alteration in:
   Abdominal pain ("intestinal angina").
9. Bowel elimination, alteration in, related to:
   A. Diarrhea; constipation.
10. Activity intolerance, potential, related to:
    A. Inadequate nutritional intake.
    B. Fatigue and exhaustion.
    C. Anemia.
11. Self-care deficit, related to:
    A. Weakness, exhaustion.
12. Sleep pattern disturbances, related to:
    A. Frequent bowel movements (diarrhea).
    B. Unfamiliar environment.
13. Coping, ineffective: individual and family, related to:
    A. Stigma of chronic disease.
    B. Impact on family lifestyle.

atherosclerosis affecting total body function. The challenge to nursing is to provide care that will ameliorate the bowel problem without causing a breakdown in another body system.

Immobility while hospitalized may predispose the patient to pressure necrosis and decubitus ulcer formation. Circulatory stasis will place the patient at risk of developing thrombophlebitis. Inadequate deep breathing and coughing exercises may predispose to atelectasis, aspiration, and pneumonia. The patient is at high risk of developing infection (nosocomial). Elderly patients become easily disoriented when removed from familiar surroundings.

## INFLAMMATORY BOWEL DISEASE

Inflammatory bowel disease is a term that encompasses the clinical disorders of *regional enteritis* (*Crohn's* disease) and *ulcerative colitis*. This grouping reflects the fact that both disorders have many similarities in their clinical and pathologic presentation.

### Regional Enteritis (Crohn's Disease) and Ulcerative Colitis

While both regional enteritis (Crohn's disease) and ulcerative colitis have many similarities clinically, some definitive distinctions do exist, which impact on treatment and management of the overall clinical course of these disorders and their prognosis. The chronic nature of these diseases has particular implications for nursing care.

### Nursing Care Considerations

The patient with inflammatory bowel disease is often faced with a chronic disease process of unknown etiology and a variable clinical course. The relationship that develops between nurse and patient is one that may be most difficult yet assumes particular importance. The elements of trust, mutual respect and understanding, sharing and caring are essential if the therapeutic interventions are to be effective.

These patients are typically young and intelligent, and probably resentful of a disease that is affecting them during the most productive period of their lives. Compassionate and sympathetic understanding is important in gradually establishing a trustful relationship, one which encourages and provides patients with the opportunity to talk about themselves, to verbalize their fears and concerns, and to ventilate anger and other pent-up feelings. The nurse with a sympathetic "listening" ear can be supportive and reassuring, while at the same time carefully evaluating the patient's response to therapy and scrutinizing for clues suggestive of underlying problems. Such problems may be responsible for disease exacerbations.

See Table 52-2 for a comparison of regional enteritis and ulcerative colitis, including their etiology, pathophysiology, clinical presentation, diagnosis, and treatment. Tentative nursing diagnoses pertinent to the care of the patient with inflammatory bowel disease are also listed.

## INTESTINAL OBSTRUCTION

An intestinal obstruction is defined as an interruption in the normal flow of contents through the gastrointestinal tract. It is a relatively common complication, frequently occurring postoperatively. The intestinal obstruction may be acute or chronic, partial or complete. Overall mortality for intestinal obstruction ranges from 10%-20%; in the setting of strangulated bowel obstruction, mortality may range as high as 75%. Clinically, complete obstruction of the small bowel can be life-threatening, signaling the need for early diagnosis and timely and appropriate surgical intervention.

### Classification

Mechanisms underlying intestinal obstruction include nonmechanical and mechanical. In a nonmechanical obstruction, the intestinal lumen remains unobstructed, but bowel motility is disrupted and the luminal contents cannot be moved along. This type of intestinal obstruction is commonly associated with altered autonomic nervous system control of intestinal motility. It usually develops within the small intestine after abdominal surgery. Mechanical obstruction may be caused by an intraluminal obstruction or obstruction associated with extraluminal pressure. Four types of mechanical obstruction of the bowel are defined: simple, closed-loop, strangulated, and incarcerated obstruction.[1]

A *simple* obstruction involves blockage of the bowel at 1 point only; a *closed-loop* obstruction involves obstruction at 2 points, thereby isolating a loop of bowel that cannot be decompressed. In this type of obstruction, an increase in intraluminal pressure can rapidly ensue, leading to ischemia and infarction. A *strangulated* obstruction is characterized by a blockage in a section of bowel to which some or all of the blood supply is compromised. Should the strangulated segment develop necrosis, an *incarcerated* obstruction results.

### Etiology

Causes of nonmechanical intestinal obstruction include paralytic ileus, electrolyte imbalance, neurogenic abnormalities, and thromboemboli occurring within the splanchnic vascular bed. A paralytic ileus is the most common cause of nonmechanical obstruction. It involves an inhibition of intestinal peristalsis usually involving the ileum. It occurs largely postoperatively following abdominal surgery, or procedures involving bowel manipulation. It has also been noted in patients with peritonitis.

Causes of mechanical obstruction, either partial

TABLE 52–2
**Inflammatory Bowel Disease: Regional Enteritis (Crohn's Disease) and Ulcerative Colitis**

| | Regional Enteritis (Crohn's Disease) | Ulcerative Colitis |
|---|---|---|
| ***Definition*** | A chronic, relapsing inflammatory disease of the intestinal tract characterized by granulomatous formation (i.e., nodular inflammatory lesions) especially involving the terminal ileus. | A nonspecific inflammatory disease of the large intestine characterized by alternating periods of remissions and exacerbations. |
| ***Incidence*** | • 2–4/100,000 population. | • 5–10/100,000 population. |
| ***Sex, Age (peak occurrence)*** | • Affects men and women equally.<br>• Young adults (usually white); 15–35 years of age. | • Same.<br>• Young adults (usually white); 20–40 years of age predominantly; there is a slight rise in incidence in ages 50–60 years. |
| ***Familial/Genetic Association*** | Frequently present. There is a definitive familial relationship between Crohn's disease, ulcerative colitis, and ankylosing spondylitis (arthritis of the vertebral spine). | Same. |
| ***Etiology and Pathogenesis*** | • Unknown.<br>Autoimmune phenomenon:<br>1. A hypersensitivity to a presently unidentified infectious agent; no auto-antibodies have been demonstrated.<br>2. Altered cell-mediated immune response demonstrated by lymphocyte-mediated cytotoxicity for intestinal mucosal epithelial cells.<br>3. Extracolonic manifestations of the disease are similar to other disorders associated with autoimmune phenomenon (e.g., arthritis, and pericholangitis).<br>4. Efficacy of immunosuppressive drugs (e.g., corticosteroids) in treatment of Crohn's disease.<br>• Viral origin (currently under investigation).<br>(For a discussion of the immune response, see Chapter 54, Immune System: Underlying Principles.) | • Unknown.<br>Autoimmune phenomenon:<br>1. Presence of anticolon epithelial cell antibodies in serum.<br>2. Lymphotoxic antibody has been found to damage normal colon mucosal cells in tissue culture.<br>3. Possible disturbance in cell-mediated immune response associated with disturbed T-lymphocyte function.<br>4. Concomitant association with other disorders suspected of having an autoimmune basis (e.g., erythema nodosum, arthritis, uveitis, autoimmune hemolytic anemia).<br>• Intestinal infection (causative organism(s) remain unidentified).<br>• Psychological/stress factors may play a secondary role in provoking overt disease. |
| ***Pathology*** | • The inflammatory lesions may be granulomatous in nature, consisting of granular, firm and persistent nodules containing a proliferation of macrophages.<br>• The inflammatory lesions may involve any part of the gastrointestinal tract, including the esophagus and stomach. Predominantly, there is extensive involvement of the terminal ileus.<br>• Crohn's disease is distinguished from ulcerative colitis:<br>1. Rarely involves colon and rectum.<br>2. Lesions are discontinuous with severely involved segments of bowel separated by apparently healthy bowel ("skip" lesions).<br>3. The bowel wall is significantly thickened with narrowing of the intestinal lumen which can predispose to intestinal obstruction.<br>4. The external appearance of the bowel is diseased with serositis; adhesions, internal strictures, and fistula formation commonly occur.<br>5. Crohn's disease is a transmural disease affecting all layers of the intestinal wall (see Fig. 47–4), and accounting in part for the thickening of the wall; the mucosal layer is least severely affected, but is commonly inflamed and ulcerated. Extensive fibrosis may be evident on surgery. | • A disease of the colon that usually involves the rectum and progresses proximally in a continuous manner to involve the entire colon. A pancolitis that involves the entire colon up to the ileocecal valve is sometimes seen.<br>• Ulcerative colitis does *not* involve the small intestine.<br>• Inflammatory reaction is localized to the mucosal and submucosal layers of the large intestinal wall. The primary response involves the mucosal epithelial cell both at its luminal surface, and in the crypts of Lieberkuhn (see Fig. 47–6). Early changes include congestion and dilation of capillaries. Cellular infiltration consists of lymphocytes, plasma cells, and eosinophils. Crypt abscesses may contain numerous polymorphonuclear leukocytes (PMNs).<br>• Mucosal and submucosal layers appear markedly hyperemic and hemorrhagic; mucosa especially becomes very friable, bleeds readily, and becomes susceptible to ulceration; edema of the submucosal layer usually occurs. Ulceration initially is scattered and shallow; in later stages the mucosa is lost over wide areas with a consequent significant loss of tissue, protein and blood.<br>• With continuous inflammation, there |

TABLE 52–2
**Inflammatory Bowel Disease: Regional Enteritis (Crohn's Disease) and Ulcerative Colitis *(Continued)***

| | Regional Enteritis (Crohn's Disease) | Ulcerative Colitis |
|---|---|---|
| ***Pathology (cont.)*** | 6. This disease process involves the mesentary and regional lymph nodes. | occurs loss of crypts and thinning of mucosa, which gives the appearance of being denuded.<br>• Inflammatory polyps (pseudopolyposis) may occur due to hyperplastic overgrowth of regenerating mucosa.<br>• Adhesions, internal strictures and fistula formation are rare; regional lymph nodes are uninvolved. There is minimal fibrosis. |
| ***Clinical Presentation*** | • Largely dependent upon region of gastrointestinal tract involved with the inflammatory process.<br>• Usual complaints include:<br>–Diarrhea with crampy right lower quadrant pain. There is usually a history of fatigue, weight loss, anorexia, nausea and vomiting; a low-grade fever may be detected.<br>• Clinical features usually reflect the location of inflammatory lesions and their relationship to adjacent structures.<br>• Abdominal pain may be steady and localized to the right lower quadrant; or it may be colicky and crampy, reflecting variable degrees of intestinal stenosis.<br>• Occasionally the patient may initially present with sudden onset of right lower quadrant pain suggestive of acute appendicitis. On surgical laparotomy the terminal ileum is found to be hyperemic and "boggy" with very edematous lymph nodes.<br>• Diarrhea is usually without blood.<br>• Extensive small bowel involvement may predispose to malabsorption of nutrients, vitamins and minerals; bile salt insufficiency may occur.<br>• Bacterial flora overgrowth may occur.<br>• Intestinal obstructions, fistula and abscess formation are frequent occurrences in chronic regional enteritis.<br>• Extraintestinal manifestations: See ulcerative colitis. | Classifications:<br>• Acute fulminating: Abrupt onset with severe bloody diarrhea, nausea, vomiting, high fever; with rapid depletion of fluid and electrolytes.<br>–Cardinal symptoms: Abdominal pain and bloody diarrhea (20–30 stools/day). Entire colon may be involved, with structural disruption of the mucosa with consequent loss of blood, mucus, protein, and fluid.<br>• Chronic intermittent: Insidious onset occurring over months to years; attacks (exacerbations) occur for periods of 1–3 months, with remissions between episodes.<br>–Clinically, the patient may be without fever, with nonspecific symptoms; only the distal colon may be affected.<br>• Chronic continuous: Characterized by mild diarrhea with intermittent bleeding; if diarrhea is more severe (>6 stools per day), there is consequent increased loss of blood and protein resulting in anemia and hypoproteinemia. Episodes of severe, colicky, lower abdominal pain may occur, and are somewhat relieved by defecation.<br>• Weight loss is a common occurrence in all types.<br>• Anorexia, nausea, vomiting, and hypokalemia (from chronic diarrhea) may be detected.<br>• Diarrheal stools may be of a semiformed consistency; 5–6 stools/day; or a disabling 20–30 liquid stools per day consisting of liquid fecal matter.<br>• Extraintestinal manifestations: Skin—erythema nodosum, perianal inflammation; eye—conjunctivitis, uveitis; renal—calcium oxalate calculi, ureteral obstruction.<br>–Hepatobiliary: Fatty infiltration; pericholangitis; bile duct carcinoma; chronic active hepatitis.<br>–Musculoskeletal: Peripheral arthritis; ankylosing spondylitis.<br>• Chronic course of this disease with remissions and exacerbations may be associated with depression and/or anxiety in patients who experience considerable costs in terms of time, money, and damaged careers. |
| ***Diagnosis***<br>***Clinical History***<br>***Physical Examination*** | A high degree of suspicion should accompany a clinical history of:<br>1. Intermittent diarrhea and abdominal pain.<br>2. Fever, weight loss, persistent perianal sepsis.<br>3. Extracolonic manifestations: arthritis, uveitis, pericholangitis. | Initial presentation may pose a diagnostic challenge.<br>Significant data:<br>1. History of bloody diarrhea and abdominal crampy pain.<br>2. Physical findings may be nonspecific.<br>A. More prominent abdomen.<br>B. Weight loss. |

*(continued)*

TABLE 52-2

**Inflammatory Bowel Disease: Regional Enteritis (Crohn's Disease) and Ulcerative Colitis *(Continued)***

| | Regional Enteritis (Crohn's Disease) | Ulcerative Colitis |
|---|---|---|
| ***Diagnosis Clinical History Physical Examination (cont.)*** | | C. Extracolonic manifestations may include: Ocular inflammation (uveitis, arthritis, jaundice). |
| ***Laboratory*** | Nonspecific.<br>• Stools for enteric pathogens, ova and parasites should be obtained to assist in differential diagnosis. Such studies should be conducted prior to barium studies as barium may temporarily suppress bacterial growth and interfere with their identification.<br>• Anemia: Nondeficiency; vitamin $B_{12}$ deficiency (malabsorption syndrome). | Nonspecific.<br>• Anemia (iron deficiency associated with chronic inflammation).<br>• Leukocytosis with febrile exacerbations.<br>• Hypoalbuminemia.<br>• Electrolyte disturbances.<br>• Mild increase in serum alkaline phosphatase.<br>• Elevated sedimentation rate. |
| ***Other Procedures*** | | • Proctoscopy/sigmoidoscopy: May reveal mucosal hyperemia with friable bleeding tissue and ulceration. The presence of a thick inflammatory exudate of pus, mucus, and blood may be observed.<br>• Colonoscopy: Helps to differentiate inflammatory bowel disease. Pseudopolyps and strictures may also be observed.<br>• Rectal biopsy: Provides confirmatory evidence of the inflammatory process. |
| ***Radiography*** | • Radiologic examination provides most definitive evidence in establishing diagnosis.<br>• Barium enema with reflux of barium into terminal ileum may demonstrate lesions of Crohn's disease with "skip" patterns.<br>• Barium studies should be avoided during acute episode; if necessary for diagnosis, such studies should be performed carefully, without extensive bowel preparation. | Barium enema: Helpful in assessing extent of disease process and presence of complications such as strictures, pseudopolyps, and carcinoma.<br>Such studies must be avoided during acute episodes as the combination of irritating barium and cleansing enemas may precipitate toxic megacolon. |
| ***Differential Diagnosis*** | Toxic megacolon can occur in regional enteritis but it is a more common occurrence in ulcerative colitis. | Differential diagnosis:<br>• Hemorrhoids (ruled out by sigmoidoscopy).<br>• Carcinoma (patients with colitis are at high risk of developing cancer).<br>• Amebiasis (bacillary dysentery) (ruled out by stool culture and serological studies).<br>• Laxative abuse with very voluminous, watery stools, dilated ascending colon, and loss of haustrations. A thorough history of patient's diet, bowel habits, and laxative use is essential to differential diagnosis. |
| ***Complications*** | Complications can involve adjacent or contiguous structures, or extraintestinal manifestations.<br>1. Intestinal obstruction is a frequent complication (20–30% of all patients with regional enteritis).<br>2. Fistula and abscess formation especially in the perirectal or perianal area.<br>3. Perforation, unlike ulcerative colitis, is an uncommon occurrence in regional enteritis because the bowel becomes greatly thickened in this disease process.<br>4. Extraintestinal complications include systemic disorders such as fatty liver, extensive pancreatic fibrosis, renal disease, erythema nodosum, pericholangitis, arthritis, among many others.<br>5. Carcinoma: Patients with regional enteritis are at less risk of developing a malignancy than patients with ulcerative colitis. | 1. Toxic megacolon: A severe fulminant form of the disease characterized by sudden, pronounced dilatation of the colon with accompanying abdominal distention, pain, alterations in vital signs, fluid and electrolyte imbalance.<br>Etiology of toxic megacolon includes vigorous use of cathartics, enemas, excessive use of anti-motility drugs (opiates and anticholinergics).<br>Toxic megacolon is thought to occur secondary to paralysis of motor function of transverse colon predisposing to rapid dilatation (as much as 9 cm in diameter) of that segment of bowel.<br>2. Bowel perforation: The sigmoid colon is most frequently implicated. Clinical manifestations include: Severe abdominal pain aggravated by any movement; shallow rapid respirations; rebound tenderness; |

TABLE 52–2
**Inflammatory Bowel Disease: Regional Enteritis (Crohn's Disease) and Ulcerative Colitis *(Continued)***

| | **Regional Enteritis (Crohn's Disease)** | **Ulcerative Colitis** |
|---|---|---|
| ***Complications (cont.)*** | 6. Hemorrhage associated with extensive denuding of mucosal surface, or local ulcer penetration into adjacent blood vessels of significant size. | fever, chills, nausea, vomiting, decreased urine output. Immediate treatment of toxic megacolon and/or bowel perforation is intestinal decompression and supportive fluid, electrolyte, and antibiotic therapy.<br>3. Massive hemorrhage.<br>4. Anorectal complications: Fissures, fistulae, and abscesses. Discomfort and anxiety produced by these complications are often of greater concern to patients than other colitis symptomatology.<br>5. Carcinoma: This is the most serious complication. Risk factors include: Duration of disease for >10 years; presence of pancolitis; and familial history of the disease.<br>6. Systemic complications include:<br>A. Nutritional and metabolic disturbances (malnutrition).<br>B. Thromboembolic disease.<br>C. Liver disease with fatty infiltration.<br>D. Erythema nodosum, cholangitis, joint manifestations. |
| ***Treatment*** | Goals of treatment: Same as for ulcerative colitis.<br>• Initial therapy is conservative, supportive, and palliative, aimed at attaining remission.<br>• Supportive care (see ulcerative colitis):<br>1. Medication therapy: Corticosteroids are the mainstay of treatment; azathioprine and sulfasalazine (azulfidine) may be used to control suppurative complications especially when there is large bowel involvement, and thus, promote remission.<br>2. Metamucil and Lomotil may help to reduce abdominal cramping, pain, and diarrhea.<br>• Nutritional deficiencies: In presence of malabsorption with steatorrhea, a low-fat, low-residue diet is prescribed when the patient can tolerate oral feedings.<br>– Vitamin $B_{12}$ replacement therapy.<br>– Bile acid binders such as cholestyramine may be helpful when ileal dysfunction is present.<br>Unabsorbed bile acids that reach the colon are conjugated by the bacterial flora, which in turn produces secretory diarrhea. | Goals of treatment:<br>1. Control inflammation.<br>2. Prevent malnutrition.<br>3. Relieve symptomatology.<br>4. Prevent infection and other complications.<br>5. Suppress immune response.<br>Supportive care:<br>1. Correct fluid and electrolyte imbalance. Patients with chronic diarrhea may be magnesium deficient.<br>2. Measures to "rest the bowel."<br>A. NPO.<br>B. Nasogastric suction.<br>C. Parenteral hyperalimentation.<br>3. Medication therapy.<br>A. Corticosteroid therapy: Goal of corticosteroid therapy is to reduce inflammation and suppress immune response. Efficacy of these drugs is reflected by improvement in the clinical picture: Reduction in diarrhea, abdominal pain, fever; and improvement in appetite.<br>When it can be tolerated, place patient on low-residue, high-protein, lactose-restricted diet. (Patients with lactose intolerance may develop cramps and diarrhea, symptoms that can interfere with evaluation as to the efficacy of the therapeutic regimen.)<br>B. Tincture of opium and paregoric may be used to control diarrhea.<br>C. Anticholinergic drugs may help to relieve abdominal cramps and diarrhea.<br>D. Sulfasalazine/sulfapyridine therapy.<br>4. Psychotherapy: May be especially helpful to patients with a chronic form of the disease. If a colectomy is indicated, such therapy may be crucial to assessing and strengthening coping and adaptive responses. |

*(continued)*

TABLE 52-2
**Inflammatory Bowel Disease: Regional Enteritis (Crohn's Disease) and Ulcerative Colitis *(Continued)***

| | Regional Enteritis (Crohn's Disease) | Ulcerative Colitis |
|---|---|---|
| ***Surgical Intervention*** | Surgical intervention is usually reserved for those cases in which conservative, medical therapy has been unsuccessful, or complications have occurred. Recurrences and spread of inflammatory lesions frequently follows surgical interventions.<br>Specific indications for surgery include:<br>1. Partial or complete intestinal obstruction.<br>2. Internal and/or external fistulas.<br>3. Massive hemorrhage.<br>• Resection of grossly diseased bowel with reanastomosis is the surgical procedure of choice in small bowel disease. | Surgical interventions: Development of toxic megacolon is the most urgent indication for a colectomy.<br>Other indications include:<br>1. The patient who fails to improve after 2–3 weeks of intensive supportive therapy; persistent and severe diarrhea; rectal bleeding, pain, fever, and weight loss.<br>2. Danger of life-threatening hemorrhage.<br>3. Stricture formation.<br>4. Suspicion of malignancy.<br>5. Chronic debilitating form of the disease, poorly controlled by medical management. |
| ***Prognosis*** | In some patients the disease process pursues a benign and uneventful course. In others the clinical course is dominated by a severe inflammatory process with numerous complications requiring multiple hospitalizations and vigorous therapy.<br>Probably ~ 75% of patients with regional enteritis will experience recurrences, and with each new exacerbation, the incidence or morbidity and mortality increases. | Prognosis is favorably influenced by use of anti-inflammatory drugs and parenteral nutrition; probability of inducing remissions in hospitalized patients is high. The effects of such therapy on chronic forms of the disease is more difficult to assess.<br>• Surgical interventions (total colectomy) may be curative. |
| ***Tentative Nursing Diagnosis*** | 1. Anxiety related to:<br>A. Lack of understanding regarding disease, and its impact on patient/family lifestyles.<br>B. Prescribed surgery (ileostomy, colostomy).<br>C. Uncertain prognosis.<br>2. Bowel elimination, alteration in: Diarrhea.<br>3. Fluid volume deficit, potential, related to:<br>A. Vomiting, diarrhea.<br>B. Inadequate oral fluid intake (dehydration).<br>4. Electrolytes, alteration in, potential, related to:<br>A. Vomiting, diarrhea.<br>B. Inadequate dietary intake.<br>C. Metabolic acidosis.<br>5. Comfort, alteration in: Abdominal cramping and pain.<br>6. Nutrition, alteration in: Less than body requirements, related to:<br>A. Anorexia.<br>B. Malabsorption.<br>C. Depression.<br>7. Activity intolerance, potential, related to:<br>A. Inadequate dietary intake.<br>B. Fatigue and exhaustion.<br>C. Anemia.<br>8. Mobility, impaired physical, related to:<br>A. Fear that movement will provoke abdominal pain and diarrhea.<br>9. Skin integrity, impairment of: Potential, related to:<br>A. Compromised nutrition.<br>B. Reluctance to move around in bed for fear of stimulating peristalsis and consequent abdominal cramping and pain.<br>10. Knowledge deficit, related to:<br>A. Therapeutic regimen (diet, medications, activity).<br>B. Care of ileostomy, colostomy.<br>11. Self-care deficit, related to;<br>Ostomy care.<br>12. Coping, ineffective individual, related to:<br>A. Chronic disease.<br>B. Potential need for ileostomy or colostomy.<br>C. Depression; emotional instabillity.<br>D. Unidentified support system.<br>13. Sleep pattern disturbance, related to:<br>A. Frequent bowel movements (diarrhea).<br>B. Unfamiliar environment.<br>C. Anxiety.<br>14. Self-concept, disturbance in, related to:<br>A. Physiological changes associated with long-term steroid therapy.<br>B. Embarrassment associated with diarrhea; ostomy care.<br>C. Stigma of chronic disease.<br>D. Dependence upon others for self-care. | |

or complete, are most commonly associated with adhesions and strangulated hernias usually involving the small intestine. Carcinomas, especially in middle-aged and older population, are the most common cause of large bowel obstruction. Other causative disorders include *intussusception* (i.e., an invagination of one section of bowel into the next section) and *volvulus* (i.e., a twisting of the intestine on its self). The former occurs largely in young children, the latter predominately in the elderly population.

## Pathophysiology

Whether an intestinal obstruction is mechanical or nonmechanical, the underlying pathophysiologic events are similar. Proximal to the obstruction, an accumulation of fluid, swallowed air, and gas causes the bowel to become progressively distended. Initially, peristalsis becomes accentuated as the bowel attempts to move its contents through the obstruction. With progressive distention, intraluminal pressure rises and peristalsis ceases. There occurs an accumulation of water and electrolytes within the proximal bowel as the absorptive capability of the intestinal mucosa becomes compromised. Because 8–10 liters of fluid (saliva, gastric and intestinal juices, and biliary and pancreatic secretions) are secreted into the lumen every 24 hours, nonabsorption leads to rapid accumulation of intra-luminal fluids. The consequent continuing distention of the bowel triggers a vicious cycle characterized by decreased absorption and increased secretion into the bowel. A profound fluid and electrolyte imbalance evolves.

Pressure of the distended bowel compromises blood circulation to the intestines, predisposing to ischemia. The consequent disruption of cellular membrane permeability causes stagnant, bacteria-laden fluid and toxins to pass into the systemic circulation. Major fluid and electrolyte losses may be enhanced by vomiting or nasogastric suctioning. Upper gastrointestinal obstruction leads to metabolic alkalosis associated with fluid depletion and loss of gastric hydrochloric acid; in lower obstructions, loss of bicarbonate predisposes to metabolic acidosis. Without prompt intervention, the patient can rapidly develop hypovolemic shock.

## Clinical Presentation

The clinical presentation depends on whether there is a small or large bowel obstruction. The cardinal symptoms of small bowel obstruction include cramplike abdominal pain, usually occurring in waves. A colicky pain is sometimes described, particularly in the scenario of strangulated bowel or peritonitis. There may be nausea and vomiting. The vomiting of fecal contents suggests a complete small bowel obstruction. Hiccups are often present, especially in mechanical obstruction. On auscultation, bowel sounds may be of a high tinkling quality with rushes and borborygmi. On palpation, the bowel may be tender with muscle guarding and abdominal distention.

A large bowel obstruction may present clinically with constipation. Abdominal pain, often colicky and continuous, may be described. There is abdominal distention. Nausea may be reported early; possible vomiting of fecal material may occur later in the course. Respiratory complications (atelectasis, compromised alveolar ventilation, and pneumonia) may occur, associated with decrease in respiratory excursion. Overall, the patient's clinical presentation is marked by significant fluid, electrolyte, and acid–base imbalances (see Chaps. 23 and 30, respectively).

## Diagnosis

The diagnosis of intestinal obstruction is confirmed on x-ray, which reflects the presence and location of intestinal gas and fluid. In small bowel obstruction, there is a typical pattern of gas throughout the large intestine but with little or no gas in the small intestine. A barium enema usually indicates a distended, barium-filled large intestine. Distention of a closed loop of sigmoid may be revealed.

Laboratory data reflect underlying hydration, electrolyte, and acid–base imbalance. An increase in the WBC count suggests possible peritonitis and/or strangulation with necrosis of a section of bowel. An increase in serum amylase may reflect pancreatitic irritation.

## Treatment

Treatment of intestinal obstruction involves the timely and aggressive correction of fluid, electrolyte, and acid–base imbalance, and shock, if present; decompression of distended bowel by use of nasogastric or Miller-Abbott tube; treatment of peritonitis or other infection; and removal of the obstruction. If the patient does not improve with conservative management, surgery is necessary. Surgical resection with end-to-end anastomosis is performed. Resection of the large bowel may involve creating a colostomy or ileostomy.

## Nursing Care Considerations

Nursing care of the patient with partial or complete bowel obstruction involves ongoing vigilant assessment and skillful supportive care. Vital signs require close monitoring, and the nurse must keenly observe for signs of shock (cool, clammy skin, pallor, and hypotension, altered state of consciousness); acid–base imbalance (altered breathing pattern, altered sensorium, abnormal arterial blood gases); and electrolyte imbalance (altered serum sodium, potassium, chloride and bicarbonate levels, elevated BUN in the presence of dehydration). Fever, chills, and leukocytosis, with a shift to the left (i.e., an increase in the number of immature WBCs), are reflective of infection. Muscle guarding or boardlike abdomen on palpation suggests peritonitis.

A strict intake and output should be maintained, and daily weight should be determined. These activities assist in monitoring the patient's fluid status. Measurement of abdominal girth can also assist in detecting progressive distention.

Meticulous mouth care is essential. Significant dehydration may cause the lips to become cracked, the tongue thickened and swollen, and the mucous membranes dry. Vomiting of foul, fecal-like fluid can be especially distressful to patient and family. Special care to the nares is essential if a nasogastric tube is in place.

A semi-Fowler's position should be maintained to facilitate respiratory excursion in the presence of significant abdominal distention. Coughing and deep breathing are necessary to ensure adequate alveolar ventilation. If a weighted nasogastric or intestinal tube has been placed, it may be necessary to help the patient to change positions to help facilitate passage of the tube. Keep the family and patient advised as to the patient's progress. Provide necessary support and reassurance.

### *Tentative Nursing Diagnoses and Possible Etiologies*

Tentative nursing diagnoses and their etiologies in the care of the patient with partial or complete intestinal obstruction may include the following:

1. Alteration in comfort: Pain, related to intestinal obstruction and altered bowel function.
2. Fluid volume deficit, related to:
   A. NPO status.
   B. Vomiting.
   C. Nasogastric decompression.
3. Cardiac output, alteration: Decreased, related to:
   A. Reduced circulating blood volume.
   B. Third-spacing of fluid within the peritoneal cavity or distended bowel.
4. Breathing pattern, ineffective, related to reduced respiratory excursion associated with abdominal distention.
5. Bowel elimination, alteration in, related to intestinal obstruction.
6. Nutrition, altered: Less than body requirements, related to:
   A. NPO status.
   B. Hypoproteinemia associated with peritonitis.
7. Tissue integrity, impaired: Oral mucous membranes, related to:
   A. NPO status.
   B. Dehydration.
   C. Mechanical injury associated with intestinal decompression.
8. Coping, ineffective, family and individual, related to sudden illness possibly requiring major surgery.

## REFERENCE

1. McConnell, EA: Meeting the challenge of intestinal obstruction. Nursing '87 17(7):34, July 1987.

CHAPTER 53

# Nutritional Support of the Critically Ill Patient

*Joanne M. Farley*

## CHAPTER OUTLINE



## LEARNING OBJECTIVES

**At the end of this chapter, you should be able to:**

1. Explain the mechanisms for energy use.
2. Identify at least 2 results of malnutrition in the critically ill.
3. Outline key elements of a nutritional assessment.
4. List the 6 nutrients required by the critically ill patient.
5. Discuss the 2 major therapeutic modalities used in the treatment of patients with an altered nutritional status.

During the initial stages of a critical illness, nutrition is generally not afforded top priority. While this may be appropriate amid life-saving efforts, too often nutrition is the afterthought that could have saved the patient's life. Florence Nightingale recognized the importance of nutrition in 1859, in her book *Notes on Nursing.*[1] She commented that "thousands of patients are annually starved in the midst of plenty."[1] In the 1980s, there exists a 50% incidence of malnutrition among hospitalized patients.[2]

While technology in nursing has increased by leaps and bounds, some basic problems are unresolved. The critical care nurse needs a sound scientific basis from which to assess, deliver, and evaluate nutritional support. This chapter will review the mechanisms of energy use, nutritional assessment, and therapeutic modalities in the treatment of the patient with an altered nutritional status.

## MECHANISMS OF ENERGY USE

The critically ill patient who has undergone a period of starvation initially uses fuel from body stores. This fuel is derived from 3 sources: carbohydrates, protein, and fat. Carbohydrate is stored as glycogen. It is an inefficient source, however, because each gram of glycogen yields approximately 1–2 kcal/g. This discrepancy is due to the fact that carbohydrate found in glycogen is packed with water. A total of 600–900 kcal are derived from this source and are usually exhausted by normal persons within 1 day.

Protein is not actually meant to be used as fuel because each protein carries out a specific function necessary for the continued existence of the body. If protein is used as an energy source, it is to the detriment of many basic functions of life. For this reason, we attempt to *spare* protein. Protein found in excess of that needed for bodily processes is quickly metabolized and excreted.

Fat, on the other hand, is a rather abundant source of energy because it yields 9.4 kcal/g. Unfortunately, the brain cannot use fat for its metabolism, so the body searches for other means to supply the needed fuel.

One of these means is through the *phosphogluconate* pathway. Through this pathway, glycerol is converted to glucose, yielding up to 20 g (based on the energy use of a 70-kg man; Fig. 53–1).

The Cori cycle takes lactate and pyruvate from the glycolytic or Embden-Meyerhof pathway, recycles it in the liver and kidney, and produces up to 30 g of glucose. Gluconeogensis is the process by which glucose is supplied through the breakdown of protein. Approximately 125 g of glucose are supplied in this way. The brain then receives its supply of energy from the pool of 180 g of glucose provided by all 3 of these mechanisms. The brain uses about 145 g from this total.

One protective mechanism of the body during starvation is the conversion of tissues outside of the central nervous system (CNS) to the exclusive use of fatty acids, thus sparing protein from catabolism. In an effort to further reduce fuel requirements, normal persons reduce their metabolic rate. This, however, is not an option for the critically ill patient who may be hypermetabolic as a result of the disease state.

## RESULTS OF MALNUTRITION IN THE CRITICALLY ILL

The critically ill patient often suffers from a multiplicity of problems. The picture can be further complicated should he/she develop any of several complications of malnutrition. The results of malnutrition may involve any one of the following end-organ effects[3] (Fig. 53–2):

- Delayed wound healing.
- Predisposition to intraoperative hemorrhage.
- Infection.
- Cardiac failure unresponsive to inotropic agents.
- Difficulty in refeeding.
- Pneumonia.

It is the critical care nurse's responsibility to assess patients who may be at risk for developing these problems.

## NUTRITIONAL ASSESSMENT

A comprehensive nutritional assessment supplies the nurse with invaluable information regarding the patient's nutritional status. This assessment should be completed as soon after admission to the hospital as possible. Periodic assessments are made throughout the hospitalization to evaluate the effect of the prescribed nutritional therapy. A nutritional assessment consists of several components: *a dietary history, anthropometric measurements, diagnostic tests*, and *physical examination*. No single parameter can be used in isolation, but multiple parameters are used to determine an individual's nutritional state.

### Dietary History

It is often not feasible to obtain a dietary history from the critically ill patient. Other sources, such as family and friends, can provide the necessary information. The history often provides clues as to the cause and degree of malnutrition. The components of a dietary history are listed in Table 53–1. The registered dietitian is trained to perform dietary histories and assess the adequacy of the patient's diet in meeting the recommended dietary allowances (RDAs).

Calorie counts are often employed to evaluate and monitor a patient's intake. Each day, the nurse accurately records all foods and fluids consumed by the patient and specifies type and amount. The registered dietitian calculates the protein and calories consumed daily. It is critical to perform calorie counts during weaning from parenteral nutrition or tube feedings to an oral diet.

### Anthropometric Measurements

Anthropometry is the measurement of a part or whole of the body. Because growth and development depend on nutrition, these measurements are used as criteria in a nutritional assessment. The most commonly used indices are height, weight,

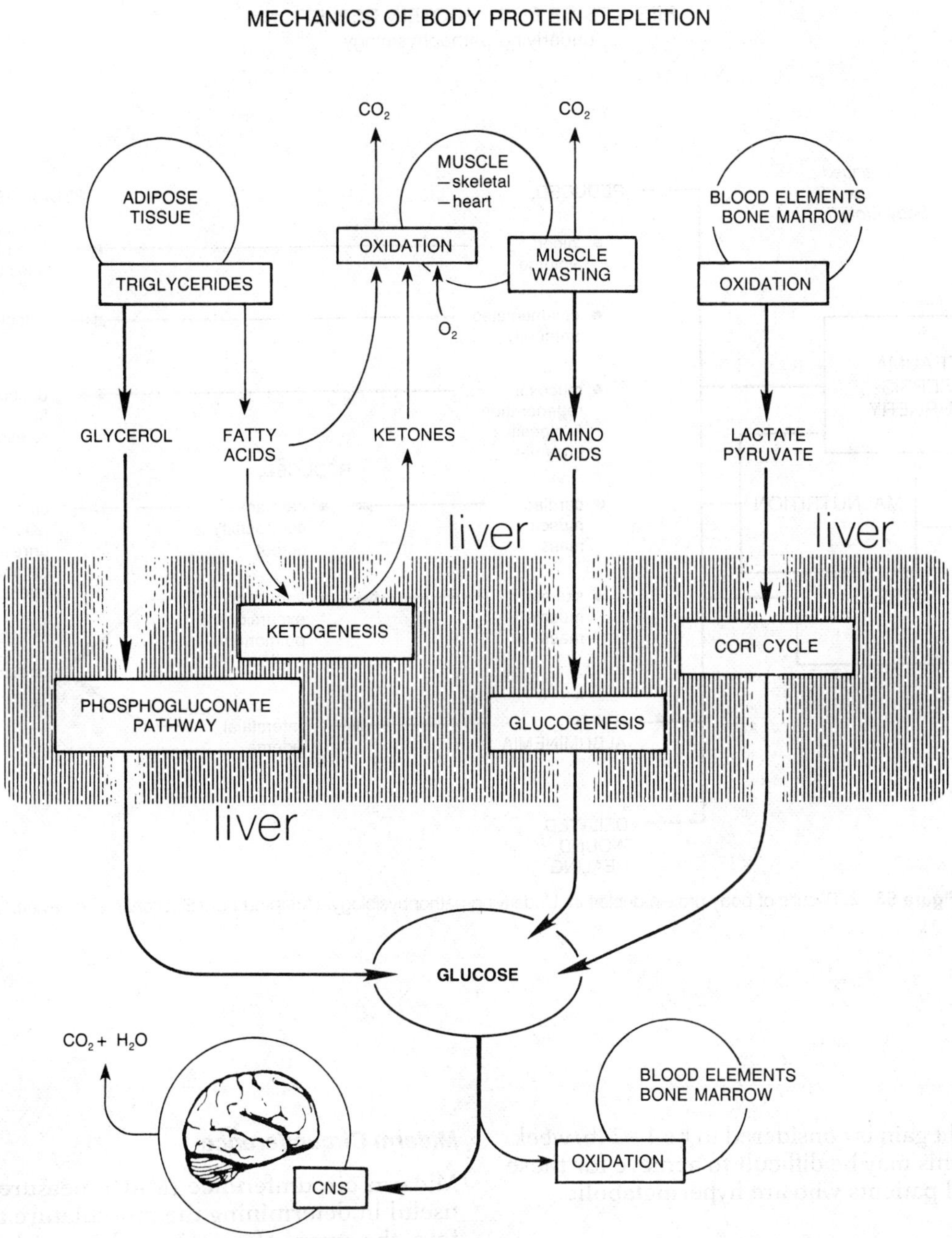


**Figure 53–1.** Mechanics of body protein depletion. (Adapted from Buchanan and Levine.[3])

skinfold thickness, midarm circumference, and midarm muscle circumference.

An initial height and weight are taken on admission whenever possible (Table 53–2). Serial weights provide helpful information related to the protein–calorie status of the person. A loss in weight may indicate a loss in lean body mass, while a weight gain may indicate a gain in lean body mass. It should be noted, however, that a weight gain or loss due to dynamic fluid movement may interfere with interpretation of these data. That is why it is so important that daily weights be taken at the same time each day. Many hospitalized patients lose weight at an alarming rate due to NPO status for tests, procedures, surgery or unpalatable meals; anorexia secondary to disease, fever, medications, chemotherapy, and so forth; as well as an atmosphere inconducive to eating. Serial weights are the *single most important* parameter available to monitor the nutritional status of a patient. This objective measurement will enable rapid nutritional support intervention.

A recent involuntary weight loss of 10% or more indicates a patient who is at risk nutritionally. Opti-

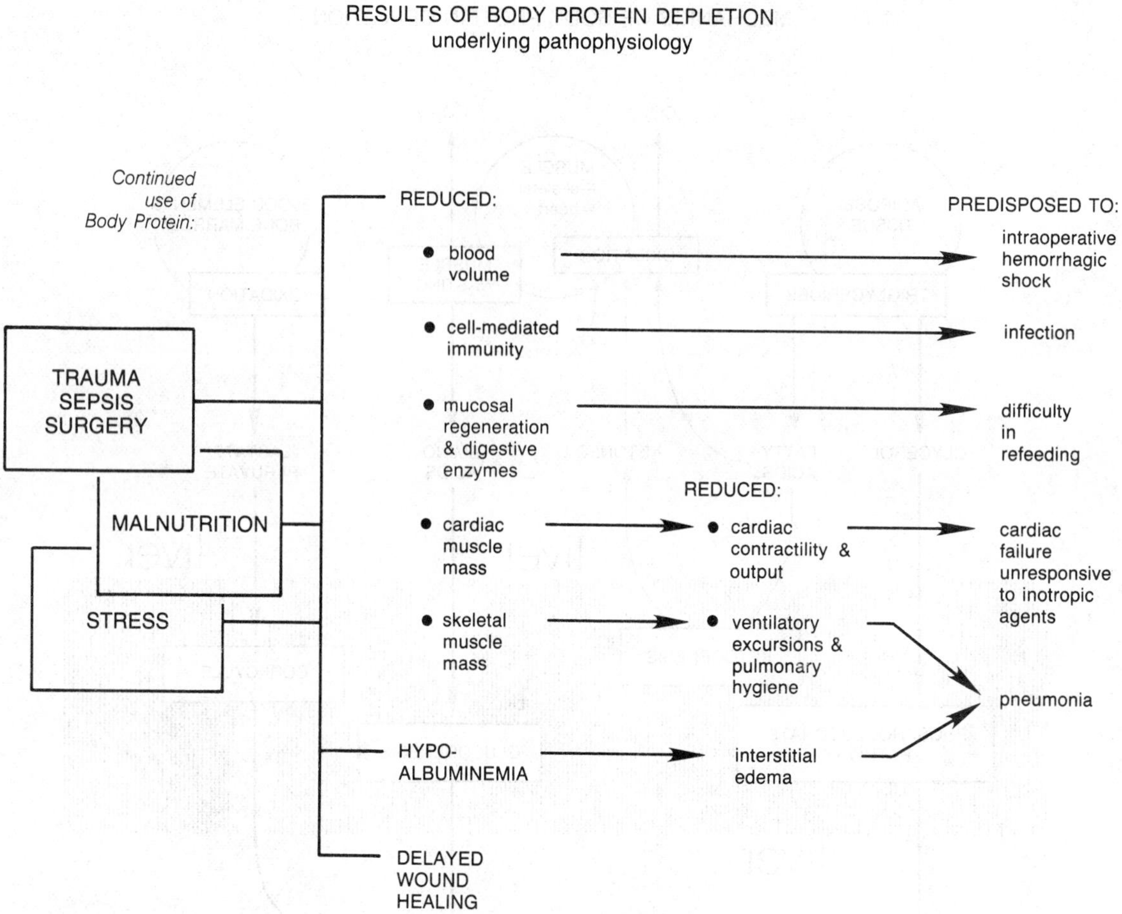


**Figure 53–2.** Results of body protein depletion. Underlying pathophysiology. (Adapted from Buchanan and Levine.[3])

mum weight gain is considered to be 1–2 lb/week. However, this may be difficult to achieve for those critically ill patients who are hypermetabolic.

### Skinfold Measurements

The measurement of triceps skinfold thickness (TSF) is the most inexpensive and simple means for assessing body fat. Skinfold measurements are indicative of subcutaneous fat, thus they are also indicative of caloric status. The measurement is taken on the nondominant arm by means of a caliper (Fig. 53–3). The caliper is placed over a pinched fold of skin on the posterior aspect of the arm over the triceps muscle. Two to three readings are obtained, and the average of these is calculated. The number in millimeters is converted to a percent standard using a simple formula (see Fig. 53–3), which is then compared with the population norm (Table 53–3).

### Midarm Circumference

Midarm circumference (MAC) measurements are useful in determining the musculature and, therefore, the extent of protein–calorie malnutrition. A measuring tape calibrated in centimeters is placed around the nondominant arm at its midpoint. The measurement is compared with the standard values for the variable (Table 53–4).

### Midarm Muscle Circumference

Midarm muscle circumference (MAMC) is a more useful criterion for assessing muscle mass reflecting available somatic protein. It is calculated by using both the TSF and MAC (see Fig. 53–3). This measurement is important in the critically ill patient because it also reflects the degree of usage of certain muscle groups. This number is also converted to a percent standard and compared with

TABLE 53-1
**Components of a Dietary History**

| Component | Description |
|---|---|
| Dietary intake | Include patient's usual dietary pattern and any recent changes in this pattern. |
| Appetite | State whether there has been a recent loss in appetite, noting the extent and any identified causative factors. |
| GI disturbances | Note whether the patient has been suffering from any of the following symptoms: Loss of appetite, heartburn, nausea, vomiting, diarrhea/constipation, bloating, gas, or distention. |
| Mechanical problems | State whether the patient has properly fitting dentures, available number of teeth to eat, or any difficulty in chewing or swallowing. |
| Food allergies/intolerance | Describe any adverse reaction the patient has in response to a particular food or food group. |
| Medications | State any medications that the patient was taking prior to admission that may interfere with nutrient uptake, or cause GI disturbances. |
| Food likes/dislikes | List foods that the patient especially likes or dislikes. State any ethnic preferences, religious, or medical restrictions. |

population norms. Because there are wide individual differences in anthropometric measurements, they are most informative when persons are used as their own norm over an extended period of time (Table 53-5).

ANTHROPOMETRIC MEASUREMENTS

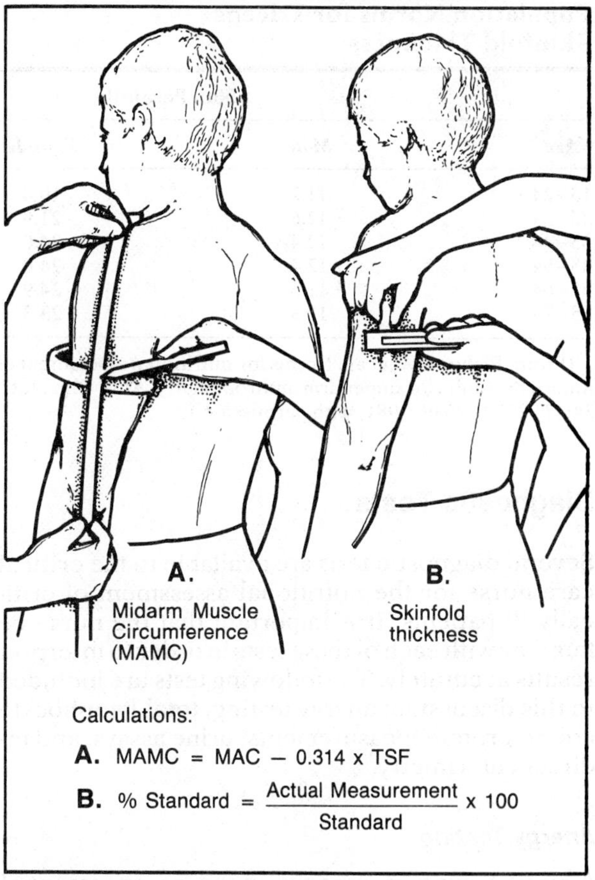


**Figure 53-3.** Anthropometric studies and calculations. Midarm circumference, and skinfold thickness. (Calculations adapted from Weinsier, RL and Butterworth, CE: Handbook of Clinical Nutrition. CV Mosby, St. Louis, 1981.)

TABLE 53-2
**1983 Metropolitan Height and Weight Tables**

| Men | | | | | Women | | | | |
|---|---|---|---|---|---|---|---|---|---|
| *Height* Feet | *Height* Inches | *Small Frame* | *Medium Frame* | *Large Frame* | *Height* Feet | *Height* Inches | *Small Frame* | *Medium Frame* | *Large Frame* |
| 5 | 2 | 128-134 | 131-141 | 138-150 | 4 | 10 | 102-111 | 109-121 | 118-131 |
| 5 | 3 | 130-136 | 133-143 | 140-153 | 4 | 11 | 103-113 | 111-123 | 120-134 |
| 5 | 4 | 132-138 | 135-145 | 142-156 | 5 | 0 | 104-115 | 113-126 | 122-137 |
| 5 | 5 | 134-140 | 137-148 | 144-160 | 5 | 1 | 106-118 | 115-129 | 125-140 |
| 5 | 6 | 136-142 | 139-151 | 146-164 | 5 | 2 | 108-121 | 118-132 | 128-143 |
| 5 | 7 | 138-145 | 142-154 | 149-168 | 5 | 3 | 111-124 | 121-135 | 131-147 |
| 5 | 8 | 140-148 | 145-157 | 152-172 | 5 | 4 | 114-127 | 124-138 | 134-151 |
| 5 | 9 | 142-151 | 148-160 | 155-176 | 5 | 5 | 117-130 | 127-141 | 137-155 |
| 5 | 10 | 144-154 | 151-163 | 158-180 | 5 | 6 | 120-133 | 130-144 | 140-159 |
| 5 | 11 | 146-157 | 154-166 | 161-184 | 5 | 7 | 123-136 | 133-147 | 143-163 |
| 6 | 0 | 149-160 | 157-170 | 164-188 | 5 | 8 | 126-139 | 136-150 | 146-167 |
| 6 | 1 | 152-164 | 160-174 | 168-192 | 5 | 9 | 129-142 | 139-153 | 149-170 |
| 6 | 2 | 155-168 | 164-178 | 172-197 | 5 | 10 | 132-145 | 142-156 | 152-173 |
| 6 | 3 | 158-172 | 167-182 | 176-202 | 5 | 11 | 135-148 | 145-159 | 155-176 |
| 6 | 4 | 162-176 | 171-187 | 181-207 | 6 | 0 | 138-151 | 148-162 | 158-179 |

(From: Metropolitan Life Insurance Company, New York, with permission.)

TABLE 53-3
**Population Norms for Triceps Skinfold Thickness**

| | 50th Percentile | |
|---|---|---|
| *Age* | *Male* | *Female* |
| 18-24 | 11.2 | 19.4 |
| 25-34 | 12.6 | 21.9 |
| 35-44 | 12.4 | 24.0 |
| 45-54 | 12.4 | 24.0 |
| 55-64 | 11.6 | 24.9 |
| 65-74 | 11.8 | 23.3 |

(From: Bishop CW, et al.: Norms for nutritional assessment of American adults for upper arm anthropometry. Am J Clin Nutr, 34(11):2530-2539, 1981, with permission.)

## Diagnostic Tests

Several diagnostic tests are available to the critical care nurse for the nutritional assessment of critically ill patients. It is important that the nurse be familiar with each of these tests in order to interpret results accurately. The following tests are included in this discussion: anergy testing, total lymphocyte count, protein measurements, urine assays, and indirect calorimetry.

### Anergy Testing

Anergy testing is recommended as an essential component of a complete nutritional assessment. *Anergy* is defined as the lack of immune response to an antigen. A person who is malnourished is not able to mount an immunologic response to an antigen, because proper nutrition is key to an intact immune system.

Their test involves the intradermal injection (0.1 ml) of each of the following antigens on the volar surface of the forearm: *Candida*, *Trichophyton*, mumps, tuberculin, and streptodornase. The diameter of induration at each injection site is measured in millimeters, 24 and 48 hours following injection. A skin test is considered positive if the induration is 5 mm or greater.[4] A patient who does not respond to 2 of the antigens is considered anergic and, therefore, possibly malnourished. This test is not definitive for malnourishment because false negatives can occur with advanced age, recent surgery or trauma, cancer, or immunosuppressive therapy.[4-6]

### Total Lymphocyte Count

Total lymphocyte count (TLC) is also a measure of the body's immune response. A low count indicates a depressed immune status reflecting protein-calorie malnutrition (Table 53-6). A false negative may be seen with this test as with the antigen skin tests.

TABLE 53-4
**Population Norms for Midarm Circumference**

| Age Group, Years | Age Midpoint, Years | Midarm Circumference Percentiles, mm, 50th |
|---|---|---|
| ***Males*** | | |
| 0.0-0.4 | 0.3 | 106 |
| 0.5-1.4 | 1 | 123 |
| 1.5-2.4 | 2 | 127 |
| 2.5-3.4 | 3 | 132 |
| 3.5-4.4 | 4 | 135 |
| 4.5-5.4 | 5 | 141 |
| 5.5-6.4 | 6 | 146 |
| 6.5-7.4 | 7 | 151 |
| 7.5-8.4 | 8 | 158 |
| 8.5-9.4 | 9 | 161 |
| 9.5-10.4 | 10 | 168 |
| 10.5-11.4 | 11 | 174 |
| 11.5-12.4 | 12 | 181 |
| 12.5-13.4 | 13 | 195 |
| 13.5-14.4 | 14 | 211 |
| 14.5-15.4 | 15 | 220 |
| 15.5-16.4 | 16 | 229 |
| 16.5-17.4 | 17 | 245 |
| 17.5-24.4 | 21 | 258 |
| 24.5-34.4 | 30 | 270 |
| 34.5-44.4 | 40 | 270 |
| ***Females*** | | |
| 0.0-0.4 | 0.3 | 104 |
| 0.5-1.4 | 1 | 117 |
| 1.5-2.4 | 2 | 125 |
| 2.5-3.4 | 3 | 128 |
| 3.5-4.4 | 4 | 132 |
| 4.5-5.4 | 5 | 138 |
| 5.5-6.4 | 6 | 140 |
| 6.5-7.4 | 7 | 146 |
| 7.5-8.4 | 8 | 151 |
| 8.5-9.4 | 9 | 157 |
| 9.5-10.4 | 10 | 163 |
| 10.5-11.4 | 11 | 171 |
| 11.5-12.4 | 12 | 179 |
| 12.5-13.4 | 13 | 185 |
| 13.5-14.4 | 14 | 193 |
| 14.5-15.4 | 15 | 195 |
| 15.5-16.4 | 16 | 200 |
| 16.5-17.4 | 17 | 196 |
| 17.5-24.4 | 21 | 205 |
| 24.5-34.4 | 30 | 213 |
| 34.5-44.4 | 40 | 216 |

(Adapted from Frisancho A: Triceps skinfold and upper arm muscle size norms for assessment of nutritional status. Am J Clin Nutr 27:1052, 1974.)

### Serum Protein Measurements

Several serum protein measurements may be monitored as indicators of nutritional status. Currently these include *albumin*, *transferrin*, and *prealbumin*. Albumin and transferrin levels are the most widely used for clinical purposes.[7] Unfortunately, these levels lack specificity and sensitivity due to their prolonged serum half-life (Table 53-7).

Along with the confounding effect of disease and medications, some of the medical conditions other

TABLE 53-5
**Population Norms for Midarm Muscle Circumference**

| | 50th Percentile | |
|---|---|---|
| *Age* | *Male* | *Female* |
| 18-24 | 27.4 | 20.9 |
| 25-34 | 28.3 | 21.7 |
| 35-44 | 28.8 | 22.5 |
| 45-54 | 28.2 | 22.7 |
| 55-64 | 27.8 | 22.8 |
| 65-74 | 26.8 | 22.8 |

Reprinted with permission from Bishop CW, et al.: Norms for Nutritional Assessment of American adults for upper arm anthropometry. Am J Clin Nutr 34(11):2530-2539, 1981.

than malnutrition that may lower protein levels include malabsorption syndrome, liver failure, renal failure, infection, cancer, recent surgery, burns, wounds, and overhydration.[8] Despite their problems, these protein levels are frequently obtained because they are readily available and easy to perform.

Several serum proteins with shorter half-lives have been investigated. One of these is prealbumin (thyroxine-binding prealbumin), which has a half-life of 2 days. Use of this protein in serum evaluations could potentially lead to a more rapid patient assessment and earlier intervention. Normal values for each of the serum proteins discussed are listed in Table 53-7. Values below the normal range may indicate protein-calorie malnutrition.

### *Urine Assays*

Urine assays can be obtained to measure the urinary excretion of creatinine and urea. A urine creatinine level provides an estimate of lean body mass because creatinine production is directly related to skeletal muscle mass. A *creatinine-height index (CHI)* is calculated by using the results of the urine creatinine clearance test. The CHI is the ratio of the observed creatinine to that expected for a normal adult of the same sex and height.

TABLE 53-6
**Total Lymphocyte Count: A Measure of Nutritional Deficiency**

| TLC | Nutritional Deficiency |
|---|---|
| 1200-1500 mm$^3$ | Mild |
| 800-1200 mm$^3$ | Moderate |
| 800 mm$^3$ | Severe |

Adapted from Silberman H and Eisenberg D: Parenteral and Enteral Nutrition for the Hospitalized Patient. Norwalk, Connecticut, Appleton-Century-Crofts, 1982, p 40.

TABLE 53-7
**Protein Measurements**

| Protein | Half Life | Normal Level |
|---|---|---|
| Albumin | 14-20 days | 3.5-5.5 gm/dl |
| Transferrin | 7-9 days | 200-400 mg/dl |
| Prealbumin | 2 days | 20-40 mg/dl |

A decreased CHI is one of the most reliable measures of skeletal muscle catabolism. Unlike body weight, the creatinine-height index is not affected by fluid retention. According to Blackburn and associates, CHI values of 60%-80% represent moderate skeletal muscle depletion, whereas values of 40%-50% signify severe depletion.[9]

The *urine urea nitrogen (UUN)* represents the end-product of protein metabolism, which is nitrogen. The 24-hour urine collection for UUN is used to calculate the balance between nitrogen intake and nitrogen output. The nitrogen intake is determined by a simultaneous 24-hour accurate calorie count. A negative balance reflects protein catabolism. The goal is always a positive nitrogen balance.

A 24-hour sample for UUN and CHI is collected in a container with preservative. It is no longer necessary to keep the specimen on ice during or immediately after collection.[10] These levels are a fairly accurate indicator of nutritional status, provided renal function is normal and the specimen is collected properly. But 24-hour urine specimens are difficult to obtain. Errors in interpretation of results frequently occur due to spillage or inadvertent discarding of the specimen.

## Physical Examination

The final phase of a nutritional assessment is the physical examination. Through this examination, physical findings indicative of deficiency states can be detected. Such findings reflect not only protein-calorie malnutrition, but vitamin and mineral deficiencies as well. These deficiencies can affect nearly every body system. Table 53-8 contains a list of physical findings and the deficiency states they represent.

Once a thorough nutritional assessment has been conducted and an actual or potential state of malnutrition has been identified, the caloric requirements of the particular patient must be calculated.

# CALORIC REQUIREMENTS OF THE CRITICALLY ILL

As has been mentioned previously, critically ill patients are often hypermetabolic due to their disease state. Energy expenditure in such patients is

TABLE 53–8
**Physical Findings Associated with Deficiency States**

| Physical Findings | Associated Deficiencies |
|---|---|
| ***Hair, Nails*** | |
| Flag sign (transverse depigmentation of hair) | Protein, copper |
| Hair easily pluckable | Protein |
| Hair thin, sparse | Protein, biotin, zinc |
| Nails spoon-shaped | Iron |
| Nails lackluster, transverse riding | Protein-calorie |
| ***Skin*** | |
| Dry, scaling | Vitamin A, zinc, essential fatty acids |
| Flaky paint dermatosis | Protein |
| Follicular hyperkeratosis | Vitamins A, C; essential fatty acids |
| Nasolabial seborrhea | Niacin, pyridoxine, riboflavin |
| Petechiae, purpura | Ascorbic acid, vitamin K |
| Pigmentation, desquamation (sun-exposed area) | Niacin (pellagra) |
| Subcutaneous fat loss | Calorie |
| ***Eyes*** | |
| Angular blepharitis | Riboflavin |
| Corneal vascularization | Riboflavin |
| Dull, dry conjunctiva | Vitamin A |
| Fundal capillary microaneurysms | Ascorbic acid |
| Scleral icterus, mild | Pyridoxine |
| ***Perioral*** | |
| Angular stomatitis | Riboflavin |
| Cheilosis | Riboflavin |
| ***Oral Cavity*** | |
| Atrophic lingual papillae | Niacin, iron, riboflavin, folate, vitamin $B_{12}$ |
| Glossitis (scarlet, raw) | Niacin, pyridoxine, riboflavin, vitamin $B_{12}$, folate |
| Hypogeusesthesia (also hyposmia) | Zinc, vitamin A |
| Magenta tongue | Riboflavin |
| Swollen, bleeding gums (if teeth present) | Ascorbic acid |
| Tongue fissuring, edema | Niacin |
| ***Glands*** | |
| Parotid enlargement | Protein |
| Sicca syndrome | Ascorbic acid |
| Thyroid enlargement | Iodine |
| ***Heart*** | |
| Enlargement, tachycardia, high output failure | Thiamine ("wet" beriberi) |
| Small heart, decreased output | Calorie |
| Sudden failure, death | Ascorbic acid |
| ***Abdomen*** | |
| Hepatomegaly | Protein |
| ***Muscles, Extremities*** | |
| Calf tenderness | Thiamine, ascorbic acid (hemorrhage into muscle) |
| Edema | Protein, thiamine |
| Muscle wastage (especially temporal area, dorsum of hand, spine) | Calorie |
| ***Bones, Joints*** | |
| Bone tenderness (adult) | Vitamin D, calcium, phosphorus (osteomalacia) |

TABLE 53–8
**Physical Findings Associated with Deficiency States *(Continued)***

| Physical Findings | Associated Deficiencies |
|---|---|
| ***Neurologic*** | |
| Confabulation, disorientation | Thiamine (Korsakoff's psychosis) |
| Decreased position and vibratory senses, ataxia | Vitamin $B_{12}$, thiamine |
| Decreased tendon reflexes, slowed relaxation phase | Thiamine |
| Ophthalmoplegia | Thiamine, phosphorus |
| Weakness, paresthesias, decreased fine tactile sensation | Vitamin $B_{12}$, pyridoxine, thiamine |
| ***Other*** | |
| Delayed healing and tissue repair (e.g., wound, infarct, abscess) | Ascorbic acid, zinc, protein |

Reprinted with permission from Morgan J: Nutritional assessment of critically ill patients. Focus on Critical Care 11(3):32–33, 1984.

often double the normal rate. Indirect calorimetry is a tool used to determine energy expenditure. The *resting metabolic expenditure (RME)* is calculated using the Harris-Benedict equation (HBE; Fig. 53–4).

The RME reflects the average minimal metabolism for nighttime and for those periods of the day when there is no exercise or exposure to cold. For a given patient, the total energy requirement to achieve energy balance is the product of the RME and applicable correction factors (Table 53–9).

For example, the 24-hour energy/caloric requirements for a patient with sepsis following elective surgery and confined to bed would be:

$$\text{kcal/day} = \text{RME} \times 1.2 \times 1.4 \times 1.0$$

Table 53-10 lists the caloric requirements necessary for weight maintenance in a variety of clinical settings. After reviewing this table, it is easy to understand the problems nurses encounter in attempting to meet these caloric needs. A critically ill patient who may require 4200 kcal/day may also have difficulty in taking in such a high caloric load

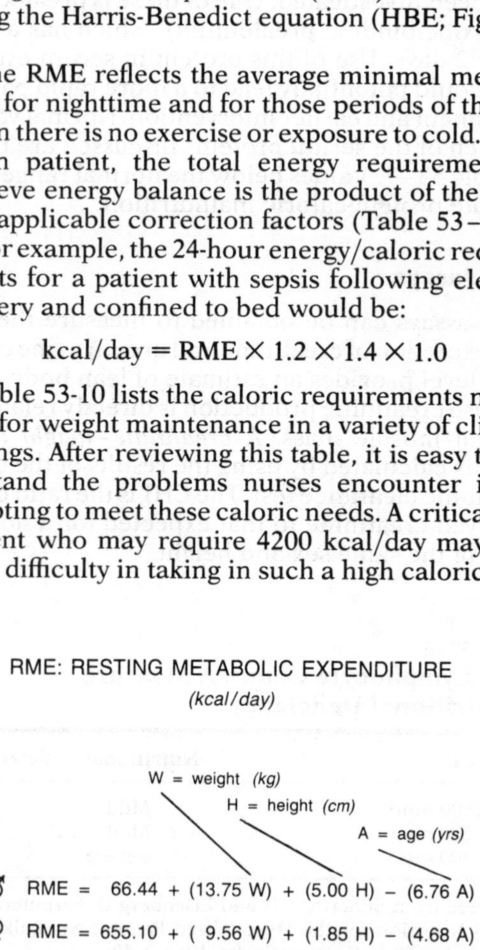

RME: RESTING METABOLIC EXPENDITURE
(kcal/day)
W = weight (kg)
H = height (cm)
A = age (yrs)
♂ RME = 66.44 + (13.75 W) + (5.00 H) − (6.76 A)
♀ RME = 655.10 + ( 9.56 W) + (1.85 H) − (4.68 A)


**Figure 53–4.** Metabolic expenditures (male and female).

TABLE 53-9
**Correction Factors for Predicting Energy Requirements in Hospitalized Patients***

| Clinical Condition | Correction Factor† |
|---|---|
| Physical activity | |
| Confined to bed | 1.2 |
| Out of bed | 1.3 |
| Fever | 1.0 + 0.13 per °C |
| Elective surgery | 1.0-1.2 |
| Peritonitis | 1.2-1.5 |
| Soft tissue trauma | 1.14-1.37 |
| Multiple fractures | 1.2-1.35 |
| Major sepsis | 1.4-1.8 |
| Thermal injury‡ | |
| 0-20% | 1.0-1.5 |
| 20-40% | 1.5-1.85 |
| 40-100% | 1.85-2.05 |
| Starvation (adults) | 0.70 |

*Total energy requirement is predicted by product of correction factors × RME (or BMR).

†Correction factors apply to men and women; figures represent maximum increases and must be adjusted as recovery and convalescence proceeds.

‡Percent body surface burned.

Adapted from Silberman H and Eisenberg D: Parenteral and Enteral Nutrition for the Hospitalized Patient. Norwalk, Connecticut, Appleton-Century-Crofts, 1982, p 60.

due to maxillofacial injuries, loss of appetite, or a nonfunctioning GI tract.

The rest of this chapter will focus on the nutrient requirements and methods for feeding patients who are not able to eat in the usual manner.

## NUTRIENT REQUIREMENTS

There are 6 categories of nutrients the body requires to maintain an adequate nutritional status. These include protein, carbohydrate, fat, electrolytes, vitamins, and trace elements. Energy requirements can be met through the administration of carbohydrate and fat. Protein should not be used to meet caloric needs. It should be spared for the synthesis of body tissues. Utilization of protein for calories is both an expensive and inefficient use of the product.

TABLE 53-10
**Caloric Requirements of the Critically Ill**

| Clinical Setting | Caloric Requirements kcal/kg wt | 70 kg man |
|---|---|---|
| Normal ambulation | 32 | 2240 |
| Elective surgery | 40 | 2800 |
| Trauma, sepsis | 50-60 | 3500-4200 |
| Extensive burns; maximum stress | 70-80 | 4900-5600 |

(Adapted from Hoppe MC: Nutritional management of the trauma patient. Critical Care Quarterly, p 5, June 1983. Reprinted with permission of Aspen Publishers, Inc.)

### Protein

To ensure that protein needs are met, the quality, as well as quantity of protein should be considered. The quality is determined by the amount of essential amino acids contained in the protein supplement. In order for anabolism to occur, both essential and nonessential amino acids must be present in appropriate amounts.

Albumin is a protein that is administered on a frequent basis in critical care. It is rarely administered, however, as a protein source because it is expensive and of limited biologic availability.[11] It is primarily used for the restoration of intravascular volume in the hypovolemic patient or the correction of malabsorption in the malnourished patient.[11] By normalizing serum colloidal osmotic pressure, vascular fluids remain in the intravascular compartment and are less likely to leak into surrounding tissue.

### Carbohydrates

Carbohydrates comprise the major source of calories, supplying 40%-50% of the caloric requirements. Nutritional supplementation of less than that amount could result in metabolic and hormonal derangements.[12-14] There are, however, several problems associated with carbohydrate administration. Increasing the glucose intake also *increases* the $CO_2$ production, because carbohydrates are broken down into $CO_2$ and $H_2O$. This offers grave implications for the respiratory patient, especially during periods of weaning from mechanical ventilation.[15]

Excess glucose administration can also lead to what is termed the "fatty liver" syndrome. Glucose not required for body energy is converted to fat, some of which is stored in the liver. Fat infiltrations in the liver can lead to liver abnormalities.[16] Other problems associated with increased amounts of carbohydrate include hyperglycemia and hyperosmolarity.

### Fat

Fat provides an obvious solution to the problems associated with the administration of high glucose loads. The administration of fat in amounts that supply 30%-50% of the calories results in a decrease in $CO_2$ production and may help to avoid other metabolic complications.[17,18]

Fat administration is also important for the delivery of *essential* fatty acids such as linoleic and lino-

TABLE 53–11
**Essential Fatty Acid Deficiency (EFAD): Signs and Symptoms**

- Dermatitis (eczematous and desquamative)
- Hair loss
- Hepatic dysfunction
- Thrombocytopenia
- Anemia
- Impaired wound healing

lenic acid. Essential fatty acids are those that cannot be synthesized in the body but are necessary for normal growth and development as well as the proper functioning of many physiologic processes. *Linoleic acid* is necessary as a precursor of prostaglandins, a regulator of cholesterol metabolism, and as an integral part in maintaining the integrity of cell walls. Less is known about *linolenic acid*. However, it is thought to be necessary for normal neuronal tissue development and maintenance, as well as prostaglandin formation. Without sufficient amounts of either of these fatty acids, the body begins to show signs of essential fatty acid deficiency (EFAD; Table 53–11).

## Electrolytes

Electrolytes are essential for the maintenance of water balance and proper functioning of the cardiac and neuromuscular systems. A depletion of the one electrolyte is usually accompanied by a depletion of several others. (For a more detailed discussion of electrolytes, see Chap. 23.)

## Vitamins

Vitamins are organic compounds that are required in minute amounts for normal growth, maintenance, and reproduction. They cannot be synthesized by the body in sufficient amounts, therefore, they must be provided in the diet. The various physiologic functions of each vitamin along with a listing of clinical signs of deficiency can be found in Table 53–12.

## Trace Elements

Trace elements were once thought to be of little importance because they exist in such small amounts within the body. We have since learned that trace elements are essential to human survival. The physiologic functions of each of the trace elements along with clinical signs of deficiency can be found in Table 53–13.

# THERAPEUTIC MODALITIES IN THE TREATMENT OF PATIENTS WITH AN ALTERED NUTRITIONAL STATUS

## Choosing a Therapeutic Modality

Persons who are unable to eat a regular diet have two other alternatives, parenteral or enteral nutrition. Enteral nutrition has certain advantages over parenteral. It is less expensive[19] and more physiologic.[20] It is easier to achieve a positive nitrogen balance, and it makes full use of any intact absorptive gastrointestinal tract. If a functioning GI tract exists, it should be used; otherwise, the parenteral route is indicated.

## Enteral Nutrition

### *Approaches to Enteral Feeding*

Several approaches may be used to deliver enteral feedings. These include the nasogastric, nasoduodenal, gastrostomy, jejunostomy, and needle catheter jejunostomy. A large bore or small bore tube may be employed for nasogastric feedings. See Table 53–14 for a detailed description of both these tubes.

Small bore tubes require the assistance of the bowel's own peristalsis to carry the tip through the pyloric opening into the duodenum. The tube should reach the duodenum within 24 hours of insertion. The patient can be positioned on his/her right side and/or administered metoclopramide (Reglan) to facilitate passage of the tube.

It is often difficult to ensure the placement of a soft bore tube other than by direct visualization on x-ray. Auscultation can be attempted, however, the tube may be lying in the bronchus, and the sound produced by instillation of air (20 ml) may be heard in the epigastric area. This can lead to false verification of tube placement. Attempts at aspiration of stomach or intestinal contents to check tube placement may also prove futile because the negative pressure applied may collapse the tube.

As mentioned in Table 53–14, small bore tubes are prone to occlusion from formula or medications. Several methods can be used to prevent tube occlusion. One method is to flush the tube after each feeding or medication instillation with 50–150 ml of water or 20–50 ml of cranberry juice.[21] If that is not effective, then crushed pancreatic enzyme can be placed down the tube, clamping for several hours, and then aspirating the contents.[21,22]

Gastrostomy and jejunostomy sites require a surgical approach, which is usually followed by the insertion of a large bore tube. They are indicated when enteral feedings are required for an extended period of time, or when there is a preexisting risk for aspiration, recent maxillofacial injury, or sur-

TABLE 53-12
## Vitamins: Physiological Function and Clinical Signs of Vitamin Deficiency

| Vitamin | Physiologic Function | Clinical Signs of Deficiency |
|---|---|---|
| A (Retinol)<br>RDA = 4000-5000 I.U. | Retinal function.<br>Epithelial tissue.<br>Fertility and reproduction.<br>Growth.<br>Immune function.<br>Glycoprotein synthesis. | Night blindness.<br>Conjunctival xerosis.<br>Bitot's spots.<br>Corneal xerosis.<br>Keratomalacia.<br>Xerophthalmic fundus.<br>Hyperkeratosis. |
| D<br>RDA = 400 I.U. | Stimulates intestinal absorption of Ca and P.<br>Plays a role in parathyroid hormone bone reabsorption.<br>Supports bone growth and mineralization. | Bone pain and tenderness.<br>Proximal muscle weakness.<br>Skeletal deformity. |
| E (Tocopherol)<br>RDA = 12-15 I.U. | Antioxidant.<br>Neutralizes free radicals.<br>Plays a role in selenium metabolism.<br>Plays a role in liver microscomal enzyme activity.<br>Influences neuromuscular function.<br>Influences biosynthesis of heme products. | Retinal degeneration.<br>Neuronal axonopathy.<br>Myopathy. |
| K<br>No RDA available | Blood clotting.<br>Possible role in either bone calcification or demineralization. | Bleeding, hemorrhage.<br>Prolonged clotting time. |
| $B_1$ (Thiamine)<br>RDA = 1.0-1.5 mg | Cardiovascular, neurological, and muscular function as precursor of thiamine pyrophosphate; coenzyme in energy metabolism, particularly carbohydrate metabolism.<br>Plays a role in enzymatic reactions. | Peripheral neuropathy.<br>Beriberi heart disease.<br>Wernicke's encephalopathy.<br>Alcoholic polyneuritis.<br>Korsakoff's syndrome. |
| $B_2$ (Riboflavin)<br>RDA = 1.1-1.7 mg | Integral part of several oxidative enzyme systems necessary for electron transport. | Angular stomatitis.<br>Glossitis.<br>Seborrheic dermatitis.<br>Corneal neovascularization. |
| $B_3$ (Niacin)<br>RDA = 13-19 mg | Nicotinamide plays a part in coenzymes NAD (H) and NADP (H), which are essential for glycolysis, fat synthesis, energy production. | Pellagra (dermatitis, dementia, diarrhea) |
| $B_5$ (Pantothenic Acid)<br>No RDA available | Vital to all energy-requiring processes within the cell as it is an integral part of coenzyme A.<br>Plays a role in immunity. | Headache, fatigue.<br>Impaired motor coordination, paresthesia, muscle cramps.<br>Intermittent vomiting and diarrhea.<br>Decreased antibody formation. |
| $B_6$ (Pyridoxine)<br>RDA = 1.6 to 2.0 mg | Metabolism of CNS.<br>Amino acid metabolism.<br>Heme synthesis.<br>Involved in glycogen phosphorylase activity. | CNS problems.<br>Peripheral neuritis.<br>Seborrheic dermatitis.<br>Glossitis.<br>Angular stomatitis.<br>Cheilosis. |
| Folic Acid (Folacin)<br>RDA = 400 $\mu g$ | Serves as a coenzyme involved in DNA synthesis. | Macrocytic anemia.<br>Megaloblastosis of bone marrow.<br>Thrombocytopenia.<br>Leukopenia.<br>Diarrhea.<br>Glossitis.<br>Weight loss. |
| Vitamin $B_{12}$ (Cyanocobalamin)<br>RDA = 3.0 $\mu g$ | Essential to the proper functioning of all body cells.<br>Involved in DNA synthesis.<br>Serves as a coenzyme in protein, fat, and carbohydrate metabolism. | Pernicious anemia.<br>Neurologic problems.<br>GI problems. |

*(continued)*

TABLE 53-12
**Vitamins: Physiological Function and Clinical Signs of Vitamin Deficiency *(Continued)***

| Vitamin | Physiologic Function | Clinical Signs of Deficiency |
|---|---|---|
| Biotin<br>No RDA available | Required for normal activity of numerous carboxylase enzyme systems involved in CHO, protein, and fat metabolism.<br>Participates in activation of folate to its coenzyme forms. | Seborrheic dermatitis.<br>Muscle pain, paresthesia.<br>Anorexia, nausea.<br>Hypercholesterolemia.<br>ECG changes. |
| C (Ascorbic Acid)<br>RDA = 60 mg | Essential to a variety of biologic oxidation processes.<br>Role in collagen synthesis.<br>Essential for normal protein and amino acid metabolism.<br>Plays a role in carbohydrate metabolism. | Scurvy.<br>Impaired wound healing. |

gery and other instances for which the transnasal route is contraindicated. The jejunostomy may be preferred for those persons at high risk for aspiration because such a risk is minimal using this route. It is also preferred for feeding during the early postoperative period, because an elemental formula can be started 12-24 hours after surgery.[23] A particular type of jejunostomy is the needle catheter jejunostomy. This approach involves the insertion of a 16-gauge catheter during abdominal surgery. Feeding can be started in the recovery room by a continuous drip infusion. It has minimized the complications of traditional jejunostomies, such as skin erosion and wound infection.[24]

### Methods of Enteral Administration

There are 3 methods by which enteral nutrition can be delivered: *bolus*, *intermittent*, or *continuous* infusion. Table 53-15 lists each of these methods, outlining their particular advantages and disadvantages. Continuous drip feeding has been found to be most tolerated by the critically ill because it allows for greater absorption time as it passes through the intestine.[25-27]

### Enteral Formulas

There are 6 different categories of enteral formulas currently on the market (Table 53-16). The type of formula selected depends on the condition of the patient and the amount of absorptive GI tract available.

*Blenderized* formulas are table food, which is either commercially or noncommercially prepared. The commercial formulas are recommended for use due to problems of bacterial contamination found with noncommercial formulas.[28] They are as close to a normal diet as can be achieved. These formulas are nutritionally complete, yet they contain intact protein requiring full digestion. The high viscosity of this formula necessitates the use of a large bore tube.

*Meal replacement* formulas are nutritionally complete, have a low viscosity, and are generally well tolerated by the majority of patients. This group of formulas is one of the most widely used.

*Elemental* or *chemically defined* formulas (as they are otherwise called) are similar to a clear liquid diet. They are generally nutritionally complete, containing some nutrients in a partially digested form, allowing easier digestion. These formulas are lactose free. Their low viscosity allows for the use of a small bore tube.

*High calorie, high protein* formulas are similar to meal replacement formulas, however, they contain more calories per milliliter. This is ideal for those patients requiring a fluid restriction or those that are catabolic and need more calories. One disadvantage is that the greater the caloric content, the greater the osmolarity. An increased osmolarity may not be tolerated by the critically ill.

*Specialty* formulas are of 3 basic types: formulas designed for those with a specific organ failure (hepatic, renal failure), those designed for the hypermetabolic patient (sepsis, trauma), and those designed for fat malabsorption or conditions requiring fat restriction. The *hepatic* formulas contain a greater ratio of branched chain to aromatic amino acids, while restricting total amino acid concentrations. The *renal* formulas contain mostly essential as opposed to nonessential amino acids. They too contain a restricted total amount of amino acids. The *hypermetabolic* formulas contain high concentrations of branched chain amino acids. These specialized formulas are often nutritionally incomplete, necessitating vitamin and electrolyte supplements. The lack of sufficient electrolytes may be considered an advantage when feeding renal failure patients. Electrolytes can then be given as their metabolic state dictates. The fat malabsorption formula provides a high percentage of

TABLE 53–13
**Trace Elements: Physiological Function and Clinical Signs of Mineral Deficiency**

| Trace Element | Physiologic Function | Clinical Signs of Deficiency |
|---|---|---|
| Iron | Oxygen transport as part of hemoglobin.<br>Skeletal muscle function.<br>Leukocyte function and host defense.<br>Cognitive function and alertness.<br>Component of iron metalloenzymes. | Pallor.<br>Fatigue.<br>Exertional dyspnea.<br>Tachycardia.<br>Headache.<br>Paresthesias.<br>Burning sensation on the tongue.<br>Altered attention span. |
| Zinc | Cell growth and proliferation.<br>Sexual maturation and reproduction.<br>Dark adaptation and night vision.<br>Gustatory acuity.<br>Wound healing.<br>Host immune defenses.<br>Hemostasis. | Growth retardation.<br>Alopecia.<br>Dermatitis.<br>Abnormalities of taste and smell.<br>Anorexia.<br>Diarrhea.<br>Mental depression.<br>Impaired wound healing.<br>Glucose intolerance. |
| Copper | Erythropoiesis, leukopoiesis.<br>Skeletal mineralization.<br>Elastin and collagen synthesis.<br>Myelin formation.<br>Catecholamine metabolism.<br>Oxidative phosphorylation.<br>Thermal regulation.<br>Antioxidant protection.<br>Cholesterol metabolism.<br>Lymphocyte function.<br>Cardiac function.<br>Glucose metabolism. | Anemia.<br>Leukopenia.<br>Neutropenia.<br>Pallor.<br>Depigmentation of hair.<br>Glucose intolerance.<br>Mental confusion.<br>Peripheral neuropathy with ataxia. |
| Manganese | Functions in antioxidant protection and energy metabolism.<br>Formation of connective tissue.<br>Functions as a cofactor in certain metabolic reactions.<br>Fertility and reproduction. | Clinical deficiency states have not yet been identified. |
| Selenium | Antioxidant | Muscle tenderness.<br>Myalgia.<br>*Cardiac myopathy.<br>*Increased RBC fragility.<br>*Pallor of fingernails and nailbeds.<br>*Pancreatic degeneration. |
| Chromium | Potentiates action of insulin.<br>Participates in regulation of lipoprotein metabolism. | Glucose intolerance.<br>Peripheral neuropathy with ataxia.<br>Metabolic encephalopathy. |
| Molybdenum | Important in oxidative metabolism of purines and sulfur-containing compounds into forms excreted by kidneys. | Clinical deficiency states have not yet been identified. |
| Iodine | Formation of thyroid hormone. | Goiter. |

*Studies not yet conclusive for these findings.

medium chain triglycerides (MCT) to facilitate absorption of fat. Low fat formulas may be indicated for pancreatitis or in diseases associated with lymphatic obstruction that impairs fat transport.

*Modular* formulas supply a single nutrient: fat, carbohydrate, or protein. These modules can be used singularly as diet supplements or combined to yield a unique formula designed for a specific patient's needs. If modules are combined, it should be done under aseptic conditions.

TABLE 53–14
## Large Bore vs. Small Bore Feeding Tubes

| Type of Tube | Size | Type of Material | Advantages | Disadvantages |
|---|---|---|---|---|
| Large bore | 10–18F | Rubber or polyvinyl chloride. | 1. Ease in administration of highly viscous fluids.<br>2. Simple insertion. | 1. Increased incidence of the following complications:<br>• Esophageal sphincter incompetence.<br>• Nasal or esophageal ulceration.<br>• Pharyngitis.<br>• Tracheal fistula. |
| Small bore | 6–12F (36–45 inches in length) | Polyurethane or silicone with a mercury or tungsten tip. | 1. More comfortable for the patient.<br>2. Able to deliver feeding to the duodenum or jejunum. | 1. Insertion may be complicated and time consuming.<br>2. Difficult to assure correct placement without x-ray.<br>3. More prone to occlusion.<br>4. Increased incidence of the following complications:<br>• Pneumothorax if guide wire used for insertion.<br>• Bronchopleural feeding if tube misplaced. |

TABLE 53–15
## Method of Enteral Administration

| | Bolus | Intermittent | Continuous |
|---|---|---|---|
| Amount delivered | 250–400 ml administered over 10–15 min. | 250–400 ml administered over 30 min to 1 hr. | 25–100 ml/hr administered by continuous infusion. |
| Frequency | 4–8 times/day | 4–8 times/day | Continuous infusion over a 16- or 24-hr period. |
| Advantages | 1. Inexpensive. Does not require the use of a feeding pump.<br>2. Convenient | 1. Inexpensive. Does not require the use of a feeding pump.<br>2. Convenient.<br>3. May be more physiologic as it more closely simulates normal feeding pattern. | 1. Best suited to the critically ill for following reasons:<br>• Allows for greater absorption time via intestine.<br>• Decreased incidence of high gastric residuals.<br>• Duodenal and jejunal feedings well tolerated. |
| Disadvantages | 1. Often accompanied by bloating, cramping, nausea, diarrhea and/or aspiration.<br>2. Not tolerated well when given through the duodenum or jejunum. | 1. Not tolerated well when given via the duodenum or jejunum. | 1. More expensive than bolus or intermittent methods as a feeding pump is required.<br>2. Less convenient for the following reasons:<br>• System must be interrupted every 4 hr to check gastric residuals and tube placement.<br>• Continuous use of feeding pump limits patient's mobility.<br>3. May lead to persistently elevated insulin levels. |

TABLE 53-16
**Enteral Formulas**

| Classification/Product Name | kcal/ml | mOsm/kg | Protein g/1000 cc | Fat g/1000 cc | CHO g/1000 cc |
|---|---|---|---|---|---|
| ***Blenderized Diet*** | | | | | |
| Compleat—Modified (Sandoz) | 1.0 | 300 | 43 | 37 | 141 |
| Compleat—Regular (Sandoz) | 1.0 | 405 | 43 | 43 | 128 |
| Vitaneed (Biosearch) | 1.0 | 310 | 35 | 40 | 125 |
| ***Meal Replacement*** | | | | | |
| Ensure (Ross) | 1.0 | 470 | 37.2 | 37.2 | 145 |
| Enrich (Ross) | 1.1 | 480 | 39.7 | 37.2 | 162 |
| Entri-Pak (Biosearch) | 1.0 | 300 | 35 | 35 | 136 |
| Isocal (Mead Johnson) | 1.0 | 300 | 34 | 44 | 130 |
| Osmolite (Ross) | 1.1 | 300 | 37.2 | 38.5 | 145 |
| Travasorb (Travenol) | 1.1 | 488 | 33 | 35 | 136 |
| Precision Isotonic (Sandoz) | 1.0 | 300 | 29 | 30 | 144 |
| ***Defined/Elemental*** | | | | | |
| Criticare HN (Mead Johnson) | 1.0 | 650 | 36 | 3 | 210 |
| Vital (Ross) | 1.0 | 500 | 42 | 10.8 | 185 |
| Vivonex Standard (Norwich Eaton) | 1.0 | 550 | 20 | 1.4 | 230 |
| Vivonex HN (Norwich Easton) | 1.0 | 810 | 42 | 0.9 | 210 |
| Vivonex T.E.N. (Norwich Eaton) | 1.0 | 300 | 46 | 3.3 | 246.8 |
| ***Specialized Formulas*** | | | | | |
| Precision HN (Sandoz) | 1.1 | 525 | 44 | 1.3 | 216 |
| Precision LR (Sandoz) | 1.1 | 505-549 | 26 | 1.6 | 248 |
| Amin-Aid (American McGraw) | 2.0 | 1125 | 19 | 70 | 324 |
| Hepatic-Aid (American McGraw) | 1.1 | 560 | 44.1 | 36.2 | 169 |
| Traum-Aid (American McGraw) | 1.0 | 675 | 56 | 12.4 | 166 |
| Trauma Cal (Mead Johnson) | 1.5 | 490 | 83 | 68 | 143 |
| Travasorb-Hepatic (Travenol) | 1.1 | 690 | 28.6 | 14.3 | 209 |
| Travasorb-Renal (Travenol) | 1.35 | 590 | 22.9 | 17.7 | 271 |
| Pulmocare (Ross) | 1.5 | 490 | 62.6 | 92.1 | 105.7 |
| Portagen (Mead Johnson) | 1.0 | 320 | 35 | 48 | 115 |
| ***High Calorie, High Protein*** | | | | | |
| Osmolite HN (Ross) | 1.0 | 300 | 44.4 | 36.8 | 141 |
| Ensure HN (Ross) | 1.0 | 470 | 44.4 | 35.5 | 141 |
| Ensure Plus (Ross) | 1.5 | 690 | 55 | 53 | 200 |
| Isocal HN (Mead Johnson) | 2.0 | 650 | 75 | 91 | 225 |
| Magnacal (Organon) | 2.0 | 590 | 70 | 80 | 250 |
| **Classification/Product Name** | **kcal/tbsp** | **mOsm/kg** | **g/tbsp** | **g/tbsp** | **g/tbsp** |
| ***Modular Formulas*** | | | | | |
| *Protein* | **kcal/tbsp** | | **g/tbsp** | **g/tbsp** | **g/tbsp** |
| Pro Mod (Ross) | 16 | — | 3.0 | 0.3 | 0.3 |
| Propac (Organon) | 16 | — | 16 | 0.3 | — |
| Casec (Mead Johnson) | 17 | — | 4 | — | — |
| *Carbohydrate* | | | | | |
| Cal-Powder (General Mills) | — | — | 0.6 | — | — |
| Moducal (Mead Johnson) | 90 | — | 0 | 0 | 23 |
| Polycose (Ross) | 23 | — | 0 | 0 | 6 |
| Sumacal (Organon) | 19 | — | 0 | 0 | 4.8 |
| *Fat* | | | | | |
| Lipomul (Upjohn) | 36 | — | 0 | 4 | 0 |
| MCT OIL (Mead Johnson) | 115 | — | 0 | 14 | 0 |
| Microlipid (Organon) | 36 | 80 | 0 | 4 | 0 |

### Advancement of Feeding

*Intermittent* feedings are usually begun with the infusion of 100 ml of formula every 3-4 hours, while continuous feedings are begun at a rate of 50 ml/hour. In the absence of gastrointestinal side effects, intermittent feedings are advanced every 12-24 hours by increments of 50-100 ml up to a total of 350 ml of formula (an additional 50 ml is given to flush the feeding tube after completion of the feedings).

*Continuous* feedings are increased by 25-

50 ml/hour until a total of 100 ml/hour is reached. The formula may initially be diluted to one half strength and increased as per patient tolerance. This regimen is controversial for all but duodenal and jejunal feedings.[21] Studies have demonstrated that the administration of a dilute formula for several days prior to giving a full strength diet is not necessary when delivered to the stomach.[29,30] The rate and strength of formula should never both be increased at the same time.

### *Complications of Enteral Nutrition*

There are several complications associated with the administration of enteral nutrition. They can be divided into 4 categories: *gastrointestinal, mechanical, metabolic,* and *psychosensory* complications. Gastrointestinal complications account for the largest percentage of these, with diarrhea the most frequently encountered.[31] Diarrhea is defined as having greater than 3 loose bowel movements/day.[32] Diarrhea is usually a symptom of a much bigger problem. Too often, however, we attempt to treat the symptom and not its cause.

Table 53–17 outlines some of the causes of diarrhea and their treatment. Agents that decrease intestinal motility should only be used as a last resort. These agents include paregoric, codeine, Lomotil, and atropine. One must be certain to check bowel sounds at least 2 times/shift because these agents can cause a paralytic ileus.

High gastric residuals can also be problematic for the patient receiving enteral feedings. Residuals should be checked prior to each bolus or intermittent feeding and every 4 hours during continuous feedings. A *high gastric residual* is defined as being greater than 50 ml or one half the amount given. Should this problem be encountered, one of several interventions can be implemented. One method is to hold the feeding and check the residual in 1 hour. This procedure can be repeated every 1–2 hours until feedings can be resumed. Once the feedings

TABLE 53–17
**Possible Causes of Diarrhea in the Tube-Fed Patient and Their Treatment**

| Cause | Rationale | Treatment |
|---|---|---|
| Recent ↑ in the amount or rate of feeding. | ↑ amount/rate may ↑ GI transit time and ↓ absorption of formula. | ↓ amount or rate of feeding. |
| Recent ↑ in formula osmolarity. | ↑ osmolarity of formula pulls fluid from intestinal capillaries into bowel. This ↑ fluid content of stool, which ↑ transit time. | ↓ formula osmolarity. |
| Lactose intolerance. | Lactase, needed for digestion of lactose, is often depleted in adults, especially critically ill adults. | Use a lactose-free formula. |
| Hypoalbuminemia. | Low albumin (protein) levels ↓ the colloid osmotic pressure causing leakage of fluid from intestine to stool. The ↑ fluid content of stool ↑ transit time. | Administer parenteral protein by TPN. |
| Lack of bulk. | Lack of bulk in stool may ↑ transit time. | Add bulk to diet through the administration of cellulose (e.g., Metamucil) or formulas containing cellulose (Enrich [Ross]). |
| Fat intolerance. | ↓ ability to digest fat is often present in those who are critically ill, have pancreatic disease and/or recently underwent gastric surgery. | ↓ dietary intake of fat. |
| Antibiotic therapy. | Antibiotics may destroy the normal bowel flora, leading to a superinfection. | ↓ the dose or eliminate antibiotic if possible.<br>Administer lactobacillus along with antibiotic. |
| Concomitant administration of other medications: | The medications listed may cause diarrhea through the following mechanisms: | |
| • Antacids. | •↑ gastric pH, which is effective medium for bacteria to proliferate. | |
| • Antiarrhythmics. | •↑ GI motility. | |
| • Aminophylline. | •↑ GI motility. | |
| • Cimetidine. | •↑ gastric pH. | |
| • Potassium chloride. | •↑ osmolarity. | |
| Bacterial contamination of feedings. | Bacterial contamination ↑ GI motility. | Use aseptic technique in the preparation and delivery of feedings. |

are resumed, it should be done at a reduced rate and/or a diluted concentration.

Another approach is to give the feeding at one half the rate or amount without delaying the feeding. Gastric emptying problems usually resolve within 2–8 hours. Should this be a recurring problem, metoclopramide (Reglan) can be used to increase gastric motility, however, this can lead to abdominal cramping and diarrhea.

Nausea and vomiting is yet another complication that may be experienced by the tube-fed patient. In fact, as many as 10%–20% of all tube-fed patients exhibit this problem.[33] Too rapid a rate of administration has been implicated as one of the causative factors.[34] A decrease in the rate, with a gradual return to the optimal rate, may help alleviate this problem.

Nausea and vomiting may also be the result of the odor of many of the enteral formulas.[34] Flavoring additives may be used to lessen any unpleasant formula odors. Lactose intolerance may also produce nausea and vomiting. Switching to one of many lactose-free formulas is the best method for managing this problem.[35] A diet high in fat may also lead to nausea and vomiting. The total caloric intake of fat should not exceed 40%–50% when provided enterally.[33]

*Mechanical* complications from feeding tubes are related mostly to the size and position of the tube. The causes, prevention, and treatment of various mechanical complications are outlined in Table 53–18.

The *metabolic* complications of enteral nutrition are rather frequent, yet easily treated. Among these are *overhydration*, *dehydration*, and *hyperglycemia*. Persons at risk for developing overhydration are those suffering from cardiac, renal, or hepatic disease. Overhydration is usually associated with the administration of sodium and water to persons deprived of this nourishment for extended periods of time.[36] Overhydration is usually adequately managed by decreasing the rate of enteral administration. Advancement of the feeding rate is accomplished through careful monitoring of the patient's physiologic status.

Dehydration is apt to occur when a formula of high osmolarity and high protein content is administered without benefit of supplemental water. This is particularly important for persons who may not be able to convey a feeling of thirst. In order to anticipate the amount of supplemental water needed by the patient, the nurse should know the amount of free water available in the product being used and the patient's fluid status.

Hyperglycemia is a metabolic complication that occurs due to a lack of insulin in the tube-fed patient. Those most likely to develop this complication are diabetics or those who were previously borderline diabetics. Careful metabolic monitoring of tube-fed patients often alleviates this problem. One is cautioned to use serum and not urine sugar measurements because urine levels have been shown to be inaccurate.[37] Hyperglycemia is corrected through the administration of insulin or oral hypoglycemia agents. The flow rate of the formula may initially be decreased and later advanced as per patient tolerance.

The *psychosensory* complications encountered by the tube-fed patient is seldom discussed. The most distressing psychosensory experiences that have been documented include those related to feelings of thirst, being deprived of tasting food, and having an unsatisfied taste for food.[38]

Various measures may be employed by the nurse to help minimize these problems. Adequate hydration can be ensured by adding additional water to the feeding regimen as needed. The patient can be allowed to rinse his mouth with water or a saline solution, chew gum, or suck on lemon candy. Mouthwashes should be avoided because the alcohol content has an astringent effect on the oral mucous membrane. Obligatory mouth breathing due to the presence of a nasal feeding tube may also enhance the sensation of dryness. The use of a small-bore tube may help to resolve this problem. Lubricating the lips with petroleum jelly or lanolin also adds to the patient's comfort.

Another common physical complaint of patients is that of a sore throat or nose. Chloraseptic lozenges or spray may help to alleviate a sore throat, while proper taping of nasoenteral tubes may help relieve an uncomfortable nose. Tape the tube so that neither traction nor pressure is applied to the naris.

### Drug Additive Compatibility

The compatibility of enteral formulas with various drug additives has recently been explored. Whenever drugs are added directly to enteral products, there exists the potential for the drug and/or enteral products to undergo degradation and/or inactivation. Furthermore, drugs mixed with enteral products alter the drug's bioavailability and therapeutic effectiveness.[39]

When possible, it is advisable to administer therapeutic agents in single bolus doses directly into the enteral tube, followed by a water rinsing. Flushing the enteral tube before and after each feeding serves a variety of purposes: (1) tube patency is ascertained, (2) the tube is cleared for better drug delivery, and (3) the drug is aided in getting to the intestine. Unless otherwise indicated, medications should be delivered 1 hour prior to or 2 hours following an intermittent tube feeding to ensure optimal absorption. Continuous feedings present a special problem in that they need to be interrupted for drug administration.

When administering medication by an enteral tube, one must take into consideration the internal

TABLE 53–18
**Mechanical Complications Associated with Enteral Feeding Tubes**

| Mechanical Complication | Cause | Prevention | Treatment |
|---|---|---|---|
| Incorrect tube placement. | • Incorrect tube insertion.<br>• Inadvertent dislodgement. | • Verify tube placement every 4 hr.<br>• Anchor tube securely. | • Reposition tube. |
| Occlusion of feeding tube. | • Feeding particles. | • Flush feeding tube with 50–150 cc $H_2O$ or 20–50 cc cranberry juice after each feeding.<br>• Thoroughly crush all medications placed down tube and flush tube prior to and after each medication instillation. | • Place a small amount of crushed pancreatic enzyme down the tube, clamp for several hours, then aspirate the contents. |
| Aspiration of feeding. | • Incorrect tube position. | • Maintain head elevation at 30° or higher during and 1 hr after feeding. | • Early detection of aspiration can be aided by testing pulmonary secretions for the presence of glucose via glucose dipstick. |
| | • High gastric residuals. | • Verify tube placement every 4 hr. | • Thorough endotracheal and orotracheal suctioning in the case of witnessed aspiration. |
| | • Incompetent esophageal sphincter. | • Use small-bore instead of a large-bore feeding tube. | • Supportive therapy such as intravenous fluids, close monitoring of vital signs, and positive pressure ventilation as indicated. |
| | • Decreased ability of glottic closure (ETT or trach tube). | • Check gastric residuals every 4 hr and treat appropriately.<br>• Feed below the pylorus when possible. | |
| Tracheoesophageal fistula. | • Under pressure on anterior esophageal wall caused by feeding tube along with pressure exerted on the posterior wall of the trachea by a tracheostomy or endotracheal tube. | • Use a small-bore instead of a large-bore feeding tube.<br>• Use a gastrostomy or jejunostomy site for feedings. | • Alleviate pressure being exerted on tracheal and esophageal walls where possible. |
| Acute sinusitis. | • Occlusion of sinus tracts by feeding tube. | • Use a small-bore instead of a large-bore feeding tube.<br>• Use a gastrostomy or jejunostomy site for feedings. | • Removal of nasal feeding tube.<br>• Bed rest.<br>• Application of hot compresses to the face.<br>• Administration of analgesics. |
| Otitis media. | • Pressure on eustachian tube by feeding tube. | • Use a small-bore instead of a large-bore feeding tube.<br>• Periodically change position of a nasal feeding tube to the other nostril.<br>• Use a gastrostomy or jejunostomy site for feedings. | • Removal of nasal feeding tube.<br>• Bed rest.<br>• Administration of antibiotics as appropriate. |

diameter of the tube. Large bore nasogastric, gastrostomy, or jejunostomy tubes permit the administration of larger drug particles and more viscous solutions than do small bore tubes. A commercially prepared liquid medication should always be used when it is available. Consider the use of granule formulations, effervescent tablets, and other solid dosage forms when preformulated liquid preparations are not available.

Solid oral dosage forms must first be compounded to liquid form before their instillation into an enteral tube (Table 53–19). Not all solid dosage forms, however, are suitable for compounding into liquid dosage form. Pulverizing an enteric-coated or slow-release compound may destroy the integrity of the drug if it is administered into the stomach or intestine.[40] An equivalent generic solid dosage form should be used in these circumstances.

TABLE 53-19
**Compounding Solid Oral Dosage Forms to Liquid Dosage Forms**

- Establish the correct drug dosage.
- Using a mortar and pestle, pulverize the correct amount of solid dosage form.
- Wash the utensils with 5-10 ml of $H_2O$ to extract residual drug.
- Transfer the pulverized drug and washings to a plastic medicine cup.
- Add a nonabsorbing liquid such as alcohol, glycerine or propylene glycol to the mixture. This will decrease the clumping of drug particles and stablize their dispersion in the liquid.
- Transfer the suspension into a feeding syringe for bolus administration.
- Thoroughly wash mixing utensils.

(Adapted from Melnick, G and Wright K: Pharmacologic aspects of enteral nutrition. In Rombeau, JL and Caldwell, MD (eds): Enteral and Tube Feeding. WB Saunders, Philadelphia, 1984.)

## Parenteral Nutrition

### *Venous Access*

Parenteral nutrition is administered by a *peripheral* or *central* venous access. The choice for the route of administration depends on such factors as: (1) fluid viscosity, (2) volume to be infused, and (3) available sites. The central route is preferred for the infusion of hypertonic solutions and solutions in large volumes. Superficial peripheral veins are used for short-term therapy of isotonic solutions.

Short, semirigid catheters are used for peripheral veins. These catheters have a life span of 2-5 days.[41] Central catheters can be used for either short-term or long-term therapy. Short-term access to the central venous system is primarily obtained by the internal jugular and subclavian veins. Materials currently available for catheterization include polyvinylchloride, Silastic, polyurethane, and heparin-coated catheters. These catheters have a life span of 5-14 days. Some are available as double and triple lumen catheters.[41] They allow the infusion of a carbohydrate and protein solution by one port and lipids by another. This alleviates any need for piggybacking lipid emulsions. When a third port is available, it can be used for the infusion of antibiotics or other intravenous additives.

Long-term (months to years) therapy presents special problems related to catheter infection and displacement. These catheters are made of silicone rubber (Silastic). They are much longer (approximately 90 cm) than short-term catheters so that they can reach the right atrium and can also be tunneled under the skin of the chest. Dacron cuffs are positioned so they may be placed in the subcutaneous tissues to anchor the catheter in place. The most commonly used of this type are the *Broviac* and *Hickman* catheters.

### *Site Care*

Techniques and protocols for site care vary from hospital to hospital with apparent success in minimizing catheter-related sepsis. The only absolute agreement in methods of site care is that *strict adherence to aseptic principles* is essential. Handwashing remains the single most effective measure for the prevention of infection. Initial preparation of the skin must be meticulous. Any disruption of the skin's integrity provides an opportunity for the entrance of bacteria or fungi. Shaving the skin at the catheter insertion site should be avoided because cuts in the skin can occur. Trimming excessive hair or using depilatory cream is preferable to shaving.[42]

Numerous antiseptics are available for cleansing the skin and any remaining hair (Table 53-20). Controversy exists as to whether skin should be defatted. Until this issue is resolved, many clinicians are hesitant to discontinue the use of defatting agents. The use of antibiotic and antiseptic ointments has also come under closer scrutiny. It seems that their effectiveness is generally diminished within 12 hours of application.[43]

Intravenous site dressings serve 2 purposes: to minimize the risk of infection and to secure the catheter. Several different materials are currently being used, including gauze sponges, elastoplast, and transparent semipermeable dressings. The transparent semipermeable dressings have gained popularity because they allow direct visualization of the intravenous site and, due to their biocclusive nature, require less frequent dressing change. It has been recommended that gauze dressing changes be made every 48 hours on critically ill patients.[44] Commercially prepared dressing kits usually contain acetone-alcohol preparation swab sticks, providone-iodine solution swabs sticks and

TABLE 53-20
**Commonly Used Antiseptics and Their Mode of Action**

| Antiseptic | Mode of Action |
|---|---|
| Isopropyl alcohol 70% | • Denaturation of proteins.<br>• Disinfectant activity—high level. |
| Hydrogen peroxide 3% | • Destruction of membrane lipids, DNA, and other cell components.<br>• Disinfectant activity—high level. |
| Acetone 10-100% | • Loosening of horny layer of epidermis.<br>• Disinfectant activity—intermittent level. |
| Indophor 1-2% | • Penetration of cell wall of microorganism, with disruption of protein and nucleic acid structure and synthesis.<br>• Disinfectant activity—intermittent level. |

(Adapted from Forlaw, L and Torosian, M.[68])

ointment, sterile gauze sponges, sterile gloves, and other dressing materials as the hospital specifies.

### Inline Filters

The use of filters during the administration of intravenous fluids also remains confusing to many. Filters are intended to remove particulate matter and air, reduce the incidence of phlebitis, and prevent sepsis. It has been recommended that a 0.22-micron filter be used in conjunction with total parenteral nutrition (TPN) and changed every 24 hours.[45] These filters can become obstructed by blood and blood products, emulsions, and suspensions. For this reason, lipid emulsions need to be infused *below* the filter.

### Infusion Devices

To avoid problems stemming from the incorrect flow rate of parenteral nutrition, it is advisable to use some form of mechanical control for regulating intravenous administration. *Mechanical infusion devices* are recommended due to their accuracy in flow rate, ability to infuse viscous fluids, and alarm system. Mechanical devices containing the following alarms are desirable: alarms that monitor for occlusion, air in the line, empty solution container, infiltration, loss of power, broken or disconnected tubing, and rate variations.

Two major types of mechanical devices are on the market, *controllers and pumps*. Controllers have no moving components, work by gravity, and count drops electronically. Pumps are usually of either the piston (syringe) or peristaltic type. Pressure is exerted to expel the fluid. Pumps are best suited for the administration of viscous fluids such as parenteral nutrition.

### Parenteral Solutions

Parenteral nutrition consists of the administration of carbohydrate, protein, lipids, electrolytes, vitamins, and trace elements. These nutritional components are available as combined or single products.

Carbohydrates are supplied in the form of dextrose. It is the most commonly used substrate for parenteral nutrition. Dextrose is available in concentrations ranging from 5%–70%, however, admixed solutions (those mixed with other substances such as protein or lipids) rarely exceed 50% as a final concentration (Table 53–21). Dextrose solutions greater than 10% require a central vein for administration due to its osmolarity and acidic pH.

Protein is supplied in the form of amino acids which can be used directly for protein synthesis. These formulas contain a combination of both essential and nonessential amino acids. Some solutions even contain premixed electrolytes. Commercially prepared formulas are available in concentrations ranging from 3.5%–10% with a final concentration of 3.5%–5% following admixture. Solutions within the 3.5% range are considered isotonic; higher concentrations are hypertonic.

TABLE 53–21
**Characteristics of Various Dextrose Solutions**

| Concentration | kcal/liter | mOsm/liter |
|---|---|---|
| 10% | 340 | 505 |
| 20% | 680 | 1010 |
| 50% | 1700 | 2525 |

(Adapted from Louie, N and Niemiec, PW: Parenteral nutrition solutions. In Rombeau, JL and Caldwell, MD (eds): *Parenteral Nutrition*. WB Saunders, Philadelphia, 1986.)

Lipid emulsions serve as a source of energy and essential fatty acids. Solutions are prepared from soybean oil or a combination of soybean and safflower oil. Safflower oil contains a greater percentage of the essential fatty acid, linoleic, and very little of the other essential fatty acid, linolenic; soybean oil contains a better balance of both fatty acids. Lipid formulas are isotonic and may, therefore, be infused by way of a peripheral vein.

A test dose of fat emulsion is recommended prior to the full infusion. In adults, 10% fat should be infused at a rate of 1 ml/minute for the first 15–30 minutes; 20% fat should be infused at a rate of 0.5 ml/minute for the first 15–30 minutes. Traditionally, 10% solutions are usually infused over 4–6 hours, and 20% solutions are infused over 6–8 hours. It has recently been suggested that all lipid emulsions be infused over 24 hours to decrease the incidence of fat-overloading syndrome.[46]

Ten percent solutions yield a caloric content of 1.1 kcal/ml; 20% solutions yield 2.0 kcal/ml. The administration of a 20% solution has the advantage of supplying twice as many calories/ml as the 10% solution. This is of particular importance in the fluid-restricted patient.

Electrolytes are infused either as a component already contained in the amino acid solution or as a separate component. Electrolytes are available in several salt forms (Table 53–22). Their administration is based on the patient's metabolic status.

Malnutrition, specific disease states, and drug therapy may predispose some patients to vitamin deficiencies, for which additional vitamin supplementation is essential. Parenteral multivitamin products and individual vitamins are available to provide additional vitamin therapy.

Trace elements such as zinc, copper, chromium, and manganese are present routinely in parenteral solutions. Recommendations for the administration of other elements such as selenium, iodide, and

TABLE 53-22
**Electrolyte Salt Forms**

- Sodium chloride
- Sodium acetate
- Sodium bicarbonate
- Sodium lactate
- Sodium phosphate
- Potassium chloride
- Potassium acetate
- Potassium phosphate
- Magnesium sulfate
- Calcium chloride
- Calcium gluconate
- Calcium gluceptate

Reprinted with permission from Louie, N and Niemiec, PW: Parenteral nutrition solutions. In Rombeau, JL and Caldwell, MD (eds): Parenteral Nutrition. Philadelphia, WB Saunders, 1986, p. 281.

molybdenum have been made, although required levels are not yet well defined.

### Parenteral Nutrition Additives

Many different types of additives are currently being used in parenteral nutrition. It is important that the critical care nurse understand the indications for their use and the degree of *compatibility* with the parenteral solution.

Insulin is considered to be chemically stable in parenteral nutrition solutions. Its addition provides a continuous supply of the hormone, an important consideration during glucose administration. It is known that insulin is responsible for the adequate metabolism of carbohydrates. In addition to this, insulin has a lipolytic effect and increases the muscle's uptake of amino acids.

A certain degree of absorptive loss of insulin to the solution container, tubing, and filter has been demonstrated in several studies.[47,48] Some have suggested the addition of albumin to the solution in order to decrease these losses. It has been found, however, that serum glucose levels can be managed adequately without the use of albumin.[49]

Heparin in doses of 1000-3000 units/liter has been routinely used to decrease the incidence of subclavian vein thrombus. Recent studies have disputed this claim.[50,51] Larger doses of heparin, perhaps as much as 20,000 units/liter, may be needed to reduce the risk of thrombosis.[52] Such doses, however, may carry an increased risk of bleeding complications. Heparin is compatible in parenteral nutrition solutions in amounts up to 20,000 units/liter.[51]

Cimetidine is routinely added to TPN in some hospitals as a prophylactic measure against the development of stress ulcers. It has been found that concentrations of 900-1300 mg/liter are compatible with parenteral nutrition solutions.[53] Cimetidine may not, however, be compatible with iron, aminophylline, or antibiotics.[54]

The addition of aminophylline to parenteral nutrition solutions is most beneficial for the pulmonary patient who requires a continuous infusion, yet is also fluid restricted. Concentrations of up to 1500 mg/liter have been found to be chemically stable in parenteral nutrition solutions.[55]

Antibiotics added to a parenteral nutrition solution are also beneficial for the fluid-restricted patient. Such a practice would also be helpful in situations in which the availability of intravenous sites is limited. Information, however, is not yet available on several aspects of this practice. It is not known at this time whether: (1) most antibiotics are physically compatible with TPN; (2) 24-hour infusions are stable; (3) a 24-hour infusion is as effective as an intermittent infusion in combatting microorganisms. For these reasons, antibiotic admixture to TPN should be practiced on a limited basis.

Little is currently known regarding the admixture of corticosteroids to parenteral nutrition solutions. The preferred method of administration continues to be intravenous push or co-infusion. (The reader should appreciate that examples of drugs used as additives, their dosages and frequency of administration as discussed in this section reflect possible approaches to the treatment of patients receiving TPN. For definitive discussion of this topic, see appropriate texts on TPN therapy and References beginning on p. 1148.)

### 3-in-1 Solutions

A relatively new product, 3-in-1 solutions, combines fat, amino acids, and dextrose in one container. Stability of various amino acid and fat solutions and electrolyte and mineral additives is variable. Bacterial growth may be enhanced by admixture of fat emulsions with dextrose and amino acid solutions. However, this form of nutritional support has been demonstrated to be more efficient and cost-effective.[56]

### Specialized Parenteral Formulas

Various parenteral formulas have been designed to meet the needs of patients with specific disease states (Table 53-23). Formulas available for use in

TABLE 53-23
**Specialized Parenteral Formulas**

| Specific Disorder | Parenteral Formulas |
|---|---|
| Renal failure | Nephramine 5.4% (McGaw)<br>Aminosyn RF 5.2% (Abbott)<br>Renamin (Travenol) |
| Liver disease | Hepatamine 8% (McGaw) |
| Trauma | FreAmine HBC 6-9% (McGaw) |

renal failure contain high amounts of essential amino acids. It is believed that high amounts of essential amino acids increase nephron repair in renal failure.[57] A particular amino acid, L-histadine, appears to enhance amino acid utilization in uremia.[57] Some studies, however, have indicated that solutions high in essential amino acids do not necessarily decrease the need for dialysis or alter the outcome. They have suggested the use of standard formulations in acute renal failure.[58]

Solutions high in branched-chain amino acids (BCAA) have been formulated for patients with liver disease. Patients with chronic liver disease are often found to have elevated levels of aromatic amino acids and depressed levels of branched-chain amino acids. This disproportion in amino acid levels is believed by some to be an etiologic factor in hepatic encephalopathy.[59] The administration of formulas high in BCAA would seem to be beneficial, however, controversy exists in this area. A recent study failed to demonstrate any clinical or laboratory improvement with BCAA infusions.[60]

Formulas high in BCAA have also been recommended in the care of the trauma patient. It is believed that this group of patients has a predilection to break down BCAA in muscles.[61] The administration of BCAA is thought to replenish those depleted stores; BCAA are also more easily metabolized than aromatic amino acids. Further study, however, needs to be conducted before widespread use of this product.

### *Complications of Parenteral Nutrition*

Much research has been done in the area of parenteral nutrition in the hope of enhancing tolerance and minimizing complications. Advances have been made that have significantly decreased the morbidity associated with this form of therapy. Complications, however, still occur and may be divided into two groups: *catheter-related* and *metabolic*. Table 53–24[61–67] contains an outline of the various complications along with measures for their prevention and treatment.

TABLE 53–24
**Complications of Parenteral Nutrition**

| Complication | Prevention | Treatment |
|---|---|---|
| | ***Catheter Related*** | |
| Pneumothorax | • Place patient in Trendelenburg position prior to central line insertion. | • A small pneumothorax may be self limiting.<br>• Insertion of chest tube by physician with underwater seal drainage. |
| Air embolus | • Place patient in Trendelenburg position prior to central line insertion. | • Should a disconnection occur, immediately place a finger over the exposed end of the catheter until the tubing can be reconnected. |
| | • Check the intravenous connections periodically during shift to be certain that they are secure. Tape connections for added protection against disconnection.<br>• Change intravenous tubing during expiratory phase of respiratory cycle.<br>• Apply an occlusive dressing over the site after the catheter has been removed. | • Place patient in Trendelenburg in a left side lying position. |
| Subclavian vein thrombosis | • Use a catheter that has proven to be the least thrombogenic (Silcone).<br>• Administer heparin as ordered by a physician. | • Assist physician with removal of catheter.<br>• Administer heparin as ordered by a physician. |
| Catheter position displacement | • Securely tape intravenous dressing and tubing in place.<br>• Check dressing at least every 4 hr for signs of inadvertent displacement.<br>• Assist with obtaining periodic chest x-rays for visualization of catheter placement. | • Notify physician immediately if catheter is displaced. |
| Catheter occlusion | • Check intravenous fluid for proper infusion rate at least every 2 hr.<br>• Check intravenous tubing for any kinks or bends in the tubing every 2 hr.<br>• Do not give blood transfusions through a catheter that is also being used for TPN infusion.<br>• Do not withdraw blood through catheter for blood specimens. | • Have patient cough and/or change body position.<br>• Attempt to aspirate clot with a syringe.<br>• Notify physician if the above measures do not alleviate the problem. |
| Infection | • Do not add any additives to the TPN solution on the nursing unit.<br>• Avoid the intravenous injection or "piggyback" of any medications to the TPN set-up.<br>• Avoid the use of stopcocks. | • Obtain blood cultures.<br>• Administer antibiotics as ordered by a physician.<br>• Assist physician with removal of catheter if so necessitated. |

TABLE 53-24
**Complications of Parenteral Nutrition *(Continued)***

| Disease State | Treatment Plan | Rationale for Treatment |
|---|---|---|
| Infection *(cont.)* | • Tape all connections securely.<br>• Use a biocclusive dressing.<br>• Change dressing and tubing every 48 hr. | • Send catheter for culture upon its removal |
| | ***Metabolic*** | |
| Hyperglycemia | • Monitor serum glucose levels frequently.<br>• Do not increase the rate of infusion even if it is behind schedule. | • Administer insulin as ordered by a physician.<br>• Adjust flow rate of infusion as ordered by a physician. |
| Hypoglycemia | • Monitor serum glucose levels frequently.<br>• Do not discontinue the infusion suddenly. | • Administer dextrose as ordered by a physician. |
| Allergic reaction | • Administer a test dose of lipid emulsions prior to initiating the infusion at the rate ordered.<br>• Monitor patient closely during the first 30 minutes of infusion of TPN (allergic reactions have been reported with lipids, iron dextran, heparin and insulin). | • Administer benadryl and/or steroids per physician's order.<br>• Avoid the use of TPN products to which the patient demonstrates hypersensitivity. |
| Burns | • Administer fluids based on patient's clinical status.<br>• Administer electrolytes based on patient's clinical status, especially sodium, potassium, chloride, calcium, magnesium, and phosphorus. | • Thermal injury results in destruction of the skin barrier leading to evaporative water loss.<br>• Electrolytes are depleted along with water via evaporative and renal losses.<br>• Some substances used in burn wound care deplete electrolytes (e.g., silver nitrate, mafenide acetate).<br>• Increased carbohydrate intake necessitates higher quantities of phosphorus. |
| Sepsis | • Administer formulas high in branched-chain amino acids (BCAA).<br>• Administer lipids as 30–50% of the total nonprotein calories.<br>• Administer insulin based on patient's clinical status.<br>• Restrict the administration of iron. | • Sepsis increases energy needs. BCAA supply energy to the heart, liver, and skeletal muscle.<br>• Lipid administration is vital during sepsis as there is an increased breakdown of this substrate.<br>• Hyperglycemia occurs in response to stress.<br>• Insulin may inhibit protein breakdown and stimulate its synthesis.<br>• Iron is essential for the growth of numerous bacteria. Iron administration during the acute phase of sepsis may increase its severity. |

TABLE 53-25
**Special Considerations for Specific Disease States**

| Disease State | Treatment Plan | Rationale for Treatment |
|---|---|---|
| Renal failure | • Administer formulas high in essential amino acids (EAA).<br>• Administer electrolytes based on patient's clinical status.<br>• Restrict fluids based on patient's clinical status. | • Formulas high in EAA may increase nephron repair.<br>• Electrolyte derangements are a common complication in renal failure.<br>• Fluid overload is a common complication in renal failure. |
| Liver disease | • Administer formulas high in branched-chain amino acids (BCAA).<br>• Restrict total protein intake in encephalopathy.<br>• Restrict fluids and sodium based on patient's clinical status. | • BCAA are depressed in severe liver disease. This may lead to encephalopathy.<br>• Protein metabolism is decreased in severe liver disease.<br>• Fluid overload, including the development of ascites, is a common complication in liver failure. |
| Cardiac disease | • Provide nutrients in as high a concentration as possible without precipitating fluid overload.<br>• Administer intravenous lipid emulsions cautiously in severe cardiac disease.<br>• Restrict fluids and sodium based on patient's clinical status.<br>• Administer electrolytes based on patient's clinical status, especially potassium and magnesium. | • Protein-calorie malnutrition is a common sequelae of severe cardiac disease.<br>• Free fatty acids can be detrimental during periods of acute myocardial ischemia because they have negative inotropic effects and increase heart size.<br>• Fluid overload is a common complication of cardiac disease.<br>• Renal excretion of potassium and magnesium may occur as a result of the potent diuretics commonly used in the treatment of cardiac disease. |

*(continued)*

TABLE 53–25
**Special Considerations for Specific Disease States *(Continued)***

| Disease State | Treatment Plan | Rationale for Treatment |
|---|---|---|
| Pulmonary disease | • Nonprotein calories should be supplied in the following amounts:<br>–Carbohydrates 40–50%.<br>–Lipids 30–50%. | • Carbohydrates supplied in amounts greater than those recommended may lead to the increased production of $CO_2$. Increased $CO_2$ levels can decrease respiratory drive. |
| | • Administer fluids and sodium cautiously so as not to cause fluid overload. | • Excess lung water can hamper effective breathing. |
| | • Administer electrolytes based on patient's clinical status, especially phosphorus, magnesium, potassium, and calcium. | • Adequate amounts of these electrolytes are required for normal pulmonary function. |
| Trauma | • Administer formulas high in BCAA. | • Trauma causes preferential breakdown of BCAA in muscles. |
| | • Administer insulin based on patient's clinical status. | • Hyperglycemia occurs in response to trauma.<br>• Insulin may inhibit protein breakdown and stimulate its synthesis. |
| | • Administer fluids and sodium cautiously (after the resuscitation period) so as not to cause fluid overload. | • In response to injury, there is an increase in sodium and water retention. |
| Burns | • Administer higher concentrations of carbohydrates than lipids (e.g., carbohydrates = 60% nonprotein calories; lipids = 40% nonprotein calories) | • Administration of higher concentrations of carbohydrate than fat in the hypermetabolic burned patient is thought to spare proteins for muscle synthesis. |
| | • Administer formulas high in amino acids. | • Formulas high in amino acids accelerate protein synthesis. |
| | • Administer insulin based on patient's clinical status. | • Hyperglycemia occurs in response to trauma.<br>• Insulin may inhibit protein breakdown and stimulate its synthesis. |
| | • Administer fluids based on patient's clinical status. | • Thermal injury results in destruction of the skin barrier leading to evaporative water loss. |
| | • Administer electrolytes based on patient's clinical status, especially sodium, potassium, chloride, calcium, magnesium, and phosphorus. | • Electrolytes are depleted along with water through evaporative and renal losses.<br>• Some substances used in burn wound care deplete electrolytes (e.g., silver nitrate, mafenide acetate).<br>• Increased carbohydrate intake necessitates higher quantities of phosphorus. |
| Sepsis | • Administer formulas high in BCAA. | • Sepsis increases energy needs. BCAA supply energy to the heart, liver, and skeletal muscle. |
| | • Administer lipids as 30–50% of the total nonprotein calories. | • Lipid administration is vital during sepsis because there is an increased breakdown of this substrate. |
| | • Administer insulin based on patient's clinical status. | • Hyperglycemia occurs in response to stress.<br>• Insulin may inhibit protein breakdown and stimulate its synthesis. |
| | • Restrict the administration of iron. | • Iron is essential for the growth of numerous bacteria. Iron administration during the acute phase of sepsis may increase its severity. |

## SPECIAL CONSIDERATIONS FOR SPECIFIC DISEASE STATES

The preceding sections of this chapter have contained a detailed description of the nutritional requirements of the critically ill patient and the therapeutic modalities available. There are patients, however, with specific conditions who require special nutritional considerations. Specific disease states are presented in Table 53–25,[68–71] along with a specially designed treatment plan.

## SUMMARY

Nutritional support for the critically ill patient is the foundation from which he/she is able to combat illness and maintain wellness. Because critically ill patients are usually hypermetabolic, relying on body stores to supply their needs, it is important that nutritional therapy be instituted as soon after admission as possible. Patients not able to eat in the usual way are afforded two other methods to receive the needed nutrients, enteral or parenteral nutrition. Methods of delivery and tips for enhancing tolerance of both parenteral and enteral nutrition have been explored. In the final assessment, the nurse plays a key role in the nutritional support of the critically ill patient.

## REFERENCES

1. Nightingale, F: Notes on Nursing: What It Is and What It Is Not. New York, Appleton and Company, 1860.
2. Bistrain, B: Prevalence of malnutrition in general medical patients. JAMA 235:1567–1570, 1976.

3. Buchanan, RT and Levine, NS: Nutritional support of the surgery patient. Ann Plast Surg 10(2):159–166, 1983.
4. Rose, SG et al: Problems with interpretation of repeat antigen skin tests in the surgical patient. NSS 6(5):14–21, 1986.
5. Glucroft, J: Skin test update. NSS 6(5):16, 1986.
6. Grossman, J et al: The effect of aging and acute illness on delayed hypersensitivity. J Allergy Clin Immunol 55:268–275, 1975.
7. Katz MD, Lor, E, and McGhan WF: Comparison of serum prealbumin and transferrin for nutritional assessment of TPN patients: A preliminary study. NSS 6(8):22–24, 1986.
8. Forse, RA and Shizgal, HM: Serum albumin and nutritional status. JPEN 1(2):89–96, 1986.
9. Blackburn, GL et al: Nutritional and metabolic assessment of the hospitalized patient. JPEN 1:11–22, 1977.
10. Konstantinides, F et al: 24-hour urine collection for nitrogen balance: Is iced collection necessary? NSS 5(9):34–37, 1985.
11. Brennan, EL: Albumin: A role in nutritional support. NSS 6(5):15, 1986.
12. Ekman, L and Wretlind, A: The glucose–lipid ratio in parenteral nutrition. NSS 5(9):26–31, 1985.
13. Elwyn, DH: Nutritional requirements of adult surgical patients. Crit Care Med 8:9–19, 1980.
14. Olson GB, Teasley KM, and Cerra FB: Balanced parenteral nutrition. NSS 5(6):16–20, 1985.
15. Askanazi, J et al: Respiratory distress secondary to increased carbohydrate load: A case report. Surgery 87:596–598, 1980.
16. Burke, JF et al: Glucose requirements following burn injury. Ann Surg 190:274–285, 1979.
17. Askanazi, J et al: Nutrition for the patient with respiratory failure. Glucose vs. fat. Anesthesiology 54:373–377, 1981.
18. O'Neil JA, Caldwell MD, and Meng HC: Essential fatty acid deficiency in surgical patients. Ann Surg 185:535–542, 1977.
19. Hoppe, M: Nutritional management of the trauma patient. Crit Care Q June:1–16, 1983.
20. Heymsfield, SB et al: Enteral hyperalimentation: An alternative to central venous hyperalimentation. Ann Intern Med 90:63–71, 1979.
21. Konstantinides, N and Shronts, E: Tube feedings: Managing the basics. Am J Nurs 83(9):1312–1320, 1983.
22. Crowley, R and Dunham, C (eds): Shock Trauma/Critical Care Manual. Baltimore, University Park Press, 1982.
23. Patterson, RS and Andrassy, RT: Needle-catheter jejunostomy. Am J Nurs 83(9):1325–1326, 1983.
24. Hoover CH, Ryan, JA, and Fischer, JE: Nutritional benefits immediate postoperative jejunal feeding of an elemental diet. A J Surg 139:153–159, 1980.
25. Orr, G et al: Alternatives to total parenteral nutrition in the critically ill patient. Crit Care Med 8:29–34, 1980.
26. Randall, HT: Enteral feeding. In Ballinger WF (ed): Manual of Surgical Nutrition. Philadelphia, WB Saunders, 1975.
27. Rombeau, JL and Jacobs, DO: Nasoenteric tube feeding. In Rombeau, JL and Caldwell, MD (eds): Enteral and Tube Feeding. Philadelphia, WB Saunders, 1984.
28. Fason, MF: Controlling bacterial growth in tube feedings. Am J Nurs 67:1246–1247, 1967.
29. Rees, RG et al: Tolerance of elemental diet administered without starter regimen. Brit Med J 290:1869–1870, 1985.
30. Russell, RI: Elemental diets. Gut 18:68–79, 1975.
31. Kelly TW, Patrick MB, and Hillman KM: Study of diarrhea in critically ill patients. Crit Care Med 11:7–9, 1983.
32. Cataldi-Betcher, E et al: Complications occurring during enteral nutrition support: A prospective study. JPEN 14:32–42, 1983.
33. Bernard, M and Forlaw, L: Complications and their prevention. In Rombeau JL, Caldwell MD (eds): Enteral and Tube Feeding. Philadelphia, WB Saunders, 1984.
34. Haynes-Johnson, V: Tube feeding complications: Causes, prevention and therapy. NSS 6:17–18, 1986.
35. Glaser, D and Mason, AT: Lactose intolerance in patients taking oral nutrient supplements. NSS 5:42, 1985.
36. Russel, RI: Progress report: Elemental diets. Gut 16:68–79, 1975.
37. Valenta, CL: Urine testing and home blood glucose monitoring. Nurs Clin North Am 18:645–659, December 1983.
38. Padilla, et al: Subjective distresses of nasogastric tube feeding. JPEN 13:53–57, 1979.
39. Altman E, Cutie AJ, and Schwartz M: Compatibility of enteral products with commonly employed drug additives. NSS 12(4):8–17, 1984.
40. Melnick G and Wright, K: Pharmacologic aspects of enteral nutrition. In Rombeau JL, Caldwell MD (eds): Enteral and Tube Feeding. Philadelphia, WB Saunders, 1984.
41. Parsa, MH and Shoemaker, WC: Nutritional failure. In Shoemaker WC, Thompson WL, and Holbrook PR (eds): The Society of Critical Care Medicine: Textbook of Critical Care. Philadelphia, WB Saunders, 1984.
42. Hamilton HW, Hamilton KR, and Lone FJ: Preoperative hair removal. Can J Surg 20:269, 1977.
43. Jarrard, M and Freeman, J: The effects of antibiotic ointments and antiseptics on the skin flora beneath subclavian catheter dressings during intravenous hyperalimentation. J Surg Res 22:521, 1977.
44. Jarrard MM, Olson CM, and Freeman JF: Daily dressing change effects on skin flora beneath subclavian catheter dressing during total parenteral nutrition. JPEN 4:391, 1980.
45. Millan, DA: Final inline filters. Am J Nurs 79:1272, 1979.
46. Berge, H et al: Clearance of fat emulsions in severely stressed patients. NSS 4(12):18–26, 1984.
47. Weber S, Wood W, and Jackson E: Availability of insulin from parenteral nutrient solutions. Am J Hosp Pharm 34:353, 1977.
48. Petty, C and Cunningham, N: Insulin absorption by glass infusion bottles, polyvinyl chloride infusion containers, and intravenous tubing. Anesthesiology 40:400, 1974.
49. Semple P, White C, and Manderson W: Continuous intravenous infusion of small doses of insulin treatment of diabetic ketoacidosis. Br Med J 2:694, 1974.
50. Ruggiero, R and Aisenstein, T: Central catheter fibrin sleeve-heparin effect. JPEN 7:270, 1983.
51. Brismar, B et al: Reduction of catheter-associated thrombosis in parenteral nutrition by intravenous heparin therapy. Arch Surg 117:1196, 1982.
52. Kobayaski, N and King, S: Compatibility of common additives in protein hydrolysate/dextrose solutions. Am J Hosp Pharm 34:589, 1977.
53. Tsallas, G and Allen, L: Stability of cimetidine hydrochloride in parenteral nutrition solutions. Am J Hosp Pharm 39:484, 1982.
54. Yuhas, E et al: Cimetidine hydrochloride compatibility. III: Room temperature stability in drug admixtures. Am J Hosp Pharm 38:1919, 1981.
55. Niemiec, P et al: Stability of aminophylline injection in three parenteral nutrition solutions. Am J Hosp Pharm 38:377, 1981.
56. Green, BA and Baptista, RJ: Nursing assessment of 3-in-1 TPN admixture. NITA 8:530–532, 1985.
57. Abel R, Abbott W, and Fischer J: Intravenous essential L-amino acids and hypertonic dextrose in patients with acute renal failure. Am J Surg 123:632–638, 1972.
58. Blumenkrantz, M et al: Total parenteral nutrition in the management of acute renal failure. Am J Clin Nutr 31:1831–1840, 1978.
59. Fischer, JE et al: The effect of normalization of plasma amino acids on hepatic encephalopathy in man. Surgery 80:77–91.
60. Wahren, J et al: Is intravenous administration of branched chain amino acids effective in the treatment of hepatic encephalopathy? A multicenter study. Hepatology 3:475–480, 1983.
61. Schmitz JE, Ahnefeld FW, and Burri C: Nutritional support of the multiple trauma patient. World J Surg 7:132–142, 1983.

62. Abel, RM: Nutritional support in the patient with acute renal failure. J Am Coll Nutr 2:33–44, 1983.
63. Maddrey, WC: Branched-chain amino acid therapy in liver disease. J Am Coll Nutr 4:639–650, 1985.
64. Wilson DO, Rogers RM, Hoffman RM: Nutrition and chronic lung disease. Ann Rev Respir Dis 132:1347–1365, 1985.
65. Armstrong, JN: Nutrition and the respiratory patient. NSS 6(3):8–32, 1986.
66. Krevsky, B and Godley, J: Nutritional support in advanced liver disease. NSS 5(8):8–17, 1985.
67. Wolk, RA and Swartz, RD: Nutritional support of patients with acute renal failure. NSS 6(2):38–46, 1986.
68. Forlaw, L and Torosian, MH: Central venous catheter care. In Rombeau, JL and Caldwell, MD (eds): Parenteral Nutrition. WB Saunders, Philadelphia, 1986.
69. Ang, SD and Daly, JM: Potential complications and monitoring of patients receiving total parenteral nutrition. In Rombeau, JL and Caldwell, MD (eds): Parenteral Nutrition. WB Saunders, Philadelphia: 1986.
70. Sheldon, GF and Baker, C: Complications of nutritional support. Crit Care Med 8(1):35–37, 1980.
71. Udall, JN and Richardson, DS: Allergic reactions to parenteral nutrition solutions. NSS 6(4):20–22, 1986.

# UNIT SEVEN

# Bibliography


Cohn, O: Complications of portal hypertension. Curr Hepatol 1(119):1980.

Eastwood, GL: Core Textbook of Gastroenterology. JB Lippincott, Philadelphia, 1984.

Goldenberg, DA: Management of bleeding esophageal varices. Crit Care Q 5(2):September 1982.

Goldrick, B: Infection control in the ICU. In Emanuelsen, K and Rosenlicht, JM (eds): Handbook of Critical Care Nursing. John Wiley & Sons.

Granger, D, Barrowman, JA, and Kvietys, P: Clinical Gastrointestinal Physiology. WB Saunders, Philadelphia, 1985.

Johnson, LR: Gastrointestinal Physiology, ed 2. CV Mosby, St Louis, 1981.

Kelton, JG: Management of the bleeding patient. In Sibbald J (ed): Synopsis of Critical Care, 2. Williams & Wilkins, Baltimore, 1984.

Malkiewicz, J: For a really thorough abdominal exam. . . . RN October 1982.

Martin, D and Galambos, J: Fulminant Hepatic Failure. Crit Care Q 5(2):September 1982.

McConnell, EA: Meeting the challenge of intestinal obstruction. Nursing 87 17(7):34, July 1987.

Nasrallah, SM: The management of acute pancreatitis. Crit Care Q 5(2):September 1982.

Nurse's Clinical Library: Gastrointestinal disorders. In Nursing 85 Books. Springhouse Corporation, Springhouse, PA, 1985.

Ranson, JH, Ritkind, KM, and Turner, JW: Prognostic signs and nonoperative peritoneal lavage in acute pancreatitis. Surg Gynecol Obstet 143(2):August 1976.

Ranson, JH and Spencer FC: The role of peritoneal lavage in severe acute pancreatitis. Ann Surg 187:(5)565, 1978.

Schwarz, T: Is it "acute abdomen"? RN July 1982.

Sinclair, DM: Upper gastrointestinal tract bleeding and liver failure. In Cane D and Shapiro, BA (eds): Case Studies in Critical Care Medicine. Yearbook Medical Publishers, Chicago, 1985.

# UNIT EIGHT

# Immune System

Diseases of or involving the immune system have become of great importance in recent years. This stems, in part, from substantial advances in the understanding of this component of the mammalian organism; in part, from rapid technologic strides in therapy that relate to immunologic function, such as transplantation; and in part (and unfortunately a most frightening part), due to the appearance of a truly new disease, acquired immunodeficiency syndrome (AIDS), which, to a major extent, involves cells of the immune system.

It is not possible in a work of this type to cover the subject of immunology comprehensively. Rather, the intent here is to present basic information regarding the organization and functioning of the immune system and then to consider three areas that impact on critical care: immunodeficiency with a consideration of AIDS, transplantation, and immunotherapy, with some reference to autoimmunity and tumors of the immune system (e.g., lymphoma and myeloma).

Because a major thrust of molecular biology has had its origin in the study of the cells of the immune system, a comprehensive grasp is not possible without knowledge of modern biology. In this treatise, explanations that involve biochemistry beyond the exposure of the majority of readers will be avoided. References for those who seek more rigorous basis are provided.

In conjunction with the discussion of immunodeficiency, transplantation, and immunotherapy, emphasis is placed on assessing immunologic function and on examining the nursing process in the clinical management of the immunosuppressed patient. A case study concerned with the psychologic perspectives in the care of the patient with AIDS is also included.

## UNIT OUTLINE

## UNIT OUTLINE—*CONTINUED*

CHAPTER 54

# Immune System: Underlying Principles

*Frederick Miller*
*Gail Habicht*

## CHAPTER OUTLINE



## LEARNING OBJECTIVES

**At the end of this chapter, you should be able to:**

1. Describe the overall organization of the immune system including the organs that comprise it and its cellular and humoral components.
2. Explore the major functions of the immune system in terms of total body physiology.
3. Define *immunogenicity* and its key determining factors.
4. Distinguish subpopulations of lymphocytes and their functions.
5. Differentiate types of immune responses: humoral versus cellular.
6. Examine the physiologic role of the serologically defined histocompatibility antigens (HLA-A, HLA-B, and HLA-D) in the regulation of immune responses, and the implications for transplantation therapy.
7. Explain how the phenomenon of immunologic memory allows serologic diagnosis of an ongoing infection.
8. Discuss the significance of tolerance as a primary characteristic of the immune response.
9. Discuss pathophysiologic mechanisms underlying autoimmune responses.
10. Explain the concept of specificity and its significance in terms of immunologic responses.
11. Differentiate the basic effector mechanisms underlying immunoresponsiveness.
12. Explain the immunologic mechanism underlying adverse (allergic) reactions to penicillin.
13. Compare/contrast types I (atopy), II (cytotoxic reactions), and III (circulating immune complexes) effector mechanisms in terms of specificity, underlying pathophysiology, immediacy of response, and clinical manifestations of specific disease entities.
14. Examine immune processes underlying delayed hypersensitivity or cell-mediated reactions (type IV) as occurs, for example, in contact dermatitis or in a granulomatous process such as tuberculosis.

# IMMUNE SYSTEM: ANATOMY AND PHYSIOLOGY

The immune system can be defined at two levels, anatomically or functionally. For the first, it consists of those organs largely devoted to the maintenance or maturation of the cells that comprise the system, *and* those tissues and organs where these cells reside. In contrast to the circulatory system, which is very circumscribed, the immune system is diffuse. It includes the thymus, the lymph nodes (including the tonsils), and the spleen. A large immune function also resides in the bone marrow, but it is not the only function of the marrow that gives rise to erythrocytes and platelets. These do not play a role, at least not directly, in immune phenomena.

Because lymphocytes are essential components of the immune system, those tissues where these cells reside in large numbers must also be included. These include the blood, lymphatics, the submucosa of the respiratory tract, and the lamina propria (i.e., the loose connective tissue beneath the epithelial lining of the gastrointestinal tract), which, by virtue of numbers of cells, is the single largest lymphoid organ in the body (see Fig. 47–4). Lymphocytes, being by nature wandering cells, pervade many other areas on a regular basis, and, thus, such organs as skin, for example, could be included in part as components of the immune system.

Also included as part of the immune system are a variety of soluble components. These include such products as *antibodies*, which act at distances from the cells that elaborate them; and substances such as *complement*, a family of proteins in the blood, which interacts with the immune system so closely that the components of the complement system are generally treated as an important subject in immunology.

*Phagocytic* cells, such as *macrophages*, are an integral part of the immune system. These cells function to process foreign substances prior to "recognition" by the immunocytes (a general term for cells that are part of the immune system; e.g., lymphocytes), or they "execute" their directives in certain effector functions, such as the delayed hypersensitivity response critical to our defense against organisms such as the tubercle bacillus. All of these cells are parts of the immune defense system, as are neutrophils and eosinophils, occasionally, endothelial cells, and certain monocytic derivatives such as Kupffer's cells of the liver.

Function is perhaps a more easily handled subject. The immune system is that component of the body that ensures maintenance of genetic integrity, that is to say it preserves "self." It functions to (1) identify and destroy foreign invaders such as bacteria, fungi, and viruses—possibly its oldest role in the phylogenetic sense; (2) assist in the removal of injured and senescent body components; and (3) provide a possible line of defense against the emergence of cells that do not conform to the plan encoded in our DNA (i.e., cancer). One of the best ways to understand immune function is to look at persons who by virtue of hereditary disease or environmental insults (e.g., radiation exposure) are deprived of the beneficial aspects of the immune system. It is for this very reason that AIDS, while becoming the scourge of our time and perhaps equaling cancer as a disease to be feared, has evoked such interest.

In this chapter, the foundations for clinical applications will be established. Initially, some important definitions pertaining to the immune system are considered, followed by a review of the organization of the system with brief vignettes of its major components. A discussion of the concepts of specificity, memory, regulation and genetic relationships will follow. Lastly, several effector mechanisms by which it accomplishes its goals will be explored.

## Definitions: Antigens and Antibodies

### *Antigens*

Bacteria, parasites, viruses, cells, or molecules that are capable of inducing an immune response are called *antigens*. Antigens are usually foreign to their host in order for them to be immunogenic. However, not all foreign substances are capable of inducing an immune response, and, conversely, nonforeign or "self" molecules may become immunogenic in a person with autoimmune disease. Most antigens have a stable, rigid structure, and most are large. In general, proteins and polysaccharides are good antigens, while lipids and nucleic acids are not. There are, however, important exceptions to these generalizations. Animal insulins, although relatively small molecules, may be immunogenic in some diabetics. Persons with autoimmune diseases have partially lost the ability to distinguish self from nonself, and, consequently, they mount immune responses against their own body constituents. Patients with systemic lupus erythematosus (SLE), one of the most common autoimmune diseases, make antibody responses against a variety of antigens associated with the cell nucleus including nucleic acids.

Small molecules that are not by themselves immunogenic may be rendered so by coupling them to larger carrier molecules. In this case, the small molecule is called a *hapten*, and the combination is referred to as a *hapten–carrier complex* (Fig. 54–1). An example of a small molecule that frequently induces immune responses is penicillin. Approximately 10% of the U.S. population is allergic to pen-

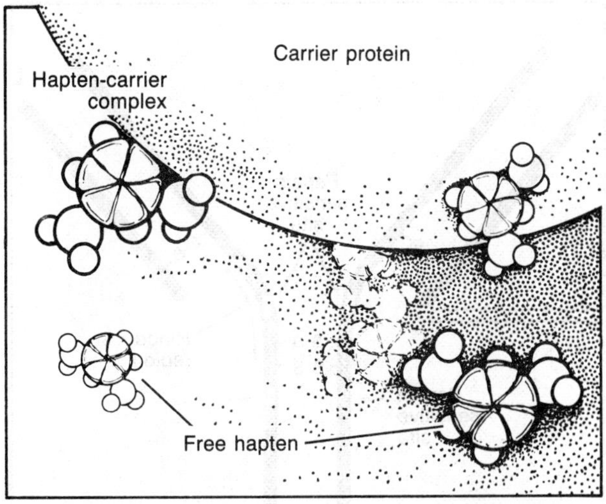


**Figure 54-1.** Small molecules, molecular weight of 1000 or less, are not usually immunogenic by themselves. They may be excreted by the kidney, or they may pass unnoticed by antigen-processing macrophages. However, when small molecules are chemically coupled to larger, carrier molecules, they may become immunogenic. They are then called haptens, and the combination is known as a hapten-carrier complex.

icillin because of immune responses specific for this hapten. Some of the metabolic breakdown products of injected penicillin are sufficiently reactive to couple themselves to carrier molecules supplied by the host. As part of a hapten-carrier complex, the penicillin becomes *immunogenic*.

**Antigenic Determinants and Crossreacting Antigens.** Even though most antigens are large molecules, only a small portion of the surface of the molecule stimulates or reacts with the products of an immune response. This portion is called an *antigenic determinant*. Thus, a single protein molecule may have several different antigenic determinants, while a polysaccharide, because of its polymeric nature, may have the same determinant repeated hundreds of times. Sometimes 2 different antigens will share antigenic determinants; these antigens are said to be *crossreacting* (Fig. 54-2). Shared antigenic determinants may be important in the induction of autoantibody formation (i.e., antibodies that react against host self-constituents).

**Immunogenicity: Determining Factors.** Immunogenicity is not an inherent property of a molecule. There are many factors that determine whether or not and to what extent a molecule is immunogenic. *Genetic* factors determine whether a person is a good or poor responder to a particular antigen. The *amount* of an antigen and the *route of exposure* also determine immunogenicity. The use of materials known as *adjuvants* in conjunction with antigen may enhance the immune response to that antigen. *Alum* is an adjuvant used in human vaccines to enhance the immunogenicity of toxoids.

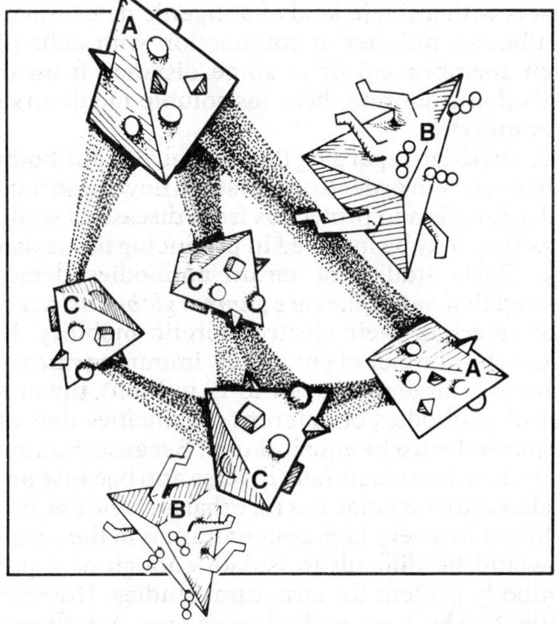


**Figure 54-2.** Proteins and other large molecules express a variety of antigenic determinants on their surfaces. When 2 molecules share antigenic determinants, they are said to be crossreacting. For example, serum albumins from 2 different species are crossreacting: antibodies against bovine serum albumin produced in a rabbit will react with determinants on human serum albumin.

**Two Arms of Immunoresponsiveness.** Antigens are capable of inducing immune responses, which may take one of two forms. The *humoral* immune response consists of the formation of *antibodies*. Antibodies belong to a family of proteins, the *immunoglobulins*, which is distributed throughout the fluid spaces of the body including the external secretions. Alternatively, exposure to an antigen may induce a *cellular* immune response mediated by the actions of living cells. Humoral and cellular immune responses are not mutually exclusive; indeed, a *mixed* response may occur. However, antigens that are soluble in the body fluids tend to induce antibody formation, while antigens found on the surfaces of cells, for example, molecules expressed on the membranes of virus infected cells, tend to induce cellular immunity. Nonetheless, it should be remembered that antibodies are also the products of living cells, the *plasma cells*. The distinction between humoral and cellular immunity lies in the fact that antibodies are active in the *absence* of cells.

### *Antibodies*

*Antibodies* are proteins produced by the humoral immune system in response to an antigen. They are very *specific* in that they can distinguish between the configurations of closely related foreign molecules. Each antibody molecule is specific for and reacts with a single kind of antigenic determinant. Antibodies may act in conjunction with cells (on their membranes) or at some distance from the cells that elaborate them (as soluble mediators of immunity).

Knowledge regarding the structure of antibodies is necessary in order to understand how these molecules function to protect us from disease as well as how they may be involved in producing tissue damage. Early studies of serum antibodies demonstrated that antibodies are *gamma globulins*, a term that refers to their electrophoretic mobility. Because the number of potentially immunogenic substances is large (perhaps 1 to 10 million), the number of antibodies of different specificities that can be formed must be equally large. Because immunoglobulins are structurally diverse and because antibodies are so specific it is rare that any one antibody is found in a very high concentration in the serum, it would be difficult to isolate enough of a pure antibody protein for structural studies. However, patients who have *multiple myeloma*, a malignant proliferation of plasma cells, synthesize large amounts of a single homogeneous immunoglobulin. Much of what we know about immunoglobulin structure derives from studies of these homogeneous antibodies (Fig. 54–3).

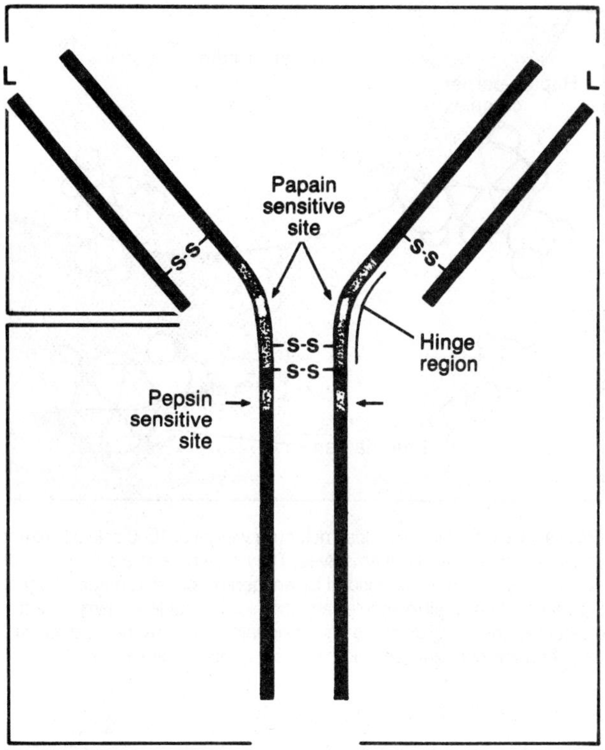


**Figure 54–3.** The basic structure of immunoglobulin consists of 4 polypeptide chains. Two H (heavy) chains are linked to each other by 1 or more disulfide bonds. One L (light) chain is joined to each H chain by a single disulfide bond. The molecule is drawn as a "Y" to reflect the flexibility of the H chain in the "hinge region." The hinge region is particularly susceptible to cleavage by papain, pepsin, and other proteolytic enzymes. The Fab and Fc fragments resulting from cleavage by papain are shown.

**Monoclonal Antibodies.** Malignant plasma cells from mice with multiple myeloma have been used in another fashion to add to our knowledge of antibodies. Some malignant plasma cells fail to secrete any immunoglobulin. These nonsecreting cells can be fused with an antibody-forming cell from an immunized mouse to confer upon the resulting hybrid cell, called a *hybridoma*, properties from both original cell types. That is, the hybrid cell proliferates as did the malignant cell and it produces the antibody originally produced by the normal cell. Appropriate selection techniques are then employed to choose the clone of cells secreting the antibody of interest. The immunoglobulins secreted by a clone of hybrid cells are identical, that is, they are *monoclonal antibodies*. This technology has allowed the production of large quantities of antibodies of a known specificity, which may be studied themselves or which may be used as tools in molecule biology or in the clinical laboratory.

**Classes of Immunoglobulins: Structural Relationships.** All immunoglobulins are structurally related. There are 5 recognized classes of immunoglobulins, which share a common subunit structure consisting of 4 polypeptide chains linked together covalently by disulfide bonds (Fig. 54–4). There are 2 pairs of chains for each molecule–1 pair of *heavy or H chains* of molecular weight ranging from 50,000 to 75,000 daltons each, depending on the class of immunoglobulin, and 1 pair of *light or L chains* of molecular weight 23,000 daltons. The important features of this structure are twofold. The *antibody-combining site* is made of portions of both the heavy and light chains, and because there are 2 pairs of these chains, antibodies are *bivalent*, that is, they can bind 2 antigen molecules at one time. The antigen-combining sites are located on the *Fab* portions of immunoglobulin molecule. The remaining portion is known as the *Fc* portion; this part of the molecule varies among classes of immunoglobulins and determines the *biologic activities* of the class of antibodies.

**Classes of Antibodies: Specific Characteristics.** Of the 5 classes of antibodies, the most abundant is *IgG*. It is found throughout the fluid spaces of the body and is unique in that it is the only class of immunoglobulin to be transported across the placenta. This transplacental movement is very important in that it provides the newborn infant with a wide variety of antibodies specific for pathogenic organisms to which the mother has been exposed. This is the most important immunity the newborn has because its own ability to form antibodies develops gradually over the first few years of life. On the other hand, transplacental transfer of IgG antibodies specific for the Rh antigen may have harmful

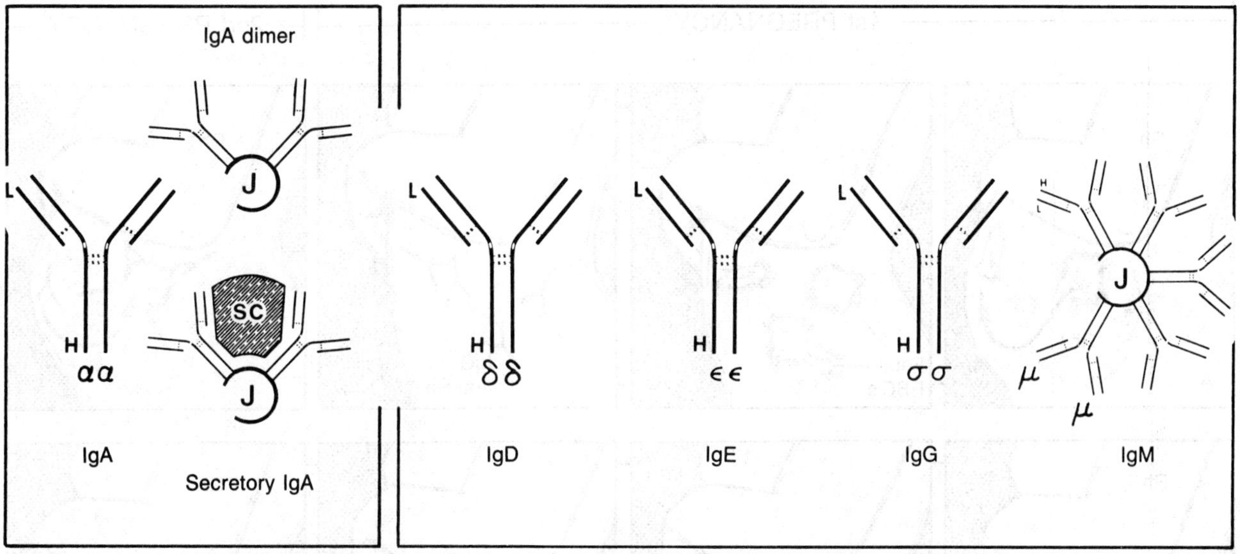


**Figure 54–4.** The arrangement of the polypeptide chains in the 5 classes of immunoglobulins is shown here. Dashed lines represent disulfide bonds. All classes of immunoglobulin have the same light chains, namely, kappa or lambda. However, the H chains are named using the Greek letter corresponding to the class name. The J or joining piece is found in IgM and polymeric IgA. The SC polypeptide or secretory component is associated with IgA in external secretions, such as tears and saliva.

effects on the unborn child resulting in erythroblastosis fetalis (Fig. 54–5).

Another important biologic function associated with the Fc portion of IgG is the ability to fix or activate complement. *Complement* is a group of serum proteins that act to enhance or amplify the effects of antibodies on living cells. This will be discussed at length later in this chapter. The activation of complement produces *cell lysis* as well as a number of cellular and tissue changes related to inflammation.

*IgM* antibodies can also activate complement. This immunoglobulin is the largest antibody, and, because of its size, it is largely restricted to the intravascular space. IgM is a pentamer of the basic immunoglobulin subunit, and it has a functional valence of 5 (see Fig. 54–4). Because of its high valence, IgM is a good *agglutinating* antibody (i.e., it is very effective at making particles or cells clump together).

*IgA* is the *secretory* immunoglobulin. It is found in the external secretions of the body where it forms part of the "first line of defense" against invasion by microorganisms. IgA is very efficient at agglutination so that IgA-coated bacteria and viruses are no longer able to adhere to surfaces through which they would otherwise gain access to the body. This immunoglobulin does not fix complement as effectively as IgG or IgM and does not participate in the lysis of cells or microorganisms. IgA antibodies are formed in response to antigens, which enter the body across the mucosal surfaces. They are found in colostrum and breast milk. Once ingested, because of an additional polypeptide chain called the *secretory piece* which protects the IgA molecule from degradation by acid in the stomach, the IgA molecules enter the infant's small intestine. Here the IgA is very effective at preventing intestinal infections, which are so devastating to a neonate.

*IgE* antibody is found only in minute concentrations in the body, but its presence is easily revealed by its powerful biologic activities. IgE, also known as homocytotropic antibody, binds to *Fc receptors* on mast cells found in the skin and mucosal linings and basophils found in the blood. Fc receptors bind the Fc portion of an antibody molecule and are specific for a particular class of immunoglobulin. By binding antibody, these receptors allow the cell to express the specificity encoded in the Fab portion of the bound antibody. Mast cells (secretory cells, present in many tissues usually near small blood vessels, capable of synthesizing histamine and similar substances) and basophils (the counterpart of the mast cell, which is present in circulating blood in small numbers) possess granules that contain a number of potent vasoactive substances. When antibodies bound to the Fc receptor react with their antigens, the contents of the granules are discharged and other potent factors are synthesized and released. These substances act on smooth muscle of the vascular and respiratory systems producing many of the symptoms commonly known as *allergy* (see the section entitled "Type I Mechanisms: Atopy," below). IgE antibodies are important components of host defenses against parasites, especially intestinal worms.

*IgD* antibodies are also found in low concentration in serum; their main function may be as mem-

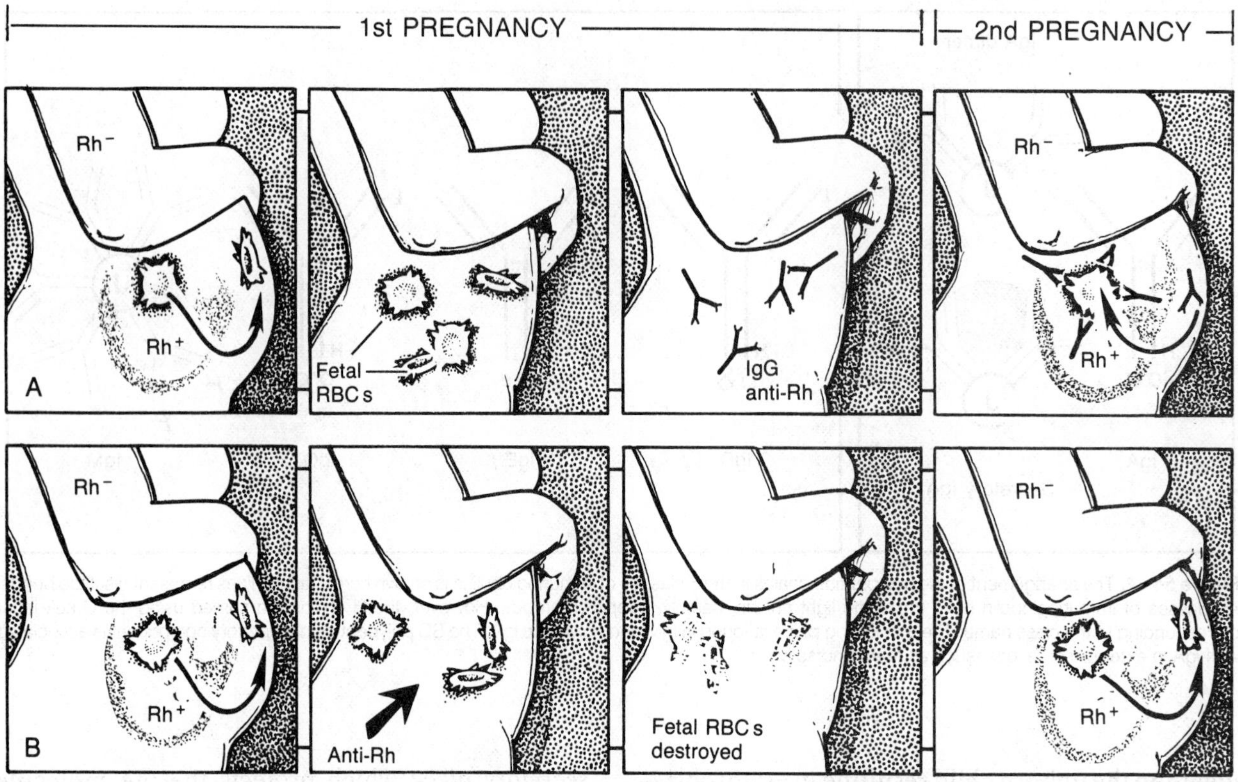


**Figure 54-5.** (*A*) Maternal antibodies of the IgG class can cross the placenta. When these antibodies react with a fetal antigen, damage to the fetus may result. This occurs in Rh disease or erythroblastosis fetalis in which an Rh-negative mother, immunized as a result of a previous pregnancy with an Rh-positive fetus, produces anti-Rh antibodies, which cross the placenta and destroy fetal erythrocytes. (*B*) Rh disease has largely been eliminated by successful immunotherapy. Just after delivery or either spontaneous or induced abortion of a possible Rh-positive fetus to an Rh-negative mother, the mother is treated with anti-Rh containing human immunoglobulin. These antibodies react with any fetal cells that have entered the maternal circulation and destroy them before they interact with the maternal immune system.

brane receptors for antigen on B-lymphocytes. They are not known to have clinical significance.

## ORGANIZATION OF THE IMMUNE SYSTEM

### Immune Response: Product of Living Cells

The specific immune response is the product of living cells. The primary cell type involved in immunoresponsiveness is the small round lymphocyte found in the blood and in various lymphoid organs. Monocytes and macrophages, however, are usually the first cells to encounter an antigen. The macrophage is the tissue form of the monocyte, which is present only in marrow and blood. These cells ingest and digest the antigen and then display the processed antigen on their cell membranes in a form suitable for stimulating lymphocytes. Antibodies are synthesized by *plasma cells,* which are derived from a class of lymphocytes known as *B cells.*

### Divisions of Immunoresponsiveness

All of the formed elements of the blood, including lymphocytes and monocytes, are derived from the bone marrow. When the lymphocytes fail to develop, the affected individuals suffer from *immunodeficiency diseases.* It was the study of persons with 2 different immunodeficiencies that led to the conclusion that there are 2 divisions of immunoresponsiveness. In the first case, an immunodeficiency characterized by frequent bacterial infections and agammaglobulinemia (Bruton's agammaglobulinemia) was shown to be due to a lack of lymphocytes in germinal centers of lymph nodes and spleen. However, the ability to make cell-mediated immune responses was retained. This suggested that the *humoral* immune response and *cell-mediated* immunity were carried out by separate populations of lymphocytes.

A second immunodeficiency characterized by near normal serum immunoglobulin levels and antibody responses but no cell-mediated immunity was found (DiGeorge syndrome). These persons suffered from recurrent viral and fungal infections. They were found to have a congenital defect in which the thymus failed to develop. In addition, the cellularity of the spleen and lymph nodes was reduced. Thus, it was recognized that the thymus is the seat of the cellular immune response. Lymphocytes that mature in the thymus are known as *T cells.* A second class of lymphocytes, missing in persons with agammaglobulinemia, complete their maturation in the bone marrow and are known as *B cells.*

### *T-Lymphocytes and B-Lymphocytes*

Although T-lymphocytes and B-lymphocytes are indistinguishable by microscopy, they may be classified according to *markers* on their cell membranes. These markers correspond to recognizable structures that have antigenic and functional properties. Human T-lymphocytes are characterized by the presence of a membrane receptor for sheep erythrocytes. In a mixture of lymphocytes and sheep erythrocytes, the red cells will bind to the T cells to form rosettes (Fig. 54-6). By counting the numbers of rosetting and nonrosetting lymphocytes, the percentage of T cells in a mixed population may be determined. B cells, on the other hand, are characterized by the presence of membrane immunoglobulin, which may be detected by immunofluorescence.

While these are the classic markers distinguishing T-lymphocytes from B-lymphocytes, the advent of monoclonal antibodies has made it possible to recognize many subpopulations, especially of T cells. By using monoclonal antibodies to select or destroy specific populations, it has been possible to assign functions to the various subpopulations of lymphocytes (Table 54-1). In addition, the ontogeny of T-lymphocytes has been characterized with respect to the appearance and disappearance of membrane molecules as the pre-T cell arrives in thymus, matures, and is exported to the peripheral blood and lymphoid tissues (Table 54-2). Characterization of lymphocytes according to their membrane markers is done by immunofluorescence and analyzed by use of a cytofluorograph. This instrument, also called a *fluorescence-activated cell sorter* (*FACS*), replaces the fluorescence microscope for enumerating the numbers of fluorescent cells in a mixed population. It has made rosette counting obsolete.

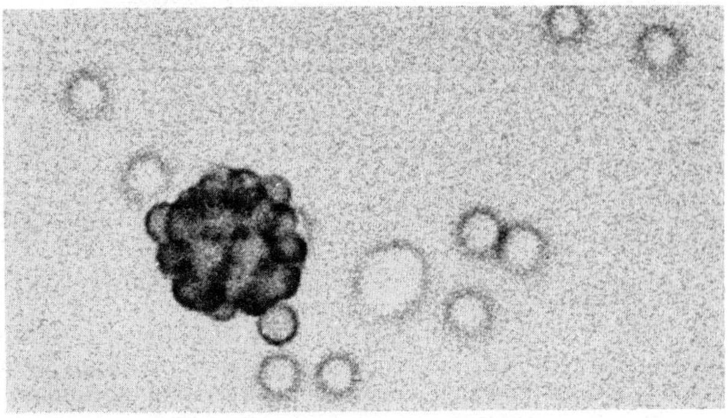

**Figure 54-6.** Human T-lymphocytes form rosettes with sheep erythrocytes. The receptor for sheep erythrocytes is a membrane protein known as T11. In a normal individual 60%-80% of peripheral blood lymphocytes are T cells (i.e., they form rosettes with sheep erythrocytes or react with monoclonal anti-T11 antibodies).

### *Subpopulations of Lymphocytes: Distinguishing Functions*

It is not always sufficient to know the numbers of lymphocytes of various subpopulations in a patient. Sometimes it is useful to know how well they function. To measure function, lymphocytes are exposed to antigens or a variety of substances derived from plants and bacteria. These substances, known as *mitogens*, stimulate DNA synthesis and cell division. B-lymphocytes respond to pokeweed mitogen, while T cell responsiveness is usually elicited with concanavalin A or phytohemagglutinin. These responses are measured by following the uptake of a radioactive precursor of DNA or by simply counting the numbers of dividing cells. While more time-consuming and expensive than counting lymphocytes, measurement of DNA synthesis provides much more specific and useful information.

TABLE 54-1
**Human Peripheral Blood Lymphocytes**

| Cells | Membrane Antigen | % of Normal Blood Lymphocytes | Function |
|---|---|---|---|
| B cells | Immunoglobulin | 10-15 | Production of antibody |
| T cells | | | |
| Total | CD2 | 60-80 | Cell mediated immunity: Immunoregulation |
| Helper T | CD4 | 15-30 | Helper/inducer |
| Suppressor T | CD8 | 40-60 | Suppressor/cytotoxic |

TABLE 54–2
**Maturation of T Lymphocytes**

| Cell | Markers | Anatomic Location |
|---|---|---|
| Early thymocyte | $CD5^+$, $CD2^+$, $HLA^+$, $TdT^+$, $PNA^+$ | Thymus (cortex) |
| Common thymocyte | $CD1^+$, $CD5^+$, $CD2^+$, $CD4^+$, $CD8^+$, $PNA^+$, $TdT^+$, $HLA^+$ | Thymus (cortex) |
| Mature thymocyte | $CD5^+$, $CD3^+$, $CD4^+$, $CD8^+$, $CD2^+$, $PNA^-$, $TdT^-$, $HLA^+$ | Thymus (medulla) |
| Inducer/Helper T cells | $CD5^+$, $CD3^+$, $CD4^+$, $CD2^+$, $PNA^-$, $TdT^-$, $HLA^+$ | Blood, spleen, lymph nodes |
| Suppressor/Cytotoxic T cells | $CD5^+$, $CD3^+$, $CD8^+$, $CD2^+$, $PNA^-$, $TdT^-$, $HLA^+$ | Blood, spleen, lymph nodes |

CD2 and CD5 are found on all T cells. CD1 is a marker of immature T cells as are receptors for peanut agglutinin (PNA) and the presence of terminal transferase (TdT) in the cytoplasm. Mature T cells express either CD4 or CD8, but not both. CD3 is closely associated with the T cell receptor for antigen and is found on mature thymocytes and peripheral T cells.

## Humoral Immunity

### *Antibody Formation*

Antibody formation and cell-mediated immune responses involve complex interactions between lymphocytes belonging to different classes and subpopulations. While early clues to these interactions came from the studies of patients with immunodeficiencies, most of what we know about the cells involved in immunoresponsiveness has come from investigations with cultured cells. Although B cells stimulated with antigen give rise to antibody-producing plasma cells, antigen stimulation alone will not result in antibody formation to most antigens. The B cell needs help, and this is provided by an antigen-specific *helper T* cell by mechanism that is not fully understood (Fig. 54–7).

Helper T cells must be stimulated with antigen presented to them in a suitable molecular environment on the surface of a macrophage. In order to excite the helper T cell, the macrophage, upon interaction with antigen, secretes a factor known as *interleukin-1* (IL-1). IL-1 acts on the helper T, causing it to do 2 things: first, it expresses membrane receptors for *interleukin-2 (IL-2)*; and, second, it secretes IL-2. IL-2 acts as a growth factor for T cells and was formerly known as T cell growth factor. This combination of events results in the proliferation of the antigen-specific helper T cells, thereby amplifying their ability to help B cells make antibody.

Helper T cells, in turn, are regulated by another subpopulation of T lymphocytes known as *suppressor T cells.* Helper T cells are characterized by the membrane molecule known as CD4, while suppressor T cells bear the *CD8* marker (see Table 54–1). These markers are recognized by monoclonal antibodies, and the ratio of helper to suppressor cells may be determined by use of the cytofluorograph (FACS).

A number of other surface markers enable us to identify additional subpopulations and to determine the maturity of lymphocytes. In a normal person, the ratio of helper to suppressor T cells in the blood is about 2 : 1. This ratio may be greatly altered in either immunodeficiency disease (e.g., AIDS) where it is decreased to less than 1 or in autoimmune disease states where the ratio is elevated. A normal immune response is the result of a delicate balance between helper and suppressor cells. T and B cells can secrete several types of small molecules called *lymphokines.* IL-2 is one and gamma interferon, which plays a role in macrophage activation, is another. They have profound effects in very, very low concentrations.

## TRANSPLANTATION AND HISTOCOMPATIBILITY

Within the last 45 years the surgical techniques for transplanting a number of organs, including the kidney and the heart, have been perfected. However, almost all transplants between genetically unrelated persons are doomed to failure resulting from an immunologic rejection of the transplanted tissue. The chief means by which transplants are rejected early in their course is through *cell-mediated* immune mechanisms. Such rejection can often be blocked by immunosuppressive drugs. Antibody plays a role only in chronic or long-term rejection, and at present there is really no effective counter measure.

### Major Histocompatibility Complex (MHC)

Tissue undergoing rejection is infiltrated with T-lymphocytes derived from the host. What is it that the T-lymphocytes recognize on the donor tissue? Just as the red blood cell surface can be characterized by the presence or absence of A or B antigens, other cells of the body are characterized by antigens on their surfaces. These antigens, referred to as *histocompatibility antigens*, differ from one person to the next. There is 1 gene complex responsible for determining the most important histocom-

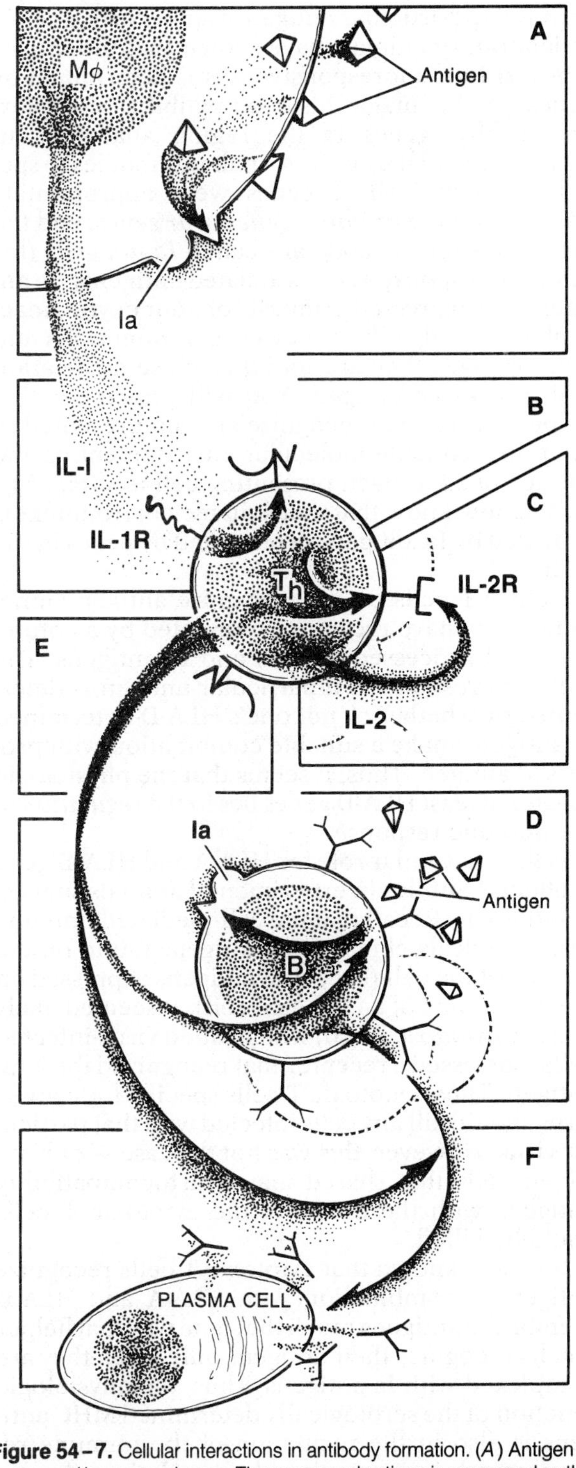


**Figure 54-7.** Cellular interactions in antibody formation. (*A*) Antigen is processed by macrophages. The processed antigen is expressed on the cell membrane in close association with Ia antigen. (*B*) The T-cell receptor for antigen recognizes a combination of Ia and antigen. The macrophage secretes interleukin 1 (IL-1), which is recognized by T-helper cell receptors for IL-1 (IL-1R). (*C*) When the T-helper cell is stimulated by IL-1 and antigen it expresses the IL-2 receptor (IL-2R) and it secretes IL-2. Interaction of IL-2 with the IL-2R causes the T-helper cell to proliferate. (*D*) B cells bind antigen through the Fab portion of the membrane immunoglobulin. The antigen is processed and reexpressed on the cell membrane with Ia. (*E*) The T-helper cell receptor recognizes the antigen–Ia complex and secretes factors that cause the proliferation and differentiation of B cells to plasma cells. (*F*) The plasma cell, which does not normally proliferate, secretes antibodies that are reactive with a determinant on the antigen.

patibility antigens, and it is referred to as the *major histocompatibility complex* (*MHC*). In humans this complex is known as the *HLA* (*human leukocyte antigen*) *gene complex* (Fig. 54–8).

Within this gene complex there is sufficient DNA to code for several hundred proteins. Three of these are expressed on the surfaces of all nucleated cells and are known as *HLA*, *HLA-B*, and *HLA-C*. These antigens, recognized by their reactions with antibodies, are also known as the *serologically defined* or *class I* major histocompatibility antigens. Each of these has many different *alleles* or alternative forms. For example, alternative alleles at the A locus are designated A-1, A-2, A-9, and so forth, while alternative alleles at the B locus are designated B-5, B-7, and so forth. One complete set of antigens is inherited from each parent (Fig. 54–9). Because of the large number of different alleles that could be inherited at each locus it is very unlikely that 2 persons would have the same histocompatibility types unless they came from the same family. Thus, among other uses, histocompatibility typing has been used to settle disputed paternity cases.

Although monoclonal antibodies are now employed to define alleles of the *HLA-D* or *class II* subregion of the MHC, these products originally defied definition by serologic techniques. Rather, they were characterized by their ability to stimulate a *mixed lymphocyte reaction* (*MLR*). The MLR is the

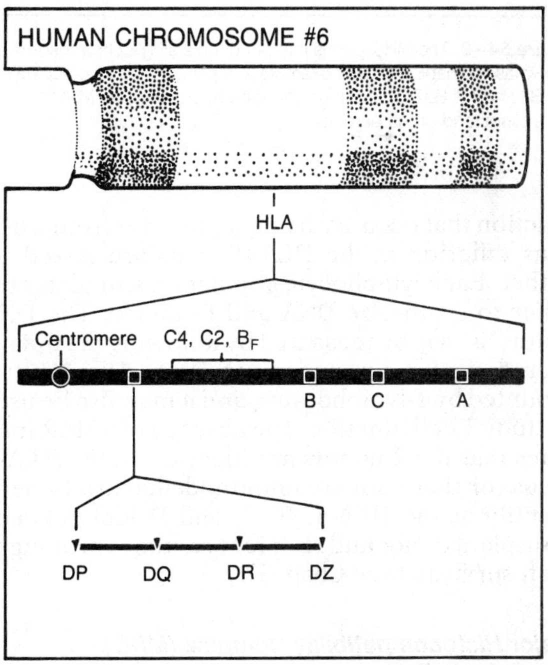


**Figure 54-8.** The human major histocompatibility complex (MHC) known as HLA (human leukocyte antigen) is found on chromosome 6. It consists of 5 regions. The D region is subdivided into 4 parts, DP, DQ, DR, and DZ, which code for membrane Ia antigens. These products are also known as MHC class II molecules. Between D and B there are genes for 3 proteins of the complement system, C4, C2, and factor B. B, C, and A, but especially A and B, are genes for the serologically defined MHC class I antigens expressed on all nucleated cells and platelets.

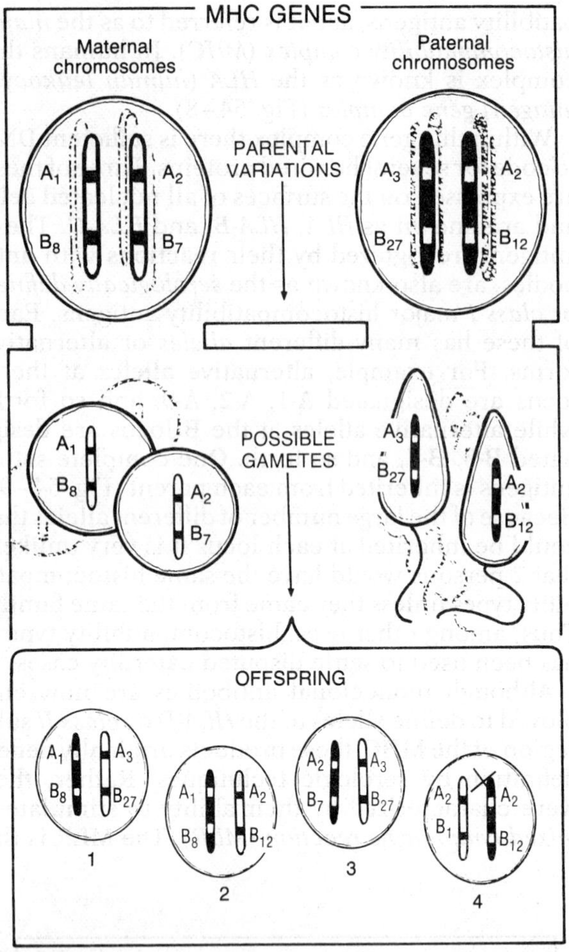


**Figure 54–9.** The MHC genes that occur on a single chromosome are known as the haplotype. For example, offspring #1 has the haplotypes A1, B8 and A3, B27. This can be deduced by studying the MHC types of the siblings and of the parents.

reaction that occurs when lymphocytes from 2 persons differing at the HLA-D locus are mixed together. Each lymphocyte population stimulates the other to synthesize DNA and to divide. The DNA synthesis may be measured by following the uptake of radioactive precursors of DNA. The MLR is mounted by T-lymphocytes, and it may also be used to study T cell function. The absence of a MLR indicates that the 2 donors are identical at the HLA-D locus (or that both are immunodeficient). Genetic identity at the HLA-A, B, C, and D loci between transplant donor and recipient results in prolonged graft survival. (See Chap. 57.)

### *Major Histocompatibility Complex (MHC): Physiologic Role*

What is the physiologic role of the MHC? Surely it was not designed to frustrate the transplant surgeon. Why do we need histocompatibility antigens, and why are there so many alleles? The ability to respond to particular antigens is inherited. Studies in laboratory animals have shown that the inheritance of immunoresponsiveness is determined by genes in the major histocompatibility complex. Specifically, genes in the region analogous to HLA-D control the ability to make antibodies to specific antigens. These genes were appropriately named *immune response genes* or *Ir genes*, and the molecules they encode are called *Ia antigens* (for immune response gene associated antigens). Ia antigens are expressed primarily on monocytes, macrophages, and B-lymphocytes. On monocytes and macrophages they are found in close association with *processed* antigen. You will remember that helper T cells only recognize antigen presented to them in a suitable molecular environment on the surface of an antigen presenting cell (see Fig. 54–7). We now know that that suitable environment is provided by Ia antigens determined by genes in the MHC.

Helper T cells do not recognize antigen alone, rather they have receptors stimulated by a combination of processed antigen and Ia antigens. The ability to respond to a particular antigen is determined by whether or not one's HLA-D-determined Ia antigens make a suitable combination with processed antigen. Thus, it seems that the physiologic role for at least HLA-D genes lies in the *regulation* of the immune response.

Is there a similar role for HLA-A and HLA-B gene products? Studies in experimental animals suggest that there is. Recall that the cell-mediated immune response deals chiefly with antigens found on the surface of the cell (e.g., viral antigens expressed on the membrane of an infected cell). It seemed likely that the *cytotoxic T* cell, which killed virus-infected cells, possessed a receptor that recognized the viral antigen. Thus, cytotoxic T cells specific for a given virus should kill any cells infected with that particular virus. However, this was not the case — only infected cells that shared major histocompatibility antigens with the donor of the cytotoxic T cells could be killed.

It is now known that cytotoxic T cells recognize antigen in combination with HLA-A and HLA-B membrane antigens much the same way that helper T cells recognize their antigens only when they are complexed with Ia antigens. Thus, the physiologic function of the serologically determined MHC antigens is also in the regulation of the immune response and, in particular, the regulation of cytotoxic T cells.

Why are there so many alleles for each HLA locus? Both class I (A, B, and C) and class II (D) gene products determine the ability of an individual to mount an immune response to certain antigens. When these antigens are pathogens, possessors of certain HLA alleles have a survival advantage. Although each person possesses only 2 alleles at any one HLA locus, the existence of many different alleles in a heterogeneous population assures that some persons will possess the alleles that confer the ability to mount an effective immune response against a pathogen. Thus, the great diversity of HLA alleles provides a mechanism whereby the species survives attack from a variety of pathogenic microorganisms. In this regard, it is interesting to note that some diseases, especially those with an immune system component, are associated with certain histocompatibility genes and that determination of the HLA type may be part of the differential diagnosis.

## IMMUNOLOGIC MEMORY

Most immune responses are characterized by the induction of immunologic memory. The induction of an immune response takes time. First, the macrophages must process the antigen, and then the interactions between T cells, B cells, and macrophages must take place. These are followed by the differentiation and proliferation of cells giving rise to plasma cells producing antibody or to cytotoxic T-lymphocytes, depending on whether humoral or cellular immunoresponsiveness is being measured. Thus, when a person is exposed to an antigen there is a lag period, usually of 7–10 days before antibodies begin to appear in the serum (or a cell-mediated immune response becomes apparent). First IgM appears and then IgG. The amount of antibody in the serum (i.e., the *antibody titer*) gradually increases until it reaches a peak about 21 days after the exposure to antigen. After this, the titer gradually declines until it reaches levels that are undetectable. This is called a *primary* immune response.

When a person is exposed to an antigen for a second, third, or subsequent time, the response is quantitatively different. First, the lag period is considerably shortened so that antibodies may be detected in the serum 3 or 4 days after the injection. The peak titer is reached within 7–10 days, and this peak is much greater than that seen during the primary immune response. The IgM component remains the same as in the primary response while the great increase in antibody is due to increased IgG. Antibody production continues for a considerably longer period of time, and in some cases antibodies may be detected in the serum years after a secondary exposure to an antigen. Thus, the *secondary* immune response, also called the *anamnestic* response, is faster, reaches a higher peak and lasts longer than the primary response.

These characteristics constitute *immunologic memory*. This phenomenon allows serologic diagnosis of an ongoing infection. If a patient has just encountered a foreign organism, there would be a weak response, mostly of the IgM type. As the immune response progresses, IgG appears and increases in titer. In the fully immune person, the IgG level is elevated and relatively constant. By examining 2 (paired) serum samples, we can determine if there has been no contact, recent contact, or immunity.

## TOLERANCE

One of the primary characteristics of the immune response is the ability to distinguish self from nonself, that is, to be able to recognize those molecules that are foreign. A person is said to be *tolerant* of his self constituents. This immunologic tolerance of self is acquired during embryogenesis. At some point, the immune system takes inventory of self constituents, and those clones (families of cells derived from one stem cell) of lymphocytes that would have been able to react against the self constituents are either inactivated or eliminated.

In theory, it should be possible to trick the immune system into accepting a foreign substance as self by introducing it during the critical time in development; in fact, this has been achieved experimentally to produce acquired immunologic tolerance. It would be useful to be able to induce tolerance in persons about to receive a tissue transplant so that they would not reject the foreign tissue. While it is not yet possible to induce tolerance to foreign histocompatibility antigens in human transplant recipients, animal experiments have been successful.

## AUTOIMMUNITY: UNDERLYING PATHOPHYSIOLOGIC MECHANISMS

When natural immunological tolerance to self antigens breaks down, a state of *autoimmunity* may ensue. Autoimmune responses may develop in 1 of 2 ways. First, there could be a change in the population of immunologically tolerant lymphocytes so that they lose their tolerant state. A second possibility, one that has been substantiated by experimental evidence, is that subtle changes in self antigens make them no longer recognizable as *self* and allow them access to the immune system. Subsequent immune responses are directed against both the new antigenic determinants and the old, self determinants.

There are several ways in which self antigens could be altered so that they induce autoimmune responses. For example, new antigens expressed on virus-infected or malignant cells may induce immune responses that crossreact with antigens expressed on normal cells of the same type. Thus, both normal and abnormal cells could be destroyed. Drugs and chemicals encountered in the environment may also induce changes in self molecules or self cell membranes that render them immunogenic.

Some self antigens may be normally hidden from the immune system such that the system is neither tolerant nor immune to the antigen. Injury or infection may unmask these hidden antigens and expose them to the immune system where they would not be recognized as self. For example, injuries that fragment the lens of the eye release antigens that induce an autoimmune reaction leading to chronic inflammation of both the injured and normal eyes. For this reason, it is necessary to remove an injured eye promptly to protect the normal eye from autoimmune attack.

Dysfunction of other immunoregulatory pathways may also result in autoimmune disease. For some potential autoantigens self tolerance may be maintained by active suppressor cells. Should these cells fail, autoimmunity may result. Suppressor cells, in turn, must be induced by a *suppressor inducer* cell—a sort of helper cell for the suppressor system. Both suppressor cells and their inducers are of the T cell lineage. If the suppressor inducers malfunction, autoimmunity is a possible outcome.

Another network of cells, also T cells, regulates the actions of suppressor cells. These cells belong to a family known as the *contrasuppressors*. As their name implies, contrasuppressors down-regulate suppressor function. Should they become overactive, suppression of autoimmunity would be abrogated and a disease state could result.

Another network also regulates immune function—the *idiotypic network*. When an antigen induces an immune response, the antibodies formed will have unique combining sites for the antigen. To the immune system these combining sites may appear to be new, nonself antigenic determinants. These antigenic determinants are called *idiotypes*. As a result, antibodies, designated anti-idiotypic antibodies, reactive with the combining site (idiotype) may be formed (Fig. 54-10). These new antibodies would compete with the original antigen for binding to the combining site of the first antibody.

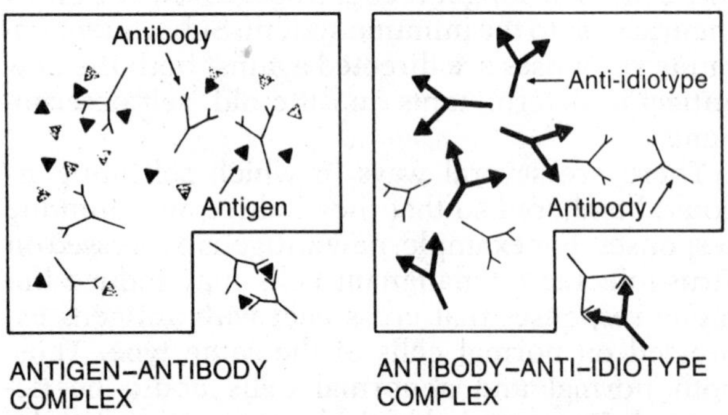


**Figure 54-10.** An idiotype is the unique antigenic determinant conferred on an antibody by its combining site. An idiotypic determinant may induce the formation of anti-idiotypic antibodies, which can regulate the immune response to the oriringinal antigen.

Anti-idiotypic antibodies may be important in regulating or neutralizing the ability of autoantibodies to react with their autoantigens. Patients with some autoimmune diseases undergo remissions when titers of anti-idiotypic antibodies, capable of neutralizing autoantibodies, rise in their blood.

## EFFECTOR MECHANISMS

Once the immune system has processed "foreign" material and then has recognized it as different from "self," the effector mechanisms operate to inactivate or dispose of the remaining antigen(s). These effects can be examined in 2 ways.

First, they can be related to the 2 arms of the immune system.

Humoral immunity (i.e., the production of antibody) can have direct effects. Antibody can bind to a bacterium and facilitate *phagocytosis*; it might interact with its flagellum to render it immobile; it might activate other systems, such as *complement*, which could lyse it through enzymatic or other actions; it can act to direct (by binding to the Fc receptor) cells to guide them to the antigen, after which those cells can use additional mechanisms to destroy the parasite; or it might bind to a toxin and directly neutralize it. More recently we have also learned that antibodies might themselves modulate the immune response by feeding back on receptors on antibody producing or accessory (T-helper cells, macrophages) cells to influence the extent of their activity.

The *cellular* immune system is more obscure. It clearly plays an important role in regulating the system through help and suppression. It may also directly destroy cells through cytotoxic T-lymphocytes, and, in this way, it serves to eliminate (usually indirectly) intracellular parasites. The cellular immune system also has the capacity to recognize and eliminate, directly through cytotoxicity and indirectly through lymphokines, "foreign" tissue whether these be senile, injured, transplanted, or neoplastic (at least so we believe in some cases). It can recruit macrophages to deal with antigens by phagocytosis, again through the elaboration of cytokines (chemotactic, immobilizing, and proliferation-inducing molecules secreted by these cells that work at very minute concentrations).

It should be clear that lymphocytes of T cell type are responsible for the specificity of the cellular reaction in much the same way that antibody directs the action of complement. While these cells can at times kill foreign invaders by the elaboration of lymphotoxin or by insertion of a complement like molecular array (as is done by *killer T cells*), in most cases they recruit other cells, macrophages for example, which nonspecifically eliminate the intruder, acting in the vicinity of the orchestrating lymphocyte. This is a very important point because sometimes host tissues or cells are injured because they are mistakenly recognized as foreign, or because they are so closely associated with an antigen that the reaction against the antigen spills over and affects them, despite the fact that they are only "innocent bystanders."

The second way of considering immune effector responses is by categorizing them in a manner related to basic mechanism. This proposal, advanced by Gell and Coombs over 20 years ago is more advantageous for our purposes because it is more closely related to therapeutic intervention than the approach noted above. Four types of reactions are commonly recognized:

Type I: Atopic or anaphylactic
Type II: Cyto (or tissue) toxic
Type III: Antigen-antibody complex medicated
Type IV: Delayed hypersensitive or cell mediated.

Each of these mechanisms is examined in some detail, and examples of diseases that relate to them are provided. It is important to remember that *rarely does only a single mechanism apply but commonly a disease is a composite of several mechanisms with perhaps one preeminent.*

## Type I: Atopy

The group of entities that have type I mechanisms are identified by several features: (1) they all are related to increased IgE on mast cells; (2) they are very rapid in onset; (3) they result from soluble mediators, which act on smooth muscle (largely in the lung and blood vessels) and, as a consequence, are amenable to several therapeutic approaches; and (4) they tend to have strong hereditary components. The diseases include certain types of asthma, hayfever, urticaria (hives), and eczema. Contact rashes that take hours to develop, such as poison ivy, are in the type IV group.

### Pathophysiology

The basic problem in most atopic or allergic patients is that they produce too much of a particular or several particular IgE antibodies. While there is uncertainty about the reason for this overproduction, most investigators believe that the group of T cells that regulate IgE production are genetically deficient and do not suppress the elaboration of IgE against certain *allergens.*

It is important to remember 2 facts about atopy. The first is that it is *specific.* One person is allergic to a certain food, another to a certain pollen, a third to an antigen in cat saliva. One is not allergic to everything. The second is that while family history is commonly positive, it is not always manifest in the same way. For example, the child has eczema, his mother is allergic to bee venom (and may be subject to *anaphylaxis*—the sudden *systemic* outpouring of mediators, which result in hypotension and severe bronchospasm), his brother has hayfever, and an aunt develops hives after eating shrimp. Degrees of illness vary, and, in a given family, many may be unaffected.

### Treatment

**Active (Immunologic) Therapy.** Therapy is of 2 types: *active,* involving immunologic intervention; and *passive,* involving pharmacologic intervention. Active therapy is aimed at *desenitization.* This may be separated into 2 situations. In the case of a person allergic to penicillin who for 1 reason or another must receive this drug (e.g., infective endocarditis), the antibodies can be "removed" and a tolerant state induced. This is achieved by *very carefully* giving tiny doses of the drug, pretreating the patient (see below) to minimize symptoms, and increasing the allergen until all antibody has been consumed. The continuing high levels of penicillin, given intravenously, will induce a state of tolerance that will last while therapy is administered. Once we stop giving the antigen to the patient in very large amounts (as would be the case in such instances where its use was essential, like bacterial endocarditis), the antipenicillin antibodies become apparent and the patient is as allergic as before desensitization was carried out.

The second form of active therapy is more familiar—a long series of injections given intramuscularly by an allergist. Here the allergen (antigen) is injected by a route and in a form in which it will induce T-suppressor cells specific for the allergen in question. Unfortunately, this does not always work well, and, frequently, it must be continued indefinitely to maintain the nonallergic state. Many patients find this unpleasant and expensive. They may choose a passive approach that does not alter the immune response, but works to minimize the mast cell responses.

In this context we must remember that IgE provides the mast cell with its specificity. The IgE binds to its surface of the cell through IgE-specific Fc receptors (present only on mast cells and basophils) and remains for long periods. If antigen is encountered, IgE specific to it is bound and the cell is activated to discharge its granules and secrete mediators. This process is under the regulation of cell surface receptors (adrenergic and cholinergic) and is modulated by the intracellular levels of cyclic nucleotides (cAMP retards the release and cGMP enhances it).

The mediators are of essentially 2 types: (1) those that are in granules, like histamine, which are extruded through a microfilament-microtubular interaction; and (2) those that are synthesized after antigen interacts with IgE on the surface of the mast cell such as leukotrienes (e.g., SRS-A or slow-react-

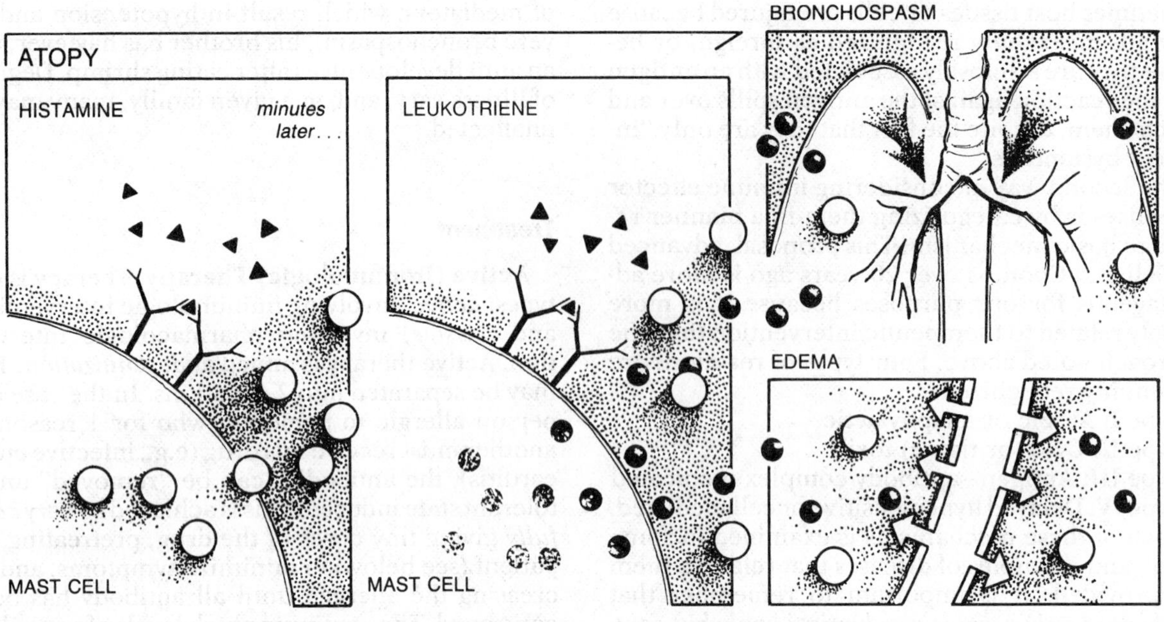


**Figure 54-11.** The time course of an atopic reaction. The antigen, perhaps a fragment of a pollen grain, reaches the surface of a mast cell in the nasal mucosa, as in the patient with hay fever. The antigen, being multivalent, crosslinks 2 or more IgE antibodies on the surface of the cell. Very rapidly this triggers 2 events. The first occurs in minutes and results in the release of preformed granules containing histamine (and other substances). In the second frame, the second event, the production, de novo, of leukotrienes by processing of cell surface lipids is shown. These substances require time to be released, but through their continued production and longer duration of action account for the long-lasting symptoms of a disease such as asthma. Both sets of mediators affect smooth muscle but in different ways depending on type and location. In the third frame (*top right*), bronchoconstriction is noted. In the final frame (*bottom right*), enhanced vascular permeability is seen. This last change may be predominant in such conditions as urticaria (hives).

ing substance of anaphylaxis) and perhaps, certain prostaglandins (Fig. 54-11).

The difference between preformed and synthesized mediators is critical to understanding the therapeutic approach to modulating atopic reactions. When the mast cell is activated by an immune reaction (or even physical stimuli such as cold, e.g., cold urticaria; or trauma, e.g., welts), the granules are immediately released and substances like histamine are extruded. The response is quick and not sustained. More granules can be made or other cells stimulated to extend this first phase or increase its intensity. On the other hand, synthesized mediators such as the leukotrienes are derived from cell surface lipids such as those containing arachidonic acid. Their production *begins* with antigen combining with and crosslinking surface IgE. They are released after a delay rather than immediately, their production continues over a longer period, and their duration of action is extended well beyond that of histamine. Therefore, they account for the lengthy bronchospasm (or vascular leakage) that may occur in some atopic diseases (e.g., extrinsic alleric asthma).

**Passive (Pharmacologic) Therapy.** Passive therapy does not alter the immune response but modifies the release or effect of mediators. *Antihistamines* do not interfere with the IgE antibody production, they do not block interaction of antigen with sensitized mast cells, and they do not interfere with mediator release. Rather they work at the end organ level by competing with histamine for receptors on smooth muscle cells. If an antihistamine has occupied a site on bronchial smooth muscle, histamine reaching that muscle can no longer initiate constriction.

*Xanthines*, like theophylline, work quite differently. They prevent the degradation of cyclic AMP. In turn, this impairs granule release, and the amount of mediators of atopic reactions are diminished. Agents like epinephrine act similarly. They are associated with an increase in the synthesis of cAMP, and, in turn, the ratio of cAMP : cGMP is increased and release is lessened. Sodium cromoglycolate (Cromolyn) prevents both release of histamine and synthesis of leukotrienes, possibly by interfering with calcium transport into the mast cells. Finally, corticosteroids are effective, but they act at so many different levels that the critical aspect of their pharmacology in allergic disorders is not yet understood with precision.

## Type II: Cytotoxic Reactions

In this type of an effector reaction, attack is directed against a cell or tissue component. Because *tissue constituents* (e.g., basement membrane) may be the target, the terminology, *cyto*toxicity is somewhat inaccurate. However, the concept of antibody (with

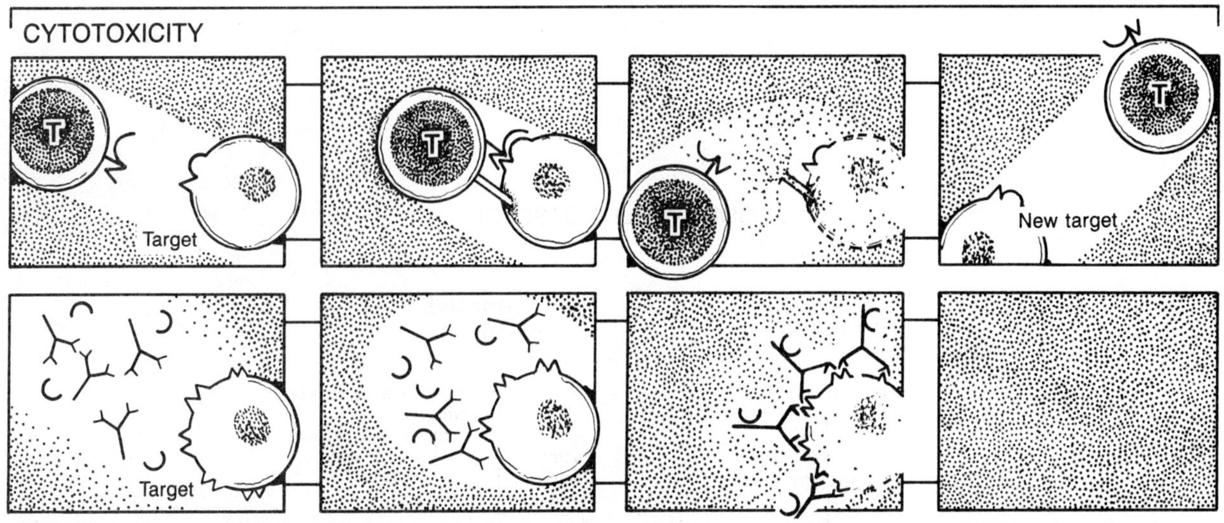


**Figure 54-12.** Two pathways for cytotoxicity. In the upper series of frames, a lymphocyte with its receptor approaches a foreign target, a cell in a transplanted organ or perhaps a tumor cell. The lymphocyte's receptor is normally directed towards altered self, and, therefore, the "antigen" is some perturbation of a class I molecule, a product of the MHC (see text). In the case of the transplanted tissue, this would be a different MHC antigen, but in the case of the tumor cell, it might represent a small change in the normal "self" marker. The cytotoxic lymphocyte recognizes the target and then inserts a channel into it, which has an effect much like complement component C9 (see Fig. 54-13 and text). As a result, the cell membrane is rendered permeable and the contents of the cell diffuse into the environment leading to cell death. The lympocyte moves off in frame 3, and in frame 4 is seen attacking another target while the prior target, in frame 3, is undergoing lysis. In the lower series of pictures, the same effect is brought about by antibody and complement. Two important differences should be noted: no effector cell is involved, and there is no genetic (MHC) restriction. This latter point is important because the same antibodies will work for any person while the cytotoxic T cell is effective only in a histocompatible person like an identical twin. Notice that complement is bound to the Fc portion of the immunoglobulin and has no specificity of its own. The final empty frame (*bottom right*) serves to indicate both cell death and the nonrepetitive nature of the antibody and complement involved in the death of the initial target. New antibody and complement must be available for other targets to be attacked in contrast to the situation with the cytotoxic lymphocyte.

or without complement) or an immunospecific cell eliminating a target by lysis, physiologic inactivation, or phagocytosis is central (Fig. 54-12).

In many of these reactions, the class of the antibody is IgG or IgM and complement is involved. *Complement* is a group of about 20 proteins circulating in the blood, which form a cascade much like that which controls coagulation (see Chap. 61). Many of these proteins are proteolytic enzymes or their inhibitors. The system, spoken of collectively as complement, is activated through either of 2 pathways (Fig. 54-13). One called the *"alternative pathway"* is initiated nonspecifically by polysaccharide, either as aggregated immunoglobulin such as IgA (which is rich in sugars that are attached to its heavy chains), bacterial cell walls, a variety of polysaccharides, and even certain enzymes as well as radiographic contrast material—something seemingly quite unrelated. The other, the *classic pathway*, is initiated by the immunologically specific interaction between IgG or IgM antibodies and their respective antigens. The alternative pathway is phylogenetically older, and it is presumed that it arose (in evolution) to deal with invading pathogens *before* antibody was elaborated. Because the classic pathway requires antibody for its initiation, there will be an inevitable lag in bringing it to operate on a bacterium or other organisms. Furthermore, in as much as it relies on the specific immune interaction between antibody and antigen, it is much more efficient and less prone to injure tissues proximate to the offending agent.

In complement activation, in a manner analogous to coagulation, there is activation, in a stepwise manner, of enzymes that cleave a small fragment of the peptide chain from the next component in the series. This activates that component and so on. The 2 pathways converge to a common point, and the terminal elements are common. The last sequence has the capacity to create holes in membranes and in such a way *lyse* cells and bacteria. The several fragments generated along the paths can enhance phagocytosis, call forth inflammatory cells, increase permeability of blood vessels, and assist in other aspects of the inflammatory process.

More specifically, the classic pathway can be examined in detail to get an idea of how complement works (see Fig. 54-13). Suppose an antibody of the IgM class is directed against a gonococcus. The antibody combines with the specific determinant on the bacterial surface. This causes a change in the structure of the antibody, which enables C1, the first component of complement, to bind to it, and, in turn, the surface of the bacterium. In turn, 2 enzymatic components of C1, C1r and C1s, are activated. This enables the molecular complex, activated C1, to cleave C4 and C2. Peptides are released (e.g., C4a), which can activate mast cells. The larger

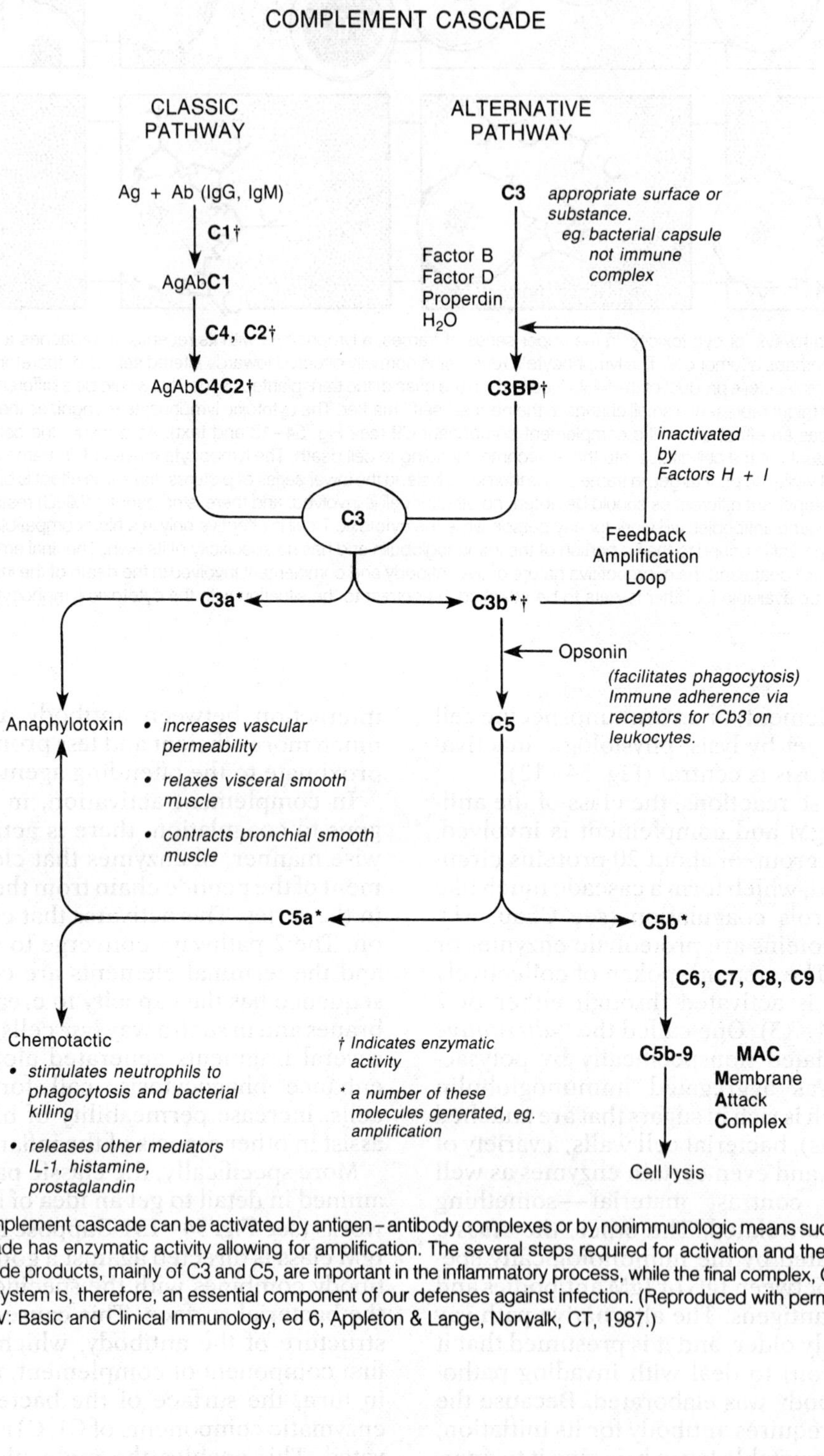


**Figure 54–13.** The complement cascade can be activated by antigen–antibody complexes or by nonimmunologic means such as bacterial or fungal cell surfaces. The cascade has enzymatic activity allowing for amplification. The several steps required for activation and the existence of inhibitors permit control. The peptide products, mainly of C3 and C5, are important in the inflammatory process, while the final complex, C5b-9, can directly lyse cells. The complement system is, therefore, an essential component of our defenses against infection. (Reproduced with permission from Stites, DP, Stobo, JD, and Wells, JV: Basic and Clinical Immunology, ed 6, Appleton & Lange, Norwalk, CT, 1987.)

parts of C4 and C2, C2a and C4b, can combine to form a new enzyme, which will cleave C3. A liberated peptide, C3a, can cause vascular permeability to increase and thus allow more antibody and more complement to enter the tissue to react with the pathogen. As before, the larger piece resulting from the enzymatic attack, C3b, combines with C2a and C4b to form still another enzyme, which can go on to cleave C5. That event will release a peptide that can attract neutrophils (C5a) and another (C5b) that will allow the formation of a complex of C6, C7, C8, and C9, which can lyse the gonococcus.

The last step, the incorporation of C9 is of interest. When C9 is acted on by preceding components, it forms a polymer. This polymer has been visualized as a channel or tunnel through the cell membrane. This allows cellular contents to leak out much as air would escape from a balloon if a hollow needle were introduced through its rubber skin. The introduction of a channel or hole as a lytic mechanism is also applicable to cellular injury as will be noted in type IV or delayed hypersensitivity mechanisms.

The complexity of the complement system is purposeful. Because several steps are enzymatic, 1 molecule acting on many others, amplification is facilitated. The several steps are each matched with an inhibitor so that regulation is possible. Complement can orchestrate aspects of inflammation by helping to alter blood flow and induce edema, attract cells capable of phagocytosis and killing, and by actually destroying pathogens (see Fig. 54–13).

The system is tightly controlled, and its inappropriate triggering can be as severe in its consequences to the host as would the absence of the whole system, a situation in which early death from infection is likely. Indeed, as there are diseases associated with the lack of certain complement components, so there are also diseases due to the lack of a complement inhibitory protein. One such entity is hereditary angioedema, a disease due to a lack of C1 inhibitor, a protein present in the circulation of normal individuals, which inhibits the activation of the first component of the classic pathway (as well as components of the kinin and coagulation cascades). In this condition, there may be sudden swelling of any part of the body, most seriously of the larynx, due to the action of complement (and kinin) peptides in enhancing vascular permeability and leading to edema.

### *Pathophysiology*

**Cytotoxic Reactions: Humoral.** The presence of an antibody against a cell or component, with or without the activation of complement, can lead to disease. Consider the case of a reaction directed against a drug, to which a patient responds immunologically (e.g., alpha-methyldopa or quinidine), that is bound by its physiochemical properties to the surface of an erythrocyte. The following sequence of events can occur: antibody attaches, complement is activated, and the cell is lysed . . . and we have an immune anemia.

The antibody itself, without complement, is sufficient to produce cell death. In Rh disease, erythroblastosis fetalis, or certain transfusion reactions, complement is not activated but cells in the spleen of the macrophage-monocyte family recognize the antibody attached to the red cell. Because they have receptors for the Fc portion of antibody, they "recognize" this portion of the antibody protruding from the surface of the erythrocyte. They can then phagocytose the erythrocyte and destroy it. In other diseases, the antibody may be directed against a structural element, the basement membrane of the kidney (Goodpasture's syndrome), the skin (pemphigoid), or the acetylcholine receptor of the neuromuscular junction (myasthenia gravis). In each of these situations, profound functional disturbances may occur: loss of filtration function, severe blistering, or weakness in each of the preceding examples, respectively. Not only macrophages but neutrophils, eosinophils, certain killer lymphocytes, and natural killer cells possess Fc receptors and can participate in reactions of this type.

**Cytotoxic Reactions: Cell Mediated.** In cytotoxic reactions, the assault need not only be by antibody. Cells may directly damage tissue. Lymphocytes of the T-cell lineage may destroy other cells in the body, or macrophages may accomplish the same end using antibodies with abnormal specificities produced by B cells. These autoantibodies adhere to receptors on the macrophage (or other cell) membrane and "direct" them to targets, which are, in turn, injured by oxygen radicals, enzymes, or other substances released by the macrophages. This cellular attack in which antibodies provide the direction is appropriately termed *antibody-dependent cell-mediated cytotoxicity* (ADCC).

These type II reactions (see Fig. 54–12) are quite specific and tend to result in specific symptom complexes referable to the loss of the target cell or tissue.

### *Treatment*

Treatment is directed at removing (by dialysis) or suppressing (by drug therapy) the immune component responsible. It would seem that a good number of these conditions may be initiated by external agents, drugs, chemicals, bacteria, or viruses, which in one way or another create a situation in which the immune system recognizes a body constituent as foreign and endeavors to eliminate it.

One exception to the point regarding specificity must be made and that refers to a specific group of effector cells that are *cytotoxic*, which have recently achieved a degree of notoriety. These are the so-called natural killer cells. The "killer" phraseology is obvious, but the "natural" modifier implies that, in contrast to *immune* mechanisms, these cells, which resemble lymphocytes but have granules and more cytoplasm, are present from the start and do not display memory. They are a heterogeneous population and their greatest claim to popular fame is their possible role in tumor destruction, particularly leukemias. This reaction should not really be grouped with the immune effector mechanisms because it lacks the degree of specificity that we associate with immunity. These *natural killers* or *NK* cells can respond to a variety of "foreign" cells.

## Type III: Circulating Immune (Antigen–Antibody) Complexes

The group of diseases in which type III mechanisms play a major role differ significantly from type I and II in that their signs and symptoms tend to be much more diverse. In type III mechanisms, the vessels of the circulatory system principally are injured and the disease picture is determined by the set or sets of vessels affected. One can imagine that a fundamental difference between type III reactions and those of types I and II is that the III reactions are commonly manifest in multisystem-multisymptom disease.

### *Pathophysiology*

In type III reactions, the symptoms depend on the set(s) of blood vessels involved and the degree of compromise. In this setting, disturbances of renal, neural, dermal, gastrointestinal, and/or other function occur in varying combinations. The antigen gains access to the circulation as an infectious agent, serum, drug, or other foreign material (Fig. 54–14). It circulates, stimulates antibody formation, and then combines with the resulting antibody at a time when the antigen(s) is in *excess*. This antigen excess keeps the immune complexes small so that phagocytic cells in the liver and spleen do not remove them from the circulation rapidly. In such a manner they are able to deposit in vessels, usually small arteries and capillaries, and commonly at

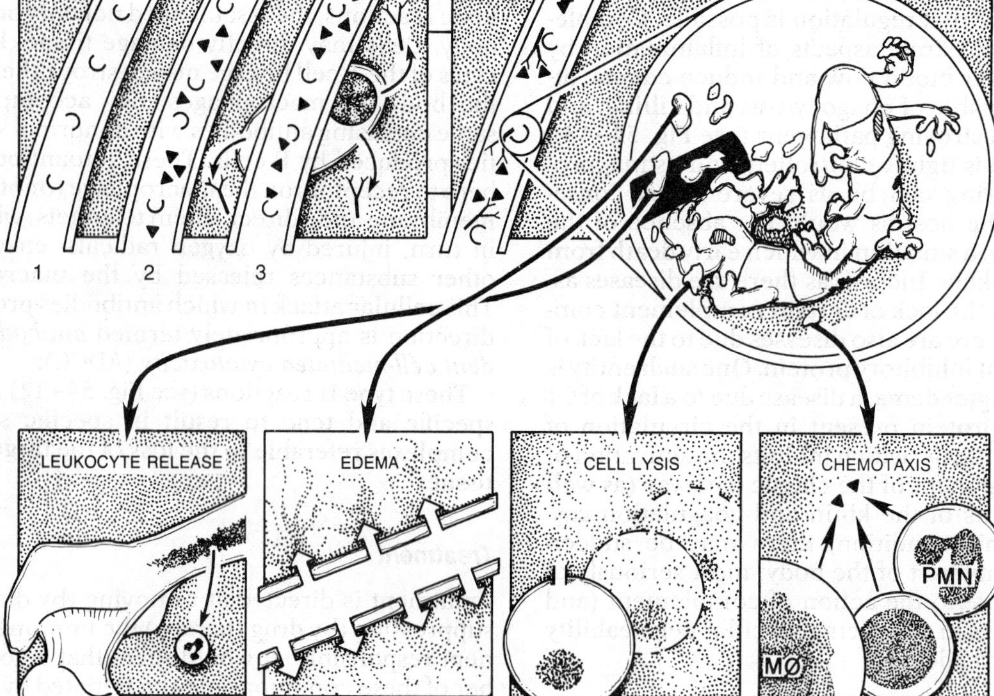


**Figure 54–14.** Serum sickness type reactions depend on circulating immune complexes. In the first panel, we see the plasma of the non-immunized person in which we have depicted inactive complement molecules (C). In the second inset, an antigen is introduced, perhaps the product of an infection somewhere in the body. A plasma cell, in the background of the third inset, the product of B-cell maturation and multiplication, begins to produce antibody. In the second picture, the antibody combines with antigen-activating complement. This series of proteins is an enzymic cascade in which one component digests a fragment of the next and so on. Each fragment may produce a discrete biologic event. These are shown in the lower frames and include liberation of neutrophils from the bone marrow accounting for leukocytosis and a "shift to the left" (the appearance of immature forms) in the blood, increased vascular permeability resulting in edema, cell lysis causing destruction of the pathogen, and positive chemotaxis permitting the accumulation of a variety of leukocytes at the site of injury.

points (bifurcations) where there is turbulence. Certain vascular beds, in the kidney and nervous system and possibly also the skin, are particularly receptive to deposition. This receptivity may result from their filtration function, variations in their endothelium, or other factors as yet unknown.

The complexes activate complement, which causes local increase in vascular permeability, thereby facilitating more deposits. Complement fragments also attract neutrophils and other phagocytic cells, which attempt to remove these complexes. It is thought that the geometry of the deposit makes phagocytosis inefficient, and some of the enzymes and oxygen radicals generated by the phagocytic cell important in the destruction of microorganisms escape and injure the vessel.

When vessels are injured, thrombosis commonly follows. This, or the destruction of the vessel wall leads to an inability to perfuse the tissue formerly served by the artery or capillary. Loss of function follows, and a symptom appears related to the structures involved: glomerulonephritis in the case of the kidney, neurologic deficits in the case of the brain, and so forth. Frequently neighboring but not directly involved structures will be damaged by the nospecificity of the ultimate effectors, proteinases, or free radicals. In many diseases, a single immune effector mechanism may predominate but not be entirely responsible for tissue injury. In lupus erythematosus, a prototype disease in this group, cytotoxic injury also occurs.

One of the more difficult to understand aspects of some autoimmune diseases is the variability of symptoms from patient to patient. It is felt that the pattern of symptoms—arthritis and glomerulonephritis in one group of patients, thrombocytopenia and rashes in another, and all of these in a third—are due to genetic predispositions. Work with humans and mice has indicated that there are genes that determine whether a given person will have a hemolytic anemia or arteritis or splenomegaly. The combination of these genes governs the symptom complex in a specific individual.

To a greater extent than in cytotoxic hypersensitivity, *complement activation* by the classical pathway is an essential part of type III reactions. It should be noted that the measurement of complement is frequently employed to follow disease activity. Because it functions as a mediator, its activation will precede symptoms. This is done in 1 of 2 ways. One can determine the amount of complement components by immunologic assay just as one measures chorionic gonadotrophin in a pregnancy test. Usually we measure C3 and C4—C3 because it is common to both pathways and is present in largest amount in plasma and C4 because it would indicate classic pathway (and therefore antigen-antibody interaction) and is additionally very sensitive. It is important to remember that this type of test measures a protein or other molecule by virtue of a certain chemical configuration (determinant) that the radioactive or labeled antibody combines with and not by its function. On occasion we use functional tests, a $CH_{50}$ or hemolytic test. In such cases, we determine if complement actually works by testing its ability to lyse red cells that have been combined with an appropriate antibody. The $CH_{50}$ measures the ability of serum complement to lyse 50% of a standard suspension of red cells.

## Type IV: Cell-Mediated or Delayed Hypersensitivity Reactions

Some processes of immune injury are caused by the ingress of specific lymphocytes into tissues. Unlike the other types of immune effector mechanisms, antibodies play no role. The specificity, closely resembling that of antibody, is encoded in a receptor on the surface of the lymphocyte. Because delayed hypersensitivity is mediated by cells, which must migrate to the antigen, the reaction takes longer to develop than type I, II, or III discussed above. Symptoms or signs take from 1 to a number of days or longer to appear. The reactions that categorize this group range from contact hypersensitivity of the poison ivy or jewelry or cosmetic type, to tuberculin (tine) or other skin tests, to graft rejection, and the reaction against certain organisms such as mycobacteria (tuberculosis or leprosy), fungi, and others.

### *Pathophysiology*

The antigens involved are persistent and poorly soluble. Metals, like alloys in jewelry, or waxes, as in the tubercle bacillus, are good examples. Frequently they are reactive and bind to our tissues (e.g., skin) and are recognized as a form of "altered" self. The oil that is the antigen in such plants as poison ivy works in this manner. It reacts with keratin to form a complex capable of inducing cell-mediated immunity.

Only a very small percentage of the cells present at the reaction site are specific (able to interact with the antigen). The remainder are recruited by *lymphokines*, small molecules elaborated by the specifically sensitized cells and able to act at minute concentrations. This allows for great amplification without requiring every cell to have a receptor for the specific antigen initiating the reaction. These lymphokines can attract phagocytic cells, cause tissue injury, protect cells (by interferon, which is a member of this group), and activate the coagulation cascade (Fig. 54-15.)

One type of tissue reaction, characterized in many cases by this type of immune response, is termed *granulomatous*. This name is derived from

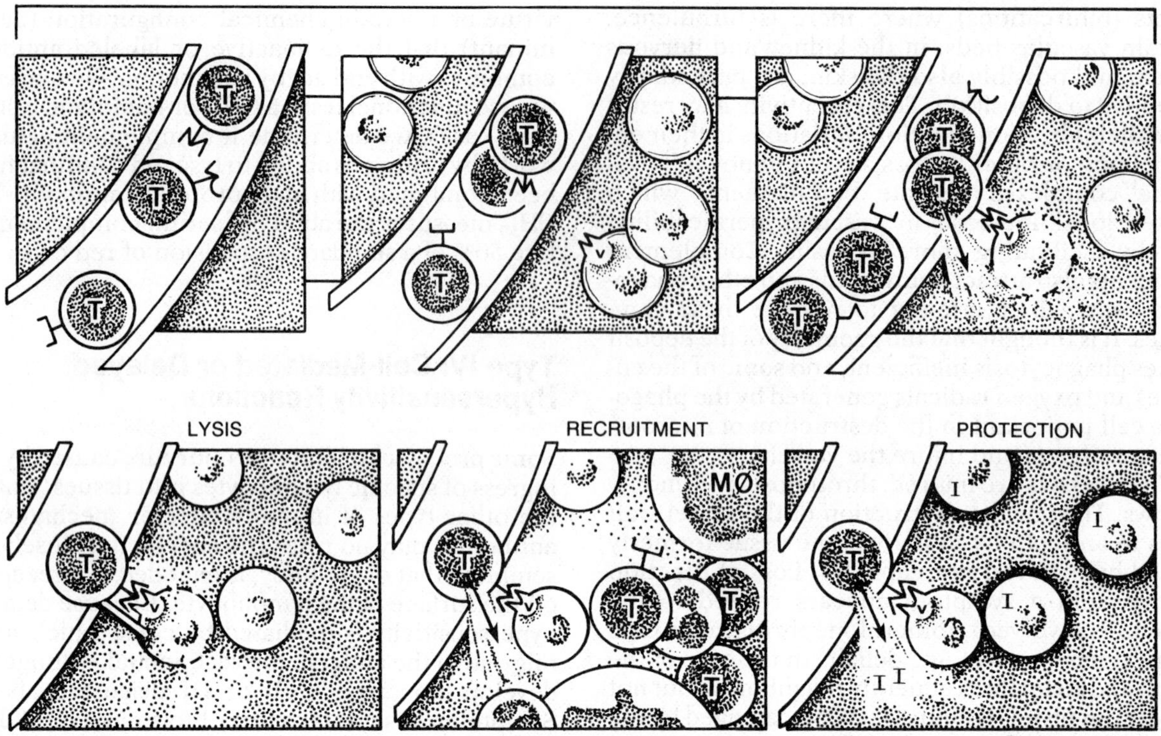


**Figure 54-15.** This series illustrates delayed hypersensitivity type reactions. In the first picture, lymphocytes move through the circulation (and other tissues as well), each having different specificities. These specificities commonly involve the recognition of altered self by virtue of reacting to a determinant linked to an MHC class I product (Ia antigen). The detail of the determinant-Ia linkage is not shown (see text), however, it should be evident that each lymphocyte carries 1 specificity on its surface and that many different antigens can be recognized by the host. The resulting response is initiated by 1 or at most only a few cells. A cell infected with virus, in the second frame, expresses a viral antigen (plus Ia) on its surface, which is recognized by an appropriate lymphocyte (third picture). Two circumstances may then occur. If the cell is a cytotoxic or killer lymphocyte, lysis can take place as in a cytotoxic reacton (*bottom left frame*). Of greater importance is the production of lymphokines, which recruit many more cells (e.g., macrophages, lymphocytes; *bottom, center frame*), which nonspecifically destroy the infected cells, protect other cells through the elaboration of interferon (a lymphokine designated "I," *bottom right frame*) and initiate a number of other reactions that result in abrogation of the infected state (if successful). Death of target cells may result, therefore, from immunospecific cytotoxic T-cell lysis, nonspecific phagocytosis by recruited cells, action of products of recruited cells (e.g. enzymes and oxygen radicals released by macrophages) or by the action of lymphokines themselves.

the nodular appearance of the tissue (granulomatous from granules). Recognition of this pattern allows the pathologist to implicate delayed hypersensitivity as a cause for the disease in question. Reactions of the delayed type may also be important in viral disease and tumor destruction.

Finally, 2 points must be made in closing. If the discriminatory receptor (*T-cell antigen receptor*) is directed against a component of the body, then injury will result. This is frequently the case when transplanted tissue is placed in a host who is not entirely *histocompatible*. Under such circumstances, *rejection* of the graft may occur (see Chaps. 27 and 57). The second point relates to the vigor of the reaction. Because amplification is a very important part of this mechanism, just a few organisms (tubercle bacilli) can elicit a potent reaction. On occasions, the reaction so exceeds the stimulus that injury to the host by his or her own immune system may greatly outweigh the likely damage that could have resulted from the pathogen.

## SUMMARY

The *recognition* and *effector* mechanisms are present to combat disease. Injury to self results form either genetic or environmental factors that deregulate the finely tuned discrimination of pathogen from self. Only then do immunocytes or antibodies depart from their preassigned beneficial roles.

## SUGGESTED READINGS

There are many references, but space allows for listing only a few.

## Clinical Orientation

Parker, CW (ed): Clinical Immunology. WB Saunders, Philadelphia, 1980.

Sampter, M, (ed): Immunological Diseases, ed 3. Little, Brown, New York, 1978.

Stites, DP, et al (eds): Basic and Clinical Immunology, ed 6. Appleton & Lange, Norwalk, CT, 1987.

## Basic Orientation

Clark, WR: (ed): The Experimental Foundations of Modern Immunology, ed 3. John Wiley & Sons, New York, 1986.

Hood, LE, et al (eds): Immunology, ed 2. Benjamin/Cummings, Menlo Park, CA, 1984.

Immunology: Readings from Scientific American. WH Freeman, San Francisco, 1976 (and recent articles in that journal to the present date).

Paul, WE (ed): Fundamental Immunology. Raven Press, New York, 1984.

## Nursing Perspective

Abernathy, E: How the immune system works. Am J Nurs 87(4):456, April 1987.

Griffin, JP: Hematology and Immunology, Concepts for Nursing. Appleton-Century-Crofts, Norwalk, CT, 1986.

Hood, L: Interferon, getting in the way of viruses and tumors. Am J Nurs 87(4):459, April 1987.

Jassak, PF and Spiewak, PL: Interleukin-2. Am J Nurs 87(4):464, April 1987.

Kemp, D: Development of the immune system. Critical Care Quarterly 9(1):1–6, June 1986.

CHAPTER 55

# Assessment of Immunologic Function

*Marc G. Golightly*
*Joan T. Dolan*

## CHAPTER OUTLINE



## LEARNING OBJECTIVES

**At the end of this chapter, you should be able to:**

1. Associate clinical data (patient history and physical examination) and laboratory testing with specific immune dysfunction including:
   a. Cell-mediated system.
   b. Humoral system.
   c. Phagocytic system.
   d. Complement deficiencies or abnormalities.

An intact immune system is essential for survival. It serves as a first line of defense, protecting persons from potential pathogenic organisms that surround them, as well as defending against cancer and neoplastic processes.

As we have seen in Chapter 54, the immune system is diffuse both anatomically and functionally; it is organized in a highly complex fashion with the *cell-mediated, humoral, phagocytic*, and the *complement cascade* systems all being linked together by a network of regulatory and synergistic interactions. The complexity and the interactions of each arm of the immune system are such that a tremendous number of possibilities for defects and dysfunction exist. When a defect does occur in 1 branch it often affects another branch primarily or secondarily. The resultant clinical symptoms are likewise dependent on which of these arms and interactive relations are affected. Often, disorders of the immune system produce multiorgan and multisystemic effects.

The diagnostic assessment and evaluation of immunologic function require a thorough clinical history and physical examination of the patient, as well as a variety of laboratory tests available to assess the immune system both quantitatively and functionally.

## CLINICAL HISTORY

When eliciting the patient's history and examining the patient, it is important to remember that the clinical presentation of suspected immunodeficient patients often suggests the type of immune dysfunction present. For example, patients with a defective *cell-mediated* immunity are more susceptible to infection by fungal, viral, and protozoan organisms (especially in the form of pneumonia, chronic skin, and mucous membrane infections). A history of recurrent bacterial infections, particularly bacterial (pus-forming) pneumonia, and otitis media suggests a *humoral* immune defect. *Phagocytic* dysfunctions are suggested by skin and systemic infections with pyogenic bacteria. Often the systemic infection is by bacteria of normally low virulence. *Complement* deficiencies are also associated with recurrent pyogenic infections.

While these associations between clinical presentation and specific immune defects generally do occur, it should be noted that they are not without exceptions. For example, a patient with a humoral deficiency may have a fungal infection. (These associations, with respect to individual deficiencies, will be examined in detail in Chap. 58.)

## Chief Complaint/History of Present Illness

The chief complaint reflects the major reason as to why the patient/family have sought health care at this point in time. The history of present illness serves to elaborate the details of the chief complaint and should include the *onset*, the *course since onset*, and the *current status*. The SLIDT tool (see Table 7-1) assists in discerning the characteristics of the patient's complaint or problem.

There are no definitive cardinal signs and symptoms reflective of an underlying immune disorder. Rather, it is important to recognize immune-related symptomatology. *Fatigue* and *weakness*, for example, while present in a variety of clinical circumstances, are commonly also present in most patients with immune defects.

*Fever* is a frequent complaint. Information elicited in this regard should include the degree of temperature elevation; whether it is constant, intermittent, or recurring; and the degree of fluctuation over what time period. Spiking temperatures (>103°F; 39.4°C), may reflect acute infection, allergy, or serum sickness; recurring fevers may suggest an immune disorder characterized by rapid cell proliferations; a temperature elevation recurring every few days is characteristic of Hodgkin's disease.

*Joint pain* frequently occurs in the setting of an autoimmune disease (e.g., rheumatoid arthritis, systemic lupus erythematosus). Characteristics of the pain should be elicited using the SLIDT tool (see Table 7-1). Associated factors such as redness and swelling around joints should be noted, as well as any limitations in performing activities of daily living that are attributed to the pain.

Any complaints regarding *lymphadenopathy* (i.e., "swollen glands") should be followed up in the physical examination. Swollen or inflamed lymph nodes suggest an infection or inflammation in the area of the body drained by the particular lymph nodes. For example, tonsilar, submaxillary, superficial, and deep cervical chains of lymph nodes drain portions of the mouth and pharynx, and superficial facial areas (see Fig. 48-1).

Any complaints of *bleeding* (e.g., hematuria, melena, unexplained ecchymotic areas or petechiae) should be explored in detail. Such complaints suggest an altered clotting mechanism and/or thrombocytopenia. The patient may experience a consequent anemia, which may underlie complaints of fatigue and weakness.

## Functional Health Patterns

### Health Perception-Health Management

Inquire as to the patient's prior health status. How does patient view his/her health status? Is there evidence of chronic disease (e.g., rheumatoid arthritis, systemic lupus erythematosus)? Is there a history of malignancy or cancer? Has the patient experienced recent fatigue or weakness? When was this first noticed? What were the surrounding circumstances? How does this affect the patient's ability to perform activities of daily living? Fulfill job responsibilities? Has there been recent stress in the patient's life? Illness? Job-related? Marital? Familial? Immunodeficiency disorders are frequently associated with stress, infection, malignancy, and autoimmune phenomena.

### Nutrition-Metabolic

Inquire as to the patient's drug usage. What drugs are taken by the patient? Are they prescribed or over-the-counter? For what reasons are they taken? Drugs such as antibiotics, corticosteroids, and chemotherapeutic agents have immunosuppressive effects. Does the patient take illegal drugs such as heroin, cocaine, or other such drugs? Does the patient share needles and syringes for self-administration of these drugs? There is a high incidence of acquired immunodeficiency syndrome (AIDS) and hepatitis among drug users.

Does the patient have any allergies to food, drugs, or allergens such as pollens, animal dander, and so forth? Have the patient/family describe the reaction, including the patient's signs and symptoms, their severity, duration, and what is done to treat the reaction. *Anaphylaxis* (*type I atopy*) occurs in response to specific allergens in sensitized persons; *cytotoxic humoral* responses (type II) are implicated in those circumstances in which the patient responds immunologically to a drug (e.g., quinidine, methyldopa) or in certain transfusion reactions. It is necessary to ascertain if the patient has received any transfusion of blood or blood products. When, how much, and for what reason? Recipients of blood and blood products (including hemophiliacs receiving factor concentrates) are at high risk for AIDS.

#### *Sexuality–Reproductive*

The patient's sexual orientation or preference may place the patient at risk for AIDS. At risk partners include but are not limited to homosexual and bisexual men. Heterosexual partners of AIDS patients are likewise at higher risk. The incidence of AIDS is rapidly increasing, as is the number of children borne of AIDS-stricken mothers. Working with the patient to assist in identifying partners increases case finding of this frightening new disease.

#### *Self-Perception/Self-Concept*

Many immune-related illnesses (e.g., systemic lupus erythematosus, rheumatoid arthritis, scleroderma) are associated with changes in physical appearance and capabilities; the ability to maintain desired lifestyle; how the person views self, and the patient's perception of how he/she is viewed by others. Inquire as to what impact the illness has had on the individual and family, economically, socially, and psychologically. What changes have occurred in the role of family members as a result of the disease in question? What progress has the patient and family made in terms of understanding the illness and its prognosis?

#### *Coping–Stress–Tolerance*

Immunodeficiency disease, such as AIDS, and a host of autoimmune diseases, such as multiple sclerosis, myasthenia gravis, as well as those mentioned previously, can have disastrous effects on the individual and family. Ascertain how the illness has impacted on family members, individually and collectively, and how they are coping. Help the family to identify coping mechanisms that were effective in meeting needs during stressful periods in the past. Assist them in identifying family strengths and resources and in setting short-term goals during the acute phase of the illness. Referrals to a psychiatric liaison nurse, social worker, continuity of care nurse, and community resources should be initiated early on as indicated by the nature of the illness and the needs of the family as a whole.

### Past Medical History

When eliciting the patient's past medical history, prior illnesses or surgeries should be noted, as well as episodes of poor wound healing. These may include recurring infections, fungal, viral, and protozoan (*cell-mediated*), and bacterial (*humoral*); bleeding disorders (e.g., hemophilia, thrombocytopenia, others); anemia; malignancies; autoimmune diseases (e.g., systemic lupus erythematosus, rheumatoid arthritis, scleroderma), and certain neurologic illnesses (e.g., myasthenia gravis, multiple sclerosis, amyotrophic lateral sclerosis, others); asthma, and allergies to food, drugs, and identified allergens; renal disease (e.g., Goodpasture's syndrome); and disorders of the skin (e.g., pemphigus), among others.

An inquiry should be made of diseases that reflect a *delayed hypersensitivity* or *cell-mediated* immune mechanism. Examples of these include contact dermatitis of jewelry or cosmetic use, contact hypersensitivity to poison ivy, tuberculosis, fungi infections, and others. Graft rejections are also included in delayed hypersensitivity reactions.

The patient's surgical history may be contributory. Thymectomy or prior organ transplantation are significant clinical occurrences. Previous transfusions of blood or blood products, and the occurrence of any transfusion reactions are especially notable. Patients requiring blood components, as for example, administration of factor VIII to hemophiliacs, are at high risk for AIDS.

The presence of cancer or malignancy should be established. Use of chemotherapy, corticosteroid therapy, or other immunosuppressives severely depresses the immune response. Radiation therapy likewise compromises immune function. The patient's occupational history becomes especially important if the person is exposed to toxic materials, hazardous waste, or radiation. For example, veterans of the Vietnam War who have been exposed to Agent Orange are at high risk of developing subsequent malignancies. Finally, it is essential to establish the presence of congenital or acquired, primary or secondary immunodeficiency disorders (see Chap. 58).

### Family History

It is important to determine the existence of any familial patterns of the disorders mentioned in the section entitled "Past Medical History," above. Such patterns, if present, may indicate a genetic predisposition to certain illnesses placing individuals within the family at greater risk.

## PHYSICAL EXAMINATION

The physical examination of a suspected immunodeficient patient should include a search for evidence of past or present, severe and/or chronic infection. The skin should be assessed for unusual pallor (e.g., pernicious anemia) or jaundice (e.g., hemolytic anemia, liver/biliary dysfunction); skin texture, evidence of pretibial edema (e.g., myxedema); scars from previous skin infections or current allergic skin reactions (e.g., erythematous rash of dermatomyositis; the characteristic weeping and dry scales of eczema); or subcutaneous nodules of rheumatoid arthritis.

Special attention must be given to the presence of lymphoid tissue. This would include possible palpable lymphoid tissue, including nodal chains in the head and neck, and in axillary, epitrochlear (i.e., inside elbow), inguinal, and popliteal regions. The examiner should be familiar with the areas drained by each group of lymph nodes and examine these areas carefully for signs of infection or inflammation (see Fig. 48-1). The tonsils, if present, should be examined, and the chest x-ray should be carefully viewed for a thymic shadow, as well as for present or past pulmonary involvement (e.g., lung abscesses, evidence of tuberculosis, pneumonia, pneumocystic carinii of AIDS, others).

Careful percussion and auscultation of the chest may help to discern pulmonary disease: dullness on percussion in pneumonia, or the hyperresonance associated with the air trapping of an asthmatic attack; the presence of abnormal or adventitious breath sounds such as bronchial sounds over the consolidated lung of pneumonia, or pneumocystic carinii, or the wheezes associated with the early phase of an acute asthmatic attack (in the later stages, breath sounds may become distant or barely audible).

The presence of a cough should be assessed. If productive, the sputum should be examined for color, consistency, odor, and amount, and should be cultured.

The abdomen should be evaluated for the presence of hepatomegaly, splenomegaly, or palpable masses. Abdominal tenderness suggests the presence of inflammation and infection. The presence of ascites suggests possible liver disease or malignancy.

## LABORATORY TESTS OF IMMUNOLOGIC FUNCTION

Many laboratory tests are available to assess the immune system both quantitatively and functionally. Unfortunately, a single screening test for most major immunodeficiencies does not exist, and laboratory immunology evaluations tend to be rather extensive. Generally, the *quantitative* tests are run first, followed by the *functional* tests. The various tests used to examine the arms of the immune system are described below. The expected findings of these tests as they relate to the different immunodeficiency states is discussed in their respective sections in Chapter 58.

### Evaluation of the Humoral Immune System

The laboratory evaluation of the humoral immune system should start with the quantitation of the immunoglobulin levels, specifically, IgG, IgA, and IgM. This should then be followed by an examination of the *functional* immunoglobulin. The clinical significance of functional studies is that a patient may be able to make immunoglobulin but it may not be directed against the proper antigen. It has been noted that normal to low levels of immunoglobulins may exist in the face of an inability to mount a specific response. Functional immunoglobulin can be assessed by determining isohemagglutination titers (mostly IgM) and the Schick test or tetanus toxoid titers (mostly IgG), in appropriately immunized persons. These tests will expose most humoral defects.

Once a defect has been found, it can be further characterized by B-cell quantitations by surface immunoglobulin, monoclonal antibodies, and *in vitro* immunoglobulin synthesis studies. Many in this group of tests are only performed by highly specialized laboratories. It has become apparent by this second group of tests that some of the previous B-cell deficiencies are not due to a defect in the B cell itself, but rather, a defect in the T cells regulating the B-cell response.

### Evaluation of the Cell-Mediated Immune System

In the evaluation of the cell-mediated immunity (T cells), like the humoral assessment, the simple quantitative tests would be performed first. One would start with a determination of the absolute *lymphocyte count.* Counts consistently below 1200/mm$^3$ may indicate a T-cell deficiency (recall that the majority of the circulating lymphocytes are T cells).

T-cell quantitation should be done next. This is helpful even in the presence of normal lymphocyte counts, inasmuch as there may be an imbalance in the various T-cell regulatory subsets (i.e., helper/inducer cells versus suppressor/cytotoxic cells) without being, or before it is evident in absolute total lymphocyte numbers. This is especially true in AIDS (see Chap. 58).

Following the quantitations, T-cell *functional* studies would then be in order. These may be done either by *in vivo* delayed hypersensitivity skin tests or by *in vitro* mitogen (i.e., a substance that stimulates mitosis and lymphocyte transformation) and antigen blastogenesis assays. (*Blastogenesis* refers to the transformation of small lymphocytes of human peripheral blood in tissue culture, into large, morphologically primitive blastlike cells capable of undergoing mitosis).

The skin testing, while being fairly good for the overall assessment of cellular immunocompetence, and inexpensive, does have several drawbacks: (1) it is of little value in the first years of life (no previous exposure to many of the test antigens); (2) it gives no indication of where the cellular defect is, and (3) it depends on patient cooperation (i.e., the patient must come back for follow-up examination in a specified time interval).

The *in vitro* blastogenesis test, while being more expensive and only available in large institutions and reference laboratories, does not suffer from the above restrictions. This test examines the ability of purified patient mononuclear cells to respond and proliferate to a variety of stimuli. These commonly include, but are not limited to, such mitogens as phytohemagglutinin (PHA), conconavalin A (Con A), pokeweed mitogen (PWM), and the antigens—tetanus toxoid and *Candida albicans*.

## Evaluation of the Phagocytic System

In the examination of the phagocytic system only the white blood cell count with a differential quantifying the total number of neutrophils and monocytes is generally available. The functional tests of the various phagocytic cell activities are, like most of the previously mentioned functional tests, often only found in the major institutions and reference laboratories. The most common of these tests is the nitroblue tetrazolium (NBT) dye reduction test, which ultimately indicates the ability of the polymorphonuclear cells to produce hydrogen peroxide and oxygen radicals necessary for intracellular killing.

The other tests used to assess various phagocytic cell functions are chemiluminescence, quantitative intracellular *in vitro* killing curves, and chemotactic and nonchemotactic migration tests. (A detailed discussion of these tests is to be found in the sources listed in Suggested Readings.)

## Immunodeficiencies: Evaluation of Complement Abnormalities

Immunodeficiencies associated with primary complement abnormalities are usually detected in the laboratory by decreases in the functional hemolytic complement assay ($CH_{50}$). When a decrease in the $CH_{50}$ assay is found in a suspected immunodeficient patient, the individual components of the complement system should then be quantified. If necessary, functional assays can also be performed on the individual components.

Of the above mentioned tests, only the C3 and C4 are readily available in most hospital laboratories. Although primary immunodeficiencies involving C3 and C4 are extremely rare, significant decrease in C3 and C4 are associated with many secondary immunodeficiencies, including various autoimmune diseases.

While it is unfortunate that there are no simple screening tests for most immunodeficiencies, many of the basic tests required to start the often extensive laboratory evaluation are readily available. In fact, most immunodeficient patients should be referred to the larger institutions before the more sophisticated tests are required in the diagnostic process and procedure.

## SUGGESTED READINGS

Griffin, P: Hematology and Immunology, Concepts for Nursing. Appleton-Century-Crofts, Norwalk, CT, 1986.

Lind, M: The immunologic assessment: A nursing focus. Heart Lung 9(4):658–661, Jul-Aug 1980.

Nyamathi, A and van Servellen, G: Maladaptive coping in the critically ill population with acquired immunodeficiency syndrome: Nursing assessment and treatment. Heart Lung 18(2):113, March 1989.

Sher, PP: Laboratory Medicine. American Society of Clinical Pathology, Chicago, November 1986.

CHAPTER 56

# Immunomodulation: Therapeutic Manipulation of the Immune System

*Raymond J. Dattwyler*

## CHAPTER OUTLINE



## LEARNING OBJECTIVES

**At the end of this chapter, you should be able to:**

1. Define *immunomodulation* and its role in today's health care.
2. Explain the immunologic principles underlying antigen-specific immune stimulation or vaccination.
3. Define *immunosuppression*, the mechanism of action of specific immunosuppressants, and their adverse reactions:
   a. Antimetabolites.
   b. Alkylating agents.
   c. Radiation therapy.
   d. Corticosteroids.
   e. Antibodies.
   f. Cyclosporine.
4. Examine other immunotherapies including apheresis and bone marrow transplantation.
5. Delineate the nursing process in caring for the immunosuppressed patient including:
   Assessment
   Nursing diagnoses
   Planning: Patient outcomes
   Desired nursing interventions/rationales.

## IMMUNOMODULATION: AN OVERVIEW

Over the past century, knowledge of human disease has increased greatly. Less than 100 years ago, epidemics of polio, smallpox, and other infectious diseases ravaged the population. Today, these diseases are virtually unknown as a result of advances in the field of immunology.

It has become clear that the immune system protects the population from the sea of microorganisms within which people live, in addition to defending against cancer and neoplastic processes. Unfortunately, it is also clear that this system, which does so much to protect the person, can cause disease by reacting against the host, or to use the common vernacular, *against self*. Unaltered, the immune system can thwart the ability to transplant organs in anyone but identical twins.

Manipulation of the immune system, inducing or enhancing responses that are deemed desirable and suppressing responses that are deemed undesirable, has become possible. Although one frequently does not think of it as such, manipulating or altering immune responses has become an everyday occurrence in modern health-care practice.

An understanding of the various ways in which the immune system can be manipulated is critical to the optimal care of patients. This chapter will discuss immunostimulation and immunosuppression. Transplantation will not be discussed here (see Chap. 57).

## ANTIGEN-SPECIFIC IMMUNE STIMULATION

While the focus of this chapter is to discuss *nonspecific* immunosuppression, it is important to reiterate the clinical significance of antigenic-*specific* immune stimulation. No other area of immunology has had the impact on human health that antigen-specific stimulation has had.

Antigen-specific immune stimulation is nothing more than *vaccination* or *immunization*. It had long been noted that persons who recovered from smallpox, typhoid, or any other *infectious* diseases acquired resistance to the specific illness. That knowledge has only been put to use recently in historic terms.

Vaccination was probably first carried out in the Arab world, but was unknown to the Western world until Lady Montague, the wife of the British ambassador to Turkey, introduced person-to-person vaccination to Britain in the early 18th century. Jenner made vaccination practical in 1796 by eliminating the need for person-to-person contact when he introduced a smallpox vaccine produced in cattle.

Real progress did not occur until Pasteur, who, little more than 100 years ago, demonstrated that disease could be caused by microorganisms, and that by attenuating or altering those microbes, a vaccine could be produced that could confer *immunity* against the specific illness caused by those microbes. Today, almost no one in our modern society has not been immunized against one or, more commonly, many infectious diseases.

### Vaccination: Underlying Principles

The concept underlying vaccination is very simple. When a person is vaccinated (immunized), a specific immune response that has been deemed to be desirable is stimulated. The type of immune response produced depends on a number of variables. These include (1) the route of administration; (2) whether the microorganism is live or not; (3) whether it is a metabolic product of the microbe, or some altered product; and (4) individual variables associated with the specific agent.

Generally, certain rules apply: (1) after immunization, both T-cell and B-cell responses are generated; (2) if an antigen is introduced into the host through a mucosal surface such as the gastrointestinal tract, a local specific IgA response will predominate; (3) if the antigen is injected, the predominant antibody response will be IgG; (4) if the microbe multiples within the host, the immunity produced will usually be long-lasting; and (5) protein antigens provoke a more vigorous, longer lasting immune response than either carbohydrate or lipid antigens.

Using these general principles, one can see why some vaccines produce life-long protection while others only produce short-lived weak immunity.

## IMMUNOSUPPRESSANTS

Having briefly reviewed the clinical significance of antigen-*specific* immunostimulation, we now turn to a discussion of immunosuppression and *non-specific* immunostimulation. Simply defined, an *immunosuppressant* is a substance that diminishes or limits the immune response. This definition is accurate but does not by any means convey the complex and varied effects that immunosuppressive agents have on the immune response. Although, immunosuppressive agents can be categorized in a number of different ways, for the purpose of this chapter, they will be grouped by their *mechanism of action* into antimetabolites, alkylating agents, ionizing radiation, corticosteroids, antibodies, and other biologicals.

Unfortunately, none of the immunosuppressive agents is by any means ideal. The therapeutic index for every one of the current immunosuppressive regimens is extremely narrow. Each is effective at or very near levels that can cause significant adverse effects. Complicating matters further, variations in each person's metabolism make it impossible to predict with certainty the optimal dose for any of these agents in a given patient. Furthermore, it is important to note that while many of these agents are prescribed to treat autoimmune diseases or prevent transplant rejection, others are not meant to be therapeutically immunosuppressive, as for example, in the treatment of cancer, but this may be an unfortunate side effect.

The cytotoxic regimens affect all rapidly dividing cell populations, especially cells of the immune system, the bone marrow, and the gastrointestinal tract. In addition to the ever-present risk of infection, most patients who receive long-term immunosuppressive therapy have a marked increase in their risk of developing a malignancy, frequently non-Hodgkin's lymphoma or acute leukemia.

## Antimetabolites

*Antimetabolites* (substances that compete with naturally occurring metabolites) act primarily within a discrete phase of the cell cycle to inhibit DNA synthesis. Many antimetabolites have been synthesized in the effort to find anticancer drugs. Two of these medications have become widely used as immunosuppressive agents. Azathioprine (Imuran), a thiopurine analogue of hypoxanthine, is converted to 6-thioinosine intracellularly, which competes with inosine as a substrate in the purine metabolic pathway.

The other major antimetabolite used as an immunosuppressant is methothrexate, a folic acid analogue. It acts by competitively inhibiting the enzyme, dihydrofolate reductase, producing an intracellular deficiency of folate coenzymes and the interruption of DNA and RNA synthesis.

Because antimetabolites act primarily on cells during DNA synthesis, one would predict that these agents would exert their effects mainly on actively proliferating cells. Experimental evidence supports this in that the best time to administer both these agents is about 24 hours after antigen challenge. This is a time when lymphocytes that were resting have been activated and are beginning to synthesize new DNA. These agents have little effect on mature cells like plasma cells or effector T cells because these cells no longer have the capacity to replicate. In light of this, it is not surprising that established immune responses are not affected as much as new responses.

For azathioprine, T cells seem to be the major target. In humans, T cell-related phenomena, like graft rejection and delayed hypersensitivity reactions, are sensitive to the effects of azathioprine at doses of 3–5 mg/kg/day or less, while antibody production is not significantly altered until doses of 5–6 mg/kg/day are given.

The increased sensitivity of T cells to azathioprine may not be entirely due to inhibition of DNA synthesis. It has been demonstrated that, even in resting cells, azathioprine can inhibit the ability of T-lymphocytes to form sheep rosettes, implying that it may directly interfere with T-cell surface receptors (markers; see section on T-lymphocytes and B-lymphocytes in Chap. 54). Methotrexate, unlike azathioprine, inhibits both cellular and humoral response to a similar degree.

In addition to their immunosuppressive effects, both of these antimetabolites have significant anti-inflammatory effects. This latter effect is due in part to the reduction in the numbers of monocytes and neutrophils induced by these drugs.

### Adverse Effects of Antimetabolites

Both these agents share a number of side effects. Azathioprine and methotrexate have the ability to produce significant bone marrow depression, especially severe leukopenia in a dose-dependent fashion. Less commonly, each can cause alopecia, stomatitis, or gastrointestinal disturbances including nausea and vomiting.

Each drug also has unique side effects. A small percentage of patients receiving azathioprine will develop a flulike illness, which frequently resolves if the drug can be discontinued. An allergic hepatitis has also been reported secondary to azathioprine therapy. Concomitant use of allopurinol and azathioprine causes a marked decrease in the metabolism of azathioprine, resulting in a dangerous enhancement of its effects. Therefore, if the 2 drugs are given together, the dose of azathioprine should be *reduced* by 75%.

Severe liver damage, including cirrhosis, has been associated with the prolonged use of methotrexate. Because this problem can be difficult to detect, some have suggested that patients receiving methotrexate for prolonged periods of time have a liver biopsy.

## Alkylating Agents

*Alkylating agents* are the most potent chemical immunosuppressants. Interestingly, these medications, which are so useful in the treatment of cancer and as immunosuppressants, were first developed as weapons of war. During World War I, it was noted that exposure to mustard gas produced leukopenia and dissolution of lymphoid tissue, in addition to its vesicant action on the skin, in the eyes, and respiratory tract. Early observations of the activities of agents such as these contributed significantly to the modern era of cancer chemotherapy.

Alkylating agents work by forming covalent bonds with nucleic acids, crosslinking the cell's DNA. They also form bonds with enzymes and other proteins critical to cell function. Both resting cells and dividing cells are susceptible to the actions of these compounds. However, because their major effect is on DNA, actively proliferating cells are killed at a significantly higher rate than resting cells.

Cyclophosphamide is the most commonly used drug of this group. Its major immunosuppressive effect is on B cells, and it can induce a significant drop in both total immunoglobulin levels and in specific antibody titers. Although less effected than B cells, T cells do not escape its effects, and alterations in T-cell functions are noted. An explanation for the selectivity for B-lymphocytes is that B cells have a higher rate of metabolic activity than T cells. Also, it has been suggested that B cells cannot repair their crosslinked DNA as rapidly as T cells.

In animals, it has been demonstrated that cyclophosphamide is most effective if given just prior to antigen administration. Giving the drug at that time kills the maximum number of immunoreactive cells because those cells stimulated by antigen to proliferate have not had sufficient time to repair the cyclophosphamide-induced lesions in their DNA.

Clinically, cyclophosphamide has proved to be most useful in the treatment of the so-called autoimmune diseases (e.g., Wegener's granulomatosis, polyarteritis nodosa, severe rheumatoid arthritis, and the nephritis of systemic lupus erythematosus). It has not proved to be very effective in preventing transplantation rejection and is felt to have little or no role in this area.

The other alkylating agent sometimes used as an immunosuppressant is chlorambucil. It has the same mechanism of action, but it is slower acting and has fewer side effects than cyclophosphamide. Unfortunately, chlorambucil is felt by some to be only weakly immunosuppressive, and it is only very rarely used for this purpose.

#### Adverse Effects of Alkylating Agents

Like the antimetabolites, alkylating agents cause bone marrow depression, especially leukopenia, in a dose-dependent fashion. With prolonged use, the dose required to produce marrow depression decreases. Therefore, any patient on 1 of these agents must have a complete blood count and differential white count at regular intervals. Nausea and vomiting are very common when large doses of these drugs are given, as is alopecia.

Cyclophosphamide causes hemorrhagic cystitis in 5% – 10% of the patients receiving it. This complication occurs as a direct result of active metabolic breakdown products, which are excreted by the kidney at concentrations that can directly affect the epithelial cells lining the bladder. All patients receiving cyclophosphamide should be encouraged to maintain a generous fluid intake and to void frequently. Bladder fibrosis and bladder carcinoma have been associated with this agent.

With prolonged use, or with high doses, cyclophosphamide can cause hypospermia, aspermia, and sometimes gonadal failure in males, and sterility, ovarian failure, and premature menopause in females. At a dose of 50 mg/kg or greater, cyclophosphamide can be associated with the syndrome of inappropriate secretion of ADH (see Chap. 16). An increased incidence of some hematologic malignancies, especially acute myelogenous leukemia, has been associated with the use of alkylating agents. This complication only occurs after many years.

### Radiation Therapy

Ionizing radiation produces lymphopenia and shrinkage of lymphoid tissue. Both x-rays and gamma rays cause the formation of free radicals, which react with DNA, RNA, and other intracellular macromolecules. Like alkylating agents, ionizing radiation affects both resting and proliferating cells but has its greatest effect on proliferating cell populations. Both total body and total nodal irradiation produces profound immunosuppression.

*Total nodal irradiation* is fractionated radiation delivered to all major lymph node areas usually over the course of a few weeks. It is better tolerated by the patient than total body irradiation, because important nonlymphoid tissues like the gastrointestinal tract and the central nervous system can be spared some of the direct effects of radiation.

Radiation produces long-lasting lymphopenia, with marked decreases in both B cells and T cells. Functionally, both T-cell and B-cell responses are significantly impaired and can remain so for years after treatment.

#### Adverse Effects of Radiation Therapy

The adverse effects of radiation therapy are, for the most part, dose-dependent. The bone marrow and the gastrointestinal tract are the most sensitive organ systems. Leukopenia and thrombocytopenia are very common. Small lymphocytes disappear rapidly from the circulation, with granulocytes and platelets reaching their nadir approximately 3 weeks after treatment. Nausea occurs about 2 hours after treatment, and vomiting can follow rapidly. Approximately 50% of patients will develop vomiting after a 2-gray dose of radiation to the gastrointestinal tract (1 gray is equal to 100 rads). Radiation also has well-known *mutagenic* effects and raises the long-term risk of a neoplastic disease, especially hematologic malignancies.

## Corticosteroids

There has been a great deal of confusion as to the immunosuppressive potency of corticosteroids. Most of the early studies of the immunosuppressive effects of corticosteroids were done in mice and other rodents. In these species, corticosteroids cause lympholysis and profound immunosuppression. It has been found that, relative to mice, humans are resistant to the immunosuppressive effects of corticosteroids, and that, at the usual doses given, corticosteroids are mainly acting as anti-inflammatory agents. That is not to say that corticosteroids are not immunosuppressive in humans. The dose required to alter immune responses is just greater than in steroid-sensitive species like mice.

Within 6 hours of their administration in humans, corticosteroids produce a significant lymphopenia. This lymphopenia is not due to destruction of lymphocytes but is secondary to an alteration in the distribution of lymphocytes into extravascular sites, and a change in their circulation patterns. Both T cells and B cells are affected, but the reduction in the number of circulating T cells is greater. The number of T-helper cells is diminished to a greater extent than is the number of T-suppressor cells.

Accompanying this alteration in the numbers of circulating lymphocytes is an increase in the number of neutrophils and a decrease in both monocytes and eosinophils. These changes are also secondary to changes in the distribution of these cells.

The precise mechanism of action of corticosteroids at the cellular level is incompletely understood. *In vitro* experiments using cultured spleen cells have demonstrated that corticosteroids can reduce the production of IgG. Other studies have shown that chronic corticosteroid administration can reduce the total concentration of IgG and perhaps IgA and IgM to a lesser extent. Because established immune responses are more resistant to alteration, it has been difficult to assess whether specific antibody titers are significantly diminished secondary to the direct actions of corticosteroids or as a result of their anti-inflammatory effects.

Cellular immune responses are markedly impaired both by chronic administration of corticosteroids, and by their acute administration in high doses (e.g., 500–1000 mg of methylprednisolone). Cytotoxic T cells are especially sensitive to inhibition by corticosteroids.

Corticosteroids also impair cellular immune responses by decreasing the release of interleukin-1 from monocytes (macrophages), diminishing the production of interleukin-2 from T-helper cells, and by blunting the migration of both T cells and monocytes into areas where they can interact with antigens. (See Fig. 54–7 and section entitled "Antibody Formation" in Chap. 54.)

It has been demonstrated that some, but not all, of the suppressive effects of corticosteroids can be abrogated by the addition of interleukin-2 cell cultures. This suggests that, at least in part, corticosteroids exert their effects by blocking interleukin-2 production or release, although this by no means fully explains the effects of corticosteroids on the immune system.

### *Adverse Effects of Corticosteroid Therapy*

The adverse side effects of corticosteroids cannot be underestimated. All too frequently the administration of high-dose daily corticosteroids for prolonged periods of time leads to greater morbidity and mortality than does the use of cytotoxic agents, or even no treatment at all. Prolonged use of corticosteroids produces multiple complications, which commonly include changes in calcium, sodium, potassium, lipid and glucose metabolism; hypercoagulable states; myopathy; psychologic disorders; cataracts and growth inhibition in children. One of the few things that corticosteroids may not do is cause peptic ulcer disease for, despite the folklore, the connection between ulcers and steroid administration is controversial. (See Appendix A for nursing implications when administering corticosteroid therapy.)

## Antibodies

*Antilymphocyte serum* (ALS) is produced by immunizing an animal with human lymphocytes, inducing formation of antilymphocyte antibodies. When injected into a patient, this crude mixture of antibodies causes destruction of lymphocytes, significant lymphopenia, and suppression of cellular immune functions. Patient antibody production is also depressed, but the degree of suppression is highly variable.

In the past, the major use of antilymphocyte serum has been in organ transplantation, but the clinical results have been mediocre and it is rarely used today. The disappointing clinical results associated with antilymphocyte serum led to attempts at refining the idea of using antibodies directed against lymphocytes to produce immunosuppression.

The first refinement tried was the production of *antithymocyte globulin* (ATG). Antithymocyte globulin is prepared by immunizing animals with human thymocytes, thus inducing antibodies mainly directed against T cells. Although this is an improvement over antilymphocyte serum, the results of this therapy have been variable. (See the section entitled "Polyclonal and Monoclonal Antibodies" in Chap. 57.)

It is doubtful that any approach that uses heterogeneous antibody mixtures produced in animals will ever become an important method to induce immunosuppression. Any time an *in vivo* system is used to produce antibodies, there is significant batch-to-batch variability in titer and, more importantly, in the effects of the antiserum. In addition, because these antisera are made in heterologous species, sensitization virtually always occurs, leading to the possibility of serum sickness or anaphylaxis (hypersensitivity reactions).

A more promising approach is the use of specific *monoclonal antibodies* that can only interact with one subset of lymphocytes. Because monoclonal antibodies are the product of a single clone, they are uniform in their specificity. Antibodies that recognize unique cell surface antigens on various lymphocyte subpopulations have been produced. (When injected into an individual, these antibodies bind to a specific surface antigen and can produce phagocytosis of the antibody-coated cell, or complement activation and lysis of the antibody-coated lymphocyte.)

Unfortunately, monoclonal antibodies binding to surface receptors can produce unexpected results. CD-3, an antigen associated with the T cell antigen receptor is found on all T-lymphocytes. It was postulated that because T cells are the major effector cells involved in transplantation rejection, that rejection could be controlled by injecting anti-CD-3 monoclonal antibodies, thus causing the elimination of T-lymphocytes.

Although completely logical, the results of infusing anti-CD-3 are quite variable. When anti-CD-3 binds to the CD-3 antigen, it can act as a mitogen, *stimulating* T cells. Thus, instead of improving the patient's status, it can create significant problems by causing release of immune mediators. Nonetheless, this approach remains very promising, and other monoclonal antibodies that recognize specific T cell antigens yet do not appear to up-regulate these lymphocytes are undergoing trials with some initial success. In the future, the use of this approach will undoubtedly increase, especially when human antibodies become available. (See section entitled "T-Lymphocytes and B-Lymphocytes" in Chap. 54 for further remarks pertaining to monoclonal antibodies.)

## Cyclosporine

Cyclosporine is a biologic product produced by *Tolyplocadium inflatum*, a species of fungi. It is composed of 11 amino acids and has mild antifungal activity. The effects of this unique peptide on the immune system are profound. Specifically, it inhibits T-lymphocytes, especially T-helper cells. At the same time, it has no significant effect on macrophage or monocyte function, resting T cells, T cell numbers, neutrophils, or hematopoiesis. It is not a cytotoxic agent, and it has no antimitotic activity. Patients treated with this agent do *not* become anemic, granulocytopenic, or thrombocytopenic.

Exactly how cyclosporine inhibits T-cell function is unknown. There are 2 leading possibilities. One is that cyclosporine inhibits activation by blocking expression of the interleukin-2 receptor (see Fig. 54–7). The other is that cyclosporine inhibits the production or secretion of interleukin-2. In either case, cyclosporine has proved to be a major advance in immunosuppressive therapy.

Because cyclosporine mainly inhibits T-helper cell function, its major use has come in the area of transplantation. It has allowed better graft survival with less infectious complications, and lower corticosteroid dosage schedules. Cyclosporine is clearly more efficacious than azothioprine in suppressing graft rejection. Its role in the treatment of autoimmune diseases has not been defined. Cyclosporine does not directly affect B cells, and its effects on antibody production are variable and only mediated through its effect on T-helper cells.

### *Adverse Effects of Cyclosporine Therapy*

Despite cyclosporine's many advantages, there is a price. Cyclosporine can induce a wide variety of side effects, including hypertension, nephrotoxicity, hirsutism, gum hypertrophy, hyperanesthesia, tremor, gastrointestinal intolerances, and hepatic dysfunction including abnormal liver function tests, cholestasis, and focal necrosis.

However, the development of non-Hodgkin's lymphoma associated with high doses of this agent has been the most worrisome side effect by far. Fortunately, reduced dosage schedules have limited the incidence of this complication. Nonetheless, cyclosporine will continue to play an important role in transplantation. Its overall place as an immunosuppressive agent will be defined as more clinical trials are reported. (See Appendix A for nursing implications when administering cyclosporine therapy.)

## NONSPECIFIC IMMUNOSTIMULATION

Although the ability to immunosuppress patients appropriately is primitive, the ability to enhance overall immune responsiveness remains even less well developed. No single approach to the problem of how to nonspecifically stimulate the immune system has met with widespread acceptance. Bacterial products (bacille Calmette Guérin [BCG], *Corynebacterium parvum*, and muramyl peptides), lymphokines (IL-2, interferon) and monokines, thymic or lymphocyte extracts (thymosin, transfer factor), and drugs (levamisole, isoprinosine) have been tried, but, at this point, the use of every one of these agents remains experimental.

Nonetheless, producing immunoenhancement in cancer, old age, or other states where the immune system is depressed or down-regulated, is an area of active interest, which in the future may yield important developments.

The use of bacterial products as *immunopotentiators* grew out of the observation that animals injected with an antigen that developed an inflammatory response or abscess at the injection site had a more intense antibody response.

This observation has led to the development and use of *adjuvants* (i.e., a vehicle used to enhance antigenicity) like Freund's adjuvant, an emulsion of oil and water with killed mycobacteria, to increase antibody production when immunizing animals to produce specific antisera. The slow release of the antigen to the host's immune system from the oil and water emulsion, in combination with a number of bacterial products, has been demonstrated to play a role in increasing the immune response.

Unfortunately, the use of this type of adjuvant in humans has not proved to be feasible because of the intensity of the local inflammatory reaction and the risk of the development of tumors at the injection site.

As part of another approach, BCG, *Corynebacterium parvum*, and other bacteria in either processed or unprocessed form, have been shown to produce immunopotentiation when injected with an antigen or, at times, by themselves. In patients with cancer, numerous experiments have been carried out, especially with BCG, but despite initial reports of significant benefits, the usefulness of BCG and other agents remains questionable. Refinement of this approach may still yield benefits, however.

*Levamisole* and *isoprinosine* are 2 drugs that possess the ability to up-regulate some immune functions. Originally developed as an antihelminthic, levamisole has been found to restore or increase T-cell responses as measured by delayed hypersensitivity skin tests, and to increase the number of circulating T cells. Several side effects, including granulocytopenia and aplastic anemia, associated with its prolonged use have limited this drug's usefulness.

Isoprinosine was developed as an antiviral agent. It is a broad-spectrum immunoenhancer with the ability to increase natural killer cell activity, interleukin-1 and interleukin-2 production, in addition to increasing T-cell numbers and enhancing lymphocyte responses to antigens and to mitogens (i.e., an agent that stimulates mitosis and lymphocyte transformation). Its lack of significant side effects offers the promise of a potentially useful medication.

Trials on the use of interferons, thymic extracts, transfer factor, lymphokines (i.e., lymphocyte products that modulate immune responses), and monokines (i.e., monocyte products that modulate the immune responses) are currently underway. Although none of these agents has been definitively proven to be clinically useful, it is very likely that one or more of these agents will find a role in clinical immunomodulation.

## OTHER IMMUNOTHERAPIES

### Apheresis

Apheresis is a therapeutic approach prescribed for some patients with an autoimmune disease (e.g., rheumatoid arthritis, systemic lupus erythematosus). It allows the selective removal of unwanted components of blood (e.g., antibodies against self basement membrane). *Plasma*pheresis is the removal of all plasma and substances included therein; *leuka*pheresis involves the removal of cellular elements. The red blood cells and remaining blood components are returned to the patient.

The procedure, which involves special apheresis equipment and requires nurses trained to implement the procedure, removes selected components from the patient's blood and returns the red blood cells and remaining components to the patient. The nurse remains with the patient throughout the procedure. Complications include hypocalcemia (as a result of a calcium binding to citrate), hypokalemia, cardiac dysrhythmias, air embolism, hypotension associated with too rapid removal of blood, thrombophlebitis, infection, and equipment malfunction, among others.

### Bone Marrow Transplantation

Bone marrow transplantation is designed primarily to reconstitute hematologic and immunologic function in patients who have not responded to conventional therapy. Such treatment is indicated in aplastic anemia, refractory leukemias and lymphomas, and some immunodeficiency disorders. Types of bone marrow transplantation include *syngeneic* (i.e., donor and recipient are perfectly matched, as in identical twins); *HLA-matched allogeneic* (i.e., donor and recipient compatibility, as in siblings); *HLA-mismatched allogeneic* (i.e., donor and recipient incompatibility); and *autologous* (i.e., the patient's own marrow is frozen and stored for reinfusion after chemotherapy or radiation therapy).

In the case of HLA *in*compatibility between donor and recipient, harmful mature T-lymphocytes are removed from the donor marrow by special agglutination procedure.

Meticulous preparation is employed prior to transplantation to prevent *graft-versus-host disease (GVHD)*, that is, rejection of the host by the immunocompetent cells in the graft. The recipient undergoes intensive immunosuppression and/or total nodal irradiation. Efforts are employed to eliminate bacteria. These include having the patient bathe with an anti-infective twice daily for several days to cleanse the skin and the administration of antibiotics to sterilize the gastrointestinal tract. Women receive intravaginal treatment with an antifungal, anti-infective agent such as clotrimazole.

Post-bone marrow transplantation, the patient is especially vulnerable to infection during the initial 2–4 weeks as a result of the intensive immunosuppressant therapy prior to the transplantation procedure. Efforts are made to control the patient's immediate environment. Room isolation is provided, ideally, with laminar airflow; and the patient is provided with sterilized clothing, bedding, and food.

Complications after transplantation include graft-versus-host disease, infection (commonly, stomatitis), bleeding associated with thrombocytopenia, and psychologic disturbances (e.g., depression). Cardinal symptoms of graft-versus-host disease include a red, maculopapular rash that occurs initially over face, palms, and soles, spreading eventually to the trunk; jaundice; hepatosplenomegaly; gastrointestinal disturbances (e.g., diarrhea); the appearance of pulmonary infiltrates on chest x-ray; central nervous system irritability; and cardiac dysrhythmias. These signs and symptoms may appear within a week to 2 weeks after transplantation. Should graft-versus-host disease occur, the prognosis for survival is not very good (see Chap. 57).

## NURSING CARE OF THE IMMUNOSUPPRESSED PATIENT

Caring for the immunosuppressed patient presents a formidable challenge to nurses and other health-care providers. This is particularly so in a setting where the outcome of the illness can be catastrophic to patient, family, and/or significant others, as is the case with acquired immunodeficiency syndrome (AIDS).

The science of immunology is still in its developmental stages. Thus, while there has been a proliferation of research and new knowledge, inspired in large part by the new disease, AIDS, much remains unknown. The "unknown" becomes a limiting factor in terms of diagnosis and treatment of patients with altered immunologic responses. A case in point is AIDS, wherein the disease ravages those stricken while health-care providers stand by, seemingly helpless to avert the ultimate demise of the individual, at least at this point in time.

The investigational nature of immunology has specific implications for nurses as they care for immunosuppressed patients, whether the underlying cause be primary or secondary, congenital or acquired (see Chap. 58). Immunodeficiency disorders are known to involve defects in one or more of the components of the immune system including the cell-mediated, humoral, phagocytic, and complement systems. Frequently, they involve multiorgan systems. To be effective in caring for the immunosuppressed patient, it is essential that nurses understand the basic principles underlying immunologic function and apply these principles in clinical practice.

In the war against diseases of the immune system, nurses must possess keenly honed assessment skills, a high level of suspicion, and an anticipatory approach to patient care. Nurses must be able to associate a variety of signs and symptoms, and laboratory findings that appear often to be unrelated, with specific immunologic dysfunction. Thorough, ongoing meticulous assessment helps to detect variable, and often subtle signs and symptoms of immunologic dysfunction. This is especially important when one considers that significant variation exists in immunologic responses from one person to the next.

Establishing *baseline* function and explicitly documenting the data are essential so that the patient's subsequent responses to therapeutic intervention can be more closely evaluated. Precise documentation of all findings is crucial for valid data interpretation of therapeutic results.

A major responsibility of nurses in caring for the patient with altered immunologic function is to remain current and aware of the recent research and technological advances. Almost daily, new evidence is presented regarding the workings of the immune system. Bedside nurses are in a pivotal position to contribute to that new evidence as they most closely interact with the patient/family/significant other in the clinical milieu. Scrupulous documentation of their observations contributes to the overall analysis and interpretation of clinical data, which, in turn, may impact on the diagnosis and treatment of diseases of the immune system.

### Therapeutic Goals

Patients who are immunosuppressed may include those with a primary or secondary immunodeficiency disorder. *Primary* indicates that the origin of the immunologic dysfunction lies within the immune system itself, whether the condition is *congenital* (i.e., existing at birth) or *acquired* (thereafter).

*Secondary* indicates that the immunodeficiency occurs as a result of disease in another organ system. It may occur as a side effect to aggressive treatment for another disease (e.g., use of chemotherapeutic agents or radiation therapy in the treatment of some cancers) or in conjunction with the clinical use of immunosuppresants in transplantation therapy. Secondary immunodeficiency is the most common form, and, very importantly, it is the most common cause of nosocomial infections, a fact that has significant implications for nursing care.

Analysis and interpretation of the patient's overall assessment data obtained by thorough clinical history, meticulous physical examination, as well (*text continues on p. 1203*)

## TABLE 56-1. CARE PLAN FOR THE IMMUNOSUPPRESSED PATIENT

| Nursing Diagnoses | Desired Patient Outcomes | Nursing Interventions | Rationales |
|---|---|---|---|
| ***Nursing Diagnosis #1*** Potential for infection, related to:<br>1. Immunosuppression. Possible etiologies:<br>• Acquired Immune Deficiency Syndrome (AIDS).<br>• Transplantation.<br>• Chemotherapy.<br>• Corticosteroid Therapy.<br>• Radiation Therapy.<br>• Malnutrition.<br>(See Table 49-7, Potential for Infection: Nursing Care Considerations.) | Patient will:<br>1. Maintain body temperature within acceptable range ~98.6°F (37°C).<br>2. Maintain white blood count: ~5000–10,000 mm³.<br>3. Remain without signs/symptoms of infection: Pain, swelling, erythema, suppuration.<br>4. Maintain lungs clear to auscultation; chest x-ray without infiltrates.<br>5. Maintain negative cultures: Blood urine, sputum, wound, incision, intravenous sites. | • Associate specific immunological dysfunction with consequent risk of infection: | • Secondary immunodeficiency is the most common cause of nosocomial infections. |
| | | ○ Altered cell-mediated immunity. | ○ Increased susceptibility to fungal and viral infections; and protozoan organisms (especially in the form of pneumonia, chronic skin and mucous membrane infections). |
| | | ○ Altered humoral immunity. | ○ Increased susceptibility to bacterial infections (e.g., bacterial pneumonia, otitis media). |
| | | ○ Altered phagocytic function. | ○ Increased susceptibility to skin and systemic infections caused by pyogenic bacteria. |
| | | ○ Complement deficiencies. | ○ Associated with infections caused by pyogenic bacteria.<br>– Clinically, more than one type of immune defect may exist in the patient concurrently. |
| | | • Define major risk fctors for nosocomial infections:<br>○ Altered immune response. | |
| | | ○ Malnutrition.<br>○ Chemotherapy.<br>○ Corticosteroid therapy. | ○ Malnutrition hinders lymphocyte production especially T cells; compromised T-cell function may also occur. |
| | | ○ Stress. | ○ Stress profoundly inhibits the body's immune response through its associated rise in endogenous corticosteroids and catecholamines. |
| | | ○ Antibiotic/antimicrobial therapy. | ○ Antibiotic therapy may disrupt normal bacterial flora, increasing risk of infection by *opportunistic* organisms; resistant strains of microorganisms may emerge. |
| | | ○ Use of invasive devices/therapies: Pressure monitoring devices; intravascular catheters (e.g., parenteral nutrition; intravenous medication regimens); urinary catheters; respiratory therapy equipment (e.g., endotracheal intubation with suctioning equipment). | |
| | | ○ Underlying chronic or debilitating disease; aging. | ○ Aging increases susceptibility to injury and infection; there is an increased vulnerability to autoimmune disease and malignancies. |

*(continued)*

**TABLE 56–1. CARE PLAN FOR THE IMMUNOSUPPRESSED PATIENT *(Continued)***

| Nursing Diagnoses | Desired Patient Outcomes | Nursing Interventions | Rationales |
|---|---|---|---|
| ***Nursing Diagnosis #1 (cont.)*** | | | |
| | | • Assess for signs and symptoms of infection:<br>◦ Fever, chills, tachycardia; general status: Weakness, fatigue, listlessness; burning on urination, cloudy, foul-smelling urine; or development of localized pain (abscess formation).<br>◦ Productive cough; abnormal breath sounds; adventitious sounds. Monitor productive cough for amount, color, consistency, odor. | • In the presence of leukopenia or lymphopenia, classic signs and symptoms of infection and inflammation may not be manifested; fever, if present, may be the only clinical evidence of infection in the immunosuppressed patient.<br>◦ Immunosuppressed patients with a *cell-mediated* defect are at high risk for infection especially in the form of pneumonia, and mucous membrane infection. Immunosuppressed patients with a *humoral* defect are also at high risk of developing pneumonia. |
| | | ◦ Vulnerable areas: Skin, mouth, mucous membranes, pharynx, axillae, perineum, vagina, and rectal areas.<br>◦ Invasive sites, wounds or skin lesions (e.g., associated with herpes zoster).<br>◦ Complaints of pain and painful areas as indicated by patient. | |
| | | • Evaluate hematology profile, establish *baseline* values: | • Enables status of bone marrow function to be monitored, and the patient's response to therapy to be evaluated. |
| | | ◦ Complete blood cell count with differential; platelets; hematocrit, hemoglobin.<br>◦ Sedimentation rate (ESR). | ◦ Bone marrow suppression is usually dose-related.<br>◦ The erythrocyte sedimentation rate (ESR) reflects the composition of plasma and the relation of RBCs to plasma. A rise in ESR accompanies most acute inflammatory disease whether localized or systemic; an increase in the ESR also accompanies exacerbations of chronic conditions such as rheumatoid arthritis and tuberculosis. This test is therefore useful in monitoring the course of, and therapy for, such chronic conditions. |

| | |
|---|---|
| • Obtain cultures using appropriate technique:<br>○ Blood, urine, sputum, cerebrospinal fluid, drainage from pleural effusion, ascites, wound drainage, invasive line insertion sites; culture of catheter tips, if indicated.<br>• Monitor chest x-rays for pulmonary infiltrates.<br>• Implement measures to minimize risk of infection. | |
| ○ Practice rigorous handwashing and teach patient/family/significant others proper handwashing technique. | ○ Activities involving the use of the hands are a common method of cross-contamination. Handwashing should be performed prior to and after contact with patient. |
| ○ Institute use of private room, reverse isolation, or room with laminar air flow as indicated, and as available. | ○ Reduces risk of exposure to a variety of organisms; a laminar air flow environment provides a nearly germ-free environment for severely immunosuppressed patients. |
| ○ Use gown, mask and gloves as indicated for all visitors and personnel; teach personnel/visitors regarding use of these precautions.<br>○ Keep patient's bedside uncluttered; retain only necessary equipment. Germicide may be used to cleanse bedside furniture/equipment. | |
| ○ Limit number of visitors. | ○ Persons (including personnel or visitors) who have colds or other infection should not be allowed into patient's immediate environment. |
| ○ Provide sterile eating utensils and well-cooked foods; avoid uncooked foods.<br>• Monitor physiological status: | |
| ○ Monitor fever if present and treat conservatively if possible, using tepid sponges, light bedding/clothing. Maintain comfortable room temperature. | ○ Use of antipyretic medication should be employed cautiously because such therapy may mask fever, thus impairing a valuable indicator of the course/status of the patient's infection. |
| • Monitor fluid and electrolyte status: Maintain strict intake and output; estimate insensible losses (via perspiration and lungs); maintain hydrated state as prescribed. | • It is essential to maintain fluid and electrolyte balance to prevent drying of skin and mucous membranes; this could result in fissuring and cracking of lips and mucous membranes, increasing the risk of infection; an increase in blood viscosity places the bedridden, immobilized patient at risk of developing deep venous thrombosis or hypercoagulable state. |

(continued)

**TABLE 56-1. CARE PLAN FOR THE IMMUNOSUPPRESSED PATIENT** *(Continued)*

| Nursing Diagnoses | Desired Patient Outcomes | Nursing Interventions | Rationales |
|---|---|---|---|
| ***Nursing Diagnosis #1 (cont.)*** | | | |
| | | • Monitor renal function.<br>○ BUN, creatinine, uric acid. | • Patients receiving immunosuppressive drugs are at increased risk of renal disease (e.g., acute tubular necrosis, nephrotoxicity, uric acid calculi).<br>○ Use of cyclophosphamide can cause hemorrhagic cystitis; administration of this drug must be accompanied by high fluid intake, and the patient should be encouraged to void frequently.<br>○ Methotrexate likewise requires a hydrated state as this drug may deposit within the renal tubules. |
| ***Nursing Diagnosis #2***<br>Oral mucous membranes, alteration in, related to:<br>1. Immunosuppression.<br>2. Dehydration.<br>3. Malnutrition. | Patient will:<br>1. Maintain integrity of mucous membranes:<br>• Mucous membranes moist.<br>• Lips without cracking or fissures.<br>• No evidence of stomatitis. | • Maintain intact mucous membranes.<br>○ Assist patient/family in performing oral hygiene therapy. | • Immunosuppressed patients are at increased risk of developing stomatitis; use of immunosuppressant agents disrupts rapidly dividing mucosal epithelial cells. |
| | | ○ Teach use of normal saline, dilute solution of hydrogen peroxide, or sodium bicarbonate and water, to cleanse mouth. | ○ Sodium bicarbonate usage is limited because of its high sodium content; monitor serum electrolytes. |
| | | ○ Avoid use of alcohol-containing mouthwashes. | ○ Alcohol has a drying effect on mucous membranes. |
| | | ○ Keep lips lubricated with petroleum jelly.<br>○ Stress necessity of oral hygiene after meals and snacks, and in between meals; if stomatitis develops, increase frequency of oral care. | |
| | | ○ Maintain hydrated state; sterile water may be used in severely immunosuppressed patient. | ○ Hydration helps to maintain mucous membranes in moist state. |
| | | ○ Avoid intake of foods or drinks that may be irritating to mucous membranes.<br>○ Use soft bristle toothbrush. | ○ Patient may have a bleeding tendency related to depressed bone marrow function (thrombocytopenia); abrasions of gums and mucous membranes may be predispose to infection. |
| | | ○ Provide meticulous perineal care. | |

| | | | |
|---|---|---|---|
| Skin integrity, impairment of: Potential, related to:<br>1. Immunosuppressed state.<br>2. Dehydration.<br>3. Malnutrition. | Patient will:<br>1. Maintain skin intact, no breaks, lesions, irritations or signs of infection; good skin turgor. | • Prevent impairment of skin integrity:<br>∘ Assess the skin over body meticulously for any lesions or breaks. | • Immunosuppressed, malnourished states increase risk of skin breakdown, and the incidence of decubitus ulcer formation.<br>∘ Skin impairment may occur through delayed hypersensitivity reactions following skin tests. |
| | | ∘ Turn patient q 2 hr; encourage frequent position changes. | ∘ If reddened areas do not blanch within 20–30 minutes of a position change, increase frequency of position changes. |
| | | ∘ Implement measures to redistribute pressure (e.g., alternating pressure mattress; egg-crate mattress, sheepskin, elbows and heel protectors).<br>∘ Keep skin well lubricated.<br>∘ Treat any skin breakdown meticulously; follow unit protocol for pressure ulcer therapy.<br>∘ Closely monitor effectiveness of therapy. | ∘ Underlying goal of skin care is to maximize tissue perfusion. |
| | | ∘ Monitor dietary intake; consult with dietitian as indicated. | ∘ Malnourishment reduces tissue healing (i.e., protein synthesis and repair). |
| | | (See Table 49–7, Potential for Infection: Nursing Care Considerations, for information regarding the following activities:)<br>• Monitor for urinary tract infection (UTI).<br>• Monitor for intravascular infection.<br>∘ Risk factors for IV-catheter-related infections.<br>∘ Signs and symptoms of intravascular cannula-related infection.<br>∘ Precautions for the insertion and maintenance of intravenous line.<br>∘ Precautions for the insertion and maintenance of pressure monitoring system.<br>• Monitor for respiratory tract infection (RTI).<br>• Appreciate significance of widespread antimicrobial use as a contributing factor in the selection of resistance strains of microorganisms. | |

*(continued)*

**TABLE 56-1. CARE PLAN FOR THE IMMUNOSUPPRESSED PATIENT** *(Continued)*

| Nursing Diagnoses | Desired Patient Outcomes | Nursing Interventions | Rationales |
|---|---|---|---|
| ***Nursing Diagnosis #4***<br>Anxiety related to:<br>1. Potential terminal illness.<br>2. Use of investigative drugs.<br>3. Increased risk of developing a malignancy associated with long-term immunosuppressive therapy (e.g., non-Hodgkin's lymphoma, or acute leukemia). | Patient will:<br>1. Verbalize feelings and concerns about underlying condition, its anticipated course, and prognosis.<br>2. Verbalize understanding of treatment protocols and expectations of therapy.<br>3. Verbalize relief of anxiety: Demonstrate relaxed demeanor.<br>4. Verbalize signs/symptoms of anxiety, and causative factors underlying its occurrence.<br>5. Demonstrate anxiety-reducing behaviors and/or activities. | • Establish baseline patient/family/significant others assessment data regarding level of anxiety or fear, mood, coping skills, and available resources. | • Such baseline data provide a measure with which to evaluate subsequent responses to therapy, and to plan care. |
| | | ○ Assess situation predisposing to anxiety. Ascertain knowledge and understanding of underlying disease, its expected course, and overall prognosis.<br>○ Determine impact of individual and familial roles and lifestyle, and their previous experiences with illness. | ○ It is important to be cognizant that no one becomes ill in a vacuum, rather, the illness of one member of a family may reflect illness involving all members of the family. Thus, treatment, to be effective, requires active participation by other family members. |
| | | ○ Identify previous coping skills and their effectiveness; ability to problem-solve; feelings regarding illness and its ramifications in terms of life goals, personal and familial resources. | ○ May help to reassure by identifying activities or behaviors that were effective for the patient in the past.<br>○ Long-term, or catastrophic illness may seriously tax family resources. Referral to outside agencies may be indicated. |
| | | • Implement measures to reduce anxiety:<br>○ Establish a rapport with patient/family/significant others. Utilize a caring attitude; spend time with patient/family; listen attentively.<br>○ Orient to hospital and unit protocols: Introduce to staff members participating in patient's care; provide a calm, reassuring environment; minimize stressors.<br>○ Encourage verbalization of fears and concerns. | ○ Fosters feelings of security and comfort. |
| | | ○ Reassure that it is normal to feel anxious. Assist to identify signs/symptoms of anxiety, and situations or concerns that predispose to anxiety. | ○ Assists patient/family/significant others to accept their feelings, "It's okay to have such feelings." |
| | | ○ Keep informed regarding all tests and therapies, and the expectations of the patient. | ○ Knowing what to expect can relieve anxiety. |
| | | ○ Instruct in method of relaxation. Encourage family or significant others to participate; reinforce positive behaviors.<br>○ Assist in problem-solving and strategizing short-term goals. | ○ Energy-releasing activities enable the patient to maintain some control of anxious state. |
| | | ○ Encourage patient to participate in self-care as much as possible. | ○ Enables patient to maintain some control over his/her care. |

| | | | |
|---|---|---|---|
| ***Nursing Diagnosis #5***<br>Knowledge deficit, related to:<br>1. Immunosuppression associated with:<br>A. Primary or secondary immunodeficiency disease.<br>B. Transplantation therapy.<br>C. Chemotherapy.<br>D. Corticosteroid therapy. | Patient will:<br>1. Verbalize knowledge regarding diagnosis and prognosis of illness and expectations as to its course.<br>2. Discuss treatment regimen and how to implement it:<br>• Medication regimen.<br>• Measures to reduce risk of infection.<br>3. Explain importance of maintaining optimal nutrition and hydration status.<br>4. Verbalize responsibility for follow-up care. | • Perform overall assessment of patient/family/significant others regarding this illness episode: | |
| | | ○ Assess understanding of underlying illness, expectations regarding prognosis, and disease course. | ○ Assists in ascertaining baseline knowledge regarding illness, and its impact on individual and collective family lifestyle; assists in clarifying any misunderstandings or preconceptions regarding the nature of the illness. |
| | | ○ Assess readiness to learn. Estimate how much information can be handled effectively at any one time. | ○ Overwhelming patient/family/significant other with information can increase anxiety and compromise learning. |
| | | ○ Minimize stress by answering questions as they arise; provide support and reassurance; remain accessible to answer questions as they arise; be honest. | ○ Stress can further compromise immune function through the increase in secretion of endogenous corticosteroids and catecholamines triggered by stress. |
| | | • Instruct regarding implementation of treatment regimen and necessity for follow-up care: | • Information presented accurately and precisely will allay fears and anxieties, and foster learning and compliance. |
| | | ○ Review prescribed medication regimen: Specific medication, or combination of medications to take; and overall treatment protocols; dose and routine of administration; mechanism of drug action. | ○ Appropriate administration of specific immunosuppressant(s) is necessary to achieve maximum benefit.<br>○ Coordination of immunotherapy around other therapies (e.g., radiation, surgery) helps to assure maximum benefit of the overall treatment regimen. |
| | | ○ Teach patient and family regarding specific adverse effects, and actions to be taken should they occur: Nausea/vomiting; bleeding (ecchymosis, petechiae, melena, bleeding gums, hematuria); coughing, dyspnea; fever, anorexia, weakness, fatigue; weight loss, signs of dehydration; numbness, tingling, tremors, etc. | ○ Patient/family/significant other should be familiar with all adverse drug effects, and know what resources are available should a problem arise. |
| | | ○ Advise avoidance of self-treatment, (e.g., use of over-the-counter drugs) unless cleared with the physician. | ○ Such drugs may predispose to undesirable drug interactions; or aggravate an underlying condition such as bleeding (e.g., use of aspirin heightens the risk of bleeding).<br>○ Investigational nature of some drugs may cause the patient to question the efficacy of the treatment regimen. |
| | | ○ Provide supportive care: Praise patient for compliance with treatment regimen; reinforce benefits of treatment; provide written directions regarding treatment when possible. | |
| | | ○ Stress importance of mandatory serial hematology testing in conjunction with immunosuppressant therapy. | |

*(continued)*

**TABLE 56-1. CARE PLAN FOR THE IMMUNOSUPPRESSED PATIENT** *(Continued)*

| Nursing Diagnoses | Desired Patient Outcomes | Nursing Interventions | Rationales |
|---|---|---|---|
| *Nursing Diagnosis #5 (cont.)* | | | ○ Immunosuppressant agents can depress bone marrow function; presence of leukopenia (lymphopenia) suggests severe bone marrow depression, which necessitates a reassessment of overall treatment regimen (e.g., adjustment in medication protocol; or possibly, institution of reverse isolation precautions may be recommended). |
| | | • Assess baseline psychological status: Monitor for changes in behavior, mood, affect. | • Baseline data provides a measure with which to evaluate subsequent responses and behavior. Patients with chronic, often terminal illness, may experience serious emotional upsets. Depression may contribute to the immunosuppressed state. |
| | | • Review measures to reduce risk of infection:<br>○ Encourage patient/family to explain and/or demonstrate measures/precautions to reduce the risk of infection. | • Bone marrow depression with leukopenia places patient at great risk of developing infection.<br>○ (See Nursing Diagnosis #1, above.) |
| | | • Instruct patient/family/significant others regarding need to maintain nutrition and fluid intake:<br>○ Have patient verbalize ways to improve appetite: Eat frequent, small meals instead of three main meals/day; maintain high-protein, high-caloric diet as prescribed. | |
| | | ○ Teach patient to perform meticulous oral hygiene prior to and after meals. | ○ Helps to eliminate undesirable taste in the mouth; minimizes risk of infection (stomatitis). |
| | | ○ Have patient verbalize ways to cope with nausea including good oral hygiene.<br>○ Advise patient to eat dry foods in small amounts should nausea occur, avoiding spicy, fatty foods. | ○ Foods with an overwhelming aroma, should be cooked by someone else if possible; spicy, fatty foods may precipitate nausea. |
| | | ○ Have patient verbalize need for increase in fluid intake (up to 2000–2500 ml/24 hr, if not contraindicated). | ○ High content of uric acid filtered at the glomerulus in conjunction with cytotoxic effect of some immunosuppressants can predispose to uric acid stone formation. Patients receiving methotrexate must be well hydrated because of risk of deposition of drug in renal tubules. |
| | | ○ In addition to large fluid intake, the patient should be encouraged to void frequently.<br>○ Encourage participation of family/significant others in treatment regimen. | ○ Hemorrhagic cystitis is associated with use of cyclophosphamide. |

| | | | |
|---|---|---|---|
| ***Nursing Diagnosis #6***<br>Nutrition, alteration in: less than body requirements, associated with:<br>1. Anorexia, nausea, vomiting, stomatitis related to immunosuppressant therapy, or immunosuppressed state. | Patient will:<br>1. Maintain ideal body weight.<br>2. Remain infection-free.<br>• body temperature: ~98.6°F (~37°C).<br>3. Maintain usual strength and activity tolerance.<br>4. Maintain laboratory values within acceptable range for patient:<br>• BUN, creatinine, glucose, total protein, albumin, serum calcium.<br>• Hematology profile. | • Collaborate with nutritionist and physician in assessing dietary needs.<br>○ Assess the following parameters: General health status, strength, activity tolerance; body weight; triceps skinfold measurement.<br>○ Laboratory profile: Serum chemistries—BUN, creatinine, electrolytes, calcium, total protein, albumin; Hematology profile: Complete blood count with differential, hematocrit, hemoglobin, platelets.<br>○ Assess reasons for inadequate nutritional intake: Anorexia, nausea/vomiting associated with immunosuppressant therapy; altered taste capacity; presence of stomatitis. | • Baseline assessment assists in determining dietary regimen; provides a measure with which to evaluate the patient's response to therapy. (See appropriate tables in Chapter 53 for other details regarding the dietary assessment and needs of the critically ill patient.) |
| | | • Implement measures to improve/maintain optimal nutrition:<br>○ Treat underlying stomatitis as prescribed.<br>○ Implement measures to relieve nausea and vomiting. | ○ Immunosuppressant therapy frequently causes disruption of gastrointestinal function because of rapid turnover of mucosal epithelial cells. |
| | | ○ Encourage meticulous oral hygiene prior to and after meals.<br>○ Encourage intake of smaller meals rather than three main meals/day.<br>○ Encourage dry foods if nausea occurs; limit fluid intake with meals. | ○ May help to relieve disagreeable taste; reduces risk of infection especially in patients with compromised cell-mediated immune response. |
| | | ○ Avoid spicy, tangy foods, which may be irritating to oral mucous membranes and gastric mucosa.<br>○ Avoid cooking foods that have a pungent odor or aroma. | ○ May precipitate nausea and vomiting. |
| | | ○ Implement plan to meet caloric and protein needs. Serve foods with high protein content; add sweeteners as tolerated.<br>○ Encourage family members or significant others to bring in the patient's favorite foods.<br>○ Maintain a relaxed setting conducive to eating. | ○ Milk and milk products are an excellent source of protein and calories, and can be used in cooking and preparing desserts. |
| | | ○ Encourage family and significant others to socialize with patient during mealtimes.<br>○ Allow adequate rest periods before meals, and enough time for the patient to eat comfortably during mealtimes. | ○ Provides a more normal setting, which may increase the patient's appetite. |

*(continued)*

**TABLE 56–1. CARE PLAN FOR THE IMMUNOSUPPRESSED PATIENT** *(Continued)*

| Nursing Diagnoses | Desired Patient Outcomes | Nursing Interventions | Rationales |
|---|---|---|---|
| ***Nursing Diagnosis #6 (cont.)*** | | • Reassess all parameters indicative of nutritional status and reevaluate the patient's response to therapy. | |
| | | ◦ Supplement patient's dietary intake with enteral/parenteral feedings as indicated, if the patient is unable to meet dietary needs. | ◦ (See appropriate sections in Chapter 53, Nutritional Support of the Critically Ill Patient.) |
| ***Nursing Diagnosis #7***<br>Bowel elimination, alteration in: diarrhea, related to:<br>1. Effect of cytotoxic drugs on rapidly replicating mucosal epithelial cells of gastrointestinal tract.<br>2. Anxiety. | Patient will:<br>1. Maintain usual bowel elimination pattern. | • Assess patient's usual elimination pattern. | • Baseline function provides a measure with which to evaluate current status of bowel elimination. |
| | | ◦ Assess signs/symptoms of *diarrhea* including: Frequency of stool, consistency, amount, type or quantity; presence of blood or mucus; duration of diarrheal problem; associated factors such as abdominal pain, cramping; factors that ameliorate the diarrhea; factors that aggravate the diarrhea; (e.g., anxiety, eating certain foods, etc.). | ◦ Use SLIDT tool to ascertain characteristics of diarrheal problem (Table 7–1). |
| | | ◦ Perform abdominal assessment including auscultation of bowel signs, percussion and palpation. Note especially any signs of tenderness. | ◦ For details regarding the gastrointestinal assessment, see Chapter 48.) |
| | | • Implement measures to treat/control *diarrhea:*<br>◦ Monitor frequency and characteristics of stool; auscultate and examine abdomen periodically.<br>◦ Identify foods (e.g., foods with high fat content, or gas-producing foods, or spicy foods) associated with precipitating or aggravating the diarrhea. | • Diarrhea commonly occurs in conjunction with administration of cytotoxic medications in response to drug effects on rapidly replicating mucosal epithelial cells. |
| | | ◦ Avoid all foods that fit this category (e.g., onions, cabbage, beans, chili; also carbonated beverages and foods/drinks high in caffeine, etc.)<br>◦ Administer prescribed medications to decrease bowel motility.<br>◦ Provide frequent small meals with low residue content.<br>◦ Monitor response to dietary and medication therapy. | ◦ Poorly digested foods, or those that act as an irritant to the gastrointestinal mucosa, should be avoided. |

| | | | |
|---|---|---|---|
| | | ○ Monitor hydration, serum electrolyte, and acid-base status. Provide parenteral fluid replacement as prescribed. | ○ Severe diarrhea can result in electrolyte imbalance with loss of potassium; loss of bicarbonate can predispose to metabolic acidemia and hyperchloremia (see Chapter 30, Acid-Base Physiology and Pathophysiology). |
| Bowel elimination, alteration in: constipation, related to:<br>1. Inadequate dietary fiber intake.<br>2. Reduced physical activity. | Patient will:<br>1. Maintain usual bowel elimination pattern. | • Assess patient's usual elimination pattern.<br>○ Assess for signs/symptoms of *constipation* (see signs/symptoms of diarrhea in the above, for parameters to be assessed). Also investigate complaints of abdominal fullness, cramping, pressure in rectum. Record bowel sounds that may indicate a pattern of decreasing frequency. | |
| | | • Implement measures to treat/prevent *constipation.*<br>○ Encourage patient to respond to urge to defecate: Provide necessary privacy, positioning (e.g., semi-Fowler's) to facilitate defecation. | • Constipation in the immunosuppressed patient must be avoided as any insult to the bowel and rectum places the patient at risk for bleeding and infection (e.g., abscess or fistula formation). |
| | | ○ Review dietary intake of foods high in fiber.<br>○ Stress the need for high fluid intake 2000–2500 ml/day (unless contraindicated).<br>○ Should constipation occur, follow prescribed therapy: Use of laxative, suppositories, oil retention enema. Administer stool softener and monitor the effectiveness of these modalities. | ○ Prevents stool from becoming dried out and impacted.<br>○ If hemorrhoids are present, constipation can aggravate and exacerbate the condition, leading to bleeding and infection. |
| | | ○ Monitor frequency and consistency of stool, and the presence of diarrhea. Avoid any unnecessary rectal invasion; avoid taking rectal temperature, and administering enemas if at all possible. | ○ Diarrhea may indicate presence of fecal impaction. Fecal impaction can injure the intestinal mucosa, predisposing to bleeding in patients with severely depressed bone marrow function (thrombocytopenia); and infection in patients with leukopenia (lymphopenia). |
| ***Nursing Diagnosis #8***<br>Self-concept, disturbance in, related to:<br>1. Immunosuppressant therapy–related changes in physical appearance (e.g., weight loss, alopecia).<br>2. Altered role and lifestyle necessitated by underlying illness. | Patient will:<br>1. Verbalize feelings about body changes.<br>2. Explore thoughts and feelings regarding perceptions of self and self-worth.<br>3. Identify self-strengths.<br>4. Verbalize positive realistic perceptions of self. | • Determine how patient feels about self, and about changes in self-image, roles, and lifestyle, necessitated by underlying illness. | • Understanding patient's perceptions and feelings forms the basis for a trusting rapport and constructive relationship. It is necessary to know where an individual is coming from, in order to assist him/her to move on, within the constraints of the patient's illness. |
| | | ○ Explore patient/family value system, previous coping capabilities; expectations, short-term and long-term goals. Help patient/family identify strengths and weaknesses; family and personal resources. | ○ Family/significant other support systems may function to increase patient's self-esteem and self-worth. |

*(continued)*

**TABLE 56-1. CARE PLAN FOR THE IMMUNOSUPPRESSED PATIENT *(Continued)***

| Nursing Diagnoses | Desired Patient Outcomes | Nursing Interventions | Rationales |
|---|---|---|---|
| ***Nursing Diagnosis #8 (cont.)*** | | | |
| | 5. Participate actively in social activities and in self-care. | ○ Encourage patient to verbalize feelings of anger and frustration. Reassure that such feelings are normal, and that it is okay to feel the way the patient feels. | ○ Changes in bodily appearance and function associated with immunosuppressant therapy can be especially distressing to patient/family/significant others. |
| | | • Discuss how illness/treatment impacts on personal and familial lifestyles.<br>○ Evaluate support system and resources. Provide opportunity for patient to verbalize concerns regarding role within family constellation: Who is the decision-maker? What role did the patient play prior to illness? Expectations of future? | ○ Concerns regarding changes in role, or in patient's perceptions as to whether he/she can fulfill the role because of illness, need to be explored because they may create problems that interfere with the treatment and progress of the patient healthwise, and socially. |
| | | ○ Encourage to identify self-perceptions. Help to identify differences between perceived and actual self. Encourage to be honest and straightforward in interactions with others. | ○ Helps patient to develop realistic view of self. |
| | | ○ Encourage participation in activities and interactions with others. Assist to become aware of responses of others. Encourage to be honest in presenting self to others. | ○ Such activities provide the opportunity for patient to become independent, and to develop self-esteem. |
| | | ○ Encourage positive feelings about self. Offer praise for accomplishments, and adjustments necessitated by illness. | ○ Increases self-acceptance and self-confidence. |
| | | ○ Encourage some initial exploration of short- and long-term goal-setting. | ○ Adjustments in goals made prior to illness may be necessary, but these goals may still be able to be pursued. |
| ***Nursing Diagnosis #9***<br>Coping, ineffective: individual, related to:<br>1. Uncertainty of underlying disease, and/or course of illness. | Patient will:<br>1. Demonstrate willingness to participate in self-care activities.<br>2. Demonstrate ability to problem-solve, and to make decisions.<br>3. Identify resources and support systems.<br>4. Identify strengths.<br>5. Identify effective coping mechanisms. | • Establish an atmosphere of mutual trust and caring. Encourage constructive expression of feelings.<br>• Assess for signs/symptoms of ineffective coping:<br>○ Ineffective coping may be reflected by the following: Disturbances of sleep; inability to concentrate; complaints of fatigue, restlessness, inability to relax.<br>○ Assist patient to identify stressors. Work with patient to explore alternative options and strategies of dealing with stressors. | • Establishing rapport with patient/family/significant others facilitates communication, and verbalization of fears and concerns. |

| | | | |
|---|---|---|---|
| | | • Implement measures to assist patient to cope:<br>○ Reduce level of anxiety (see Nursing Diagnosis #4, above.)<br>○ Provide opportunities for participating in problem-solving, decision-making process regarding care.<br>○ Set limits on number of choices.<br>○ Set limits on inappropriate behaviors.<br>○ Assist patient in exploring short-term goals.<br>○ Reinforce positive behaviors; support patient's adaptations and adjustments to current status.<br>○ Encourage patient to share with others factors that will assist him/her to cope.<br>○ Encourage verbalization of feelings, perceptions, and concerns.<br>○ Encourage continued emotional support from family/significant others. | ○ Involving patient in decisions regarding care enables the patient to experience some control over his/her care. This builds self-confidence and self-esteem.<br>○ Prevents patient from feeling overwhelmed; helps to focus/channel energies on constructive activities.<br>○ Unaddressed fears and concerns can retard progress toward independence and self-reliance. |
| ***Nursing Diagnosis #10***<br>Potential for injury: bleeding disorders, related to:<br>1. Thrombocytopenia, associated with bone marrow depression, which may occur with use of immunosuppressants or in conjunction with radiation therapy. | Patient will not experience unusual bleeding:<br>1. Mental status: Alert, oriented to person, place, date.<br>2. Vital signs within acceptable physiological range.<br>3. Absence of petechiae or ecchymosis.<br>4. Absence of frank or occult blood:<br>• Epistaxis, hemoptysis.<br>• Vomitus (hematemesis), gastric aspirate.<br>• Stool (melena).<br>• Urine (hematuria).<br>• Cervical/vaginal secretions.<br>5. Absence of abdominal tenderness, distention, or increase in abdominal girth. | • Assess for signs/symptoms of unusual bleeding:<br>○ Vital signs: Blood pressure (hypotension), tachycardia, rapid, thready pulse.<br>○ Skin color: Pallor, mottling, cyanosis; skin temperature, turgor, moisture.<br>○ Evidence of bleeding: Arterial or venule puncture sites; intravenous insertion, injection sites, epistaxis, hemoptysis, sputum; hematuria; hematemesis, melena, gastric aspirate; peritoneal aspirate (ascites); incision sites or open wounds/drainage.<br>• Assess neurological function: Mental status, orientation; complaints of headache, blurred vision; twitching or seizure activity; restlessness, agitation; lethargy.<br>• Assess abdomen: Evidence of abdominal distention; increase in abdominal girth. | ○ Changes in skin color, temperature and moisture (cold and clammy) suggest reduced peripheral perfusion associated with reduced cardiac output and hypotension.<br>• Changes caused by intracerebral bleeding can be subtle and may go unnoticed until such time as there is a symptomatic increase in intracranial pressure.<br>• Increases in abdominal girth may be the only evidence of intra-abdominal bleeding in the scenario of slow or gradual bleeding over time, which is not of the volume to disturb cardiovascular dynamics. |

*(continued)*

## TABLE 56–1. CARE PLAN FOR THE IMMUNOSUPPRESSED PATIENT *(Continued)*

| Nursing Diagnoses | Desired Patient Outcomes | Nursing Interventions | Rationales |
|---|---|---|---|
| ***Nursing Diagnosis #10 (cont.)*** | | | |
| | 6. Stable hematologic and coagulation profiles:<br>• Hematocrit, hemoglobin, platelets (count, aggregation).<br>• Prothrombin time, activated partial thromboplastin time; bleeding time. | • Assess laboratory data:<br>○ Hematologic profile: Hematocrit, hemoglobin, platelets (count and aggregation).<br>○ Coagulation profile: Prothrombin time; activated thromboplastin time, thrombin time. | ○ In patients receiving large quantities of blood, the hematocrit may not be a reliable parameter early post-transfusion because the blood may not have evenly distributed throughout the body. In this instance, blood pressure and pulses may be more reliable parameters to assess. |
| | | • Monitor (ongoing) body functions for evidence of frank or occult blood as above. | • High-risk patients (e.g., immunosuppressed) should be identified and carefully monitored for evidence of bleeding. |
| | | • Implement measures to prevent bleeding:<br>○ Avoid unnecessary arterial or venous puncture or injections. Apply firm, continuous, and prolonged (>5 minutes) pressure to all puncture and injection sites.<br>○ Avoid unnecessary blood pressure readings; do not overinflate cuff.<br>○ Avoid use of rectal thermometer. | ○ Patients with thrombocytopenia have compromised bleeding and clotting times; consequently, any disruption of body surfaces can result in significant blood loss.<br>○ Frequent and excessive pressure on fragile capillaries can cause bleeding with formation of petechiae.<br>○ Fragile mucous membranes bleed easily. |
| | | • Instruct patient/family in activities that may reduce the risk of bleeding:<br>○ Use electric razor, soft bristle toothbrush; avoid rigorous nose-blowing.<br>○ Take stool softeners as prescribed; follow diet prescribed including necessary bulk-forming foods. Maintain hydration status.<br>○ If bleeding occurs, apply pressure if possible; maintain fluid volume; notify physician. Offer reassurance to patient/family. | ○ Constipation is to be avoided to reduce risk of bleeding within the gastrointestinal tract.<br>○ For a discussion of hemorrhagic, hypovolemic shock, see Chapters 46 and 63. |

as laboratory findings, provide the basis for diagnosing and planning care (see Chap. 55).

In treating immunosuppressed patients, major areas of concern include: increased risk of developing infection, or exacerbation and spread of existing infection; knowledge deficit on the part of patient/family/significant others regarding the underlying disease; anxiety regarding its treatment, potential complications (e.g., increased risk of malignancy), and prognosis; impact of underlying pathophysiology or its treatment on total body functioning (e.g., cardiopulmonary function, fluid and electrolyte status, gastrointestinal function, bleeding potential); alteration in nutritional status; overall impact of stress on the patient/family/significant other's ability to cope; and psychologic implications (e.g., disturbance in self-concept and self-image).

Whatever the underlying cause of the immunosuppressed state, implementation of nursing process in the care of the immunosuppressed patient, the family and/or significant others revolves around the following therapeutic goals:

1. Establish a thorough, comprehensive database including:
   a. Clinical history, including functional health patterns.
   b. Physical examination.
   c. Laboratory data.
2. Prevent infection, impairment of integrity of skin and mucous membranes.
3. Provide emotional and psychologic support to patient/family/significant others.
4. Initiate health education to assist patient/family/significant others in achieving optimal level of health desired.
5. Provide nutritional support.
6. Monitor fluid and electrolyte balance and renal function.
7. Monitor for possible bleeding.
8. Monitor use of cytotoxic or immunosuppressant agents including method of administration, dosage, mechanism of action, potential side effects, patient education.
9. Minimize discomfort, and promote rest and relaxation.

### Care Plan for the Immunosuppressed Patient

Pertinent nursing diagnoses, desired patient outcomes, and nursing interventions and rationales in the care of the immunosuppressed patient are presented in Table 56–1. Psychologic perspectives in the nursing care of the patient with acquired immunodeficiency syndrome (AIDS) are included in the Case Study presented in Chapter 58.

## CONCLUSION

Although great progress has been made in the ability to modulate the human immune system and to care for patients receiving immunomodulation, it is clear that research remains at a very primitive stage. The future holds great promise in the areas of transplantation, control of autoimmunity, cancer, aging, and immunodeficiency, to name just a few. As overall knowledge of the working of the immune system increases, so the ability to manipulate the immune system in an effective, yet safe, manner will also increase, as will the implications for the nursing care.

## SUGGESTED READINGS

Arnold, AN, et al: Effect of renal allograft dysfunction upon cyclosporine through levels in host blood. Transplantation 40:605, 1985.

Goldstein, G, et al: A randomized clinical trial of $OKT_3$ monoclonal antibody for acute rejection of cadaveric renal transplants. N Engl J Med 3134:337, 1985.

Griffin, JP: Hematology and Immunology, Concepts for Nursing. Appleton-Century-Crofts, Norwalk, CT, 1986.

Jarowenko, MV, et al: Treatment of steroid resistant rejection in patients receiving cyclosporine. Transplantation 41:578, 1986.

Matas, AJ, et al: Treatment of steroid resistant rejection in patients receiving cyclosporine. Transplantation 41:579, 1986.

Mathewson, MK: Pharmacotherapeutics, A Nursing Process Approach. FA Davis, Philadelphia, 1986.

Webb, DR and Winkelstein, A: Immunosuppression, immunopotentiation, and anti-inflammatory drugs. In Stites, DP, et al (eds): Basic and Clinical Immunology, ed 6. Appleton & Lange, Norwalk, CT, 1987.

CHAPTER 57

# Clinical Application: Clinical Organ Transplantation

*Wayne C. Waltzer*

## CHAPTER OUTLINE



## LEARNING OBJECTIVES

**At the end of this chapter, you should be able to:**

1. Define *allotransplantation*.
2. Discuss the significance of tissue matching in terms of tissue compatibility between donor and recipient and, thus, the best outlook for successful transplantation.
3. List key factors to be considered when evaluating a person/family as a potential recipient for organ transplantation.
4. Describe potential donor sources and key assessment considerations in donor selection.
5. List criteria for brain death in the clinical practice setting.
6. Describe major considerations in managing the patient during the post-transplant course.
7. Discuss the impact of available immunosuppressive drug therapy on clinical transplantation, and the special problems and concerns associated with specific immunosuppressive agents.
8. Examine classic presenting signs and symptoms and laboratory findings in kidney transplant rejection.

## HISTORY

Over the past decades, transplantation has evolved from being an experimental procedure to a practical, everyday, and clinically accepted means of the treatment of end-stage organ disease.

In 1902, Carrel described the successful transplant of an autogenous kidney to the neck vessels of a dog by means of vascular suture.[1] His experiments showed that while autogenous organs survived after vascular anastomosis and were able to function, unknown biologic factors caused failure in allogenic (i.e., of different species) organ grafts.

Following decades of experimental work, it was discovered that the survival of grafted organs depends on similarities in the *genetic* constitution of the donor and recipient. Dausset[2] first described the human leukocyte antigen, Mac, later known as HLA-2. This was defined by the presence of antibody in the sera of multiple transfused patients and later was shown to be part of the major histocompatibility complex (MHC) in humans.

The MHC, known as the HLA (human leukocyte antigen) gene complex in humans, is responsible for encoding the expression of specific antigens present on the surface of most nucleated cells. It is also the chromosomal segment where histocompatibility-linked immune response (Ir) genes are located. Thus, the HLA not only controls the synthesis of antigens of concern to transplantation and graft rejection, but also influences immune responses to infection and susceptibility to the development of immunologically mediated diseases.[3]

Advances in immunology, anesthesia, organ preservation, antibiotics, the use of heparin, and later, extracorporeal circulation made feasible a new phase of surgical activity and the rebirth of transplantation. In the 1950s there were major efforts to accomplish successful kidney transplantation in humans. In 1954, the first syngeneic human kidney transplant was successful; the exchange of kidneys was between monozygotic twins (i.e., twins derived from a single, fertilized ovum).

After failure of nonimmunosuppressed allotransplants,* the discovery of 6-mercaptopurine, steroids, and x-ray irradiation proved to be critical in controlling allograft rejection. With the discovery of the HLA system in humans, the possibility of getting optimally compatible combinations between donors and recipients was enhanced. The success of allotransplants improved, and by 1986, over 65,000 kidney transplants had been performed worldwide.

The introduction of cyclosporine, an even more effective means of suppressing host immune reactivity, has allowed the rapid clinical proliferation of transplantation of heart, liver, lungs, pancreas, bone marrow, and intestine. Thus, most patients with irreversible organ damage are now potential candidates for transplantation.

## TISSUE MATCHING: HISTOCOMPATIBILITY

Histocompatibility testing determines the degree of tissue compatibility between donor and recipient. The discovery of the human major histocompatibility complex (MHC) occurred in the 1950s when antibodies were found in the sera of multiple transfused patients and multiparous females. Subsequent research suggested that these antibodies could detect alloantigens (i.e., antigens present on the cells of individuals of a given species), which were products of a polymorphic genetic locus.

The HLA is a single, complex genetic locus located on the short arm of the C-6 chromosome.[4] Based on results from family studies, the antigens are grouped into 2 main divisions or subloci. The 2 divisions are called class I (HLA-A, B and C) and class II (HLA-D, DR) antigens. The names assigned to antigens are uniform throughout the world to allow correlation of data and exchange of blood and tissue samples. Such antigens are characteristic of an individual and stimulate rejection of tissue allografts.

Each pair of HLA antigens (termed haplotype) is inherited from 1 parent. One antigen of the pair is from class I and the other from class II. Within a family there is a 1-in-4 possibility that 2 siblings have identical HLA types. The perfect match (4 antigens) or HLA identical match offers the best outlook for successful transplantation.

### Blood Group Matching: ABO System

*ABO typing* is used for blood group determination (O, A, B, and AB) and is the first hurdle to successful transplantation.[5] The same rules apply to organ transplantation as to blood transfusion with regard to the ABO system. Blood cell proteins cause an immune reaction if they are administered to a recipient of a different or incompatible blood group.

Because of the lack of cell proteins responsible for immune reactions, type O organs may serve as a universal *donor* (i.e., type O allografts may be transplanted to any other blood type without a reaction). Because both A and B cell proteins are represented on the cell surface, type AB is known as the universal *recipient*. Group A and B, because of their respective cell proteins, may only receive a transplant from their own group or group O. Thus, only organs from same ABO groups will be considered for transplantation, otherwise incompatibility will result in immediate graft rejection.

### Crossmatching

*Crossmatching* is a histocompatibility technique that identifies the presence of preformed circulating antibodies in the recipient against antigens on the tissue of a potential donor. The presence of these antibodies is a strong contraindication to transplantation. Patients who have been presensitized by blood transfusion, pregnancy, or previous transplants are thus eliminated.

The test is done by mixing a sample of the recipi-

*Allotransplantation is the removal of tissue from a person and grafting it into a genetically different recipient.

ent's serum with donor lymphocytes in the presence of complement. If cell agglutination or lysis occurs, this is a positive crossmatch. If this reaction occurs, transplantation generally cannot be performed.

*HLA tissue typing* is performed by exposing lymphocytes from both donor and recipient to antisera containing known HLA specificities.[4] In this manner, it is possible to identify the antigens present on donor and recipient tissue. HLA typing is important in the selection of renal allograft recipients; however, it has a limited role in cadaveric heart, liver, or pancreas transplantation.

### Mixed Leukocyte Culture (MLC)/Mixed Leukocyte Reaction (MLR)

Mixed leukocyte reaction (MLR) measures the degree of compatibility between donor and recipient without defining the antigens responsible for these results, although this reaction is most likely controlled at the HLA-D locus.[6]

The mixed leukocyte culture is performed by mixing lymphocytes from recipient and donor, and culturing them for 5 days. Antigenic stimulation of T-lymphocytes responding to foreign histocompatibility antigen on unrelated lymphocytes causes this reaction. DNA synthesis is then measured as a reflection of cellular response.

The mixed leukocyte culture is useful in the selection of living, related donors because it aids in predicting outcome of transplants between donor and recipient. Unfortunately, it cannot be used for matching cadaver donors because organs cannot be preserved for the 5–6 days necessary to perform the test. (See the section entitled "Transplantation and Histocompatibility" in Chap. 54).

## TYPES OF ORGAN TRANSPLANTATION

### Renal Transplantation

Kidney transplantation has become an accepted form of therapy for patients with end-stage renal disease. Most people are eligible for transplantation if they meet the following criteria: (1) they are under the age of 60, (2) they have permanent irreversible renal failure, (3) they have a functional lower urinary tract, and (4) they are free from serious vascular, cardiac, or neurologic complications of uremia. Many high-risk patients, who were previously excluded, are now included in the growing lists of recipients awaiting renal allografts. Such high-risk patients include those with diabetes, abnormal lower urinary tract, prior malignancy, coronary artery disease, cystinosis, collagen vascular disease (e.g., systemic lupus erythematosus), or persistent hepatitis B antigenemia (i.e., antigen in the blood).

Transplantation remains contraindicated for the management of renal failure secondary to *oxalosis* (i.e., widespread deposition of calcium oxalate crystals in the kidney), as well as in patients with active infections, uncontrolled or recently treated malignancies, or severe extrarenal disease making the risks of surgery or anesthesia prohibitive. Patients less than age 1 or greater than age 60 are considered acceptable on an individualized basis.

Transplantation is usually not performed until the patient with end-stage renal disease has been stabilized on hemodialysis. Transplantation is recommended, however, as early as possible in patients with diabetic nephropathy, in order to try to prevent extrarenal manifestations such as diabetic retinopathy and neuropathy. In young patients with chronic renal failure who are seen prior to the institution of dialysis, and who have HLA identical siblings, transplantation may be scheduled for the same time when the patient would otherwise require the institution of dialysis.

### Cardiac Transplantation

Selection of appropriate cardiac transplant recipients is crucial to the outcome of transplantation. These are patients with New York Heart Association class IV end-stage heart failure (see Table 38–2) whose disease is not amenable to conventional medical or surgical therapy. Most patients have cardiomyopathy, usually idiopathic or of viral origin (50%). Another large group of patients consists of those with ischemic cardiomyopathy (40%).[7] (See Chap. 44).

Transplant recipients must have no evidence of infection, cancer, or recent pulmonary infarction, because the infarcted area serves as an excellent locus for opportunistic pulmonary infection. Pulmonary hypertension manifested by significantly increased pulmonary vascular resistance contraindicates transplantation because acute failure of the normal donor right ventricle usually will occur. A relative contraindication for transplantation is age over 50 years, because older patients are less likely to tolerate such a major operation and the associated complications of infection and rejection.

Survival following heart transplantation has improved dramatically over the past years. At Stanford University, the 1-year survival rate is 80%, compared with 22% in 1963.[7] At least half of the patients are expected to be alive with good quality of life 5 years following transplantation. These improvements reflect better patient management, improved immunosuppressive therapy with cyclosporine, and the use of cardiac biopsy for the preclinical diagnosis of early acute graft rejection.

### Liver Transplantation

Pioneering advances by Starzel[7] in liver transplantation have obtained >65% 1-year graft survival in this high-risk procedure. It is reserved for patients with irreversible chronic liver disease, most commonly in adults with nonalcoholic cirrhosis, including chronic active hepatitis. The indications include primary liver tumors and alcoholic cirrhosis. In children, biliary atresia and congenital metabolic abnormalities are the most common indications for hepatic transplantation.

Absolute contraindications to transplantation include ongoing alcoholism, poor cardiopulmonary or renal function, patient age over 55 years, portal vein thrombosis, and metastatic cancer. Hepatitis is a relative contraindication because not all such patients reinfect the donor liver. On the other hand, patients who are both HB-surface and core-antigen positive inevitably reinfect the donor liver and must not receive a transplant.

### Pancreatic Transplantation

Currently, methods of delivering exogenous insulin to diabetic patients have not proved effective in maintaining normal carbohydrate metabolism or in preventing microvascular disease. Thus, the aim of pancreas transplantation is to achieve perfect metabolic control and to stop the progression of these microvascular changes.[7] Pancreative transplantation is unlikely to be of great value in persons with microvascular disease so far advanced that metabolic correction would not be expected to affect the course.

The first pancreas transplant was performed in 1966. Initially, the pancreas was transplanted with the duodenum, but, owing to complications related to the duodenum (i.e., leakage, fistula formation), pancreatoduodenal transplantation had largely been abandoned. However, it has recently had a resurgence of interest. Subsequent techniques have used (1) islet cells injected into the portal vein or small bowel mesentery (though this method never totally controlled diabetes); (2) segmental pancreas transplantation using half of the gland (body and tail), with vascular anastomosis between the donor splenic artery and splenic vein and the recipient iliac vessels; and (3) whole pancreas transplantation using the entire gland. The pancreatic duct can either be injected with a polymer or, alternatively, the duct can be anastomosed to be a defunctionalized limb of small bowel or the urinary bladder. Approximately one third of the grafts are functioning at 1 year; rejection and interstitial fibrosis and vascular thrombosis account for the majority of failures.[7]

## RECIPIENT EVALUATION

Prior to transplantation, the referring physician sends a complete medical history and physical examination and results of diagnostic studies and laboratory tests to the transplant center. These studies are designed to identify problems that may be amenable to correction or contravene transplantation, and thus to eliminate postoperative problems.

An assessment of the patient's psychologic status is also made. The patient and family may be referred to a psychiatrist whose impressions are added to those of the referring doctor. The candidate must have emotional stability as well as physical stamina to tolerate the stress of transplant experience. The social worker and dialysis nursing staff should also send a summary of pertinent patient/family information to foster continuity of care between the patient's dialysis center and the transplant center.

The patient, family, and any potential living donors are then interviewed by the transplant surgeon. During the interview, they hear about transplantation, the risks of the procedure, and possible complications. To give informed consent for the procedure, the person must have both knowledge and understanding of transplantation and its implications.

After the interview, the recipient and all potential donors undergo histocompatibility studies. The patient without a compatible related donor must wait for a kidney from a cadaveric donor source. A schema for the patient who develops end-stage renal disease is presented in Table 57-1.

## DONOR SOURCES

The number of patients who can receive transplants is limited severely by the availability of donor organs. Because of this scarcity, in the United States in 1986, only 7,800 kidney transplants were performed, while there are approximately 65,000 patients on maintenance hemodialysis.[8]

The paradox of this situation is that, while the number of potential donors far exceeds the number of organs needed for transplantation, most of the potential donors will never be considered. This is primarily because of insufficient efforts and/or awareness by physicians, nurse, and the public of the need for cadaveric organs. Because more than two thirds of patients with end-stage renal disease do not, by current criteria, have a suitable living, related donor, transplant programs increasingly depend on utilization of cadaveric organs.

To treat all patients with end-stage renal disease in a geographic area, an ongoing transplantation program must have an adequate supply of cadaveric organs in its own region.[8] Although sharing of cadaveric kidneys has received much attention, an

TABLE 57-1
**Recipient Evaluation: A Schema for the Patient with End-Stage Renal Disease**

1. Patient enters program.
   A. Irreversible renal failure.
   B. Biopsy.
   C. Clinical course.
2. Medical, dietary management.
3. Vascular access for hemodialysis or peritoneal dialysis.
4. Dialysis.
5. Plans for transplantation.
   A. Family psychological evaluation.
   B. Tissue typing.
      • ABO blood groups.
      • HLA genotypes.
      • Mixed lymphocyte culture.
   C. Donor workup.
6. Urological assessment of patient's status.
   A. Voiding cystourethrogram.
   B. Cystoscopy.
   C. Cystometrics.
   D. Urologic reconstruction.
7. Surgical procedures (if indicated).
   A. Parathyroidectomy.
   B. Splenectomy.
   C. Vagotomy/pyloroplasty.
8. Living related donor.
9. Transplantation.

active transplant center cannot depend primarily on the sharing of organs from other programs.[8] Efforts to develop cadaveric donor sources have focused on increasing public awareness, encouraging physicians to participate in identification of potential donors, and physician participation in efforts to enact legislation that would increase the number of organ donors.[8]

## DONOR SELECTION

Assessing the suitability of a donor begins when the referring hospital gives notification that a potential donor exists. At this time, the medical history of the donor, the circumstances and extent of the present injury, and the patient's immediate condition are evaluated. If a patient has not yet met the criteria for brain death, the patient should be managed without regard for his or her status as a potential donor, even if this management includes treatment with agents potentially detrimental to donor organ function. Specific questions on the suitability of such donors may be addressed at this time by the transplantation team. However, throughout the process of donor identification, members of the transplantation team do not play a role in the management of the patient, certification of brain death, or in obtaining consent for organ donation. If brain death occurs and organ donation is feasible, a final decision regarding donor suitability is made.[8]

Kidneys from cadaveric donors older than 55 years of age generally do not tolerate the insults of nephrectomy, preservation, and transplantation as well as those from younger donors. Therefore, cadaveric donors are usually less than 55 years of age; pediatric donors are also used and are generally greater than 1 year of age. Kidneys from these donors will provide life-sustaining function even if transplanted as a single organ in an adult.

Careful evaluation of the medical history of the cadaveric donor is critical. Patients with malignant skin lesions or primary central nervous system lesions, because of low tendency for dissemination and metastases, are not eliminated as potential donors. However, the organs of donors with malignant lesions elsewhere in the body, despite the absence of documented metastases, should not be used for transplantation. That the organ graft may serve as a source of malignant cells transferred from the donor to the immunosuppressed host has been reported.[8] The absence of neoplastic disease in the donor should not be assumed until there has been a thorough evaluation of the intra-abdominal cavity or a complete postmortem examination.

The cadaveric donor with injuries involving several organ systems frequently will have had a previous procedure such as laparotomy, craniotomy, or orthopedic repair. These donors are acceptable unless the earlier operation showed bowel perforation, gangrenous changes of any intra-abdominal organs, or other conditions that may cause bacterial contamination of the kidneys, liver, or pancreas.

As an isolated finding, gross or microscopic hematuria does not contraindicate organ retrieval. These findings are often associated with pelvic fractures, urinary bladder contusions, or retroperitoneal hematomas, whereas the kidneys, ureters, and associated vascular structures remain normal. Occasionally, a single kidney can be used, despite a traumatized contralateral kidney. Significant elevations of the prothrombin time or partial thromboplastin time are no barrier to organ donation, provided the cause is not disseminated intravascular coagulation secondary to sepsis or carcinoma.

Organs from donors who have evidence of septicemia, an abscess, viral or fungal disease are not used because the transfer of infection to the immunosuppressed host may have serious consequences. Low cytomegalovirus (CMV) titers do not rule out a donor; however, any evidence of HTLV III antibody excludes an organ donor. The presence of tracheobronchitis or bacteriuria (i.e., presence of bacteria in urine) does not contraindicate organ donation, because cadaveric donors with an endotracheal tube or urinary catheter often will have these findings without the kidneys being involved. An active pneumonia of any bacterial cause, as well as aspiration pneumonia associated with trauma, do not entirely rule out organ donation. Many centers will procure kidneys from these donors provided blood and urine cultures are nega-

TABLE 57-2
**Brain Death Criteria**

- Absence of induced hyperthermia and central nervous system depressant drugs.
- Generalized flaccidity, no spontaneous muscle movement, and no evidence of postural activity or shivering.
- Absent cranial nerve reflexes.
  - Pupils light-fixed and dilated.
  - No corneal reflexes.
  - No response to upper and lower airways stimulation.
  - No ocular response to head turning and cold calorics.
- Absence of spontaneous breathing movements for 3 minutes.
- Isoelectric electroencephalogram.
- No blood flow seen on angiogram or brain scan.

TABLE 57-3
**Sequence of Organ Retrieval Process**

- Identification of the potential donor.
- Notification of the transplant team by the referring hospital of a potential donor.
- Evaluation of donor's suitability.
- Discussion with the patient's family and physician.
- Consent obtained from the next of kin.
- Discussion with the medical examiner and district attorney, if necessary.
- Continued observation and maintenance of the donor.
- Pronouncement of donor death by 2 physicians according to protocol.
- Notification by the transplant coordinator of surgeon, operating room, and time for organ procurement.
- Notification of eye bank, skin bank, and other specialty areas.
- Surgery.
- Perfusion and preservation of organs.
- Transportation of organs.
- Tissue typing of organs.
- Identification of recipients.
- Transplantation of organs.

tive. Of course, such would not be suitable for a heart or lung donor. Thus, the basic rule in organ procurement is that any disease process that potentially could cause irreversible organ damage and could be transferred to the transplant recipient eliminates the possibility of organ donation.

## Brain Death Criteria

The concept of brain death, or irreversible coma, has been extensively reviewed, and generally accepted criteria are now present throughout the United States. The legal recognition that a patient can be declared dead although circulation is temporarily maintained by artificial means has been of great significance to organ transplantation. This fact has allowed procurement of organs under accepted legal and ethical guidelines.

The diagnosis of brain death is a clinical diagnosis and can be made without ancillary investigation other than a detailed clinical examination. If the cause or extent of injury are unknown, it is essential that an electroencephalogram, brain scan, or arteriogram be performed.

When organs are to be removed for transplantation, 2 physicians must pronounce the donor brain dead. One of these physicians ordinarily is a neurologist or neurosurgeon because the electroencephalogram commonly used in these circumstances is a specific diagnostic tool of these specialists and should be evaluated by them. The interval between 2 successive examinations (usually 6-24 hours) is determined by the examining physicians. Table 57-2 shows the criteria that are generally agreed on as guidelines for brain death; however, these may differ from institution to institution.

# RETRIEVAL PROCESS

The retrieval process should include the orderly sequence of events shown in Table 57-3. Only through a systematic approach can an organ procurement team function effectively.

# LEGAL ISSUES

Many physicians fear the consequences of pronouncing brain death and being involved with organ donation. This is so because the donor has often died after the perpetration of a crime resulting in legal issues. Questions are raised as to whether the doctor is liable for taking a patient off a respirator and how the doctor's liability could affect the question of who is responsible for the patient's injury.[8] The legal system now recognizes that brain death criteria are legitimate, and the physician cannot be accused of either taking the patient's life or being an accomplice to a crime. Consultation with the medical examiner usually clarifies the issues involved and serves to protect the physician. (For additional information regarding ethical/legal issues in this regard, see Chap. 70).

# SURGICAL ASPECTS OF THE KIDNEY TRANSPLANTATION PROCEDURE

A hockey stick-shaped incision is made either in the right or left lower quadrant. This is carried through the skin and subcutaneous tissue until a pocket is developed in the retroperitoneal space by mobilizing the peritoneum medially. The external iliac vein is dissected sharply, and either the internal iliac artery or external iliac artery is used for the arterial anastomosis. Subsequently, the renal allograft vein is anastomosed end-to-side to the external iliac vein, and the transplant renal artery is anastomosed either end-to-end to the internal iliac artery or end-to-side to the external iliac artery (see Fig. 27-2). After the completion of this procedure and the release of the vascular clamps, the kidney usually obtains a firm and pinkish appearance indicating good vascular perfusion to the kidney.

The bladder is then mobilized and opened by a midline incision. The ureter is brought through the bladder and passed through a submucosal tunnel and anastomosed near the medial aspect of the ipsilateral ureter near the trigone (bladder base); this is called a ureteroneocystostomy. The bladder is then closed, and the wound is irrigated copiously with antibiotic solution. The wound is then carefully closed to prevent any post-transplant wound herniation.

Complications of this procedure can include infection, hematoma, ureteral obstruction, gross hematuria, arterial or venous thrombosis, ureteral necrosis, hydrocele (scrotal swelling) or lymphocele (lymphatic swelling).

## RENAL PRESERVATION

Organ preservation is a key part of any kidney transplantation program. The ultimate function of a transplant organ is highly dependent on the quality of procurement and preservation. The inadequate supply of cadaver organs in the United States and worldwide places further emphasis on these goals. Ischemic injury and deterioration during storage leading to damage may severely impair the recovery of function and ultimately may lead to failure of procured kidneys.[9]

Relevant features for effective preservation are support of blood pressure and fluid volumes to maintain adequate renal perfusion and diuresis, and support of metabolic needs to avoid vasospasm and nephrotoxins.[10] Mannitol should be administered to promote an osmotic diuresis. Renal vasospasm can be managed by giving Dibenzyline, an alpha-adrenergic blocker. Isoproterenol can be given for hypotension unresponsive to fluid challenge; however, kidneys obtained from such donors give inferior results.

There are 2 methods of renal preservation—simple *cold storage*, which has the advantage of simplicity, low cost and ease of transportation, and *pulsatile perfusion*, which has the advantage of extended preservation as well as the possibility of monitoring the degree of ischemic damage and quality of the kidney. Both methods are currently in use in the United States and throughout the world.

## POST-TRANSPLANT COURSE

### Fluid and Electrolyte Balance

The patient's early postoperative urinary output may be somewhat unpredictable and may range from complete anuria to polyuria. Each must be noted, and the fluid replacement must be adjusted accordingly. As a general rule, anuria and oliguria require replacement of the urine output volume per volume in addition to daily insensible loss replacement. Diuretics should be considered only after a *fluid challenge* (i.e., rapid infusion of 500 ml normal saline solution) has failed to increase the urine output.

A difficult problem in clinical transplantation is *anuria*, which infrequently occurs in the absence of any other signs or symptoms during the early postoperative phase. The central differential diagnosis of early anuria include (1) acute tubular necrosis, (2) acute rejection, (3) urinary tract obstruction (technical), and (4) renal arterial or venous thrombosis.

Anuria requires immediate attention because all drugs excreted by the kidney system are now recirculating in the recipient. As a consequence, the required therapeutic levels for antibiotics, for example, are significantly lower, and the continued administration of myelosuppressive agents, such as Imuran, can readily lead to marrow suppression and overwhelming infection. Recent evidence indicates that cyclosporine excretion is impaired in the presence of renal dysfunction.

Blood chemistries must be followed with great care, with particular regard to serum potassium levels. Dietary and/or intravenous potassium chloride (KCl) replacement must be stopped, and any serum potassium levels exceeding 6.0 mEq/liter must be managed immediately by the administration of cation exchange resins (Kayexalate), by enema or orally. Hemodialysis is usually required in such patients no later than the third postoperative day if they were dialyzed on the day of operation, or the second postoperative day if they were dialyzed on the day preceding transplantation. Decisions on hemodialysis are made in conjunction with the nephrology staff.

When anuria occurs, investigative procedures should include (1) technetium DPTA scan of the kidney, which provides evidence of the intactness of the renal vascular supply; (2) ultrasound of the transplanted kidney, which may exhibit blurring of the corticomedullary junction characteristic of rejection or hydronephrosis indicative of urinary obstruction; (3) cyclosporine levels by radioimmune assay (RIA); and (4) transplant core needle biopsy or fine needle aspiration biopsy (FNAB).[11–13]

### Immunosuppressive Therapy

All clinical transplantation would cease if immunosuppressive drugs were removed from the therapeutic armamentarium (see Chap. 56). On the other hand, such drugs must be considered with the utmost care because of the potentially life-endangering side effects their use entails. The key agents in use today are prednisone, Imuran (azathioprine), and cyclosporine.[14]

### Prednisone

The drug shown to be of paramount importance in clinical transplantation is prednisone—a corticosteroid, which is administered orally in doses of 2–2.5 mg/kg/24 hours on the day of transplantation, with gradual tapering of this dosage to a level of 1.5 mg/kg/24 hours by the end of the first week. The dose is then continuously tapered (in daily decrements of 5–10 mg) if untoward problems or a rejection crisis do not arise. Under such circumstances, the eventual maintenance dose upon discharge will be approximately 15–20 mg daily.

During prednisone therapy, special caution must be given to the possible development of peptic ulceration, esophagitis, osteoporosis, pseudodiabetes, or infection.

Recent evidence suggests that the corticosteroids may exert their immunoregulatory function through primary inhibition of interleukin-1 (IL-1) production by macrophages, with secondary inhibition of helper T cell function (see section entitled "Antibody Formation" in Chap. 54). These properties indirectly suppress interleukin-2 (IL-2) production, the proliferation and differentiation of cytotoxic T-lymphocytes, B-cell function, and the release of lymphokines important in delayed hypersensitivity reactions. Corticosteroids may be further capable of lysing activated T-lymphocytes (see Fig. 27–1). (See Appendix A for nursing implications.)

### Imuran (Azathioprine)

Imuran is an *antimetabolite*, which is broken down into 6-mercaptopurine and urea by the liver. It has myelosuppressive effect (see Fig. 27–1), and excessive doses will result in hemopoietic ablation, associated with loss of the host's defenses against microorganisms. A specific program of therapy and close follow-up of key hematologic and physiologic indices is therefore required if this agent is to be used with a relative degree of safety.

Generally, Imuran is first given to the recipient on the day before, or at the time of transplantation, with a total oral dose of 2.5–3 mg/kg/24 hours. The daily dose is then reduced to 2 mg/kg/24 hours. It must be noted that the maximal effects of a given dose of Imuran may not be exerted until 48 hours after administration.

The dose of Imuran given at each period is determined by blood indices (hematocrit, white blood cell count and differential, platelet count). Any significant decline in the leukocyte count, or platelet count, or the appearance of liver dysfunction, skin eruption, or evidence of infection, requires immediate changes in the dose of Imuran ordered or complete discontinuance of the drug. In uncomplicated cases, the usual maintenance dose of Imuran is 75–150 mg/day.

### Cyclosporine

Cyclosporine, a fungal cyclic peptide, has a high degree of specificity for T-lymphocytes and can prevent early T-cell activation in 3 ways: (1) by inhibiting T-cell help to accessory cells that normally produce interleukin-1 (IL-1); (2) by preventing interleukin-2 producing T cells from expressing receptors for interleukin-2, so that they cannot produce IL-2; and (3) by rendering cytotoxic T cells unresponsive to IL-2 (see Figs. 27–1 and 54–7).

Nephrotoxicity is the most important side effect. Unlike Imuran (azathioprine), there is no simple laboratory test to detect toxicity, and patients taking cyclosporine must therefore have blood drug levels checked periodically. A whole-blood level of 100–200 ng/ml is sought for renal transplantation recipients, and a level of 250–350 ng/ml is achieved in heart, liver, and pancreas transplant patients.

**Cyclosporine Nephrotoxicity.** In clinical practice, there appears to be 2 forms of cyclosporine nephrotoxicity. One form is dose-dependent, and prompt recovery usually occurs when the dose is decreased before irreversible renal damage occurs. The other form of nephrotoxicity develops in susceptible patients despite "normal" levels of cyclosporine. These patients usually benefit from substitution of azathioprine for cyclosporine once rejection is excluded by renal biopsy.

Another side effect that may require substitution of conventional therapy is tremor and behavioral changes unresponsive to dose adjustments. Other side effects include hirsutism, hypertension, hyperkalemia, and dose-dependent hepatoxicity. There is probably no increase in the incidence of lymphoma. Low-dose cyclosporine combined with low-dose prednisone and azathioprine (triple drug therapy) is a promising approach to preventing rejection and may be associated with fewer drug-related side effects. (See Appendix A for nursing implications.)

## Allograft Rejection

Acceptance of a kidney transplant is the end result of a delicate balance between the attempts of the host to reject the foreign tissues and the success of immunosuppressive drug therapy in inhibiting such a response. When the balance is tilted in the direction of the immunosuppressive drugs, the organ is tolerated and functions well, sustaining the life of the host. If, for a variety of reasons, the balance is tilted in the opposite direction, however, rejection ensues. Prompt recognition and management of such crises are essential in protecting the function and survival of the transplanted kidney. The classic presenting signs and symptoms include (see Table 27-1):

1. Fever.
2. Hypertension.
3. Tenderness at site of transplant.
4. Decreased urinary output.
5. Weight gain.

The most common laboratory findings include:

1. Rise in serum BUN, creatinine, and fall in creatinine clearance.
2. Leukocytosis.
3. Technetium DPTA scan showing decreased renal perfusion.
4. Ultrasound demonstrating significant increase in the size of the transplanted kidney.

As noted earlier, there is a significant variety of other situations that may mimic rejection, including acute tubular necrosis (good vascular perfusion, but kidney is not enlarged and enzymes not usually elevated), renal arterial or venous thrombosis (with typical nonperfusion of the transplanted renal cortex), urinary tract obstruction due to extrinsic pressure (e.g., hematoma or lymphocele, which may be detectable by x-ray or by ultrasound scanning), or as a result of technical factors (ureteral obstruction), which may require cystoscopy and retrograde pyelogram. In addition, drug nephrotoxicity must be considered because cyclosporine[15] antibiotics and $H_2$ antagonists (e.g., ranitidine)[16] can all contribute to renal dysfunction.

Once the diagnosis has been established, rejection constitutes an *emergency* and should be managed immediately. A general approach includes methylprednisolone therapy, 1 g intravenously, daily for 3-5 days.

### *Polyclonal and Monoclonal Antibodies*

Heterologus *antilymphocyte globulin (ALG)* and *antithymocyte globulin (ATG)* are potent immunosuppressive agents of value in preventing and reversing acute rejection.[17] Most often, ALG is used with azathioprine and prednisone. ALG causes lysis of circulating lymphocytes (see Fig. 27-1) as well as depletion of T cells from the paracortical regions of the lymph nodes. The B cells in the medullary regions and germinal center of the nodes are less effected. The absolute T-cell count in the peripheral blood remains low up to 2 weeks after a course of ALG/ATG.

Recently, *OKT3*, a biochemically purified IgG2a immunoglobin, which reacts with the T3 (CD3) antigen on the surface of all mature T-lymphocytes has been developed.[18,19] This causes inhibition of signal transduction, essential for the T-lymphocyte. It blocks the generation and function of cytotoxic T cells, which is most probably the mechanism of reversing acute cellular allograft rejection. OKT3 has been successfully used in treating primary renal allograft rejection and as a second line of treatment in steroid-resistant allograft rejection. Such specific therapy holds great promise for the future of allotransplantation.

## NURSING CARE CONSIDERATIONS

For a discussion of end-stage renal disease and nursing care considerations for the patient with end-stage renal disease, see Chap. 26.

For a discussion of nursing care considerations in the scenario of renal transplantation, see Chap. 27 and Tables 26-1 and 27-2.

## REFERENCES


1. Carrel, A: Techniques and remote results of vascular anastomosis. Surg Gynecol Obstet 14:246, 1912.
2. Hamilton, D: A history of transplantation. In Morris, PJ (ed): Tissue Transplantation. Grune & Stratton, New York, 1984, pp 1-13.
3. Bellanti, JA: Immunology Basic Processes, ed 2. WB Saunders, Philadelphia, 1985, p 56.
4. Schwartz, BD: The human major histocompatibility complex. In Stites, DP, et al (eds): Basic and Clinical Immunology, ed 6. Appleton & Lange, Norwalk, CT, 1987, pp 55-68.
5. Mackintosh, P: ABO matching in kidney graft survival. Nature 250(5464):351, July 1974.
6. Opelz, G and Terasaki, PI: Significance of mixed leukocyte culture testing in cadaver kidney transplantation. Transplantation 23:375, 1977.
7. Simmons, RL and So, SK: Clinical transplantation. In Stites, D, et al (eds): Basic and Clinical Immunology, ed 6. Appleton & Lange, Norwalk, CT, 1987, pp 491-499.
8. Waltzer, WC: Procurement of cadaveric kidneys for transplantation. Ann Intern Med 98:536, 1983.
9. Miller, HC, Alexander, JW, and Nathan, P: Effects of warm ischemic damage on intrarenal distribution of flow in preserved kidneys. Surgery 72:193, 1972.
10. Lambert, R, et al: Glomerular damage after kidney preservation. Transplantation 42:125, 1986.
11. Rosano, TG, et al: Immunosuppressive metabolites of cyclosporine in the blood of renal allograft recipients. Transplantation 42:262, 1986.
12. Matas, AJ, et al: The value of needle renal allograft biopsy III: A prospective study. Surgery 98:922, 1985.
13. Hayry, P and von Willebrand, F: Transplant aspiration cytology. Transplantation 38:7, 1984.
14. Webb, DR and Winkelstein, A: Immunosuppression, immunopotentiation, and anti-inflammatory drugs. In Stites, DP, et al (eds): Basic and Clinical Immunology, ed 6. Appleton & Lange, Norwalk, CT, 1987, pp 55-68.
15. Arnold, AN, et al: Effect of renal allograft dysfunction upon cyclosporine through levels in host blood. Transplant 40:605, 1985.
16. Jarowenko, MV, et al: Ranitidine, cimetidine and the cyclosporine treated patient. Transplantation 42:311, 1986.
17. Matas, AJ, et al: Treatment of steroid resistant rejection in patients receiving cyclosporine. Transplantation 41:579, 1986.
18. Cosimi, AB, et al: A randomized clinical trial comparing OKT3 and steroids for treatment of hepatic allograft rejection. Transplantation 43:91, 1987.
19. Goldstein, G, et al: A randomized clinical trial of OKT3 monoclonal antibody for acute rejection of cadaveric renal transplants. N Engl J Med 3134:337, 1985.

CHAPTER 58

# Clinical Application: Immunodeficiency Disorders

*Marc G. Golightly*

## CHAPTER OUTLINE



## LEARNING OBJECTIVES

**At the end of this chapter, you should be able to:**

1. Differentiate between primary and secondary immunodeficiency disorders.
2. Describe clinical presentation of primary immunodeficiency diseases with possible pathophysiologic mechanisms underlying the immunologic dysfunction.
3. Explain why recurrent pyogenic infections in a child diagnosed to have a combined T- and B-cell immunodeficiency disorder generally do not manifest prior to 6 months of age.
4. Explain why strict T-cell immunodeficiencies in which the humoral immune system is not secondarily affected are very rare.
5. Examine the pathophysiologic mechanism(s) underlying the acquired immunodeficiency of AIDS including the causative agent and its primary target.

The immune system is organized in a highly complex fashion with the cell-mediated, humoral, phagocytic, and the complement components being linked through complex interactions. Upon review of some of these interactions (see Chap. 54), it can be appreciated that the extreme complexity of the immune system, in turn, affords a tremendous number of possibilities for dysfunction and defects to occur.

When a defect does occur in one branch, it often affects another branch primarily or secondarily. The resultant clinical symptoms likewise depend on which of these arms and interactive relations are affected. Due to this fact, the clinical presentation of suspected immunodeficient patients often suggests the type of immune dysfunction present. For example, patients with a defective *cell-mediated* immunity are more susceptible to infection by fungal, viral, and protozoan organisms (especially in the form of pneumonia, chronic skin infection, and mucous membrane infections). A history of recurrent bacterial infections, particularly bacterial pneumonia and otitis media, suggests a *humoral* defect. *Phagocytic* dysfunctions are suggested by skin and systemic infections with pyogenic (pus-forming) bacteria. Often the systemic infection is by bacteria of normally low virulence. *Complement* deficiencies are also associated with recurrent pyogenic infections.

While these associations generally do occur, it should be noted that they are not without exceptions. For example, a patient with humoral deficiency may have a fungal infection. Furthermore, the type of immunologic dysfunction present may range from no notable clinical symptoms to severe illness and even death. These associations will be examined with respect to the individual immunodeficiencies discussed later in this chapter.

## IMMUNODEFICIENCIES: CLASSIFICATION

Immunodeficiencies are generally classified into 2 groups: *primary* immunodeficiencies and *secondary* immunodeficiencies. Primary immunodeficiencies are, as the name implies, inherent in the immune system itself as the primary cause of the immunologic dysfunction. These deficiencies are often congenital and may have a genetic component to them. They can occur at varying ages ranging from infancy to adulthood. While the cause of the defect(s) responsible for primary immunodeficiencies in many cases is known (e.g., embryologic abnormality or enzyme deficiencies), in many cases it is not. However, in most primary immunodeficiencies, the dysfunction can usually be identified (e.g., T-cell defect). Primary immunodeficiencies are known to occur in all 4 of the components of the immune system previously mentioned. These defects occur either alone or in combination with each other (Table 58–1). However, primary immunodeficiencies with relatively few exceptions (e.g., selective IgA deficiency) are uncommon.

TABLE 58–1
**Primary Immunodeficiency Diseases**

| |
|---|
| **Combined B-Cell and T-Cell Immunodeficiencies** |
| Severe combined immunodeficiency |
| Wiskott-Aldrich syndrome |
| Hereditary ataxia-telangiectasia |
| Nezelof's syndrome |
| Others |
| **B-Cell and Antibody Immunodeficiencies** |
| X-linked infantile agammaglobulinemia |
| Transient hypogammaglobulinemia of infancy |
| Common, variable immunodeficiency |
| Selective immunoglobulin deficiencies |
| Others |
| **T-Cell Immunodeficiencies** |
| Thymic hypoplasia |
| Chronic mucocutaneous candidiasis |
| Others |
| **Primary Phagocytic Deficiencies** |
| **Primary Complement Deficiencies** |

In contrast, secondary immunodeficiencies are much more common and are often transient in nature. Secondary immunodeficiencies, as the name implies, may also occur secondary to a primary disease. They are associated with a variety of primary diseases or conditions such as infection, malignancy, autoimmune diseases, protein losing (wasting) states, immunosuppressive therapy, and a long list of other disorders (Table 58–2). Secondary immunodeficiencies often resolve when the primary disorder is successfully treated or corrected, and, like primary disorders, are also known to affect the

TABLE 58–2
**Secondary Immunodeficiency Diseases**

| |
|---|
| **Infection** |
| Rubella |
| Measles |
| Leprosy |
| Tuberculosis |
| HIV (AIDS) |
| Coccidioidomycosis |
| Chronic infection |
| Acute viral infection |
| Multiple or repeated viral infections |
| CMV |
| **Neoplastic Disease** |
| Hodgkin's disease |
| Acute leukemia |
| Chronic leukemia |
| Nonlymphoid malignancy |
| Myeloma |
| **Autoimmune Disease** |
| SLE (Systemic Lupus Erythematosus) |
| Rheumatoid Arthritis |
| **Protein-Losing States** |
| Nephrotic syndrome |
| Protein-losing enteropathy |
| **Other Disorders** |
| Diabetes |
| Alcoholic cirrhosis |
| Chronic active hepatitis |
| Malnutrition |
| Burns |
| Sarcoidosis |
| Splenectomy |
| Sickle cell anemia |
| Uremia |
| Subacute sclerosing panencephalitis |
| Down's syndrome |
| Premature infants |
| **Immunosuppressive Treatment** |
| Corticosteroids |
| Cytotoxic drugs |
| Antithymocyte globulin |
| Radiation |
| Cyclosporin A |
| Phenytoin, penicillamine |
| **Anesthesia** |
| **Aging** |

Adapted from Stites, DP, Stobo, JD, and Wells, JV (eds): Basic and Clinical Immunology, ed 6. Appleton & Lange, Norwalk, CT, 1987.

cellular, humoral, phagocytic, or the complement systems. While the underlying mechanisms of many of the secondary immunodeficiencies are also still in question, it is important to recognize the association of this group of immunologic dysfunctions with the various primary diseases and disorders for supportive and diagnostic purposes.

This chapter is devoted to the discussion of primary and secondary immunodeficiencies with respect to their basic defects, pathogenesis, and treatment. While an examination of all of the immunodeficiencies is beyond the scope of this chapter, it is hoped that those presented will provide insight and the basis to understand most immunodeficiency diseases and the problems faced by patients with these diseases.

## PRIMARY IMMUNODEFICIENCIES

In this section we will consider some of the classic primary immunodeficiencies. Combined B- and T-cell defects will be discussed first, followed by separate B-cell and T-cell defects. Finally, this section will end with a brief mention of phagocytic and complement primary deficiencies.

### Combined B- and T-Cell Immunodeficiencies

Immunodeficiencies of this type are variable in both their degree of severity and in their cause. The survival of patients with these disorders is likewise highly variable ranging from less than a year of age in severe combined immunodeficiency to well into adulthood in partial combined immunodeficiency. The symptoms begin early in infancy in most of these patients. As might be expected, these patients are susceptible to a wide range of bacterial, fungal, viral, and protozoal infections. The basic defect of many of the combined immunodeficiencies is not known; however, there have been associations with enzyme deficiencies, genetic components, short-limbed dwarfism, and thymoma. These deficiencies require extensive immunologic laboratory workups.

#### *Severe Combined Immunodeficiency*

Severe combined immunodeficiency (SCID) is the most extreme of all immunodeficiency diseases. It is characterized by severe defects of both B-cell and T-cell immunity. This is evident by the scarcity of lymphoid tissue and the marked depressions in the numbers and/or functions of T and B cells. SCID should not be thought of as a single disease but rather a collection of disorders, all of which are manifested by a compromised cellular and humoral immunity. As such, SCID exhibits variable patterns of inheritance and different degrees of severity (albeit all are extremely serious and life-threatening). The forms of inheritance in SCID are autosomal recessive (the Swiss type lymphopenic agammaglobulinemia) and X-linked recessive type. Both of these forms are clinically similar.

SCID is basically a disorder of infants. The true incidence of SCID is difficult to determine because these patients usually die within the first 1–2 years of life, often before the diagnosis can be made. These patients fail to thrive, suffer from chronic diarrhea, and, as mentioned, are susceptible to a wide range of microbial infections. The infections are usually of skin, respiratory, and gastrointestinal tracts. However, during the first few months of life, they may be protected from bacterial infections and, to some extent, viral infections, by the maternal IgG transferred *in utero*.

Vaccination with live attenuated vaccines should never be attempted in these patients because death from progressive viremia is most likely. In addition, transfusions with nonirradiated blood should never be given to an infant suspected of SCID, or any other immunodeficiency for that matter. This is because of the graft-versus-host reactions (Chap. 56) that would occur in SCID patients, and that may occur in other immunodeficient patients.

**Pathogenesis.** The pathogenesis of SCID has not been fully elucidated. This is most likely due to the fact that SCID is a heterogeneous group of disorders. In some forms of SCID, it appears that there is a defect in the pluripotential lymphoid stem cells' ability to differentiate into mature lymphocytes (see Fig. 61–1). In other forms, it may be a defect in the thymus that prevents proper maturation of regulatory T cells. In yet others, there is an association with a defective enzyme, adenosine deaminase, which may allow the buildup of a metabolite toxic to lymphocytes.

**Treatment.** Treatment of SCID by bone marrow transplantation, fetal liver transplantation, and fetal thymus transplantation, have all been tried with varying success. Following successful transplantation, survivals of 10 years and greater have been reported, depending on the procedure. Some of the treatment protocols are still too new to fully evaluate.

#### *Wiskott-Aldrich Syndrome (Immunodeficiency with Thrombocytopenia and Eczema)*

Wiskott-Aldrich syndrome (WAS) is another disorder in which both the T- and the B-cell arms of the immune system are affected. It is characterized by severe thrombocytopenia, often with bleeding, recurrent infections with a wide range of microbial organisms, and eczema. B cells are present in normal numbers; however, they are unable to respond to polysaccharide antigens. Consequently, serum levels of IgM are usually decreased. On the other hand, serum IgA and IgE are frequently elevated.

The cellular responses are also abnormal (normal mitogen responsiveness, little or no antigen responsiveness). The T-cell immunity may deteriorate both quantitatively (T-cell numbers) and functionally with increasing age. WAS is inherited in an X-linked fashion.

The recurrent infections do not generally begin prior to 6 months of age; however, thrombocytopenia usually begins at birth. By the first year of life, eczema is evident and often becomes infected. Episodes of pneumonias, meningitis, and septicemia become more prevalent as time passes, and survival rarely exceeds the first decade of life. As with most immunodeficiencies, there is an increase in the frequency of lymphoreticular malignancies (as high as 30% in WAS patients).

**Pathogenesis.** The pathogenesis of WAS is largely unknown. However, increased Ig catabolism, regulatory cell failure, and a defective major glycoprotein in the T-cell membrane have all been implicated as having a role.

**Treatment.** Bone marrow transplantation has been performed to treat patients with WAS, with varying success. In addition, transfer factor has been used, but not enough data have been collected to evaluate this treatment adequately.

#### *Hereditary Ataxia-Telangiectasia with Immunodeficiency*

This disorder is primarily neurologic but also severely affects the immune, vascular, and endocrine systems. It is an autosomal recessive disorder characterized by ataxia (incoordination), telangiectasia of the eye (red lesions caused by dilated venules), and recurrent sinopulmonary infections. These infections dominate the clinical picture.

Both T and B cells are affected in a variable fashion. While the B-cell numbers are relatively normal to slightly increased, these patients exhibit absent or decreased levels of serum and secretory IgA. IgE deficiencies have also been noted. T cells may be reduced in both absolute numbers, percentage, and functional ability.

Patients with this disorder are noted to have ataxia beginning in infancy, with the telangiectasia occurring later. The increased number of infections usually begins early in the first decade. If the recurrent infections begin before the ataxia and telangiectasia, it may be difficult to distinguish from other combined immunodeficiencies with abnormal Ig production and selective IgA deficiency (discussed below).

As the patient ages, the neurologic and immunologic functions progressively deteriorate, until approximately the second or third decade, when death from chronic respiratory infection or lymphoreticular malignancy is common. The pathogenesis of this disorder is still not clearly defined. DNA repair defects and defective germ-line tissue have been postulated.

#### *Miscellaneous Combined Immunodeficiencies*

The above immunodeficiencies are the major disorders that have been traditionally classified as primary combined immunodeficiencies. Others, such as Nezelof's syndrome (characterized by cellular immunodeficiency with abnormal immunoglobulin synthesis), seem to be a collection of disorders with T- and B-cell abnormalities to varying degrees that do not seem to be able to be classified into any of the groups discussed above.

It should be noted that, as our ability to elucidate the basic defects in immunodeficiency disorders increases, the distinction between combined T-cell, B-cell immunodeficiencies will also change. This will be evident in the later discussion of certain B-cell deficiencies that are now known to actually be the result of defective T-cell regulation.

### B-Cell and Antibody Immunodeficiencies

Like the combined immunodeficiencies, the B-cell or antibody immunodeficiencies exhibit a wide range of extremes both in the defects and the resultant symptoms. The defects range from a complete lack of all immunoglobulin classes to a selective deficiency of an immunoglobulin subclass. The symptoms are closely linked to the type and extent of the immunoglobulin deficiency and range from severe recurrent infections to no apparent clinical symptoms.

The age at which symptoms appear depends on the severity of the antibody deficiency (the more severe the earlier) and the age of onset of the deficiency (which is not necessarily at birth). With prompt diagnosis and institution of proper therapy, usually gammaglobulin, many of these patients do extremely well. The defects have been attributable to inherent B-cell abnormalities at the various stages of B-cell maturation, and misregulation by T cells. Most of the laboratory workup for the detection of these B-cell deficiencies can be performed by the majority of hospital laboratories.

#### *X-Linked Infantile Agammaglobulinemia (Bruton's Type Agammaglobulinemia)*

X-linked infantile agammaglobulinemia is the most severe of the B-cell deficiencies. It is, as the name implies, inherited in an X-linked recessive pattern and has an incidence of approximately 1 per 100,000. This disorder is characterized by a lack of circulating B cells and plasma cells. These patients do, however, have pre-B cells in the bone marrow and in the circulation, but they do not secrete immunoglobulin.

As a result, the immunoglobulin levels are drastically reduced: IgG typically is less than 100 mg/dl, IgA and IgM less than 1% of normal. T-cell quantitations and functional analysis are normal. These patients are subject to recurrent pyogenic infections, but usually handle the common viral diseases of childhood without much sequelae.

Infants with Bruton's disorder usually remain well during the first months of life due to the passive transfer of maternal antibodies. As these antibodies wane, however, an excessive susceptibility to infection becomes evident. These patients develop sinusitis, dermatitis, pneumonia, otitis media, sepsis, and meningitis. The most common infecting organisms are streptococci, staphylococci, and *Hemophilus influenza*. These infections normally are easily controlled with appropriate antibiotic therapy.

The patient's quick response to treatment in these infections, however, may actually be unfortunate because it may delay the early diagnosis of Bruton's. Early diagnosis and institution of treatment are extremely important to the successful long-term maintenance of most immunodeficient patients. As mentioned previously, the therapy for most patients with B-cell immunodeficiencies is gammaglobulins, which can now be administered intravenously.

**Pathogenesis.** The pathogenesis of X-linked agammaglobulinemia was thought to be attributable to a lack of the stem cells that give rise to the B cells. However, pre-B cells have been found in the bone marrow and circulation of some of these patients so the defect may be in the maturation of these pre-B cells into mature B cells.

### *Transient Hypogammaglobulinemia of Infancy*

A normal infant begins to synthesize IgM at birth, IgA within approximately 3 weeks, and IgG by 6 to 8 weeks. At around age 5–6 months, the infant's serum concentration of IgG is at its lowest. This is because maternally transferred IgG has been almost completely catabolized at this point and the infant's own IgG has not yet offset the loss of maternal antibody. At this time, normal infants are more susceptible to those infections associated with lower IgG levels. Typically, this is soon corrected.

However, in infants with *transient hypogammaglobulinemia*, the production of IgG (occasionally IgM and IgA as well) is delayed by up to 2 years, and these individuals remain hypogammaglobulinemic. These infants do have circulating B cells, which distinguishes them from infants with congenital hypogammaglobulinemia. The cellular immunity is intact.

Infants with transient hypogammaglobulinemia are prone to recurrent respiratory tract and skin infections. These eventually decrease as the patient's delayed immunoglobulin synthesis begins. Some patients may exhibit the same severity and type of infections as X-linked hypogammaglobulinemia and should be treated similarly.

**Pathogenesis.** Two different mechanisms for the pathogenesis of this disorder have been postulated: (1) the passive transfer of maternal anti-IgG antibody, which could, in turn, suppress the production of IgG in the infant; and (2) a transient deficiency in the number and/or function of the T-helper cells required for proper immunoglobulin production.

### *Common Variable Immunodeficiency (Primary Acquired Agammaglobulinemia)*

Common variable immunodeficiency (CVI), like many of the deficiencies previously discussed, is a heterogeneous population disorder with similar features (in this case, *acquired* agammaglobulinemia). It is characterized by a clinical presentation similar to X-linked agammaglobulinemia except that the onset of the disorder may occur at any age, although usually between 15 and 35 years. There is no definitive inheritance pattern; however, there are familial cases reported, and there does seem to be a high incidence of immunologic abnormalities in the families of these patients.

The majority of CVI patients have circulating B cells. The immunoglobulin levels in these patients are slightly better than the X-linked disorder; however, they are still extremely reduced.

The T-cell immunity in a large number of these patients does demonstrate some quantitative and functional abnormalities, which, in time, may actually worsen. These patients also have a higher-than-normal incidence of collagen vascular diseases and malignancy.

The clinical manifestations, as mentioned, are similar to the X-linked agammaglobulinemia and are essentially treated the same way. The long-term prognosis of treated patients is good.

**Pathogenesis.** Because this is a group of similar disorders, it might be expected that the pathogenesis would be variable. Indeed, this is the case. Intrinsic B-cell defects, enzymatic abnormalities, increased activated suppressor T cells, and decreased helper T cells have all been demonstrated as causes of this disorder.

### *Selective Immunoglobulin Deficiencies*

In contrast to all or many of the immunoglobulin classes being deficient, these disorders lack only one immunoglobulin class or subclass with the rest being present in normal concentrations. *Selective IgA deficiency* is the most common of all immunodeficiencies occurring in approximately 1 in 600 persons. The clinical presentations range from recurrent sinopulmonary infections and/or sepsis, to being asymptomatic (most selective IgA deficients are asymptomatic). The treatments also vary from no gammaglobulin in IgA deficiencies to gammaglobulin in some of the other class and subclass deficiencies. The pathogenesis is not known but is speculated to be a defect in the terminal differentiation of the B cell.

## T-Cell Immunodeficiencies

Strict T-cell immunodeficiencies in which the humoral immune system is not secondarily affected are very rare. This is because of the dependency of the humoral immune system on the regulatory T cells to mount a proper antibody response. There are, however, a few cases where T-cell deficiencies occur in the face of normal to near normal antibody production. These individuals suffer from severe recurrent infections with opportunistic fungal, viral, and protozoal organisms.

### *Thymic Hypoplasia (DiGeorge's Syndrome)*

DiGeorge's syndrome is a congenital malformation that occurs early in gestation (in the third and fourth pharyngeal pouches). It is characterized at birth by multiple anomalies including abnormal facial structures, congenital heart defects, hypoparathyroidism, and a reduced or absent thymus. The cellular immune defect varies with the severity of the thymic defect. The lymphocyte counts are usually low. While the percentage of T cells and the responsiveness to the mitogens is reduced, the B-cell percentages may actually be increased with somewhat normal function. Immunoglobulin quantitations are of little value at birth because the majority of immunogloublin will be of maternal origin when these infants present.

In these infants it is not the cellular immune defect but rather the congenital heart defects and hypocalcemia that are the first manifestations of this syndrome requiring attention. These infants must first survive correction of these immediate life-threatening defects before the chronic recurrent infections become apparent. The cellular immunity has been known either to recover spontaneously or deteriorate further, if left untreated. Fetal thymus transplants have been used successfully to reconstitute the T-cell immunity, resulting in long-term survival.

The cause of this congenital defect is not known and it does not appear to occur generally in an inherited fashion. However, there appears to be an increased incidence of DiGeorge's syndrome in infants of alcoholic mothers.

### *Chronic Mucocutaneous Candidiasis*

Chronic mucocutaneous candidiasis is a relatively restricted T-cell immunodeficiency. It is characterized by a selective inability to mount a cellular immune response against *Candida albicans* and related fungi. For the most part, the response against viral, protozoal, bacterial, and other fungal infections remains intact. There are varying forms of the disorder, including autosomal recessive inheritance, association with endocrine abnormalities, early onset, and late onset forms. The B-cell immunity and immunoglobulin levels are normal. The lymphocyte count is generally normal. Skin tests and blastogenesis assays are not responsive to *Candida*; however, the response to other antigens and mitogens is, for the most part, normal.

The clinical manifestations of this disorder range from a very mild involvement of a single fingernail to a severe infection of the mucous membranes and skin. Life-threatening infections do not usually occur, and these patients do relatively well. Treatment, including antifungal agents and various *immunostimulatory* techniques, have had limited success (see Chap. 56).

**Pathogenesis.** Various models have been put forth to explain the pathogenesis of this disorder. These include genetic response restrictions, tolerance, specific suppressor cells, and monocyte/macrophage defects.

## Phagocytic Deficiencies

A major proportion of primary phagocytic dysfunctions all are related to the inability of the phagocytic cell to kill microorganisms. Usually this is the result of an enzymatic defect or deficiency. The clinical manifestations of these disorders, like many of the immunodeficiencies, vary widely. They range from recurrent mild bacterial infections to severe systemic fatal infections. Because T- and B-cell systems are intact in these patients, problems with viral and protozoal infections are not generally encountered.

## Complement Deficiencies

Primary complement deficiencies are extremely rare, and, when they do occur, they are often associated with various autoimmune diseases. In addition, not all complement deficiencies are associated with an increased vulnerability to infections. This is surprising in light of what we know about complement's involvement in the microbial killing process and attests to the remarkable versatility of the immune system. A detailed treatment of these deficiencies is beyond the scope of the text (see Suggested Readings at the end of this chapter).

## SECONDARY IMMUNODEFICIENCIES

As stated previously, secondary immunodeficiencies may be caused by an extremely wide range of primary disorders such as infection, malignancy, autoimmunity, protein-losing states, immunosuppressive therapy, and a long list of others (see Table 58-2). The recognition of these associations is important because it often explains the increased susceptibility to infection seen in these disorders.

The immunologic abnormalities that occur in secondary immunodeficiencies are highly variable and range from being limited to very extensive. An exhaustive discussion of all of these disorders is beyond the scope of this chapter; a representative sampling of some of the more frequently encountered secondary immunodeficiency groups will be described. Specifically, acquired immunodeficiency syndrome (AIDS), immunodeficiency in malignancy, and immunodeficiency associated with autoimmune disease will be examined.

### Acquired Immunodeficiency Syndrome (AIDS)

Acquired immunodeficiency syndrome (AIDS) is by far the most well-known immunodeficiency to both the health professional and the layperson. The incidence of AIDS among the *high-risk groups* ranges from 168-350/100,000 population in the United States.

AIDS has characteristics of both a primary and secondary immunodeficiency. The most severe manifestation of this disease is its profound effect on the immune system; however, this effect is *secondary* to, and induced by infection with the *human immunodeficiency virus (HIV)*, formerly designated HTLVIII or LAV. Therefore, it is included here as a secondary immunodeficiency.

The effects of HIV infection on the immune system range from an asymptomatic immunodeficiency to the extreme immunodeficiency with its associated opportunistic infections and malignancies seen in classic AIDS. Virtually all arms of the immune system may be affected by HIV infection; however, the *primary* target seems to be the T-helper cell.

In clinical AIDS, there is usually a decrease in the lymphocyte count, with marked reductions in the percentage and absolute numbers of *T-helper* cells. This results in the classic inversion of the T-helper to T-suppressor cell ratio, which is typically approximately 2 to 1.

Early in the disease, the number and percentage of T-suppressor cells may actually increase. All of these lymphocyte values (including the T-suppressor cells) eventually deteriorate as the disease progresses. Antigen proliferation responses are decreased, and, as the disease progresses further, the mitogen proliferation responses are affected as well. Immunoglobulin levels are frequently elevated due to a polyclonal B-cell activation.

Late in the disease course these immunoglobulin (Ig) levels also deteriorate, most likely because of an obliteration of the lymphoid tissue germinal centers. Other cells of the immune system, such as macrophages and natural killer cells, are also adversely affected. The majority of these defects may be linked to the primary HIV-induced impairment and destruction of the T-helper cells as well as the monocyte/macrophages also infected with the virus. Again, one only has to refer to the multitude of interactions and secreted regulatory factors involving the T-helper cell to understand the majority of these defects (see Chap. 54 for a review of some of these interactions).

The clinical manifestations of HIV infection, like the immunologic abnormalities vary considerably. One end of the spectrum is an asymptomatic carrier. This is followed by the AIDS-related complex (ARC), which includes abnormalities that may be predictive of AIDS. Finally, at the other end, is the full-blown AIDS. The first clinical symptoms in patients infected with HIV include fever, night sweats, lymphadenopathy, and fatigue. This may then be followed by extreme weight loss, diarrhea, opportunistic infections, and malignancies (Kaposi's sarcoma and lymphoma). The most common infection in AIDS is *Pneumocystis carinii* pneumonia. However, toxoplasmosis, cryptosporidiosis, fungal, bacterial, and concominant viral infections also occur. These infections are the prime cause of death in patients with AIDS. Treatment for HIV and the induced immunodeficiency is still experimental with several clinical trials underway. The majority of these include the inhibitors of HIV replication (specifically—reverse transcriptase) such as azidothymidine (AZT), phosphonoformate, suramin, and HPA-23.

#### Pathogenesis

The pathogenesis is essentially related to the effects of HIV on the various cells that it infects. The main target for HIV is the T-helper cell in which rapid viral replication and cell death occur shortly after infection. Under certain conditions, a chronic viral infection may also be established. There are also reports suggesting that B cell and macrophages may become infected.

#### Nursing Care of the Patient with AIDS

Of utmost importance in caring for the immunosuppressed patient diagnosed as having AIDS-related complex (ARC; i.e., a condition attributed to the human immunodeficiency virus, in which the person tests positive for AIDS and demonstrates symptomatology, although less severe than in classic AIDS) or classic AIDS is to implement measures that prevent the transmission of HIV in the clinical setting, and to focus on minimizing exposure of the immunosuppressed person to exogenous organisms. Toward this end, each health-care provider should be familiar with the "Universal Precautions" set forth by the Centers for Disease Control (CDC)* and should incorporate these recommendations into daily practice. Such precautions are essential in caring for *all* patients because HIV-infected patients are not always reliably diagnosed based on clinical history and physical examination.

Handwashing may provide the most important barrier to transmission of disease, and it should be performed meticulously using appropriate technique. Patients and family/significant others should be taught the need for and the appropriate technique in handwashing. Raising the consciousness and awareness of patient and visitors in this regard may help to impact on their overall perceptions of health and how health is managed.

When exposure or contact with blood and body fluids is anticipated, *all such fluids should be considered to be infective*. Gloves should be worn, and articles in contact with such fluids should be disposed of in containers labeled "infectious waste." Handwashing before and after use of gloves and handling of such materials should be diligently performed. Care should be taken to avoid contaminating the outside of these receptacles.

For purposes of obtaining blood samples or administering parenteral medications, only disposable needles and syringes should be used and properly discarded in puncture-resistant containers. Recapping of needles after use should be *avoided* because of the risk of self-puncturing. Meticulous care of invasive lines should be provided. Acceptable practice is to use aseptic technique during insertion of lines and dressing changes. Sites of invasive lines should be assessed for any signs of infection (redness, swelling, pain, warmth). Use of indwelling urinary catheters should be avoided, if at all possible, because urinary tract infection is a major source of infection in hospitalized patients. If catheterization is necessary, scrupulous perineal care should be provided. Thorough mouth care and personal hygiene should be provided to prevent stomatitis. The skin should be assessed for signs of impairment, and special skin care should be provided to prevent breakdown of this first line of defense against opportunistic organisms.

In general, nurses caring for the immunosuppressed patient must adhere to high standards of practice in implementing personal hygiene, treatments, and procedures. It is essential to be thorough in assessing patients and to have a high degree of suspicion because these patients are especially at high risk of developing nosocomial infections.

For a detailed nursing care plan for the immunosuppressed patient, see Table 56–1. Additional nursing care considerations regarding the potential for infection are included in Table 49–7. See the case study at the end of this chapter for a depiction of a nursing approach, specifically psychologic perspectives in the treatment of the patient with AIDS.

## Immunodeficiency Secondary to Malignant Disease

Immunodeficiency is very often associated with malignancy. In fact, this is such a common occurrence that excessive opportunistic infections are not only a risk to the diagnosed cancer patient but are also grounds to suspect an underlying malignancy. This is especially true of cancer involving the cells of the immune system.

B-cell malignancies such as Burkitt's lymphoma, most chronic lymphocytic leukemia (CLL), multiple myeloma, and Waldenström's macroglobulinemia often demonstrate hypogammaglobulinemia (excluding any monoclonal spikes) and a decrease *in vivo* antibody response to antigenic stimulation (vaccine, organisms, etc.). Often the cellular responses are also decreased. In CLL, the malignant B cells do not often secrete immunoglobulin and the defective humoral response seems to lie in a reduced immunoglobulin synthesis. In plasma cell malignancies such as multiple myeloma and Waldenström's macroglobulinemia, the malignant cells do produce immunoglobulin. In fact, the levels in the blood may become so high that the serum actually becomes viscous. However, the immunoglobulin is monoclonal (only one specificity), and these patients have very little polyclonal functional immunoglobulin. It has been suggested that this decrease in normal immunoglobulin may result from maturational block or inhibition of B cells by host suppressor monocytic cells.

The T-cell malignancies such as T-cell acute lymphocytic leukemia and Sézary syndrome (mostly a T-helper cell malignancy) have variable defects in both the humoral and cellular system. This often depends on whether the malignant cells are functional or not.

It should be noted that if the malignancy itself does not cause an immunodeficiency, very often the treatment will. This is because most cancer chemotherapy and radiation therapy are immunosuppressive.

*Centers for Disease Control: Recommendations for prevention of HIV transmission in health care settings. HHS Pub. No. (CDC) 87-8017. MMWR CDC Surveill Summ 36(25): August 21, 1987.

## Miscellaneous Secondary Immunodeficiencies

It should be realized that although the discussed secondary immunodeficiencies are among some of the more common ones encountered, the complete list is extremely large and cannot be included due to space limitations. Furthermore, equally as large as the number of secondary immunodeficiencies is the range of immune abnormalities that occur in them.

## SUMMARY

Immunodeficiency disorders are by no means rare, and they are constantly being encountered by the health professional in one form or another, depending on the specific defect. It is hoped that this overview of the defects encountered in the immune system will enable the reader to appreciate the tremendous complexity and interactions of the immune system and the consequences of any errors or abnormalities that may occur.

## CASE STUDY WITH SAMPLE CARE PLAN: PATIENT WITH ACQUIRED IMMUNODEFICIENCY SYNDROME (AIDS): PSYCHOLOGIC PERSPECTIVES*

Mr. W.B. is a 33-year-old white male, admitted to the Medical Unit with a chief complaint of increasing shortness of breath over a 1-week period. The patient states he is a lifelong homosexual whose ex-lover died last night of AIDS. Their last encounter was 3 years ago.

Mr. W.B. reported that the shortness of breath occurs while at rest, increasing significantly upon exertion. It is associated with a dry, unproductive cough and chest pain across the sternum. This pain is aggravated upon inspiration.

The patient also complains of dizziness at times, but admits to not eating well over the past 2 weeks because he has had no appetite. Mr. W.B. denies fever, chills, night sweats, or any other associated complaints.

Mr. W.B.'s past medical history includes hepatitis 7 years prior to this admission; gonorrhea, 11 years prior to this admission, which was treated effectively with tetracycline; and herpes zoster, which developed about 4 months ago and was treated with acyclovir. A lesion attributed to the herpes infection is still evident on the patient's forehead.

Mr. W.B.'s sexual history reveals that he has been exclusively a homosexual, active since age 14. He states that his last sexual contact was a year and a half ago. Prior to that, he had 5 partners; he estimated that he has had fewer than 50 partners over the last 19 years. He was active with his most recent lover about 3 years ago. The ex-lover was diagnosed as having AIDS about 2 years ago and died last night at a city hospital.

Socially, Mr. W.B. has a history of cigarette smoking of about 18 pack years; he quit smoking altogether about 2 months prior to this admission. He describes himself as an occasional drinker. Mr. W.B. denies intravenous drug use; he admits to using recreational drugs including cocaine, mescaline, and Quaalude.

Mr. W.B. reports that he was fired from his job as a manager of a store selling women's garments. He offered no explanation regarding the circumstances of his firing. Mr. W.B. states that he has no medical/health insurance and limited personal funds. Mr. W.B. denies having had blood transfusions; he has not traveled outside of the United States.

Significant family history reveals that the patient's father died at age 72 from heart disease; his mother is alive and well at age 71. There are 5 siblings, including 3 brothers and 2 sisters, all alive and well. Two of Mr. W.B.'s brothers and one sister are gay.

On physical examination, the patient presents as a well-developed white male in no acute distress. A herpes lesion is evident on the forehead, and thrush is noted on left lateral surface of the tongue. On auscultation, breath sounds are decreased bilaterally. Examination of lymph nodes reveals anterior cervical nodes about 1 – 2 cm in size and nontender; posterior cervical and inguinal nodes are also palpable and, likewise, 1 – 2 cm in size and nontender bilaterally.

Psychologically, the patient has experienced undue stress. He has had actual sexual contact with known AIDS victims; he has witnessed 10 close friends die of AIDS over the past 3 years.

Laboratory data of significance: Arterial blood gases on admission indicated: pH 7.45, $PaCO_2$ 36, $PaO_2$ 62 mmHg (room air). A bronchoscopy performed on admission confirmed the diagnosis of *Pneumocystis carinii* pneumonia associated with AIDS. Bactrim therapy was initiated.

On the second hospital day following admission, Mr. W.B. expressed a desire for his family to be informed regarding his status. The family was subsequently advised of his diagnosis in his presence, as he requested. On the third hospital day, the patient requested "no resuscitation," should this become an issue. The request was made based on his knowledge of AIDS and its prognosis. At this time, the patient was experiencing increasing dyspnea upon speaking, thus limiting his ability to commu-

*This case study and sample care plan were contributed by Kathleen Daley White and Margaret Connelly.

## SAMPLE CARE PLAN FOR THE PATIENT WITH ACQUIRED IMMUNODEFICIENCY SYNDROME (AIDS): PSYCHOLOGIC PERSPECTIVES

| Nursing Diagnoses | Desired Patient Outcomes | Nursing Interventions | Rationales |
|---|---|---|---|
| ***Nursing Diagnosis #1*** Fear of death and dying, related to: 1. AIDS diagnosis. | Patient will be able to: 1. Verbalize fear regarding AIDS. 2. Identify support systems to deal effectively with AIDS. | • Assess patient's perceived fear as expressed in his own words. | |
| | | • Help to identify factors he feels he has control over, and those he does not. | • Separating those items which are able to be controlled, and those which are not, gives the patient an area where he can focus his energies toward resolution of the fear. |
| | | • Utilize support persons and resources to help patient in sorting out and dealing with fear. ○ Interview family members and identify those who are positive in their attitude and approach to the patient; encourage their participation in his care. ○ Investigate patient's background to identify available support resources; contact these resources to help in creating a supportive environment in which the patient can verbalize fear. | • By working within the patient's own framework, support systems and resources can be used more effectively in assisting the patient to deal with his fear. |
| | | • Document patient's questions, and responses in progress notes, so as to communicate the patient's goals, progression, as well as regression in working toward goals. • Document any key characteristic behavior exhibited by patient, and reflective of his underlying fear; use these to help the patient deal effectively with his fear. | • Documentation assists in providing continuity of care. |
| | | • Encourage family participation in patient care activities. | • Clarifying the status of AIDS, including what it is, what can be done to treat it, its prognosis, and expected course, for the patient and family members, ultimately will strengthen the effectiveness of the patient-family-health team, support system. • It is essential to be honest and straightforward. |

| | | | |
|---|---|---|---|
| ***Nursing Diagnosis #2***<br>Body image, disturbance, related to:<br>1. Actual bodily changes. | Patient will:<br>1. Verbalize feelings regarding body changes.<br>2. Demonstrate positive attitude regarding self:<br>• Identify strengths.<br>• Express interest in self-care activities.<br>• Involve family in care. | • Assess thoughts and feelings regarding body changes. | • Underlying immune defect of cell-mediated immunity in AIDS places these patients at high risk of developing fungal and other opportunistic infections. Such infections can be physically unsightly, and emotionally difficult for the patient to cope with. |
| | | • Ask patient to identify these changes. | • If patient can identify body changes that particularly distress him, the nurse may help him to understand why the infections occur and what can be done to minimize the risk of infection. For example, frequent and meticulous oral hygiene, handwashing. |
| | | • Help patient to become aware of the support systems that surround him and who accept him as he is regardless of body changes. | • By identifying his support system, the patient may begin to realize his acceptance by those caring for him in spite of his body changes; he may realize that his body image in no way threatens their friendship, love, and support for him. |
| | | • Provide personalized nursing care; touch the patient, and care for the patient in a manner you would care for any patient while implementing appropriate precautions. | • Nurses are able to demonstrate their acceptance of him by personalizing care; use of touch therapy is especially reassuring to the patient; furthermore, it sets an example for the family members and significant others to follow. Utilizing this type of approach in caring for the patient reassures him that he is accepted in spite of his own perceptions and self-doubts. |
| | | • Work with family to help them be aware of patient's misgivings about body changes; help them to identify grooming habits important to patient, and to implement a plan of care: Haircut and shave; manicure; use of favorite cologne. | • Involving family in patient's care may enable them to feel positive about contributing in some way. By arranging for special grooming activities, the patient may be made to feel more positive about himself, and his acceptance by others. |
| | | • Document patient's response to care and progress made toward accepting self; update and revise the care plan accordingly. | • Documentation assists in continuity of patient's care as efforts of all health care providers can be focused on identified goals and the achievement of desired patient outcomes. |
| ***Nursing Diagnosis #3***<br>Social isolation, related to:<br>1. Diagnosis of AIDS.<br>2. Necessary isolation precautions. | Patient will:<br>1. Explain the reasons for isolation precautions.<br>2. Inform family and significant others as to need for precautions. | • Explain need for and underlying rationales for instituting isolation precautions. | • Patient, family, and staff must understand what the disease AIDS entails, and implications as to precautions to prevent its transmission to others. This is true not only within the hospital setting, but in daily activities of living. |

*(continued)*

## SAMPLE CARE PLAN FOR THE PATIENT WITH ACQUIRED IMMUNODEFICIENCY SYNDROME (AIDS): PSYCHOLOGIC PERSPECTIVES *(Continued)*

| Nursing Diagnoses | Desired Patient Outcomes | Nursing Interventions | Rationales |
|---|---|---|---|
| ***Nursing Diagnosis #3 (cont.)*** | | | |
| | 3. Demonstrate specific precautions in self-care. | • Implement isolation techniques involving patient and family in performing specific procedures according to hospital protocol. | |
| | | • Assess patient's previous social lifestyle and social interactions. | • If patient has been active socially and enjoys people, this should not change because of AIDS. Patient's preferences should be respected and made known to all who interact with the patient. Maintaining some control over his life fosters self-confidence and self-esteem. |
| | | • Maintain socialization process on patient's behalf, and within the patient's activity tolerance.<br>◦ After conferring with patient, encourage visitors when appropriate.<br>◦ Keep door to patient room open except when he is sleeping.<br>◦ Encourage timely use of television and radio to keep abreast of events.<br>◦ Hang up pictures, cards and other decorations with meaning to patient. | • Socially withdrawing could lead to a situational depression, or be reflective of depression already present. If patients see the staff as "over-isolating," or perceive a "repugnance" on the part of the staff and/or visitors, they may become depressed, and socially withdraw. |
| | | • Enlist family's help in determining important social situations in patient's life (e.g., birthday, holiday, anniversary, etc.). Work with support system to bring a part of each of these to the patient. | • For patients on isolation, special efforts should be made so that important events or interactions are not left unnoticed. |
| | | • Encourage staff to carry out necessary isolation techniques, but caution not to "over-isolate." | • Patients on isolation precautions sometimes feel they are missing something; such feelings as "being left out" can predispose to a depressive reaction and may delay progress in the patient's improvement. |

| | | | |
|---|---|---|---|
| ***Nursing Diagnosis #4***<br>Verbal communication, impaired, related to:<br>1. CPAP mask.<br>2. Constant tachypnea.<br>3. Fatigue. | Patient will be able to communicate with family, staff and significant others to make his needs known, and to enjoy interacting with others. | • Assess the patient's ability to communicate.<br>◦ Work with patient to identify the problem underlying his inability to communicate. | • Patients who have had a terminal disease confirmed have a great deal of processing to go through intellectually, emotionally, and psychologically. If the patient needs to verbalize his thoughts and feelings in this regard, an inability to communicate can cause the patient to feel isolated and alone. |
| | | • Work with patient to devise a communication tool to meet his needs:<br>◦ Use of chalk or alphabet board.<br>◦ Use of "frequent words used" sheet.<br>◦ Lip-reading.<br>◦ Anticipate needs; remain accessible. | • Inability to communicate can be extremely frustrating particularly when it concerns the "small" needs that people in general take for granted. Aggravation associated with small concerns can become exaggerated, and expand into major problems. |
| | | • Document key likes and dislikes so that the entire staff can anticipate patient's needs. For example, ice in water; call bell in left hand. | • If the patient who is already distressed and compromised must use remaining strength and energy requesting the same thing over and over again, or needs to continually make explanations regarding his needs, then the "therapeutic" milieu provided for the patient needs to be reassessed, and a revised plan of care implemented accordingly. |

nicate fully with family, nurses, social worker, priest, or other health-care provider.

On day 5 of this admission, Mr. W.B.'s arterial blood gas studies were as follows: pH 7.46, $PaCO_2$ 34, and $PaO_2$ 46, $HCO_3^-$24. He was transferred to the intensive care unit (ICU) and placed on continuous positive airway pressure (CPAP) at +5 cm/$H_2O$. The patient refused intubation. Subsequently, arterial blood gases were: pH 7.41, $PaCO_2$ 36, $PaO_2$ 107, $HCO_3^-$ 28. The patient remained extremely tachypneic.

Over the next 24 hours, Mr. W.B.'s condition remained unchanged. He confirmed: "I don't want to spend the rest of my life on a machine to breathe." Siblings were supportive of his decision and proud of his "bravery." The patient's mother was having a difficult time agreeing with her son's decision, but siblings were supportive to her.

On the eighth day after admission, the patient's body temperature rose to 103°F. Bactrim was discontinued, and pentamidine (Pentam) therapy was initiated. Patient reaffirmed, "no heroics." Entire family seemed at peace with this decision.

Twenty-four hours later, the patient became unresponsive, and apneic at times. The health team continued the treatment plan, hopeful that the patient could be supported until pentamidine would be effective. On consultation with an infectious disease expert, large doses of intravenous corticosteroids were recommended because there have been instances of abrupt reversal of fully fulminating *Pneumocystis carinii* pneumonia with this approach.

The patient's mother and sister were upset with the steroidal therapy as they viewed this treatment as an "heroic" measure, one that was prolonging the patient's life in opposition to his request. When all siblings were called to the bedside, there was not full agreement by the family regarding the use of steroids. Following the administration of the first dose of intravenous steroidal therapy, the mother and one sister became so irate that further doses were discontinued. The patient appeared obtunded; body temperature remained at 103°F.

Over the next 18 hours following initial steroidal therapy, the patient became alert, oriented, and afebrile. He was agreeable to further steroidal therapy. Over the next 24 hours, Mr. W.B. had improved so that the CPAP was discontinued. The mother and one sister thought "a miracle had occurred."

On the 13th day following admission, the patient was able to celebrate his birthday with family and friends. He verbalized that his recovery and positive attitude were a result of the support from family, friends, and members of the health team.

Over the next 10–12 days, the patient continued to improve with a treatment regimen of pentamidine, steroids, and increased nutrition. He was subsequently transferred to an acute Medical Unit. During the ensuing 2 weeks, the patient established a new support system in religion, and he received his first holy communion as a Roman Catholic.

The patient continued to progress slowly and was discharged to his mother's home with referral to the AIDS Clinic, approximately 46 days following his admission.

### Initial Nursing Diagnoses

1. Fear of death and dying, related to diagnosis of AIDS.
2. Body image, disturbance in, related to actual bodily changes including herpetic lesion, *Candida* infection (stomatitis), and cachexia (10-lb weight loss).
3. Social isolation, related to diagnosis of AIDS and necessary isolation precautions.
4. Verbal communication, impaired, related to continuous positive airway pressure (CPAP) mask and constant tachypnea and consequent fatigue.

### Additional Nursing Diagnoses

5. Coping, ineffective, family (mother, sister), related to exhaustion of supportive capacity and questionable knowledge about AIDS.
6. Sleep pattern disturbance, related to dyspnea, febrile state, ICU setting.
7. Depression, reactive (situational), related to perceived powerlessness of future with AIDS.
8. Self-esteem, disturbance in, related to loss of job, loss of financial independence.
9. Anticipatory grief, related to prognosis of AIDS diagnosis.
10. Knowledge deficit.

## SUGGESTED READINGS


Bellanti, JA: Immunology III. WB Saunders, Philadelphia, 1985.

Bellanti, JA: Immunology Basic Processes, ed 2. WB Saunders, Philadelphia, 1985.

Centers for Disease Control: Recommendations for prevention of HIV transmission in health care settings. HHS Pub. No. (CDC) 87-8017. MMWR CDC Surveill Summ 36(25): 1987.

Lewandowski, AJ: The immunopathogenesis of AIDS. J Med Technol 3:145–149, 1986.

Mathewson, MK: Pharmacotherapeutics, A Nursing Process Approach. FA Davis, Philadelphia, 1986.

Nyamathi, A and van Servellen, G: Maladaptive coping in the critically ill population with acquired immunodeficiency syndrome: Nursing assessment and treatment. Heart Lung 18(2):113, March 1989.

Stites, DP, Stobo, JD, and Wells, JV (eds): Basic and Clinical Immunology, ed 6. Appleton and Lange, Norwalk, CT, 1987.

# UNIT EIGHT

# Bibliography


Abernathy, E: How the immune system works. Am J Nurs 87(4):456, April 1987.

Abernathy, E: Biological response modifiers. Am J Nurs, 87(4):458, April 1987.

Arnold, AN, et al: Effect of renal allograft dysfunction upon cyclosporine through levels in host blood. Transplantation 40:605, 1985.

Bellanti, JA: Immunology III. WB Saunders, Philadelphia, 1985.

Bellanti, JA: Immunology Basic Processes, ed 2. WB Saunders, Philadelphia, 1985.

Carrel, A: Techniques and remote results of vascular anastomosis. Surg Gynecol Obstet 14:246, 1912.

Clark, WR: The Experimental Foundations of Modern Immunology, ed 3. John Wiley & Sons, New York, 1986.

Cosimi, AB, et al: A randomized clinical trial comparing OKT3 and steroids for treatment of hepatic allograft rejection. Transplantation 43:91, 1987.

Goldstein, G, et al: A randomized clinical trial of OKT3 monoclonal antibody for acute rejection of cadaveric renal transplants. N Engl J Med 3134:337, 1985.

Griffin, JP: Hematology and Immunology: Concepts for Nursing. Appleton-Century-Crofts, Norwalk, CN, 1986.

Hamilton, D: A history of transplantation. In Morris, PJ (ed): Tissue Transplantation. Grune & Stratton, New York, 1984.

Hayry, P: vonWillebrand F. Transplant aspiration cytology. Transplantation 38:7, 1984.

Hood, LE: Interferon, getting in the way of viruses and tumors. Am J Nurs 87(4):459, April 1987.

Hood, LE, et al (eds): Immunology, ed 2. Benjamin/Cummings Publishing, Menlo Park, CA, 1984.

Immunology: Readings from Scientific American. WH Freeman and Co., San Francisco, 1976 (and recent articles in that journal to the present date).

Jarowenko, MV, et al: Treatment of steroid resistant rejection in patients receiving cyclosporine. Transplantation 41:579, 1986.

Jassak, PF and Spiewak, PL: Interleukin-2, turning on the system. Am J Nurs 87(4):464, April 1987.

Kemp, D: Development of the immune system. Crit Care Q 9(1):1, June 1986.

Lambert, R, et al: Glomerular damage after kidney preservation. Transplantation 42:125, 1986.

Mackintosh, P: ABO matching in kidney graft survival. Nature 250(5464):351, July 1974.

Matas, AJ, et al: Treatment of steroid resistant rejection in patients receiving cyclosporine. Transplantation 41:579, 1986.

Matas, AJ, et al: The value of needle renal allograft biopsy III. A prospective study. Surgery 98:922, 1985.

Mathewson, MK: Pharmacotherapeutics: A Nursing Process Approach. FA Davis, Philadelphia, 1986.

Miller, HC, Alexander, JW, and Nathan, P: Effects of warm ischemic damage on intrarenal distribution of flow in preserved kidneys. Surgery 72:193, 1972.

Nyamathi, A and van Servellen, G: Maladaptive coping in the critically ill population with acquired immunodeficiency syndrome: Nursing assessment and treatment. Heart Lung 18(2):113, March 1989.

Opelz, G and Terasaki, PI: Significance of mixed leukocyte culture testing in cadaver kidney transplantation. Transplantation 23:375, 1977.

Parker, CW: Clinical Immunology. WB Saunders, Philadelphia, 1980.

Paul, WE: Fundamental Immunology. Raven Press, New York, 1984.

Rosano, TG, et al: Immunosuppressive metabolites of cyclosporine in the blood of renal allograft recipients. Transplantation 42:262, 1986.

Sampter, M: Immunological Diseases, ed 3. Little, Brown & Co, Boston, 1978.

Schwartz, BD: The human major histocompatibility complex. In Stites, DP, et al (eds): Basic and Clinical Immunology, ed 6. Appleton & Lange, Norwalk, CT, 1987.

Sher, PP: Laboratory Medicine. American Society of Clinical Pathologists, Chicago, November 1986.

Simmons, RL and So, SK: Clinical transplantation. In Stites, DP, et al (eds): Basic and Clinical Immunology, ed 6. Appleton & Lange, Norwalk, CT, 1987.

Stiehm, ER and Fulginiti, VA: Immunologic Disorders in Infants and Children, ed 2. WB Saunders, Philadelphia, 1980.

Waltzer, WC: Procurement of cadaveric kidneys for transplantation. Ann Intern Med 98:536, 1983.

Webb, DR and Winkelstein, A: Immunosuppression, immunopotentiation, and antiinflammatory drugs. In Stites, DP, et al (eds): Basic and Clinical Immunology, ed 6. Appleton & Lange, Norwalk, CT, 1987.

Weir, DM (ed): Handbook of Experimental Immunology. Volume 2: Cellular Immunology. Blackwell Scientific Publications, Oxford, 1986.

UNIT NINE

# Oncologic Critical Care Nursing

While cancer remains a prevalent disease, major advances in its diagnosis and treatment over the past 2 decades have resulted in a steady rise in the survival rate. For many patients who remain in remission, treatment protocols (e.g., surgery, radiation therapy, and/or chemotherapy) have increased the length of survival of many patients until advanced stages of the disease.

As a consequence, the incidence of oncologic emergencies has risen appreciably. Such emergencies are frequently associated with treatment-related problems, as, for example, immunosuppression induced by chemotherapy and/or radiation therapy, or they may be associated with the pathophysiologic effects of advanced stages of cancer on overall body functioning.

Care of the critically ill oncology patient has special implications for nursing. Successful patient outcomes depend on early recognition of high-risk patients; on thorough, accurate, and rapid assessment; and on timely therapeutic interventions. Decisions regarding care must be determined based on the overall therapeutic goals. Such decision-making requires knowledge of the underlying disease status and its effect on body function, the patient's nutritional state, and prior anticancer therapy.

Despite the steady rise in the rate of survival, a diagnosis of cancer continues to trigger such perceptions as fear, pain, loss, and death in many patients, as well as their family and/or significant others. In this regard, nurses are not only instrumental in treating the underlying pathophysiology of cancer, but, very importantly, nurses play a key role in identifying and establishing the psychologic support systems so vital to the recovery and rehabilitation of the patient and family. In the setting of terminal illness, such support may be crucial in assisting the patient and family/significant others in resolving and eventually accepting the ultimate outcome, that is, death.

In the chapters to follow, specific oncologic emergencies are examined, including the identification of patients at risk, clinical presentation, diagnosis, and treatment. Nursing process is addressed in terms of nursing diagnoses, patient outcomes, and nursing interventions, and is reflected in the nursing care plans.

The discussion of medical oncologic emergencies includes cardiac tamponade, septic shock, spinal cord compression, syndrome of inappropriate secretion of antidiuretic hormone (SIADH), superior vena cava syndrome, hypercalcemia, and pain. Case studies are also included in certain instances to assist the reader to integrate underlying physiologic principles with the clinical circumstances, and to more closely appreciate the approach to treatment and nursing care.

In the discussion concerned with the surgical treatment of cancer, nursing care is addressed with respect to surgical intervention involving the head and neck and surgical treatment of esophageal carcinoma. Nursing care plans reflect the nursing process.

## UNIT OUTLINE

CHAPTER 59

# Nursing Care of Patients with Neoplastic-Related Medical Emergencies

*Merri Walkenstein and Deborah Rodzwic*

## CHAPTER OUTLINE



## LEARNING OBJECTIVES

**At the end of this chapter, you should be able to:**

1. Identify patients at risk for developing neoplastic emergencies including:
   a. Cardiac tamponade.
   b. Septic shock.
   c. Spinal cord compression.
   d. Syndrome of inappropriate secretion of antidiuretic hormone (SIADH).
   e. Superior vena cava syndrome (SVCS).

## LEARNING OBJECTIVES—*CONTINUED*

f. Hypercalcemia.
g. Pain
2. List tentative etiologies for each of these oncologic emergencies.
3. Discuss pathophysiology underlying these oncologic emergencies.
4. Recognize the clinical presentation of these oncologic emergencies.
5. Discuss the clinical diagnosis and treatment of these oncologic emergencies.
6. Identify pertinent aspects in the nursing care of the patient with an oncologic emergency including:
   Assessment
   Diagnosis
   Planning: Desired patient outcomes
   Nursing interventions/rationales.

The conditions covered in this chapter are reflective of those medical oncologic emergencies commonly encountered in critical care settings. They do not encompass all the medical oncologic emergencies, but they do reflect the kind of nursing care required by these patients.

## NEOPLASTIC CARDIAC TAMPONADE

### Etiology and Pathophysiology

Cardiac tamponade is a life-threatening condition caused by an accumulation of fluid within the inelastic parietal pericardial space leading to a decrease in cardiac output with subsequent shocklike symptoms. This fluid accumulation, referred to as a pericardial effusion, results from a variety of neoplastic syndromes. *Neoplastic* cardiac tamponade, which accounts for the majority of pericardial effusions,[1] implies that the cause of this fluid accumulation is cancer related.

Malignant pericardial effusions potentially can cause cardiac tamponade. Cancers most likely associated with this process include: (1) malignant tumors that invade the mediastinum blocking the normal resorption of pericardial fluid, (2) malignant tumors that metastasize to the heart, and (3) constrictive pericarditis that results from the effects of radiotherapy to the pericardium or mediastinum. For some patients, symptoms of cardiac tamponade are the initial presentation of cancer, especially when the primary cancer or metastases to other sites are limited.[2]

The accumulation of fluid causes an increase in the pressure around the heart, thereby preventing the ventricles from completely filling during diastole (see Fig. 59–1). As a result, cardiac output (CO) is markedly impaired. This rise in pericardial pressure may be rapid or gradual with fluid accumulation between 50 and 2500 ml. If the fluid accumulation is gradual, the patient is often able to tolerate several hundred milliliters of fluid before symptoms occur.[3] If the fluid accumulation is rapid, acute symptoms of decreased CO are apparent.

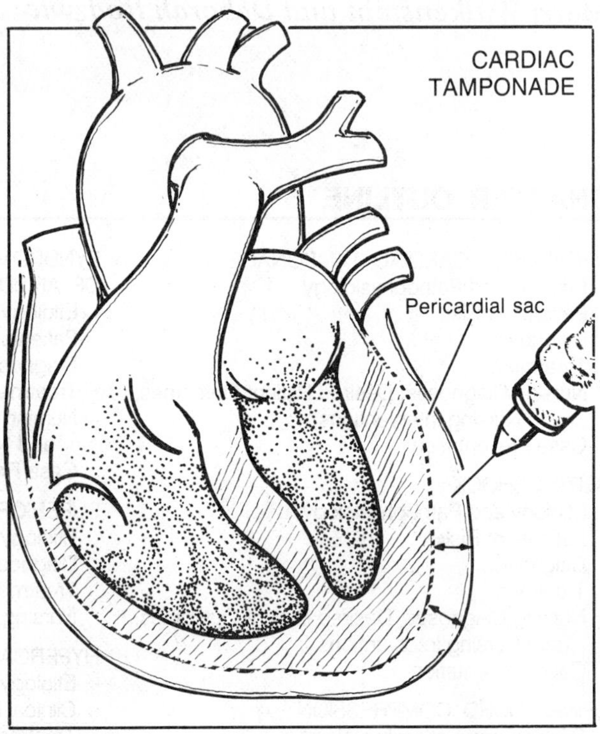


**Figure 59–1.** Cardiac tamponade. A pericardiocentesis, performed by introducing a needle into the pericardial sac, confirms the diagnosis of cardiac tamponade.

### Patients at Risk

Approximately 20% of patients with cancer will have metastases involving the pericardium and, to a lesser extent, the myocardium.[4] Patients at the highest risk for developing neoplastic tamponade include those diagnosed with melanoma, leukemia, lymphoma, and metastatic tumors of the lung and breast. Cancers of the lung and breast have the highest incidence of tamponade,[4,5] which is related, in part, to the lymphatic drainage of the heart, lungs, and breast.[2] Patients treated with large doses of radiotherapy to the chest may also develop this condition.

## Diagnosis

Although the clinical symptoms of cardiac tamponade may appear gradually, the signs and symptoms must be recognized immediately or death may ensue rapidly. Diagnosis of cardiac tamponade is made by evaluating the patient's clinical signs and symptoms, as well as evaluating x-rays and hemodynamic invasive monitoring values using a pulmonary artery (PA) flow-directed balloon-tipped catheter.

Common signs and symptoms of cardiac tamponade include tachycardia, muffled heart sounds, hypotension, a narrow pulse pressure, and Kussmaul's sign. A weak, tachycardic pulse is a compensatory mechanism resulting from the decreased cardiac output. Heart sounds on auscultation are muffled because the heart is now surrounded by fluid. Hypotension with classic shocklike symptoms are apparent and related to the decreased cardiac output. A narrowing pulse pressure is indicative of a decreased stroke volume with arterial constriction. One of the classic signs of tamponade is distended neck veins or Kussmaul's sign. This sign is present when the patient is lying with the head of the bed at a 60-degree angle, and on inspiration the neck veins distend, indicating an increase in right atrial pressure.

Other signs and symptoms of tamponade include a pulsus paradoxus of greater than or equal to 10 mmHg (see Fig. 38–2). This paradox is characterized by a decline in systolic arterial pressure with normal inspiration and is usually absent if the patient's pressure is below 50 mmHg. Additional manifestations of cardiac tamponade are apprehension and restlessness (often the first signs indicating impaired cerebral oxygenation). Cool, pale, and diaphoretic skin, shortness of breath, cough, and decreased urine output are other accompanying symptoms.

More definitive diagnostic measures that the nurse monitors include values obtained by using a PA catheter. These values include elevation of central venous pressures, pulmonary artery systolic and diastolic pressures, and pulmonary capillary wedge pressures (PCWP). Conversely, the cardiac output will be decreased. An echocardiogram, CT scan, and chest x-ray often show an enlarged heart with fluid accumulation. Continuous cardiac monitoring is essential because the electrocardiogram (ECG) may demonstrate ST–T wave changes and/or electrical alternans (alternating large and small QRS complexes or altered direction of the complexes). This may indicate a diseased pericardium and is not commonly seen in other conditions.

A pericardiocentesis confirms the diagnosis of cardiac tamponade. This procedure involves the physician inserting a large bore needle into the pericardial space to withdraw the fluid (Fig. 59–1). The fluid is tested for cytologic identification of malignant cells. Complications of this diagnostic procedure include perforated ventricles, lacerated coronary arteries, air embolism, punctured lung, and infection. The nurse must anticipate these problems and be prepared to employ emergency measures.

## Treatment

The patient and family/significant others need to be aware that the treatment for cardiac tamponade is often palliative. This therapy is generally aimed at restoring fluid volume and cardiac output, relieving pressure around the heart, and enhancing oxygen perfusion of tissues. Fluid volume and cardiac output are improved with administration of whole blood, colloids, and/or inotropic agents such as isoproterenol and dobutamine, which increase the heart rate, myocardial contractility, and stroke volume while decreasing the systemic vascular resistance. The pressure around the heart is decreased by performing a pericardiocentesis, in which case 20–50 ml of fluid will usually improve the patient's status (elevated blood pressure and cardiac output). A pericardial catheter may be inserted for repeated drainage of fluid and for instillation of chemotherapy or sclerosing agents (see Fig. 59–1). In addition, a pericardiectomy may be surgically performed to allow subsequent drainage to escape from the pericardial space, increasing the patient's survival time.[2] Tissue perfusion, maintenance of cardiopulmonary function, and comfort are achieved by the administration of supplemental oxygen.

## Nursing Diagnoses, Desired Patient Outcomes, and Nursing Interventions

For nursing diagnoses, desired patient outcomes, and nursing interventions in the care of the patient with cardiac tamponade, refer to the Care Plan in Table 59–1.

## Case Presentation

The following case study illustrates the classic signs and symptoms, diagnostic studies, and therapy related to neoplastic cardiac tamponade. Although not all patients present with every symptom mentioned in this particular case, clinical manifestations such as dyspnea on exertion, tachycardia, ECG changes, jugular vein distention, and pulsus paradoxus are almost universally present.[5]

Ms. C. is a 55-year-old woman with metastatic adenocarcinoma of the lung. She is admitted to the hospital complaining of shortness of breath, dyspnea on exertion, and right lateral chest pain. She is

**TABLE 59–1. CARE PLAN FOR THE PATIENT WITH NEOPLASTIC CARDIAC TAMPONADE**

| Nursing Diagnoses | Desired Patient Outcomes | Nursing Interventions | Rationales |
|---|---|---|---|
| ***Nursing Diagnosis #1***<br>Alteration in cardiac output: decreased, related to:<br>1. Elevated intrapericardial pressure. | Patient will:<br>1. Maintain hemodynamic stability:<br>• Heart rate: <100 beats/minute.<br>• CVP: 0–8 mmHg.<br>• PAP: <25 mmHg.<br>• PCWP: 8–12 mmHg.<br>• CO: 4–8 liters/minute. | • Assess heart rate, and blood pressure q 15 minutes until stable. Note pulse pressure difference.<br>• Assess for pulses paradoxus with each blood pressure.<br>• Assess for neck vein distention with the head of bed elevated 60° q 2 hr.<br>• Assess dependent areas for edema q 4 hr.<br>• Assess hemodynamic pressure measurements q 1 hr (CO and PCWP q 4 hr).<br>• Administer inotropic agents as prescribed and monitor response.<br>• Administer fluid volume replacements as prescribed and monitor response. | • Cardiac output can become significantly compromised as fluid accumulates within the pericardium. |
| | | • Assess heart and breath sounds q 1 hr. | • As fluid accumulates within the pericardium, heart sounds become distant on auscultation. |
| | | • Measure urine output q 1 hr.<br>• Palpate peripheral pulses for presence and strength q 4 hr.<br>• Maintain patient in low Fowler's position.<br>• Assist with pericardiocentesis.<br>• Assess hemodynamic changes after pericardiocentesis.<br>• Monitor for cardiac irregularities related to needle placement. | • Reduced cardiac output compromises renal perfusion, reducing glomerular filtration. |
| ***Nursing Diagnosis #2***<br>Impaired gas exchange, related to:<br>1. Decreased cardiopulmonary perfusion. | Patient will:<br>1. Maintain effective cardiopulmonary function.<br>A. Stable arterial blood gases:<br>• pH 7.35–7.45.<br>• $PaCO_2$ 35–45 mmHg.<br>• $PaO_2$ >60 mmHg.<br>2. Remain oriented to person, place, and date. | • Administer oxygen as prescribed.<br>• Assess blood pressure and heart rate q 15 minutes until stable.<br>• Assess for evidence of respiratory distress. | • Mediastinal fluid accumulation can compromise lung expansion and respiratory mechanics. |
| | | • Perform neurological assessment as it relates to mental status and level of consciousness.<br>• Assess arterial blood gas results. | • Changes in mental status and orientation may reflect decreased cerebral perfusion. |

| | | | |
|---|---|---|---|
| ***Nursing Diagnosis #3***<br>Alteration in fluid and electrolytes, related to:<br>1. Decreased renal perfusion. | Patient will:<br>1. Have a balanced fluid intake and output.<br>2. Maintain serum electrolytes, BUN, creatinine and total protein within the physiologically normal range. | • Measure intake, output and specific gravity q 1 hr.<br>• Assess skin turgor q shift.<br>• Palpate for peripheral edema q 4 hr.<br>• Assess for Kussmaul's sign q 2 hr.<br>• Auscultate breath sounds q 1 hr.<br>• Daily weights.<br>• Assess related lab work q 4 hr or as reported. | • Fluid overload may enhance fluid accumulation within the pericardium, further complicating the patient's clinical status.<br>• Crackles (rales) on auscultation may reflect pulmonary congestion.<br>• Daily weight is best measure of fluid status. |
| ***Nursing Diagnosis #4***<br>Fear related to:<br>1. Severity of illness. | Patient/significant others will:<br>1. Verbalize fears and concerns. | • Assess knowledge regarding condition.<br>• Encourage verbalization of fears.<br>• Help patient/significant others identify resources.<br>• Refer to chaplain, social service, for additional support. | • Patient/significant others may have preconceived perceptions of cancer.<br>• Myths about cancer may include that it is a "death sentence"; extremely painful or mutilating; or that it is contagious. |
| ***Nursing Diagnosis #5***<br>Anxiety related to:<br>1. Decreased cerebral oxygenation.<br>2. Underlying diagnosis of cancer. | Patient will:<br>1. Verbalize and demonstrate feelings of relaxation. | • Assess for signs and symptoms of anxiety.<br>• Monitor oxygen therapy for effectiveness.<br>• Orient patient to relaxation techniques.<br>• Remain with patient during stressful periods; provide a "listening ear."<br>• Medicate as prescribed and monitor response. | • Anxiety can further compromise respiratory status; tachypnea associated with anxiety can significantly compromise alveolar ventilation. |
| ***Nursing Diagnosis #6***<br>Alteration in comfort:<br>1. Dyspnea and chest pain. | Patient will:<br>1. Verbalize feeling pain-free.<br>2. Exhibit eupneic pattern of breathing. | • Administer pain medications as prescribed and monitor response.<br>• Monitor output from pericardiocentesis and evaluate effect on symptoms.<br>• Monitor output from pericardial catheter.<br>• Administer oxygen as prescribed.<br>• Position patient in low Fowler's. | • Goal is to prevent pain. Analgesics should be given in adequate amounts and at appropriate intervals to prevent recurrence or worsening of pain.<br>• Acknowledge that patients are the authority on their pain. |

*(continued)*

## TABLE 59-1. CARE PLAN FOR THE PATIENT WITH NEOPLASTIC CARDIAC TAMPONADE *(Continued)*

| Nursing Diagnoses | Desired Patient Outcomes | Nursing Interventions | Rationales |
|---|---|---|---|
| ***Nursing Diagnosis #7***<br>Knowledge deficit, related to:<br>1. Emergency procedures. | Patient and/or significant other will:<br>1. Verbalize understanding of procedures such as pericardiocentesis, pericardial window, and/or pericardial catheter. | • Clarify/reinforce explanations of procedures for patient/significant other.<br>• Assess patient's/significant other's understanding of procedure. | |

restless and apprehensive. Her skin is cool, moist, and pale. Further assessment reveals hypotension with a narrowing pulse pressure and a pulsus paradoxus of 22 mmHg. Her neck veins are engorged, and she has a positive Kussmaul's sign. She is tachycardic with weak peripheral pulses and distant heart sounds.

Shortly after she is admitted to the Intensive Care Unit, a flow-directed balloon-tipped catheter is inserted to provide continuous monitoring of her hemodynamic status. The nurse caring for Ms. C. finds that she has an elevated right atrial pressure, elevated pulmonary artery systolic and diastolic pressures during expiration, an increased PCWP, and a decreased CO. The ECG reveals electrical alternans of the P waves and QRS complexes and ST–T wave changes. She is scheduled for an echocardiogram, which shows a collapsed right ventricle and confirms the suspected diagnosis of cardiac tamponade. Ms. C.'s low CO is treated with volume expanders and inotropic agents in preparation for a pericardiocentesis.

The pericardiocentesis is performed for 2 reasons: it confirms the diagnosis of cardiac tamponade, and it relieves the pressure around the heart, allowing for increased ventricular filling. During the procedure, 850 ml of grossly bloody pericardial fluid is obtained. A specimen for cytologic identification is sent and reveals the presence of malignant cells consistent with adenocarcinoma of the lung. This confirms a neoplastic etiology, allowing for appropriate therapy to be initiated. A pericardial window is performed, at which time a portion of the fifth rib is removed. This procedure allows for a decrease in pressure around the heart. A pericardial catheter is inserted for instillation of thiotepa (used as a sclerosing agent and a cytotoxic drug) and for continued drainage of pericardial fluid.

Because the nurse assessed this patient quickly, appropriate measures were taken. Ms. C.'s vital signs returned to normal within several hours, and her complaints subsided almost immediately. Although the therapy instituted did not change the overall prognosis of her disease, it allowed her to continue to receive further palliative therapy (see Table 59–1 for nursing care considerations).

## SEPTIC SHOCK

### Etiology and Pathophysiology

Septic shock is an oncologic emergency, which must be recognized and treated in the early stages. Neoplasms, immunosuppressive therapy, and invasive procedures make a patient more prone to developing septic shock. Sepsis often begins with a bacterial invasion secondary to a major infection such as pneumonia or peritonitis.[6] Although the gram-negative and gram-positive organisms are responsible for the majority of cases of septic shock, viral, fungal, and protozoal infections may also be responsible.[7]

Septic shock is associated with systemic vasodilation leading to a decreased CO and tissue perfusion. The end result is cellular hypoxia, acidosis, and the potential for death. The patient initially responds to this process with mild hypotension, increased CO, hyperthermia or hypothermia, chills, mental confusion, tachycardia, and tachypnea. As the process progresses, capillary leakage and vasoconstriction occur, leaving the patient with cool skin, peripheral edema, and oliguria. Without treatment, the condition worsens, causing further hypovolemia and the formation of microthrombi. At this point, the patient appears cold and clammy, has severe hypotension, and may develop multiple organ failure exhibited by adult respiratory distress syndrome (ARDS), renal failure, and disseminated intravascular coagulation (DIC). (For a more detailed discussion of the pathophysiology underlying septic shock, see Chap. 66.)

### Patients at Risk

Any patient who succumbs to an overwhelming infection is at risk for developing septic shock. However, patients with cancer are especially prone because of a variety of factors that compromise immune function. These include such factors as altered mucous membranes and skin integrity secondary to invasive lines, chemotherapy, radiation therapy, and predominantly surgical intervention. Fistula formation can potentially occur in patients who have had abdominal surgery as a result of poor healing, tumor invasion, or a past history of radiotherapy to the abdomen.

In addition, alterations in total white blood cell counts predispose patients with cancer to infection. Likely causes of myelosuppression in patients with cancer include malignant tumor invasion of the bone marrow (often seen with leukemias, lymphomas, and certain solid tumors) and bone marrow suppression from systemic chemotherapy and radiation therapy to the bone marrow reserves in the iliac crest, spine, or sternum. The total neutrophil count is an important determinant in assessing infection risk. (See Chap. 66 for other risk factors and laboratory data related to sepsis.) Cancers commonly treated by chemotherapy and radiotherapy include lung, breast, and colon cancer. Table 59–2 lists some cytotoxic agents that cause immunosuppression. (See Chap. 56 for a brief review of some immunosuppressant agents.)

### Diagnosis

Once it has been determined that a shock state is in existence (i.e., significantly decreased blood pressure and cardiac output, tachycardia, and poor tis-

TABLE 59-2
**Cytotoxic Agents Causing Immunosuppression**

| |
|---|
| Busulfan |
| Methotrexate |
| Doxorubicin (Adriamycin) |
| Cisplatin |
| Etoposide (VP-16) |
| 5-Fluorouracil (5-FU) |
| Cyclophosphamide (Cytoxan) |
| Vinblastine sulfate (Velban) |
| Mitomycin |

sue perfusion), the type of shock must be identified based on its underlying etiology and presenting symptomatology (e.g., cardiogenic, neurogenic, anaphylactic, hypovolemic, or septic). The diagnosis of septic shock is based on a careful history and physical examination. Diagnosis, age, prior surgery, and other treatment modality are essential factors to be considered. Their presence may constitute a significant risk for the occurrence of septic shock. Other data to be evaluated include the white blood cell count, coagulation studies, body temperature, and the results of blood cultures.

Vital signs, hemodynamic measurements including cardiac output, pulmonary artery wedge pressures, and urine output are monitored frequently along with assessment of peripheral blood flow and tissue perfusion. The patient's oxygenation status is assessed including mental status and arterial blood gases (ABGs). The patient is continuously monitored for signs of respiratory failure (see Chap. 31).

## Treatment

The source of the infection must be identified rapidly so that appropriate antibiotic therapy can be administered promptly.[6] Efforts are made to conserve the patient's energy so that vital functions are maintained despite the anaerobic metabolic state resulting from cellular hypoxia. Limiting activity, promoting rest, and reducing environmental stimuli may be helpful in this regard. Ventilation may need to be supported by a mechanical ventilator to conserve the patient's energy and improve ABGs.

Intravascular fluid volume is replaced based on the PCWP and urine output. Blood pressure may be maintained by administering an inotropic and/or vasoactive agent such as dopamine, dobutamine, or isoproterenol.[8] Temperature regulation is managed by using a warming or cooling blanket, iced saline gastric lavages, or ice packs to the groin. If complications such as ARDS, disseminated intravascular coagulation (DIC), or acidosis appear, they are treated accordingly.

The best therapy when dealing with septic shock is prevention, or the recognition of signs and symptoms of septic shock early in its course. Preventative measures may include:

- Strict handwashing technique.
- Identifying patients at risk.
- Using meticulous aseptic technique.
- Teaching patients and families how to care for wounds and tubes and the importance of handwashing.
- Assessing a patient's baseline mental and physical status so that subtle changes can be noted.
- Being alert to the signs and symptoms of impending shock so that they can be recognized and treated early.

## Nursing Diagnoses, Desired Patient Outcomes, and Nursing Interventions

For nursing diagnoses, desired patient outcomes, and nursing interventions in the care of the patient in septic shock, refer to the Care Plan in Table 59-3. For a detailed discussion of septic shock, see Chapter 66. For nursing diagnoses, patient outcomes, and nursing interventions in the care of the patient with septic shock, see also the Care Plan in Table 66-4.

The following case study includes some of the classic signs and symptoms, diagnostic studies, and therapy related to septic shock.

## Case Presentation

Mrs. G. is a 78-year-old woman with adenocarcinoma of the colon with metastasis to the liver. She is admitted to the hospital 2 years after diagnosis with a persistent cough, chills, and urinary frequency. She has decreased breath sounds, a systolic pressure of 70 mmHg, a pulse of 135/minute, respirations of 30/minute and a temperature of 36.9°. She has 3 plus bilateral pretibial pitting edema. Her peripheral pulses are barely palpable. Her white blood cell count is 13,600/$mm^3$ with a normal differential. Her hemoglobin is 12 g/100 ml; platelets are 60,000/mm; prothrombin time is 31 seconds; partial thromboplastin time is 56 seconds; and arterial blood gasses are pH 7.47, $PCO_2$22 mmHg, and $PO_2$ 82 mmHg.

Several months ago she had been hospitalized with malignant ascites, at which time a paracentesis was done and a subclavian line inserted. She had a sigmoidcolectomy with a resulting colostomy and was receiving 5-Fluorouracil by an Infusaport. Mrs. G. has a high risk for developing an infection, which could lead to septic shock because of her compromised immune function, invasive lines, and the antineoplastic drugs she is on.

To compensate for her falling blood pressure and platelet count, she is hydrated with normal saline and transfused with fresh frozen plasma and plate-

## TABLE 59-3. CARE PLAN FOR THE PATIENT WITH SEPTIC SHOCK

| Nursing Diagnoses | Desired Patient Outcomes | Nursing Interventions | Rationales |
|---|---|---|---|
| ***Nursing Diagnosis #1***<br>Alteration in cardiac output: decreased, related to:<br>1. Systemic arterial hypotension associated with vasodilation of vasculature. | Patient will:<br>1. Maintain hemodynamic stability.<br>• Heart rate 60–80/minutes; rhythm regular sinus.<br>• Blood pressure within 10 mmHg of baseline.<br>• CVP 0–8 mmHg.<br>• PCWP 8–12 mmHg.<br>2. Maintain hourly urine output greater than 30 ml/hr.<br>3. Maintain intact neurological function:<br>• Mental status alert; oriented to person, place, and date. | • Assess heart rate and blood pressure q 15 minutes until stable.<br>• Assess dependent areas for edema q 4 hr.<br>• Assess hemodynamic pressure measurements q 1 hr (CO, PCWP, q 4 hr).<br>• Administer inotropic and/or vasopressor agents as prescribed and monitor response to therapy.<br>• Administer fluid volume replacements as prescribed.<br>• Measure urine output q 1 hr.<br>• Palpate peripheral pulses for presence and strength q 4 hr. | • Signs/symptoms of early septic shock reflect the body's compensatory response to reduced perfusion: There is increase in heart rate and peripheral vascular resistance.<br>• Monitoring cardiac output and PCWP is essential to evaluate fluid needs, and the patient's response to therapy.<br>• Monitoring urine output hourly is essential to determine status of renal perfusion. |
| ***Nursing Diagnosis #2***<br>Impaired gas exchange, related to:<br>1. Hypoxic respiratory failure. | Patient will:<br>1. Maintain a $PaO_2 > 60$ mmHg. | • Assess mental status and level of consciousness.<br>• Assess ABGs as prescribed.<br>• Provide frequent rest periods.<br>• Follow appropriate procedure for endotracheal suctioning.<br>• Administer oxygen therapy as prescribed.<br>• Monitor patient for acute respiratory failure. | • Changes in mental status and neurological function may reflect decreased cerebral perfusion related to reduced cardiac output. |
| ***Nursing Diagnosis #3***<br>Alteration in tissue perfusion, related to:<br>1. Capillary leakage and vasoconstriction. | Patient will:<br>1. Maintain a viable peripheral circulatory status.<br>• Easily palpable pulses.<br>• Brisk capillary refill.<br>• Usual skin color, absence of mottling and cyanosis. | • Assess peripheral pulses q 4 hr.<br>• Assess for peripheral edema q 4 hr.<br>• Maintain hydration to compensate for decreased CO.<br>• Assess skin for color and warmth.<br>• Instruct patient to avoid positions that compromise blood flow. | • Altered endothelial permeability allows blood albumin to leak into the interstitium reducing the capillary oncotic pressure and predisposing to peripheral edema. |

*(continued)*

**TABLE 59–3. CARE PLAN FOR THE PATIENT WITH SEPTIC SHOCK *(Continued)***

| Nursing Diagnoses | Desired Patient Outcomes | Nursing Interventions | Rationales |
|---|---|---|---|
| ***Nursing Diagnosis #4***<br>Activity intolerance related to:<br>1. Cellular hypoxia. | Patient will:<br>1. Conserve energy for vital functions.<br>• Verbalize feeling rested.<br>• Demonstrate relaxation techniques. | • Assess patient's vital signs related to activity.<br>• Assist patient with all activities to conserve energy.<br>• Explain importance of energy conservation to patient/significant others. | |
| ***Nursing Diagnosis #5***<br>Knowledge deficit related to:<br>1. Infection control. | Patient/significant others will:<br>1. State measures effective in reducing the risk of infection. | • Instruct patient/significant others on proper infection control measures.<br>• Follow procedures for patient on WBC precautions. | • For detailed information on infection control refer to the following:<br>– Chapter 56, Table 56–1, Nursing Diagnoses #1, #2, and #5.<br>– Chapter 49, Table 49–7 for the nursing diagnosis: Potential for Infection. |
| ***Nursing Diagnosis #6***<br>Alteration in body temperature, related to:<br>1. Impaired temperature regulation. | Patient will:<br>1. Maintain a core body temperature within normal limits. | • Assess for hypothermia/hyperthermia q 1 hr.<br>• Alter the environment to control temperature.<br>• Administer antipyretics as prescribed and monitor response. | |
| ***Nursing Diagnosis #7***<br>Infection related to:<br>1. Immunosuppressed state.<br>2. Altered nutritional intake. | Patient will:<br>1. Be free from the clinical manifestations of infection.<br>• Baseline body temperature (37°).<br>• WBC within acceptable range.<br>• Negative blood cultures.<br>• Chest x-ray at baseline. | • Monitor temperature q 1 hr.<br>• Monitor WBC and report abnormalities.<br>• Obtain and monitor cultures when indicated.<br>• Assess for additional signs of sepsis, i.e., tachycardia, hypotension, changes in CO, tachypnea, altered mental status, DIC.<br>• Administer antibiotics as prescribed and monitor response.<br>• Use aseptic technique as indicated.<br>• Restrict visitors and number of personnel coming in contact with patient. | |

lets. Because a positive culture has not been obtained yet, she is started on broad-spectrum antibiotics. A dopamine infusion is started to increase her CO, and a Foley catheter is inserted to provide accurate urine measurements.

As she becomes more hypoxic and hypovolemic, Mrs. G. becomes increasingly lethargic, her nailbeds become cyanotic, and her urine output and blood pressure begin to fall.

A flow-directed balloon-tipped catheter is inserted to monitor continuously her hemodynamic status. Her CO and PCWP are below normal from the massive vasodilation. Her respiratory status continues to deteriorate, requiring intubation and mechanical ventilation. In order to maintain a $PO_2$ of 60 mmHg, the ventilator is set at an $FiO_2$ of 70% and 10 cm of positive and expiratory pressure (PEEP).

The rapid assessment and implementation of nursing and physician orders led to the stabilization of Mrs. G. (See Tables 59–3 and 66–4 for nursing care considerations.)

## SPINAL CORD COMPRESSION

### Etiology and Pathophysiology

Compression of the spinal cord from a neoplasm in the epidural space is classified as an oncologic emergency because a successful patient outcome depends on *accurate* and *rapid* assessment, diagnosis, and treatment. Cancer-induced spinal cord compression differs from trauma-induced injury not only in the etiology of the emergency, but also in the incidence of occurrence and the survival rates. Cancer-induced spinal cord compression occurs more often than traumatic injury and has a lower survival rate.[9]

Spinal cord compression can occur when a tumor reaches the extradural space by direct extension from vertebral bony metastases, by growth through the intravertebral foramina, or by hematogenous spread. The neurologic symptoms associated with the compression are related to vascular compromise, ischemia, hemorrhaging, or direct compression by the tumor.[10] Any portion of the spinal cord may be invaded; however, the most commonly seen sites are in the thoracic and lumbar region, particularly $T_8$, $T_{12}$ and $L_5$.[11] The location of spinal metastases can be summarized as 10% in the cervical spine, 70% in the thoracic spine, and 20% in the lumbosacral region.[10]

### Patients at Risk

Spinal cord compression is one of the most common neurologic complications of metastatic cancer. Approximately 5% of patients with systemic

TABLE 59–4
**Incidence of Spinal Cord Compression by Site of Primary Tumor[10]**

| Site | Percentage |
|---|---|
| Lung | 16 |
| Breast | 12 |
| Unknown | 11 |
| Lymphoma | 11 |
| Myeloma | 9 |
| Sarcoma | 8 |
| Prostate | 7 |
| Kidney | 6 |
| GI | 4 |
| Thyroid | 3 |

cancer have epidural metastasis resulting in spinal cord compression.[9] The cancer most commonly associated with spinal compression is lung cancer. In one large study, it accounted for 20%–30% of all cases.[12] In women, spinal cord compression is associated most commonly with metastatic breast cancer with an incidence of 70% documented in advanced disease.[11] Table 59–4 lists the incidence of spinal cord compression by primary tumor.

The *clinical* presentation depends on the level at which the spinal cord is compressed, rather than the location of the primary tumor. Patients generally present late in their metastatic disease. Neurologic symptoms may be what initially brings the patient into the hospital for evaluation, especially in the case of rapidly growing metastatic tumors.[13] Table 59–5 lists the most common symptoms associated with spinal cord compression.

Back pain is the initial symptom in the majority of patients. It can be described as local or may radiate to the chest, abdomen, or extremities.[10] It may be described as persistent and intense and is often made worse by movement. Coughing or Valsalva's maneuver may also aggravate the pain.[14] The pain may be worse when lying down. The patient, therefore, may often find it more comfortable to sleep sitting up.

Other symptoms commonly encountered include weakness, autonomic dysfunctions, and sensory dysfunctions. The location and extent of weakness depend on the level and degree of spinal cord compression. An initial complaint of unilateral weakness may progress to paraplegia. Autonomic

TABLE 59–5
**Symptoms Associated with Spinal Cord Compression**

| |
|---|
| Back Pain |
| Weakness |
| Paraplegia |
| Autonomic dysfunction |
| Sensory loss |

dysfunctions, which include urinary retention or hesitancy, bowel and bladder incontinence, and sexual impotence, are other common symptoms of a compressed spinal cord (see Tables 12–10 and 12–11). Sensory dysfunctions may include loss of light touch, pain, and thermal sensation. There may also be loss of proprioception and deep pressure. (See Chap. 7 for details regarding neurologic assessment.)

## Diagnosis

Early detection and treatment of spinal cord compression are instrumental in maintaining the patient's current neurologic status and/or preventing further nerve damage. Patients with known or suspected malignancies complaining of back pain should have spinal cord compression ruled out, even if the neurologic assessment is normal.[15] Diagnosis is confirmed with skeletal x-ray, bone scan, computed tomographic (CT) scan, myelogram, or, most recently, magnetic resonance imagery (MRI). The MRI is felt to be the best noninvasive study for diagnosing the location and extent of spinal cord injury.[16]

## Prognosis

Prognosis is determined, for the most part, by the patient's status prior to receiving any treatment for the compression. For example, if the patient is ambulatory when first diagnosed with spinal cord compression, the chance of maintaining an ambulatory status after therapy is 60%.[10] If the patient is paraplegic at diagnosis, there is only a 7% chance that ambulation can be regained after therapy.[10] Other prognostic indicators include how rapidly the neurologic symptoms appear, whether there is loss of sphincter control, and where the compression is located.[10,17] The median survival time for patients with spinal cord compression is 40 days.[12]

## Treatment

The choice of treatment for spinal cord compression consists of corticosteroid administration, surgery alone, radiotherapy alone, or surgery followed by radiotherapy. Therapy may be aimed at either preventing neurologic complications or treating symptoms already present. The type of therapy selected often depends on the type of tumor, what level of the cord is compressed, and how rapidly the symptoms appear.[12,17]

The urgency of the therapy may depend on where the cord is compressed. For example, a cervical compression would demand emergency therapy to prevent respiratory paralysis. Early treatment is essential in order to prevent neurologic damage. Although therapy may alleviate pain, it rarely corrects any preexisting neurologic impairment.[12]

## Nursing Diagnoses, Desired Patient Outcomes, and Nursing Interventions

Nursing diagnoses, patient outcomes, and nursing interventions in the care of the patient with spinal cord compression are presented in the Care Plan in Table 59–6. Table 12–7 presents essential information related to nursing care of the patient with spinal cord injury.

## Case Presentation

The following case study illustrates how a patient with a spinal cord compression may present and be diagnosed and treated.

Mr. K. is a 62-year-old man with cancer of the colon. He is admitted to the hospital, ambulating, with rapidly increasing numbness in his legs of 18 hours' duration. His history includes a diagnosis of cancer several years ago, a colon resection, and treatment with chemotherapy. The cancer recurred several months later. He has had severe pain, which has been managed with oral narcotics.

Mr. K. is well-nourished and is in no apparent distress. He has marked weakness of his lower extremities, which is more severe on the left side. He has a moderate decrease in pain sensation around $T^{10}$. There are no reports of incontinence at this time.

An emergency myelogram reveals a complete block at $T^{10}$ with partial obstruction of the lumbar region. An emergency radiotherapy consult is obtained, and radiotherapy is started immediately along with high-dose steroids to decrease the inflammation around the spinal cord. Mr. K.'s neurologic and pain status are evaluated frequently for any changes.

Mr. K.'s condition remains stable with gradual return of his motor and sensory function. He is discharged, ambulating, and treated for his recurring colon cancer on an outpatient basis. (See Tables 59–6 and 12–7 for nursing care considerations.)

# SYNDROME OF INAPPROPRIATE SECRETION OF ANTIDIURETIC HORMONE (SIADH)

## Etiology and Pathology

This syndrome of inappropriate secretion of antidiuretic hormone (SIADH) implies that there is continuous release of antidiuretic hormone (ADH) that

**TABLE 59–6. CARE PLAN FOR THE PATIENT WITH SPINAL CORD COMPRESSION**

| Nursing Diagnoses | Desired Patient Outcomes | Nursing Interventions | Rationales |
|---|---|---|---|
| ***Nursing Diagnosis #1***<br>Potential for injury, related to:<br>1. Sensory deficits. | Patient will:<br>1. Remain free from injury while hospitalized. | • Keep siderails up at all times.<br>• Have call light and personal items within patient's reach.<br>• Instruct patient to call for assistance if desiring to get out of bed.<br>• Assess level of consciousness as indicated.<br>• Assess sensory level q shift. | • Patients receiving narcotics for pain relief may have an altered sensorium.<br>• Loss of sensation places patient at increased risk of injury. |
| ***Nursing Diagnosis #2***<br>Alteration in comfort: Acute pain, related to:<br>1. Damaged spinal cord. | Patient will:<br>1. Utilize measures effective in managing pain.<br>2. Verbalize relief from pain.<br>3. Present relaxed facies and overall demeanor. | • Assess patient for intensity, radiation, and character of pain.<br>• Inform patient and/or significant others of available methods of pain relief.<br>• Administer pain medication as requested and prescribed. Assess for effect in 10–20 minutes.<br>• Explain importance of pain medication in patient's progress.<br>• Collaborate with physician and patient in altering pain medication as needed.<br>• Suggest alternate positions.<br>• Log roll when needed.<br>• Position on eggcrate mattress or other pressure relief device. | • Pain associated with spinal cord compression may be especially severe.<br>• Patient should be encouraged to request pain medication early on instead of waiting until the pain becomes unbearable. |
| ***Nursing Diagnosis #3***<br>Alteration in bowel and urinary elimination: incontinence and/or constipation, related to:<br>1. Nerve disruption.<br>2. Immobility.<br>3. Narcotic administration. | Patient will:<br>1. Maintain regular bowel elimination without constipation or fecal impaction. | • Explain need for scheduled bowel elimination program.<br>• Monitor intake and output q shift.<br>• Instruct patient on need for good hydration.<br>• Force fluids as necessary unless contraindicated. | • It is essential for the patient to establish and maintain regular bowel elimination. The patient's usual bowel habits should be assessed and incorporated into daily schedule.<br>• Patient/family should be able to explain the importance of hydration and diet high in fiber, in terms of overall bowel function.<br>• Patient/family should be aware of signs and |

*(continued)*

**TABLE 59–6. CARE PLAN FOR THE PATIENT WITH SPINAL CORD COMPRESSION** *(Continued)*

| Nursing Diagnoses | Desired Patient Outcomes | Nursing Interventions | Rationales |
|---|---|---|---|
| ***Nursing Diagnosis #3 (cont.)*** | | | symptoms suggestive of constipation: Abdominal fullness or distention, loss of appetite, nausea, headache, feeling of fullness in rectum.<br>• Appearance of diarrheal stool may suggest the presence of fecal impaction. |
| | | • Administer stool softeners/laxatives as needed and prescribed.<br>• Consult dietician to increase fiber in foods. | |
| | 2. Adhere to a bladder control program. | • Offer fluids to patient q 2 hr.<br>• Offer bedpan or assist patient to bathroom q 2 hr. | |
| | | • Palpate bladder for distention. | • Urinary retention can predispose to infection. |
| | | • Explain importance of bladder program. | • Patient/significant others should be able to check for urinary retention of which the patient may not be aware. |
| ***Nursing Diagnosis #4***<br>Potential impairment of skin integrity, related to:<br>1. Decreased mobility. | Patient will:<br>1. Be free from skin breakdown. | • Inspect patient's skin integrity q shift. | • Loss of mobility and sensation, immunosuppressed state, and altered nutrition place patient at greater risk of skin breakdown.<br>• Meticulous surveillance of pressure areas is essential to maintain skin integrity. |
| | | • Encourage/assist patient to turn q 2 hr while in bed.<br>• Apply lotion to dry skin q shift.<br>• Apply eggcrate mattress or sheepskin to bed.<br>• Force fluids as necessary unless contraindicated. | |

| | | | |
|---|---|---|---|
| ***Nursing Diagnosis #5***<br>Impaired physical mobility, related to:<br>1. Motor neuron damage. | Patient will:<br>1. Maintain muscle tone and coordination.<br>• Demonstrate active range of motion of all extremities.<br>• Verbalize importance of exercise and avoidance of fatigue. | • Inspect muscles of arms and legs for atrophy and involuntary movements.<br>• Assess for muscle coordination.<br>• Perform active and/or passive ROM exercises to all extremities qid.<br>• Encourage activity as prescribed/tolerated.<br>• Collaborate with Rehabilitation Department regarding mobility and an individualized exercise plan. | • A baseline assessment should be performed to establish the patient's physical capabilities.<br>• Actions should be performed to maintain muscle strength, and mobility.<br>• Family participation in exercise regimen should be encouraged. |
| ***Nursing Diagnosis #6***<br>Alteration in self-concept, related to:<br>1. Incontinence and immobility. | Patient and/or significant other will:<br>1. Begin accepting the change in usual functions.<br>• Verbalizes feelings.<br>• Initiates discussion of disease and impact on lifestyle. | • Explain to patient and/or significant others reasons for changes in muscle control.<br>• Assess patient's/significant other's usual coping mechanisms, encouraging positive ones.<br>• Encourage patient and/or significant other to discuss their feelings regarding these changes. | • Recognizing one's feelings and emotions is the first step in dealing with them.<br>• Observing patient/family/significant other interactions may assist in determining strengths and effective coping capability. |

cannot be explained by normal stimuli. Normal or appropriate stimuli for secretion of ADH include:[18]

- Increased extracellular fluid osmolality, which may occur when a person becomes dehydrated or given large volumes of hyperosmolar solutions.
- Decreased plasma volume as related to hemorrhage or capillary leakage.
- Reduced central blood pressure as may be seen in patients in cardiogenic or septic shock.

(For a detailed discussion of the physiology and pathophysiology of ADH, see Chap. 16).

The end result of SIADH is excessive water retention, decreased serum osmolality, hyponatremia and increased urine sodium and urine osmolality.[19,20]

If SIADH is not discovered and treated early, the complications of hyponatremia and water intoxication may lead to severe neurologic complications that may ultimately end in coma and death. Many diseases and medications are associated with the development of SIADH. *Cancer-related* causes are listed in Table 59–7.

It is believed that some neoplasms synthesize, store, and release ADH identical to the ADH produced in the hypothalamus.[18,21] However, even in patients with cancer, most cases of SIADH are attributed to "abnormal regulation of the hypothalamo-neurohypophyseal system."[20]

The mechanism by which drugs produce SIADH is not known. Some drugs may increase hypothalmic ADH production and release. Others may act on the renal tubules, increasing their sensitivity to circulating ADH. Some cytotoxic agents (listed in Table 59–7) may produce SIADH by acting either directly on the osmoreceptors in the supraoptic nucleus of the hypothalamus (see Fig. 16–1), or indirectly, by causing nausea, which stimulates ADH secretion.[18,20]

Regardless of the underlying cause of SIADH, patients experience defects in the normal feedback mechanism of ADH. Therefore, patients become hypervolemic with resulting dilutional hyponatremia and hypo-osmolality. As the kidneys conserve water, there is an increase in the urine sodium and urine osmolality. The plasma volume expands, which increases blood pressure. As water retention progresses, patients demonstrate signs and symptoms of water intoxication (listed in Table 59–8). Serum sodium drops from the hemodilution and increased renal excretion of sodium resulting in signs of hyponatremia (listed in Table 59–9). In both cases, the symptoms are related to how low the serum sodium is and how quickly it is restored to appropriate physiologic range.[22]

TABLE 59–7
**Cancer Related Causes of SIADH[18,19,20,21]**

| Carcinomas | Cytotoxic Drugs |
|---|---|
| Lung | Vincristine |
| Pancreas | Vinblastine |
| Duodenum | Cyclophosphamide |
| Prostate | |
| Bladder | |
| Thymoma | |
| Lymphoma | |

TABLE 59–8
**Signs and Symptoms of Water Intoxication[19]**

| | |
|---|---|
| Anorexia | Confusion |
| Nausea | Hypothermia |
| Vomiting | Aberrant respirations |
| Diarrhea | Coma |

## Patients at Risk

Cancer-related factors responsible for SIADH are outlined in Table 59–7. Other causes of SIADH are indirectly related to cancer, such as severe pain, emotional stress, nausea, and morphine administration. Other related factors seen in the oncology patient that can cause SIADH are central nervous system disorders, such as infection or seizures, and pulmonary disorders, such as pneumonia. (See Chap. 16 for further explanations of how these disorders cause SIADH and additional conditions associated with the syndrome.)

## Diagnosis

Diagnosis of SIADH depends on several criteria being present (Table 59–10). The syndrome should be suspected in any patient who is hyponatremic and has urine that is hypertonic in relation to plasma osmolality.[23]

A *water loading* test may also be used to diagnose SIADH. The water loading test is initiated by giving the patient 20–25 ml water/kg body weight over 15–20 minutes. Urine is collected and measured hourly for 5 hours. Patients with SIADH have concentrated urine versus the normal person who will excrete 80% of the fluid given by the fifth hour.[23]

TABLE 59–9
**Signs and Symptoms of Hyponatremia[22]**

| | |
|---|---|
| Headache | Nausea |
| Lethargy | Vomiting |
| Mental confusion | Seizures |
| Anorexia | Coma |
| Muscle cramps | Death |
| Weakness | |

TABLE 59-10
**Diagnosis of SIADH[18,20]**

| |
|---|
| Hyponatremia. |
| Decreased serum osmolality. |
| Inappropriately increased urine osmolality. |
| Increased urine sodium. |
| Normal renal, cardiac, and adrenal function. |
| No known defect in circulating volume or free water generation. |

Another diagnostic test includes measuring serum ADH levels. Serum levels of ADH can be measured with the use of radioassay.

## Treatment

Before treatment is begun, one should consider the cause of SIADH, the degree of water intoxication, and, subsequently, the extent of hyponatremia.[18]

Treatment of SIADH includes a free water restriction with approximately 500–1000 ml fluid/day.[19,21,23] In mild cases, water restriction may be all that is required. In more severe cases of water intoxication, when confusion, seizures, or coma is present, hypertonic (5%) saline solution may be given to restore plasma osmolality and serum sodium.[22,23] It is possible, however, that this effect is only transient because the sodium may continue to be excreted in the urine.[20,21] If fluid overload is excessive, the patient is monitored closely for symptoms of congestive heart failure, and diuretics are administered.

When SIADH is the result of a neoplasm, attempts are made to remove the tumor surgically or treat it with radiation or chemotherapy. This treatment may not necessarily cure the cancer, but may alleviate the life-threatening symptoms of SIADH.[23] If SIADH occurs as a result of chemotherapy, therapy may be discontinued or other chemotherapeutic agents may be administered. When SIADH is chronic, as may be the case with oncology patients, drugs that inhibit ADH in addition to a water restriction may be instituted. Demeclocycline is an antibiotic that inhibits the response of the renal tubules to ADH causing nephrogenic diabetes insipidus.[21]

## Nursing Diagnoses, Desired Patient Outcomes, and Nursing Interventions

Nursing diagnoses, desired patient outcomes, and nursing interventions in the care of the patient with inappropriate secretion of ADH are presented in Table 59-11. (See also Tables 16-1, 16-2, and 16-4.)

## Case Presentation

Mr. J. is a 64-year-old man with small cell cancer of the lung. While Mr. J. is being treated with vincristine, he notices that both of his feet and ankles are swollen. He contacts the nurse, reporting symptoms of fatigue, restlessness, and slight confusion. He is admitted to the hospital with a blood pressure of 188/106 mmHg, and a pulse of 94–140/minute with occasional premature atrial contractions. A serum sodium is drawn, and a level of 128 mEq/liter is reported. Careful urine output reveals an average of 18 ml/hour, with a specific gravity of 1.030. Mr. J.'s hematocrit is 32%.

Within hours, his sodium falls to 116 mEq/liter. His nurse immediately places Mr. J. on seizure precautions and explains to his family the importance of maintaining a strict fluid restriction. Mr. J. becomes more confused and begins hallucinating. Within minutes, he experiences a hyponatremic seizure and is diagnosed as having SIADH. He is immediately started on demeclocycline, intravenous (IV) sodium replacement, and IV furosemide. His chemotherapy regimen was revised to eliminate vincristine. The therapy is continued, and he is observed closely for, and instructed to report, additional signs and symptoms of SIADH.

With continued therapy, his sodium returns to 143 mEq/liter, and symptoms of SIADH are temporarily relieved. Before discharge, Mr. J. and his family are instructed regarding the importance of the prescribed therapy, the relationship between his tumor and SIADH, and signs and symptoms of hyponatremia and water intoxication, which must be reported. (See Tables 59-11 and 16-4 for nursing care considerations.)

# SUPERIOR VENA CAVA SYNDROME

## Etiology and Pathophysiology

Superior vena cava syndrome (SVCS) is a clinical diagnosis that refers to either an external or intraluminal compression of the superior vena cava resulting in impaired venous drainage. This condition is observed in patients with bronchogenic and breast cancers, malignant lymphomas, and various other tumors. As the incidence of lung cancer steadily rises, an increase in SVCS is projected. Therefore, knowledge of the signs and symptoms, patients at risk, and therapeutic interventions is necessary to prevent the serious consequences of this syndrome.

The superior vena cava is the principal vein draining the upper portion of the body, which includes the head, neck, arms, and upper trunk. This vessel empties into the right atrium and is surrounded by lymph nodes, pericardium, and the right lung. Because of its low intravascular pres-

**TABLE 59–11. CARE PLAN FOR THE PATIENT WITH SYNDROME OF INAPPROPRIATE ANTIDIURETIC HORMONE SECRETION**

| Nursing Diagnoses | Desired Patient Outcomes | Nursing Interventions | Rationales |
|---|---|---|---|
| ***Nursing Diagnosis #1***<br>Alteration in fluid volume: excess, related to:<br>1. Overproduction of ADH.<br>(Note: See Table 16–4.) | Patient will:<br>1. Be free from signs and symptoms of water intoxication.<br>• Serum sodium 135–145 mEq/liter.<br>• Serum osmolality 285–295 mOsm/kg water. | • Maintain water restriction as indicated.<br>• Daily weights.<br>• Monitor for, and teach patient to report anorexia, nausea, vomiting, or diarrhea.<br>• Assess patient for confusion, hypothermia and aberrant respirations.<br>• Assess for changes in blood pressure and respiratory status.<br>• Administer diuretics and ADH inhibiting drugs as prescribed, and monitor response to therapy. | • Water intake is severely restricted to prevent aggravating state of water intoxication and hyponatremia.<br>• Altered neurological function reflects severe hyponatremia.<br>• Diuretics enhance water excretion. |
| ***Nursing Diagnosis #2***<br>Potential for injury, related to:<br>1. Hyponatremia. | Patient will:<br>1. Be free from hyponatremic-related injury.<br>• Serum sodium: 135–145 mEq/liter.<br>• Serum osmolality: 285–295 mOsm/kg water.<br>• Urine osmolality: 50–1400 mOsm/kg water.<br>• Urine sodium: 80–180 mEq/liter/24 hr.<br>• Urine specific gravity: 1.010–1.025. | • Assess blood work for sodium level.<br>• Monitor for, and teach patient to report, headache, anorexia, muscle cramps, nausea, vomiting, or weakness.<br>• Assess for lethargy, confusion, and seizures.<br>• Administer hypertonic saline solution, as prescribed, and monitor response.<br>• Maintain patient on seizure precautions. | • Serial electrolytes, serum and urine osmolality should guide therapy.<br>• Hypertonic saline increases serum sodium rapidly, and assists to relieve seizures and other neurological dysfunction. |

| | | | |
|---|---|---|---|
| ***Nursing Diagnosis #3***<br>Knowledge deficit regarding SIADH and its treatment. | Patient and/or significant others will:<br>1. Verbalize an understanding of SIADH and its treatment. | • Assess patient's/significant other's knowledge of SIADH.<br>• Explain the relationship between cancer and this syndrome.<br>• Explain the importance of water restrictions.<br>• Teach patient/significant other to report any of the symptoms of SIADH to a health professional.<br>• Explain the importance of taking ADH inhibiting drugs. | • Patient/significant other should be able to explain the relationship between underlying pathophysiology and occurrence of SIADH.<br>• Patient/significant other should be able to describe symptoms reflective of hyponatremia, and actions to take to relieve the problem.<br>• Patient/significant other should understand the significance of strict intake/ouput measurements, and daily weights.<br>• Efforts should be made to help patient/significant other to remain responsible for self-care. |

sure, the superior vena cava is extremely vulnerable to external compression caused by tumors.

Obstruction to venous return in the superior vena cava causes a selective increase in upper body venous pressure. The pressure forces blood to return from this region to the right atrium by collateral vascular channels. The resulting venous hypertension and all its complications constitute the signs and symptoms of SVCS.

The clinical picture ranges from the insidious onset of signs and symptoms to the acute onset. Often, patient complaints develop over a period of 2–8 weeks. Given the time frame of clinical symptom development, early detection is quite probable.

Symptomatology of acute SVCS is fairly obvious. Shortness of breath, facial edema, and arm and trunk swelling are the 3 major symptoms. Cough, chest pain, and dysphagia are less common. Other complaints include a ruddy complexion, cyanosis, headache, and visual disturbances. Thoracic vein distention may be present but not universally observed.

### Diagnosis

The diagnosis of SVCS is made based on clinical findings. A chest x-ray may be useful to confirm SVCS, however, in many circumstances it is normal. A biopsy must be done to establish a tissue diagnosis. Invasive diagnostic procedures are generally avoided due to hazards created by the elevated venous pressure in the chest and arms. The patient with SVCS is also prone to bleeding and respiratory problems.

### Treatment

Radiation therapy is the standard treatment for SVCS. Three to 6,000 rads over 3 weeks is common. Most patients will feel subjective relief from their symptoms after 72 hours. A decrease in edema is noted after approximately 7 days of therapy.

Roughly 70% of patients with lung cancer who experience SVCS will have their obstruction controlled with radiation therapy. Ninety-five percent of patients with lymphoma will experience the same. The patient with lung cancer is more prone to experience the emergency again. Recurrence of symptoms after treatment for patients with lymphoma is rare.

### Nursing Management

Nursing management includes the identification of patients at risk for SVCS. Patient positioning is very important. An upright position to promote drainage by gravity and prevent fluid accumulation in the upper body is essential. Administration of oxygen, diuretics, and steroids is also indicated. The provision of emotional support in what is a frightening scenario for the patient can be of utmost importance. Patient and family must be taught to recognize future signs and symptoms.

## HYPERCALCEMIA

Hypercalcemia, defined as an elevated serum calcium greater than 11 mg/100 ml, is a common complication of certain malignancies. Because an increase in calcium causes many potentially life-threatening effects, prompt diagnosis and treatment are necessary. Otherwise, approximately 50% of patients who go untreated will die.

### Etiology and Pathophysiology

The serum calcium level is regulated by 3 major factors. The equilibrium between calcium intake, turnover, and the loss of calcium is a result of a sensitive regulatory mechanism involving parathyroid hormone (PTH), calcitonin, and vitamin D (see Chap. 24). A disturbance in the absorption of calcium from the gastrointestinal tract, renal excretion of calcium, or resorption of calcium in the bones may all result in a hypercalcemic episode. Calcium maintains cellular permeability. Excitability of nervous tissue and contractibility of cardiac, smooth, and skeletal muscle are altered by changes in the calcium level.

Oncology patients are commonly at risk for developing hypercalcemia. Cancers of the lung and breast, multiple myeloma, hypernephroma, and head and neck tumors are the most frequent etiologies.

### Clinical Presentations

Symptoms of hypercalcemia may be observed in the central nervous, renal, gastrointestinal, cardiovascular, and ocular systems. Central nervous system symptoms include fatigue, weakness, hyporeflexia, lethargy, apathy, stupor, and coma. Renal complaints may range from polyuria, polydipsia, and renal insufficiency to renal calculi and failure. Patients with gastrointestinal symptoms experience anorexia, nausea, vomiting, constipation, and abdominal cramping. Cardiovascular problems include dysrhythmias, electrocardiogram changes (increased PR interval and shortened QT interval [see Fig. 40–53]), and a risk for digoxin toxicity. Conjunctivitis and corneal calcifications result from the effects of calcium deposition in the ocular system.

### Treatment

The treatment for hypercalcemia depends on the signs and symptoms and degree of calcium elevation. The goals of treatment are reducing bone resorption of calcium and enhancing the excretion of calcium from the body.

Hydration with large volumes of saline is indicated. The usual rate is 3–5 liters/24 hours. When large volumes of saline are administered, the patient is monitored for fluid overload and electrolyte imbalances. Nursing measures include daily weights, intake and output, central venous pressure measurements, if applicable, and monitoring electrolytes.

Oral phosphates are occasionally used for long-term management of hypercalcemia but may cause severe diarrhea. Nonthiazide diuretics may be used to increase calcium excretion. Caution is required in maintaining hydration in order to prevent hypovolemia. Depending on the acuteness of the situation, glucocorticoids, mithramycin, and calcitonin may be administered. Steroids are used in treating hypercalcemia associated with breast cancer and malignant melanoma. The efficacy of glucocorticosteroids may be explained by the direct effect of these drugs on the tumor, or by the increase in bone resorption of calcium.

Mithramycin, an antineoplastic agent, is used in very symptomatic cases of hypercalcemia. Myelosuppression may result with prolonged use. Hypocalcemia is also associated with the use of mithramycin. Therefore, patients are also monitored for low serum calcium levels.

Calcitonin, a polypeptide hormone secreted by the thyroid gland, lowers calcium by inhibiting bone resorption. It is usually not effective by itself.

When hypercalcemia is evident from tumor activity, serum calcium is best controlled with effective antitumor treatments. For many patients, hypercalcemia is a true emergency, and treatment is critical.

### Nursing Diagnoses, Desired Patient Outcomes, and Nursing Interventions

Nursing interventions are directed toward preventing fluid overload, electrolyte imbalances, and cardiac abnormalities. (For specific nursing diagnoses, desired patient outcomes, and nursing interventions/rationales in the care of the patient with hypercalcemia, see Table 24–3).

## PAIN

Pain related to cancer is said by some professionals to be the newest of the oncologic emergencies. Prolonged, unrelieved pain is a pathologic state, which often limits one's ability to perform every day tasks of daily living, severely compromising the person's quality of life. The cancer pain experience not only involves physiologic processes, but also has psychologic, intellectual, interactional, and spiritual components. It is a multidimensional and highly subjective experience. Therefore, pain is defined in terms of the patient's description. Health professionals must uphold the notion that the patients are the authority on their pain.

Even though not all patients with cancer experience pain, approximately two thirds do. Multiple concurrent pains are common, and it is thought that 25% of all cancer patients throughout the world are without relief from severe pain.

### Types of Pain

There are two types of cancer pain: acute and chronic.

#### *Acute Pain*

Acute pain is related to specific underlying tissue damage. It has an immediate onset and signals the body to stimulate action to eliminate or relieve the cause of pain. Acute pain is usually caused by injury or illness and commonly subsides as healing takes place. The sympathetic nervous system responds to acute pain by increasing respirations, heart rate, blood pressure, and muscle tension. Most patients will groan or cry and openly express the experience. Thus, acute pain is often associated with increased anxiety. Postoperative pain and discomfort related to procedures such as wound care and dressing changes are examples of acute pain.

#### *Chronic Pain*

Pain that persists for longer than 6 months is deemed *chronic*. Unlike acute pain, chronic pain is not always directly related to any specific underlying damage. It is of long duration, and relief may not depend on cure or reverse of underlying pathology. Chronic pain may begin as acute, recur regularly, or be continuous. Many patients describe their chronic pain as a "nightmare." Often the pain becomes the central focus of one's life, interfering with the ability to participate in activities of daily living. As a result, chronic pain can cause anger, depression, and withdrawal.

### Pain Management

The goals of pain management are: identify the cause, prevent the pain, maintain an unclouded sensorium, and minimize side effects. The first goal

**TABLE 59–12. CARE PLAN FOR THE PATIENT WITH NEOPLASTIC-RELATED PAIN**

| Nursing Diagnoses | Desired Patient Outcomes | Nursing Interventions | Rationales |
|---|---|---|---|
| ***Nursing Diagnosis #1***<br>Alteration in comfort: Pain.<br>(See Table 60–2, Nursing Diagnosis #6). | Patient will:<br>1. Be free from pain.<br>• Verbalizes pain relief.<br>• Demonstrates relaxed facies and overall demeanor. | • Acknowledge that patient has pain.<br>• Administer pain medication around the clock.<br>• Be alert for possible side effects of narcotics: Constipation, nausea, and drowsiness. Promote measures that prevent and control them.<br>• Suggest nonpharmacologic methods of pain control such as relaxation and distraction.<br>• Evaluate and document effectiveness of pain relief measures.<br>• Encourage verbalization about the pain experience.<br>• Include family members and significant others in teaching. | • Recognize that patients are the authority on their own pain.<br>• This will prevent pain and erase the pain memory.<br>• These can be used in addition to medications. |
| ***Nursing Diagnosis #2***<br>Potential for alteration in sensorium (drowsiness), related to:<br>1. Narcotics. | Patient will:<br>1. Not knowingly become injured as a result of taking pain medication.<br>2. Verbalize potential side effects of pain medication. | • Inform patient/significant others that drowsiness is transient and should dissipate within 36–72 hr.<br>• Promote safety measures:<br>◦ Assistance with ambulation.<br>◦ Night lights.<br>◦ Siderails.<br>◦ Call bell within reach. | • This reassurance will encourage patients to continue taking their medication without fear of somnolence. |
| ***Nursing Diagnosis #3***<br>Potential for alteration in elimination, related to:<br>1. Narcotic-induced constipation. | Patient will:<br>1. Not become constipated.<br>2. Resume usual bowel routine. | • Be alert for the possibility of constipation with administration of narcotics.<br>◦ Encourage a preventive mode.<br>◦ Administer stool softeners and laxatives at the onset of administration of narcotics.<br>◦ Encourage patient to eat bulky foods and to increase fluid intake (when feasible).<br>◦ Record all stools.<br>◦ Check for impaction if no stool for three days. | • Preventing constipation is simpler than remedying it once it has occurred. |

is to identify the cause. If the cause is treatable, such as local infection or hemorrhoids, efforts to manage the source of pain become a priority. If the pain is related to the primary cancer, antitumor therapy is initiated. When neither the tumor nor other source of pain can be managed, therapy aimed at alleviating the pain through analgesic interventions is tried.

A second important aim is to prevent the pain. Medications are given in adequate amounts and at appropriate intervals to prevent recurrences or worsening of the pain. Pain medicine is administered around the clock and not "as needed." Ineffective administration leads to increased confusion, disorientation, and sedation, but *not* pain relief.

The maintenance of an unclouded sensorium is another aim. Sedation usually occurs upon initiation or an increase in narcotics but dissipates after 48–72 hours. In most instances, as the pain worsens and narcotics are safely escalated, sedation is rarely a long-term problem. Of utmost importance in any pain management regimen is to promote maximum participation in activities of daily living and to allow the patient to remain as alert as possible.

A last goal of any pain management program is to prevent physical side effects from the medication. Side effects are anticipated and prevented or minimized. Relief of one symptom should not be traded for the presence of another. The nurse who is knowledgeable about the pharmacology and clinical use of analgesics can have significant impact on the analgesic plan.

A variety of drugs are currently available for pain management. For mild pain, aspirin or acetaminophen can be used. For moderate pain, Percocet, Percodan, or acetaminophen (Tylenol) with codeine are effective drugs. Morphine, dilaudid, and methadone in various dosages can be given to patients who complain of severe to very severe pain. For excruciating pain, all of the aforementioned drugs can be prescribed along with extra measures such as nerve blocks. Meperdine, although sometimes used for cancer pain, should be avoided. Its short duration of action (2–3 hours) and decreased analgesic potency when given by mouth deem it unsuitable for patients with cancer pain. In addition, safe dosage escalations beyond normal dosages are virtually impossible due to the accumulation of meperdine's toxic metabolite, normeperidine.

Patients with cancer pain may be on extremely high doses of medication. Many clinicians remain afraid of the risk of addiction in these patients. Because addiction is a behavior pattern of abusing a narcotic for its psychic effects rather than medical reasons, it is not a problem for the overwhelming majority of patients with cancer.

In addition to administering medication, nurses should also consider nonpharmacologic approaches to pain management. Distraction is the use of activity or other measures to move a patient's focus from the pain on to something else. Simple conversation, music, television, and reading are examples of this technique. Progressive muscle relaxation is another useful tool. Although learning how to relax the body takes practice by both the nurse and patient, it is very therapeutic for episodic, acute pain. For example, a patient about to undergo a bone marrow biopsy would benefit from muscle relaxation. Guided imagery is also helpful for patients with both acute and chronic pain. This technique involves either a nurse "leading" a patient "somewhere else" by the use of dialogue or by the patient doing it alone. Guided imagery has undergone scrutiny for its therapeutic effectiveness as well as psychologic benefits. Therapeutic touch has also been investigated for use in other areas in addition to pain control. In its simplest form, it involves the transfer of energy between practitioner and patient. All other nonpharmacologic measures of pain management are useful tools; however, they should be used in conjunction with medication, not in place of it.

## Nursing Diagnoses, Desired Patient Outcomes, and Nursing Interventions

Nursing diagnoses, desired patient outcomes, and nursing interventions in the care of the patient with pain attributed to neoplastic disease are presented in Table 59–12.

## REFERENCES


1. Concilus, E and Bohachick, P: Cancer: Pericardial effusion and tamponade. Cancer Nursing 7:391, October 1984.
2. Fraser, R, Viloria, J, and Wang, N: Cardiac tamponade as a presentation of extracardiac malignancy. Cancer 45:1697, April 1980.
3. Glancy, D: Myocardial, endocardial and pericardial disease. In Wenger, N, et al (eds): Cardiology for Nurses. McGraw-Hill, New York, 1980, p 476.
4. Gilbert, I and Henning, R: Adenocarcinoma of the lung presenting with pericardial tamponade: Report of a case and review of the literature. Heart Lung 14:83, January 1985.
5. Adenle, D and Edwards, J: Clinical and pathological features of metastatic neoplasms of the pericardium. Chest 81:166, February 1982.
6. Schumer, W: Septic shock. JAMA 242:1906, October 1979.
7. McConnell, E: Septic shock. Nursing Life 3:34, Sept/Oct 1983.
8. Karakusis, P: Considerations in therapy of septic shock. Med Clin North Am 70:933, July 1986.
9. Murray, P: Functional outcome and survival in spinal cord injury secondary to neoplasia. Cancer 55:197, January 1985.

10. Bruckman, J and Bloomer, W: Management of spinal cord compression. Semin Oncol 5:135, June 1978.
11. Harrison, K, et al: Spinal cord compression in breast cancer. Cancer 55:2839, June 1985.
12. Pedersen, A, Bach, F, and Mclgaard, B: Frequency, diagnosis, and prognosis of spinal cord compression in small cell bronchogenic carcinoma: A review of 817 consecutive patients. Cancer 55:1818, April 1985.
13. Klein, P: Neurologic emergencies in oncology. Semin Oncol Nurs 1:278, November 1985.
14. Donoghue, M: Spinal cord compression. In Yasko, J (ed): Guidelines for Cancer Care, Symptom Management. Reston, Reston, VA, 1983, p 353.
15. Rodichok, L, et al: Early diagnosis of spinal epidural metastases. Am J Med 70:1181, 1981.
16. Bleck, T and Klawans, H: Neurologic emergencies. Med Clin North Am, 70:1167, September 1986.
17. Kornblith, P and Cassady, J: Central nervous system emergencies. In DeVita, V, et al (eds): Cancer: Principles and Practice of Oncology, Vol 2, Ed 2. JB Lippincott, Philadelphia, 1985, p 1860.
18. Rice, V: problems of water regulation: Diabetes insipidus and syndrome of inappropriate antidiuretic hormone. Crit Care Nurse 3:64, Jan/Feb 1983.
19. Johndrow, P and Thornton, S: Syndrome of inappropriate antidiuretic hormone. Focus Crit Care 12:29, October 1985.
20. Zerbe, R: Inappropriate antidiuretic hormone secretion. Hosp Med 20:241, January 1984.
21. Zucker, A and Chernow, B: Diabetes insipidus and the syndrome of inappropriate antidiuretic hormone release. Crit Care Q 6:63, December 1983.
22. Arieff, A and Schmidt, W: Fluid and electrolyte disorders and the central nervous system. In Maxwell, M and Kleeman, C (eds): Clinical Disorders of Fluid and Electrolyte Metabolism Ed 3. McGraw-Hill, New York, 1980, p 1409.
23. Streeton, D, Moses, A, and Miller, M: Disorders of the neurohypophysis. In Petersdorf, R, et al (eds): Harrison's Principles of Internal Medicine, Ed 10. McGraw-Hill, New York, p 612.

## SUGGESTED READINGS

### Superior Vena Cava Syndrome

Morse, L, Heery, M, and Flynn, K: Early detection to avert the crisis of superior vena cava syndrome. Cancer Nurs 8(4):228, August 1985.

Rahko, P and Shaver, J: Superior vena cava syndrome. Hosp Med, July 1985, pp 83–86.

### Hypercalcemia

Doogan, R: Hypercalcemia of malignancy. Cancer Nurs 4(4):299, August 1981.

Elbaum, N: With cancer patients, be alert for hypercalcemia. Nursing '84 14(8):58, August 1984.

Poe, C and Radford, A: The challenge of hypercalcemia in cancer. Oncol Nurs Forum 12:29, 1985.

Valentine, A and Stewart, J: Oncologic emergencies. Am J Nurs 83(9):1283, September 1983.

### Pain Management

Anderson, J: Nursing management of the cancer patient in pain. A review of the literature. Cancer Nurs 5(1):33, February 1982.

Levine, J: Pain and nanalgesia: The outlook for more rational treatment. Ann Intern Med 100:269, 1984.

Foley, K: The treatment of cancer pain. N Engl J Med 313:84, 1983.

Hauck, S: Pain: Problem for the person with cancer. Cancer Nurs 9:66, 1986.

Johnson, L and Gross, J (eds): Handbook of Oncology Nursing. Wiley, New York, 1985, pp 145–147.

CHAPTER 60

# Nursing Care of Patients with Neoplastic-Related Surgery

*Janet Donnard and Deborah Rodzwic*

## CHAPTER OUTLINE



## LEARNING OBJECTIVES

**At the end of this chapter, you should be able to:**

1. Identify key nursing care considerations for patients with surgery for cancer of the head and neck.
2. Discuss symptomatology closely associated with esophageal carcinoma.
3. Describe surgical procedure for esophagogastrectomy and implications for nursing care.
4. Identify major complications of esophagogastrectomy surgery and pertinent preventive and therapeutic interventions.
5. Examine implications for nursing care based on implementation of nursing process:
   Assessment
   Specific nursing diagnoses
   Planning: Patient outcomes and nursing interventions/rationales.

## THERAPEUTIC MODALITIES IN THE TREATMENT OF CANCER

Cancer is a prevalent disease in our society. Public awareness of cancer has increased over the years, which has led to early detection, prompt treatment, and improved survival. Today, the 7 warning signals of cancer (Table 60-1) are widely publicized. Comprehensive cancer treatment centers are now available to those seeking diagnosis and treatment.

The 3 most common modalities in the treatment of cancer are surgery, radiation therapy, and chemotherapy. Tumor staging and cell type determine which methods are used. Table 60-2 lists the principles of surgery. Surgery is the most common initial therapy used either to diagnose a malignant tumor or remove it for purposes of cure or palliation. However, surgical recovery is likely to be complicated by the addition of radiation or chemotherapy. The latter 2 forms of treatment are used to eradicate residual tumor cells by either focusing on the primary malignant tumor site or treating it systemically. Both radiation therapy and chemotherapy may impair wound healing, cause fistula formation, or alter immunologic functioning necessary to guard against infection.

Patients with head and neck carcinoma and esophageal carcinoma face the possibilities of receiving a combination of cancer therapies, experiencing a variety of complications, and requiring intensive nursing care. For these reasons, these 2 types of cancers are used in this chapter as representatives of the radical surgical techniques often

TABLE 60-1
**Cancer's Seven Warning Signals**

1. Change in bowel or bladder habits.
2. A sore throat that does not heal.
3. Unusual bleeding or discharge.
4. Thickening or lump in breast or elsewhere.
5. Indigestion or difficulty in swallowing.
6. Obvious change in wart or mole.
7. Nagging cough or hoarseness.

Source: The American Cancer Society.

necessary in the treatment of patients with cancer and of the sophisticated nursing care required. This chapter provides information with respect to the use of myocutaneous flaps in head and neck surgery and the chest and abdominal surgery required in the treatment of esophageal neoplasms. Both topics include nursing care plans, which provide the nurse with desired patient outcomes, specific nursing interventions, and associated rationales.

## SURGERY FOR CANCER OF THE HEAD AND NECK

Head and neck cancers constitute approximately 5% of all malignancies. Yet the aesthetic, emotional, and functional difficulties encountered by patients with these cancers heighten their significance. The pharynx as a pathway for deglutition and respiration, visibility of the features of the head and neck, and deficits encountered after treatment all increase the magnitude of the problem.

### Nursing Management

The nurse caring for patients with head and neck cancer faces many challenges. The radical changes in the patient's body image and self-concept make coping with this type of surgery difficult. Therefore, thorough assessment of the patient's current body image is performed preoperatively. Potential changes in normal body structures and ventilation are discussed based on the patient's ability to understand these changes as well as the patient's level of anxiety. Whenever possible, realistic hope is offered.

After a patient undergoes extensive surgery for head and neck cancer, recovery usually occurs in a critical care setting. The following guidelines are offered to assist the nurse with the management of patients who undergo these surgical procedures (see Tables 60-3 and 60-4). Surgical time, especially if reconstruction is involved, is often long and arduous. Because the patient is anesthetized for an extended period of time, close observation and careful assessments are done.

It is essential that the nurse understand the extent of surgery and the permanent and temporary alterations that are present. Immediate postoperative care is aimed at maintaining a patent airway, preventing and monitoring for complications, and assessing the surgical site for signs of bleeding or swelling. If reconstructive surgery using myocutaneous skin flap is performed, flap viability is a major consideration.

After surgery, the patient's head is elevated without a pillow at 30 degrees. Most patients have a prophylactic tracheostomy and require humidified oxygen to keep secretions moist. Respiratory status is assessed at least every 4 hours including auscultation of lung sounds, respiratory rate, and arterial blood gases. Neurologic status is also assessed because changes in level of consciousness result from decreased oxygenation.

If drains have been inserted in the neck and chest area to extract accumulated fluid, clear fluid from drains usually indicates improper placement into lymph channels. Drainage is measured and recorded accurately. Other assessments of fluid balance such as intake and output and drainage from other tubes are performed. A Foley catheter is usually inserted intraoperatively to measure urine output accurately and prevent distention of the bladder. Lastly, a feeding tube is in place, initially to drain stomach contents and later to maintain adequate nutrition. Depending on the location of the surgical site, the patient may either have an esophagogastric (EG) or nasogastric (NG) tube.

The circulatory system requires careful monitoring. The threat of a cerebral vascular accident (CVA) postoperatively is possible due to the severing of major and minor vessels during surgery. Blood pressure and pulse are assessed at least every 4 hours. Range-of-motion exercises of unaffected extremities are performed to prevent venous stasis. Tracheostomy ties are tied loosely to prevent decreased circulation to flaps. Excessive dressings over the neck and chest areas are avoided to improve visibility of the side.

TABLE 60-2
**Principles of Surgery**

1. Biopsy—microscopic proof of malignancy.
   A. Needle aspiration.
   B. Incisional—removing a portion of the mass.
   C. Excisional—removing the entire mass.
2. Staging.
   A. Stage I—neoplasm confined to original site.
   B. Stage II—metastases to regional lymph nodes.
   C. Stages III and IV—distant metastatic spread.
3. Types of oncology surgery.
   A. Local resections—wide excisions.
   B. Radical resection—includes tumor, surrounding muscle, and lymphatics.
   C. Palliation—surgery that is performed to relieve symptoms without attempting to cure the patient.

Impaired skin integrity and signs of local or systemic infection are assessed frequently. Any swelling or discoloration in the neck and chest area is immediately recorded and reported to the physician. Incisions may be cleansed as per physician or institutional protocol.

#### *Nursing Diagnoses, Patient Outcomes, and Nursing Interventions*

Nursing diagnoses, patient outcomes, and nursing interventions in the postoperative nursing care of the patient undergoing surgery for head and neck cancer are presented in Table 60–3.

## ESOPHAGEAL CARCINOMA

### Incidence

Tumors of the esophagus account for 1% of new cases and 8,800 deaths each year.[1] The most frequently found forms include squamous cell carcinoma and adenocarcinoma.[2] The majority of cases are found in men, the median age being 60 years. Risk factors include cigarette smoking and alcohol consumption.

### Symptomatology

The symptoms of the esophageal cancer in their order of incidence include: dysphagia, weight loss, substernal epigastric pain or burning, vomiting, hoarseness, coughing, choking, aspiration pneumonia, and palpable cervical lymph nodes. Diagnosis is based on findings from a number of different sources including esophagastroscopy with biopsy, barium swallow, computed tomography (CT) scan,[2] or nuclear magnetic resonance imaging (MRI) scans.[3]

### Surgical Procedure— Esophagogastrectomy

An understanding of the surgical procedure is needed to use the nursing process and successfully accomplish a patient's goals. There are several approaches to the surgical treatment of esophageal neoplasms. The type of procedure chosen depends in part on tumor location, the presence or absence of metastasis, and the surgeon's preference. For the purposes of this chapter, the esophagogastrectomy approach will be discussed. The goal of such extensive surgery is curative. The procedure is as follows[4] (Fig. 60–1):

A midline abdominal incision is carried out from the xiphoid to the umbilicus. The abdominal cavity is examined for any metastatic disease. If the examination is benign for tumor, the stomach and esophagus are freed up from accessible organs by releasing the major blood vessels that feed them. This allows the stomach to be pulled up into the thoracic cavity. A pyloroplasty or stretching of the pyloric sphincter is performed. Lymph nodes from this area will be sent to pathology for frozen section determination.

Attention is then turned to the jejunum. A feeding jejunostomy consisting of a #18 Levine tube is placed approximately 1½ feet distal to the ligament of Traitz. A drainage tube is placed through a separate stab wound in the left upper quadrant. The abdominal incision is closed.

The patient is then turned on the side, and a thoracotomy is performed through the fifth or sixth intercostal space. The ribs are gently spread with a rib retractor, although rib resections are occasionally required. The parietal pleura overlying the esophagus is divided. An incision is made in the diaphragm for placement of the stomach in the chest. The esophagus is freed from its posterior mediastinal bed, the neoplasm is located and transected completely. The specimen is sent to pathology to ensure that the margins are free of tumor. Once established, the 2 ends are anastomosed by either hand sewing or use of the end-to-end circumferential anastomosic (EEA) stapler.[5] An NG tube is inserted into the remaining esophagus, through the anastomosis, and into the remaining stomach. Two chest tubes are placed through separate stab wounds, one laterally at the anastomosis and the second midway up the thorax. The chest is then closed.

### Postoperative Care: Nursing Management

The nursing management of the surgical oncology patient is very challenging. The patient's preoperative physical status is often compromised by side effects of the disease, treatment of the disease, or both.

People with esophageal cancer most commonly present with malnutrition due to dysphagia. Unfortunately, esophageal carcinoma is associated with a poor prognosis. It is often not diagnosed until the neoplasm has occluded 50% of the esophagus.[6] The chance that tumor cells may have spread to lymph nodes or by direct invasion through the muscle wall is increased by this late finding.[5] This knowledge often prompts physicians to prescribe radiation therapy preoperatively to decrease tumor burden or postoperatively to eradicate tumor cells outside of the surgical area.

**TABLE 60-3. CARE PLAN FOR THE PATIENT WITH NEOPLASTIC-RELATED SURGERY OF THE HEAD AND NECK**

| Nursing Diagnoses | Desired Patient Outcomes | Nursing Interventions | Rationales |
|---|---|---|---|
| ***Nursing Diagnosis #1***<br>Alteration in breathing pattern, related to:<br>1. Postoperative tracheostomy. | Patient will:<br>1. Maintain adequate respiratory function:<br>A. Respiratory rate <25/minutes.<br>B. Tidal volume 5–7 ml/kg.<br>C. Arterial blood gases:<br>• pH 7.35–7.45.<br>• $PaCO_2$ 35–45 mmHg.<br>• $PaO_2$ >60 mmHg.<br>2. Maintain intact neurological function:<br>A. Mental status alert and oriented to person, place, and date. | • Note preoperative respiratory status and history from records.<br>• Assess respiratory status q 4 hr. Include auscultation of anterior and posterior chest, respirations, and arterial blood gases (as indicated).<br>• Tracheostomy care q 4 hr (as per institutional guidelines).<br>• Encourage coughing, turning, and deep breathing q 2 hr.<br>• Encourage use of incentive spirometer.<br>• Administer humidified air/oxygen.<br>• Keep head of bed elevated 30°.<br>• Assess neurological status q 4 hr and PRN. | • May already be compromised.<br><br><br><br><br>• To mobilize secretions.<br><br>• To moisten secretions.<br>• Note physician recommendations.<br>• Changes in level of consciousness may result from decreased oxygen. |
| ***Nursing Diagnosis #2***<br>Potential for alteration in hemodynamics and tissue perfusion, related to:<br>1. Manipulation of major vessels in neck intraoperatively. | Patient will:<br>1. Maintain presurgical circulatory status.<br>• Heart rate 60–80/minute.<br>• Rhythm: Regular sinus.<br>• Blood pressure within 10 mmHg of baseline.<br>• Hemodynamic parameters within acceptable range (arterial pressure, pulmonary artery and pulmonary capillary wedge pressures).<br>• Usual skin color, skin warm to touch.<br>• Brisk capillary refill. | • Note preoperative circulatory status and history from records.<br>• Assess pulse and blood pressure q 4 hr.<br>• Encourage range of motion to unaffected extremities q 2 hr with assistance.<br>• Note color and temperature of extremities PRN and record.<br>• Observe for signs and symptoms of phlebitis every shift.<br>• Encourage early ambulation.<br>• Keep tracheostomy ties loosely applied.<br>• Avoid use of excessive dressings on neck and chest as per physician recommendations. | • May have history of circulatory problem (e.g., carotid arterial insufficiency, risk of cerebral vascular accident).<br>• Will prevent venous stasis.<br><br><br><br>• Will prevent decreased circulation to flaps.<br>• Improves visibility of area and facilitates assessment. |

| | | | |
|---|---|---|---|
| ***Nursing Diagnosis #3***<br>Alteration in fluid balance, related to:<br>1. Surgical procedure. | Patient will:<br>1. Maintain balanced intake and output, and body weight within 5% of baseline.<br>2. Maintain stable laboratory values:<br>• Serum osmolality 285–295 mOsm/kg.<br>• Serum electrolytes within acceptable range.<br>• Urine specific gravity: 1.010–1.025. | • Assess present fluid balance.<br>• Record accurate intakes and outputs and report imbalances.<br>• Administer intravenous fluids/blood products as prescribed.<br>• Note and record color and type of drainage from drains, EG and NG tubes.<br>• Begin tube feedings when indicated. | • Note estimated blood loss, insensible losses, urine output, intravenous infusions, blood products, gastric and wound drainage. Clear fluid from drains may indicate improper placement into lymph channels. |
| ***Nursing Diagnosis #4***<br>Impaired skin integrity, related to:<br>1. Surgical incision.<br>2. Poor wound healing. | Patient will:<br>1. Not experience an infection at surgical sites.<br>2. Have skin become/remain intact. | • Note preoperative skin integrity from history.<br>• Assess skin integrity q 4 hr.<br>• Assess unaffected areas in neck and chest area for swelling and discoloration.<br>• Cleanse incisions as per institutional protocol. | • May already be compromised. |
| ***Nursing Diagnosis #5***<br>Alteration in body image, related to:<br>1. Surgical procedure. | Patient will:<br>1. Verbalize feelings about body image changes.<br>2. State ways to adapt to body alterations. | • Discuss potential changes in body image preoperatively.<br>• Encourage patient to voice feelings, comments, and questions about surgery.<br>• Answer questions and reinforce information given by physician.<br>• Encourage support from family or significant others.<br>• Offer realistic hope whenever possible.<br>• Refer patient for additional professional help when indicated. | • Important to assess previous problems, adjustment difficulties, or coping mechanisms. |

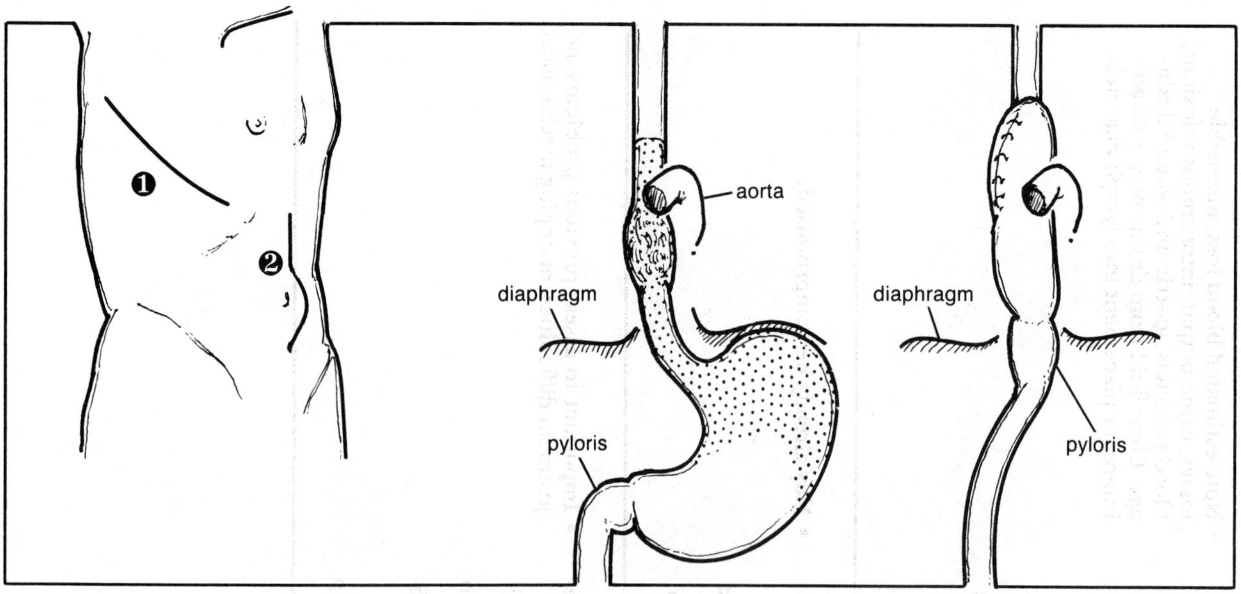


**Figure 60-1.** Esophagogastrectomy; a surgical approach for the treatment of esophageal carcinoma is a two-step approach involving (*1*) an initial abdominal incision, followed by (*2*) thoracotomy. (See text for details.)

### *Complications of Respiratory Function*

Due to the nature of the surgical procedure, potential complications involving the respiratory system often exist. It is therefore important for the nurse to keep in mind any preexisting health problems identified in the nursing history. For example, the combination of smoking or pulmonary disease[6] along with the manipulation of the lungs at the time of surgery potentiate postoperative complications. In a study done by Galandiuk and associates at the Cleveland Clinic, the most common complication was atelectasis followed by pneumonia.[6]

The nurse can provide support to the patient by evaluating the effectiveness of pain control and instructing the patient to splint incisions while coughing and deep breathing. Other measures implemented to maintain an adequate respiratory status include placing the patient in a semi-Fowler's position and turning every 2 hours. The necessity for oxygen therapy is determined by arterial blood gas and/or pulse oximetry, which monitors the oxygen saturation of available hemoglobin. Lung expansion is enhanced by 2 chest tubes, and progress is checked daily by chest film. Lungs are auscultated every 4 hours during the acute period, and the quality/quantity of sputum production is noted. (For additional details related to assessment of respiratory function, see Chap. 29.)

### *Complications of Cardiovascular Function*

Closely involved with the pulmonary system is the cardiovascular system. The patient's cardiac history is noted so that baseline data can be used as a form of comparison. The patient undergoing chest surgery is at greater risk for the development of dysrhythmias, most commonly atrial fibrillation.[7] Etiology is unknown, although studies suggest an increased incidence with an increase in the patient's age. If the patient develops this dysrhythmia postoperatively, the nurse should be aware of potential complications such as increased oxygen demands, decreased cardiac output, and emboli formation.

Increased oxygen demands may tax or stress an already compromised cardiopulmonary system, causing cardiac ischemia/dysrhythmias. The nurse notes the ventricular rate and the regularity of the apical pulse. An increased rate is associated with increased oxygen consumption. In a nonacute setting, the nurse promotes rest and administers antianxiety agents as prescribed and monitors the patient's response to therapy.

The second complication, a 20%–30% decrease in cardiac output occurs when the atria do not function properly. This directly affects coronary, cerebral, and renal perfusion. The nurse performs an ongoing cardiovascular assessment, comprised of continuous cardiac and hemodynamic monitoring. (For details related to cardiac assessment and hemodynamic monitoring, see Chaps. 38 and 41.) The lungs are auscultated for the presence of rales (crackles), a sign of fluid overload. Neck vein distention and pedal edema also indicate heart failure. An altered level of consciousness may be suggestive of cerebral hypoxia. Serum electrolytes, BUN, creatinine, and hourly urine output are monitored to observe for abnormalities of renal perfusion.

Finally, 30% of all patients who develop atrial fibrillation experience systemic or pulmonary emboli.[8] An increase in patient activity will decrease venous stasis, a precurser to emboli formation. Such activity includes sitting in a chair within the first 24 hours after surgery and range-of-motion exercises to extremities. (See Chap. 35 for the signs, symptoms, medical and nursing management of pulmonary embolisms.)

Treatment of atrial fibrillation will depend on the clinical status of the patient. Therapy for one who is experiencing cardiac decompensation consists of synchronized cardioversion. A conservative approach with medications may be used for those patients who experience dysrythmias without major sequelae. This form of treatment includes the use of conventional drugs such as digoxin, verapamil, propranolol, and quinidine.[8]

### *Complications of Gastrointestinal Function and Nutrition*

The most serious complication of esophagogastrectomy is dehiscence of the anastomotic site. This problem accounts for high mortality and morbidity.[9] Poor nutritional status and preoperative radiation therapy are likely factors linked to the separation of the esophagus–gastric union. When tumor is present in the margins of resection or if the surgical technique is less than optimal, breakdown of the site of anastomosis may occur. The use of stapling devices over a hand-sewn anastomosis significantly reduces the incidence of this complication.[5]

Nursing care requires prudent attention to the drainage catheters. Should the NG tube become dislodged from its original placement, the surgeon may be hesitant to replace it. Reinsertion has the potential to disrupt the anastomosis.

Observation of the color and amount of drainage is equally important. Should the chest tube or sump begin to drain either bile or "coffee-ground" drainage, the physician should be notified and specimens should be sent for analysis.

Once a leak occurs, gastric secretions are emptied into the mediastinum, causing thoracic empyema, mediastinitis, cardiopulmonary dysfunction, and general sepsis.[10] The patient may present with chest pain, dysrhythmias, an elevated WBC count, and fever. Diagnosis is often made by gastrografin swallow and analysis of the drainage from the chest tubes or sump. Treatment is aimed at draining the site of the leakage to promote healing and management of related symptoms.[11]

Several aspects of nursing care are employed in coping with this problem. The patient with a negative nitrogen balance preoperatively is placed on total parenteral nutrition (TPN). TPN is a hypertonic solution consisting of dextrose, fat emulsions, and L-amino acids. Attempts to restore an adequate nutritional state have been shown to enhance the patients' immunologic capabilities.[9]

Calories are gradually increased until a therapeutic level is reached as determined by the physician or nutritional support service. This enables the pancreas to adjust its insulin production in response to the increased glucose load. The patient's serum glucose level is checked at least daily during this period of adjustment. Urine testing may be done every 6 hours to determine the need for insulin coverage. More commonly, serial blood glucose monitoring is performed and reflects more definitively the need for insulin coverage.

The nurse who is monitoring a patient receiving TPN should be cognizant of the potential for infection. The high glucose concentration is a good medium for bacterial growth. The central line catheter provides a ready access for systemic sepsis. Once dedicated for TPN use, infusions of additional medications, central venous pressure (CVP) readings, or blood sampling should be avoided. Special attention to vital signs and white blood cell counts is prudent at this time. The central venous line site care is performed according to the institution's policy. A transparent dressing allows the nurse to assess the site for signs of redness, swelling, pain, or drainage. (For additional nursing care related to a patient on TPN, see Chap. 53.)

During the operative procedure, the patient will have a feeding tube placed in the jejunum (J-tube). If the GI tract is able to absorb nutrients, it is the preferred route for nutrition. Gastrointestinal motility is evidenced by auscultated bowel sounds or the presence of flatulence. Feedings are initiated and gradually increased according to the patient's tolerance. The nutritional support service will determine caloric intake and will gradually wean the patient off TPN. Intolerance may be evidenced by residual feeding that is not emptying from the stomach or the development of diarrhea. Medications such as metroclopramide (Reglan), which stimulates gastric and intestinal emptying, or paregoric, which decreases gastrointestinal motility, are often used to treat such problems.

In summary, a person with a malignancy requiring surgical intervention who has been previously treated with chemotherapy and radiation therapy has the potential for poor wound healing. When such complications do not respond to conservative medical management, the patient may require surgical repair with an associated poor prognosis. This demonstrates the importance of understanding the surgical procedure, potential complications, and the essential role of the nurse.

### *Nursing Diagnoses, Desired Patient Outcomes and Nursing Interventions*

A comprehensive nursing care plan for the patient with cancer of the esophagus treated by surgery is presented in Table 60–4. Included in the table are pertinent nursing diagnoses, desired patient outcomes, and nursing interventions/rationales.

## TABLE 60-4. CARE PLAN FOR THE PATIENT WITH CANCER OF THE ESOPHAGUS TREATED BY SURGERY

| Nursing Diagnoses | Desired Patient Outcomes | Nursing Interventions | Rationales |
|---|---|---|---|
| ***Nursing Diagnosis #1*** Alteration in cardiac output: decreased, related to:<br>1. Altered hemodynamics associated with thoracic/abdominal surgery.<br>***Nursing Diagnosis #2*** Alteration in tissue perfusion: cardiopulmonary. | Patient will:<br>1. Maintain presurgical cardiovascular function as manifested by:<br>A. Stable hemodynamics.<br>• Blood pressure within 10 mmHg of baseline.<br>• Heart rate <100 beats/minute.<br>• Cardiac output ~5 liters/minute.<br>• CVP: 0–8 mmHg.<br>• CWP: 8–12 mmHg.<br>B. Absence of: Extreme weakness or fatigue, peripheral edema, neck vein distention or chest pain.<br>C. Absence of cardiac dysrhythmias. | • Perform ongoing cardiovascular assessment:<br>◦ Continuous cardiac monitoring. Establish baseline rate, rhythm and ectopy.<br>◦ Continuous hemodynamic monitoring when indicated. Establish baseline CVP and PCWP measurements.<br>◦ Auscultate lungs q 4 hr.<br>◦ Auscultate heart sounds—presence of S3.<br>◦ Assess for fatigue, neck vein distention? sacral edema?<br>◦ Monitor arterial blood gases. | • Chest surgery may cause cardiac irritability. Many patients develop atrial fibrillation. This dysrhythmia may decrease cardiac output by 20–30%.<br>◦ Rales (crackles) are an indication of fluid overload.<br>◦ Diagnostic sign for congestive heart failure. |
| | 2. Maintain intact neurological status:<br>• Mental status: Alert and oriented. | • Perform neurological assessment.<br>◦ Level of consciousness.<br>◦ Behavior. | • Compromised hemodynamics and hypoxemia predispose to cerebral hypoxia with altered cerebral function. |
| | 3. Maintain fluid and electrolyte balance.<br>• Stable body weight.<br>• Balanced intake and output.<br>• Hourly urine output >30 cc/hr. | • Assess fluid and electrolyte status.<br>◦ Daily weight.<br>◦ Intake and output with hourly urine outputs.<br>◦ Serum electrolytes, BUN, creatinine. | • Reduced blood volume will further compromise venous return and cardiac output; blood volume may need to be expanded with use of colloids or fluids.<br>◦ Reduced cardiac output may diminish renal perfusion, placing patient at risk of developing acute renal failure. |

| | | | |
|---|---|---|---|
| ***Nursing Diagnosis #3***<br>Impaired gas exchange, related to:<br>1. Pulmonary congestion associated with surgical manipulation of intrathoracic structures and altered by lymphatic drainage.<br>2. Atelectasis. | Patient will:<br>1. Maintain effective respiratory function:<br>• Rate <25/minute.<br>• Rhythm eupneic.<br>• Breath sounds clear on auscultation.<br>• Mental status: Alert and oriented.<br>• Usual skin color.<br>• Arterial blood gases at baseline. | • Monitor and report signs and symptoms of altered respiratory function:<br>∘ Presence of rapid, shallow, or irregular respirations; dyspnea, orthopnea; use of accessory muscles.<br>∘ Presence of adventitious breath sounds on auscultation.<br>∘ Presence of restlessness, irritability, confusion, or somnolence.<br>∘ Presence of dusky red, mottled, or cyanotic skin color.<br>• Monitor arterial blood gas values and report abnormal results. | |
| | | • Monitor pulse oximetry. Obtain ABGs for saturation of hemoglobin. | • Monitors the oxygen saturation of available hemoglobin. |
| | | • Monitor hemoglobin/hematocrit. | • Anemia provokes tissue hypoxia. |
| | | • Implement measures to maintain adequate respiratory function:<br>∘ Maintain semi-Fowler's position.<br>∘ Maintain prescribed $O_2$ therapy and monitor response.<br>∘ Encourage coughing and deep breathing q 1–2 hr.<br>∘ Assist in turning q 2 hr.<br>∘ Instruct to splint incision when coughing.<br>∘ Encourage use of pain medication as prescribed and monitor response. | ∘ Due to extent of surgery, patient will "guard" incision, which leads to decreased lung expansion, atelectasis and poor gas exchange. |
| ***Nursing Diagnosis #4***<br>Alteration in bowel elimination, related to:<br>1. Surgical trauma, stress, and enteral tube feedings. | Patient will:<br>1. Regain peristaltic activity and presurgical bowel function. | • Maintain nasogastric tube to low suction. Irrigate with 30 cc normal saline solution q 4 hr or as prescribed.<br>∘ **Do not reposition or reinsert.** | • Maintains patency and prevents gastric distention which may cause stress to suture line and lead to an anastomotic leak.<br>∘ The tube is placed during surgery. Care must be taken to avoid harm to the anastomosis. Physician will determine benefit risk, and method of replacement. |
| | | • Assess for presence of abdominal distention and auscultate for bowel sounds every shift. | • Distention may indicate malfunctioning NG and stress to the anastomosis.<br>• Bowel sounds indicate that the intestines have regained peristaltic activity. |

*(continued)*

**TABLE 60-4. CARE PLAN FOR THE PATIENT WITH CANCER OF THE ESOPHAGUS TREATED BY SURGERY (Continued)**

| Nursing Diagnoses | Desired Patient Outcomes | Nursing Interventions | Rationales |
|---|---|---|---|
| ***Nursing Diagnosis #4 (cont.)*** | | • Inquire as to the presence or absence of flatulence.<br>○ Encourage ambulation when indicated. | |
| | | • Monitor daily intake and output, weight, and electrolyte balance. | • Fluid loss after gastrointestinal surgery may approach 2 liters or more. Fluid and electrolyte replacement may be required with the loss of large amounts of fluids. |
| | | • Assess character and frequency of stool. | • Diarrhea may result in wasting of $Mg^{++}$ and $Ca^{++}$. Observe for muscle weakness or tetany. |
| ***Nursing Diagnosis #5***<br>Impairment of skin integrity, related to:<br>1. Surgical incision with potential for impaired wound healing due to:<br>A. Preoperative radiation therapy.<br>B. Poor nutrition.<br>C. Infection.<br>2. Irritation or breakdown related to:<br>A. Contact of skin with wound drainage.<br>B. Stress from drainage tubes.<br>C. Use of tape. | Patient will:<br>1. Experience normal healing of surgical wounds. | • Position patient to reduce stress on suture lines.<br>• Maintain NG tube patency.<br>• Splint wounds while coughing. | • Prevents gastric distention.<br>• Equalizes pressure to the wounds. Reduces the possibility of dehiscence. |
| | | • Change dressings frequently and perform aseptic wound care.<br>• Note type and amount of drainage. Obtain culture if indicated and monitor results.<br>• Note drainage tube sites. Provide anchoring tape to prevent tensions or "pulling" at insertion sites.<br>○ Consider use of Montgomery straps. | • Minimizes skin irritation from drainage and prevents nosocomial infections.<br>○ Prevents skin abrasions due to frequent tape changes. |
| | | • Monitor laboratory values for signs of anemia, decreased albumin levels, or an increased leukocyte count. | • Anemia will result in decreased oxygenation. Low albumin level: Indicates a decrease in the colloidal osmotic pressure, which will lead to edema and interference with healing. A leukocytosis may indicate an infectious process. |
| ***Nursing Diagnosis #6***<br>Alteration in comfort level: pain, related to:<br>1. Surgical procedure. | Patient will:<br>1. Utilize measures effective in managing pain.<br>2. Verbalize pain relief. | • Determine pain "tolerance." Assess patient's willingness to use pain medication vs. stoic behavior.<br>• Assess for physical manifestations of pain.<br>○ Restlessness, reluctance to move, guarding | • Many people fear they will become addicted to narcotics. |

| | | | |
|---|---|---|---|
| | 3. Exhibit relaxed demeanor:<br>• Relaxed facial expression and body posturing.<br>• Ease of breathing. | incision, clenched fist.<br>○ Diaphoresis, rapid shallow breathing, tachycardia, hypertension.<br>• Assess complaints of pain including severity, location/radiation, duration, and quality (i.e. sharp, dull, knifelike).<br>• Collaborate with physician and patient in titrating pain medication as needed.<br>• Suggest alternate position changes. | |
| ***Nursing Diagnosis #7***<br>Alteration in nutrition: less than body requirements, related to:<br>1. Presence of a neoplasm in the GI tract preoperatively, and NPO status postoperatively.<br>(See Chapter 53, Nutritional Support of the Critically Ill Patient.) | Patient will:<br>1. Meet the estimated nutrients:<br>• Calories per day<br>• Grams of protein per day as established by the nutritional support service.<br>2. Maintain body weight within 5% of baseline.<br>3. Maintain laboratory data within acceptable range: BUN, creatinine, electrolytes, glucose, albumin, and transferrin levels. | *Parenteral nutrition*<br>• Monitor daily intake and output, calorie count, and weights. Notify physician for weight gain greater than 2 lb in 24 hr. | • Monitors effectiveness of therapy. |
| | | • Monitor blood glucose levels and ketone levels in urine q 6 hr. | • The increased glucose load may overtax the pancreas and its ability to produce insulin. Patient may require regular insulin coverage. |
| | | • Monitor lab values (while on TPN):<br>○ Hematology profile.<br>○ Serum glucose and electrolytes, calcium, phosphorus.<br>○ BUN and creatinine.<br>○ Liver profile.<br>○ Serum cholesterol, triglycerides.<br>○ Total protein and serum albumin, transferrin.<br>○ Coagulation profile. | • Obtain full compliment of blood work prior to initiation of TPN for baseline values. Repeat weekly.<br>○ Monitors adequacy of replacement therapy. |
| | | • Maintain a constant IV infusion via infusion pump. Should therapy be interrupted, run dextrose 10W at the TPN rate. | • Allows pancreas to adjust to a high glucose level. |
| | | • Administer vitamin K 20 mg IM once per week as prescribed.<br>• Infuse lipids (10 or 20%) and amino acids daily as prescribed. | • Provides nutritional supplement. |
| | | *Enteral tube feedings*<br>• Monitor daily intake and output, caloric counts.<br>○ Weigh patient 3 times per week.<br>○ Monitor serum glucose and ketone levels in urine q 6 hrs. | • Monitors effectiveness of therapy. |
| | | • Monitor laboratory values: CBC with differential, albumin, and TIBC, electrolytes, BUN, and glucose. | • Obtain full complement weekly. |

*(continued)*

**TABLE 60–4. CARE PLAN FOR THE PATIENT WITH CANCER OF THE ESOPHAGUS TREATED BY SURGERY *(Continued)***

| Nursing Diagnoses | Desired Patient Outcomes | Nursing Interventions | Rationales |
|---|---|---|---|
| ***Nursing Diagnosis #7 (cont.)*** | | • Place continuous tube feeding on infusion pump. Keep head of bed elevated 30°. Check residual volume of feeding q 4 hr. If > 150 cc, discontinue feeding for 1 hr. If feeding held for more than 2 hr, notify physician.<br>○ Irrigate feeding tube with at least 20 cc water q 4 hr. | ○ Patients receiving enteral nutrition in high osmolar concentrations require free water to prevent dehydration. |
| | | • Notify physician if patient develops diarrhea. | • Indicates patient's intolerance to glucose and/or osmolar concentration. May require either a decrease in rate or concentration. Patient may require antidiarrheal medication to prevent fluid and electrolyte imbalance. |
| | | • Administer formula at room temperature. Discard unused feeding q 4 hr.<br>• Provide frequent mouth care. | • Asthetically pleasing to patient. Keeps mucous membranes moist and intact. |
| ***Nursing Diagnosis #8***<br>Potential for infection, related to:<br>1. Central line and TPN infusion.<br>(See also Table 56–1, Nursing Diagnoses #1, #2, and #3; Table 49–7.) | Patient will:<br>1. Be free from catheter and infusion-related infections. | • Monitor for symptoms of infection, i.e. fever, tachycardia, increased WBC count.<br>• Perform central venous line site care as per unit protocol. The area is cleansed with acetone and betadine and redressed with a transparent, occlusive dressing.<br>• Assess dressing integrity and catheter site q shift for redness, swelling, pain, or drainage. Obtain cultures as needed. Tubing changes are done daily. TPN bottles are discontinued after 24 hours. | • Patients receiving TPN are susceptible to infection due to high glucose concentration.<br>• TPN solution is a media for bacterial growth. The central line allows for systemic access into the patient. |
| | | • Note: Once a central line is dedicated for TPN use, it *should not* be used for additional medication, infusions, CVP readings, or blood aspiration. | • Allows for additional entry of bacteria into system. |
| ***Nursing Diagnosis #9***<br>Social isolation related to prolonged hospital stay. | Patient will:<br>1. Maintain social contacts developed prior to surgery. | • Encourage verbalization regarding social contacts.<br>• Consult social service when indicated.<br>• Promote privacy for patients and visitors. | • Identifies contacts that the nursing staff may make on behalf of the patient while in ICU. |

## REFERENCES


1. American Cancer Society: Cancer statistics. 35:12, 1985.
2. Skinner, DB et al: Selection of operation for esophageal cancer based on staging. Ann Surg 204:391, October 1986.
3. DeMeester, TR, et al: Surgery and current management for cancer of the esophagus and cardia: Part I. Curr Probl Surg 25:492, July 1988.
4. Data compiled from patient records at the Fox Chase Cancer Center, Philadelphia.
5. Goodwin, D: Editorial. Eur J Surg Oncol 12:105, June 1986.
6. Galandiuk, S, et al: Cancer of the esophagus: The Cleveland Clinic Experience. Ann Surg 203:101, January 1986.
7. Kirsh, M, et al: Complications of pulmonary resection. Ann Thorac Surg 20:219, August 1975.
8. Andreoli, KC, et al (eds): Comprehensive Cardiac Care: A Test for Nurses, Physicians, and Other Health Practitioners, ed 6. CV Mosby, St Louis, 1987, p 208.
9. Riboli, EB, et al: Treatment of esophageal anastomotic leakages after cancer resection. The role of total parenteral nutrition. JPEN J Parenter Enteral Nutr 10:82, January/February 1986.
10. Sons, HU: Aortic rupture in manual dissection of the esophagus: A rare complication during palliative esophagectomy performed on account of radiated esophageal cancer. A pathologic-anatomic view. J Surg Oncol 31:13, January 1986.
11. Ofek, B and Hoffman, J: Noninvasive treatment of esophagogastric anastomotic leakage. Arch Surg 12(1):124, January 1986.

# UNIT NINE

# Bibliography

## Neoplastic Cardiac Tamponade


Bear, P and Moodie, D: Malignant primary cardiac tumors. Chest 92:860, November 1987.

Chernecky, C and Ramsey, P: Neoplastic pericardial effusion and tamponade. In Chernecky, C: Critical Nursing Care of the Client with Cancer. Appleton-Century-Crofts, Norwalk, CT, 1984, p 88.

Ewer, M and Ali, M: Critical cardiologic considerations in the cancer patient. Crit Care Clin 4:41, January 1988.

Hiller, G: Cardiac tamponade in the oncology patient. Focus on Critical Care 14:19, August 1987.

Langfitt, D: Pulmonary embolism and chest trauma. In Critical Care Certification, Preparation and Review. Appleton & Lange, Norwalk, CT, 1984.

Patel, A, et al: Catheter drainage of the pericardium. Chest 92:1018, December 1987.

Polomano, R and Miller, E (eds): Understanding and Managing Oncologic Emergencies. Adria Laboratories, Columbus, Ohio, 1987.

Press, O and Livingston, R: Management of malignant pericardial effusion and tamponade. JAMA 257:1088, February 1987.

Pursley, P: Acute cardiac tamponade. AM J Nurs 83:1414, October 1983.

Roberts, S: Physiological Concepts and the Critically Ill Patient. Prentice-Hall, Englewood Cliffs, NJ, 1985, p 101.

Spodnick, D: Acute pericardial disease. Heart Lung 14:599, November 1985.

Spodnick, D: The technique of pericardiocentesis. Journal of Critical Illness 2:91, July 1987.

Stein, L, Shubin, H, and Weil, M: Recognition and management of pericardial tamponade. JAMA 225:503, July 1973.

Sulzbach, L: Management of pulsus paradoxus. Focus on Critical Care 16:142, April 1989.

Valentine, A and Stewart J: Oncologic emergencies. Am J Nurs 83:1283, September 1983.

Yasko, J: Guidelines for Cancer Care: Symptom Management. Reston Publishing, Reston, VA, 1983, p 343.


## Spinal Cord Compression


Bruetman, D and Harris, J: Oncologic emergencies, Part I: SVC syndrome and spinal cord compression. Journal of Critical Illness 3:31, September 1988.

Chernecky, C and Ramsey, P: Spinal cord compression. In Chernecky, C: Critical Nursing Care of the Client with Cancer. Appleton-Century-Crofts, Norwalk, CT, 1984, p 195.

Pederson, A, et al: Frequency, diagnosis, and prognosis of spinal cord compression in small cell bronchogenic carcinoma. Cancer 55:181, April 1985.

Rate, W, Solin, L, and Turrisi, A: Palliative radiotherapy for metastic malignant melanoma: Brain metastases, bone metastases and spinal cord compression. Int J Radiat Oncol Biol Phys 15:859, October 1988.

Valentine, A and Stewart, J: Oncologic emergencies. Am J Nurs 83:1283, September 1983.


## Septic Shock


Bary, S: Septic shock: Special needs of patients with cancer. Oncology Nursing Forum 16:31, January/February 1989.

Callender, D: Infections in neutropenic cancer patients: Your general approach. Journal of Critical Illness 3:17, February 1988.

Chang, J: How to differentiate neoplastic fever from infectious fever in patients with cancer. Heart Lung 16:122, March 1987.

Chernecky, C and Ramsey, P: Neutropenic and nonneutropenic sepsis. In Chernecky, C: Critical Nursing Care of the Client with Cancer. Appleton-Century-Crofts, Norwalk, CT, 1984, p 147.

Ersek, M: The adult leukemia patient in the intensive care unit. Heart Lung 13:183, March 1984.

Kahn, R: Shock as a complication of cancer. Critical Care Clinics 4:129, January 1988.

Keely, B: Septic shock. Crit Care Q 7:59, March 1985.

Lamb, L: Think you know septic shock? Nursing 12:34, January 1982.

Langfitt, D: Septic shock. In Critical Care Certification Preparation and Review. Appleton & Lange, Norwalk, CT, 1984.

Root, R and Sande, M (eds): Septic Shock. Churchill Livingstone, New York, 1985.

Yasko, J: Septic shock. Guidelines for Cancer Care: Symptom Management. Reston Publishing, Reston, VA, 1983.


## Syndrome of Inappropriate Secretion of Antidiuretic Hormone


Chernecky, C and Ramsey, P: Secretion of inappropriate antidiuretic hormone. In Chernecky, C: Critical Care of the Client

with Cancer. Appleton-Century-Crofts, Norwalk, CT, 1984, p 46.
Goldberg, M: Hyponatremia. Med Clin North Am 65:251, March 1981.
Kopec, I and Groeger, J: Life-threatening fluid and electrolyte abnormalities associated with cancer. Critical Care Clinics 4:81, January 1988.
Tilkian, S, Conover, M, and Tilkian, A: Clinical Implications of Laboratory Tests, Ed 2. CV Mosby, St. Louis, 1979.

## Neoplastic-Related Surgery

Goldfaden, D, et al: Adenocarcinoma of the distal esophagus and gastric cardia. J Thorac Cardiovasc Surg 91:242, February 1986.
Kratz, JM, et al: A comparison of endoesophageal tubes. J Thorac Cardiovasc Surg 97:19, 1989.
Pradhan, GN, et al: Left thoracotomy approach for resection of carcinoma of the esophagus. Surg Gynecol Obstet 168:49, 1989.
Sato, T, et al: Small cell carcinoma (non-oat cell type) of the esophagus concomitant with invasive squamous cell carcinoma and carcinoma in situ. Cancer 57:328, 1986.

UNIT TEN

# Hematologic System

Hematology is the science concerned with blood and blood-forming products. The blood functions in a variety of capacities vital to the preservation of life. It is the primary vehicle by which gases, nutrients, and metabolic products are exchanged at the cellular level. Thus, the blood plays a strategic role in the bodily processes of respiration, nutrition, and elimination, respectively. Through its role in the distribution and dissipation of heat, blood functions to assist in the regulation of body temperature. The flow of blood through specialized sensory receptors affords selective physiologic responses on a moment-to-moment basis to such variables as oxygen tension, pH, blood volume, electrolyte concentrations, osmolality, and hormonal levels. Thus, the blood also plays a key role in fluid, electrolyte, and acid–base balance.

The cellular and humoral components of blood provide essential constituents of the body's immunologic defense system. Lymphocytes, immunoglobulins (antibodies), complement, and phagocytic cells all play an integral part in the immune response (see Chap. 54). Components of the blood also play a major role in hemostasis (i.e., the process by which the body spontaneously arrests bleeding while maintaining the blood in a fluid state within the vascular system).

In the discussion that follows, two aspects of hematologic physiology will be addressed, namely, hematopoiesis (i.e., the formation of blood cells), and the hemostatic mechanism, including the interaction of the vascular system, platelets, and the plasma systems of coagulation and fibrinolysis. Emphasis is placed on reviewing the essential components of the assessment of hematologic function. The discussion of hematologic pathophysiology includes the syndrome of disseminated intravascular coagulation (DIC). Nursing process in the management of the patient with DIC is examined, including the use of pertinent nursing diagnoses. A Nursing Care Plan based on nursing diagnoses and including desired patient outcomes and specific nursing interventions and their rationales is presented.

## UNIT OUTLINE

CHAPTER 61

# Anatomy and Physiology of the Hematologic System: Hematopoiesis and Hemostasis

## CHAPTER OUTLINE



## LEARNING OBJECTIVES

**At the end of this chapter, you should be able to:**

1. Define *hemostasis* in terms of the interaction among blood vessels, platelets, and the plasma systems of coagulation and fibrinolysis.
2. Describe the reaction of blood vessels to vascular injury.
3. Examine the role of platelets in the hemostatic process.
4. Distinguish the coagulation pathways and their clinical significance.
5. Explain the function of the fibrinolysis system.
6. Outline the major control mechanisms of hemostasis.
7. Describe the activities of the inflammatory response in terms of the interrelationship among coagulation, fibrinolysis, and other humoral systems within the body including the kinin and complement cascades.

## HEMATOPOIESIS: CELLULAR COMPONENTS OF BLOOD

Hematopoiesis refers to the formation and development of the various types of blood cells from the hematopoietic stem cell. The bone marrow maintains an environment conducive to proliferation and maturation of blood cell formation (with the probable exception of lymphocyte production). Marrow stem cells are considered to be pluripotent in that they give rise to progenitor multipotential myeloid stem cells needed for erythropoiesis, leukopoiesis, and megakaryocytopoiesis, and the lymphoid stem cell essential for lymphopoiesis (Fig. 61–1).

### Erythropoiesis

Mature erythrocytes, or red blood cells (RBCs), are derived from erythroid progenitor cells through a series of mitotic divisions and maturation phases. Erythropoietin, a humoral agent produced primarily by the kidney in response to tissue hypoxia, stim-

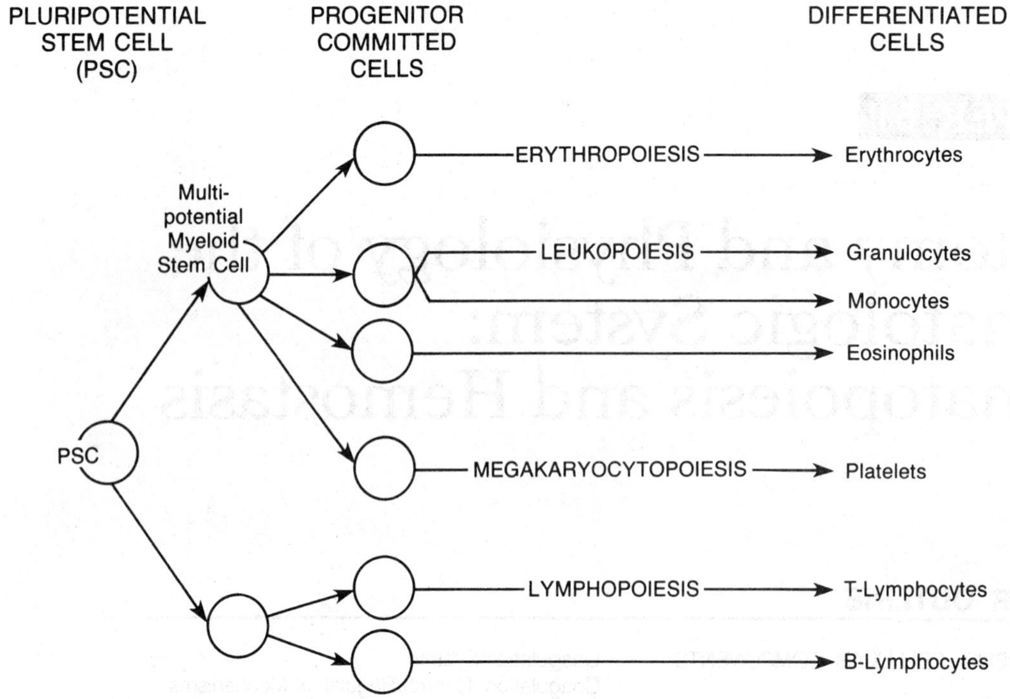


**61–1.** Hematopoiesis: differentiated cells.

ulates the erythropoietic process by acting on erythroid stem cells to induce proliferation and differentiation of RBCs (see Fig. 61–1). RBCs, in turn, function as an intermediary in the exchange of oxygen and carbon dioxide between the lungs and the tissues.

### *Red Blood Cells (Erythrocytes)*

Maturation of RBCs occurs in the bone marrow over a period of 4–5 days. During this time there are successive morphologic alterations in the nucleated cells initially, followed in later stages in non-nucleated cells. The reticulocyte stage, which precedes that of the mature RBC, is characterized by active hemoglobin synthesis, and it is at this stage that the non-nucleated reticulocyte is released into the circulation. Reticulocytes circulate in the blood for approximately 24 hours before maturing.

The normal mature RBC is a biconcave disk that is 7–8 $\mu$ in diameter. It is described as being highly flexible and pliable, features that facilitate passage through tiny capillaries while also affording optimal exposure of surface area for the exchange of oxygen and carbon dioxide. RBCs have an average lifespan of approximately 120 days. Most senescent or damaged RBCs are removed from the circulation by the spleen by a process referred to as *extra*vascular destruction. A small percentage of senescent RBCs are also destroyed normally within the circulation by a process termed *intra*vascular destruction.[1]

The normal RBC count is 4.5–5.5 million cells. Of this number, approximately 0.2–2.0% are reticulocytes. The reticulocyte count is of particular clinical significance because it is a parameter that reflects the RBC production rate and it is a good indicator of the erythropoietic response.[2] An elevated reticulocyte count is associated with hemolytic anemias.

### *Hemoglobin*

The major constituent of RBCs is hemoglobin. This molecule is largely responsible for oxygen transport to the tissues and carbon dioxide transport from the tissues to the lungs. In addition, by virtue of its high concentration and ubiquitous status, hemoglobin is considered to be the most effective body buffer (see section entitled "Chemical Buffering Systems" in Chap. 30).

Structurally, hemoglobin consists of the protein, globin (2 pairs of polypeptide chains), and 4 heme groups, each of which contains a protoporphyrin ring, plus iron ($Fe^{++}$). Oxygen specifically binds to the iron atom found within each of the heme groups. The amount of oxygen bound to hemoglobin is a function of the partial pressure of oxygen. This quantitative relationship between oxygen bound and the partial pressure of the gas is characterized by the oxyhemoglobin dissociation curve (see Fig. 28–15).

The unique structure of the hemoglobin molecule accounts for the unusual affinity this molecule has for oxygen. When the concentration of oxygen is high, as in the lungs, oxygen readily binds with hemoglobin; when the concentration of oxygen is low, as in the tissues, oxygen is readily released. The affinity of hemoglobin for oxygen is modified by several factors. The presence of acidemia, hyperthermia, and an increase in certain organic phosphates (especially 2,3-diphosphoglycerate, 2, 3-DPG) reduces hemoglobin's affinity for oxygen, thereby increasing the amount of oxygen released to the tissues. Conversely, alkalemia, hypothermia, and reduced levels of 2, 3-DPG increase hemoglobin's affinity for oxygen, thereby reducing the amount of oxygen released to the tissues (see section entitled "Transport of Oxygen" in Chap. 28).

## Leukopoiesis

Leukopoiesis refers to the production of white blood cells or leukocytes. Six types of circulating white blood cells have been identified. These include the granulocytes — neutrophils, eosinophils, and basophils; monocytes; lymphocytes, and plasma cells. Granulocytes, monocytes, and a few lymphocytes are formed in the bone marrow; remaining lymphocytes and plasma cells have their origin in lymphoid tissue. Overall, granulocytes and monocytes are responsible for phagocytosis; lymphocytes and plasma cells play key roles in the immune response, including cell-mediated and humoral immunity, respectively.

### *Granulopoiesis*

Granulopoiesis or myelopoiesis refers to the production of granulocytes including neutrophils, eosinophils and basophils, and monocytes (see Fig. 61-1). In general, granulocytes are essential components of the body's defense system. They function specifically in phagocytosis (i.e., the ingestion and digestion of bacteria and particles), chemotaxis (i.e., movement of neutrophils to a site of injury or inflammation in response to a chemical stimulus or messenger), and microbial killing.

Granulocytes also possess considerable biologic activity in other areas. They are active in the production of kinins. Kinins influence smooth muscle contraction inducing vasodilatation; they increase vascular permeability; and they exert a chemotactic effect, thereby attracting granulocytes to an area of inflammation. Granulocytes are also thought to produce pyrogens, fever-producing substances. In general, most granulocytic functions take place extravascularly.

**Neutrophils.** Neutrophils are the most numerous of the granulocytes normally representing 50-70% of the total number of WBCs. *Band* neutrophils, an immature form, account for approximately 3% of the total WBC count. A "shift to the left" describes an increase in the number of band and other immature neutrophils and is usually reflective of an underlying infectious process. The greater the shift, the more severe the infection.

Neutrophils are produced in the bone marrow from committed myeloid progenitor cells. They are stored in bone marrow, released to enter the blood for approximately 7-10 hours, and then exit the blood to enter the tissues. Normally, the rate at which neutrophils enter the blood and the rate of egress from the blood are in equilibrium. As these cells exit the blood for the tissues, they are replaced by other neutrophils from the bone marrow.

The key role of neutrophils in the body's defense system is phagocytosis. Specific events involved in this process include the migration of neutrophils to a site of infection or inflammation in response to chemotactic factors released from such sites; recognition; and phagocytosis with killing and digestion of invading microorganisms. Neutrophils are particularly efficient in phagocytizing bacteria coated with antibody.[1]

Corticosteroids induce an increase in the number of neutrophils, however, the number of *mature* neutrophils is decreased. Because only the mature neutrophil engages in phagocytosis, patients who receive pharmacologic doses of corticosteroids are more prone to develop significant infections.

**Eosinophils.** Eosinophils represent 1-3% of the total peripheral WBC count. They are described as having large, round secondary granules that have an affinity for the acid eosin stain. Mature eosinophils are stored in the bone marrow for several days prior to appearing in the blood. These cells migrate from the blood to tissues, and it is within the tissues that eosinophils largely reside.

Eosinophils function as part of the body's defense system. In this regard, the function of eosinophils is similar to that of neutrophils in that they can migrate into sites of infection and inflammation. These cells are able to ingest bacteria, but their phagocytic and microbial killing capabilities are less efficient than those of neutrophils.

Eosinophils are thought to play a key role in the detoxification of foreign protein. For example, the total number of circulating eosinophils increases during an allergic response as these cells collect at sites of antigen-antibody reactions and remove the resulting immune complexes from the blood. Eosinophils are also present in large numbers in the mucosal lining of the gastrointestinal and respiratory tracts, potential sites of entry of antigens into the body. Eosinophilia (i.e., the presence of increased numbers of eosinophils in the blood) has been associated with drug reactions (e.g., penicillin), allergic reactions (e.g., asthma), and parasitic infections (e.g., trichinae). Increased numbers of eosinophils have also been associated with skin diseases (e.g., exfoliative dermatitis), neoplasms (e.g., Hodgkin's disease), infections (e.g., tuberculosis), and the syndrome, periarteritis nodosa. Corticosteroids significantly decrease the number of eosinophils.

**Basophils.** Basophils constitute less than 2% of the normal WBC count. These cells are produced in the bone marrow arising from a multipotential precursor stem cell as do other granulocytes. Basophils differ from neutrophils in that they are not phagocytic. Rather, these cells play a significant role in acute systemic allergic reactions owing to the fact that basophilic granules contain histamine, serotonin, and heparin. If released in massive amounts, these agents can precipitate anaphylaxis (i.e., an allergic sensitivity reaction of the body to a foreign protein or drug).

Basophilic granules also contain a substance called eosinophil chemotactic factor, which attracts eosinophils when released during immediate hypersensitivity reactions. Endogenous secretion of heparin by basophils plays a vital role in clot formation. Increased numbers of basophils have been associated with such states as asthma, inflammatory bowel disease, carcinoma, post-splenectomy, and chronic inflammation. Inflammation has a coagulant effect on RBCs. Thus, the reason for an increase in heparin-rich basophils at inflammatory sites may be explained by the body's need for more heparin to prevent the coagulation process from consuming RBCs. Blood basophils are functionally related to their tissue counterparts, commonly called *mast* cells.

### *Monocytes and Macrophages*

Monocytes are phagocytic leukocytes that play a key role in the body's defense against pathogenic organisms and the invasion of foreign cells. Monocytes, which account for 1–6% of normal blood leukocytes, are immature cells released into the blood from the bone marrow. These cells then migrate into tissues and mature into active macrophages. Macrophages are present in all tissues but are especially concentrated in filter organs such as the liver, spleen, lungs, and lymph nodes.

The monocyte-macrophage system (i.e., the reticuloendothelial system, RES) plays a key role in host defense. Macrophages very efficiently entrap and phagocytize pathogenic microorganisms, ingest and degrade noxious exogenous agents, and engulf and process antigen. The processed antigenic substances are then passed on to cells of the lymphocytic-plasmocytic system responsible for cell-mediated immunity and for the synthesis of antibodies.

Phagocytic cells play a key role in removing hemoglobin-containing RBCs, injured and dead cells, hemosiderin granules, as well as red and white cell fragments and debris from the blood. Insoluble particles, activated clotting factors, and antigen–antibody complexes are also cleared from the blood by phagocytic cells. By the scavenger function of *motile* macrophages, which escape between epithelial cells of the respiratory tract, gastrointestinal, and renal/genitourinary organs, the body is cleared of additional unnecessary debris. These cells are found at sites of inflammation and in body fluids (e.g., peritoneal, pleural, synovial, and others). *Fixed* macrophages (or histiocytes) exert their phagocytic effect in the bone marrow, lymph nodes, spleen, sinusoids of the liver, lungs, and endothelial cells of the vascular system.

Macrophages also serve as secretory cells. Together with lymphocytes, they function in the immune response. Upon interaction with an antigen, the macrophage secretes a factor known as interleukin-1 (IL-1), which, in turn, induces T-cell proliferation (see Fig. 54–7). Macrophages also serve as secretory cells by elaborating prostaglandins, which function as mediators in the inflammatory response. Monocytes are especially sensitive to corticosteroids exhibiting impaired chemotaxis and phagocytic activity upon exposure to small doses of these substances.

### *Lymphopoiesis*

Lymphopoiesis refers to the formation of lymphocytes or of lymphoid tissue. Lymphocytes are the second most numerous of the white blood cells in blood with a range of 20–40%. Lymphocytes are concerned primarily with maintaining the body's immune defense system.

**Lymphocytes.** Lymphocytes originate from a lymphoid stem cell in bone marrow (see Fig. 61–1) and undergo sequential development into lymphoblasts, prolymphocytes, and mature lymphocytes. Differentiation into mature lymphocytes occurs in the thymus or the bursa-equivalent organs. Thymus-derived or T-lymphocytes are responsible for cell-mediated immune responses; bursa-equivalent or B-lymphocytes, upon appropriate antigenic stimulation, differentiate into antibody-producing cells or plasma cells (humoral immune response). Lymphocytes and plasma cells are essential in the body's defense against bacteria, viruses, and other microorganisms. For a detailed discussion of the role played by lymphocytes and plasma cells in the body's immune response, see Chapter 54.

## Megakaryocytopoiesis

The megakaryocyte is a giant bone marrow precursor cell, which, in the presence of the hormone, thrombopoietin, gives rise to fragments of cytoplasm called platelets (or thrombocytes). Thus, megakaryocytopoiesis refers to the production of platelets (see Fig. 61–1). Platelets are the smallest of the formed elements of the blood, and they exhibit a unique ability to adhere to injured blood vessel walls and to aggregate with other platelets, thereby forming hemostatic plugs (see below). The normal platelet count ranges between 150,000 and 350,000/mm$^3$. At any given moment, 80% of platelets occur in circulating blood, and 20% are pooled in the spleen. In the presence of splenomegaly, up to 80% of platelets released from bone marrow may be pooled in the spleen.

## HEMOSTASIS

Hemostasis, simply defined, means prevention of blood loss. It is a process by which the body spontaneously arrests bleeding while maintaining the fluidity of blood within the vascular compartment. Hemostasis is achieved by the interaction of several interrelated mechanisms that are initiated almost immediately upon vessel injury, highly localized to the site of injury, and precisely controlled. The major systems within the body involved in maintaining hemostasis include the vascular system, platelets, coagulation system (fibrin-forming), and the fibrinolysis system (fibrin-lysing).

### Vascular Mechanisms of Hemostasis

Blood normally flows within a continuous monolayer formed by overlapping endothelial cells. Within the capillaries, this continuous lining of overlapping endothelial cells is tightly anchored to supportive basement membrane. Larger vessels of the microcirculation (arterioles and venules) consists structurally of 3 components. The *intima,* or inner surface, includes the endothelium and subendothelium (i.e., basement membrane, elastic tissue, and collagen fibers); the *media,* or middle layer, is composed of smooth muscle cells, collagen fibers and occasional fibroblasts; and the *adventitia,* or outer layer, consists of fibroblasts, collagen fibers, extracellular connective tissue, and, depending on the size of the vessel, small blood vessels and, occasionally, nerves.

Because of their position as the cells interfacing between the vessel lumen and the blood, endothelial cells play a key role in maintaining the delicate balance between hemostasis and thrombosis, (i.e., localized process of vascular occlusion involving components from circulating blood). Endothelial cells perform several critical functions. It is across this layer of cells that metabolic exchange occurs. Endothelial cells function to maintain the integrity of the vessel wall preventing egress of blood cells, plasma proteins, macromolecules, and particulate material. Gaps that occur in the endothelial lining are sealed over by the barrier function of endothelial cells in conjunction with underlying vascular connective tissue and platelets.

A basic characteristic of intact, normal endothelium, and one of utmost importance in maintaining the fluidity of blood, is its nonreactivity to platelets, leukocytes, and coagulation factors. This thromboresistant characteristic of endothelium is achieved in part by several mechanisms.[3] These include, among others, the synthesis and release of prostacyclin ($PGI_2$), a prostaglandin that potently inhibits platelet adhesion and aggregation (see below); and the secretion of plasminogen activators that may protect against fibrin formation. These cells also synthesize/metabolize mediators that regulate the interaction between the vessel wall and blood components (e.g., factor VIII/von Willebrand's factor, collagen, fibronectin, and proteoglycans). Heparin sulfate, a proteoglycan, provides a surface that is nonthrombogenic. The connective tissue matrix produced by the endothelium functions to modulate vascular permeability and provides the principal stimulus to thrombosis post-vessel injury.[3]

Endothelial cells also process a number of vasoactive mediators such as bradykinin, serotonin, and norepinephrine. These cells are involved in the mediation of vascular repair processes such as cell migration, proliferation, and thrombolysis. Additionally, endothelial cells may play a role in the processing of antigen in cellular immunity.[4]

Disruption of the endothelium activates directly the major systems involved in maintaining hemostasis (Fig. 61-2):

1. In response to vessel injury, a rapid and direct vasoconstriction (vasospasm) occurs involving the injured vessel as well as adjacent structures. That consequent reduction of blood loss ensures a more effective contact/activation of platelets and coagulation.
2. Platelets adhere immediately upon exposure to subendothelial collagen and connective tissues and endothelial tissue thromboplastin. The release of thromboxane $A_2$ and vasoactive amines (e.g., serotonin, epinephrine) by adhering and aggregating platelets, in turn, enhances vasoconstriction.
3. Coagulation is initiated by both the intrinsic and extrinsic systems (see below).
4. Fibrinolysis follows with the release of plasminogen activators from the vascular wall. The fibrolytic process is essential to reestablishing vascular patency (see below).

Vessel size and the extent of tissue injury determine, in part, the relative importance of these reactions. Blood vessels having a more definitive media, or muscle layer (e.g., large arteries, veins, and arterioles), have the capacity to achieve a greater degree of vasoconstriction or vasospasm. Smaller arterioles and venules, once ruptured, become occluded with a platelet plug (see below). Capillaries, which have no muscle layer, are unable to vasoconstrict in response to injury and, therefore, rely primarily on platelets for hemostasis.

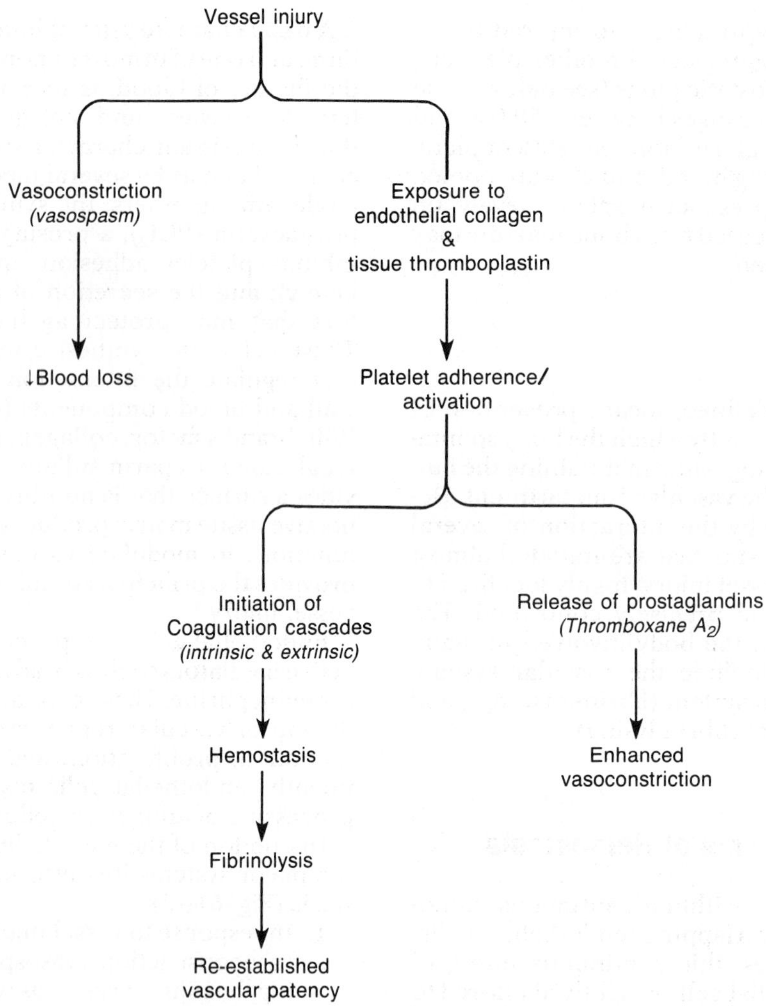


**Figure 61-2.** Vessel Injury: triggering event.

The extent of vessel injury also increases the degree of vasospasm achieved. Thus, a sharply cut blood vessel usually bleeds more initially than does a vessel sustaining a more extensive crushing-type injury.

Clinically, bleeding from capillaries and smaller arterioles and venules results in pinpoint hemorrhages or *petechiae;* bleeding from larger vessels results in soft tissue bleeding termed *ecchymoses.* Vascular spasm can last from less than a minute to several minutes. During this time, the second event in hemostasis is initiated, that is, the formation of the platelet plug.

## Cellular Mechanism of Hemostasis: Platelet Activation

Platelets play a key role in maintaining vascular integrity. When activated in response to vessel injury (see Fig. 61-2), platelets function to initiate primary hemostasis by the formation of the platelet plug. The platelet plugging mechanism is extremely important to close the minute ruptures in very small vessels and capillaries. Injury to larger vessels requires the formation of a blood (hemostatic) clot superimposed on the platelet plug to stop the bleeding. Platelets also contribute to the process of fibrin formation, which stabilizes the hemostatic plug.

Several processes are involved in the initial formation of the platelet plug, including platelet adhesion, platelet aggregation, and platelet release reaction. Following the formation of the platelet plug, there is consolidation of the plug into a dense thrombus, and stabilization of the clot by fibrin formation.

### *Platelet Adhesion*

Exposure of platelets to damaged endothelial cells, to subendothelial connective tissue such as collagen fibers, and to thromboplastin released by endothelial cells, is the triggering or initiating event in hemostasis, causing platelet adhesion.

### Platelet Aggregation

Adherent platelets, as well as damaged endothelial cells, release adenosine diphosphate (ADP), a potent initiator of platelet aggregation. ADP acts on nearby circulating platelets, causing them to undergo a transformation in their shape and ultrastructure. Among other things, this causes them to become very sticky. The stickiness of these adjacent platelets causes them to adhere to the initial platelet layer at the site of injury and to each other. This promotes additional aggregation, and it is this ongoing accumulation of increasing numbers of aggregating platelets that results in the formation of a loose, *primary* platelet plug. Such a plug is usually effective in preventing further blood loss if the site of the vessel rupture is small.

### Release Reaction

The release reaction is the process by which platelets exude the contents of their granules, which are essential to the hemostatic process. Important substances secreted by platelets include vasoactive amines (e.g., epinephrine, serotonin), which contribute to vasospasm of the injured vessel(s); ADP, which is essential for platelet adhesion and aggregation; calcium, which is necessary for the platelet release reaction and for the functional integrity of the coagulation pathways; and platelet factor (PF3), which is essential for thrombin production by the coagulation pathways. Among other functions, thrombin is necessary for irreversible binding or fusion of platelets to each other, thus forming the *secondary* platelet plug.

**Release Reaction: Action of Aspirin.** The release reaction is mediated in part by the action of prostaglandins. Prostaglandins, hormonelike substances that generate a potent localized effect, are derived from the conversion of platelet membrane phospholipid to arachidonic acid. Arachidonic acid is subsequently converted to prostaglandin by the enzyme, cyclooxygenase. Once available, platelet prostaglandin stimulates platelets to release calcium. Calcium, in turn, by its action on contractile proteins and microfilaments, triggers the release reaction.

Aspirin exerts its anticoagulant effect by blocking the action of the enzyme, cyclooxygenase, thus preventing the formation of platelet prostaglandin. Platelets exposed to aspirin are therefore unable to undergo the release reaction and to extrude their many substances necessary for the hemostatic process.

## Coagulation System

The purpose of the blood coagulation system is the formation of a fibrin clot on the surface of activated platelets (i.e., the platelet plug). As discussed above, vessel injury with disrupted endothelium initiates the process of hemostasis. In response, platelets adhere and aggregate to form the platelet plug, thereby reducing bleeding while also providing the framework for tissue repair. This is followed by the formation of a fibrin clot by the activation of the coagulation system (see Fig. 61–2).

The blood coagulation process involves a series of biochemical reactions that, ultimately, by converting soluble fibrinogen to fibrin, transforms circulating blood into an insoluble gel or clot. In vascular trauma that is minor, clot formation is initiated in 1–2 minutes. In more severe trauma, the actual clot begins to form in 15–20 seconds.

As the clot forms, an interlacing network of fibrin threads entraps platelets, RBCs, and plasma to form a stable clot. As the clot occludes the entire vessel lumen, additional blood loss is prevented. Within minutes, the clot retracts thereby pulling the edges of the vessel together, further ensuring hemostasis while exuding serum. (Because serum does not contain clotting factors and fibrinogen, it cannot clot.)

The coagulation system consists of 2 distinct pathways, both of which share a *common* pathway leading to the production of fibrin. These pathways involve a number of discrete molecules, or proenzymes, and clotting factors. These substances, together with platelets, phospholipid and calcium, participate in the coagulation process.

Both coagulation pathways require an initiating event, leading to subsequent activation of various coagulation factors in a cascading fashion. This means that each coagulation factor is activated by the preceding reaction. This system has the capacity for enormous acceleration and amplication, requiring specific controls. The acceleration phenomenon is caused by *autocatalysis,* whereby certain products formed in the coagulation process actually catalyze the reactions by which they themselves were formed. Thrombin is a principal autocatalyst (see p. 1280).

### Sources and Characteristics of Coagulation Factors

The coagulation factors are designated by Roman numerals assigned according to the sequence of discovery and not to the point of interaction in the coagulation cascade. Table 61–1 lists the coagulation factors and their most commonly used designations. With the exception of factor IV, calcium, all other coagulation factors are proteins; and except for factors V, VIII, and calcium, other coagulation factors, when activated, have very specific *enzymatic* activity. Factors V and VIII are cofactors rather than enzymes and function to accelerate enzymatic reactions involved in the coagulation process.

Synthesis of coagulation factors occurs in the liver except for factors VIII and XIII. Factor VIII

TABLE 61-1
**Nomenclature of Coagulation Factors**

| | |
|---|---|
| Factor I | Fibrinogen |
| Factor II | Prothrombin |
| Factor III | Tissue thromboplastin (tissue factor) |
| Factor IV | Calcium |
| Factor V | Labile factor |
| Factor VI | Not assigned |
| Factor VII | Stable Factor |
| Factor VIII | Antihemophilic factor (AHF) |
| Factor IX | Christmas factor |
| Factor X | Stuart-Prower factor |
| Factor XI | |
| Factor XII | Hageman factor |
| Factor XIII | Fibrin stabilizing factor (FSF) |

may be synthesized by endothelial cells. Factors II, VII, IX, and X are described as the vitamin K-dependent coagulation factors because synthesis of these factors by the liver requires the presence of vitamin K. Drugs that act as antagonists to vitamin K inhibit the activity of these factors. The anticoagulant effect of warfarin is exerted in this way.

Clinically, patients with a vitamin K deficiency exhibit a decreased production of these factors. The 2 major sources of vitamin K include ingested foods and an active bacterial flora in the distal small intestine. Thus, patients receiving parenteral feedings without vitamin K supplements, or patients receiving high doses of intravenous antibiotics, are at risk of developing a vitamin K deficiency with a bleeding diathesis. Liver disease, wherein the synthesis of coagulation factors is disrupted, may also present clinically, with a bleeding problem.

In the scenario of a bleeding diathesis, factor assay may help to distinguish liver dysfunction as a cause of bleeding, from another problem, for example, disseminated intravascular coagulation (DIC; see Chap. 63).

### *Coagulation Pathways: Extrinsic and Intrinsic*

The coagulation system consists of 2 pathways that evolve to a common final pathway of factor X activation with consequent clot formation. These include the extrinsic and intrinsic pathways.

The term "extrinsic" reflects the fact that this pathway is initiated by a substance not found in the blood. Factor III (or tissue thromboplastin) enters the vascular system from the injured tissues, and it provides the phospholipid component essential to the initiation of the extrinsic system.

The term "intrinsic" reflects the fact that all factors necessary for the coagulation process are found within the vascular compartment, that is, within the circulating blood. The phospholipids required by the intrinsic pathway are provided by the activated platelet membrane.

**Extrinsic Pathway.** In the extrinsic pathway, factor VII is activated to VIIa in the presence of calcium and tissue factor (factor III) released from injured tissue. The interaction of these 3 factors is sufficient to activate factor X to Xa, which, in turn, activates the common pathway (Fig. 61-3). The activities of the extrinsic pathway provide a means of rapidly generating small amounts of thrombin. Thrombin acts on fibrinogen (factor I) to convert it to fibrin; thrombin generated by the extrinsic pathway, in turn, accelerates the intrinsic pathway by enhancing the activity of cofactors V and VIII. In the laboratory, the prothrombin time (PT) is used to monitor the extrinsic pathway measuring factors VII, X, V, II, and I.

**Intrinsic Pathway.** Following exposure to foreign substances as, for example, subendothelial collagen, factor XII is activated to XIIa, thus initiating coagulation by the intrinsic pathway (see Fig. 61-3). The next reaction involves the activation of factor IX to IXa, in the presence of calcium. Activated factor IX (IXa) participates along with cofactor VIII, in the presence of calcium and platelet factor 3 (PF3; the latter providing the source of phospholipids necessary for activation), to activate factor X, thus triggering the common pathway. In the laboratory, the activated partial thromboplastin time (aPTT) is used to evaluate the intrinsic pathway measuring factors XII, XI, X, IX, VIII, V, II, and I.

**Common Pathway.** The common pathway is initiated when factor X is activated to Xa either by the extrinsic pathway (i.e., VIIa in the presence of tissue thromboplastin [factor III]) and calcium, or by the intrinsic pathway (i.e., IXa in the presence of cofactor VIII), calcium, and platelet factor three (PF3). After the formation of Xa, this activated factor, in the presence of cofactor V, calcium, and PF3, converts factor II, prothrombin, to the activated enzyme, thrombin. The complex of Xa, V, calcium, and PF3 assembles on the surface of the activated platelets.

### *Thrombin: The Pivotal Molecule*

Once generated by the common pathway, thrombin functions to amplify the coagulation process. Major functions of thrombin include the following: (1) stimulates platelet aggregation, release reaction, and fusion into the secondary platelet plug; (2) enhances the activity of cofactors V and VIII; (3) activates factor XIII to XIIIa; (4) converts fibrinogen to fibrin; and (5) initiates the conversion of plasminogen to plasmin (i.e., the fibrinolysis system).

The fibrin monomer produced by the action of thrombin on fibrinogen is held together by weak hydrogen bonding. The action of activated factor XIII (XIIIa) on fibrin converts it to a stronger, more stable clot. By using the prothrombin time (PT) and partial thromboplastin time (PTT) laboratory test results, it is possible to identify defects or deficien-

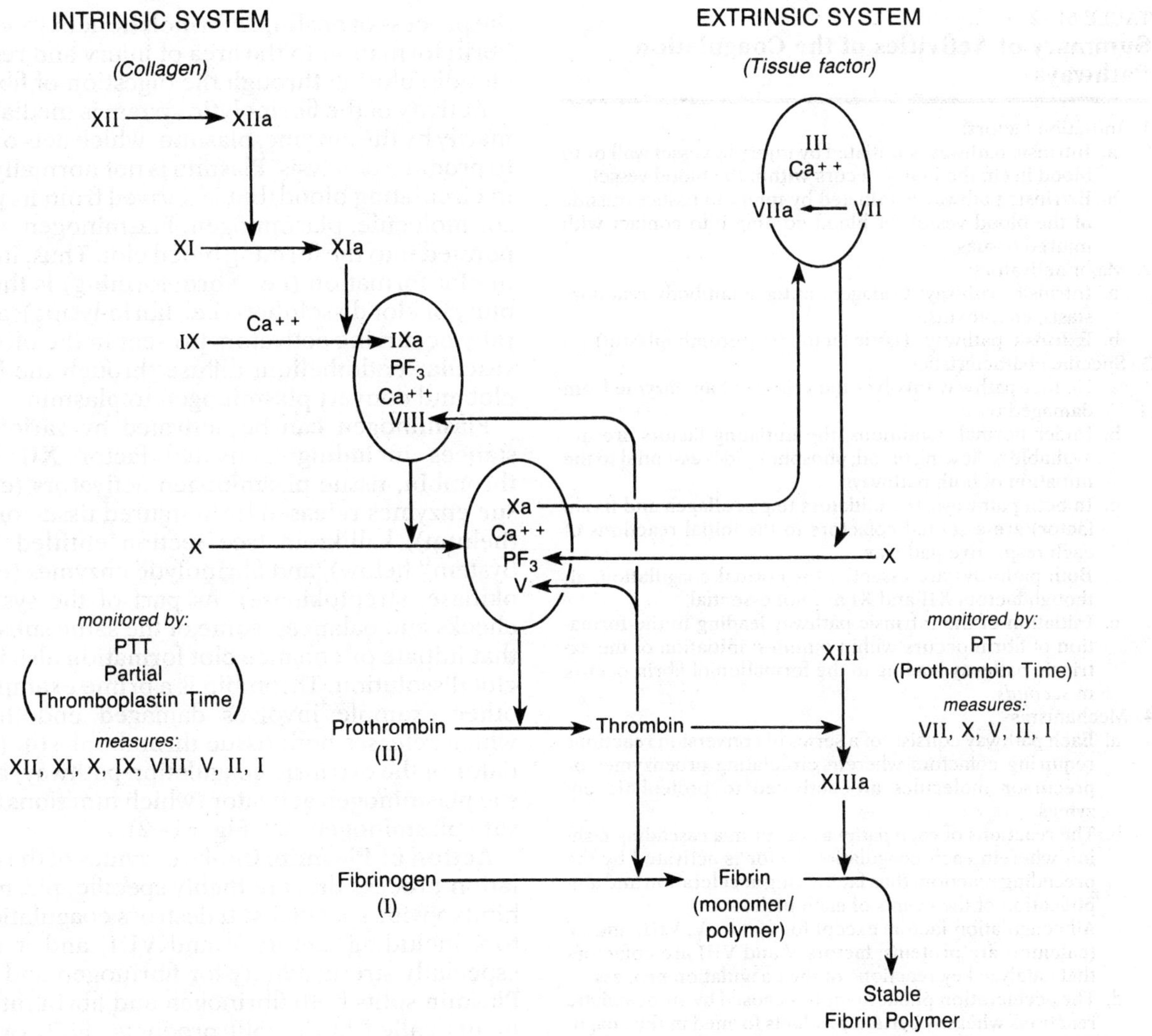


**Figure 61–3.** Coagulation pathways.

cies in the extrinsic, intrinsic or common pathways of blood coagulation. Table 61–2 summarizes the key activities of the coagulation system.

## Coagulation: Control/Regulatory Mechanisms

A delicate system of checks and balances exists within the body to allow necessary localized clotting to repair injury on the one hand, while maintaining the fluidity of the blood on the other. The significance of such a system can be appreciated when one considers that sufficient thrombin can be generated from a milliliter of blood to coagulate the fibrinogen in 3 liters of blood within 15 seconds.[5]

The fibrinolysis system is the major system involved in fibrin clot dissolution. In addition, other anticoagulant forces include blood flow, the role of antithrombin III, and various positive and negative feedback mechanisms.

### *Fibrinolysis System*

The activities of both the coagulation and fibrinolytic systems are intimately related. When both systems are in balance, a normal response to injury occurs wherein fibrin is formed, tissue is repaired, and fibrin is gradually digested and removed from the circulation by the cells of the monocyte-macrophage system (reticuloendothelial system). In this normal response, the processes of fibrin formation and fibrin degradation proceed simultaneously, the latter at a somewhat slower rate than the former. The slow dissolution of the clot allows time for repair of damaged tissue. The action of the fibrinolytic system reestablishes blood flow in vessels oc-

TABLE 61-2
**Summary of Activities of the Coagulation Pathways**

1. Initiation factors:
   a. Intrinsic pathway is initiated by injury to vessel wall or to blood itself; the injury occurs within the blood vessel.
   b. Extrinsic pathway is initiated by injury to tissues outside of the blood vessel; or blood coming into contact with injured tissues.
2. Major activators:
   a. Intrinsic pathway: Collagen, antigen-antibody reaction, stasis, endotoxins.
   b. Extrinsic pathway: Tissue factor III (thromboplastin).
3. Specific characteristics:
   a. Neither pathway involves the release of an enzyme from damaged tissue.
   b. Under normal conditions, the initiating factors are unavailable to flowing blood; phospholipid is essential to the initiation of both pathways.
   c. In both pathways, the initiators (e.g., collagen and tissue factor) are essential cofactors to the initial reactions of each respective pathway.
   d. Both pathways are essential for normal coagulation, although factors XII and XI are not essential.
   e. Initiation of the intrinsic pathway leading to the formation of fibrin occurs within *minutes*; initiation of the extrinsic pathway leading to the formation of fibrin occurs in *seconds*.
4. Mechanisms:
   a. Each pathway consists of a series of conversion reactions requiring cofactors wherein circulating proenzymes or precursor molecules are activated to proteolytic enzymes.
   b. The reactions of each pathway occur in a cascading fashion wherein each coagulation factor is activated by the preceding reaction, thus facilitating acceleration and amplification of the events of each pathway.
   c. All coagulation factors except for factors V, VIII, and IV (calcium) are proteins; factors V and VIII are cofactors that catalyze key reactions of the coagulation process.
   d. The acceleration phenomenon is caused by autocatalytic reactions whereby certain products formed in the coagulation process actually catalyze the reactions by which they themselves were formed. Thrombin is a principal autocatalyst.
   e. Vitamin K-dependent factors (VII, IX, X and II) function in the tight binding of coagulation factors to calcium and phospholipid. This activity raises the localized concentrations of the reactants and increases the speed of reactions leading to the amplification effect.
   f. Thrombin is the pivotal molecule in these reactions with the following key functions:
      (1) Stimulates platelet aggregation, release reaction and fusion into the secondary platelet plug that forms the basis for the interaction of coagulation factors.
      (2) Enhances the activity of cofactors V and VIII, which accelerate the coagulation process.
      (3) Converts fibrinogen to fibrin, which forms the basis for the clot.
      (4) Activates factor XIII to XIIIa, which converts fibrin into a stable clot.
      (5) Initiates the fibrinolysis system.

cluded by a clot and facilitates the healing process following injury.

The fibrinolysis system is essential in (1) removing fibrin from sites of vascular injury, (2) reestablishing patency of blood vessels, and (3) facilitating the process of healing. Fibrinolytic activity restricts fibrin formation to the area of injury and results in clot dissolution through the digestion of fibrin.

Activity of the fibrinolytic system is mediated primarily by the enzyme, plasmin, which acts on fibrin to produce clot lysis. Plasmin is not normally found in circulating blood, but is derived from its precursor molecule, plasminogen. Plasminogen is incorporated into the forming blood clot. Thus, inherent in clot formation (i.e., fibrin-forming) is the capability of clot dissolution (i.e., fibrin-lysing), as naturally occurring activators present in the blood and vascular endothelium diffuse through the formed clot and convert plasminogen to plasmin.

Plasminogen can be activated by various substances including: activated factor XII (XIIa), thrombin, tissue plasminogen activators (e.g., tissue enzymes released from injured tissue or endothelium), kallikrein (see section entitled "Kinin System" below), and fibrinolytic enzymes (e.g., urokinase, streptokinase). As part of the system of checks and balances, some of the same substances that initiate or enhance clot formation also initiate clot dissolution. Thrombin is a prime example. Another example involves damaged endothelium, which releases both tissue thromboplastin (an initiator of the extrinsic coagulation pathway) and tissue plasminogen activator (which functions to activate plasminogen; see Fig. 61-2).

**Action of Plasmin.** Unlike enzymes of the coagulation process that are highly specific, plasmin exhibits a wide specificity. It destroys coagulation factors including factors V and VIII, and it has an especially strong affinity for fibrinogen and fibrin. Plasmin splits both fibrinogen and fibrin into fragments called fibrin split products (FSP) or fibrin degradation products (FDP). Clinically, these degradation products are important because they can increase vascular permeability and interfere with the clot-forming activities of platelets, thrombin, and fibrinogen. Thus, they are potent anticoagulants. Fibrin degradation products can be measured and monitored. Enhanced fibrinolysis may be observed in various coagulopathies, as well as traumatic injury, major surgery, or liver disease, among others.

**Control of Fibrinolysis.** As has been discussed, the activity of the fibrinolytic system plays a major role in controlling blood coagulation. In turn, the fibrinolytic system, likewise, is controlled so as to prevent unusual bleeding. Plasmin is rapidly inhibited in the circulation by 2 major inhibitors. These include alpha$_2$ macroglobulin and alpha$_2$ plasmin inhibitor. In addition, plasminogen is adsorbed by fibrin, leading to its decreased availability.

### Blood Flow

Blood flow provides a major mechanism for the control of coagulation. The smooth endothelial lining reduces turbulence and facilitates blood flow; its layer of negatively charged proteins minimizes the interaction between vessel and blood. The circulating blood rapidly dilutes or disperses formed activated coagulation factors preventing their accumulation. In this way, blood flow ensures that coagulation reactions remain localized to the site of injury. Circulation of blood through the liver and reticuloendothelial system facilitates the removal of activated factors by these organs, thus providing another mechanism that prevents unwanted accumulation of these clotting factors. Finally, because blood normally lacks phospholipids, the coagulation cascades are not activated.

#### *Role of Antithrombin III*

Antithrombin III is a plasma protein that inhibits all activated clotting factors except VIIa and XIIIa. It is the molecule through which the drug, heparin, exerts its anticoagulant effect. Alpha$_2$ macroglobulin is similar to antithrombin III in that it likewise combines with the proteolytic coagulation factors.

#### *Feedback Mechanisms*

Feedback mechanisms controlling coagulation include both positive and negative feedback systems. The feedback of thrombin on platelets to enhance platelet aggregation and release reaction is an example of a positive feedback loop; as is the feedback of Xa on factor VII, thus enhancing the production of thrombin by the extrinsic pathway (see Fig. 61-1).

Previously, the role of platelet prostaglandin (inducer) in mediating the platelet release reaction was discussed. Similarly, endothelial prostaglandin (inhibitor) acts to inhibit the release reaction. Without a source of platelet factor three (PF3), the coagulation process is prevented. The activation/inactivation of factors V and VIII by thrombin is another example of the role of feedback mechanisms in controlling the coagulation process.

#### *Additional Control Mechanisms*

Other controls include the adsorption of thrombin to fibrin, which decreases the availability of thrombin. In the absence of thrombin, the formation of fibrin from fibrinogen is prevented. The sequestation of plasminogen within the forming clots, where it can be activated to plasmin by thrombin, was mentioned earlier. This facilitates clot dissolution by the fibrinolysis system. In addition, fibrin split (degradation) products exert a potent anticoagulant effect. Fibrin split products compete with thrombin for fibrinogen, and they prevent the polymerization of fibrin into a stable clot.

## INTEGRATED REACTIONS AMONG HEMOSTATIC COMPONENTS

As has been discussed, the vascular endothelium, platelets, coagulation, and fibrinolytic systems interrelate by numerous mechanisms. In addition, components of these systems also implicate other physiologic mechanisms involving the kinin and complement systems and, to some extent, the inflammatory response.

### Kinin System

The kinin system, of importance to the inflammatory response, vascular permeability, and chemotaxis, is activated by both the coagulation and fibrinolytic systems. The precursor, prekallikrein, is activated to the enzyme, kallikrein, by the action of XIIa (Hageman factor) and plasmin. Kallikrein, in turn, acts on plasma kininogens converting them to kinin. Bradykinin is an example of a kinin, and it functions to increase vascular permeability, contract smooth muscle, dilate blood vessels, induce inflammation, and cause the release of prostaglandins from tissues.[6] The kinin system, in turn, is involved in the activation of the intrinsic pathway. For example, the activation of factor XII to XIIa requires the presence of the enzyme, killikrein.

### Complement System

The complement system is composed of approximately 22 serum proteins, which, working together with antibodies and clotting factors, play an important role as mediators of both the immune and allergic responses.[6] Activated by 2 independent pathways (see Fig. 54-13), these proteins play an especially significant role in the cell membrane lysis of antibody-coated target cells. Plasmin, an important activator of complement factors, plays a key role in interactions between the fibrinolysis and complement systems. (For additional information regarding the activities of the complement system, see Chap. 54.)

### Inflammatory Process

In response to trauma, infection, or other insult, a complex of sequential changes occurs at the site of tissue damage that constitutes the inflammatory process (Table 61-3). Implicated in these changes are a number of important mediators involving the coagulation, fibrinolysis, kinin, and complement systems. The key factor that seems to bridge the interrelationships of these systems is activated factor XII, or Hageman factor.

The impact of Hageman factor may be direct or

TABLE 61–3
**Phases of the Inflammatory Process**

"Rubor et tumor cum calore et dolore" by Cornelius Celsus, Roman writer, First Century, AD.
Phases of the inflammatory process include the following:

A. The release by injured cells of enhanced amounts of chemical substances including histamine, bradykinin, and serotonin; proteolytic enzymes; and prostaglandins.
B. The occurrence of a vascular response mediated by these chemical substances and characterized by:
   - A transient vasodilation increasing local blood flow to the injured tissues (Rubor = erythema) (Calore = heat or warmth)
   - An immediate increase in vascular permeability resulting in transudative extravasation of fluid from intravascular to interstitial space (Tumor = swelling or edema) (Dolore = pain)
C. The occurrence of a cellular response facilitated by the vascular changes and characterized by:
   - Migration of leukocytes (initially neutrophils followed by monocytes, and later by lymphocytes) from the circulation into the area of damaged tissues where they trigger several important processes:
     - **Chemotaxis**—Force of attraction on circulating leukocytes facilitating their movement to area of tissue injury.
     - **Phagocytosis**—Force exerted by neutrophils involving destruction of pathologic antigen by engulfment and/or intracellular killing
     - **Immune Response**—Force exerted by neutrophils and macrophages wherein the pathologic antigen is captured for presentation to lymphocytes with triggering of the immune response by cell-mediated or humoral (antibodies) mechanisms.
     - **Complement System Activation**—Potent mediators of inflammatory response, triggered by antibody and non-antibody-dependent events.
D. The occurrence of wound healing by:
   - Tissue regeneration: Replacement of lost cells with similar cell types.
   - Tissue repair: Replacement of lost cells with connective tissue, usually with scar formation.

indirect. Among others, it has been associated with coordinating the following activities:

1. Activated Hageman factor triggers the intrinsic coagulation cascade leading to the formation of fibrin. In turn, certain products derived from fibrin also act as vasoactive mediators of inflammation.
2. The plasminogen pathway of fibrinolysis is activated by activated Hageman factor liberating plasmin. This activated enzyme not only lyses fibrin, but also activates the complement system. Several components of the complement system function as important mediators of inflammation, some exerting potent chemotaxic effects.
3. Activated Hageman factor also activates the conversion of prekallikrein to kallikrein, an active proteolytic enzyme (see above). The action of this enzyme on plasma kininogen causes the liberation of bradykinin. Bradykinin is a potent vasodilator that also increases vascular permeability. The consequent vasodilation at the site of injury accounts for the erythema and warmth; the increase in vascular permeability underlies the edema and pain associated with the inflammatory process.

## REFERENCES


1. Pittiglio, DH: Clinical Hematology and Fundamentals of Hemostasis. FA Davis, Philadelphia, 1987, p 7.
2. Griffin, J: Hematology and Immunology Concepts for Nursing. Appleton-Century-Crofts, Norwalk, CT, 1986, p 25.
3. Thompson, A and Harker, L: Manual of Hemostasis and Thrombosis, ed 3. FA Davis, Philadelphia, 1983, p 5.
4. Hirschberg, H, Bergh, O, and Thorsby, E: Antigen presenting properties of human vascular endothelial cells. J Exp Med 152:249, 1980.
5. Griffin, JP: Hematology and Immunology Concepts for Nursing. Appleton-Century-Crofts, Norwalk, CT, 1986, p 62.
6. Pittiglio, DH: Clinical Hematology and Fundamental of Hemostasis. FA Davis, Philadelphia, 1987, p 343.


## SUGGESTED READINGS


Beck, WS (ed): Hematology, ed 4. MIT, Cambridge, MA, 1985.
Griffin, JP: Hematology and Immunology Concepts for Nursing. Appleton-Century-Crofts, Norwalk, CT, 1986.
Pittiglio, DH: Clinical Hematology and Fundamentals of Hemostasis. FA Davis, Philadelphia, 1987.
Pittiglio, DH: Modern Blood Banking and Transfusion Practices. FA Davis, Philadelphia, 1983.
Rifkind, R, et al: Fundamentals of Hematology, ed 3. Yearbook Medical Publishers, Chicago, 1986.
Thompson, A and Harker, L: Manual of Hemostasis and Thrombosis, ed 3. FA Davis, Philadelphia, 1983.

CHAPTER 62

# Assessment of Hematologic and Hemostatic Function

## CHAPTER OUTLINE



## LEARNING OBJECTIVES

**At the end of this chapter, you should be able to:**

1. Describe cardinal signs and symptoms of hematologic and hemostatic dysfunction.
2. Explain the clinical significance of a "shift to the left" in white blood cell differential.
3. Define *bleeding diathesis* and its manifestations, purpura, petechiae, and ecchymosis.
4. Describe the impact of hematologic and hemostatic dysfunction on a person's functional health patterns.
5. Discuss the significance of a thorough drug history in patients suspected of having a hematologic and/or hemostatic disorder.
6. Identify familial disorders of importance in hematologic and hemostatic function and dysfunction.
7. Outline key findings in the physical examination of patients with, or suspected of having, a hematologic and/or hemostatic disorder.
8. List tests of hematologic function and the usual ranges of normal.
9. List tests of hemostatic function and the usual ranges of normal.
10. Relate abnormalities in tests of hematologic and hemostatic function to the overall clinical presentation of the patient/family, including the clinical history and physical examination.

Disorders of hematologic function (i.e., the function of blood and blood-forming tissues) can be extremely complex. Until recently, many diseases in this realm of medicine remained unfamiliar; others have yet to be defined. Some have been diagnosed in the course of treating another underlying problem. Frequently, hematologic problems occur as a complication of another organ system disease or as a consequence of a specific course of therapy (e.g., chemotherapy).

Valid assessments are crucial to diagnosis (and differential diagnosis), treatment, and/or prevention of hematologic disease or complications. Symptoms reflective of underlying hematologic dysfunction can be subtle, easily overlooked or unrecognized, or even misleading. As the bedside health-care provider who interacts most intimately with patient and family, the nurse must make necessary ongoing and continuous assessments, establish baseline function, and assess for actual or potential problems. Such assessments assist in defining/refining the underlying problem, determining the course of therapy, and evaluating the patient's response to therapy.

The diagnostic assessment and evaluation of hematologic function require a thorough history and physical examination of the patient, as well as a variety of laboratory tests that assist in pinpointing the underlying problem. The emphasis here will be to provide a brief overview of the hematologic assessment, and then to concentrate more closely on the assessment of hemostasis and coagulation.

## CLINICAL HISTORY

The clinical history affords the patient and family/significant others the opportunity to verbalize their problems and concerns as to why they have chosen to seek health-care assistance at this point in time (subjective data); it enables the nurse to observe closely for any overt or covert cues that may be helpful in diagnosing and planning care (objective data). The sequence and detail of the assessment process will vary according to the nurse's judgment about the patient's status. The extent and comprehensiveness of the initial history and examination should be modified accordingly.

### Components of the Clinical History

#### *Chief Complaint/History of Present Illness*

The chief complaint reflects the major concern or symptom experienced by the patient and family/significant others, and it should be documented in their very words. The events surrounding the complaint should be elicited, including its onset, the course since onset, and the current status of the patient. Use of the SLIDT tool (see Table 7-1) assists in eliciting pertinent details regarding the patient's underlying complaint and general health status.

#### *Cardinal Signs/Symptoms of Hematologic and Hemostatic Dysfunction*

***Anemias — Red Blood Cell Disorders.*** *Anemia* is a condition in which there is a reduction in the number of circulating red blood cells, the amount of hemoglobin, or the volume of packed red cells. It exists when hemoglobin content is less than that required to meet the oxygen demands of body tissues.

Anemia is classified on the basis of (1) mean corpuscular volume (MCV) calculated as the volume of packed cells divided by the RBC count, and includes *microcytic* (characterized by abnormally small RBCs), *normocytic* (wherein the size and hemoglobin content of RBCs remain normal), and *macrocytic* (marked by abnormally large RBCs); (2) mean corpuscular hemoglobin (MCH) calculated as the hemoglobin concentration of whole blood divided by the number of red cells present, and includes *hypochromic* (wherein there is a hemoglobin deficiency and mean corpuscular hemoglobin concentration is less than normal), *normochromic* (wherein the RBCs contain the normal amount of hemoglobin), and *hyperchromic* (characterized by a mean corpuscular hemoglobin concentration greater than normal); and (3) etiologic factors, such as excessive blood loss, excessive RBC destruction or hemolysis, or decreased red blood cell synthesis. (For specific tests and their usual ranges, see Table 62-2).

***Leukopenia and Leukocytosis: White Blood Cell Disorders.*** White blood cells, or leukocytes, are classified as granulocytes (i.e., those possessing granules) and agranulocytes (i.e., those lacking granules). Granulocytes, in turn, are classified according to their staining properties and morphology, and include neutrophils, basophils, and eosinophils. Agranulocytes include lymphocytes and monocytes.

*Leukopenia* is an abnormal decrease in the number of white blood cells (usually under 5000/mm$^3$). *Leukocytosis* is an abnormal increase in the number of white blood cells (usually over 10,000/mm$^3$). In addition to their total numbers, a differential white blood cell count reflects the percentage of each type of white blood cell. Abnormal morphology may provide a clue as to the underlying disease process. For example, it is abnormal for more than 8-10% of circulating neutrophils to be in *band* form (i.e., immature). When immature granulocytes become prominent in the differential white blood cell count, it is sometimes referred to as a "shift to the left."

A *neutro*philia (i.e., an increase in the number of circulating neutrophils), accompanied by a "shift to the left" (i.e., an increase in morphologically immature white cells), is usually indicative of an underlying bacterial infection. *Eosino*philia (i.e., an increase in circulating eosinophils) is associated with allergic conditions and parasitic infections; *baso*philia (i.e., an increase in circulating basophils) occurs in hypersensitivity reactions, in stressful states, and chronic inflammatory processes.

*Lymphopenia* (*lymphocytopenia*), a deficiency of lymphocytes in the blood, is associated with immunodeficiency disorders, severe, debilitating diseases (e.g., renal failure), or with defects in lymphatic circulation (e.g., disorders of intestinal mucosa or thoracic duct drainage). *Lymphocytosis*, an excess of lymph cells in the blood, is commonly associated with infectious diseases (bacterial and viral) and chronic inflammatory conditions (e.g., ulcerative colitis), among others. (For specific tests and their usual ranges, see Table 62-2.)

**Bleeding Diathesis.** Presenting complaints reflective of underlying hemostatic dysfunction may involve recent excessive or prolonged bleeding episodes. Purpura, petechiae, and ecchymosis are classic signs of an underlying bleeding disorder.

***Purpura.*** Purpura, bleeding or extravasation of blood into tissues (e.g., skin, mucous membranes, internal organs, and others), is considered to be the cardinal sign of hemostatic dysfunction, although its occurrence may reflect conditions with diverse causes. Its actual cutaneous appearance varies with the duration of the lesion and the acuteness of onset. Typically, in an acute episode, the color of the skin is initially red; it gradually becomes darkened and somewhat purple, fading finally to brownish-yellow before disappearing over a 2-3 week period.

***Petechiae.*** Petechiae are minute hemorrhagic spots about the size of a pinpoint. Their presence suggests a possible platelet dysfunction as capillaries and tiny blood vessels, lacking the capacity for vascular spasm, depend largely on platelet plugging for hemostasis.

***Ecchymosis.*** Ecchymosis reflects a purplish area reflective of bleeding into the soft tissues and skin. It differs from petechiae only in the size of the patches.

**Other Symptomatology.** In addition to the cardinal signs and symptoms, patients may present with complaints of epistaxis, persistent hoarseness, hematemesis, melena, hematuria, or mennorrhagia. Occasionally, such complaints may be related to a known underlying condition (e.g., liver disease, blood dyscrasias, or clotting disorders). Visual disturbances or tinnitus may be associated with an underlying bleeding disorder. Cough, hemoptysis, dyspnea, or anginal-type pain may reflect pulmonary pathology (e.g., pulmonary embolism) associated with an underlying thromboembolic disorder.

Patients on long-term anticoagulant therapy may present unsuspectingly with a bleeding diathesis. Such patients may not manifest obvious bleeding but, rather, subtle symptomatology reflective of underlying internal bleeding. For example, alterations in neurologic function, such as recent changes in behavior or personality, or altered state of consciousness, may actually be caused by intracranial bleeding associated with the anticoagulant therapy.

Many patients present with nonspecific complaints such as unusual fatigue, general malaise, anorexia, and weight loss. Fever, chills, night sweats, and poor wound healing are not uncommon.

### Functional Health Patterns

Patients experiencing alterations in hematologic and hemostatic function may present with changes in their functional health patterns. Assessment of these patterns is essential to nursing diagnosis, treatment, patient/family education, and discharge planning.

**Health Perception-Health Maintenance.** The patient's perception of his/her overall health status needs to be ascertained. What level of health is desired and how motivated are the patient/family to achieve and maintain health and well-being? What are their expectations of health care? Decisions regarding health rest with the patient and family. Nurses support the patient/family and help them to get through the crisis situation, encourage them in self-care activities, and assist in planning for the patient's eventual return to the home/community setting. Care is guided by the concern as to what were the circumstances in which illness occurred, and how can interventions be implemented to ameliorate those factors that caused the illness? The goal is not only to restore the patient to wellness, but to assist in ensuring that the wellness state will be maintained upon discharge, at the optimal level as desired by the patient/family.

What is the patient's health status? Is there evidence of acute or chronic illness? Have subtle changes in the patient's behavior or personality been observed by family members/significant others? Unexplained irritability, inability to concentrate, apathy, and depression often accompany hematologic disorders, which may not otherwise be apparent or even suspected.

What is the patient's occupation? Depression of bone marrow hematopoiesis has been associated with exposure to toxic chemicals, radiation, and drugs.

**Nutrition/Metabolic.** Deficiencies in dietary intake over a period of time may place the patient at risk of developing hematologic dysfunction. Altered hematopoiesis may occur in the presence of depleted iron stores, and vitamin $B_{12}$ and folate deficiencies. Excessive alcohol consumption suppresses the appetite and predisposes to avitaminosis (i.e., vitamin deficiency). Alcohol may also impair platelet function leading to bleeding and coagulation defects. The patient may present with a recent, unexplained weight loss, recurrent infection, or poor wound healing, all of which may occur in the presence of a hematologic disorder (e.g., erythrocyte deficiency, leukopenia).

Altered hemostasis occurs in the presence of vitamin K deficiency. Vitamin K deficiency may be associated with inadequate dietary intake and/or overly aggressive use of intravenous antibiotics, which obliterate the gastrointestinal bacterial flora essential to vitamin K synthesis and absorption. The end result is altered hemostasis as vitamin K-dependent coagulation factors (these include factors II, VII, IX and X) become deficient.

Recent onset of anorexia, nausea, vomiting, food intolerance, and dysphagia may predispose to malnutrition, which, in turn, may compromise hematologic function. A reduction in essential nutrients disrupts vitamin synthesis. Altered metabolism (e.g., diabetes mellitus or its complication, diabetic ketoacidosis) likewise compromises hematopoiesis.

**Elimination.** Recent changes in bowel habits (e.g., diarrhea, constipation) or in the characteristics of the stool (e.g., clay-colored, tarry) may be a contributing factor to, or a reflection of, underlying hematologic dysfunction. Severe diarrhea predisposes to serious electrolyte disturbances and malabsorption of essential nutrients. Malabsorption syndromes interfere with vitamin K absorption, predisposing to altered hemostasis. Hematuria may be an initial clue as to the presence of an otherwise unsuspected bleeding problem.

**Activity/Exercise.** Weakness, exercise intolerance, and inability to carry out activities of daily living commonly accompany hematologic dysfunction. Anemia, which causes a decrease in the oxygen available to the tissues, may be a major contributory factor in this regard. Dyspnea on exertion may reflect an underlying anemia, or it may be associated with a thromboembolic disorder caused by altered hemostasis. It is important to ascertain the patient's usual exercise/rest patterns so that he or she may be assisted in setting realistic patient goals.

**Coping-Stress Intolerance/Role-Relationships.** It is important to identify the circumstances surrounding the occurrence of illness. How do the present circumstances differ from the usual pattern in lifestyle? Stressors, whether recent or ongoing, should be identified.

It may be important to have the patient/family examine past coping patterns. Has a similar problem been experienced previously? Under what circumstances? How was it handled? What can the patient/family do for themselves? How can they be motivated to assume responsibility for their own health and well-being?

Who is the decision-maker in the family? What effect does the illness have on the patient's role in the family, and on overall family dynamics? What family/community support systems are available to the patient? What changes are anticipated in terms of patient/family lifestyles as a consequence of the illness? Malignant hematologic neoplasms, such as certain leukemias, multiple myeloma (i.e., a neoplastic disorder of plasma cells), and lymphomas (e.g., Hodgkin's disease), can have far-reaching effects on overall family dynamics and resources. The acuity and/or chronicity of such illnesses, many characterized by remissions and exacerbations, places a tremendous burden on familial resources —physically, emotionally, psychologically, as well as financially. Bleeding and clotting disorders (e.g., hemophilias, von Willebrands's disease) can similarly stress patient/family resources. Patients requiring blood replacement therapy have the additional risk of developing acquired immune deficiency syndrome (AIDS).

### *Past Medical History*

It is essential to ascertain whether the patient has experienced any previous chronic or longstanding illness, a recent acute illness, major trauma, and/or surgery. Such pathophysiologic insults can predispose to hematopoietic disorders and hemostatic dysfunction. Disseminated intravascular coagulation (DIC), for example, an acute disorder of hemostasis, is a major complication associated with a variety of pathophysiologic insults (see Chap. 63). Among others, these include shock states (e.g., anaphylactic, septic, post-traumatic, hemorrhagic, or cardiogenic shock), crushing-type injuries, burns, and major surgery. Tissue injury and/or disruption of the vascular system (i.e., the blood and blood vessels) place the patient at risk of developing such a coagulopathy (or bleeding diathesis). Certain surgical patients who experience a circulatory crisis may be at especially high risk of developing a bleeding diathesis.

Major abdominal surgery (e.g., descending aortic aneurysm), cardiothoracic surgery (e.g., prosthetic heart valve replacement) and associated post-extracorporeal circulation, and splenectomy are examples of surgical procedures associated with hemostatic complications. The spleen, as part of the reticuloendothelial system, functions in the clearance of activated coagulation factors from the blood. Removal of the spleen alters this process, predisposing to higher concentrations of such activated factors in circulating blood.

Certain types of gastrointestinal surgery, such as duodenal excision or total gastrectomy, predispose to hematologic disorders. Removal of the duodenum disrupts iron absorption, which largely occurs within the duodenum. Depletion of iron stores predisposes to hematopoietic dysfunction. A total gastrectomy results in loss of gastric parietal cells (see Chap. 47), which function to synthesize intrinsic factor, necessary for vitamin $B_{12}$ absorption from the small intestine (ileum). Is there a history of pernicious anemia with parenteral vitamin $B_{12}$ supplementation?

Replacement transfusions can suppress erythropoiesis and alter vitamin $B_{12}$, folate, and iron levels. Such therapy can interfere with the interpretation of diagnostic tests. It is essential to elicit history in this regard.

The liver functions to synthesize many of the clotting factors, and it clears activated factors from the blood. The presence of underlying liver disease is a significant fact, and a thorough history in this regard is essential to differential diagnosis.

The patient's immunologic history should be ascertained. A history of immunodeficiency disease (e.g., AIDS), incompatible blood transfusion, and transplant graft rejection may provide valuable clues as to the patient's current status. Hematologic and immunologic functions are closely interrelated, and both impact on total body function. The presence of leukemia, solid tissue tumors (or recent surgical excision), radiation therapy or chemotherapy should be documented.

**Allergies/Drug History.** A thorough medication history and any allergic reactions to specific drugs or foods should be elicited. Is the patient taking medications, such as iron, vitamin $B_{12}$, folate, and pyridoxine, to treat an existing hematologic disorder (e.g., anemia)? Has the patient experienced a bleeding disorder (e.g., a hemophilia) requiring the administration of blood products such as cryoprecipitate? Is the patient taking anticoagulant therapy? If so, for what reason? Is the patient currently taking an antineoplastic or chemotherapeutic agent? If so, for what reason?

A variety of medications taken for the treatment of nonhematologic disorders may exert an untoward effect on hematopoietic function. Bone marrow depression has long been associated with the use of certain drugs. These include the antibiotic, chloramphenicol; the antibacterial agent, Bactrim; the anticonvulsants, phenytoin and carbamazepine; and certain long-standing antidysrhythmics, such as quinidine sulfate.

Long-term use of certain antihypertensives (e.g., methyldopa) and diuretics (such as chlorothiazide) has been implicated as a cause of hematopoietic dysfunction. Anti-inflammatory agents, including glucocorticoids (e.g., ACTH, prednisone), and nonsteroidal drugs such as phenylbutazone are known to depress bone marrow activity. Other drugs with a similar effect include immunosuppressives (e.g., azathioprine); the antifungal agent, amphotericin-B; and oral contraceptives (e.g., diethylstilbesterol). The use of aspirin, heparin, or coumadin products, and the reason for their use, should be ascertained. In addition, it is essential to establish what combinations of drugs are being taken. For example, taking aspirin along with warfarin may potentiate the anticoagulant effect, predisposing to bleeding. The concurrent administration of such drugs as phenobarbital and warfarin may potentiate the anticoagulant effect, predisposing to bleeding. It is also important to ascertain what the patient/family knows about the drugs being taken. Such information may help to determine the presence of a knowledge deficit requiring patient/family education prior to discharge.

### *Family History*

Genetic factors are especially influential in certain hematologic disorders. Among these are a variety of hereditary hemolytic anemias, which are classified based on whether the underlying defect is intracorpuscular (i.e., within the RBC) or extracorpuscular. *Intra*corpuscular defects include defects in the RBC membrane (e.g., hereditary spherocytosis), enzyme defects (e.g., glucose-6-phosphate dehydrogenase), hemoglobinopathies (e.g., sickle cell anemia, methemoglobinemia), and thalassemia syndromes.

*Extra*corpuscular defects underlying hemolytic anemias include:

1. Immune hemolytic anemias (e.g., *allo*immune hemolytic anemia wherein the individual develops antibodies upon stimulation by a foreign antigen such as in a transfusion reaction; and *auto*immune hemolytic anemia wherein the ability for self-recognition of the individual's own red cells is lost and the consequent autoantibodies that are formed, in turn, destroy the individual's own RBCs).
2. Nonimmune hemolytic anemias (e.g., infection-induced anemia such as occurs in malaria; anemia induced by certain chemicals, toxins, or physical agents).
3. Microangiopathic and macroangiopathic hemolytic anemias (i.e., anemias resulting from fragmentation, shearing, and/or rupture of RBCs as they circulate; turbulent blood flow, or flow through blood vessels that are damaged or partially occluded by fibrin strands are largely implicated in these anemias); examples of microangiopathic anemias include thrombotic thrombocytopenic purpura, hemolytic uremic syndrome, disseminated carcinoma, and disseminated intravascular coagulation.
4. Hypersplenism wherein a prolonged transit of blood cells through an enlarged spleen results in decreased RBC survival and pooling within the spleen.

Anemias are associated with other diseases such as infection, chronic renal disease (wherein there is a decrease in erythropoietin depressing RBC synthesis, as well as the effect of uremic toxins on RBC survival), liver and endocrine disorders, connective tissue disorders (e.g., rheumatoid arthritis and systemic lupus erythematosus), and anemias associated with malignancy.

Conditions involving white blood cell dysfunction are largely acquired. Leukemia does not appear to be inherited. Lipid (lysosomal) storage diseases, although rare, are largely inherited disorders. A familial history of Gaucher's disease,

Niemann-Pick disease, Tay-Sachs disease, and mucopolysaccharidoses (MPS) should be carefully documented.

Hereditary disorders of platelet function include Bernard-Soulier syndrome and Glanzmann's thrombasthenia. Von Willebrand's disease is an inherited condition in which all elements of the factor VIII complex are decreased. Clinically, this disorder manifests as a mixed coagulopathy/qualitative platelet defect, which results in abnormal bleeding. Defects in clotting may be transferred by heredity. Hemophilia A, a hereditary disorder characterized by a defect in factor VIII, is perhaps the most widely known of the bleeding disorders.

A family history of jaundice should be documented. Jaundice is frequently associated with increased RBC hemolysis. While familial occurrences of polycythemia vera (i.e., an excess of RBCs in peripheral blood) are rare, the presence of the disorder should be documented.

## PHYSICAL EXAMINATION

Components of the physical examination in assessing hematologic and hemostatic function include inspection, palpation, percussion, and auscultation. Meticulous techniques are required because physical findings reflective of underlying hematologic dysfunction are generally nonspecific. In some patients, however, the presenting scenario may provide key clues as to the underlying problem. For example, signs of malnutrition, accompanied by alterations in neurologic function (e.g., loss of proprioception, vibratory sense), are highly suggestive of a possible vitamin $B_{12}$ deficiency.

### Integument

Changes in skin coloration are commonly associated with hematologic and hemostatic dysfunction. A pallor or whitish tint to the skin, nailbeds, mucous membranes, and conjunctivae may reflect an underlying anemia; pallor is also a clinical feature of leukemia. Jaundice (icterus) of the skin and especially of the sclera (see Table 47–5) is frequently reflective of excessive RBC hemolysis with a consequent increase in serum bilirubin levels. Erythema or reddish tint is seen in fever; it may reflect an underlying polycythemia (i.e., an excess of RBCs). Cyanotic, cold, mottled skin reflects vascular insufficiency, which may be associated with an underlying bleeding diathesis that occurs, for example, in DIC.

Evidence of a bleeding problem is frequently manifested by the presence of purpura, petechiae, and ecchymosis. Gingival and mucosal bleeding, oozing of blood from around peripheral intravenous sites, and abnormal or prolonged bleeding from puncture sites are highly indicative of a bleeding problem. Strict surveillance of all invasive tubing (e.g., central lines, nasogastric, endotracheal, tracheostomy, and Foley catheter) is essential.

Skin turgor over forehead or sternum assists in determining fluid status and should be monitored. Extremities and dependent areas of the body should be regularly assessed for the presence of edema and signs of vascular insufficiency (Table 62–1).

### Eyes

The eyes should be examined for scleral icterus (jaundice) and retinal hemorrhages. Sunken orbits may reflect a dehydrated state. Periorbital edema may reflect underlying renal failure.

### Ears

The ears should be examined for evidence of bleeding from the external auditory canal; a bluish-colored tympanic membrane suggests the presence of blood in the middle ear.

TABLE 62–1
**Chronic Vascular Insufficiency***

| | Chronic Arterial Insufficiency (Advanced) | Chronic Venous Insufficiency (Advanced) |
|---|---|---|
| Pulses: | Decreased or absent | Normal, though may be difficult to feel through pitting edema |
| Color: | Pale, especially on elevation; dusky red on dependent position | Normal, or cyanotic in dependent position |
| Temperature: | Cool | Normal |
| Edema: | Absent or mild | Present, often marked |
| Skin changes: | Thin, shiny, atrophic skin; loss of hair over foot and toes; nail beds thickened and ridged | May show brown pigmentation around ankles; stasis dermatitis |
| Ulceration: | If present, involves toes or points of trauma on feet | If present, develops at sides of ankle |
| Gangrene: | May develop | Does not develop |

*Source: Bates, B: A Guide to Physical Examination, ed 3, JB Lippincott Co, Philadelphia, 1983, p 318.

## Mouth/Pharynx

The mouth, tongue, and mucous membranes are examined for coloration (e.g., pallor) and bleeding; the presence of a smooth tongue is frequently associated with hematologic dysfunction. The lips and mucous membranes should be examined for cracks and fissures (i.e., cheilosis), "fever blisters," vascular spots such as hemangiomas or telangiectasias, firm white plaques, ulcerations, or masses.

## Head/Neck

Superficial lymph nodes should be assessed for lymphadenopathy. The location, size, texture, mobility, tenderness, or pain, if present, should be noted. Lymph nodes frequently reflect underlying pathophysiology. They are frequently enlarged in acute infections (in the areas that they drain). Changes in lymph nodes often accompany metastatic cancer or leukemia. In these circumstances, they may feel firm or hard on palpation, with an irregular shape; when these changes occur unilaterally, they may reflect an acute infection. Lymph nodes larger than 1 cm should be viewed with suspicion.

The neck should also be auscultated for carotid bruit.

## Respiratory

The respiratory rate, rhythm, and breathing pattern (e.g., tachypnea, dyspnea, orthopnea) should be determined. Dyspnea, if present, may be associated with an underlying anemia, or it may be due to a pulmonary embolus associated with a thromboembolic disorder. Evidence of hemoptysis should be noted. Symmetry of chest expansion, diaphragmatic excursion, and use of accessory muscles should be documented.

The thorax should be carefully auscultated for the presence of abnormal breath sounds and adventitious sounds. Patients with compromised hematologic function are at increased risk of developing pulmonary complications (e.g., pulmonary effusion, pulmonary embolus). The chest should be palpated for sternal and/or rib tenderness.

## Cardiovascular

The heart rate and rhythm, and the quality of peripheral pulses should be ascertained. Tachycardia is a common finding in anemias because there is an increased cardiac workload to meet the oxygen demands of the cells. Peripheral pulses may feel full and bounding when associated with a high cardiac output; weak, thready pulsations may be indicative of significant bleeding. Heart sounds should be evaluated for extra heart sounds, systolic murmurs, and pericardial friction rub.

The patient should be assessed for postural hypotension. Baseline hemodynamic parameters should be established and monitored. Neck vein distention and systemic (pitting) edema suggest right heart failure.

## Gastrointestinal

The abdomen should be inspected for skin texture, lesions, scars, any discoloration, or bruises; abdominal distention and/or bulging of the flanks frequently reflect ascites. If ascites is present, the abdominal girth should be determined and assessed regularly at the level indicated on the skin with a marking pencil. Pulsations of the abdominal wall may be normally visualized in a thin-walled abdomen; in the distended abdomen, such pulsations may reflect an underlying ascites. Bowel sounds should be auscultated carefully in all quadrants.

The abdomen should be percussed and palpated for masses, pulsations, hepatosplenomegaly, and tenderness. Splenomegaly is associated with a variety of hemolytic anemias and other hematologic disorders; the liver, as part of the reticuloendothelial system, may also become enlarged in these instances. The liver is also the site of bilirubin metabolism. The presence of elevated bilirubin levels may reflect increased RBC hemolysis or altered liver function. The liver may also be implicated in altered hemostatic function because it not only synthesizes most clotting factors, but is responsible for the clearance of activated factors from the circulating blood and their eventual metabolism. The stool should be examined for the presence of occult blood, because gastrointestinal bleeding, whether due to stress or to a bleeding diathesis, frequently complicates the patient's underlying condition.

## Genitourinary

Hematuria and back/flank pain may appear as presenting signs and symptoms; or they may occur in the course of a hematologic or hemostatic problem. Oliguria may suggest renal failure. Menorrhagia (i.e., excessive menstrual bleeding) is frequently associated with compromised hemostasis.

## Musculoskeletal

Bones and joints should be assessed for swelling, tenderness, pain, and mobility (i.e., range of motion). Hemarthrosis (i.e., bloody effusion into joints) frequently underlies joint and bone pain associated with some hematologic disorders, such as sickle cell anemia, and some leukemias.

## Neurologic

Seemingly subtle changes in mental status, behavior, and neurologic function may, in the patient with, or at risk of developing a bleeding diathesis, signal ominous clues as to the presence of underlying intracranial bleeding. Patients may complain of headache or a feeling of lightheadedness. They may experience visual disturbances (associated with retinal hemorrhages); aphasia (i.e., absence or impairment of the ability to communicate by speech); and paresthesias (e.g., numbness, tingling, altered proprioception and vibratory sense).

Changes in the patient's mental status (i.e., inability to remember, alteration in mood and affect) and level of consciousness may become apparent. The patient may become restless, irritable, and lethargic. Motor coordination may become impaired, and deep tendon reflexes may be altered.

The status of cranial nerve function in patients with altered level of consciousness entails close monitoring of pupillary equality, size, shape, and reactivity; ptosis of the upper eyelid on the affected side reflects compromise of occulomotor nerve function; a drooping of the lower eyelid or of the face suggests facial nerve dysfunction. Neurologic findings may reflect intracranial bleeding or an increase in intracranial pressure caused by such bleeding. (See Chap. 7 for a detailed discussion of the neurologic assessment.)

## Immunologic

Assessment of immunologic function entails the inspection and palpation of all superficial lymph nodes (see section entitled "Head/Neck" above). It is necessary to look for signs of infection, such as an increase in body temperature, and the presence of any inflammatory areas (i.e., areas of erythema, swelling, warmth, and pain or tenderness; see also Chap. 55). Laboratory indices assist in differential diagnosis (see section that follows).

# LABORATORY TESTS/STUDIES OF HEMATOLOGIC AND HEMOSTATIC FUNCTION

The laboratory assessment of hematologic function includes an examination of the cellular elements of blood and the physical relationship between these elements and the blood volume, and between RBCs and plasma.

## Hematopoiesis

Hematopoiesis (i.e., the production and development of blood cells) occurs largely in the bone marrow, except for some lymphocytes produced in lymphoid tissues.

### *Bone Marrow: Aspiration and Biopsy*

Hematopoietic activity can be evaluated by examining bone marrow tissue obtained by aspiration or biopsy. Cells normally present in bone marrow include granulocytes and erythrocytes, which occur in all stages of maturation, and megakaryocytes, which give rise to platelets. Bone marrow examination is diagnostic for patients with multiple myeloma and in most cases of leukemia. It may also be performed to diagnose the presence of lymphoma or metastatic carcinoma in bone marrow.

Prior to the procedure, appropriate explanations should be made to the patient/family, and a consent must be signed. Meticulous aseptic technique is necessary to avoid infection and potential septicemia. After the biopsy needle is withdrawn, application of firm pressure to the site is necessary to prevent hemorrhagic complications.

## Laboratory Tests of Hematologic Function

Laboratory tests of hematologic function include an examination of whole blood for a complete blood count with differential and peripheral smear. The complete blood count (CBC) includes the red blood cell (RBC) and white blood cell (WBC) counts. The usual range for these and other tests are included in Table 62–2. Specific blood tests include:

### *Hemoglobin (Hgb)*

Hemoglobin laboratory test measures the oxygen-carrying capacity of the blood and reflects the total amount of hemoglobin in peripheral blood.

### *Hematocrit (Hct)*

Hematocrit laboratory test reflects the proportion of whole blood contributed by red blood cells. Changes in plasma volume are reflected by changes in both the Hgb and Hct. Overhydration results in decreases in these parameters; dehydration causes these parameters to be fictitiously high.

### *Red Cell Indices*

**Mean Corpuscular Volume (MCV).** This index reflects the relative size of red blood cells. An increase in the MCV reflects red blood cells that are abnormally large (i.e., *macro*cytic); a decrease in the MCV reflects *micro*cytic or abnormally small red blood cells seen commonly in iron deficiency anemia or in thalassemias.

TABLE 62-2
**Laboratory Values: Hematologic and Hemostatic Function***

| Test | Normal Range |
|---|---|
| ***Hematologic Function*** | |
| Red blood cell count (RBCs) | 4.2-5.9 million/mm³ |
| Hemoglobin (Hgb) | Male: 13-18 gm/100 ml<br>Female: 12-16 gm/100 ml |
| Hematocrit (Hct) | Male: 45-52%<br>Female: 37-48% |
| Red cell indices: | |
| Mean corpuscular volume (MCV) | 80-94 cu microns |
| Mean corpuscular hemoglobin (MCH) | 27-32 picograms (pg) |
| Mean corpuscular hemoglobin concentration (MCHC) | 32-36% |
| White blood cell count (WBCs) | 4300 to 10800/cu mm |
| WBC differential: | |
| Neutrophils (PMNs) | 39-79% |
| Eosinophils | 0-5% |
| Basophils | 0-2% |
| Monocytes | 3-8% |
| Lymphocytes | 10-40% |
| Reticulocyte count | 0.5-2.0% of total RBC |
| Erythrocyte sedimentation rate (ESR) | Male: 1-13 mm/hr<br>Female: 1-20 mm/hr |
| Total iron-binding capacity (TIBC) | 250-410 $\mu$g/dl |
| Coombs' test: | |
| Direct | Negative |
| Indirect | Negative |
| ***Hemostatic Function*** | |
| Bleeding time | 3-9 minutes |
| Platelet function: | |
| Platelet count | 150,000-350,000/mm³ |
| Clot retraction | 50-100%/2 hr |
| Aggregation | Full response to ADP, epinephrine, and collagen |
| Platelet factor 3 | 33-57 sec |
| Vitamin $B_{12}$ | 90-280 pg/ml |
| Coagulation tests: | |
| Prothrombin time (PT) | <2 sec deviation from control; normally 11-13 sec |
| Partial thromboplastin time (PTT) | 25-37 sec |
| Thrombin clotting time (TCT) | 8-12 sec (Control ±5 sec) |
| Plasma fibrinogen levels | 200-400 mg/100 ml |
| Fibrin degradation products (FDP) | <10 $\mu$g/ml |
| Euglobulin clot lysis time | 90 min to 6 hr (no lysis within initial 90-120 min) |

*Source: Scully, RE. (ed): Case Records of the Massachusetts General Hospital, N Engl J Med 314:39-49, 1986.

**Mean Corpuscular Hemoglobin (MCH).** This index reflects the average amount of hemoglobin in red blood cells as calculated by dividing the hemoglobin concentration of whole blood by the number of red blood cells present.

**Mean Corpuscular Hemoglobin Concentration (MCHC).** This index reflects the average concentration of hemoglobin in a single RBC and is derived by dividing the hemoglobin (Hgb) by the hematocrit.

### *Peripheral Smear*

Peripheral smear allows for a more exact evaluation of red blood cell size, shape, and composition. It is especially useful in diagnosing anemias (see section on Anemias on p. 1286).

### *White Blood Cells*

White blood cells are distinguished from circulating red blood cells by the presence of a nucleus. Fully mature circulating white cells include granulocytes, lymphocytes, and monocytes.

**White Blood Cell Count (WBC).** White blood cell count reflects the total number of white cells, or leukocytes, in circulating blood. It is important to appreciate that white cells found in the blood may be in a penultimate stage of maturation. White blood cells serve no function within the vascular system but, rather, are enroute to another location as triggered by a chemotactic factor, for example (see Table 61-3).

**White Blood Cell Differential.** White blood cell differential reflects the percentage of each type of white cell. These include neutrophils (polymorphonuclear, PMNs), eosinophils, basophils, lymphocytes, and monocytes. The absolute count of each specific type of white cell is important to differential diagnosis. Elevated neutrophil count is associated with infection. These cells are frequently seen in their immature stage (i.e., as band cells). An increase in band neutrophils is referred to as "a shift to the left" and is associated with acute infection.

An elevation in the eosinophil count may be seen in allergic reactions, parasitic infections, eczema, leukemia, and some autoimmune diseases. A decrease in eosinophils is associated with corticosteroid therapy.

An increase in lymphocytes (i.e., lymphocytosis) is seen in some bacterial or viral infections, infectious mononucleosis, lymphocytic leukemia, and multiple myeloma. A reduction in lymphocytes (i.e., lymphopenia) occurs in immunodeficiency diseases, sepsis, chemotherapy, and in certain leukemias.

### *Reticulocyte Count*

Reticulocyte count reflects the number of immature red blood cells circulating in the blood and provides a measure of bone marrow function.

### *Erythrocyte Sedimentation Rate (ESR)*

Erythrocyte sedimentation rate reflects the composition of plasma and the relation of red cells to plasma. A rise in the ESR accompanies most inflammatory diseases, whether localized or systemic, acute or chronic. The ESR is especially helpful in monitoring response to therapy for chronic conditions such as rheumatoid arthritis and tuberculosis. A very high ESR is associated with multiple myeloma; a less marked increase may accompany solid tumors.

## Additional Tests of Hematologic Function

### *Total Iron Binding Capacity Test (TIBC)*

This test reflects a direct, quantitative measurement of transferrin, the globulin that binds iron and transports it in the blood. Reduced levels of iron and TIBC are frequently associated with iron deficiency anemias.

### *Coombs' Tests*

These tests differentiate types of hemolytic anemias and detect immune antibodies.

- Direct Coombs' test: Measures antibodies (IgG) attached to RBCs.
- Indirect Coombs' test: Measures antibodies (IgG) in the serum.

Both the direct and indirect Coombs' tests are read as normally negative.

A discussion of other specific tests of hematologic function and dysfunction (e.g., hemolysis, red cell survival, red cell fragility, enzyme defects, hemoglobinopathies, and special leukocyte studies) is beyond the scope of this text and the reader is referred elsewhere.

## Laboratory Tests of Hemostasis

### *Tests of Platelet Activity*

**Bleeding Time.** A prolonged bleeding time is the single best indication of platelet deficiency, and it is seen in thrombocytopenia of any cause.

**Platelet Count.** This is the least accurate approach to assessing platelet function. In general, the bleeding time becomes prolonged when the platelet count falls below 100,000/mm$^3$. Bleeding time is prolonged by aspirin therapy. Aspirin interferes with platelet aggregation (see section entitled "Platelet Aggregation" in Chap. 61).

**Clot Retraction.** Clot retraction reflects the process wherein platelets contract and serum is expressed from the clot leaving only red blood cells enmeshed in the fibrin mass. Platelet contraction is fundamentally necessary for this process of clot retraction. Patients with thrombocytopenia or abnormally functioning platelets will demonstrate altered clot retraction. Patients with polycythemia (i.e., an excess of RBCs) or low fibrinogen levels (i.e., fibrinopenia), likewise, demonstrate altered clot retraction.

### *Coagulation Tests*

**Prothrombin Time (PT).** Prothrombin time evaluates the function of the extrinsic coagulation pathway (see Fig. 61–3). A firm fibrin clot normally occurs in 11–13 seconds. This test reflects the presence of adequate levels of fibrinogen and factors X, V, VII, and II.

**Partial Thromboplastin Time (PTT).** Partial thromboplastin time evaluates the function of the intrinsic coagulation pathway. The normal range for clot formation is about 25–37 seconds. Factors XII, XI, IX, and VIII must all be present and at adequate levels to have a normal PTT time. Factors X and V, prothrombin and fibrinogen, are likewise reflected by normal PTT. This test does not reflect factor VII because it bypasses the extrinsic coagulation pathway.

**Thrombin Clotting Time.** Thrombin clotting time reflects the conversion of fibrinogen (Ø) to fibrin, or the final phase of coagulation. The thrombin clotting time (TCT) is prolonged in the presence of reduced levels of fibrinogen (<100 mg/100 ml) or if the fibrinogen is functionally abnormal.

**Plasma Fibrinogen Levels.** This test evaluates the level of fibrinogen (Ø) in blood plasma. The normal range is 200–400 mg/100 ml.

**Fibrin Degradation Products.** Results of this test reflect the products of fibrin cleavage or breakdown. Whenever fibrin undergoes fibrinolysis, low levels of degradation products enter the circulation and are cleared by the liver and reticuloendothelial system. In the presence of increased fibrinolysis, fibrin degradation products (FDP) (also called fibrin split products, FSP) may circulate in the plasma at levels high enough to cause serious hemostatic complications. FDP interfere with the conversion of fibrinogen to fibrin and further compromise clotting by interfering with the formation of the platelet hemostatic plug. The presence of FDP also reflects the activity of the fibrinolysis system, specifically the activity of plasmin, the major factor that degrades fibrin.

**Euglobulin Clot Lysis Time.** Results of this test reflect the presence of excessive fibrinolytic activity and, thus, provide a measure of the activity of the fibrinolytic system. Euglobulins are proteins found in the plasma and include fibrinogen, plasminogen, and plasminogen activator. Addition of thrombin to a euglobulin solution converts fibrinogen to fibrin and activates plasminogen. The time measured from clot formation to clot lysis is referred to as the euglobulin clot lysis time.

**Coagulation Factor Concentration Tests.** Tests are now available to measure the concentration of specific clotting factors including factors XI, IX, X, VIII, VII, and II (prothrombin).

## BLOOD TYPING AND Rh DETERMINATION

See an appropriate text for a discussion of blood typing and Rh factor determination.

## SUGGESTED READINGS

Beck, WS (ed): Hematology, ed 4. MIT, Cambridge, MA, 1985.
Cahill, M, Di Carlantonio, M, and Leibrandt, T (eds): Diagnostics: Patient Preparation, Interpretation, Sources of Error, Post-Test Care. Intermed Communications, Horsham, PA, 1981.
Fishbach, FT: A Manual of Laboratory Diagnostic Tests, ed 2. JB Lippincott, Philadelphia, 1984.
Griffin, JP: Hematology and Immunology Concepts for Nursing. Appleton-Century-Crofts, Norwalk, CT, 1986.
Pittiglio, DH: Modern Blood Banking and Transfusion Practices. FA Davis, Philadelphia, 1983.
Rifkind, R, et al: Fundamentals of Hematology, ed 3. Yearbook Medical Publishers, Chicago, 1986.

CHAPTER 63

# Nursing Management of the Patient with Disseminated Intravascular Coagulation

## CHAPTER OUTLINE



## LEARNING OBJECTIVES

**At the end of this chapter, you should be able to:**

1. Explain the pathophysiologic changes that occur in DIC.
2. Identify patients at risk of developing DIC.
3. Describe the clinical presentation of DIC.
4. Interpret laboratory data reflective of the diagnosis of DIC.
5. Describe approaches to medical treatment and management of DIC.
6. Delineate the nursing process in the care of the patient with DIC including:
   Assessment
   Diagnosis
   Planning: Desired patient outcomes
   Nursing interventions/rationales.

## DISSEMINATED INTRAVASCULAR COAGULATION: DEFINED

Disseminated intravascular coagulation (DIC) is a pathophysiologic process caused by the presence of thrombin in the systemic circulation. The emphasis here is on *systemic* because, unlike normal clotting, which occurs as a *localized* reaction to vascular injury, the clotting of DIC occurs throughout the circulatory system and is characterized by widespread coagulation followed by excessive, diffuse fibrinolysis in an effort to bring about clot dissolution.

Thrombin is the key factor triggering these events. The actions of this proteolytic enzyme result in the formation of fibrin, consumption of specific plasma proteins, irreversible platelet aggregation with a consequent depletion of platelets, and activation of fibrinolysis. The combination of these effects predisposes to the clinical manifestations of DIC, which include diffuse hemorrhage and fibrin thrombus formation. Bleeding is ultimately the major underlying clinical problem—not clotting. Therein lies the paradox, because it all begins as excessive clotting.

The syndrome of DIC is known by many titles including consumption coagulopathy, defibrination syndrome, diffuse intravascular clotting, and intravascular coagulation. Its onset may be insidious or rapid; its symptoms may be mild or severe. It may produce mild, occult bleeding, or widespread hemorrhage.

## DIC: Pathophysiology

DIC is triggered by the presence of some unusual agent or substance in the bloodstream that initiates the clotting cascade (see Fig. 61–3). The clotting mechanism can be initiated by:

1. Direct stimulation of the intrinsic pathway by injury to the endothelial cells.
2. Stimulation of the extrinsic pathway by the release of thromboplastin (i.e., tissue factor) into the circulation by procoagulants such as bacterial toxins, cancer, tissue fragments, free hemoglobin, placental tissue fragments, hypoxia, and acidosis.
3. Stasis or pooling of blood.
4. Defective clearing of the activated clotting factors by the reticuloendothelial system.
5. Defective fibrinolysis.

Regardless of the initiating mechanism for clotting, the end result is the activation of thrombin. The excess thrombin, in turn, activates fibrinogen, causing fibrin to be deposited in the microcirculation. Platelet aggregation or adhesiveness is increased, thereby enabling fibrin clots to form. As the clots continue to form, red blood cells are trapped in the fibrin strands and destroyed. The resultant sluggish circulation of blood reduces the flow of nutrients and oxygen to the cells. This leads to tissue ischemia, injury, and necrosis, if untreated.

Concurrent with these events is the overutilization of platelets, prothrombin, fibrinogen, and other clotting factors. As these factors are used up, a deficiency of these factors ensues, compromising coagulation and predisposing to bleeding. The excessive clotting at the microcirculatory level activates the fibrinolytic system, causing production of fibrin degradation products (FDP; i.e., fibrin split products). FDP compete with fibrinogen for thrombin and interfere with the formation of the stable fibrin clot, thereby perpetuating systemic bleeding.

To summarize, DIC is a condition characterized by a depletion of clotting factors, particularly fibrinogen, and factors V and VIII; the presence of FDP released by the activity of the fibrinolytic system; diffuse hemorrhage or bleeding; and fibrin thrombus formation with diffuse microthrombi causing ischemia, injury, and possible multiorgan dysfunction.

## Etiologic Factors in DIC

Fifty percent of all DIC cases occur in patients with obstetric problems, 35% in patients with cancer. The remaining 15% occur in patients with sepsis, autoimmune reactions, and tissue injuries (Table 63–1).

More specifically, etiologic factors can be examined according to the manner in which clotting is initiated. Conditions that cause activation of the *intrinsic* coagulation pathway include hemolytic processes such as transfusion of mismatched blood, or acute hemolysis from infection or immunologic disorders; endothelial tissue damage from extensive burns and trauma, transplant rejections, heat

TABLE 63–1
**Predisposing–Etiologic Factors in DIC**

| Obstetric Conditions | Cancer | Sepsis | Autoimmune Reactions | Tissue Injuries |
|---|---|---|---|---|
| Abortions<br>Abruptio placenta<br>Amniotic fluid emboli<br>Eclampsia<br>Placenta previa<br>Retained placental tissue<br>Stillbirths | Leukemias<br>Lymphomas<br>Solid tumors<br>Metastasis | Viral<br>Bacterial, especially gram negative<br>Meningoccemia<br>Mycotic histoplasmosis<br>Mycotic aspergillosis<br>Rickettsial<br>Herpes<br>Rubella<br>Smallpox<br>Hepatitis<br>Reye's syndrome | Acute pancreatitis<br>Allograft rejection<br>Anaphylaxis<br>Drug reaction or hypersensitivity<br>Immune complex diseases | External:<br>Burns<br>Giant capillary hemangiomatosis<br>Head injury<br>Heat stroke<br>Hypovolemic or hemorrhagic shock<br>Major surgery<br>Snake bites<br>Trauma or crush syndrome<br>Internal:<br>Acute glomerulonephritis<br>Acute hemolysis<br>ARDS<br>Mismatched transfusions<br>Vascular aneurysms especially dissecting aortic aneurysms |

stroke, or in surgery, particularly when extracorporeal circulation is used because this results in destruction of RBCs; fat emboli, because this provides a source of lipid necessary to initiate clotting; circulatory crisis (e.g., shock state, septicemia); and acute pancreatitis.

Conditions that cause the *extrinsic* coagulation pathway to become activated include obstetric and gynecologic conditions such as abruptio placentae, amniotic fluid embolism, retained dead fetus, and septic abortion; neoplastic processes such as prostatic cancer, acute leukemias, giant hemangiomas, and bronchogenic carcinoma; and chemotherapy.

Conditions in which the activating mechanism is not known include acute bacterial and viral infections (the effect of endotoxins may be to disrupt the endothelium); glomerulonephritis, purpura fulminans (large foci of skin necrosis), thrombotic thrombocytopenic purpura, cirrhosis, defects in the reticuloendothelial system, pulmonary embolism, adult respiratory distress syndrome, and shock states.

Although there are many predisposing or etiologic factors, a common denominator occurring among patients with DIC is some type of circulatory crisis. Arterial hypotension, with its consequent systemic vasoconstriction and capillary dilatation, leads to stagnation of blood in the microvasculature. Such compromised circulation leads to hypoxemia and acidemia because tissues, experiencing a reduction in the supply of oxygen and nutrients, must turn to anaerobic metabolism with a consequent increase in lactic acid production. Hypoxemia and acidemia, as procoagulants (i.e., precursors) initiate the onset of the clotting mechanism at the cellular level.

Etiologic factors of DIC share another common denominator—they all act by triggering mechanisms that eventually liberate free thrombin into the systemic circulation and subsequently lead to blood clotting. Nurses must be aware of the patient's underlying condition and be able to identify patients at risk of developing DIC. Patients need to be assessed constantly for signs of its development, and appropriate measures must be implemented to prevent or control it.

Major areas of concern for nursing care include observing for pulmonary emboli, adult respiratory distress syndrome (ARDS), renal failure, and gastrointestinal necrosis. Unrestrained clotting may predispose to neurologic deficits associated with cerebral emboli. The possibility of hemorrhage throughout the body is great, especially along the gastrointestinal tract and at the site of any open wounds, incisions, or abrasions. Patients need to be assessed for signs of decreased cardiac output, which may be related to dysrhythmias and myocardial infarction. These clinical phenomena may occur secondary to either clotting and/or hemorrhage.

## Clinical Presentation

Major signs and symptoms of DIC including bleeding, as reflected by the presence of purpura, petechiae and ecchymoses; gastrointestinal bleeding (including hemetemasis, melena, or tarry stools); genitourinary bleeding (e.g., hematuria, menorrhagia in women); wound bleeding, bleeding and oozing from puncture sites and around invasive catheters and lines; hematoma formation, pulmonary hemorrhage, purpura fulminans (i.e., large foci of skin necrosis resulting from tissue injury and necrosis associated with compromised circulation); and acrocyanosis (i.e., cyanosis of hands and feet associated with vasomotor and circulatory disturbances).

In addition to bleeding, the syndrome of acute multiorgan dysfunction may occur. The syndrome is characterized by hypotension, oliguria, dyspnea, confusion, convulsions, coma, abdominal pain, diarrhea, and other gastrointestinal symptomatology.

The onset of symptoms may be slow or sudden. Through astute listening and observational skills the nurse can assess the patient for changes early in the course of DIC. Table 63-2 lists subjective and objective symptoms of DIC. Usually the subjective signs are so vague that they are frequently overlooked by the patient, nurse, and other health-care providers.

The nurse should be aware of early signs of impaired tissue perfusion. This includes subtle mental changes such as restlessness, confusion, and inappropriate behavior. Early physical signs include hypotension, especially orthostatic hypotension, dyspnea, tachypnea, syncope, and decreased urinary output. The possibility of DIC may be over-

TABLE 63-2
**Signs and Symptoms of DIC**

| Subjective | Objective |
|---|---|
| Angina | Abdominal girth |
| Dyspnea | Acrocyanosis |
| Fatigue | Bleeding at venipuncture sites, surgical incisions |
| Headache | Coma |
| Malaise | Confusion |
| Nausea and vomiting | Convulsions |
| Palpitations | Cutaneous petechiae, ecchymosis, hematomas |
| Severe pain in the abdomen, back, muscles, joints, and bones | Epistaxis |
| Sudden vision changes | Hematuria |
| Vertigo | Hemoptysis |
| Weakness | Hyper-hypothermia |
| | Irritability |
| | Orthostatic hypotension |
| | Pale yellow skin or sclera |
| | Peripheral thromboemboli |
| | Scleral or conjunctival hemorrhages |
| | Shock |

looked because these signs are nonspecific alone. But in the presence of bleeding, whether overt or occult, they become substantiating data.

Overt bleeding may be reflected by oozing of blood from mucous membranes, needle puncture sites, or incisions. Hemorrhagic bullae, hematomas, ecchymosis, or petechiae may be observed. Occult bleeding can be suspected or documented by the presence of positive guaiac stools or emesis, abdominal distention, or hematuria. Jaundice of the skin and sclera, hemorrhages of the conjunctiva, air hunger, orthopnea, tachypnea, headache, and altered sensorium may all be reflective of an underlying bleeding problem.

## Diagnosis

Astute assessment and diagnosis of DIC require (1) identifying the patient at risk of developing DIC, (2) implementing sophisticated assessment skills and observation to detect subtle changes that may forewarn of the presence of DIC, and (3) interpretating and evaluating clinical and laboratory data to detect DIC, and to follow its course and the patient's response to therapy.

The clinical history for patients at risk of developing DIC should include any history of bleeding tendencies, coagulation disorders, intake of medications that may alter the coagulation mechanism (e.g., anticoagulants), liver abnormalities, bruising tendencies, hematuria, and menorrhagia. Also important is the history of any recent insult to the circulatory system such as shock or vascular injury. (See Chap. 62 for a detailed examination of the assessment of hematologic and hemostatic function.)

### *Laboratory Data: Interpretation and Analysis*

Numerous bleeding disorders mimic DIC. Diagnosis may be difficult because bleeding is not always obvious. In general, when a patient has a disease known to be capable of eliciting or predisposing to DIC, DIC is probably present if bleeding appears suddenly.

Indications for specific laboratory tests include (1) bleeding in a patient with no history of bleeding; (2) the presence of acrocyanosis, and generalized diaphoresis, with cold, mottled fingers and toes; petechiae or purpura; and the patient who seems to be "going sour" for no obvious reason.

There is no test pathognomonic of DIC. Diagnosis requires a clinical suspicion elicited by thorough history, physical examination, and laboratory studies. Because of the need for rapid diagnosis when dealing with a severe bleeding diathesis, it is important to use reliable, although unsophisticated, tests. The major screening tests for DIC include platelet count, prothrombin time and partial thromboplastin time, and fibrinogen level. Confirmatory tests include the concentration of fibrin degradation products (FDP), thrombin time, euglobulin clot lysis time, and factor assays. Factor assays are not routine procedures because they require sophisticated personnel and equipment. Results of assays may vary depending on the methods used.

A cardinal diagnostic finding in most patients with DIC is a significant decrease in the platelet count.[1] Other findings include a decrease in fibrinogen levels and an increase in fibrinolytic activity. Diagnosis of DIC is frequently difficult if multiple transfusions have been given, because they may dilute clotting factors and platelets. Diagnosis may also be difficult in the presence of liver disease with portal hypertension because the disease process causes a decrease in the synthesis of clotting factors, with a reduction in the clearance of activated clotting factors. Thrombocytopenia and activation of the fibrinolytic system may further complicate the clinical picture. See Table 63–3 for the laboratory tests and findings in DIC.

## Treatment and Management

Successful treatment and management of patients with a disorder of the hemostatic mechanism depend on an accurate diagnosis. The objectives of medical management are to halt the coagulation process and to correct the underlying cause. Other therapeutic approaches include (1) the use of heparin to inhibit the effects of thrombin, (2) replacement of deficient clotting factors, and (3) correction of other processes that may hinder clotting mechanism, as for example, administration of vitamin K and folate.

The use of heparin in the treatment of DIC is controversial. While the drug does not have any effect on formed clots, it is thought to inhibit the formation of new clots, thereby slowing down the consumption of clotting factors. Heparin exerts its action through the molecule, antithrombin III, which inactivates thrombin. The drug causes increased amounts of thrombin to be *ad*sorbed by fibrin, which decreases the amount of thrombin available to convert fibrinogen to fibrin.

In association with albumin factors, heparin is thought to inhibit the action of thrombin on fibrinogen, thereby preventing conversion of fibrinogen to fibrin. It may prevent the formation of prothrombin activator by the intrinsic pathway. Specifically, it prevents the reaction between activated factor XI and factor IX, which is catalyzed by thrombin.

Heparin is most effective when given early in the course of DIC. The preferred route is by continuous intravenous drip, although it can be given in intermittent intravenous doses or subcutaneously. Heparin is frequently given in therapeutic doses, but the dose should be adjusted according to the patient status, especially with the presence of both renal

TABLE 63–3
**Laboratory Findings in DIC[1–3]**

| Test | Normal Values | Values in DIC |
|---|---|---|
| Platelets | 150,000–400,000 μl | <50,000 μl |
| Fibrinogen | 200–400 mg/100 ml | <100 mg/100 ml |
| Prothrombin time (PT) | 11–15 sec | >15 sec |
| Partial thromboplastin time (PTT) | 40–100 sec | >100 sec |
| Activated partial thromboplastin time (APTT) | 30–40 sec | >46 sec |
| Thrombin time | 10–15 sec ± 3 sec | >18 sec |
| Bleeding time | 2–8 min (template method) | >8 sec |
| Fibrin Degradation Products (FDP) | 2–8 μg/ml | >10 g/ml |
| Platelet adhesion | 50–90% (glass bead method) | <50% |
| Antithrombin III (AT III) | 18–40 mg/100 ml | <18 mg/100 ml |
| Euglobin Lysis Time | >2 hr | <2 hr |
| Factors V | 70–140% | Very low |
| VIII | 50–200% | Low |
| XII | 60–170% | Low with sepsis |
| X | 70–140% | Low |
| VII and IX | 60–170% | Decreased |
| Paracoagulation Tests: | | |
| Fi Test | Negative | Positive |
| Protamine Sulfate Test | Negative | Strongly positive |
| Hemoglobin | M—14–18 g/100 ml<br>F—12–16 g/100 ml | <10 g/100 ml |
| Hematocrit | M—40–54%<br>F—37–47% | <33% |
| Peripheral smear | | Fragmented RBCs, large platelets |
| Electrolytes: $K^+$ | 3.5–5.5 mEq/liter | <3.5 mEq/liter |
| BUN | 6–20 mg/100 ml | >25 mg/100 ml |
| Creatinine | 0.8–1.5 mg/100 ml | >1.3 mg/100 ml |
| ABG: pH | 7.35–7.45 | <7.35 |
| Bicarbonate | 22–26 mmol/liter | <22 mmol/liter |
| EKG | | Arrhythmias may be present |
| Chest x-ray | | Interstitial edema with diffuse deposition of microemboli in the lungs |

Note: Normal laboratory findings may vary among institutions due to the technique used. Always check your facility's laboratory manual if in doubt.

and hepatic impairment where the half-life of heparin is prolonged. Heparin is continued until the underlying cause of DIC has been corrected and the clinical and laboratory findings demonstrate a reversal of the abnormalities.

Blood and blood replacement therapy is still controversial. When used, it should be given after heparin therapy has been initiated, otherwise the replacement components are consumed rapidly in the DIC process. Whole blood, platelets, and fresh frozen plasma may be given for severe depletion of platelets and coagulation factors. Cryoprecipitate is given for depletion of factors V and VIII.

A treatment still under investigation is the antithrombin III concentrate. The purpose of this treatment is to replenish depleted stores of antithrombin.

Effectiveness of treatment and management is monitored by serial fibrinogen levels and platelet counts. An increase in either parameter signals that clotting and depletion of clotting factors are normalizing.

## Nursing Care of the Patient with DIC

### *Therapeutic Goals*

Major goals of nursing care include detection of occult bleeding, prevention of further bleeding, correct measurement/estimate of blood loss, and support of the patient/family in other needs. Nursing care should be careful, planned, and gentle.

### *Nursing Diagnoses, Desired Patient Outcomes, and Nursing Interventions*

Nursing diagnoses, desired patient outcomes, and nursing interventions/rationales in the care of the patient with DIC are presented in the Care Plan in Table 63–4.

**TABLE 63–4. CARE PLAN FOR THE PATIENT WITH DISSEMINATED INTRAVASCULAR COAGULATION**

| Nursing Diagnoses | Desired Patient Outcomes | Nursing Interventions | Rationales |
|---|---|---|---|
| ***Nursing Diagnosis #1***<br>Tissue perfusion, alteration in: Decreased cerebral, peripheral, renal, gastrointestinal, related to:<br>1. Intravascular coagulation with thrombosis in the microcirculation.<br>2. Hypotension. | Patient will:<br>1. Remain alert, and oriented to person, place and date.<br>2. Maintain peripheral pulses that are strong proximally and distally; skin normal pink in color, warm and dry to touch.<br>3. Maintain urine output >30 ml/hour.<br>4. Maintain negative values for occult blood in body secretions and drainage. | • Assess neurologic status.<br>◦ General cerebral functions: Mental status; level of consciousness; monitor for confusion, lethargy, obtundation, coma, seizures, behavioral changes, headache, dizziness.<br>◦ Cranial nerve function:<br>◦ Assess pupillary reaction to light and accommodation; drooping upper eyelid.<br>◦ Assess for drooping lower eyelid and facial drooping.<br>◦ Ability of patient to talk; presence of protective reflexes: Cough, gag.<br>◦ Sensorimotor function: Assess movement and strength of all extremities.<br>◦ Assess for the presence of paresthesias, numbness, tingling. | • Ongoing assessment of neurologic status is essential because of risk of possible cerebral emboli/thrombi, intracranial bleeding, cerebral anoxia related to cerebral edema, hypoxemia.<br>◦ Alterations in cranial nerve function reflect brainstem involvement.<br>◦ Signals oculomotor nerve involvement.<br>◦ Signals facial nerve involvement.<br>◦ Reflect function of cranial nerves IX, X. Airway must be protected especially in the compromised patient.<br>◦ Peripheral thrombosis compromises systemic circulation.<br>◦ Deep retroperitoneal bleed may cause pressure on lumbar nerve roots. |
| ***Nursing Diagnosis #2***<br>Cardiac output, alteration in: Decreased, related to:<br>1. Fluid volume deficit<br>2. Myocardial infarction<br>3. Dysrhythmias | Patient will:<br>1. Maintain stable hemodynamics:<br>• BP within 10 mmHg of baseline.<br>• Heart rate <100/beats/min.<br>• Central venous pressure ~0–8 mmHg.<br>• PAP ~25 mmHg.<br>• PCWP ~8–12 mmHg.<br>• Cardiac output: 4–8 liters/min. | • Assess cardiovascular status.<br>◦ Assess vital signs: BP and heart rate; heart sounds: gallop rhythms, murmur; CVP, PAP, PCWP, CO; monitor for dysrhythmias.<br>◦ Assess for chest pain.<br>◦ Assess peripheral vascular status:<br>◦ Degree of peripheral or dependent edema; peripheral pulses; capillary refill.<br>◦ Monitor skin color and temperature of arms and legs. Monitor for signs of thromboemboli: Homan's sign. | • Ongoing assessment assists in identifying potential underlying bleeding, and helps to evaluate the patient's response to fluid and blood replacement therapy.<br>◦ Sluggish circulation predisposes to cardiac ischemia.<br>◦ Edema may occur with altered capillary permeability and osmotic pressure dynamics.<br>Note quality of peripheral pulses both proximally and distally; monitor refill time.<br>◦ Presence of acrocyanosis reflects microthrombi within peripheral vasculature. |

*(continued)*

**TABLE 63–4. CARE PLAN FOR THE PATIENT WITH DISSEMINATED INTRAVASCULAR COAGULATION *(Continued)***

| Nursing Diagnoses | Desired Patient Outcomes | Nursing Interventions | Rationales |
|---|---|---|---|
| ***Nursing Diagnosis #3***<br>Fluid volume deficit, related to:<br>1. Bleeding/hemorrhaging (see Tables 23–2 and 23–3). | Patient will:<br>1. Remain without signs of rebleeding:<br>• Without hemetemesis, melena.<br>• Without hematuria.<br>• Without oozing around invasive lines and wounds.<br>2. Maintain balanced intake and output.<br>• Skin turgor good; warm to touch.<br>3. Maintain stable laboratory parameters:<br>• RBC and WBC counts.<br>• Hgb: 12–18 g/100 ml.<br>• Hct: 37–54%.<br>• BUN, creatinine, electrolytes, calcium, and glucose all within acceptable levels.<br>4. Maintain normovolemia.<br>• Body weight within 5% of baseline.<br>5. Achieve resolution of impaired coagulation.<br>6. Achieve resolution of underlying cause. | • Initiate activities to detect the presence of occult bleeding.<br>◦ Assess skin and mucosal membranes for pallor, cyanosis, jaundice, petechiae: observe sclera and conjunctiva; gingival bleeding? epistaxis? ecchymosis? purpura?<br>◦ Determine overall status: presence of fatigue, weakness, malaise.<br>◦ Myalgia, hemarthrosis (i.e., bloody effusion into joint cavity).<br>◦ Presence of visual disturbances.<br>◦ Measurement of blood loss: All body fluids and secretions: Stool (especially if diarrheal), hematochezia (i.e., stool containing red blood); urine; emesis, nasogastric drainage; sputum and/or hemoptysis; diaphoresis, wound drainage, drains.<br>– Bandages and lines should be weighed; sanitary napkins counted.<br>◦ Sequential measurement of extremity circumference as well as abdominal girth.<br>– Observe arterial and venipuncture sites for oozing of frank blood.<br>◦ Monitor laboratory parameters: Hemoglobin and hematocrit.<br>• Administer prescribed fluid/blood replacement therapy. | ◦ Acrocyanosis reflects microemboli within peripheral circulation; presence of jaundice suggests extensive hemolysis associated with underlying coagulopathy.<br>◦ Bleeding into joint cavities may underlie joint/bone pain.<br>◦ Retinal hemorrhages may underlie vision disturbances.<br>◦ Multi-organ system involvement in some patients with DIC requires a delicate balance between hypovolemic shock on the one hand, and overhydration from overly aggressive fluid/blood replacement therapy on the other. The key to therapy is accurate measure of all fluid and blood losses.<br>◦ Persistent oozing or increase in bloody drainage may indicate a developing/increasing coagulopathy.<br>◦ These parameters are chief indicators as to the presence of bleeding; however, the patient's hydration status must be considered when evaluating these values; blood administration may also alter these values.<br>◦ Early identification of bleeding enables timely initiation of therapy to minimize and/or prevent bleeding.<br>• Adequate tissue perfusion requires an adequate intravascular blood volume. |

| | |
|---|---|
| ◦ Administer lactated Ringer's/saline solutions; albumin and other plasma expanders. | ◦ Massive fluid resuscitation is frequently necessary to maintain intravascular volume at levels to maintain optimal cardiac output and blood pressure to meet the oxygen and nutrient needs of body tissues. |
| ◦ Blood/blood products replacement therapy.<br>– Whole blood, platelets and fresh, frozen plasma may be given for severe depletion of platelets and coagulation factors.<br>– Cryoprecipitate is given for depletion of factors V and VIII. | ◦ Blood replacement therapy remains controversial. When utilized, it should be initiated after heparin therapy has been administered to prevent rapid consumption of blood products through the underlying disease process. |
| ◦ Nursing care considerations: Monitor vital signs before, during, and after administration; double-check product with patient's identification, and with donor's type and cross-match. | ◦ For nursing care considerations and precautions to be taken when administering blood/blood products, see Tables 49–2 and 49–3. |
| ◦ Monitor patient for transfusion reaction. Note: Hives, chills, fever, facial flushing, headache, palpitations, tachycardia, chest pain, dyspnea. | ◦ Patient should be closely monitored for the initial 30 minutes. |
| ◦ Use blood administration set with a filter and large gauge needle (19 gauge). Infuse blood products with normal saline. | ◦ Helps to remove injured cells and other debris in blood that may be antigenic. Minimizes injury to red blood cells. Dextrose solutions will cause RBCs to clump. |
| ◦ Allow blood products (e.g., platelets) to warm to room temperature before administering. | ◦ Infusion of chilled blood/blood products may induce hypothermia. However, blood/blood products should be administered within 15 minutes of arrival on unit to minimize bacterial contamination/colonization. |
| • Initiate actions to prevent further bleeding.<br>◦ Gentleness is the rule of thumb when caring for the patient with DIC. Use an electric razor. | ◦ Gentle care minimizes injury to fragile tissues, which may predispose to further bleeding. |
| ◦ Gentle tooth brushing; cleansing of mouth with cotton swabs. | ◦ Use of mild saline solution, bicarbonate, and peroxide as a rinse are recommended instead of a mouthwash; if a mouthwash is used, dilute it 1 : 1. |
| ◦ Skin protection through gentle handling; special attention to skin and mucous membranes especially around catheters, endotracheal tubes, and other invasive lines and catheters. | |
| ◦ Orotracheal suctioning should be performed only when absolutely essential, and with meticulous aseptic technique. | ◦ Careful and timely suctioning minimizes injury to mucosal lining, reducing the risk of bleeding and infection. |
| ◦ Blood pressure cuffs should be used as infrequently as possible. | ◦ To avoid rupture of superficial capillaries with further bleeding. While an arterial line is invasive, it may be preferred to monitor vital signs and to obtain blood samples. |

*(continued)*

**TABLE 63-4. CARE PLAN FOR THE PATIENT WITH DISSEMINATED INTRAVASCULAR COAGULATION *(Continued)***

| Nursing Diagnoses | Desired Patient Outcomes | Nursing Interventions | Rationales |
|---|---|---|---|
| ***Nursing Diagnosis #3 (cont.)*** | | | |
| | | ○ Administer prescribed medications and monitor response: Oral medications should be given whenever possible; parenteral medications should be administered using the smallest gauge needle and applying pressure to the puncture site for a 5 to 10 minute period. | |
| | | ○ Stool softeners should be given. | ○ Help to prevent constipation with straining at stool. |
| | | ○ Aspirin preparations contraindicated. | ○ Aspirin interferes with platelet aggregation thus inhibiting coagulation. |
| | | ○ Heparin therapy via continuous infusion pump or intermittently (via minidose protocol). | ○ Controversy regarding use of heparin in treatment of DIC.<br>– Heparin is most effective when given early in the course of DIC.<br>– Preferred route of administration is continuous intravenous drip. Doses are adjusted according to patient's overall status.<br>– Heparin therapy is usually continued until clinical and laboratory data indicate patient's condition is stabilizing. |
| | | ○ Vasopressors (e.g., dopamine). | ○ Vasopressors may be indicated if blood pressure does not stabilize with full hydration. |
| | | • Monitor hematopoietic function.<br>○ Assess the following: Bleeding—estimate loss; presence of petechiae, ecchymosis, purpura, hematoma; note size and location.<br>○ Monitor hemoglobin, hematocrit, coagulation studies especially platelets, prothrombin time, partial thromboplastin time, fibrin degradation products, and bleeding time. | • Changes in laboratory values are indicative of the patient's status and response to therapy; they afford the capability of following trends in the patient's condition that enable timely and appropriate therapy to be instituted. |
| | | ○ Monitor for exacerbation of bleeding. | ○ Exacerbation of bleeding in patients receiving heparin therapy longer than eight days may be indicative of antiplatelet antibody formation. |

| | | | |
|---|---|---|---|
| ***Nursing Diagnosis #4***<br>Gas exchange, impaired, related to:<br>1. Increased pulmonary capillary permeability, pulmonary embolism, ARDS, with increased pulmonary shunting. | Patient will:<br>1. Maintain respiratory rate <30/min.<br>2. Maintain adequate ventilation as gauged by the work of breathing and arterial blood gases:<br>• PaO2 >60 mmHg (room air).<br>• PaCO2 ~35–45 mmHg.<br>• pH 7.35–7.45.<br>3. Maintain breath sounds clear to auscultation. | • Assess pulmonary function.<br>○ Respiratory rate and breathing pattern.<br>○ Breath sounds.<br>○ Adventitious sounds: Rales, rhonchi, stridor.<br>○ Chest pain: pleuritic causes.<br>○ Sputum production; hemoptysis.<br>○ Monitor arterial blood gases.<br>• Initiate precautionary/supportive therapy.<br>○ Teach patient to cough, sneeze, and blow nose gently.<br>○ Avoid sudden Valsalva maneuver.<br>○ Provide humidified supplemental oxygen.<br>○ Encourage to breathe deeply at regular intervals.<br>○ Encourage use of incentive spirometer. | • Onset of respiratory distress suggests intravascular clotting and/or bleeding into pulmonary tissues.<br>○ Tachypnea, orthopnea, tachycardia reflect effort to maintain tissue oxygenation.<br>○ Hemoptysis suggests possible pulmonary emboli.<br>○ Altered pulmonary vascular dynamics predisposes to pulmonary shunting with compromised gas exchange and consequent hypoxemia.<br>○ Reduce risk of dislodging clots and causing rebleeding.<br>○ Humidification helps to keep secretions moist and easier to mobilize and remove; helps avoid infection.<br>○ Helps to expand the lungs and prevent areas of atelectasis. |
| ***Nursing Diagnosis #5***<br>Urinary elimination, alteration in, related to:<br>1. Hematuria.<br>2. Hypovolemia.<br>3. Renal dysfunction associated with microemboli.<br>4. Hemoglobinopathy. | Patient will:<br>1. Maintain urinary output >30 ml/hour.<br>2. Maintain urine without red blood cells/hemoglobin/protein.<br>3. Maintain renal function studies at baseline.<br>• BUN, creatinine. | • Assess renal status.<br>○ Hydration: Intake and output; urine specific gravity; body weight.<br>○ Hematuria.<br>○ Monitor renal function studies: BUN, creatinine; urine glucose, acetone; renal calculi, if bedrest is prolonged.<br>• Monitor urinary function.<br>○ Assess for hematuria, burning on urination, urgency, frequency.<br>○ Maintain sterility of closed urinary system if Foley catheter is in place.<br>○ Use leg strap to secure the tubing to the leg to prevent pulling.<br>○ Maintain hydration. | • Urine output less than 30 ml/hour suggests dehydration, hypovolemic state, or possible microemboli within the kidneys.<br>○ Oliguria may be associated with renal insufficiency or acute tubular necrosis.<br>○ Massive fluid resuscitation may be necessary to maintain intravascular volume.<br>○ Major complication is urinary infection.<br>○ Tugging on the catheter can cause injury to the urinary meatus and urinary tract. |

*(continued)*

**TABLE 63-4. CARE PLAN FOR THE PATIENT WITH DISSEMINATED INTRAVASCULAR COAGULATION *(Continued)***

| Nursing Diagnoses | Desired Patient Outcomes | Nursing Interventions | Rationales |
|---|---|---|---|
| ***Nursing Diagnosis #6***<br>Bowel elimination, alteration in, related to:<br>1. Bleeding potential. | Patient will:<br>1. Remain without signs of intra-abdominal bleeding:<br>• Without abdominal distention and pain.<br>• Stable abdominal girth.<br>• Without nausea and vomiting.<br>• Negative for occult blood in nasogastric drainage, emesis, stools.<br>• Bowel sounds appropriate.<br>• Vital signs stable. | • Assess gastrointestinal function.<br>○ Assess for signs of distention and increasing abdominal girth; abdominal cramps or pain; nausea/vomiting.<br>○ Assess bowel sounds.<br>○ Presence of paralytic ileus.<br>○ Hematest for occult blood: Nasogastric secretions; emesis, stools.<br>• Implement precautionary/supportive measures.<br>○ Maintain good oral hygiene.<br>○ Avoid loose fitting dentures. Keep lips lubricated.<br>○ Monitor patient's response to antacid protocol: Cimetidine; ranitidine; Maalox.<br>○ Avoid use of rectal temperatures.<br>– Avoid use of suppositories.<br>○ Avoid use of aspirin and steroids. Administer stool softeners as prescribed. | ○ Bleeding into peritoneal cavity should be suspected in the presence of increasing abdominal girth.<br>○ Presence of microthromboemboli within splanchnic circulation may underlie mesenteric ischemia and/or necrosis.<br>○ Helps patient to feel good and reduces the risk of infection.<br>○ Potential for injury to oral mucosa causing bleeding.<br>○ Reduce secretion and deleterious effects of HCl acid (gastric).<br>○ May irritate friable rectal tissues, resulting in bleeding.<br>○ These drugs compromise hematologic and immunologic functions leading to potential bleeding and infection. |
| ***Nursing Diagnosis #7***<br>Nutrition, alteration in: Less than body requirement, related to:<br>1. NPO status in the presence of potential bleeding.<br>2. Anorexia, fatigue. | Patient will:<br>1. Maintain body weight within 5% of baseline.<br>2. Maintain plasma protein levels 6–8 gm/100 ml.<br>3. Maintain triceps skinfold and midarm circumference measurements within acceptable range. | • Collaborate with nutritionist in assessing nutrition status.<br>○ Implement prescribed dietary feeding or hyperalimentation.<br>– Maintain strict intake and output.<br>○ Encourage liquids and soft foods as tolerated.<br>– Avoid use of hot, spicy foods/fluids.<br>○ Encourage carbonated beverages as tolerated. | • Dietary regimen must meet tissue protein needs to promote healing.<br>○ Avoids oral mucosal irritation and gingival bleeding.<br>○ Carbonated beverages help to loosen crusts around mouth and oral cavity without bleeding. |

| | | | |
|---|---|---|---|
| | 4. Maintain blood chemistries within acceptable range.<br>• BUN, creatinine.<br>• Serum glucose.<br>• Serum electrolytes including calcium, phosphorus, magnesium, sodium, potassium, chloride. | | |
| ***Nursing Diagnosis #8***<br>Mobility, impaired, related to:<br>1. Pain caused by bleeding into muscle and joints.<br>2. Debilitated state.<br>3. Increased risk of rebleeding. | Patient will:<br>1. Be able to resume pre-illness activity. | • Assess mobility.<br>◦ Assess movement of all extremities.<br>◦ Assess for the presence of joint/muscle pain; hemarthrosis. Assess extremities and joints for swelling and tenderness. | ◦ Thrombosis/bleeding into muscle and joints may necessitate restriction of movement to minimize further trauma. |
| | | • Institute precautionary measures:<br>◦ Utilize a bed cradle.<br>◦ Immobilize affected areas.<br>◦ Treat bone/joint pain with hot or cold compresses as prescribed.<br>◦ Maintain proper body alignment.<br>◦ Provide gentle passive range of motion. | • Goal is to protect the patient from further trauma; minor injury/stress may potentiate bleeding. |
| | | ◦ Utilize extra assistance when moving patient; use draw sheet to *lift* patient. | ◦ This avoids dragging the patient, as for example, when moving the patient up in bed; such action could cause skin abrasions and other trauma increasing potential for bleeding. |
| | | • Monitor all peripheral pulses, color of skin, and temperature of skin. | |
| ***Nursing Diagnosis #9***<br>Skin integrity, impaired, related to:<br>1. Capillary fragility, bleeding sites.<br>2. Inadequate dietary intake.<br>3. Immobility. | Patient will:<br>1. Maintain skin intact, no breaks, lesions, irritations, or signs of infection; good skin turgor.<br>2. Without signs of acrocyanosis or tissue necrosis. | • Assess integrity of skin and mucous membranes.<br>• Institute precautionary measures.<br>◦ Avoid unnecessary intramuscular and subcutaneous injections; if necessary, use small-gauge needle, rotate sites, and apply steady pressure for 5–10 minutes. | ◦ Reduces the risk of bleeding. |
| | | ◦ Implement use of pressure relief device (e.g., air mattress). | ◦ Reduces pressure points which can predispose to skin breakdown especially in the compromised patient. |
| ***Nursing Diagnosis #10***<br>Oral mucous membranes, alteration in. | Patient will:<br>1. Maintain integrity of mucous membranes.<br>• Mucous membranes moist. | ◦ Implement turning and positioning schedule.<br>◦ Identify pressure areas: Include stage and depth of ulcer if present.<br>◦ Review patient's nutritional status. | ◦ Helps to maximize tissue perfusion.<br>◦ Dietary intake should ensure adequate sources of protein for tissue repair. |

*(continued)*

**TABLE 63–4. CARE PLAN FOR THE PATIENT WITH DISSEMINATED INTRAVASCULAR COAGULATION *(Continued)***

| Nursing Diagnoses | Desired Patient Outcomes | Nursing Interventions | Rationales |
|---|---|---|---|
| ***Nursing Diagnosis #10 (cont.)*** | | | |
| | • Lips without cracking/fissuring.<br>• No evidence of bleeding.<br>• No evidence of infection (stomatitis). | ◦ Keep skin well lubricated.<br>◦ Provide meticulous skin and wound care.<br>◦ Be gentle with patients. Discourage scratching; removing scabs; keep nails trimmed. | ◦ To avoid dryness and cracking which can predispose to skin breakdown and infection.<br>◦ To prevent infection.<br>◦ To avoid trauma. |
| ***Nursing Diagnosis #11***<br>Anxiety, fear, related to:<br>1. Knowledge deficit regarding bleeding and status of condition.<br>2. Altered level of body function and capability for carrying out self-care activities. | Patient will:<br>1. Verbalize fear about bleeding.<br>2. Exhibit relaxed facial expression and overall demeanor.<br>3. Heart rate at baseline for patient. | • Assess level of anxiety/discomfort.<br>◦ Signs and symptoms: Verbalization of fear and anxiety; body posture: Clenched fists, restlessness, irritability, insomnia; evaluate pain.<br>• Provide comfort measures.<br>• Monitor response to pain medication.<br>• Promote rest and sleep periods.<br>• Offer necessary explanations regarding condition and therapy. | • Relaxation affords comfort.<br>• Assist in conserving strength.<br>• Prevents unnecessary anxiety and concern on the part of patient and family. |
| ***Nursing Diagnosis #12***<br>Coping, ineffective: Individual/family. | Patient/family will:<br>1. Verbalize feelings regarding underlying disease and prognosis.<br>2. Identify strengths and coping mechanisms.<br>3. Make decision of importance to the patient/family. | • Assess patient/family's prior coping methods.<br>◦ Identify family/community resources.<br>• Evaluate patient/family's understanding of illness: Anticipate needs; be accessible; make necessary explanations.<br>• Provide emotional and psychological support. | • Identifying past coping capabilities may assist patient/family in dealing with current illness; familiarity breeds self-confidence.<br>• Knowledge of underlying problem may be especially helpful in coping with a bleeding disorder. The sight of even a little blood can be frightening. |

| | | | |
|---|---|---|---|
| | 4. Identify familial and community resources. | • Assist in self-care activities. | • Encourages patient/family to assume responsibility for their own health. This is especially important in those instances where the bleeding problem is a chronic problem. |
| ***Nursing Diagnosis #13***<br>Potential for infection, related to:<br>1. Debilitated state.<br>2. Stagnation of blood.<br>3. Open wounds.<br>4. Impaired skin integrity.<br>(See Table 49–7, Potential for Infection.) | Patient will remain without signs and symptoms of infection.<br>1. Body temperature at baseline.<br>2. Hematology profile within acceptable limits. | • Assess patient for signs and symptoms of possible infection: Monitor temperatures; productive cough with rust-colored or purulent sputum; purulent drainage from open wounds, incisions; redness, swelling, and pain at catheter sites.<br>• Implement protocols in the event of infection: Cultures/sensitivity of body secretions and excretions—sputum, blood, urine, wounds, catheter tips. | • Patients in a compromised, debilitated state are at increased risk of developing infection and sepsis.<br>• Sepsis may be the underlying cause of DIC.<br>• See Table 49–7 for nursing care considerations in the patient with or at risk of infection. |

## REFERENCES

1. Griffin, JP: Be prepared for the bleeding patient. Nursing '86 16(6):34–42, 1986.
2. Cahill, M, DiCarlantonio, M and Leibrandt, T (eds): Diagnostics: Patient Preparation, Interpretation, Sources of Error, Post-Test Care. Intermed Communications, Horsham, PA, 1981, pp 50–65.
3. Fishbach, FT: A Manual of Laboratory Diagnostic Tests, ed 3. JB Lippincott, Philadelphia, 1984, pp 69–74.

## SUGGESTED READINGS

Cahill, M, DiCarlantonio, M and Leibrandt, T (eds): Diagnostics: Patient Preparation, Interpretation, Sources of Error, Post-Test Care. Intermed Communications, Horsham, PA, 1981, pp 50–52, 57, 58, 62, 63, 65.

Fishbach, FT: A Manual of Laboratory Diagnostic Tests, ed 2. JB Lippincott, Philadelphia, 1984, pp 69–74.

Griffin, JP: Be prepared for the bleeding patient. Nursing '86 16(6):34–42, 1986.

Lewis, SM and Collier, IC: Medical-Surgical Nursing: Assessment and Management of Clinical Problems. McGraw-Hill, New York, 1983.

Long, BC and Phipps, WJ: Essentials of Medical-Surgical Nursing: A Nursing Process Approach. CV Mosby, St Louis, 1985.

McGillick, K: DIC: The deadly paradox. RN 45(8):41–43, 1982.

Patrick, ML, et al: Medical-Surgical Nursing: Pathophysiological Concepts. JB Lippincott, Philadelphia, 1986.

# UNIT TEN

# Bibliography

Beck, WS (ed): Hematology, ed 4. MIT, Cambridge, MA, 1985.
Cahill, M, DiCarlantonio, M, and Leibrandt, T (eds): Diagnostics: Patient Preparation, Interpretation, Sources of Error, Post-Test Care. Intermed Communications, Horsham, PA, 1981.
Fishbach, FT: A Manual of Laboratory Diagnostic Tests, ed 2. JB Lippincott, Philadelphia, 1984.
Griffin, JP: Be prepared for the bleeding patient. Nursing '86 16(6):34–42, 1986.
Griffin, JP: Hematology and Immunology Concepts for Nursing. Appleton-Century-Crofts, Norwalk, CT, 1986.
Kelton, JG: Management of the bleeding patient. In Sibbald W (ed): Synopsis of Critical Care, ed 3. William & Wilkins, Baltimore, 1988.
McGillick, K: DIC: The deadly paradox, RN 45:8, 1982.
Pittiglio, DH: Clinical Hematology and Fundamentals of Hemostasis. FA Davis, Philadelphia, 1987.
Pittiglio, DH: Modern Blood Banking and Transfusion Practices. FA Davis, Philadelphia, 1983.
Rifkind, R, et al: Fundamentals of Hematology, ed 3. Yearbook Medical Publishers, Chicago, 1986.
Thompson, A and Harker, L: Manual of Hemostasis and Thrombosis, ed 3. FA Davis, Philadelphia, 1983.

# UNIT ELEVEN

# Trauma and Emergencies

Trauma, including head and spinal cord injury (see Chaps. 10 and 12), thoracic, abdominal and long bone trauma (see Chap. 64), and emergencies, including burn (thermal) injury (see Chapter 65), anaphylaxis (see Chap. 67), and acute poisoning (see Chap. 68), collectively, constitute a major health problem in the United States today accounting for the majority of deaths occurring during the first 3 decades of life. Overall, trauma and emergencies rank as the fourth leading cause of death preceded only by heart disease, cancer, and stroke, and the incidence of trauma and emergencies is increasing yearly.

As a major health problem, trauma and emergencies account for a major expenditure of health-care dollars and manpower each year. Such insults commonly involve long-term disability, with decreased productivity, and an inestimable reduction in the quality of life for the individual, family, and/or significant others.

Several factors contribute to the trend of increasing morbidity and mortality associated with trauma and emergencies. One major factor is the expanding population of drivers of motor vehicles and, in particular, the increasing numbers of persons driving while intoxicated. Automobile accidents alone kill more Americans each year than were lost during the entire Korean War. Of those who survive, many remain permanently disabled.

The proliferation of new chemicals and drugs has heightened the problem of acute poisoning. Most poisoning is by ingestion, especially accidental ingestion of a household chemical by an unsupervised child. The increased availability of drugs, including prescribed, over-the-counter, illegal drugs (marijuana, hashish, cocaine, crack), and alcohol has contributed to an increased incidence of drug abuse and drug overdose, whether accidental or intentional. The consequent alteration in sensorium and neurologic function associated with such drug usage, in turn, places the person at greater risk of sustaining an insult resulting in major trauma, acute poisoning, or other emergency.

A variety of socioeconomic factors also impact on the incidence of trauma and emergencies. The instability of the nuclear family as reflected by the high divorce rate, the need for dual "bread winners" in families to subsidize the cost of living expenses, job-related stress, among others, all influence our daily lives and environments. Unsupervised children of a working parent, as mentioned previously, are at increased risk for acute poisoning from ingestion of household chemicals. Burn injuries associated with playing with matches, smoking cigarettes, or cooking, also contribute to the incidence of medical and traumatic emergencies in children.

Elderly people are at especially high risk for trauma and emergencies. Failing eyesight and motor incoordination are major contributing factors. Many elderly persons live alone on fixed incomes, which do not keep pace with the rising cost of living. Thus, they are compelled to cut living costs. Many do so by trying to cut fuel costs, for example. The use of kerosene stoves or other heating devices that are not entirely safe, places these individuals at risk for injury from fire, the inhalation of toxic fumes, or undetectable gases (e.g., carbon monoxide).

The increasing incidence of trauma and emergencies, and their consequent complex pathophysiologic and psychosocial alterations in the life processes of the body, has created the need for improved and sophisticated knowledge, techniques, and systems designed to increase survival, prevent further damage, maintain optimal function, and preserve quality of life.

Trauma, Burn and Poison Control Centers evolved from professional and community concerns relating to acute medical and traumatic emergencies. It was recognized that an organized, multidisciplinary approach in specialty areas would streamline care and decrease morbidity and mortality in the identified injured populations. Such centers, through the efforts of highly skilled and dedicated health-care professionals, the availability of equipment and materials of the latest technology, and sophisticated communication and transport systems, have afforded quality on-site care almost immediately after injury.

Critical care nurses are an integral part of this multidisciplinary and collaborative approach. The timeliness, appropriateness, and efficiency of the initial assessment and management during the prehospital and resuscitation phase, have increased survival of the trauma patient, and, increasingly, these patients are being cared for in the critical care setting. Aggressive management during the critical phase may largely determine the overall patient outcome. Such management requires that critical care nurses be current in their knowledge and skills related to trauma care, and sensitive and caring in their approach to trauma patients and their family/significant others.

The chapters that follow examine those medical and traumatic emergencies seen most commonly in the critical care setting. These include thoracic, abdominal, and orthopedic trauma; burns; anaphylaxis; and acute poisoning. A chapter concerned with septic shock, a major complication in trauma patients, is also included. In each case, emphasis is placed on integrating basic knowledge of underlying anatomy, physiology, and pathophysiology with respect to the specific trauma/emergency. Medical and/or surgical management of the patient with a medical and/or traumatic emergency, is examined. Nursing care plans reflective of nursing process are included.

## UNIT OUTLINE

## UNIT OUTLINE—*CONTINUED*

CHAPTER 64

# Nursing Management of the Patient with Thoracic, Abdominal, and Orthopedic Trauma

*K. Sue Hoyt and Gary Sparger*

## CHAPTER OUTLINE



## LEARNING OBJECTIVES

**At the end of this chapter, you should be able to:**

1. Identify patterns of trauma associated with thoracic, abdominal, and long bone trauma.
2. Describe the pathogenesis and pathophysiologic changes underlying trauma to the chest, abdomen, and long bones.
3. Describe the initial assessment considerations in patients presenting with trauma of the chest, abdomen, and long bones.
4. Discuss therapeutic modalities indicated in specific types of trauma including chest, abdominal, and long bone trauma.
5. Discuss why treatment is provided simultaneously with the diagnostic process in the management of the trauma victim.

## LEARNING OBJECTIVES—*CONTINUED*

6. Discuss implications for nursing management based on nursing process:
   Assessment
   Diagnoses
   Planning: Desired patient outcomes
   Nursing interventions/rationales.

# INTRODUCTION TO TRAUMA SYSTEMS

## Current Statistics

Trauma has been coined the "neglected disease of modern society" and is viewed as the epidemic of the '80s. Traumatic injury accounts for over 140,000 deaths per year in the United States, and 1 person in 3 suffers a nonfatal injury. Additionally, for every death, another 2 persons are permanently disabled. Trauma is the leading cause of death for individuals up to 44 years of age. It is the fourth overall cause of death for all individuals, exceeded only by cardiovascular disease, cancer, and stroke. Trauma affects predominantly young individuals, with its peak incidence in the 15–24 age group. It is the leading killer of children. Annual trauma-related costs, nationally, equal $75–100 billion.

## Regionalization of Systems Approach

Regionalization of trauma care (i.e., the concentration of care for the critically injured into designated specialty centers) is being implemented and has been shown to decrease the mortality and morbidity related to accidental injury. A major goal of trauma systems is to limit the number of facilities involved in the care of major trauma victims and to triage critically injured individuals to designated trauma centers.

Institutions are designated as trauma centers if they have the resources available to provide, on a consistent basis, the services necessary to meet the special needs of victims of trauma. Trauma center designation may occur as a result of local, county, state, or federal legislation.

## Blunt Versus Penetrating Trauma

Trauma is an injury resulting from external forces. Injury occurs when energy is dissipated or transferred to body tissues. The etiology may involve blunt or penetrating forces, with blunt trauma occurring more frequently. Motor vehicle accidents, falls, and sporting accidents are examples of blunt trauma. Penetrating trauma results largely from gun shot injuries and stabbings. Penetrating injuries may also be related to sporting events, or they may occur in conjunction with blunt injuries.

## Patterns of Trauma

Patterns of trauma have been identified to assist the trauma team to anticipate specific injuries based on the mechanism of injury. Table 64–1 lists frequently occurring mechanisms of injury and the predictable associated injuries. The details of the accident and knowledge of patterns of trauma help the trauma team accurately assess and plan the care for the trauma patient during the initial phase.

## Initial Assessment

The patient who sustains major trauma presents a special challenge to the health-care team. Often the injuries are life-threatening, yet not immediately evident on initial assessment. During the initial assessment of the trauma patient, a systematic approach is used to identify the patient's status. Lifesaving interventions are implemented as indicated. Immediate interventions are concerned with the ABCs (airway, breathing, and circulation) of trauma care. A patent airway is established and maintained, and supportive ventilation and oxygenation are provided. Cervical spine stabilization should be ensured at this time. Fluid volume replacement therapy is initiated to maintain effective cardiac output and tissue perfusion to vital organs. Insertion of a nasogastric tube and urinary catheter is usually indicated in severe trauma.

Once advanced life support is underway, a comprehensive assessment is performed *simultaneously* as diagnostic procedures and stabilization occur. At this time, decisions are made about the course of therapy, whether conservative medical treatment or surgical intervention should be undertaken.

## Critical Care Phase

Once the patient has been diagnosed and stabilization has occurred, the critical care nurse must be especially vigilant for injuries not evident on the initial examination. A knowledge of predictable patterns of trauma will assist the nurse to anticipate the special needs of the critically injured patient. An ongoing assessment of airway, breathing, and circulatory status continues, and findings are documented accurately. Frequent and accurate documentation is an essential element of patient care

TABLE 64-1
**Patterns of Trauma**

| Mechanism of Injury | Force | Associated Injury |
|---|---|---|
| I. Occupant | | |
| A. Frontal impact Down and under pathway | Forward movement, knees strike dash; energy transferred along axis of femur | Patellar fractures; ligamentous injury; mid-shaft femur fracture; posterior dislocated hip |
| | If feet are braced on floor with legs trapped below dash | Femur fracture; ligamentous injury of knee—occult |
| Up and over pathway | Body movement and energy transfer is up and over dash; head strikes windshield | Maxillofacial trauma (Le Fort fracture—with high speed impact) |
| | Neck may be compressed, hyperextended or flexed; | Cervical spine injuries |
| | Chest hits steering wheel or dash | Rib/sternal fractures; myocardial contusion; aortic tear; pneumothorax |
| B. Rear impact | Body pushed forward excluding head | Cervical strain of anterior ligaments |
| C. Lateral impact | Impact by car door; moves body out from under head | Cervical strain of lateral ligaments |
| | Side chest impact | Rib fractures; pulmonary contusion; fractured humerus |
| | Femur head driven through acetabulum | Genitourinary trauma |
| D. Rollovers and combination rotational impacts | Multiple forces | Constellation of injuries |
| II. Pedestrian | | |
| A. Extremity triad | Victim turns sideways to avoid impact | Fractured femur, tibia, and fibula |
| | Lateral impact applied by hood and/or bumper | Ligamentous knee injury to opposite side (often missed) |
| B. Waddell's triad | Car impacts femur and chest and/or torso | Fractured femur, blunt chest and/or abdominal trauma |
| | Victim thrown to ground by impact | Contrecoup head injury |
| III. Falls/jumpers | | |
| A. Don Juan syndrome (Triad) | Victim jumps or falls from great height | Bilateral wrist (Colles) fractures |
| | Victim lands on heels | Bilateral calcaneal fractures |
| | Twisting motion during fall | Lumbosacral fractures (L-1 and L-2) |

NOTE: See also Tables 12-3 and 12-4 for vertebral and spinal cord injuries.

because it provides a most reliable method to communicate trends in the patient's condition and the response to therapy. Thorough documentation is essential to the continuity of patient care.

# THORACIC TRAUMA

## Anatomy and Physiology

The thoracic cavity extends from above the clavicles to the level of the diaphragm. It contains the left and right pleural spaces and the mediastinum. The mediastinal cavity is located between the pleural spaces and houses the heart, aortic arch, and other great vessels, including the pulmonary arteries, and the superior and inferior vena cavae (see Fig. 37-1). Other structures included are the esophagus, trachea, thymus, and the vagus nerves. The lungs are contained within the pleural cavities (see Figs. 29-5, 29-6, and 29-7).

## Pathogenesis

Chest injuries can result in a variety of insults to cardiopulmonary function. These include airway impairment, derangement of chest wall mechanics, changes in intrathoracic pressures, and compromised cardiac function. These derangements, in turn, can result in impaired gas exchange with hypoxemia, alterations in cardiac output and tissue perfusion, and a depleted intravascular volume.

## Pathophysiology: Hypovolemic Shock

Chest trauma patients frequently present in hypovolemic shock. Shock is a profound alteration in tissue perfusion, which results in a cellular oxygen demand that exceeds the supply (see Chap. 46). Without timely intervention, the shock state may become irreversible leading to cellular death.

In response to the shock state, various bodily compensatory mechanisms are activated in an effort to maintain perfusion to vital organs, including the heart, brain, and liver. For a time, this is done at the expense of blood flow to the splanchnic circulation, kidneys, lungs, and the skin.

### *Compensatory Mechanisms*

The body responds to an insult to bodily functions by various compensatory mechanisms including the sympathetic response, baroreceptor activity, fluid shifts, activation of the renin–angiotensin–aldosterone system, and enhanced secretion of antidiuretic hormone.

**Sympathetic Response.** An initial generalized response to the loss of circulating volume is stimulation of the sympathetic nervous system. Epinephrine and norepinephrine, circulating catecholamines, when released into the blood, initiate arterial and venous vasoconstriction. This, in turn, increases systemic vascular resistance with a consequent increase in arterial blood pressure. Additionally, increased levels of circulating epinephrine enhance glycogenolysis. Additional glucose is made available to support cellular metabolism in the presence of the shock state.

**Baroreceptor Response.** Baroreceptors, located in the carotid sinus and aortic arch, respond to changes in arterial blood pressure. As blood pressure decreases, these pressure receptors respond by generating impulses that travel by afferent (sensory) neurons to the vasomotor center in the medulla. Among others, responses elicited include an increase in heart rate and myocardial contractility, and enhanced vasoconstriction of the systemic vasculature, thereby further increasing the systemic vascular resistance. As a result of these activities, mean arterial blood pressure is reestablished within the acceptable physiologic range for the patient.

**Fluid Shifts.** Fluid comprises about 60% of body weight, or about 40 liters in the average adult. Of this amount, approximately 25 liters are found within the intracellular compartment; the remaining 15 liters make up the extracellular fluid compartment. The extracellular compartment, in turn, contains 12 liters of fluid in the interstitial space (i.e., the fluid bathing each cell) and about 3 liters in the intravascular space. In a state of hypovolemic shock, the body compensates for a depleted intravascular volume (i.e., the blood volume) by shifting fluid from the interstitial space into the blood vessels. The fluid in the interstitial compartment acts as a buffer, allowing fluid to move into the intravascular space when blood volume is depleted, and receiving fluid from the intravascular space when blood volume is adequate. In this way, the blood volume, essential for tissue perfusion, is maintained.

**Renin–Angiotensin–Aldosterone System.** Renin is an enzyme that is activated in response to hypoperfusion and ischemia of the kidneys, as in hypovolemic shock. The consequent diminished pulse pressure triggers the conversion of renin to angiotensin by a series of enzymatic reactions (see Fig. 21–9). The renin–angiotensin mechanism helps to maintain effective cardiac output in the presence of shock. Once formed, angiotensin stimulates secretion of aldosterone by the adrenal cortex. This hormone acts on cells of the distal tubules to increase the reabsorption of sodium and, thus, water. In this way, aldosterone functions to increase the circulating blood volume and cardiac output.

**Secretion of Antidiuretic Hormone (ADH).** Antidiuretic hormone (ADH), also called vasopressin, secreted from the posterior pituitary gland in response to an increase in serum osmolality, acts on the epithelial cells of the distal tubules and collecting ducts to increase the reabsorption of water (see Fig. 21–10). The increase in serum osmolality is reflective of a relative increase in solutes that accompanies the loss of plasma. Receptors in the right atrium, stimulated in response to a decreased venous return to the heart associated with the hypovolemic state, also contribute to an increased secretion of ADH. The consequent reabsorption of water functions to expand the intravascular volume. Additionally, ADH exerts a potent vasopressor effect on the systemic vasculature, thereby increasing blood pressure and enhancing tissue perfusion.

## Clinical Presentation

Typically, the initial signs and symptoms experienced by the chest trauma patient will reflect anxiety; pain with associated dyspnea and tachypnea; tachycardia and signs reflective of a hypovolemic state with reduced tissue perfusion, including a decreased pulse pressure with declining arterial pressure, delayed capillary refill, decreased urinary output; pale, cool, clammy skin with poor turgor; and dry mucous membranes. Arterial blood gases may reflect hypoxemia ($PaO_2 < 80$ mmHg), and hypocapnia ($PaCO_2 < 35$ mmHg) initially; followed by hypercapnia ($PaCO_2 > 45$ mmHg), with a consequent acidemia (pH <7.35). Depending on the extent of injury, only a few or all of the above signs and symptoms may be present.

## Diagnostic Considerations

The diagnosis of specific chest trauma is based on clinical history, including mechanisms of injury, precipitating events, and assessment of pulmonary and cardiovascular status. The patient's clinical presentation and acuity status will determine the appropriateness of diagnostic studies. Specific diagnostic studies include laboratory, radiographic, and electrocardiographic. Table 64–2 lists normal and abnormal values for commonly prescribed laboratory studies of significance in the chest trauma patient. Radiographic studies of diagnostic importance are included in Table 64–3. Serial electrocardiographic (ECG) studies may be especially helpful in patients with trauma, particularly in patients who sustain a blunt chest trauma such as that associated with steering wheel impact.

TABLE 64-2
**Laboratory Values Associated with Shock**

| Lab Value | Normal Lab Value | Lab Value in Shock |
|---|---|---|
| 1. Hematocrit | 37-45% | 30% |
| 2. Arterial blood lactate level | 5-20 mg/dl | >20 mg/dl |
| 3. Arterial $PaO_2$ (room air) | 100 mmHg | <70 mmHg |
| 4. Arterial pH | 7.35-7.45 | <7.30 |
| 5. Arterial $PaCO_2$ | 35-45 mmHg | Variable |
| 6. Urine output | 30-50 ml/hr | <30 ml/hr |
| 7. Urine specific gravity | 1.010-1.020 | >1.025 |
| 8. Serum osmolality | 285-295 mOsm/kg water | >300-310 mOsm/kg water |

NOTE: This is a simplistic representation of laboratory values in shock. It should be appreciated that laboratory values may differ with the specific type of shock and/or the stage of shock.

Significant ECG findings may vary from the presence of peaked T waves to life-threatening ventricular dysrhythmias.

## Treatment

Effective treatment of chest trauma requires ongoing efforts to diagnose and treat the underlying injury while maintaining optimal respiratory and cardiovascular function. Of immediate concern is the stabilization of a patent airway to afford adequate alveolar ventilation. Arterial blood gases are serially monitored closely to determine the adequacy of ventilation. In the scenario of severe hypoxemia ($PaO_2$ <60 mmHg on room air), initiation of mechanical ventilation with positive end-expiratory pressure (PEEP) may be indicated. Such therapy helps to ensure adequate alveolar ventilation, maximize ventilation/perfusion matching, and minimize shunting. (For an indepth discussion of ventilation/perfusion ratio and pulmonary shunting, see appropriate sections in Chap. 28.)

Hemodynamic monitoring (using pulmonary artery catheter) affords ongoing assessment of left heart pressures and hydration status. Analysis of mixed venous oxygen tensions ($SvO_2$) affords assessment of tissue oxygen availability and uptake, and overall tissue perfusion. (Hemodynamic monitoring is discussed in detail in Chap. 41).

Aggressive fluid resuscitation is initiated as indicated. Severe chest injuries may be accompanied by hypovolemic, hemorrhagic shock associated with hemothorax and/or hemomediastinum. The use of autotransfusion (autologous blood transfusions) has been used effectively in salvaging blood from life-threatening traumatic hemothorax.[1] Cardiac output measurements help to determine cardiovascular dynamics.

Recent technologic advances in fluid volume resuscitation, including the rapid infusion system (RIS) and rapid solution administration set (RSAS), are under investigation.[2,3] Such systems afford rapid fluid volume replacement of up to 1500-2000 ml/min by a venous access, without high pressures or the need for multiple infusion lines. The clinical

TABLE 64-3
**Common Radiologic Procedures Performed in Chest Trauma**

| Radiologic Procedure | Injury Suspected | Diagnostic Findings |
|---|---|---|
| Supine/upright chest (PA and lateral) | Any abnormality | Fractured ribs, flail chest, pneumothorax, hemothorax |
| | Ruptured diaphragm | Free air below the diaphragm |
| Chest x-ray | Aortic disruption | Widened mediastinum, fractures of 1st or 2nd ribs; obliteration of aortic knob; presence of pleural cap; obliteration of space between pulmonary artery and aorta; tracheal deviation to the right; depression of left mainstem bronchus; elevation and rightward shift of left bronchus |
| Aortogram | (Performed if patient is stable) | Aortic disruption/tear can be confirmed |
| Serial chest x-rays | *Pulmonary contusion, *atelectasis | "White out," infiltrates |
| | *Missed or developing pneumothorax | Partial or total lung collapse |

*Changes may develop over hours or several days.

TABLE 64–4
**Categories of Cardiothoracic Trauma**[4]

| Classification | Specific Trauma |
|---|---|
| 1. Bony thoracic structure disruption | Rib and sternal fractures<br>Flail chest |
| 2. Parenchymal tissue disruption | Myocardial contusion<br>Pulmonary contusion |
| 3. Cardiothoracic dynamic disruption | Cardiac tamponade<br>Tension pneumothorax<br>Massive hemothoraces<br>Sucking chest wounds (open pneumothorax)<br>Simple pneumothorax<br>Hemothorax |
| 4. Conducting airway disruption | Tracheobronchial injuries |
| 5. Accessory structure disruption | Aortic rupture and other great vessel disruption |

advantages of these systems over conventional intravenous therapy have yet to be determined.

Cardiothoracic trauma can be divided into 5 general categories[4] (Table 64–4):

1. Bony thoracic structure disruption
2. Parenchymal tissue disruption
3. Cardiothoracic dynamic disruption
4. Conducting airway disruption
5. Accessory structure disruption.

Life-threatening forms of chest trauma requiring emergent intervention include cardiac tamponade, tension pneumothorax, and massive hemothoraces. These forms of chest trauma are considered *life-threatening*, and they require treatment simultaneously with the diagnosing.

### *Cardiac Tamponade*

Cardiac tamponade results from a blunt or penetrating injury to the heart, which causes fluid to accumulate in the pericardial sac (see Fig. 59–1). This accumulation impairs ventricular filling, decreasing cardiac output. Clinical presentation is that of Beck's triad, which consists of jugular venous distention, muffled heart sounds, and pulsus paradoxus (see Fig. 38–2). Life-saving intervention is pericardiocentesis or emergency thoracotomy if the patient is in cardiopulmonary arrest. The patient is taken to surgery to correct the underlying problem.

### *Tension Pneumothorax*

Tension pneumothorax occurs when air enters the pleural space but cannot escape. This is known as a *one-way valve effect.* Accumulating pressure in the pleural cavity causes a shifting of mediastinal structures to the unaffected side, thereby compromising the unaffected lung along with mediastinal structures. These dynamics impair venous return, resulting in cardiovascular collapse. Signs and symptoms include severe dyspnea, hypotension, tracheal deviation to the side opposite the injury as a result of shifting of intrathoracic structures to the unaffected side, and displacement of heart sounds. Distended neck veins are usually present unless severe hypovolemia exists. Cyanosis is a late, extremely ominous sign.

Treatment must be immediate. It consists of needle thoracentesis at the second intercostal space, midclavicular line on the affected side (see Fig. 29–2 for landmarks). This life-saving intervention will relieve the pressure in the pleural space as trapped air is allowed to exit. Chest tube insertion always follows needle thoracentesis in the case of tension pneumothorax. (For nursing care considerations related to thoracentesis and chest drainage, see Tables 36–2 and 36–3, respectively.)

### *Massive Hemothoraces*

Massive hemothoraces represent another form of life-threatening chest trauma resulting from the severe hypovolemia that ensues with this type of injury. A hemothorax is caused by either blunt or penetrating trauma lacerating the lungs, heart, diaphragm, or other vessels. Blood accumulates in the pleural cavity, causing partial or total lung collapse. Venous return is impaired if a mediastinal shift occurs. Clinical manifestations are those consistent with shock, namely, hypotension with narrowing pulse pressure (i.e., a decrease in the numerical difference between systolic and diastolic blood pressures reflective of tone of arterial walls), thready pulse, flat neck veins, and pale, cool skin.

Treatment of massive hemothoraces consists of rapid fluid resuscitation with warmed crystalloids (i.e., a low molecular weight solute such as sodium, glucose, or urea) and blood products (packed red blood cells). Autotransfusion of the patient's own blood (discussed above) is another alternative to rapid blood replacement. Chest tube placement should occur *after* fluid resuscitation because chest tube thoracostomy prior to adequate fluid and blood administration may lead to irreversible shock. This is so because the chest cavity can pool up to 4 liters of blood at any given point in time.

Other potential life-threatening chest injuries include aortic rupture and/or disruption of the integrity of other great vessels; sucking chest wounds; myocardial and/or pulmonary contusion; flail chest; tracheobronchial injuries; and thoracoabdominal trauma (see Table 64–4).

### *Aortic Rupture/Tears to Great Vessels*

Aortic rupture or tears to great vessels are usually associated with blunt trauma, and they are fatal in about 90% of all cases. Individuals sustaining these types of injuries usually die immediately of exsanguination. The most common cause of aortic rupture is a rapid deceleration or acceleration injury (e.g., steering wheel impact), resulting in the application of differential forces to intrathoracic structures. Penetrating wounds or punctures from fractured ribs and vertebrae have been cited as precipitating factors.

Diagnostic findings in patients with aortic rupture include asymmetric peripheral pulses, with an increased pulse amplitude and blood pressure in the upper extremities, and a decreased pulse amplitude and blood pressure in the lower extremities. A classic finding on x-ray is a widening mediastinum. Obliteration of the aortic knob and space between the pulmonary artery and aorta may also be present on x-ray. Clinically, if patients are conscious, they may complain of chest pain; they usually appear anxious and frightened, restless and agitated. Hemothorax is usually present. Definitive diagnosis is made on aortography, if time and the patient's condition permit.

Treatment requires an emergency thoracotomy to correct the underlying pathology. Pharmacologic treatment may involve administration of nitroprusside, a potent vasodilator, to decrease preload and afterload, thereby preventing complete disruption of the involved vessel. Use of the military antishock trousers (MAST; also referred to as pneumatic antishock garment, PASG) may be initiated in patients in shock (see Chap. 46). This special garment can be applied quickly. It consists of inflatable compartments that, when filled with air, compress the lower extremities and abdomen, thereby preventing pooling of blood and fluid in the tissues. Its use remains controversial because, while it raises blood pressure in hypotensive individuals, it does so primarily by increasing afterload. In patients with compromised cardiac output, increasing the afterload may further diminish cardiac output.

### *Sucking Chest Wounds/Open Pneumothorax*

Sucking chest wounds are commonly the result of penetrating chest trauma and/or puncture wounds attributed to fractured ribs. In an open pneumothorax, an opening in the chest wall creates a *two-way valve effect* where air is sucked in and out with each respiration. There is equilibration of intrathoracic and atmospheric pressures. If the defect is greater than two thirds the diameter of the trachea, total lung collapse is inevitable. The diagnosis is usually straightforward because the chest wound is visible.

Clinical manifestations of an open pneumothorax range from severe dyspnea to respiratory distress. Subcutaneous emphysema may be palpated in the neck and upper chest. Tracheal deviation to the unaffected side may be evident. Auscultation reveals diminished or absent breath sounds on the affected side. On chest percussion, a hyperresonance will be elicited due to the presence of air in the pleural cavity.

Prompt treatment involves placement of an occlusive dressing over the defect in the chest wall with impregnated gauze. The nurse must reassess the patient frequently after this dressing has been applied because an open pneumothorax covered with a petroleum jelly dressing may convert to a tension pneumothorax (see above). The overall treatment is chest thoracostomy or operative intervention to repair the defect in the chest wall.

### *Pneumothorax and Hemothorax*

A pneumothorax is the result of blunt or penetrating chest trauma. Air enters the pleural cavity causing partial or total lung collapse. With a hemothorax, blood occupies the pleural space instead of air, but the result is the same. Typical findings are shortness of breath, tachypnea, and respiratory distress. With a pneumothorax, there will be hyperresonance upon percussion attributed to the air in the pleural cavity; with a hemothorax, there will be dullness on percussion. Confirmation of the diagnosis of either pneumothorax or hemothorax is by chest x-ray. Treatment is tube thoracotomy. To treat a pneumothorax, the chest tube is usually inserted into the second intercostal space; in treating a hemothorax, the chest tube is placed in the fifth intercostal space at the midaxillary line (see Figs. 29–2 and 29–4 for landmarks). Underwater chest tube drainage is then initiated (see Table 36–3).

### *Myocardial Contusion*

Myocardial contusion, a bruise to the muscular layer of the heart, occurs as the result of blunt trauma to the chest commonly sustained during a motor vehicle accident. It has often been identified in drivers unrestrained with seat belts who experience an impact with the steering wheel.

This potentially lethal injury is difficult to diagnose because the clinical presentation varies from patient to patient. Observe for bruises to the anterior chest or seat belt ecchymosis, and evaluate any chest pain carefully. Some patients will complain of retrosternal angina. The patient may even display signs of cardiogenic shock (see Table 44–8). ECG findings may be observed in some patients, ranging from ST and T wave changes suggestive of myocardial ischemia to cardiac dysrhythmias (e.g., sinus tachycardia, heart block). A pericardial or pleural friction rub may be auscultated (see Chaps. 38 and 29, respectively). Laboratory data may reveal elevation of isoenzymes (CPK-MB). These enzymes as well as electrocardiograms are usually ordered serially. Treatment is generally supportive and similar to that of the patient with a myocardial infarction (see Tables 43–6 and 43–7).

### Pulmonary Contusion

Pulmonary contusion, a bruise sustained by the lung parenchyma, is potentially a lethal type of chest trauma. There is a direct insult to the lungs from blunt trauma, penetration, or puncture injury associated with fractured ribs, flail chest, or sudden compression of the thoracic cavity. Tissue anoxia occurs from leakage of blood and fluid into lung interstitium secondary to increased capillary permeability.

The clinical picture may progress to that of adult respiratory distress syndrome (ARDS, see Chap. 34). The patient is observed for dyspnea, tachypnea, hemoptysis, ineffective cough with copious secretions, tachycardia, and restlessness and anxiety in the conscious individual. Rales (crackles) may be heard on auscultation. Diagnosis is made on chest x-ray, although definitive findings may not be apparent on x-ray for the first 48–72 hours.

Treatment of pulmonary contusion involves fluid restriction and diuretics to decrease interstitial edema. Hemodynamic monitoring assists in determining hydration status. Trends in cardiopulmonary dynamics assist in evaluating the patient's response to therapy. Intubation and initiation of mechanical ventilation therapy may be indicated in patients with severe hypoxemia ($PaO_2$ <60 mmHg on 40% $FIO_2$) unresponsive to supportive therapy. PEEP therapy in conjunction with mechanical ventilation may be implemented. In the scenario of ARDS, PEEP therapy maintains airway opening pressure at end-expiration above atmospheric pressure. This distending airway pressure increases lung volumes including functional residual capacity (FRC); it prevents collapse of airways, enhances gas exchange and oxygen transport, and helps to reduce right to left shunting. (For nursing considerations in caring for the patient with pulmonary contusion complicated by ARDS, see Table 34–3.)

### Flail Chest

Flail chest refers to a fracture of two or more ribs in two or more places, usually as a result of blunt trauma. Severe flail injuries can disrupt pulmonary ventilatory mechanics as reflected by paradoxical respirations (i.e., a collapse of the chest wall on inspiration and an expansion of the chest wall on expiration). The patient may appear dyspneic and in obvious respiratory distress. Some patients may experience stridor (a high-pitched noisy respiration, like the blowing of the wind). In severe cases, cyanosis may be noted. The patient may complain of severe chest pain; shallow respirations with poor tidal volume, and splinting are commonly observed. Subcutaneous emphysema may be present, and diminished breath sounds will be heard on auscultation. There is usually point tenderness at the location of injury, and crepitus may be heard or palpated over the fracture sites.

Initially, treatment of flail chest may involve manual stabilization of the flail segment by application of pressure during expiration or by sandbagging. This latter approach is controversial because an increase in atelectasis has been associated with the pressure applied to the chest by this approach. Mechanical ventilation with PEEP therapy has been successful in the treatment of flail chest. Such therapy helps to maintain chest wall expansion, thereby preventing the chest cage from becoming smaller as healing progresses.

Another approach employed is the use of thoracic epidural analgesic therapy for pain control. On occasions, this technique has eliminated the need for intubation because patients will breathe more efficiently and splint less if their pain is relieved. Intercostal nerve blocks have also been used with minimal success.

### Rib Fractures

Rib fractures are the most common chest injury. Such injuries can seriously compromise alveolar ventilation as a result of splinting of the ribcage secondary to pain. Puncture injury of the lung parenchyma may become potentially life-threatening. Patients usually complain of severe pain, and point tenderness over the fracture is frequently noted. Rib fractures can often be palpated. Patients will also be observed to splint the chest when they breathe, thereby compromising the ventilatory effort and predisposing to atelectasis. Diagnosis is confirmed on chest x-ray. Treatment usually involves adequate pain control so as to ease the work of breathing and depth of respirations.

### Sternal Fractures

Sternal fractures are frequently the result of steering wheel injuries. They commonly occur in drivers who use seat belts, who would otherwise have sustained a more serious injury (e.g., myocardial or pulmonary contusion, severe flail chest) had seat belts not been used. Diagnosis is confirmed by x-ray. Treatment is supportive.

### Tracheobronchial Injuries

Tracheobronchial injuries are caused when a shearing force is exerted to the trachea or bronchial structures. Blunt trauma is the primary cause for this injury, although penetrating trauma is also a mechanism of injury. Severe tracheobronchial injuries are almost always fatal because they lead to complete airway collapse. Efforts to ventilate the patient mechanically are compromised by air leaks associated with the injuries. Subcutaneous emphysema is almost always present. Tension pneumothorax may be seen in conjunction with a tracheobronchial injury, further complicating the clinical picture and treatment options.

Treatment is directed toward establishing and maintaining an adequate airway. A patent airway may be established and maintained by positioning an endotracheal tube beyond the point of bronchial injury. Creation of a surgical opening by cricothyrotomy or tracheotomy is frequently the only method available to establish a patent airway in patients who have sustained injury to the trachea, larynx, and bronchi (see Fig. 28–1). Definitive treatment is performed in the operating room and is directed at correction of the underlying pathophysiology.

#### Thoracoabdominal Trauma

Thoracoabdominal trauma is defined as trauma that involves both the thoracic and abdominal cavities. It is also *torsotrauma*. Injuries include esophageal trauma, diaphragmatic rupture, and other associated abdominal organ injuries. The clinical presentation varies depending on the structures involved. The nurse must be cognizant of the fact that a chest injury also implies the presence of an abdominal injury, especially in penetrating trauma, as for example, a stab wound. Involvement of the diaphragm is always a possibility because the diaphragm rises during expiration.

## Nursing Care of the Patient with Chest Trauma

Nursing care in chest trauma is first directed toward use of an *anticipatory* approach to intervene in the immediate life-threatening types of chest trauma. Knowledge of the mechanism of injury, initial clinical status, and patient history are helpful in providing appropriate, timely and continuous care.

In severe cases of thoracic trauma, the multidisciplinary team treats the patient *simultaneously* while diagnosing. This is especially true of patients with severe tension pneumothorax, pericardial tamponade, and massive hemothoraces (see above). In about 85% of all chest trauma cases, however, the patient can be managed with a simple procedure such as the insertion of a chest tube. Only about 15% of all thoracic trauma victims require immediate surgical intervention. These are the patients who require rapid assessment and quick intervention if death or permanent sequelae are to be prevented. It is the responsibility of the critical care nurse to recognize these facts when caring for the chest trauma patient.

The critical care nurse assumes many other responsibilities in the overall care of the patient with thoracic trauma. As diagnosis and stabilization occur, the nurse continues with a comprehensive ongoing assessment to determine patient needs, emotional as well as physiologic, and their priorities. Subtle changes in patient status may be significant in detecting complications or previously undetected injuries in these patients. Serial reassessments of the patient include airway and ventilatory status, vital signs, and neurologic status. Hemodynamic parameters are continuously monitored. Serial arterial blood gas analyses reflect status of gas exchange and oxygenation.

The patient's hydration status is monitored meticulously. Outputs, including nasogastric, urinary, and chest tube drainage, are documented carefully. Fluid resuscitation is prescribed to maintain cardiac output and circulatory support. Exsanguination is a major concern in any patient with trauma to the thorax. A patient who drains excessive amounts of blood by way of a chest tube may require surgical intervention. Chest tube output of greater than 300–500 ml/hour, or an output of greater than 200 ml/hour for 3–4 hours consecutively, suggests massive hemorrhage and the need for immediate surgery.

#### Complications in Thoracic Trauma

Patients who have sustained serious chest trauma are at high risk of complications involving other organ systems, in addition to cardiopulmonary function. Many of these patients are victims of multisystem trauma requiring vigilant assessment and monitoring. Hemorrhage is always a major complication of chest trauma. Bleeding associated with a coagulopathy (i.e., a defect in blood clotting mechanism), induced by either the injury sustained or from massive transfusions in its treatment, is a common occurrence in patients with severe chest or multisystem trauma. ARDS, pulmonary emboli, and respiratory failure often compound the clinical picture. The occurrence of renal and liver dysfunction is not unusual. The critical care nurse must be especially vigilant to detect subtle clues and to recognize trends that suggest underlying pathophysiology. Early recognition and timely institution of appropriate interventions may help to avert reversible pathophysiology from becoming *ir*reversible.

#### Therapeutic Goals

Overall management of the trauma patient begins with the ABCs (airway, breathing, and circulation). Therapeutic goals for the patient with chest trauma involve the following:

1. Establish and maintain a patent airway (Chap. 32).
2. Support alveolar ventilation and oxygenation to relieve hypoxemia.
3. Provide hemodynamic support to maintain adequate cardiac output and tissue perfusion (Table 33–2, Nursing Diagnoses #4, 5, and 6).
4. Monitor/maintain fluid and electrolyte balance (Chap. 23).
5. Monitor/maintain acid–base balance (Chap. 30).

6. Recognize clues of underlying pathophysiology associated with ARDS, pulmonary embolism, hemorrhage (Chaps. 34, 35, and 49).
7. Provide nutritional support (Table 33-2, Nursing Diagnosis #9; Chap. 53).
8. Prevent infection (Table 33-2, Nursing Diagnosis #10; Table 49-7).
9. Provide pain control and promote patient comfort.
10. Prevent impairment in skin integrity related to immobility and stress.
11. Provide emotional and psychologic support to patient and family (Chaps. 3 and 5).

#### *Nursing Diagnoses, Desired Patient Outcomes, and Nursing Interventions*

Implementation of the nursing process in the care of the patient with thoracic trauma centers around the therapeutic goals listed above. Nursing diagnoses, desired patient outcomes, and nursing interventions and their rationales are outlined in Table 64-5.

## ABDOMINAL TRAUMA

### Blunt Versus Penetrating Abdominal Trauma

Abdominal trauma results from blunt and penetrating forces. Trauma resulting from blunt impact is the most common. Blunt injuries frequently are the result of motor vehicle accidents and physical assault. Penetrating abdominal trauma is usually associated with violent acts such as gunshot wounds and stabbings. Victims of multiple trauma often experience abdominal injury as a life-threatening component. Chest and pelvic trauma should be suspected in association with abdominal trauma, and a high index of suspicion must be maintained.

The severity of blunt injury is directly related to the force of impact, the amount of time the force is applied, and anatomical area where force is applied. The abdominal wall offers minimal support and protection from injury as compared to the protection provided by the skull and bony thorax (see Chap. 10). Abdominal trauma may result in massive blood loss with subsequent hemorrhagic shock, or peritoneal contamination with subsequent peritonitis. Abdominal injuries, therefore, may lead to fluid volume deficit, alteration in tissue perfusion, alteration in comfort, and alteration in bowel and urinary elimination.

The abdomen is the portion of the trunk located between the diaphragm and the pelvis. It consists of three sections, the intrathoracic abdomen, the pelvic or true abdomen, and the retroperitoneal space.

The abdominal viscera contains both hollow and solid organs, with solid organs frequently injured by blunt force and hollow organ injuries resulting from penetrating trauma. The hollow organs include the stomach, gallbladder, intestines, bladder, and a portion of the esophagus (see Fig. 47-1). The liver, spleen, pancreas, kidneys, and uterus comprise the solid organs, with the liver and spleen being the most frequently injured abdominal organs. When the stomach, bladder, or intestines are filled with fluid, they act as solid organs in response to severe impact or force. The major vessels in the abdominal area include the aorta and the inferior vena cava.

### Clinical Presentation

The initial signs and symptoms exhibited by the abdominal trauma patient may be as severe as those indicative of profound hypovolemia or as subtle as no signs of injury or complaint of pain. Typical initial signs and symptoms include those associated with shock and abdominal pain. The major life-threatening concern in abdominal injuries is severe blood loss and the resulting hemorrhagic shock (see Chaps. 46 and 49).

Clinical signs, in addition to those related to shock, may include abdominal ecchymosis, decreased or absent bowel sounds, muscular rigidity and involuntary guarding, and rebound tenderness. Left shoulder pain, referred to as Kehr's sign, is a classic finding in patients with splenic rupture and is caused by blood below the diaphragm irritating the phrenic nerve.

### Diagnostic Considerations

Specific information regarding the mechanism of injury, events preceding the incident, location of the patient at the time of injury, and force of impact provide significant data for diagnosis of abdominal injury. Diagnostic studies must occur as life-saving intervention is initiated. As with chest trauma, initial diagnostic efforts should address airway, breathing, and circulatory status.

The most important diagnosis in abdominal trauma or suspected abdominal trauma is whether or not the patient will require immediate surgical intervention to prevent death or disability. During the early resuscitation and stabilization phases of care, the actual diagnosis of specific intra-abdominal injuries may not be of prime importance. However, the timely decision to move the patient to the surgical suite is of great importance.

#### *Laboratory Studies*

The patient with abdominal trauma requires many of the same laboratory studies as the chest trauma

**TABLE 64–5. CARE PLAN FOR THE PATIENT WITH MULTISYSTEMS TRAUMA: THORACIC, ABDOMINAL AND LONG BONE (ORTHOPEDIC)**

| Nursing Diagnoses | Desired Patient Outcomes | Nursing Interventions | Rationales |
|---|---|---|---|
| ***Nursing Diagnosis #1*** Alteration in tissue perfusion related to:<br>1. Hypovolemia,<br>2. Impaired blood supply, and/or<br>3. Vascular compromise from fracture. | Patient will maintain:<br>1. Skin temperature, color, and moisture—pink, warm, and dry.<br>2. Capillary refill of <2 seconds.<br>3. Normal neurovascular assessment of extremities: Sensorimotor function intact.<br>4. Urinary output of 30–50 ml per hour. | • Perform patient assessment and monitoring (includes ABCs with C-spine, and hemorrhage control).<br>• Perform "mini" neuro exam (Glasgow Coma Score, and pupils).<br>• Note vital signs (including temperature) at frequent intervals (every 15 minutes unless patient condition dictates more frequent vitals, then every 1–5 minutes).<br>• Perform capillary refill checks with vital signs.<br>• Assess neurovascular function of immobilized extremity (pain, pulse, pallor, puffiness, paralysis, paresthesias). | • Complete patient assessment and monitoring aids the nurse in discovering overt/covert changes in patient status at frequent intervals in those with multisystem trauma.<br>• Early recognition of these changes results in timely care and the appropriate interventions to decrease trauma patient morbidity and mortality.<br>• Reflects status of tissue perfusion. |
| ***Nursing Diagnosis #2*** Impaired gas exchange related to:<br>1. Disruption of alveolar-capillary membrane,<br>2. Decreased tissue perfusion, and/or<br>3. Other complication (e.g., fat emboli). | Patient will maintain:<br>1. Arterial blood gases:<br>• $PaO_2 > 80$ mmHg (room air)<br>• $PaCO_2$ 35–45 mmHg; pH 7.35–7.45.<br>2. Minimum pulmonary function:<br>• Tidal volume >7–10 ml/kg<br>• Vital capacity >15 ml/kg<br>3. Cardiac ouput of 4–8 liters/minute.<br>4. Respiratory rate of 12–20/minute, eupneic.<br>5. $SvO_2$ within normal limits. | • Ensure patent airway via appropriate route (chin lift, jaw thrust, without neck hyperextension).<br>• Provide high flow oxygen at 6–10 liters/minute (use mask or cannula, or oral or nasal adjuncts).<br>• Give ventilatory support as needed $FIO_2$ of 100% (endotracheal or nasotracheal intubation; cricothyrotomy or tracheotomy, if indicated, for obstructed airway).<br>• Monitor serial arterial blood gases (ABGs) per physician.<br>• Obtain serial chest x-rays per physician.<br>• Cover sucking or open chest wounds.<br>• Observe for tension pneumothorax. | • Establishing a patent airway provides the initial route for adequate intake of oxygen.<br>• Oxygen delivery in the proper amount via the appropriate method assists in the maintenance of adequate tissue oxygenation.<br>• Serial blood gas measurements accurately reflect gas exchange requirements in impaired patients with decreased tissue perfusion.<br>• Serial chest x-rays provide for ongoing monitoring for potential or missed lung injury (i.e., pulmonary contusion).<br>• Covering sucking or open wounds provides for more effective gas exchange until the defect can be repaired. |

*(continued)*

**TABLE 64–5. CARE PLAN FOR THE PATIENT WITH MULTISYSTEMS TRAUMA: THORACIC, ABDOMINAL AND LONG BONE (ORTHOPEDIC)** *(Continued)*

| Nursing Diagnoses | Desired Patient Outcomes | Nursing Interventions | Rationales |
|---|---|---|---|
| ***Nursing Diagnosis #3***<br>Fluid volume deficit related to:<br>1. Blood loss. | Patient will maintain:<br>1. Wedge pressure (PCWP) of 8–12 mmHg.<br>2. Systolic B/P of >100 mmHg (including orthostatic B/P).<br>3. Pulse pressure of >30 mmHg.<br>4. Strong, palpable peripheral pulses of 2+ bilaterally.<br>5. No external bleeding noted.<br>6. Normal skin turgor.<br>7. Level of consciousness: Alert, awake, and oriented ×3.<br>8. Absence of signs of internal bleeding (hematochezia, periumbilical ecchymoses). | • Control external bleeding with direct pressure.<br>• Position patient in Trendelenburg if not contraindicated.<br>• Assess for signs of occult bleeding frequently (i.e., rigid abdomen, stools for guaiac).<br>• Start IVs with large bore 14–16 gauge needles; crystalloids, colloids, and blood may be administered.<br>○ Fluid replacement therapy:<br>– Crystalloids: 3 ml/1 ml blood loss.<br>– Blood: 1 ml/1 ml blood loss.<br>• Assist with cutdowns or central lines as needed.<br>• Prepare for autotransfusion if indicated with chest injuries.<br>• Consider use of antishock garment (controversial). Monitor response: Blood pressure in hypotension; assess trouser pressure in bleeding; monitor ventilatory response as pressure over abdomen can compromise chest excursion.<br>• Splint and immobilize extremities, prevent gross movement.<br>• Provide hemodynamic monitoring for critical patients.<br>• Monitor serial hematocrits (as per physician). | • Controlling external bleeding prevents exsanguinating hemorrhage—direct pressure is the best method.<br>• Trendelenburg aids in venous return to augment B/P. Contraindicated in possible head injury, impedes blood flow from cranium.<br>• Assessment for occult bleeding is necessary to prevent missed injuries and to note the changing status of the patient.<br>• Large bore IVs with crystalloids, colloids, and/or blood help replace fluid volume deficit.<br>• Cutdowns or central venous lines provide quick fluid access to central circulation.<br>• Autotransfusion provides an immediate autologous blood transfusion to the patient.<br>• Antishock trousers enhance peripheral resistance, perform arterial tamponade, promote shunting of blood to vital organs, and splint fractures to decrease blood loss. (See Chap. 46 for discussion of antishock trousers.)<br>• Immobilization of fractures prevents further hemorrhage; reduces risk of fat emboli.<br>• Hemodynamic pressure monitoring assists in determining fluid requirements in patients with fluid volume deficit.<br>• Serial Hcts determines the amount of packed red cells found in the blood. |

| | | | |
|---|---|---|---|
| ***Nursing Diagnosis #4***<br>Alteration in cardiac output (decreased) related to:<br>1. Hemorrhage shock.<br>2. Cardiac injury. | Patient will maintain:<br>1. Normal electrocardiogram.<br>2. Heart sounds S1 and S2 normal without extra sounds.<br>3. Cardiac output of 4–8 liters/minute.<br>4. Normal skin temperature, color, and moisture (as noted above).<br>5. Pulse rate of 60–100 beats/minute.<br>6. Signs of adequate tissue perfusion (e.g., brisk capillary refill). | • Obtain 12-lead electrocardiogram (per physician).<br>• Perform continuous ECG monitoring.<br>• Consider antishock garment (controversial)<br>• Monitor hemodynamic status to titrate fluids (see Nursing Diagnosis #3, above).<br>• Obtain serial labwork (Hgb, Hct, chemistries, and enzymes). | • 12 lead-ECG provides baseline electrocardiographic data.<br>• Continuous EKG monitoring is performed to note potential cardiac dysrhythmias since they are a complication of impaired gas exchange and alteration in cardiac output.<br>• Antishock garment enhances peripheral resistance (see Nursing Diagnosis #3, above)<br>• Hemodynamic monitoring defects status of cardiopulmonary function and measures cardiac output.<br>• Maintaining hematocrit within normal range assures tissue oxygenation. |
| ***Nursing Diagnosis #5***<br>Impaired skin integrity related to:<br>1. Open wounds from fractures,<br>2. Penetrating trauma,<br>3. Abrasions, contusions, lacerations, edema, or<br>4. Neurovascular compromise. | Patient will maintain:<br>1. Absence of bacterial infection and secondary infections.<br>2. Intact skin surfaces.<br>3. Proper wound healing and reduced inflammatory response.<br>4. Absence of sepsis or other systemic reactions.<br>5. Body temperature at baseline: 98.6°F (37°C). | • Stabilize all impaled objects prior to operative removal.<br>• Cleanse and irrigate all open wounds with solution of choice.<br>• Cover all open wounds with sterile dressings. Perform sterile dressing changes as needed. Note amount, color, and consistency of drainage from wounds.<br>• Cover "sucking" wounds with impregnated (petroleum jelly) gauze.<br>• Provide antibiotic therapy as ordered (IV, IM, or oral).<br>  ○ Obtain specimens for culture and sensitivity (as appropriate).<br>• Give tetanus toxoid or tetanus immunoglobulin (per physician).<br>• Turn and position q2hr; range of motion exercises (as indicated). | • Stabilization of impaled objects prevents further injury.<br>• Cleansing and irrigation of open wounds removes debris and decreases bacteria, which cause infection.<br>• Covering wounds maintains sterile environment.<br>• Covering sucking wounds with impregnated gauze temporarily restores skin integrity and may reduce chest wall defect.<br>• Antibiotic therapy inhibits and/or kills microorganisms and the growth of anaerobic Gram-positive and Gram-negative organisms.<br>• Tetanus toxoid and tetanus immune globulin prevent tetanus.<br>• Maximizes perfusion, reduces risk of thrombophlebitis and pressure ulcer in immobilized patient. |

*(continued)*

**TABLE 64–5. CARE PLAN FOR THE PATIENT WITH MULTISYSTEMS TRAUMA: THORACIC, ABDOMINAL AND LONG BONE (ORTHOPEDIC)** *(Continued)*

| Nursing Diagnoses | Desired Patient Outcomes | Nursing Interventions | Rationales |
|---|---|---|---|
| ***Nursing Diagnosis #6***<br>Impaired physical mobility related to:<br>1. Chest, abdominal, and/or long bone trauma. | Patient will:<br>1. Demonstrate mobility to pre-injury capacity, or to optimal level of restored function. | • Remove all constrictive clothing and jewelry. | • Removing constrictive clothing and jewelry provides for enhanced mobility and increased circulation to promote healing. |
| | | • Splint and immobilize all extremities above and below joints. | • Immobilization and splinting allow for increased mobility and the prevention of further injury. |
| | | • Provide gait training and crutches during limited mobility. | • Proper gait training prevents injury, and crutch walking provides a method of early ambulation in patients with long bone trauma. |
| | | • Assist with cast, traction, pin, and/or fixator application if indicated. | • Casting, pin insertion, external and/or internal fixators, and/or traction promote alignment of bone, restore tissue function, and increase circulation to the affected area to promote healing. |
| | | • Encourage early ambulation in multisystem trauma patients. | • Early ambulation prevents other complications (i.e., pulmonary). |
| ***Nursing Diagnosis #7***<br>Alteration in comfort (pain) related to:<br>1. Tissue, nerve, or vessel disruption from penetrating, blunt, or extremity trauma. | Patient will:<br>1. Verbalize that pain is diminished or that pain relief has occurred (if conscious).<br>2. Display relaxed musculature, no facial grimace, and minimal signs of combativeness. | • Provide position of comfort for patient as permitted by patient's clinical status.<br>• Provide pain medication via proper route and monitor response.<br>• Use other pain reduction techniques if alternative therapy indicated (biofeedback, TENS, distraction, guided imagery). | • Providing position of comfort for patients in pain may alleviate or reduce discomfort.<br>• Pain medication binds to receptor sites, which function to reduce perception of pain.<br>• Pain reduction techniques alter pain perception and/or sensation. |
| | | • Splint and immobilize all injured extremities. | • Splinting of injured extremities brings about immobilization, which reduces edema, restores circulation and therefore, tissue perfusion, to reduce or eliminate pain. |
| | | • Cover all wounds. | • Dressings to wounds decrease pain to the injured site and reduce risk of infection. |

| | | | |
|---|---|---|---|
| ***Nursing Diagnosis #8***<br>Alteration in elimination (bowel or urinary) related to:<br>1. Decreased circulating volume.<br>2. Associated hypoperfusion from multisystem organ failure, gastrointestinal injury, or renal trauma. | Patient will maintain:<br>1. Urinary output of 30–50 ml/hour (ml/kg).<br>2. Urine specific gravity of 1.010–1.025.<br>3. Normal color, amount, consistency of urine.<br>4. Decreased gastric distention.<br>5. Expected nasogastric drainage (if NG tube is in place).<br>6. Abdomen, soft and non-tender.<br>7. Normal bowel sounds, bowel movement if appropriate. | • Insert continuous urinary drainage catheter. Monitor urinary output. Note color, amount, consistency, and specific gravity.<br>• Insert nasogastric or orogastric tube.<br>• Monitor gastric drainage (to suction if indicated).<br>• Note color, amount, and consistency of drainage. | • Continuous urinary drainage allows for monitoring of potential alterations in urinary and/or renal function.<br>• Continuous gastric drainage allows for monitoring of gastrointestinal function and potential bleeding; decompressed stomach allows for full chest excursion and lung expansion; minimizes risk of aspiration in patients with an altered level of consciousness. |
| ***Nursing Diagnosis #9***<br>Knowledge deficit related to:<br>1. Lack of information regarding injury or illness. | Patient/family comprehends treatment regimen through verbalization and resultant compliance in self-care. | • Assess for readiness of the learner(s).<br>• Provide for patient and family education.<br>• Give one-to-one teaching regarding specific aspects of care.<br>• Teach to level of patient/family. | • Assessing for learner readiness provides information as to the patient/family level of comprehension.<br>• Patient/family education may promote an understanding of the injury and therefore greater acceptance and compliance with treatment regimens.<br>• One-to-one teaching may result in enhancing absorption of information and reinforcement.<br>• Teaching to the level of the patient allows for greater retention and understanding. |
| ***Nursing Diagnosis #10***<br>Ineffective coping patterns (patient and/or family or significant others) to stress of trauma. | Patient/family will:<br>1. Exhibit effective coping mechanisms.<br>2. Verbalize feelings.<br>3. Identify/access support systems (persons, institutions, associations).<br>4. Identify past coping mechanisms that have been successful. | • Assess for life-threatening injury or illness and/or patient and family perceptions of such illness.<br>• Communicate and develop trusting relationship with patient/family.<br>• Act as patient/family advocate.<br>• Encourage patient/family to verbalize feelings. | • Assessing for life-threatening injuries may assist in relating patient prognosis information to patient/family, and clarifying patient's overall clinical status.<br>• Development of a trusting relationship increases communication thereby giving clear messages to the client.<br>• Acting as patient/family advocate may assist in patient support.<br>• Verbalization of feelings encourages dealing with perceptions about the injury, and known/unknown fears. |

*(continued)*

### TABLE 64–5. CARE PLAN FOR THE PATIENT WITH MULTISYSTEMS TRAUMA: THORACIC, ABDOMINAL AND LONG BONE (ORTHOPEDIC) *(Continued)*

| Nursing Diagnoses | Desired Patient Outcomes | Nursing Interventions | Rationales |
|---|---|---|---|
| ***Nursing Diagnosis #10 (cont.)*** | 5. Be able to set short-term goals and objectives.<br>6. Eventually be able to set long-term goals, and a plan of action for the future. Anxiety reaction, if present, will be appropriate to crisis or event. | • Assist patient/family to identify past coping mechanisms.<br>• Help patient/family define immediate areas where decision making is involved.<br>• Provide emotional and verbal support during crisis.<br>• Involve patient/family in as many decisions as possible (includes care activities, short- and long-term decisions).<br>• Encourage the development of new coping mechanisms where past mechanisms have proven ineffective for problem-solving.<br>• Initiate referral system as needed. | • Identifying past coping mechanisms may help in knowing which techniques were helpful.<br>• Patient/family participation is imperative for future well-being and overall health care management.<br>• Providing emotional support during crisis may decrease anxiety.<br>• Involving patient/family in decisions about care allow them to assume responsibility for actions and promotes dignity and patient self-esteem.<br>• Encourging the use of new coping methods may strengthen patient/family and assist them in identifying effective coping mechanisms.<br>• Utilization of a referral system (social service, pastoral care, psychological counseling) will be of significance in planning total, comprehensive, holistic patient care during acute phase, and rehabilitation. |
| ***Nursing Diagnosis #11***<br>Alteration in nutritional status, decreased from multisystem trauma. (See appropriate tables in Chapter 53, Nutritional Support of the Critically Ill Patient.) | Patient will maintain:<br>1. Adequate nutritional intake via oral, IV, and/or parenteral or enteral route (regular diet or diet to tolerance).<br>2. Positive nitrogen balance will be achieved. | • Provide nutritional support via appropriate route (oral, parenteral or enteral route as indicated).<br>• Obtain serial electrolytes per physician.<br>• Assess skin turgor and mucous membranes during complete patient assessment.<br>• Monitor nitrogen balance in critically injured patients. | • Nutritional support is necessary for the repair of injured tissue and the promotion of health.<br>• Serial electrolytes provide baseline data for the monitoring of the patient's nutritional and overall status.<br>• Skin turgor assessment detects dehydration or overhydration status of the patient.<br>• Positive nitrogen balance is imperative for the multisystems trauma patient in a compromised, catabolic state due to injury. |

| | | | |
|---|---|---|---|
| | 3. Normal serum electrolytes:<br>• Potassium 3.5–5.0 mEq/liter<br>• Sodium 135–145 mEq/liter<br>• Chloride 100–106 mEq/liter<br>• $CO_2$ content 24–30 mEq/liter<br>• Glucose 70–110 mg/100 ml<br>• Creatinine 0.6–1.5 mg/100 ml<br>• BUN 8–25 mg/100 ml<br>4. Normal skin turgor present. | | |
| ***Nursing Diagnosis #12***<br>Alteration in body image related to:<br>1. Traumatic incident,<br>2. Disfigurement, or<br>3. Perceived body image disturbance. | Patient will:<br>1. Be able to discuss body image disturbance if present and verbalize feelings about self, including positive comments.<br>2. Demonstrate signs of acceptance of self in actions like dress and performance of the ADL. | • Assess patient coping style.<br>• Discuss with patient body image perceptions.<br>• Offer praise and accomplishment when appropriate.<br>• Establish open lines of communication.<br>• Make appropriate referrals as needed. | • Assessment of patient coping styles assists in discovering successful methods of dealing with body image crises.<br>• Verbalizing feelings regarding body perceptions may reduce anxiety and fears and help patients overcome disturbances.<br>• Offering praise and support when appropriate creates feelings of enhanced human dignity, self-worth, and self-esteem.<br>• Open lines of communication allows for verbalization of body image concerns.<br>• Making appropriate referrals will assist in patient well-being. |

victim. Early determination of hemoglobin and hematocrit, electrolytes, urinalysis, and arterial blood gases is essential to direct resuscitative measures, as well as to establish baseline data for ongoing assessment and comparison. Table 64–2 lists normal and abnormal values for commonly used laboratory data. Actual or potential abdominal injury may require transfusion of blood products; therefore, a type and screen, or type and cross-match should be obtained as part of initial laboratory studies.

Additional laboratory studies specific to abdominal trauma may include determination of amylase, BUN, and creatinine. Although often obtained, controversy exists as to their actual value in identifying significant injury. Guaiac of stool and gastric contents may indicate injury and bleeding.

#### Radiographic Studies

Radiographic studies vary depending on severity of injury and institutional and community attitudes. Prior to the use of computerized axial tomography (CAT) in assessing abdominal trauma, abdominal films were routinely obtained. With increasing use of the CAT scan to determine significant injury, a decrease in the use of abdominal films is evident.

The following radiographic studies may be indicated in abdominal trauma. An upright abdominal film may reveal air below the diaphragm, indicating disruption of a hollow organ or abnormal densities associated with bleeding from solid organs (less than 800 ml of blood may not be visualized on x-ray). A lateral decubitus film may reveal disruption of hollow organs through air along the lateral aspects of the abdomen. An intravenous pyelogram (IVP) may be used to determine extravasation of contrast media, indicating injury to the kidney, ureters, or bladder. Computerized axial tomography may be used to determine actual sites of bleeding and to quantify bleeding in the abdominal cavity both intraperitoneally and extraperitoneally.

#### Peritoneal Lavage

The peritoneal lavage is used to determine the presence of intra-abdominal bleeding. The accuracy of the peritoneal lavage is approximated to be 95% and is most useful in the assessment of blunt abdominal trauma. Controversy exists regarding the effectiveness and accuracy of peritoneal lavage versus computerized axial tomography. Current modalities indicate a rise in popularity of the CAT scan determination of abdominal injuries, but the peritoneal lavage continues to be the procedure of choice in the clinically unstable patient.

Prior to initiation of the peritoneal lavage, a nasogastric (NG) or orogastric tube and urinary catheter should be inserted. The NG tube is both diagnostic and therapeutic because it decompresses the stomach, prevents aspiration, and minimizes gastric content contamination of the abdominal cavity. The urinary catheter is inserted to empty the bladder, thereby decreasing the risk of puncturing the bladder during the procedure. It further allows monitoring of urine output and analysis of urine for gross or occult blood.

Saline solution or Ringer's lactate should be infused into the peritoneal cavity and should be warmed to prevent the risk of hypothermia induced by the infusion of cold or room temperature fluids. If frank blood is not initially aspirated, 1000 ml (10 ml/kg) of fluid should be infused over 10–15 minutes. The fluid then drains by gravity and is analyzed.

Laboratory analysis of peritoneal fluid is performed to determine the presence of blood cells, bile, amylase, urine, or feces, all indicative of intra-abdominal injury. Table 64–6 depicts positive peritoneal lavage findings.

TABLE 64–6
**Positive Peritoneal Lavage Findings**

- Frank, non-clotting blood
- Red blood cells: 100,000 red cells/mm$^3$ (blunt trauma)
- Red blood cells: 1,000–100,000 red cells/mm$^3$ (penetrating trauma)
- Hematocrit: >2%
- White blood cells: >500 white cells/mm$^3$
- Amylase: >200 Somogyi units
- Presence of bile
- Presence of fecal material, bacteria, or urine

Frequently, a quick method will be used to determine the need for immediate surgical intervention when evaluating peritoneal lavage fluid. The statement made is that, if newsprint can be read through the lavage return, the peritoneal lavage is negative. This rule may not always be accurate, and immediate laboratory analysis of lavage fluid is necessary to assure appropriate treatment.

## Therapeutic Interventions

#### Critical Care Phase

Critical life-saving interventions should include activities to support or reestablish vital physiologic functions. Immediate interventions must be directed toward ensuring a patent airway, providing high-flow oxygen, and supporting effective ventilation. Airway patency requires continual assessment, optimal positioning with cervical spine stabilization, and suctioning as indicated. Volume replacement, initially with warmed crystalloids or colloids, should begin immediately with peripheral intravenous catheters. A generally accepted principle for volume replacement with crystalloids is to infuse 3 ml for every 1 ml of blood loss, a 3 : 1 ratio.

Blood products should be transfused as indicated to maintain adequate perfusion and oxygenation of vital organs. Fluid replacement with blood is obtained by infusing 1 ml blood for each milliliter of loss, a 1 : 1 ratio.

Ongoing assessment by the critical care nurse should continue as diagnostic procedures and stabilization occur. Throughout this process, preparation for immediate transport and surgical intervention must be considered. Insertion of a nasogastric or orogastric tube and urinary catheter, although not life-saving, should occur during stabilization of the patient.

One approach to abdominal trauma is conservative management with surgical intervention indicated only when injury includes perforation or rupture of abdominal contents, or when the attainment of hemodynamic stability is not possible. The conservative approach views surgical intervention as an immediate treatment modality only in life-threatening situations. This modality requires close monitoring through ongoing assessment. The critical care nurse should observe for subtle changes in level of consciousness, respiratory and circulatory status, and pain response to determine alterations indicating a need for immediate surgery.

Abdominal injury resulting from penetrating trauma requires special attention. Impaled or foreign objects should be stabilized as they are and should not be removed until the patient is in the surgical suite. Removal of such objects may result in massive bleeding once the tamponading agent has been removed.

Important concerns for the patient with abdominal trauma are hemodynamic stability, recognition and identification of occult injuries, risk of sepsis, nutritional support, and psychosocial support for the patient and significant others. A high index of suspicion must be maintained for intra-abdominal injuries and other injuries commonly associated with a particular mechanism of injury or pattern of trauma.

#### *Sepsis: Perforated Viscus with Peritonitis*

Sepsis is of major importance for any victim of trauma but particularly when injury results in perforation of a hollow organ. The perforation produces leakage of gastrointestinal contents into the peritoneum. This contamination of the abdominal cavity results in peritonitis and the potential for septic shock. To minimize complications, all open wounds or eviscerated viscera should be covered with sterile dressings moistened with normal saline. Prophylactic antibiotics should be administered as prescribed by the trauma surgeon during the stabilization of the patient. Tetanus immunization status should be determined because trauma results in open and contaminated wounds, which tend to be tetanus prone. (For a detailed discussion of septic shock, see Chap. 66.)

#### *Nutritional Support*

Adequate nutrition is necessary to promote wound healing and prevent loss of body mass. An assessment of the patient's nutritional requirements should be completed within the first 24 hours after admission to the critical care unit. Nutritional support is best attained through the use of a multidisciplinary approach, involving medical and surgical staffs, a nutritional support team, pharmacists, and, above all, appropriately trained critical care nursing staff. (For a detailed discussion of nutritional support of the critically ill patient, see Chap. 53.)

## Nursing Care of the Patient with Abdominal Trauma

Critical life-saving interventions are instituted immediately and include activities to support or reestablish vital physiologic functions. Immediate intervention must be geared toward ensuring a patent airway and providing for adequate alveolar ventilation and oxygenation. Airway patency requires ongoing assessment, optimal positioning with cervical spine stabilization, and suctioning as indicated.

Fluid resuscitation should begin immediately because the major concern in abdominal trauma is massive blood loss and subsequent hypovolemia. Initial circulating volume replacement should be provided through large-bore (14–16 gauge) peripheral intravenous catheters. Warmed crystalloids or colloids should be infused as indicated by patient status and estimation of blood loss. Blood products should be available for immediate use as indicated (see Tables 49–1 through 49–4). The pneumatic antishock garment (PASG) should be considered to provide circulatory support only as an adjunct when volume cannot be quickly infused.

As diagnostic procedures and stabilization evolve, the critical care nurse should continue ongoing assessment and prepare for immediate transport to surgery if indicated. Insertion of the nasogastric or orogastric tube and urinary catheter should be performed during stabilization of the patient.

Interventions related specifically to the patient with abdominal trauma may include stabilization of foreign or impaled objects. As mentioned earlier, such objects should never be removed prior to surgery because of the risk of massive bleeding that might occur once the tamponading object is removed. To minimize complications, all open wounds or eviscerated viscera should be covered with sterile dressings, moistened with normal saline as indicated.

Tetanus immunization status and the need for

antibiotics should be determined during the resuscitation and stabilization of the trauma victim. Antibiotics are indicated if intra-abdominal organs have been perforated and leakage of contents has occurred. The risk of peritonitis and sepsis is great in this event.

#### *Documentation*

Documentation of care, diagnostic procedures, therapeutic interventions, and patient responses is a responsibility of critical care and trauma resuscitation nurses. During the initial resuscitation, a nurse *scribe* is frequently used to ensure accurate documentation of specific responses of team members, time, and chronology of events. In the critical care unit, the use of an extensive nursing flowsheet is ideal for documenting appropriate and necessary information.

#### *Therapeutic Goals*

Effective treatment of abdominal trauma requires immediate attention to airway, breathing, circulatory status, and a high index of suspicion for severe injury. Therapeutic goals for the patient with abdominal trauma should include the following:

1. Establish a comprehensive database.
2. Establish and maintain a patent airway.
3. Provide necessary ventilatory support and oxygenation to relieve hypoxemia, hypercapnia, and consequent acidemia.
4. Provide hemodynamic support to ensure adequate cardiac output and tissue perfusion.
5. Maintain fluid, electrolyte, and acid–base balance (Chaps. 23 and 30).
6. Prevent impairment to skin integrity.
7. Provide nutritional support (Chap. 53).
8. Prevent infection.
9. Provide emotional and psychologic support to patient/family.
10. Provide pain relief.

#### *Nursing Diagnosis, Desired Patient Outcomes, and Nursing Interventions*

Implementation of the nursing process in the care of the patient with an abdominal injury revolves around the therapeutic goals listed above. Nursing diagnoses, desired patient outcomes, and nursing interventions and their rationales are outlined in Table 64–5.

## SELECTED ABDOMINAL TRAUMA

### Lacerated Liver

The liver is one of the most frequently injured abdominal organs. Liver injuries frequently occur as a result of blunt trauma to the abdomen from motor vehicle crashes. A bleeding liver laceration requires immediate control of blood loss. Packing around the liver often is used to initiate hemorrhage control.

Signs and symptoms specific to liver injury include right upper quadrant abdominal pain, abdominal wall musculature spasms, involuntary guarding, and signs of hypovolemic shock. Fracture of the lower right ribs and ecchymosis of the right upper quadrant are often associated with liver injury.

### Splenic Injury

Blunt abdominal trauma often results in injury to the spleen, with the spleen and liver being the most frequently injured abdominal organs. Conservative management of splenic injuries requires frequent CAT scan assessment and continual monitoring of patient status and vital signs.

Ecchymosis of the left upper quadrant and fractures of the lower left ribs are associated with splenic injuries. Pain radiating to the left shoulder, Kehr's sign, occurs when the intra-abdominal bleeding irritates the phrenic nerve. Additional signs and symptoms include point tenderness, involuntary guarding, and absent bowel sounds.

### Kidney Injury

Trauma to the kidney frequently is a result of blunt trauma. The kidney does not tolerate impact well, with multiple lacerations and fragmentation of the tissue. IVP may be used to assess kidney injuries. Kidney injury often requires removal of the injured organ.

Ecchymosis over the involved flank area, tenderness on palpation, and gross hematuria are signs and symptoms associated with kidney trauma. The kidney is located retroperitoneally, therefore, the peritoneal lavage is not used to diagnose kidney injuries.

### Rupture of the Hollow Viscus

The hollow organs frequently are injured in blunt trauma to the abdomen but may also be damaged by penetrating trauma. The hollow organs when full are more likely to be injured by blunt forces. Surgical intervention is often necessary to repair or resect the damaged tissue and to remove contaminants from the peritoneal cavity.

Signs and symptoms include rebound tenderness, abdominal rigidity, involuntary guarding, and possibly hematuria, depending on the actual injury.

TABLE 64–7
**Patterns of Associated Trauma for Extremity Injuries**

| Traumatic Injury | Associated Injury |
|---|---|
| Fractured humerus (distal 1/3) | Radial nerve palsy |
| Fractured humerus (supracondyle) | Compressed brachial artery; radial and/or median nerve injury |
| Anterior shoulder dislocation | Compressed axillary artery, nerve, vein |
| Wrist | Elbow or shoulder fracture |
| Calcaneal (heels) | L-1 or L-2 vertebral fractures |
| Anterior knee fracture | Hip fracture/dislocation |
| Knee dislocation | Compression of popliteal vessel |
| Hip | Dislocated opposite hip |
| Posterior hip dislocation | Sciatic nerve compression; aseptic necrosis of femoral head |
| Fractured tibia (epiphysis) | Popliteal artery laceration |
| (proximal 1/3 tibia) | Anterial tibial artery and/or nerve compression, compartment syndrome |
| Fractures of femur | Dislocated hip |
| (distal 1/3) | Femoral artery laceration |
| Supracondyle | Popliteal artery, nerve, vein injury |
| Ankle dislocation | Compression of pedal artery |

## ORTHOPEDIC (LONG BONE) TRAUMA

Extremity trauma is rarely life-threatening. There are, however, instances in which musculoskeletal trauma assumes priority in the multisystem trauma patient. Complete neurovascular compromise, joint dislocation, and amputation take precedence once the ABCs of emergency care have been performed. These injuries can lead to significant morbidity and mortality. In the case of an amputation, which results in severe hemorrhagic shock, the loss of limb and life from circulatory collapse make this type of orthopedic trauma an immediate consideration. Joint dislocations and neurovascular injury or compromise can lead to permanent disability.

### Anatomy and Physiology

The musculoskeletal system is made up of muscles, bones, joints, tendons, and ligaments. The primary function of this system is to provide structure and form to the human body. Bones, the most dense connective tissue in the body, give the skeletal system a framework and protect the underlying organs from injury. They are composed of three tissue layers, the periosteum (outermost layer), the bone itself, and the cancellous or spongy bone (innermost layer). Bones act as a storehouse of calcium. Blood vessels and nerves also make up the musculoskeletal system. The bone marrow, which forms the cancellous bone matrix, produces and stores red blood cells.

### Pathogenesis

Musculoskeletal injuries frequently result from blunt forces. Motor vehicle accidents, falls, and sports injuries account for the majority of extremity trauma. Child and adult abuse, known as nonaccidental trauma (NAT), can also involve a form of blunt trauma. Statistics confirm the fact that NAT continues to be a major contributor to extremity trauma. Orthopedic trauma can also be caused by penetrating injury. These mechanisms include stab wounds, gunshot wounds, missile and blast injuries.

Associated injuries often found in combination with long bone trauma are listed in Table 64–7. Understanding these patterns of trauma based on the mechanism of injury provides the nurse with valuable information that can be used to predict and anticipate orthopedic problems that may be present or may arise secondarily.

Certain types of extremity trauma, although single system, carry with them additional risks. The patient with a femur fracture, for example, may be in profound hypovolemic shock because the average femur fracture in an adult can result in a loss of up to 3 units of blood. Table 64–8 lists the approximate blood loss associated with each type of orthopedic trauma (see Table 49–1 for signs and symptoms associated with approximate blood losses).

TABLE 64–8
**Blood Loss Associated with Various Fractures**

| Fracture | Approximate Blood Loss |
|---|---|
| Fractured humerus | 1/2–1 unit |
| Fractured tibia | 1–2 units |
| Fractured femur | 2–3 units |
| Pelvic fractures | 1 unit/fracture |

TABLE 64-9
**Classic Fracture Patterns**

| A. Type of Fracture | Definition/Description |
|---|---|
| Open | Skin integrity over or near fracture site disrupted |
| Closed | Skin integrity over or near fracture site intact |
| Complete | Total interruption of bony continuity |
| Incomplete | Incomplete interruption of bony continuity |
| Comminuted | Splintering of bone into fragments |
| Greenstick | Bone buckles; bends, but still securely hinged on one side |
| Impacted | Bone broken and wedged into other break |
| Overriding | Bone edges slip past one another out of alignment |
| **B. Direction of Fracture** | **Fracture Line Description** |
| Longitudinal | Parallel to bone axis |
| Transverse | Crosses bone at right angle to axis |
| Oblique | Crosses bone at a slanted angle to axis |
| Spiral | Runs through bone in a spiral direction |

## Pathophysiology

In long bone trauma, the pathophysiology presents itself in the form of tissue deformity and ischemia. Fractures are categorized in a number of ways. One such classification is presented in Table 64-9.

Orthopedic trauma can result in many kinds of disruptions. Bone can crack, bend, or break, and the skin surfaces may be bruised, abrased, or lacerated. Ligaments, the tissue that attaches bone to bone, may be sprained or torn from their attachments. Tendons, those structures that attach muscle to bone, may be pulled, stretched, or even sheared from their points of insertion. Nervous tissue disruption predisposes to inflammation and peripheral neuropathy (e.g., paresthesias). Such disruptions cause muscle strain and bony discontinuity leading to diminished sensory and motor function. Extremity trauma can result in impaired mobility and severe pain.

In long bone trauma, the blood supply may be partially or completely disrupted by torn or sheared vessels, altering circulation to the affected extremity. The extremity may become edematous from hematoma formation and leakage of cellular contents into the surrounding tissues. The vascular status of the extremity therefore, is, disrupted, causing decreased blood flow, decreased tissue oxygenation, and, at times, cellular anoxia and death. The repair of these torn vessels, tendons, ligaments, skin, and nervous tissue occurs in a timely fashion in conjunction with bone realignment, and results, eventually, in restoration of function.

## Clinical Presentation

The overriding clinical presentation of a disrupted bone is the subjective complaint of pain. Even if a closed fracture has occurred and a deformity is not readily apparent, the chief complaint of pain alerts the nurse to the possibility of an extremity injury. The six "Ps" of fracture assessment are listed in Table 64-10. Other factors to be assessed include the presence of deformity, swelling, discoloration, and associated wounds.

## Diagnostic Considerations

Along with the history and physical examination, radiologic and laboratory assessment is undertaken. Radiologic studies should consist of anterior, posterior, and lateral views of the injured extremity. These views are necessary because a fracture, not obvious in one, may be seen in another view. It is important to x-ray above and below all injured areas because other fractures may be missed. Oblique films may also be ordered. Magnetic resonance imaging (MRI) has been an especially significant adjunct in the diagnosis of musculoskeletal injury. Information regarding soft tissue injury, as for example, tendon and ligament tears, can be obtained by this method.

Stress x-rays may also be done to view bones and joints in various positions. In some fractures, especially those in the pediatric patient, it may be necessary to obtain comparison views to diagnose the fracture. Postreduction films are always performed.

Arteriography is performed when there is suspicion of an injured vessel. Doppler studies have also been done to detect flow rates.

Laboratory studies are those performed on any trauma patient with a single system injury. They include, but are not limited to, complete blood

TABLE 64-10
**Assessment of Limb Fractures: Six "P's"**

| |
|---|
| Pain |
| Point tenderness |
| Pulses—distal to the fracture site |
| Pallor (skin color) |
| Paresthesias (numbness or tingling) |
| Paralysis |

count, type and cross match, blood chemistries, coagulation studies, and urinalysis. Blood alcohol level may also be obtained as indicated.

## Nursing Care of the Patient with Long Bone Trauma

### Initial Management

As with the care of all trauma patients, the ABCs of care take precedence in the patient with a long bone injury. The overall goal for the patient with long bone trauma is to relieve pain and to restore limb function to pre-injury status, or to an optimal level of functioning. This also requires the restoration of tissue perfusion and maintenance of skin integrity during the course of therapy.

Pain is generally relieved by alignment of the fracture. Relief from pain is provided by intramuscular or intravenous injection of a narcotic analgesic. Later, oral medication can be administered for pain control. Diminished pain response is validated by patient comfort and verbalization that relief has been achieved.

Once the ABCs are assessed and stabilized, and the affected extremity has been properly aligned and immobilized, a second survey or head-to-toe examination is performed to determine the presence of any additional injury not readily apparent. This assessment should include a meticulous neurologic examination, particularly of sensory and motor function of the extremities, and a careful check of peripheral pulses, color, and temperature in all extremities. Monitoring of vital signs may be helpful in determining the presence of any internal injuries and bleeding.

Fracture care includes the use of soft and rigid splints, plaster or fiberglass casts, skin and skeletal traction, internal and external fixators. Closed and open reduction methods by operative intervention, when indicated, are important adjuncts to promote proper healing of the injured extremity and to restore motor and sensory function to the affected limb.

Minor fractures can be easily treated with immobilization, limb elevation, and ice to reduce swelling. Moist heat may be applied, once edema has subsided, to increase circulation and promote healing.

### Critical Care Phase

The control of external hemorrhage is an important consideration in the care of the patient with a long bone injury. Elevation of the limb may be initially employed to control bleeding. *Manual pressure* is, however, the best method to control bleeding. Direct pressure over the palpated pulse or at the site of injury can prevent exsanguination from extensive blood loss.

The PASG has also been used to control arterial bleeding (see section on chest trauma, above, and Chap. 46). Use of this modality has become controversial because patients have been known to continue to bleed under the suit. The PASG has been used to splint femur fractures in addition to controlling arterial bleeding. Use of tourniquets is reserved as a last resort measure because their use results in amputation. Although their use may not be *limb*-saving, they are a *life*-saving alternative.

Adequate fluid replacement during all phases of care, provided hypovolemia exists, is an essential treatment considered in the care of the patient with long bone trauma. Immediate measures to correct fluid and blood loss must be initiated to prevent hypoperfusion to the affected extremity. Fluid resuscitation is initiated with insertion of large-bore (14–16 gauge) angiocaths. Ringer's lactate and normal saline are the crystalloids of choice. Colloids and blood are used when blood loss exceeds 20% of the patient's total blood volume. The fluid/blood product should be warmed to prevent hypothermia.

A compromised patient status is inevitable if volume restoration is not a part of the total regimen for the trauma patient (see section entitled "Complications," below). Many polytrauma patients, who typically include those with long bone fracture, continue to be underresuscitated. Therefore, in the treatment of the patient with an orthopedic injury, the use of crystalloids at a replacement ratio of 3 : 1 and blood replacement at a 1 : 1 ratio are important considerations in the treatment of the patient with associated bleeding from an orthopedic injury.

Critical interventions may be necessary in orthopedic patients with a joint dislocation or neurovascular compromise. Early supportive measures to prevent permanent disability include immediate manual maneuvers to realign dislocated joints or operative intervention for neurovascular compromise to restore limb function.

Normal function is evident when mobility without pain returns. Tissue integrity is apparent when the skin temperature is warm and dry, and when the color of the extremity is its usual pink. Normal sensation, palpable pulses, and normal capillary refill (less than 2 seconds when the nailbed or fingertip is blanched) are other ways to assess for optimal function and normal tissue perfusion.

### Complications

General nursing management of the patient with orthopedic trauma requires that the nurse have an understanding of the pathophysiology of the injury and the rationales on which treatment is based. Nursing care is directed toward performing a thorough assessment, implementing appropriate nursing interventions, and documenting these activities. The overall goal is to prevent further injury or permanent disability, and to maintain the injured limb in a manner that will afford optimal function post-healing and rehabilitation.

Management of the patient with extremity trauma includes ongoing monitoring of the patient's vital signs and hemodynamic status, laboratory data, and diagnostic studies performed and their results. This information gives the nurse a complete picture of the patient's overall clinical status. Attention to the affected limb and use of the six "Ps" in assessment (see Table 64–10) will provide the critical care nurse with a complete database to evaluate comprehensively the patient and his/her response to therapy.

As is the case with chest and abdominal trauma (discussed above), the nurse must be ever vigilant for complications. Complications seen in the care of the patient with long bone trauma include wound infections, compartment syndrome, fat emboli, and osteomyelitis.

**Wound Infections.** Wound infections are usually the result of a break in the skin noted at the time of injury. Wounds include lacerations, abrasions, avulsions, puncture wounds, and even wounds from foreign objects or missiles.

Vigilance by the critical care nurse who continually observes for signs of inflammation (heat, pain, redness, swelling, compromised function) is crucial in the care of the patient with a long bone injury. Frequent assessment with adequate lighting, proper cleansing of the affected area with removal of debri, application of dry, sterile dressings as per Unit protocol, and administration/monitoring of prescribed antibiotic, both topically and systemically, will hasten wound healing.

**Compartment Syndrome.** Compartment syndrome, a state of excessive pressure within a muscle compartment due to edema formation and bleeding, is seen in conjunction with arterial vascular injuries or when there is massive swelling of the closed-space tissue compartment associated with impairment of distal blood flow. If the antimicrobial therapy is ineffective, or the swelling cannot be minimized by a surgical technique known as a fasciotomy (see Chap. 65), then the affected limb must be amputated. Usual sites for compartment syndrome phenomenon are the forearm, lower leg, and thigh.

The role of the nurse in the care of the patient with compartment syndrome is *early* detection of this complication. The patient who continually complains of pain unrelieved by the use of narcotic analgesics is a classic example of a patient who may be developing compartment syndrome. Other signs and symptoms include loss of motor function, hyperesthesia, diminished pulses in the affected extremity, and palpable compartment tension.

Compartment pressures can be measured by the use of a slit or wick catheter device. Readings can easily be obtained by inserting an 18-gauge needle, connected to a water manometer, into the suspected compartment. Normal pressure readings range from 9–15 mmHg. Compartment pressure readings of greater than 30 mmHg are diagnostic of compartment syndrome.

**Fat Emboli.** The etiology of fat embolization syndrome (FES) is still unknown. There are two widely accepted theories based on the pathophysiology of FES. The *extra*vascular theory states that FES occurs from disruption of fat-containing tissues, resulting in the flow of fat globules into the microcirculation. The *intra*vascular theory states that, fat, in some way, is altered in the bloodstream, forming large droplets and occluding small vessels. The result is the same and predisposes to ARDS and pulmonary embolism (see Chaps. 34 and 35, respectively).

Most orthopedic patients will develop symptoms within 2 days post-injury. Clinical manifestations include severe dyspnea, tachycardia, restlessness, agitation, petechiae on the chest and in skinfolds, and even seizures and coma in severe cases. Laboratory diagnosis of FES includes lipuria, elevated serum lipase, thrombocytopenia (platelet count <150,000), and a decreased $PaO_2$. Chest x-ray findings are consistent with ARDS; ECG findings may reflect ischemia (ST segment and T wave changes).

Treatment is supportive. The critical care nurse must be cognizant of the fact that frequent manipulation of the involved extremity may increase the incidence of FES. Immediate immobilization, prompt stabilization of the fracture, adequate blood and fluid replacement, and prevention of hypotension are critical measures to be employed in the care of the patient with long bone trauma.

Mortality from fat emboli is greater in patients with long bone fractures involving the tibia and femur. These rates can be reduced by implementing the aforementioned nursing measures.

**Osteomyelitis.** Another significant complication of long bone trauma is osteomyelitis. Osteomyelitis, an inflammation of the bone, is usually the result of a secondary infection. It is most common in patients who have undergone surgery for the repair of long bone fracture. Nursing considerations include prevention of infection and the administration of prescribed antibiotic therapy.

### Therapeutic Goals

Nursing management considerations in caring for the patient with long bone trauma are focused on the following therapeutic goals:

1. Establish a thorough comprehensive database.
2. Establish and maintain a patent airway with adequate alveolar ventilation.
3. Provide necessary circulatory support to ensure adequate tissue perfusion.
4. Maintain fluid, electrolyte, and acid–base balance (Chaps. 23 and 30).

5. Maintain skin integrity.
6. Provide nutritional support (Chap. 53).
7. Prevent complications of immobility including thromboembolic and pulmonary embolic phenomena (Chaps. 35 and 63).
8. Provide emotional and psychologic support to patient and family (Chaps. 3 and 5).
9. Monitor patient's expectation of therapy and concerns associated with body image and self esteem.

### *Nursing Diagnoses, Desired Patient Outcomes, and Nursing Interventions*

Implementation of the nursing process in the care of the patient with an extremity fracture centers around the above mentioned therapeutic goals. Specific diagnoses, desired patient outcomes, nursing interventions and their rationales are presented in Table 64–5.

## REFERENCES

1. Barriot, P, Riou, B, and Viars, P: Prehospital autotransfusion in life-threatening hemothorax. Chest 93:522, 1988.
2. Dunham, C, et al: Rapid infusion system: The MIEMSS experience. In Proceedings of the 10th National Trauma Symposium, Baltimore, MD, November 1987.
3. Satiani, B, Fried, S, Zeeb, P: Normothermic rapid volume replacement in traumatic hypovolemia. Arch Surg 122:1044, 1987.
4. Mann, J and Oakes, A: Critical Care Nursing of the Multi-Injured Patient, American Association of Critical Care Nurses. WB Saunders, Philadelphia, 1980, p 61.

CHAPTER 65

# Nursing Management of the Patient with Burns

*Patricia M. Orr*

## CHAPTER OUTLINE



## LEARNING OBJECTIVES

**At the end of this chapter, you should be able to:**

1. Discuss pathophysiology underlying burn (thermal) injury and its impact on total body function.
2. Identify key assessment factors in establishing the severity of burn injury.
3. Examine the major complications of burn injury and implications for nursing care.
4. Delineate therapeutic goals in the management of burn injury during the emergency and acute phases.
5. Describe the major considerations underlying effective wound management and the implications for nursing care.
6. Describe therapeutic modalities used to enhance wound healing.
7. Discuss the nursing process in caring for the patient with burn injury including
   Assessment.
   Nursing diagnoses.
   Planning: Desired patient outcomes
   Nursing interventions/rationales.

## BURN (THERMAL) INJURY

### Description

An energy transfer from a heat or cold source to the body will result in burn injury. The causes of this energy transfer are listed in Table 65-1. The amount of heat transfer can be decreased by the thickness of the skin; the surface pigmentation; the presence of hair, dirt, natural skin oils; surface cellular water content; and the peripheral circulation in the area of contact. The temperature of the burning agent and the duration of exposure to this agent can increase the severity of the injury.

### Pathophysiology

#### *Local Skin Response*

Heat transfer denatures cellular protein, inactivates or blocks thermolabile enzymes, and interrupts vascular supply. Three zones of injury have been identified (Fig. 65-1).

TABLE 65-1
**Causes of Injury**

| **Thermal Injuries** | | |
|---|---|---|
| ***Dry Heat*** | | |
| Flame | → | most common injury |
| Flash | → | sudden ignition or explosion of short duration |
| ***Contact*** | | |
| Tar | → | splatter type injuries. Temperature >400°F |
| Metals | → | industrial injuries. Temperature usually >200°F |
| Grease | → | household injury. Temperature >200°F. |
| ***Moist Heat*** | | |
| Steam | → | under pressure, trauma is greater |
| Scald | → | third degree burns occur in 1 second if the temperature is 156°F |
| ***Chemicals*** | → | 25,000 products marketed are used in industry, agriculture, and in the home, and are capable of producing burns |
| ***Electrical*** | → | low-voltage direct current creates less damage than low-voltage alternating current. High-voltage direct current creates more hazard than high-voltage alternating current. |
| Lightning | → | uncommon injury with extremely variable trauma |

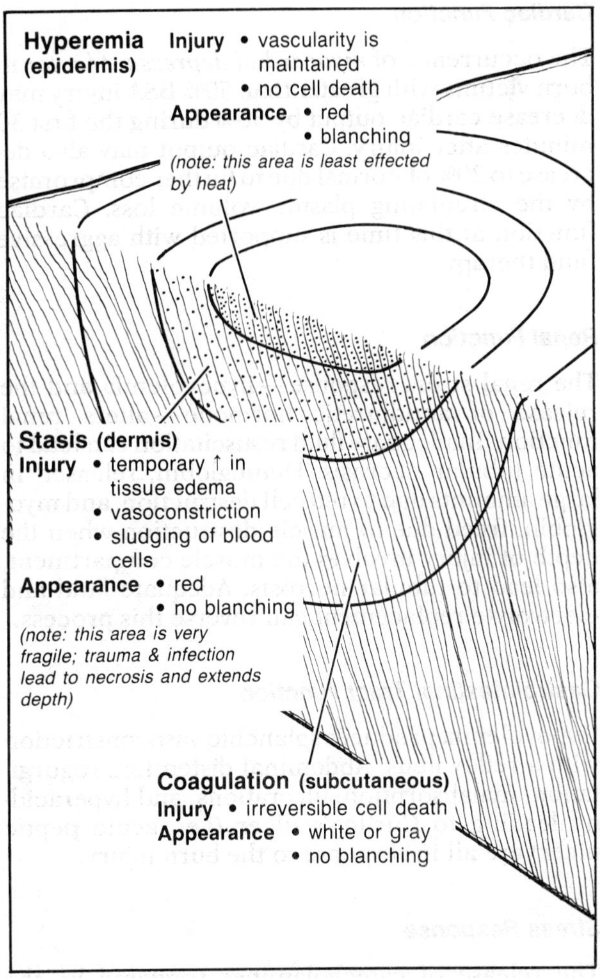


**Figure 65-1.** *Hyperemia* (Epidermis): this area is least effected by heat. Vacularity is maintained with no cellular death. Skin is red and blanches. *Stasis*(Dermis): damage to this layer is due to temporary lack of good blood supply. Vasoconstriction occurs leading to sludging of the blood cells and an increase in tissue edema. Appearance is red with no blanching. This area is very fragile as trauma and infection lead to necrosis and extends depth. *Coagulation* (Subcutaneous): innermost area. Cellular death is an irreversible process. Appearance is white or gray, with no blanching. Size will increase with heat intensity and exposure time.

### *Systemic Response*

Altered functional capacity of the skin affects all body systems either directly or indirectly due to the interdependence of all body systems.

**Hemodynamics.** After a burn injury occurs, increased capillary permeability leads to the extravasation of water, electrolytes, albumin, and protein into the interstitial and intracellular compartments leading to the formation of edema. Beginning immediately after the burn occurs, this process can lead to a 60% loss of intravascular volume because the capillary response extends to unburned tissues if the burn injury is greater than 30% body surface area (BSA). An increase in the body's metabolic rate will lead to further water loss through the respiratory system. Insensible water loss through burn wounds can range between 90 and 350 ml/hour. Impaired circulation and decreased peripheral perfusion lead to metabolic acidosis.

*Burn shock* (hypovolemic) causes a decrease in blood pressure, blood flow, and polycythemia due to hemoconcentration. Blood viscosity leads to sludging in the vasculature. This vascular volume depletion can continue up to 36 hours after injury, although capillary integrity is generally restored after 24 hours.

### *Cellular Response*

Similar to an inflammatory response (see Table 61-3), neutrophils converge in the area of injury and phagocytosis of bacteria occurs. An increase of monocytes, which convert to macrophages in tissues, continues to act on residual wound debris. Interference with cellular enzyme processes leads to red blood cell destruction in the area of injury and partial destruction of those red cells on the periphery of the wound. Disseminated intravascular coagulopathy (DIC) may occur due to a decrease in platelet and fibrinogen levels; these levels return to normal within 24 to 36 hours. (DIC is discussed in detail in Chap. 63.)

### Cardiac Function

The occurrence of *myocardial depressant factor* in burn victims with greater than 50% BSA injury may decrease cardiac output by 30% during the first 30 minutes after injury. Cardiac output may also decrease to 20% of normal due to further compromise by the circulating plasma volume loss. Cardiac function at this time is supported with aggressive fluid therapy.

### Renal Function

The renal stress response—hypovolemia and the release of antidiuretic hormone—alters renal function. Inadequate fluid resuscitation can lead to acute tubular necrosis. Hemoglobin, released in large amounts due to red cell destruction, and myoglobin, freed due to muscle destruction when the depth of injury involves the muscle compartment, also lead to tubular necrosis. Adequate fluid and electrolyte replacement can reverse this process.

### Gastrointestinal Tract Function

Hypovolemia produces splanchnic vasoconstriction with a reflex ileus. Abdominal distention, regurgitation, malabsorption, ulcerations, and hyperacidity leading to Curling's ulcer (i.e., acute peptic ulcer) are all in response to the burn injury.

### Stress Response

The release of catecholamines triggered by the stress response increases the release of norepinephrine out of proportion to other traumas. A blood sugar increase is secondary to adrenal hormone release with a decrease in insulin effectiveness. Acceleration of the metabolic rate is directly proportional to the size and depth of the burn injury, evaporative water loss through burned tissue, and increased protein losses. Hypoglycemia, unique in the pediatric age group, is due to inadequate glycogen stores in the liver.

### Immune Response

Severe burns cause an immediate depression of the immunoglobins, IgA, IgG, and IgM. With host defenses depressed, bacterial invasion at the site of injury can quickly lead to a septic episode. (The immune response is discussed in detail in Chap. 54.)

## Assessment: Severity of Injury

The following factors influence the severity of burn injury:

1. Depth of injury.
2. Size of the burn.
3. Age of the patient.
4. Past medical history.
5. Location of burn injury.
6. Associated trauma.

### Depth of Injury

Factors that influence which layers of tissue are involved are the temperature of the burning agent and the duration of contact.

Depth of injury is classified as *partial-thickness* injury, which affects the epidermal layer and from one half to seven eighths of the dermal layer of skin; and *full-thickness* injury, which can involve all epidermis and dermis, subcutaneous tissue, muscle, and bone (Table 65-2).

Partial-thickness injuries can easily convert to

TABLE 65-2
**Classification of Burn Depth**

| Classification | Formerly | Areas Involved | Appearance | Sensitivity | Healing Time |
|---|---|---|---|---|---|
| Partial thickness Superficial | 1°-2° | Epidermis<br>Papillae of dermis | Bright red to pink. Blanches to touch. Serum-filled blisters. Glistening, moist. | Sensitive to air, temperature, and touch. | 7-10 days |
| Partial thickness Deep | 2° | Epidermis, ½-⅞ of dermis.<br>Appendage usually present. | Blisters may be present. Pink to light red to white. Soft and pliable. Blanching present. | Pressure may be painful from exposed nerve endings. | 14-21 days. May need grafting to decrease scarring. |
| Full thickness | 3°-4° | Epidermis<br>Dermis<br>Tissue<br>Muscle<br>Bone | Snowy white, gray, or brown. Texture is firm and leathery. Inelastic. | No pain as nerve endings are destroyed. | Needs grafting to complete healing. |

full-thickness injuries when ice is used initially to cool the wound, which leads to vasoconstriction in the zone of stasis. The drying effects of air and infection of the wound can also convert a partial-thickness wound to full-thickness injury.

### Size of the Burn

The size of the wound must be determined correctly in order to determine accurately fluid requirements during resuscitation. There are 3 methods to determine the extent of the injury. The *Palmer* method is a quick assessment that uses the palm of the hand to represent 1% of the BSA. This method is inaccurate and is used to assess smaller wounds. The *rule of nines* method, most commonly used in emergency departments, is the simplest calculation method. The total body is divided into nine sections or multiples of nine as indicated in Fig. 65–2. This method is quick and convenient but is not accurate, especially in children, due to the head size.

The *Lund and Browder* method is the most accurate way to assess the size of a burn wound because it allows for age-related size differences. However, this is a very time-consuming method (Fig. 65–3).

### Age of the Patient

Children less than 2 years of age and adults older than 65 years of age are the populations at risk for burn injury. Poor antibody response in the very young results in early infection leading to septicemia. Preexisting illness and the inability of the aged body to handle stress leads to increased mortality in elderly persons.

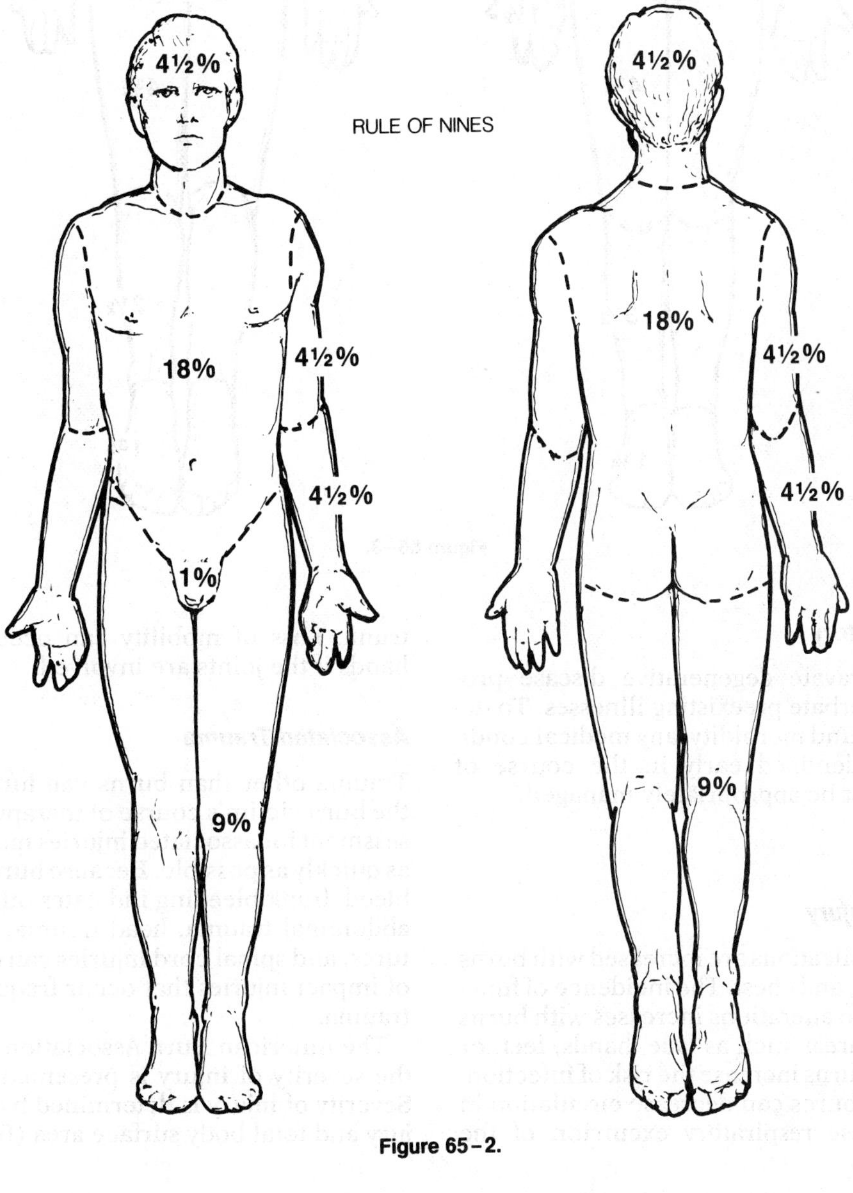


**Figure 65–2.**

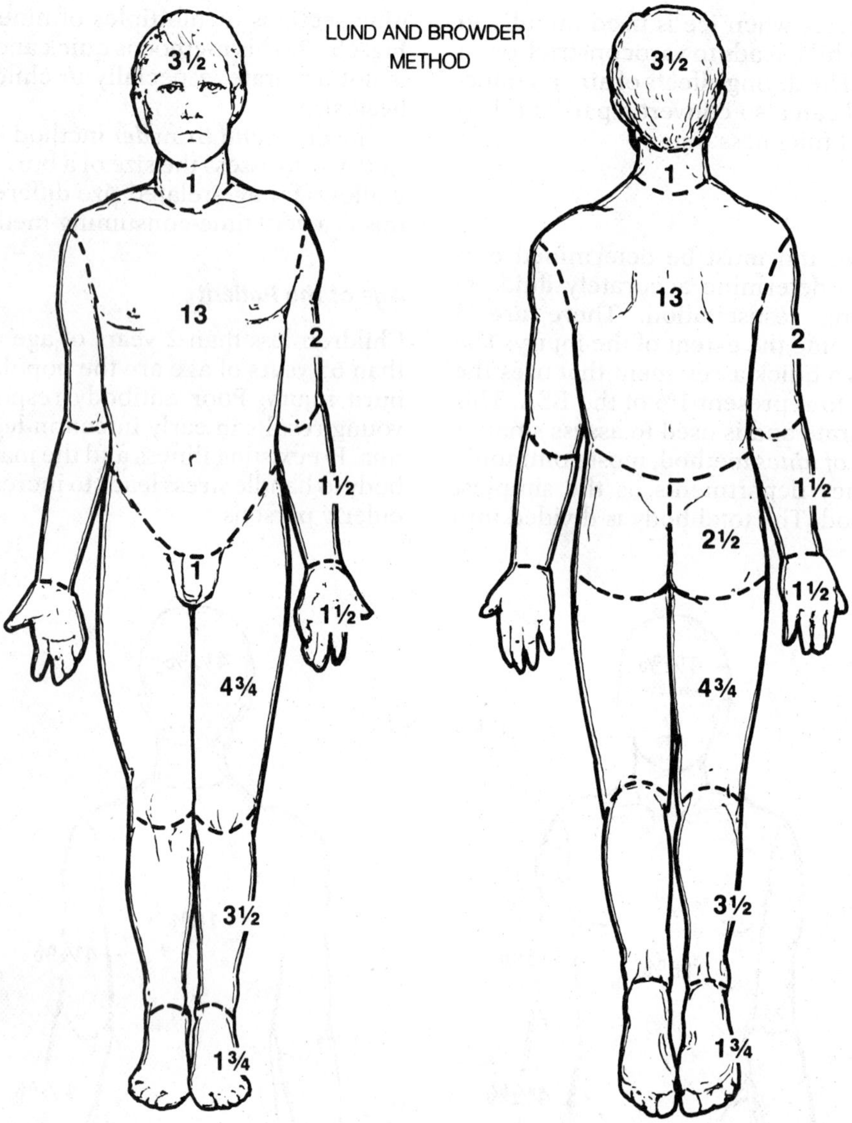


**Figure 65-3.**

#### Past Medical History

Burns can aggravate degenerative disease processes and exacerbate preexisting illnesses. To decrease mortality and morbidity, any medical condition must be identified early in the course of therapy and must be appropriately managed.

#### Location of the Injury

Pulmonary complications are increased with burns of the head, neck, and chest. The incidence of functional or cosmetic alterations increases with burns in critical body areas such as face, hands, feet, or joints. Perineal burns increase the risk of infection. Circumferential burns can decrease circulation in limbs or decrease respiratory excursion of the trunk. Loss of mobility can occur, especially in hands if the joints are involved.

#### Associated Trauma

Trauma other than burns can further complicate the burn victim's course of therapy. A thorough assessment for associated injuries must be completed as quickly as possible. Because burn wounds do not bleed, frank bleeding indicates other injury. Intra-abdominal trauma, head trauma, long bone fractures, and spinal cord injuries can occur as a result of impact injuries that occur frequently with burn trauma.

The American Burn Association classification of the severity of injury is presented in Table 65-3. Severity of injury is determined by the depth of injury and total body surface area (BSA) involved.

TABLE 65-3
**American Burn Association Classification Severity of Injury**

**Minor Injury**
1. Second-degree injury less than 15% BSA in adults, less than 10% in children.
2. Third-degree injury of less than 2% BSA, not involving eyes, ears, face, and genitalia, in both adults and children.

**Moderate Injury**
1. Second-degree injury of 15-25% BSA in adults, 10-20% in children.
2. Third-degree injury of 2-10% BSA, in both adults and children.

**Major Injury**
1. Second-degree injury of 25% BSA in adults, 20% in children.
2. Third degree of at least 10% BSA in both adults and children.
3. If hands, face, eyes, ears, feet, perineum are involved.
4. Inhalation injury is present.
5. All electrical injuries.
6. Poor risk patients due to other preexisting conditions.
8. Child abuse is suspected.

## Complications of Burn Injury

### *Pulmonary Injury*

The most immediate threat to life associated with burns is *inhalation* injury. Carbon monoxide poisoning and smoke inhalation are the greatest killers at the scene of the fire and are the leading cause of death in admitted patients. Of the 50,000 fire victims admitted to hospitals per year, smoke or thermal damage to the respiratory tract may occur in approximately 30%. Smoke inhalation influences survivability of fire victims by doubling the mortality for a burn of any size. The four types of pulmonary injury are presented in Table 65-4.

### *Sepsis*

The burn wound is an excellent culture medium for bacterial growth. The incidence of serious infection in burn patients increases with the size of the burn wound. The burn wound flora must be monitored carefully for signs of colonization and infection. Bacterial growth greater than $10^5$ colonies/gram of tissue can predict a septic episode. The use of topical agents on the burn wound can control the number of bacteria sufficiently to prevent invasive infection. Types of infection are presented in Table 65-5.

When sepsis is suspected, prompt identification of the offending organisms is essential, and antibiotic therapy should be instituted. Wound care must be meticulous and constant with evaluation of topical antimicrobials for their effectiveness against the offending organisms.

### *Neurovascular Compromise*

Full-thickness burns form an inelastic thick tight eschar over the wounds. With edema formation due to the capillary leak, this eschar forms tight constricting bands on injured limbs creating pressure on underlying structures and decreasing blood flow to areas distal to the burned area.

Signs and symptoms of diminished blood flow begin 1 hour post burn injury. Assess pulses hourly using an ultrasonic Doppler. Elevate the affected limb. In the absence of pulses and with positive symptoms of decreased perfusion, an escharotomy must be performed to release the constriction and increase blood flow to compromised limbs.

## Management of the Patient with Burns: Implications for Nursing Care

### *Emergency Management*

Critical management of the wound is essential at the time of injury. The burning process must be halted and the wound must be cooled to decrease depth and extent of the injury. This is followed by the ABCs (airway, breathing, circulation) of trauma resuscitation (see Chap. 64). Every attempt must be made to stabilize the patient, control any hemorrhage, fractures or suspected injuries. Inhalation injury is suspected if the fire occurred in a closed space, if the face and neck are burned, if the nares or buccal mucosa are singed, if vocal changes are present, and if the patient is coughing carbonaceous particles. Treatment for hypovolemic shock is begun using the formulas in Table 65-6. The burn wound should not be treated at this time. The wound should be covered with clean blankets in an attempt to decrease the amount of contamination of the wound. Body temperature should be maintained.

As soon as possible, an accurate history should be obtained of how the injury occurred, what the burning agent was, and what occurred at the scene. This accurate account can aid in determining the severity of injury and any associated trauma. An accurate medical history at this time must also include allergies, current medications, past and present illness, and substance abuse. Crisis intervention and emotional support for the patient/family unit begins as the victim arrives in the emergency care facility. Burn care treatment modalities are explained, and the need for admission to a burn care facility is discussed.

### *Acute Phase*

The acute phase of burn care begins with stabilization of the burn victim after injury, usually 48-72 hours, and continues until wound healing is com-

TABLE 65-4
## Types of Pulmonary Injury

**CARBON MONOXIDE POISONING**

Carbon monoxide (CO) is a colorless, odorless, tasteless, non-irritating gas given off by nearly everything that burns.

The biologic effects are due to tissue hypoxia as the carbon monoxide molecule replaces the oxygen molecule on the hemoglobin sites.

The victim is usually trapped in an enclosed or poorly ventilated smoke-filled area.

***Signs and Symptoms***

Toxicity depends on the concentration of CO in the inspired air, the length of exposure, and the individual victim's response.
Carboxyhemoglobin (CO + Hgb) produces the following symptoms:

| | |
|---|---|
| <10% | Does not cause symptoms. |
| 10–20% | Complaints of headaches, nausea, vomiting, loss of manual dexterity. |
| 21–40% | Confusion, lethargy, may show depressed ST segment on ECG. This level can be lethal because the victim loses both the interest and the ability to flee the smoke. |
| 41–60% | Ataxia, convulsions, coma with respiratory failure. |
| >60% | Usually fatal. |

***Treatment***

Restoration of adequate oxygenation is the primary goal. Since there is 50% reduction in the CO Hgb level in the first 20 minutes in the presence of 100% oxygen, this therapy must be initiated as quickly as possible with an established airway.

**SMOKE OR CHEMICAL INHALATION INJURY**

Injury to lung mucosa from the inhalation of smoke is primarily a chemical injury.

The chemical composition of smoke depends on the type of materials being burned, listed as follows:

Cyanide→nylon carpets, polyurethane carpets, chair cushions.

Hydrochloric acid→burning or smoldering vinyl. When inhaled, this very strong acid corrodes lung and throat tissue.

Aldehydes→acrylics such as curtains and drapes.

Two hundred-eighty separate toxic products have been found in wood smoke.

Fire history is very important. Suspect this injury if the victim was in a closed space, if it was a smoky fire, or there is the smell of smoke on the victim's clothes. Question the rescuers or the victim on the type of items burning, the length of time the victim was exposed to smoke, and the condition of the victim on rescue.

***Signs and Symptoms***

*Initial response:*
1. Immediate loss of bronchial cilia. (See Chap. 28 for discussion of anatomy and physiology of respiratory tract and lungs.)
2. Decrease in alveolar surfactant.
3. Atelectasis.
4. Mucosal edema in small airways.
5. Wheezing and air hunger.

*12–24 hours' response:*
1. Tracheal and bronchial epithelium begins to slough and hemorrhagic tracheobronchitis develops.
2. Patients may expectorate mucosa and bronchial casts.

*24–48 hours' response:*
1. Interstitial edema becomes prominent, resulting in a typical ARDS pattern.
2. Pulmonary macrophages are destroyed, leading to bacterial pneumonia.

Suspect this injury if the following are present.
1. Facial burns.
2. Intraoral burns.
3. Singed nasal hair.
4. Soot in the oropharynx.
5. Carbonaceous sputum.
6. Hoarseness and wheezing.
7. Hypoxemia with an elevated $CO_2$ level and CO present on blood gas analysis.
8. Positive bronchoscopy that shows mucosal erythema, hemorrhage, ulceration, edema, and carbonaceous particles in the lower airways.

***Treatment***

In the presence of increasing laryngeal edema, establishment of a patent airway is indicated; usually endotracheal intubation is required.

Mechanical ventilation or humidified $O_2$.

Vigorous pulmonary toilet.

Bronchodilators as needed.

Sputum cultures.

Management of IV fluids to decrease the incidence of pulmonary edema; and to maintain hemodynamic stability without compromising pulmonary function.

Treatments completed aseptically to prevent pneumonia, a lethal complication of burns.

**UPPER AIRWAY INJURY**

Direct exposure to superheated air at temperatures >150°F can cause burns of the face, nose, oropharynx, and larynx above the trachea.

Reflex closure of the glottis prevents further injury to the lower airway.

Superheated steam is capable of burning the respiratory tract to the bronchioles as it has a greater heat-carrying capacity (4000 times greater than air).

TABLE 65-4
**Types of Pulmonary Injury** (*Continued*)

***Signs and Symptoms***

Heat injury to the mucosa results in erythema, ulcerations, and edema. When associated with face and neck burns, airway obstruction increases due to increased edema.

Suspect this injury if physical examination shows:

1. Burns of the face and neck.
2. Carbon deposits in mouth and throat.
3. Inflammation of nasal and buccal mucosa with posterior pharyngeal swelling.
4. Tachypnea, respiratory distress, hoarseness, cough, anxiety, stridor, disorientation, and combative behavior.

***Treatment***

Early endotracheal intubation is indicated. Airway edema forms in the first hour post-injury leading to difficulty in intubation as signs of tracheal edema worsen.

**RESTRICTIVE DEFECT**

This defect is caused by third-degree or circumferential burns of the chest and/or neck.

The inelastic quality of the eschar and splinting effect of the edema in the burn area prohibit lung expansion.

***Signs and Symptoms***

Abdominal respirations.

Severely restricted respiratory excursion.

Inability to ventilate with an endotracheal tube in place.

***Treatment***

Escharotomies may have to be performed in order to allow for proper respiratory excursion and adequate ventilation.

plete. A multidisciplinary approach to care begins, and complex care is provided. Major energies of the burn team are directed at managing the burn wound. Therapeutic goals include (1) providing pain relief; (2) providing adequate nutritional support; (3) maintaining fluid, electrolyte, and acid-base balance; (4) ongoing monitoring for complications; (5) providing emotional support to the patient and family; and (6) planning for rehabilitation and discharges.

### Wound Management

Regardless of the etiology or extent of burn wound injury, the principles of wound care remain the same. Immediate stopping of the burning process is the first priority in emergency care. Specific wound care is never initiated prior to stabilization of the burn injured patient. Upon stabilization of the patient's condition, wound care begins. The 4 goals of wound care are (1) contain bacterial growth; (2) provide comfort; (3) facilitate the healing process; and (4) promote restoration and function.

#### Stages of Repair

***Inflammatory Phase.*** Inflammation begins immediately and lasts approximately 72 hours after injury. The immediate response is vasoconstriction with fibrin clot formation. Damaged cells release histamine, serotonin, and intracellular enzymes, which disrupt endothelial membranes and increase capillary permeability. This results in a leakage of

TABLE 65-5
**Types of Infection**

| | Noninvasive | Invasive Without Bacteremia | Invasive With Bacteremia |
|---|---|---|---|
| | Stays on the surface of the wound, can grow and divide. | Granulation area of burn wound that was healing deteriorates as organisms invade viable tissue. | Both colonizing and invading bacteria may enter the lymphatic system and systemic circulation. |
| **Signs and Symptoms** | Bacterial count is $10^3-10^5$. Low-grade but spiking fever. Mild leukocytosis. Patient is awake and alert. | Invaded tissue is edematous, pale and progresses to dry, crusty, and necrotic. Persistent temperature elevation. Bacterial count is $10^6-10^8$. Leukocytosis. Patient becomes less responsive, may progress to coma. | Same as invasive without bacteremia. Bacterial count is $10^9-10^{12}$. If caused by Gram-negative organisms, the temp may fall and WBCs may be depressed. Septicemia is followed by septic shock and death. |

TABLE 65-6
**Fluid Resuscitation Formulas**

| | Crystalloids | Colloid | 5% D/W | Urine Output |
|---|---|---|---|---|
| **First 24 Hours** | | | | |
| Evans | Lactated Ringer's 1 ml/kg wt/% burn | 1 ml/kg wt/% burn | 2000 ml | 30-50 ml/hr (adult) |
| Brooke | Lactated Ringer's 1.5 ml/kg wt/% burn | 0.5 ml/kg wt/% burn | 2000 ml | 30-50 ml/hr (adult) |
| Parkland | Lactated Ringer's 4 ml/kg wt/% burn | None | None | 50-70 ml/hr (adult) |
| | Rate of infusion for all formulas listed is: ½ of the total in the first 8 hours; ¼ of the total in the second 8 hours; ¼ of the total in the third 8 hours | | | |
| **Second 24 Hours** | | | | |
| Evans | Lactated Ringer's 0.5 ml/kg wt/% burn | 0.5 ml/kg wt/% burn | 1500-2000 ml | 30-50 ml/hr (adult) |
| Brooke | Lactated Ringer's 0.75 ml/kg wt/% burn | 0.25 ml/kg wt/% burn | 1500-2000 ml | 30-50 ml/hr (adult) |
| Parkland | None | 700 to 2000 ml (adult) | Sufficient to maintain urine output | 30-50 ml/hr (adult) |

fluid and hydrophilic protein molecules into the interstitial space leading to edema formation and intravascular volume depletion. Polymorphonuclear leukocytes (PMNs) move into the interstitial space. Monocytes convert to macrophages. PMNs and macrophages begin the repair process by attacking the foreign material, digesting this debris, and transporting it from the wound site.

***Destructive Phase.*** The *destructive* phase lasts from day 1 to day 6. The PMNs and macrophages clear the wound of debris. Macrophages attract more macrophages to the wound site, which facilitates the healing process. These macrophages stimulate formation and multiplication of fibroblasts. With increased cellular activity, more enzymes are released to debride unwanted fibrin and necrotic material. Edema increases as protein is released from digested cells.

***Proliferative Phase.*** In the *proliferative* phase, from day 3 to day 24, healing is evident. Fibroblasts, stimulated by an acidic environment, begin synthesis of collagen, the principal component of connective tissue, and mucopolysaccharides. Early collagen synthesis is disorganized, and the quality of the synthesis will depend on tissue vascularity and perfusion. The increased cellular and chemical activity results in the formation of granulation tissue along fragile capillary loops supported by collagen fibers. Granulation tissue will remain highly vascular, fragile, and dusky red in color.

***Maturation Phase.*** The *maturation* phase begins on day 24 and lasts for years. Progressively, vascularity of the scar decreases. Fibroblasts exit the wound, and collagen fibers strengthen and reorient. The wound changes from a dusky red of vascular granulation to a pale, white avascular scar.

TABLE 65-7
**Topical Antibiotic Agents**

| Agent | Dressings | Advantages | Disadvantages |
|---|---|---|---|
| Silver Sulfadiazine 1% cream | Buttered on. With light dressings once to twice a day. | Broad spectrum. Low toxicity. Painless, easy to apply and remove. | Intermediate penetration of eschar; leukopenia. |
| Mafenide Acetate (Sulfamyalon) | Buttered on. Open exposure method. Applied 3-4 times daily. | Broad spectrum. Rapid, deep penetration. Rapid excretion. | Pain on application. Pulmonary toxicity. Metabolic acidosis. Inhibits wound healing. Hypersensitivity. |
| Silver-Nitrate Solution 0.5% | Wet dressings. Change bid. Re-soak every 2 hours. | Broad spectrum. Non-allergenic. Low toxicity. Inexpensive. Does not interfere with healing. | Poor penetration of eschar. Ineffective on established wound infections. Electrolyte imbalance. Discoloration of wound and environment. |
| Povidone-Iodine | Buttered on. Used with or without dressing 1-2 times daily. | Broad spectrum. Low toxicity. Eases debriding by tanning of eschar. | Poor penetration of eschar. Pain on application. Iodine sensitivity. Metabolic acidosis. Absorption of iodine. |
| Bacitracin | Buttered on. Reapply every 4-6 hours. | No pain. Clear, odorless. Useful for face burns. Softens eschar. | Poor penetration of eschar. Not effective in reducing sepsis in large burns. Occasional allergic sensitivity. |

TABLE 65-8
**Dressing Types**

| Method | Advantage | Disadvantage |
|---|---|---|
| Open exposure | Wound is always visible for inspection.<br>Less nursing care of the wound needed.<br>Bacterial growth is suppressed by the drying effect of air. | Increased heat loss.<br>Requires strict isolation<br>Requires frequent linen changes.<br>Open to both direct and indirect transmission of contamination. |
| Semi-open exposure | Light dressings.<br>Patient is more mobile.<br>Frequent observation of the wound.<br>Patient can be treated on an outpatient basis. | May be painful.<br>On an outpatient basis, dressings must be changed at least 3 times a week.<br>Requires skilled personnel. |
| Closed-occlusive | Decreased pain.<br>Decreased exposure to bacterial contamination.<br>Can be treated on an outpatient basis with minimal dressing changes. | Decreased effectiveness of topical agents.<br>Limitation of mobility.<br>Decreased wound observation may delay diagnosis of wound infection.<br>Partial-thickness injury may convert to full-thickness injury. |

Gradually, the skin softens and tissues flatten. During this phase, hypertrophic scar or keloid formation becomes evident and may require surgical intervention or preventive measures to control the scar formation.

### Other Healing Processes

***Contracture.*** Wound healing by *contracture* is especially important when there is a great deal of tissue loss. Healing occurs from wound edges converging at the center of the wound. Myofibroblasts are necessary for this type of wound closure, which begins on the fourth day. Cell viability at the edge of the wound contributes to the ability of contracture to heal the wound.

***Epithelialization.*** *Epithelialization* occurs by the migratory effort of new cells over live epithelial cells in the wound, usually around the skin appendages not totally destroyed in the injury. Epithelial cells usually form under eschar as the healing progresses. In large wounds, eschar or a dressing can protect these fragile cells from trauma.

Other fractures that influence the healing process are (1) hemostasis; (2) hypovolemia; (3) infection; (4) inadequate nutrition; and (5) dressing type.

### *Definitive Wound Care*

Cleansing and debridement of the burn wound must be a daily procedure to promote healing and decrease the risk of infection. The wound is inspected for suspect areas, and wound cultures are obtained. Confirmed invasive burn wound sepsis mandates aggressive therapies with the use of topical antimicrobials and systemic antibiotics.

Wound cleansing can be accomplished by tubbing, using a Hubbard tank; by showering, using a shower trolley or shower chair; and bedside dressing changes.

**Debridement.** Debridement of eschar from the burn wound controls infection and prepares the wound for skin grafting. *Mechanical* debridement involves a cutting away of dead tissue from viable granulation bed. *Chemical* debridement, with the use of proteolytic enzymes, aids in the initial debridement before a patient can tolerate surgery. Easily applied, these agents selectively digest necrotic soft tissue without harming viable tissue. These agents are not bactericidal, may cause bleeding, and may be irritating to the wound or surrounding tissues; therefore, dressings need to be changed more frequently, at least every 8 hours.

**Selection of Burn Dressing.** Selection of a burn dressing includes selection of a method of treatment, a topical agent, and design of the dressing. Many topical agents are used in burn wound care. Table 65-7 presents those most frequently used. Dressing types are influenced by area, extent, and depth of injury (Table 65-8).

Dressing design depends on the status of the wound. Protective dressings are used on clean, healing wounds. If mechanical debridement is needed, dressings can be used to cleanse the surface of the wound. Bulky dressings can be based on the need for absorption of fluids from the wound. Some principles of burn wound dressings are listed in Table 65-9.

TABLE 65-9
**Principles of Burn Wound Dressing**

1. Wound surfaces must not be wrapped together.
2. Limit the bulk of dressing to facilitate maximum mobility.
3. Individualize dressing based on the need for absorption, debridement, or protection.
4. Wrap extremities distal to proximal to promote venous return.
5. Ace-wrap dependent areas to limit edema formation and bleeding and to facilitate graft take.

## TABLE 65-10. CARE PLAN FOR THE THERMALLY INJURED PATIENT

| Nursing Diagnoses | Desired Patient Outcomes | Nursing Interventions | Rationales |
|---|---|---|---|
| ***Nursing Diagnosis #1*** Impairment of skin integrity related to: 1. Thermal injury: dry/moist heat, chemical or electrical. | The patient has: 1. Had the burning process halted. 2. A skin pH near normal. 3. No complaints of burning on the wound. 4. A decrease in the degree of corneal ulcerations and eye infection. | • Assess burning process. If fire or scald injury and heat are evident on the wound, cool the area with tap water. | • Depth of injury increases due to length of exposure to the burning agent. |
| | | • Remove clothing and jewelry. | • Clothing, jewelry, belts, etc., retain heat and can increase depth of injury. |
| | | • Do not apply ice. | • Vasoconstriction occurs, damaging the surrounding tissues. Core temperature decreases. |
| | | • Cover patient with clean sheet or blanket. | • Prevents excessive heat loss. Body heat is lost through the burned area. • Decreases pain from exposure to air. • Protects from emergency room contamination. |
| | | • Obtain history of the burning agent. | • Provides information on agent as extent and depth of injury are directly related to the concentration, activity, and penetrability of the chemical; also, duration of contact and the resistance of tissues impact on severity of injury. |
| | | • Initiate extensive lavage with cool water for all chemical burns along with simultaneous removal of contaminated clothing. Brush off dry chemicals before lavage. | • Dilution of the chemical and removal of the chemical from the injured tissues will halt the burning process. Although some chemicals create heat when united with water, copious lavage can dissipate that heat away from the body. (Health care workers must protect themselves from exposure to chemicals.) |
| | | • If eyes are affected, lavage with a minimum of 2–3 liters of NSS. If blepharospasm occurs during irrigation, apply topical ophthalmic anesthetic agent as prescribed. | • Important to remove all chemicals from the eyes to preserve sight. (Blepharospasm refers to a twitching or spasm of orbicularis oculi muscle.) |
| ***Nursing Diagnosis #2*** Impaired gas exchange related to: 1. Upper airway edema. 2. Carbon monoxide poisoning. 3. Smoke inhalation injury. 4. Disruption of alveolar-capillary membrane. | The patient will: 1. Have a carbon monoxide level less than 10%. 2. Maintain a patent airway. 3. Maintain acceptable blood gas parameters: • pH ~ 7.35–7.45. | • Assess for signs or symptoms of tracheal obstruction and respiratory distress as indicated in Table 65-4. • Establish an airway. Administer humidified oxygen at 100%. | • Upper airway edema with smoke inhalation can cause a rapid, progressive airway obstruction leading to respiratory arrest. |
| | | • Monitor arterial blood gases and carbon monoxide level. | • Carbon monoxide and acute airway obstruction are the greatest threats to life immediately after burn injury. Carbon monoxide level of more than 10–20% is indicative of carbon monoxide poisoning. |

| | | | |
|---|---|---|---|
| | • $PaO_2 > 60$ mmHg (room air)<br>• $PaCO_2$ ~35–45 mmHg<br>4. Be responsive, awake, and cognizant of the surroundings. | • Assess arterial pH. | • Patient will demonstrate a metabolic acidosis due to decreased tissue perfusion. |
| | | • Assess chest x-ray. | • This may initially be negative but may demonstrate inflammation or pulmonary edema in 12–24 hours after burn injury. |
| | | • Prepare for endotracheal intubation and mechanical ventilation with positive signs and symptoms of inhalation injury. | • Early intubation prior to the development of airway obstruction is preferred over tracheostomy due to the increased chance of infection from tracheostomy. |
| | | • Assess breath sounds for abnormalities: Wheezing. | • Wheezing is heard across all lung fields due to edema and inflammation caused by carbon deposits and damage to the airways. |
| | | ◦ Rales. | ◦ Rales can occur 12–24 hours after injury. |
| | | • Prepare for bronchoscopy. | • Bronchoscopy will be diagnostic for inhalation injury. |
| | | • Administer prescribed bronchodilators as indicated.<br>• Begin vigorous pulmonary toilet. | • Frequent suctioning of smoke inhalation victims is necessary to clear the airway of copious secretions and carbon deposits.<br>◦ This must be completed aseptically to prevent the lethal complication of pneumonia. |
| | | • Assess chest wall excursion and the use of accessory muscles for breathing. | • For severe burns of the neck and chest, eschar and edema formation create a splinting effect that prohibits lung expansion. |
| | | • With positive signs of restrictive defect, prepare for escharotomy. | • Eschar is released by cutting the eschar on both sides of the chest and from the zyphoid process and/or sternal notch to the outer chest wall. |
| ***Nursing Diagnosis #3***<br>Fluid volume deficit related to:<br>1. Capillary leak—loss of plasma proteins.<br>2. Insensible water loss. | The patient will be maintained with adequate circulating volume and cardiac output as evidenced by:<br>1. Urine output of 50 ml/hour. If hemochromogens* are in the urine, an output of 100 ml/hour is maintained.<br>2. Adequate blood pressure as evidenced by an arterial systolic pressure approximately 100 mmHg, and urine output is maintained as above. | • Monitor for signs and symptoms of hypovolemia including: Hypotension, tachycardia, tachypnea, extreme thirst, restlessness, disorientation. | • Fluid volume is lost through increased capillary permeability, which begins at the time of injury. Insensible fluid loss through the burn wound contributes to decreasing circulation volume. |
| | | • Administer IV fluids according to fluid resuscitation formulas in Table 65–6. Insert large-bore IV catheter. | • IV placement should be in large vessels for the rapid delivery of fluid.<br>◦ Difficulty of peripheral IV insertion is due to vasoconstriction and volume depletion. |
| | | ◦ Prepare for the insertion of subclavian catheters and arterial lines. | ◦ With the insertion of subclavian catheters, hemodynamics can be more accurately assessed and monitored. |
| | | ◦ Send blood specimens for determination of: Hematocrit and hemoglobin, electrolytes, prothrombin/partial thromboplastin times, blood sugar, BUN, and creatinine. | ◦ Hemodyamic status is also assessed through the laboratory data.<br>◦ Increased potassium ($K^+$) is due to cellular trauma, which releases $K^+$ into extracellular fluid. |

(continued)

**TABLE 65–10. CARE PLAN FOR THE THERMALLY INJURED PATIENT** *(Continued)*

| Nursing Diagnoses | Desired Patient Outcomes | Nursing Interventions | Rationales |
|---|---|---|---|
| ***Nursing Diagnosis #3 (cont.)*** | | | |
| | 3. Heart rate: ~100/min<br>4. Hemoglobin and hematocrit within normal range. | | ○ Sodium is lost from the circulation as edema forms.<br>○ Metabolic acidosis results from the loss of bicarbonate ions with the sodium. |
| | 5. Stabilized body weight. | • Insert indwelling urinary catheter. | • Most effective measurement of volume replacement at this time is a urine output of 50–100 ml/hour. |
| | | ○ Monitor urine for amount, specific gravity, and the presence of hemochromogens. | ○ Specific gravity can predict the volume replacement.<br>○ Myoglobin is released in the bloodstream from muscle damage, especially in electrical injuries. Hemoglobin is released through the destruction of RBCs. These hemochromogens can cause renal-tubular obstruction. Osmotic diuretics can aid in reversing this process. |
| | | ○ Administer osmotic diuretics as ordered and monitor response to diuretic therapy. | ○ Decreased urinary output can be a result of: Decreased renal blood flow; increased secretion of ADH; increased adrenocortical activity. |
| | | • Monitor serum pH. Administer prescribed sodium bicarbonate. | • Correct the metabolic acidosis that results from vasoconstriction and tissue ischemia. |
| | | • Continue to monitor hourly for the effectiveness of fluid resuscitation. | • Hypervolemia will lead to increased edema and pulmonary congestion. |
| | | • Assess gastrointestinal function: Absence of bowel sounds. | • Splanchnic constriction as a result of hypovolemia leads to paralytic ileus. |
| | | ○ Insert a nasogastric tube and attach to suction. | ○ Paralytic ileus occurs in burn victims with a >20–25% total body surface burn. |
| | | ○ Monitor gastric pH every 1–2 hours. Administer antacids via nasogastric tube as prescribed to maintain a gastric pH >5. | ○ Antacids help neutralize gastric secretions. Antacids decrease the risk of Curling's ulcer related to stress. |

* Hemochromogens—compounds containing heme and a nitrogen-containing substance such as a protein.

| | | | |
|---|---|---|---|
| ***Nursing Diagnosis #4*** Alteration in comfort: pain. | The patient will:<br>1. Receive assistance in controlling the pain.<br>2. Verbalize that the pain is tolerable.<br>3. Receive validation that the pain exists. | • Assess the degree and duration of pain during painful procedures.<br>• Decrease the anxiety of the patient through the use of relaxation, distraction, or music. | • Validate pain during therapeutic modalities, such as wound care and exercise.<br>• Relaxation can reduce intensity.<br>○ Acute anxiety can be related to anger or guilt about the accident and the chance of survival. |
| | | • Acknowledge the presence of pain. Explain the causes of pain in burn injury. | • In partial-thickness injury, the presence of prostaglandins and histamines in and around the injured area stimulates peripheral pain receptors and intensifies central perceptions of discomfort. Full-thickness burns initially are painless but as the nerve endings regenerate, pain occurs due to exposure to air. |
| | | • Provide privacy for painful therapies. | • Patients feel a loss of control during painful modalities. |
| | | • Decrease the fear associated with pain and the use of narcotics.<br>• Motivate the patient to participate in noninvasive methods to reduce the intensity of pain. | • Patients frequently will not ask for medication for fear of becoming addicted to a drug.<br>• Patients exhibit wide variability in both pain perception and response to pain, attributed to sociological background and previous pain threshold.<br>○ How the injury occurred also contributes to the patient's response. |
| | | • Administer narcotic analgesics as prescribed to provide optimal relief:<br>○ Administer IV narcotics during the emergent phase. | ○ Due to the capillary leak, IM medications are not absorbed adequately to provide acute pain relief. |
| | | ○ Administer narcotics as often as necessary during the acute phase especially prior to dressing change and exercise. | ○ Inadequate narcotic doses are frequently prescribed due to the fear by the medical professionals of producing respiratory depression or addiction to a narcotic. |
| | | ○ Assess adequate doses of drugs. Assess the patient's response to the medication. Recommend increasing prescribed doses as necessary. | ○ Careful titration of narcotic doses can provide adequate pain relief. |
| | | • Decrease the amount of narcotic analgesia as the burn wound heals. | • At the time of discharge, the patient's pain should be adequately controlled with oral agents. |

*(continued)*

## TABLE 65–10. CARE PLAN FOR THE THERMALLY INJURED PATIENT *(Continued)*

| Nursing Diagnoses | Desired Patient Outcomes | Nursing Interventions | Rationales |
|---|---|---|---|
| ***Nursing Diagnosis #5***<br>Potential for alteration in peripheral perfusion related to:<br>1. Circumferential eschar.<br>2. Compartment syndrome. | The patient will have:<br>1. Pulses present and of good quality distal to burn area on limbs.<br>2. Extremities warm to touch.<br>3. Edema minimized to prevent vascular compromise. | • Assess pulses on burned extremities every 15 min. Use the ultrasonic Doppler as necessary. Assess capillary refill.<br>• Assess for numbness, tingling, and increased pain in the burned extremity.<br>• Elevate burned extremities<br>• Apply burn dressing loosely.<br>• Assess muscle compartment pressure.<br>◦ If signs and symptoms of circulatory impairment and inadequate deep tissue perfusion are present, prepare the patient for escharotomy and/or fasciotomy. | • As edema forms on circumferential burns, eschar forms a tight constricting band, decreasing the circulation to the limb distal to the circumferential site.<br>• Increasing pain in extremities can be predictive of increasing pressure from tight bands.<br>• Elevation of the limb promotes venous return and decreases edema.<br>• To allow for expansion as edema forms.<br>• Increasing pressure readings from muscle compartments are indicative of decreased tissue perfusion.<br>◦ These surgical procedures will release constricting eschar bands and improve deep tissue perfusion. |
| ***Nursing Diagnosis #6***<br>Potential for sepsis related to: Wound infection.<br>(Refer to the following:<br>Table 49–7<br>Table 56–1, Nursing Diagnosis #1<br>Table 65–5) | The patient will have:<br>1. Healthy granulation tissue on unhealed areas with $<10^5$ colonies of bacteria as demonstrated on wound culture.<br>2. Absence of clinical manifestation of infection (body temperature, WBC).<br>3. Skin graft sites that have taken.<br>4. Donor sites that are free of infection. | • Use sterile technique when caring for the burn wound.<br>• Maintain protective isolation with good handwashing technique.<br>• Administer immunosupportive medications as prescribed: Tetanus, gamma globulin.<br>• Perform wound care as prescribed:<br>◦ Inspect and debride wounds daily; culture wounds 3 times a week or at any sign of infection; shave all burned areas, especially the scalp and perineum; assess carefully any invasive line site for inflammation especially if the line is through a burn area.<br>• Monitor the patient constantly for signs and symptoms of sepsis: Temperature; sensorium; vital signs; increase/decrease in bowel sounds; decreased output; fluid translocation; positive blood/wound cultures.<br>• Administer systemic antibiotics as prescribed and monitor response to therapy. | • Burn wound is a culture medium for bacterial growth.<br>• Prevent the spread of bacteria from patient to patient.<br>• Immunoglobulins are depressed at the time of severe burn injury.<br>• Quick identification of bacterial wound invasion can decrease the incidence of septic episodes.<br>• The burn patient will experience several septic episodes during hospitalization until the burn wound is healed.<br>• Judicious use of antibiotics can decrease the incidence of drug-resistant organism development. |

| | | | |
|---|---|---|---|
| ***Nursing Diagnosis #7***<br>Alteration in nutrition related to:<br>1. Inadequate intake due to inability to eat, therapeutic regimen, or multiple surgeries.<br>2. Increased metabolic demands.<br>(Also refer to appropriate tables in Chapter 53, Nutritional Support of the Critically Ill Patient) | The patient is:<br>1. Maintained within 10% of pre-burn weight.<br>2. Healing burn wound.<br>3. In a positive nitrogen balance. | • Institute enteral feedings as soon as bowel sounds are present.<br>• Ensure required caloric and protein intake by:<br>◦ Having a dietitian calculate caloric needs.<br>◦ Accurate calorie counts; accurate intake and output; daily weights.<br>• If tube feedings are needed to supplement caloric needs: Insert a feeding tube; assess patency and placement every 4 hours; place patient in a semi-Fowler's position;<br>◦ Assess for gastric residuals at least every four hours.<br>◦ Assess bowel sounds every 2–4 hours.<br>◦ Increase feeding regimen as prescribed.<br>◦ Monitor for adverse side effects such as diarrhea or gastric distention.<br>◦ Accurately document amount of feeding administered. | • The burn patient may require up to 4000 calories per day.<br>• Formulas have been developed to assess necessary caloric needs utilizing total body surface area burn (see Chapter 53).<br>◦ Maintenance of protein mass is critical to survival.<br>• Burn victims frequently require more calories than they are able to eat.<br>• Frequent treatment modalities and surgeries interrupt feeding schedules.<br>◦ Absence of bowel sounds is frequently the first sign of impending sepsis.<br>◦ If the patient is unable to tolerate enteral feedings, hyperalimentation may need to be considered. |
| ***Nursing Diagnosis #8***<br>Impairment of activity related to:<br>1. Reformation of collagen.<br>2. Excisional wound therapy.<br>3. Auto-grafting. | The patient will:<br>1. Maintain positioning as prescribed during multiple surgeries.<br>2. Be able to perform activities of daily living.<br>3. Be ambulatory with no assistive devices.<br>4. Retain full range of motion of all affected joints. | • Assess the need for positioning and/or splinting.<br>◦ Consult occupational therapy.<br>◦ Apply splints and check frequently for fit or areas of pressure.<br>◦ Clean splints at least every shift. Evaluate the need for continuous splinting or night-time use only.<br>◦ Encourage patient to exercise burned limbs, and to actively participate in as many ADLs as possible.<br>• Observe the burn wound closely for any exposed tendons, unresolved edema, peripheral neuropathies, or points of pressure.<br>• Assess problem areas:<br>◦ Position patient with neck burns in extension. Use no pillow.<br>◦ Inspect ears frequently.<br>◦ Position patient with axilla burns in 90° shoulder abduction and 10° elbow flexion.<br>◦ Use special skin care and topical agent of choice after each voiding or defecation.<br>◦ For facial injuries elevate head of the bed. Lubricate lips every 4 hours.<br>• Inspect the burn wound for early signs of webbing, contracture, banding, or keloid formation. | • Attempt to maintain neutral positioning of burned areas.<br>• Maintain a stretch of skin to decrease the pull of contracture.<br>◦ As edema subsides, splints might need revision.<br>◦ Decrease contamination of the burn wounds.<br>• Rapid identification of problem areas helps to decrease additional injury to burned areas.<br>◦ Prevent the development of neck contractures.<br>◦ Pressure can cause necrosis and bending can cause chondritis.<br>◦ Prevent the formation of scar bands in the axilla.<br>◦ Prevent infection or contamination of the burn wound.<br>◦ Decrease edema formation. Avoid lips that crack and bleed.<br>• Quick identification of defects can lead to reversal through the use of splints or pressure. |

*(continued)*

## TABLE 65-10. CARE PLAN FOR THE THERMALLY INJURED PATIENT *(Continued)*

| Nursing Diagnoses | Desired Patient Outcomes | Nursing Interventions | Rationales |
|---|---|---|---|
| ***Nursing Diagnosis #9***<br>Ineffective coping of individual/significant others related to:<br>1. Trauma of burns.<br>2. Family loss.<br>3. Lack of knowledge of the disease process.<br>4. Surgical procedures.<br>5. Expected outcomes. | The patient/significant other will:<br>1. Demonstrate acceptance of the accident with a decreased level of anxiety.<br>2. Verbalize fears, grief, and acceptance of an altered body image.<br>3. Verbalize treatment modalities, process of skin healing and scar/contracture formation.<br>4. Develop supportive behaviors. | • Assess patient/significant other for level of understanding of burn treatment.<br>• Describe the pathophysiology of the burn process and what the patient will experience.<br>• Explain the precautionary isolation of the victim. | • At high stress times, repetition is necessary for understanding.<br>• Attempt to enlist the support of the family to help the patient cope with pain and disfigurement. |
| | | • Assist and identify the coping mechanisms of both patient/significant other. Provide time for questions and discussion of feelings and fears. | • This event is disruptive to patient/significant other lifestyles, relationships, careers, and finances. |
| | | • Be honest. Do not protect the patient/significant other from necessary emotional experiences. | ◦ Frequently there are other injuries or deaths at the scene. Burn victims will ask about the outcome of loved ones. These concerns must be dealt with to enable the patient to cope with his/her injury. |
| | | • Keep patient and significant others informed of the progress of the patient. | • If the burn is severe, the death and dying process needs to be instituted. |
| | | • Explain all procedures and enlist the patient's cooperation. | • Painful procedures preclude patient cooperation. |
| | | • Develop a contract with the patient/significant other and set realistic short-term goals. Allow the patient to make decisions and choices when possible. | • Allows the patient to have some control over his/her environment.<br>(Contracting is discussed in Chap. 4) |
| | | • Approach and administer care in a consistent, positive manner. Carry out your part of the contract regardless of the patient's behavior.<br>• Administer sedatives and analgesics as needed.<br>• Provide adequate rest time.<br>• Encourage discussion of feelings, family, and future plans. | • The patient will be cognizant of the inability to manipulate staff. Burn patients frequently become combative, argumentative and resistant to therapeutic modalities due to the pain. |
| | | • Support and encourage the patient to participate in self-care. Provide assistive devices.<br>• Recommend a psychiatric consult if the patient/significant other need help in order to cope.<br>• Refer the patient/significant other to appropriate resources for aid: Burn support groups; social services; rehabilitation centers; financial services. | • Patients will experience a positive self-image as ADLs increase.<br>• Patient/significant others frequently need help in dealing with body disfigurement and the long-term care needs. |

### *Wound Healing: Therapeutic Modalities*

The overall goal of wound care in burn therapy is wound closure with minimal scarring. This is accomplished with autografting, beginning within 48–72 hours post injury when stabilization of the patient is complete. The grafts used for burn wound closure are split thickness skin grafts (STSG), which are a partial thickness of epidermis and dermis.

STSG may be applied as a meshed graft, which can be expanded 1½ to 9 times its original size to cover a large wound, or as a sheet graft for cosmetic effect. The STSG is nourished by an osmotic exchange of tissue nutrients until healing is complete. Graft take is complete in 3–5 days when collagen strands have attached the graft to the base supporting tissues and an effective blood supply develops.

Cadaver skin; synthetics, such as Op Site; semisynthetics such as Biobrane or artificial skin; and biological dressings, such as pigskin, may be used as temporary wound covering over clean partial and full thickness injuries. These dressings can decrease pain, evaporative water loss, bacterial proliferation, and dessication of a viable wound surface. These skin substitutes can be used to maintain a wound surface until healing occurs or the wound is in condition for autografting as donor skin becomes available.

## Rehabilitation

Survival in any burn victim is the immediate goal post injury. The scarring process and the potential for severe deformity, however, cannot be overlooked or accepted on the basis of burn severity. Rather, aggressive treatment of burns should begin during the acute phase, once the patient's condition is stabilized, and such therapy should continue throughout the rehabilitative phase.

During the rehabilitative phase two, observations of the burn wound must be made: (1) the position of comfort is the position of contracture; and (2) the burn wound will shorten until it meets an opposing force. Contractures can be avoided by starting patients on an active exercise program within 24–48 hours post burn injury. Gentle sustained stretching with the use of splinting devices can be used to maintain a range of motion. Effective therapeutic positioning requires a full team effort and support. These critically ill immobile victims require frequent repositioning to achieve rehabilitative results.

## Nursing Diagnoses, Desired Patient Outcomes, and Nursing Interventions

Nursing diagnoses, desired patient outcomes, nursing interventions, and rationales for the management of the thermally injured patient/family through the phases of care are presented in Table 65–10.

CHAPTER 66

# Nursing Management of the Patient with Septic Shock

*Carol F. Evans*

## CHAPTER OUTLINE



## LEARNING OBJECTIVES

**At the end of this chapter, you should be able to:**

1. Define *septic shock*.
2. Identify causative microorganisms and their portal of entry.
3. List patients at high risk of developing septic shock.
4. Examine the pathophysiology underlying septic shock.
5. Differentiate between early and late signs and symptoms of septic shock based on the underlying pathophysiology.
6. Discuss approach to treatment of septic shock and its prevention.
7. Delineate the nursing process in caring for the immunosuppressed patient including:
   Assessment
   Nursing diagnoses
   Planning: Desired patient outcomes
   Nursing interventions/rationales.

## SEPTIC SHOCK

### Definition

Septic shock, like other forms of shock, is a syndrome characterized by inadequate tissue perfusion and impaired cellular function. The difference between septic shock and other forms of shock syndrome lies in its etiology, pathophysiology, and clinical presentation.

Unlike cardiogenic and hypovolemic shock (see Chaps. 44 and 46), the initial hemodynamic effects of septic shock are *low* systemic vascular resistance and *high* cardiac output. However, in the last stage the effects are about the same; *high* systemic vascular resistance and *low* cardiac output. The ultimate outcome of uncompensated and untreated septic shock is multisystem organ failure and death.

### Etiology

Septic shock is caused by the effects of toxins, produced by pathogenic microorganisms, on the vascular, coagulation, and immune systems. It is precipitated by sepsis or septicemia, defined as the presence of pathogens and their toxins in the circulating blood.

Although gram-negative bacilli are most frequently associated with sepsis and septic shock,

TABLE 66-1
**Common Microorganisms Associated with Sepsis[2]**

| Genus (Species) | Form | Gram Stain Reaction | Type of Respiration |
|---|---|---|---|
| Bacteroides (fragilis) | Bacilli | Negative | Anaerobic |
| Clostridium | Bacilli | Positive | Anaerobic |
| Enterobacter | Bacilli | Negative | Aerobic or anaerobic |
| Escherichia (coli) | Bacilli | Negative | Aerobic or anaerobic |
| Klebsiella (pneumoniae) | Bacilli | Negative | Aerobic or anaerobic |
| Neisseria (meningitidis) | Cocci | Negative | Aerobic |
| Proteus (mirabilis, vulgaris) | Bacilli | Negative | Aerobic or anaerobic |
| Pseudomonas (aeruginosa) | Bacilli | Negative | Aerobic |
| Serratia (marcescens) | Bacilli | Negative | Aerobic or anaerobic |
| Staphylococcus (aureus) | Cocci | Positive | Aerobic or anaerobic |
| Streptococcus (pneumoniae) | Cocci | Positive | Aerobic or anaerobic |

gram-positive cocci and bacilli also have been implicated. Moreover, shock syndrome may develop secondary to systemic infection by the fungus *Candida albicans*.[1]

Table 66-1 contains a list of microorganisms commonly associated with sepsis and septic shock. Pathogens may be part of the patient's normal body flora or may be endemic to the hospital environment. Species of staphylococci and streptococci constitute the normal flora of the skin and mucous membranes. *Enterobacter, Proteus, Escherichia,* and *Bacteroides* are flora of the gastrointestinal tract. *Pseudomonas* species are commonly found in water and soil.

Debilitated hospitalized patients are extremely prone to bacterial invasion, especially after surgery and other invasive procedures. The risk of septic shock is increased in the elderly population and in patients with a compromised immune system.

The most common portal of entry for microorganisms is the urinary tract. Other avenues of entry and related conditions are listed in Table 66-2. The frequent use of urinary catheters, intravenous therapy, invasive monitoring devices, and mechanical ventilators in critical care areas increases the risk of sepsis in the critically ill patient.

TABLE 66-2
**Common Portals of Entry of Microorganisms[3]**

| Entrance Point | Related Conditions |
|---|---|
| Urinary tract | Urinary catheters<br>Suprapubic tubes<br>Cystoscopic examination |
| Respiratory tract | Endotracheal tubes<br>Tracheostomy tubes<br>Mechanical ventilation<br>Suctioning<br>Inhalation therapy<br>Aspiration |
| Gastrointestinal tract | Peritonitis<br>Abdominal abcess<br>Cirrhosis<br>Ascites<br>Peptic ulcers |
| Skin | Surgical wounds<br>Burns<br>Traumatic injury<br>Intravenous catheters<br>Intra-arterial catheters<br>Invasive monitoring<br>Decubitis ulcers |
| Female genital tract | Postpartum<br>Post-abortion |

## Pathophysiology

The pathophysiology of septic shock is complex and not completely understood. Effects on hemodynamic variables, coagulation factors, and the immune system are attributed to endotoxin, a lipopolysaccharide released from the cell walls of dead gram-negative bacilli.

Gram-positive bacilli and cocci do not produce endotoxin. However, they can produce a shock state similar to gram-negative shock, although not as profound. Despite the absence of endotoxin in some forms of septicemia, the effects of endotoxin are used as a model to explain the physiologic changes in septic shock.

### *Effects of Endotoxin*

A summary of the effects of endotoxin is presented in Figure 66-1. Endotoxin causes cellular damage through a variety of mechanisms. Initially there is direct damage to the endothelial lining of the small blood vessels. The vasculature of the kidneys and the lungs are most susceptible to this damage.[4]

Cellular damage stimulates the release of vasoactive proteins (kinins) and activates factor XII of the coagulation cascade. Vasoactive kinins promote peripheral vasodilation and increase capillary permeability. Activation of the coagulation cascade leads to the production of multiple intravascular thrombi.

Endotoxin affects immune response by directly activating the alternative complement pathway.

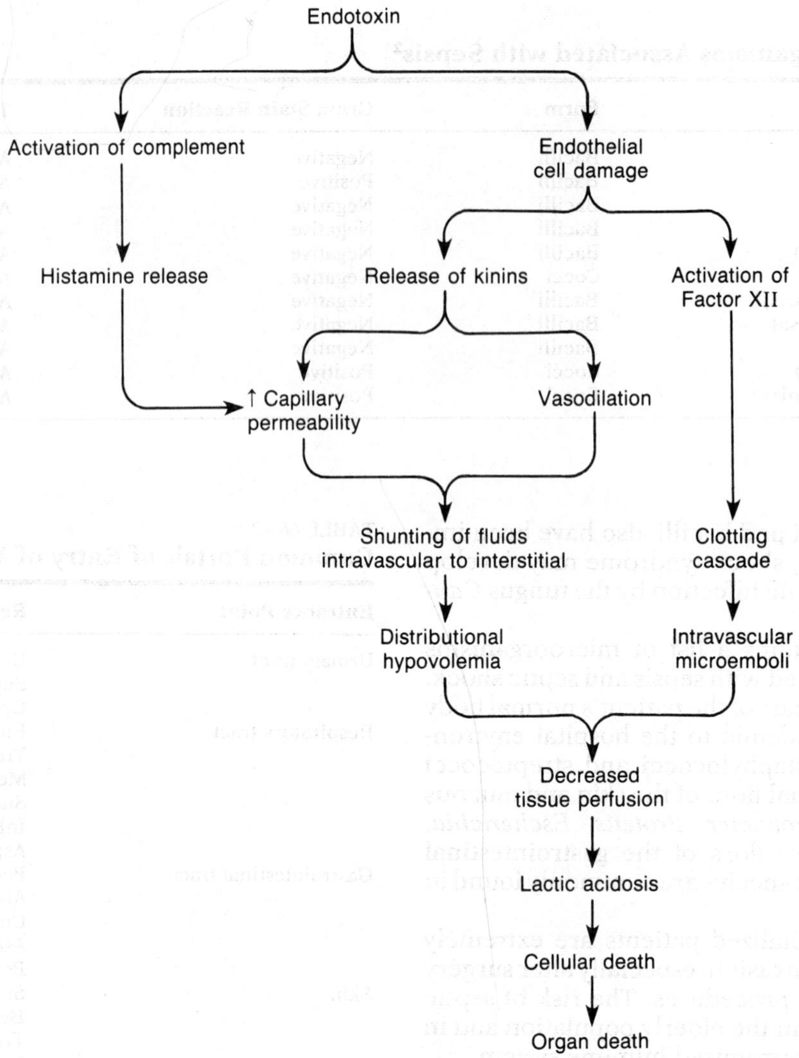


**Figure 66-1.** Summary of the pathophysiologic effects of endotoxin (see text for discussion).

The inflammatory response triggered by complement further stimulates the production of kinins and accelerates the coagulation cascade.[5]

Fluids are shunted from the intravascular to the interstitial space because of increased capillary permeability, with consequent disruption of osmotic gradients, and peripheral vasodilation. Decreased tissue perfusion is the result of distributional hypovolemia, coupled with intravascular coagulation. The decrease in oxygen and nutrients provided to the peripheral tissues leads to anaerobic metabolism, lactic acidosis, and cellular death.

**Disseminated Intravascular Coagulation.** Through the intrinsic coagulation pathway (factor XII), fibrin clots are produced in the microcirculation. Fibrin formation and vascular wall damage enhance platelet aggregation. Moreover, platelets are directly damaged by endotoxin.

The cumulative result is thrombocytopenia, a decrease in circulating clotting factors, and activation of the fibrinolytic system. Disseminated intravascular coagulation (DIC), characterized by clotting in the microcirculation and bleeding from larger vessels, may occur in advanced cases of septic shock (see Chap. 63).

## Clinical Presentation

It is generally accepted that septic shock can be divided into two distinct phases: early (hyperdynamic) septic shock and late (hypodynamic) septic shock. Signs and symptoms of the two phases of septic shock are listed Table 66-3.

### *Early Septic Shock*

Early septic shock is usually characterized by high fever, chills, weakness, and warm, flushed skin. The hemodynamic response is attributed to decreased systemic vascular resistance (afterload) secondary to profound peripheral vasodilation. With de-

TABLE 66-3
**Signs and Symptoms of Early and Late Septic Shock[6]**

| | Early Septic Shock (Hyperdynamic) | Late Septic Shock (Hypodynamic) |
|---|---|---|
| General | Hyperthermia, chills, weakness, and warm flushed skin | Normothermia or hypothermia, and cool, pale skin |
| Neurological | Alert and oriented, anxiety | Altered level of consciousness |
| Respiratory | Rapid, deep breathing | Rapid, shallow breathing |
| Acid-base | Respiratory alkalosis | Metabolic acidosis |
| Renal | Normal urine output | Oliguria or anuria |
| Gastrointestinal | Nausea, vomiting, and diarrhea | |
| Cardiovascular | Normotension or hypotension | Hypotension |
| | ↓Afterload (SVR) | ↑Afterload (SVR) |
| | ↓Preload (PCWP) | ↓Preload (PCWP) |
| | ↑Cardiac output | ↓Cardiac output |
| | ↓Central venous pressure | ↓Central venous pressure |
| | Tachycardia | Tachycardia, ventricular arrhythmias |

creased afterload, cardiac work is reduced, promoting an increase in cardiac output. However, the patient may become hypotensive secondary to decreased vascular resistance and hypovolemia.

### Late Septic Shock

As fluids are shunted into the interstitial space and hypovolemia develops, compensatory mechanisms are activated. Activation of the sympathetic nervous system produces tachycardia, vasoconstriction, and increased myocardial contractility. There may be an initial increase in cardiac output; however, increased afterload and decreased venous return ultimately lead to a decrease in cardiac output. Cardiac failure in late septic shock is related to the aforementioned hemodynamic changes and to the damaging effects of endotoxin on the myocardium.

The clinical presentation of late septic shock is similar to that of cardiogenic shock (see Chap. 44). The patient is cold, diaphoretic, oliguric or anuric, and manifests mental changes such as disorientation and altered level of consciousness. These signs and symptoms are related to decreased tissue perfusion, low cardiac output, and vasoconstriction.

The patient ultimately succumbs to heart, respiratory, and/or renal failure. Respiratory distress syndrome develops as a result of the effects of endotoxin and the shock state on the pulmonary tissue (see Chap. 34). Acute tubular necrosis develops because of hypovolemia, decreased perfusion, and microthrombi in the renal circulation (see Chap. 25).

### Laboratory Findings

Laboratory data are useful in the diagnosis and management of septic shock. Positive blood cultures identify the causative agent and direct appropriate antibiotic therapy. However, the presence of viable bacteria in the blood may be transient. Negative blood cultures, therefore, do not rule out the possibility of septicemia.

The most common hematologic variation is leukocytosis, with a white cell count of greater than 15,000/mm$^3$ and a shift of bands to the left.[7] However, some patients may have normal leukocyte counts or leukopenia. Thrombocyte (platelet) count is reduced, and coagulation studies may be elevated. Fibrin split products are increased in the presence of DIC.

Acid–base balance varies according to the stage of septic shock. Respiratory alkalosis is evident during the early phase due to compensatory hyperventilation. In late septic shock, after tissue perfusion is reduced, metabolic acidosis develops.

## Treatment

Early recognition of the signs and symptoms of septic shock is important. Prompt therapy may prevent early shock from progressing to late shock. Initial therapeutic interventions include fluid volume replacement, antibiotic therapy, and identification and removal (if possible) of the focus of the infection.[4]

### Fluid Replacement

Fluid replacement with crystalloid and/or colloid helps to correct hypovolemia and to improve tissue perfusion. Colloids are needed to increase osmotic pressure, thus promoting the retention of fluids within the intravascular space. Colloid replacement with packed red blood cells, if indicated, has the added benefit of improving oxygen transport to the tissues.

### Antibiotic Therapy

Antibiotic therapy is based on the results of positive cultures that indicate the sensitivities of the invading organism(s). Usually, the physician will order 2 antibiotic agents, 1 of which is an aminoglycoside,

**TABLE 66–4. CARE PLAN FOR THE PATIENT WITH SEPTIC SHOCK**

| Nursing Diagnoses | Desired Patient Outcomes | Nursing Interventions | Rationales |
|---|---|---|---|
| ***Nursing Diagnosis #1*** Fluid volume deficit related to: 1. Distributional volume loss; shift to interstitial space. 2. Increased insensible loss with high fever. | Patient will: 1. Maintain adequate circulating blood volume and stable hemodynamic variables: • Heart rate 60–100/min when resting. • Systemic arterial blood pressure adequate for tissue perfusion. • Normal pulmonary capillary wedge pressure 8–12 mmHg. • Normal central venous pressure 0–8 mmHg. | • Assess for signs and symptoms of septic shock (see Table 66–3) | • Baseline assessment data is needed to establish the phase of septic shock: Early or late. Baseline data is useful in determining changes in patient status and evaluating response to therapy. |
| | | ○ Assess for early signs of septic shock: Hyperthermia, warm, dry, flushed skin; chills; weakness; nausea, vomiting, diarrhea. | ○ Early recognition of septic shock is important in order to institute prompt measures to prevent late or irreversible shock. |
| | | ○ Assess neurological status: 1. Altered level of consciousness. 2. Anxiety. | ○ Neurologic assessment is a way to gauge cerebral perfusion. Orientation and anxiety are indicative of early septic shock, when cerebral perfusion is not as yet compromised. Confusion, disorientation, and coma may indicate decreased perfusion as seen in late septic shock. |
| | | ○ Assess cardiovascular status: Hypotension; tachycardia; character of pulse. | |
| | | ○ Observe for ventricular dysrhythmias. | ○ Dysrhythmias may indicate decreased coronary perfusion, as seen in late septic shock. |
| | 2. Maintain normal body temperature. | ○ Note color and character of the skin: Cool, pale, diaphoretic. | ○ Cool, pale skin is a sign of decreased perfusion and peripheral vasoconstriction. |
| | 3. Maintain adequate urine output $>30$ ml/hour (ml/kg). 4. Maintain baseline and/or optimal neurological status. | ○ Assess renal function: Urine output; urine specific gravity, urinary sodium. | ○ Reduced renal perfusion will reduce glomerular filtration, causing a decrease in urine output. A decrease in urinary sodium is indicative of hypovolemia secondary to aldosterone release. |
| | 5. Maintain fluid and electrolyte balance as demonstrated by laboratory data within normal limits: • Electrolytes. • Hemoglobin and hematocrit. • BUN and creatinine | ○ Obtain baseline laboratory data: Cultures: Urine, sputum; wound (if applicable). | ○ Determination of the portal of entry and focus of infection is crucial to successful treatment. |
| | | ○ Blood cultures—two specimens from different sites by venipuncture. | ○ Bacteremia may be transient. Blood cultures should not be obtained through indwelling venous or arterial catheters, as they may be colonized with bacteria not responsible for the septicemia. |
| | | ○ Electrolytes. ○ Coagulation factors and clotting times; fibrin split products. ○ Hemoglobin and hematocrit. | ○ These data will be helpful in monitoring fluid replacement therapy and in identifying complications such as DIC. |
| | | ○ White cell count with differential. | ○ Elevated leukocyte count with a left shift is frequently observed in septic shock; indicative of acute infection. |

| | | | |
|---|---|---|---|
| | | • Assist with the insertion of hemodynamic monitoring devices.<br>○ Arterial catheters: Blood pressure; arterial blood gases.<br>○ Pulmonary artery catheter: Central venous pressure; pulmonary artery pressure; cardiac output, $SvO_2$ (mixed venous gases). | • Hemodynamic variables (CVP, PCWP, CO, SVR, $SvO_2$, A-a$DO_2$, $VO_2$) are important in determining the effectiveness of fluid replacement therapy and in determining the phase of septic shock.<br>○ Reduction in oxygen tension (<40 mmHg) in mixed venous gases ($SvO_2$) is indicative of compromised tissue perfusion. |
| | | • Administer and monitor prescribed fluid replacement therapy:<br>○ Monitor hemodynamic variables (as above). | ○ Higher than normal central venous pressure, pulmonary artery pressure, and wedge pressure may indicate a too rapid infusion of fluids and impending fluid overload. |
| | | ○ Monitor hourly urine output. | ○ Urine output of greater than 30 cc/hour indicates adequate renal perfusion. |
| | | ○ Assess respiratory status: Respiratory rate; rhythm of breathing; presence of adventitious breath sounds: Crackles, wheezes. | ○ Tachypnea and crackles may indicate fluid overload. |
| | | • Institute measures to control body temperature. | • High body temperature increases the metabolic rate of the tissues and may exacerbate tissue ischemia and hypoxia. |
| | | ○ Monitor body temperature every 2 hours if the patient is febrile.<br>○ Administer antipyretic drugs as ordered; evaluate response to therapy.<br>○ Apply hypo-hyperthermia blanket as prescribed:<br>– Manual mode.<br>○ Automatic cooling mode using rectal probe. | ○ Insensible fluid loss may increase when the patient is febrile.<br><br>○ Continuous measurement of temperature while the patient is on a cooling blanket will prevent excessive cooling and chills. |
| ***Nursing Diagnosis #2***<br>Potential impaired gas exchange related to:<br>1. Hypovolemia resulting in reduced pulmonary perfusion (ventilation/perfusion mismatch).<br>2. Altered alveolar-capillary membrane. | Patient will:<br>1. Maintain acceptable blood gas parameters:<br>• pH 7.35–7.45<br>• $pO_2 > 60$ mmHg<br>• $pCO_2 \sim 35-45$ mmHg<br>2. Maintain baseline and/or optimal neurological status. | • Assess respiratory status.<br><br>○ Respiratory rate and rhythm.<br><br>○ Breath sounds. | • Respiratory distress syndrome may occur in septic shock secondary to decreased perfusion and endotoxin damage to the pulmonary vasculature (see Chap. 34).<br>○ Altered respiratory patterns such as hyperventilation and tachypnea occur secondary to fever and sympathetic nervous system stimulation.<br>○ Development of abnormal breath sounds such as crackles indicates fluid overload and pulmonary edema. |

(continued)

**TABLE 66-4. CARE PLAN FOR THE PATIENT WITH SEPTIC SHOCK *(Continued)***

| Nursing Diagnoses | Desired Patient Outcomes | Nursing Interventions | Rationales |
|---|---|---|---|
| ***Nursing Diagnosis #3***<br>Breathing pattern, ineffective, related to:<br>1. Tachypnea, hyperventilation.<br>(See Nursing Diagnosis #1 and #2, Table 34-3) | Patient will:<br>1. Achieve effective alveolar minute ventilation (arterial blood gas values as above).<br>2. Verbalize ease of breathing. | ○ Monitor arterial blood gases and pH. | ○ Decreased $PaO_2$ <60 mmHg, and increased $PaCO_2$ >50 mmHg (room air) are signs of impending respiratory failure. |
| | | • Maintain patent airway. | • Patients with septic shock may require endotracheal intubation. |
| | | • Administer and monitor oxygen and respiratory therapy.<br>○ Monitor arterial blood gases.<br>○ Observe for increased peak inspiratory pressures during mechanical ventilation. | ○ In the patient requiring mechanical ventilation, increased inspiratory pressures indicate decreased lung compliance observed in respiratory distress syndrome. |
| | | • Assess neurological status. | • Changes in mental status may indicate cerebral hypoxia. |
| ***Nursing Diagnosis #4***<br>Alteration in cardiac output: decreased, related to:<br>1. Decreased venous return (late septic shock). | Patient will:<br>1. Demonstrate stable hemodynamic variables:<br>• Blood pressure >90 mmHg systolic.<br>• Pulmonary capillary wedge pressure 8-12 mmHg.<br>• Cardiac output >4 liters/min.<br>• Systemic vascular resistance 800-1400 dyne-seconds/cm⁵.<br>3. Maintain adequate urine output >30 ml/hour (ml/kg).<br>4. Maintain adequate respiratory status: | • Assess hemodynamic status.<br>○ Cardiac output.<br>○ Pulmonary capillary wedge pressure.<br>○ Systemic vascular resistance. | • Increased cardiac output and decreased systemic vascular resistance are observed in early septic shock; however in late septic shock, cardiac output is reduced and systemic vascular resistance is high. Monitoring these variables will determine the effectiveness of therapeutic interventions. |
| | | • Assess neurological status. | • Changes in neurological status may indicate decreased cerebral perfusion secondary to decreased cardiac output. |
| | | • Assess respiratory status:<br>○ Rate and rhythm of breathing.<br>○ Adventitious breath sounds. | • Acute respiratory failure may develop secondary to cardiac failure. Baseline data are needed in order to monitor the effectiveness of therapeutic interventions. |
| | | • Administer and monitor the effects of prescribed medical interventions: Vasodilators; positive inotropes; antiarrhythmics. | |

| | | | |
|---|---|---|---|
| | • Respiratory rate <30/min.<br>• Absence of adventitious breath sounds.<br>• Arterial blood gases within acceptable limits.<br>5. Demonstrate adequate peripheral tissue perfusion:<br>• Warm, dry skin.<br>• Absence of cyanosis.<br>• Absence of skin breakdown.<br>6. Maintain baseline/optimal neurological function:<br>• Level of consciousness: Oriented to person place, time.<br>• Deep tendon reflexes brisk. | | |
| ***Nursing Diagnosis #5***<br>Potential impairment of skin integrity, related to:<br>1. Immobility.<br>2. Decreased tissue perfusion. | Patient will:<br>1. Demonstrate skin integrity as evidenced by the absence of skin breakdown and pressure ulcers. | • Assess skin condition frequently.<br>• Perform passive range of motion exercises.<br>• Provide pressure relief device.<br>• Teach the patient to shift position frequently.<br>• Establish a turning schedule of every 1–2 hours depending on the patient's condition. | • To improve peripheral circulation.<br>• Pressure ulcers may be prevented by reducing the amount and duration of pressure to a given area. |
| ***Nursing Diagnosis #6***<br>Potential for reinfection. | Patient will:<br>1. Re-establish and maintain normal body temperature.<br>2. Remain without new evidence of infection. | • For specific nursing interventions and rationales, see Table 49–7 and Table 56–1, Nursing Diagnosis #1. | |

*(continued)*

**TABLE 66-4. CARE PLAN FOR THE PATIENT WITH SEPTIC SHOCK *(Continued)***

| Nursing Diagnoses | Desired Patient Outcomes | Nursing Interventions | Rationales |
|---|---|---|---|
| ***Nursing Diagnosis #7***<br>Anxiety related to:<br>1. Intensive care environment.<br>2. Septic shock. | Patient will:<br>1. State that he/she feels less anxious.<br>2. Verbalize feelings about illness and care in the intensive care unit.<br>3. Perform relaxation techniques. | • For specific nursing interventions and rationales, see Table 35-3, Nursing Diagnosis #1. | |
| ***Nursing Diagnosis #8***<br>Sleep pattern disturbance related to:<br>1. Intensive care environment.<br>2. Anxiety.<br>3. Assessments and treatments. | Patient will:<br>1. State that he/she feels rested.<br>2. Verbalize feelings about illness. | • Plan nursing care activities such as assessment, treatments, and tests to allow for rest periods. | • Longer periods of rest can be provided when nursing care is organized. |
| | | • Determine the patient's normal sleep pattern. | • Knowledge of the patient's normal sleep pattern is useful to determine the timing and length of rest periods.<br>○ Patients in ICU may sleep up to 50% of their limited sleep time during the day; little or no sleep may occur at night due to frequent awakenings and anxiety. |
| | | • Assess the duration and quality of sleep as perceived by patient. | |
| | | • Administer prescribed sedatives and hypnotics.<br>○ Monitor for signs of respiratory depression: Significantly decreased respiratory rate (<8 spontaneous breaths/min); evidence of reduced alveolar hypoventilation. | |
| | | ○ Monitor trends in $PaCO_2$ and $PaO_2$. | ○ A rising $PaCO_2$ and decreasing $PaO_2$ may suggest ventilatory compromise. |

in order to expand the spectrum of antibacterial action. Initially, large doses are administered, and the intravenous route is preferred.[8]

*Identification* of the *focus of entry* of infection is important in order to prevent the recurrence of septicemia. If a surgical wound or abcess is at fault, it must be drained or excised. Suspect venous or arterial catheters must be removed and replaced in another site. If the urinary tract is the focus of infection, the decision whether to remove or avoid a urinary catheter must be weighed against the need for monitoring urinary output.

### Additional Interventions

Additional interventions are directed toward the prevention and treatment of complications such as hypotension, acidosis, respiratory failure, and cardiac failure. Medical interventions include inotropic agents, vasopressors, and corticosteroids. Inotropic agents, such as dobutamine, are recommended in the treatment of low cardiac output in late septic shock.[9] The use of vasopressors, such as dopamine, may be indicated if hypotension cannot be alleviated by fluid replacement, correction of metabolic imbalances, and inotropic agents.[10] Steroid therapy may be beneficial by inhibiting the effects of endotoxin on complement and by decreasing pulmonary vascular resistance.[8,11]

## Nursing Care

The critical care nurse has an important role in the prevention, recognition, and management of septic shock. Prevention of infection is a primary goal in the care of all critically ill patients. Nursing care considerations in the patient with potential for infection are described in Table 49–7 (see also Table 56–1, Nursing Diagnosis #1).

Early recognition of septic shock is enhanced through careful patient assessment coupled with knowledge of the signs and symptoms of septic shock and infection. Baseline assessment data assist the nurse to identify and interpret subtle changes, which may indicate decreased cerebral or peripheral perfusion. Changes in hemodynamic variables must be monitored as well.

### Therapeutic Goals

Therapeutic goals in the care of the patient with septic shock are as follows:

1. Promote adequate tissue perfusion.
2. Support ventilation and oxygenation.
3. Maintain hemodynamic stability.
4. Prevent reinfection and/or superimposed infection.
5. Prevent and/or monitor for complications of septic shock, including DIC, respiratory failure, renal failure, and cardiac failure.
6. Prevent injury and breakdown of the skin and soft tissues.
7. Promote patient comfort and provide psychologic support for the patient and family.

### Nursing Diagnoses, Desired Patient Outcomes, and Nursing Interventions

Nursing diagnoses, desired patient outcomes, and nursing interventions/rationales in the management of the patient with septic shock are presented in Table 66–4 (see also Table 56–1).

## REFERENCES

1. Riccardi, KP: Septic shock and the mechanism of tissue injury. In Guthrie, M (ed): Contemporary Issues in Critical Care Nursing, Vol 2, Shock. Churchill Livingstone, New York, 1982, p 33.
2. Brown, WJ: A classification of microorganisms frequently causing sepsis. Heart Lung 5:397, 1976.
3. Gorbach, SL, Bartlett, JG, and Nichols, RL (eds): Manual of Surgical Infections. Little, Brown & Co., Boston, 1984, p 180.
4. Petersdorf, RG and Dale, DC: Gram-negative bacteremia and septic shock. In Isselbacher, KJ, et al (eds): Harrison's Principles of Internal Medicine, ed 9. McGraw-Hill, New York, 1980, p 562.
5. Riccardi, KP: Septic shock and the mechanism of tissue injury. In Guthrie, M (ed): Contemporary Issues in Critical Care Nursing, Vol 2, Shock. Churchill Livingstone, New York, 1982, p 35.
6. Bordicks, KJ: Patterns of Shock—Implications for Nursing Care. Macmillan, New York, 1980, p 262.
7. Petersdorf, RG and Dale, DC: Gram-negative bacteremia and septic shock. In Isselbacher, KJ, et al (eds): Harrison's Principles of Internal Medicine, ed 9. McGraw-Hill, New York, 1980, p 563.
8. Gorbach, SL, Bartlett, JG, and Nichols, RL (eds): Manual of Surgical Infections. Little, Brown & Co., Boston, 1984, p 181.
9. Zaritsky, AL and Chernow, B: Catecholamines, sympathomimetics. In Chernow, B and Lake, CR (eds): The Pharmacologic Approach to the Critically Ill Patient. Williams & Wilkins, Baltimore, 1983, p 495.
10. Shoemaker, WC: Pathophysiology and therapy of shock syndromes. In Shoemaker, WC, Thompson, WL, and Holbrook, PR (eds): Textbook of Critical Care. WB Saunders, Philadelphia, 1984, p 70.
11. Shoemaker, WC: Pathophysiology and therapy of shock syndromes. In Shoemaker, WC, Thompson, WL, and Holbrook, PR (eds): Textbook of Critical Care. WB Saunders, Philadelphia, 1984, p 71.

## SUGGESTED READINGS

Bellanti, JA (ed): Immunology, Basic Processes. WB Saunders, Philadelphia, 1985.

Carpenito, LJ: Nursing Diagnosis, Application to Clinical Practice, ed 2. JB Lippincott, Philadelphia, 1987.

Cowley, RA and Trump, BF (eds): Pathophysiology of Shock, Anoxia and Ischemia. Williams & Wilkins, Baltimore, 1982.

Rice, V: Shock, a clinical syndrome, Part II: Stages of shock. Crit Care Nurse, 1(4): 4, May-June 1981.

# CHAPTER 67

# Nursing Management of the Patient with Anaphylactic Shock

*Lorraine Fallon and Jeannette Waterman*

## CHAPTER OUTLINE



## LEARNING OBJECTIVES

**At the end of this chapter, you should be able to:**

1. Define *anaphylaxis.*
2. Identify etiologic factors and patients at risk for anaphylactic shock.
3. Examine pathophysiology underlying anaphylactic shock including the actions of chemical mediators released in this immune response.
4. Identify key factors of importance to assessment and diagnosis of anaphylactic shock including the patient's past history and the clinical presentation.
5. Outline key considerations in the emergent care of the patient with anaphylactic shock.
6. Delineate the nursing process in caring for the patient with anaphylactic shock including:
   Assessment
   Nursing diagnoses
   Planning: Desired patient outcomes
   Nursing interventions/rationales.

## ANAPHYLACTIC SHOCK

Anaphylaxis (type I, atopy) is one of four basic immune mechanisms underlying host responses to foreign substances (i.e., antigens). The other mechanisms are listed in Table 67-1, and include: Cytotoxic responses (type II) immune complexes (type III), and delayed hypersensitivity (cell-mediated, type IV). (See Chap. 54 for a detailed examination of these mechanisms.) This chapter is concerned with anaphylaxis, or type I immune response.

Anaphylactic shock is an immediate systemic normovolemic vasogenic reaction that occurs when an antigen interacts with the preformed antibody (immunoglobulin IgE) that is found on the surface of mast cells and basophils. The interaction between the antigen and the antibody causes the release of chemical mediators from mast cell granules. These mediators trigger the life-threatening clinical manifestations that we call anaphylactic shock. Unless treatment is immediately given, the results of this shock can be fatal.

### Pathophysiology

Anaphylactic shock is a 2-phase reaction. The first phase occurs when persons are exposed to a foreign substance (antigen) and their body produces specific IgE antibodies against this antigen. These IgE

TABLE 67-1

**Effector Mechanisms Underlying Immune Responses***

**Type I. Atopy (Anaphylaxis)**

Type I mechanism is characterized by an increase in IgE antibody bound to mast cells, by a rapid onset, and by release of chemical mediators from mast cells that catalyze reactions underlying the anaphylactic response. There is a strong hereditary component to this type of immune response.

Examples of Type I immune responses (see Fig. 54-11) include:

1. Anaphylactic shock.
2. Allergic asthma.
3. Atopic reactions (dust, molds, pollen, etc.).

**Type II. Cytotoxic Response**

Type II mechanisms involve reactions wherein an attack is directed against a cell or tissue component by an antibody, with or without complement (humoral), or by antibody-dependent cell-mediated cytotoxicity. The target is eliminated by cell lysis, physiologic inactivation, or phagocytosis.

Examples of Type II immune responses (see Fig. 54-12) include:

1. Rh disease, erythroblastosis fetalis, or certain transfusion reactions.
2. Goodpasture's syndrome, pemphigoid, myasthenia gravis.
3. Drug-related hemolytic anemias, leukopenias, etc.

**Type III: Circulating Immune (Antigen-Antibody) Complexes**

Type III reactions are characterized by an antigen-antibody reaction at a time when the antigen is in excess. This results in immune complexes that are so small that phagocytic cells in the liver and spleen do not remove them from the circulation rapidly. These complexes become deposited in small arteries and capillary beds particularly in the kidney, nervous system, and possibly the skin. Complement is activated and the consequent inflammatory response predisposes to tissue injury, and thus, disease.

Examples of Type III responses (see Fig. 54-14) include:

1. Acute glomerulonephritis.
2. Rheumatoid arthritis.
3. Sytemic lupus erythematosus.

**Type IV. Delayed Hypersensitivity or Cell-Mediated reactions**

Type IV reactions are characterized by the egress of specific lymphocytes into tissues where processes of injury are initiated. These reactions do not involve antibodies, but are exclusively cell mediated. Since the lymphocytes migrate to the antigen, this reaction takes longer to occur and therefore, it is *delayed*.

Examples of Type IV immune responses (see Fig. 54-15) include:

1. Contact dermatitis (e.g., poison ivy).
2. Transplant organ rejection.
3. Delayed hypersensitivity to bacteria, fungi, and viruses (e.g., tuberculosis, herpes and other viral diseases).

*See Chapter 54 for a more detailed discussion of these immune mechanisms.

antibodies bind with mast cells found in connective tissue of the lungs, uterus, spleen, liver, omentum, kidneys, heart, skin, as well as in the connective tissues that surround the blood vessels. IgE also binds with basophils, the counterparts of mast cells found in blood plasma. Once the person's immune system has become sensitized to that specific antigen (i.e., he/she has antigen specific IgE antibodies on the surface of mast cells), phase 1 is completed and the person is now at risk for anaphylactic shock.

Phase 2 occurs when the person is again exposed to the specific antigen. The antigen now reacts with the *preformed* IgE antibodies attached to the mast cells and basophils. The consequent reaction causes cellular integrity to become disrupted with the release of chemical mediators from within intracellular granules. These chemical mediators, upon release, catalyze the sequence of reactions that underlie anaphylactic shock.

An anaphylactoid syndrome, having clinical manifestations nearly identical to those of anaphylactic shock, has been recognized.[1] In this anaphylactoid reaction, however, there is no prior sensitization, and preformed IgE antibodies are not involved. In other words, there is no immune mechanism involved. The chemical agent causes a direct mediator release triggering the anaphylactoid reaction. Such agents as radiographic contrast materials, nonsteroidal anti-inflammatory drugs, and opiates have been identified as causative agents, and these reactions are dose-related.

Other anaphylactoid reactions have been associated with vigorous exercise. Three patterns have been identified.[2] The first reaction is exercise-induced unrelated to eating. The second reaction occurs during exercise after eating a specific food (e.g., shellfish, nuts, and celery). The last pattern has occurred in patients who exercised within 2 hours of having eaten (any foods). Speculation has implicated changes in blood volume distribution during the digestive/absorptive phase as a possible etiologic factor. Perhaps some unexplained deaths of runners and swimmers are related to exercise-induced anaphylaxis.

### *Antigens*

Many different antigens (allergens) have been implicated as possible causes of anaphylactic shock. They fall basically into 3 categories often classified by how they enter the body. The major categories include injections, ingestions, and bites/stings, and examples of each are listed in Table 67-2.

Because of the unpredictable pathogenesis, morbidity, and mortality associated with anaphylactic shock, attempts to identify persons at increased risk of experiencing anaphylaxis have been unsuccessful. For example, it has been discovered that persons who suffer with ragweed hay fever also frequently have a local anaphylactic reaction to melons and bananas. This *local* reaction is manifested by acute swelling, burning, and itching of the mouth. This reaction is IgE-mediated but is not to be confused with *systemic* anapylactic shock. An allergy to fish products or iodine may predispose individuals to an untoward reaction when contrast medias are used in diagnostic testing. Yet, individ-

TABLE 67–2
**Etiology of Anaphylactic Shock**

| | |
|---|---|
| Injection or Ingestion: | |
| Drugs:* | Antibiotics (e.g., penicillin, sulfonamides) |
| Sera | Foreign proteins (e.g., vaccines or medications made from animal serum such as insulin, tetanus antitoxin, rabies antitoxin, snakebite antitoxin) |
| | Local anesthetics (e.g., Novocain) |
| | Salicylates (e.g., aspirin compounds) |
| | Diagnostic contrast media |
| | Plasma expanders, blood and blood products |
| | Barbiturates and narcotics (e.g., codeine, Demerol) |
| | Muscle relaxants (e.g., Robaxin) |
| Foods: | Legumes (soybeans, peanuts) |
| | Nuts and seeds |
| | Shellfish (lobster, shrimp, clams, crabs) |
| | Egg albumin |
| | Cereals (wheat, corn) |
| | Fish (salmon, cod) |
| | Milk products |
| | Chocolate |
| | Fruits (berries, bananas, oranges) |
| Additives: | Food coloring agents |
| | Preservatives (e.g., sodium bisulfite, monosodium glutamate, tartrazine, and sodium benzoate) |
| Bee Stings/Insect Bites: | Honey bee, wasp, hornet, yellow jacket, fire ant, and deer fly |
| Snake vemon: | Pit vipers (e.g., rattlesnakes, cottonmouths, and copperheads) |
| Environmental Factors: | Sunlight, cold, exercise, heat, pollens, molds, and spores. |

*Drugs administered by the parenteral route rank highest as the causes of anaphylactic shock. Anaphylaxis to penicillin is a well-known phenomenon, but fatal reactions to oral penicillin are rare. Beta-blockade can apparently potentiate anaphylactic reactions to penicillin and unusually aggressive treatment may be necessary to reverse the shock state.[6]

uals with general allergies and/or asthma are not necessarily at greater risk for anaphylactic shock.

While *prevention* of anaphylaxis would be the best defense, it is difficult to recognize high-risk groups. After surviving 1 reaction, the individual must create an environment with limited or no exposure to that allergen. Health histories are beneficial in identifying persons who have had previous reactions, but they will not help to distinguish the remaining high-risk persons in our general population.

### Chemical Mediators

The degranulation of mast cells releases chemical mediators into the tissues and circulation. The major mediator is histamine, which is released in large doses. Histamine causes smooth muscles to contract, blood capillaries to dilate, and capillary permeability to increase. The resulting fluid shift and vascular dilation progress to a sudden and severe drop in blood pressure and cardiac output. The contraction of smooth muscle results in constriction of the bladder, uterus, intestines, and bronchioles of the lungs. Respiratory distress, bronchospasm and laryngospasm, and severe abdominal cramps ensue. The increased capillary permeability leads to a shift of fluid, blood, plasma proteins, and leukocytes from the vascular system into the interstitial space. While this change in permeability is beneficial to promote healing in tissue injuries, the degree seen in anaphylactic shock causes so great a response that it becomes a threat to life itself.

Serotonin is another mediator released from mast cells. It also increases capillary permeability, particularly in the lungs. As plasma leaks into the alveoli, the integrity of the alveolar–capillary membrane (see Figs. 28–5, and 28–11) becomes disrupted, impairing gas exchange. Unless the process can be reversed quickly, hypoxemia and hypercapnia will ensue. Leakage of plasma into the alveoli also precipitates pulmonary edema (see Fig. 34–1), which can quickly become fatal if not arrested.

Other substances released from mast cells include bradykinins, platelet-activating factor, eosinophil chemotactic factor, and prostaglandins (see Table 61–3). A list of chemical mediators and their physiologic activity is presented in Table 67–3.

The slow-reacting substance of anaphylaxis (SRS-A) has similar effects on the body as does histamine, except that it is slower and more prolonged. This slower response follows the more rapid histamine response and must be considered when treating patients in anaphylactic shock (i.e., a relapse can result if the patient is discharged prematurely). Thus, patients require not only adequate treatment, but extended observation.

## Diagnosis

A carefully elicited history is essential to the diagnosis and treatment of the patient with anaphylac-

TABLE 67-3
**Chemical Mediators: Actions and Physiologic Effects**

| Mediator | Actions/Physiologic Effects |
|---|---|
| 1. Histamine | • Increases vascular permeability causing fluid shifts from the circulation to the interstitial space.<br>• Decreased cardiac output associated with diminished circulating blood volume, decreased venous return, and altered cardiac contractility.<br>• Hypotension caused by fluid shifts and vasodilation.<br>• Dysrhythmias associated with decreased coronary artery perfusion and hypoxia.<br>• Smooth muscle contraction resulting in bronchospasm.<br>• Pulmonary edema.<br>• Urticaria and pruritus. |
| 2. Slow-reacting substance of anaphylaxis (SRS-A) (Leukotriene) | • Increases vascular permeability that predisposes to fluid shifts from the intravascular to interstitial space resulting in: Hypotension, decreased venous return, and decreased cardiac output.<br>• Causes smooth muscle contraction resulting in bronchospasm. |
| 3. Platelet activating factor. | • Triggers platelet aggregation with release of histamine and serotonin. |
| 4. Eosinophil chemotactic factor of anaphylaxis (ECF-A) | • Stimulates unidirectional migration of eosinophils to the tissue sites involved in allergic inflammation.<br>• Exact role of ECF-A remains unclear. |
| 5. Prostaglandins (D and F) | • Cause smooth muscle contraction and vasodilation resulting in bronchospasm and hypotension. |
| 6. Serotonin (5-hydroxytryptamine) | • Increases capillary permeability especially in the lungs; predisposes to noncardiogenic pulmonary edema. |
| 7. Bradykinin | • Causes smooth muscle contraction and increases capillary permeability. |

tic shock. An attempt should be made to identify the following: (1) the specific allergen; (2) the patient's initial exposure to the allergen; (3) the type of reaction triggered by the allergen including signs and symptoms, and the interval of time between the exposure and the initial symptoms; and (4) what was done to treat the problem.

Typically, the patient with atopy relates a history of a previous reaction to a specific antigen. A family history of allergies is commonly positive, although the clinical presentation in each member may vary.

Characteristically, most cases of anaphylaxis have a rapid onset occurring within minutes of exposure to an allergen. Occasionally, the response may not develop for as long as an hour post-exposure. It is imperative that nurses monitor anyone who has been in contact with a potential allergen, for at least 1 hour. This observation period should be employed when high-risk patients have received any known allergen, as, for example, the administration of medications or an x-ray contrast medium. Patients who are victims of insect stings or who have ingested a food allergen must likewise be observed.

For patients with life-threatening food allergies, avoidance may be difficult. Many food offenders, such as peanuts and fish, are used as food extenders, thickeners, and taste enhancers. For these potential victims, anaphylaxis may begin as the food allergen passes into the intestinal mucosal surface. The reaction may also be biphasic (i.e., the initial symptoms are immediate, and, as the food is digested, the symptoms reappear 6–8 hours later).[3]

A reaction may occur after the first contact with the allergen, although the individual will usually relate a history of slight reaction from a previous exposure. A nursing history is mandatory before administering any medications or other suspected allergens. Specific symptomatology may include complaints of a new rash, pruritus, hoarseness, difficulty breathing, and apprehension. Urticaria, either localized or diffuse, may be evident on physical examination. Pitting edema and angioedema may also be observed. (Angioedema describes a condition characterized by urticaria and the development of edematous areas of the skin and mucous membranes.) Respiratory distress associated with laryngospasm or severe bronchospasm may be reflected clinically as strider or severe wheezing, respectively (see Chap. 29). Hypotension and vascular collapse occur in profound anaphylaxis.

## Clinical Presentation

### *Early Phase*

Initially, the patient may be observed to be restless, apprehensive, uneasy, or fearful. Minor complaints may include lightheadedness and/or paresthesias (e.g., abnormal sensations of burning or tingling). Pruritus may develop with local or generalized urticaria. As fluid shifts between intravascular and interstitial spaces occur, angioedema may become evident. Edema may be observed particularly in the face (lips and eyelids), tongue, and hands, as well as feet, and possibly the genitalia.

### *Intermediate Phase*

With progression to the intermediate phase, patients experiencing laryngospasm and bronchospasm may be observed to be increasingly dyspneic and wheezing. They may also appear exhausted from the increased work of breathing. As fluid shifts progress, pulmonary edema develops along with abdominal cramps, diarrhea, and vomiting. Smooth muscle contraction may lead to incontinence of urine and, in women, uterine bleeding.

#### Advanced Phase

As fluid shifts continue, the circulatory system experiences a marked decrease in blood volume. Hypotension, tachycardia, and ECG changes that mimic myocardial infarction may occur. These changes include ST segment elevation and T wave flattening (see Chap. 43). Respiratory distress occurs as laryngeal edema obstructs the airway and severe pulmonary edema prevents adequate gas exchange. The respiratory complications and circulatory collapse contribute to the high death rate associated with anaphylaxis.

## Therapeutic Management

The best treatment for anaphylactic shock is *prevention*. The initial emergent treatment is to halt the spread of the antigenic agent. In the case of an insect sting on an extremity, for example, obstructing the venous and lymph circulation with a tourniquet will help reduce the allergen's entry into the systemic circulation. The tourniquet must be loosened every 15 minutes until definitive treatment (e.g., intravenous fluids and vasopressors, if necessary) is available. Application of ice to the affected area may also assist in preventing spread of the allergen by the circulation.

In the scenario of an insect sting, scraping off the stinger from the epidermis will also diminish absorption of the antigen. Never try to pinch or pull out the stinger with the fingertips or tweezers because this may only squeeze or inject more of the venom or toxin into the wound. The patient may display only early clinical manifestations of anaphylactic shock if the initial interventions have been successful. An antihistamine, such as diphenhydramine (Benadryl), is frequently administered as part of the initial treatment.

Should the anaphylactic shock state progress to an advanced stage, maintaining a patent airway becomes the majority priority. The leading cause of death from anaphylaxis is laryngeal edema with airway obstruction. For patients experiencing upper airway (e.g., laryngeal edema or spasm) and/or lower airway (e.g., bronchospasm) obstruction, epinephrine administered subcutaneously is the drug of choice. This drug counteracts the adverse effects of histamine. If there is a delay in establishing an intravenous access, this medication can be instilled directly into the tracheobronchial tree by the endotracheal route. When antigen exposure occurs in an extremity, one third of the initial epinephrine dose may be given directly into the wound site.[4] Table 67-4 may be used as a reference guide for epinephrine dosages, but it should be understood that it is only a *guide*. Considerable controversy exists as to specific dosages and administration of epinephrine. In addition to dosage and route of administration, this table also includes mechanism of action of epinephrine and nursing implications in its use.

Other medications are frequently given in conjunction with epinephrine or to patients whose conditions are refractory to treatment (see Table 67-4). Intravenous aminophylline (theophylline) is usually administered to relieve bronchospasm. Corticosteroids may also be prescribed, but their effect is not beneficial immediately. Respiratory support with mechanical ventilation and oxygenation may be necessary. In the scenario of unstable hemodynamics and vascular collapse, oxygen therapy, intravenous fluid administration, and intravenous epinephrine therapy are initiated. Benadryl and other antihistamines are useful only to control local itching, if present, and edema. Such drugs are not effective in the treatment of bronchospasm or airway obstruction. (See Appendix A for information related to adverse reactions and implications for nursing care of the above mentioned drugs, namely, epinephrine, aminophylline, and corticosteroids.)

#### Therapeutic Modalities

In addition to drug therapy, other therapeutic modalities that function synergistically to raise blood pressure are employed. Intravenous fluids are administered aggressively to restore the circulating blood volume so as to maintain perfusion to vital organs. Fluid resuscitation, initially, may not reverse the vasogenic hypovolemia. However, the concomitant administration of epinephrine, which exerts its sympathomimetic effect by increasing peripheral vascular resistance, heart rate, and stroke volume, functions synergistically to augment blood pressure.

In patients who are already intubated, a simple measure to treat hypotension, although controversial, is to place the patient in a supine position and elevate the leg. This increases venous return to the heart, thus increasing cardiac output with a consequent increase in systemic blood pressure and tissue perfusion. A similar goal is achieved with use of the pneumatic antishock garment (PASG). This treatment modality, likewise controversial, continues to be used in treating hypotensive patients with bee-sting anaphylaxis with some success, and it has been useful in other forms of "low-flow" shock[5] (see Chap. 46).

Vasopressors (e.g., dopamine) may be necessary

TABLE 67-4
**Drugs Used to Treat Anaphylaxis**

| | |
|---|---|
| **Epinephrine** | |
| ***Clinical Manifestations*** | Dosage* |
| Early | • 0.1–0.5 ml of 1 : 1000 SQ, or IM. SQ doses may be repeated at 10–15 min intervals as necessary. The site should be massaged vigorously to increase absorption.<br>• The SQ route may be safer because it is absorbed more slowly. If the patient is experiencing hives and bronchospasm, but can still maintain a patent airway, SQ or IM dosages can be continued. If the patient's condition deteriorates, or if the blood pressure falls, the IV route may be indicated. |
| Severe | • 0.1–0.25 ml of 1 : 1000 or 1.0–2.5 ml of 1 : 10,000 IV. Any patient who is unconscious should be treated by this route.<br>• A SQ injection given to a patient who is in shock may not be effective because of poor absorption and impaired circulation.<br>• Epinephrine has a rapid antagonistic effect on histamine. The patient needs close monitoring for the alpha and beta agonist properties of this drug. Too much alpha stimulation can elevate the blood pressure to the point of causing cerebral hemorrhage, while too much beta stimulation can lead to myocardial ischemia, angina, and dysrhythmias.<br>• Benadryl (diphenhydramine), a drug commonly prescribed for the atopic patient, will not prevent histamine release, or neutralize circulating histamine. It will compete with released histamine at the receptor binding sites and block further absorption. This drug may be given with epinephrine and may be all the treatment the patient requires. |
| **Supplemental Drugs, and Drugs Used to Treat Refractory Anaphylaxis** | |
| Aminophylline | • Loading dose: 6 mg/kg administered over 30 min; not to exceed 25 mg/min.<br>• Maintenance dose: 0.5–0.7 mg/kg/hr (nonsmoking adult).<br>• Desired effect is to reduce bronchospasm.<br>• Adverse effects include hypotension and tachydysrhythmias. |
| Hydrocortisone | • 100 mg IV, q 6 hr.<br>• Inhibits the formation of preformed mediators. Decreases severity of symptoms. Increases the number of receptor sites available for sympathomimetic interaction.<br>• Controversy exists surrounding its benefits. |
| Atropine | • 0.4–0.6 mg IV or IM, may be repeated every 4–6 hr.<br>• Relaxes bronchial smooth muscle and inhibits tracheal secretions.<br>• The absolute clinical benefits are yet to be determined. |
| Dopamine | • 2–5 mcg/kg/min IV; may be increased gradually up to 20 to 50 mcg/kg/min, if necessary.<br>• Clinical effects include alpha and beta adrenergic stimulation.<br>• Adverse effects include headache, tachydysrhythmias, anginal pain, and dyspnea, among many others. |
| Levophed | • 4–8 mcg/kg/min continuous IV. Dosage is highly individualized according to patient's response.<br>• A potent, direct acting sympathomimetic that maintains blood pressure.<br>• Adverse effects include several hypertension, cardiac dysrhythmias, and extravasation necrosis. |
| Benadryl | • 25–50 mg PO, IM, or IV.<br>• Inhibits already released histamine effect.<br>• Contraindicated in acute asthma and narrow-angled glaucoma. |

*Source: Govoni and Hayes: Drugs and Nursing Implications, ed 5. Appleton-Century-Crofts, Norwalk, Connecticut, 1985.
*Note:* Dosages and strengths indicated here are only meant to be a guide. Actual doses administered depend upon the physician's prescription, hospital protocol, and response of patient to therapy.

to stabilize the patient hemodynamically and to increase cardiac output. Corticosteroids (e.g., Solu-Medrol) may be administered to stabilize lysosomal membranes, maintain intravascular volume, and preclude further fluid imbalances. However, as mentioned previously, the effects of corticosteroid therapy may not be immediately nor definitely apparent.

Once ventilation and circulation are restored, comfort measures and education can be employed. The patient and family/significant others must be taught preventive strategies and emergency interventions before discharge. Post-anaphylactic shock, patients need instructions to eliminate the allergen from their surroundings. If this is impossible due to the patient's lifestyle, immunotherapy (hyposensitization) is initiated. Cutaneous tests are used to evaluate the immune system's ability to respond to known allergens.

### Hyposensitization

The basic problem in most atopic or allergic patients is that they produce too many IgE antibodies. Therefore, a goal of hyposensitization or desensitization therapy is to reduce the amount of IgE antibody produced within the body in response to a specific allergen (antigen). This is accomplished by administering a long series of injections of the allergen, beginning initially with low doses, and gradually increasing the amount until the patient's tolerance increases. The resulting tolerance may be induced by increasing the population of T-suppressor cells specific for the allergen in question.

The mechanism underlying this form of immunotherapy is thought to involve a proliferation of the population of T-suppressor cells specific for the allergen in question. Unfortunately, this is not always effective. Injections may be given throughout the year or beginning 3–6 months before the season starts, depending on the type of allergen. Treatments may continue for years or until the patient is free of allergic symptomatology. (For a discussion of T-suppressor cells, see Chap. 54.)

### *Patient Teaching and Prevention*

Patients with a known history of hypersensitivity should be instructed to wear a Medic-Alert bracelet. Any individual who experiences a severe systemic reaction from a bee sting, a bite, or other various causes needs an allergy referral for further evaluation and care. Patients who have had or who are presently undergoing hyposensitization therapy should be reminded that immunotherapy is not a cure, but can provide protection against further exposure to the particular allergen(s).

Instruction regarding continuity of care post-anaphylactic shock should be individualized according to each patient's particular allergy history and may include some of the discharge instructions and follow-up recommendations listed in Table 67–5. The patient and at least one family member should be able to verbalize emergency first aid measures that should be performed should the patient develop anaphylaxis. Commercial kits, available for this purpose, can readily be purchased with a physician's prescription. The patient and family member will need guidance and instruction in its appropriate use. Should the patient be apprehensive about self-injection, pocket pressure nebulizers are available, but these are less effective than the more rapid injectable methods available.

Effective immunotherapy for insect sting prophylaxis is specific venom therapy. However, the patient's history may not reveal what the causative insect was that precipitated the attack. If the patient can bring the dead vector to the treatment center, absolute identification and treatment with the appropriate antidote may be possible. If the causative vector is unknown, a mixture of venoms may be administered.

Upon discharge following an anaphylactic episode, the patient must be instructed to avoid any medication or activity that induces a state of vasodilatation. Therefore, after anaphylaxis treatment, patients must avoid vasodilator drugs and alcoholic beverages. They should also avoid strenuous exercise and hot showers or baths for at least 24–36 hours.

TABLE 67–5
**Patient Teaching: Prophylaxis**

The following include key nursing considerations for patient/family instruction regarding follow-up and preventative care:

1. The patient must be responsible for informing all health care personnel of specific medications, foods, etc., that elicit a hypersensitivity response. It is highly recommended that the patient wear a "medic alert" bracelet or tag.
2. As an outpatient, the patient can expect to wait 30–60 minutes after any injection so that direct observation can guarantee the patient is allergy-free.
3. At least one member of the family should be versed in emergency first aid measures in the event the patient develops anaphylaxis.
4. Patient/family must be aware of high-risk situations, and have access to information regarding insect-breeding areas, and characteristics of vectors.

**Insect Anaphylaxis: Self-Protective Measures**

1. Caution is needed when near insect habitats such as flowering and fruit shrubbery or fields.
2. Clothing can be sprayed with repellent, and long-sleeved shirts, long pants, and shoes should be worn whenever possible for outings.
3. Insects are attracted to dark and bright clothing, as well as shiny jewelry.
4. Avoid aromatics such as fragrances and scented cosmetics.
5. Remain calm and still if insects swarm. Realize that warm weather increases insect numbers.
6. Avoid stings around the face and neck as these areas are vascular and the sting more threatening. Lie on the ground and/or cover the face with arms and hands.
7. Keep windows up in cars and use air conditioning whenever possible.

**Household Preventative Measures**

1. Limit shrubs and plants in and around the house. Keep screens and doors in good repair.
2. Consider hiring a professional gardener, or assign another family member to perform the garden chores.
3. Exterminate all nests and hives in the vicinity.
4. Wear garden gloves for all outdoor work.
5. Keep trash cans clean and sprayed with insecticide.

## Nursing Diagnosis, Desired Patient Outcomes, and Nursing Interventions

The case study that follows provides the assessment data used as the basis for care planning. See the Sample Care Plan for the patient with anaphylactic shock, for specific nursing diagnoses, desired patient outcomes, and nursing interventions.

## CASE STUDY WITH SAMPLE CARE PLAN: PATIENT WITH ANAPHYLACTIC SHOCK

J.P. is a 25-year-old housewife and dental hygienist who has a history of sulfonamide allergy and allergies to dust, pollen, molds, and mildew. Her medical history reveals a diagnosis of rheumatoid arthritis within the last 3 months. Tonight, 10 minutes

## SAMPLE CARE PLAN FOR THE PATIENT WITH ANAPHYLACTIC SHOCK

| Nursing Diagnoses | Desired Patient Outcomes | Nursing Interventions | Rationales |
|---|---|---|---|
| ***Nursing Diagnosis #1*** Airway clearance, ineffective: actual or potential related to:<br>1. Bronchospasm, laryngospasm.<br>2. Increased pulmonary secretions in response to release of chemical mediators from degranulated mast cells. | Patient will:<br>1. Maintain adequate alveolar ventilation and oxygenation:<br>• $PaCO_2 \sim 35-45$ mmHg (room air).<br>• $PaO_2 > 60$ mmHg.<br>• pH 7.35–7.45.<br>2. Verbalize ease of breathing; breath sounds clear on auscultation; absence of adventitious breath sounds.<br>3. Verbalize reduced anxiety; perform relaxation exercises: demonstrate a relaxed demeanor. | • Assess respiratory function:<br>○ Respiratory parameters: Respiratory rate, rhythm; diaphragmatic excursion; use of accessory muscles; | • It is essential to establish baseline function to facilitate evaluating the patient's response to therapeutic measures. |
| | | ○ Presence of abnormal or adventitious breath sounds on auscultation. | ○ Adventitious sounds are noted with special emphasis placed on the presence of stridor and wheezing. Inspiratory wheezes and stridor are ominous signs. |
| | | ○ Neurological parameters: Mental status: Orientation to person, place, and date. | ○ A deterioration in the level of consciousness may be the first warning sign of inadequate oxygenation and tissue perfusion. |
| | | ○ Cardiovascular parameters: Vital signs.<br>○ Arterial blood gas parameters. | |
| | | • Implement measures to assure a patent airway:<br>○ Maintain upright position. | ○ Upright position allows for chest wall expansion and diaphragmatic excursion; accessory muscles can be utilized to the fullest. |
| | | ○ Place suction and intubation equipment at the bedside. | ○ Suction equipment, etc., is needed for prophylactic readiness in case laryngospasm or edema compromises the airway. |
| | | ○ Initiate oxygen therapy as prescribed (e.g., nasal cannula at 2 liters/min). | ○ Oxygen prevents hypoxia and consequent respiratory acidemia. |
| | | ○ Obtain baseline arterial blood gases (room air) prior to initiating oxygen therapy.<br>○ Monitor serial arterial blood gas parameters. | ○ Monitoring of arterial blood gases provides a direct indication as to the effectiveness of therapeutic measures in assisting the patient to maintain adequate gas exchange. |
| | | • Administer medication regimen as prescribed:<br>○ Anticipate subcutaneous injection of epinephrine. | ○ Subcutaneous route may be safer because it is more slowly absorbed. There are fewer adrenergic side effects. Epinephrine will help to control bronchospasm, and improve ventilation. |
| | | ○ Implement Alupent treatments in conjunction with the Respiratory Therapy department as per physician. | ○ Alupent, a frequently used adrenergic agent, stimulates beta receptors and thus exerts the following effects: Bronchodilation, positive inotropic and chronotropic cardiac activity, and decreased synthesis and release of chemical mediators by mast cells. |

*(continued)*

## SAMPLE CARE PLAN FOR THE PATIENT WITH ANAPHYLACTIC SHOCK *(Continued)*

| Nursing Diagnoses | Desired Patient Outcomes | Nursing Interventions | Rationales |
|---|---|---|---|
| ***Nursing Diagnosis #1 (cont.)*** | | • Provide restful and calm environment to reduce tensions and anxiety.<br>∘ Spend time at the patient's bedside.<br>∘ Keep abreast of progress.<br>∘ Instruct regarding relaxation exercises.<br>∘ Provide periods of uninterrupted rest and/or sleep. | |
| ***Nursing Diagnosis #2***<br>Fluid volume deficit, actual or potential, related to:<br>1. Vasodilation.<br>2. Increased capillary permeability with increased third-spacing (angioedema). | Patient will:<br>1. Maintain stable vital signs:<br>• Blood pressure within 10 mmHg of baseline.<br>– Heart rate < 100 beats/min.<br>2. Remain without evidence of third-spacing (e.g., no angioedema or pitting edema). | • Monitor vital signs, particularly blood pressure and heart rate.<br>• Monitor intake and output hourly.<br>• Implement prescribed fluid regimen.<br>∘ Initiate intravenous therapy with lactated Ringer's solution (fluids may need to be infused wide open).<br>∘ Anticipate repeated doses of SQ epinephrine, followed by intravenous administration if there is no clinical improvement. | • An increase in blood pressure and decrease in heart rate may be indicative of restoring circulatory volume and cardiac output.<br>• Renal function parallels normal cardiac output and normovolemia. Urine output should be maintained at > 30 ml/hour.<br>• Initial fluid challenges must be monitored in relation to patient's clinical status.<br>∘ Ringer's lactate is the most compatible physiologic (isotonic) solution and can be infused at a rapid rate in an attempt to stabilize intravascular volume.<br>∘ Epinephrine is an endogenous catecholamine that stimulates both alpha and beta receptors. It will increase the heart rate and myocardial contractility; it will increase systemic vascular resistance and thereby increase arterial blood pressure. It may be necessary to give epinephrine intravenously since peripheral perfusion may be inadequate for SQ or IM injection if the shock state progresses. The intravenous route is fast and efficacious, but when this route is unavailable, epinephrine may be instilled directly into the endotracheal tube after intubation (as prescribed). |

| | | | |
|---|---|---|---|
| ***Nursing Diagnosis #3***<br>Anxiety related to:<br>1. Respiratory distress (hypoxia and dyspnea stimulate flight/fight responses and emotional distress).<br>2. Hypotensive state. | Patient will:<br>1. Verbalize ways to reduce stress and avoid panicking.<br>2. Assume a relaxed demeanor. | • Implement measures to assist patient/family to maintain control and react appropriately in the event of an emergency.<br>∘ Assist patient to assume a position of comfort — may try orthopnea.<br>∘ Allow patient decision-making alternatives.<br>∘ Speak in a calm, soothing voice.<br>∘ Offer optimistic reassurances.<br>∘ Do not leave patient unattended.<br>∘ Keep patient/family informed of treatments and progress.<br>∘ Consider the sedative effects of drugs such as Benadryl to assist in managing anxiety. | ∘ Facilitates ease of breathing and may relieve respiratory distress.<br>∘ Anxiety may be decreased when patients are permitted decision-making power.<br>∘ Choices facilitate autonomy and self-control.<br>∘ There are positive psychological benefits derived from reassurances.<br>∘ Fear is perpetuated when patient is left alone. The patient's condition may deteriorate rapidly.<br>∘ Fear of the unknown is alleviated.<br>∘ Benadryl can be used as an adjunct epinephrine therapy, after the acute symptoms are controlled. |
| ***Nursing Diagnosis #4***<br>Skin integrity, impairment of, related to:<br>1. Severe urticaria with pruritus | Patient will:<br>1. Avoid scratching.<br>2. Demonstrate ways to avoid scratching (e.g., massaging with prescribed lotion).<br>3. Maintain intact skin, with absence of angioedema. | • Implement measures to relieve itching and maintain skin integrity:<br>∘ Apply cool compresses to affected areas, PRN.<br>∘ Remove all unnecessary clothing/bedding.<br>∘ Instruct patient to avoid scratching; if all else fails, instruct patient to use fingertips rather than nails, and to use a massaging motion.<br>∘ Administer Benadryl as prescribed.<br>∘ A prescription may be given upon discharge that includes oral Benadryl and/or a topical cream. | ∘ Cool temperatures reduce the discomfort that coincides with pruritus and angioedema.<br>∘ Removal of clothing sometimes relieves itching and feelings of constriction.<br>∘ Scratching disrupts skin integrity, the first line of defense against infection.<br>∘ Benadryl competes with histamine for the histamine receptor sites. It effectively controls localized itching.<br>∘ Since some chemical mediators (e.g., SRS-A) have slower and more prolonged action, an antihistamine and local, topical agents may be prescribed to counteract the annoying skin eruptions (urticaria). |

*(continued)*

## SAMPLE CARE PLAN FOR THE PATIENT WITH ANAPHYLACTIC SHOCK *(Continued)*

| Nursing Diagnoses | Desired Patient Outcomes | Nursing Interventions | Rationales |
|---|---|---|---|
| ***Nursing Diagnosis #5*** Knowledge deficit related to:<br>1. Inability to identify allergen (allergen was disguised as a preservative).<br>2. Delay in receiving treatment (driving to distant hospital rather than the one nearby; this may have exacerbated the shock-state). | Patient will:<br>1. Review sources of sulfur preparations.<br>2. Discuss cross-reactivity with allergens.<br>3. Verbalize need to expedite emergency treatment upon exposure to allergen(s). | • Assess patient/family knowledge regarding allergic status: Known allergens; precautions taken to avoid exposure to allergen(s); emergency care with onset of allergic reaction. | • Assessing patient/family knowledge base regarding anaphylaxis assists in determining essential information to include in patient/family instruction; it may also help to discern misunderstandings that might complicate the patient's care. |
| | | • Assess readiness to learn.<br>○ Identify support system in family. | • It is imperative that one or more family members be versed in emergency first-aid measures should the patient develop anaphylactic shock. |
| | | • Implement patient/family education program:<br>○ Teach the importance of reading all labels. | ○ Sulfiting agents (e.g., sulfur, sodium or potassium bisulfate or sodium sulfite) are commonly used as antioxidants and food preservatives. Potatoes, shellfish, and wines are just a few items that contain sulfites. |
| | | ○ Reinforce responsibility to notify all health professionals of specific allergies. | ○ Patients are active participants as well as recipients of interdisciplinary health care. |
| | | ○ Encourage patient to wear a "medic alert" tag/bracelet. | ○ Identification of the allergen or anaphylactoid reaction may be lifesaving, especially if only minutes can be spared. |
| | | ○ Recommend an allergy referral. | ○ Clients who experience severe systemic reactions need a referral for further evaluation and care. |
| | | ○ Inform patient/family that treatment must be sought immediately as subsequent reactions may be more severe. | ○ Phase two reactions cause chemical mediators to be released into the blood, since the patient is already sensitized (i.e., has preformed IgE antibody from initial exposure). Treatment must be solicited at *nearest* hospital, via ambulance if necessary. |

NOTE: Effective August 1987, the FDA has banned the use of sulfite agents on fruits and vegetables intended for raw consumption. Also, effective January 1987, foods and nonalcoholic beverages must be labeled when sulfites are present in detectable amounts. Individuals can now test for sulfites right at the table just by dipping a test strip into the suspect food or drink. A simple color change indicates the presence of sulfites.[7]

after eating dried apricots, she developed warmth, flushing, and a maculopapular rash that quickly became generalized. She read the container label and discovered the apricots were preserved with a sulfur preparation.

Her husband drove her to the emergency department about 20 miles away, although another hospital was within a 5-mile distance from their home. On arrival, she presents with shortness of breath, diaphoresis, no fever, pulse 110/min and regular, respirations 28/min, and blood pressure 150/86. Ms. P. is anxious, and between breaths blurts out that she thought that she would never make it to the hospital. "I cannot catch my breath; my throat feels tight." Angioedema is seen on her lips and hands. Five minutes later, she becomes hypotensive.

## Initial Nursing Diagnoses

1. Airway clearance, ineffective, related to:
   a. Bronchospasm, laryngospasm.
   b. Increased pulmonary secretions.
2. Fluid volume deficit, related to:
   a. Vasodilation.
   b. Increased capillary permeability.
3. Anxiety, related to:
   a. Respiratory distress.
   b. Hypotensive state.
4. Skin integrity, impairment of, related to severe urticaria.
5. Knowledge deficit, related to:
   a. Inability to identify allergen.
   b. Delay in receiving treatment.

## REFERENCES

1. Dickerson, M: Anaphylaxis and anaphylactic shock. Crit Care Nurs Q 11(1):68, 1988.
2. Allergic to what he eats. Emerg Med 19(2):22, 1987.
3. Hill, J: Emergency anaphylaxis. Hosp Med 23(1):19, 1987.
4. Maybee, J: Anaphylaxis an emergency medicine overview. Emerg Med 10(11):17, 1986.
5. Suit up against anaphylaxis. Emerg Med 17(7):127, 1985.
6. Beta blockers and penicillin anaphylaxis. Nurses' Drug Alert 10(5):38, 1986.
7. A continuing education service for physicians and nutritionists. Nutrition and the M.D. 12(10):1, 1986.

CHAPTER 68

# Nursing Management of the Patient with Acute Poisoning

*Thomas E. Kearney*

## CHAPTER OUTLINE



## LEARNING OBJECTIVES

**At the end of this chapter, you should be able to:**

1. Discuss the incidence of acute poisoning, populations at high risk, and its impact on health-care resources.
2. Define *poisoning exposure* and its specific characteristics in terms of duration of exposure, reasons for exposure, route of exposure, and adverse reactions.
3. List major categories of substances involved in acute poisoning.
4. Identify community and governmental resources available to prevent or control the incidence of acute poisoning, and to treat it, should it occur.
5. Describe the major components of the assessment of the poison victim and implications for nursing care.
6. Examine mechanisms of toxicity of the most common toxic agents.
7. Define *decontamination* as a therapeutic modality for acute poisoning and indications for its use.
8. Differentiate therapeutic approaches and implications for nursing care in the decontamination of the following: dermal and ocular exposures, inhalations, and ingestion.
9. Delineate the nursing process in the care of a patient with acute poisoning, including:
   Assessment
   Diagnosis
   Planning: Desired patient outcomes
   Nursing interventions/rationales.

Poisonings are a major health problem in the United States, resulting in long-term disability, major expenditures in health-care dollars and manpower, and even deaths. The causes of poisoning are continually changing due to the proliferation of new chemicals and drugs, the reformulation of household products, environmental contamination, as well as to a variety of socioeconomic factors such as the stability of the nuclear family, dual-career families, job-related stress, an aging society, cost-containment of health care, and a myriad of other factors that may influence our daily environments. Health-care professionals must appreciate the factors that interplay in the problem as a whole, to improve readiness and heighten awareness to deal with this complex issue.

The poisoning problem requires a multidisciplinary team approach to manage a diverse set of issues ranging from prevention of poisoning accidents in the home to supporting a critically ill poisoned patient in the Intensive Care Unit. Nursing professionals have played an integral role in poisoning as educators, poison information specialists employed in Regional Poison Control Centers, and in the provision of care to poisoned victims in outpatient and inpatient settings. An understanding of the epidemiology, resources, assessment, pathophysiology, and treatment concepts for poisonings is important to enhance the delivery of adequate and appropriate care to the poisoned patient.

Many recent major advances have occurred in the field of clinical toxicology in the areas of prevention, epidemiology, the development of new pharmacologic antagonists, increased understanding of the mechanisms of toxicity of chemicals and drugs, new technologic advances in extracorporeal removal of toxins and analytical methodologies, use of antibodies in the treatment of poisonings (immunotoxicology), the emergence of new areas of research in clinical toxicology such as toxicokinetics (the study of the absorption, distribution, and excretions of poisons), the recognition of activated charcoal in the therapeutic armamentarium for poisoning and its use to enhance the elimination of toxins by "gastrointestinal dialysis," improved supportive care of the poisoned patient, the recognition of clinical toxicology as a discipline, as well as the nationwide development of sophisticated networks of expertise to manage the poisoning problem through organizations known as Regional Poison Control Centers.

It has been suggested that the morbidity and mortality of poisoning in the United States has decreased over the past 25 years.[1] This may be attributable to any or all of these advances in the prevention and treatment of poisonings. However, many traditional viewpoints or dogmas on the approach to the poisoned patient have undergone recent scrutiny, especially in the area of first aid for poisoning.

## EPIDEMIOLOGY

The National Data Collection System of the American Association of Poison Control Centers (AAPCC) has emerged as the most comprehensive epidemiologic data collection system on poisonings to date. This system has the advantages of being standardized in a format amenable to rapid computer analysis, and is comprised of human poisonings reported to Poison Control Centers across the United States. In 1985, this data system had tabulated 900,513 human poisoning exposures.[2] It has been estimated, based on the experience of this system and others, that anywhere from 4.8 to 10 million poisonings occur each year in the United States.[2,3]

To review and assess poison epidemiologic data, it is important to consider the definition of a poisoning exposure, as well as other terminology used in these epidemiologic databases. Specific terminology and definitions are included in Table 68–1.

Most of the poisonings can be characterized as acute, accidental, occurring in the home, and involving children less than 5 years of age. The circumstances in which poisonings occur may vary considerably. While most involve exposures to substances ingested by children in the home, some situations may include drug abuse, attempts at suicide, industrial workers exposed to toxic chemicals in the workplace, or entire communities exposed to hazardous waste, toxic fumes, and chemical spills.

The types of substances involved in poisonings can span the entire range of products within the

TABLE 68–1
**Poisoning Exposure: Terminology**

**Poisoning exposure:** Any suspected contact with any substance which when ingested, inhaled, absorbed, applied to, injected into, or developed within the body may cause damage to the structure or disturbance of function to living tissue.

*Duration of Exposure:*

**Acute:** A single exposure occurring over a relatively short period of time, usually within a period of 8 hours.

**Chronic:** A repeated exposure to the same substance, or single exposure lasting longer than 8 hours.

*Reasons for Exposure:*

**Accidental:** An unintended poisoning exposure; commonly involves situations where children gain access to a toxic substance in the home, where it is obvious that they did not realize the potential danger of their actions.

**Intentional:** Implies a purposeful action with an exposure that results from an inappropriate use of a substance for self-destructive, or manipulative reasons, such as a suicide gesture, or the improper use of a substance in an attempt to gain a psychotropic effect.

**Adverse reaction:** An unexpected reaction to a drug, food, or other agent; or the patient experiences an unwanted effect, which is usually due to either an allergic, hypersensitive, or idiosyncratic response at a normal dose, or with normal use of a substance.

*Routes of Exposure:*

**Oral:** Exposures to substances occurred because they were ingested into the gastrointestinal tract.

**Inhalation:** Exposure to gaseous or vaporized agents into the airways and lungs.

**Ocular:** Due to substances splashed directly into the eye.

**Dermal:** Contact with substances that may involve the skin, hair, fingernails, and clothing where direct irritation or percutaneous absorption may occur.

**Bites or stings:** Exposures resulting from the bite or sting of either an animal or insect, such as a bee, wasp, or hornet.

**Parenteral route:** An exposure resulting from the injection of a substance into the body, such as the intravenous administration of heroin.

home environment and community. Substances most frequently involved in poisonings also tend to be the ones most commonly available in the home environment. The substances involved in poisoning include a vast array of pharmaceutical and nonpharmaceutical products. The ranking of categories of substances according to their frequency of involvement in poisonings, as reported by the 1985 Annual Report of the AAPCC National Data Collection System,[2] lists pharmaceuticals, which include prescription and nonprescription drugs, most notably the over-the-counter analgesics such as aspirin and acetaminophen, as the major category of substances involved in poisoning. This substance category constituted approximately 40% of the total number of substances involved in poisoning. Ranking of additional categories involved in poisonings is presented in Table 68–2.

Although most poison victims are children, all age groups and socioeconomic levels are affected. More than 60% of poisonings involve children less than 5 years of age; approximately 8% involve adults. It has been recently observed[4,5] that due to the aging of our society, and special risks inherent with the elderly, the problem of geriatric poisoning has grown significantly and will probably continue to do so.

TABLE 68–2
**Common Categories of Substances Involved in Poisonings**

| Substance | Ranking: % of Total Number of Poisonings |
|---|---|
| **Cleaning substances** Household bleach, ammonia, cleansers, washing and laundry detergents | 9.5% |
| **Plants** Within home, in the yard, or in the wild | 8.3 |
| **Cosmetics and personal care products** Mouthwashes, aftershaves, colognes, perfumes, shampoos, nail polish | 5.8 |
| **Bites and envenomations** Snakes, spiders and stinging insects | 3.4 |
| **Pesticides and rodenticides** Agents to kill rodents and insects in the home environment; highly concentrated industrial agents used by professional exterminators | 2.9 |
| **Pharmaceuticals** Prescription and nonprescription (over-the-counter) drugs (e.g., aspirin, acetaminophen) | 40.0 |

## RESOURCES

### The Regional Poison Control Center Movement

During the 1950s, poisonings were recognized as a major pediatric problem, and health-care professionals became increasingly aware of the need to provide expertise during such emergencies.[6] Following a collaborative effort among local, state, and federal government officials, and other health-care interests, the first poison control center emerged in Chicago in 1953. Since that time, hundreds of others have been developed throughout the country. Unfortunately, many of these poison control centers were developed very haphazardly. There were no standards nor consistency in the qualifications of personnel, frequency of calls received, response procedures, or types of records maintained. As a result, the services they provided were erratic and unpredictable.

This fragmented, nonstandardized development of poison centers led to the regional poison control center movement, fostered by the AAPCC and the American College of Emergency Physicians (ACEP). These professional groups have established criteria for certification of regional poison control centers, which require that a Regional Poison Control Center offer services to a population base of at least 1 million people, and not greater than 10 million people. A Regional Poison Control Center must be open around the clock; staffed by trained, dedicated personnel; licensed in either pharmacy, nursing or medicine; and it must have a host of comprehensive resources and consultants to assist in the delivery of care to the poisoned patient.

The Regional Poison Control Center must understand and be able to interface with all health-care facilities and emergency transport systems throughout the region served. In addition, they provide functions such as interfacing with local, state, and federal agencies regarding hazards to the community. These may include product recalls, contaminated foods, widespread applications of pesticides, and chemical spills. In addition, a major responsibility of a Regional Poison Control Center is to provide education programs to inform the general public on how to use the poison center, what to do if a poisoning occurs, and how to prevent a poisoning from occurring. Education is also made available to physicians, nurses, pharmacists, paramedics, and other personnel involved in the treatment of poisoned patients.

It is important for all those in practice in a given region to identify their closest Regional Poison Control Center. Often, resources such as textbooks on poisoning or medicine are outdated and are unable to evolve with the recent advances in toxicology and the medical management of the poisoned victim. Poison centers have attempted to consolidate the expertise for a region, as well as keep abreast of the latest treatment, diagnostic, and analytical methodologies for poisoning.

## ASSESSMENT OF THE POISON VICTIM

The assessment of the poison victim entails the solicitation of a poisoning history, the physical examination of the poison patient, response to pharmacologic antagonists, as well as analysis of gastric contents, blood, and urine from the poison victim. It should be noted, especially with intentional exposures (drug abuse or suicide gestures), the agent involved in the poisoning is frequently unknown so that all four components of assessment as listed above, must be considered collectively.

### History

Often the initial contact with the poisoning will be from the site of the exposure when either the victim or the person managing the poison victim calls either a poison center, hospital, outpatient clinic, or other emergency service. Obtaining a complete and accurate poisoning history will be necessary to assess the immediacy of the situation and the toxic potential of the exposure, to identify medical treatments needed for the poison victim to support the patient's hemodynamic and respiratory systems, and to minimize the extent of the exposure. A thorough poison history is essential to triage decision-making for the poisoned patient. In addition, understanding the basic elements of a poison history will enhance the ability of the health-care professional to interface with the poison control center. Table 68–3 contains key questions and elements of the poison history.

### Physical Examination

The physical examination can determine the necessity for immediate supportive care measures and can confirm evidence of the poisoning. Following the physical examination, the findings must be viewed collectively to define a characteristic constellation of symptoms reflective of a particular toxic substance or group of substances. These characteristic constellations of symptoms are known as "toxidromes." For instance, anticholinergic poisoning from an agent such as atropine will cause a characteristic set of symptoms. A device to remember this toxidrome is: The patient with atropine poisoning will be "dry as a bone," "mad as a hatter," "red as a beet," and "blind as a bat." Table 68–4 lists the physical finding on examination and

TABLE 68–3
**Elements of a Poison History**

The following include basic questions and elements of a poison history:

**1. What was involved in the poisoning?**
This information may be difficult to ascertain because the substance involved in the poisoning may not be in the original container, products are frequently reformulated, and many poisonings are unsupervised. If possible, information regarding the substance should be obtained from the label on the container from which the substance was derived. Any patient transported to a hospital should be accompanied by the container with the substance involved in the poison incident.
At the site of exposure, it should be noted whether other substances could have been available to the poisoning victim, any evidence of open medicine containers and household products, or if there were any characteristic smells or odors.

**2. Who was involved in the poisoning?**
Characteristics of the poisoning victims such as age, weight, and past medical history are important components of the poisoning history. Poisonings involving older children, teenagers, and adults are more likely to be the result of an intentional exposure, in comparison with a victim less than 5 years of age. Weight can also be helpful because, for many toxins, the dose of the toxin in relation to the weight of the patient can be calculated to provide an expected range of toxicity.

**3. When did the poisoning occur?**
Knowing when the poisoning occurred helps to establish a causal relationship between a poison exposure and symptoms the patient is manifesting, as well as predicting upcoming symptomatology.

**4. Where did the poisoning occur?**
Knowing where the poisoning occurred is especially important for children, to assist with the determination of what product was involved. For instance, a child found in the bathroom may have access to a set of substances normally found in that area of the home such as toilet bowl cleaners, bleaches, medications in the medicine cabinet, versus a poisoning occurring in the yard, or the garage, where substances such as automotive products, pesticides, or garden care products are available.

**5. How much of the substance was involved in the poisoning?**
This question is important especially when a substance has been ingested. This can provide an estimation of the dose of a toxin that a victim was exposed to, which will allow an estimation of the toxic potential of the poisoning incident.

**6. What was the route or routes of exposure?**
In addition to ingestions, poisons may also be inhaled, come in direct contact with the eye, splashed on the skin, or be rejected. There are a significant number of poisons that do involve multiple routes of exposure. Each route of exposure requires a specialized decontamination procedure. Also, for each route, those tissues exposed to a toxin may incur direct injury, or may become a route of administration for systemic absorption.

**7. What symptoms has the patient had?**
Is the patient conscious? Is the patient breathing? Does the patient have a pulse? Are the symptoms likely to be related to the exposure?

**8. What was the reason for exposure?**
It is important to differentiate between an accidental versus an intentional exposure. As previously noted, many intentional exposures involve multiple drugs, have worse outcomes in terms of morbidity and mortality, and are often accompanied by inaccurate or incomplete histories. Therefore, they may require more aggressive therapy and monitoring.

**9. What first aid has been performed?**
It is important to determine whether or not the patient has had an adequate decontamination procedure performed. Many first-aid procedures can complicate the poisoning, such as the use of salt water as an emetic in children, which has resulted in fatalities due to hypernatremia.[7]

*(continued)*

TABLE 68–3
**Elements of a Poison History *(Continued)***

**10. What current medications is the patient on?**
The substances involved in a poisoning may interact with another medication that a patient is chronically administered for a therapeutic purpose. For example, a patient taking an MAO inhibitor who ingests a therapeutic dose of a sympathomimetic or decongestant, such as phenylpropanolamine, could develop a life-threatening hypertensive crisis.[8]

**11. What allergies does the patient have?**
Some patients are at risk for hypersensitivity reactions to medications, chemicals, and venoms. A patient who has previously been exposed and sensitized to hymenoptera venom may be at greater risk for an acute anaphylactic reaction when stung by a honey bee, wasp, or hornet (see Chap. 67).

**12. What other chronic disease states does the patient have?**
Many times, patients with chronic disease states will be at higher risk for severe toxicity to exposures of certain substances. For instance, elderly patients with cardiovascular disease are more sensitive to the effects of, and respond poorly to, exposures to carbon monoxide.[9,10]

**13. What is the race of the poison victim?**
A poison victim with an enzyme deficiency such as a G6PD deficiency, will be at greater risk for an acute hemolytic episode after ingestion of a mothball containing naphthalene than a patient without this enzyme deficiency.[11] It has been determined that certain populations such as blacks, or those of Mediterranean origin, have a higher incidence of this enzyme deficiency.[12]

the possible corresponding etiologic agents for each listed finding.

## Laboratory Studies

The laboratory can be a useful adjunct to the other forms of assessment. Qualitative screening tests for drugs and other substances are routinely run on urine samples. Quantitative tests are performed on blood, serum, or plasma samples. Analysis of gastric contents may allow the clinician to determine what was acutely ingested and to confirm exposure to a drug or chemical in some cases before significant systemic absorption has occurred. In some circumstances, a quantitative analysis of substances from the blood of the patient, such as methanol, ethylene glycol, acetaminophen, salicylate, iron, lead, arsenic, and mercury, may be necessary to determine if the substances are at toxic levels in the patient, and if the patient will require specialized therapies. For most other substances, a toxicology analysis is only necessary as confirmatory evidence of the substances ingested. It is of extreme importance to understand what toxicology tests are performed by your institution, as well as the turnaround time for their results.

## X-Ray Examination

An x-ray (radiograph) of the poison patient can provide an assessment of secondary complications from a poisoning episode, such as using a chest

TABLE 68–4
**Expected Physical and Laboratory Findings for Poisonous Substances**

| Finding | Substance |
|---|---|
| ***Blood Pressure*** | |
| Hypotension | Sedative-hypnotics (barbiturates, glutethimide), theophylline, iron, cyclic antidepressants, antihypertensives (Aldomet, clonidine). |
| Hypertension | Amphetamines, cocaine, phencyclidine, anticholinergics (atropine), black widow spider venom |
| ***Respirations*** | |
| Slowed rate-apnea | Opiates, alcohols, sedative-hypnotics |
| Hyperpnea, tachypnea | Salicylates, theophylline, dinitrophenol, CNS stimulants |
| ***Electrocardiogram (ECG)*** | |
| Bradyarrhythmia | Beta-blockers, clonidine, organophosphate insecticides, calcium channel blockers (verapamil) |
| Tachyarrhythmias | Amphetamines, cocaine, caffeine, theophylline, anticholinergics (atropine), cyclic antidepressants, nicotine |
| Conduction defects (PR, QRS, QT prolongation) | Cyclic antidepressants, quinidine, arsenic, mercury, propoxyphene, propranolol |
| ***Temperature*** | |
| Hyperthermia | Salicylates, amphetamine, cocaine, anticholinergics, dinitrophenol, phencyclidine |
| Hypothermia | Opiates, ethanol, sedative-hypnotics, phenothiazines |
| ***Pupils*** | |
| Miosis | Organophosphate insecticides, phenothiazines, chloral hydrate, clonidine, sedative-hypnotics, opiates |
| Mydriasis | Anticholinergics, cyclic antidepressants, cocaine, LSD, amphetamine |
| Nystagmus | Phenytoin, barbiturates, phencyclidine |
| ***Bowel Sounds*** | |
| Increased | Organophosphate insecticides, sympathomimetics |
| Decreased | Anticholinergics (atropine, cyclic antidepressants), sedative-hypnotics |
| ***Muscular System*** | |
| Muscle tremor | Amphetamines, cocaine, caffeine, theophylline, lithium, alcohol and sedative-hypnotic withdrawal |
| Muscle flaccid/paralysis | Opiates, clonidine, sedative-hypnotics, botulism |

*(continued)*

TABLE 68-4
**Expected Physical and Laboratory Findings for Poisonous Substances *(Continued)***

| Finding | Substance |
|---|---|
| ***Muscular System*** | |
| Muscle rigidity | Strychnine, tetanus, phencyclidine, haloperidol, methaqualone, phenothiazines |
| Fasciculations | Organophosphate insecticides, nicotine, lithium, phencyclidine |
| Myoclonus | Cyclic antidepressants, carbamazepine, phenytoin, methaqualone |
| ***Integumentary System*** | |
| Dry skin | Anticholinergics, vitamin A |
| Sweaty skin (diaphoresis) | Organophosphate insecticides, nicotine, sympathomimetics |
| Cyanosis (slate-blue discolorations) | Methemoglobin producers (nitrates, phenazopyridines, aniline) |
| Alopecia | Thallium, antineoplastic agents |
| Fingernails (Mees-Aldrich lines; transverse leukonychia) | Arsenic, thallium |
| ***Acid-Base Disorders*** | |
| Respiratory acidosis | Sedative-hypnotics, opiates |
| Metabolic acidosis | Salicylates, methanol, paraldehyde, iron, isoniazid, ibuprofen, ethanol, ethylene glycol, carbon monoxide, cyanide |
| Respiratory alkalosis | Salicylates |
| Metabolic alkalosis | Sodium bicarbonate |

x-ray to determine if aspiration has occurred, or using an abdominal x-ray to determine the presence of a radiopaque substance in the gastrointestinal tract. Radiopaque substances may include agents such as chloral hydrate, heavy metals (i.e., lead, arsenic, mercury, iron), iodide, phenothiazines, cyclic antidepressants, enteric-coated tablets, solvents, and other miscellaneous foreign objects, such as disk batteries, or coins.[13] The x-ray can be used to localize the substance ingested to assist with retrieval from the GI tract.

## Diagnostic Trials

The administration of certain pharmacologic antagonists or antidotes as presumptive therapy, such as naloxone therapy for a suspected narcotic overdose in a comatose patient, may be an extremely useful diagnostic tool in a poisoned patient. If a patient responds to this presumptive therapy (awakens after administration of naloxone), then this becomes a key diagnostic element in the assessment of the poisoned patient. However, a few toxins are antagonized by pharmacologic "antidotes." A list of the more commonly used pharmacologic antagonists with their respective uses is provided on Table 68-5.

TABLE 68-5
**Pharmacological Antagonists Used in Poisoning**

| Agent | Uses |
|---|---|
| Antivenin | |
| (Crotalidae) polyvalent | Pit viper snake bites (rattlesnakes, water moccasins, copperheads) |
| (Latrodectus mactans) | Black widow spider bites |
| (Micrurus fulvius) | Coral snake bites |
| Atropine | Organophosphate and carbamate insecticide poisonings |
| Calcium gluconate | Calcium-channel blocker (verapamil) poisonings, hydrofluoric acid burns |
| Cyanide antidote kit (amyl nitrite, sodium nitrite, sodium thiosulfate) | Cyanide poisonings |
| Deferoxamine | Iron poisoning |
| Dimercaprol (BAL) | Arsenic, gold, lead and mercury poisoning |
| Diphenhydramine | Phenothiazine and butyrophenone-induced dystonias |
| Edetate calcium disodium (EDTA) | Lead poisoning |
| Ethanol | Ethylene glycol and methanol poisoning |
| Fab fragments (Digibind) | Digoxin and digitoxin poisoning |
| Glucagon | Beta-blocker (propranolol) poisoning |
| Methylene blue | Drug and chemical-induced methemoglobinemias |
| N-Acetylcysteine | Acetaminophen poisoning |
| Naloxone | Opiate poisoning |
| Physostigmine | Anticholinergic poisoning |
| Pralidoxime | Organophosphate insecticide poisoning |
| Pyridoxine | Isoniazid, hydrazine-containing mushrooms |

## PATHOPHYSIOLOGY AND MECHANISMS OF TOXICITY

The mechanisms for toxicity of many toxins are quite varied in nature and involve complex imbalances of physiologic systems. The morbidity and mortality secondary to poisons are often attributed not to the direct mechanism of toxicity of a substance, but to secondary complications from the poisoning, especially those involving the respiratory system. For instance, many sedative-hypnotics may cause a loss of consciousness and the gag reflex in the patient. This may predispose the patient to aspiration of gastric contents, which can result in an aspiration pneumonitis.[14] In addition, patients who have been either unconscious for a prolonged period of time, develop seizures, or who have suffered crush injuries may be predisposed to destruction of muscle cells resulting in rhabdomyolysis. This releases myoglobin into the urine and may result in acute renal failure.[15]

It is important to realize that any substance could be potentially toxic at a given dose. The famous 15th century Swiss physician and alchemist, Paracelsus, provided a definition of poison: "All substances are poisons; there is none which is not a poison. The right dose differentiates a poison and a remedy."[16] A substance such as table salt may be used on a daily basis without causing any difficulty, but in larger amounts it could result in fatal hypernatremia.[7] In the assessment of acute human poisonings it is best to obtain, if available, the minimum toxic dose of a substance. These are usually derived from individual case histories of poisonings, or case series of poisonings, and may not be available for a wide variety of substances.

Some poisons mediate their toxic effects directly, while others mediate through the production of toxic metabolites, as is the case with methanol, ethylene glycol, and acetaminophen.[17,18] Poisons may cause immediate effects or damage such as with exposures to alkaline corrosives, resulting in a liquefaction necrosis of tissue within seconds of contact,[19] while others may be delayed in their effects, such as with exposures to the herbicide, paraquat, which can result in pulmonary fibrosis 1–2 weeks following contact.[20] Also, the duration of exposure has a bearing on the toxic potential of many agents in the overall outcome of the poisoning. This is exemplified by chronic salicylism due to repeated intake of high doses of aspirin over a period of days associated with a higher incidence of severe symptoms and death than acute salicylism due to a one-time ingestion.[21]

The following is a list of seven categories of mechanisms of actions of the most common toxic agents. It should be noted that this is not an all-inclusive list and that certain substances may mediate their effects by multiple mechanisms.

1. *Direct surface or cellular injury*—This may be exemplified by agents that cause denaturation of proteins or cellular necrosis upon surface contact. These may include the caustic acids and alkalis or snake and hymenoptera venoms, which mediate their efforts through enzymatic degradation or digestion of tissue.[22]
2. *Enzyme inhibitors*—Most heavy metals, such as arsenic, lead, and mercury, mediate their toxic effects by binding sulfhydryl groups of enzymes, thereby inhibiting enzyme function.[23] Cyanide binds the enzyme cytochrome oxidase, thus inhibiting oxygen utilization and ATP production.[24]
3. *Neurotransmitter potentiation and inhibition*—This is one of the major mechanisms by which various pharmaceutical substances, venoms, and other chemicals mediate their toxic effects. Many effects of these substances can be predicted on the basis of their influence on the autonomic nervous system (the parasympathetic and sympathetic nervous systems; see Chap. 6). The substances may act on one of the following mechanisms:
   a. Blockade of the postsynaptic receptors—The effects of atropine poisoning are mediated by competitive blockade of acetylcholine at muscarinic receptors of the parasympathetic nervous system.[25]
   b. Blocking reuptake of the neurotransmitter into the presynaptic neuron—This results in an excess of the neurotransmitter in the synaptic cleft, and thereby enhances neurotransmission. This is exemplified by the cyclic antidepressants and cocaine. They both result in increased neurotransmission of the sympathetic nervous system by blockade of norepinephrine uptake into the presynaptic neuron.[26,27]
   c. Increasing the release of the neurotransmitter—Black widow spider venom can cause an increase in the neurotransmitter release in neurons innervating skeletal muscle, resulting in severe neuromuscular symptoms.[28]
   d. Inhibition of the breakdown of the neurotransmitter—This is exemplified by organophosphate pesticides, which inhibit the enzyme acetylcholinesterase, which is responsible for the breakdown of acetylcholine and the termination of neurotransmission. This results in an excess of acetylcholine in the synaptic cleft, which stimulates cholinergic receptors.[29]
   e. The mimicking of the neurotransmitter—This is exemplified by tobacco poisoning through the ingestion of cigarettes. Nicotine is absorbed and can directly stimulate nicotinic receptors of the autonomic nervous system.[30]
   f. Sensitization of the effector tissue to the neurotransmitter—This is exemplified by the effects of halogenated hydrocarbons such as freon. The myocardium may be sensitized to epinephrine after inhalation exposure to freon, which can result in a life-threatening cardiac arrhythmia.[31]
   g. Impaired production of the neurotransmitter—This can be exemplified by isoniazid poisoning, which inhibits the synthesis of GABA (gamma-aminobutyric acid). A decrease in the CNS levels of the inhibitory neurotransmitter, GABA, results in an imbalance of excitatory neuronal activity manifested as seizures in an isoniazid poisoned patient.[32]
   h. Inhibition of release of the neurotransmitter—Botulinum toxin from the

bacteria, *Clostridium botulinum*, mediates its effects through inhibition of the release of acetylcholine from the presynaptic neurons that innervate skeletal muscle, resulting in muscular paralysis.[33]

4. *Derangements of metabolic and respiratory processes*—Some toxins compete with normal substrates necessary for respiratory and metabolic processes to produce ATP. This occurs during carbon monoxide poisoning, which has 240 times greater binding affinity for hemoglobin than oxygen, and thus results in oxygen deprivation.[34] Other agents uncouple oxidative phosphorylation, which inhibits ATP production through the electron transport system. Substances such as aspirin and wood preservatives (dinitrophenol) mediate their effects by this mechanism.[35,36] Patients with poisonings from these agents develop a characteristic hyperthermia because heat is produced as an end-product of metabolism, instead of ATP.
5. *Agents with target organ specificity*—Certain toxins may have a propensity for a particular organ system due to either their avid binding affinity for certain tissues, production of an organ-specific toxic metabolite, or due to the sensitivity of cellular components of an organ system to the toxin. The primary effect of acetaminophen poisoning is hepatocellular damage due to the accumulation of a toxic metabolite within liver cells.[18] The herbicide, paraquat, can result in pulmonary fibrosis, which is often fatal. This may be attributed to the availability of oxygen within pulmonary tissue, which aids in the production of superoxides and free radicals, resulting in membrane damage and fibrosis of lung tissue.[20]
6. *Alteration of cellular and/or tissue function*—Some toxins may alter the capability of specialized cells or tissue to perform physiologic functions by inducing structural or chemical alterations. Examples of substances in this category may include a host of methemoglobin producers, which are substances that oxidize the iron core of the hemoglobin molecule from the ferrous($Fe^{+2}$) to the ferric form($Fe^{+3}$).[37] The newly formed ferric core of methemoglobin is incapable of transporting oxygen, thus rendering a nonfunctional erythrocyte pigment.
7. *Inhibition of anabolic processes*—Some toxins have an effect on cell replication or on the production of various physiologic proteins in the body. These may constitute some of the most toxic agents involved in poisonings. The toxic effects from poisonings with the cyclopeptide mushrooms, of the amanita species, as well as from poisonings of seeds from other plants, such as the castor bean, containing ricin, and the rosary pea, containing abrin, are mediated by inhibition of protein synthesis.[38–40] This results in severe damage to the liver, kidneys, and in tissues with the highest rate of cell replication, such as the gastrointestinal system.

## TREATMENT

In the treatment of the poisoned patient, good, supportive care is of paramount importance and may be most responsible for the decrease in morbidity and mortality secondary to poisonings. Of the supportive care measures, the maintenance of the ABCs (airway, breathing, circulation) is crucial for any severely poisoned patient. Once this has been achieved, then other therapeutic options, such as the use of pharmacologic antagonists, decontamination, and enhancement of elimination, should be considered for the poisoned victim. This discussion will be limited to the decontamination procedures for the poisoned patient.

### Decontamination

The general premise for decontamination is to remove the substance involved in the poisoning exposure from the victim to decrease the amount of local tissue damage, as well as limit the amount of the substance absorbed into the body. The decontamination procedure used should be based on the amount of substance involved, its potential for local and systemic toxicity, and the routes of exposure. The routes may include, as previously discussed, the skin, the eye, the lungs, or by ingestion.

#### *Dermal Exposures*

Many toxins can cause direct irritation or burns to the skin, as well as be absorbed systemically into the body by this route, which is known as *percutaneous absorption*. For example, a primary route of exposure through the skin is observed with the organophosphate insecticides. Therefore, it is important to decontaminate exposed skin immediately upon exposure to one of these agents to prevent severe systemic toxicity.

In addition, during the decontamination procedure, it is important to protect the decontaminator. Often the persons performing the decontamination may, themselves, become contaminated with the poisonous substance. So, the decontaminator, if using liquid, should wear gloves, an apron, and a mask if necessary when fumes have evolved.

The exposed patient should be washed from head to toe, including the hair and under the nails. Because some agents, such as the organophosphate insecticides, are fat-soluble, they may require special washing solutions, such as tincture of green soap (alcohol-based soap solution), to decontaminate the victim. The patient should be first rinsed with cold water, then with warm water, and finally with hot water. The reason to commence with cold water is to avoid causing peripheral vasodilation, thereby minimizing systemic absorption. It is extremely important to decontaminate a poisoned patient at the site of exposure, rather than "scoop and run." In addition, it is important to remove all clothing from the victim. Certain clothing articles, such as leather products, absorb pesticides and are difficult to decontaminate.

### Ocular Exposures

Following ocular exposures to substances, it is important to irrigate the substance from the eye as soon as possible.[41] This should be done, preferably, at the site of exposure. Proper irrigation of the eye or of the affected eye or eyes should consist of a continuous irrigation for a period of at least 15–20 minutes. The irrigation solution may include tap water if at the home, or sterile saline in an emergency room.

Eyedroppers and irrigating syringes are worthless. In the home, the irrigation may be performed on a patient by holding his or her head back over a sink and pouring tap water from a large pitcher, liter bottle, or running faucet at low pressure about 6 inches from the eye. To avoid cross contamination of the eyes, the irrigant should be poured from the bridge of the nose to the outward portion of the eye. Always avoid direct high pressure irrigation. The irrigant can be just poured on the eye, even with children, because the eyes will usually open and close.

In addition, especially in the home setting, it may be useful to wrap a child in a sheet or a towel as a restraint. Other important tips to remember are that the victim should never place any form of medication, such as eyedrops or neutralizers, into an infected eye. Symptoms may not be good indicators of ocular injury, especially in the setting of alkaline corrosive exposures.

### Inhalation

Frequently, victims exposed to fumes or gases will also require measures to decrease the amount of exposure and alleviate local irritation. With exposures involving the respiratory tract, measures, such as having the victim breathe fresh air or, in many cases, humidified air, will alleviate local irritation of the mucous membranes and upper airway. If the patient is cyanotic due to asphyxiation or to an impairment of gas exchange or delivery of oxygen through the pulmonary system, then oxygen administration to the patient is required. It should be noted that patients exposed to fumes or gases may incur injury to the eyes as well as the upper and lower airways; therefore, it is always important to consider the possibility of multiple routes of exposure, and that the decontamination procedure be targeted towards each route.

### Ingestion

The most common route of exposure for poisonings is by ingestion. The approach taken by the clinician to decontaminate the gastrointestinal tract of the poisoned victim has been an issue of ongoing controversy. The premise for GI decontamination is to prevent absorption of a toxin that has a potential for systemic effects. There are many options in the area of gastrointestinal decontamination, such as the induction of emesis, gastric lavage, use of activated charcoal, cathartics, and even in some circumstances, endoscopy and surgery.

Gastrointestinal dilution with water or milk has long been touted as a first-aid procedure for poisonings. This maneuver, if done inappropriately, can complicate a poisoning. For instance, milk used as the dilution fluid may delay the ability to induce emesis with syrup of ipecac, or if a drug has been ingested, oral administration of water may enhance the dissolution of the tablets or capsules,[42] thereby facilitating systemic absorption and possibly resulting in faster onset of toxic effects from the drug. Administration of water is appropriate, though, for a toxic ingestion that produces local tissue irritation or is a caustic. This results in decreasing the contact time between the toxin and the exposed tissue, as well as the concentration of the caustic agent, thereby decreasing the amount or degree of irritation and injury.[19]

The use of neutralizers after acid or alkaline caustic ingestion is not recommended because of the production of heat during the neutralization process. This first-aid measure is still recommended on the labels of commercially packaged products and first-aid charts. A policy statement regarding the gastrointestinal dilution with water as a first-aid procedure in poisoning has been issued by the AAPCC.[42] Their recommendations include the following:

1. Oral dilution with water should *not* be used as a general first-aid measure to treat ingestions of medications.
2. Following the ingestion of a caustic or corrosive substance, the immediate oral administration of water or milk is recommended.
3. Water is the appropriate fluid to administer in conjunction with syrup of ipecac.

It has been demonstrated that the first-aid recommendations on labels of commercial products are often times hazardous, inappropriate, and inaccurate.[43] There are reported cases of patients developing severe toxicity, not from a substance initially involved in the poisoning, but from the first-aid procedure.[7]

Another modality of therapy is to empty the stomach after ingestion of a poison. Two primary options to accomplish gastric emptying are to induce vomiting or emesis, or with the use of a large-bore orogastric tube to perform gastric lavage. It should be noted that studies assessing the outcome of poisonings have not clearly demonstrated the beneficial effect on patients who are provided gastric-emptying procedures. In fact, many ongoing studies have failed to show a beneficial effect of gastric emptying on the outcome of the poisoned victim.[44] However, it is commonly observed that during these procedures the substance that was ingested is retrieved as evidenced by pill fragments or retrieval of a colored fluid.

In making the decision to perform gastric emptying, the clinician should be cognizant of the pitfalls and contraindications for these procedures, as well as situations in which their use is deemed appropriate. A variety of agents, such as salt water, mustard, and copper sulfate, have been previously used and recommended as emetics in the treatment of poisoning, but most of these are no longer used due to their ineffectiveness or potential hazards associated with their use.[45,46] Apomorphine, a morphine derivative with central-acting emetic properties, has been considered an effective emetic that produces a rapid onset of emesis. However, this agent has fallen into disuse due to a number of disadvantages: the necessity for parenteral administration, difficulty in preparation of dosage form, its effect on the CNS with the potential for respiratory depression, and its potential ineffectiveness in a patient who has ingested an antiemetic, such as a phenothiazine.[47]

Ipecac syrup, due to its safety, efficacy, and oral route of administration, is considered by most to be the emetic of choice in poisonings. Ipecac is derived from a plant, *Cephaelis ipecacuanha*, and contains a mixture of alkaloids, such as emetine, psychotrine, and cephaeline.[48] Ipecac has both local and central emetic properties. Cardiotoxicity, resulting in fatalities, has been attributed to the use of fluid extract of ipecac, which is 14 times more concentrated than ipecac syrup, and due to chronic abuse (of ipecac syrup) by bulimics.[49–51] Ipecac syrup is shown to induce emesis in approximately 96% of the patients to whom it was administered, and the onset of emesis will usually occur in 20–30 minutes.[52]

Contraindications to the induction of emesis include those situations in which the risk of pulmonary aspiration in the poisoned patient is high, in the comatose or seizing patient, or after the loss of gag reflex; in which the induction of emesis could precipitate severe gastrointestinal injury, the patient who has ingested a strong acid or base, or solid objects, such as razor blades, or nails; or in patients predisposed to hemorrhagic diathesis, such as patients with cirrhosis and esophageal varices or thrombocytopenia. As previously noted, removal of the ingested toxin from the GI tract is based on the assertion that there is a significant risk for systemic absorption with significant toxicity once absorbed.

Certain hydrocarbons, such as gasoline, kerosene, or mineral seal oil, may mediate their toxicity primarily through direct aspiration into the lungs (rather than by absorption from the stomach). Therefore, in those settings, it is not advisable to induce vomiting due to the increased risk of aspiration during the procedure, unless the hydrocarbon is aromatic, such as benzene, or halogenated, such as carbon tetrachloride, or is contaminated by another toxic substance, such as a pesticide, because of their potential for systemic absorption and toxicity. Also, due to the delayed onset of emesis with ipecac syrup, an assumption must be made that the clinical status of the patient will not change sufficiently as to contraindicate the induction of emesis during that time period. If substances are ingested that are rapidly absorbed with a fast onset action and that can produce seizures, such as camphor or strychnine, the induction of emesis is not recommended. Other ingestions, such as cyclic antidepressants, may also produce a rapid unpredictable onset of seizures and coma, and, therefore, the induction of emesis in that setting may be hazardous as well.

The other procedure used to empty the stomach is gastric lavage. This requires the use of a large-bore orogastric tube. Lavage should be performed in those situations where induction of emesis with syrup of ipecac is contraindicated, such as the patient who is seizing or comatose. The use of nasogastric tubes to remove contents from the stomach is essentially worthless. The patient must be placed in the left lateral decubitus position, and, if severely obtunded or comatose or if the patient has a loss of the gag reflex, the airway should be protected with a cuffed endotracheal tube, prior to the lavage procedure. Then a lavage solution, usually saline, in 200-ml aliquots in adults or 10 ml/kg in a child, is instilled into a lavage tube and then removed by aspiration or gravity suction. This should be continued until several liters of lavage fluid have been used or until the lavage fluid is clear. The tube then can be used for the instillation of activated charcoal and cathartic. It should be noted that there are limitations with gastric lavage. Large pill fragments may be unable to travel through the tube, especially those used for children, because of the size of the bore.

Gastric emptying is most effective if performed soon after the poisoning. However, the rate at which a substance is absorbed is quite variable and depends on a variety of patient-related and toxin-related parameters: the presence of food, the patient's intrinsic gastrointestinal motility, the amount of substance ingested, the effect of a substance on gastric emptying time, the time since ingestion, and the physical properties of the substance. Ingestion of substances with anticholinergic properties, which decrease gastric motility and increase gastric emptying time, may be amenable to gastric emptying procedures even a day after ingestion.

Activated charcoal is another useful adjunct to the treatment of poisoning substance that has been provided growing attention and has been identified as the primary line of therapy.[53,54] Activated charcoal is made from the destructive distillation or burning of organic materials, such as wood, coconut, bones, and rice starch. It is activated by treatment with oxidizing gases such as steam. Activated charcoal, itself, is a fine, black, odorless, and tasteless powder comprised of extremely small and porous particles. This porosity provides a large surface area to adsorb a large quantity of a substance. One gram of activated charcoal has a surface area ranging from 1000–3000 $m^2$. Substances that are adsorbed by charcoal are those that are un-ionized and have a large molecular weight. These will include most medications, as well as a wide variety of other chemicals and natural toxins. Other substances poorly adsorbed by activated charcoal include small ionic compounds, such as cyanide and caustic acids or alkalis, or small organic molecules, such as methanol.

Another therapeutic modality used to prevent gastrointestinal absorption of toxins is the administration of cathartics. Cathartics such as magnesium sulfate and citrate, sorbitol, and sodium sulfate have all been used in the treatment of poisonings.[55] It is important that activated charcoal, in most cases, be accompanied by the use of a cathartic to facilitate transport of the charcoal-drug complex. It should also be noted that there is no scientific basis to substantiate the use of cathartics alone. In addition, cathartics are contraindicated and may cause problems in the following situations: small children in whom it may result in fluid and electrolyte imbalances, very old patients, those with preexisting renal disease following the ingestion of nephrotoxic substances and caustics, and patients with recent bowel surgery, absent bowel sounds, hypertension, or congestive heart failure.

Another method used to decrease absorption of a compound from the gastrointestinal tract is to administer complexation agents, which chemically react with a toxin, resulting in an insoluble, nonabsorbable complex. Examples include the administration of a calcium-containing compound to the patient who has ingested fluoride,[56] which results in an insoluble, neutralized calcium fluoride complex; and the use of bicarbonate for an iron poisoning,[57] where a bicarbonate solution is either administered orally or instilled through a lavage tube following an iron ingestion, which results in the production of insoluble iron salts, such as ferrous carbonate.

Another less frequent mode of removal of a toxic product from the gastrointestinal tract is by endoscopy and/or surgery. Certain products when ingested may either lodge in parts of the gastrointestinal tract or form tenaciously adhering concretions. These are difficult to remove by either lavage or emesis or other methods for GI decontamination and, if left in contact with the GI mucosa, may result in not only systemic absorption, but severe damage to the lining of the gastrointestinal tract. Examples of such substances are: ingestion of iron, especially those with perinatal ferrous sulfate tablets, and disk batteries, both of which can be removed by either endoscopy or surgery.[58,59]

## CASE STUDY WITH SAMPLE CARE PLAN: PATIENT WITH ACUTE POISONING

A 5-year-old boy is brought into the Emergency Department at 6:00 P.M. by his mother. She is concerned about his "congestion" and sleepiness which began that morning and worsened over the ensuing 9 hours. He was a previously healthy child.

At the triage station of the Emergency Department, it is immediately apparent that the child is obtunded and in respiratory distress. Drooling, stertorous respirations, tachypnea, retraction, and cyanosis were also noted.

The boy's respiration became less labored and the cyanosis disappeared after oxygen was administered with airway positioning and suctioning. On 35% $O_2$, the patient's arterial blood gases are as follows: pH = 7.34, $PCO_2$ = 40, $PO_2$ = 62, and $O_2$ saturation of 90%. He is responsive only to tactile stimuli as the IV line is placed. The child is then undressed, and a physical examination is performed. The physical examination reveals the following:

VS. T = 36°C
RR = 52/min
HR = 140/min
BP = 148/98 mmHg

General—obtunded, eyes open at times, responds briefly with purposeful movements to painful stimuli, some spontaneous vocalization.

Head—atraumatic.

Eyes—pupils 1 mm, minimally reactive; EOMs full; fundi—not visualized.

ENT—mouth—unremarkable except for copious secretions.

Neck—supple, no adenopathy.

Chest—coarse rhonchi, occasional wheezes and inspiratory rales.

Heart—R R, no murmur.

Abdomen—soft, no organomegaly or mass. Active bowel sounds.

Genitalia—normal; underpants stained with diarrheal stool behind and wet in front.

Skin—profuse sweating.

## SAMPLE CARE PLAN FOR THE PATIENT WITH ACUTE POISONING

| Nursing Diagnoses | Desired Patient Outcomes | Nursing Interventions | Rationales |
|---|---|---|---|
| ***Nursing Diagnosis #1***<br>Ineffective breathing pattern (tachypnea, stertorous breathing) related to:<br>1. Altered state of consciousness.<br>2. Muscle weakness/paralysis (associated with organophosphate poisoning). | Patient will maintain:<br>1. Respiratory rate $<30$/min; regular rhythm and depth.<br>2. Adequate chest excursion.<br>3. Tidal volume $>5-7$ ml/kg with spontaneous breathing.<br>4. Mental status: alert; oriented to name. | • Perform overall assessment.<br>◦ Assess respiratory function: Respiratory rate, rhythm, depth; chest excursion, tone of respiratory musculature.<br>◦ Breath sounds/presence of adventitious sounds (crackles). | • Establishes a baseline with which to evaluate the response to therapy.<br>◦ Organophosphate poisoning can precipitate muscle weakness and paralysis.<br>◦ Enhanced cholinergic stimulation predisposes to excessive bronchial secretions. |
| ***Nursing Diagnosis #2***<br>Ineffective airway clearance related to:<br>1. Excessive secretions associated with enhanced cholinergic stimulation caused by organophosphate poisoning. | Patient will:<br>1. Demonstrate ability to cough and expectorate secretions. | ◦ Assess serial arterial blood gases.<br>◦ Assess neurologic function: Mental status, level of consciousness; sensorimotor function; and deep tendon reflexes.<br>◦ Assess cardiovascular function: (see Nursing Diagnosis #5, below). | ◦ Excessive alveolar and pulmonary interstitial fluid predisposes to impaired gas exchange and hypoxemia.<br>◦ Disruption of CNS function can be an ominous sign in acute poisoning. |
| ***Nursing Diagnosis #3***<br>Impaired gas exchange related to:<br>1. Pulmonary alveolar and interstitial congestion. | Patient will maintain arterial blood gases as follows:<br>• $PaO_2 > 60$ mmHg (room air)<br>• $PaCO_2 \sim 35$ to 45 mmHg<br>• pH 7.35–7.45 | • Implement measures to support alveolar ventilation/oxygenation.<br>◦ Initiate endotracheal intubation and mechanical ventilation.<br>◦ Initiate oxygen therapy.<br>◦ Teach use of incentive spirometer when indicated.<br>• Implement measures to maintain patent airway:<br>◦ Timely aseptic suctioning.<br>◦ Aggressive pulmonary toilet: Postural drainage; chest physiotherapy. | • Patients with acute organophosphate poisoning are at risk of developing hypoxemia.<br>◦ Altered state of consciousness and neuromuscular impairment compromise respiratory function.<br>• Excessive secretions occur as a result of the enhanced cholinergic response associated with organophosphate poisoning. |

*(continued)*

## SAMPLE CARE PLAN FOR THE PATIENT WITH ACUTE POISONING *(Continued)*

| Nursing Diagnoses | Desired Patient Outcomes | Nursing Interventions | Rationales |
|---|---|---|---|
| ***Nursing Diagnosis #4***<br>Potential for poisoning related to inadvertent intake of organophosphate chemical (Dursban). | Patient will recuperate from poisoning episode without any obvious sequelae; patient will maintain:<br>1. Mental status: Alert; states name.<br>2. Usual personality (as per parents).<br>3. Respiratory function within acceptable parameters. Breathing easy; breath sounds clear to auscultation. | • Assess potential/actual poisoning:<br>∘ What/who was involved in the poisoning?<br>∘ What was the route of exposure and how much of the agent was taken?<br>∘ What were the signs and symptoms?<br>∘ What medications or other emergent actions were taken? | • Thorough assessment including history, physical examination, and laboratory testing are essential to timely diagnosis and treatment (see Table 68–4). |
| | | • Implement antagonistic treatment as prescribed: | • Timely treatment is essential to reverse the effects of the poisoning agent before irreversible pathophysiologic changes occur. |
| | | ∘ Initiate gastric lavage. | ∘ Controversy exists as to the clinical efficacy of this modality. The decision to initiate lavage therapy is based on the time of exposure; the more recent the occurrence (30 to 60 min), the more effective the outcome. |
| | | ∘ Assure ET tube cuff is inflated. | ∘ An inflated cuff will help to prevent aspiration in the comatose patient.<br>∘ Gastric lavage is contraindicated in the scenario of a caustic ingestate (e.g., lye). |
| | | ∘ Administer activated charcoal as prescribed and monitor response to therapy. | ∘ Activated charcoal decreases toxicity by adsorbing chemical to its surface. Efficacy depends on timing of administration (most effective within 30 to 60 min, but may be effective up to 24 hr). |
| | | ∘ Auscultate for bowel sounds prior to administration. | ∘ Activated charcoal is not given if bowel sounds are absent. |
| | | ∘ Monitor gastric pH. | ∘ Food in stomach may decrease effect of charcoal. |
| | | ∘ Administer prescribed dosage of activated charcoal. | ∘ Inadequate dose may induce *desorption**: a reversible process in which an adsorbed chemical is removed from the charcoal causing free chemical to again be available to exert its untoward effects. |
| | | ∘ Administer cathartic therapy (e.g., magnesium citrate). | ∘ Cathartic maintains bowel motility to hasten elimination of drug/chemical/charcoal complex. |
| | | ∘ Administer prescribed anticholinergic (atropine). | ∘ Atropine competes with acetylcholine for cholinergic receptor sites thereby exerting its anticholinergic effect. |
| | | ∘ Administer prescribed organophosphate antagonist, pralidoxime | ∘ Pralidoxime reactivates the enzyme cholinesterase, inhibited by the organophosphate; the enzymatic breakdown of acetylcholine reduces the overall cholinergic effect. |

*(continued)*

| | | | |
|---|---|---|---|
| ***Nursing Diagnosis #5*** Fluid volume deficit related to:<br>1. Profuse diaphoresis, lacrimation, salivation, bronchorrhea, associated with enhanced cholinergic stimulation. | Patient will:<br>1. Maintain stable vital signs.<br>• Blood pressure within 10 mmHg of baseline for patient.<br>• Heart rate <100/min.<br>2. Exhibit usual skin color, without cyanosis or mottling; capillary refill brisk.<br>3. Maintain balanced intake/output: Urine output >30 ml/hr.<br>4. Maintain body weight within 5% of baseline.<br>5. Exhibit good skin turgor and moist mucous membranes.<br>6. Maintain laboratory data within acceptable range: BUN, serum creatinine, serum electrolytes, hematocrit, hemoglobin; urine specific gravity. | • Assess hydration and cardiovascular status:<br>◦ Heart rate, blood pressure, skin color, temperature, moisture, capillary refill, peripheral pulses.<br>◦ Assess intake and output.<br>◦ Weigh daily.<br>◦ Monitor serum electrolytes and acid-base balance.<br>• Implement fluid replacement therapy (as per physician). | • Excessive loss of fluid associated with enhanced cholinergic activity places the patient at risk for hypovolemia.<br>◦ Assessment parameters should include those indicative of peripheral perfusion.<br>◦ A meticulous record of intake/output and daily weight provides the best measure as to the patient's hydration status.<br>• Aggressive fluid replacement therapy is necessary to maintain adequate circulating blood volume. |
| ***Nursing Diagnosis #6*** Ineffective family coping related to:<br>1. Feelings of guilt. | Family will:<br>1. Verbalize feelings about poisoning episode and the circumstances under which it occurred.<br>2. Verbalize actions to be taken to prevent a recurrence. | • Assess the circumstances within which the poisoning exposure occurred.<br>◦ Allow the family the opportunity to verbalize their feelings.<br>• Instruct family in precautions that need to be taken to prevent future such crises.<br>◦ Have family verbalize the telephone number of the local branch of the Poison Control Center.<br>◦ Have family verbalize emergency measures to be taken if such an episode would inadvertently recur. | • It is essential to evaluate how the poisoning occurred so that measures may be taken to prevent a recurrence.<br>◦ Verbalizing their feelings may help them to cope with this family crisis.<br>• Family may need to assess how household chemicals are handled in their home setting.<br>◦ It is essential for all households to have the telephone number of the Poison Control Center.<br>◦ In the event of an emergency, it is essential that the family not panic, but follow the necessary steps to get help immediately. Minutes can mean the difference between life and death. |

*Kinney, MR, Packa, DR, and Dunbar, SB: AACN's Clinical Reference for Critical-Care Nursing, ed 2. McGraw-Hill, New York, 1988, p 1603.

Neuro—obtunded, no focal findings. DTRs 1 + / 4+ and symmetric.

Laboratory studies reveal the following:

Na = 143 mEq/liter
Cl = 106 mEq/liter
Serum creatinine = 0.6 mg/dl
K = 3.3 mEq/liter
Glucose = 222 mg/dl
BUN = 15 mg/dl
Hgb = 14.3
Hct = 43.6
WBC = 12,000

On admission, chest x-ray showed patchy hilar areas. The nurse who undressed the child smelled a "solvent"-like odor on the child's shirt. The mother is taken aside in order to provide some reassurance and questioned more closely about the events of the day. The mother then states that her son was left with a sitter (his aunt) for the morning. When she arrived home at 2:00 P.M., she found her son in bed. The aunt said the child had been fine until 10:00 A.M. when he complained of a stomachache and vomited twice. The child then became tired and went to bed. The aunt thought these symptoms may have been due to some milk that the child ingested at 9:00 A.M. She commented that it may have gone bad, because it smelled "funny."

Shortly after the physical examination, the child becomes cyanotic again, with secretion gurgling in his mouth and oropharynx. He no longer vocalizes or moves. His arms and legs are flaccid, DTRs cannot be elicited. Muscle fasciculations are noted on his abdominal wall.

The mother then contacted her sister and together they realized that the "bad" milk was in fact a diluted solution of Dursban, an organophosphate insecticide used to kill roaches. This had been stored in an empty milk container and then inadvertently placed in the refrigerator.

The child underwent endotracheal intubation, then was treated with gastric lavage, activated charcoal, magnesium citrate, IV atropine, and IV pralidoxime. He was then managed in the Intensive Care Unit where he made steady improvement with continued atropine and pralidoxime therapy. His muscular strength increased and respiratory status improved with percussion, postural drainage, and incentive spirometry coupled with the pharmacologic management. He was extubated after 3 days and discharged without apparent sequelae after 6 days.

It was further revealed that the child was a premature infant weighing 2 lb at birth and required supportive care in an Intensive Care Unit for 4 months after delivery. He has mild mental retardation and hyperactivity. The family, consisting of his mother and 3 siblings, lives in a chronically roach-infested apartment in an older part of the inner city with low-income housing.

## Nursing Diagnoses

Ineffective breathing pattern, related to:
1. Altered state of consciousness.
2. Muscle weakness (paralysis).

Ineffective airway clearance, related to excessive secretions.

Impaired gas exchange, related to pulmonary alveolar and interstitial congestion.

Potential for poisoning, related to inadvertent intake of organophosphate chemical (Dursban).

Fluid volume deficit, related to profuse diaphoresis, lacrimation, salivation, bronchorrhea.

Ineffective family coping, related to feelings of guilt.

## REFERENCES


1. National Poison Prevention Week. 25th Anniversary Observance. MMWR 35(10):149, 1986.
2. Litovitz, TL, Normann, SA, and Veltri, JC: Annual report of the American Association of Poison Control Centers National Data Collection System. Am J Emerg Med 4(5):427, 1986.
3. Temple, AR: Poison prevention education. Pediatrics 74(Suppl):964, 1984.
4. Klein-Schwartz, W and Oderda, GM: Poisoning in the elderly. J Am Geriatr Soc 31(4):195, 1983.
5. Oderda, GM and Klein-Schwartz, W: Poison prevention in the elderly. Drug Intell Clin Pharm 18(3):183, March 1984.
6. Manoguerra, AS and Temple, AR: Observations on the current status of Poison Control Centers in the United States. Emerg Med Clin North Am 2(1):185, 1984.
7. Barer, J, et al: Fatal poisoning from salt used as an emetic. Am J Dis Child 125:889, 1973.
8. Smookler, S: Hypertensive crisis resulting from an MAO inhibitor and an OTC appetite suppressant. Ann Emerg Med 11(9):482, 1982.
9. Aronom, WS and Isbell, MW: Carbon monoxide effect on exercise-induced angina pectoris. Ann Intern Med 79:392, 1973.
10. Grace, TW and Platt, FW: Subacute carbon monoxide poisoning. Another great imitator. JAMA 246(15):1698, 1981.
11. Shannon, K and Buchanan, GR: Severe hemolytic anemia in black children with glucose-6-phosphate dehydrogenase deficiency. Pediatrics 70(3):364, 1982.
12. Piomelli, S and Vora S: G6PD deficiency and related disorders of the pentose pathway. In Nathan DG and Oski, FA (eds): Hematology of Infancy and Childhood, ed 2. WB Saunders, Philadelphia, 1981, p 608.
13. O'Brien, RP, et al: Detectability of drug tablets and capsules by plan radiography. Am J Emerg Med 4(4):302, 1986.
14. Bertino, JS and Reed, MD: Barbiturate and nonbarbiturate sedative hypnotic intoxication in children. Pediatr Clin North Am 33(3):703, 1986.
15. Frymoyer, PA, et al: Technetium Tc 99m medronate bone scanning in rhabdomyolysis. Arch Intern Med 145:1991, 1985.
16. Doull, J, Klaassen, CD, and Amdur, MO: In Doull, J, Curtis, D, Klassen, M, and Amdur, O (eds): Cassarett and Doull's Toxicology: The Basic Science of Poisons, ed 2. Macmillan, New York, 1980.
17. Litovitz, T: The alcohols: Ethanol, methanol, isopropanol, ethylene glycol. Pediatr Clin North Am 33(2):311, 1986.
18. Rumack, BH: Acetaminophen overdose in children and adolescents. Pediatr Clin North Am 33(3):691, 1986.
19. Rothstein, FC: Caustic injuries to the esophagus in children. Pediatr Clin North Am 33(3):665, 1986.

20. Mofenson, HC, et al: Paraquat intoxication: Report of a fatal case. Discussion of pathophysiology and rational treatment. J Toxicol Clin Toxicol 19(8):821, 1982–83.
21. Gaudreault, P, Temple, AR, and Lovejoy, FH, Jr: The relative severity of acute versus chronic salicylate poisoning in children. Pediatrics 70:566, 1982.
22. Kunkel, DB, et al: Reptile envenomations. J Toxicol Clin Toxicol 21(4&5):503, 1983–84.
23. Chisolm, JJ: Poisoning from heavy metals (mercury, lead, and cadmium). Pediatr Ann 9(12):28, 1980.
24. Vogel, SN and Sultan, TR: Cyanide poisoning. Clinical Toxicology 18(3):367, 1981.
25. Weiner, N: Atropine, scopolamine, and related antimuscarinic drugs. In Gilman, AG, et al (eds): Goodman and Gilman's The Pharmacological Basis of Therapeutics, ed 7. Macmillan, New York, 1985, p 132.
26. Gay, GR: Clinical management of acute and chronic cocaine poisoning. Ann Emerg Med 11(10):562, 1982.
27. Pentel, PR and Benowitz, NL: Tricyclic antidepressant poisoning. Med Toxicol 1:101, 1986.
28. Rauber, H: Black widow spider bites. J Toxicol Clin Toxicol 21(4&5):473, 1983–84.
29. Mortensen, ML: Management of acute childhood poisonings caused by selected insecticides and herbicides. Pediatr Clin North Am 33(2):421, 1986.
30. Oberst, B and McIntyre, R: Acute nicotine poisoning. Pediatrics 11:338, 1953.
31. Baselt, RC and Cravey, RH: A fatal case involving trichloromonofluoromethane and dichlorodifluoromethane. J Forensic Sci 13:407, 1968.
32. Messing, RO, Closson, RG, and Simon, RP: Drug-induced seizures: A 10-year experience. Neurology 34:1582, 1984.
33. Dowell, VR: Botulism and tetanus: Selected epidemiologic and microbiologic aspects. Rev Infect Dis 6(Suppl 1): S202, 1984.
34. Zimmerman, SS and Traxal, B: Carbon monoxide poisoning. Pediatrics 68(2):215, 1981.
35. Temple, AR: Acute and chronic effects of aspirin toxicity and their treatment. Arch Intern Med 141:364, 1981.
36. Gosselin, R, Smith, R, and Hodge, H: Clinical Toxicology of Commercial Products (Section III, Therapeutics Index), ed 5. Williams & Wilkins, Baltimore, 1984, p III–156.
37. Smith, RP and Olson, MV: Drug-induced methemoglobinemia. Semin Hematol 10(3):253, 1973.
38. Davis JH: *Abrus precatorius* (rosary pea): The most common lethal plant poison. J Fla Med Assoc 65(3):189, 1978.
39. Wedin, GP, et al: Castor bean poisoning. Am J Emerg Med 4(3):259, 1986.
40. Olson, KR, et al: Amanita phalloides-type mushroom poisoning. West J Med 137:282, 1982.
41. Rost, KM, Jaeger, RW, and deCastro, FJ: Eye contamination: A poison center protocol for management. Clinical Toxicology 14(3):295, 1979.
42. American Association of Poison Control Centers: Policy statement, gastrointestinal dilution with water as a first-aid procedure in poisoning. Vet Hum Toxicol 25(1):55, 1983.
43. Alderman, D, Burke, M, and Cohan, B: How adequate are warnings and first-aid instructions on consumer product labels? An investigation. Vet Hum Toxicol 24:8, 1982.
44. Kulig, K, et al: Management of acutely poisoned patients without gastric emptying. Ann Emerg Med 14(6):562, 1985.
45. Chin, L: Induced emesis—A questionable procedure for the treatment of acute poisoning. Am J Hosp Pharm 29:877, 1972.
46. Oderda, GM and Manoguerra, AS: Poisoning. In Katcher, BS, Young, LE, and Koda-Kimble, MA (eds): Applied Therapeutics, ed 3. Applied Therapeutics, San Francisco, p 1531.
47. Corby, DG, et al: Clinical comparison of pharmacological emetics in children. Pediatrics 42:361, 1968.
48. Manno, BR and Manno, JE: Toxicology of ipecac, a review. Clinical Toxicology 10(2):221, 1977.
49. Miser, JS and Robertson, WO: Ipecac poisoning. West J Med 128:440, 1978.
50. Smith, RP and Smith, DM: Acute ipecac poisoning. N Engl J Med 265(11):523, 1961.
51. Brotman, MC, et al: Myopathy due to ipecac syrup poisoning in a patient with anorexic nervosa. Canadian Medical Association Journal 125:453, 1981.
52. Manoguerra, AS and Krenzelok, EP: Rapid emesis from high-dose ipecac syrup in adults and children intoxicated with antiemetics or other drugs. Am J Hosp Pharm 35:1360, 1978.
53. Derlet, RW and Albertson, TE: Activated charcoal—Past, present and future. West J Med 145(4):493, 1986.
54. Park, GD, et al: Expanded role of charcoal therapy in the poisoned and overdosed patient. Arch Intern Med 146:969, 1986.
55. Reigel, JM: Use of cathartics in toxic ingestions. Ann Emerg Med 10(5):254, 1981.
56. Monsour, PA, et al: Acute fluoride poisoning after ingestion of sodium fluoride tablets. Med J Aust October, 13:503, 1984.
57. Czajka, PA, Konrad, JD, and Duffy, JP: Iron poisoning: An in-vitro comparison of bicarbonate and phosphate lavage solutions. J Pediatr 98(3):491, 1981.
58. Venturelli, J, et al: Gastrotomy in the management of acute iron poisoning. J Pediatr 100(5):768, 1982.
59. Litovitz, TL: Button battery ingestions, a review of 56 cases. JAMA 249(18):2495, 1983.

## SUGGESTED READINGS

### Trauma

American College of Surgeons Committee on Trauma: Advanced Trauma Life Support Course for Physicians. Award Printing Corporation, Chicago, 1989.
Barriot, P and Viars, P: Prehospital autotransfusion in life-threatening hemothorax. Chest 93:522, 1988.
Bires, B and Sparger, G: Multiple trauma: Chest trauma, orthopedic and abdominal trauma. In Holloway, N (ed): Nursing the Critically Ill Adult, ed 3. Addison-Wesley, Menlo Park, CA, 1988.
Cardona, V and Hurn, P: Trauma Nursing: From Resuscitation Through Rehabilitation. WB Saunders, Philadelphia, 1988.
Dunham, C, et al: Rapid infusion system: The MIEMSS experience. In Proceedings of the 10th National Trauma Symposium, Baltimore, MD, 1987.
Howell, E, Widra, L, and Hill, G: Comprehensive Trauma Nursing Theory and Practice. Scott, Foresman, Glenview, IL, 1988.
Hoyt, KS: Chest assessment. Trauma Quarterly: Pulmonary Trauma. 2(2). Aspen, Rockville, MD, 1986.
Hoyt, KS and Sparger, G: Chest trauma. In Sommers, L (ed): Difficult Diagnoses in Critical Care. Aspen, Rockville, MD, 1988.
Knezevich, B: Trauma Nursing: Principles and Practice. Appleton-Century-Crofts, Norwalk, CT, 1986.
Mann, J and Oakes, A: Critical Care Nursing of the Multi-Injured Patient. American Association of Critical Care Nurses. WB Saunders, Philadelphia, 1980.
Rea, R: Trauma Nursing Core Course Provider Manual. Award Printing Corporation, Chicago, 1987.
Richardson, J, Polk, H, and Flint, L: Trauma: Clinical Care and Pathophysiology. Yearbook Medical Publishers, Chicago, 1987.
Satiani, B, Fried, S, and Zeeb, P: Normothermic rapid volume replacement in traumatic hypovolemia. Arch Surg 122:1044, 1987.
Siegel, J: Trauma Emergency Surgery and Critical Care. Churchill Livingstone, New York, 1987.
Strange, J: Shock Trauma Care Plans. Springhouse Corporation, Springhouse, PA, 1987.
Wiener, S and Barrett, J: Trauma Management for Civilian and Military Physicians. WB Saunders, Philadelphia, 1986.

## Burns


Artz, CP, Moncrief, JA, and Pruitt, BA: Burns: A Team Approach. WB Saunders, Philadelphia, 1979.
Bernstein, NR and Robson, MC: Comprehensive Approaches to the Burned Person. Medical Examination Publishing, New York, 1983.
Finlayson, L: Emergency care of the burn patient. Crit Care Update 7(10):18, 1980.
Finn, KL: Rebuilding skin: A successful graft may be up to you. RN 40(10):41, Oct 1977.
Garner, JS and Simmons, BP: Guidelines for isolation precautions in hospitals. Infection Control 4(4):245, 1983.
Gatson, SF and Schumann, LL: Burn wound management. Crit Care Update 7(10):5, 1980.
Heimbach D: Smoke inhalation: Current concepts. In Wachtel, T, Kahn, V, and Frank, H (eds): Current Topics in Burn Care. Aspen, Rockville, MD, 1983.
Helm, PA: Burn injury: Rehabilitation management in 1982. Arch Physical Medicine and Rehabilitation: 63(1):6, 1982.
MacMillan, BG: Surgical and Medical Support for Burn Patients. Publishing Sciences Group, Littleton, MA, 1982.
Marvin, JA: Planning home care for the burn patient. Nursing 83 13(8):65, Aug 1983.
Salisbury, RE, Newman, NM, and Dingeldein, GP: Manual of Burn Therapeutics. Little, Brown & Co, Boston, 1980.
Wagner, M: Care of the Burn Injured Patient: A Multidisciplinary Approach. Publishing Sciences Group, Littleton, MA, 1980.
Wilkens, EW: Textbook of Emergency Medicine, ed 2. Williams & Wilkins, Baltimore, 1982.


## Septic Shock


Bellanti, JA: Immunology, Basic Processes. WB Saunders, Philadelphia, 1985.
Bordicks, KJ: Patterns of Shock: Implications for Nursing Care. MacMillan, New York, 1980.
Brown, WJ: A classification of microorganisms frequently causing sepsis. Heart Lung 5(3):397, May-June 1976.
Cowley, RA and Trump, BF: Pathophysiology of Shock, Anoxia and Ischemia. Williams & Wilkins, Baltimore, 1982.
Gorbach, SL, Bartlett, JG, and Nichols, RL: Manual of Surgical Infections. Little, Brown & Co, Boston, 1984.
Riccardi, KP: Septic shock and the mechanism of tissue injury. In Guthrie, M (ed): Contemporary Issues in Critical Care Nursing, Vol 2, Shock. Churchill Livingstone, New York, 1982.
Rice, V: Shock: A clinical syndrome, Part II: Stages of shock. Crit Care Nurse 1:4–14, May-June 1981.
Shoemaker, WC: Pathophysiology and therapy of shock syndromes. In Shoemaker, WC, Thompson, WL, and Holbrook, PR (eds): Textbook of Critical Care. WB Saunders, Philadelphia, 1984.
Zaritsky, AL and Chernow, B: Catecholamines, sympathomimetics. In Chernow, B, and Lake, CR (eds): The Pharmacologic Approach to the Critically Ill Patient. Williams & Wilkins, Baltimore, 1983.


## Anaphylactic Shock


A continuing education service for physicians and nutritionists. Nutrition and the MD 12(10):1, Oct 1986.
Allergic to what he eats. Emerg Med 19(2):22, Jan 30, 1987.
Beta blockers and penicillin anaphylaxis. Nurses' Drug Alert 10(5):38, May 1986.
Dickerson, M: Anaphylaxis and anaphylactic shock. Crit Care Nursing Q 11(2):68, June 1988.
Hill, J: Emergency anaphylaxis. Hosp Med 23(1):19, Jan 1987.
Maybee, J: Anaphylaxis, an emergency medicine overview. Emerg Med 10(11):17, Nov 1986.
Suit up against anaphylaxis. Emerg Med 17(7):127, April 1985.


## Acute Poisoning


Alderman, D, Burke, M, and Cohan, B: How adequate are warnings and first-aid instructions on consumer product labels? An investigation. Vet Hum Toxicol 24:8, 1982.
American Association of Poison Control Centers, Policy statement: Gastrointestinal dilution with water as a first-aid procedure in poisoning. Vet Hum Toxicol 25(1):55, 1983.
Aronom, WS and Isbell, MW: Carbon monoxide effect on exercise-induced angina pectoris. Ann Intern Med 79:392, 1973.
Barer, J, et al: Fatal poisoning from salt used as an emetic. Am J Dis Child 125:889, 1973.
Bertino, JS and Reed, MD: Barbiturate and nonbarbiturate sedative hypnotic intoxication in children. Pediatr Clin North Am 33(3):703, 1986.
Chin, L: Induced emesis: A questionable procedure for the treatment of acute poisoning. Am J Hosp Pharm 29:877, 1972.
Davis, JH: *Abrus precatorius* (rosary pea): The most common lethal plant poison. J Fla Med Assoc 65(3):189, 1978.
Derlet, RW and Albertson, TE: Activated charcoal—Past, present and future. West J Med 145(4):493, 1986.
Dowell, VR: Botulism and tetanus: Selected epidemiologic and microbiologic aspects. Rev Infect Dis 6(Suppl 1):S202, 1984.
Gay, GR: Clinical management of acute and chronic cocaine poisoning. Am Emerg Med 11(10):562, 1982.
Grace, TW and Platt, FW: Subacute carbon monoxide poisoning. Another great imitator. JAMA 246(15):1698, 1981.
Klein-Schmartz, W and Oderda, GM: Poisoning in the elderly. J Am Geriatr Soc 31(4):195, 1983.
Knukel, DB, et al: Reptile evenomations. J Toxicol Clin Toxicol 21(4 & 5):503, 1983–84.
Kulig, K, et al: Management of acutely poisoned patients without gastric emptying. Ann Emerg Med 14(6):562, 1985.
Litovitz, TL, Norman, SA, and Veltri, JC: Annual Report of the American Association of Poison Control Centers National Data Collection System. Am J Emerg Med 4(5):427, 1986.
Manno, BR and Manno, JE: Toxicology of ipecac, a review. Clin Tox 10(2):221, 1977.
Manoguerra, AS and Temple, AR: Observations on the current status of poison control centers in the United States. Emerg Med Clin North Am 2(1):185, 1984.
Messing, RO, Closson, RG, and Simon, RP: Drug-induced seizures: A 10-year experience. Neurology 34:1582, 1984.
Miser, JS and Robertson, WO: Ipecac poisoning. West J Med 128:440, 1978.
Mofenson, HC, et al: Paraquat intoxication: Report of a fatal case. Discussion of pathophysiology and rational treatment. J Toxicol Clin Toxicol 19(8):821, 1982–83.
O'Brien, RP, et al: Detectability of drug tablets and capsules by plan radiography. Am J Emerg Med 4(4):302, 1986.
Park, GD, et al: Expanded role of charcoal therapy in the poisoned and overdosed patient. Arch Intern Med 146:969, 1986.
Pentel, PR and Benowitz, NL: Tricyclic antidepressant poisoning. Med Toxicol 1:101, 1986.
Reigel, JM: Use of cathartics in toxic ingestions. Ann Emerg Med 10(5):254, 1981.
Rost, KM, Jaeger, RW, and deCastro, FJ: Eye contamination: A poison center protocol for management. Clin Tox 14(3):295, 1982.
Rumack, BH: Acetaminophen overdose in children and adolescents. Pediatr Clin North Am 33(3):691, 1986.
Shannon, K and Buchanan, GR: Severe hemolytic anemia in black children with glucose-6-phosphate dehydrogenase deficiency. Pediatrics 70(3):364, 1982.
Smith, RP and Olson, MV: Drug-induced methemoglobulinemia. Semin Hematol 10(3):253, 1973.
Smookler, S: Hypertensive crisis resulting from an MAO inhibitor and an OTC appetite suppressant. Ann Emerg Med 11(9):482, 1982.
Temple, AR: Poison prevention education. Pediatrics 74 (Suppl):964, 1984.
Temple, AR: Acute and chronic effects of aspirin toxicity and their treatment. Arch Intern Med 141:364, 1981.
Vogel, SN and Sultan, TR: Cyanide poisoning. Clin Tox 18(3):367, 1981.

UNIT TWELVE

# Critical Care Nursing: Humanness and Professionalism

The essence of critical care nursing involves, on the one hand, the *humanness* of the patient-nurse interaction, wherein participants in the interaction share a little of themselves as they strive to meet each other's needs and to maintain the life processes of each individual in a state of dynamic equilibrium. As a result of this exchange, each participant has the opportunity to gain a keener sense of self and an appreciation for the importance of sharing and feeling in human interactions.

On the other hand, *professionalism* is integral to critical care nursing. Each nurse, in the course of his/her practice, makes decisions based on underlying ethical and legal principles and within the framework of acceptable standards of care. In the complexity of today's health-care scene, the critical care nurse assumes ever-increasing responsibilities for decision-making in daily patient care. In the intensive care unit, where the scope of nursing and the scope of medicine may not always be clearly delineated, critical care nurses often question if they are practicing medicine. Consequently, it is necessary for each nurse to become well versed in those principles involving ethics and the law as they pertain to the practice of nursing.

Chapter 69 explores the humanness of the patient-nurse interaction from the perspective of the critical care nurse. Through highly descriptive and poignant vignettes, emphasis is placed on how the sharing of feelings provides the critical care nurse with a basis for continuing personal and professional growth.

Chapter 70 emphasizes the ethical theories that most closely affect critical care nursing practice. Laws that regulate nursing practice are examined to enhance the nurse's understanding of how such laws impact on the decision-making process and on the nurse's potential legal liability. A distinction is made between ethics and law.

## UNIT OUTLINE

# CHAPTER 69

# Sharing Feelings

*Adrienne Coppola and*
*Mary Amendolari*

In caring for critically ill patients and their families, all of whom must try to cope intellectually, emotionally, and physically with what may be a life-threatening illness, critical care nurses themselves experience many moods and emotions. Included among these are feelings of satisfaction and fulfillment that are realized when the patient and family perceive that, as a result of the patient-nurse interaction, a beneficial change has occurred and that the interaction has made a difference in the outcome, be it a return to a quality lifestyle, or to the acceptance of the ultimate outcome, that is, death, with respect and dignity.

Other feelings experienced by critical care nurses include the anxiety and fear that accompanies caring for patients with life-threatening illnesses whose recovery and eventual return to a quality lifestyle may depend largely on the professional nursing care rendered during the acute phase. Often critical care nurses experience feelings of helplessness, powerlessness, and frustration, when, despite all their effort and that of other health-care providers, they witness the demise of the patient and the grief of the family with whom they feel a close bond.

In the patient-nurse interactions described in the vignettes that follow, the focus is on the humanness of the critical care nurse, both as a caregiver and as an individual. Through candid sharing of thoughts and feelings experienced by these critical care nurses, one is able to become involved in the intimacy of the patient-nurse interaction and how the process that is nursing intertwines with the life processes of the patient and family. As a result of these human interactions, there evolves within each individual an ever-increasing awareness and understanding of self and of one's integrity.

"I have just arrived home after a really busy night in our ICU, a night that has left me physically and emotionally drained. I was called last evening to help out with the workload in what was an especially busy night in the unit. As the Nursing Care Coordinator, that is, the charge nurse in the unit, the staff looked to me for assistance, reassurance, and relief. So I said, OK, and I was on my way.

"As I look back at the events that transpired in the ICU this night, I realized that it was one of those nights when you have mixed emotions and feelings. At one point, I found myself questioning what it was I was doing. I have been a critical care nurse for nearly 11 years now, and I wondered—is it really worth it? Is it really worth all the stress and anguish? Should I do something less stressful and demanding of one's energies? On the other hand, I felt I did my best to help out, to help make people feel what they had to feel and needed to feel. Maybe that's what it's all about, I mean, to experience a fine balance between one's feelings, and when you feel you've got to have a break just to sit back and reflect.

"Let me tell you a little bit about the night. There was a young, handsome guy, about 20 years old, whose name was Peter. He was admitted the day before for a small bowel resection secondary to a bowel obstruction. Clinically, there were many problems. On admission, he had a low hemoglobin, hematocrit, and platelet count. Nevertheless, an exploratory laparotomy with a small bowel resection was performed. Upon his return to the ICU, a pulmonary artery catheter was inserted to assist in monitoring his fluid status. Some difficulty was encountered in stabilizing Peter's vital signs while he was in the recovery room. So it was imperative to monitor his overall status closely, and in particular, his hydration status, postoperatively. In addition, Peter was in a highly agitated state.

"Peter was a tall, strong, rugged guy. If you looked at him, you'd say to yourself, how can this guy be sick? Yet, here he was vented, with a pulmonary catheter and arterial line, and hooked up to a variety of monitors. Anyone looking at Peter would be bewildered by all these lines and equipment.

"When I approached Peter's bedside I found him

loosely restrained to prevent him from dislodging his airway or intravenous lines. I went over to him and noticed this look of fear in his expression. I tried to talk softly to him, to explain to him what was going on, why he had the tube in his mouth. I felt very concerned and uncomfortable. I wanted him to relax, but I didn't want to sedate him. I felt it was very important to Peter to know what was going on, because I felt he needed to know. I tried to hold his hand to calm him down. It worked for awhile, but we ended up having to give him some Valium. He seemed to relax a bit, and his vital signs remained stable.

"Meanwhile, while I was trying to comfort Peter, the patient in bed 5, Mrs. M, was asking for the bedpan. A woman in her early fifties admitted with a rule-out inferior wall myocardial infarction, she seemed almost apologetic asking for the bedpan, saying, 'You're all so very busy, I hope I'm not bothering you.' I tried not to show my anxiety, which is something difficult to do, especially when the pace is so hectic. While she was probably the least sick of all our patients, I took the time to try to show her that we were there to meet her needs. Inwardly, I recognized that feeling of impatience with her, especially because I was so concerned about Peter. I knew I had to be especially careful not to be abrupt with her, with so many other things on my mind.

"I also realized, however, that I did not want Mrs. M to sense my anxieties because that's something that brushes off on people and patients, especially in an ICU. Allowing patients to sense one's anxieties may, in turn, precipitate other patient problems, as, for example, chest pain in someone of Mrs. M's status. Mrs. M went on to say, 'How can you be running around so quickly, and you're doing so much. It's really busy in here, what's going on with the man next door?' I just told her that he was a young man who had just had surgery. I reassured Mrs. M, gave her the bedpan and the call bell, and told her to call when she was finished with its use and we would assist her.

"In the meantime, in bed 1, was Ms. T, a woman in her early forties, admitted with an acute anteroseptal wall myocardial infarction. She was in the process of having a pulmonary catheter inserted. She appeared ashen, and her skin felt cool, moist, and clammy. She was also experiencing a lot of chest pain not entirely controlled with morphine. We initiated a nitroglycerin drip, and she seemed to be doing better. However, at that point, we experienced equipment failure with her bedside monitor. The physician was at the bedside agitating about how do we get this monitor to work? The graph wouldn't come on the oscilloscope, and we couldn't get a pulmonary artery pressure reading. I tried fiddling around with the buttons but was still unable to get a reading.

"I placed a call to the evening supervisor who responded immediately. With Ms. T's condition so acute and unstable, it warranted a one-to-one nurse-patient ratio. So I had the nurse caring for Ms. T continue to monitor her closely, while the evening supervisor and I attempted to deal with the equipment failure. We could have moved Ms. T from bed 1 to bed 3, but we felt that she was too unstable to be moved. So we ended up disengaging the patient from the entire system, and with a trusty screwdriver and some logistical maneuvering, we were able finally to hook the patient up to another monitor, and it worked.

"Things went pretty smoothly afterwards, and I had time to reflect on what had transpired. I knew I felt panicky inside. I didn't want to take a chance on moving this patient to another bed because she was so sick. It was kind of hard to deal with the physician at this time. I knew he wanted to get the pulmonary artery catheter inserted as soon as possible. I also sensed the anxieties he was experiencing. I had worked with this physician for quite some time, and when you get to know someone well enough, and this person usually had a mellow-type personality, I just knew by looking at him that he felt panicky and we had to get the job done.

"With Ms. T's condition stabilizing, before I left her bedside, I took the time to reassure Linda, Ms. T's nurse. I briefly reviewed significant events and what could be learned from these events; while also consoling her and verbalizing the anxieties and fears I knew she was experiencing, I let Linda know that it was all right to feel panicky or extremely anxious. We were able to get the job done by working together, as a team.

"I went back to Peter's bedside and was just standing there, kind of helping out with turning and repositioning, when suddenly his eyes rolled back. I quickly looked at the monitor and noted that both his blood pressure and wedge pressure readings were falling. Within moments, Peter went into cardiac arrest and we called a code. While I was resuscitating him with the Ambu bag, I remember thinking to myself that here is a guy but 20 years old. Usually, our patients are much older. Somehow, having such a young patient involved in a code situation just brings about different feelings that ordinarily would not be experienced. Peter is young and such a strong guy—why should this be happening to him? I remember thinking that we *must* bring him back, he has his whole life ahead of him.

"The code team worked on Peter for over an hour, using every therapy at our command. You name it and we tried it. Pharmacologically, we used epinephrine, calcium chloride, dopamine, levophed, and sodium bicarbonate. A pacemaker wire was inserted, but we couldn't get it to capture. I don't think his heart muscle was intact, and later on, we found out that there were other things involved in his illness.

"As I gazed around and took note of people's expressions, some had tears in their eyes. We all kind of had tears in our eyes. As the code progressed unsuccessfully, the more intense everybody became. My fellow nurses were saying to me, 'We've got to do something else. We need to do *something*.' The physician directing the code, a cardiologist, and one I have high regard for, tried everything possible, but we just weren't getting any results. The expression on everyone's face looked like their very hearts were sinking along with Peter's.

"I remember thinking to myself, maybe there was something else we could do, or perhaps should have done earlier. I began second-guessing myself. Maybe there was something I could have done to prevent this from happening; maybe something else was going on with Peter that I didn't see on the monitor; or maybe we were just so busy and so stressed that we weren't paying closer attention to Peter. So many things were going through my mind. I think down deep inside I felt we did the best we could. But there are just so many mixed feelings.

"Other questions and concerns began to enter my mind. What's going to happen when Peter's mother arrives? The physician called his mother. In the meantime, we all just stood around the bedside as nurses, touching one another, and I guess, you could say we all just stood there, crying. I know I cried. It had really been a long time since I remember crying. But this interaction with Peter, it really upset me.

"Peter's mother arrived about 20 minutes after the physician declared his death. She came into the center of the ICU in front of his curtain. We had closed Peter's curtain and, in so doing, perhaps provided him with a final moment of solitude. The physician explained to his mother that we tried everything humanly possible, but Peter just didn't make it. She suddenly was overwhelmed with the magnitude of this reality, bursting into tears and sobbing uncontrollably with her hands covering her face. She was just sobbing so helplessly.

"As Peter's mother, the physician, and I were standing together, I was thinking to myself, what can I really do to ease her burden, what could I say? Here's a woman who just lost her 20-year-old son. I suddenly found myself putting my arm around her, and I said to her 'I really want you to know that we tried everything we could to save Peter. He was very special to each one of us. I truly wish there was something else that we could do to help you.' I gave her a glass of water and some tissues, and we sat down, my arm around her shoulder.

"Meanwhile, Peter's 18-year-old younger brother came into the unit, and after he saw the closed curtains and his mother crying, he just ran out of the unit. I wanted to run after him, but I realized that it was necessary to let the family handle this burden in their own way. I continued to console Peter's mom, and when his dad arrived, they consoled one another.

"In retrospect, I was comforted by the thought that I was able to comfort Peter's family at least somewhat in their hour of need. As for the staff, we were all drained emotionally, mentally, and physically. My nurses were so drained there was nothing else that they could give of themselves. It's as if they functioned on pure instinct the remainder of the shift. I was also glad that I could be there for my staff, to offer support and to provide reassurance. Having worked with these nurses, being familiar with their personalities, I had a good idea as to how they were feeling. The special bond that exists among critical care nurses, the sharing of feelings —this helps each of us to gain some insight into who we really are, what makes us tick, and, yes, to muster our energies for yet another day.

"We were informed subsequently that, at autopsy, Peter was found to have mitral valve vegetation, some myocardial damage, and severe liver disease. Other factors were identified as possibly contributory to his demise, including a history of drug and alcohol abuse. And so, we laid Peter to rest."

"Let me share with you my interaction with Mr. D, a 60-year-old man with a longstanding history of COPD. Mr. D had been hospitalized on numerous occasions with an exacerbation of his disease, and both he and his wife were aware that his emphysema was severe. At this time, it was necessary to intubate Mr. D and initiate mechanical ventilation to ensure adequate alveolar ventilation.

"When I approached Mr. D's bedside I was impressed with the look of fear on both his face, and that of his wife, who was at his bedside. I found myself likewise experiencing some of their fear as I asked myself, how could I help this loving couple? How could I relieve their anxiety? Their anxiety seemed to rub off on everyone. It may have been caused by the alarm on his ventilator, which seemed to be sounding constantly.

"In an ICU, people are especially tuned in to the sounds created by various monitors, ventilators, and other equipment. I found myself thinking as I responded to Mr. D's ventilator alarm, I wonder how many of us tend to concern ourselves more with the equipment rather than directly with the patient? Perhaps, some of us are more comfortable concentrating on the machinery, 'treating' the sounds rather than having to interact with the patient or family. Sometimes you just have so many mixed feelings about caring for patients, especially when you know their prognosis for recovery isn't very positive. I find it's often difficult to deal with these feelings. Perhaps we concentrate more on the equipment rather than on the patient and family as a defense mechanism, as if to insulate our own feelings from surfacing.

"Another mechanism we may employ in caring for patients whose alarms are constantly going off is to sedate these patients, which is what we did with

Mr. D. Don't get me wrong, I know that he really needed sedation at this point in time and it did slow down his heart rate a little, but I also know that sedation may not always be necessary. Rather, taking the time to talk to a patient, and touching the patient—holding the patient's hand, placing your hand on the shoulder, or caressing the head—these types of therapies may be sufficiently effective as to negate the need for sedation. This approach can be used even when the patient is experiencing an altered level of consciousness and is unable to respond. They may, nevertheless, hear and feel.

"I remember observing Mr. D's wife on one of her frequent visits, how she took his hand and his eyes closed, and he seemed to relax, if but for a moment. I went over to Mr. D's bedside and introduced myself to both him and his wife and told them I would be taking care of Mr. D during the rest of the evening. I told them that I would stop by to talk with them and would try to anticipate their needs. I suggested to Mr. D that perhaps he could calm down and relax a little bit because this would probably help him with breathing. I rubbed his forehead with my hand, and he seemed comforted by this. I explained to Mr. D that his hands were loosely restrained because he might inadvertently pull out his endotracheal tube while he was sleeping, and he seemed to understand. I did give him some Zanax, which he had been taking at home.

"As I reviewed Mr. D's chart, it was evident that Mr. D's disease was progressive, and his ventilatory and gas exchange capabilities were severely compromised. It occurred to me that perhaps both Mr. D and his wife were concerned that he was going to die and that this, at least in part, underlay their extreme anxiety. I think Mr. D knew that he was really very sick. His wife told me that he had never been intubated so quickly during his previous hospitalizations. She explained that he really stopped breathing at home before the ambulance arrived. She said she was afraid he was going to die.

"The many days I took care of Mr. D, I tried to bring out his feelings. I remember one day in particular when I took his hand and I just said to him, 'I know you're afraid.' I really wanted to say to him that I knew he was afraid that he was going to *die*. But I guess that I was afraid myself of the thought of him dying. Yet, I knew I had to help him work through what he was feeling. The fear of dying is really something each critical care nurse must work out within himself or herself. Sometimes it is good just to come out and say it—are you afraid to die? It is important to involve the family in this process if possible, so they can all try to work through their feelings and to deal with them together.

"In retrospect, there was one thing I regret not having done, and this was to give Mr. D the choice of whether or not he wanted to be a Do Not Resuscitate patient. There was time to address this with him earlier in this hospitalization when he was much more alert and oriented. Later on, his condition deteriorated and his level of consciousness became altered. I did bring it up to Mrs. D. I think she wanted this in the beginning, but she never really pursued it with him. I don't think, I really don't know—maybe it's just my feelings of guilt that I didn't emphasize this enough, so that maybe, if I did, Mr. D would have had the choice.

"When Mr. D's time came and he had to be resuscitated, his wife wanted everything to be done. She became almost fanatical about the need to *bring him back*. I tried to explain to her what the situation was and what we were trying to do. I felt that this was important to her. But, at one point, Mrs. D made me feel as if we weren't doing enough, that there should be other things that we should be doing. When I looked back and thought about Mrs. D, it occurred to me that she was probably using denial to cope. What concerned me was that I may have lost my objectivity in this circumstance and perhaps in so doing did not recognize that Mrs. D was having difficulties resolving the fact that her husband was dying.

"Well, Mr. D did die. He had his wife at his bedside, which I really felt was important to both of them. Caring for Mr. D helped me to deal with some of my own feelings about death and dying, despite the fact that I have been a critical care nurse for over 10 years. I guess there's always a patient who touches you deeply. I guess in caring for Mr. D some of these thoughts and feelings surfaced. Mr. D, although he was vented, was still alert. He could still choose certain things, or at least be informed of certain things. Mr. D was a very intelligent man. It was especially difficult for Mrs. D and the family to accept his death, particularly because Mr. D was only in his early sixties and had so much to live for.

"About a week later, Mrs. D sent all the nurses, uniforms and a big box of cookies. She thanked us. Believe it or not, about a year later, she, herself, was admitted to our ICU with a diagnosis of angina. When I went to her bedside, there was just something about her, I said, 'Mrs. D, how are you doing?' I took care of her that night. I just felt such a close bond with her probably because we did share a lot of inner feelings about her husband."

"As I mentioned earlier, I have been a nurse for about 11 years. I have always worked in an ICU except for a few months early on after graduation from nursing school, when I worked in Med-Surg. But basically, I'm a critical care nurse. I think it's true when it is said that you have to be a special type of person to work in an ICU. I have worked with nurses who came to realize that the tempo and demands of an ICU were not for them. Others I have worked with just burnt out. Still other critical care nurses have worked in an ICU for such a long time, I don't think they have taken the time to think about their feelings, and whether or not they still feel they can function productively and are not just going through the motions.

"Basically, to be an effective critical care nurse, you need to be knowledgeable, you need to really keep up-to-date and on top of things. For myself, I really enjoy attending continuing education offerings, especially when I don't know about something. For example, when thrombolytic therapy with tPA and streptokinase was initiated in our ICU, I realized that this treatment modality was one that I knew very little about. I was able to attend a continuing education program that helped me to learn the essentials of caring for a patient receiving thrombolytic therapy. Now, this therapy is frequently implemented in our ICU.

"It's essential for critical care nurses to seek out information when they are doubtful or uncertain about anything. I especially stress to my nurses that they should consult the policy and procedure manuals initially, and then consult with one of the other nurses, or myself, as the resources in the unit. Critical care nurses also need to use their common sense. Often, one's instincts, experience, and common sense are all that is needed to intervene effectively.

"Psychomotor skills and dexterity are a must for the critical care nurse. Critical care nurses deal constantly with a lot of equipment and instruments. Often, it is necessary to assist physicians with procedures. Even more often, it is the critical care nurse who helps physicians maintain aseptic technique.

"Working with physicians in the ICU can be especially challenging. Over time, you eventually get to know the personalities of the ICU physicians, and this can be very helpful in the day-to-day workings of the ICU. Basically, every physician has his/her own way of performing procedures (e.g., inserting a Swan-Ganz catheter or pacing wire) and of dealing with patients. Often, critical care nurses must be assertive with physicians to ensure that the patient's needs are met. As the patient's nurse, the critical care nurse may be in the best position to determine what the patient's needs are and what type of therapy may be appropriate, and to evaluate the patient's response to therapy. At times, the critical care nurse may not agree that a particular therapy is appropriate for the patient. In the ICU, it is important to bring this to the physician's attention, including the rationales supporting your stance. Critical care nurses, with their level of knowledge essential to caring for the critically ill patient, should not hesitate to question a physician's order if it is felt to be inappropriate. In fact, it is the responsibility of the nurse to do so. It is also the responsibility of each nurse to question another nurse if he/she is observed to be doing something inappropriate when caring for a patient.

"An essential characteristic, required of nurses to be effective bedside nurses is simply to be caring. Not only caring for patients, but, very importantly, caring for each other as nurses. Some of my most satisfying and fulfilling experiences as a critical care nurse include those when I'm working and interacting with my fellow nurses, knowing that they care. You know they care because everyone is in tune with each other's feelings and, no matter how someone reacts to stress, they can ventilate their feelings knowing someone is listening and really cares.

"Occasionally, in our ICU, one of the nurses becomes really stressed, and she'll suddenly snap at someone. Basically, what I do is to kind of let her be for awhile, give her some space. Eventually, I go to her and say, 'Is there something bothering you? What's going on?' Or I might say, 'How can I help you? Is there something I can do for you?' Or I try to anticipate her needs much as I do with my patients. Often, when I can, I'll go over and tell her to take a break, and I'll monitor her patients for awhile.

"The *esprit de corps* that exists in our ICU is perhaps best illustrated at those times when a patient goes bad, or when we are getting an admission from the Emergency Department, for example. Everyone gets together and pitches in. This togetherness and caring are seen when someone needs a break. Sometimes it is necessary to say to a fellow nurse, 'You look awfully tired, you've really been working a lot. Maybe you need to take a break.' I know there are times when I need a break. I think it occurs at least once a month, I really need a day when I'm totally not thinking of the unit.

"I think my experiences as a critical care nurse have affected my overall view of life. Somehow, when one deals with life and death on a daily basis, when you see people suffering and become cognizant of the terrible problems that beset them, so many things seem trivial in comparison. Having this perspective, you can handle your own life a little better. I know I have become much more organized in my own life. Although, I do know some critical care nurses who are so very organized at work and yet are totally disorganized in their home life. After being a critical care nurse for so long, I believe what you do at your job, how you perform, and how you interact with people are really a reflection of the kind of person you really are. You can't be a phony in an ICU. You have to be down to earth, you need to be realistic, you have to deal with problems effectively, and you need to be able to accept criticism as well as other people.

"I think *touch* is a very important component in dealing with people in general, and with patients, in particular. I recently read an article in *Heart & Lung* that discussed how important touch is when performing procedures and caring for patients. It's the way you are with patients, it's a part of caring.

"Let me share my real feelings—how I feel about ICU. I guess I really do love it. I thought about doing other things. I'm sure I probably will in the future. Perhaps I'll attempt to do something different. Of course there have been other occasions when I have thought about this, yet I still end up working in the critical care setting. I think I have gotten the most satisfaction from my practice as a critical care nurse because I go in and care for my patients knowing that, in some small way, I can affect them and can make a difference for them and their families.

"Of course, the most rewarding feeling occurs when you know that the patient is going to improve. Recently, we had a 40-year-old patient admitted with an anterior wall myocardial infarction. He was treated with tPA, and we were able to reverse a lot of the injury to his myocardium. He stopped by to visit us about a month after his discharge. How good it felt to see him, knowing that in some small way we had influenced his life. It's these little things that happen that become meaningful. They recharge the batteries and give us the strength to tackle the next challenge.

"What evolves from experiences in the ICU is a critical care nurse *practitioner*. You consider what you do to be your *practice*, rather than just a job. I've become a member of the American Association of Critical Care Nurses (AACN), the professional organization of critical care nurses. I've tried to encourage my colleagues to join by setting an example. It is such a pleasure observing nurses on their break to be scanning through *Heart & Lung* or *Focus on Critical Care*. (These are the two journals of the AACN.) Even more satisfying is observing nurses starting to apply new knowledge to patient care. I mean it is just such a good feeling to see other nurses grow as professionals and as individuals. Often, people expect a lot of things in return. As for me, like I said, if you can find satisfaction in these little things—just watching people grow, and you know you've done the best job you can, that's basically all I've ever needed."

"Elizabeth was a special lady, well-known to us in the ICU. It was just about a year ago that she was brought into the Emergency Department after having a cardiac arrest. She was intubated and transferred to our unit.

"She was under a great deal of stress at the time. She was caring for her husband who was riddled with cancer, and, in addition, she was caught up in the activities, excitement, and tensions of her daughter's wedding. In fact, we didn't know then if Elizabeth would make it, and we all prayed that she wouldn't die before the wedding. Well, she persevered, and, although she remained on the ventilator, Elizabeth did see her daughter dressed in her wedding gown. Her daughter came into the ICU to show her mom what a beautiful bride she was to be. How hard it must have been for the family and for Elizabeth. I couldn't even begin to imagine how they must have felt.

"Although Elizabeth did sustain considerable damage to her myocardium, her condition stabilized and she was discharged on medications, and on limited activity.

"Now, a year later, I again met Elizabeth who was admitted to the ICU, this time with acute congestive heart failure and complaints of chest pain. Her husband had since died, and, on the positive side, she had her first grandson. Knowing that people are especially vulnerable to illness during the first year after a spouse's death, I wondered if perhaps this was true in Elizabeth's case, and I thought about the stress she was experiencing, what she must be going through.

"I requested to care for Elizabeth because I felt close to her, some sort of a bond with her. It was difficult to see her again on the ventilator and the multiple IV drips that were necessary to maintain her. Everyday, I would tell her how she was doing and try to set goals with her. I knew it was important to be honest and realistic with Elizabeth. I knew she knew how she was doing. So many times, patients just don't know what's going on. Others may be afraid to know. But I feel that if patients aren't informed or don't get any positive feedback, how can they help themselves?

"One day, a few hours after she was extubated, Elizabeth complained of difficulty breathing. Her vital signs were stable, and as I assessed her, I couldn't find any underlying reasons for her respiratory distress, except her anxiety, which was causing her to hyperventilate. The results of her arterial blood gases confirmed my suspicions, and I shared the results with Elizabeth. I explained to her that the results of her gases were within normal limits, that she was understandably anxious, but doing quite well off the ventilator. I stayed with her and comforted her until she, herself, believed that she was, in fact, fine.

"As Elizabeth slowly progressed, she was placed on a waiting list for coronary artery bypass surgery at New York University Medical Center. She was of such high risk that this was her only hope.

"Elizabeth's daughters came in to see their mom faithfully, 2–3 times a day. They were so supportive and caring. I could see that they couldn't bear to think of losing their mother.

"Whenever I had a few moments, I would sit with Elizabeth and hold her hand. We would talk, laugh, and sometimes, cry. She knew her prognosis was guarded, and she worried about what her daughters would do without her. Her face would light up and she had a sparkle in her eyes when she spoke about her little grandson. I made sure Elizabeth got to see him, knowing it was very likely for the last time.

"One day, when I asked her how she really felt she was doing, she said, 'Not so good,' with a sad look in her eyes. I asked her if there was anything I could get for her, and she smiled and said, 'A pastrami on rye with mustard.' She was getting so very weary. Without saying it, Elizabeth knew she wasn't getting any better. As her wait became longer (due to lack of a bed), I found myself becoming more frustrated and angry. This was, after all, her only hope. I became very involved with the family and tried to help them sort out their feelings and to be realistic in their expectations. I tried to prepare them for what no one wanted to face, Elizabeth's death.

"I remember waking her one morning to take her vital signs. She had been in a deep sleep and woke up startled and uneasy. Realizing that something was wrong, I pursued it with Elizabeth. She explained to me that she had been dreaming and she felt 'so tired,' as if she had been 'working all night.' She told me that she dreamed that her daughters were moving furniture in her house and that her husband was breaking down a wall.

"It was at this time that her daughters came to visit their mother, and they told her to stop talking about their father and to stop wanting to be with him. I tried to explain to them that this was a normal part of grieving and that Elizabeth needed to talk about her husband, their father. But I could see that they were uncomfortable with this.

"I, however, found myself being very uncomfortable with Elizabeth's dream. I knew right away that something was going to happen that day. I shared these thoughts with an intern who believed in dreams also, and she confirmed my feelings.

"That night, Elizabeth developed severe chest pain and was put back on multiple IV drips. Her condition steadily worsened, and I could see that she started to withdraw. I tried to comfort her, stroking her forehead and holding her hand, but she continued to get worse. I remember praying that when the time came, and Elizabeth was to die, I didn't want to be there. I felt that I might lose it emotionally. I had gotten so very close to her. I was afraid that, the way I felt about Elizabeth, I wouldn't be able to function.

"My prayers were answered. The day Elizabeth was to die, I was on call and I got called in. As I approached the hospital, one of the nurses informed me that an extra nurse came in by mistake and that I could go home. And so I did. That night Elizabeth coded and died.

"After hearing about Elizabeth's death, I was very upset and tears filled my eyes. After so many years of nursing, it doesn't seem easier—the pain and the hurt are still there when a patient dies, and you feel such a loss.

"Her dream still haunted me, and I was angry with myself for not having looked up its meaning. When I finally did, I sat in disbelief. The dream interpretation was 'being surrounded by loved ones' and 'conclusion of all affairs.' Elizabeth had dreamed her own death!

"For days thereafter, I would look for her in the bed she had occupied for such a long time. I had tried to come to terms with her death, wondering if she needed more time than I had spent with her, to verbalize her fears and feelings. Had I really done enough? So many feelings were awakened in me. Why did I go into nursing? Was it worth it? Was it worth having my emotions played with all the time? But I know deep down that this is my calling in life, and I could never do anything else. Nothing else could give me the sense of satisfaction I feel. I knew that I had helped Elizabeth even if but in some small way. And despite the fact that I kept asking myself if there was something else that I could have done for her, I knew I had touched her heart, just as she had touched mine."

## SUGGESTED READINGS

Barker, RK: You made a difference. Focus Crit Care 15(1):38, 1988.
Edwards, LW: Thanks Floyd. Focus Crit Care 12(4):52, 1985.
Estabrooks, C: Touch: A nursing strategy in the intensive care unit. Heart Lung 18(4):392, 1989.
Levine, S, Wilson, S, and Guido, G: Personality factors of critical care nurses. Heart Lung 17(4):392, 1988.
Schoenhofer, S: Affectional touch in critical care nursing: A descriptive study. Heart Lung 18(2):146, 1989.
Schunior, C: Close to bull's horns. Focus Crit Care 14(2):19, 1987.

CHAPTER 70

# Ethical and Legal Principles Affecting Decision-Making in Critical Care Nursing

*Ginny Wacker Guido*

## CHAPTER OUTLINE

SELECTED ETHICAL THEORIES
- Theories of Obligation
- Theories of Value

APPLICATION OF ETHICAL THEORIES

DISTINCTION BETWEEN ETHICS AND LAW

LEGAL CONCEPTS

LAWS AFFECTING THE PRACTICE OF NURSING
- Nonintentional Torts
- Intentional Torts
- Quasi-Intentional Torts
- Vicarious Liability

EXPANDED ROLES AND THE CRITICAL CARE NURSE

SPECIFIC LEGAL CONCERNS
- Consent
- Do-Not-Resuscitate Issues
- Staffing Issues
- Life-Support Measures

CONCLUSIONS

## LEARNING OBJECTIVES

**At the end of this chapter, you should be able to:**

1. Describe selected ethical theories and the basic premise on which the theory is based.
2. Differentiate theories of obligation and theories of value.
3. Apply ethical theories to everyday nursing practice by describing the practical value of ethical theories in practice.
4. Distinguish between law and ethics.
5. Examine the various elements of malpractice/negligence and the significance that each element has for the nurse.
6. Discuss intentional torts and defenses to each in the professional setting.
7. Discuss quasi-intentional torts and defenses to each in the professional setting.
8. Analyze the concepts of vicarious liability and expanded roles within critical care nursing.
9. Discuss specific legal concerns, including informed consent, do-not-resuscitate issues, staffing issues, and application of life-support measures.

Ethical theories and legal principles guide many of the decisions that critical care nurses make daily in their professional practice. Because nurses have an increasing responsibility for decision-making, an understanding of ethical principles allows the nurse to give order to moral situations and to provide a systematic basis for making nonarbitrary decisions. An understanding of the laws that regulate nursing practice is essential to ensure that decision-making is consistent with applicable legal principles and to protect the nurse from potential legal liability.

## SELECTED ETHICAL THEORIES

Many different theories have evolved to justify existing moral consensus or particular moral principles. Some theories are based on theological premises while other theories have their roots in the historical, sociological, or psychological sciences.

### Theories of Obligation

Theories of obligation define decision-making based on a given action. What makes an action right or wrong? Good or bad? Several different theories of obligation exist today.

#### *Natural Law Theory*

The natural law theory is the oldest of the known ethical theories and is difficult to separate from traditional religious beliefs. Both the Greeks and the Romans argued that the world is rationally intelligible because it exists as an ordered whole, governed by rational laws. Human reason, therefore, is but part of Divine Reason, which is the basis of the rational order; human reason can understand that order and live in accordance with that order.[1]

This theory allows a standard by which to measure rightness and wrongness and is above society and one's temporal concerns.[2] The natural law theory looks at what theologians have taught and what has been handed down through God's teachings in determining whether an action is good or bad. The natural law theory has had a tremendous effect on the development of legal and social institutions. When the U.S. Supreme Court attempts to test the validity of the U.S. Constitution, the 9 Justices speak of principles of justice that are more universal than statutory law. Patient's bills of rights and professional codes of ethics also have their foundations in the natural law theory.

#### *Utilitarian Theories*

Utilitarian theories look to an overall goal or sense of direction or purpose in nature. Humans have a tendency to strive toward fulfillment as a human being; the goal that governs this striving is the pursuit of happiness, both in personal well-being and fulfillment as well as the well-being of all of society. Ethics that interpret this pursuit of happiness are called utilitarian because the value of the action/deed is determined by whether it aids human happiness. Taken to its fullest extent, utilitarian ethics seek the greatest happiness for the greatest number of persons in society.

Frankena[3] carries this theory of utilitarianism to a principle of beneficence: there is an obligation to maximize the balance of good over evil because one is obligated to do good and prevent harm. There are 4 concepts to his theory: (1) one ought not to inflict evil or harm, (2) one ought to prevent evil or harm, (3) one ought to remove evil, and (4) one ought to do or promote good.

Utilitarian ethics may be subdivided into rule utilitarianism and act utilitarianism. Rule utilitarianism seeks the greatest happiness for all; it appeals to public agreement as a basis for objective judgment about the nature of happiness. Act utilitarianism does not invoke a universal rule, but tries to determine in a particular situation which course of action will bring the most happiness, or the least harm and suffering, to a given individual. As such, act utilitarianism makes happiness subjective.

### Theories of Value

The following theories look at what makes an action morally good or evil not at whether it is good or bad. "What is the motivating factor or driving force that compels a person to act as he/she does?" is the question raised.

**Agapeistic ethics** base moral principles and decision-making on love: the most important value in human life is love. Thus, one acts based on what is the most loving thing to do given a specific set of circumstances.

**Situation ethics** have developed from this basic love premise. The nurse who ascribes to this theory is, in effect, saying that decision-making takes into account the unique circumstances of each patient, the nature of the caring relationship between the nurse and the patient, and what is the most loving thing to do in the situation. Thus, one could disconnect the ventilator from a ventilator-dependent patient and allow the patient a natural death.

**Deontological ethics** look not to the end/consequences of an action, but to the intention of the action. It is one's good intentions, the intentions to do a moral duty, that ultimately determine the praiseworthiness of an action. Four principles may be included in this approach to ethics: autonomy, nonmaleficence, beneficence, and justice.

*Autonomy* is personal liberty of action, implying independence, self-reliance, and the ability to make decisions. One cannot be autonomous in a vacuum; this principle must be respected and acknowledged by others. Autonomy is frequently discussed in the health-care delivery system when health-care providers "allow" the patient the right to decide against further therapy and to die a natural death.

*Nonmaleficence* is the duty to do no harm and implies that one also has a duty to prevent, or at least limit, the risk of harm. This concept usually arises in health-care delivery when a patient is facing major surgery or an invasive diagnostic procedure. The health-care provider then faces a dilemma: should one encourage the procedure or surgery knowing its risks or discourage the medical action knowing that the patient's health will deteriorate without the intervention?

*Beneficence* is the active promotion of good; it is the conferring of health benefits to patients. But with this duty comes a requirement that there is a balancing of benefits over harm, and one is left facing a similar choice as that faced with nonmaleficence.

*Justice* is (1) treating people according to their needs, (2) dealing with people according to their merits or "just deserts," or (3) treating all people as equals in the sense of distributing good and evil equally.[4] Applying justice frequently becomes a balancing act—the balancing of one's rights and claims with those of another.

The principle of justice usually comes to the forefront in deciding how to allocate scarce resources. With only one donor liver, who should be the recipient? Although the nurse may not realize it, this ethical principle may be the guiding factor one uses in making common, everyday decisions. For example, 2 patients are in need of medications at the same time or 2 patients should have their vital signs checked at the same moment. Principle, not emotion, guides the nurse in his/her choice of whom to medicate first and which patient can wait until second.

**Conscientiousness** is the ethical theory that defines the sense of duty motivating a person to act. One acts according to duty to family, duty to self, duty to employer, and the like. This duty to act is seen by some ethicists as all one needs to act in a virtuous manner.

## APPLICATION OF ETHICAL THEORIES

Regardless of the ethical theory or theories that one chooses to follow, the practical value of ethical theories is that they allow for agreement and objective decision-making. Making decisions and then acting on those decisions are essential for the practice of nursing. Such decision-making must be based on rational thinking: a process that requires consideration of options, resolutions, and judgment. And the judgment involves an ethical component.

Each ethical theory produces arguments for how one conducts oneself in a given situation. Ultimately, in ethical dilemmas, one is faced with a choice between what should be done (theories of obligation) and a judgment about the chosen course of action (theories of value). This blending of the broad categories of ethics provides the framework for understanding responsible ethical choices.

Perhaps the nurse most consciously uses these principles and theories when serving on hospital ethics committees. With the increasing numbers of legal and ethical dilemmas in medicine today, health-care providers have implemented such committees to (1) provide structure and guidelines for potential problems, (2) serve as an open forum for discussion, and (3) function as a true patient advocate by placing the patient at the core of committee discussions.

Wlody and Smith[5] describe 3 models on which to structure a hospital ethics committee. The autonomy model seeks to aid the competent patient to make decisions about his/her care. The patient benefit model facilitates decision-making for the incompetent patient and seeks to include family members as much as possible in the decision-making process. The social justice model looks at institutional issues rather than individual patient issues. Most institutions use a combination of the 3 models.

## DISTINCTION BETWEEN ETHICS AND LAW

Ethics are subject to philosophical, moral, and individual interpretations. There are 2 systems of right and wrong in any given health-care delivery dilemma—those of the health-care providers and those of the health-care recipients. Ethics is, thus, internal in respect to the given person; it is based on the values of an individual. Ethics concerns one's motives and attitudes and looks to answer the question of why one acts as he/she does. Ethics are enforced through ethics committees and looks to the good of the individual within a given society.

Laws are founded on rules and regulations of a society; laws bind the society in a formal manner. Although man-made and capable of change, laws provide the general foundation that guides health-care givers, regardless of the health-care givers' personal views and value system. Laws are external to oneself, and they tend to benefit the entire population rather than the individual in society. Laws are enforced through the legislature and judiciary; law concerns one's conduct and actions—what did the person do or fail to do as opposed to why one acted as he/she did.

## LEGAL CONCEPTS

Several key legal concepts may aid the nurse in decision-making in critical care areas. As our society has become more litigious, more nurses are being named as defendants in medical malpractice suits. Understanding and applying legal principles may help protect the nurse from future lawsuits.

Although the number of reported lawsuits naming critical care nurses as defendants is relatively few, this does not ensure the critical care nurse against a potential lawsuit. Several factors, including (1) low nurse-patient ratios, (2) increased communications with patients and their families, and (3) better consumer education on health-care issues and expectations, have been cited as possibly influencing the small number of lawsuits.

## LAWS AFFECTING THE PRACTICE OF NURSING

Most of the laws that affect the professional practice of nursing can be grouped under the general classification of civil law. Civil laws involve the rights of individuals as opposed to criminal laws, which regulate conduct that is harmful or offensive to society as a whole.

Under this general classification of civil law comes tort law. A tort describes a legal wrong committed against the person or property of another. Torts may be intentional or nonintentional in nature; that is, I may intend to do a certain action that interferes with another person or his/her property or I might harm another merely by a negligent action.

### Nonintentional Torts

#### *Negligence and Malpractice*

Most of the lawsuits encountered in clinical practice involve the area of nonintentional torts and may be classified as either negligence or malpractice. Often used interchangeably, the 2 terms are not synonymous.

Negligence denotes conduct lacking in due care; it is an act or failure to act that leads to the injury of another. In its simplest definition, negligence is carelessness. Negligence may be attributed to either a professional or nonprofessional person; anyone who fails to perform to the standard of care that a reasonable person would meet in a particular set of circumstances may be guilty of negligence.

Malpractice is a more specific term and looks to the standard of care as well as to the professional status of the caregiver. Courts have defined malpractice as any professional misconduct, unreasonable lack of skill or fidelity in professional or judiciary duties, or illegal or immoral conduct.[6] In a more modern legal definition, malpractice is the failure of a professional person to act in accordance with the prevailing professional standards or failure to foresee consequences that a professional person, having the necessary skills and education, should foresee.

**Elements of Negligence and Malpractice.** The injured party bringing a lawsuit charging negligence or malpractice must prove to the court that the health-care giver or health-care institution was truly at fault. To meet this requirement, there are 6 elements that the injured party must show: duty owed the patient, breach of duty owed the patient, foreseeability, causation, injury, and damages.

**Duty owed the patient** involves the manner in which the health-care giver conducts himself/herself. The nurse has a duty to use reasonable care in his/her interactions with a patient. The standard of care owed is that of the reasonably prudent critical care nurse under similar circumstances—how would a reasonable, prudent critical care nurse with the same skills and educational level as the defendant nurse have acted under the same or similar circumstances? If the reasonable critical care nurse would have acted in the same manner as did the defendant critical care nurse, then no malpractice exists and no damages are due the injured party, no matter how substantial his/her injuries.

The applicable *standard of care* is possibly the most difficult portion of the lawsuit to show. Standards of care may be viewed as a level or degree of quality considered adequate by a given profession; standards of care are the skills and learning commonly possessed by members of a specific profession. Standards of care are derived from various sources: professional nursing organizations, state nurse practice acts, hospital policy and procedure manuals, protocols and/or standing orders, certification standards, job descriptions, and precedent court decisions. Above all, the standard of care of a given practitioner is set by his/her education and experience; the more education that one has and the greater one's professional skills, the more liable one becomes for failure to perform at an acceptable standard of care.

At trial, the acceptable standard of care is outlined by the use of expert witnesses. This role of expert witness exists to aid the jury and/or judge in determining the acceptable standard of care. The expert witness ideally has no prior connection with the persons involved in the lawsuit or with the claim. The sole function of the expert witness before the court is to help interpret evidence for the jury, clarify the care that was given, and establish appropriate standards of care. The expert witness testifying for the critical care nurse has a thorough understanding of the necessary skills and clinical expertise at the time of the alleged malpractice; the expert witness would then establish the standard of care to which the defendant nurse is accountable.

**Breach of the duty owed the patient** involves the showing of a deviation from the standard of care that was owed the injured party. Usually the deviation from the standard of care is termed ordinary negligence, implying professional carelessness either in an action performed or in the omission of a required action. The nurse, though, may be found to be grossly negligent, implying that the nurse willfully or consciously ignored a risk known to be harmful to the patient.

**Foreseeability**, the third element of malpractice, involves the concept that certain events may foreseeably cause specific results. For example, the omission of an ordered insulin injection to a known diabetic patient will foreseeably result in an abnormally high serum glucose level. The injured party must show that the action or omission of a required action by the nurse could foreseeably result in the actual happening.

**Causation** means that the injury must have resulted directly from the negligent action or negligent omission of a required action. It is not sufficient that an undesirable outcome occurred; the outcome must be directly related to the commission or omission of an action. Not every unusual occurrence is the result of a negligent action; for example, the injured party must show that the fall he sustained or the complication he incurred was directly caused by a health-care giver's negligent action.

**Injury** is the fifth element of malpractice. The injured party must demonstrate that some type of physical, financial, or emotional injury resulted from the breach of duty owed the patient. For example, the critical care nurse may be negligent in failing to raise the side rails on the bed of a disoriented, combative patient, but unless some injury actually occurs (the patient falls to the floor because there is no side rail to prevent his/her falling), there is no liability in a court of law for the substandard care.

**Damages** are awarded to compensate the injured party and to restore the patient to his/her original position as far as is financially possible. For example, the patient who becomes brain dead at age 30 because of substandard cardiopulmonary resuscitation measures will receive damages that include future medical costs for the rest of the patient's life. The damages would be less if the patient failed to survive the substandard cardiopulmonary resuscitation efforts because no future medical costs are then included.

The health-care provider must understand that damages in malpractice suits are not disciplinary in nature. The goal of awarding damages is truly to compensate the injured party and not to punish the defendants for their substandard care.

The more common areas of negligence in critical care settings today include: patient falls, medication errors, failure of the nurse to assess the patient adequately, and failure of the nurse to notify the primary health-care provider of changes in the patient's status.

## Intentional Torts

The nurse may also encounter intentional torts in the critical care setting. All intentional torts share 3 common elements: (1) there must be a volitional action by the defendant, (2) the person so acting must intend to bring about the consequences or appear to have intended to bring about the consequences, and (3) there must be causation in that the action must be a substantial factor in bringing about the consequences. Unlike negligence, the injured party does not have to show actual damages to be successful in his/her lawsuit; the law infers liability for intentional torts because the defendant intended to act as he/she did.

The most commonly seen intentional torts within the critical care setting are assault, battery, and false imprisonment. Although assault and battery are usually pled together, they are 2 separate torts.

An **assault** is any action that places another person in apprehension of being touched in a manner that is offensive, insulting, or physically injurious without consent or authority. No actual touching of the person is required; the action or motion must create a reasonable apprehension in the other person of immediate harmful or offensive contact with the defendant.

A **battery** involves a harmful or unwarranted contact with the patient without his/her permission. The patient need not be injured by the unwarranted contact nor does he/she need to even be aware of the unwarranted contact. For example, a battery occurs when a patient is restrained for the purpose of giving a medication, whether the patient is conscious or not. In most situations, a battery is averted because the health-care provider has consent to proceed with the treatment or therapy prior to its implementation. In fact, most of the case law in this area has focused on the consent issue.

**False imprisonment** is the unjustifiable detention of a person without legal warrant to confine the person. The nurse falsely imprisons the patient when he/she confines the patient or restrains the patient in a confined, bounded area with the intent to prevent the patient from freedom. The nurse may also falsely imprison the patient if he/she refuses to return to the patient his/her clothes, car keys, or personal belongings.

For the nurse to be liable in a court of law for false imprisonment, the patient must show that he/she was aware of the confinement. Confused, disoriented persons who are restrained for their own protection or to protect others from them will not be successful in a lawsuit for false imprisonment. Care, caution, and reasonableness are the prerequisites in the use of restraints.

Other possible defenses to intentional torts include consent and self-defense. No tort exists if the patient has given valid consent prior to the touching of his/her person. And a health-care provider may use necessary force to prevent a patient from either harming himself/herself or others in the area.

## Quasi-Intentional Torts

The law also recognizes what it terms quasi-intentional torts. This type of tort lacks the intent that is so crucial to intentional torts, but a volitional action and causation still must be shown so that the tort is more than mere negligence. The two quasi-intentional torts seen in critical care settings are invasion of privacy and defamation.

The right to protection against unreasonable and unwarranted interferences with the individual's solitude is well recognized. The tort of **invasion of privacy** includes the protection of personality as well as the protection against interference with one's right to be left alone. Usually, this tort is encountered in the critical care setting when confidential information is revealed without permission to someone not entitled to the information. For example, pictures are taken of the patient and used without his/her expressed authority or, more commonly, information about a patient's diagnosis and condition is given out over the telephone to interested callers.

Nurses are to be cautioned in releasing information concerning patients within their units. Remember, even family members do not have a right to such information without the patient's prior approval. Before releasing information over the telephone, the nurse should know what information may be given to the caller and the nurse should verify who the person is who is seeking the information. The caller may be instructed to check with family members if he/she is not one of the persons that the patient has authorized to receive such information.

A second area where invasion of privacy becomes a potential issue is with walking reports. Frequently, pertinent patient information is given by one shift of nurses to the oncoming shift at the patient's bedside. Family members or other patients may well be able to hear what is said at that report, and the possibility of invasion of privacy is great. The nurse is cautioned to either ask the family members to leave or to give the information to the oncoming nurses in a more private environment.

**Defamation** is the tort of wrongful injury to the reputation of another. This tort involves the written or oral communication to someone other than the person defamed of matters concerning a living person's reputation. A claim of defamation may arise from inaccurate or inappropriate release of medical information or from untruthful statements.

Caution is the key advice in this tort. The nurse should be careful about any reference made in charting about the patient's actions or reputation. For example, chart the behavior that the patient is exhibiting rather than that the patient is "crazy."

## Vicarious Liability

The issue of who is liable when a patient comes to harm is an increasing concern for nurses and hospitals alike. One always has personal accountability; no matter how many other persons might also be liable to the patient for his/her untoward outcome, the individual nurse retains personal accountability. Put more simply, one never losses personal accountability because someone else is also at fault.

The hospital may incur liability under the doctrine of *respondeat superior* or "let the master answer." This legal doctrine serves to impute liability to an employer because the employer has the right to both hire and fire an employee and, thus, has accountability for placing a given person within the setting. For the hospital to be liable, the nurse must have been within the scope of his/her employment when the incident occurred. For example, when a patient is negligently allowed to fall by the nurse assigned to his/her care, the employing hospital may also be found liable in the ensuing lawsuit.

The hospital may also incur liability through the doctrine of corporate liability. Suppose that a patient is harmed while hospitalized and the injured party's attorney is unable to show negligence against the nurses who cared for the injured party. The hospital would not be liable because the doctrine of *respondeat superior* is not applicable. The hospital may be liable, though, if the injured party can show that the hospital failed to meet the standards of the Joint Commission for the Accreditation of Hospitals (JCAH) or failed to evaluate its employees periodically. This doctrine of corporate liability makes the hospital directly liable to the injured party.

The hospital and a supervising physician may jointly be liable for a nurse's actions. Frequently referred to as a dual servant role, this type of situation is most often encountered in critical care settings during cardiopulmonary resuscitation efforts. Because one person is directly in charge of the resuscitation efforts, the nurse may be said to be acting as an employee to that individual. The nurse is also, though, accountable to the employing institution and is charged with following the hospital's policies and procedures. A negligent action by the nurse could potentially make both the hospital and the ordering physician liable.

# EXPANDED ROLES AND THE CRITICAL CARE NURSE

As the scope of nursing and the scope of medicine become more intertwined and less capable of exact delineation, critical care nurses question if they are practicing medicine. This is especially true in situations that demand immediate action and that require advanced technology. For example, a coronary care patient suddenly begins having frequent, paired premature ventricular contractions and short bursts of ventricular tachycardia. Lidocaine is readily available in its intravenous form; does the coronary care nurse practice medicine when he/she administers 100 mg of lidocaine intravenously through a previously placed intravenous line? Or, as Roth and Daze[7] contend, are nurses who accept this increased responsibility merely practicing good nursing?

To answer this dilemma, several factors must be addressed. The courts have long recognized the individual judgment of nurses and have held the nurse accountable to this independent judgment.[8] This type of court interpretation provides the basis for expanding roles in nursing.

Second, the state nurse practice act gives guidance for expanding roles and expanded nursing practice. Several of the individual nurse practice acts now allow for nursing diagnosis and treatment. A nurse so acting could be said to be acting on the nursing assessment of the patient and responding appropriately.

Third, individual hospital protocols may give the nurse guidance. If the acceptable standard of care is that the nurse in the intensive care unit may institute appropriate measures to alleviate a patient's presenting symptomatology in emergency situations, then to act accordingly is not considered practicing outside the scope of nursing practice. These hospital protocols should be established by a joint committee representing medicine and nursing and be reviewed and updated frequently. This latter provision allows the protocols to remain current in light of changing technological advances and standards of care.

JCAH guidelines also provide excellent standards of care. These guidelines are unit-specific and nationally based, and they provide evidence of reasonable nursing care should a subsequent lawsuit be filed.

Fourth, the presence of an emergency situation may give the experienced critical care nurse more standing to initiate appropriate therapy. Before initiating any standing protocols, a nurse should (1) ensure that this is an emergency situation and that the patient's life or physical well-being is imminently threatened, (2) ensure that the nurse's level of expertise and skills is not exceeded, and (3) ensure that a physician is not readily available before proceeding. What is allowable in an emergency situation is usually determined based on whether the nurse acted in a reasonable manner and in accordance with sound nursing principles.

Certification, the process of granting recognition to individuals who have attained a specific level of knowledge and expertise in a given field of a profession, may also aid the nurse in proving that he/she had the necessary skills and expertise to act in a specific situation. Advanced certification credentials may weigh favorably in the event of a lawsuit.

## SPECIFIC LEGAL CONCERNS

Additionally, the critical care nurse faces several specific concerns on a day-to-day basis. Some of the commonly encountered concerns are patient consent issues, do-not-resuscitate issues, staffing issues, and life-support issues.

### Consent

As explained previously, all patients have the right to be consulted and give consent before caregivers may proceed with ordered treatments and interventions. Once the patient or his/her legal representative gives consent, the health-care provider may proceed without fear that a suit for battery will ensue.

Informed consent, a more current issue, indicates that the patient or his/her legal representative has had treatments and procedures explained to him/her and that the person has been given sufficient information on which to base an informed choice. The duty to see that informed consent is obtained prior to initiating treatments and procedures usually falls on the physician or the primary health-care practitioner.

The nurse's role in this area of the law is still evolving. Some hospitals through policy make the nurse accountable for seeing that the patient signs informed consent forms; other hospitals have policies that mandate valid informed consent forms be obtained by the primary health-care practitioner and that the nurse may sign as a witness only. Some hospitals may require a signed form for each procedure and therapy, while other hospitals rely on documentation of the patient's consent in the medical chart.

Generally, the nurse is responsible for informing the physician and the hospital administration if there is a problem with informed consent. For example, the patient asks the nurse about a surgical procedure and it becomes clear to the nurse that the patient was either not informed by the physician or that the information given was incomplete; the nurse then has a duty to see that valid informed consent is obtained prior to the scheduled surgery.

Informed consent may be implied in limited situations. For example, the health-care provider may intervene to save a patient's life in a life-threatening situation without first obtaining consent for the proposed treatment and procedures. Implied consent is often relied on in critical care settings.

### Do-Not-Resuscitate Issues

Cardiopulmonary resuscitation for all patients, unless noted otherwise, has been fairly standard since the mid-1960s. The issue for nursing has usually not been whether one could or should order a no-code for a given patient, but whether a verbal order was sufficient for the manner in which the code was to be implemented.

It has always been the best course of action for nursing to have a written and documented no-code order. And most hospitals by policy now require that the attending physician write such an order before the patient will be no-coded. Absent policy or state statutes, a verbal no-code order is valid, although it may be more difficult to prove in a court of law. It is also recommended that written orders be resigned and re-evaluated every 24–72 hours.[9]

If cardiopulmonary resuscitation is to be initiated, a "slow code" or a "partial code" (one in which the nurses move slowly or fail to respond in a timely manner) should never be permitted because such actions fall below the minimal standard of care. The nurse should either code the patient in a competent manner or press for a no-code so that no resuscitative measures need be initiated.

## Staffing Issues

An issue that frequently arises is that of the float nurse in a critical care setting. What standard of care is required of the float nurse, one who typically works either on a general floor of the hospital or one who is unfamiliar with the policies and procedures of the unit? Generally speaking, the float nurse will be held to the same standard of care of the experienced critical care nurse if the float nurse fails to inform the charge nurse of his/her lack of critical care skills and accepts responsibility for patients as a critical care nurse.

There are some things that the float nurse and the charge nurse may do to protect the float nurse: (1) ask the float nurse exactly what his/her expertise is and assign the float nurse to patients requiring care that he/she is competent to give; (2) serve as a resource to the float nurse and ensure that his/her expertise is not exceeded; (3) request that administration initiate classes to cross-educate nurses so that the float nurse can competently give care to patients in critical care settings.

## Life-Support Measures

What constitutes life-support measures, when will they be initiated and how may they be terminated are issues that have been raised in various court cases, beginning with the New Jersey Supreme Court in 1976.[10] The law will continue to evolve in this area as each jurisdiction continues to create its own guidelines. Consequently, there are no set answers for the nurse within the legal sphere. This is perhaps still an area where the nurse must look at ethical decision-making and do what he/she can to best help the patient and/or his/her family members.

## CONCLUSIONS

This chapter has explored both ethical theories and legal principles in an effort to aid the individual nurse in effective decision-making within critical care settings. Although written in 2 distinct parts, there is no such division between legal and ethical dilemmas in most critical care settings. Having mastered this content, the nurse must make his/her own decisions.

## REFERENCES

1. Thompson, IE, Melia, KM, and Boyd, KM: Nursing Ethics. Churchill Livingstone, New York, 1983, p 130.
2. Thompson, IE, Melia, KM, and Boyd, KM: Nursing Ethics. Churchill Livingstone, New York, 1983, p 131.
3. Frankena, WK: Ethics, ed 2. Prentice Hall, Englewood Cliffs, 1973, pp 45–47.
4. Frankena, WK: Ethics, ed 2. Prentice Hall, Englewood Cliffs, 1973, p 49.
5. Wlody, GS and Smith, S: Ethical dilemmas in critical care: A proposal for hospital ethics advisory committees. Focus Crit Care 12(5):41, 1985.
6. *Napier v Greenzweig*, 256 F.196 (2d. Cir.1919) and *Forthofer v Arnold*, 60 Ohio App. 436, 21 N.E.2d. 869 (1938).
7. Roth, MD and Daze, AM: Are nurses practicing medicine in the ICU? Dimensions of Critical Care Nursing, 3(4):230, July–Aug 1984.
8. See generally, *Fraijo v Hartland Hospital*, 160 Cal. Rept. 246, 99 Cal. App. 3d. 331 (1979) and *Cooper v National Motor Bearing Company*, 288 P. 2d. 581 (California 1955).
9. Greenlaw, J: Orders not to resuscitate: Dilemma for acute care as well as long term care facilities. Law, Medicine, and Health Care 10(1):30, Feb 1982.
10. *In Re Quinlan*, 70 N.J.10, 355 A. 2d. 647 (1976).

# Glossary

**Absorption** Movement of particles across a cellular membrane from a body compartment toward the blood or intravascular compartment.

**Absorptive state** Period during which nutrients are being absorbed from the gastrointestinal tract into the bloodstream.

**Abulia** Lack of spontaneity; inability to make a decision.

**Accommodation** Adjustments within the eye for viewing distances by changes in the shape of the lens, pupillary constriction, and convergence of eyeballs.

**Acetone** Ketone body produced from metabolism of acetyl CoA during prolonged fasting, or in diabetic ketoacidosis.

**Acetylcholine** Neurotransmitter released at neuromuscular junctions, preganglionic synapses, and cholinergic synapses of parasympathetic nervous system.

**Acetylcholinesterase** Enzyme that degrades acetylcholine.

**Acid** Substance capable of releasing hydrogen ions in a solution; a solution having a hydrogen-ion concentration greater than that of water (i.e., pH <7.0).

**Acidemia** Reflects an increase in the concentration of hydrogen ions in the blood resulting in a pH <7.35.

**Acidosis** Any circumstances in which the hydrogen-ion concentration in blood is in the process of becoming increased, thereby lowering the pH <7.35.

**Acquired immune deficiency syndrome (AIDS)** Caused by the human immunodeficiency virus (HIV). The immunologic defect is due to the effect the virus has in making T4 lymphocytes ineffective.

**ACTH** Adrenocorticotropic hormone secreted by the anterior pituitary gland.

**Action potential** Reversal in the polarity of the membrane potential in which the inside of the cell momentarily becomes positive with respect to the outside; the electrical signal conducted over nerve and muscle cells.

**Active hyperemia** Increased blood flow through tissues in response to metabolic activity.

**Active transport** An energy-requiring, carrier-mediated transport system in which molecules can be moved across a membrane against an electrochemical gradient.

***Primary active transport*** in which chemical energy is transferred directly from ATP to carrier proteins.

***Secondary active transport*** The energy released during the transmembrane movement of one substance from a higher to lower concentration is transferred to the simultaneous movement of another substance from lower to higher concentrations (coupled facilitated diffusion).

**Adenosine diphosphate (ADP)** Two-phosphate product from the breakdown of ATP.

**Adenosine monophosphate (AMP)** Monophosphate derivative from the breakdown of ATP.

**Adenosine triphosphate (ATP)** Major molecule that accepts energy from the breakdown of fuel molecules during formation from ADP and Pi.

**Adenylcyclase** Enzyme that catalyzes the transformation of ATP to cyclic AMP.

**Adrenal cortex** Endocrine gland that forms the outer perimeter of each adrenal gland; secretes glucocorticoids (cortisol), mineralocorticoids (aldosterone), and androgens.

**Adrenal medulla** Endocrine gland that forms the inner core of each adrenal gland and secretes mainly epinephrine and, to a lesser extent, norepinephrine.

**Adrenergic** Term applied to nerve fibers that when stimulated release epinephrine at their axon endings; sympathetic nervous system response.

**Adrenocorticotropic hormone (ACTH)** Hormone secreted by the anterior pituitary, essential to the growth, development, and continued function of the adrenal cortex.

**Aerobic** Living only in the presence of oxygen.

**Affect** Emotional reactions associated with an experience.
**Afferent neuron** Neuron that transmits impulses from receptors in the periphery to the central nervous system (brain and spinal cord).
**Afferent pathway** Series of afferent (sensory) neurons that transmit impulses from receptors in the periphery to the integrating centers and primary sensory centers in the brain.
**Affinity** Attraction between molecules.
**Afterload** Load against which the heart muscle must exert its contractile force.
**Agonist** Molecule that binds to a receptor site and triggers the same response as the true chemical messenger.
**Aldosterone** Mineralocorticoid hormone secreted by adrenal cortex that stimulates reabsorption of sodium by distal tubule cells.
**Alkalemia** Decrease in hydrogen-ion concentration of the blood (pH >7.45).
**Alkaline** Having a hydrogen-ion concentration lower than that of water (pH >7).
**Alkalosis** Any state in which the hydrogen-ion concentration of arterial blood is reduced (pH >7.45).
**All or none** Event that occurs maximally or not at all.
**Allergy** Acquired hypersensitivity to a substance (antigen, allergen) that does not normally evoke an immune response.
**Alpha-adrenergic receptor** A site in autonomic nerve pathways wherein excitatory responses occur when adrenergic agents such as norepinephrine and epinephrine are released. Alpha-adrenergic and beta-adrenergic receptors are distinguished from one another by the type of response elicited.
**Alpha cells** Glucagon-secreting cells of the pancreatic islets of Langerhans.
**Alternate complement pathway** Sequence for complement activation that is initiated nonspecifically and is not antibody-dependent.
**Alveolar–arterial oxygen difference (A–a gradient)** Difference between alveolar and arterial oxygen tensions.
**Alveolar deadspace** Volume of inspired gas that reaches the alveoli but is not involved in gas exchange (i.e., deadspace unit).
**Alveolar ventilation** Volume of inspired gas that reaches the alveoli and participates in gas exchange.
**Ammonia** Produced by breakdown of amino acids; converted to urea in the liver.
**Amphipathic molecule** Molecule containing a polar or ionized group at one end and a nonpolar group at the other.
**Amylase** Enzyme that breaks down starch into disaccharides.
**Anabolism** Constructive phase of metabolism wherein cells take nutrients from the blood for the growth and repair of tissue.
**Anaerobic** In the absence of oxygen.
**Analgesia** Pain relieving.
**Anaphylaxis** Sudden, acute allergic hypersensitivity reaction to an antigen or drug.
**Anatomic deadspace** Volume of inspired gas that occupies the space in the upper airways and tracheobronchial tree (i.e., the conducting zone) that does not participate in gas exchange.
***Alveolar deadspace*** Alveoli that are fully ventilated but do not receive adequate perfusion to facilitate gas exchange.
***Physiologic deadspace*** Deadspace ventilation equal to the anatomical deadspace plus the alveolar deadspace.
**Anemia** Condition characterized by a reduction in the number of circulating red blood cells and total hemoglobin in the blood.
**Anemic hypoxia** State in which the $PaO_2$ is normal, but the total oxygen content of the blood is reduced due to reduction in total blood hemoglobin.
**Aneurysm** Abnormal localized dilatation of a blood vessel usually associated with the weakening of the vessel wall.
**Angiotensin I** Vasopressor substance formed in the blood by the interaction of renin and angiotensinogen (a plasma precursor).
**Angiotensin II** Potent vasopressor substance formed from angiotensin I by the action of converting enzyme; stimulates secretion of aldosterone from adrenal cortex.
**Anion** Negatively charged ion (e.g., $Cl^-$, $HCO_3^-$).
**Anosognosia** Lack of awareness as to the presence of neurologic deficits.
**Anoxia** Absence of oxygen.
**Antagonist** Molecule that binds to a receptor site and triggers a response opposed to that elicited by the true chemical messenger.
**Antibody** Protein substance synthesized and secreted by plasma cells in response to, and interacting specifically with, an antigen.
**Antibody-mediated immunity** Specific immune response in which circulating antibodies play a central role (see *humoral immunity*).
**Antidiuretic hormone (ADH)** Hormone synthesized in the hypothalamus and released from the posterior pituitary; increases the permeability of cells of the distal renal tubules and collecting ducts to water; also called vasopressin.
**Antigen** Foreign molecule, usually a protein, that stimulates a specific immune response when introduced into the body.
**Antihistamine** Chemical that blocks the action of histamine.
**Antrum (gastric)** Lower portion of the stomach (i.e., the region closest to the pyloric sphincter).
**Aphasia (dysphasia)** Absence or impairment of the ability to communicate by formulating or understanding oral or written language; recep-

tive (sensory) reflects the inability to understand spoken or written word; expressive (motor) reflects inability to speak one's thoughts.

**Apnea** Cessation of respiration.

**Apraxia** Disturbance in the execution of learned movements or the manipulation of objects in space.

**Arachidonic acid** Fatty acid that is the major precursor of prostaglandins.

**Arrhythmia (dysrhythmia)** Any variation from the usual rhythm of the heartbeat.

**Arteriolar resistance** Resistance to the flow of blood offered by the arterioles.

**Asterixis** See *tremor*.

**Asthenia** Debilitated, loss of strength, extreme weakness.

**Astigmatism** Defect in vision due to irregularities in the curvation of the cornea and/or lens of the eye.

**Atelectasis** Collapse of alveoli; failure of expansion or resorption of gas (resorptive atelectasis).

**Atherosclerosis** Pathologic process characterized by a thickening of the arterial wall associated with accumulation of lipids, cholesterol, platelets, and calcium deposits, and by infiltration of abnormal smooth muscle and connective tissue cells.

**Athrombia** Impairment in blood clotting due to thrombin deficiency.

**Atmospheric pressure** The air pressure of the environment at sea level (760 mmHg).

**Atom** Smallest unit of matter that has unique chemical characteristics.

**ATPase** Enzyme that breaks down ATP to ADP and inorganic phosphate.

**Autoimmune disease** Disease produced by antibodies or T cells acting against the body's own cells, resulting in alteration of cellular function.

**Automaticity** Capable of self-excitation.

**Autonomic dysreflexia** Clinical emergency characterized by an exaggerated sympathetic response occurring below the level of the spinal cord lesion and resulting in uncontrolled paroxysmal hypertension.

**Autonomic nervous system** Component of the efferent division of the peripheral nervous system that innervates cardiac muscle, smooth muscle and glands; consists of the parasympathetic and sympathetic subdivisions.

**Autoregulation** Ability of individual organs and tissues to alter their vascular resistance so as to maintain a relatively constant blood flow to meet their oxygen and nutrient needs.

**Axon terminals (synaptic knob)** Network of fine branches at the end of each axon, each branch ending at a synapse or neuromuscular junction.

**Azotemia** Renal dysfunction characterized by a progressive accumulation and retention of nitrogenous waste.

**B cells** Immune system: Lymphocytes that upon activation proliferate and differentiate into antibody-secreting plasma cells. Endocrine system: Insulin-secreting cells in the islets of Langerhans of the pancreas.

**Baroreceptor** Sensory nerve endings located in the carotid sinus, *vena cava*, and aortic arch, and sensitive to pressure or the degree of stretch.

**Basal ganglia** Nuclei deep in the cerebral hemispheres that relay information associated with the control of body movements.

**Base** Any molecule that can combine with a hydrogen ion.

**Basement membrane** Thin proteinaceous layer of extracellular material associated with the plasma membranes of many cells.

**Beta-adrenergic receptor** Receptor within the sympathetic nervous system to which epinephrine and norepinephrine bind, thereby triggering a sympathetic response. Alpha-adrenergic and beta-adrenergic receptors are distinguished from one another by the type of response elicited.

**Bile** Fluid secreted by the liver containing bile salts, cholesterol, lecithin, bile pigment, and other end-products of organic metabolism.

**Bile canaliculi** Tiny, intercellular, biliary vessels that channel bile into bile ducts.

**Bile duct** Conveys bile from the liver to the hepatic duct, which joins the cystic duct carrying bile from the gallbladder, to form the common bile duct. The common bile duct conveys bile to the duodenum.

**Bile pigments** Colored substances derived from the breakdown of the heme group of hemoglobin and secreted in the bile.

**Bile salts** Steroid molecules secreted by the liver in the bile that promote solubilization and digestion of fat in the small intestine.

**Bilirubin** Yellow substance resulting from the breakdown of heme excreted in the bile as a bile pigment.

***Direct*** Bilirubin conjugated by the liver cells to form water-soluble bilirubin diglucuronide.

***Indirect*** Fat-soluble unconjugated bilirubin present in blood.

**Biliverdin** Greenish pigment formed in bile by the oxidation of bilirubin.

**Binding site** A region on the surface of a protein that has a chemical group/conformation that molecules interact with and specifically bind.

**Blood–brain barrier** Barrier membrane between circulating blood and the brain interstitium which closely controls the kinds of substances (and the rate at which they enter) allowed to enter the brain's substance.

**Blood types** Classification of the blood determined by the presence of antigens of the A, B, C, or AB types on the plasma membranes of erythrocytes, and by the presence in the plasma of anti-A or anti-B antibodies (or both, or neither).

**Bone marrow** Highly vascular cellular substance of the central cavity of some bones; site of synthesis of RBCs, WBCs, and platelets.

**Bradykinin** Molecule formed by the action of the enzyme, kallikrein, on a protein precursor; a potent vasodilator that increases capillary permeability.

**Bruit** Adventitious sound of venous or arterial origin heard on auscultation.

**Buffering** Reversible binding of hydrogen ions by various compounds; these reversible reactions tend to minimize changes in acidity of a buffered solution when acid is added or removed.

**Bulk flow** Movement of fluids or gases from a region of higher pressure to one of lower pressure.

**Calcitonin** Hormone secreted by parafollicular cells of the thyroid gland; involved in calcium regulation.

**Calcium antagonist** Calcium-blocking agents that inhibit transmembrane flow of calcium ions.

**Calmodulin** Intracellular protein that binds calcium and mediates many of calcium's second messenger functions.

**Calorie (cal)** Unit in which heat energy is measured; the amount of heat needed to raise the temperature of 1 g of water 1 °C.

**Carbon monoxide (CO)** Gas that reacts with the same iron-binding sites on hemoglobin as does oxygen but with a much greater affinity than oxygen; decreases the oxygen-carrying capacity of blood.

**Carbonic anhydrase** Enzyme that catalyzes the reaction in which $CO_2$ and $H_2O$ combine to form carbonic acid ($H_2CO_3$).

**Carcinogen** Any of a number of agents (radiation, viruses, certain chemicals) that can induce the cancerous transformation of cells.

**Cardiac cycle** One episode of contraction–relaxation of the heart muscle.

**Cardiac output** Volume of blood pumped by each ventricle each minute.

**Carotid sinus** Dilated area at the bifurcation of the common carotid that is richly supplied with sensory nerve endings sensitive to pressure and degree of stretch (baroreceptors).

**Carrier** Integral membrane protein capable of combining with specific molecules and facilitating their passage through a membrane.

**Catabolism** Degradative phase of metabolism wherein cells break down complex substances into their simpler parts usually with the release of energy.

**Catalyst** Substance that accelerates chemical reactions but does not itself undergo any net chemical change during the reaction.

**Catechol-O-Methyltransferase** Enzyme that breaks down catecholamine neurotransmitters.

**Catecholamines** Neurotransmitters that have a similar chemical structure, including dopamine, epinephrine, and norepinephrine; they have marked effects especially on the nervous and cardiovascular systems, smooth muscle, cardiac muscle, and glands.

**Cation** Ion having a net positive charge.

**Cell-mediated immunity** Type of immune response mediated largely by cytotoxic T lymphocytes.

**Central venous pressure** Blood pressure in large veins of the thorax (superior, inferior vena cavae) and right atrium.

**Cephalic phase (gastrointestinal control)** Initiation of the neural and hormonal reflexes regulating gastrointestinal functions by stimulation of the receptors in the head—sight, smell, taste.

**Cerebral edema** Increase in water content of brain parenchyma.

**Cerebral perfusion pressure** Driving force underlying cerebral blood flow; determinants include mean arterial blood pressure minus intracranial pressure.

**Cerebrospinal fluid (CSF)** Fluid that fills the cerebral ventricles and subarachnoid space surrounding the brain and spinal cord.

**Chemical equilibrium** System in which the rates of the forward and reverse components of a chemical reaction are equal (i.e., no net change in the concentrations of the reactants or products occurs).

**Chemical specificity** Property of a protein binding site such that only certain molecules or ions can bind with it.

**Chemoreceptor** *Peripheral:* Sensory receptors or sensory nerve endings stimulated by and react to concentrations of certain chemicals (outside of the central nervous system); chemoreceptors in the carotid body and aortic arch are sensitive to changes in serum oxygen, $CO_2$, and hydrogen-ion concentration. *Central:* Sensory receptors in the brain stem that respond to changes in hydrogen-ion concentration in the brain extracellular fluid.

**Chemotaxis** Orientation and movement of cells in a specific direction in response to a chemical stimulus (i.e., movement of neutrophils to area of inflammation).

**Cholecystokinin (CCK)** Hormone secreted by cells in the upper small intestine regulates several gastrointestinal activities including motility of and secretion by the stomach, gallbladder, contraction, and enzyme secretion by the pancreas.

**Cholesterol** Steroid molecule that is the precursor of the steroid hormones and bile salts; a component of plasma membranes.

**Cholinergic** Substance that acts like acetylcholine.

**Chylomicron** Lipid droplet comprised of phospholipid, cholesterol, triacylglycerol, free fatty acids, and proteins, which is released from the intestinal epithelial cells and enters the lacteals during fat absorption.

**Cilia** Hairlike projections from the surface of specialized epithelial cells; they sweep back and forth in a synchronized manner to propel material along the cell surface.

**Classical complement pathway** Antibody-dependent system for activating complement.

**Coagulation** Process of clotting.

**Coagulopathy** Disturbance in blood-clotting mechanisms.

**Collagen** Fibrous protein that has great strength; functions as a structural element in the interstitium of various types of connective tissues (i.e., tendons and ligaments).

**Collateral circulation** Circulation of small anastomosing blood vessels connecting branches of the same vessels and other blood vessels.

**Collateral ventilation** Movement of air between alveoli through pores in the walls separating the alveoli.

**Colloid** Large molecule to which the capillaries are relatively impermeable (i.e., a plasma protein).

**Compensatory mechanisms** Activities that function to make up for a deficiency or defect, and to restore/maintain a central function; compensatory mechanisms usually have limitations beyond which they are no longer effective.

**Complement** A group of plasma proteins that upon activation kill microbes directly and facilitate the inflammatory process. (See Table 61–3; see *alternate complement pathway* and *classical complement pathway*.)

**Compliance** Measure of the ease with which a structure or substance may be deformed (e.g., compressed, expanded, distended).

**Concentration gradient** Gradation in concentration that occurs between two regions having different concentrations.

**Conjugate gaze** Both eyes move together so that one image is perceived.

**Contralateral** Originating in or affecting the opposite side of the body.

**Control system** Collection of interconnected components that function to keep a physical or chemical parameter within a predetermined range of values.

**Converting enzyme** Enzyme that catalyzes the reaction in which angiotensin I is changed to angiotensin II.

**Corpus callosum** Large wide band of myelinated nerve fibers that connects the two cerebral hemispheres.

**Corticotropin-releasing hormone (CRH)** Hypothalamic hormone that stimulates ACTH secretion by the anterior pituitary.

**Cortisol** Glucocorticoid steroid hormone secreted by the adrenal cortex that regulates various aspects of cellular metabolism and has many other actions.

**Countercurrent multiplier system** Mechanism associated with the loops of Henle that creates within the medullary interstitium a high fluid osmolality.

**Creatine phosphate** Molecule that transfers phosphate and energy to ADP to generate ATP.

**Creatinine** Waste product derived from muscle creatine.

**Cross-bridge** Projection extending from a thick filament in muscle; a portion of the myosin molecule capable of exerting force on the thin filament and causing it to slide past the thick one (see Fig. 37–11).

**Crystalloid** Low-molecular-weight solute (e.g., $Na^+$, glucose, or urea).

**Current** Movement of electrical charge achieved by the movement of ions.

**Cyclic AMP (cAMP)** Cyclic 3′,5′-adenosine monophosphate; a cyclic nucleotide that serves as a second messenger for many hormones and neurotransmitters.

**Cytotoxic T cells** Class of T lymphocytes that, upon activation by specific antigens, directly attack the cell bearing that type of antigen.

**D cells** Somatostatin-secreting cells of the islets of Langerhans of the pancreas.

**Deamination** Removal of an amino ($-NH_2$) group from a molecule such as amino acid.

**Decerebrate** Pattern of abnormal posturing/rigidity in which an abnormal extensor response occurs in both upper and lower extremities.

**Decorticate** Pattern of abnormal posturing/rigidity in which an abnormal flexor response occurs in the upper extremities, and an abnormal extensor response occurs in the lower extremities.

**Decussation** Crossing over of nerve tracts to the side opposite their origin.

**Deoxyhemoglobin (Hb)** Hemoglobin not combined with oxygen; reduced hemoglobin.

**Deoxyribonucleic acid (DNA)** Nucleic acid that stores and transmits genetic information; consists of a double strand (double helix) of nucleotide subunits that contain the sugar deoxyribose.

**Depolarization** Change in the value of the membrane potential toward zero due to an increase in membrane permeability to sodium.

**Dermatomes** Segments of skin innervated by the various spinal cord segments.

**Desmosome** Type of cell junction whose function is to hold cells together.

**Diastole** Period of the cardiac cycle when ventricular muscle fibers are not contracting; ventricular relaxation.

**Diastolic pressure** Minimum blood pressure during the cardiac cycle; ventricular end-diastolic pressure is the pressure in the ventricles just prior to ventricular systole, ventricular contraction.
**Diffusion** Movement of molecules from a region of higher concentration to one of lower concentration because of random molecular motion.
**Diffusion equilibrium** State during which the diffusion fluxes in opposite directions are equal.
**2,3-diphosphoglycerate (DPG)** Substance produced by red blood cells (RBCs) that binds reversibly with hemoglobin, decreasing hemoglobin's affinity for oxygen, thereby allowing oxygen to be released to the tissues.
**Diplopia** Double vision.
**Diuretic** Any substance that inhibits fluid reabsorption in the renal tubule causing an increase in the volume of urine excreted.
**Dominant hemisphere** Cerebral hemisphere that controls the hand used most frequently for intricate tasks (i.e., left hemisphere in a right-handed person).
**Dopamine** Catecholamine neurotransmitter; a precursor of epinephrine and norepinephrine.
**Dorsal** Posterior, toward the back.
**Dual innervation** Innervation of an organ or gland by both sympathetic and parasympathetic nerve fibers.
**Dysarthria** Speech impairment due to a disruption of the muscles of the tongue and other muscles essential to speech.
**Dyskinesia** Alteration in movement; loss of functional integrity related to movement.

**Ectopic focus** Region of the heart other than the SA node that assumes the role of the cardiac pacemaker.
**Edema** Accumulation of excess fluid in the interstitial space.
***Vasogenic*** Fluid accumulation in interstitial space (extracellular edema).
***Cytotoxic*** Fluid accumulation within the cells (intracellular edema).
**Effector** Structures, including nerves, muscle, and glands through which the response of the central nervous system to sensory input is actualized; results in response or altered activity.
**Efferent neuron (motor)** Neuron that carries information away from the central nervous system to muscle cells, glands, and other neurons.
**Efferent pathway** Motor neurons that transmit impulses from the receptive/integrating unit within the brain and spinal cord, to the periphery where the response to the CNS is evoked by muscles and glands.
**Elastance** Measure of the tendency of a structure to return to its original form after removal of a deforming force.
**Electric force** Force that causes the movement of charged particles toward regions having an opposite charge and away from regions having a similar charge.
**Electrochemical gradient** Force determining the magnitude of the net movement of charged particles; a combination of the electrical gradient (as determined by the voltage difference between 2 points) and the chemical gradient (as determined by the concentration differences between the same 2 points).
**Electrode** A probe to which electrical charges can be added (or from which they can be removed) to cause changes in the electrical current flow to a recorder.
**Electrolyte** Substance that dissociates into ions when in solution.
**Embolus** Foreign body, such as a fragment of blood clot, or an air bubble, circulating in the blood.
**Emulsification** Fat-solubilizing process in which large, lipid droplets are broken into smaller droplets.
**End-diastolic volume (EDV)** Amount of blood in a ventricle of the heart just prior to systole.
**End-systolic volume (ESV)** Amount of blood remaining in the heart after ejection.
**Endocytosis** Method of cellular digestion of a foreign body; a process in which the plasma membrane invaginates and the invaginations become pinched off, forming small, intracellular membrane-bound vesicles that enclose a volume of material.
**Endogenous pyrogen** Protein secreted by monocytes and macrophages, which acts in the brain to cause fever.
**Endorphins** Chemical substances synthesized within the brain that act as opiates and produce analgesia by binding to opiate receptor sites; beta-endorphins are highly active endorphins with morphinelike effect.
**Endothelium** Thin layer of cells that lines the cavities of the heart and the vasculature.
**Enkephalin** Peptide that functions as a neurotransmitter at synapses activated by opiate drugs.
**Enterohepatic circulation** Recycling pathway for bile salts and other substances by reabsorption from the intestines, passage to the liver by way of the hepatic portal vein, and passage back to the intestines by way of the bile duct.
**Enzyme** Protein that accelerates specific chemical reactions but does not itself undergo any net change during the reaction; a biochemical catalyst.
**Eosinophil** Granulocyte leukocyte whose granules stain readily with red dye eosin; involved in allergic responses and destruction of parasitic worms.
**Epinephrine** Hormone secreted by the adrenal medulla and involved mainly in the regulation of metabolism; a catecholamine neurotransmitter.

**Equilibrium potential** Voltage difference at which there is zero net flux of an ion between two compartments.
**Erythropoietin** Hormone that stimulates red blood cell production in bone marrow.
**Essential amino acids** Amino acid that cannot be formed by the body at all and, therefore, must be obtained from the diet.
**Excitability** Ability to produce action potentials.
**Excitation–contraction coupling** Mechanisms in muscle fibers linking depolarization of the plasma membrane with generation of force by the cross bridges.
**Excitatory synapse** Response of the postsynaptic membrane to the chemical neurotransmitter released by the presynaptic neuron is depolarization (i.e., moving the resting membrane potential toward threshold potential).
**Exocytosis** Process in which the membrane of an intracellular vesicle fuses with the plasma membrane, the vesicle opens, and the vesicle contents are liberated into the extracellular fluid (e.g., release of chemical neurotransmitter at cholinergic and adrenergic synapses).
**Expiratory reserve volume (ERV)** Volume of air that can be exhaled by maximal active contraction of the expiratory muscles at the end of a normal expiration.
**Extracellular fluid** Fluid surrounding cells; includes interstitial fluid and intravascular blood volume.
**Extrasystole** Heartbeat that occurs before the normal time in a cardiac cycle.
**Extrinsic clotting pathway** Formation of fibrin clots by a pathway using tissue thromboplastin.

**Facilitated diffusion** Simple: Carrier-mediated transport system that moves molecules from high to low concentration across a membrane; energy is not required, and equilibrium is reached when the concentration on the two sides of the membrane become equal. Coupled facilitated diffusion: See *active transport, secondary* and Fig. 21–10.
**Fasciculations** Involuntary contraction or muscle twitching.
**Fat-soluble vitamins** Vitamins that are soluble in nonpolar solvents and insoluble in water; vitamins A, D, E, and K.
**Feedback control system** Type of control system in which the output of the system (response) influences the input.
**Ferritin** Iron-binding protein that is the storage form for iron.
**Fibrillation** Extremely rapid contraction of myocardial fibers in an unsynchronized repetitive manner, which compromises the pumping action of the heart, thereby reducing cardiac output.
**Fibrinolysis** Dissolution of fibrin by plasmin (fibrinolysin).
**Fight or flight response** Overall activation of the sympathetic nervous system in response to stress.
**Filtration** Movement of essentially protein-free plasma across the walls of a capillary out of its lumen as a result of a pressure gradient across the capillary wall.
**Fluid mosaic model** Molecular structure of cell membranes consists of proteins embedded in a bimolecular layer of phospholipids; the phospholipid layer has the physical properties of a fluid, allowing the membrane protein to move laterally within the lipid layer.
**Flux** An excessive flow or discharge from an organ or cavity of the body.
**Functional residual capacity (FRC)** Equal to the sum of the expiratory reserve volume plus the residual volume. The FRC is the volume of gas that remains in the lungs at end-expiration during quiet breathing to ensure gas exchange continues uninterrupted.
**Functional unit** Subunit of which an organ is composed; all subunits have similar structural and functional properties.

**Gammaglobulin** Immunoglobulin G (IgG), the most abundant class of plasma antibodies.
**Ganglion (ganglia)** Cluster of neuronal cell bodies; generally restricted to neuronal clusters located outside the central nervous system.
**Gap junction** Type of cell junction allowing ions and small molecules to flow between the cytoplasm of adjacent cells by way of small channels or gaps.
**Gastric phase (gastrointestinal control)** Initiation of neural and hormonal reflexes controlling gastrointestinal function by stimulation of the wall of the stomach.
**Gastrin** Hormone secreted by the antral region of the stomach that stimulates gastric acid secretion.
**Gastroileal reflex** Physiologic relaxation of the ileocecal valve resulting from food in the stomach.
**Globulin** One of the types of protein found in blood plasma.
**Glomerular filtration** Movement of an essentially protein-free plasma through the capillaries of the renal glomeruli into Bowman's capsule.
**Glomerular filtration rate (GFR)** Volume of fluid filtered through the renal glomerular capillaries into Bowman's capsule per unit time.
**Glucagon** Hormone secreted by the A cells of the islets of Langerhans of the pancreas; its action on target cells leads to a rise in plasma glucose.
**Glucocorticoid** One of several steroid hormones produced by the adrenal cortex having major effects on glucose metabolism.
**Gluconeogenesis** Formation of glucose from

noncarbohydrate sources, including amino acids, fatty acids, pyruvate, and lactate.

**Glycogen** Major form of carbohydrate storage in the body, composed of thousands of glucose subunits.

**Glycogenolysis** Breakdown of glycogen.

**Glycolysis** Metabolic pathway that breaks down glucose to form 2 molecules of pyruvate (in the presence of oxygen) or 2 molecules of lactate (in the absence of oxygen).

**Granuloma** Mass or growth consisting of numerous layers of lymphoid or epithelial cells at the center of which may be a microbe or potentially harmful nonmicrobial substance, all enclosed in a fibrous capsule, which isolates the substance from healthy tissue.

**Growth hormone (GH)** Hormone secreted by the anterior pituitary; stimulates the release of somatomedins; stimulates body growth by means of its action on carbohydrate and protein metabolism; somatotropin.

**Growth hormone-releasing hormone (GH-RH)** Hypothalamic hormone that stimulates the secretion of growth hormone by the anterior pituitary.

**Halo sign** Presence of dark or bloody drainage encircled by a yellow stain on dressing or linen. Highly suggestive of CSF leak. Presence of glucose detected by testing drainage with a Dextrostix confirms the presence of CSF; CSF contains glucose, while mucus is glucose-free.

**Hapten** Small molecule that does not itself elicit an immune response but can attach to an existing antigen and thereby acquire the ability to trigger an immune response.

**Heat exhaustion** Acute reaction to heat exposure characterized by a state of hypotension precipitated by a depletion of intravascular volume associated with extreme diaphoresis, and extreme vasodilation of cutaneous blood vessels; thermoregulatory centers are still intact.

**Heat stroke** Condition characterized by impairment of thermoregulatory centers caused by a positive feedback state wherein the heat gain is greater than the heat loss causing body temperature to become extremely elevated.

**Helper T cells** Class of T cells that enhances antibody production and cytotoxic T-cell function.

**Hematochezia** Passage of stools containing red blood rather than tarry stools.

**Hematocrit** Percentage of total blood volume occupied by blood cells.

**Hematoma** Collection or mass of blood confined to an organ, tissue, or space and associated with injury to a blood vessel (e.g., epidural, subdural, and subarachnoid hematomas).

**Hematomyela** Bleeding into spinal cord parenchyma.

**Hematopoiesis** Production and growth of red blood cells in bone marrow.

**Heme** Iron-containing organic molecule bound to each of the 4 polypetide chains of a hemoglobin molecule.

**Hemetemesis** Vomiting of blood.

**Hemianesthesia** Loss of sensation of one side of the body.

**Hemianopia hemianopsia** Loss of one half of the field of vision in one or both eyes.

***Homonymous hemianopsia*** Loss of sight in corresponding halves of both eyes.

***Bitemporal hemianopsia*** Loss of temporal half of visual field in each eye.

**Hemiparesis** Weakness to slight paralysis affecting only one side of the body.

**Hemiplegia** Paralysis of one side of the body.

**Hemoglobin** Red protein located in erythrocytes; transmits most of the oxygen in the blood.

**Hemostasis** Cessation of bleeding from damaged vessel.

**Hepatic portal vein** Vein that conveys blood from the capillary beds in the intestines to the capillary beds in the liver.

**Herniation** Protrusion of an organ, or part of any organ, through the wall of the cavity that normally compartmentalizes it (i.e., brain herniation, protrusion of uncal portion of temporal lobe into tentorial notch, see Fig. 8–7).

**Histamine** Inflammatory mediator released mainly by mast cells; exerts a vasodilatory effect on blood vessels resulting in flushing of skin and reduction in blood pressure; stimulates gastric secretion.

**Histamine-2 antagonist** Drugs that block the effect of histamine on its receptors.

**Histocompatibility antigens** Tissue antigens present on the surface of all nucleated cells. They are controlled by genes at several loci termed the major histocompatibility complex (MHC).

**Histotoxic hypoxia** Hypoxia in which the quantity of oxygen reaching the tissues is normal, but the cell is unable to use the oxygen because a toxic agent has interfered with its metabolism (e.g., cyanide poisoning).

**Homeostasis** State of dynamic equilibrium of the internal environment and maintained by various feedback and regulatory mechanisms.

**Hormone** Chemical messenger synthesized by a specific endocrine gland in response to certain stimuli and secreted into the blood, which carries it to the other cells in the body where its actions are exerted.

**Humoral immunity** Type of specific immune response in which circulating antibodies play a central role.

**Hydrogen ion ($H^+$)** Single free proton; the concentration of hydrogen ions in a solution determines the pH of the solution.

**Hydrolysis** The breaking of a chemical bond

with the addition of water to the products formed; a hydrolytic reaction.

**Hydrostatic pressure** Pressure exerted by a fluid (e.g., blood).

**Hypercapnia** Increased carbon dioxide concentration in the blood (>45 mmHg); hypercarbia.

**Hyperemia** Increased blood flow.

**Hyperesthesia** Increase in sensitivity to sensory stimuli such as touch, pain, vibration.

**Hyperglycemia** Plasma glucose concentrations increased above normal levels (serum glucose >110 mg/100 ml).

**Hyperplasia** Excessive proliferation of normal cells in a tissue or organ whereby the bulk of the part or the organ is increased.

**Hyperpolarization** Change in the membrane potential so that the inside of the cell becomes more negative than its resting state; associated with efflux of potassium ions from the cell.

**Hypersensitivity** An acquired reactivity to an antigen which can result in bodily damage upon subsequent exposure to that particular antigen.

**Hyperthermia** Body temperature above normal; hyperpyrexia; fever.

**Hypertonic** Having a higher concentration and thus a higher osmotic pressure than a compared solution (e.g., blood).

**Hypertrophy** Increase in size; enlargement of tissue or organ that results from an increase in cell size rather than in cell number.

**Hyperventilation** Ventilation greater than that needed to maintain normal plasma $PaCO_2$.

**Hypervolemia** Abnormally increased blood volume.

**Hypocalcemic tetany** Skeletal muscle spasms due to a low extracellular calcium concentration.

**Hypoesthesia** Reduced sensitivity to touch, tactile stimuli.

**Hypoglycemia** (serum glucose <70 mg/100 ml) Low blood sugar (glucose concentration).

**Hypothalamic releasing hormones** Hormones released from hypothalamic neurons into the hypothalamo-pituitary portal vessels to control the release of anterior pituitary hormones.

**Hypothermia** Body temperature below normal.

**Hypotonic solution** Having a lesser concentration and thus a lower osmotic pressure than a compared solution (e.g., blood).

**Hypoventilation** Ventilation insufficient to maintain normal plasma $PaCO_2$.

**Hypoxemia** Insufficient oxygenation of the blood.

**Hypoxia** Reduction in tissue oxygen concentration (see also *anemic hypoxia, histotoxic hypoxia,* and *ischemic hypoxia*).

**Hypoxic hypoxia** Hypoxia due to decreased arterial $PO_2$.

**Idiopathic** Of undetermined cause.

**Ileogastric reflex** Reflex reduction in gastric motility in response to a distention of the ileum.

**Immunity** Physiologic mechanisms that allow the body to recognize foreign or abnormal substances (i.e., antigen) and to neutralize and/or eliminate them; allows the body to recognize and protect/maintain what is "self."

**Immunoglobulin** Antibody: includes five classes IgG, IgM, IgA, IgE, IgD.

**Immunologic tolerance** Ability of the body to recognize those molecules that are foreign; to distinguish self from non-self.

**Infarction** Area of necrotic tissue resulting from localized ischemia due to diminished blood supply.

**Inflammation** Local response to tissue injury characterized by swelling, heat, redness, and pain.

**Inhibitory synapse** Response of the postsynaptic neuron to the chemical neurotransmitter released by the presynaptic neurons causes the membrane potential to become more negative, that is, moving away from threshold potential.

**Inotropic** Pertaining to the heart's contractile state; factor influencing force of myocardial contractility.

**Insensible loss** Imperceptible loss of water (e.g., by evaporation from cells of the skin or respiratory tract).

**Inspiratory reserve volume** Maximum volume of air that can be inspired over and above the resting tidal volume.

**Insulin** Hormone secreted by B cells of islets of Langerhans of the pancreas, which facilitates uptake of glucose and amino acids by most cells.

**Intercalated disks** Low resistance pathways between adjacent cardiac muscle cells.

**Interferon** Protein or proteins formed when cells are exposed to viral or other foreign nucleic acids; important to immune function and have antitumor activity (esp. in hairy cell leukemia).

**Interleukin-1 (IL1)** Substance secreted from macrophages that stimulates activated B cells to proliferate, and the T cells to secrete interleukin-2 (see Fig. 54-7).

**Interleukin-2 (IL2)** Protein (lymphokine) secreted by helper T cells that causes activated T cells to proliferate (secretion of interleukin-2 is stimulated by interleukin-1).

**Internal environment** Includes interstitial fluid that bathes each cell, and the blood plasma.

**Interstitial fluid** Extracellular fluid surrounding cells.

**Interstitium** Space between cells containing extracellular (interstitial) fluid.

**Intestinal phase (gastrointestinal control)** Initiation of neural and hormonal reflexes controlling gastrointestinal functions by stimulation of the walls of the gastrointestinal tract.

**Intrapleural pressure** Pressure within the pleural space generated by the tendency of the lungs and chest wall to pull away from each other.

**Intrinsic clotting pathway** Intravascular sequence of fibrin formation initiated by Hageman factor (factor XII).

**Intrinsic factor** Substance normally secreted by cells of the stomach and essential for the absorption of vitamin $B_{12}$ in the ileum.

**Ion** Particle or small molecule carrying an electrical charge in solution.

**Ipsilateral** Pertains to the same side; affecting the same side of the body.

**Ischemia** Reduced blood supply to a tissue or organ.

**Ischemic hypoxia** Hypoxia in which the underlying defect is too little blood flow to tissues to ensure adequate oxygen supply.

**Isometric contraction** Contraction of muscles under conditions in which they develop tension but do not change length.

**Isotonic contraction** Contraction of a muscle under conditions in which a load on the muscle remains constant but the muscle length shortens.

**Isotonic solution** Solution in which the concentration and, thus, the osmotic pressure are equivalent to the solution to which it is being compared (i.e., blood).

**Isovolumetric ventricular contraction** Early phase of systole when myocardial tension increases but both the atrioventricular and semilunar valves remain closed.

**Isovolumetric ventricular relaxation** Early phase of diastole when myocardial tension is decreasing but both the atrioventricular and semilunar valves remain closed.

**Ketone bodies** Certain products of fatty acid metabolism, including acetoacetic acid, acetone, and beta-hydroxybutyric acid, that accumulate in the blood and contribute to the metabolic acidosis of diabetic ketoacidosis (DKA).

**Kinesthesia** Ability to sense the extent, direction, and weight of movement.

**Kinins** Group of peptides derived from kininogens that have considerable biologic activity, that facilitate vascular changes associated with inflammation including an increase in blood flow and capillary permeability, and that stimulate pain receptors.

**Laryngospasm** Spasm of laryngeal muscles; major concern is closing off of airway.

**Lecithin** Phospholipid.

**Leukotrienes** Group of chemical mediators of inflammation; stimulate contraction of bronchiolar smooth muscle (related to prostaglandins).

**Lipoproteins** Protein molecules that combine with lipids (including cholesterol, phospholipids, and triglycerides) and transport lipids in the blood. Lipoproteins are classified as high density (HDL), low density (LDL), and very low density (VLDL) lipoproteins.

**Local current flow** Movement of positive ions from a membrane region with a high positive charge directly through the cytoplasm or extracellular fluid toward a membrane region of more negative charge; and the simultaneous movement of negative ions in the opposite direction; in this way adjacent segments of membrane become depolarized (see Fig. 6–3).

**Lung compliance** Change in lung volume caused by a given change in pressure difference across the lung wall (i.e., the greater the lung compliance, the more easily the lungs can be expanded).

**Lymphokines** Substances (non-antibody) released by sensitive lymphocytes when in contact with specific antigens that contribute to cellular immunity by stimulating macrophages and monocytes.

**Lysosome** Cell organelle containing digestive enzymes and surrounded by a limiting membrane. These enzymes are capable of breaking down proteins, some carbohydrates, and, if released into the cytoplasm, can digest components of the cell itself.

**Macrophage** Cell of the reticuloendothelial system that functions as a phagocyte in many tissues, processes and presents antigen to lymphocytes, and secretes chemicals involved in the proliferation of activated lymphocytes in the inflammatory processes and in the body's overall response to infection.

**Major histocompatibility complex (MHC)** Group of genes that codes for many proteins important for immune responses including HLA, or histocompatibility antigens, present on the surface of all nucleated cells.

**Mast cells** Connective tissue cell that releases histamine and other chemicals in response to local tissue injury.

**Maximum tubular capacity (Tm)** Maximum rate of mediated transport of a substance, (e.g., glucose) across the membrane of renal tubule cells.

**Mean arterial blood pressure** "Average" blood pressure during the cardiac cycle and equal to diastolic pressure plus one third the pulse pressure.

**Mediated transport** Movement of molecules across membranes by binding to protein carrier molecules located within the membrane (see *active transport* and *facilitated diffusion*; see Fig. 21-10).

**Melanosis** Disorder of pigment metabolism resulting in abnormal dark brown or brown/black pigmentation of various tissues or organs.

**Membrane potential** Voltage difference between the inside and outside of the cell due to the separation of charge across the membrane.

**Memory cells** B and T lymphocytes produced after initial exposure to an antigen that respond expeditiously during a subsequent exposure to the same antigen.

**Metabolic acidosis** Associated with an accumulation of acid by-products of metabolism other than carbon dioxide (lactate production during exercise; ketone formation in DKA).

**Metabolic alkalosis** Reduction in the hydrogen-ion concentration in the body associated with mechanisms other than the respiratory removal of carbon dioxide (loss of hydrogen ions from stomach due to vomiting or continuous nasogastric suctioning).

**Metabolic rate** Reflects total energy expenditure in the body per unit time.

**Micelle** Soluble cluster of amphipathic molecules in which the polar regions of the molecules line the surface of the micelle, the nonpolar regions are oriented toward the middle of the micelle. Formed during digestion of fats in the small intestine (see Fig. 47-5).

**Microvilli** Small hairlike projections from the surface of some epithelial cells, which greatly increase the absorptive surface area of the cell.

**Micturition** Urination.

**Mineralocorticoids** Steroid hormones synthesized and secreted by the adrenal cortex having their major effect on sodium and potassium balance, (e.g., aldosterone).

**Mitochondria** Intracellular organelles that produce ATP.

**Mixed venous blood** Status of the oxygen and carbon dioxide tensions of blood in the pulmonary artery as a reflection of the total extraction of oxygen from circulating blood by all tissues within the body.

**Monoclonal antibodies** Identical immunoglobulins secreted by a clone of hybrid cells.

**Muscarinic receptors** Acetylcholine receptors that can be stimulated by the drug, muscarine; occur primarily at postganglionic synapses in the parasympathetic branches of the autonomic nervous system.

**Myelin** Insulating substance containing lipid and protein that forms a sheath around axons of certain nerves; presence of nodes of Ranvier facilitates rapid impulse transmission by saltatory conduction (see Fig. 6-3).

**Myenteric plexus** Network of nerve cells lying between muscle layers in the gastrointestinal tract.

**NA-K-ATPase** Primary active transport carrier protein present in all plasma membranes, which releases energy used to pump sodium ions out of the cell in exchange for potassium ions.

**Natriuretic factor** A hormonelike substance secreted by cells especially in right atrium that enhances renal excretion of sodium. Concomitant with sodium loss, extracellular fluid volume and intravascular blood volume decrease slightly.

**Natural killer (NK) cells** Cells, probably lymphocytes, that bind relatively nonspecifically to cells exhibiting foreign surface antigens, and kill them directly; no prior exposure to the antigen is required.

**Negative balance** State wherein the loss of a substance from the body is greater than that gained, and the total concentration of that substance in the body is decreased.

**Negative feedback** System wherein a series of changes are initiated to return a factor that has become excessive or depleted, back toward a certain mean value; type of feedback wherein an increase in the output of the system results in a decrease in the input.

**Neuroglycopenia** Presence of adrenergic and CNS alterations in the presence of serum glucose levels <55 mg/100 ml.

**Neurotransmitter** Chemical messenger released at chemical synapses through which the electrical activity of the presynaptic neuron influences the activity of the postsynaptic neuron, (e.g., norepinephrine, acetylcholine).

**Nicotinic receptors** Acetylcholine receptors that respond to the drug, nicotine; primarily occurs at neuromuscular junctions and ganglia in the autonomic nervous system.

**Nystagmus** Continuous involuntary movement of the eyeball in any direction.

**Oncogene** Gene in a virus that appears to be able to induce a cell to become malignant. Oncogenes have been identified in human tumors.

**Onycholysis** Loosening of nails, usually beginning at the free border with detachment from the nailbed.

**Ophthalmoplegia** Paralysis of ocular muscles.

**Opisthotonos** Tetanic spasm causing the head and heels to bend backwards and the trunk to bow forward.

**Osmolality** Osmotic concentration, the characteristic of a solution determined by the ionic concentration of dissolved particles per unit of solvent expressed as osmoles per kilogram of water.

**Osmolarity** Concentration of osmotically active particles in solution.

**Osmole** The amount of substance that dissociates in solution to form one mole of osmotically active particles.

**Osmosis** Net diffusion of water from a region of high water concentration to one of low water concentration across a membrane; water moves from regions of low solute concentration (high water concentration) to a region of high solute concentration (low water concentration).

**Osmotic pressure** Pressure that develops when two solutions of different concentrations are separated by a semipermeable membrane; or pressure that must be applied to a solution on one side of a membrane to prevent osmotic flow of water into the solution from a source of pure water on the opposite side of the membrane.

**Otorrhea** Drainage or discharge from the ear; suspect CSF leakage in the scenario of head injury.

**Oxidative phosphorylation** Process by which energy derived from the reaction between hydrogen and oxygen (to form water) is transferred to ATP during its formation from ADP and inorganic phosphate; this reaction occurs in mitochondria.

**Oxyhemoglobin** Hemoglobin combined with oxygen.

**Oxyhemoglobin dissociation curve** Reflects that the amount of oxygen bound to hemoglobin is a function of the partial pressure of oxygen (see Fig. 28–15).

**Paralytic ileus** State of complete atony of the small bowel with an absence of peristalsis; associated with abdominal surgery/trauma.

**Parasympathetic nervous system** Division of the autonomic nervous system whose preganglionic fibers leave the brain and sacral region of the spinal cord; most of its postganglionic fibers release the neurotransmitter, acetylcholine.

**Parasympathomimetic** Drug that produces effects similar to those of the parasympathetic nervous system.

**Parenchyma** Essential substance or components of an organ concerned with its function.

**Paresthesia** Heightened sensitivity; sensations of prickling, tingling, numbness.

**Parietal cells** Gastric gland cells that secrete hydrochloric acid and intrinsic factor (oxyntic cell) (see Fig. 47–3).

**Partial pressure** Pressure exerted by the molecules of one specific gas; (e.g., $PO_2$, the partial pressure of oxygen, is that part of total atmospheric pressure attributed to oxygen molecules).

**Permissiveness** Situation whereby a small quantity of one hormone is required in order for a second hormone to exert its effect.

**pH** Measure of the acidity or concentration of hydrogen ions of a solution; as acidity increases, pH decreases.

**Phagocytosis** Form of endocytosis or pinocytosis involving the engulfment and digestion of bacteria and particles by phagocytic cells (e.g., leukocytes, macrophages).

**Phospholipid** Lipid molecules containing phosphorus, fatty acids, and a nitrogenous base (e.g., lecithin).

**Phosphorylation** Addition of a phosphate group to an organic molecule.

**Pinocytosis** Cellular process of engulfing liquid.

**Plasma** Fluid, noncellular portion of the blood, comprising about 3% of total extracellular fluid.

**Plasma cells** Cells derived from activated B lymphocytes that secrete antibodies.

**Plasma proteins** Include albumin, globulins, and fibrinogens present in blood plasma.

**Plasmapheresis** Process of plasma exchange wherein blood is removed from the body and centrifuged in order to separate the cellular components from the plasma. Undesired components, (e.g., autoantibodies) can be removed and the remainder of the blood can be returned to the patient.

**Plasmin** Fibrinolytic enzyme derived from its precursor, plasminogen; functions to decompose fibrin and, thereby, to dissolve blood clots.

**Plethora** Hypervolemia: excess of any body fluid; expanded blood volume.

**Polarized** Having 2 electric poles, one positive, the other negative.

**Polydipsia** Excessive thirst.

**Polyunsaturated fatty acid** Fatty acid that contains more than one double bond.

**Portal vessels** Blood vessels that link 2 separate capillary networks, (e.g., hypothalamic–hypophyseal portal system).

**Postabsorptive state** Period between meals during which nutrients are not being absorbed by the gastrointestinal tract and energy must be supplied by the body's endogenous stores.

**Postganglionic neuron** Neuron of the autonomic nervous system whose cell body lies in a ganglion and whose axon endings terminate in effector organs (i.e., neuromuscular junction, glands).

**Postsynaptic neuron** Neuron that conducts impulses away from a synapse (see Fig. 6–4).

**Postural (orthostatic) hypotension** Reduction in blood pressure upon assuming an erect position or upon standing.

**Postural reflexes** Those reflexes that maintain or restore upright, stable posture.

**Potential (potential difference)** Voltage differences between two points.

**Precapillary sphincter** Ring of smooth muscle around a capillary at the point at which it exits from an arteriole.

**Preganglionic neuron** Neuron of the autonomic nervous system whose cell body lies in the CNS and whose axon terminals lie within a ganglion; conducts impulses from the CNS toward a ganglion.

**Preload** Distending force stretching the ventricular muscle fibers just prior to contraction.

**Presynaptic neuron** Neuron that conducts impulses toward a synapse (see Fig. 6–4).

**Proprioception** Awareness of posture and the knowledge of position and weight in relation to the body.

**Prostaglandins** Large group of biologically active, unsaturated fatty acids derived from arachidonic acid. Biologic effects are short-lived and are not mediated by the blood. They exert their effects locally, in the tissues within which they are formed. Physiologic activities influenced by prostaglandins include platelet aggregation, local blood flow, fluid balance, lypolysis, and neurotransmission, among others.

**Proteolysis** Breakdown of proteins into simpler substances; amino acid components.

**Pulse pressure** Difference between systolic and diastolic arterial blood pressures.

**Raynaud's phenomenon** Intermittent attacks of pallor followed by cyanosis, then redness of digits, before return to normal.

**Reactive hyperemia** Transient increase in blood flow following the release of occlusion of the blood supply to a tissue or organ; attributed to the vasodilatory effects of chemical mediators released by ischemic tissues.

**Receptor** Specialized peripheral ending of an afferent (sensory) neuron, or distinct cell intimately related to it that detects changes in the environment; receives stimulus or detects an alteration in environmental conditions.

**Receptor site** Specific protein binding site with which a chemical mediator or neurotransmitter combines to exert its effect.

**Reciprocal innervation** Inhibition of motor neurons activating those muscles whose contraction would oppose the intended movement (e.g., inhibition of flexor motor neurons during extensor motor neuron activation).

**Recommended daily allowance (RDA)** Daily intake of nutrients considered sufficient to prevent nutritional insufficiency in most healthy persons.

**Reduced hemoglobin** See *deoxyhemoglobin.*

**Reflex** Involuntary response when a stimulus is linked with a response and mediated by a reflex arch composed of neural and/or hormonal elements.

**Reflex arc** Components that mediate a reflex; comprised of a receptor, afferent pathway, integrating center, efferent pathway, and effector.

**Refractory period** Time period during which an excitable membrane does not respond to a stimulus.

***Absolute refractory period*** Timeframe during which an excitable membrane is unable to generate another action potential in response to any stimulus.

***Relative refractory period*** Time during which an excitable membrane will produce an action potential only in response to stimuli of greater strength than the usual threshold strength.

**Releasing hormones** Hormones secreted by the hypothalamus that control the release of hormones by the anterior pituitary.

**Renin** Enzyme secreted by the kidneys that acts on angiotensinogen in the blood to form angiotensin I (see Fig. 21–9).

**Repolarization** Return of the value of the transmembrane potential to its resting state.

**Residual volume** Volume of air remaining in the lungs after maximal expiration.

**"Resistance" vessels** Vessels that offer the greatest frictional resistance to blood flow (arterioles).

**Respiratory acidosis** Acidosis resulting from the failure of the lungs to eliminate carbon dioxide as rapidly as it is produced (hypoventilation).

**Respiratory alkalosis** Alkalosis resulting from the elimination of carbon dioxide from the lungs faster than it is produced (hyperventilation).

**Respiratory "pump"** Effect of the changing intrathoracic and intra-abdominal pressures associated with breathing on the venous return to the heart.

**Respiratory quotient (RQ)** Ratio of carbon dioxide produced to oxygen consumed during metabolism.

**Resting membrane potential** Voltage differences across a plasma membrane between the inside and outside of a resting cell.

**RH factor** Group of antigens that may (RH positive) or may not (RH negative) be present on the plasma membrane of red blood cells.

**Rhinorrhea** Thin, watery discharge from nose; suspect CSF leakage in scenario of head injury, basal skull fracture, and/or dural tear.

**Rostral-to-caudal** Head to toe.

**Saltatory conduction** Conduction that occurs along myelinated axons in which the myelin sheath is interrupted by the nodes of Ranvier, the action potential skips from node to node enhancing the rapidity of impulse conduction (see Fig. 6–3).

**Saturated fatty acid** Fatty acid whose carbon atoms are all linked by single covalent bonds.

**Saturation** Degree to which binding sites are occupied by specific molecules; if all sites are occupied, the binding sites are fully saturated; adding more of the substance will not increase its concentration.

**Secretin** Hormone secreted by cells in the upper part of the small intestine; stimulates pancreas to secrete bicarbonate into the small intestine; bicarbonate neutralizes the acid chyme entering the duodenum.

**Semipermeable membrane** Membrane permeable to some substances but impermeable to other substances.

**Serotonin** Chemical mediator with potent vasoconstrictor effects present in platelets, gastrointestinal mucosa, and mast cells; a monoamine neurotransmitter thought to be involved in neuromechanisms associated with sensory perception and sleep.

**Serum** Blood plasma from which fibrinogen has been removed as a result of clotting.

**"Shift to the left"** Increase in band neutrophils indicative of acute infection.

**Shunt**

***Right-to-left shunt*** Mixing of deoxygenated blood with oxygenated blood; passage of blood from right to left side of the heart.

***Left-to-right shunt*** Mixing of oxygenated blood with deoxygenated blood; passage of blood from left to right side of the heart.

**Skeletal muscle "pump"** Pumping action of contracting skeletal muscles especially in the lower extremities that assists venous return to the heart.

**Sliding filament theory** Process of muscle contraction wherein shortening occurs as a result of the sliding of thick (myosin) and thin (actin) filaments past each other.

**Sodium inactivation** Closing of sodium channels in the plasma membrane at the peak of an action potential when the membrane is depolarized.

**Solubility coefficient** Refers to the extent that molecules of gas are physically and chemically attracted to water molecules.

**Solute** Molecules dissolved in a liquid.

**Solution** Liquid containing dissolved molecules or ions.

**Solvent** Liquid in which molecules or ions are dissolved.

**Somatomedin** Group of growth-stimulating hormones released primarily from the liver in response to growth hormone.

**Somatosensory (somesthetic) cortex** Strip of cerebral cortex in the parietal lobe where nerve fibers transmitting somatic (i.e., pertaining to the body) sensations (i.e., touch, temperature, vibration) synapse. It provides a representation of senses from various segments of the body.

**Somatostatin** Hormone that inhibits release of somatotropin (growth hormone) and thyrostimulating hormone (TSH) from the anterior pituitary. This hormone is also secreted by D cells of the pancreatic islets of Langerhans and stomach, inhibiting secretion of insulin and gastrin.

**Specificity** Ability of a protein-binding site to react with one type, or a limited type, of structurally related molecules.

**Spinal cord syndrome** Incomplete spinal cord injuries having different patterns of neurologic dysfunction.

**Spinal shock (neurogenic shock)** Sudden complete transection of the spinal cord causing immediate loss of motor, sensory, reflex, and autonomic function below the level of the injury; spinal shock may also occur in incomplete transection of the cord.

**Starling's law of the heart** States that, within limits, an increase in the end-diastolic volume of the heart (i.e., increasing stretch of muscle fibers) increases the force of cardiac contraction.

**Stimulus** Any change in the environment detectable by a receptor (sensory).

**Stroke volume** Volume of blood ejected by a ventricle during each beat of the heart.

**Submucosa** Connective tissue layer underlying the mucosa in the walls of the stomach and intestines.

**Substrate** Reactant in an enzyme-mediated reaction.

**Suppressor T cells** Class of T lymphocytes that inhibit antibody production and cytotoxic T cell function.

**Surface tension** Unequal attractive forces at the surface of a liquid in contact with a gas or another liquid, wherein the attraction of the molecules to each other results in a net force that acts to reduce the surface area.

**Surfactant** Phospholipid agent produced by type II pneumocytes that markedly reduces surface tension within the alveoli. This reduces the tendency of the alveoli to collapse, thereby minimizing atelectasis.

**Sympathetic nervous system** Division of autonomic nervous system whose preganglionic fibers leave the thoracolumbar region of the spinal cord; most of the postganglionic neurons release the neurotransmitter, norepinephrine.

**Sympathetic trunk** One of a paired chains of interconnected sympathetic ganglia that lie on either side of the vertebral column

**Sympathomimetic** Drug that produces effects similar to those of the sympathetic nervous system.

**Synapse (chemical)** Anatomically specialized junction between 2 neurons where the electrical activity in one neuron (presynaptic) influences the excitability of the second neuron (postsynaptic) by a chemical neurotransmitter (see Fig. 6–4).

**Synaptic cleft** Narrow extracellular space separating the presynaptic and postsynaptic neurons at a chemical synapse.

**Synergistic** Enhancement of the activity of one molecule by the activity of another producing an effect that neither could produce alone; or the total effect may be greater than the summation of each substance functioning by itself.

**Systemic (peripheral) vascular resistance**

Resistance to blood flow offered by the systemic vasculature, including, in particular, that offered by the arterioles and metarterioles.

**Systole** Period when the ventricles of the heart are contracting.

**Systolic pressure** Maximum arterial blood pressure reached during the cardiac cycle.

**T cells (T lymphocytes)** Lymphocytes derived from precursors in the thymus (see also *cytotoxic T cells*, *helper T cells*, and *suppressor T cells*).

**Thick filaments** Filaments in muscle cells consisting of myosin molecules.

**Thin filaments** Filaments in muscle cells consisting of actin, troponin, and tropomyosin molecules.

**"Third spacing"** Shift of fluid from intravascular space to transcellar spaces (e.g., ascites).

**Thoroughfare channel** Capillary that connects arterioles and venules directly and from which capillaries branch to comprise the capillary bed.

**Threshold (renal)** Plasma levels at which a substance begins to appear in the urine.

**Threshold (threshold potential)** Membrane potential to which an excitable membrane must be depolarized in order to initiate an action potential.

**Threshold stimulus** Stimulus capable of depolarizing the membrane to threshold potential.

**Thrombin** Enzyme that catalyzes the conversion of fibrinogen to fibrin.

**Thrombosis** Formation, presence, or development of a blood clot (thrombus) that obstructs a blood vessel, partially or completely, or occurs in a cavity of the heart.

**Thyroglobulin** Large iodine-containing protein synthesized by the thyroid gland and stored within its colloid substance to which thyroid hormones bind and are stored.

**Thyroid hormone** Hormones synthesized and secreted by the thyroid gland; include thyroxine ($T_4$) and tri-iodothyronine ($T_3$); these hormones increase the metabolic rate of most cells.

**Thyroid-stimulating hormone (TSH; thyrotropin)** Hormone secreted by the anterior pituitary that induces its target gland, the thyroid gland, to secrete thyroid hormones.

**Thyrotropin-releasing hormone (TRH)** Hormone released by hypothalamus that stimulates thyrotropin (TSH) by the anterior pituitary

**Tidal volume** Volume of air entering and leaving the lungs during a single spontaneous breath.

**Tight junction** Type of junction formed between adjacent epithelial cells in some tissues that restrict diffusion of molecules across a layer of epithelial cells by way of the extracellular space between cells (e.g., blood–brain barrier in which two adjacent ependymal cells are fused together; see Fig. 6–11).

**Tissue thromboplastin** Extravascular enzyme capable of initiating the extrinsic clotting cascade leading to the formation of a fibrin clot.

**Total lung capacity** Equal to the sum of the vital capacity plus the residual volume.

**Tract** Large bundle of myelinated nerve fibers in the CNS (brain and spinal cord).

**Transudation** Passage of fluid or solute through a membrane as a result of hydrostatic and osmotic pressure gradients.

**Transverse tubule (T tubule)** Tubule extending from the sarcolemma (i.e., the delicate membrane surrounding the muscle fiber) into the fiber interior; conducts action potentials into the muscle fibers (see Figs. 37–9 and 37–10).

**Tremor** Involuntary, quivering type movement of a part or parts of the body associated with alternate contractions of opposing muscles.

***Intention*** Tremor when voluntary movement is attempted.

***Resting*** Presence of tremor at rest, but absent or diminished when movement is attempted.

***Flapping*** Coarse tremor seen in outstretched arm or hand and associated with hepatic coma and other diseases that cause encephalopathy (asterixis).

**Tropomyosin** Regulatory protein associated with the actin filament that is capable of reversibly covering the binding sites on actin, thereby preventing myosin heads from binding to actin to form cross-bridges.

**Troponin** Regulatory protein that attaches to both actin and tropomyosin.

**Tubular reabsorption** Transfer of substances from lumen of kidney tubule to the peritubular capillaries.

**Tubular secretion** Transfer of substances from the peritubular capillaries to the lumen of the renal tubules.

**Ultrafiltrate** Fluid that is essentially protein free; formed by plasma as it is forced through capillary walls by a pressure gradient.

**Unsaturated fatty acid** Fatty acid containing one or more double bonds.

**Uremia** Complex multisystem alterations that occur when the level of kidney function can no longer support the internal milieu.

**Valsalva's maneuver** Maneuver wherein an attempt is made to exhale forcibly against a closed glottis, thereby increasing intrathoracic pressures; this, in turn, decreases venous return to the heart; associated vagal stimulation results in slowing of the heart rate.

**Vapor pressure** Pressure exerted by water molecules as they escape from the fluid surface.

**Vasoconstriction** Decrease in diameter of blood vessels caused by vascular smooth muscle contraction.

**Vasodilation** Increase in diameter of blood

vessels caused by vascular smooth muscle relaxation.

**Velocity** Rate of fluid movement per unit time expressed as $cm^3$/second.

**Venous capacitance** Ability of veins to accommodate large volume increases without large increases in pressure.

**Venous return** Volume of blood filling the ventricles during diastole; preload.

**Ventilation** Bulk flow exchange of air between atmosphere and alveoli.

***Alveolar minute ventilation*** Equal to the number of breaths per minute (i.e., the respiratory rate) times the tidal volume minus the anatomical deadspace volume (i.e., alveolar volume).

***Minute ventilation*** Total volume of gas inspired each minute; equal to the respiratory rate times the tidal volume.

**Ventilatory dyscoordination** Disruption of the orderly sequence of contraction of muscles of inspiration and expiration associated with extreme weakness or fatigue.

**Ventilation–perfusion ratio ($\dot{V}/\dot{Q}$)** Reflects the relationship between alveolar ventilation and pulmonary capillary blood flow. (Normally the ratio is about 0.8.)

**Ventral** Anterior, towards the front.

**Villi** Projections of the highly folded surface of the mucosal lining of the small intestine; increases surface area for digestive and absorptive activities (see Fig. 47–4).

**Viscosity** Property of a fluid that makes it resist flow, caused by the frictional interactions between its molecules.

**Vital capacity** Volume of gas that is maximally expired following a maximal inspiration.

**Vitiligo** Appearance upon otherwise normal skin of loss of pigment with white skin patches of varied sizes, frequently symmetrically distributed.

**Voltage** Measure of the potential of separated electric charges to do work, expressed in volts.

**Water intoxication** State of excess water and sodium retention.

**Weak acid** Acid whose molecules do not completely ionize to form hydrogen ions when dissolved in water.

**Work of breathing** Energy or work required to expand the lungs and thorax so as to provide for a given volume of ventilation; effort generated by the contraction of expiratory musculature.

APPENDIX A

# Drugs Commonly Used in the Critical Care Setting

*Gene D. Morse, Steven B. Meisel*

## INTRODUCTION TO PHARMACOKINETICS

A drug dosage administered to a patient undergoes absorption, distribution, metabolism, and finally, elimination — these principles are collectively known as pharmacokinetics and they determine the concentration of the drug at its site of action. As this concentration increases, the intensity of the drug's pharmacologic effect also increases. In order to know the proper dose, dosage form, and route of administration of a given drug, understanding these pharmacokinetic principles is essential.

### Absorption

When a drug is administered intravenously, the entire amount is available immediately in the bloodstream for distribution to its sites of action. However, when a drug is administered by other routes, it first passes across cell membranes to reach the bloodstream. The absorption may be delayed or inhibited by a number of barriers. Only molecules that are in solution are able to cross cell membranes. Therefore, *intramuscular* absorption depends on the solubility of the drug in the muscular environment. For example, diazepam is very lipid soluble and will precipitate out of solution when administered intramuscularly. The absorption of the drug may be delayed for hours or even days after administration.

Other factors that affect the solubility of the drug include its relative acidity. For example, phenytoin is a weak acid with a pKa of 8.3. When it comes in contact with the more neutral pH of the muscle it will precipitate out of solution, consequently, intramuscular absorption may be slow and erratic.

Intramuscular absorption also depends on the blood supply to the injection site. If it is a poorly vascularized area, or if the patient's cardiac output is compromised, too little blood will be delivered to the drug-administration site for effective absorption to occur, in which case intravenous administration is usually preferred.

*Oral* absorption is further complicated by the following factors:

1. **Gastrointestinal (GI) motility** If a patient's gastric emptying time is rapid, the drug is in contact with the cell membranes responsible for its absorption for a short time. Patients with slow GI motility may absorb drugs more thoroughly.

2. **Gastric pH** Some drugs, such as ampicillin, are partially destroyed by the presence of acid. If a patient's gastric pH is increased, less drug will be destroyed and more will be available for absorption. Conversely, states of hyperacidity may cause more destruction of the drug and less systemic absorption.

3. **Co-administered medications or food** A number of drugs, as well as food, may affect GI motility or gastric pH, thereby influencing drug absorption. Also, some drugs, such as tetracycline, may be physically bound to food, antacids, or other drugs

with a resultant decrease in absorption. This may influence when a drug should be administered with respect to meals.

4. **The "first-pass" effect** As a drug is absorbed by the gut, it is delivered via the portal vein directly to the liver. If a drug is rapidly metabolized, only a fraction of the amount absorbed will appear in the systemic circulation. This is known as the first-pass effect and accounts for significant variability in the pharmacologic activity of orally administered drugs.

5. **Pharmaceutical factors** Inherent properties of the drug manufacturing process will influence the disintegration and dissolution of tablets and capsules. Although most brands of a given drug are designed to be absorbed to the same degree as other brands, some variability does exist among generic brands of some drugs. This also accounts for some of the variability in pharmacologic activity of orally administered drugs.

*Bioavailability* is the degree of absorption of a drug after oral administration. If a drug is 50% bioavailable, only half of the administered dose is delivered to the systemic circulation. Therefore, drugs low in bioavailability must be given in higher doses orally than intravenously in order to achieve a similar clinical effect. The bioavailability of a drug is particularly important when converting a patient's dose from intravenous to oral therapy.

### Distribution

As the drug enters the bloodstream, it immediately becomes distributed to the various parts of the body. An equilibrium is established between the bloodstream and other body tissues. This distribution is affected by a number of factors:

1. **Lipid solubility** If a drug is insoluble in lipid, it will not be able to penetrate tissues with high lipid content such as the central nervous system, adipose, breast milk and placenta.

2. **Water content of tissues** If a drug is highly water soluble, it will tend to be distributed to parts of the body that have a high water content. Therefore, if a patient has ascites, a water soluble drug such as gentamicin will be diluted by the excess fluid. Higher doses will be needed to achieve therapeutic amounts in other parts of the body.

3. **Size of the drug molecule** Small molecules are able to cross cell membranes more effectively than large molecules. Therefore, drugs with large molecular weights, such as hetastarch, will not cross cell membranes and will not distribute outside the systemic circulation.

4. **Protein binding** Most drugs are relatively insoluble in plasma. They must be transported through the systemic circulation by carrier proteins (usually albumin). Drugs are only partially bound to plasma proteins; only the fraction that is unbound (free) is available for distribution to other tissues and able to exert a pharmacologic effect. As the free drug is distributed and metabolized, more drug will become released from the plasma proteins. Therefore, protein binding serves as a reservoir for drug distribution and pharmacologic activity.

A patient's ability to bind drugs depends on the quantity and quality of available plasma proteins. If there is a deficiency in serum albumin due to malnutrition, for example, then less drug will be bound and more will be free for drug distribution. Consequently, the same total serum concentration of the drug will contain a higher free fraction, have more drug available for distribution, and exert a greater pharmacologic effect. Other factors that influence protein binding include renal failure, the pH of the blood, and competition from other highly bound drugs.

A drug's *volume of distribution* represents the theoretical amount of fluid to which the drug is distributed.* It is the volume of distribution that determines the concentration of the drug in the serum. The volume of distribution and serum drug level can be calculated from equation 1 and equation 2 as follows:

1. Volume of distribution = dose administered ÷ measured serum level.
2. Serum level = dose administered ÷ volume of distribution.

---

*Since some drugs are greatly concentrated by certain tissues, the theoretical, or apparent, volume of distribution may exceed the total body mass.

For example, if 100 mg of gentamicin is distributed to 10 liters of fluid, it will give a serum concentration of 10 mg/l. If the volume of distribution were 20 liters, the serum concentration would be only 5 mg/l. Therefore, patients who have higher volumes of distribution, as might be seen in ascites, must be given larger doses to achieve comparable serum levels.

## Metabolism

Most drugs are considered by the body as toxins. Therefore the body will convert the drug to more water soluble metabolites that are easier for the body to eliminate. Most metabolism occurs in the liver, but metabolism may also take place in the kidney, spleen, lung, and gut.

Most metabolites of a drug are less pharmacologically active than the parent drug. However, some drugs are inactive when administered but are converted by the body to a pharmacologically active substance. An example of this is prednisone, which must be converted by the liver to prednisolone. In the case of liver failure, it would be preferable to administer the active moiety, prednisolone, to the patient.

Metabolism depends on the capacity of the liver to process the drug as well as delivery of other drug to the site. The capacity of the liver may be decreased by other drugs, such as cimetidine, or increased by drugs such as phenobarbital, phenytoin, or cigarette smoking. The delivery of the drug to the liver may be compromised by such patient factors as cirrhosis or congestive heart failure, or by drugs such as propranolol and cimetidine. Therefore, the metabolic rate of the drug in an individual patient will vary along with the presence or absence of these intervening variables.

## Elimination

Both parent drug and its metabolites are eventually eliminated from the body. While most elimination occurs in the kidney, some drug may be lost in the feces, breath, perspiration, saliva, tears, breast milk, and even hair and nails.

The kidney will eliminate drugs both through glomerular filtration and by secretion of the drug through the renal tubules. Therefore, the elimination rate depends on the innate capacity of the kidney as well as on renal blood flow. As the glomerular filtration rate (measured by creatinine clearance) declines, the kidney becomes less able to eliminate the drug from the body.

The *half-life* of a drug is the time it takes for a blood level of a drug to fall by 50 percent. Half-life is dependent upon both the metabolic and elimination rate of the drug and the volume of distribution. The half-life of a drug is an important characteristic used to determine the optimal interval between doses.

## Drug Accumulation

As a drug is administered in repetitive doses, its concentration increases in the bloodstream until an equilibrium is established between the amount administered and the amount metabolized and eliminated. The time it takes to achieve this equilibrium, known as *steady-state*, strictly depends on the half-life of the drug.

Steady-state conditions are achieved after the same dose of a drug has been administered for a period of five half-lives. Therefore, a drug such as dopamine, with a half-life of just a few minutes, will achieve steady-state conditions within 10 minutes of adjusting the dose. On the other hand, digoxin, with a normal half-life of 36 hours, will not achieve steady-state blood levels for a week after starting therapy. Therefore, the full pharmacologic or toxic effects will not be seen until the patient has received the drug for a period equivalent to five half-lives.

If immediate pharmacologic effects are needed and the half-life is long, a large *loading dose* may be administered. When this is done, therapeutic blood levels are rapidly achieved. These blood levels are then maintained by administering a regular *maintenance dose* at specified intervals.

## Interpretation of Serum Levels

It is often useful to know the concentration of a drug at its site of action. Unfortunately, this is not usually practical or possible since the site of action is often deep within a body's tissues. What is relatively easy to measure, however, is the concentration of the drug in the serum. After distribution occurs, the serum concentration will be proportional to the concentration in other body organs and at the receptor sites.

To accurately reflect the concentration of the drug at the receptor site, sufficient time must be allowed after administration for complete distribution to occur. Serum levels drawn before the completion of the distribution phase will be clinically meaningless. For most drugs this occurs within 20 minutes of an intravenous dose. Other drugs, such as digoxin, have a distribution time as long as 6 hours or more. Therefore, it is important to know a drug's distribution time before deciding when to draw a serum level after a dose.

When interpreting a serum level it is also important to know how the timing of the assay relates to steady-state conditions. A serum level drawn before the achievement of steady-state conditions will underestimate the long-term serum levels that will be achieved once steady-state is reached.

It is also important to interpret the serum level in relation to the desired "therapeutic range." The usual therapeutic range of phenytoin, for example, is 10 to 20 mcg/ml. However, if protein-binding is altered, as might be the case in renal failure, a serum level range of 7 to 13 mcg/ml might provide similar activity. If a patient such as this is dosed to achieve a serum level of 20 mcg/ml, toxicity may occur.

Finally, it is important to realize that serum levels are but one tool useful to assess a patient's response to therapy. It is not the only tool, however, and should not replace sound clinical judgment. For example, if a patient has a theophylline level of 7 mcg/ml (therapeutic range: 10 to 20 mcg/ml) but is responding well, the dose should not be increased merely to increase the serum level to the therapeutic range. Conversely, higher than expected serum level in the absence of side effects does not necessarily mean that the dose should be reduced. Rather, the dose should be adjusted based upon the therapeutic needs of the patient.

## DRUG CLASSIFICATION: AMINOGLYCOSIDES

| Drug Name | Dosage |
|---|---|
| Gentamicin *(Garamycin, Apogen, Jenamycin, Bristagen)* | 3–6 mg/kg/day IM or IV in 2–4 divided doses |
| Tobramycin *(Nebcin)* | 3–6 mg/kg/day IM or IV in 2–4 divided doses |
| Netilmicin *(Netromycin)* | 3–6 mg/kg/day IM or IV in 2–4 divided doses |
| Amikacin *(Amikin)* | 7.5 mg/kg IM or IV q 12 hr |

### Nursing Implications

1. **Nephrotoxicity** Decreased renal function, as reflected by increased serum creatinine or increased BUN should be monitored daily. Nephrotoxicity may be additive with other nephrotoxic drugs (i.e., amphotericin B, cisplatin, cyclosporine). If nephrotoxicity develops, the dosage of other drugs that are renally excreted should be adjusted.
2. **Ototoxicity** Related to dose and duration of therapy. Toxicity may be cochlear (tinnitus, loss of high frequency range first) or vestibular (intense headache, nausea, vomiting, vertigo). In either case the drug should be discontinued, at this stage the damage is reversible. Concurrent use of other ototoxic drugs should be monitored closely (i.e., furosemide, ethacrynic acid).
3. **Dosing and blood-level monitoring** Dosage is based on age, lean body weight, renal function; blood-level measurement also is used to guide therapy. Peak concentrations, obtained 30 min after the infusion, and trough concentrations obtained just prior to dose. Exact time of blood collection and dose should be indicated on tube. If patient is also receiving carbenicillin or ticarcillin, the tube should be placed on ice and sent immediately to the lab to decrease inactivation of aminoglycoside.

4. **Intravascular volume status** Hypotensive states and diseases which manifest a decrease in renal blood flow (i.e., congestive heart failure, cirrhosis with ascites) will increase the risk of nephrotoxicity. Monitor blood pressure, urine output, BUN/Cr ratio, urinary sodium, mucous membranes, and sunken eyes for evaluating intravascular volume status.
5. Use with caution in patients receiving neuromuscular blockers or general anesthetics because of an increased risk of **neuromuscular blockade**.
6. Drug is **incompatible** with penicillins and cephalosporins. Do not mix in the same container.

## DRUG CLASSIFICATION: PENICILLINS

| Drug Name | Dosage |
|---|---|
| **First Generation** | |
| Penicillin G | 1–40 million units in 3–8 doses/day |
| **Extended Spectrum** | |
| Ampicillin | 2–16 g in 3–8 doses/day |
| **Penicillinase-Resistant** | |
| Oxacillin | 4–12 g in 4–6 doses/day |
| Methicillin | 4–12 g in 4–6 doses/day |
| Nafcillin | 4–12 g in 4–6 doses/day |
| **Anti-Pseudomonal** | |
| Carbenicillin | 8–40 g in 3–8 doses/day |
| Ticarcillin | 6–18 g in 3–8 doses/day |
| Mezlocillin | 8–18 g in 3–8 doses/day |
| Piperacillin | 6–18 g in 3–8 doses/day |
| Azlocillin | 8–18 g in 4–6 doses/day |

### Nursing Implications

1. **Hypersensitivity reactions** Allergic responses (skin rashes, angioedema, anaphylaxis, serum sickness, hepatitis, fever) can occur in patients previously exposed to any member of the penicillin family, and in a small percentage of patients with a previous reaction to a cephalosporin.
2. **Neurotoxicity** High doses of penicillins can induce seizures especially in patients with a previous seizure focus and poor renal function (↑ Cr, ↑ BUN). Direct IM injection can cause nerve damage.
3. **Nephrotoxicity** Penicillins can induce a syndrome of acute interstitial nephritis which presents with decreased renal function. Patients often have one or more of the following symptoms: Fever, rash, eosinophilia, eosinophiluria.
4. **Hypokalemia** High doses of penicillins (primarily antipseudomonal) can increase renal excretion of potassium. Patients with cardiac arrhythmias or who are receiving digoxin should have their serum potassium monitored closely. Hypokalemia may be worsened by concurrent diuretic therapy.
5. **Inactivation of aminoglycosides** High concentrations of penicillins (primarily antipseudomonal penicillins) can inactivate aminoglycosides. When aminoglycoside peaks and trough values are measured in a patient receiving high-dose penicillin therapy, the tube should be placed on ice and sent to the lab as soon as possible. These drugs should not be mixed in the same IV container.
6. **Sodium overload** Antipseudomonal penicillins, when administered in high doses, provide a sodium load and patients on sodium restricted diets should be monitored closely. (Carbenicillin 4.7 mEq/g, Ticarcillin 5.2 mEq/g, Mezlocillin 1.9 mEq/g, Piperacillin 2.0 mEq/g, Azlocillin 2.2 mEq/g)
7. **Coagulation abnormalities** High dose penicillin therapy (primarily antipseudomonal) can alter coagulation by decreasing platelet aggregation or by promoting hypothrombinemia.
8. **Gastrointestinal** The development of antibiotic-inducd diarrhea or pseudomembranous colitis can occur in patients receiving prolonged penicillin therapy.

## DRUG CLASSIFICATION: CEPHALOSPORIN ANTIBIOTICS

| Drug Name | Dosage (IM, IV) |
|---|---|
| **First Generation** | |
| Cefazolin *(Ancef, Kefzol)* | 0.5–1.0 g q 8 hr |
| Cephalothin *(Keflin, Seffin)* | 0.5–2.0 g q 4–6 hr |
| **Second Generation** | |
| Cefamandole *(Mandol)* | 0.5–2 g q 4–8 hr |
| Cefonicid *(Monocid)* | 0.5–1 g q 24 hr |
| Cefuroxime *(Zinacef)* | 0.75–3.0 g q 6–8 h |
| Cefotetan *(Cefotan)* | 0.5–2 g q 12 hr |
| Cefoxitin *(Mefoxin)* | 1–2 g q 4–6 hr |
| **Third Generation** | |
| Cefoperazone *(Cefobid)* | 1–2 g q 8–12 hr |
| Cefotaxime *(Claforan)* | 1–2 g q 4–12 hr |
| Ceftazidime *(Fortaz, Tazidime, Tazicef)* | 1–2 g q 8–12 hr |
| Ceftizoxime *(Cefizox)* | 0.5–4 g q 8–12 hr |
| Ceftriaxone *(Rocephin)* | 1–2 g q 12–24 hr |
| Moxalactam *(Moxam)* | 0.5–2 g q 8–12 hr |

### Nursing Implications

1. Use caution in patients with documented history of **hypersensitivity reactions** to penicillins or cephalosporins.
2. Most cephalosporins require a component of **renal excretion** for elimination from the body. Dosage and/or interval should be adjusted according to estimates of renal function (serum creatinine, creatinine clearance).
3. Cephalosporins can induce **seizures** when high dosages are given to patients with impaired renal function and in patients with an underlying seizure focus.
4. **Acute interstitial nephritis** may occur, and is often associated with nephrotoxicity (reflected by an ↑ serum creatinine or BUN), rash, fever, eosinophilia, eosinophiluria.
5. **Diarrhea and/or colitis** may occur with prolonged use.
6. **Hypoprothrombinemia** may be induced by prolonged use, especially in nutritionally depleted patients. Vitamin K 5 mg should be given daily during moxalactam therapy.
7. May cause **false-positive urine glucose reactions** with clinitest tablets, Fehling's or Benedict's reagent.
8. Should not be admixed in the same container with aminoglycosides.
9. Alcohol-containing products should be avoided in patients receiving moxalactam, cefotetan, cefobid to avoid a **disulfiram reaction.**

## DRUG CLASSIFICATION: MISCELLANEOUS ANTIBIOTICS

| Drug Name | Dosage |
|---|---|
| Aztreonam *(Azactam)* | 2–8 g IM or IV q 6–12 hr |
| Imipenem/Cilastatin *(Primaxin)* | 2–4 g IM or IV q 6 hr |

### Nursing Implications

1. Caution when used in patients with a previous history of **hypersensitivity** to penicillins or cephalosporins.
2. **Renal function** is required for elimination from the body; dose and/or interval should be adjusted in relation to the decrease in renal function as noted by serum creatinine or creatinine clearance.
3. **Seizures** may be induced when patients with decreased renal function are given standard dosages.

4. **Nausea and vomiting** during IV infusion can be minimized by decreasing the infusion rate.

---

| **Drug Name** | **Dosage** |
|---|---|
| Erythromycin *(Ilotycin)* | Oral: 0.25–0.5 g 3–4 × daily<br>IV: 15–20 mg/kg in 4 divided doses |

**Nursing Implications**

1. **Thrombophlebitis** may occur at the IV infusion site. This can be minimized by diluting the drug in 100–250 ml of fluid and using a 1 hr infusion period.
2. **Hepatotoxicity** should be monitored by measuring liver function tests during therapy.
3. **Ototoxicity** may occur at high doses; patients receiving other ototoxic drugs (i.e., aminoglycosides, vancomycin, furosemide) should be evaluated routinely for hearing loss.
4. **Decreased metabolism of other drugs** (i.e., theophylline, cyclosporine) may occur during erythromycin therapy; dosages of these agents should be adjusted accordingly.

---

| **Drug Name** | **Dosage** |
|---|---|
| Clindamycin *(Cleocin)* | IV: 2.4–2.7 g in 3–4 doses<br>Oral: 150–450 mg q 6 hr |

**Nursing Implications**

1. **Gastrointestinal** disturbances including: diarrhea, cramps, colitis may occur at usual doses. After discontinuation of the drug, anti-diarrheals should be avoided and if colitis is present, vancomycin or metronidazole may be prescribed.

---

| **Drug Name** | **Dosage** |
|---|---|
| Trimethoprim—Sulfamethoxazole *(TMP—SMX, Cotrimoxazole, Bactrim, Septra)* | **In terms of trimethoprim:** 8–10 mg/kg IV in 2–4 doses<br>For **Pneumocystis carinii** pneumonia: 15–20 mg/kg IV or PO in 3–4 divided doses. |

**Nursing Implications**

1. **Hypersensitivity** reactions, including rash, anaphylaxis, serum sickness, photosensitivity may occur in patients with a history of sulfonamide allergy.
2. **Nephrotoxicity** (as indicated by ↑ serum creatinine or ↑ BUN) may occur if patients are not well-hydrated. In patients with renal impairment the dose and/or interval must be adjusted.
3. **Hematologic toxicity** including anemia, neutropenia, or thrombocytopenia may occur and is reversible if drug is discontinued.
4. Patients concurrently receiving **warfarin, phenytoin**, or **cyclosporine** should be monitored closely for enhanced pharmacologic effects when TMP—SMX is added.

---

| **Drug Name** | **Dosage** |
|---|---|
| Chloramphenicol *(Chloromycetin, Mychel-S)* | 50–100 mg/kg/day IV or PO in 4 divided doses |

**Nursing Implications**

1. **Hematologic toxicity** may present as either reversible or irreversible bone marrow suppression. Patients should be monitored with CBC and platelet count for anemia, leukopenia, or thrombocytopenia with clinical monitoring for bleeding or bruising.

2. Requires **hepatic** metabolism, dosage adjustments are required in neonates, patients with liver disease and renal disease.
3. **Inhibits hepatic metabolism** of other drugs (i.e., phenytoin, phenobarbital, tolbutamide, chlorpropamide, cyclosphosphamide), therefore, monitor for enhanced effects of these agents.

---

| Drug Name | Dosage |
|---|---|
| Metronidazole *(Flagyl, Metryl, Protostat)* | 15 mg/kg IV loading dose; then 7.5 mg/kg IV or PO q 6 hr |

**Nursing Implications**

1. **Neurotoxicity**, patient should be followed closely for signs of peripheral neuropathy or seizures.
2. **Disulfiram-like reaction** may occur if patient is exposed to alcohol (up to 3 days after discontinuation).
3. **Requires hepatic metabolism** and dosage adjustment in patients with liver disease.

---

| Drug Name | Dosage |
|---|---|
| Pentamidine *(Pentam 300)* | 4 mg/kg IV or IM daily |

**Nursing Implications**

1. Pain or abscess at injection site should be looked for daily and blood pressure should be checked during and following administration.
2. **Nephrotoxicity** as indicated by an ↑ serum creatinine, caution when patients are receiving other nephrotoxins (aminoglycosides, amphotericin). Dosage should be decreased in patients with impaired renal function.
3. **Hyper- or Hypoglycemia** requires routine evaluation of serum glucose.

---

| Drug Name | Dosage |
|---|---|
| Vancomycin *(Vancocin, Vancoled)* | 1–2 g IV; IM 2–4 divided doses; 125–500 mg PO q 6 hr (for pseudomembranous colitis only) |

**Nursing Implications**

1. **Infusion reactions** may occur when given over <1 hr. Monitor for rash, pruritis, hypotension.
2. **Nephrotoxicity** (noted by ↑ serum creatinine) especially in patients receiving aminoglycosides.
3. **Ototoxicity** may occur at higher serum concentrations; caution with other ototoxic drugs (aminoglycosides, furosemide). Monitor for tinnitus or hearing loss.
4. **Requires renal excretion** and dosage must be adjusted in relation to the extent of renal impairment.
5. **Monitor serum concentrations** to maintain peaks approximately 30–40 mcg/ml and troughs ≤10/mcg/ml.

---

| Drug Name | Dosage |
|---|---|
| Ciprofloxacin *(Cipro)* | 250–750 mg bid PO |
| Norfloxacin *(Noroxin)* | 400 mg bid PO |

**Nursing Implications**

1. **Gastrointestinal intolerance** may present as nausea, cramping, diarrhea.
2. **Central Nervous System** effects may include dizziness, headache, lightheadedness, and infrequent seizures.
3. **Coadministration with antacids** should be avoided to avoid decreased antibiotic absorption.
4. **Theophylline** plasma levels should be monitored closely when these agents are added to a patient previously stabilized on theophylline.

| Drug Name | Dosage |
|---|---|
| Amphotericin B *(Fungizone)* | 1 mg IV test dose; up to 0.5 – 1 mg/kg/day |

**Nursing Implications**

1. **Infusion reactions** including pain, phlebitis, fever, chills, hypotension should be followed daily during administration.
2. **Nephrotoxicity** may lead to an increased serum creatinine or BUN, hypokalemia, hypomagnesemia, or metabolic acidosis and should be monitored with routine clinical chemistries. Electrolyte abnormalities may be worse in patients receiving diuretics.
3. **Anemia** may occur and is followed with CBC.
4. **Hepatotoxicity** requires monitoring of liver enzymes.

| Drug Name | Dosage |
|---|---|
| Ketoconazole *(Nizoral)* | 200 – 400 mg once or twice daily |

**Nursing Implications**

1. **Gastrointestinal** (nausea, vomiting, constipation) effects are dose-related, while potential **hepatotoxic** affects should be monitored with hepatic enzyme levels.
2. **Endocrine** effects may include gynecomastia or inhibition of cortisol synthesis, and should be monitored in patients with pre-existing endocrine abnormalities.
3. **Drug interactions** (cyclosporine, theophylline, phenytoin, methylprednisolone, warfarin) may occur due to the inhibitory effect of ketoconazole on hepatic metabolism. Also, histamine antagonists and antacids may decrease ketoconazole absorption.

## DRUG CLASSIFICATION: ANTIVIRAL AGENTS

| Drug Name | Dosage |
|---|---|
| Acyclovir *(Zovirax)* | 5 mg/kg IV q 8 hr; 200 mg PO or topically 5 times daily |

**Nursing Implications**

1. **Nephrotoxicity** secondary to crystalluria (noted by ↑ serum creatinine) requires maintenance of good hydration and infusion (≤7 mg/ml) over 1 hr.
of good hydration and infusion (≤7 mg/ml) over 1 hr.
2. **Requires renal excretion** and appropriate dosage adjustment in patients with renal impairment.
3. **Probenecid** prolongs the serum half-life of acyclovir.
4. **Neurotoxicity** at high concentrations including lethargy, confusion, tremors, hallucinations, seizures.
5. **Thrombophlebitis** during IV infusion.

| Drug Name | Dosage |
|---|---|
| Vidarabine *(Adenosine, arabinoside, Ara-A, Vira-A)* | 10 – 15 mg/kg/day infused over 12 – 24 hr |

**Nursing Implications**

1. **Anorexia, nausea, vomiting** during administration.
2. **Neurotoxicity** including tremor, dizziness, hallucinations, confusion, headache.

| Drug Name | Dosage |
|---|---|
| Zidovudine *(Retrovir)* | 100 – 300 mg PO q 4 hr while awake |

**Nursing Implications**

1. **Hematologic** effects (anemia, neutropenia) should be monitored closely.

2. **Neurologic** (headache, dizziness) and *muscular* (myositis myalgia) may occur during acute and chronic dosing.
3. **Gastrointestinal** effects (nausea, abdominal pain, diarrhea) may require dosage reduction.

## DRUG CLASSIFICATION: ANTIARRHYTHMIC DRUGS

| Drug Name | Dosage |
|---|---|
| Amiodarone *(Cordarone)* | 0.8–1.6 g PO daily × 1–3 weeks, then 0.6–0.8 g PO daily × 4 weeks, then 0.2–0.6 g daily (with food or as multiple doses to decrease GI upset) |

**Nursing Implications**

1. **Neurotoxicity** malaise, fatigue, tremor, poor coordination and gait, peripheral neuropathy may be reversed by dose reduction.
2. **Pulmonary toxicity** should be monitored for on physical examination (dyspnea, cough) and with pulmonary function tests and chest x-rays during therapy.
3. **Corneal deposits** may be asymptomatic and the drug should be discontinued if blurred vision or halos develop.
4. **Drug interactions** may lead to increased serum levels of digoxin, quinidine, procainamide, flecainide, and warfarin requiring a 33–50% dosage reduction of these drugs.
5. **Half-life** of this drug is ≈ 53 days.
6. **Hypothyroidism or hyperthyroidism** should be monitored for during therapy.

| Drug Name | Dosage |
|---|---|
| Atropine | *Asystole*: ≈ 1 mg rapid IV, then q 5 min<br>*Bradycardia*: 0.5 mg IV q 5 min up to 2 mg |

**Nursing Implications**

1. **CNS effects** (hyperpyrexia, disorientation, insomnia, delirium, coma) at high doses.
2. **Other anticholinergic effects** are dry mouth, blurred vision, tachycardia.

| Drug Name | Dosage |
|---|---|
| Bretylium *(Bretylol)* | *Ventricular fibrillation*: 5 mg/kg rapid IV, then 1–4 mg/min by continuous infusion (pump or controller). Bolus may be repeated with 10 mg/kg q 15 min up to a total dose of 30 mg/kg<br>*Ventricular tachycardia*: 5 mg/kg IV (in 50 ml D5W over 8–10 min), then 1–4 mg/min or 5–10 mg IM q 6–8 hr |

**Nursing Implications**

1. **Hypotension** rapid bolus doses may drop blood pressure and induce emesis; monitor rhythm and blood pressure and keep patient supine to avoid dizziness, syncope, vertigo.
2. **IM tissue damage** may be avoided by frequently rotating sites.
3. **Contraindicated** if arrhythmia is due to digitalis toxicity.

| Drug Name | Dosage |
|---|---|
| Calcium Chloride | *Asystole*: 0.5–1.0 g IV push or intraventricular during CPR. *Other indications*: 0.2–1 g IV or IM p.r.n. |

**Nursing Implications**

1. **Cardiovascular effects** may result; bradycardia, cardiac standstill, hypotension, digitalis toxicity.
2. **Preparations**: Calcium gluconate contains 4.5 mEq of calcium and calcium chloride contains 13.6 mEq of calcium.

---

| Drug Name | Dosage |
|---|---|
| Digoxin *(Lanoxin, Lanoxir caps)* | 0.5–1.25 mg IV (over 5 min) IM or PO loading dose divided in 3–6 equal doses over 24 hr; then 0.0625–0.375 mg daily |

**Nursing Implications**

1. **Cardiac effects** (bradycardia, AV block, CHF, ventricular irritability) require frequent clinical monitoring of vital signs. Cardiac effects can be potentiated by hypokalemia, hypomagnesemia, and hypercalcemia (i.e., during diuretic therapy), as well as hypothyroidism.
2. **Requires renal excretion** and appropriate dosage and/or prolonged dosing interval in patients with renal dysfunction.
3. **Serum levels** (6 hr after a dose) should be maintained between 0.8–2.2 ng/ml. Levels may be **decreased** by concurrent administration with kaolin-pectin, antacids, cholestyramine or colestipol. Levels may be **increased** by flecainide, quinidine, verapamil and nifedipine therapy and may require a 30–50% digoxin dose reduction.
4. **CNS effects** (nausea, vomiting, anorexia, yellow-green halos) require a dosage reduction.

---

| Drug Name | Dosage |
|---|---|
| Disopyramide *(Norpace, Norpace-CR)* | 200–300 mg loading dose; then 100–200 mg q 6–8 hr; (Norpace-CR given q 12 hr). |

**Nursing Implications**

1. **Cardiac effects** (worsening CHF, hypotension, abnormal ECG) require close monitoring of vital signs clinical status. Widening QRS or QT > 25% prolongation requires dose reduction or discontinuation.
2. **Anticholinergic** effects such as dry mouth, blurred vision, urinary retention, and constipation should be looked for closely.
3. **Requires renal excretion** and appropriate dosage-adjustment in relation to the degree of renal dysfunction.

---

| Drug Name | Dosage |
|---|---|
| Flecainide *(Tambocor)* | 100 mg PO q 12 hr; up to 600 mg daily dose (dosage increases should be made >4 days after the previous change) |

**Nursing Implications**

1. **Cardiac effects** (worsening CHF, abnormal ECG, heart block) require dosage reduction or discontinuation. May increase digoxin levels 25%.
2. **Serum levels** should be maintained from 0.2–1.0 mcg/ml.
3. **CNS effects** (dizziness, blurred vision, headache, nausea) may occur.

---

| Drug Name | Dosage |
|---|---|
| Lidocaine *(Xylocaine)* | 1 mg/kg IV bolus dose (≤50 mg/min) then 1–4 mg/min infusion (pump or controller); additional bolus dose (0.5 mg/kg) may be given q 10 min up to a total dose of 3 mg/kg |

**Nursing Implications**

1. **Cardiac effects** are monitored with frequent evaluation of rhythm, pulse, and blood pressure.
2. **CNS effects** (lightheadedness, drowsiness, dizziness, slurred speech, blurred vision, vomiting, twitching, seizures, respiratory depression) require constant monitoring and may require dosage reduction.
3. **Dosage reduction** for CHF patient: decrease load and maintenance dose 50%; liver failure: usual load, decrease maintenance dose 50%. If infusion lasts > 24 hr decrease rate by 50%.
4. **Serum levels** maintained between 1.5–5.5 mcg/ml. Cimetidine and beta-blockers may increase lidocaine levels.

---

| Drug Name | Dosage |
|---|---|
| Mexiletine *(Mexitil)* | 200–400 mg PO q 8 hr; with food if GI upset occurs |

**Nursing Implications**

1. **Cardiac effects** (bradycardia, atrial fibrillation, worsened ECG, hypotension) require close monitoring of vital signs and rhythm.
2. **CNS effects** (tremor, dizziness, lightheadedness, ataxia, confusion, blurred vision, nausea, vomiting) may require dosage reduction.
3. **Serum levels** maintained from 0.5–2.0 mcg/ml. Phenytoin may increase mexiletine levels.
4. **Drug-induced SLE** may present with rash, positive antinuclear antibodies, and requires decreased dose or discontinuation.

---

| Drug Name | Dosage |
|---|---|
| Procainamide *(Pronestyl, Pronestyl-SR, Procan-SR)* | **Acute arrhythmias**: 50–100 mg (25 mg/min) slow IV push q 5 min until rhythm normalizes or adverse effects occur, up to a total dose of 1 g; then 1–4 mg/min infusion (pump or controller)<br>**Chronic**: 3–6 g PO in 4–8 divided doses; sustained-release forms given q 6 hr) |

**Nursing Implications**

1. **Cardiac effects** (hypotension, worsened ECG, heart block) require frequent vital signs and rhythm checks; wide QRS or QT > 25% of baseline may require dose reduction or discontinuation.
2. **CNS effects** (nausea, vomiting, anorexia, insomnia, fatigue, tremor, fever) require dose reduction.
3. **Serum levels** maintained from 4–10 mcg/ml for procainamide and N-acetylprocainamide (an active metabolite).

---

| Drug Name | Dosage |
|---|---|
| Quinidine *(Quinidex, Cin-Quin, Quinora, Duraquin, Quinaglute, Cardioquin)* | **Acute supraventricular tachycardia:** 400–600 mg IM (not IV) q 2 hr until dysrhythmia resolves or side effects occur<br>**Chronic arrhythmia:** 200–300 mg quinidine base tid–qid. Sustained release formulations: bid–tid |

**Nursing Implications**

1. **Cardiac effects** (hypotension, worsened ECG) require frequent vital signs and rhythm checks. Wide QRS or QT > 25% of baseline may require dose reduction or discontinuation. *Quinidine syncope*, an atypical ventricular fibrillation, is associated with these ECG changes and may lead to sudden death. Rhythm and blood pressure should be monitored closely during therapy.

2. **Quinidine salts** Sulfate: 83% quinidine base; Quinidex, Cin–Quin, Quinora, Gluconate salt: 62% quinidine base; Duraquin, Quinaglute, Polygalacturonate salt: 60% quinidine base; Cardioquin.
3. **Gastrointestinal effects** (nausea, vomiting, diarrhea, anorexia) may require dosage reduction or discontinuation.
4. **Hypersensitivity reactions** (allergy, rash, hemolytic anemia, hepatitis, thrombocytopenia) requires monitoring of CBC and patient history for bruising, bleeding, or jaundice during therapy.
5. **Serum levels** maintained between 2–5 mcg/ml. Higher levels may be associated with ECG changes, tinnitus, diarrhea. Digoxin levels will be increased when quinidine is added, and may require a 30–50% decrease in digoxin dose.

| Drug Name | Dosage |
|---|---|
| Tocainide *(Tonocard)* | 400–600 mg bid–tid |

**Nursing Implications**

1. **Cardiac effects** (worsened ECG, CHF, hypotension, bradycardia, chest pain) requires close monitoring of ECG and vital signs during therapy. This agent should be used cautiously in patients receiving beta-blocking drugs because of additive decreases in cardiac contractility.
2. **Neurologic effects** (lightheadedness, paresthesias, tremors, confusion, restlessness, blurred vision, uncoordination, headache) should be evaluated closely and may require dosage reduction.
3. **Gastrointestinal effects** (nausea, vomiting, anorexia, diarrhea) may be minimized if administered with food.
4. **Hypersensitivity reactions** (allergies, positive antinuclear antibodies with systemic lupus erythematosus, pulmonary fibrosis, blood dyscrasias) requires that a CBC and chest x-ray be obtained every three months.
5. **Serum levels** maintained between 4–10 mcg/ml.

| Drug Name | Dosage |
|---|---|
| Verapamil *(Calan, Isoptin)* | **Acute supraventricular tachycardia:** 0.075–0.15 mg/kg (5–10 mg) IV push over 2 min. Repeat 0.15 mg/kg (10 mg) in 30 min if needed.<br>**Subacute management:** 1–10 mcg/kg/min as a continuous infusion (pump or controller).<br>**Angina:** 80–120 mg orally tid–qid |

**Nursing Implications**

1. **Cardiac effects** (hypotension, bradycardia, A-V block, worsened CHF) require close monitoring of vital signs and ECG during parenteral administration. Symptomatic hypotension is usually transient (20–30 min) and can be treated by repositioning the patient in the Trendelenburg position.
2. **CNS effects** (headache, nausea, fatigue, dizziness) may require a dose reduction.
3. **Mixtures for continuous infusion** should be protected from light and not admixed with alkaline solutions or drugs.
4. **Drug interactions** with verapamil may lead to elevated levels of digoxin and theophylline, with corresponding dose reductions needed if indicated.

| Drug Name | Dosage |
|---|---|
| Nifedipine *(Procardia)* | 10–30 mg PO 2–3 times daily; infrequently used sublingually for immediate effect (puncture capsule first) |

**Nursing Implications**

1. Adverse effects are relatively uncommon, however **hypotension with dizziness** may occur in elderly patients; use with caution in patients with congestive heart failure, especially in those patients already taking a beta-adrenergic blocker.

| Drug Name | Dosage |
|---|---|
| Diltiazem *(Cardiazem)* | 30–90 mg PO 3–4 times daily |

**Nursing Implications**

1. Generally well-tolerated; use with caution in patients with previous rhythm abnormalities.

## DRUG CLASSIFICATION: DIURETICS

| Drug Name | Dosage |
|---|---|
| Acetazolamide *(Diamox)* | 250–500 mg IV daily (≤500 mg/min) |

**Nursing Implications**

1. **Renal effects** (diuresis, glycosuria, urinary frequency, renal calculi, crystalluria, increased potassium excretion, increased bicarbonate excretion) require close clinical and urine evaluation. Daily weight, blood pressure, intake/output should be routinely recorded. **Potassium losses** may lead to hypokalemia requiring supplementation (caution in patients already receiving digoxin). **Metabolic acidosis,** which decreases the diuresis, requires that the drug be discontinued for 1–2 days. Urinary alkalinization may decrease the elimination of quinidine, while increasing the clearance of salicylates, lithium, and methotrexate.
2. **Hypersensitivity reactions** (allergies, photosensitivity) may require discontinuation. This drug is a sulfonamide derivative and will cross-react in patients with sulfonamide allergy.
3. **CNS effects** (fatigue, nervousness, drowsiness, depression, dizziness, tinnitus) requires a dose reduction or discontinuation.

| Drug Name | Dosage |
|---|---|
| **Loop Diuretics** | |
| Bumetanide *(Bumex)* | **Edema:** 0.5–1.0 mg IV, IM, PO, repeat 1–2 mg in 2–3 hr if needed |
| Ethacrynic Acid *(Edecrin)* | 0.5–1.0 mg/kg slow IV injection, 50–200 mg PO daily |
| Furosemide *(Lasix)* | 20–40 mg IM, slow IV or PO, doses of up to 2000 mg have been given.<br>**Hypertension:** 40–160 mg orally in 1 to 4 divided doses. |

**Nursing Implications**

1. **Renal effects** (overdiuresis, electrolyte losses: $Mg^{++}$, $Ca^{++}$, $K^{+}$, $Na^{+}$, $Zn^{++}$, $Cl^{-}$) may lead to hypotension, muscle cramps, headache, decreased serum electrolytes: hypokalemia, hyponatremia, hypocalcemia, hypomagnesemia, hypozincemia. Routine clinical examination and serum chemistry monitoring are required during diuretic therapy especially in patients receiving digoxin. Elevations in serum glucose, uric acid, creatinine, and blood urea nitrogen may also occur and should be followed with scheduled lab tests. Peak diuresis occurs in 15–45 min, and lasts up to 8 hr.
2. **Ototoxicity** may be additive in patients already receiving aminoglycoside antibiotics or vancomycin. Also, **rapid IV infusion should be avoided** to decrease ototoxicity; use > 2–4 min infusion period (furosemide ≤ 4 mg/min); tinnitus precedes hearing loss.
3. **Hypersensitivity reactions** to furosemide and ethacrynic acid may occur in patients with a previous sulfonamide allergy. Bumetanide is not a sulfonamide derivative and is an alternative for these patients.
4. **Dosages and administration**: 40 mg furosemide is equivalent to 1 mg of bumetanide; ≈ 50–60% of an oral furosemide dose is absorbed. Therefore, con-

version from IV furosemide may require higher oral doses for the same effect. Ethacrynic acid may require IV site rotation if thrombophlebitis occurs.

| Drug Name | Dosage |
|---|---|
| **Thiazide and thiazide-like diuretics:** | |
| Chlorothiazide *(Diuril)* | 0.5–2.00 g IV or oral once or twice daily |
| Hydrochlorothiazide *(Hydrodiuril, Esidrex)* | 50–200 mg oral once daily |
| Chlorthalidone *(Hygroton)* | 12.5–100 mg once daily |
| Metolazone *(Diulo, Zaroxolyn)* | 2.5–20 mg oral once daily |

**Nursing Implications**

1. **Renal effects** (overdiuresis, electrolyte losses: $Na^+$, $K^+$, $Cl^-$, $Mg^{++}$, $Zn^{++}$) may lead to hypotension, muscle cramps, headache, decreased serum electrolytes: hypokalemia, hyponatremia, hypochloremia. Routine clinical evaluation of weight, blood pressure, intake/output and serum chemistry monitoring are required during diuretic therapy with these agents, especially in patients receiving digoxin. Elevations in serum glucose, uric acid, calcium, creatinine, blood urea nitrogen, lipids may also occur and should be followed with lab tests.
2. **Hypersensitivity reactions** caution in patients with a previous sulfonamide allergy since these diuretics are similar chemical derivatives. Acute hypersensitivity reactions (nephritis, pancreatitis, anemia, thrombocytopenia) may occur in any patient.
3. **Optimal diuresis** requires that patients have a creatinine clearance ($Cl_{cr}$) > 25 ml/min. If $Cl_{cr}$ < 25 ml/min loop diuretics (see above) should be used.

| Drug Name | Dosage |
|---|---|
| **Osmotic Diuretics** | |
| Mannitol *(Osmitrol)* | Acute renal failure: 0.2 g/kg test dose over 3–5 min, then 50–100 g IV push<br>Intracranial pressure lowering: 1.5–2 g/kg over 30–60 min (as a 15, 20, or 25% solution) |

**Nursing Implications**

1. **Renal effects** (overdiuresis, electrolyte losses) may lead to hypotension, dehydration, electrolyte imbalances (i.e., hypokalemia). Blood pressure, daily weights, intake/output, and serum electrolytes should be followed frequently during osmotic diuresis, especially in patients receiving digoxin.
2. **Cardiovascular effects** may result from increased serum osmolality (circulatory overload, pulmonary edema, congestive heart failure) and should be evaluated closely by physical examination. Increased thirst, nausea, and vomiting may also occur. Mannitol should not be given to anuric patients since it requires renal excretion.
3. **Intravenous administration** requires an IV set with a filter; dissolution of crystalized solutions via immersion in hot water. Extravasation will cause tissue damage.
4. When **decreasing intracranial pressure,** a pressure reduction should be noticed within 15 min, however a rebound increase in pressure may occur 12 hr later.

| Drug Name | Dosage |
|---|---|
| **Potassium Sparing Diuretics** | |
| Spironolactone *(Aldactone)* | 25–400 mg oral daily in 1–4 divided doses; |
| Triamterene *(Dyrenium)* | 50–100 mg oral twice daily |
| Amiloride *(Moduretic)* | 5–20 mg oral daily in 1–2 divided doses |

**Nursing Implications**

1. **Renal effects** (overdiuresis, electrolyte losses) may lead to hypotension, dehydration, and electrolyte imbalances. Blood pressure, daily weight, intake/output, and serum electrolytes should be followed frequently. $K^+$-sparing diuretics should not be given to patients with renal dysfunction because fatal hyperkalemia may develop.
2. **Drug interactions** that result in hyperkalemia may occur if these diuretics are given to patients receiving $K^+$ supplements, beta-blockers, angiotensin converting enzyme inhibitors, or nephrotoxic drugs. Spironolactone may interfere with certain digoxin assays causing a falsely elevated digoxin level.

## DRUG CLASSIFICATION: PLASMA VOLUME EXPANDERS

| Drug Name | Dosage |
|---|---|
| Normal Serum Albumin *(Albuminar, Abutein, Buminate, Plasbumin)* | 5% solution: 250–1000 ml IV daily<br>25% solution: 50–200 ml IV daily |

**Nursing Implications**

1. **Administration** should be at 4 ml/min (5% solution) or 1 ml/min (25% solution) (except in emergencies) with an in-line filter administration set; contains 130–160 mEq of sodium per liter.
2. **Cardiovascular effects** may fluctuate between intravascular overload and hypotension depending on the clinical setting and the rate of infusion. Blood pressure, pulse, and respiratory status should be monitored continuously during administration.

| Drug Name | Dosage |
|---|---|
| Hetastarch *(Hespan)* | 6% solution: 500–1500 ml IV daily |

**Nursing Implications**

1. **Administration** should be at ≥ 20 ml/kg/hour (except in emergencies); contains 154 mEq of sodium per liter.
2. **Cardiovascular effects** may fluctuate between intravascular overload and hypotension depending on the clinical setting and the rate of infusion. Blood pressure, pulse, and respiratory status should be monitored continuously during administration.
3. **Hypersensitivity** reactions may occur (uncommon).

| Drug Name | Dosage |
|---|---|
| Plasma Protein Fraction *(Plasmanate, Plasma-Plex, Plasmatein, Proteanate)* | 5% solution: 250–1000 ml IV daily |

**Nursing Implications**

1. **Administration** should be at ≤ 8 ml/min (except in emergencies) with an in-line filter administration set. Contains 130–160 mEq of sodium per liter.
2. **Cardiovascular effects** may fluctuate between intravascular overload and hypotension depending on the clinical setting and the rate of infusion. Blood pressure, pulse, and respiratory status should be monitored continuously during administration.
3. **Hypersensitivity** reactions may occur (uncommon).

## DRUG CLASSIFICATION: SYMPATHOMIMETICS

| Drug Name | Dosage |
|---|---|
| Amrinone *(Inocor)* | Loading dose (IV push over 2–3 min): 0.75 mg/kg IV (repeat × 1 if indicated |

after 30 min), maintenance infusion (pump or controller) of 5–10 mcg/kg/min; daily dose should not exceed 10 mg/kg.

**Nursing Implications**

1. **Cardiovascular effects** (cardiac output, arrhythmias, blood pressure) should be evaluated by monitoring vital signs, ECG, urine output, and Swan-Ganz catheter readings.
2. **Thrombocytopenia** may occur and is monitored by repeated platelet counts, and by observing the patient for bleeding and bruising. Platelet count < 150,000 may require discontinuation.
3. **IV administration** in dextrose solutions or with furosemide should be avoided. Discard solutions > 24 hr old.

---

| Drug Name | Dosage |
|---|---|
| Dobutamine *(Dobutrex)* | 2.5–10 mcg/kg/min IV infusion (pump or controller) |

**Nursing Implications**

1. **Cardiovascular effects** (tachycardia, arrhythmias, hypertension, angina, reflex vasodilation) require close monitoring of vital signs, ECG, urine output, and Swan-Ganz catheter readings (if available). Excessive heart rate or new arrhythmias require a decrease in the infusion rate.
2. **IV administration** in alkaline solutions should be avoided; discard solutions >24 hr old.

---

| Drug Name | Dosage |
|---|---|
| Dopamine *(Intropin)* | 2–20 mcg/kg/min IV infusion (pump or controller) |

**Nursing Implications**

1. **Cardiovascular effects** (hypertension, tachycardia, arrhythmia, angina) require close monitoring of vital signs, ECG, urine output, and Swan-Ganz catheter readings (if available). At 2–5 mcg/kg/min increased renal perfusion may increase urine output. At higher infusion rates (5–10 mcg/kg/min) direct cardiac stimulation occurs while at > 10 mcg/kg/min direct peripheral vasoconstriction is evident.
2. **IV administration** in alkaline solutions should be avoided. Discard solutions >24 hr old. If IV infiltrates, phentolamine 5–10 mg diluted in 10–15 ml of normal saline can be injected subcutaneously into the site of infiltration.

---

| Drug Name | Dosage |
|---|---|
| Epinephrine *(Adrenalin)* | Shock: Continuous IV infusion (pump or controller) of 0.1–1.5 mcg/kg/min<br>Cardiac arrest: 0.5–1 mg IV or intracardiac<br>Anaphylaxis asthma: 0.1–0.5 mg IV or SC every 10–30 min as needed. |

**Nursing Implications**

1. **Cardiovascular effects** (tachycardia, hypertension, arrhythmias, angina) require close monitoring of vital signs, ECG, urine output, and Swan-Ganz catheter readings (if available).
2. **Neurologic and endocrine effects** (nervousness, tremor, headache, disorientation, hyperglycemia) reflect excessive catecholamine action and may require dosage reduction.

3. **IV administration** in alkaline solutions should be avoided. Discard solutions >24 hr old. If IV infiltrates, phentolamine 5–10 mg diluted in 10–15 ml of normal saline can be injected subcutaneously into the site of infiltration.

---

| **Drug Name** | **Dosage** |
|---|---|
| Isoproterenol *(Isoprel)* | Bradycardia: 0.02–0.06 mg rapid IV push<br>Shock: 0.5–1.0 mcg/min continuous infusion (pump or controller) |

**Nursing Implications**

1. **Cardiovascular effects** (tachycardia, palpitation, hypotension, angina) require close monitoring of vital signs, ECG, urine output, and Swan-Ganz catheter readings (if available); when used for AV block, a heart rate ≈ 60 beats/min is desired.
2. **Neurologic and endocrine effects** (nervousness, tremors, nausea, hyperglycemia) reflect excessive catecholamine action and may require dosage reduction.
3. **IV administration** in alkaline solutions should be avoided. Discard solutions >24 hr old.

---

| **Drug Name** | **Dosage** |
|---|---|
| Metaraminol *(Aramine)* | Continuous infusion: 20 mcg/min (pump or controller) |

**Nursing Implications**

1. **Cardiovascular effects** (tachycardia, hypertension, arrhythmias, palpitations) require close monitoring of vital signs, ECG, urine output, and Swan-Ganz catheter readings (if available). Hypotension, due to norepinephrine depletion, may occur following discontinuation of this drug.
2. **Neurologic and endocrine effects** (headache, flushing, nausea, hyperglycemia) reflect excessive catecholamine action and may require dosage reduction.
3. **IV administration** in alkaline solutions should be avoided. Discard solutions >24 hr old. If IV infiltrates, phentolamine 5–10 mg diluted in 10–15 ml of normal saline can be injected subcutaneously into the site of infiltration.

---

| **Drug Name** | **Dosage** |
|---|---|
| Norepinephrine, Levarterenol *(Levophed)* | Initially, 2 mcg/min continuous infusion (pump or controller), titrated to blood pressure |

**Nursing Implications**

1. **Cardiovascular effects** (hypertension, decreased urine output, cold extremities, decreased cardiac output, arrhythmias, angina) require close monitoring of vital signs, ECG, urine output, and Swan-Ganz catheter readings (if available).
2. **Neurologic and endocrine effects** (headache, paresthesias, hyperglycemia) reflect excessive catecholamine action and may require dosage reduction.
3. **IV administration** in alkaline solutions or in nondextrose-containing solutions should be avoided. Discard solutions > 24 hr old. If IV infiltrates, phentolamine 5–10 mg diluted in 10–15 ml of normal saline can be injected subcutaneously into the site of infiltration.

---

| **Drug Name** | **Dosage** |
|---|---|
| Phenylephrine *(Neo-Synephrine)* | Shock: 0.1–0.5 mg IV push, continuous infusion of 20–180 mcg/min (pump or controller) |

**Nursing Implications**

1. **Cardiovascular effects** (hypertension, decreased urine output, cold extremities,

decreased cardiac output, arrhythmias, angina) require close monitoring of vital signs, ECG, urine output, and Swan-Ganz catheter readings (if available).
2. **Neurologic effects** (headache, paresthesias) reflect excessive catecholamine action and may require dosage reduction.
3. **IV administration** in alkaline solutions should be avoided and solutions > 24 hr discarded.

| Drug Name | Dosage |
|---|---|
| Terbutaline *(Bricanyl, Brethine, Brethaire)* | 0.25–0.5 mg SC (lateral deltoid area), 2.5–5.0 mg orally or 2 puffs of inhaler q 6–8 h. |

**Nursing Implications**

1. **Cardiovascular effects** (tachycardia, arrhythmias, palpitations) require close monitoring of vital signs and ECG.
2. **Neurologic and endocrine effects** (nervousness, tremors, headache, vomiting, sweating, anxiety, hyperglycemia) reflect excessive catecholamine action and may require dosage reduction.

## DRUG CLASSIFICATION: VASCULAR RESISTANCE LOWERING DRUGS

| Drug Name | Dosage |
|---|---|
| **Centrally Acting Agents** | |
| Clonidine *(Catapres)* | 0.1 mg PO bid, increased in 0.1 mg increments up to 2.4 mg daily. Topical patch: 2.5–7.5 mg patch (0.1–0.3 mg per day) once weekly<br>Opiate detoxification: 0.4–0.8 mg daily in 2–3 divided doses |
| Methyldopa *(Aldomet)* | 0.25–1.0 g IV q 6 hr or 0.5–3 g PO in 2–4 divided doses |
| Reserpine | Hypertensive crisis: 0.5–1 mg IM, then 2–4 mg q 3 hr if needed (up to 4 mg maximum dose); Hypertension: 0.1–0.25 mg daily |

**Nursing Implications**

1. **Cardiovascular effects** (hypotension, orthostasis, rebound hypertension, bradycardia, worsening congestive heart failure) are monitored by weight, pulse, repeated blood pressure measurements (supine and standing if possible). Abrupt discontinuation may result in rebound hypertension (primarily with clonidine). Clinical evaluation of cardiac status is essential in patients with heart failure that receive these agents.
2. **Central neurologic effects** (drowsiness, sedation, nightmares, insomnia, depression, dizziness, headache, fatigue) are common and may require dosage reduction. These effects are potentiated by ethanol and other centrally acting drugs (i.e., sedatives).
3. **Peripheral neurologic effects** (dry mouth, nasal congestion, Raynaud's disease, impotence, urinary retention, dry eyes) reflect the normal actions of these drugs, however, they may subside with dose reduction in some patients.
4. **Hypersensitivity reactions** (hemolytic anemia, thrombocytopenia, hepatitis) occur primarily with methyldopa and requires drug discontinuation.

| Drug Name | Dosage |
|---|---|
| Trimethophan *(Arfonad)* | 2–4 mg/min (in D5W only) continuous infusion only (pump or controller), titrated to blood pressure |

**Nursing Implications**

1. **Cardiovascular effects** (hypotension, orthostasis, tachycardia) require close monitoring of vital signs, ECG, and urine output. Onset of effect is very rapid and disappears quickly.
2. **Neurologic effects** (urinary retention, dry mouth, weakness, restlessness, pupillary dilation) may require dosage reduction.
3. **Hypersensitivity reaction** (urticaria, rash) occur secondary to histamine release and are usually self-limiting.

| Drug Name | Dosage |
|---|---|
| Prazocin *(Minipres)* | 1 mg PO at bedtime, then 2–20 mg PO daily in 2–3 divided doses |

**Nursing Implications**

1. **Cardiovascular effects** (syncope, dizziness, orthostasis) are a direct result of the vasodilating action. *First-dose syncope* can be avoided by administering the initial dose with the patient in bed. Blood pressure (supine and standing) and pulse should be monitored regularly.
2. **Neurologic effects** (headache, drowsiness, weakness, impotence, priapism, dry mouth) may require dosage reduction.

| Drug Name | Dosage |
|---|---|
| **Direct-acting Vasodilators** | |
| Hydralazine *(Apresoline)* | Hypertensive crisis: 5–40 mg IM or IV (over 3–10 min) q 4–6 hr<br>Hypertension: 40–600 mg PO daily in 2–4 divided doses |

**Nursing Implications**

1. **Cardiovascular effects** (palpitation, tachycardia, angina, orthostasis) may occur as a result of a reflex response to direct vasodilation. Blood pressure (supine and standing), pulse, intake/output, and weight should be monitored regularly. Use with caution in patients with coronary artery disease.
2. **Hypersensitivity and immunologic effects** [allergic reactions, hepatitis, blood dyscrasias, systemic lupus erythematosis (at doses > 400 mg/day)] require discontinuation of the drug.

| Drug Name | Dosage |
|---|---|
| Minoxidil *(Loniten)* | 5–100 mg daily PO in 1–4 divided doses |

**Nursing Implications**

1. **Cardiovascular effects** (tachycardia, fluid retention, heart failure, ECG changes, pericardial effusion, and tamponade) occur frequently and require close monitoring of blood pressure, pulse, weight, intake/output, ECG, and physical examination of the heart. Excessive lowering of blood pressure may initially cause underperfusion of the kidneys with resultant elevated creatinine or BUN. Use with caution in patients with coronary artery disease.
2. **Hypertrichosis** (increased hair growth) will occur in most patients during chronic therapy.

| Drug Name | Dosage |
|---|---|
| Diazoxide *(Hyperstat, Proglycem)* | 1–3 mg/kg (maximum 150 mg) rapid IV push over ≤30 sec. Repeat at 5–15 min intervals; or 300 mg IV push q 4–6 hr |

**Nursing Implications**

1. **Cardiovascular effects** (hypotension, orthostasis, fluid retention, congestive

heart failure) result from direct vasodilation and may require the addition of a diuretic. Blood pressure, pulse, and ECG should be monitored closely during administration.
2. **Biochemical effects** (hyperglycemia, increased BUN or creatinine, hyperuricemia) may occur and should be monitored with repeated lab tests.

| Drug Name | Dosage |
|---|---|
| Nitroglycerin *(Nitrol, Nitrostat, Tridil, Nitrobid, Nitrodur, Nitrodisc, Transderm-Nitro)* | Antihypertensive, preload reduction: 5 mcg/min continuous infusion (pump or controller) in glass containers (adheres to plastic)<br>Anti-anginal: 0.15–0.6 mg q 5 min until relief or three doses; 5–15 mg patch once daily or one-half inch to 5 inches of ointment q 4–6 hr |

**Nursing Implications**

1. **Cardiovascular effects** (tachycardia, hypotension, orthostasis, headache, fluid retention) occur as a result of vasodilation and require close monitoring of blood pressure (supine and standing), pulse, weight, intake/output, and clinical evaluation of volume status. Upon discontinuation, decrease infusion rate 5 mcg/min q 5 min to avoid return of pretherapy symptoms. Tolerance to headache usually develops with time.
2. **IV, topical, and oral administration** provide systemic delivery of drug. SL tablets should elicit a tingling or burning under the tongue to indicate potency, while topical application sites should be rotated to avoid local inflammation. Application of ointment is over a 6 × 6 inch thin uniform area wrapped with plastic and adhesive. Topical patches may be worn in shower.

| Drug Name | Dosage |
|---|---|
| Nitroprusside *(Nipride, Nitropress)* | 0.5–10 mcg/kg/min continuous IV infusion (pump or controller), titrate to blood pressure. |

**Nursing Implications**

1. **Cardiovascular effects** (hypotension, palpitations, tachycardia) require close monitoring of vital signs, rhythm, urine output, and intake/output. Effects are rapidly increased or decreased by infusion rate changes.
2. **Metabolic effects** (thiocyanate toxicity, cyanide toxicity) may present as tinnitus, blurred vision, delirium, or metabolic acidosis. Thiocyanate serum levels should be maintained $< 100$ mcg/ml. Patients with renal failure are more prone to develop these effects. Hydroxycobalamin may be administered if the drug must be continued in the presence of toxicity.
3. **IV administration** of highly colored nitroprusside solutions should be avoided and a new bottle (covered with protective wrapping) should be hung every 24 hr.

| Drug Name | Dosage |
|---|---|
| Nifedipine *(Procardia, Adalat)* | 30–180 mg PO daily in 3–4 divided doses; in hypertensive emergencies 10 mg SL may be given (squeeze contents of capsule under tongue). |

**Nursing Implications**

1. **Cardiovascular effects** (hypotension, fluid retention, orthostasis, tachycardia, palpitations, syncope) occur due to direct vasodilation and require close monitoring of vital signs, urine output, and body weight. May increase serum digoxin levels in patients receiving both drugs.
2. **CNS effects** (dizziness, lightheadedness, headache, flushing, weakness, nausea,

nervousness, sleep disturbances) occur due to excessive lowering of blood pressure and may require a dosage reduction.

| Drug Name | Dosage |
|---|---|
| **Angiotensin Converting Enzyme Inhibitors** | |
| Captopril *(Capoten)* | 25–450 mg PO daily in 1–3 divided doses |
| Enalapril *(Vasotec)* | 5–40 mg PO daily in 1–2 divided doses |

**Nursing Implications**

1. **Cardiovascular effects** (hypotension, orthostasis) occur as a result of vasodilation and require close monitoring of vital signs during therapy. Hypotension occurs more commonly in patients who were previously taking diuretics or were salt-restricted. Liberalized salt-intake and low initial doses will avoid this problem.
2. **Renal effects** (proteinuria, nephrotic syndrome, potassium retention) must be monitored closely during therapy with clinical assessment for edema as well as laboratory testing of serum and urine for protein, albumin, and potassium. Hyperkalemia may result in patients taking these drugs with $K^+$-supplements or $K^+$-sparing diuretics.
3. **Hematologic (neutropenia) and sensory (taste loss) effects** should be monitored for during therapy and the drug discontinued if noted.

## DRUG CLASSIFICATION: SYMPATHOLYTICS

| Drug Name | Dosage | |
|---|---|---|
| **Beta-Adrenergic Receptor Blockers** | | |
| ***Nonselective*** | ***Arrhythmia*** | ***Hypertension*** |
| Propranolol *(Inderal)* | SVT: 1 mg slow IV push | 30–320 mg PO daily in 1–4 divided doses |
| Timolol *(Blocadren)* | MI: 10 mg bid | 10–20 mg once/twice daily |
| ***Beta-1 Selective*** | | |
| Metoprolol *(Lopressor)* | MI: 5 mg slow IV push | 100–450 mg PO daily in |
| Atenolol *(Tenormin)* | q 2 min × 3 doses | 1–3 divided doses |
| ***Short Acting*** | | |
| Esmolol *(Brevibloc)* | SVT: 500 mcg/kg over 1 min, then 100–200 mcg/kg/min | |
| ***With Intrinsic Sympathomimetic Activity*** | | |
| Pindolol *(Visken)* | | 200–800 mg PO in divided doses 1–2 times daily |

**Nursing Implications**

1. **Cardiovascular effects** (hypotension, bradycardia, congestive heart failure, heart block, peripheral vasoconstriction) require close monitoring of vital signs, urine output, ECG, and clinical evaluation of cardiac status.
2. **Central neurologic** (dizziness, drowsiness, depression, insomnia, nightmares) may require dosage reduction. These effects are additive with other CNS depressants (i.e., sedatives).
3. **Peripheral neurologic effects** (GI upset, impotence, hypoglycemia) occur due to beta-blockade in other organs. Tolerance to these effects may develop; however, some patients may require a dosage reduction.

| Drug Name | Dosage |
|---|---|
| Phentolamine *(Regitine)* | Pheochromocytoma: Diagnosis: 5 mg rapid IV push, treatment: 5 mg IM or IV |

1–2 hr before surgery or 50–100 mg PO q 4–6 hr
Prevent tissue necrosis from alpha-adrenergic stimulants: 5–10 mg diluted in 10 ml saline. Left ventricular failure: 0.17–0.4 mg/min continuous infusion.

**Nursing Implications**

1. **Cardiovascular effects** (hypotension, orthostasis, tachycardia, arrhythmias, angina) require close monitoring of vital signs and ECG.

## DRUG CLASSIFICATION: SEDATIVES

| Drug Name | Dosage |
|---|---|
| **Benzodiazepines** | |
| Lorazepam *(Ativan)* | Anxiety: 2–3 mg PO or hs daily in 2–3 divided doses<br>Insomnia: 0.5–4 mg PO at bedtime<br>Withdrawal: 0.3–2 mg IV or IM |
| Chlordiazepoxide *(Librium, A-Poxide, Sk-Lygen, Libritabs)* | Anxiety: 5–25 mg PO 3–4 times daily<br>Insomnia: 5–25 mg PO at bedtime<br>Withdrawal: 25–100 mg IM or IV q 2–6 hr |

**Nursing Implications**

1. **Central neurologic effects** (drowsiness, respiratory depression, ataxia, confusion, sedation, lethargy, fatigue, dizziness, stupor, coma) occur in a dose-related manner and are additive with other CNS depressants (i.e., ethanol). Patients should be closely monitored for signs of CNS and respiratory depression.
2. **IV administration** (reconstitute with saline or water for injection) may be associated with phlebitis at the injection site, and IM injections are painful. Absorption injection (reconstitute with commercially supplied diluent) is slow and erratic and should not be used when a rapid effect is desired.
3. **Hepatic metabolism** is more extensive for chlordiazepoxide and is decreased by concurrent administration with cimetidine. Therefore, lower doses may be needed.

| Drug Name | Dosage |
|---|---|
| Paraldehyde *(Paral)* | 2–10 ml IM or IV q 2–6 hr or 10–30 ml PO or PR q 2–6 hr |

**Nursing Implications**

1. **Mucosal irritation** occurs commonly following PO, IV, or PR administration. Oral doses should be diluted in large amounts of juice or milk; IV doses diluted 20-fold in normal saline (infused at ≤ 1 ml/min), while rectal doses should be dissolved in 200 ml normal saline, olive oil, or cottonseed oil.
2. **CNS effects** (CNS depression, respiratory depression, coma) must be closely monitored with vital signs, and are additive with other CNS depressants.
3. **Problems associated with IV administration** (pulmonary edema, circulatory collapse, respiratory distress) and **IM administration** (sterile abscesses) require daily checks. IM injections should be given deep into the gluteus maximus away from nerve endings. Parldehyde reacts with plastics, is light-sensitive, flammable, addicting, and causes a foul-breath odor.

| Drug Name | Dosage |
|---|---|
| Pentobarbital *(Nembutal)* | **Reduce intracranial pressure:** Loading dose: 10–15mg/kg IV over 30–60 min, then 2–3 mg/kg/hour. |

| | |
|---|---|
| | **Seizures:** 100–500 mg slow IV push (≤50 mg/min)<br>**Sedative:** 50–100 mg IM, PO, PR as needed. |

### Nursing Implications

1. **CNS effects** (somnolence, agitation, confusion, CNS depression, respiratory depression) must be closely monitored with vital signs and clinical examination of mental status. Excessive CNS depression may require dosage reduction.
2. **When used to induce coma**: (1) Patients must be mechanically ventilated. Pupils will be small and minimally reactive and the patient will be unresponsive to painful and verbal stimuli. (2) The dose may be titrated to produce an isoelectric EEG < 2 uV potentials. Therapeutic serum levels are 25 to 40 mcg/ml. (3) Intracranial pressure, cerebral perfusion pressure (CPP), and hemodynamic monitoring is required. Desirable ICP is < 15 mmHg; desirable CPP is > 50 mmHg; desirable mean arterial pressure = 90 to 120 mmHg. (4) Pentobarbital is highly alkaline; extravasation may cause local tissue injury. (5) Prepare solutions for IV infusion in D5W. Concentrations under 25 mg/ml are stable for 12 hrs.
3. **Drug interactions** may occur due to the ability of this drug to induce the hepatic metabolism of warfarin, tricyclic antidepressants, phenytoin, estrogen, digitoxin, and corticosteroids. Increased doses of these agents may be required.

## DRUG CLASSIFICATION: NARCOTICS AND NARCOTIC ANTAGONISTS

| Drug Name | Dosage |
|---|---|
| Codeine | 15–60 mg PO, IM, IV, or SC q 4–6 hr |
| Meperidine *(Demerol)* | 50–100 mg IM, SC, or PO q 2–4 hr, or 12.5–50 mg IV q 2–4 hr |
| Morphine | 4–10 mg IV push or 5–20 mg PO, IM, or SC q 3–6 hr |

### Nursing Implications

1. **CNS effects** (drowsiness, dizziness, depression, respiratory depression, euphoria, sedation, coma, nausea, vomiting, cerebral hypoxia with increased CSF pressure, constriction of the pupil, dependence) are dose- and duration-related. Close evaluation of neurologic and mental status changes is important during therapy with these analgesics. These effects are additive with those of other drugs that depress CNS function.
2. **Peripheral neurologic effects** (biliary spasm, urinary retention, flushing, sweating) may occur at doses that are required for analgesia. Dose-reduction and/or adjunctive treatment (i.e., stool softeners) may be needed to overcome these effects.
3. **Cardiovascular effects** (peripheral vasodilation, bradycardia, orthostasis) are the basis for the use of morphine in patients with acute myocardial infarction, CHF, and pulmonary edema.
4. **Analgesic effects** may be achieved more consistently if a regular dosing schedule is used instead of a p.r.n. (as needed) schedule.

| Drug Name | Dosage |
|---|---|
| Naloxone *(Narcan)* | 0.4–2.0 mg IV, IM, or SC; repeat in 3 min if needed (up to 10 mg total dose) |

### Nursing Implications

1. **Reversal of narcotic-induced effects** is achieved rapidly and lasts up to 2 hrs. The patient should be observed closely for reversal of CNS or respiratory depres-

sion. Repeated doses or a continuous infusion (0.1–0.5 mg/hour) may be required to prolong the reversal.

## DRUG CLASSIFICATION: ANTICONVULSANTS

| Drug Name | Dosage |
|---|---|
| Diazepam *(Valium)* | **Seizures:** 5–10 mg IV push (≤5 mg/min), repeat in 10–15 min as needed up to a total dose of 30 mg.<br>**Anxiety:** 2–10 mg IV or IM q 3–4 hr or 2–10 mg PO 3–4 times daily<br>**Withdrawal:** 5–10 mg IV q 15–30 min until calm<br>**Amnesia:** 5–15 mg IV prior to procedure |

**Nursing Implications**

1. **CNS effects** (drowsiness, ataxia, confusion, sedation, lethargy, fatigue, dizziness, stupor, respiratory depression, coma, nausea, vomiting) are cumulative and dose-related. Anticonvulsant activity diminishes within 15–30 min. Patients must be observed closely for beneficial effect versus adverse effects with repeated evaluation of vital signs, mental, neurologic, and respiratory status.
2. **IV administration** may be accompanied by phlebitis at the injection site. This drug is also very irritating and care should be taken to prevent extravasation. Diazepam is insoluble in many IV fluids and binds to plastics. IM absorption is slow and erratic and should be avoided if rapid effects are desired.
   **Drug interactions** occur with other agents that depress CNS function. Cimetidine inhibits the metabolism of diazepam and lower doses may be needed in patients receiving both drugs.

| Drug Name | Dosage |
|---|---|
| Phenobarbital *(Luminal)* | **Seizures:** Acute: 200–600 mg IM or IV (≤60 mg/min); chronic: 100–300 mg PO daily at bedtime or in 2–4 divided doses<br>**Sedation:** 30–120 mg PO or IM daily in 2–3 divided doses<br>**Insomnia:** 100–320 mg PO at bedtime |

**Nursing Implications**

1. **CNS effects** (somnolence, agitation, confusion, CNS depression, respiratory depression) require close monitoring of vital signs, mental, neurologic, and respiratory status. Anticonvulsant effect may be delayed 15–30 min following IV administration. CNS effects are additive with other drugs that depress CNS function.
2. **Drug interactions** occur in patients receiving warfarin, tricyclic antidepressants, phenytoin, estrogens, digitoxin, and corticosteroids, due to the ability of phenobarbital to induce the hepatic metabolism of these agents; dosage adjustments may be necessary. Therapeutic serum levels for anticonvulsant activity ranges from 10–40 mcg/ml.

| Drug Name | Dosage |
|---|---|
| Phenytoin *(Dilantin)* | 10–15 mg/kg slow IV infusion (≤50 mg/min in saline, < 6 mg/ml), then 3–7 mg/kg/day PO, IV, or IM in 1–3 divided doses (Dilantin brand only)<br>Loading doses may also be given as 1000 mg in divided doses over 6 hr |

**Nursing Implications**

1. **CNS effects** (nystagmus, ataxia, diplopia, drowsiness, lethargy, asterixis, nausea, vomiting) occur in a serum concentration-dependent manner and require a dosage reduction. Therapeutic blood levels range from 10–20 mcg/ml (except in dialysis patients where it is lower). Close monitoring of vital signs, mental and neurologic status is required. Phenytoin will potentiate the CNS effects of other drugs.
2. **IV administration** may result in phlebitis and tissue necrosis at the injection site and should not exceed 50 mg/min (to avoid circulatory collapse). IM absorption is slow and erratic, and this route is not recommended.
3. **Other adverse reactions** (loss of taste, gingival hypertrophy, hypertrichosis, lymphadenopathy, folic acid deficiency, osteomalacia, hyperglycemia) should be monitored for clinically and with CBC, platelet-count, and liver-function tests. Gingival hyperplasia may be minimized with good oral hygiene.
4. **Altered metabolism** of numerous other drugs may occur when phenytoin is added. Phenytoin may stimulate the metabolism of corticosteroids, disopyramide, and quinidine while inhibiting warfarin metabolism. In addition, barbiturates, carbamazepine, valproic acid, folic acid, and antacids may decrease serum levels of phenytoin.

## DRUG CLASSIFICATION: DRUGS AFFECTING IMMUNE FUNCTION

| Drug Name | Dosage |
|---|---|
| **Corticosteroids** | |
| Dexamethasone *(Decadron, Dexone, Hexadrol)* | 0.5–9 mg IM or IV daily in 2–3 divided doses<br>Cerebral edema: 10–20 mg IM or IV, then 4 mg IM or IV q 6 hr<br>Shock: 1–6 mg/kg IV or 40 mg IV q 2–6 hr |
| Hydrocortisone *(Hydrocortone, A-Hydrocortef, Solu-Cortef)* | 100 mg–8 g IV (over 15–60 min) or IM in 2–12 divided doses<br>Shock: 50 mg/kg (or 500 mg–2000 mg) IV; repeat in 4 hr |
| Methylprednisolone *(A-Methapred, Solu-Medrol)* | 40–500 mg IV or IM daily in 4–6 divided doses<br>Shock: 30 mg/kg IV over 10–20 min; repeat q 4–6 hr |

**Nursing Implications**

1. **Immunologic effects** (fungal infections, impaired wound healing, anergy) occur at clinically effective doses. Patients should be monitored for infections with temperature, CBC, and clinical evaluation.
2. **Metabolic and endocrine effect** (hirsutism, amenorrhea, cushingoid state, Addisonian crisis upon withdrawal, glucose intolerance, protein breakdown, weight gain, hypokalemia, osteoporosis, muscle weakness) occur at clinically effective doses and may require dosage reduction. Monitor $K^+$ closely in patients receiving diuretics or digoxin, as well as blood pressure.
3. **CNS effects** (euphoria, dysphoria, hallucinations, confusion, depression, insomnia, irritability) are dose-related and may require dosage reduction. Monitor closely in patients receiving other drugs that elicit CNS effects.
4. **Drug interactions** related to the stimulation of the metabolism of other drugs (theophylline) or the metabolism of steroids by drugs such as barbiturates, phenytoin, rifampin.

| Drug Name | Dosage |
|---|---|
| Cyclosporine *(Sandimmune)* | 2–5 mg/kg (in 20–100 ml of diluent) IV over 4–12 hr; then 10–155 mg/kg/day in a glass of juice or milk; adjust to trough concentrations |

**Nursing Implications**

1. **Renal effects** (acute renal dysfunction, chronic nephrotoxicity, hyperkalemia, hyperuricemia) are blood concentration-dependent and requires a dosage reduction. Close monitoring of blood pressure, urine output, serum creatinine, blood urea nitrogen, serum uric acid, and electrolytes is essential during cyclosporine therapy. Nephrotoxicity is additive with other nephrotoxic drugs (aminoglycosides, amphotericin).
2. **Other systemic effects** (hypertension, muscle weakness, hepatotoxicity, hirsutism, gingival hyperplasia) may require dose reduction or discontinuation. Blood pressure and liver function tests should be obtained during therapy. Anaphylaxis or pulmonary edema may occur if the IV formation is infused too rapidly.
3. **Trough blood levels** of cyclosporine are usually maintained from 100–300 mg/ml (depending on the type of assay used). Cyclosporine levels may be increased by ketoconazole or cimetidine, while they may be reduced by phenytoin, barbiturates, or rifampin.

## DRUG CLASSIFICATION: GASTROINTESTINAL DRUGS

| Drug Name | Dosage |
|---|---|
| Antacids | 5–60 ml PO q 1–6 hr; when given NG the tube should be clamped for 15 min |

**Nursing Implications**

1. **Gastrointestinal effects** (anorexia, nausea, constipation, diarrhea) are primarily related to the ingredients in a particular product. Aluminum-containing antacids tend to be constipating while magnesium-containing formulations cause diarrhea. Some products contain both aluminum and magnesium in an attempt to balance the GI effects.
2. **Electrolyte abnormalities** may result in patients with renal failure who get large amounts of antacids. Both magnesium and aluminum will accumulate in patients with renal dysfunction. In addition, certain antacids contain large amounts of sodium and should be avoided.
3. **Drug Interactions** result from the decreased absorption of certain drugs (tetracycline, cimetidine, phenothiazines, iron, digoxin, phenytoin, quinidine, warfarin) due to altered gastric pH.

| Drug Name | Dosage |
|---|---|
| **Histamine Antagonists** | |
| Cimetidine *(Tagamet)* | **Active ulcer:** 300 mg IV (≤150 mg/min), IM, PO q 6 hr or 200 mg tid and 400 mg hs; or 400 mg bid; or 800 mg at bedtime<br>**Chronic:** 400 mg PO at bedtime<br>**Hypersecretory states:** 500 mg q 4 hr up to 2400 mg/day |
| Ranitidine *(Zantac)* | Active Ulcer: 50 mg IM or IV (50–100 ml diluent over 15–60 min) q 6–8 h or 150 mg PO bid; or 300 mg at bedtime<br>Chronic: 150 mg PO at bedtime<br>Hypersensitivity states: up to 6 g per day |

**Nursing Implications**

1. **CNS effects** (primarily cimetidine) (drowsiness, confusion, hallucinations, delirium) occur more commonly in the elderly, patients with liver disease or kidney disease and require dosage reduction. Close monitoring of mental status and avoidance of other drugs that act in the CNS is recommended.
2. **Drug interactions** (primarily cimetidine) occur that lead to decreased metabolism of other drugs (theophylline, lidocaine, warfarin, phenytoin, propranolol, metoprolol, diazepam, chlordiazepoxide) and may require reduced dosages of these agents.
3. **Other systemic effects** (primarily cimetidine) (bradycardia, impotence, reduced sperm count, gynecomastia, neutropenia) are uncommon but should be monitored for in certain patients.
4. **Gastrointestinal effects** (nausea, vomiting, diarrhea) and the ulcer-healing process require routine assessment of the patient's clinical status. The elevated gastric pH that results from these agents may allow bacterial overgrowth in the stomach, and theoretically alter the absorption of certain drugs.

| Drug Name | Dosage |
|---|---|
| Sucralfate *(Carafate)* | 1 g po qid; NG administration requires dissolution in 15–30 ml of water |

**Nursing Implications**

1. **Gastrointestinal effects** (constipation, diarrhea, nausea) may occur during therapy and may require dosage reduction or discontinuation. This agent may interfere with the absorption of other drugs given concomitantly, but this has not been well-studied.

| Drug Name | Dosage |
|---|---|
| Metoclopramide *(Reglan)* | 10–20 mg PO, IM, IV (slow infusion) q 6 hr; Antiemetic: up to 2 mg/kg as needed |

**Nursing Implications**

1. **Neurologic effects** (drowsiness, restlessness, lassitude, extrapyramidal reactions, anxiety, depression, headache, nausea) require close patient observation. For changes in mental or neurologic status, especially dystonia, akathisia, parkinsonian-like reactions, muscle rigidity, and involuntary movements.
2. **Gastrointestinal effects** (diarrhea, altered GI transit time, altered gastric emptying rate) may require dose reduction. Drug interactions may occur in which absorption decreases (digoxin) or increases (acetaminophen, tetracycline, cyclosporine).

## DRUG CLASSIFICATION: DRUGS AFFECTING HEMOSTASIS

| Drug Name | Dosage |
|---|---|
| **Fibrinolytic Agents** | |
| Streptokinase *(Kabikinase, Streptase)* | 250,000 u IV over 30 min, then 100,000 u/hr, acute MI: 1–1.5 million units IV over 1–2 hr, or intracoronary 5–20 thousand units/min continuous intracoronary infusion up to 250,000 units total dose. Catheter patency: 5–20 thousand units instilled for 5–60 min. A-V canula: 250,000 u instilled. |
| Urokinase *(Abbokinase)* | 4400 units/kg IV over 10 min, then 4400 u/kg/hr; Acute MI: 600 u/min to a maximum of 500,000 u. Catheter Patency: 5000 u instilled for 5–60 min. |

**Nursing Implications**

1. **Hematologic effects** (hemorrhage) must be monitored closely with clinical observation for bleeding gums, nose bleeds, hematuria, melena, and hematemesis. Other drugs which alter hemostasis (heparin, aspirin, dipyridamole, dextran, extended-spectrum penicillins, warfarin, moxalactam) with extreme caution. Lab tests during therapy include thrombin time, hematocrit, and platelet count. Heparin therapy, for subsequent anticoagulation, should not be started until the thrombin time is < 2 × control. Effects of these agents are reversed by administering aminocaproic acid or fresh frozen plasma.
2. **IV administration** should be via a volumetric infusion pump only. Hypersensitivity responses can be treated with hydrocortisone and/or diphenydramine. Avoid IM injections, central line placement, arterial punctures, and unnecessary venipunctures in patients receiving these drugs.

| Drug Name | Dosage |
|---|---|
| Heparin *(Lipo-Hepin, Liquaemin, Calciparine)* | **Acute:** 5000-15,000 u IV bolus, then 500-3000 u/hr via continuous infusion; or 3000-10,000 u IV bolus q 4 hr<br>**Prophylaxis:** 5000 u SC q 8-12 hr |

**Nursing Implications**

1. **Hematologic effects** (bleeding, thrombocytopenia) are minimized by maintaining the activated partial thromboplastin time or the whole blood clotting time to 1.5-2 and 2.5-3 × control, respectively. These tests along with hematocrit and platelet count should be monitored daily. Use with caution in patients receiving aspirin, extended-spectrum penicillins, moxalactam, dextran, or dipyridamole. Observe patient routinely for bruising, bleeding gums, nose bleeds, hematuria, melena, or hematemesis. Overdoses of heparin can be treated with protamine (1 mg protamine will inactivate 100 u of heparin).
2. **IM administration** should never be used due to the risk of hematoma formation.
3. **SQ administration** sites should be rotated frequently to minimize the development of ecchymoses or tissue necrosis (area above the ileac crest or into abdominal fat layer are the optimal sites).

| Drug Name | Dosage |
|---|---|
| Protamine | 1 mg IV (over 1-3 min) for every 100 u of heparin to be neutralized, (maximum dose: 500 mg IV 10 min) |

**Nursing Implications**

1. **Hypersensitivity reactions** (hypotension, anaphylaxis, dyspnea, pulmonary edema) can be minimized by administering the IV dose slowly and avoiding the use of this drug in patients allergic to salmon or other fish.
2. **Anticoagulation** may occur due to the release of heparin from the protamine-heparin complex. Observe patients closely for bleeding for up to 18 hr after the dose of protamine.

| Drug Name | Dosage |
|---|---|
| Aminocaproic Acid *(Amicar)* | **Acute:** 4-5 g IV over 1 hr, then 1-1.5 g/hr continuous infusion until bleeding is controlled<br>**Chronic:** 5-30 g/day PO in 4-8 divided doses |

**Nursing Implications**

1. A variety of **nonspecific adverse effects** (nausea, cramping, diarrhea, dizziness, headache, rash, hypotension, malaise, seizures, allergic reactions, and phlebitis) are associated with treatment with this drug. However, patients who require aminocaproic acid are usually critically ill and these effects are tolerated.

## DRUG CLASSIFICATION: MISCELLANEOUS DRUGS

| Drug Name | Dosage |
| --- | --- |
| Pancuronium *(Pavulon)* | 0.06–0.1 mg/kg IV, then 0.01–0.015 mg/kg at 30–60 min intervals to maintain muscle paralysis |

**Nursing Implications**

1. **Pulmonary function** must be maintained by mechanical ventilation during pancuronium therapy. Close monitoring of arterial blood gases is imporant to evaluate oxygen balance. Respiratory muscle paralysis occurs within 2–3 min of an IV dose, and lasts for 35–45 min. The effects can be reversed by pyridostigmine or neostigmine.
2. **Possible drug interactions** may occur if the patient receiving other medications that potentiate the neuromuscular blockade (inhaled anesthetics, aminoglycosides).

| Drug Name | Dosage |
| --- | --- |
| Sodium Bicarbonate | **Acidosis:** 1–5 mEq/kg IV over 4–8 hr<br>**Cardiac Arrest:** 1 mEq/kg IV bolus, repeat 0.5 mEq/kg q 10 min as needed |

**Nursing Implications**

1. **Electrolyte effects** (metabolic alkalosis, sodium and water retention, hypokalemia) following sodium bicarbonate administration must be monitored closely with arterial blood gases and serum electrolytes.
2. **IV admixture** with many emergency drugs (epinephrine, dopamine, dobutamine, norepinephrine, calcium chloride) should be avoided due to incompatibility. Extravasation during IV administration may cause a chemical cellulitis.

| Drug Name | Dosage |
| --- | --- |
| Theophylline | **Acute:** 2.5–6 mg/kg IV loading dose over 30 min, then 0.1–0.9 mg/kg continuous infusion (pump or controller)<br>**Chronic:** 2.4–21 mg/kg/day in 2–3 divided doses (sustained-release) or 3–6 divided doses (rapid-release) |

**Nursing Implications**

1. **Neurologic effects** (nausea, vomiting, diarrhea, abdominal cramps, headache, irritability, restlessness, nervousness, insomnia, seizures, palpitations, tachycardia) occur in a serum-concentration dependent manner and are usually reversible if the drug is stopped, and then restarted at a lower dose. Close monitoring of vital signs, rhythm, and pulmonary status are essential during theophylline therapy.
2. **Theophylline dosage** must be decreased in patients with liver disease, congestive heart failure, pulmonary edema, or advanced age while younger patients tend to require higher doses.
3. Theophylline **serum levels** are used to guide therapy. The therapeutic range is 10–20 mcg/ml with signs of toxicity usually occurring at > 20 mcg/ml.
4. **Drug interactions** occur when patients receive certain drugs (cimetidine, erythromycin, propranolol, verapamil) that decrease theophylline metabolism. As well, theophylline metabolism may be increased by concurrent treatment with phenytoin, carbamazepine, phenobarbital, corticosteroids, and rifampin.
5. **Theophylline salts:** Aminophylline contains 75–86% theophylline; Oxtriphylline contains 64% theophylline. (The theophylline content must be considered when switching patients between formulations).

| **Drug Name** | **Dosage** |
| --- | --- |
| Vasopressin *(Pitressin)* | **Diabetes insipidus:** 5–10 u IM or SQ 2–4 times daily<br>**GI hemorrhage:** 0.1–0.4 u/min continuous IV infusion or intra-arterial infusion (pump or controller). |

**Nursing Implications**

1. **Fluid and electrolyte effects** (overhydration, hyponatremia) occur as a result of the hormonal actions of this agent. Fluid intake/output, weight, serum and urine electrolytes should be monitored during therapy. Clinical assessment of mental status (drowsiness, listlessness, headache, confusion) should be followed closely to prevent water intoxication.
2. **Cardiovascular effects** (hypotension, bradycardia, angina, excessive vasoconstriction resulting in gangrene or ischemic colitis) reflect excessive vasoconstriction and require dose-reduction. Clinical monitoring of vital signs, urine output, and examination of extremities are important to detect these effects.
3. **Neuromuscular effects** (tremor, sweating, vomiting, diarrhea, uterine cramping) may also require dose reduction, depending on the patient's clinical status.

APPENDIX B-1

# NANDA-Approved Nursing Diagnoses

Activity intolerance
Activity intolerance, potential for
Adjustment impaired
Airway clearance, ineffective
Anxiety (specify)
Aspiration, potential for

Body image disturbance
Body temperature, altered potential
Breastfeeding, ineffective
Breastfeeding, effective*
Breathing pattern, ineffective

Cardiac output, altered: decreased
Comfort, altered (see Pain)
Communication, impaired: verbal
Constipation
Constipation, colonic
Constipation, perceived
Coping, defensive
Coping, ineffective individual

Decisional conflict (specify)
Denial, ineffective
Diarrhea
Disuse syndrome, potential for
Diversional activity, deficit
Dysreflexia

Family coping, compromised
Family coping, disabling
Family coping, potential for growth
Family processes, altered

Fatigue
Fear
Fluid volume deficit (1) [regulatory failure]
Fluid volume deficit (2) [active loss]
Fluid volume deficit, potential
Fluid volume, excess

Gas exchange, impaired
Grieving, anticipatory
Grieving, dysfunctional
Growth and Development, altered

Health maintenance, altered
Health seeking behaviors (specify)
Home maintenance management, impaired
Hopelessness
Hyperthermia
Hypothermia

Incontinence, bowel
Incontinence, functional
Incontinence, reflex
Incontinence, stress
Incontinence, total
Incontinence, urge
Infection, potential for
Injury, potential for

Knowledge deficit [learning need] (specify)

Mobility, impaired physical

*Diagnosis proposed for approval at NANDA Conference, 1990.
Bracketed material designates author recommendations. *Taxonomy 1, Revised*, 1989.

Noncompliance, specify [Compliance, altered, specify]
Nutrition, altered: less than body requirements
Nutrition, altered: more than body requirements
Nutrition, potential for more than body requirements

Oral mucous membrane, altered

Pain
Pain, chronic
Parental role conflict
Parenting, altered
Parenting, altered: potential
Personal identity disturbance
Poisoning, potential for
Post-trauma response
Powerlessness
Protection, altered*

Rape-trauma syndrome
Rape-trauma syndrome: compound reaction
Rape-trauma syndrome: silent reaction
Role performance, altered

Self-care deficit, bathing/hygiene, dressing/grooming, feeding, toileting
Self-esteem, chronic low
Self-esteem, situational low
Self-esteem disturbance in
Sensory-perceptual alterations (specify): visual, auditory, kinesthetic, gustatory, tactile, olfactory
Sexual dysfunction
Sexuality patterns, altered
Skin integrity, impaired: actual
Skin integrity, impaired: potential
Sleep pattern disturbance
Social interaction, impaired
Social isolation
Spiritual distress (distress of the human spirit)
Suffocation, potential for
Swallowing impaired

Thermoregulation, ineffective
Thought processes, altered
Tissue integrity, impaired
Tissue perfusion, altered (specify: cerebral, cardiopulmonary, renal, gastrointestinal, peripheral)
Trauma, potential for

Unilateral neglect
Urinary elimination, altered
Urinary retention [acute/chronic]

Violence, potential for: directed at self/others

---

*Diagnosis proposed for approval at NANDA Conference, 1990.
Bracketed material designates author recommendations. *Taxonomy 1, Revised*, 1989.

APPENDIX B-2

# NANDA-Approved Nursing Diagnoses: Definitions*

**Activity intolerance**
The state in which an individual has insufficient physiologic or psychologic energy to endure or complete required or desired daily activities.

**Activity intolerance, potential for**
The state in which an individual is at risk of experiencing insufficient physiologic or psychologic energy to endure or complete required desired daily activities.

**Adjustment, impaired**
The state in which an individual is unable to modify his/her lifestyle/behavior in a manner consistent with a change in health status.

**Airway clearance, ineffective**
The state in which an individual is unable to clear secretions or obstructions from the respiratory tract to maintain airway patency.

**Anxiety**
A vague, uneasy feeling, the source of which is often nonspecific or unknown to the individual.

**Aspiration, potential for**
The state in which an individual is at risk for entry of gastric secretions, oropharyngeal secretions, or exogenous food or fluids into tracheobronchial passages due to dysfunction or absence of normal protective mechanisms.

**Body-image disturbance**
Disruption in the perception of one's body image.

**Body temperature, potential altered**
The state in which an individual is at risk for failure to maintain body temperature within normal range.

**Breastfeeding, ineffective**
The state in which a mother, infant, and/or family experiences dissatisfaction or difficulty with the breastfeeding process.

**Breathing pattern, ineffective**
The state in which an individual's inhalation and/or exhalation pattern does not enable adequate ventilation.

**Cardiac output, altered: decreased**
The state in which the blood pumped by an individual's heart is sufficiently reduced that it is inadequate to meet the needs of the body's tissues.

**Comfort, altered**
(see Pain)

**Communication, impaired verbal**
The state in which an individual experiences a decreased or absent ability to use or understand language in human interaction.

---

*Adapted from Kim, MJ, McFarland, GK, and McLane, AM: Pocket Guide to Nursing Diagnoses. ed. 3. CV Mosby, St. Louis, 1989, with permission.

**Constipation**
The state in which an individual experiences a change in normal bowel habits characterized by a decrease in frequency and/or passage of hard, dry stools.

**Constipation, colonic**
The state in which an individual's pattern of elimination is characterized by hard, dry stool that results from a delay in passage of food residue.

**Constipation, perceived**
The state in which an individual makes a self-diagnosis of constipation and ensures a daily bowel movement through use of laxatives, enemas, and suppositories.

**Coping, defensive**
The state in which an individual experiences falsely positive self-evaluation based on a self-protective pattern that defends against underlying perceived threats to positive self-regard.

**Coping, ineffective individual**
Impairment of adaptive behaviors and problem-solving abilities of a person in meeting life's demands and roles.

**Decisional conflict (specify)**
A state of uncertainty about the course of action to be taken when choice among competing actions involves risk, loss, or challenge to personal life values. (Specify focus of conflict, e.g., choices regarding health, family relationships, career, finances, or other life events.)

**Denial, ineffective**
A conscious or unconscious attempt to disavow the knowledge or meaning of an event to reduce anxiety/fear to the detriment of health.

**Diarrhea**
The state in which an individual experiences a change in normal bowel habits characterized by the frequent passage of loose, fluid, unformed stools.

**Disuse syndrome, potential for**
The state in which an individual is at risk for deterioration of body systems as the result of prescribed or unavoidable inactivity.

**Diversional activity deficit**
The state in which an individual experiences a decreased stimulation from, or interest or engagement in, recreational or leisure activities.

**Dysreflexia**
The state in which an individual with a spinal cord injury at T-7 or above experiences, or is at risk of experiencing, a life-threatening uninhibited sympathetic response of the nervous system to a noxious stimulus.

**Family coping, compromised**
Insufficient, ineffective, or compromised support, comfort, assistance, or encouragement usually by a supportive primary person (family member or close friend); client may need it to manage or master adaptive tasks related to his/her health challenge.

**Family coping, disabling**
Behavior of significant person (family members or other primary person) that disables his/her own capacities and the client's capacities to effectively address tasks essential to either person's adaptation to the health challenge.

**Family coping, potential for growth**
Effective managing of adaptive tasks by family member involved with the client's health challenge, who now is exhibiting desire and readiness for enhanced health and growth in regard to self and in relation to the client.

**Family processes, altered**
The state in which a family that normally functions effectively experiences a dysfunction.

**Fatigue**
An overwhelming sense of exhaustion and decreased capacity for physical and mental work regardless of adequate sleep.

**Fear**
Feeling of dread related to an identifiable source that the person validates.

**Fluid volume deficit (1) [Regulatory failure]**
The state in which an individual experiences vascular, cellular, or intracellular dehydration related to failure of regulatory mechanisms.

**Fluid volume deficit (2) [Active loss]**
The state in which an individual experiences vascular, cellular, or intracellular dehydration related to active loss.

**Fluid volume deficit, potential**
The state in which an individual is at risk of experiencing vascular, cellular, or intracellular dehydration.

**Fluid volume excess**
The state in which an individual experiences increased fluid retention and edema.

**Gas exchange, impaired**
The state in which an individual experiences an imbalance between oxygen uptake and carbon dioxide elimination at the alveolar-capillary membrane gas exchange area.

**Grieving, anticipatory**
The state in which an individual grieves before an actual loss.

**Grieving, dysfunctional**
The state in which actual or perceived object loss (object loss is used in the broadest sense) exists. Objects include people, possessions, a job, status, home, ideals, parts and processes of the body, etc.

**Growth and development, altered**
The state in which an individual demonstrates deviations in norms from his/her age group.

**Health maintenance, altered**
Inability to identify, manage, and/or seek out help to maintain health.

**Health-seeking behaviors (specify)**
The state in which a client in stable health is actively seeking ways to alter personal health habits and/or the environment in order to move toward optimal health. (*Stable health status* is defined as age-appropriate illness prevention measures achieved; the client reports good or excellent health, and signs and symptoms of disease, if present, are controlled.)

**Home maintenance management, impaired**
Inability to independently maintain a safe growth-promoting immediate environment.

**Hopelessness**
The subjective state in which an individual sees limited or no alternatives or personal choices available and is unable to mobilize energy on own behalf.

**Hyperthermia**
The state in which an individual's body temperature is elevated above his/her normal range.

**Hypothermia**
The state in which an individual's body temperature is reduced below his/her normal range but not below 35.6°C (rectal).

**Incontinence, bowel**
The state in which an individual experiences a change in normal bowel habits characterized by involuntary passage of stool.

**Incontinence, functional**
The state in which an individual experiences an involuntary, unpredictable passage of urine.

**Incontinence, reflex**
The state in which an individual experiences an involuntary loss of urine occurring at somewhat predictable intervals when a specific bladder volume is reached.

**Incontinence, stress**
The state in which an individual experiences a loss of urine of less than 50 ml occurring with increased abdominal pressure.

**Incontinence, total**
The state in which an individual experiences a continuous and unpredictable loss of urine.

**Incontinence, urge**
The state in which an individual experiences involuntary passage of urine occurring soon after a strong sense of urgency to void.
**Infection, potential for**
The state in which an individual is at increased risk for being invaded by pathogenic organisms.
**Injury, potential for**
The state in which an individual is at risk of injury as a result of environmental conditions interacting with the individual's adaptive and defensive resources. *See also* Poisoning, potential for; Suffocation, potential for; Trauma, potential for.
**Knowledge deficit [Learning need] (specify)**
The state in which specific information is lacking.
**Mobility, impaired physical**
The state in which an individual experiences a limitation of ability for independent physical movement.
**Noncompliance (specify)**
A person's informed decision not to adhere to a therapeutic recommendation.
**Nutrition, altered: less than body requirements**
The state in which an individual experiences an intake of nutrients insufficient to meet metabolic needs.
**Nutrition, altered: more than body requirements**
The state in which an individual is experiencing an intake of nutrients that exceeds metabolic needs.
**Nutrition, potential for more than body requirements**
The state in which an individual is at risk of experiencing an intake of nutrients that exceeds metabolic needs.
**Oral mucous membrane, altered**
The state in which an individual experiences disruptions in the tissue layers of the oral cavity.
**Pain**
The state in which an individual experiences and reports the presence of severe discomfort or an uncomfortable sensation.
**Pain, chronic**
The state in which an individual experiences pain that continues for more than 6 months.
**Parental role conflict**
The state in which a parent experiences role confusion and conflict in response to a crisis.
**Parenting, altered, potential**
The state in which the ability of nurturing figure(s) to create an environment that promotes the optimum growth and development of another human being is altered or at risk.
**Personal identity disturbance**
Inability to distinguish between self and oneself.
**Poisoning, potential for**
Accentuated risk of accidental exposure to, or ingestion of, drugs or dangerous products in doses sufficient to cause poisoning.
**Post-trauma response**
The state in which an individual experiences a sustained painful response to (an) overwhelming traumatic event(s).
**Powerlessness**
Perception of one's own action will not significantly affect an outcome; a perceived lack of control over a current situation or immediate happening.
**Rape-trauma syndrome**
Forced, violent sexual penetration against the victim's will and consent. The trauma syndrome that develops from this attack or attempted attack includes an acute phase or disorganization of the victim's life-style and a long-term process of reorganization of life-style.
**Rape-trauma syndrome: compound reaction**
An acute stress reaction to a rape or attempted rape, experienced along with

other major stressors, that can include reactivation of symptoms of a previous condition.

**Rape-trauma syndrome: silent reaction**
A complex stress reaction to a rape in which an individual is unable to describe or discuss the rape.

**Role performance, altered**
Disruption in the way one perceives one's role performance.

**Self-care deficit, bathing/hygiene**
The state in which an individual experiences an impaired ability to perform or complete bathing/hygiene activities for oneself.

**Self-care deficit, dressing/grooming**
The state in which an individual experiences an impaired ability to perform or complete dressing and grooming activities for oneself.

**Self-care deficit, feeding**
The state in which an individual experiences an impaired ability to perform or to complete feeding activities for oneself.

**Self-care deficit, toileting**
The state in which an individual experiences an impaired ability to perform or complete toileting activities for oneself.

**Self-esteem, chronic low**
Long-standing negative self-evaluation/feelings about self or self-capabilities.

**Self-esteem, situational low**
Negative self-evaluation/feelings about self that develop in response to a loss or change in an individual who previously had a positive self-evaluation.

**Self-esteem disturbance in**
Negative self-evaluation/feelings about self or self-capabilities, which may be directly or indirectly expressed.

**Sensory-perceptual alterations (specify): (visual, auditory, kinesthetic, gustatory, tactile, olfactory)**
The state in which an individual experiences a change in the amount or patterning of incoming stimuli accompanied by a diminished, exaggerated, distorted, or impaired response to such stimuli.

**Sexual dysfunction**
The state in which an individual experiences a change in sexual function that is viewed as unsatisfying, unrewarding, or inadequate.

**Sexuality patterns, altered**
The state in which an individual expresses concern regarding his/her sexuality.

**Skin integrity, impaired: actual**
The state in which an individual's skin is adversely altered.

**Skin integrity, impaired: potential**
The state in which an individual's skin is at risk of being adversely altered.

**Sleep pattern disturbance**
Disruption of sleep time causes discomfort or interferes with desired life-style.

**Social interaction, impaired**
The state in which an individual participates in an insufficient or excessive quantity or ineffective quality of social exchange.

**Social isolation**
Aloneness experienced by an individual and perceived as imposed by others and as a negative or threatened state.

**Spiritual distress (distress of the human spirit)**
Disruption in the life principle that pervades a person's entire being and that integrates and transcends one's biological and psychosocial nature.

**Suffocation, potential for**
Accentuated risk of accidental suffocation (inadequate air available for inhalation).

**Swallowing, impaired**
The state in which an individual has decreased ability to voluntarily pass fluids and/or solids from mouth to stomach.

**Thermoregulation, ineffective**
The state in which an individual's temperature fluctuates between hypothermia and hyperthermia.

**Thought processes, altered**
The state in which an individual experiences a disruption in cognitive operations and activities.

**Tissue integrity, impaired**
The state in which an individual experiences damage to mucous membrane or corneal, integumentary, or subcutaneous tissue. See also Oral mucous membrane, altered.

**Tissue perfusion, altered (specify: cerebral, cardiopulmonary, renal, gastrointestinal, peripheral)**
The state in which an individual experiences a decrease in nutrition and oxygenation at the cellular level due to a deficit in capillary blood supply.

**Trauma, potential for**
Accentuated risk of accidental tissue injury (e.g., wound, burn, fracture).

**Unilateral neglect**
The state in which an individual is perceptually unaware of and inattentive to one side of the body.

**Urinary elimination, altered**
The state in which an individual experiences a disturbance in urine elimination. See also *Incontinence (functional, reflex, stress, total, urge).*

**Urinary retention [acute/chronic]**
The state in which an individual experiences incomplete emptying of the bladder.

**Violence, potential for: directed at self/others**
The state in which an individual experiences behaviors that can be physically harmful either to self or others.

APPENDIX C-1

# Functional Health Patterns*

**Health Perception - Health Management**
**Nutritional - Metabolic**
**Elimination**
**Activity - Exercise**
**Sleep - Rest**
**Cognitive - Perceptual**
**Self-Perception - Self-Concept**
**Role - Relationship**
**Sexuality - Reproductive**
**Coping - Stress Tolerance**
**Value - Belief**

*From Gordon, M: Nursing Diagnosis: Process and Application. ed. 2. McGraw-Hill, New York, 1987, with permission.

APPENDIX C-2

# Functional Health Patterns: Definitions

### Health Perception–Health Management

Describes the client's perceived pattern of health and well-being and how his or her health is managed. Includes the individual's perception of health status and its relevance to current activities and future planning. Also included is the individual's general level of health-care behavior, such as adherence to mental and physical prevention health practices, medical or nursing prescriptions, and follow-up care.

### Nutritional–Metabolic

Describes patterns of food and fluid consumption relative to metabolic need and pattern indicators of local nutrient supply. Includes the individual's patterns of food and fluid consumption, daily eating times, the types and quantity of food and fluids consumed, particular food preferences, and the use of nutrient or vitamin supplements. Reports of any skin lesions and general ability to heal are included. The condition of skin, hair, nails, mucous membranes, and teeth and measures of body temperature, height, and weight are included.

### Elimination

Describes patterns of excretory function (bowel, bladder, and skin) of individuals. Includes the individual's perceived regularity of excretory function, use of routines or laxatives for bowel elimination, and any changes or disturbances in time pattern, mode of excretion, quality, or quantity. Also included are any devices employed to control excretion. Includes family or community waste disposal pattern when appropriate.

### Activity–Exercise

Describes pattern of exercise, activity, leisure, and recreation. Includes activities of daily living requiring energy expenditure, such as hygiene, cooking, shopping, eating, working, and home maintenance. Also included are the type, quantity, and quality of exercise, including sports, which describe the typical pattern. (Factors that interfere with the desired or expected pattern for the *individual*, such as neuromuscular deficits and compensations, dyspnea, angina, or muscle cramping on exertion, and, if appropriate, his or her cardiac/pulmonary classification, are included.) Leisure patterns are included and describe the recreational activities undertaken with others or alone. Emphasis is on activities of major importance to the client.

### Sleep–Rest

Describes patterns of sleep, rest, and relaxation. Includes the patterns of sleep and rest/relaxation periods during the 24-hour day. Includes the perception of the quality and quantity of sleep and rest, and perception of energy level. Included also are aids to sleep such as medications or night-time routines that are employed.

### Cognitive – Perceptual

Describes sensory – perceptual and cognitive pattern. Includes the adequacy of sensory modes, such as vision, hearing, taste, touch, or smell, and the compensation or prostheses utilized for disturbances. Report of pain perception and how pain is managed are also included when appropriate. Also included are the cognitive functional abilities, such as language, memory, and decision making.

### Self-Perception – Self-Concept

Describes self-concept pattern and perceptions of self. Includes the attitudes about self, perception of abilities (cognitive, affective, or physical), image, identity, general sense of worth, and general emotional pattern. Pattern of body posture and movement, eye contact, voice, and speech patterns are included.

### Role – Relationship

Describes pattern of role engagements and relationships. Includes perception of the major roles and responsibilities in current life situation. Satisfaction or disturbances in family work, or social relationships and responsibilities related to these roles are included.

### Sexuality – Reproductive

Describes patterns of satisfaction or dissatisfaction with sexuality; describes reproductive pattern. Includes the perceived satisfaction or disturbances in sexuality or sexual relationships. Included also is the female's reproductive stage, pre- or postmenopause, and any perceived problems.

### Coping – Stress Tolerance

Describes general coping pattern and effectiveness of the pattern of stress tolerance. Includes the reserve or capacity to resist challenges to self-integrity, modes of handling stress, family or other support systems, and perceived ability to control and manage situations.

### Value – Belief

Describes patterns of values, goals, or beliefs (including spiritual) that guide choices or decisions. Includes what is perceived as important in life and any perceived conflicts in values, beliefs, or expectations that are health-related.

APPENDIX D

# Classification of Nursing Diagnoses by Functional Health Patterns

**Health perception – health management**

Altered health maintenance
Noncompliance (specify)
Potential for infection
Potential for injury
Potential for trauma
Potential for poisoning
Potential for suffocation
Health-seeking behaviors (specify)

**Nutritional – metabolic**

Altered nutrition: potential for more than body requirements
Altered nutrition: more than body requirements
Altered nutrition: less than body requirements
Ineffective breastfeeding
Effective breastfeeding
Potential for aspiration
Impaired swallowing
Altered oral mucous membrane
Potential fluid volume deficit
Fluid volume deficit (1)
Fluid volume deficit (2)
Fluid volume excess
Potential impaired skin integrity
Impaired skin integrity
Impaired tissue integrity
Potential altered body temperature
Ineffective thermoregulation
Hyperthermia
Hypothermia

**Elimination**

Constipation
Perceived constipation
Colonic constipation
Diarrhea
Bowel incontinence
Altered patterns of urinary elimination
Functional incontinence
Reflex incontinence
Stress incontinence
Urge incontinence
Total incontinence
Urinary retention

**Activity – exercise**

Potential activity intolerance
Activity intolerance
Impaired physical mobility
Potential for disuse syndrome
Fatigue
Bathing/hygiene self-care deficit
Dressing/grooming self-care deficit
Feeding self-care deficit
Toileting self-care deficit
Diversional activity deficit
Impaired home maintenance management
Ineffective airway clearance
Ineffective breathing pattern
Impaired gas exchange
Decreased cardiac output
Altered (specify type) tissue perfusion

*From Gordon, M: Nursing Diagnosis: Process and Application. ed. 2. McGraw-Hill, New York, 1987, with permission.

(renal, cerebral, cardiopulmonary, gastrointestinal, peripheral)
Dysreflexia
Altered growth and development

**Sleep-rest**

Sleep pattern disturbance

**Cognitive-perceptual**

Pain
Chronic pain
Sensory perceptual alterations (specify) (visual, auditory, kinesthetic, gustatory, tactile, olfactory)
Unilateral neglect
Knowledge deficit (specify)
Altered thought processes
Decisional conflict (specify)

**Self-perception-self-concept**

Fear
Anxiety
Hopelessness
Powerlessness
Body image disturbance
Personal identity disturbance
Self-esteem disturbance
Chronic low self-esteem
Situational low self-esteem

**Role-relationship**

Anticipatory grieving
Dysfunctional grieving
Altered role performance
Social isolation
Impaired social interaction
Altered family processes
Potential altered parenting
Altered parenting
Parental role conflict
Impaired verbal communication
Potential for violence: self-directed or directed at others

**Sexuality-reproductive**

Sexual dysfunction
Altered sexuality patterns
Rape-trauma syndrome
Rape-trauma syndrome: compound reaction
Rape-trauma syndrome: silent reaction

**Coping-stress tolerance**

Ineffective individual coping
Defensive coping
Ineffective denial
Impaired adjustment
Post-trauma response
Family coping: potential for growth
Ineffective family coping: compromised
Ineffective family coping: disabling

**Value-belief**

Spiritual distress (distress of the human spirit)

APPENDIX E

# Monograph: Assessment of the Critically Ill Cardiovascular Patient*

*Cathy Rodgers Ward*

## OUTLINE



## LEARNING OBJECTIVES

**At the end of this monograph you should be able to:**

1. Explain the significance of a valid assessment in formulating nursing diagnoses and rendering patient care.
2. Identify and define the human response patterns.
3. Differentiate subjective and objective assessment data.
4. Incorporate the human response patterns as a guide to patient/family assessment.
5. Formulate nursing diagnoses based on clusters of assessment data and cues reflective of human responses.

A basic premise in the nursing process is that valid assessment is essential in order to diagnose a patient's problem and, once having diagnosed the problem, to develop and implement a plan of care. In the care of the critically ill patient there is the added dimension of continuously assessing for potential problems which may never occur. Nevertheless, such *anticipatory* assessments are essential to prevent potential, possibly life-threatening complications from occurring, or should they

*Based on a nursing framework of nine human response patterns (from *NANDA Taxonomy*).

occur, to enable timely and appropriate intervention to be initiated so as to ensure a favorable outcome.

In less acute settings the nurse may have the opportunity to sit down to interview the patient and to proceed with the physical examination. In the intensive care setting, however, the rapidly changing patient condition, and the intensity of care required over short periods of time, preclude this approach to assessment. Often, patients exhibit an altered state of consciousness requiring critical care nurses to be ever vigilant in their assessment and monitoring of the patient's overall clinical status. In assessing the critically ill patient the nurse integrates the collection of subjective and objective data, prioritizes the patient's needs, and initiates a plan of action in an appropriate and timely manner.

This will serve as a guide for assessing critically ill patients, particularly those with cardiovascular dysfunction, as for example the patient with a myocardial infarction or postcardiac surgery.

## HUMAN RESPONSE PATTERN ASSESSMENT GUIDE

The assessment guide presented in this work is based on a nursing framework of nine human response patterns which were developed by nurse-theorists and introduced as a means of classifying nursing diagnoses by the North American Nursing Diagnosis Association (NANDA). The intent of this guide is to assist the critical care nurse to assess the patient for information relevant to nursing using the NANDA taxonomy. The categories and descriptions under each of the nine patterns have been adapted specifically for the assessment of the cardiovascular patient.

The order of assessment may vary according to the nurse's judgment about the patient's condition but *all* patterns should be included in a comprehensive assessment. It is recognized that the collection of subjective and objective data is frequently integrated and is not necessarily sequential.

Subjective data include those assessment cues obtained from verbal indications by the patient and/or family in response to direct questioning or those voluntarily expressed. Examples of questions for the critical care nurse to ask are cited in the assessment guide (see Table 2), verbalizations from the patient and/or family are also noted.

Objective data are those assessment cues the critical care nurse observes or can tangibly identify. Although the physical assessment techniques of inspection, palpation, percussion, and auscultation are necessary in collecting objective data, the assessment guide presented here provides a more comprehensive approach to accurately reflect assessment activities routinely performed by the critical care nurse. Examples include checking the functioning of a pacemaker, or confirming the dosage of an inotropic infusion.

Cues may occur in the assessment guide more than once to be assessed under more than one pattern. This reflects the fact that cues are assimilated into various cluster groups to formulate different nursing diagnoses. For example, the critical care nurse may observe changes in mental status as a sign of *sensory/perceptual alteration* in the *perceiving* pattern, while also assessing for changes in mental status when evaluating the patient for *alteration in cardiac output* in the *exchanging* pattern. Each pattern is defined in Table 1, and discussed below as it applies to the

### Assessment of the Critically Ill Patient with Cardiovascular Dysfunction

**TABLE 1: Definitions of Human Response Patterns**

1. **Exchanging** A human response pattern involving mutual giving and receiving
2. **Communicating** A human response pattern involving sending messages
3. **Relating** A human response pattern involving establishing bonds
4. **Valuing** A human response pattern involving the assigning of relative worth
5. **Choosing** A human response pattern involving the selection of alternatives
6. **Moving** A human response pattern involving activity
7. **Perceiving** A human response pattern involving the reception of information
8. **Knowing** A human response pattern involving the meaning associated with information
9. **Feeling** A human response pattern involving the subjective awareness of information

## Assessment of the Critically Ill Patient With Cardiovascular Dysfunction

**TABLE 2: Human Response Pattern-Assessment Guide**

| *Possible Cues and Parameters* | *Possible Nursing Diagnosis (Actual/Potential)* |
|---|---|
| **EXCHANGING** | |
| I. Circulation | |
| A. Cardiac | Alteration in Cardiac Output: Decreased |
| Subjective data | |
| Orientation to person, place, time? | |
| Can you tell me where you are? | |
| What day is today? month? | |
| Any palpitations or fluttering in your chest? | |
| Objective data | |
| Heart rate: assess heart rate and rhythm | |
| Heart sounds: $S_1$, $S_2$, murmurs, extra heart sounds | |
| Pacemaker settings and function | |
| 12-lead ECG: evidence of infarction | |
| Ventricular ectopy | |
| Anti-arrhythmic medications | |
| Potassium level | |
| Afterload: systemic arterial pressure | |
| Mean arterial pressure (MAP) | |
| Diastolic arterial pressure | |
| Compare arterial line blood pressure to cuff pressure | |
| Pulse pressure | |
| Systemic vascular resistance (SVR) | |
| $SVR = \left\{\frac{\text{Mean arterial pressure} - \text{right atrial pressure}}{\text{Cardiac output in liters/minute}}\right\} \times 80$ | |
| Current afterload reducing agent, vasodilator therapy | |
| Calculate in mcg/kg/min | |
| Intra-aortic balloon pump: | |
| Ratio of ECG to counterpulsation | |
| Augmentation pressure | |
| Functioning of pump console, settings, trigger mode | |
| Ventricular assist device: flow in liters/minute | |
| Myocardial oxygen demand ($MVO_2$) | |
| Venous saturation: $SvO_2$, $PvO_2$ | |
| $AVO_2$ difference | |
| Level of muscular activity: Shivering, afebrile | |
| Preload: | |
| Right atrial pressure (RAP) | |
| Central venous pressure (CVP) | |
| Left atrial pressure (LAP) | |
| Pulmonary artery pressure (PAP) | |
| Pulmonary capillary wedge pressure (PCWP) | |
| Contractility: | |
| Cardiac output/cardiac index (cardiac output/body surface area) | |
| Amount of inotropic support: mcg/kg/minute | |
| Ejection fraction, other data from cardiac catheterization, echocardiogram | |
| Perfusion: | |
| Strength of pedal pulses (Grade 0–4) | |
| Hemoglobin | |
| Extremity temperature, color, capillary refill | |
| Toe temperature | |
| Carotid upstroke | |
| Assess arterial blood gases (ABGs) for acidemia (Base deficit $> -3$) | |
| Urine output $>30$ ml/hr | |
| Bowel sounds present | |
| Level of consciousness: alert, lethargic, restless, observed changes in mental status | |

*(continued)*

## Assessment of the Critically Ill Patient With Cardiovascular Dysfunction *(Continued)*

**TABLE 2: Human Response Pattern-Assessment Guide**

| *Possible Cues and Parameters* | *Possible Nursing Diagnosis (Actual/Potential)* |
|---|---|
| B. Vascular | Alteration in Tissue Perfusion |
| Subjective data | |
| Sensation in extremities: tingling, perceived temperature, pain | |
| Perception of change in weight, edema | |
| Objective data | |
| Peripheral pulses: Brachial, radial, femoral, popliteal, pedal | |
| Pulses equal bilaterally (Grade 0–4) | |
| Pulses palpable or by Doppler | |
| Extremity temperature and color: symmetry | |
| Bruit | |
| Pedal and/or sacral edema | Alteration in Fluid Volume: Excess |
| Jugular vein distention | |
| Intake and output (balanced?) | Alteration in Fluid Volume: Deficit |
| Urine output: assess for excessive diuresis, note less than 30 ml/hour | |
| Weight: Compare to pre-operative or previous admission weight | |
| Intravenous fluids currently receiving? | |
| Urine specific gravity: (normal: 1.010–1.025) | |
| Serum osmolality: (normal range: 285–295 mOsm/kg) | |
| Electrolytes, BUN, creatinine levels? | |
| Hematocrit? Hemoglobin? | |
| Nasogastric tube drainage: amount, color, pH, presence of heme? | |
| Chest tube drainage: amount? | |
| Clotting studies: activated clotting time | |
| Prothrombin time | |
| Partial thromboplastin time | |
| Platelets | |
| Central venous pressure, atrial pressure, pulmonary capillary wedge pressure | |
| Chest x-rays: Evidence of pulmonary edema? | |
| Mediastinal widening, cardiac tamponade | |
| Orthostatic hypotension, postural changes in BP | |
| II. Oxygenation | |
| Subjective data | Ineffective Breathing Pattern |
| Do you feel short of breath? Do you feel as if you're getting enough air? | |
| Oriented to person, place, time? | |
| Ask patient/family to compare present breathing pattern with usual breathing pattern | |
| History of pulmonary disease? | |
| Smoking history: number of pack years = packs per day times number of years? | |
| Objective data | |
| Chest excursion: equal bilaterally? | |
| Breath sounds: presence of adventitious sounds | |
| Oxygen delivery mode: nasal cannula Venturi mask, mechanical ventilation—tidal volume | |
| minute ventilation | |
| Secretions: amount, color, ability of patient to handle secretions | Ineffective Airway Clearance |
| Strength and productivity of cough? | |
| Initiation of chest physiotherapy? Incentive spirometry? | |
| Assess work of breathing: Nasal flaring, use of accessory muscles, rib retraction, tachypnea | |
| Weaning parameters: | |
| Level of alertness | |
| Vital capacity (10–15 ml/kg) | |
| Tidal volume (3–5 ml/kg) | |
| Inspiratory pressure: (−20 cm $H_2O$) | |
| Spontaneous respiratory rate | |

## Assessment of the Critically Ill Patient With Cardiovascular Dysfunction *(Continued)*

**TABLE 2: Human Response Pattern-Assessment Guide**

| *Possible Cues and Parameters* | *Possible Nursing Diagnosis (Actual/Potential)* |
|---|---|
| Chest x-ray:<br>Position of endotracheal tube above carina<br>Presence of atelectasis, pneumothorax, pleural effusions, pulmonary edema, position of pleural chest tubes, position of pulmonary artery catheter, other invasive lines | |
| Arterial blood gases: Any abnormal values? Preoperatively? On admission?<br>Pulse oximetry ($SaO_2$)<br>Color of nailbeds, circumoral areas; observed changes in mental status | Impaired Gas Exchange |
| III. Physical Regulation<br>Subjective data<br>Do you feel cold/warm?<br>History of infection? Endocarditis?<br>Verbalized knowledge of need for prophylactic antibiotics with procedures (ex. dental)<br>Objective data<br>Body temperature (rectal, core [blood, esophageal, bladder], oral, axillary) | Potential Alteration in Body Temperature<br>Ineffective Thermoregulation<br>Hypothermia |
| Skin temperature<br>Perspiration, diaphoresis<br>Shivering<br>Heating/cooling blanket settings<br>Antipyretic medication: time and dose, other antipyretic measures previously performed, and patient's response to therapy | Hyperthermia |
| Check invasive line sites: redness, warmth, swelling, pain?<br>Check intravenous line sites: redness, drainage, infiltrations?<br>Assess incisions: redness, swelling<br>Dressing changes as per unit protocol<br>IV tubing, hemodynamic line tubing changes as per unit protocol<br>Monitor WBC, CBC | Potential for Infection |
| IV. Elimination<br>Subjective data<br>Describe urinary and bowel patterns at home<br>Any problems with constipation, diarrhea, incontinence, painful urination? Relief measures used at home?<br>Verbalization knowledge of dangers associated with Valsalva maneuver?<br>Objective data<br>Urine: Amount, frequency, color, clarity?<br>Patency of urinary catheter<br>Urinary incontinence<br>Stool; Amount, frequency, color, consistency, heme positive<br>Abdominal distention, bowel sounds<br>Flatus<br>Incontinence of urine or stool: Assess factors associated with incontinence | Alteration in Urinary Elimination Pattern<br>Stress Incontinence<br>Urge Incontinence<br>Reflex Incontinence<br>Functional Incontinence<br>Total Incontinence<br>Urinary Retention<br>Alteration in Bowel Elimination:<br>Constipation<br>Diarrhea<br>Incontinence |

*(continued)*

## Assessment of the Critically Ill Patient With Cardiovascular Dysfunction *(Continued)*

**TABLE 2: Human Response Pattern-Assessment Guide**

| ***Possible Cues and Parameters*** | ***Possible Nursing Diagnosis (Actual/Potential)*** |
|---|---|
| V. Physical Integrity | Potential for Injury |
| Subjective data: | |
| Do you take Coumadin, anticoagulants? | |
| Verbalized compliance with anticoagulant therapy? | |
| History of skin breakdown, dermal ulcers? | |
| Objective data: | |
| Assess skin for bruises, petechiae | Impaired Tissue Integrity |
| Monitor: Prothrombin time | |
| Partial thromboplastin time | |
| Prescribed anticoagulant therapy: drug, dose, schedule | |
| Skin redness? Breakdown? | Impaired Skin Integrity |
| Dermal ulcer: stages | |
| I reddened area over pressure site | |
| II reddened area with breakdown of epidermis | |
| III breakdown through full thickness of skin (epidermis, dermis) | |
| IV breakdown into deeper tissues (ex. muscle, bone) | |
| Hypothermia | |
| Skin turgor | |
| Known periods of bedrest or immobility? | |
| Note time patient was last turned | |
| Spontaneous weight shifts by patient | |
| Assess wound healing: granulation tissue, need for debridement of eschar, observe for redness or drainage; approximation of wound edges; increased sternal movement with sternotomy incision | |
| VI. Nutrition | Alteration in Nutrition: |
| Subjective data | |
| Time of last food or drink intake: | Greater than Body Requirements |
| Describe usual daily diet; alcohol, sodium, caffeine, cholesterol intake? | Less than Body Requirements |
| Do you wear dentures? | |
| Major weight losses or gains recently? | |
| Appetite? | Impaired Swallowing |
| Ease or difficulty swallowing? | |
| Objective data | |
| Weight? Ideal weight? | |
| Check placement of nasogastric tube, feeding tube | |
| Hyperalimentation or tube feedings: | |
| Rate, frequency of feedings? | |
| Content of nutrients | |
| Note residual of feedings | |
| Electrolytes, trace elements | |
| Length of time without nutrition (NPO status)? | |
| Caloric intake and adequacy | |
| Abdominal distention? Bowel sounds in all quadrants? | |
| Observed eating patterns | |
| **COMMUNICATING** | |
| Subjective data | Impaired Verbal Communication |
| Do you speak English? | |
| Identify language spoken if other than English | |
| Perceived success of communicating | |
| Objective data | |
| Level of consciousness? | |
| Clarity of speech? | |
| Intubated: Nonverbal cues: | |
| Pointing, gesturing, grimacing, facial expression, touching, sign language, body language | |
| Written communication | |

## Assessment of the Critically Ill Patient With Cardiovascular Dysfunction *(Continued)*

**TABLE 2: Human Response Pattern-Assessment Guide**

| *Possible Cues and Parameters* | *Possible Nursing Diagnosis (Actual/Potential)* |
|---|---|
| **RELATING** | |
| Subjective data | |
| Identification of family/social support system: spouse, children, significant others | Alteration in Family Processes |
| Verbalizations of family/patient role conflicts | |
| What is your occupation? Verbalization of fear of disruption of lifestyle by cardiac disease | Social Isolation |
| Perceptions of sexual role | Sexual Dysfunction |
| History of angina with sexual activity? | |
| Problems in sexual relationships as a result of cardiac illness | Altered Sexuality Pattern |
| Perceived needs of family/significant others | |
| Objective data | |
| Presence of family/significant others visiting in ICU | |
| Observed patient/family interactions | |
| Overt sexual behaviors | |
| **VALUING** | |
| Subjective data | |
| Patient/family requests for religious affiliate support: clergy | Spiritual Distress |
| Any religious practices or values interrupted by illness, hospital admission? | |
| Verbalized religious beliefs | |
| Objective data | |
| Observed objects brought in by family having significant meaning to patient (such as photos, rosary, personal items) | |
| Observed cultural or religious items | |
| **CHOOSING** | |
| Subjective data | |
| Scheduled (elective) versus emergency surgery? | |
| Reactions to previous myocardial infarction, chest pain, or cardiac surgery? | |
| Verbalizations of denial of illness or circumstance | Ineffective Individual Coping |
| Verbalizations of adherence to therapeutic regimen in the past | |
| What coping mechanisms are identified by the patient/family? | Impaired Adjustment |
| Objective data | Ineffective Family Coping |
| Observed denial behavior | |
| Objective evidence of nonadherence to therapeutic regimen (Ex. decrease in prothrombin time while on Coumadin) | |
| **MOVING** | |
| I. Activity | |
| Subjective data: | |
| Any fatigue, shortness of breath, angina, claudication with activity or exercise? | Activity Intolerance |
| Perceived exertion scale with activity? | |
| Statements of concern about, or inability to perform activity | |
| Extremity weakness, soreness, immobility complaints | |
| Objective data | |
| Heart rate and blood pressure response to activity | |
| Presence of diaphoresis, pallor, cyanosis, tachypnea, work of breathing with activity? | |
| Level of assistance required for activity? | |
| Movement of all extremities; bilateral movement, hemiparesis | Impaired Mobility |
| Assessed hand grasp strength | |
| II. Rest | |
| Subjective data | Sleep Pattern Disturbance |
| Expressed deficit of sleep, rest | |
| Assess usual pattern of sleep prior to admission | |
| Angina at night? Paroxysmal nocturnal dyspnea | |
| Sleeping aids used at home? | |

*(continued)*

## Assessment of the Critically Ill Patient With Cardiovascular Dysfunction *(Continued)*

**TABLE 2: Human Response Pattern-Assessment Guide**

| *Possible Cues and Parameters* | *Possible Nursing Diagnosis (Actual/Potential)* |
|---|---|
| Objective data | |
| Patterns of sleep interruption: Awakened for therapy, noise | |
| Disorientation | |
| Irritability, fatigue, yawning, lethargy | |
| III. Activities of Daily Living | Alteration in Health Maintenance |
| Subjective data | |
| Expressed intention for nonmodification cardiac risk factors | |
| Objective data | |
| Observed evidence of not modifying risk factors: smoking, food high in sodium, cholesteral, triglycerides | |
| IV. Self-Care | Self-Care Deficit |
| Subjective data | |
| Expressed inability to perform self-care activities: feeding, bathing, dressing, toileting | |
| Objective data | |
| Body odor, general hygiene, appearance | |
| Note time of last bath | |
| Incontinence? | |
| Immobility? | |
| Anesthetized or paralyzed status? | |
| Decreased activity tolerance | |
| **PERCEIVING** | |
| I. Self-Concept | Disturbance in Self-Concept |
| Subjective data | |
| Verbalizations of self esteem changes with illness | |
| Verbalizations of self concept and identity changes with illness | |
| Perceptions of body image changes (post myocardial infarction; post cardiac surgery, for example) | |
| Objective data | |
| Facial expressions | |
| Body language (ex. reactions to viewing incisions) | |
| II. Sensory/Perceptual | Sensory Perceptual Alterations |
| Subjective data | |
| Verbalizations indicating: hallucinations, strange thoughts, delusions, disorientation. | |
| Expressed difficulty with hearing, vision, touch, smell | |
| Objective data | |
| Assess multiple environmental stimuli: noise, multiple providers, lights | |
| Length of ICU stay | |
| Length of time on cardiopulmonary bypass | |
| Mean blood pressure on cardiopulmonary bypass | |
| Assess stimuli deficit: isolation, totally quiet environment | |
| Restlessness, combative behavior | |
| Observed changes in mental status | |
| Mood swings, personality changes | |
| Medications: Amount and time of last dose of tranquilizers, anti-anxiety therapy | |
| Observed visual, audition, touch, and smell difficulties | |
| III. Meaningfulness | |
| Subjective data | |
| Verbal expressions of hopelessness versus hope for recovery | Hopelessness |
| Verbal expressions of powerlessness versus control over illness | Powerlessness |
| Expressed wish to live versus die | |
| Expressions of depression versus enthusiasm to recover | |
| Objective data | |
| Facial expressions | |
| Depressed state observed | |
| Assess level of participation in care | |
| Level of dependence versus independence | |

## Assessment of the Critically Ill Patient With Cardiovascular Dysfunction *(Continued)*

**TABLE 2: Human Response Pattern-Assessment Guide**

| *Possible Cues and Parameters* | *Possible Nursing Diagnosis (Actual/Potential)* |
|---|---|
| **KNOWING** | |
| Subjective data | Knowledge Deficit |
| Verbalized knowledge of disease process, interventions, outcomes regarding: | |
| Surgical procedure | |
| Medications | |
| Rationale for restrictions | |
| Rationale for nursing interventions | |
| Rationale for medical interventions | |
| Educational level | |
| Ability to repeat/retain information given | |
| Family's knowledge of illness | |
| Objective data | |
| Assess behavior inconsistent with verbalized knowledge | Alteration in Thought Processes |
| Nonadherence to therapy | |
| Assess what information has been given to patient by other health care providers | |
| **FEELING** | |
| I. Comfort | |
| Subjective data | Alteration in Comfort |
| Verbalization of pain, discomfort | |
| Description of anginal pain: onset, intensity, frequency, duration, location, radiation, changes in pain pattern, associated factors | |
| Usual pain relief measures and effectiveness: nitroglycerin, prophylactic nitroglycerin, number of nitroglycerin tablets taken? | |
| Objective data | |
| Assess heart rate, respiratory rate | |
| Guarding behavior of painful area | |
| Facial grimace, diaphoresis | |
| Decreased mobility of painful area | |
| Time and type of last pain medication and its effectiveness | |
| II. Emotional Integrity | |
| Subjective data | Anxiety |
| Verbalizations of anxiety, fear, worry | Fear |
| Expressions of feelings of loss, grief | Anticipatory Grieving |
| Family verbalizations of fear, anxiety, worry | Dysfunctional Grieving |
| History of anti-anxiety medications, tranquilizers | |
| Objective data | |
| Heart rate, blood pressure, pupil dilation, vasoconstriction, diaphoresis | |
| Restlessness, insomnia, nervousness, extraneous movements | |
| Crying, quivering voice, trembling | |
| Medications: anti-anxiety, tranquilizers: amount and time of last dose? | |

evaluation of the critically ill cardiovascular patient. Possible nursing diagnoses are listed in Table 2 for each corresponding pattern. The reader is encouraged to refer to the assessment guide for specific assessment cues to pursue for each pattern.

## EXCHANGING

Frequently, the priority assessment of the cardiac patient in the ICU lies within the *exchanging* pattern due to the physiologic nature of categories in this pattern including circulation, oxygenation, physical regulation, elimination, physical integrity, and nutrition. The majority of cues identified in the ICU are in these categories and therefore consume a high percentage of the nurse's time.

### Circulation

Understanding principles of physiology underlying cardiac output and thus the basis for *alteration in cardiac output: decreased,* are essential in assessing circulation in the cardiac patient. Cardiac output is known to be determined by heart rate times stroke volume. This is a very simplified definition and is limiting for the ICU nurse who has direct access to afterload and preload measurements, and who must be cognizant of tissue oxygen demand and extraction from the blood. The ICU nurse is also aware of cardiac output as a function of blood flow over a period of time and the resulting tissue/organ perfusion. The majority of cardiac critically ill patients have intracardiac monitoring which allows for direct measurement of cardiac output in liters per minute, and the cardiac index calculated in liters per minute per square meter, to produce a value not subject to varying body surface areas from patient to patient. A normal cardiac index in healthy adults ranges from 2.5 to 4.0 liters/min/$m^2$, whereas an acceptable cardiac index in postoperative cardiac surgery patients is 2.0 liters/min/$m^2$. Comparison to the preoperative or previously measured index is helpful in determining progress or deterioration in cardiac function.

**Auscultation of Heart Sounds**

Auscultation of heart sounds is an assessment measure the critical care nurse employs to detect any abnormal sounds and to establish a baseline to detect any changes in heart sounds which may develop. It is important to develop a systematic approach to listening to heart sounds. A detailed discussion of the examination of the heart is presented in Chapter 38 and includes the techniques of inspection, palpation, and auscultation. Timing of heart sounds in relation to the events of the cardiac cycle is discussed in Chapter 37 (See Fig. 37–16).

Clinically, characteristics of heart sounds are often significant parameters to be assessed by the critical care nurse. In the postcardiac surgical patient it may be important to compare postoperative heart sounds to documented preoperative sounds. Auscultation of heart sounds in the patient with a newly implanted valve may early on detect regurgitation or obstruction to blood flow within the heart, which may occur. In the postinfarction patient, detected changes in heart sounds may provide clues as to underlying pathophysiology associated with the infarction. Rupture of the ventricular septum postinfarction may produce a loud systolic murmur; a new systolic murmur postinfarction may reflect mitral regurgitation associated with rupture of a papillary muscle.

### Oxygenation

The need for oxygenation in the cardiac patient is accented by the myocardium's need for an adequate and constant supply of oxygen to prevent ischemia, injury, and infarction of cardiac tissue. Establishing and maintaining an airway, delivering oxygen, and assessing arterial blood gas parameters are crucial functions of the ICU nurse. Changes in the patient's ventilatory status whether associated with excess secretions, inability to handle secretions, or altered breathing pattern, reflect cues that support the diagnoses of *ineffective airway clearance* and *ineffective breathing pattern.*

Vigilant, ongoing assessment for signs of pulmonary edema indicative of left ventricular failure is essential in the postmyocardial infarction and postcardiac surgery patients. *Impaired gas exchange* is reflected by abnormal blood gas values. Pneumothorax is often associated with thoracic/cardiac surgery. Therefore, it is mandatory for the critical care nurse to monitor breath sounds, and to assess chest excursion for symmetry bilaterally. Maintaining the integrity of the chest drainage system is mandatory postcardiac and thoracic surgery. Aggressive pulmonary hygiene is essential to handle secretions, prevent altelectasis, and to promote and maintain adequate alveolar ventilation.

### Physical Regulation

Physical regulation in the cardiac patient includes the regulation of body temperature. All patients are hypothermic after cardiac surgery due to necessary cooling for cardiopulmonary bypass. Assessing body temperature, the progression of warming, and the presence of shivering are significant responsibilities of the critical care nurse in caring for the postcardiac surgical patient. Shivering increases myocardial oxygen consumption and is, therefore, potentially dangerous in the early postoperative period and requires immediate treatment. A rebound hyperthermia is not unusual in these patients during the first 24–48 hours post surgery. Therefore, close monitoring of body temperature is warranted. *Potential alteration in body temperature, hyperthermia and hypothermia,* are nursing diagnoses supported by cues involving the regulation of body temperature.

Another aspect of physical regulation in the cardiac patient involves the *potential for infection.* All critically ill cardiac patients have invasive monitoring lines and/or intravenous accesses which increase the risk of infection in these patients. Strict aseptic technique is essential when managing all invasive lines. Postcardiac surgical patients have the added risk of the sternotomy incision which must be assessed for any signs of infection. Patients with valvular disease are at particular risk for endocarditis postoperatively and/or postrecovery. Nurses should assess their knowledge of the need for prophylactic antibiotics with any dental or surgical procedures and patient education should be incorporated into their plan of care and implemented when the patient/family indicate a readiness to learn.

### Elimination

Elimination in the acutely ill cardiac patient is important to assess primarily as it relates to cardiovascular dynamics. For example, the patient with a myocardial infarction must be taught the importance of avoiding the Valsalva maneuver with bowel elimination to avoid abrupt changes in venous return to the heart, or a vasovagal response (i.e., an abrupt drop in blood pressure associated with vagal stimulation). Assessment of daily bowel routine may provide cues underlying *alteration in bowel elimination.* Assessment of stool specimens for the presence of occult blood is an important consideration especially in the patient receiving anticoagulant therapy. The cardiac patient who has experienced a hypotensive episode should be monitored closely for oliguria. Renal failure is often associated with low cardiac output states and the presence of cues underlying *alteration in urinary elimination* should be assessed and documented.

### Physical Integrity

Physical integrity refers to the condition of the patient's skin and soft tissues. Cardiac patients receiving anticoagulants are at risk for bleeding which may be reflected by the presence of petechiae or ecchymotic areas. Careful monitoring of prothrombin or partial thromboplastin times in conjunction with anticoagulant therapy is essential.

Cardiac patients, especially the cardiac surgical patient who may have experienced hypothermia and who may be immobile for long periods of time, are especially at high risk of compromised circulation with *impaired skin integrity.* Diligent nursing care is imperative to prevent pressure areas from breaking down.

### Nutrition

Nutrition is fundamental to the healing of all tissues. A continuous, adequate supply of essential nutrients must be made available to cardiac tissue to meet the high energy needs of myocardial muscle fibers. Often, critically ill cardiac patients may initially receive only dextrose and water. However, when one realizes that the total caloric value of 1000 ml dextrose 5% in water is but 600 calories, it is readily apparent that the critical care nurse must be tuned in to the patient's nutritional status, and for *alterations in nutrition less than body requirements.* Consultation with the patient's physician and dietician may enable a diet to be planned to meet overall needs of the patient's caloric intake, and including foods with necessary fiber to facilitate normal bowel functioning. In conjunction with the patient's hemodynamic status, *fluid volume: excess,* and *fluid volume: deficit,* are major considerations in ongoing patient assessment.

## COMMUNICATING

The critical care nurse assesses the cardiac patient for alterations in both verbal and nonverbal communication. This is especially important for patients who remain intubated for a period of time, or in patients postextubation. Laryngeal or subglottal edema postextubation may cause difficulty with speech. The occurrence of slurred speech in a patient without previous speech difficulties may suggest a cerebral embolism and such cues may support an underlying diagnosis of *impaired verbal communication.*

Nonverbal cues from the patient whose verbal communication is impaired becomes especially important to assess. Asking the patient to point to where pain is located, asking the patient to nod his/her head, yes or no, or allowing the patient to write questions/answers on a note pad, are examples of illiciting nonverbal cues.

## RELATING

The roles and relationships of the critically ill patient including the identification of a social support system is important for the nurse to ascertain so that plans and interventions can include these significant others. Family members should be assessed to determine their needs while the patient is in the critical care unit. Interventions with families have been shown to produce outcomes with cardiac patients. The nurse should also observe for negative as well as positive interactions between the patient and family members. Visiting hours provide an opportune time for such assessments and determination. *Impaired social interaction, social isolation, alteration in family processes,* are nursing diagnoses of consideration within the relating pattern.

## VALUING

Determining the patient's cultural, religious, and social values will assist the critical care nurse in maintaining an environment conducive to supporting these values. Patient or family requests for visitation by religious affiliates of their choice, verbalizing philosophical beliefs, and bringing items of personal and/or cultural value into the ICU, are examples of acknowledging the importance of values during the time of illness. Given the high acuity levels and mortality rates of critically ill cardiac patients, awareness of spiritual values and *spiritual distress* may be heightened during this phase of hospitalization so that determining the patient's or family's spiritual needs is an important activity of the critical care nurse.

## CHOOSING

Cardiac patients most likely have not had a conscious choice in the development of their disease so the nurse must assess their reactions to the illness including how well they are able to cope. Many patients use denial of their disease as a coping mechanism. This may lead to noncompliance with the therapeutic regimen, which in turn may exacerbate the underlying disease. Denial may also serve a useful purpose in that it may help the patient to cope during the hyperacute stage of the illness, thereby conserving the patient's energies during this critical period.

Discussing with the patient and/or family the specific coping mechanisms utilized during this illness can be helpful in determining whether or not the patient can be diagnosed as having *ineffective coping.* Coping response differences between those patients who undergo emergency cardiac surgery versus those electively scheduled, have not been formally studied although emergency surgery patients are certainly less prepared and may react differently than those with elective surgery. The nurse should ask if the patient has had previous cardiac surgery, previous infarctions, or prior hospitalizations for any reason, and try to help the patient/family identify what coping mechanism(s) worked for them in the past.

## MOVING

The pattern of moving includes cues related to activity tolerance, rest, activities of daily living, and self-care. Assessing the critically ill cardiac patient's response to activity is crucial as it is reflective of the workload the heart is able to perform. Asking patients about their perceptions of exertion, fatigue, shortness of breath, and angina upon walking, lifting, exercising, or with sexual activity, is important as the patient's perceptions have been found to correlate well with actual increased demands on the heart. Observing for physiologic signs of increased demand on the heart, such as an increase in heart rate and blood pressure, provides a source of vital information in determining if the patient has *activity intolerance*.

Rest in the cardiac patient is indicated for preserving maximal myocardial performance. Physical activity is restricted in the myocardial infarction patient to decrease the myocardium's demand for oxygen. The critical care nurse must assess not only the quantity of rest and sleep experienced by the patient, but also, the quality of rest and sleep as perceived by the patient within the ICU. Etiologies of any noted *sleep pattern disturbance* must be identified so that effective sleep can be restored.

Upon arrival in the ICU postsurgery, possibly still intubated and with a variety of drips being administered intravenously, the cardiac surgical patient is usually totally dependent upon the nurse for mobility and self care needs. The patient who has sustained a serious myocardial infarction, who remains unstable and on bed rest, is likewise dependent upon the nurse. It is especially important for the nurse to assess the needs of patients regarding their activities of daily living, including such items as bathing, hygiene, feeding, and toileting, as well as their perceptions as to how they feel about being dependent upon others for such functions.

## PERCEIVING

The cues included under the perceiving pattern include those related to self-concept, meaningfulness, and sensory/perceptual categories. Examining the patient for *disturbances in self-concept* includes assessing cues related to perceptions of body image, self-esteem, and personal identify. The cardiac patient may experience changes in these areas and may exhibit guilt, depression, or fear. It may be important to appraise the patient's perceptions of body image, especially when one acknowledges that the heart is a vital organ, which if damaged, can have catastrophic effects on patient and family.

*Hopelessness* and *powerlessness* are potential diagnoses in cardiac patients due to the palliative versus curative nature of treatment. Patients in ICU are also very dependent on the nurse and may experience powerlessness for this reason. The nurse must scrutinize verbal remarks and body language for signs of alterations in meaningfulness to patient and/or family.

*Sensory/perceptual alteration* occurs to some degree in the majority of patients who undergo cardiac surgery and is thought to be related to the effects of cardiopulmonary bypass and environmental stimuli. The nurse looks for verbalizations of hallucinations, disorientation, mood swings, restlessness, hostility, and changes in mental status. Myocardial infarction patients may exhibit the same symptoms but the etiology may be related to stimuli deficits in a restrictive, quiet environment, or to alterations in cerebral perfusion resulting from decreased cardiac output.

## KNOWING

Prior to initiation of patient/family education, the nurse should assess their knowledge base regarding the illness, its cause, and course of therapy. Knowledge of relevant cardiac disease processes, risk factors for coronary artery disease, prescribed medications, and other therapeutic regimens, must be investigated to some extent by the critical care nurse with follow-up by the nurse after transfer from the ICU. Cardiac surgical patients should be asked about their knowledge of the surgical procedure preoperatively, as well as their expectations postoperatively so that any misconceptions can be corrected and/or eliminated. Because many myocardial infarctions recur without previous warning, the patient may not be aware he/she has cardiac disease. *Knowledge deficit* is a common nursing diagnosis in myocardial infarction patients.

## FEELING

The feeling pattern encompasses cues for assessing comfort and emotional integrity. *Alteration in comfort: pain* is a nursing diagnosis that occurs in the majority of critically ill patients with cardiovascular dysfunction. Angina is one of the most important signs to assess in cardiac patients. A full description of the anginal pattern is required. This is especially important in the postcardiac surgical patient who may also be experiencing postoperative infarction pain. The nurse must assess the need for pain medication, factors accentuating the pain, and response to pain alleviating measures.

Emotional integrity is vulnerable during the period of critical illness for both patient and family so that signs or symptoms of *fear, anxiety,* and *grieving* must be noted by the nurse. Asking direct questions about fear of dying, or fear related to permanent disability are appropriate; often the patient will express these fears openly when asked. Objective symptoms of anxiety, including an increase in sympathetic activity, are not uncommon in cardiac patients.

## SUMMARY

Assessing the critically ill cardiovascular patient for actual or potential nursing diagnoses is a crucial role for the critical care nurse. This will guide the assessment of the critically ill patient with cardiovascular dysfunction utilizing as its nursing framework the nine human response patterns. The assessment guide presented incorporates cues to be pursued in deriving assessment data including questions to be asked and observations to be made. Collecting such subjective and objective information in a comprehensive and organized fashion yields a thorough nursing assessment and consequently an inclusive identification of risk factors for potential problems and for actual problems in these patients.

## BIBLIOGRAPHY

Alspach, JG and Williams, SM: Core Curriculum for Critical Care Nursing. WB Saunders, Philadelphia, 1985.

Braunwald, E: Heart Disease: Textbook of Cardiovascular Medicine. WB Saunders, Philadelphia, 1984.

Guzzetta, CE and Dossey, DM: Cardiovascular Nursing: Bodymind Tapestry. CV Mosby, St. Louis, 1984.

Kim, MJ and Moritz, DA: Classification of Nursing Diagnoses: Proceedings of the Third and Fourth National Conference. McGraw-Hill, New York, 1982.

Kim, MJ, McFarland, GK, and McLane, AM: Classification of Nursing Diagnoses: Proceedings of the Fifth National Conference. CV Mosby, St. Louis, 1984

Kirklin, JW and Barrett-Boyes, W: Cardiac Surgry. John Wiley & Sons, New York, 1986.

North American Nursing Diagnoses Association: Nursing Diagnosis Taxonomy 1. NANDA, St. Louis, 1986.

Nurses Clinical Library. Dracup, K (ed): Cardiovascular Disorders. Nursing 84 Books, Springhouse, PA, 1984.

Underhill, SL, Woods, SL, Sivarajan, ES, and Halpenny, CJ: Cardiac Nursing. JB Lippincott, Philadelphia, 1982.

APPENDIX F

# Normal Reference Laboratory Values*

## BLOOD VALUES

| | |
|---|---|
| Ammonia | 12–55 umol/liter |
| Amylase | 4–25 units/ml |
| Bilirubin | direct: up to 0.4 mg/100 ml<br>total: up to 1.0 mg/100 ml |
| Calcium | 8.5–10.5 mg/100 ml |
| Carbon dioxide content | 24–30 mEq/liter |
| Carcinoembryonic antigen (CEA) | 0–2.5 ng/ml |
| Chloride | 100–106 mEq/liter |
| CK isoenzymes | 5% MB or less |
| Creatinine | 0.6–1.5 mg/100 ml |
| Digoxin | 17 ± 6 ng/ml |
| Glucose | 70–110 mg/100 ml (fasting) |
| Iron | 50–150 ug/100 ml |
| Iron-binding capacity | 250–410 ug/100 ml |
| Lipase | 2 units/ml or less |
| Lipids: | |
| Cholesterol | 120–220 mg/ml |
| Triglycerides | 40–150 mg/100 ml |
| Magnesium | 1.5–2.0 mEq/liter |
| Osmolality | 280–296 mOsm/kg water |
| Oxygen saturation (Arterial) | 96–100 percent |
| $PCO_2$ | 35–45 mmHg |
| pH | 7.35–7.45 |
| $PO_2$ | 75–100 mmHg (Room air) |
| Phenobarbital | 15–50 ug/ml |
| Phenytoin | 5–20 ug/ml |
| Phosphatase (Acid) | male: total: 0.13–0.63 sigma U/ml<br>female: total: 0.01–0.56 sigma U/ml |
| Phosphatase (Alkaline) | 13–39 U/liter |
| Phosphorus (Organic) | 3.0–4.5 mg/100 ml |
| Potassium | 3.5–5.5 mEq/liter |
| Protein: Total | 6.0–8.4 g/100 ml |
| Albumin | 3.5–5.5 g/100 ml |
| Globulin | 2.3–3.5 g/100 ml |
| Sodium | 135–145 mEq/liter |
| Transaminases, SGOT (Aspartate aminotransferase) | 7–27 U/liter |
| Transaminases, SGPT (Alanine aminotransferase) | 1–21 U/liter |
| Urea nitrogen (BUN) | 8–25 mg/100 ml |
| Uric acid | 3.0–7.0 mg/100 ml |
| Vitamin A | 0.15–0.6 ug/ml |

* From Scully, RE (ed): Case Records of the Massachusetts General Hospital. New England Journal of Medicine, 314:39–49. January 2, 1986, with permission.

### Special Endocrine Tests

| | |
|---|---|
| Adrenocorticotropin (ACTH) | 15–70 pg/ml |
| Aldosterone | excretion: 5–19 ug/24 hours |
| Calcitonin | male: 0–14 pg/ml<br>female: 0–28 pg/ml |
| Cortisol: | |
| 8 AM | 5–15 ug/100 ml |
| 8 PM | <10 ug/100 ml |
| 4-hr ACTH test | 30–45 ug/100 ml |
| Overnight suppression test | <5 ug/100 ml |
| Parathyroid hormone | <25 pg/ml |
| Thyroid-stimulating hormone (TSH) | 0.5–5.0 uU/ml |
| Thyroxine-binding globulin capacity | 15–25 ug T4/100 ml |
| Total triiodothyronine (T3) | 75–195 ng/100 ml |
| Total thyroxine by RAI(T4) | 4–12 ug/100 ml |
| T3 resin uptake | 25–35 percent |
| Free thyroxine index (FT4I) | 1–4 |
| Vitamin D derivatives: | |
| 1,25-Dihydroxy vitamin D | 26–65 pg/ml |
| 25-Hydroxy-vitamin D | 8–56 ng/ml |

## URINE VALUES

| | |
|---|---|
| Acetone plus acetoacetate (Quantitative) | 0 |
| Amylase | 24–76 units/ml |
| Calcium | 300 mg/day or less |
| Catecholamines: | |
| Epinephrine | under 20 ug/day |
| Norepinephrine | under 100 ug/day |
| Copper | 0–100 ug/day |
| Creatine | under 100 mg/day or less than 6% of creatinine |
| Creatinine | 15–25mg/kg of body weight/day |
| Hemoglobin (Myoglobin) | 0 |
| pH | 5–7 |
| Phosphorus (Inorganic) | Varies with intake; average = 1 g/day |
| Protein: | |
| Quantitative | <150 mg/24 hours |
| Steroids: | |
| 17-ketosteroids | (see below) |

17-ketosteroids:

| Age | Male | Female |
|---|---|---|
| 10 | 1–4 mg | 1–4 mg |
| 20 | 6–21 | 4–16 |
| 30 | 8–26 | 4–14 |
| 50 | 5–18 | 3–9 |
| 70 | 2–10 | 1–7 |

| | |
|---|---|
| 17-hydroxysteroids | 3–8 mg/day (women lower than men) |
| Glucose | 0 |
| Urobilinogen | up to 1.0 Ehrlich U |
| Vanillylmandelic acid (VMA) | up to 9 mg/24 hours |

## HEMATOLOGIC VALUES

| | |
|---|---|
| Coagulation factors: | |
| Factor I (Fibrinogen) | 0.15–0.35 g/100 ml |
| Factor II (Prothrombin) | 60–140 percent |
| Factor VII | 70–130 percent |
| Factor X (Stuart factor) | 70–130 percent |
| Factor VIII (antihemophilic globulin) | 50–200 percent |
| Factor IX (Plasma thromboplastic cofactor) | 6–140 percent |
| Factor IX (Plasma thromboplastic antecedent) | 60–140 percent |
| Factor XII (Hageman factor) | 60–140 percent |
| Coagulation screening tests: | |
| Bleeding time | 3–9.5 minutes |
| Prothrombin time | less than 2-second deviation from control |
| Partial thromboplastin time (Activated) | 25–38 seconds |
| Whole blood clot lysis | no clot lysis in 24 hours |
| Fibrinolytic studies: | |
| Euglobin lysis | no lysis in 2 hours |
| Fibrinogen split products | negative reaction at >1:4 dilution |
| Thrombin time | control ±5 seconds |
| Complete blood count: | |
| Hematocrit | males: 45–52 percent |

| | |
|---|---|
| | females: 37–48 percent |
| Hemoglobin | male: 13–18 g/100 ml |
| | females: 12–16 g/100 ml |
| Leukocyte count | 4300–10,800/$mm^3$ |
| Erythrocyte count | 4.2–5.9 million/$mm^3$ |
| Mean corpuscular volume (MCV) | 86–98 $\mu m^3$/cell |
| Mean corpuscular hemoglobin (MCH) | 27–32 pg/RBC |
| Mean corpuscular hemoglobin concentration (MCHC) | 32–36 percent |
| Erythrocyte sedimentation rate | male: 1–13 mm/hour |
| | female: 1–20 mm/hour |
| Platelet count | 150,00–350,000/$mm^3$ |
| Platelet function tests: | |
| Clot retraction | 50–100 percent/2 hours |
| Platelet aggregation | Full response to ADP, epinephrine, and collagen |
| Platelet factor 3 | 33–57 seconds |
| Reticulocyte count | 0.5–2.5 percent red cells |

## CEREBROSPINAL FLUID VALUES

| | |
|---|---|
| Bilirubin | 0 |
| Cell count | 0–5 mononuclear cells |
| Chloride | 120–130 mEq/liter |
| Albumin | Mean: 29.5 mg/100 ml |
| Immunoglobulin G (IgG) | Mean: 4.3 mg/100 ml |
| Glucose | 50–75 mg/100 ml |
| Pressure (Initial) | 70–180 mm of water |
| Protein: | |
| Lumbar | 15–45 mg/100 ml |

## IMMUNOLOGIC TESTS

| | |
|---|---|
| Alpha-fetoprotein | undetectable in normal adult |
| Alpha-I-antitrypsin | 83–213 mg/100 ml |
| Rheumatoid factor | <60 IU/ml |
| Anti-DNA antibodies | negative at a 1 : 8 dilution of serum |
| Autoantibodies to: | |
| Thyroid colloid and microsomal antigens | negative at a 1 : 10 dilution of serum |
| Gastric parietal cells | negative at a 1 : 20 dilution of serum |
| Adrenal gland | negative at a 1 : 10 dilution of serum |
| Bence Jones protein | no Bence Jones protein detected in a 50-fold concentrate of urine |
| Complement, total hemolytic | 150–250 U/ml |
| Cryoprecipitate proteins | None detected |
| Hemoglobin A 1C | 3.8–6.4 percent |
| Immunoglobulins: | |
| IgG | 639–1349 mg/100 ml |
| IgA | 70–312 mg/100 ml |
| IgM | 86–352 mg/100 ml |

# Index

An *italic* page number indicates a figure. A "t" indicates a table.